Textbook of Ocular Pharmacology

Textbook of Ocular Pharmacology

EDITOR-IN-CHIEF

Thom J. Zimmerman, M.D., PH.D.
Professor and Chairman
Department of Ophthalmology and Visual Sciences
Professor of Pharmacology and Toxicology
University of Louisville School of Medicine
Kentucky Lions Eye Center
Louisville, Kentucky

EDITORS

Karanjit S. Kooner, M.D.
Assistant Professor
Department of Ophthalmology
Southwestern Medical School
Dallas, Texas

Mordechai Sharir, M.D., PH.D.
Chief of Glaucoma
Department of Ophthalmology
The Edith Wolfson Hospital
Tel Aviv, Israel

ASSOCIATE EDITOR

Robert D. Fechtner, M.D.
Associate Director
Glaucoma Service
Associate Professor
Department of Ophthalmology and Visual Sciences
University of Louisville School of Medicine
Kentucky Lions Eye Center
Louisville, Kentucky

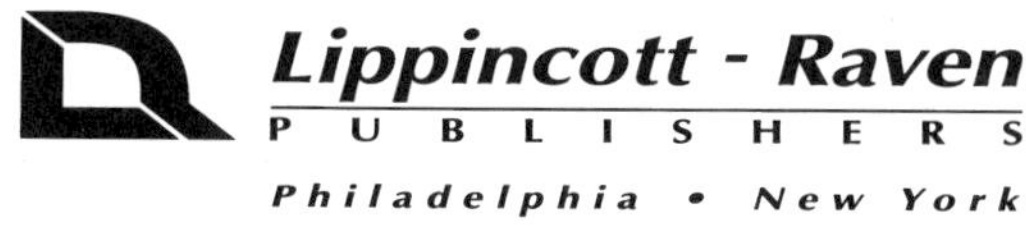

Acquisitions Editor: Vickie Thaw
Developmental Editor: Delois Patterson
Manufacturing Manager: Dennis Teston
Associate Managing Editor: Kathy Bubbeo
Production Editor: Nicholas Radhuber
Cover Designer: Susan J. Moore
Indexer: Jayne Percy
Compositor: Compset
Printer: Maple Press

Printed in the United States of America

9 8 7 6 5 4 3 2 1

Library of Congress Cataloging-in-Publication Data

Textbook of ocular pharmacology / editor-in-chief, Thom J. Zimmerman;
editors, Karanjit S. Kooner,
Mordechai Sharir, Robert D. Fechtner.
p. cm.
Includes bibliographical references and index.
ISBN 0-781-70306-9
1. Ocular pharmacology. I. Zimmerman, Thom J.
[DNLM: 1. Eye Diseases—drug therapy. 2. Eye—drug effects. WW
166 T355 1997]
RE994.T49 1997
617.7′061—dc21
DNLM/DLC
for Library of Congress 97-1434
CIP

To our respective families whose love, support and encouragement provided the impetus to complete this book.

To students, present and in the future, who wish to know more about ocular pharmacology in order to benefit their patients.

And finally, Thom J. Zimmerman wishes to dedicate this book to Tom Maren whom he considers his mentor and the father of ocular pharmacology.

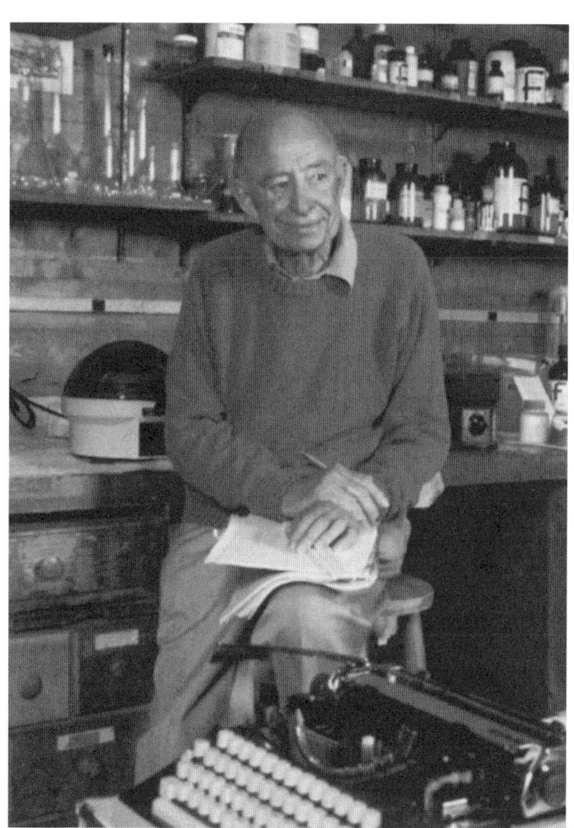

Contents

Section VIII: Diagnostic Drugs

Section Editors

Section I: General Ocular Pharmacology

Mordechai Sharir, M.D., Ph.D.
Chief of Glaucoma
Department of Ophthalmology
The Edith Wolfson Hospital
Tel-Aviv University
Holon 58100, Israel;
Assistant Professor
Department of Ophthalmology and Visual Sciences
Department of Microbiology and Immunology
University of Louisville School of Medicine
Louisville, Kentucky 40292

Thom J. Zimmerman, M.D., Ph.D.
Professor and Chairman
Department of Ophthalmology and Visual Sciences
Professor of Pharmacology and Toxicology
University of Louisville School of Medicine
Kentucky Lions Eye Center
301 E. Muhammad Ali Blvd.
Louisville, Kentucky 40292

Section II: Glaucoma

Karanjit S. Kooner, M.D.
Assistant Professor
Department of Ophthalmology
Southwestern Medical School
5323 Harry Hines Blvd.
Dallas, Texas 75235-9057

Thom J. Zimmerman, M.D., Ph.D.
Professor and Chairman
Department of Ophthalmology and Visual Sciences
Professor of Pharmacology and Toxicology
University of Louisville School of Medicine
Kentucky Lions Eye Center
301 E. Muhammad Ali Blvd.
Louisville, Kentucky 40292

Robert D. Fechtner, M.D.
Associate Professor
Department of Ophthalmology and Visual Sciences
Associate Director, Glaucoma Service
University of Louisville School of Medicine
Kentucky Lions Eye Center
Louisville, Kentucky 40292

Section III: Retina

David V. Weinberg, M.D.
Assistant Professor of Ophthalmology
Department of Ophthalmology
Northwestern University Medical School
645 N. Michigan Avenue
Suite 440
Chicago, Illinois 60611

Lee M. Jampol, M.D.
Louis Feinberg Professor and Chairman
Department of Ophthalmology
Northwestern University Medical School
645 N. Michigan Avenue
Suite 440
Chicago, Illinois 60611

Section IV: Cornea and External Diseases

George R. John, M.D.
Assistant Professor
Department of Ophthalmology and Visual Sciences
University of Louisville
301 E. Muhammad Ali Blvd.
Louisville, Kentucky 40292

Herbert E. Kaufman, M.D.
Boyd Professor of Ophthalmology and Pharmacology and Experimental Therapeutics
Head, Department of Ophthalmology
LSU Eye Center
Louisiana State University Medical Center School of Medicine
2020 Gravier, Suite B
New Orleans, Louisiana 70112

Section V: Uveitis

Albert Vitale, M.D.
21 Marlboro Street
Newton, Massachusetts 02158

C. Stephen Foster, M.D.
Professor of Ophthalmology
Director, Immunology Uveitis Service
Massachusetts Eye and Ear Infirmary
243 Charles St.
Boston, Massachusetts 02114

Section VI: Anesthesia

Martin A. Acquadro, M.D., D.M.D.
Clinical Instructor
Department of Anesthesia
Massachusetts Eye and Ear Infirmary
Harvard Medical School
243 Charles St.
Boston, Massachusetts 02114

Section VII: Pediatric

Forrest D. Ellis, M.D.
Department of Ophthalmology
Indiana University
702 Rotary Circle
Indianapolis, Indiana 46202

Section VIII: Diagnostic Drugs

Carol F. Zimmerman, M.D.
Associate Professor of Ophthalmology and Neurology
University of Texas Southwestern Medical Center at Dallas
5323 Harry Hines Blvd.
Dallas, Texas 75235-9057

Contributing Authors

Ozlem Evrem Abbasoglu, M.D.
Glaucoma Fellow
Department of Ophthalmology
University of Texas Southwestern Medical Center at Dallas
5323 Harry Hines Blvd.
Dallas, Texas 75235-9057

Future Role of Neuroprotective Agents in Glaucoma

Steven R. Abel, Pharm. D.
Professor and Head
Department of Pharmacy
Purdue University
Pharmacy Programs at Indianapolis
1001 W. 10th St., OPW U-2005
Indianapolis, Indiana 46202-2879

Effect of Disease on Drug Disposition
Effect of Age on Drug Disposition

Mark B. Abelson, M.D.
Associate Clinical Professor of Ophthalmology
Department of Ophthalmology/Immunology
Harvard Medical School/Schepens Eye Research Institute
20 Staniford St.
Boston, Massachusetts 02114

Antiallergic Therapies

Martin A. Acquadro, M.D., D.M.D.
Clinical Instructor
Department of Anesthesia
Harvard Medical School/Massachusetts Eye and Ear Infirmary
243 Charles St.
Boston, Massachusetts 02114

Anesthetic and Perianesthetic Medications
Anesthetic Considerations for Ophthalmic Surgery

Eduardo C. Alfonso, M.D.
Bascom Palmer Eye Institute
900 NW 17th St.
Miami, Florida 33136

The Tetracyclines
Erythromycin, Clarithromycin, and Azithromycin
Chloramphenicol

Hassan Alizadeh, Ph.D.
Assistant Professor of Ophthalmology
Department of Ophthalmology
University of Texas Southwestern Medical Center at Dallas
5323 Harry Hines Blvd.
Dallas, Texas 75235-9057

Amebic Disease of the Eye

R. Rand Allingham, M.D.
Assistant Professor of Ophthalmology
Duke University Department of Ophthalmology Medical Center
Erwin Rd.
Box 3802
Durham, North Carolina 27710

Medical Trabeculocanulotomy

Roger Amass, D.Ph.
Alcon Laboratories, Inc.
6201 South Freeway
Fort Worth, Texas 76134-2099

Intraocular Irrigating Solutions

James E. Arena
Department of Pharmacy
Duke University Medical Center
Erwin Road
Durham, North Carolina 27710

Rifampin

Amir Bar-Ilan, Ph.D.
Pharmos Limited
Kiryat Weizmann
Rehovot 76236, Israel

Basic Considerations of Ocular Drug-Delivery Systems

Richard J. Barohn, M.D.
Department of Neurology
University of Texas Southwestern Medical School at Dallas
5323 Harry Hines Blvd.
Dallas, Texas 75235

Drugs for the Diagnosis and Treatment of Myasthenia Gravis

Jules Baum, M.D.
16 Webster St.
Brookline, Massachusetts 02146

Penicillins and Cephalosporins

Frederick W. Benz, Ph.D.
Professor
Department of Pharmacology and Toxicology
University of Louisville School of Medicine
301 E. Muhammad Ali Blvd.
Louisville, Kentucky 40292

Pharmacodynamics: Drug–Receptor Interactions

Parimal Bhattacherjee, Ph.D.
Professor of Ophthalmology and Visual Sciences
Department of Ophthalmology and Visual Sciences
University of Louisville School of Medicine
301 E. Muhammad Ali Blvd.
Louisville, Kentucky 40292

Eicosanoid Receptors in Ocular Tissues

Laszlo Z. Bito, Ph.D.
Professor of Ophthalmology
Department of Ophthalmology, Research Division
Columbia College of Physicians and Surgeons
630 West 168th St.
New York, New York 10032

Physiologic Aspects of Glaucoma and Its Current and Future Management
Prostaglandins and Prostaglandin Analogues

William F. Buss, Pharm. D.
Clinical Pharmacist
Department of Neonatal Nursing/Pharmacy
James Whitcomb Riley Hospital for Children
Indiana University Medical Center
702 Barnhill Drive
Indianapolis, Indiana 46202

Effect of Age on Drug Disposition

Carl B. Camras, M.D.
Professor and Vice-Chairman
Department of Ophthalmology
University of Nebraska Medical Center
600 South 42nd St.
Omaha, Nebraska 68198-5540

Prostaglandins and Prostaglandin Analogues

Margaret K. L. Cheung, M.D., Ph.D.
Assistant Clinical Professor
Department of Surgery
John A. Burns School of Medicine
University of Hawaii
1960 East-West Rd.
Honolulu, Hawaii 96822

Immunosuppressive Therapy for Uveitis

Craig E. Crosson, Ph.D.
Associate Professor
Department of Ophthalmology and Pharmacology
Texas Tech University Health Sciences Center
Lubbock, Texas 79430

Cholinergics

Patricia A. D'Amore, Ph.D.
Department of Surgery and Pathology
Children's Hospital and Harvard Medical
300 Longwood Ave.
Boston, Massachusetts 02115

Angiogenesis and Growth Factors

Gerard D'Aversa, M.D.
Department of Ophthalmology
Long Island Jewish Medical Center
600 Northern Blvd.
Great Neck, New York 11021

Peptide Antibiotics: Vancomycin, Bacitracin, and Polymyxin B

Henry F. Edelhauser, Ph.D.
First Professor of Ophthalmology, Director of Ophthalmic Research
Department of Ophthalmology
Emory University
1365-B Clifton Rd.
Atlanta, Georgia 30322

Intraocular Irrigating Solutions

Forrest D. Ellis, M.D.
Department of Ophthalmology
Indiana University
702 Rotary Circle
Indianapolis, Indiana 46202

Topical Ophthalmic Preparations Used for Infants and Children
Cycloplegic Agents
Topical and Local Anesthetic Agents
Antiglaucoma Medications
Ocular Antiinflammatory Agents

Ervin N. Fang, M.D.
Department of Ophthalmology and Visual Sciences
Washington University School of Medicine
St. Louis, Missouri 63110

Epinephrine and Dipivefrin

Robert D. Fechtner, M.D.
Associate Professor
Department of Ophthalmology and Visual Sciences
Associate Director, Glaucoma Service
University of Louisville School of Medicine
Kentucky Lions Eye Center
Louisville, Kentucky 40292

Definitions and Classification of Glaucoma

C. Stephen Foster, M.D.
Professor of Ophthalmology, Director, Imunology Uveitis Service
Massachusetts Eye and Ear Infirmary
243 Charles St.
Boston, Massachusetts 02114

Pharmacology of Medical Therapy for Uveitis
Mydriatic and Cycloplegic Agents
Nonsteroidal Antiinflammatory Drugs
Immunosuppressive Chemotherapy

W. Craig Fowler, M.D.
Department of Ophthalmology
Duke University Eye Center
Box 3802
Durham, North Carolina 27710

Rifampin

B'Ann True Gabelt
Department of Ophthalmology and Visual Sciences
University of Wisconsin
600 Highland Ave., F4/328 CSC
Madison, Wisconsin 53792-3220

Direct, Indirect, and Dual-Action Parasympathetic Drugs

Steven L. Galetta, M.D.
Department of Neurology
University of Pennsylvania Medical Center
Philadelphia, Pennsylvania 19104

Drugs for the Diagnosis and Treatment of Myasthenia Gravis

Bryan M. Gebhardt, Ph.D.
Professor of Ophthalmology and Microbiology, Parasitology, and Immunology
LSU Eye Center/LSU Medical Center
2020 Gravier St., Suite B
New Orleans, Louisiana 70112-2234

Antivirals

Stephen R. Glaser, M.D.
Center for Sight - 7PHC
Georgetown University Medical Center
3800 Reservoir Rd., NW
Washington, D.C. 20007

Antiseptics and Disinfectants

Joseph R. Gussler, M.D.
Bascom Palmer Eye Institute
900 NW 17th St.
Miami, Florida 33136

Chloramphenicol

Bruce C. Henderson, M.D.
Clinical Assistant Professor of Ophthalmology
Department of Ophthalmology
Louisiana State University Medical School in Shreveport
2121 Fairfield Ave.
Shreveport, Louisiana 71104

Antifibrosis Agents: Pharmacologic Inhibition of Wound Healing

James M. Hill, Ph.D.
Professor of Ophthalmology, Pharmacology, and Experimental Therapeutics, Microbiology, and Immunology
Department of Ophthalmology
LSU Eye Center/LSU Medical Center
2020 Gravier St., Suite B
New Orleans, Louisiana 70112-2234

Antivirals

R. Nick Hogan, M.D., Ph.D.
Assistant Professor
Department of Ophthalmology and Pathology
University of Texas Southwestern Medical Center at Dallas
5323 Harry Hines Blvd.
Dallas, Texas 75235-9057

Mydriatic and Cycloplegic Drugs
Sodium Fluorescein and Other Tissue Dyes

Helen Y. How, M.D.
Assistant Professor
Department of Obstetrics and Gynecology
University of Cincinnati
Medical Sciences Bldg.
231 Bethesda Avenue
Cincinnati, Ohio 45267-0526

Effect of Pregnancy on Drug Disposition

Harrell E. Hurst, Ph.D.
Professor of Pharmacology and Toxicology
Department of Pharmacology and Toxicology
University of Louisville School of Medicine
Louisville, Kentucky 40292

Introduction to Toxicology

Robert A. Hyndiuk, M.D.
Wisconsin Eye Institute
8700 W. Wisconsin Ave.
Milwaukee, Wisconsin 53226

Aminoglycosides in Ophthalmology
Fluoroquinolones
Surgical Viscoelastic Substances

Mark J. Iacobucci
Duke University Eye Center
Box 2808
Durham, North Carolina 27710

Rifampin

Glenn J. Jaffe, M.D.
Associate Professor of Ophthalmology
Department of Ophthalmology
Duke University
Box 3802
Durham, North Carolina 27710

Proliferative Vitreoretinopathy: Biology and Pharmacology

Lee M. Jampol, M.D.
Louis Feinberg Professor and Chairman
Department of Ophthalmology
Northwestern University Medical School
645 N. Michigan Ave.
Suite 440
Chicago, Illinois 60611

Pharmacologic Therapy for Cystoid Macular Edema

George R. John, M.D.
Assistant Professor
Department of Ophthalmology
University of Louisville
301 E. Muhammad Ali Blvd.
Louisville, Kentucky 40292

Cyanoacrylate Tissue Adhesives

Mark S. Juzych, M.D.
Assistant Professor of Ophthalmology
Department of Ophthalmology
Wayne State University
Kresge Eye Institute
4717 St. Antoine Blvd.
Detroit, Michigan 48201-1423

Alpha-2 Agonists in Glaucoma Therapy
Beta-blockers

Carol L. Karp, M.D.
Assistant Professor of Clinical Ophthalmology
Bascom Palmer Eye Institute
900 N.W. 17th St.
Miami, Florida 33136

The Tetracyclines
Erythromycin, Clarithromycin, and Azithromycin
Chloramphenicol

Michael A. Kass, M.D.
Professor of Ophthalmology
Department of Ophthalmology and Visual Sciences
Washington University School of Medicine
660 South Euclid Ave.
St. Louis, Missouri 63110

Epinephrine and Dipivefrin

Adam H. Kaufman
University of Cincinnati
University Medical Arts Building
222 Piedmont Ave., Suite 1700, ML665-E
Cincinnati, Ohio 45219

Penicillins and Cephalosporins

Herbert E. Kaufman, M.D.
Boyd Professor of Ophthalmology and Pharmacology and Experimental Therapeutics, Head, Department of Ophthalmology
LSU Eye Center
Louisiana State University Medical Center School of Medicine
2020 Gravier, Suite B
New Orleans, Louisiana 70112

Paul L. Kaufman, M.D.
Professor of Ophthalmology and Visual Sciences, Director of Glaucoma Service
Department of Ophthalmology and Visual Sciences
University of Wisconsin Medical School
600 Highland Ave., F4/328 CSC
Madison, Wisconsin 53792-3220

Direct, Indirect, and Dual-Action Parasympathetic Drugs

Lisa D. Kelly, M.D., F.A.C.S.
5012 W. 128th St.
Leawood, Kansas 66209

Antiparasitic Agents

Karanjit S. Kooner, M.D.
Assistant Professor
Department of Ophthalmology
Southwestern Medical School
5323 Harry Hines Blvd.
Dallas, Texas 75235-9057

Definitions and Classification of Glaucoma
Thymoxamine (Alpha-Adrenergic Antagonist)
Future Role of Neuroprotective Agents in Glaucoma

Theodore Krupin, M.D.
David E. Shoch Professor of Ophthalmology
Department of Ophthalmology
Northwestern University
Tarry 5-715
300 E. Superior
Chicago, Illinois 60611

Hyperosmotic Agents

Prasad S. Kulkarni, Ph.D.
Professor of Ophthalmology and Visual Sciences
Department of Ophthalmology and Visual Sciences
University of Louisville School of Medicine
301 E. Muhammad Ali Blvd.
Louisville, Kentucky 40292

Steroids in Ocular Therapy

Richard Lambert, D.V.M., Ph.D.
Alcon Laboratories, Inc.
6201 South Freeway
Fort Worth, Texas 76134-2009

Intraocular Irrigating Solutions

Moshe Lazar, M.D.
Chairman
Department of Ophthalmology
Ichilov Hospital
Sackler Faculty of Medicine
Tel-Aviv University
Tel-Aviv, Israel

Drug Reactions Not Mediated via Receptors

Trang Diem Le, M.D.
Department of Ophthalmology
University of Texas Southwestern Medical Center at Dallas
5323 Harry Hines Blvd.
Dallas, Texas 75235-9057

Mydriatic and Cycloplegic Drugs

Robert E. Leonard II, M.D.
Instructor
Bascom Palmer Eye Institute
900 N.W. 17th St.
Miami, Florida 33136

Erythromycin, Clarithromycin, and Azithromycin

Anat Loewenstein, M.D.
Department of Ophthalmology
Ichilov Hospital
Sackler Faculty of Medicine
Tel-Aviv University
Tel-Aviv, Israel

Drug Reactions Not Mediated via Receptors

James P. McCulley, M.D.
Professor and Chairman
Department of Ophthalmology
University of Texas Southwestern Medical Center
Zale Lipshy Hospital
5323 Harry Hines Blvd.
Dallas, Texas 75235-9057

Amebic Disease of the Eye

Paula J. McGarr
Ophthalmic Research Associates, Inc.
863 Turnpike St.
North Andover, Massachusetts 01845

Antiallergic Therapies

Travis A. Meredith, M.D.
Retina Consultants, LTD
One Barnes Hospital Plaza, Suite 17413
St. Louis, Missouri 63110

Antibiotics and Antifungals

Joan W. Miller, M.D.
Department of Ophthalmology
Massachusetts Eye and Ear Infirmary
243 Charles St.
Boston, Massachusetts 02114

Medical Therapy for Macular Degeneration
Angiogenesis and Growth Factors

Ramana S. Moorthy, M.D.
Associated Vitreoretinal and Uveitis Consultants
8704 N. Meridian St.
Indianapolis, Indiana 46260

Antivirals in the Treatment of Retinal Diseases

Bruce A. Mueller, Pharm. D.
Associate Professor of Clinical Pharmacy
Department of Pharmacy Practice
School of Pharmacy and Pharmaceutical Practice
Purdue University
West Lafayette, Indiana 46202-2879

Effect of Disease on Drug Disposition
Effect of Age on Drug Disposition

Mark P. Nasisse, D.V.M.
Kraeuchi Professor of Ophthalmology
College of Veterinary Medicine
University of Missouri
379 E. Campus Drive
Columbia, Missouri 65211

Ethical Issues in Ophthalmic Research

George F. Nardin, M.D., M.P.H.
Private Practice
407 Uliniu St., #214
Kailua, Hawaii 96734

Antifibrosis Agents: Pharmacologic Inhibition of Wound Healing

Ron Neumann, M.D.
Pharmos Limited
Kiryat Weizmann
Rehovot 76326, Israel

Basic Considerations of Ocular Drug-Delivery Systems

Jerry Niederkorn, Ph.D.
Professor of Ophthalmology and Microbiology
Department of Ophthalmology
University of Texas Southwestern Medical Center at Dallas
5323 Harry Hines Blvd.
Dallas, Texas 75325-9057

Amebic Disease of the Eye

Gary D. Novack, Ph.D.
President
PharmaLogic Development, Inc.
17 Bridgegate Drive
San Rafael, California 94903-2181

Adrenergic Pharmacology of the Anterior Segment
Development of New Drugs for Ophthalmology
The Opthalmologist as Clinical Investigator
Alpha-2 Agonists in Glaucoma Therapy

Terrence P. O'Brien, M.D.
Ocular Microbiology Laboratory
The Wilmer Eye Institute
Johns Hopkins University School of Medicine
Baltimore, Maryland 21287-9121

Pharmacotherapy of Fungus Infections of the Eye

Richard J. O'Callaghan, Ph.D.
Professor
Department of Microbiology/Ophthalmology
LSU Medical Center
1901 Perdido St.
New Orleans, Louisiana 70112

Antivirals

Gregory S. H. Ogawa, M.D.
Assistant Professor of Ophthalmology
Department of Surgery
Division of Ophthalmology
University of New Mexico Health Sciences Center
2211 Lomas Blvd. NE
Surgery/Ophthalmology 2-ACC, UNMHSC
Albuquerque, New Mexico 87131-5341

Fluoroquinolones

Steven M. Patalano, M.D.
Medical Arts Building
236 Highland Ave.
Somerville, Massachusetts 02143

Aminoglycosides in Ophthalmology

P. Andrew Pearson, M.D.
Assistant Professor
Department of Ophthalmology
University of Kentucky
Kentucky Clinic
Lexington, Kentucky 40536

Proliferative Vitreoretinopathy: Biology and Pharmacology

Roswell R. Pfister, M.D.
Professor of Ophthalmology
Department of Ophthalmology
University of Alabama, Eye Hospital
513 Brookwood Blvd., Suite 504
Birmingham, Alabama 35209

Mitomycin Treatment of Corneal Disease

Jeffrey G. Piper, M.D.
Associate Staff/Department of Surgery
Department of Ophthalmology
Rutland Regional Medical Center
160 Allen St.
Rutland, Vermont 05701

Oral Carbonic Anhydrase Inhibitors

David E. Potter, Ph.D.
Professor/Chairman of Pharmacology and Toxicology
Department of Pharmacology and Toxicology
Morehouse School of Medicine
720 Westview Drive, S.W.
Atlanta, Georgia 30310-1495

Adrenergic Pharmacology of the Anterior Segment

Rajesh K. Rajpal, M.D.
Cornea Consultants
8133 Leeburg Pike
Suite 240
Tysons Corner, Virginia 22182

Antiseptics and Disinfectants

Lawrence I. Rand, M.D.
164 Bigelow Rd.
West Newton, Massachusetts 02165

Ocular Pharmacology of Diabetic Retinopathy

Peter Rhee, M.D.
Ocular Microbiology Laboratory
The Wilmer Eye Institute
Johns Hopkins University School of Medicine
Baltimore, Maryland 21287-9121

Pharmacotherapy of Fungus Infections of the Eye

Kevin P. Richard
Harvard Medical School/Schepens Eye Research Institute
200 Staniford St.
Boston, Massachusetts 02114

Antiallergic Therapies

Gavin J. Roberts, M.D.
Ophthalmology Consultants of Fort Wayne
7224 Engle Rd.
Fort Wayne, Indiana 46804

Surgical Viscoelastic Substances

Alan L. Robin, M.D.
Associate Professor of Ophthalmology
Johns Hopkins University and the University of Maryland Schools of Medicine
6115 Falls Rd.
Baltimore, Maryland 21209

Alpha-2 Agonists in Glaucoma Therapy

James T. Rosenbaum, M.D.
Casey Eye Institute
3375 S.W. Terwilliger Blvd.
Portland, Oregon 97201-4197

Immunosuppressive Therapy for Uveitis

Ronald D. Schoenwald, Ph.D.
Professor of Pharmaceutics
College of Pharmacy
The University of Iowa
118 Pharmacy Bldg.
Iowa City, Iowa 52242-1112

Ocular Pharmacokinetics

Gregory Schultz, Ph.D.
Departments of Ophthalmology and Gynecology
JH Miller Health Center, Box 100294
1600 SW Archer Rd.
University of Florida
Gainesville, Florida 32610

Future Developments in Corneal Therapy: Growth Factors

Johanna M. Seddon, M.D.
Associate Professor of Ophthalmology
Department of Ophthalmology
Epidemiology Unit and Retina Service
Massachusetts Eye and Ear Infirmary
Harvard Medical School
243 Charles St.
Boston, Massachusetts 02114
Associate Professor of Epidemiology
Department of Epidemiology
Harvard School of Public Health
Boston, Massachusetts

Medical Therapy for Macular Degeneration

Mordechai Sharir, M.D., Ph.D.
Assistant Professor
Department of Ophthalmology and Visual Sciences
Department of Microbiology and Immunology
University of Louisville School of Medicine
Louisville, Kentucky 40292
Chief of Glaucoma
Department of Ophthalmology
The Edith Wolfson Hospital
Tel-Aviv University
Holon 58100, Israel

The History of Ocular Pharmacology
Topical Carbonic Anhydrase Inhibitors

Kuldev Singh, M.D.
Assistant Professor of Ophthalmology
Department of Ophthalmology
Stanford University
A-157
Stanford, California 94305

Hyperosmotic Agents

Joseph A. Spinnato, M.D.
Professor and Director
Department of Obstetrics and Gynecology
Division of Maternal-Fetal Medicine
University of Louisville School of Medicine
Louisville, Kentucky 40292

Effect of Pregnancy on Drug Disposition

George A. Stern, M.D.
Department of Ophthalmology
University of Florida College of Medicine
Box 100284 JHMHC
Gainesville, Florida 32610-0284

Peptide Antibiotics: Vancomycin, Bacitracin, and Polymyxin B

Carol Toris, Ph.D.
Assistant Professor and Director of Glaucoma Research Lab
Department of Ophthalmology
University of Nebraska Medical Center
600 South 42nd St.
Omaha, Nebraska 68198-5540

Prostaglandins and Prostaglandin Analogues

Albert Vitale, M.D.
21 Marlboro St.
Newton, Massachusetts 02158

Pharmacology of Medical Therapy for Uveitis
Mydriatic and Cycloplegic Agents
Nonsteroidal Antiinflammatory Drugs
Immunosuppressive Chemotherapy

David V. Weinberg, M.D.
Assistant Professor of Ophthalmology
Department of Ophthalmology
Northwestern University Medical School
645 N. Michigan Ave.
Suite 440
Chicago, Illinois 60611

Antivirals in the Treatment of Retinal Disease

George A. Williams, M.D.
Chief, Vitreoretinal Surgery
William Beaumont Hospital
3535 West Thirteen Mile Rd.
Royal Oak, Michigan 48703
Clinical Professor of Biomedical Sciences
Eye Research Institute of Oakland University
Rochester, Michigan

Drugs Affecting the Coagulation/Fibrinolysis Pathways

Gil I. Wolfe, M.D.
Department of Neurology
University of Texas Southwestern Medical School at Dallas
5323 Harry Hines Blvd.
Dallas, Texas 75235

Drugs for the Diagnosis and Treatment of Myasthenia Gravis

Carol F. Zimmerman, M.D.
Associate Professor of Ophthalmology and Neurology
University of Texas Southwestern Medical Center at Dallas
5323 Harry Hines Blvd.
Dallas, Texas 75235-9057

Mydriatic and Cycloplegic Drugs
Drugs for the Diagnosis of Pupillary Disorders
Sodium Fluorescein and Other Tissue Dyes

Thom J. Zimmerman, M.D., Ph.D.
Professor and Chairman
Department of Ophthalmology and Visual Sciences
Professor of Pharmacy and Toxicology
University of Louisville School of Medicine
Kentucky Lions Eye Center
301 E. Muhammad Ali Blvd.
Louisville, Kentucky 40292

Beta-blockers

Preface

The study of medicine has influenced humanity since the beginning of mankind. The basic human instincts of curiosity, observation, experimentation, and improvement have shaped our destiny and our relationship to the world. The "medicine man," "faith healer," and "high priest" have enjoyed special status in past societies; but out of superstitious and crude experimentation came the desire to understand the scientific basis of diseases and therapy. The search for "miracle drugs" that cause "miracle cures" still goes on, and the marvelous technological advances after World War II were once beyond our imagination. We have come a long way, and the future looks promising and exciting.

Our knowledge of ophthalmic physiology, molecular biology, diagnostics, and therapeutics is evolving at such a rapid pace that it is difficult to keep abreast of all the relevant developments. The last 25 years have seen phenomenal growth in ocular pharmacology in particular. We have learned more about our established drugs, and a large number of new drugs have become available for the treatment of patients with cornea and external diseases, glaucoma, cataract, uveitis, endophthalmitis, retinitis, choroiditis, scleritis, optic neuritis, and orbital diseases.

The expert contributors to this book have assembled information that provides the most up-to-date knowledge on currently available ophthalmic drugs. The various sections of this book and their editors are *General Ocular Pharmacology* (Sharir and T.J. Zimmerman), *Glaucoma* (Kooner, T.J. Zimmerman, and Fechtner), *Retina* (Weinberg and Jampol), *Cornea and External Diseases* (John and Kaufman), *Uveitis* (Vitale and Foster), *Anesthesia* (Acquadro), *Pediatrics* (Ellis), and *Diagnostic Drugs* (C. Zimmerman).

In the book, each drug is considered as follows: history and source, official drug name and chemistry, pharmacology, clinical pharmacology, pharmaceuticals, pharmakinetics, therapeutic uses, side effects and toxicity, high-risk groups, drug interactions, and major clinical trials. Our aim is to provide the most authoritative source of present and emerging knowledge on ocular pharmacology. Both the basic and clinical relevance of each drug is presented in an easy-to-read and uniform format. This will help ophthalmologists and residents-in-training to comprehend various drugs and their classes and to use this updated information to treat patients. Innovative approaches to pharmacotherapy are also presented. Each chapter concludes with the most recent references, which correspond to the flow of text and contain important new primary clinical or basic data.

Thom J. Zimmerman
Karanjit S. Kooner
Mordechai Sharir
Robert D. Fechtner

Acknowledgments

We acknowledge the outstanding cooperation, encouragement, and editorial expertise of Vickie Thaw, Joyce-Rachel John, and Delois Patterson of Lippincott–Raven Publishers. For over four years they have untiringly kept the group together and have always reminded us of our goal.

SECTION I

General Ocular Pharmacology

Section Editors: Mordechai Sharir and Thom J. Zimmerman

OVERVIEW

In this section, the reader is invited to explore the basic sciences on which all our knowledge and clinical skills are based. The spectrum of works has encompassed centuries of pioneering in vitro and in vivo experimentations. Breakthrough in many fields, for example, the concept of *receptor,* coined by Paul Ehrlich, and the drug-receptor interaction and drug efficacy (pharmaco*dynamics*) has enabled the prediction of general or ocular bioavailability, absorption, distribution, tissue concentration as well as drug elimination (all included under pharmaco*kinetics*) via almost precise mathematical models and computations.

This section should serve as an introduction and a foundation to the clinical sections to follow. From the huge amount of works and publications, the authors elected to concentrate on those that have an immediate impact on the eye and the ocular tissues. Nevertheless, most of this section includes chapters that have implications in general pharmacology as well as the eye.

Following an anecdotal journey through the history of civilization and its discovery of ocular remedies (Chapter 1), some basic molecular pharmacology is reviewed (Chapters 2 and 3). Selected topics, according to drug classifications, are overviewed in Chapters 4 through 8. Cho-linergics, autacoids, steroids, adrenergic, and immunosuppressive agents separately would be topics for textbooks on their own; therefore, the avid reader is invited to explore these specific sources, listed as references, to broaden his or her knowledge.

Chapters 9 through 14 describe in detail various specific aspects of ocular pharmacokinetics. The unique and privileged position of the ocular adnexae and the ocular interior necessitates complex considerations when a medication is developed for topical application. Chapter 15 is an example of applying the principles explored in the kinetic studies toward the development of more sophisticated ocular drug delivery systems.

The second part of this section summarizes in a concise form issues that have not been dealt with in previous pharmacology textbooks but carry some importance in the dynamic and fast-growing field of preclinical and clinical ocular drug trials. Chapter 16 should be renamed "What does it take to get from an idea to a final eyedrop on the shelf?" The long, expensive and highly demanding road includes animal studies for which some ethical considerations are reviewed in Chapter 17.

Drug safety and toxicity are two major concerns that are addressed in an introduction to the discipline of ocular toxicology (Chapter 18). Because of the scope of the subject, we have chosen to introduce concepts, definitions, and designs of acute and chronic toxicity studies that have ocular implications. For the detailed side effects and toxic reactions, the reader is referred to the specific literature.

The final part of this section focuses on three special risk groups: the chronically ill, the aged, and the pregnant patient. The variations in each case and their impact on drug therapy have been extensively reviewed.

We are deeply grateful to our contributing authors. Without their enthusiasm, dedication, and expert contributions, preparation of this textbook would have been impossible. The list is long, with distinguished names, some of whom are leading authorities in their field of research. This has resulted, in our opinion, in a unique mosaic that reflects the most recent scientific data and insight. The following section has become a very fruitful interaction between basic scientists and clinicians.

Textbook of Ocular Pharmacology,
edited by T.J. Zimmerman, et al.
Lippincott–Raven Publishers, Philadelphia © 1997.

CHAPTER 1

The History of Ocular Pharmacology

Mordechai Sharir

A drug is a substance that, when injected into a rat, produces a scientific paper.

Edgerton Y. Davis, Jr.

If the whole materia medica, as now used, could be sunk to the bottom of the sea, it would be all the better for mankind—and all the worse for the fishes.

Oliver Wendell Holmes, 1860

Poisons and medicine are oftentimes that same substance given with different intents.

Peter M. Latham (1789–1875)

One should treat as many patients as possible with a new drug while it still had the power to heal.

William Osler (1849–1919)

The desire to take medicine is, perhaps, the great feature which distinguishes people from other animals.

William Osler (1849–1919)

The history of pharmacology in general, and ocular pharmacology in particular, is as long and convoluted as the history of mankind. Rather than present a dry account of documented information pertaining to the discoveries and developments in ocular pharmacology, I have elected to provide the most colorful anecdotal oddities that contributed significantly to our present state of the art in ocular pharmacology. This brief account involves a wide spectrum of witchcraft, myth, strong will, compassion, and emotional stimuli as well as charlatanism. The practice of ocular pharmacology was hazardous, as in the case of an angry husband with a sharp knife chasing a failing healer, to unpredictable locations of practice, for example, 7 Green Pea Street (better known by the sailors as Hog Lane) inside a notorious brothel.

The eye, as the focus of vision and myth, has fascinated mankind from the most remote times. In ancient nations, magic and horror were associated closely with efforts to divine the mysteries of sight and to combat the evil effects of ocular disease.

PROTOPHARMACOLOGY: THE ANCIENT EAST

From the earliest classical writers, we know that considerable medical literature was accumulated in Mesopotamia, the cradle of civilization. Ocular treatment is first mentioned in the Code of Hammurabi, a collection of civil laws promulgated by Hammurabi, the sixth king of the first dynasty of Babylon, in about 2250 B.C. Babylonian medicine was probably in the hands of the priest of healing divinity, Ea, and his son Marduk, and surgery was in the hands of a special class of skilled handworkers. For a successful operation that saves the eye of the patient, the fee would be ten sheckels of silver in the case of a "gentleman," but only five sheckels in the case of a poor man and two sheckels for a slave. The fee-for-service scale was generous. Five sheckels was equivalent to the yearly rent of a good house and represented 150 times the daily wage of a workman. The eye was sometimes held at the same value as that of life: "If a physician operate on a man and cause the man's death; or, with a bronze lancet, open an abscess in the eye of a man and destroy the man's eye, they shall cut off his fingers."

Medical treatment consisted largely of administering drugs containing a varying number of ingredients and tested substances of therapeutic value. Drugs were given in water, milk, wine, or oil, or sometimes as "Tanner's verdigris (shoemaker's vitriol), copper dust, yellow sulphide of arsenic, mix in curd and apply to the man's sick eyes."

The earliest records of Egyptian medicine date back to a period not much later than the code of Hammurabi. The Edwin Smith papyrus (ca. 1600 B.C.), the Ebers papyrus (ca. 1550 B.C.), and the Brugsch papyrus (ca. 1300 B.C.) mark significant genuine efforts to treat eye diseases rather than simply to describe them. In the Ebers papyrus, the Egyptians recognized entities such as blepharitis, chalazion, ectropion, entropion, trichiasis, pterygium, pinguecula,

M. Sharir: Department of Ophthalmology, The Edith Wolfson Hospital, Tel-Aviv University, Holon, Israel.

staphyloma, leukoma, iritis, cataract, "blood in the eye," ophthalmoplegia, inflammation, and dacryocystitis. Although the attempt at differential treatment implies a degree of differential diagnosis, medicine was still in the hands of priests. Nevertheless, there is much evidence that Egyptian ophthalmology was held in high esteem in the ancient world. The prophet Jeremiah and Herodotus were impressed by the number of physicians and their specialties: "One treats only the diseases of the eye, another those of the head, the teeth, the abdomen, or of the internal organs."

Herodotus also relates that Cambyses II of Persia sent to Amasis, the King of Egypt, for a physician to cure his beloved mother, queen Cassandane, of her eye trouble. That search ended in a war between the two nations. Ancient sources divulge that Amasis the Pharaoh ordered his most famous eye therapist, Nebenchari, "a man of learning and courtesy," against his will, to go to the court of Cambyses II to treat the eyes of the aging queen mother. He was forced to leave behind his wife, child, and what is believed to be the first textbook of ocular pharmacology, *Additional Writings on Treatment of the Diseases of the Eye, by the Great God Thoth, Newly Discovered by the Oculist Nebenchari.* Modesty at that time permitted all healing knowledge to be attributed to the gods. The only other available book about ophthalmic therapy was by the Chinese emperor Shen Nung (2737 B.C.) entitled *The Importance of Needling,* which covers almost every spot about the eyes. Although the records are not clear, it would seem that Cassandane was troubled with senile cataracts. While in exile, Nebenchari learned that his own king, who was afflicted by the same malady, preferred Pentammon, arch professional rival of Nebenchari, as his ophthalmologist. Distressed by the news of betrayal, and more intimate to Cambyses after successfully operating on his mother, Nebenchari devised a plot of demanding the beautiful Pharaoh's daughter for the Persian court. The arrival of a substitute gift was a humiliation, initiating a sequence of misunderstandings, insults, and an invasion of Egypt by the mighty Persian ruler. Hence, ophthalmology was the cause of a world war. It is assumed that in the years to follow, Nebenchari was appointed the Life President of the Persian–Egyptian Ophthalmological Society, but no sources are available to verify the whereabouts of that ancient oculist after the invasion.

Sumerian medicine (ca. 600 B.C.) was based on plants (shammu), or mineral materials (abnu). A great library of some 30,000 clay tablets was discovered in a mound near the site of Ninevah. Those that could be deciphered describe various remedies for rheumatism, cardiac disease, stomach troubles, and eye diseases. The Sumerians developed a high degree of specialization in medical practice and a clear recognition of not only pharmacists and dentists but also specialists for almost every part of the body. A joke of the period relates how one doctor asks another, "What is your specialty?" The reply was, "Eyes", to which another question was asked, "Which eye?"

The Babylonian and Egyptian captivities influenced the development of Jewish medicine. Biblical and Talmudic accounts of hygienic conditions and postmortem examinations of slaughtered animals for the determination of what was "kosher" describe pathological conditions not known to other peoples. A sleeping potion ("Samme de shina") was devised for pain relief in connection with surgical operations. Whether it was hemp or opium is not known from the sources.

Altogether the significance of the Mesopotamian peoples in regard to health affairs was great. There was probably a considerable exchange of information between the tribes and nations that later extended to faraway places, like India and China.

GREEK–ROMAN PHARMACOLOGY

Eight hundred years elapsed from the appearance of Hippocrates to the end of the fruitful Roman period. Early Greek medicine was in the hands of the divine, the cult of Asclepius, with Pallas Athene as the healer. Hygieia was worshipped as the guardian of eyesight (like St. Lucia, the patron saint of the sore-eyed today in Italy). Fragments of two stone tablets found in a temple bearing the title "Cures of Apollo and Asclepius" read:

> . . . A one-eyed [man] visited by the god in abaton during the night. [The god] applies an ointment in the empty orbit. Upon awaking, the man finds he has two sound eyes. . . . Thyson of Hermione is blind of both eyes; a temple dog licks [the organs] and he immediately regains his sight.

The medical group of Kos, of which Hippocrates (460–375 B.C.) was the most prominent member, contributed to the advancement of medical therapy primarily by taking the treatments away from the hands of the priests and instituting a professional line of healers. Knowledge then was limited to superficial anatomy, and with a lack of any understanding of physiology, therapy was limited as well. Around 400 B.C., "blepharoxysis" was a popular treatment of ocular diseases. It consisted of rubbing the inner surface of the eyelids with Milesian wool. Granulations were removed with a scoop or scratched out with a rough fig leaf. Aristotle (384–322 B.C.) was the first to provide a scientific background for the practical affairs of the health professions.

Greek medicine was widely disseminated through the Roman Empire by Greek physicians, who often were slaves. Their high intellectual standard commanded the respect of their masters, and frequently they were freed to enjoy a relatively high social status.

De re Medicina, the eight books of Celsus, are a compendium of medical practice at that time (A.D. 29) The sixth book includes a detailed anatomy of the eye and an accurate description of trachoma. Ocular therapeutics were similar to those of Hippocrates, with "collyrium" for inflammation, essentially a tiny cake or bar of medicine dissolved in water or oil. These cakes were stamped with seals displaying the name of the inventor, together with the disease it meant to cure. For a stye, Celsus recommended hot bread or a honey poultice, and for proptosis he prescribed venesection. Hypopyon was the contribution of Galen (A.D. 131–201) to ophthalmology, together with some (failing) efforts to systematize the ocular disorders and their treatments.

THE ARABIAN PERIOD

Muslim medicine carried forward the Greek–Roman tradition in a blend with old Sumarian, Egyptian, and Coptic treatment practices. Greek–Roman medicine invaded the Arab world via the Bishop of Arius, who claimed against church teachings that Jesus was no more divine than any other person and that there is only one god. The Arians settled in Persia and spread their medical practices, among other things.

Mohammed (A.D. 570–632) was a fiery Arian who so inflamed his followers that they conquered Asia Minor, North Africa, and Spain within a couple of centuries after his death. The Islamic contributions to ocular pharmacology were considerable. By A.D. 887, there was already a medical training hospital in Kairouan. In the tenth century, Isaac Ibn Soleiman, whose origin was Jewish, wrote about drugs and foods; Ziad el Moucafir later described compound drugs, including eyedrops. Ishaq Al-Kindi of Kufa (now Iraq) wrote the *Kitab fi-kimiya* (Book on Chemistry), in which prescription no. 158 using metallic ingredients for an eye salve reads:

> Collyrium of abn Muhammed for preserving the eyes. It strengthens and protects them.
>
> Tutty (impure zinc oxide) pounded and washed seven times with clear water and then put in a mortar -3 mithals (about 14 gm.)
>
> Antimony sulfide 1 mithqal
> Iron pyrite 1 mithqal
>
> It is soaked in water, then pulverized, soaked in marjoram juice and filtered over a fire. Sukk (a confection of dates, clove, cardamon and sandalwood) and one mithqal is added to it. Then it is pulverized until dry. Use then as collyrium. It is helpful, with God's aid.

FROM MEDIEVAL EUROPE THROUGH THE EIGHTEENTH CENTURY

The thousand years to follow were relatively dormant for ocular pharmacology. Medical studies shifted to the cities of Salerno and Montpellier. Constantine, an African adventurer who crossed the Mediterranean from Carthaage in the eleventh century, was first to coin the term *cataract.* He also translated Arabic writings into Latin, beginning a movement that gathered speed with the years. Ophthalmology in those days of twilight was influenced by masters like Benevenutus Grassus "of Jerusalem," who lectured in southern France and Italy for large fees and generated monumental books on eye treatments, such as *Practica Oculorum,* the earliest printed book on the eye (Ferrara, 1475). His books were written in Hebrew and translated into Latin, Old French, and Old English. Peter the Spaniard (later Pope John XXI) introduced a treatise on hygiene of the eye and medical management of various diseases. If no memorable oculists were produced, it was the versatile geniuses, like Roger Bacon and Leonardo da Vinci, who concentrated on optics and anatomy.

Ferrari of Pavia, in his advice to treat eye disease with "reserve," describes an oculist neighbor of his who, having failed to relieve his patient's agony or to save her eye (from acute glaucoma?), was pursued in the night by her infuriated husband, sword in hand.

Ocular pharmacology also found its way to the graveyard. In 1696 Dr. Walter Pope wrote his farewell note to his dearest friend and ophthalmologist, Dawbigney Turberville, the personal physician of Queen Anne. The eulogy said: "Adieu my dear friend, a rivederci, till we meet and see one another again with eyes which will never stand in need of a COLLYRIUM."

The study of anatomy during the sixteenth and seventeenth centuries paved the way for the great pathological and clinical progress of the eighteenth century, the century of cataract extraction. Italy pioneered ocular occupational medicine. It started in Professor Bernardino Ramazzini's (1633–1714) privy vault, or jakes, where his hired workers gave his office its triennial cleaning. The professor was troubled by the anxiety with which the jakes cleaners overtired themselves and asked them to slow down. Their reply was: "That none but those who tried it could imagine the trouble of staying above four hours in that place," and "It being equally troublesome as to be struck blind." When the cleaners came out of the vault, their eyes were very red and dim. Ramazzini was at a loss to explain why the eyes were the only parts to suffer. He found it hard to believe that "steams arising from the human ordure, after three years lying, assume a particular nature . . . forcing the lachrymal juice . . . noxious only to the eyes." He advised the workers to put transparent bladders over their faces or to find another occupation. In afflicted eyes, he suggested washings with muscadine wine, an excellent remedy, for it "invited the animal spirits to come from the brain and the optic nerve to return to the eyes, from whence they had been driven by the sordid and penetrating damps." It should be remembered that all was inspired when that good man stood by a dismal vault and looked down into the streaming eyes of jakes cleaners, a rare feeling of compassion of a nobleman in those times.

Toward the end of the seventeenth century, exotic tropical plant drugs were becoming known in Europe, if only by rumor, among them the ancestral sources of our modern miotics. From a West African woody climber came the feared ordeal bean, or Calabar bean (*Physostigma venenosum*), carried by slaves to the Americas for exotic use in determining guilt; if one survived ingesting it, one was innocent. From South America came another bean, jaborandi or *Pilocarpus pinnatus* or Paraguay bean. These remained curiosities until the nineteenth century, when technical methods were devised for studying their biological effects and for isolating from them the chemical substances responsible for their biological action. Eserine was isolated only in 1864 and pilocarpine in 1875. It would be 11 more years until Ludwig Laqueur, himself a glaucoma patient, would publish his findings that physostigmine (eserine) lowers intraocular tension in glaucomatous eyes.

On the "dilating end," in 1686 John Ray of England first recorded that a belladonna leaf, applied to a small abscess near the eye, caused dilation of the pupil. Only a hundred years later, three independent reports (by Daries, Loder, and Reimarus) advocated its use to facilitate cataract extraction. All this is particularly remarkable, as atropine was not isolated until 1831, almost half a century later.

The eighteenth century witnessed the first plagiarism in ocular pharmacology. William Rowley's 1790 book was copied almost verbatim from Joseph Plenck, a notorious Hungarian professor of surgery. It also carried the ridiculously long title *A Treatise on One Hundred and Eighteen Principal Diseases of the Eyes and Eyelids, etc., In Which Are Communicated Several New Discoveries Relative to the Cure of Defects in Vision; with Many Original Prescriptions. To Which Are Added Directions in the Choice of Spectacles.* Only 40 years later, William Mackenzie, an oculist of Glasgow, wrote in his textbook: "The influence of mercury alone, or combined with opium, has long been recognized. See Warner, Plenck, his plagiarist Rowley, etc." It is still not understood why Rowley, a respectable scientist on his own account, committed that felony.

The eighteenth century matured around the creation of special eye hospitals. The first eye hospital in history opened in Vienna in 1786, when Georg Beer set aside two rooms in his apartment for the treatment of eye diseases. As early as 1771, William Rowley had founded "St. John's Hospital for Diseases of the Eyes, Legs and Breasts."

OCULAR PHARMACOLOGY IN THE NINETEENTH CENTURY

The first half of the nineteenth century was a remarkable period of consolidation, and the second half brought the medical and operative treatment of various ocular diseases. The ophthalmoscope opened a world undreamt of and raised ophthalmology to the most exact of clinical disciplines.

Mydriatics gained widespread clinical application. For ocular pain, the Greeks used opium, mandragora, and hyoscyamus; the latter was also used cosmetically for blue-eyed people to induce in them black pupils.

Schmidt had used mydriatics as early as 1805 for the treatment of iritis, but his practice did not gain wide acceptance. It was largely through the advocacy of Desmarres and von Graefe in 1856 that atropine came to occupy its place in modern ophthalmology. Von Graefe also reported in 1868 the deleterious action of atropine in glaucoma, stirring a dispute over its value, until entities such as uveitis were recognized.

Miotics have a briefer history. The first systematic evaluation of the Calabar bean was in Edinburgh in 1846 and 1855. Thomas Fraser showed its miotic effect in 1862, and Argyll Robertson demonstrated its action on accommodation a year later. His first paper, titled "The Calabar Bean as a New Ophthalmic Agent," served as an introduction to its use in antiglaucoma treatment. Argyll Robertson's good looks cause his clinic to be crowded by young ladies of the time, who gladly paid his fee of two guineas to have him examine their perfect eyes so they might gaze into his. He collected his fee and allowed them to do so.

In the same year, 1863, Von Graefe studied the antagonistic effects of atropine and employed it to facilitate iridectomy in noninflammatory glaucoma. As mentioned, the active components were actually isolated only a decade later.

Francois Magendie (1783–1855) laid the foundation for modern pharmacology by introducing the concepts of dose-effect relationships, absorption, distribution, biotransformation, and elimination of drugs into and out of living material. His pupil, Claude Bernard, followed with the explanation of the site of action (neuromuscular junction for curare), specific mechanisms of action (carbon monoxide and tissue anoxia), and the relation between the chemical properties and biological activity.

Jan Purkyne (1787–1886), the brilliant Czech microscopist, studied, with Wolfgang Goethe's stimulation, the "visual flickerings" and effects of belladonna, opium, and digitalis, while in Germany, Rudolf Buchheim (1820–1897) started a systematic review book on therapeutics.

The nineteenth century also marks the coming of asepsis and anesthesia. Both had a profound impact on surgery in general and ocular procedures in particular. Before their introduction, patients and surgeons dreaded more the postoperative prospect of infection than the surgery itself.

Ocular inoculation had a disgusting start. In 1811 Henry Walker suggested inoculation with gonorrheal pus as a treatment for corneal pannus, a thought that would turn germ-conscious souls cold and loathing. The idea was based on the observation that pannus would clear in patients infected with Egyptian (neonatal) ophthalmia. In Moorfields, 170 patients were successfully treated. This phase was followed by 50 years of trial and error. "To inoculate an eye, a drop of yellow pus was placed on the inside of the lower eyelid. Within 24 hours the lid would swell and become edematous. There would be irritation, lacrimation, and photophobia. In three to four days all symptoms of acute purulent ophthalmia would be present . . . the cornea would clear over a four week period." Only one eye was inoculated at the time, the other eye "closed by hermetic collodion compress," and an ice pack was the only method to relieve pain. Dr. Elkanah Williams, of Cincinnati, pioneered this treatment in the United States and coined a new term, *Glandola,* to the remedy. Inspired by the muses and sworn to secrecy as to its composition, a grateful patient once wrote, "But, however that may be I once was blind Glandola did the work for me."

In 1872 the Wills Eye Hospital in Philadelphia was among the first to report counterirritation by a blister behind the ear, or on the arm, as a beneficial treatment for granular (trachomatous) conjunctivitis. With dense pannus, the eyes were inoculated with gonorrheal pus or a solution of jequirity bean. Venesection, leeches, potassium iodide, seclusion from light, and artificial dilatation of the pupil were common recommendations for a variety of diseases.

During that time, "Dr." Isaac Thompson's Celebrated Eye Water broke the record, having the largest sale of any topical ophthalmic preparation in the nineteenth century. With an aggressive advertising and marketing campaign, Thompson, of Connecticut, could afford a comfortable retirement from what ended up to be "1 and 1/2 grains of opium, 10% alcohol, zinc sulphate and rose water."

In 1860 Albert Neimann isolated cocaine from coca leaves. Sigmond Freud (1856–1939), the famous Viennese psychoanalyst, toyed with the central nervous system stimulating effect of cocaine and its bizarre numbing action on the tongue. By his suggestion, his friend Carl Koller carefully studied the subject and showed the effects of cocaine, the first local anesthetic. It was an actual serendipity, following a frustrating day in the laboratory with rabbits, dogs, and guinea pigs, carving the way for today's outpatient procedures. In early 1885, Koller, resenting an insult from a colleague, was challenged to a duel because of his findings, and he was the victor. His position in Vienna became precarious, however, and after a brief stay with Donders in Utrecht, he migrated to New York City in 1889. Chauncey Leake mentions his first personal account with the ophthalmologist as his patient in a handsome second-floor office on the corner of 59th Street and Madison Avenue, encouraging him to describe his discovery (3). A Johns Hopkins surgeon, William Stewart Halsted, reported in 1885 the abuse of cocaine after his own exhilarating experience following accidental ingestion of a solution he had prepared for use on others.

Epinephrine and its effect on blood vessels were discovered in 1898 by John Abel of the Johns Hopkins Hospital and independently as "adrenalin" by Takamine in Detroit in 1901. Only decades later, it was employed as an antiglaucoma medication.

TRANSITION INTO THE TWENTIETH CENTURY

Into the twentieth century, ocular pharmacology came with a rush. The tale is vast, with many distinguished scientists involved, adding to a huge jigsaw puzzle.

The foundations of modern pharmacology were laid by Paul Ehrlich (1854–1915). Influenced by methods developed by Louis Pasteur, Robert Koch, Von Behring, and others, Ehrlich introduced the "receptor" concept, a specific site for interaction with a drug. John Newport Langley (1852–1925) clearly differentiated the sympathetic and parasympathetic aspects of the autonomic nervous system. The terms *agonist* and *antagonist* also were coined.

With the dissemination of knowledge from Europe in bacteriology, biochemistry, physiology, and pharmacology, therapeutic modalities underwent a major revolution.

Under George De Schweinitz, the department of ophthalmology at the University of Pennsylvania became a focus of research and experimental ocular treatments. The classification of conjunctivitis was no longer purely descriptive but included etiological factors as well, and "under no circumstances should [the eye] be bandaged, or covered with poultices of tea-leaves, bread and milk and like." Boric acid, yellow oxide of mercury, and calomel were the usual topical medications prescribed. Optic nerve atrophy was treated with nitroglycerine, and a Turkish bath was prescribed for diabetic retinitis. More understanding of glaucoma came in the form of measuring intraocular tensions (with a Schiotz's tonometer) and the association with nerve–head excavation, changes in pupillary size and anterior chamber depth, loss of corneal transparency, and alterations in episcleral vessels. For the treatment of glaucoma, De Schweinitz preferred pilocarpine, supplemented by strychnine, nitroglycerine, and massage. For intractable cases, an iridectomy was performed. In his *Some Results of a Bacteriological Examination of Pipettes and Collyria Taken from a Treatment Case Used in Ophthalmic Practice,* De Schweinitz pointed out the importance of sterilization of solutions and instruments in clinical and surgical use.

Between the two World Wars, sulfonamides were introduced and gradually replaced leaches and yellow oxide ointments. Drs. Scheie, Sounders, and Leopold, working at the University of Pennsylvania, were among the first to study the penetration of sulfonamide compounds into the eye. The 1940s were the exciting epoque of penicillins (Fleming), streptomycin (Waksman), and chloramphenicol. Dr. Hench announced in 1949 the dramatic effects of cortisone and adrenocorticotropic hormone in rheumatoid arthritis. During the same period, Dr. Robb McDonald, under the guidance of Dr. Francis Heed Adler, studied the ocular manifestations of vitamin A deficiency as well as observations on the treatment of glaucoma with diisopropyl fluorophosphate.

In the decades to follow, more sophisticated antibiotics were synthetized. Enzymes and their specific inhibitors gained an important role in the understanding of pathological processes. Hormonal preparations, cytotoxics, and antiviral agents made their appearance. Beta-adrenoreceptor antagonists without local anesthetic properties became the first-line antiglaucoma therapy, and topical carbonic anhydrase inhibitors minimized the troublesome side effects associated with their systemic use. Novel delivery methods have made drugs safer and more efficacious, and controlled clinical studies have become the standard mode of drug evaluations. Ocular pharmacology benefited from structure-activity relationship studies as well as new prospects from molecular biology, immunology, and genetics.

The complete story is far from being told, as ocular pharmacology is now more dynamic and fascinating than ever. The following chapters are a reflection of the knowledge and skills gained throughout thousands of years of civilization, for which an almost endless list of contributors deserves credit.

REFERENCES[1]

1. Chance B. Clio Medica. A Series of Primers on the History of Medicine. XXI. Ophthalmology. New York: Paul B Hoebner, 1939.
2. Sorsby A. *A Short History of Ophthalmology.* 2nd ed. London: Staples Press, 1948.
3. Leake CD. *An Historical Account of Pharmacology to the 20th Century.* Springfield: Charles C Thomas, 1975.
4. Parnham MJ, Bruinvels J, eds. *Selections from Discoveries in Pharmacology.* Amsterdam: Elsevier, 1987.
5. Albert DM, Scheie HG. *A History of Ophthalmology at the University of Pennsylvania.* Springfield: Charles C Thomas, 1965.
6. Snyder C. *Our Ophthalmic Heritage.* Boston: Little, Brown and Company, 1967.
7. Clark FH, ed. *How Modern Medicines are Discovered.* Mount Kisko: Futura Publishing Company, 1973.
8. Parascandola J. *The Development of American Pharmacology. John Abel and the Shaping of a Discipline.* Baltimore: The Johns Hopkins University Press, 1992.
9. Ferry AP, Ferry MK. Dr. Isaac Thompson and His Celebrated Eye Water. *Ophthalmology* 1984;91:528–537.

[1]Due to the unorthodox nature of this chapter, the references are not cited in text.

Textbook of Ocular Pharmacology,
edited by T.J. Zimmerman, et al.
Lippincott–Raven Publishers, Philadelphia © 1997.

CHAPTER 2

Pharmacodynamics: Drug–Receptor Interactions

Frederick W. Benz

The purpose of this chapter is to lay the foundation for understanding the mechanisms by which drugs produce their pharmacological effects. This study of the biochemical and physiological processes underlying drug action is called *pharmacodynamics.* As will become evident, most drug action is initiated when the drug molecule noncovalently interacts with a macromolecular component of the cell. The chemical nature of this component varies among the different classes of drugs but includes proteins, nucleic acids, and possibly even the cell membrane. Of these, proteins represent, by a wide margin, the most likely target for drug interaction. Although enzymes, transporters, and structural proteins are involved in many mechanisms of drug action, the types of protein that most often represent the initiation site for drug action are those that normally interact with endogenous neurotransmitters, hormones, and other mediators of various physiological functions. These specialized functional proteins with which drugs interact are called drug *receptors.*

As with the receptor, the chemical nature of drugs can be quite varied. Typically, most drugs are relatively low-molecular-weight organic chemicals but may include metals, organometallics, peptides, proteins, lipids, the building blocks of nucleic acids, as well as nucleic acids themselves. In the not too distant future, whole genes will need to be included.

FORCES INVOLVED IN DRUG–RECEPTOR INTERACTIONS

Having considered the chemical nature of drugs and receptors and having stated that the interaction between them initiates drug action, the nature of the forces involved in the interaction is reviewed briefly. As mentioned, the chemical interaction between the drug and its receptor is usually noncovalent. The strongest noncovalent bond involves the electrostatic interaction between full and opposite charges and is called the *ionic bond.* This force acts at greater distances than other noncovalent forces but is attenuated by the dielectric constant of the medium, which, in the case of water, is quite high. In addition, the force may be diminished by the presence of relatively high concentrations of counterions present in the physiological milieu. These inhibitory factors may be mitigated by the presence in the receptor of an active site pocket with a microenvironment significantly shielded from the conditions that exist in the bulk water phase.

Other weaker electrostatic interactions are also available, for example, ion–dipole, dipole–dipole, ion–induced dipole, and so on. One special case of a dipole–dipole interaction is that of a *hydrogen bond.* Hydrogen bonds are of considerable importance in protein and nucleic acid structure as well as in drug-receptor interactions. One important feature of hydrogen bonding is the fact that it has structural constraints. The strongest hydrogen bonds are planar and linear and have an optimum distance between the two atoms that are sharing the proton between them. Thus, if hydrogen bonds form between a drug and its receptor, some information about the three-dimensional structure of the complex may be provided.

The weakest of the electrostatic forces involved in drug-receptor interactions is the *van der Waals bond,* which results from local fluctuations in electron density between the interacting partners. As the two molecules approach, the electron density of the atoms involved is polarized, and a weak electrostatic interaction ensues. The optimum distance between the atoms involved is the sum of their van der Waals radii; therefore, the drug and receptor interacting

F. W. Benz: Department of Pharmacology and Toxicology, University of Louisville School of Medicine, Louisville, Kentucky 40292.

surfaces must be highly complementary for such bonding to play an important role in the interaction. Although noncovalent bonding accounts for the vast majority of drug–receptor interactions, some drugs do form covalent bonds with their receptors. Unlike *noncovalent bonds,* which are reversible, leading to transient drug action, *covalent bonds* are usually irreversible and can lead to prolonged drug action. On occasion, such prolonged drug action may be desirable.

DRUG ACTION AT RECEPTORS

The minimal requirement for a drug to produce a pharmacological effect via its receptor is for it to bind, that is, to occupy the receptor. Consideration is now given to methods available for assessing receptor occupancy.

Law of Mass Action

The binding of a single drug molecule (A) to a single binding site on the receptor protein (R) can be described by the following scheme:

$$R + A \rightleftarrows RA$$

The strength of the interaction between the drug (*ligand*) and its receptor can be expressed by the *equilibrium dissociation constant* K_D for the above scheme, namely,

$$K_{\mathrm{D}} = \frac{[R]\,[A]}{[RA]} \qquad [1]$$

The concentrations in the numerator represent the free receptor and drug. It is typically assumed that the free drug concentration $[A]$ is equal to the total concentration of drug added $[A_T]$. This cannot hold for the receptor, however. Thus, the free concentration of receptor $[R]$ is equal to the total receptor concentration $[R_T]$ minus the concentration of bound receptor $[RA]$. Substituting this difference for $[R]$ in Eq. 1 and rearranging yields:

$$\frac{[RA]}{[R_{\mathrm{T}}]} = \frac{[A]}{[A] + K_{\mathrm{D}}} \qquad [2]$$

This equation expresses the fractional occupation of receptor sites by drug A in terms of the concentration of drug A added and the dissociation constant of the drug A-receptor complex. Expressed in this way, it is clear that the receptors will be half occupied when $[A]$ is equal to K_D.

Equilibrium Radioligand Binding

Currently, a common method for assessing the K_D of a drug for a specific receptor site in a tissue is to conduct an equilibrium radioligand binding experiment. Typical data collected in such an experiment are shown in Table 2-1. Briefly, a homogenate of the tissue containing the receptor is prepared, and a portion of the homogenate is added to pairs of test tubes, seven pairs in the current example. To each pair is added a known and increasing concentration of radioactively labeled drug (columns 1 and 2). Because it is possible for the drug to interact not only with the specific receptor site of interest but also nonspecifically with other components of the homogenate or apparatus used in the experiment, a correction for this nonspecific binding must be applied. One method used to accomplish this correction is to add to one member of each pair of tubes a high concentration of the same ligand that is not radioactively labeled. The concentration of nonlabeled drug added must be sufficient to interact with all the specific receptor binding sites; that is, they must be saturated with nonlabeled drug molecules. The pairs of tubes then are incubated for a sufficient time for the drug-receptor system to reach equilibrium. Typically, the contents of each tube then are filtered such that the receptors, containing bound drug molecules, are

TABLE 2-1. *Equilibrium radioligand binding data*

Drug A added[a]		Raw binding data (dpm)[b]			Bound[c]	Bound/free[d]	Occupancy[e]
dpm/2 ml	nM	Total	Blank	Specific	(fmol/mg)	(fmol/mg/nM)	%
3431	0.06	98	4	94	0.35	5.45	6
13440	0.25	331	19	312	1.16	4.64	20
28948	0.54	586	40	546	2.03	3.77	35
53760	1.00	855	75	780	2.90	2.90	50
99840	1.86	1153	140	1013	3.77	2.03	65
215040	4.00	1548	301	1247	4.64	1.16	80
1021440	19.00	2911	1430	1481	5.51	0.29	95

[a]Drug A (12 Ci/mmol) was incubated with 2-ml aliquots of tissue homogenate containing 10 mg of wet weight of tissue per tube. [b]Seven pairs of tubes were incubated with increasing concentrations of labeled ligand. Blank tubes also contained 10 μM unlabeled ligand to correct for nonspecific binding.

Bound radioactivity retained on the filters for the two sets of samples is tabulated. Specific binding is the difference between these pairs. [c]Moles of bound ligand were calculated from the dpm specifically bound, the specific activity of the radioactive ligand, and the weight of the tissue.

[d]Calculated by dividing the moles bound by the free concentration of ligand that produced them.

[e]Calculated by dividing the bound ligand by the B_{max}, which was 5.8 fmol/mg. (See text for details.)

retained on the filters. The amount of drug retained is assessed by liquid scintillation spectrometry. A plot of the total (column 3) and nonspecific (column 4) radioactivity on the filters against the concentration of drug added to each tube is shown in Figure 2-1A. The difference in binding between the pairs of tubes at each concentration represents the specific binding (column 5). The plot of specific binding versus drug concentration can be seen as a rectangular hyperbola as expressed in Eq. 2.

Scatchard Plot

Scatchard showed that Eq. 2 could be rearranged into the following linear form:

$$\frac{[RA]}{[A]} = -\frac{1}{K_D}[RA] + \frac{[R_T]}{K_D}$$

Figure 2-1B shows that a plot of $[RA]/[A]$ (column 7) versus $[RA]$ (column 6) yields a straight line with a slope equal to $-1/K_D$ and an intercept on the abscissa equal to $[R_T]$, often called B_{max}. In this way, the K_D of the drug-receptor complex and the receptor density in the tissue can be readily determined.

Relative Affinity

Another graphical portrayal of data of this type is shown in Figure 2-1C. Here the rectangular hyperbolic-specific binding curve of Figure 2-1A is converted into a sigmoidal curve by changing the drug-concentration axis to a logarithmic scale. The midpoint of the sigmoid curve reflects the K_D for the drug-receptor complex. A drug is said to have high *affinity* for its receptor site if it has a very low K_D. Figure 2-1C also shows similar binding data for a second drug *B*. It can be seen that drug *B* has a higher K_D than drug *A* and thus by definition has lower affinity for the receptor than drug *A*. The ratio of the two K_D values, which reflects the distance between the two curves on the log concentration axis, is a measure of the *relative affinities* of the two drugs. Drug *B* can be said to have 1/10 the affinity of drug *A* for the receptor.

ACTION OF AGONISTS

Although evaluation of the concentration dependence of drug occupancy is an important pharmacological objective, what sets the science of pharmacology apart from the other basic medical sciences is its focus on the assessment of the concentration dependence of drug effect. A drug that can interact with a receptor to produce a pharmacological response is called an *agonist.* As drugs, such agents are used primarily to mimic the effect of some endogenous compound; for example, the vasoconstrictor effects of epinephrine can be mimicked by the drug phenylephrine.

Types of Responses to Drugs that Can Be Measured

Because measurement of drug response is central to pharmacology, consideration must be given to the types of biological responses that can be measured. A *quantal response* is an all-or-none response. In the pharmacological evaluation of new drugs, toxicity testing is done in which high doses may be administered to groups of animals, and the numbers alive versus dead are measured as a function of dose; this is a quantal response. Alternatively, a drug's ability to produce ataxia may be assessed by placing groups of ten mice on a rotating rod. All nontreated animals may be able to stay on the rod for 5 minutes. The ability of groups of ten treated mice to stay on the rod for this length of time can be measured. Evaluating the number of mice that fall off and those that remain on the rod within each group as a function of drug dosage would serve as a way to quantify the ataxic potential of a drug or group of drugs. Responses of this type are also quantal responses.

More typically, however, graded responses to drugs are measured. A *graded response* is measured on a continuous

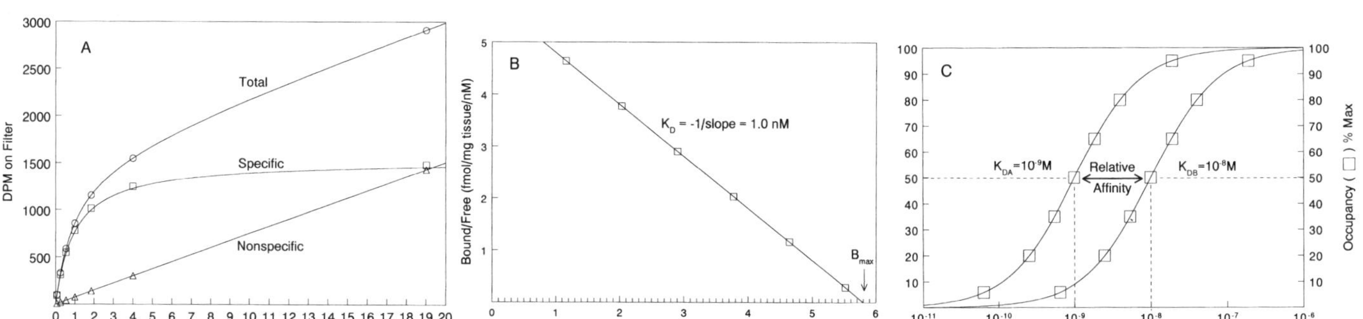

FIG. 2-1. A: Plot of equilibrium radioligand binding data from Table 2-1 on a linear concentration scale. **B:** Scatchard plot of equilibrium radioligand binding data from Table 2-1. **C:** Log concentration-occupancy curve for the equilibrium radioligand binding data for drug A from Table 2-1 and a second drug B with a lower affinity for the receptor than drug A. (See text for details.)

scale, and there is a systematic relationship between the dose administered and the magnitude of the response observed. Measurement of blood pressure, intraocular pressure, heart rate, or muscle-tension changes as a function of drug dose would be examples. Graded responses can be converted into quantal responses if one specifies a given level of graded response as being a positive response and all lower levels of graded response as being negative. An example of this conversion will be presented near the end of this chapter.

Quantitative Relationships between Drug Concentration and Response

In the following discussion of the theories of drug action, no attempt will be made to present them in the historically correct sequence. Rather, some liberties will be taken to present the pharmacological concepts in a more logical progression. In fact, this historical laxity has already been perpetrated in that the radioligand binding method of assessing receptor occupancy already presented postdates the methods of assessing response as a function of drug concentration, to be discussed subsequently.

The quantitative relationships between drug concentration and pharmacological response were initially studied using isolated tissues. A typical preparation of this sort is shown in Figure 2-2A. In this example, a section of intestinal tissue from a small animal is suspended in an oxygenated physiological salt solution. The intestinal strip is connected to a device for measuring contractile force. In the absence of added drug, the strip is placed under a basal resting tension. When an agonist drug is added to the bath,

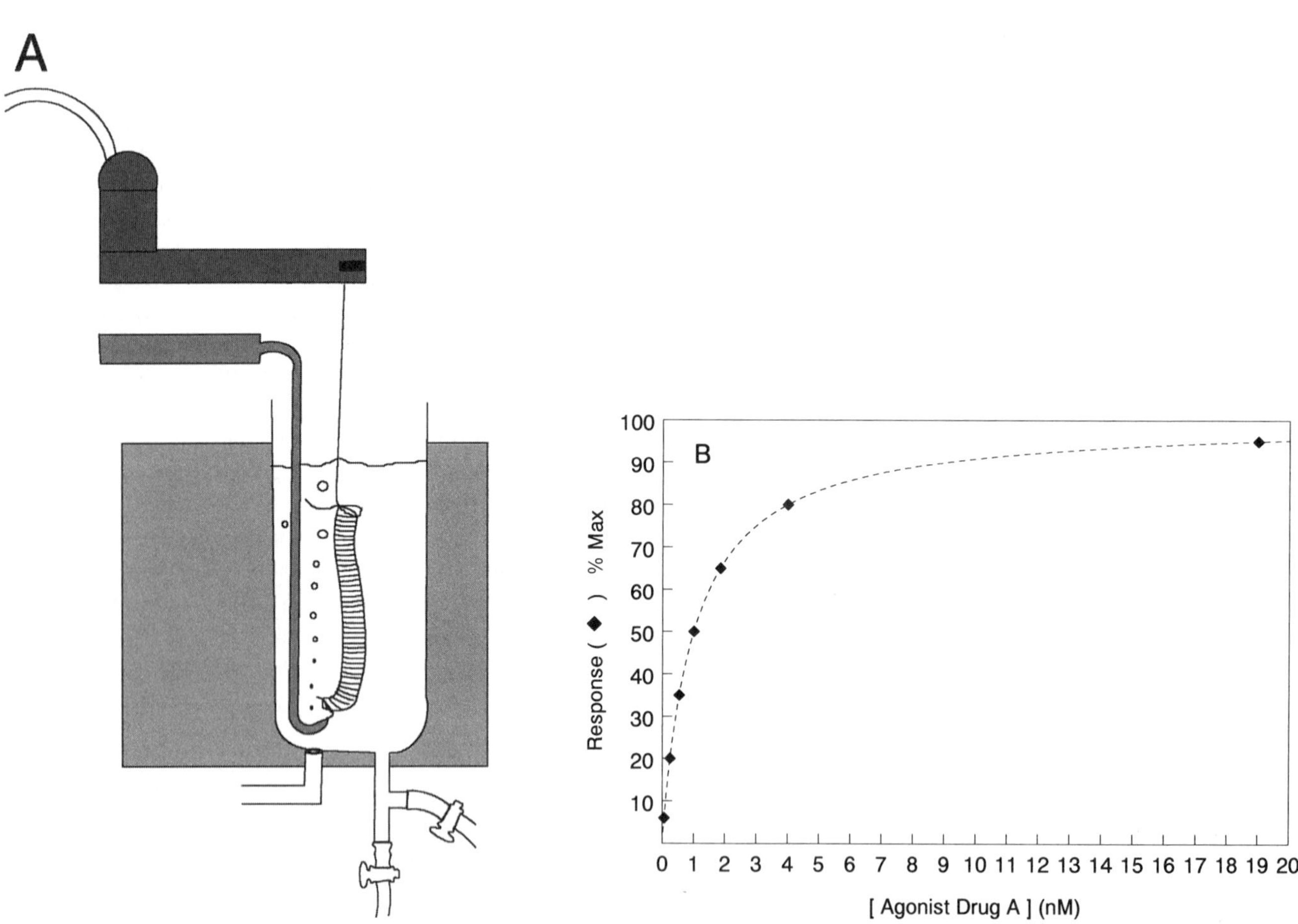

FIG. 2-2. A: Typical pharmacological preparation for studying the quantitative relationships between drug concentration and response. (See text for details.) **B:** Concentration-response curve for agonist drug A acting on the pharmacological preparation illustrated. A concentration of drug is added to the physiological salt solution bathing the tissue. When the response has reached equilibrium, the drug solution is drained from the bath and replaced with fresh medium. This sequence is repeated with other concentrations of the agonist drug until the complete concentration-response curve has been described. The response to each agonist concentration is expressed as the percent of the maximal response that the agonist can produce. The agonist concentration axis is linear.

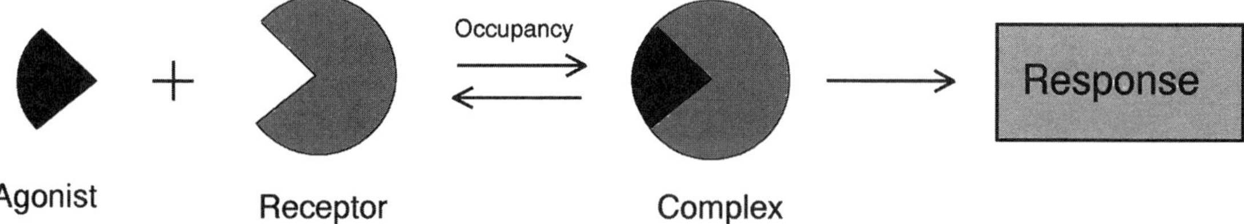

FIG. 2-3. Occupancy Model of A. J. Clarke.

it can interact with receptors in the tissue, which results in the pharmacological effect of increased contractile force. When a sufficiently high concentration of drug is added to the bath, the maximal force of which the tissue is capable is measured. When one applies concentrations of the agonist drug between no drug and the concentration that produces the maximal response, the concentration-response curve shown in Figure 2-2B is observed. The curve's shape is identical to that observed in Figure 2-1A for the occupancy of specific receptor binding sites as a function of added drug concentration.

Simple Occupancy Model ($EC_{50} = K_D$)

It should not be surprising, therefore, to discover that the earliest model that attempted to quantify the relationship between response and drug concentration was the Occupancy Model of A. J. Clarke (Figure 2-3). This model proposed drug response to be a linear function of drug occupancy of receptor sites. That is to say, 25% occupancy would yield 25% response, 50% occupancy would give 50% response, and so on. Thus, if one plots the response as a function of concentration on the same graph as the occupancy as a function of concentration, the two curves will be superimposable (Figure 2-4). Thus, an equation analogous to Eq. 2 may be written to describe the relationship between response (effect) and concentration of drug:

$$\frac{E_A}{E_{max}} = \frac{[A]}{[A] + EC_{50}} \qquad [3]$$

This equation expresses the fractional effect in terms of the concentration of drug A and the EC_{50}, which is the concentration of drug A required to produce 50% of the maximal response (E_{max}). As indicated in Figure 2-4, for the simple Occupancy Model of drug action, the concentration of drug required to produce 50% of the maximal response and the dissociation constant of the drug receptor complex are numerically identical.

Log Concentration-Response Plot

In pharmacology, it is more typical to plot the concentration-response curve of agonists on a log concentration scale (Figure 2-5). Here again, as in Figure 2-1C, the rectangular hyperbolic response curve is converted into a sigmoidal curve. The midpoint or inflection point of the sigmoid curve reflects the drug concentration required to produce 50% of the maximal response (EC_{50}). A drug is said to have *high potency* if it has a very low EC_{50}. Figure 2-5 also shows a similar log concentration-response curve

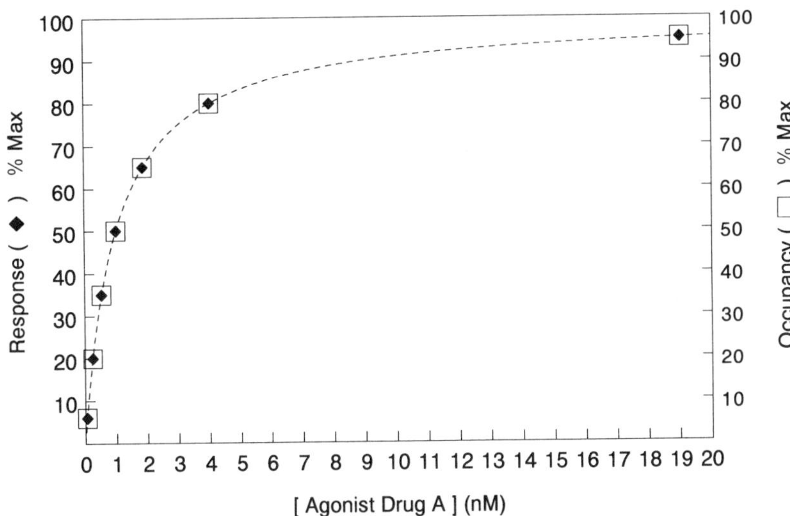

FIG. 2-4. Plot of the concentration-occupancy curve for drug A from Figure 2-1A and the concentration-response curve for the same drug from Figure 2-2B on the same linear scale. In the simple Occupancy Model of drug action, the two curves are superimposable.

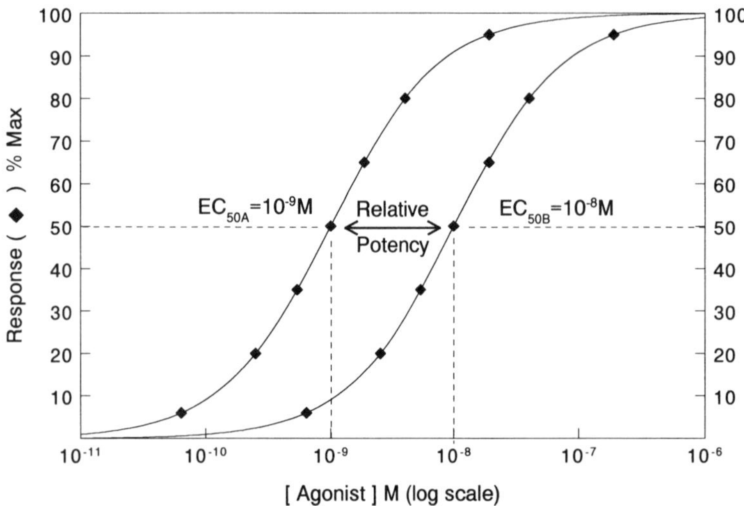

FIG. 2-5. Log concentration-response curve from the response data for drug A in Figure 2-2B and for a second drug B with a lower potency for the receptor system than drug A. (See text for details.)

for a second drug *B*. It can be seen that drug *B* has a higher EC_{50} than does drug A and thus by definition has a lower potency. The ratio of the two EC_{50} values, which reflects the distance between the two curves on the log concentration axis, is a measure of the *relative potency* of the two drugs. Drug *B* can be said to have 1/10 the potency of drug *A* for the response measured.

There are several advantages for portraying concentration-response curves on a log concentration scale. The first is that the response between approximately 15% and 85% of the maximal response is nearly linear with log concentration, meaning that if the responses of the tissue to two concentrations of agonist are known, the dose required to produce any other response within this range can be predicted. For example, if it is known that a drug produces 25% of the maximal response at 1×10^{-8} *M* and that a 50% response requires 3×10^{-8} *M*, it can be predicted that a 75% response will require 9×10^{-8} *M*. Notice that for the same increase in response (Δ=25%) between each concentration of drug, a geometric or proportional change in drug concentration is required, that is, a factor of 3 increase in this hypothetical example. The actual proportional change required in any system, of course, will depend on the actual slope of the log concentration-response curve for that system.

A second advantage of the log concentration-response curve is that, as mentioned, the position of the curves for individual drugs on the log concentration axis reflects the potency of each drug. Because of the compression of the concentration axis, when plotted on a log rather than linear scale, the relative potency of drugs that differ by several orders of magnitude may be readily portrayed. Finally, it is an axiom of pharmacology that drugs that produce their effects by the same mechanism of action, but differ only in potency, will yield parallel log concentration-response curves; that is, their slopes will be identical.

In summary, the simple Occupancy Model of drug action predicts that all agonists for a receptor will be able to produce the same maximal effect. Agonists will differ only in their ability to bind to the receptor (i.e., their affinity, a biochemical parameter, represented by K_D), which can also be expressed as the concentration of agonist required to produce a 50% response (i.e., their potency, a pharmacological parameter, represented by EC_{50}). It must be noted that this equality of K_D and EC_{50} applies only to isolated tissue experiments that can be described adequately by the simple Occupancy Model. As will be seen later, more complicated receptor systems are known where these parameters diverge. In addition, the potency of a drug in a whole-animal experiment or as used therapeutically in humans will be a function not only of the affinity of the drug for its receptor but also a function of how the drug is absorbed, distributed, metabolized, and excreted (i.e., its *pharmacokinetics*). These factors will influence the eventual concentration of the drug at its receptor and may easily play a dominant role in determining the potency of a drug in patients. In most cases, differences in relative potencies among drugs of the same class simply determine how much of a particular drug the patient must take to achieve a given pharmacological effect.

Slope of the Log Concentration-Response Plot

It can be shown for the simple Occupancy Model of drug action that the maximum slope occurs at the EC_{50} and represents a 58% change in response for a tenfold increase in drug concentration. As with the equality of K_D and EC_{50}, this theoretical slope would be observed only in isolated tissue experiments that fit this simple model. Deviations from this slope served as a clue that certain drug-receptor systems require a more complex model. In addition, in

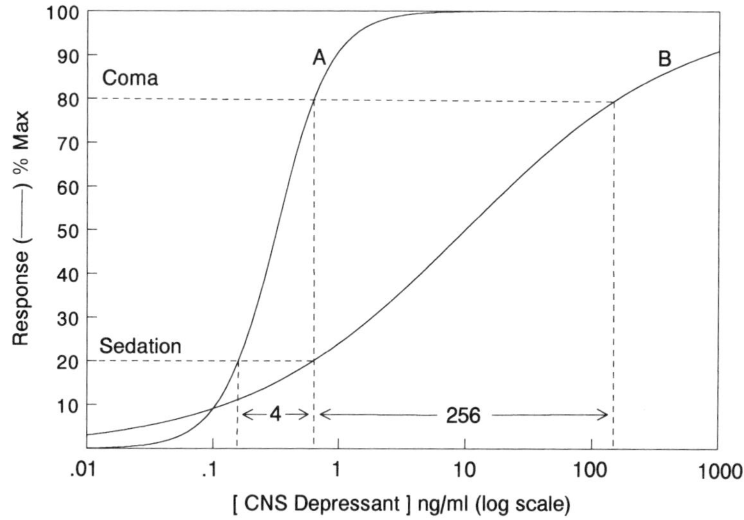

FIG. 2-6. Log concentration-response curves for two CNS depressants exhibiting considerably different slopes. (See text for details.)

whole-animal experiments or in humans, because pharmacokinetic effects may dominate, the slope could have a very different value. The relative steepness of log concentration-response curves does have therapeutic implications, however. Figure 2-6 compares hypothetical blood concentration-response curves for two agents that can produce CNS depression. If we arbitrarily assign the response equal to 20% of maximal CNS depression as sedation and 80% of maximal depression as coma, for curve *A* the concentration difference between these two responses is only a factor of 4, whereas for drug *B*, a 256-fold concentration increase would be required. Obviously, the response to drug *B* would be much easier to adjust safely than would be the case for drug *A*. In addition, the substantial slope differences between drugs *A* and *B* in this example would indicate that the two agents were producing the CNS-depressant effects by different mechanisms.

Occupancy and Intrinsic Activity Model ($EC_{50} = K_D$)

The simple Occupancy Model of Clarke had to be adjusted when it was discovered that in a series of agonists, all of which interact with the same receptor, not all agonists within the class could produce the same maximal response. This phenomenon is illustrated in Figure 2-7. For drugs *A* and *B*, both can produce the E_{max}. The response curve equals the occupancy curve for each, and the two agents would be said to differ only in potency (and affinity). For drugs *C* and *D*, however, the response curves (filled diamonds) are not superimposable on the occupancy curves (open squares), and neither drug can produce the E_{max}. Thus, these two agents differ from *A* and *B*, and from each other, not only in affinity but in some other fundamental way.

To account for agonists of this type, the simple Occupancy Model of Clarke was modified by Ariens to endow

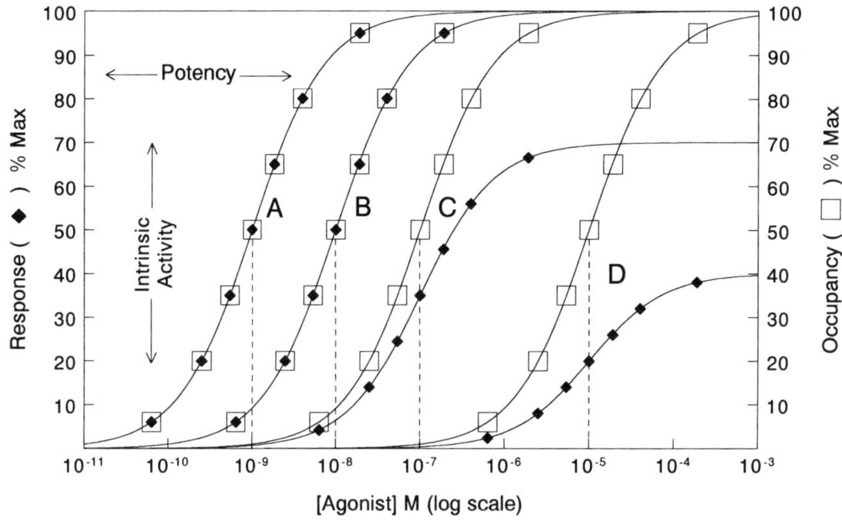

FIG. 2-7. Log concentration-response curves for a series of agonists (A–D) with different potencies and intrinsic activities. For drugs C and D, the concentration-occupancy curves and the concentration-response curves are not superimposable. (See text for details.)

each agonist with a second property that could explain the existence of drugs such as *C* and *D*. In this model, Ariens proposed that each agent not only had affinity for the receptor but also had a variable ability to "stimulate" the receptor after occupation had occurred (Figure 2-8).

In this model of drug action, there is an occupancy step that is controlled by the affinity of the drug for the receptor site and a subsequent signaling process that is controlled by the drug's *intrinsic activity*, defined as the effectiveness of the drug-receptor complex in producing a response in the tissue. The intrinsic activity α for each drug was quantified by the ratio of the maximal response produced by the drug, divided by the maximal response of which the tissue was capable via that receptor system. Thus, in Figure 2-7, drugs *A* and *B* would have an $\alpha = 1$, and drugs *C* and *D* would have $\alpha = 0.7$ and 0.4, respectively. Agonists that can produce the maximal response of which the receptor system is capable are called *full agonists* (*A* and *B*); agonists that cannot are called *partial agonists* (*C* and *D*). In this model, all full agonists would have the same intrinsic activity ($\alpha = 1$). Partial agonists would have $0 < \alpha < 1$. Drugs with $\alpha = 0$ would be *competitive antagonists* and will be discussed later.

Ariens retained the assumption of the Clarke model in that the response was still thought to be a linear function of the occupancy. What was different, however, was that the EC_{50} of each drug was now normalized with respect to the maximal response of which that drug was capable. Thus, although the response curves for drugs *C* and *D* are not superimposable with their respective occupancy curves, the normalized EC_{50} for each drug is still numerically identical to its K_D. The concentration-response curves shown in Figure 2-7 can be adequately described by Ariens' modification of Clarke's model, as represented by Eq. 4.

$$\frac{E_A}{E_{max}} = \alpha_A * \frac{[A]}{[A] + EC_{50}} \quad [4]$$

Differences in the position of the concentration-response curves on the log concentration axis represent differences in potency (and affinity since K_D still equals EC_{50} in this model), whereas differences in the maximal response produced by each agent reflect differences in intrinsic activity (see Figure 2-7). Unlike potency differences, differences in intrinsic activity between agonists of the same class are potentially therapeutically important.

Drug-Receptor Signal Transduction Mechanisms

Recognition and Transduction Steps in Agonist Action

As mentioned, agonist action can be divided into a drug-receptor recognition step followed by a signal transduction process. Before discussing further refinements in the development of drug-receptor theory, it will be helpful to consider four major signal transduction processes by which drugs may produce their pharmacological effects.

Ligand-Gated Ion Channels

Many neurotransmitters produce their effects by acting on ligand-gated ion channels. A well-characterized example of such a mechanism is the action of acetylcholine on the skeletal-muscle acetylcholine receptor. A simplified diagram of such a signal transduction mechanism is shown in Figure 2-9. The actual skeletal muscle receptor is a transmembrane protein with five subunits arranged around a central core, which forms the ion channel. In the absence of agonist, the channel is, in general, closed. Two of the subunits contain a binding site for the agonist. When both binding sites are occupied by agonist, the receptor is thought to undergo a structural change such that the channel opens and ions can flow through the channel. In the case of this particular receptor, the channel is selective for cations. Local depolarization of the membrane via this ligand-gated channel in turn activates voltage-gated sodium channels, which allow the depolarization to spread and ultimately result in skeletal muscle contraction. This process is illustrated in the scheme below:

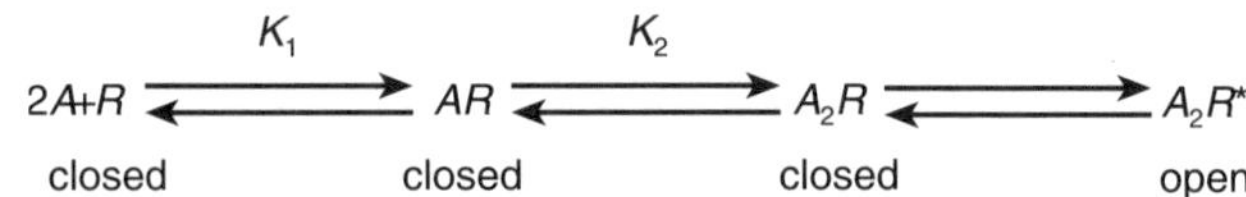

where R^* represents the activated open channel form of *R*. Binding of the first ligand is thought to affect coopera-

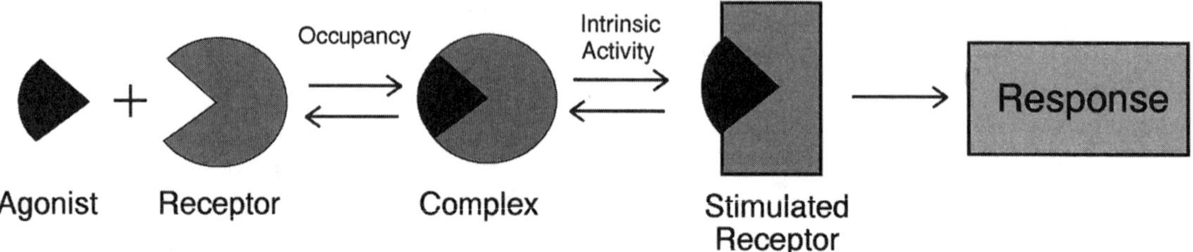

FIG. 2-8. Ariens' modification of Clarke's Occupancy Model.

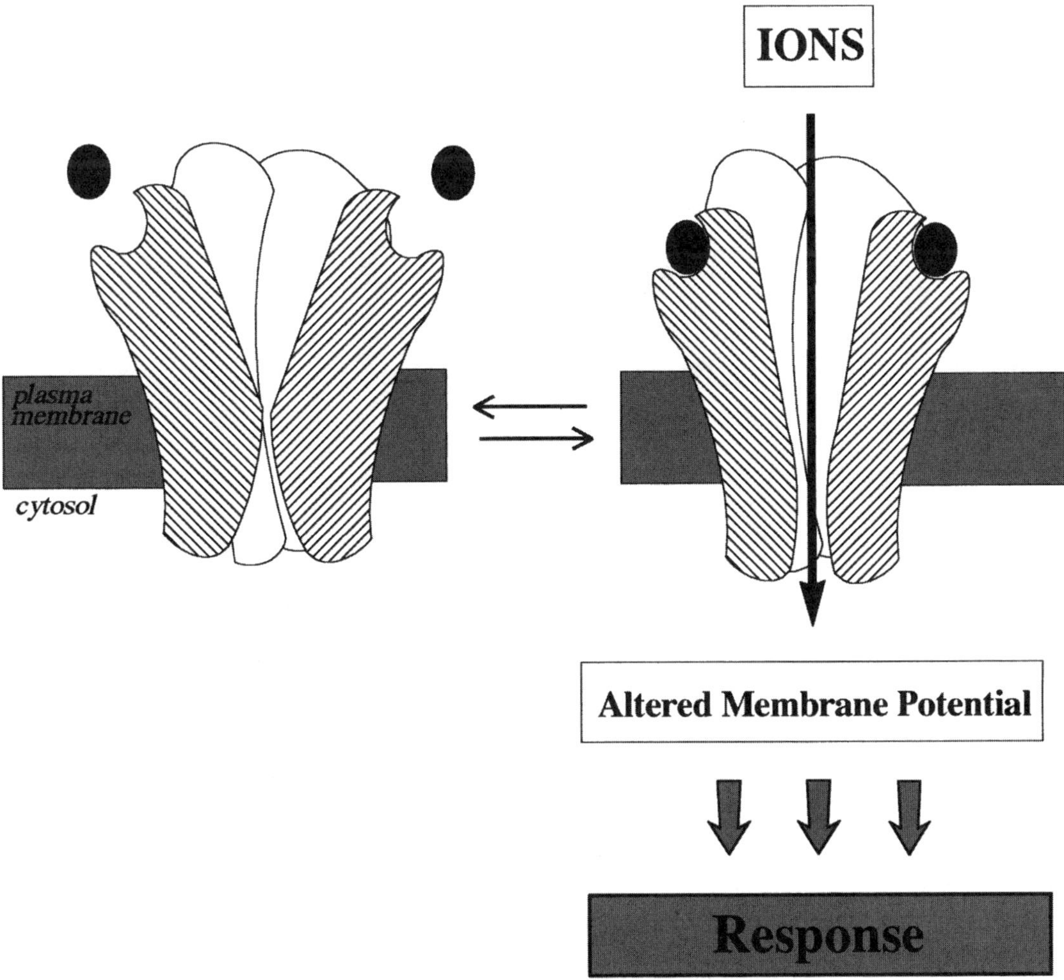

FIG. 2-9. Ligand-gated ion channel signal transduction mechanism. In the absence of ligand binding, the receptor-ion channel is closed. On binding of two molecules of agonist, the receptor undergoes a conformational change and the ion channel opens, allowing membrane depolarization and the eventual pharmacological response. (See text for details.)

tively the binding of the second. To explain such cooperative agonist binding, two-state models of drug-receptor interactions were developed and will be discussed later. Finally, other drugs use a similar signal-transduction mechanism. In some cases, the mechanism is more complex in that not only can the channel be gated by direct-acting agonists but also the gating can be modulated by other drugs acting at allosteric sites, for example the gamma-aminobutyric acid (GABA) receptor.

Receptor-Regulated Second Messengers

A second major agonist signal transduction pathway is regulation of the levels of intracellular second-messenger molecules via cell-surface receptors. Two examples are presented to illustrate this mechanism. First, the control of adenosine 3′,5′cyclic monophosphate (cAMP) levels by the regulation of adenylyl cyclase and, second, the control of the phosphatidylinositol pathway by the regulation of phospholipase C. These enzymes serve at the beginning of the effector portion of the pathway. The receptor and transducer portions of the pathway are discussed first.

Receptor-G Protein Interactions. A common feature of receptors that utilize this signal transduction mechanism is their ability to modulate the activity of enzymes involved in second-messenger synthesis or degradation via a class of *transducer proteins,* known collectively as guanine nucleotide-binding proteins or *G proteins.* Receptors that can couple to these G proteins share structural features (Figure 2-10) in that they are single-chain membrane-spanning proteins containing seven transmembrane helices with three extracellular loops and three variable intracellular loops. It has been proposed that at least two of the intracellular loops and the C-terminal tail are involved in the specificity of the receptor for a particular G protein. Surprisingly, the ligand binding site is thought not to be on the extracellular domains but rather is buried in the membrane-

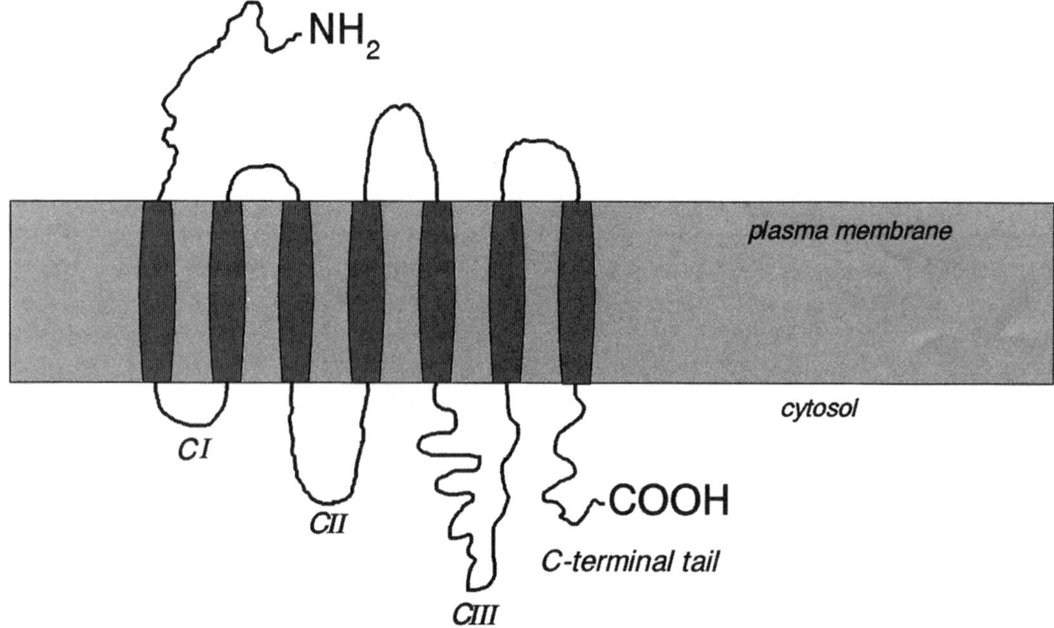

FIG. 2-10. Structural features of receptors coupled to G-protein signal transduction pathways. (See text for details.)

spanning helices. Binding of agonist to the receptor is believed to cause a conformational change, which triggers interaction with the G protein.

G proteins are heterotrimers composed of an alpha chain (G_α) and a beta-gamma complex ($G\beta_\gamma$). The alpha and gamma subunits are lipidated, which anchors the heterotrimer as well as the separated alpha and beta-gamma components to the cytoplasmic surface of the plasma membrane. The steps involved in the interaction of the receptor with a G protein are shown in Figure 2-11. The interaction cycle begins in the upper left panel and continues in a clockwise fashion. The unoccupied receptor, the G protein, and the effector to be modulated via drug action are shown. In the resting state, the alpha subunit of the heterotrimer contains one bound molecule of guanosine diphosphate (GDP). Binding of the agonist to the receptor

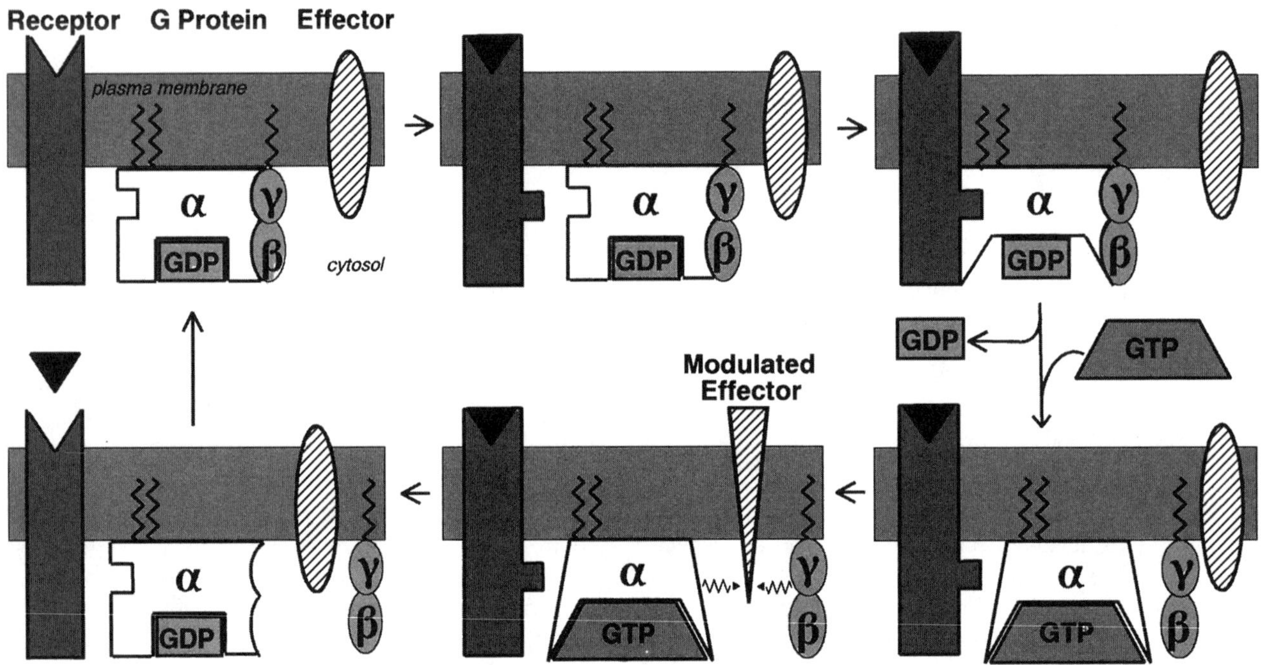

FIG. 2-11. Drug receptor-G protein-effector interaction cycle. (See text for details.)

induces a conformational change, resulting in the exposure of a portion of the receptor, which now has affinity for G_{α}. Diffusion of the receptor and the G protein in the plane of the membrane allows receptor-G protein docking. In response to receptor docking, the G protein undergoes a conformational change, which decreases its affinity for GDP and increases its affinity for guanosine triphosphate (GTP). The interaction with agonist bound receptor thus promotes GTP for GDP exchange. GTP binding causes the dissociation of the alpha subunit from the receptor and from the $G_{\beta\gamma}$ complex. Each G protein component is freely diffusible in the plane of the plasma membrane and can individually or collectively modulate the activity of a given effector. Significant amplification of the initial agonist-receptor occupation signal may occur at this point in that the released agonist-bound receptor is free to activate other G proteins. In many receptor systems, which act through this pathway, an excess of G proteins over receptors exists.

The modulation of effector activity by the G-protein component(s) is terminated when the alpha subunit, which has intrinsic guanosine triphosphatase (GTPase) activity, hydrolyzes GTP to GDP. The GTPase activity is such that the GTP-bound form persists for many seconds, providing sufficient time for prolonged modulation of the effector. Because the effector is often an enzyme, persistent enhancement of enzymatic activity through the G protein will result in considerable signal amplification. Once hydrolysis of GTP has occurred, however, the separated components of the G protein reassemble into the heterotrimer, and the system is restored to its resting state.

Effector Systems Modulated. We now return to the two examples of the effector components of second-messenger pathways. First is the modulation of the activity of adenylyl cyclase by G-protein-coupled receptors. Adenylyl cyclase catalyzes the conversion of adenosine triphosphate (ATP) into the second-messenger cAMP. In many tissues, cAMP is continually produced by the cyclase and destroyed by phosphodiesterase (PDE). As shown in Figure 2-12, both stimulatory and inhibitory drugs can modulate activity. Stimulatory drugs act via receptors coupled to stimulatory G proteins (G_s); likewise, inhibitory drugs couple to inhibitory G proteins (G_i). Drugs that are agonists for receptors coupled to G_s lead to a stimulation of adenylyl cyclase and a subsequent increase in intracellular cAMP. In turn, cAMP activates a cAMP-dependent protein kinase (PKA), which phosphorylates one or more intracellular proteins, which trigger subsequent steps in the signal transduction pathway, leading to the eventual pharmacological response.

Figure 2-13 illustrates another important receptor modulated second-messenger pathway, namely, the phos-

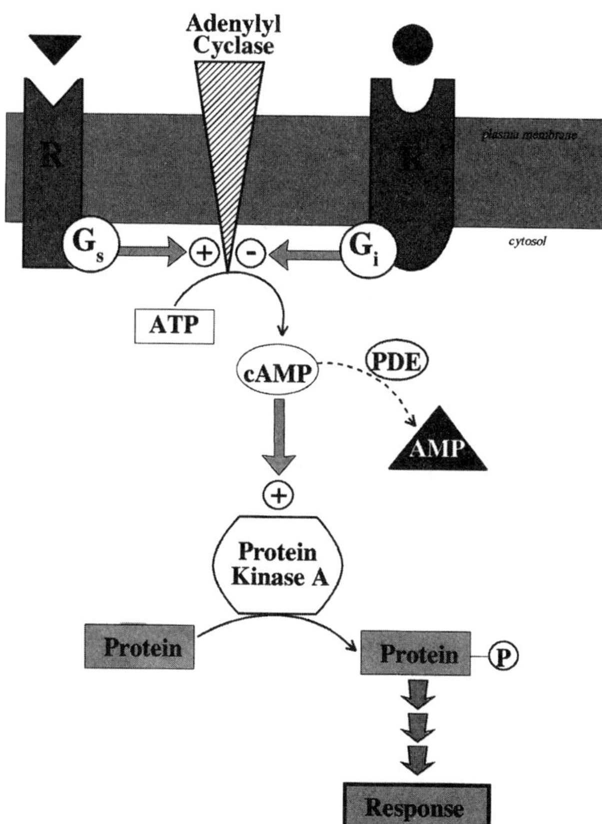

FIG. 2-12. Modulation of adenylyl cyclase activity by drugs with affinity for receptors coupled either to stimulatory or inhibitory G proteins. (See text for details.)

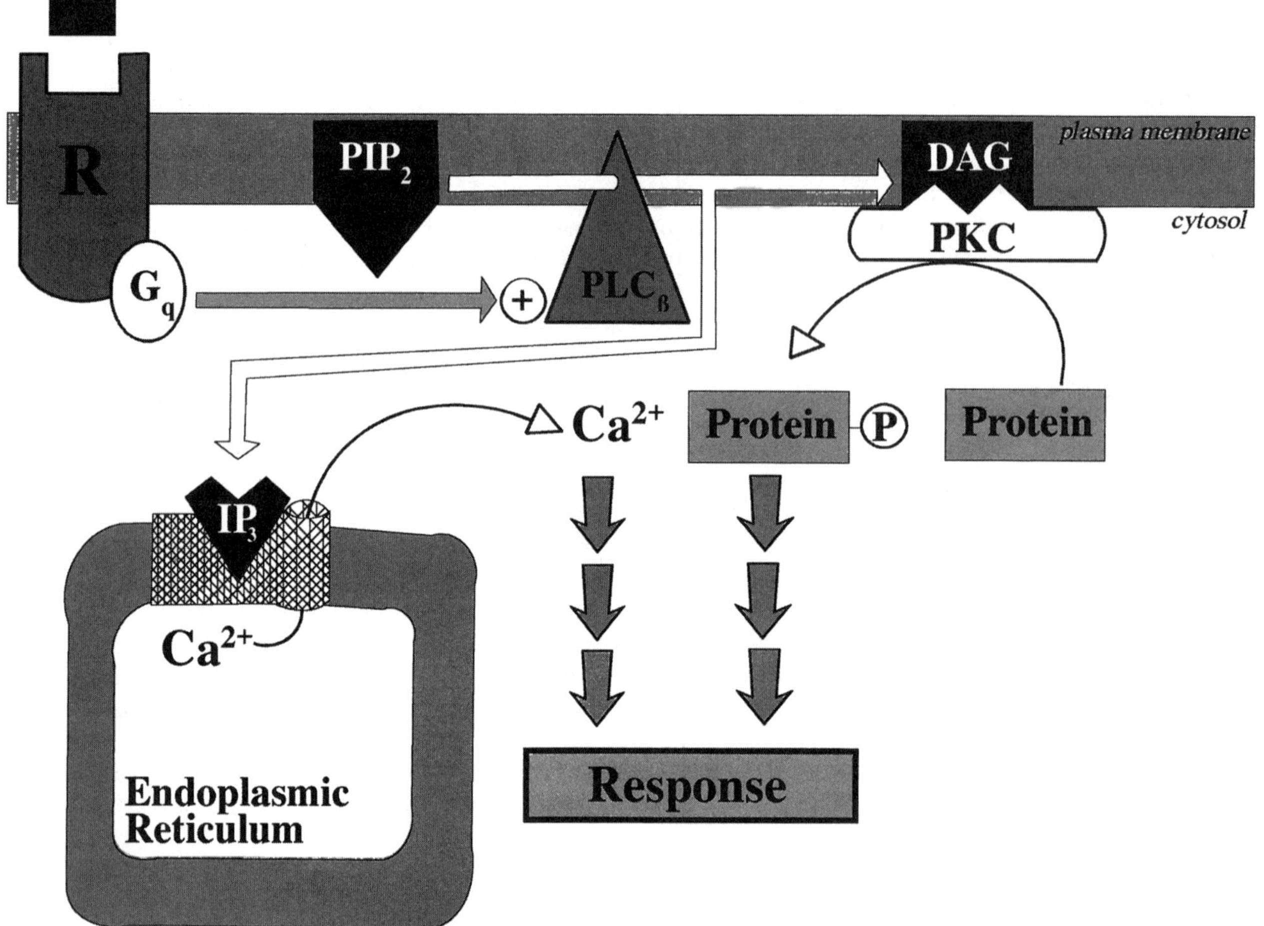

FIG. 2-13. Modulation of the phophatidylinositol signal transduction pathway by drugs with affinity for receptors coupled to G proteins which activate phospholipase C. (See text for details.)

phatidylinositol pathway. Here, agonist receptor interaction activates another type of G protein (G_q), which is coupled positively to phopholipase C_β (PLC_β). Once activated, PLC_β catalyzes the breakdown of phophatidylinositol 4,5-bisphosphate (PIP_2) into two second messengers, the hydrophilic inositol 1,4,5-trisphosphate (IP_3) and the hydrophobic diacylglycerol (DAG). The hydrophilic IP_3 diffuses through the cytosol and, in turn, binds to its receptor, which is a ligand-gated ion channel found on the membrane of the endoplasmic reticulum. The IP_3 binding causes the release of Ca^{2+} from the intracellular storage site into the cytoplasm. Similarly, the hydrophobic DAG can diffuse in the plane of the membrane and activate protein kinase C (PKC), which is also dependent on calcium and phospholipid for activity. Activated PKC carries out the phosphorylation of intracellular and membrane-bound proteins. The third messengers in this pathway, namely, calcium and the proteins phosphorylated by PKC, can activate individually or in concert the subsequent steps in signal transduction that ultimately lead to the pharmacological response.

Receptor-Regulated Transmembrane Enzymes

The third class of signal transduction pathways involves enzymes linked to cell-surface receptors. The various receptor tyrosine kinases fall into this class. In general, these receptors are transmembrane proteins that contain a ligand-binding domain facing the extracellular space and a cytosolic domain, which either can associate with cytosolic tyrosine kinases or has intrinsic tyrosine kinase (YK) activity. An example of the latter is shown in Figure 2-14. In this case, ligand binding induces receptor oligomerization, often dimerization. In some systems, the ligand itself may be a dimer that cross-links two receptor molecules. In others, the receptors normally exist as disulfide-bridged dimers.

Ligand binding activates the tyrosine kinase activity of the cytoplasmic domains. The juxtaposed kinase domains can cross-phosphorylate each other (*autophosphorylation*). The autophosphorylation can occur on tyrosines located both inside and outside the tyrosine kinase section of the cytosolic domain. Phosphorylation within the tyrosine kinase domain often results in enhancement of the kinase ac-

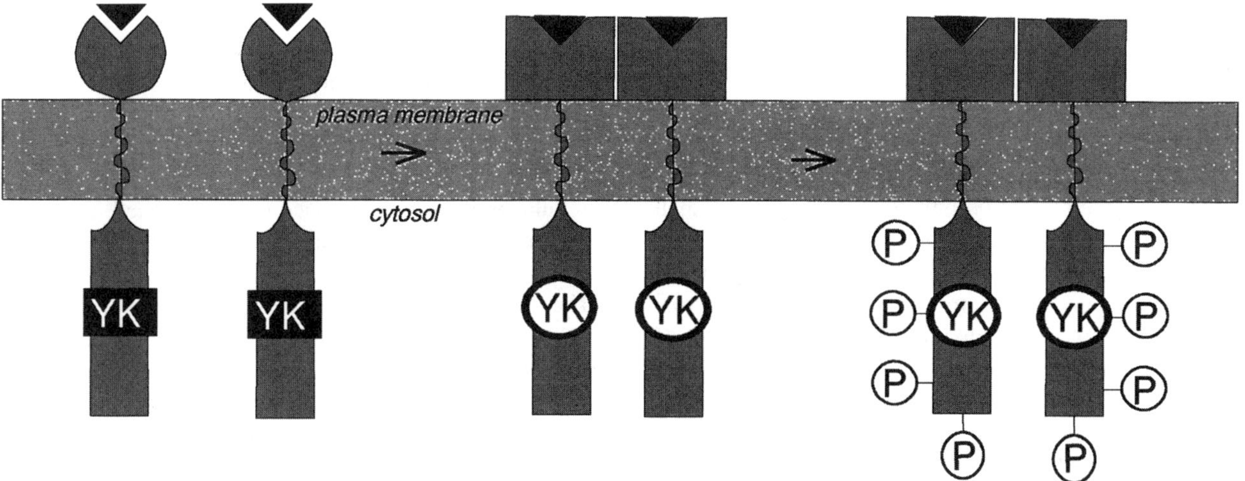

FIG. 2-14. Initial events in a receptor tyrosine kinase signal transduction pathway. Ligand binding induces receptor dimerization and subsequent autophosphorylation. (See text for details.)

tivity, which may lead to additional phosphorylation at other tyrosine sites within the cytosolic domain. Phosphorylation on tyrosines outside the kinase domain can serve as docking sites for cytosolic proteins involved in subsequent steps in signal transduction. Once the autophosphorylation is complete, the presence of ligand may no longer be necessary for continued signal transduction. Dephosphorylation of the receptor by a phosphatase is required for signal termination.

Some initial events that may follow receptor autophosphorylation are shown in Figure 2-15. Once phosphorylated, the receptor can serve as a binding site for a variety

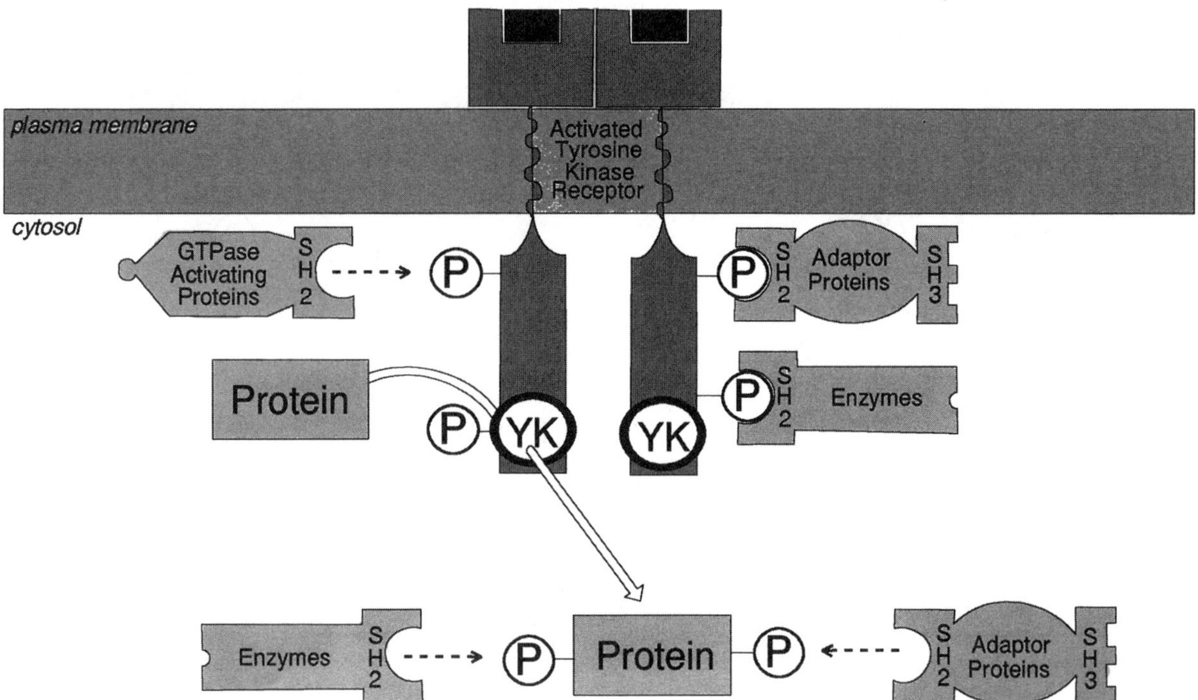

FIG. 2-15. Secondary events in a receptor tyrosine kinase signal transduction pathway. The autophosphorylated receptor serves as a docking site for a variety of cytosolic enzymes, adaptor proteins, or enzyme-activating proteins. Alternatively, the activated receptor's tyrosine kinase domain can phosphorylate various cytosolic proteins, which in turn may serve as similar docking sites. (See text for details.)

of cytosolic proteins that contain a domain that recognizes not only the phosphorylated tyrosine but also several adjacent amino acids. This domain is called a *Src homology 2* (SH2) domain after the *Src* oncogene product where it was first found. This domain may be found on a variety of cytosolic proteins, three of which are illustrated in Figure 2-15. First, it may be found on intracellular enzymes, which bind to the phosphorylated receptor and become activated. The activation may involve either a phosphorylation of the enzyme by the kinase domain of the receptor or a conformational change in the enzyme triggered by the binding of the enzyme's SH2 domain to the phosphorylated receptor. Second, other SH2-domain-containing proteins are not enzymes but rather function as adaptor proteins. These proteins contain not only an SH2 domain but also another domain known as SH3, which recognizes proline-rich areas of yet other intracellular proteins. As adaptors, these proteins can serve as a bridge between intracellular proteins involved in signal transduction, which themselves do not contain SH2 domains and therefore cannot directly interact with the phosphorylated receptor. Third, SH2 domains may be found in proteins that enhance the activity of intracellular enzymes. The GTPase-activating protein, shown in Figure 2-15, is one example of this type.

Serving as a binding site for other intracellular proteins is not the only way in which the activated receptor can promote further signal transduction. As illustrated in Figure 2-15, the tyrosine kinase domain can also phosphorylate intracellular proteins, which, once phosphorylated, can serve as docking sites for the same sort of SH2 domain-containing proteins that bound directly to the phosphorylated receptor. The imparting of the signal to a diffusible protein substrate may allow delivery of the signal to locations in the cell that are not accessible to the plasma membrane-bound receptor.

It should be clear from the previous discussion that receptor phosphorylation acts as a switch that turns on the signal transduction process. Individual receptor tyrosine kinases can couple to different combinations of SH2-domain-containing proteins or phosphorylate different intracellular protein substrates. In this way, specific pharmacological effects can be produced. The signal transduction cascade, which relays the signal to the interior of the cell, even to the nucleus, can be quite complex. As an example, one such sequence is illustrated in Figure 2-16. Here the activated tyro-

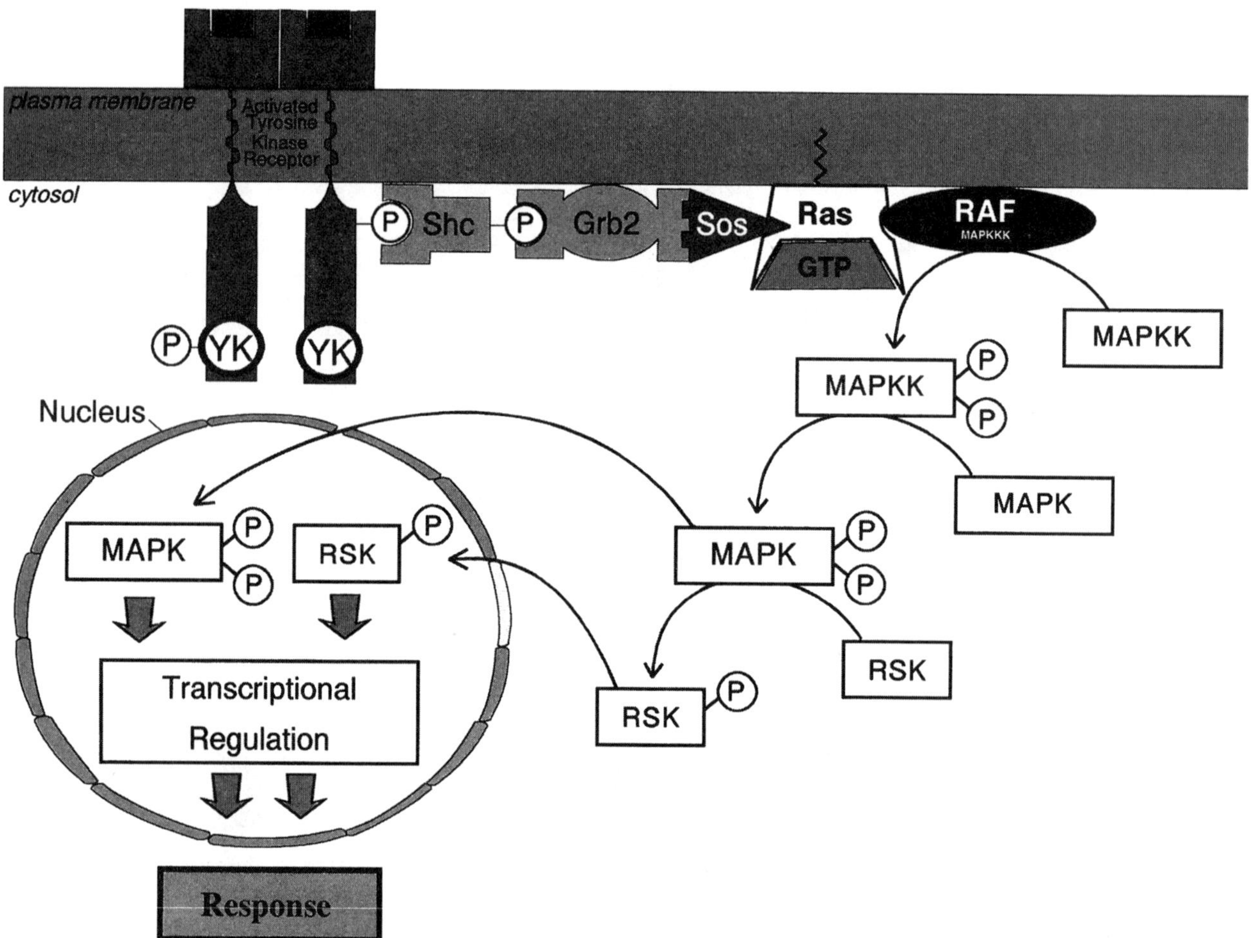

FIG. 2-16. Example of a receptor tyrosine kinase signal transduction pathway. (See text for details.)

sine kinase receptor autophosphorylates, creating a binding site for an SH2-domain-containing adapter protein, Shc. Subsequent to phosphorylation by the receptor, Shc in turn functions as a binding site for another adaptor protein, Grb2. This bifunctional adaptor contains an SH2 domain for binding to Shc and two SH3 domains for linking to a guanine nucleotide-releasing protein, Sos, which functions similarly to the receptor in the heterotrimeric G protein-coupled signal transduction pathway discussed earlier. It promotes the exchange of GTP for GDP on a small molecular mass G protein called Ras, a member of a family of monomeric GTPases. Like the heterotrimeric G proteins, it cycles between its inactive GDP and active GTP bound forms. Sos promotes Ras activation; other proteins stimulate its GTPase activity and subsequent inactivation.

Unlike Shc, Grb2, and Sos, which are sequentially recruited to the membrane by the activated receptor, Ras is anchored to the cytoplasmic side of the plasma membrane by an isoprenyl tail. In the pathway illustrated, in its activated, GTP-bound form, Ras functions to couple receptor activation to an intracellular protein kinase cascade, which eventually delivers the agonist signal to the nucleus. Ras recruits the first member of the cascade to the membrane and activates it. The protein kinase cascade is known as the mitogen-activated protein (MAP kinase) cascade. In this instance, the recruited serine/threonine kinase is called RAF and has MAP kinase-kinase-kinase activity. As such, it catalyzes the phosphorylation of MAP kinase-kinase on two serine residues, leading to activation of its enzymatic activity. Activated MAP kinase-kinase is an unusual kinase in that it can phosphorylate both serine/threonine and tyrosine residues. It is thought that MAP kinase-kinase phosphorylates MAP kinase on both threonine and tyrosine. Phosphorylation at both sites is necessary for full expression of MAP-kinase activity. Once activated, MAP kinase either can translocate to the nucleus to modulate transcription factors by phosphorylation or phosphorylate other cytosolic protein kinases (e.g., RSK), which may also migrate to the nucleus to phosphorylate transcription factors. The phosphorylated factors modulate transcription of selected genes, the protein products of which are involved in the ultimate pharmacological response of the agonist which initiated the process.

Receptor-Regulated Gene Expression

The final signal transduction pathway to be outlined in this chapter is the regulation of gene expression by intracellular receptors (Figure 2-17). The receptors for agonists acting via this pathway may be found in the cytoplasm or in the nucleus, depending on the particular agonist. Usually, they are composed of a ligand-binding domain for interaction with agonist and a DNA-binding domain for modulation of gene transcription. The DNA-binding domain is often, but not always, of the zinc-finger type. As illustrated in Figure 2-17, the lipid-soluble ligand enters the cell by diffusion. For those agonists that act via cytosolic receptors, the following scenario may occur. The cytosolic receptors are thought to exist as an aporeceptor complex with several proteins known as *chaperones.* In general, protein chaperones are involved in assisting other proteins in folding into their correct three-dimensional structure. In the case of intracellular receptors, the chaperones may also be involved in maintaining the receptor in an "agonist-sensitive" form and in masking the DNA-binding domain. Subsequent to ligand binding, the receptor undergoes a conformational change, causing the dissociation of certain chaperones and the exposure of its DNA-binding domain. These steps may be assisted by other sets of protein chaperones. The agonist-receptor complex then can translocate to the nucleus. In the case of those agonist receptors that have a nuclear localization, simple ligand binding prepares the receptor for interaction with DNA. In either case, the agonist-receptor complex interacts with distinct sequences, usually on the 5′-flanking region of the gene(s) to be regulated. These distinct sequences are called *response elements* and, on interaction with the activated receptor complex, enhance transcription of specific genes responsive to the particular agonist. The new mRNA is processed and exported to the cytoplasm for translation into protein and, ultimately, the pharmacological response.

Further Refinements of Drug-Receptor Theory

Nonlinear Relationship Between Occupancy and Response ($EC_{50} \neq K_D$)

We now return to develop drug-receptor theory further. Although the Ariens model, which incorporated receptor transduction processes, could account for the existence of full and partial agonists, it could not account for the results of additional pharmacological experimentation. Recall that in both the Clarke and Ariens models, the response and occupancy curves for a full agonist were superimposable. In order for a full agonist to produce 100% of the maximal response, it had to occupy 100% of the receptor sites. Stephenson was first to suggest that it might be unreasonable to assume that response would be linearly related to receptor occupancy. He observed that the log concentration-response curves for several drug-receptor systems had slopes far steeper than that predicted from the law of mass action. In addition, the concentration-response data Stephenson collected on a homologous series of alkyl trimethylammonium agonists acting on the guinea pig ileum suggested that the EC_{50} for contractile response and the K_D for receptor occupancy were not numerically identical for the most potent agonists in the series. Somewhat later, data were collected by others that indicated, in some agonist systems, that one could irreversibly inactivate a substantial fraction of the total population of receptor sites

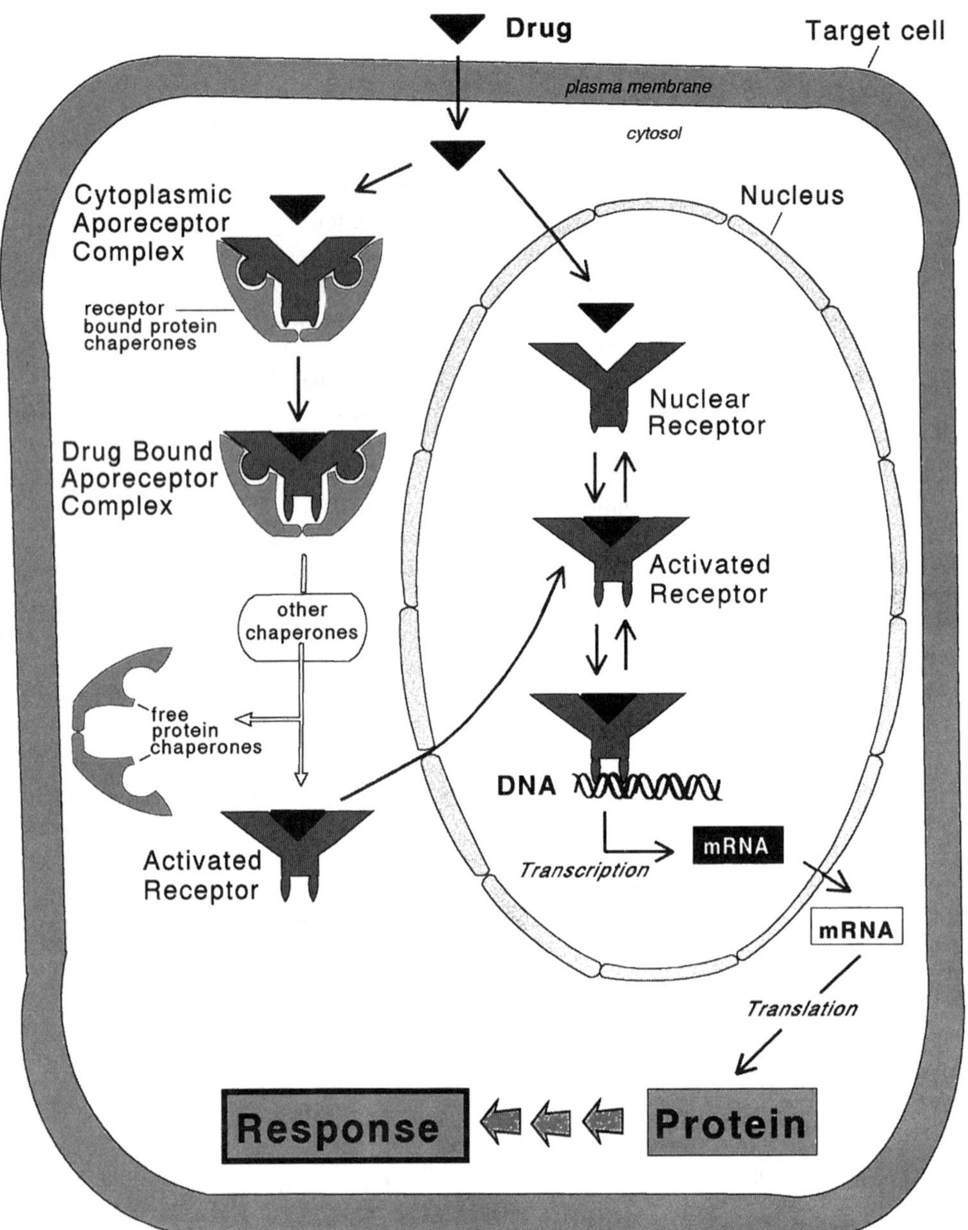

FIG. 2-17. Example of a receptor-regulated control of gene expression signal transduction pathway. (See text for details.)

in a tissue, for example, by alkylating them with a drug with which they formed a covalent bond; yet some agonists were still capable of producing the full pharmacological response E_{max}. Previous drug-receptor theories could not account for any of these experimental results.

To account for experimental observations such as these, Stephenson proposed that, in some receptor systems, the controlling factor for a full biological response may not be receptor occupancy but rather some intervening process subsequent to occupation.

$$A + R \leftrightarrows AR \rightarrow 1 \rightarrow 2 \rightarrow 3 \rightarrow 4 \rightarrow 5 \rightarrow \text{Response}$$

If 1–5 represent steps in a biochemical signal transduction sequence leading to the final pharmacological response, then one of these steps could reach its maximal level with only a small fraction of the available receptors occupied. Having just discussed the complex cascade of biochemical steps that may occur subsequent to receptor occupation, it may seem that Stephenson's postulate was intuitively obvious. At the time Stephenson made his proposal, however, what happened after receptor occupation was a complete "black box." Mathematically, the nonlinearity between occupancy and response was handled as follows: Stephenson proposed that the agonist interacted with the receptor to produce a stimulus (S). The stimulus was linearly related to occupancy according to the following equation:

$$S = e^* \frac{[A]}{[A] + K_D} \quad [5]$$

where e is a proportionality constant which Stephenson called the drug's *efficacy.* Stephenson's efficacy is different from Ariens' intrinsic activity in that it is the proportionality constant between occupancy and stimulus, not response. In Stephenson's model, the response (E) is a nonlinear function of the stimulus (S).

$$\frac{E_A}{E_{max}} = f\{S\} = f\left\{e * \frac{[A]}{[A] + K_D}\right\} \quad [6]$$

$$= f\{\text{efficacy } (e) * \text{occupancy (p)}\}$$

For the agonist action of a series of alkyl trimethylammonium agents on the guinea pig ileum, Stephenson empirically determined that there was a hyperbolic functional relationship between response and stimulus. One such hyperbolic relationship is shown in Eq. 7.

$$\frac{E_A}{E_{max}} = \frac{S}{S + 1} \quad [7]$$

Substituting for S in terms of efficacy and occupancy gives

$$\frac{E_A}{E_{max}} = \frac{p}{p + 1/e} \quad [8]$$

Concept of Agonist Signal Amplification

Concentration-response curves predicted by this model of drug action are presented in Figure 2-18. The concentration-occupancy curve, assuming an agonist $K_D = 10^{-6}$ M, is also plotted to serve as a reference point. In Stephenson's model, an agonist that needed to occupy 100% of the receptor sites to produce 1/2 E_{max} was defined as having an efficacy =1. If the K_D is fixed at 10^{-6} M and the efficacy is increased progressively by factors of 10, it can be seen that the EC_{50} gets progressively smaller as the efficacy of the agonist increases, reflecting the fact that significant amplification of the initial drug-receptor occupation signal can occur. Thus, high efficacy reflects efficient receptor-effector coupling via the signal transduction pathway.

Concept of Spare Receptors (Receptor Reserve)

Clearly, in this model, the EC_{50}, which is a measure of the agonist's potency, and the K_D, which is a measure of the agonist's affinity, are no longer numerically identical. An agonist's potency is a function not only of its affinity but also of its efficacy. An agonist that has high efficacy does not need to occupy all the receptors to produce E_{max}. Receptors that are not occupied when the agonist has produced E_{max} are called *spare receptors* or *receptor reserve* and result from the nonlinearity between occupancy and response. Unlike in Ariens' model, not all full agonists will have the same efficacy. Rather, those agonists that require the least amount of occupation to produce a given response will have the greatest efficacy. Agonist efficacy in this model can range from greater than zero to infinity. In agreement with Ariens' model, partial agonists will not be able to elicit a maximum response even when all the receptors are occupied; that is, there are no spare receptors for partial agonists. Unfortunately, this model creates ambiguity with respect to the interpretation of position and heights of concentration-response curves in terms of quantifying the affinity and the efficacy of drug-receptor interactions. If a drug's K_D and EC_{50} can be measured independently, the ratio K_D/EC_{50} will be a measure of the efficacy of the agonist. This ratio can be used to compare the *relative efficacies* of a series of agonists for the same receptor site.

Threshold Phenomenon

In some receptor systems, the reverse situation may operate. The EC_{50} could be greater than the K_D if some process in the signal transduction pathway had to achieve some threshold level before passing the signal on to subsequent steps. Systems that behave in this way would be said to display a *threshold phenomenon.*

Intrinsic Activity, Efficacy, Intrinsic Efficacy

Although as originally developed the concepts of efficacy and intrinsic activity are not identical mathematically, in a general sense, both reflect the varying abilities of agonists to "stimulate" the receptor. This concept was refined further by Furchgott into *intrinsic efficacy* (ε), which he defined as Stephenson's efficacy (e) divided by the total population of receptors in the tissue (R_T). This is analogous to the difference between V_{max} (Stephenson's efficacy) and k_{cat} (Furchgott's intrinsic efficacy) in enzymology. Thus, intrinsic efficacy would be efficacy per drug-receptor interaction.

In general pharmacological parlance, these distinctions in the terms used to convey the relative abilities of agonists to "stimulate" the receptor, although conceptionally important, are rarely made. For many, the term *efficacy* has a clinical rather than molecular connotation. In order for a drug to be approved for use in patients, both its safety and clinical efficacy must be demonstrated. As will become apparent in the following chapters, many highly efficacious drugs used clinically are competitive antagonists that by definition have a molecular efficacy = 0. Thus, a lack of efficacy in a molecular sense does not imply lack of efficacy in a clinical sense. Perhaps for this reason, the term *intrin-*

sic activity may be less ambiguous for describing this molecular property of drug action.

Two-State Model of Drug Action: Physicochemical Basis for Intrinsic Activity

Although the Stephenson model, and further refinements of it, can account satisfactorily for the observed concentration-response relationships in a wide variety of receptor systems, it fails to provide a physicochemical basis for the intrinsic activity differences among agonists interacting with the same receptor. One model that can accomplish this goal is a two-state model of drug action. Here the receptor is considered oligomeric in nature, with each subunit containing a drug binding site. This model can be represented by the following scheme:

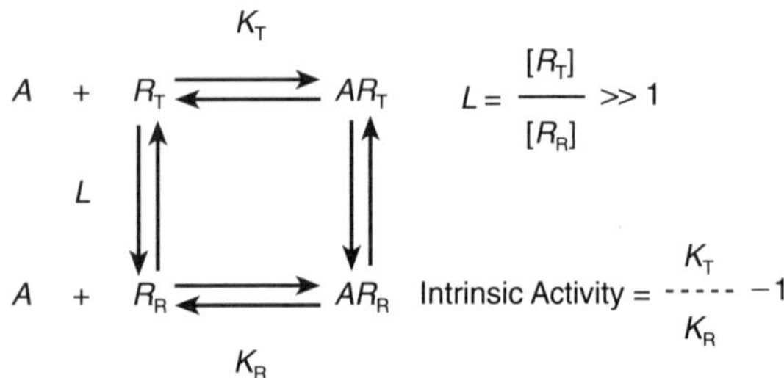

The protomers can exist in two conformational forms (*structures*), one of which is "active" = R_R, the other "inactive" = R_T. These two forms are in equilibrium, but the inactive form predominates in the absence of drug ($L >>1$). Drugs vary in their ability to bind to the two forms of the receptor, and intrinsic activity has its biochemical/molecular basis as the relative affinity of a drug for these two forms. Full agonists would have a higher affinity for the active form of the receptor ($IA >>1$) and thus perturb the equilibrium so that, in their presence, the receptor would exist predominantly in the active form. Partial agonists would have a lower affinity for the active form and thus would not be able to shift the equilibrium to the same extent. Because the effect measured is thought to be related to the amount of active form of the receptor present, partial agonists would have varying abilities to produce a response. Indeed, the same spectrum of concentration-response curves predicted by Stephenson's model by varying the efficacy (Figure 2-18) can be predicted by various two-state models by varying the ratio of the affinities of agonists for the two states of the receptor.

A competitive antagonist would be expected to have equal affinity for both forms and thus not perturb the resting equilibrium. This model would also predict the existence of drugs that could have a higher affinity for the inactive form of the receptor, and such *inverse agonists* are known to exist. The effects of inverse agonists are difficult to detect, however, unless a sufficient fraction of the receptor population exists in the active state in the absence of any drug such that a basal pharmacological response can be measured, which the inverse agonist can then decrease. This model can also account for the observation that in some receptor systems, as the response measured moves farther up the signal transduction pathway toward the receptor occupation step, sigmoidal concentration-response curves are observed when dose is plotted on a linear scale. A hyperbolic curve would be expected. This sigmoidicity is evidence for a two-state/cooperative binding model of drug action in such systems.

Terms Applicable to Agonist Action

Addition describes the effect observed when single doses of two drugs acting in the same direction produce a response that is greater than that expected for one of the drugs acting alone:

$$[A]_{25\%} + [B]_{25\%} \rightarrow 25\% < \text{response} < 50\%$$

Summation is a special case of addition in which the effect of single doses of two drugs acting in the same direction is exactly equal to the algebraic sum of the individual responses if each were given alone. The distinction between addition and summation is not often made:

$$[A]_{25\%} + [B]_{25\%} \rightarrow \text{response} = 50\%$$

Synergism describes the situation in which the effect of single doses of two drugs acting in the same direction is greater than the algebraic sum of the individual responses if each were given alone:

$$[A]_{25\%} + [B]_{25\%} \rightarrow \text{response} > 50\%$$

Potentiation occurs when the administration of one drug with no effect of its own causes the effect of a single dose of another drug to be greater than that expected if the second drug were acting alone:

$$[A]_{25\%} + [B]_{0\%} \rightarrow \text{response} > 25\%$$

Potentiation of agonist action would be anticipated in circumstances in which the second drug is an inhibitor of the removal of the agonist from the area of the receptor site, whether by metabolism or some other physiological process.

Tolerance characterizes the decreased effectiveness of an agonist with chronic use. Usually, it is reserved for decreased effectiveness, which takes days, weeks, or months to develop. The effect of tolerance on the concentration-response curves of an agonist are illustrated in Figure 2-19. The control concentration-response curve represents the sensitivity of the system at zero time. If the agonist is administered chronically for a period of time ($T1$) and then the concentration response curve is repeated, the curve can be seen to have shifted to the right; that is, the tissue is less responsive (Figure 2-19A). Now a higher concentration

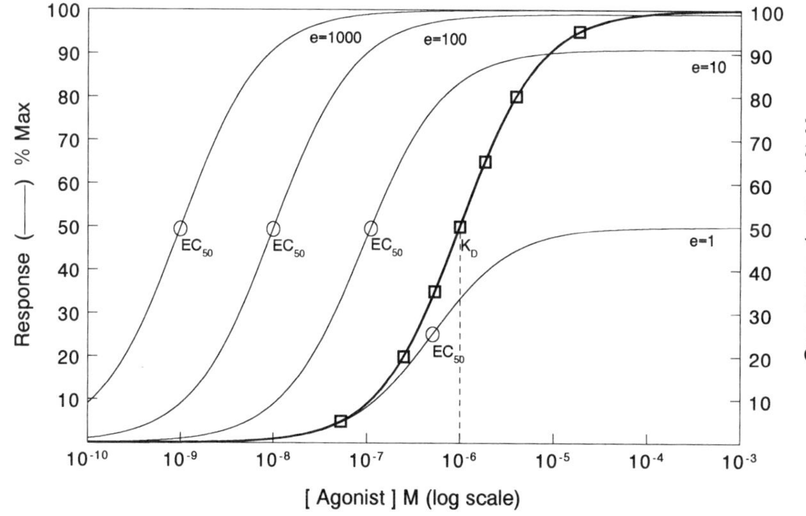

FIG. 2-18. Concentration-response curves predicted by the Stephenson model of drug action. Agonist affinity was arbitrarily set to a $K_D = 10^{-6}$ *M*, and the concentration-occupancy curve was plotted for reference. Concentration-response curves predicted for agonists with this same affinity, but different efficacies are shown. (See text for details.)

must be administered to achieve the same response as achieved previously. If the period of chronic use is increased further (*T*2), a further loss of responsiveness occurs. This loss of responsiveness may be reflected either as a shift to the right or as a decrease in the maximum response (Figure 2-19B) or a combination of both.

Tachyphylaxis describes an acute form of tolerance, which may take minutes or hours to develop. Figure 2-20 illustrates how the responses to an agonist in an isolated tissue preparation may quickly fade. In the top figure, a single high dose of agonist is added at the arrow and then washed out at the dot when the response has reached its

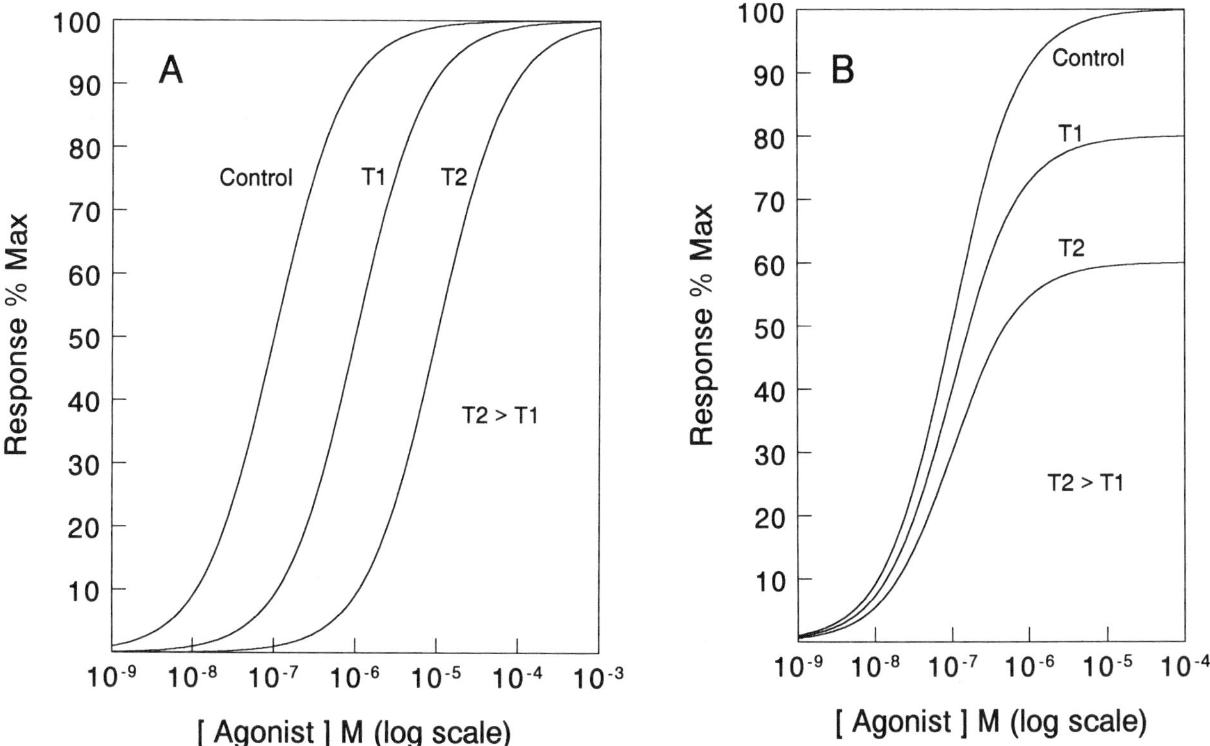

FIG. 2-19. Concentration-response curves for an agonist displaying tolerance. **A:** The control curve indicates the initial responsiveness of the receptor system. *T*1 and *T*2 represent different lengths of time of chronic use of the agonist. In this case, tolerance is characterized by a progressive shift to the right of the concentration response curve. **B:** Same as A, indicating that tolerance can also be manifested as a decrease in the maximal response to the agonist. (See text for details.)

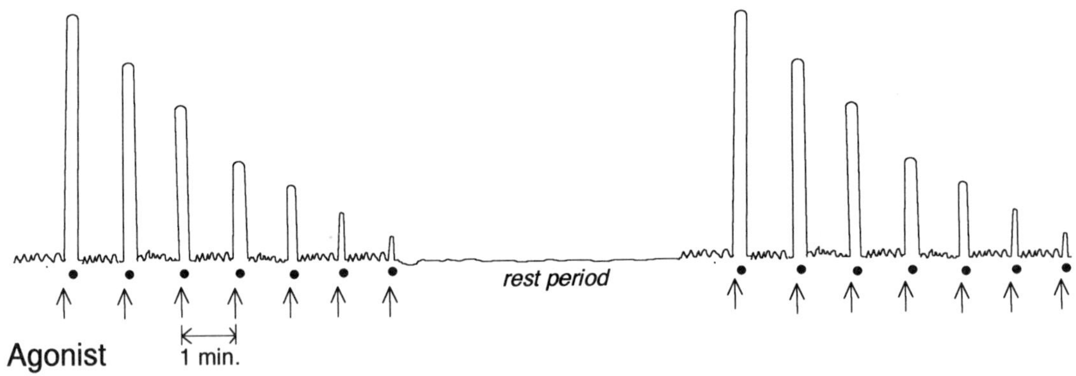

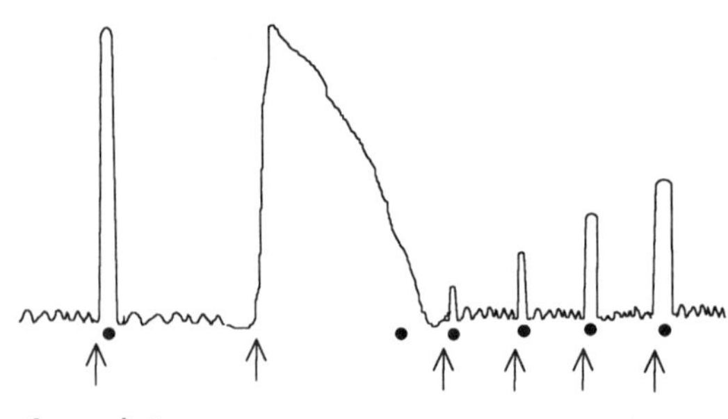

FIG. 2-20. Tissue responses to agonist action with the receptor system displaying the phenomenon of tachyphylaxis. (See text for details.)

maximum. Repeated challenges with the same concentration of the agonist cause the response to fade with each successive application. A rest period allows the system to recover, but the tachyphylaxis recurs with repetition of the sequence. The bottom figure illustrates a similar phenomenon in which a high concentration of the agonist is allowed to stay in contact with the receptors for a prolonged period. Subsequent challenge with the agonist indicates that the system has lost its sensitivity, which gradually returns with time.

Mechanisms of Tachyphylaxis or Tolerance

Pharmacodynamic

There are a number of pharmacodynamic mechanisms by which a tissue may lose its responsiveness to agonist action. A biochemical term used to describe the more rapid loss of responsiveness that may be observed is receptor *desensitization;* the term linked to mechanisms responsible for the loss of responsiveness on a more long-term basis is receptor *downregulation.* A classic example of a receptor system that illustrates receptor desensitization is the acetylcholine-gated ion channel in skeletal muscle. The scheme proposed for ion-channel activation by acetylcholine was presented earlier. The Katz and Thesleff modified version of the activation scheme, which has been used to rationalize the very rapid agonist-induced loss of responsiveness, which this system can display, is as follows:

$$
\begin{array}{ccccccc}
 & & \text{- - - - - - fast - - - - - -} & & & & \\
2A + R & \overset{K_1}{\rightleftharpoons} & AR & \overset{K_2}{\rightleftharpoons} & A_2R & \rightleftharpoons & A_2R^* \\
\text{slow } D \updownarrow & & \updownarrow & & \updownarrow & & \\
2A + R' & \underset{}{\overset{K_1'}{\rightleftharpoons}} & AR' & \overset{K_2'}{\rightleftharpoons} & A_2R' & & D = \dfrac{[R']}{[R]} \ll 1
\end{array}
$$

The upper path describes the equilibria involved in receptor activation, and the lower path accounts for desensitization. The model proposes that the receptor can exist in at least three states: the resting state (R), the activated state (R^*), and the desensitized state (R'). The equilibrium constant D defined as $[R']/[R]$ is very much less than one in the absence of ligand. The horizontal ligand binding equilibria are fast, whereas the vertical desensitization equilibria are slow. Each receptor state is thought to have a different affinity for the agonist. Agonists with a higher affinity for R' than for the other two states will be prone to induce receptor desensitization. In their presence, the receptor population will be drawn into the lower pathway, which is not directly coupled to channel opening. On removal of the agonist, the system will return to its resting state, and responsiveness to agonist will be restored.

Another receptor system that illustrates a very different mechanism of desensitization is the β-2 adrenergic receptor, which uses a G-protein signal transduction pathway (see Figure 2-11). Recall that in this pathway the agonist-occupied receptor facilitates GTP for GDP exchange on the alpha subunit of the G protein, followed by dissociation of the G-protein components, which individually or collectively modulate effector function. In the case of this particular receptor, the effector is adenylyl cyclase, and the modulation is activation. As a consequence of agonist action, therefore, the intracellular concentration of cAMP increases. The cAMP in turn activates PKA, which phosphorylates several intracellular substrates, one of which is the β-2-receptor itself. This phosphorylation occurs on sites within the third intracellular loop and on the C-terminal tail of the receptor (see Figure 2-10). Phosphorylation at these sites occurs at low ("physiological") agonist concentrations and results in a rightward shift of the concentration-response curve, as illustrated in Figure 2-19A. This rightward shift (i.e., desensitization) is due to the fact that phosphorylation of the receptor by PKA decreases the interaction of the receptor with the G protein.

At higher agonist concentrations, a second desensitization mechanism comes into operation (Figure 2-21). This mechanism also involves a protein kinase but one that is more specific for the activated form of the β-2-adrenergic receptor than PKA. This kinase is called the β-adrenergic receptor kinase, or β-ARK, and is also a serine/threonine kinase normally found in the cytoplasm. On intense agonist-induced receptor stimulation, however, β-ARK translocates to the membrane, which becomes possible because β-ARK has affinity for $G_{\beta\gamma}$, which is anchored to the membrane by virtue of its lipidated γ-subunit. Free $G_{\beta\gamma}$, from which the G_α has dissociated, would be located only at sites on the membrane where activated receptors are present. The membrane-localized β-ARK now may diffuse in the plane of the membrane and interact with the agonist-bound receptor for which it also has affinity. Then β-ARK phosphorylates the receptor on its C-terminal tail at sites different from those phosphorylated by PKA. The phosphorylated receptor now becomes a binding site for yet another protein, called β-arrestin, which interacts with the receptor and prevents further coupling of the receptor to the G protein. Subsequent to the GTP hydrolysis by the α-subunit, the G-protein heterotrimer reassembles, and modulation of the effector terminates. The desensitized state induced by β-ARK leads to a decrease in the E_{max} in the concentration-response curve for the agonist. Thus, desensitization induced by exposure of the receptor to high levels of agonist can produce both a shift to the right and a depression of the maximal response requiring the in-

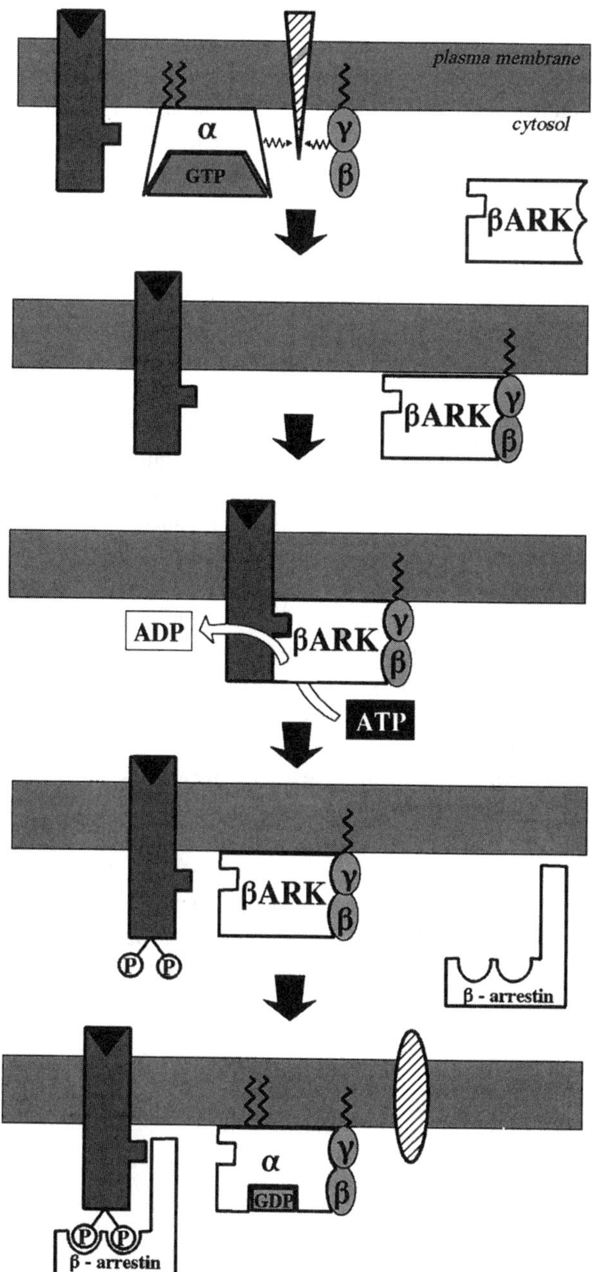

FIG. 2-21. Desensitization of the β-2-adrenergic receptor mediated by the beta adrenergic receptor kinase, β-ARK. (See text for details.)

volvement of both PKA and β-ARK. The described desensitization pathway is not unique to the β-adrenergic receptor. Rhodopsin undergoes a similar desensitization sequence under the influence of rhodopsin kinase. Additional mechanisms may be involved for a complete description of receptor desensitization. Evidence exists that exposure of a receptor to high levels of agonist may also lead to sequestration of the receptors in a membrane compartment that is not accessible to ligands that act at the cell surface. These sequestered receptors eventually may recycle to the cell surface or may be proteolytically degraded in the lysosome. The term *downregulation* is often reserved for this latter process in which the receptors, and often their bound ligand, not only are removed from the plasma membrane but subsequently destroyed. It appears that many receptors, once activated by their agonists, undergo feedback regulation via rapid internalization and downregulation.

A general rule in receptor regulation may be stated as follows: Conditions that increase or decrease agonist-receptor interactions, either chronically or acutely, result in opposing alterations in receptor sensitivity. Agonist treatment generally leads to desensitization/downregulation, whereas antagonist treatment usually leads to *supersensitivity/upregulation.* It would appear that desensitization may be a basic homeostatic mechanism that a cell can use to protect itself from excessive stimulation. Desensitization can be said to be *homologous* when it is ligand specific in that the agonist causes desensitization only of the specific receptor that it occupies. The skeletal muscle acetylcholine receptor falls into this category. *Heterologous* desensitization occurs when the agonist causes the desensitization of a different agonist receptor system as well as its own and typically would be observed when the two receptors share a signal transduction pathway.

It is important to note that tolerance does not always have to be linked to desensitization or downregulation. The tolerance observed with the opiate drugs does not seem to involve receptor downregulation. In fact, it has been shown in this system that inhibition of steps upstream in the signal transduction pathway causes upregulation of steps downstream. Removal of the inhibition by withholding the opiate allows the upregulated steps to act unabated, leading to symptoms of withdrawal.

Other Mechanisms of Tolerance

There are mechanisms by which tolerance/tachyphylaxis can result which historically have not been attributed to having a pharmacodynamic basis. One example that has been classified as having a pharmacokinetic basis is that of enzyme induction. Some drugs can induce their own metabolism, and on chronic administration, the dose required for therapeutic effectiveness typically will increase. Although metabolism, along with absorption, distribution, and excretion of drugs, is the purview of pharmacokinetics, the mechanism by which most drugs induce their own metabolism is by acting via the receptor-regulated gene-expression signal transduction pathway, as discussed earlier. Clearly, this is a pharmacodynamic mechanism; thus, the classification of tolerance produced by enzyme induction as having a pharmacokinetic basis seems arbitrary.

A final classic example of a mechanism for tachyphylaxis is that seen when indirectly acting agonists are used. Some drugs do not have significant affinity for a receptor site but instead can induce the release of the physiological agonist for that site. Drugs that can cause the release of norepinephrine from sympathetic nerve terminals fall into this category. Agonist activity of such agents is solely dependent on sufficient stores of the neurotransmitter. Repeated administration of such drugs can lead to the rapid depletion of neurotransmitter from the nerve terminal, resulting in tachyphylaxis. If time is allowed for resynthesis of the transmitter, agonist action of the indirectly acting agent is restored.

ACTION OF ANTAGONISTS

Up to this point, the discussion has been restricted to the pharmacodynamics of drugs that have the ability to "stimulate" the receptor and thereby produce their pharmacological effects (i.e., agonists). Consideration now will be given to the pharmacodynamics of antagonists. There are several mechanisms by which drugs can produce pharmacological antagonism.

Competitive Antagonism

A *competitive antagonist* (*X*) is a drug that reversibly binds to the receptor, that is, one that has affinity, but does not stimulate the receptor to produce a pharmacological response; that is, it has no intrinsic activity:

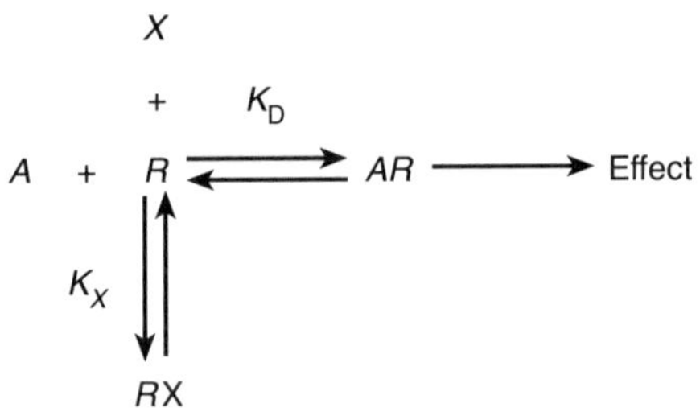

The effect of a competitive antagonist on the concentration-response curve of an agonist is illustrated in Figure 2-22. In the presence of a fixed concentration of a competitive antagonist ([*X*1]), the concentration-response curve of the agonist is shifted to the right of the curve produced by agonist alone (*control*). The amount of the shift is proportional to the concentration of antagonist ([*X*2] > [*X*1]). It is clear that all the levels of response produced by the agonist alone, including the maximal response, can be reproduced in the presence of the competitive antagonist. The only requirement is that the agonist concentration required is higher in the presence of the antagonist; that is, the EC_{50} is increased. The antagonism is therefore said to be *surmountable.* Drugs of this type would be of obvious pharmacological importance in bringing systems that are receiving excessive physiological stimulation by an agonist under control. In addition, however, although competitive antagonists have no ability to produce pharmacological ef-

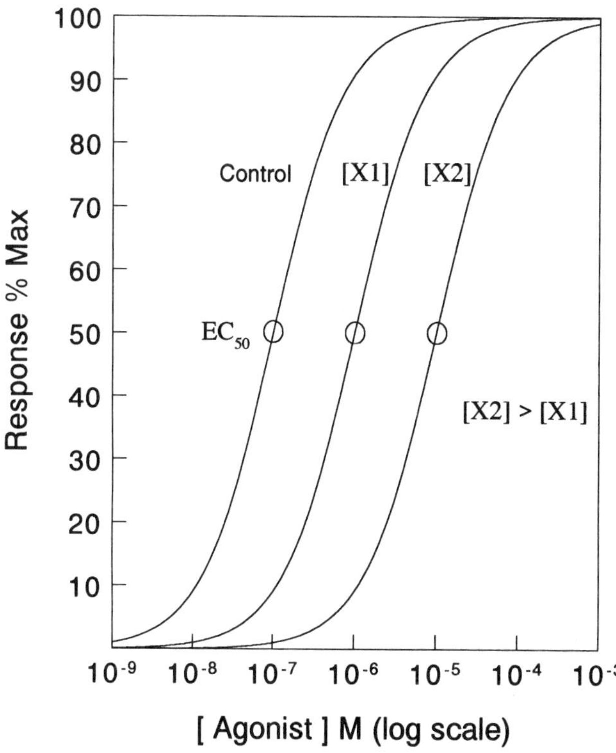

FIG. 2-22. The effect of increasing concentrations of a competitive antagonist (X) on the concentration-response curve of an agonist. (See text for details.)

fects on their own, they can produce effects in receptor systems that are under basal physiological activity or tone. The ability of a competitive antagonist of acetylcholine to dilate the pupil is an example of this type of pharmacological effect.

Noncompetitive Antagonism

The mechanisms by which a drug may produce noncompetitive antagonism are considerably more varied than for competitive antagonism. One such mechanism is illustrated as follows:

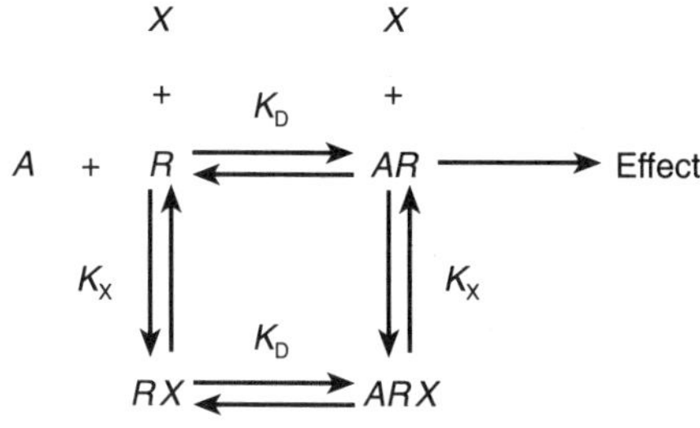

In this case, the antagonist (X) binds to the receptor at a site distinct from the agonist site such that a ternary complex forms. The ternary complex, however, is not coupled to the response. Alternatively, a noncompetitive antagonist may act distal to the agonist-receptor interaction and impair a step further down the signal transduction pathway. Independent of the exact molecular mechanism of action, the central feature of noncompetitive antagonism is that the agonist has no effect on the level of antagonism or its reversibility. Thus, unlike competitive antagonism, it is nonsurmountable. In many instances, the agonist system responds as though the total number of agonist receptors has been reduced. This is easy to understand for those antagonists whose mechanism involves the formation of a covalent bond with the agonist receptor site. Such antagonists may also be called *nonequilibrium competitive* rather than noncompetitive. The effect of noncompetitive antagonists on the concentration-response curve depends on whether or not the agonist receptor system has a receptor reserve. The effects of varying levels of noncompetitive antagonism under these two conditions are shown in Figure 2-23. In the absence of spare receptors (Figure 2-23A), the E_{max} decreases progressively, with no change in the EC_{50} as the antagonism increases. On the other hand, in the presence of spare receptors (Fig. 2-23B), the concentration-response curves show a progressive shift to the right with no decrease in the E_{max} until the level of antagonism encroaches into the minimum number of receptors required to produce E_{max}. Additional antagonism beyond this point will produce decreases in the maximal response as seen in the absence of receptor reserve. Because noncompetitive antagonists can produce a pattern of concentration-response curves in systems with receptor reserve, which, at least at moderate levels of antagonism, mimic the pattern seen with competitive antagonism, caution must be applied in the interpretation of such patterns in terms of mechanism of antagonist action. Theoretically, competitive antagonists will produce parallel shifts in the agonist concentration-response curve at all levels of antagonism, whereas noncompetitive antagonists should not. Thus, in principle, the two mechanisms may be differentiated.

Chemical Antagonism

Chemical antagonism is similar to competitive antagonism, except the antagonist interacts reversibly with the agonist instead of the receptor:

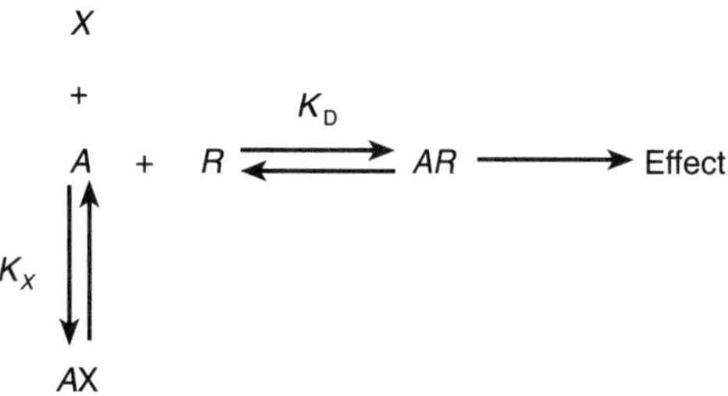

The effect of a chemical antagonist on the agonist concentration-response curves will be identical to that of a competitive antagonist. The two mechanisms may be dis-

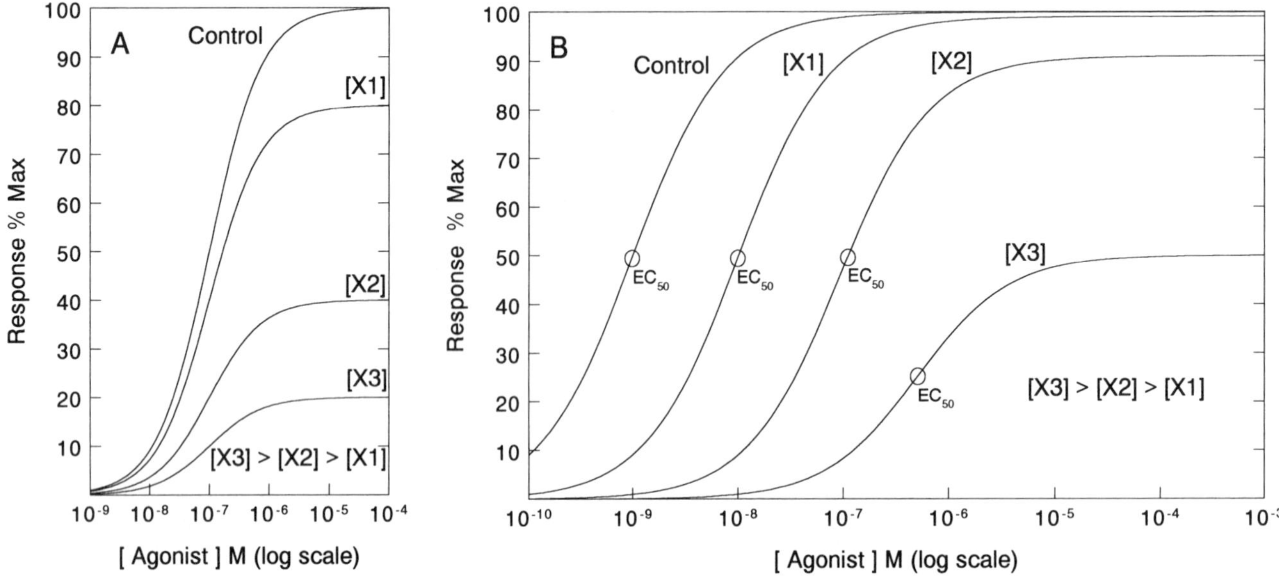

FIG. 2-23. The effect of increasing concentrations of a noncompetitive antagonist (X) on the concentration-response curve of an agonist. **A:** The effect of increasing concentrations of a noncompetitive antagonist in a system with no receptor reserve. **B:** The effect of increasing concentrations of a noncompetitive antagonist in a system with a receptor reserve. (See text for details.)

tinguishable, however, in that the effect of a competitive antagonist will be independent of the particular agonist used to stimulate the receptor. This should not be true for a chemical antagonist in that the interaction is with the agonist, and thus some specificity would be anticipated.

Functional Antagonism

Like noncompetitive antagonism, there are many molecular mechanisms by which drugs may interact functionally. In comparison to competitive antagonism, one clear example follows:

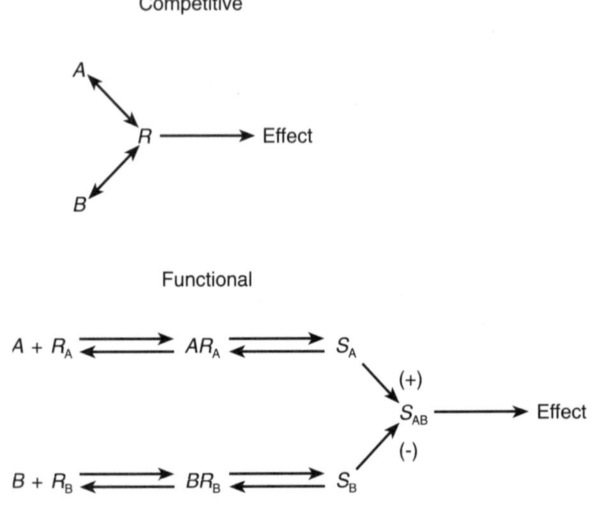

In this example, two agonists, each with its own receptor, produce opposite pharmacological effects via a common effector. Agonist A interacts with its receptor R_A to produce a stimulus S_A, which has a positive action on the effector (e.g., smooth-muscle contraction), whereas agonist B interacts with its receptor R_B to produce a negative action on the effector (e.g., smooth-muscle relaxation). Antagonism of this type is also often called *physiological antagonism.* The interaction of functional antagonists can produce complex effects on the concentration-response curves, which depend on the strengths of the individual signal transduction systems mediating the opposite responses.

BIOLOGICAL VARIATION

Up to this point, attention has been given to the molecular aspects of drug action by considering the concentration-response curves produced by agonists and antagonists in model systems. To introduce several additional pharmacodynamic concepts, the action of drugs in individual animals or humans is discussed.

Normal Distribution Curve and Cumulative Distribution Curve

It should not be surprising that all persons within a population will not require exactly the same dose to produce a given response, even if the dose has been adjusted for the individual patient's body mass. The point was made much earlier in this chapter that pharmacokinetic differences between individuals will account for some of the variation in a drug's potency within a population. Pharmacodynamic

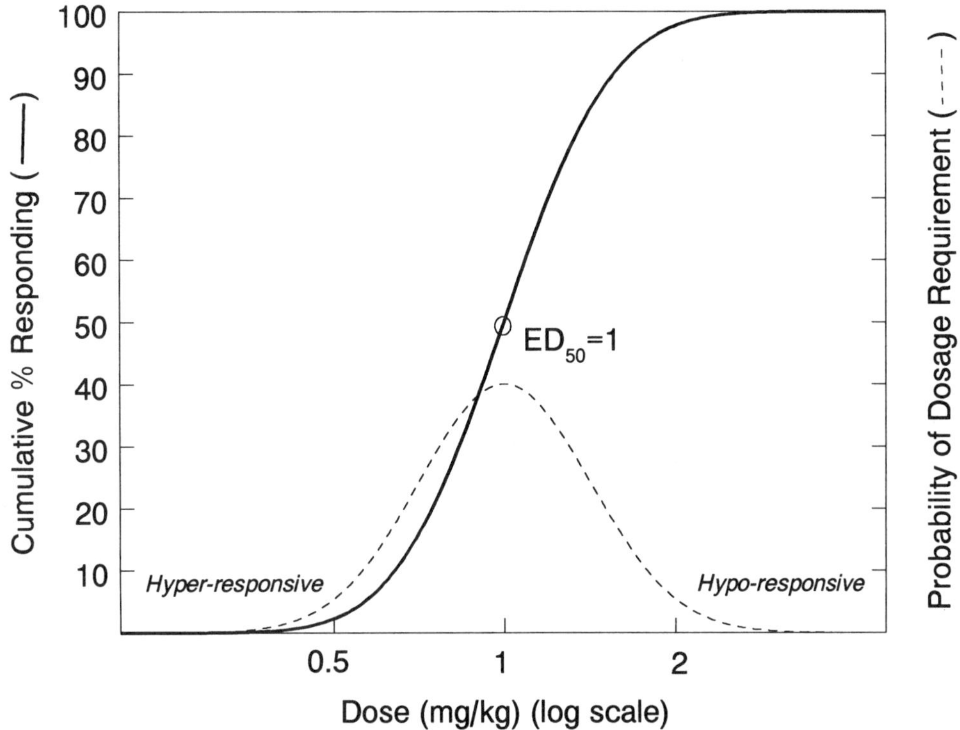

FIG. 2-24. Normal distribution curve representing the probability of a dosage requirement for the production of a specified response in a homogeneous group of individuals. Most frequently, individuals will require a dose close to the central dose. The probability that they will respond to a lower dose or require a higher dose is smaller. Superimposed on the probability curve is the cumulative response curve where the area under the probability curve is represented by the height on the cumulative curve. (See text for details.)

differences undoubtedly also play a role in the biological variability of individuals. This potency variability can be portrayed graphically in the form of the normal distribution curve. To accomplish this, the graded response of drug action in an individual patient must be converted into a quantal response, which can be achieved as follows: First, a specific response level of the drug to be measured is chosen. For example, if the drug to be administered has the ability to increase heart rate, a 50-beats-per-minute increase in heart rate may be chosen as the specified response level. Next, a given dose of the drug is administered to an individual, and one can determine whether a response equal to or greater than this specified magnitude was produced. In this way, the response measured is a quantal response; that is, the individual responded or did not respond. Whether a patient responded or not can be thought of as a measure of how responsive that individual was to the drug's effect. It would be expected that in a homogeneous population, the responsiveness would be normally distributed (Figure 2-24). Most frequently, individuals would require a dose close to the central effective dose. The probability that an individual will respond to a dose less than this (*hyperresponsive*) or will require a dose larger than this (*hyporesponsive*) is much smaller, leading to a bell-shaped probability curve. Alternatively, if one plots the cumulative percentage of responders as a function of dose, then the bell-shaped curve is transformed into a sigmoidal curve. A given area under the bell-shaped curve corresponds to a given height on the sigmoidal curve. The dose that will produce the specified response level in half of the individuals to which it is administered is called the *median effective dose,* or ED_{50}. If instead of therapeutic effectiveness lethality was the response measured, then the dose that kills 50% of the individuals to which it is administered is called the *median lethal dose,* or LD_{50}. The distance between these two sigmoid curves on the dose axis (Figure 2-25) is one measure of the relative safety of a drug and is called the drug's *therapeutic index* (*TI*).

$$\textit{Therapeutic Index} = \frac{LD_{50}}{ED_{50}}$$

As can be seen in Figure 2-25A, the TI for drug *A* is 10. Theoretically, one would expect that another drug with a *TI* higher than that of drug *A* should be safer. The potential fallacy in this expectation is illustrated in Figure 2-25B, where it can be seen that, although drug *B* has a *TI* ten times greater than drug *A,* the significant overlap of the effect curve on the lethality curve makes the higher *TI* meaningless. One measure of this relative overlap is the ratio of the *LD*1/*ED*99. The figure shows that the ratio for drug *A* is approximately one, whereas the ratio for drug *B* is much

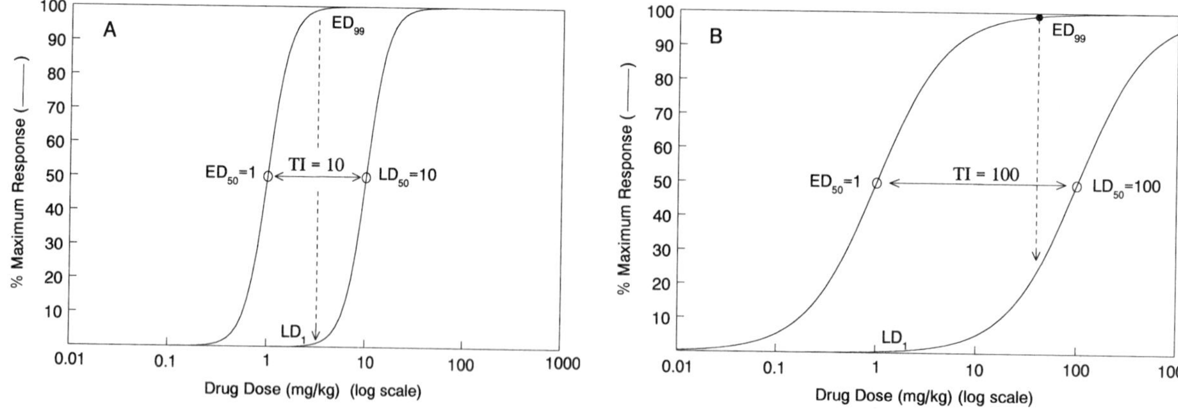

FIG. 2-25. Illustration of the determination of a drug's therapeutic index (TI) and other measures of safety. **A:** The TI for drug A is the LD_{50}/ED_{50} = 10. In addition, drug A's ED_{99} is approximately equal to its LD_1. **B:** The TI for drug B = 100; however, its ED_{99} is very much greater than its LD_1. (See text for details.)

less than one. Obviously, the higher the ratio, the greater the margin of safety.

The formal definition of the therapeutic index, as stated above, obviously precludes its determination in human subjects; however, if an appropriate animal experimental model for the drug's effectiveness is available, it is hoped that the *TI* determined in animal experimentation would provide some estimate of the potential safety in humans. In addition, a less formally defined "therapeutic index" may be measured in humans for a drug toxicity short of lethality–for example, nausea. With this in mind, it is important to note that a drug may have more than one *TI* whether formally or informally defined. If the drug has more than one clinical indication, and if the ED_{50} values for each indication are not identical, the drug will have a separate *TI* for each of its uses.

DRUG SPECIFICITY AND SELECTIVITY

Ideally, any drug administered clinically would produce only the desired effect for which it was prescribed. Unfortunately, no drug produces a single effect. It is easy to imagine that, as one increases the dose beyond the therapeutic range, toxic effects will come into play. Even at therapeutic levels, however, drugs lack specificity. Some reasons for the lack of specificity are that the receptor for the drug may be located in more than one tissue. If the drug is systemically administered, then drug responses in those tissues would be expected. The therapeutic effect would result in the target tissue, and side effects would result in the nontarget tissues. One possible way to overcome this problem would be to administer the drug locally rather than systemically. Topical application of drugs to the eye would be an excellent example. A second reason why a drug may lack selectivity is because it may have affinity for more than one receptor. Theoretically, this problem could be overcome by suitable modification of the chemical structure of the drug to enhance its selectivity for the target receptor. Selectivity and intrinsic activity are far more important than potency with respect to the successful use of drugs clinically.

REFERENCES

1. Goldstein A, Aronow L, Kalman SM. *Principles of Drug Action: The Basis of Pharmacology,* pp. 1–117. New York: John Wiley & Sons, 1974.
2. Pratt WB, Taylor P, eds. *Principles of Drug Action: The Basis of Pharmacology,* pp. 1–200. New York: Churchill Livingstone, 1990.
3. Kenakin TP. *Pharmacologic Analysis of Drug-Receptor Interaction.* New York: Raven Press, Ltd., 1993.
4. White MF, Kahn CR. The insulin signaling system. *J Biol Chem* 1994;269:1–4.
5. Birnbaumer L, Birnbaumer M. Signal transduction by G proteins: 1994 ed. *J Recept Signal Transduct Res* 1995;15:213–252.
6. Bohen SP, Kralli A, Yamamoto KR. Hold 'em and fold 'em: chaperones and signal transduction. *Science* 1995;268:1303–1304.
7. Inglese J, Koch WJ, Kazushige T, Lefkowitz RJ. $G_{\beta\gamma}$ interactions with PH domains and Ras-MAPK signaling pathways. *TIBS* 1995;20: 151–156.
8. Marshall CJ. Specificity of receptor tyrosine kinase signaling: transient versus sustained extracellular signal-regulated activation. *Cell* 1995;80:179–185.
9. Pawson T. Protein modules and signalling networks. *Nature* 1995; 373:573–580.
10. Premont RT, Inglese J, Lefkowitz RJ. Protein kinases that phosphorylate activated G protein-coupled receptors. *FASEB J* 1995;9:175–82.
11. Seger R, Krebs EG. The MAPK signaling cascade. *FASEB J* 1995;9:726–735.

Textbook of Ocular Pharmacology,
edited by T.J. Zimmerman, et al.
Lippincott–Raven Publishers, Philadelphia © 1997.

CHAPTER 3

Drug Reactions Not Mediated via Receptors

Anat Loewenstein and Moshe Lazar

The interaction of a drug with a specific constituent of the cell initiates a biochemical and physiological cascade of changes that characterizes the response to the drug: "A drug will not work unless it is bound" (Paul Ehrlich). Most drugs actually exert their effect by binding, mostly to proteins, glycoproteins, or proteolipids, and, for most, the site of action is a specific biological molecule, a *receptor.*

The term *receptive substance* or, more simply, *receptor,* can be used to label every target with which a drug molecule binds to elicit its specific effect. Alternatively, it can be restricted to a specific protein, producing an effect only after having been bound to the drug. There is general agreement, however, that the term *receptor* should be used only in the latter case. This chapter abides by this definition and deals only with pharmacological agents *not* acting by binding to specific receptor sites. Ophthalmological drugs that meet the above restrictions include: (a) drugs acting by modulating inhibiting enzymes (carbonic anhydrase, cholinesterase, collagenase, and prostaglandin synthetase inhibitors); (b) drugs acting by opening ion channels (local anesthetics); (c) drugs that do not cross membranes (hyperosmotic agents); and (d) enzymes (chymotrypsin, hyaluronidase).

The drugs discussed in this chapter will serve as illustrations of reactions not mediated via receptors. These drugs are discussed in greater detail elsewhere in the textbook.

DRUGS MODULATING THE ACTIVITY OF ENZYMES

Enzymes constitute the site of action of many drugs, with selective binding of the drug usually resulting in inhibition of catalytic activity. This inhibition may occur by a number of mechanisms: competitive inhibition, counterfeiting of the substrate, irreversible enzyme interaction, and action on enzyme cofactors. In ophthalmology, four types of drugs exert their effect by modulating enzyme activity: carbonic anhydrase inhibitors, cholinesterase inhibitors, collagenase inhibitors, and prostaglandin synthetase inhibitors.

Carbonic Anhydrase Inhibitors

Carbonic anhydrase (carbonate hydrolyase; EC 4.2.1.1.), a zinc metalloenzyme, was first discovered in the ciliary epithelium by Meldrum and Roughton (1). The enzyme catalyzes the reversible hydration of CO_2. Several isoenzyme forms exist throughout the body. Because sodium movement is isotonic and linked directly to bicarbonate synthesis (2), net fluid movement into the posterior chamber results from the carbonic anhydrase activity. The most well-studied isoenzyme II $-Zn^{++}-OH^-$, which has a complex of three histidines, exists at the active site and has a turnover rate of approximately 4×10^7 per minute (among the fastest in nature). Thus, a relatively high percentage of the enzyme must be inhibited to achieve any physiologic effect. The enzyme probably works via its active site, that is, namely, the Zn^{++} serving as a Lewis acid, thereby providing a high degree of nucleophilicity. A five-coordinate intermediate is formed eventually, and a ligand exchange is produced.

Aromatic sulfonamides were used routinely in the late 1930s as bacteriostatic agents. Southworth's serendipitous observation of metabolic acidosis in patients treated with sulfonamide antibiotics (3) led Mann and Keilin to the discovery of their carbonic anhydrase inhibitory effect (4).

The feature common to the carbonic anhydrase inhibitors is the presence of a free sulfonamide group ($-SO_2NH_2$) linked to an aromatic ring (5). This free sulfonamide group competes with the bicarbonate ion in binding to the active site of the enzyme in its acidic form, thereby inhibiting the conversion of CO_2 to HCO_3^- (6). Carbonic anhydrase inhibition reduces bicarbonate synthesis and the

A. Loewenstien and M. Lazar: Department of Ophthalmology, Ichilov Hospital, Sackler Faculty of Medicine, Tel-Aviv University, Tel-Aviv, Israel.

rate of fluid movement across the membrane. The carbonic anhydrase inhibitors reduce aqueous flow by about 30%, providing the basis for their use as antiglaucoma medications (7).

The introduction of acetazolamide, the prototype of the heterocyclic sulfonamide inhibitors (8), revolutionized research in the field. Later, methazolamide was found to be less bound to plasma protein and to have a lower rate of ionization than acetazolamide, which allows more diffusibility and greater activity on a weight-to-weight basis (9). The carbonic anhydrase inhibitors are potent agents and are relatively safe in short-term treatment. Chronic use, however, is associated with troublesome side effects (e.g., paresthesias, malaise, weight loss, and others), which are probably secondary to mixed-type acidosis.

Topical Carbonic Anhydrase Inhibitors

Most carbonic anhydrase inhibitors have poor corneal penetration. Because corneal permeability requires biphasic solubility, the conventional agents were not suitable for transcorneal movement. Acetazolamide crossed the cornea barrier in sufficient concentrations only in extreme conditions (10).

Several novel ring systems of thienothiopyran-2-sulfronamide were synthesized by Merck, Sharp and Dohme. Among them MG-417 (sezolamide), MK-507 (dorzolamide), and MK-927 had considerable potential in the treatment of glaucoma and ocular hypertension (11). The reduction in intraocular pressure and aqueous flow was more gradual than with the use of systemic agents, although the peak effects were similar (12). The prospects of targeting agents topically, thereby alleviating the side effects of systemic administration, increase the therapeutic index. More details about clinical aspects are outlined in Chapter 26.

Cholinesterase Inhibitors

Acetylcholinesterase is a ubiquitous enzyme that is found in all cell membranes examined, including red blood cells. The enzyme hydrolyzes the transmitter acetylcholine to the inactive products choline and acetic acid. Acetylcholinesterase binds the positively charged acetylcholine molecule at an anionic site, close to which is the esteradic site where hydrolysis takes place (13). Another anionic site exists wherein acetylcholinesterase is located more distal from the esteradic site and inhibits the action of the esteradic site. The inhibition of acetylcholinesterase allows individual acetylcholine molecules to repeat their effect. As a result, the half-decay time of the end plate currents increases from 1.5–2.0 to 3.0–10.0 msec (14). The acetylcholinesterase inhibitors also act by competing with acetylcholine for nonspecific binding sites, thereby increasing unbound levels of acetylcholine (15).

Inactivation by reversible inhibitors (demecarium bromide) results from binding of the drug to the cholinesterase enzyme, which then is slowly reversed by hydrolysis. Binding of cholinesterase, whatever the manner, prevents hydrolysis of acetylcholine, which accumulates at the neuromuscular junction, stimulating the parasympathetic nerve ending.

Cholinesterase inhibitors increase activity in both muscarinic and nicotinic structures. Their value in ophthalmology is mainly for their muscarinic effects. Only in the diagnosis of myasthenia gravis their nicotinic effect is used (intravenous edrophonium in the Tensilon test).

The cholinesterase inhibitors can be subdivided into carbamylating and phosphorylating agents. Physiostigmine, neostigmine, pyridostigmine, and demecarium are carbamylating agents, whereas diisopropyl fluorophosphonate (DFP) and echothiophate are phosphorylating ones. In general, the carbamylating agents are shorter acting, with demecarium the one exception. The anticholinesterase organophosphates are a group of compounds that were initially synthesized during World War II in search of materials for chemical warfare. In the 1950s, these agents were first used in the treatment of glaucoma, when it was noted that they had a very strong parasympatomimetic activity and a longer duration of action than other miotic agents. Their mechanism of action is by inactivating acetylcholinesterase and butyrylcholinesterase. The irreversible anticholinesterase agents (DFP) and phosopholine iodide (echothiophate iodide) bind to the enzyme by alkylphosophorylation to form a stable complex, which is only minimally reversible. Reactivation is possible only if the esteradic site is dephosphorylated rapidly by nucleophilic agents, such as pyridine oxime, during the first 2 hours of reaction (16). More details about clinical utility are outlined in Chapter 20.

Collagenase Inhibitors and Wound-healing Modulators

The delicate balance in the process of wound healing, shifting between the formation of collagen and its cleavage, has become a challenging pharmacological field of interest. The search for safe, effective inhibitors of collagenase started in the 1960s, when cysteine was used to prevent collagenolytic activity in human skin (17). Since then, many agents have been claimed to be effective inhibitors of collagenase and proposed to act as preventive treatment of corneal perforation. Other agents induce their effect by various mechanisms: ethylenediaminetetraacetic acid (EDTA) probably chelates the calcium necessary for collagenase activity. Cysteine and acetylcysteine (Mucomyst) have a double action: chelating calcium while simultaneously reducing a disulfide bond in the collagenase molecule (18). These agents have been proved in vivo as being effective in the prevention of corneal perforation resulting from overaction of collagenase in situations such as alkali burns (19).

In certain experimental and clinical settings, it is desirable to achieve the opposite effect, namely, to prevent collagen formation and wound healing (e.g., following glaucoma filtration surgery). Various agents have been screened as adjuvant therapy to prolong bleb survival. Although a specific "receptor" has been delineated for some agents, others exert their action on the cell membrane and cytoskeleton (e.g., taxol, colchicine, heparin) (20–22) or by disrupting collagen cross-linkage through specific inhibition of enzymes required for collagen linkage (e.g., minoxidil, beta-amino proprionitrile) (23,24). More details about clinical utility are outlined in Chapter 28.

Prostaglandin Synthetase Inhibitors

The prostaglandins are a complex group of oxygenated fatty acids that have been found in all mammalian tissues. They are important both as bioregulators and as participants in pathologic states. They are not stored in tissues but are synthesized de novo as a result of membrane changes that cause the release of free fatty acids, generally arachidonic acid, from esterified lipid sources. The free arachidonic acid then reacts with prostaglandin cyclooxygenase, the first enzyme of the prostaglandin biosynthetic cascade. Cyclooxygenase oxygenates arachidonic acid to the endoperoxide intermediate, prostaglandin G_2 (PGG_2), which then is converted to a variety of other biologically active products. Another enzymatic pathway involves the enzyme lipooxygenase. This pathway leads to the conversion of arachidonic acid to 12-hydroperoxy arachidonic acid (HPETE) and 12-hydroxy-arachidonic acid (HETE).

Substances that inhibit the synthesis or release of prostaglandins in the eye might help in the management of ocular inflammation. In addition to aspirin and indomethacin, which have been shown to prevent the synthesis or release of prostaglandins from arachidonic acid, mefenamic acid, phenylbutazone, clofibrate, perprofen, ibuprofen, fenoprofen, indoxyl, and naproxen have also been demonstrated to be efficacious.

It was found that systemic indomethacin barely penetrates the eye. Thus, its suggested efficacy in reducing the inflammation in uveitis (25) has been refuted (26). Topical application of indomethacin is capable of reducing cystoid macular edema after cataract extraction and the intraoperative pupillary miosis claimed to be induced by prostaglandin release. More details about clinical utility are outlined in the clinical Chapter 29.

DRUGS ACTING BY OPENING ION CHANNELS

Drugs that belong to this group are used in ophthalmology as local anesthetics. The prototypical compound, cocaine, an alkaloid contained in the leaves of *Erythroxylon coca,* a shrub growing in the Andes Mountains, was first isolated in 1860 by Niemann, who noted that it had a bitter taste and produced a peculiar effect on the tongue, making it numb and almost devoid of sensation. Koller, in 1895, was the first to appreciate the anesthetizing properties of cocaine and introduced it as a local anesthetic in ophthalmology.

The structure of local anesthetics contains hydrophilic and hydrophobic groups that are separated by an intermediate alkyl chain. The hydrophilic group is a secondary or tertiary amine; the hydrophobic moiety is an aromatic residue. Linkage to the aromatic group is by either the ester or amide type, a fact that determines certain pharmacological properties of these agents. The formula is as follows:

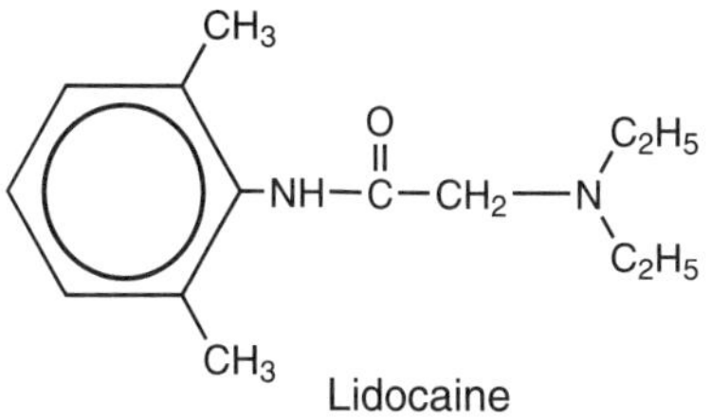

CH_3, CH_3 — (2,6-dimethylphenyl)–NH–C(=O)–CH_2–N(C_2H_5)(C_2H_5)

Lidocaine

Local anesthetics are drugs that block nerve conduction when applied locally to nerve tissue in appropriate concentrations. They act at the cell membrane to prevent the generation and conduction of nerve action potential and can induce their effect on any part of the nervous system and on every type of nerve fiber. In myelinated nerves, the anesthetic gains access only to the membrane at the nodes of Ranvier. In unmyelinated nerves, the anesthetic effect is along the entire surface of the nerve. There is no interaction with a specific "receptor" molecule.

Local anesthetics prevent the generation and conduction of nerve impulses. Their site of action is the cell membrane, where they diminish the transient increase in the permeability of excitable membranes to sodium, which is produced by a slight depolarization of the membrane. This action of local anesthetics is due to their interaction with voltage-sensitive sodium channels (27). In general, small-diameter nerve fibers seem to be more susceptible to the action of local anesthetics than large fibers. The sensation of pain is usually the first modality to disappear, followed by the loss of sensation of cold, warmth, touch, and deep pressure, although individual variations exist. Motor function disappears last. In retrobulbar anesthesia, the optic nerve is the most resistant to complete conduction block because it is the largest nerve within the orbit.

The duration of action of a local anesthetic is proportional to the time during which it is in contact with the nerve. Consequently, procedures that maintain the drug at the nerve site prolong the period of anesthesia. The addition of a vasoconstrictor localizes the anesthetic to the desired site, decreases the rate of local anesthetic absorption, and simultaneously diminishes its absorption into the circulation, thereby reducing its potential systemic toxicity.

In addition to blocking conduction in nerve axons in the peripheral nervous system, local anesthetics interfere with the function of all organs in which conduction or transmission of impulses occur, such as in the central nervous system, autonomic ganglia, neuromuscular junction, and muscles (28). Analgesia is produced by a reversible blockage of sensory nerve endings in the corneal epithelium and conjunctiva.

The local anesthetics are weak bases. The unprotonated species is necessary for diffusion through cellular membranes to reach its site of action; the cationic form is probably the active one. The local anesthetics differ in their ocular bioavailability and rate of elimination. For increased solubility, the compounds are generally marketed as water-soluble salts, usually the hydrochlorides.

The onset of sensory anesthesia following injection depends on the pKa of the anesthetic. It is also determined by the need for diffusion of the agent from its site of injection to its site of action. The duration of nerve block anesthesia depends on the physical characteristics of the local anesthetic used. Especially important are lipid solubility and protein binding. Absorption of local anesthetics from an injection site depends on the degree of tissue vascularity and blood flow. Metabolism occurs in the plasma or liver only after absorption into the vascular system, not at the injection site. Ester-linked anesthetics are hydrolyzed mainly by plasma pseudocholinesterases and liver microsomes. Hydrolysis results in an aromatic acid and one amino alcohol. Amide-linked anesthetics undergo oxidative dealkylation and hydrolysis in hepatic microsomes. The metabolic products usually are eliminated in the urine, promoted by urine acidification. In some cases, the metabolic products are excreted in bile or in the lungs as carbon dioxide.

Lidocaine is quickly absorbed after parenteral administration to the gastrointestinal tract. After completing its action, lidocaine is dealkylated in the liver by mixed-function oxidase. More details about clinical utility are outlined in Chapter 63.

HYPEROSMOTIC AGENTS

Hyperosmotic agents are solutes that are freely filtered at the glomerulus, undergo limited reabsorption by the renal tubule, and are relatively inert. They produce an increase in serum osmolarity but do not penetrate the blood-aqueous barrier. Thus, a gradient between blood and ocular fluid is produced. Intraocular water exits the eye via retinal and choroidal blood vessels, reducing vitreous volume by 3% to 4% and lowering intraocular pressure (29,30).

Sodium salts are the major solutes in the proximal tubular fluid. Because the epithelium of this segment cannot maintain a substantial osmotic gradient, sodium and water normally are reabsorbed from the tubular fluid in the same ratio as that in the glomerular filtrate. Thus, the concentration of the lumen remains essentially constant; however, a nonreabsorbable solute in the proximal tubular lumen becomes progressively concentrated as fluid is reabsorbed, a phenomenon that produces a counterforce to the normal reabsorption of water. Consequently, relatively more sodium than water is reabsorbed, and the luminal concentration of sodium begins to fall. The net reabsorption of sodium diminishes and causes an enhanced rate of urine flow associated with a relatively smaller increment in the excretion of salts. As a result, the serum osmolarity increases. Because these agents do not penetrate the blood-aqueous barrier rapidly, an osmotic gradient between the blood and ocular fluid is produced, creating an exit of intraocular water into intraocular blood vessels. Some studies have shown that changes in intraocular pressure and serum osmolarity do not always correlate; therefore, it was proposed that hyperosmotic agents might lower intraocular pressure by central effects on the hypothalamus. This was proved to occur in animals and might account for the rapid decrease in intraocular pressure before the establishment of a blood-ocular osmotic gradient (31). The decrease in vitreous volume has a greater intraocular pressure-lowering effect in glaucomatous eyes than in eyes with normal intraocular pressure (32). More details about clinical utility are outlined in Chapter 27.

ENZYMES

Chymotrypsin

Barraquer, in 1958, demonstrated the value of the enzymatic zonulolysis of chymotrypsin in facilitating intracapsular cataract extraction, and the enzyme has since been commonly used for that purpose (33). The enzyme, in dilutions of 1:5,000 to 1:10,000, rapidly produces a selective disintegration of lens zonules, characterized by fragmentation of the fibrils into uniform small segments. Its main proteolytic effect is to split peptide bonds only at the location of certain amino acids, mainly L-tyrosine, L-phenylalanine, and L-tryptophan. The potency of commercial preparations of alpha-chymotrypsin is measured in Armour proteolytic activity (APA) units. One unit releases 1 μg of tyrosine from a hemoglobin substrate. Potency varies between 750 and 1,300 APA units/mg. Solutions of alpha-chymotrypsin are relatively unstable at room temperature, but refrigeration at 2° C maintains full activity of the solution for at least 1 month (34).

Hyaluronidase (Wydase)

This enzyme is a widely used additive to local anesthetic solutions for injection. This mucolytic enzyme hydrolyzes and depolymerizes the mucopolysaccharide hyaluronic acid that binds water in interstitial spaces. When hyaluronidase is added to the anesthetic solution, the effective area of action is increased, and the induction time of the anesthesia is markedly shortened. Systemic absorption is increased, and therefore epinephrine should be added to the anesthetic solution when hyaluronidase is used (35).

REFERENCES

1. Meldrum NV, Roughton FJW. Carbonic anhydrase: its preparation and properties. *J Physiol (Lond)* 1933;80:113–142.
2. Garg LC, Oppelt WW. The effect of ouabain and acetazolamide on the transport of sodium and chloride from plasma to aqueous humor. *J Pharmacol Exp Ther* 1970;175:237–247.
3. Southworth H. Acidosis associated with administration of para-amino benzene-sulfonamide (prontylin). *Proc Soc Exp Biol Med* 1937;36: 58–61.
4. Mann T, Keilin D. Sulfanilamide as specific inhibitor of carbonic anhydrase. *Nature* 1940;146:164–165.
5. Maren TH. Relations between structure and biological activity of sulfonamides. *Annu Rev Pharmacol Toxicol* 1976;16:309–327.
6. Maren TH. The physiology of reactions catalyzed by carbonic anhydrase and their inhibition by sulfonamides. *Ann N Y Acad Sci* 1984;429:568–579.
7. Daily RA, Brubaker RF, Bourne WM. The effects of timolol maleate and acetazolamide on the rate of aqueous formation in normal human subjects. *Am J Ophthalmol* 1982;93:232–237.
8. Becker B. Diamox and the therapy of glaucoma. *Am J Ophthalmol* 1954;38:16.
9. Stone RA, Zimmerman TJ, Shin DH, Becker B, Kass MA. Low-dose methazolamide and intraocular pressure. *Am J Ophthalmol* 1977;83: 674–679.
10. Friedman Z, Allen RC, Raph SM. Topical acetazolamide and metazolamide delivered by contact lenses. *Arch Ophthalmol* 1985;103: 963–966.
11. Lippa E, Carlson LE, Ehinger B, Eriksson LO, Finnshem K, Holmin C, Nilsson SE, Nyman K, Raitha C, Ringvald A. Dose response and duration of action of dorzolamide, a topical carbonic anhydrase inhibitor. *Arch Ophthalmol* 1992;110:495–499.
12. Brechue W, Maren T. A comparison between the effect of topical and systemic carbonic anhydrase inhibitors on aqueous humor secretion. *Exp Eye Res* 1993;57:67–78.
13. Nachmanson D, Wilson IB. Enzymatic hydrolysis and synthesis of acetylcholine. *Adv Enzymol* 1951;12:259–339.
14. Del-Castillo J, Katz B. The membrane change produced by the neuromuscular transmitter. *J Physiol* 1954;125:546–565.
15. Escolona-De-Motta G, Del-Castillo J. Diffusion barrier for acetylcholine at the neuromuscular junction. *Nature* 1977;270:178–180.
16. Wilson I, Binsburg S. A powerful reactivator of aldylphosphate-inhibited acetylcholinesterase. *Biochim Biophys Acta* 1955;18:168.
17. Eisen AZ, Jeffrey JJ, Gross J. Human skin collagenase: isolation, and mechanism of attack on the collagen molecule. *Biochim Biophys Acta* 1968;637–645.
18. Evans RM, Mc Crary JA, Christensen G. Mucomyst (acetylcysteine) in the treatment of corneal alkali burns. *Annals of Ophthalmology* 1972;4: 320–328.
19. Hook C, Brown SI, Iwanij W, Nakamishi I. Characterization and inhibition of corneal collagenase. *Invest Ophthalmol* 1971;10:496–503.
20. Molteno ACB, Ancker E, Biljon GV. Surgical technique for advanced juvenile glaucoma. *Arch Ophthalmol* 1984;102:51–57.
21. Joseph JP, Grierson I, Hitchings RA. Taxol, cytochalasin B and colchicine effect of fibroblast migration and contraction: a role in glaucoma filtration surgery? *Curr Eye Res* 1989;8:203–215.
22. Jampel HD, Thbault D, Leong KW, Uppal P, Quigley HA. Glaucoma filtration surgery in nonhuman primates using taxol and etoposide in polyanhydride carriers. *Invest Ophthalmol Vis Sci* 1993;34:3076–3083.
23. Sharir M. Topical minoxidil for glaucoma filtration surgery in the rabbit. *Exp Eye Res* 1995;59:707–714.
24. Moorhead LC, Smith J, Stewart R, Kimbrough R. Effects of beta aminoproprionitrile after glaucoma filtration surgery: pilot human trial. *Annals of Ophthalmology* 1987;19:223–225.
25. Perkins ES, MacFaul PA. Indomethacin in the treatment of uveitis: a double blind trial. *Transactions of the Ophthalmological Society of the United Kingdom* 1965;85:53–58.
26. Gordon D. Discussion. In: Kaufman HE, ed. *Ocular Anti-inflam-matory Therapy.* Springfield, Illinois: Charles C Thomas, 1970;146.
27. Courtney K, Strichartz G. Structural elements which determine local anesthetic activity. In: Strichartz G, ed. *Local Anesthetics: Handbook of Experimental Pharmacology.* Berlin: Springer-Verlag, 1987;53– 94.
28. Gintant G, Hoffman B. The role of local anesthetic effects in the actions of antiarrhythmic drugs. In: Strichartz G, ed. *Local Anesthetics. Handbook of Experimental Pharmacology.* Berlin: Springer-Verlag, 1987;213–251.
29. Robbins R, Galin MA. Effect of osmotic agents on the vitreous body. *Arch Ophthalmol* 1969;82:694–699.
30. Vucicevic ZM, Tark E, Ahmad S. Echographic studies of osmotic agents. *Annals of Ophthalmology* 1979;11:1331–1335.
31. Krupin T, Podos S, Becker B. Effect of optic nerve transection on osmotic alterations of intraocular pressure. *Am J Ophthalmol* 1970;70: 214–220.
32. Drance SM. Effect of oral glycerol on intraocular pressure in normal and glaucomatous eyes. *Arch Ophthalmol* 1964;72:491–493.
33. Barraquer J. Enzymatic zonulolisis. *Proc R Soc Med* 1959;973–981.
34. Schwartz B, Schwartz JB. A review of the biochemistry and pharmacology of alpha-chymotrypsin. *Transactions of the Ophthalmological Society of the United Kingdom* 1960;64: 17–24.
35. Havener WH. *Ocular Pharmacology,* pp. 211–212. St. Louis: CV Mosby, 1978.

Textbook of Ocular Pharmacology,
edited by T.J. Zimmerman, et al.
Lippincott–Raven Publishers, Philadelphia © 1997.

CHAPTER 4

Cholinergics

Craig E. Crosson

Since the identification of acetylcholine as a chemical messenger in the nervous system, our understanding of cholinergic pharmacology has grown to include the mechanisms involved in biosynthesis, storage, release, and metabolism of acetylcholine. In addition, two families of cholinergic receptors have been identified: muscarinic and nicotinic. As a result, a number of therapeutic agents that modulate cholinergic function have been developed. In the eye, cholinergic agonists and antagonists represent some of the primary classes of drugs used for therapeutic, surgical, and diagnostic indications. This chapter reviews cholinergic neurotransmission in the anterior segment of the eye, the current status of cholinergic pharmacology, and the use of cholinergic agents in ophthalmology

OCULAR CHOLINERGIC INNERVATION

Autonomic Innervation

Efferent autonomic innervation to the anterior segment of the eye, like other organs, is supplied by two subdivisions: sympathetic and parasympathetic nervous systems. Both systems are composed of preganglionic and postganglionic nerve fibers. Preganglionic nerve fibers of sympathetic and parasympathetic division, as well as postganglionic parasympathetic fibers, secrete acetylcholine and are termed *cholinergic neurons.* Postganglionic sympathetic fibers secrete norepinephrine and are termed *adrenergic neurons* (see Chapter 7). Preganglionic sympathetic fibers originate in the upper thoracic segments of the spinal cord and enter the sympathetic chain, where they pass upward to the superior cervical ganglion. Postganglionic adrenergic fibers exit the superior cervical ganglion and innervate the anterior segment and extraocular structures of the eye.

C. E. Crosson: Department of Ophthalmology and Visual Sciences, Texas Tech University Health Sciences Center, Lubbock, Texas 79430.

Preganglionic parasympathetic fibers that originate in the Edinger-Westphal nucleus form part of the oculomotor nerve (III cranial nerve) and terminate in the ciliary ganglion. From the ciliary ganglion, parasympathetic postganglionic fibers form the short ciliary nerves that innervate the ciliary body and the sphincter muscle of the iris. Most of these neurons (97%) innervate the ciliary muscle over the iris sphincter (1). The lacrimal gland is innervated by postganglionic parasympathetic fibers that originate in the pterygopalatine ganglion, which receives preganglionic input from the lacrimatory nucleus.

Somatomotor Innervation

Motor neurons innervate the extraocular muscles and the lids. Like parasympathetic fibers, these nerves secrete acetylcholine and therefore are considered cholinergic neurons; however, these neurons form continuous connections from the central nervous system to the muscle fiber. Extraocular muscles are innervated by fibers from the oculomotor nerve (III cranial nerve), trochlear nerve (IV cranial nerve), and the abducens nerve (VI cranial nerve). The orbicularis oculi and the levator palpebrae muscles of the lids are innervated by fibers from the facial and oculomotor nerve, respectively.

When autonomic fibers terminate at their target organ, they branch diffusely over the surface and form multiple varicosities distributed along the length of these branches. Varicosities are regions where the excitatory neurotransmitter acetylcholine is released. Unlike autonomic fibers, motor neurons form a discrete junctional complex with skeletal muscle fibers, termed *muscle motor end plates.* The membrane motor end plates invaginate into the muscle and form the synaptic cleft between the nerve terminal and the motor fiber. This end plate is covered by one or more Schwann's cells. Normally, there is only one motor end-plate complex per fiber.

CHOLINERGIC NEUROTRANSMISSION

The junctional complex formed by cholinergic neurons and their respective target organs are the sites of chemical neurotransmission. For cholinergic neurons, this process involves the synthesis, storage, release, receptor activation, and metabolism of acetylcholine. Acetylcholine neurotransmission requires the synthesis of vesicles by the Golgi in the cell bodies of the neurons. The vesicles then are transported via axon transport to the nerve terminals, where they collect in numbers of about 300,000 for a single muscle motor end plate. The synthesis of acetylcholine occurs in the cytosol of the nerve terminal. The rate-limiting step in this process is the uptake of choline by a high-affinity, sodium-dependent uptake system. This choline transporter is inhibited by hemicholinium-3 (2). It should be noted that the retinal cells contain a high-affinity choline transporter that is sodium independent and not inhibited by hemicholinium-3 (3). This sodium-independent transporter in the retina is thought to be associated with supplying choline for phospholipid synthesis, and not acetylcholine production.

In the cytosol of cholinergic nerve terminals, the enzyme choline acetyltransferase catalyzes the biosynthetic conversion of choline and acetyl-coenzyme A (CoA) to the acetylester of choline (i.e., acetylcholine). The acetyl-CoA for this reaction is produced, in part, by mitochondria; however, other cytosolic sources, such as citrate and acetylcarnitine, may serve as sources of acetyl-CoA. From the cytosol, acetylcholine then is transported and concentrated in the terminal vesicles, where it is stored until released during synaptic transmission. Work using torpedo synaptic vesicles has suggested that this vesicular transport occurs via a proton pump and can be inhibited by vesimicol (4). Although this vesicular transport system has not been confirmed in mammalian systems, vesimicol treatment has been shown to deplete acetylcholine in mammalian cholinergic fibers (5). The concentration of acetylcholine in terminal vesicles has been estimated to be 1,000 to 50,000 molecules per vesicle.

Cholinergic nerves spontaneously release acetylcholine; however, this release normally is not sufficient to produce a postjunctional or postsynaptic response because of the high concentration of the enzyme acetylcholinesterase located on the postjunctional or postsynaptic membrane. With the arrival of depolarizing action potential, however, voltage-activated calcium channels are opened, and Ca^{++} levels rise in the nerve terminal, which leads to the fusion of several vesicles (i.e., exocytosis) and the release of acetylcholine into the junctional region. Once released, acetylcholine can activate receptors within the junctional complex. Various toxins and venoms act by modulating the release of acetylcholine (6). Black widow spider venom induces the release of acetylcholine, whereas botulinum toxin blocks the release of acetylcholine. In the eye, botulinum toxin has been used for the treatment of strabismus and blepharospasm.

The end of neurotransmission is accomplished by the metabolism of acetylcholine to acetate and choline by the enzyme acetylcholinesterase. The catalytic subunit of acetylcholinesterase is a protein of about 70,000 daltons and contains an anionic and esteratic subsite. The anionic site has a high affinity for the quaternary structure of choline. The esteratic site is where nucleophilic attack of the acyl carbon of acetylcholine occurs with the eventual release of choline and acetate. About half of the hydrolyzed choline is taken back up into the prejunctional terminal to be reacetylated. Hence, there is a continuous requirement for choline, which may be supplied from the blood or membrane phospholipids. A second type of cholinesterase, butyrylcholinesterase, is found only in small amounts in the nervous system, but it is found in the plasma and liver. The physiological function of butyrylcholinesterase is unknown; however, this enzyme serves as a detoxifying mechanism for exogenous compounds, such as the nicotinic antagonist succinylcholine.

CHOLINERGIC RECEPTORS

Acetylcholine activates two different types of receptors: muscarinic and nicotinic. In the peripheral nervous system, muscarinic receptors are located primarily in effector cells stimulated by postganglionic parasympathetic neurons. Studies have shown, however, that muscarinic receptors are located postsynaptically in sympathetic ganglia and prejunctionally on autonomic neurons. Nicotinic receptors are located primarily in postsynaptic membranes in sympathetic and parasympathetic ganglions and on skeletal muscles at the neuromuscular junctions.

Muscarinic Receptors

Structurally, muscarinic receptors are part of the superfamily of receptors termed *metabotropic receptors*. The convention adopted for muscarinic receptors use M_1–M_4 for pharmacologically defined subtypes and m_1–m_5 for cloned receptors. Like other metabotropic receptors, muscarinic receptors are coupled to intracellular second-messenger systems by guanine nucleotide-binding proteins (G proteins). These actions of second messengers then lead to functional change in the target system. Studies applying molecular biological techniques have demonstrated five different genes that code for putative muscarinic receptors: m_1, m_2, m_3, m_4, and m_5 (7–12). Each of these genes codes for a peptide sequence that has seven transmembrane domains (TM1–TM7) and three intracellular loops (i1–i3). Recent work has suggested that the i3 loop is involved in the binding of G proteins (13).

The stimulation of muscarinic receptors leads to a conformational change in the receptor, permitting an interaction with heterotrimeric G protein. This receptor–G protein interaction catalyzes the exchange of guanosine diphosphate (GDP) for guanosine triphosphate (GTP) on the α-subunit, which leads to the disassociation of the G protein into its α and β-γ subunits. The activated Gα-subunit then can interact with an enzyme, such as adenylate cyclase or phospholipase C (PLC), to produce intracellular second messengers, or it can interact directly with membrane proteins, such as ion channels. Disassociation of the G protein also reduces the receptor's affinity for the agonist. Termination of the intracellular response is the hydrolysis of GTP to GDP. There is also evidence that muscarinic receptors may activate via PLC through β–γ subunit interaction and that agonists may not need to disassociate from the receptor for the hydrolysis of GTP to occur (13,14).

Muscarinic receptors and associated G proteins interact primarily with two second-messenger systems: adenylate cyclase and PLC. In general, M_2 and M_4 receptors are coupled with the inhibition of adenylate cyclase (8). The inhibitory action of M_2 and M_4 receptors on adenylate cyclase activity can be blocked by pertussis toxin (PTX)-induced adenosine disphosphate (ADP)-ribosylation of G proteins. This action of PTX has been used as evidence that M_2 and M_4 receptors are coupled with $G_{i/o}$ proteins. In the CNS, M_2 receptors also appear to be coupled with G_o proteins (8). Stein et al. (15) provided evidence that M_1 and M_3 receptor activation also can inhibit adenylate cyclase by a PTX-sensitive system. The functional response in these systems likely reflects the decrease in protein kinase activity associated with the muscarinic-induced reduction in cyclic adenosine monophosphate (cAMP).

Studies have shown that M_1, M_3, and m_5 receptors are preferentially coupled with the activation of PLC. This activation is mediated by a PTX-insensitive G_q protein family (16). The products of PLC activation are inositol triphosphate (IP_3) and diacylglycerol. These second messengers in turn mediate functional responses to these receptors by elevations in intracellular Ca^{++} and the activation of protein kinase C.

Recent in situ hybridization studies by Zhang et al. (17) demonstrated that mRNA for m_2, m_3, and m_5 receptors are expressed by human ciliary muscle. Expression of m_2 and m_3 mRNAs were greater in circular regions, whereas the expression of m_5 mRNA was greater in the longitudinal region of the ciliary muscle. Northern blots also provided evidence that the ciliary muscle can also express mRNA for m_1 and m_4 receptors. Expression of m_3 mRNA was also demonstrated in the bovine iris sphincter muscle and ciliary process (18). Trace amounts of m_2 mRNA were also found in the iris sphincter muscle and ciliary process and m_4 mRNA in the ciliary process.

Muscarinic Antagonists

In general, muscarinic antagonists have little effect on nicotinic receptors. Hence, muscarinic antagonists are directed primarily at neuroeffector junctions innervated by postganglionic parasympathetic neurons. As a result, these compounds have been termed *parasympatholytic* or *antimuscarinic agents.* Muscarinic antagonists are competitive in nature and therefore can be overcome by increasing acetylcholine concentrations.

The alkaloids atropine and scopolamine, originally isolated from belladonna plants, are the best known nonselective muscarinic antagonists (Fig. 4-1). Homoatropine is a semisynthetic analog of atropine that is produced by combining the aromatic mandelic acid with the organic base tropine. These compounds each contain one chiral carbon, and the *l*-enantiomer is more active than the *d*-enantiomer. Methylation of the nitrogen produces the corresponding quaternary ammonium and methylatropine, methylscopolamine, and methylhomoatropine. In general, the quaternary amine analogs of muscarinic antagonists are more potent antagonists of muscarinic receptors; however, these agents are also more potent in inhibiting nicotinic receptors in autonomic ganglia. It should also be noted that quaternary amine analogs are more poorly absorbed across mucosal membranes and blood–brain or blood–ocular barriers.

In the eye, muscarinic antagonists, such as atropine, are used to inhibit cholinergic-mediated contraction of the iris sphincter and ciliary muscle. The functional response to the topical application of atropine is an increase in the pupil diameter (*mydriasis*) and relaxation of the ciliary muscle (*cycloplegia*). In these eyes, the pupillary light reflex is absent, and the lens shape is fixed for far vision. The duration of action following topical administration of these agents may be several days. The synthetic muscarinic antagonists tropicamide and cyclopentylate exhibit much shorter durations of action, with full reversal of mydriatic activity 6 to 24 hours after topical administration. The systemic administration of antimuscarinic compounds is used to reduce gastric acid secretion and gastric motility and also may result in the loss of lens accommodation.

The side effects associated with the topical use of antimuscarinic agents include dilation of peripheral blood vessels, dry mouth, tachycardia, restlessness, and potential delirium. In general, the topical administration of antimuscarinics does not alter intraocular pressure. In persons with narrow anterior-chamber angles, however, pupillary dilation induced by these agents may occlude the trabecular meshwork and produce an acute rise in intraocular pressure (angle-closure glaucoma).

The pharmacological characterization of muscarinic receptor subtypes has been slowed by the lack of selective antagonists. Currently, muscarinic receptors are defined by differences in equilibrium disassociation constants from binding studies or apparent disassociation constants from functional experiments. Table 4-1 provides pK_b values for some relatively selective antagonists (chemical structures are shown in Figure 4-1). The data are given as ranges to reflect the variability among different laboratories.

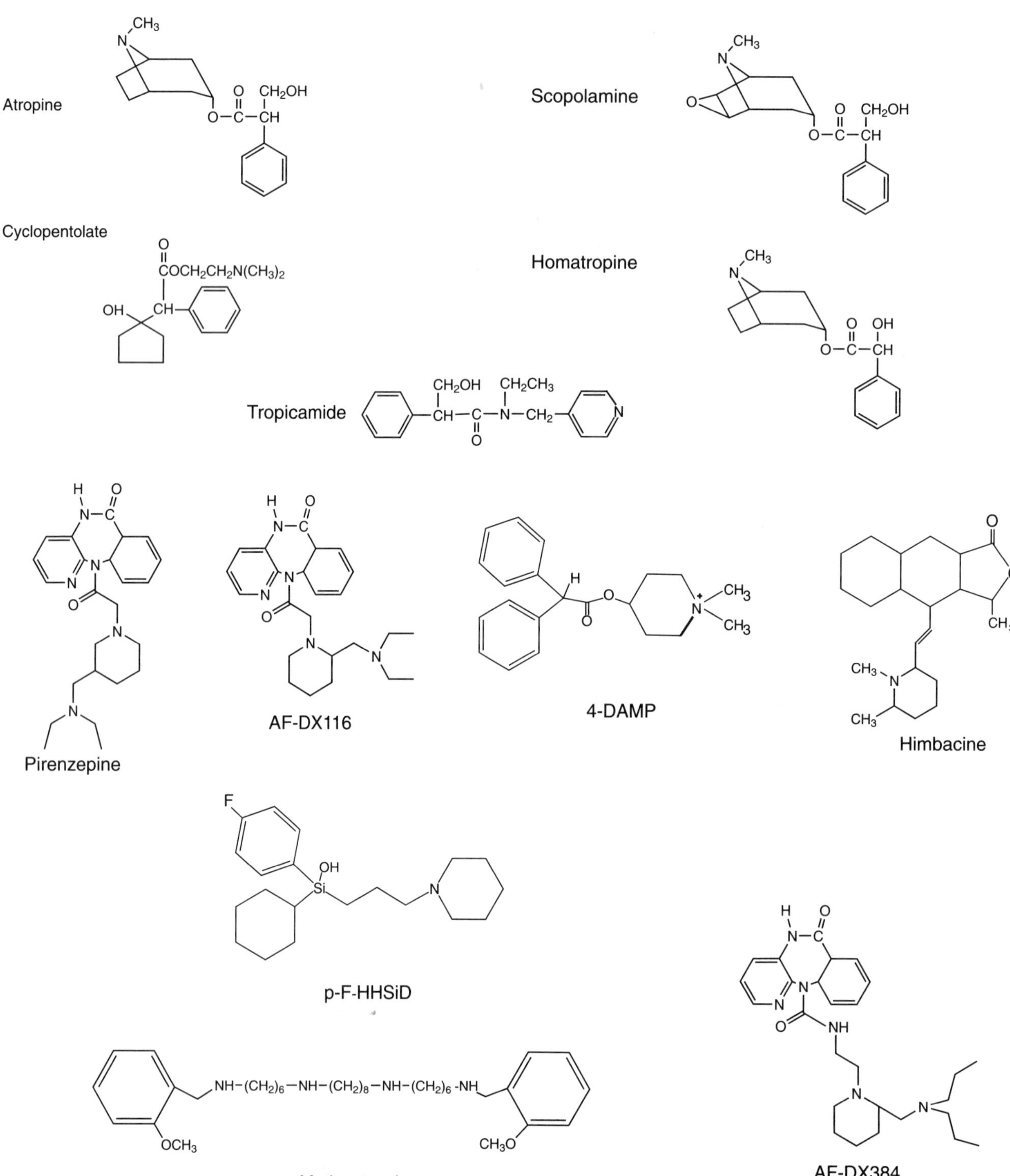

FIG. 4-1. Chemical structures of muscarinic antagonists.

Originally, M_1 receptors were defined as receptors with a high affinity for pirenzepine and a lower affinity for AF-DX-116 (19); however, pirenzepine also has significant affinity for M_4 receptors. Therefore, pirenzepine can distinguish between M_1 and M_2 or M_3 receptors. Additional antagonists, such as himbacine, must be used to discriminate between M_1 and M_4 receptors.

The M_2 receptors are characterized by a high affinity for antagonist methoetramine, 4-DAMP, and himbacine and a relatively low affinity for pirenzepine and pFHHSiD. The

TABLE 4-1. *Affinities of selected muscarinic antagonists*

Antagonist	Receptor subtype affinity (pK_b)				
	M_1	M_2	M_3	M_4	m_5[a]
Pirenzepine	7.9–8.5	6.3–6.8	6.7–7.1	7.1–8.1	6.2–7.1
AF-DX 116	6.4–6.9	7.1–7.2	5.9–6.6	6.6–7.0	6.6
Methoetramine	6.5–7.6	7.8–8.3	6.0–6.9	7.4–8.1	6.9–7.2
4-DAMP	8.6–9.2	8.0–8.5	8.9–9.3	8.9–9.4	9
Himbacine	7.0–7.2	8.0–8.3	6.9–7.6	8.0–8.8	6.3
pFHHSiD	7.2–7.7	6.0–6.9	7.8–7.9	7.5	7
AF-DX 384	7.3–7.5	8.2–9.0	7.2–7.8	8.0–8.7	6.3

Information modified from data originally presented by Caulfield, ref 16, and Eglen et al., ref 41.
[a]To date, no functional responses have been identified for the cloned m_5 receptor gene.

M_3 receptors have the characteristics of a high affinity for 4-DAMP and a lower affinity for pirenzepine. M_4 receptors exhibit a relatively high affinity for both pirenzepine and himbacine compared with other subtypes. The cloned m_5 receptor has a lower affinity for the antagonist AF-DX-384 when compared with other receptors.

In the eye, ciliary muscles and the iris sphincter muscle represent the primary target organs of the parasympathetic short ciliary nerves. Initial studies investigating the effects of the cholinergic agonist aceclidine suggested that the cholinergic-induced reduction in intraocular pressure and the miotic effects could be separated pharmacologically from the accommodative effects of cholinergic agents (20); however, studies with relatively selective antagonists indicate that the primary receptors responsible for the ciliary and iris sphincter muscles are of the M_3 subtype, and the disassociation of accommodative action from miotic and facility effects is not due to pharmacological differences in the receptors (21–23). These M_3 receptors are linked to PLC activation and an elevation in intracellular Ca^{++} (23,24). Other studies have shown that prejunctional muscarinic receptors are located on sympathetic nerve fibers in the eye, and these receptors are of the M_2 subtype (25,26).

Muscarinic Agonists

Directly acting muscarinic agonists are agents that activate muscarinic receptors via interaction with the receptor. These agonists can be divided into two general classes: choline esters and naturally occurring alkaloids. These agents act primarily at effector organs innervated by postganglionic parasympathetic fibers. Therefore, these agents often are referred to as *parasympathomimetic agents.* Structures of several nonselective muscarinic agonists are presented in Figure 4-2. Although acetylcholine is used clinically for the reversal of mydriasis following cataract surgery, its ability as a drug is limited by the rapid rate of hydrolysis by acetylcholinesterase and butyrylcholinesterase. Methacholine, carbachol, and bethanechol differ from acetylcholine primarily in their resistance to cholinesterase activity. Methacholine is hydrolyzed slowly by acetylcholinesterase and not at all by butyrylcholinesterase, whereas carbachol and bethanechol are resistant to cholinesterase activity.

Although methacholine and bethanechol are not used for ophthalmic indications, carbachol is used as a mitotic agent following cataract surgery and for the treatment of glaucoma. This agent, like other parasympathomimetics, stimulates the contraction of the iris sphincter muscle, resulting in a decrease in pupil diameter. The ability of cholinergic agonists to reduce intraocular pressure results from the contraction of muscles in the ciliary body. This contraction increases tension on the scleral spur, resulting in a change in the trabecular meshwork structure. This change in trabecular structure results in an increase in outflow facility (i.e., decreased resistance to aqueous humor outflow) and an ultimate reduction in intraocular pressure (27).

The second group of parasympathomimetics are the natural alkaloids. This group includes pilocarpine, muscarine, and arecoline. These agents have a pharmacological profile similar to the choline esters. Pilocarpine and arecoline also have some weak activity at nicotinic receptors. Pilocarpine is the primary directly acting cholinergic agent used in ophthalmology. The topical administration of pilocarpine is effective in reducing intraocular pressure. This agent, like carbachol, reduces intraocular pressure by contraction of the ciliary muscle and subsequent increases in outflow facility. The ocular hypotensive activity induced by pilocarpine is additive to other ocular hypotensive agents, such as β-adrenergic antagonists and carbonic anhydrase inhibitors.

Pilocarpine has also been used for the diagnosis of ocular parasympathetic neuropathies (i.e., Adie's syndrome). Dilute solutions (0.125%) produce pupillary constriction in patients with Adie's syndrome, whereas no constriction is normally observed in persons with intact innervation. This increased sensitivity to muscarinic agents results from denervation-induced upregulation of muscarinic receptors in the iris sphincter muscle.

Pilocarpine is also used for the treatment of angle-closure glaucoma. In patients with narrow angles, the iris can block the trabecular meshwork, producing a sudden rise in intraocular pressure. Muscarinic agents, primarily pilocarpine, can be used to lower intraocular pressure by

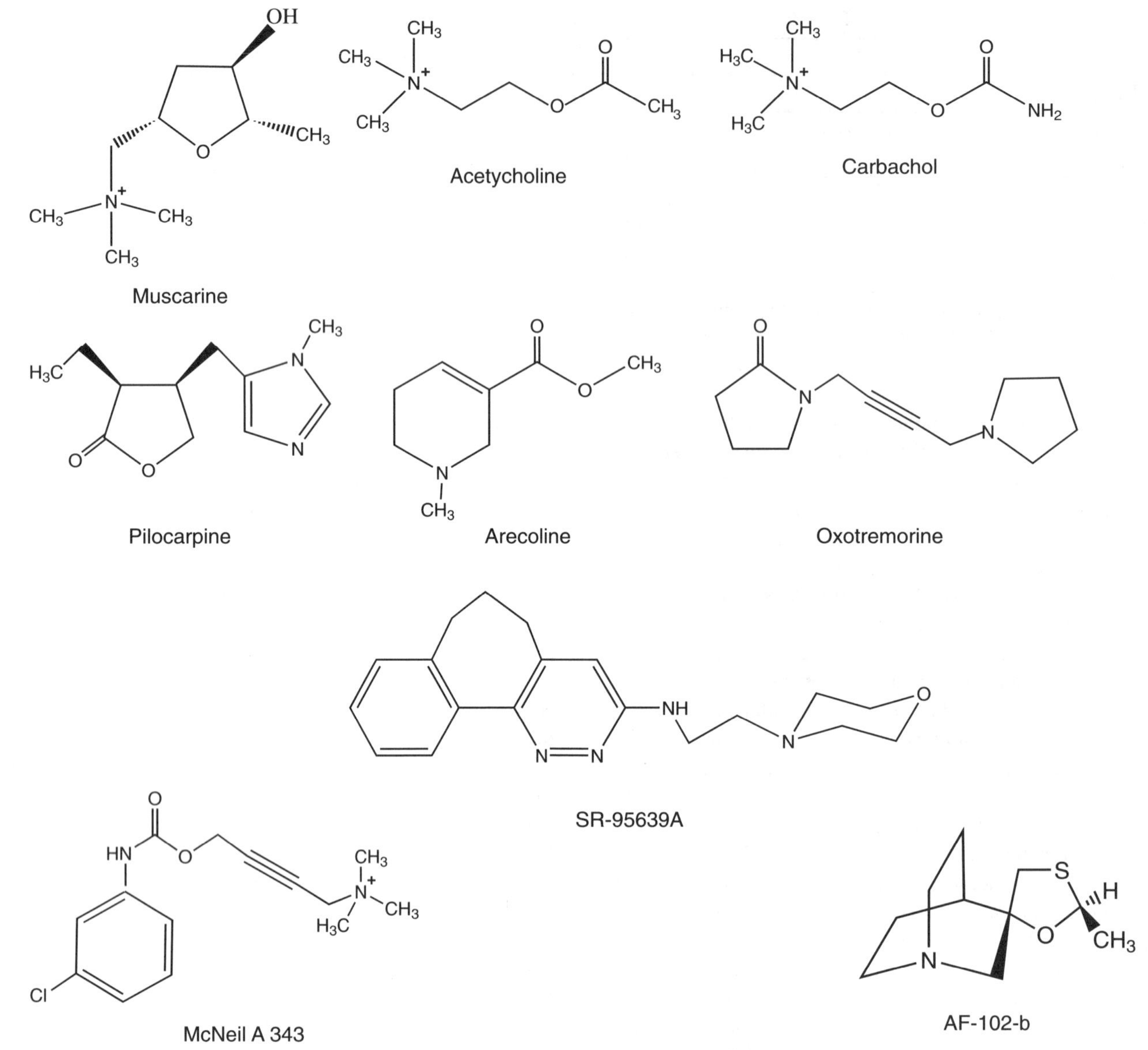

FIG. 4-2. Chemical structures of muscarinic agonists.

constricting the iris, moving it away from the trabecular meshwork, and allowing aqueous to flow out of the eye.

Local side effects of muscarinic agonists can include drug-induced myopia as a result of ciliary muscle contraction, miosis, and an accompanying decrease in vision under conditions of low illumination, brow ache, lacrimation, and hyperemia of the conjunctiva. Systemic side effects include bronchoconstriction, salivation, abdominal cramps, and diarrhea.

Attempts to identify selective muscarinic receptor agonists have not led to any general consensus, but studies have provided evidence that the spiro-oxothiolane quinuclidine derivative AF-102 is relatively selective for M_1 and M_3 receptors over M_2 receptors (28,29), whereas other studies have shown that SR-95639 is a relatively selective M_1 agonist (30). Studies of oxotremorine and oxotremorine-M indicate that these agents may have some selectivity for M_2 receptors (31,32).

Cholinesterase Inhibitors

These agents are considered indirectly acting muscarinic agonists, as they stimulate acetylcholine receptors by blocking the metabolism of acetylcholine by acetylcholinesterase at cholinergic nerve endings. As a result, junctional levels of acetylcholine rise to levels sufficient to stimulate postjunctional and postsynaptic receptors. Anticholinesterases are divided into two classes: reversible and irreversible cholinesterase inhibitors. Structures of anticholinesterases are shown in Fig. 4-3. The pharmacological response to both reversible and irreversible inhibitors is

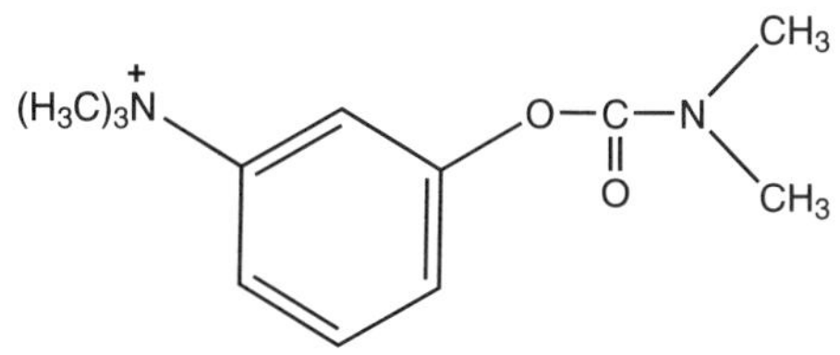

Neostigmine

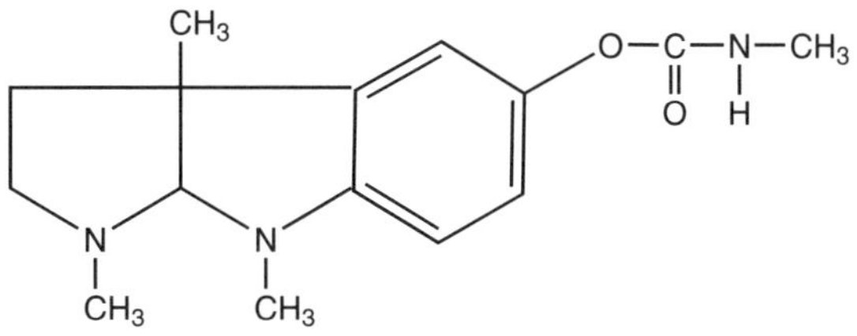

Physostigmine

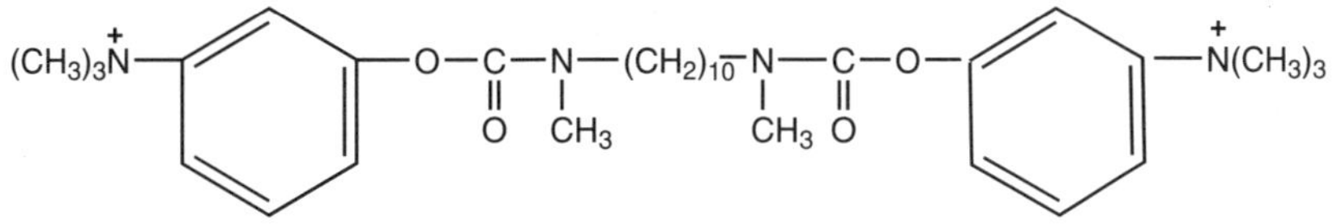

Demecarium

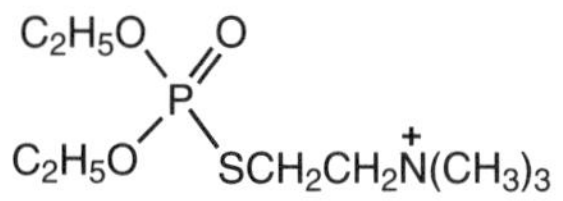

Echothiophate

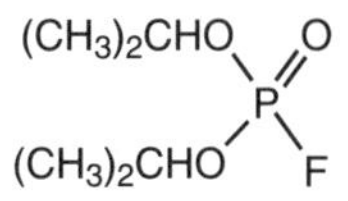

Isoflurophate

FIG. 4-3. Chemical structures of acetylcholinesterase inhibitors.

similar, with the primary difference being the duration of action. Reversible anticholinesterases typically have a duration of action of 12 to 36 hours, whereas irreversible inhibitors can have durations of action that range from days to weeks. Both classes of inhibitors block acetylcholinesterase activity by covalent modification of the active site of the enzyme. The difference in the durations of action represents the rate of deacylation to reform the active acetylcholinesterase.

Physostigmine, neostigmine, and demecarium are examples of reversible inhibitors. These compounds form carbamoyl ester intermediates with acetylcholinesterase, producing carbamoylated enzymes that cannot hydrolyze acetylcholine. In general, demecarium is more potent than other reversible inhibitors, as this agent consists of two neostigmine molecules bridged by ten methylene groups. Physostigmine is not used for any ophthalmic indication because of the hypersensitivity associated with its chronic use. Demecarium is used occasionally in the treatment of open- and closed-angle glaucoma and accommodative esotropia.

Irreversible cholinesterase inhibitors are organophosphate compounds. These agents form highly stable phosphorylated conjugates of acetylcholinesterase. As a result, the return of cholinesterase activity usually requires the synthesis of new enzyme. Like directly acting muscarinic agonists, these agents are used to increase outflow facility in glaucomatous eyes by contraction of the ciliary muscle. Normally, these agents are administered only for ophthalmic indications when directly acting muscarinic agonists are inadequate to control intraocular pressure. These agents can also be used in the treatment of accommodative esotropia as well as adjuvant treatment to eradicate lice in eyelashes.

The acute ocular side effects associated with anticholinesterases include lacrimation, dilation of conjunctival vessels, ciliary muscle spasm, brow ache, and induced myopia with blurred vision. Chronic use of anticholinesterases can produce iris cysts and lens opacities. Ocular administration of anticholinesterases also can stimulate nicotinic receptors in the skeletal muscles of the lids to produce lid twitching. Systemic side effects can include nausea, sweating, salivation, cardiac arrhythmias, abdominal cramps, diarrhea, and general fatigue.

Nicotinic Receptors

Nicotinic receptors are receptor-gated ion channels (i.e., ionotropic receptors) belonging to a superfamily of receptors that also includes gamma-aminobutyric acid-A ($GABA_A$) and *N*-methyl-D-aspartate (NMDA) receptors. Nicotinic receptors from muscle and neural origins are structurally similar and comprise five individual subunits. Each polypeptide subunit contains four transmembrane domains (M_1–M_4), a large hydrophilic region at the amino terminal end that faces the synaptic clef, and a second large hydrophilic intracellular loop between the M_3 and M_4 domains. Five general types of subunits have been identified: α, β, γ, δ, and ε(33). Muscle-type nicotinic receptors are composed of four subunit types, α_1, β_1, δ, and γ (or ε) in the ratio of 2:1:1:1. In the CNS, molecular biology studies have identified several distinct gene products for α and β subunits. Seven α-subunits, designated α_2–α_8, and three β-subunits, designated β_2–β_4, have been cloned from rat brain (34). Although the specific subunit compositions of neuronal nicotinic receptors have yet to be determined, several different subunit combinations express nicotinic activity (35).

Nicotinic agonists open ion channels by interacting with specific sites on the pentameric muscle and neuronal receptor. The cholinergic binding site appears to be associated with the α-subunit, and the M_2 transmembrane domains of each subunit line the ion channel (33). The binding of acetylcholine or other nicotinic agonists leads to the opening of cation-selective ion channels. Although nicotinic channels are cation selective, they do not distinguish between specific cations, such as Ca^{++} or Na^+. Open times vary from 0.06 to 50 msec, and channel conductance ranges from 0.4 to 50 pS (34). These measured differences in nicotinic receptors led to the idea that functional heterogeneity exists not only between muscle and neuronal receptors but also that subtypes exist within the neuronal division. These subtypes of neuronal nicotinic receptors may reflect different combinations of subunits or posttransitional modifications.

Continuous exposure of nicotinic receptors to acetylcholine produces desensitization of the receptor to additional channel openings (36). This process of desensitization appears to result from the ability of nicotinic receptors to exist in three distinct states: resting closed channel, acetylcholine-activated open channel, and a desensitized closed channel that can also bind acetylcholine. Interestingly, the desensitized receptor has a much higher affinity for acetylcholine (Kd 1 μM) than the resting state (Kd 50 μM) of the receptor (37). Studies have shown that up to 20% of nicotinic receptors may exist in this high-affinity, desensitized state in the absence of any agonist.

Nicotinic receptors may also be modulated by second messengers. Nicotinic receptors can be phosphorylated by at least four different protein kinases: cAMP-dependent protein kinase, protein kinase C, tyrosine kinase, and calcium-calmodulin protein kinase (38). Other studies suggested that phosphorylation by protein kinase C can accelerate the rate of desensitization; however, it is unlikely that phosphorylation of the receptor is responsible for the processes of desensitization.

Nicotinic Antagonists

Although nicotinic antagonists are not used specifically for ophthalmic indications, these agents can be useful as adjuvants in anesthesia for the muscle-relaxing properties. Structural formulas for selected nicotinic antagonists are shown in Fig. 4-4. Nicotinic receptor antagonists can be divided into two general classes: competitive or nondepolarizing antagonists and depolarizing antagonists. Nondepolarizing antagonists, such as *d*-tubocurarine and hexamethonium, act by competitive blockade of the nicotinic acetylcholine receptors. Although *d*-tubocurarine can act as a competitive antagonist at muscle-type nicotinic receptors, it also has some activity at postganglionic neurons in autonomic ganglia. Depolarizing antagonists, such as succinylcholine and decamethonium, produce an initial depolarization excitation. Following the excitation period, these agents produce a block of neuromuscular transmission and muscle paralysis.

Pharmacological heterogeneity of nicotinic receptors was first suggested by studies comparing the effect of decamethonium and hexamethonium. Decamethonium was more selective toward muscle nicotinic receptors, and hexamethonium was more selective for autonomic ganglia nicotinic receptors. Although complicated by pharmacokinetic concerns, this led to the designation of C10 (muscle) and C6 (neuronal) nicotinic receptors. More recent studies provided evidence that mecamylamine is a potent functional antagonist of ganglionic-type nicotinic receptors (39). Work with toxins, such as α-bungarotoxin and neuronal-

$$(CH_3)_3\overset{+}{N}-(CH_2)_6-\overset{+}{N}(CH_3)_3$$

Hexamethonium

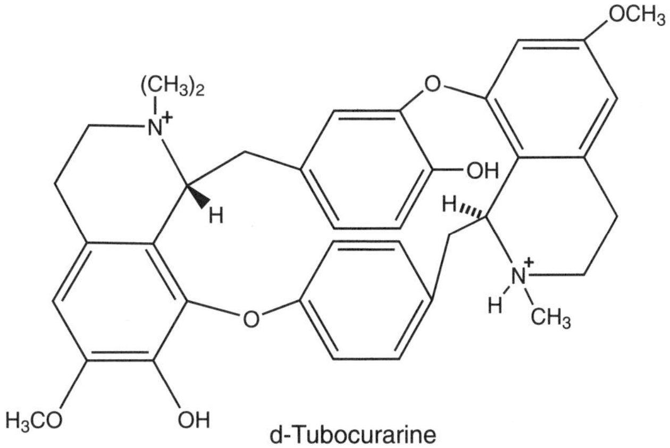

d-Tubocurarine

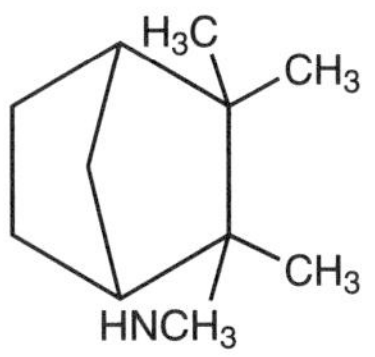

Mecamylamine

$$(CH_3)_3\overset{+}{N}CH_2CH_2O\overset{O}{\overset{\|}{C}}CH_2CH_2\overset{O}{\overset{\|}{C}}OCH_2CH_2\overset{+}{N}(CH_3)_3$$

Succinylcholine

$$(CH_3)_3\overset{+}{N}-(CH_2)_{10}-\overset{+}{N}(CH_3)_3$$

Decamethonium

FIG. 4-4. Chemical structures of nicotinic antagonists.

bungaratoxin, has also provided evidence for heterogeneity of nicotinic receptors. Most muscle-type nicotinic receptors are sensitive to α-bungaratoxin, whereas neuronal-bungaratoxin primarily affects ganglionic-type receptors. In general, nicotinic receptors in the CNS have pharmacological profiles for antagonists similar to ganglionic-type receptors; however, other studies indicated that musclelike nicotinic receptors are also present in the CNS.

A number of studies suggest that a variety of chemically diverse molecules can act as noncompetitive inhibitors by interacting with an allosteric site on nicotinic receptors. These interactions appear to block nicotinic receptor activation without altering the binding of acetylcholine (38). These compounds include histrionicotoxin, procaine, barbiturates, volatile anesthetics, chlorpromazine, and MK-801. Other studies have shown that dihydropyridines, such as nimodipine, can block Na^+ entry associated with nicotinic receptor activation.

Toxicity associated with nicotinic receptor antagonists may include prolonged apnea or respiratory paralysis and cardiovascular failure. Competitive antagonists, such as *d*-tubocurarine, can also induce histamine release in a typical wheal reaction. Toxicity of these compounds can be aggravated by coadministration with general anesthetics, antibiotics, and calcium-channel antagonists. Treatment of competitive nicotinic antagonist overdose can be accomplished by means of anticholinesterases; however, anticholinesterases are synergistic with depolarizing blockers, such as succinylcholine, as cholinesterase activity is responsible for the degradation of these agents.

Nicotinic Agonists

As stated above, nicotine and acetylcholine are potent agonists at nicotinic receptors. In the CNS, studies have shown that cystisine and azetidine analogs of nicotine and (-)-lobeline can be used to stimulate nicotinic receptors (39). The binding affinity of these agonists appears to be determined by the combination of the α- and β-subunits associated with individual nicotinic receptors. In addition to the acetylcholine binding site, other ligands, such as the cholinesterase inhibitor (physostigmine), appear to activate nicotinic receptors by binding to an alternative site (40). Ligands that bind to this alternative site are not subject to desensitization and are termed *channel activators.*

REFERENCES

1. Warwick R. The ocular parasympathetic nerve supply and its mesencephalic sources. *J Anat* 1954;88:195–203.
2. Yamamura HI, Snyder SH. High-affinity transport of choline into symaptosomes of rat brain. *J Neurochem* 1973;21:1355.
3. Masland RH, Mills JW. Choline accumulation by photoreceptor cells of the rabbit retina. *Proc Natl Acad Sci USA* 1980;77:1671–1675.
4. Marshall IG, Parsons SM. The vesicular acetylcholine transport system. *Trends Neurosci* 1987;10:174–177.
5. Cooper JR. Unsolved problems in the cholinergic nervous system. *J Neurochem* 1994;63:395–399.
6. Potter LT. Synthesis, storage, and release of acetylcholine from nerve terminals. In: Bourne GH, eds. *The Structure and Function of Nervous Tissue.* New York: Academic Press, 1972;105–128.
7. Bonner TI, Buckley NJ, Young AC, Brann MR. Identification of a family of muscarinic acetylcholine receptor genes. *Science* 1987; 237:527–532.
8. Hulme EC, Birdsall NJM, Buckley NJ. Muscarinic receptor subtypes. *Annu Rev Pharmacol Toxicol* 1990;30:633–673.
9. Kubo T, Fukuda K, Mikami A, Maeda A, Takahashi H, Mishina M, Haga T, Haga K, Ichiyama A, Kangawa K, Kojima M, Matsuo H, Hirose T, Numa S. Cloning, sequencing and expression of complementary DNA encoding in the muscarinic acetylcholine receptor. *Nature* 1986;323:411–416.
10. Kubo T, Maeda A, Sugimoto K, Akiba I, Mikami A, Takahashi H, Haga T, Haga K, Ichiyama A, Kangawa K, Matsuo H, Hirose T, Numa S. Primary structure of porcine cardiac muscarinic acetylcholine receptor deduced from the cDNA sequences. *FEBS Lett* 1986;209: 367–372.
11. Peralta EG, Ashkenazi A, Winslow JW, Smith D, Ramachandran J, Capon DJ. Distinct primary structures, ligant-binding properties and tissue-specific expression of four human muscarinic acetylcholine receptors. *EMBO J* 1987;6:3923–3929.
12. Peralta EG, Winslow JW, Peterson G, Smith DH, Ashkenazi A, Ramchandran J, Schimerlik M, Capon DJ. Primary structure and biochemical properties of an M2 muscarinic receptor. *Science* 1987;236: 600–605.
13. Jones SVP, Levey AI, Weinter DM, Ellis J, Novotny E, Yu S-H, Dörje F, Wess J, Brann MR. Muscarinic acetylcholine receptors. In: Brann M, ed. *Molecular Biology of G-protein Coupled Receptors.* Boston: Birkhauser, 1992;170–197.
14. Katz A, Wu D, Simon MI. Subunits β-γof heterotrimeric G protein activate β2 isoform of phospholipase C. *Nature* 1992;360:687–688.
15. Stein R, Pinkas-Kramarski R, Sokolovsky M. Cloned M1 muscarinic receptors mediate both adenylate cyclase inhibition and phosphoinositide turnover. *EMBO J* 1988;7:3031–3035.
16. Caulfield MP. Muscarinic receptors—characterization, coupling and function. *Pharmacol Ther* 1993;58:319–379.
17. Zhang X, Hernandez MR, Yang H, Erickson K. Expression of muscarinic receptor subtype mRNA in the human ciliary muscle. *Invest Ophthalmol Vis Sci* 1995;36:1645–1657.
18. Hankanen RE, Howard EF, Abdel-Latif AA. M3-muscarinic receptor subtype predominates in the bovine iris sphincter smooth muscle and ciliary process. *Invest Ophthalmol Vis Sci* 1990;31:590–593.
19. Mitchelson F. Muscarinic receptor differentiation. *Pharmacol Ther* 1988;37:357–423.
20. Erickson-Lamy KA, Schroeder A. Dissociation between the effect of aceclidine on outflow facility and accommodation. *Exp Eye Res* 1990;50:143–147.
21. Gabelt BT, Kaufman PL. Inhibition of aceclidine-stimulated outflow facility, accommodation and miosis in rhesus monkeys by muscarinic receptor subtype antagonists. *Exp Eye Res* 1994;58:623–630.
22. Poyer JF, Gabelt BT, Kaufman PL. The effect of muscarinic agonists and selective receptor subtype antagonists on the contractile response of the isolated rhesus monkey ciliary muscle. *Exp Eye Res* 1994;59: 729–736.
23. Woldemussie E, Feldmann BJ, Chen J. Characterization of muscarinic receptors in cultured human iris sphincter and ciliary smooth muscle cells. *Exp Eye Res* 1993;56:385–392.
24. Matsumoto S, Yorio T, DeSantis L, Pang I-H. Muscarinic effects on cellular function in cultured human ciliary muscle cells. *Invest Ophthalmol Vis Sci* 1994;35:3732–3738.
25. Bognar IT, Baumann B, Damman F, Knoll B, Meincke M, Pallas S, Fuder H. M2 muscarinic receptors on the iris sphincter muscle differ from those on iris noradrenergic nerves. *Eur J Pharmacol* 1989;163: 263–274.
26. Jumblatt JE, Hackmiller RC. M2-type muscarinic receptors mediate prejunctional inhibition of nonepinephrine release in the human iris-ciliary body. *Exp Eye Res* 1994;58:175–180.
27. Kaufman PL, Wiedman T, Robinson JR. Cholinergics. In: Sears ML, ed. *Pharmacology of the Eye. Handbook of Experimental Pharmacology,* vol 69. Berlin: Springer-Verlag, 1984;149–191.
28. Fisher A, Brandeis R, Pittel Z, et al. (±)-cis-2-Methylspiro(1,3-oxathiolane-5,3′) quinuclidine (AF102B): a new M_1 agonist attenuates cognitive dysfunctions in AF64A-treated rats. *Neurosci Lett* 1989;102:325–331.
29. Mochida S, Mizobe F, Fisher A, Kawanishi G, Kobayashi H. Selective M_1 muscarinic agonists McN-A-343 and AF102B cause dual effects on superior cervical ganglia of rabbits. *Brain Res* 1988;455:9– 17.
30. Schumacher C, Steinberg R, Kan JP. Pharmacological characterization of the aminopyridazine SR-95639A, a selective M_1 muscarinic agonist. *Eur J Pharmacol* 1989;166:139–147.
31. Potter LT, Flynn DD, Hanchett FE, Kalinoski DL, Luber-Narod J, Mash D. Independent M1 and M2 receptors: ligands, autoradiography and functions. *Trends Pharmacol Sci* 1984;5:22–31.
32. Spencer DG Jr, Horvath E, Traber J. Direct autoradiographic determination of M1 and M2 muscarinic acetylcholine receptor distribution in the rat brain: relation to cholinergic nuclei and projections. *Brain Res* 1986;380:59–68.
33. Changeux J-P, Galzi J-L, Devillers-Thiery A, Bertrand D. The functional architecture of the acetylcholine nicotinic receptor explored by affinity labeling and site-directed mutagenesis. *Q Rev Biophys* 1992;25:395–432.
34. Papke RL. The kinetic properties of neuronal nicotinic receptors: Genetic basis of functional diversity. *Prog Neurobiol* 1993;41:509–531.
35. Luetje CW, Patrick J. Both alpha- and beta-subunits contribute to the agonist sensitivity of neuronal nicotinic acetylcholine receptors. *J Neurosci* 1991;11:837–845.
36. Changeux J-P, Devillers-Thiery A, Chemouilli P. Acetylcholine receptor: an allosteric protein. *Science* 1984;225:1335–1345.
37. Heidmann T, Bernhardt J, Neumann E, Changeux J-P. Rapid kinetics of agonist binding and permeability response analysed in parallel on acetylcholine receptor rich membranes from Torpedo marmorata. *Biochemistry* 1991;22:5452–5459.
38. Lena C, Changeux J-P. Allosteric modulations of the nicotinic acetylcholine receptor. *Trends in Neuroscience* 1993;16:181–186.
39. Lukas RJ, Bencherif M. Heterogeneity and regulation of nicotinic acetylcholine receptors. *Int Rev Neurobiol* 1992;34:25–130.
40. Pereira EFR, Reinhardt-Maelicke S, Schrattenholz A, Maelicke A, Albuquerque EX. Identification and functional characterization of a new agonist site on nicotinic acetylcholine receptors of cultured hippocampal neurons. *J Pharmacol Exp Ther* 1993;265:1474–1491.
41. Eglen RM, Reddy H, Watson N, Challis RA. Muscarinic acetylcholine receptor subtypes in smooth muscle. *TIPS* 1994;15:114–119.

Textbook of Ocular Pharmacology,
edited by T.J. Zimmerman, et al.
Lippincott–Raven Publishers, Philadelphia © 1997.

CHAPTER 5

Eicosanoid Receptors in Ocular Tissues

Parimal Bhattacherjee

Eicosanoids are a family of lipids derived from arachidonic acid abundantly present in the cell membrane phospholipids. Eicosanoids are biosynthesized locally via cyclooxygenase and a number of lipooxygenases (Fig. 5-1) and act via specific receptors present in the cell membrane. The physiological, pathophysiological, and pharmacological actions of eicosanoids are diverse. They affect a large spectrum of tissues and fluids in the body; however, prostaglandins (PGs) have actions in almost every tissue examined, whereas the actions of leukotrienes (LTs) are, to a large extent, tissue specific. The ocular tissues are no exception in these respects; they respond in a particular fashion to endogenous and synthetic PGs and LTs. The known ocular responses to PGs, depending on the type and dose of PGs and the animal species, are vasodilation, increased permeability of the blood-aqueous barrier, corneal neovascularization, and modulation of the intraocular pressure (1–3); however, carefully selected doses of PGE_2, PGD_2, $PGF_{2\alpha}$ and prostacyclin reduce intraocular pressure (4,2,5). Of these, $PGF_{2\alpha}$ is the most effective in humans as an ocular hypotensive, and its analogue Latanoprost available for the treatment of glaucoma (6). The leukotriene group of compounds, which include leukotriene B_4 and cysteinyl-leukotrienes C_4, D_4, E_4 as well as other hydroxy products, are also highly biologically active. In experimental animals, these compounds are chemotactic for polymorphonuclear leukocytes and eosinophils (7–9), cause conjunctival and uveal edema, and probably modulate functions of immune processes either on their own or in conjunction with cytokines (10–13).

Eicosanoids, in common with other biologically active molecules, elicit cellular responses via stimulation of distinct receptors. Prostanoids were the first group of arachidonic acid metabolites to be actively investigated for their role in physiological and pathological conditions in the 1970s, a time when the knowledge of prostanoid receptors and their characteristics was lacking. In the early 1980s, Coleman's group (14,15) proposed a system of classification of PG and thromboxane (TX) receptors based on the responses of the smooth-muscle preparations to five prostanoids, PGD_2, PGE_2, $PGF_{2\alpha}$, PGI_2, and thromboxane A_2. The nomenclature for receptors proposed by Coleman was *P receptors,* with a preceding letter indicating the natural prostanoid to which each receptor is most sensitive. Thus, the receptors were termed DP, EP, FP, IP, and TP, respectively (16). Table 5-1 shows the selectivity of PG agonists for PG receptors in decreasing order.

The classification of prostanoid receptors has facilitated the understanding of their biological actions; however, progress has not been as significant as that with LT receptors because of a lack of selective agonists and antagonists, with the exception of DP and TP receptors. The availability of highly selective antagonists of LT receptors helped to provide a better characterization of these receptors. Consequently, their roles underlying various physiological and pathological processes are well understood. The nomenclature for LT receptors has been proposed by a working group headed by Coleman (16). According to their proposal, LTB_4 receptors have provisionally been termed OH-LTRs and those for cysteinyl leukotrienes as Cys-LTRs, which exist as subtypes Cys-LTR-1 and Cys-LTR-2. Studies of the past two decades established a linkage of a number of biological actions of eicosanoids to specific PG or LT receptors, some of which are listed in Table 5-2.

AGONISTS AND ANTAGONISTS

In tissues where a receptor population of neurotransmitters, hormones, and autocoids is expressed in low densities, it is often difficult to identify the receptors and to characterize their kinetics in vitro and biological actions in vivo using the conventional ligand-binding and biochemi-

P. Bhattacherjee: Department of Ophthalmology and Visual Sciences, University of Louisville School of Medicine, Louisville, Kentucky 40292.

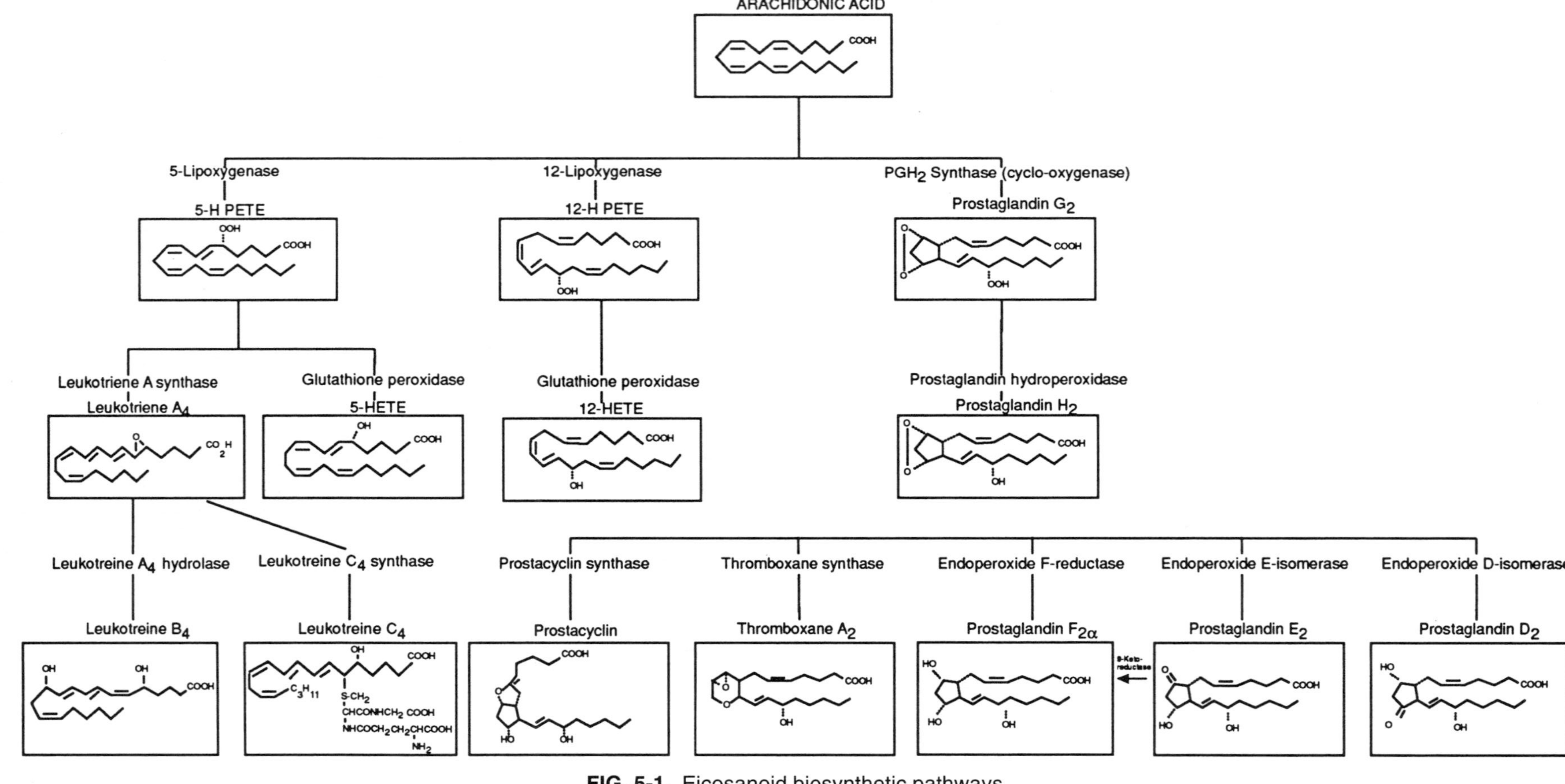

FIG. 5-1. Eicosanoid biosynthetic pathways.

TABLE 5-1. *PG receptor agonists and their relative potencies*

Receptors	Agonist potency in decreasing order	Selective agonists
DP	$PGD_2 > PGE_2, PGF_{2\alpha}, PGI_2, TXA_2$	BW245C
EP	$PGE_2 > PGI_2, PGF_{2\alpha}, PGD_2 >$ U-46619	PGE_2
FP	$PGF_{2\alpha} > PGD_2 > PGE_2$, U-46619 $> PGI_2$	Fluprostenol, cloprostenol
IP	$PGI_2 > PGD_2, PGE_2, PGF_{2\alpha}, TXA_2$	Cicaprost
TP	$TXA_2 > PGD_2 > PGF_{2\alpha}, PGI_2 > PGE_2$	U-46619, STA_2, I-BOP

PG, prostaglandin; TX, thromboxane.

cal approaches. This is especially true of prostanoid receptors in the ocular tissues of all the species studied so far and is probably true for other tissues. In such situations, highly selective agonists and antagonists are powerful tools in identifying and characterizing receptor properties. The structure–activity, rank–order potency, and functional studies have identified potent and selective LT receptor antagonists. The selectivity of PG receptor agonists and antagonists, however, is not as great as that of LT receptors; this is the principal problem in studying PG receptor kinetics and PG-receptor-mediated biological actions, particularly when highly selective antagonists for most PGs are not available. It is outside the scope of this section to discuss all the agonists and antagonists for eicosanoid receptors; only the most well-characterized ones will be discussed (for an extensive review, see refs. 17 and 18). Figure 5-2 shows the chemical structures of some of the eicosanoid agonists and antagonists.

EP RECEPTORS

To date, EP receptors are known to have at least four subtypes (19,20). At the molecular level, recombinant EP_3 receptors were recently shown to exist in four isoforms, differing in the carboxy-terminal domains in ocular and nonocular tissues. The agonist potency and antagonists of EP-receptor subtypes are shown in Table 5-3. There are no EP_1, EP_2, EP_3, and EP_4 highly selective agonists; the difference in the selectivity of the available agonists between the EP-receptor subtypes is not great. Prostaglandin E_2 and 16,16-dimethyl PGE_2 (DME) are mixed EP-receptor agonists with affinities for the EP_1, EP_2, and EP_3 receptor subtypes; 16,16-dimethyl PGE_2 is more selective for EP_1 and EP_3 than EP_2 subtypes, as classified by its action on vascular and nonvascular smooth-muscle preparations (21). In the ocular tissues of a number of species, including humans, and in SV-40-transformed ciliary nonpigmented or pigmented epithelial cells, 16,16-dimethyl PGE_2 consistently stimulated adenylyl cyclase (22–25). The EP_2 and EP_4 receptors are coupled to adenylyl cyclase. Therefore, it is most likely that in ocular tissues and cells, 16,16-dimethyl PGE_2 is a more selective agonist for EP_2 or EP_4 than either EP_1 and EP_3 receptors.

The expression and distribution of EP_1 receptors in the ocular tissues have not yet been studied in depth. ODMCl-2, a human nonpigmented ciliary epithelial cell line, has been reported to express EP_2 but not EP_1 receptors (25). All ocular tissues and cultured cells, including those from humans, express EP_2 receptors (22–26). In the eye, EP_3 receptors appear to be presynaptic (27) and are thought to be involved in the diurnal control of intraocular pressure;

TABLE 5-2. *PG receptor-mediated biological actions*

Receptors	Biological actions	Receptors	Biological actions
DP	Vasodilatation Myometrial relaxation Modification of hypothalamic/pituitary hormone release Reduction of intraocular pressure	**EP_4**	Relaxation of dog and pig saphenous vein
EP_1	Gastrointestinal contraction Contraction of vascular and nonvascular smooth muscles Miosis	**FP**	Lueolysis Myometrial contraction Bronchoconstriction Reduction of intraocular pressure
EP_2	Stimulation of intestinal fluid secretion Disruption of the blood–aqueous barrier Vasodilation Bronchodilation Gastrointestinal relaxation	**IP**	Vasodilatation Inhibition of platelet aggregation Reduction of intraocular pressure
EP_3	Gastrointestinal relaxation Inhibition of autonomic neurotransmitter release Reduction of intraocular pressure Secretion/cytoprotection	**TP**	Vasoconstriction Bronchoconstriction Platelet aggregation

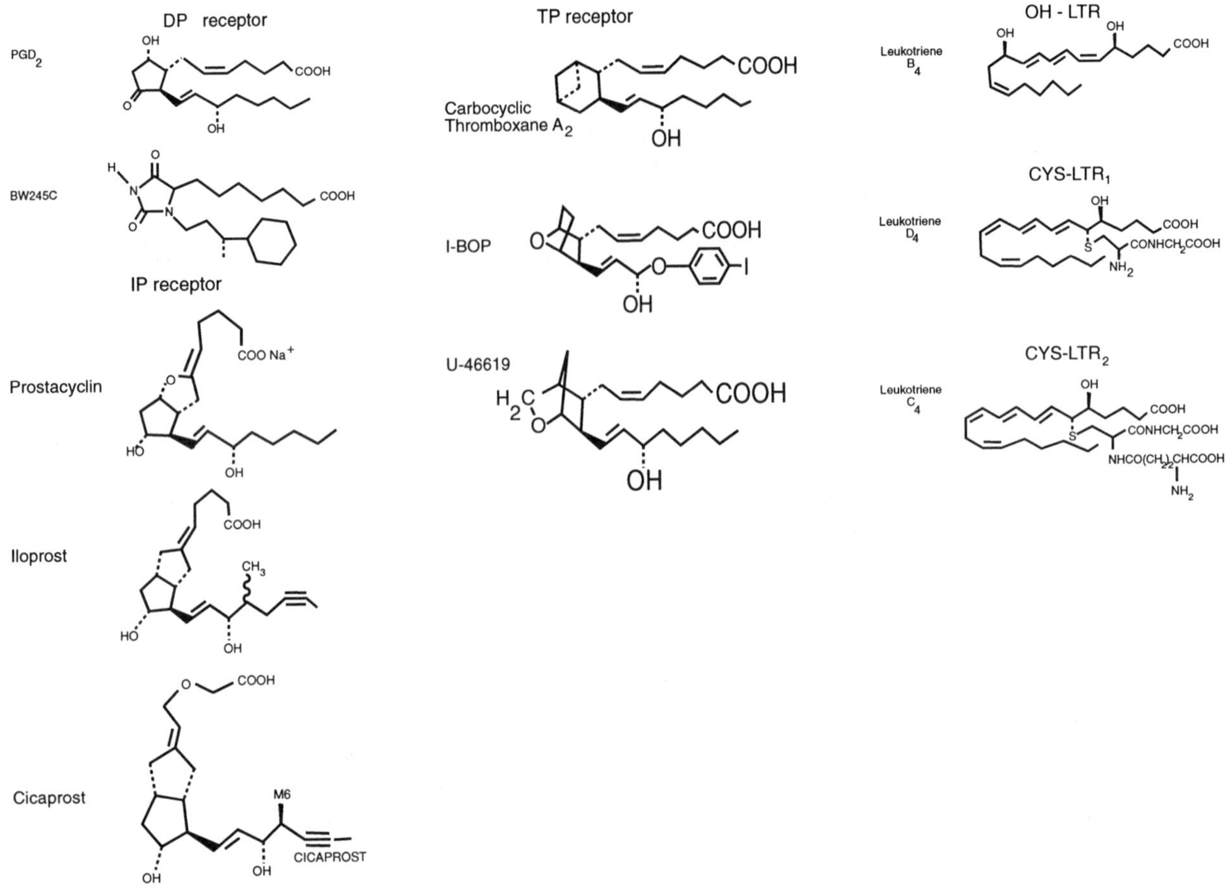

DP receptor

PGD_2

BW245C

IP receptor

Prostacyclin

COO Na^+

Iloprost

Cicaprost

CICAPROST

TP receptor

Carbocyclic Thromboxane A_2

I-BOP

U-46619

OH - LTR

Leukotriene B_4

CYS-LTR_1

Leukotriene D_4

CYS-LTR_2

Leukotriene C_4

A

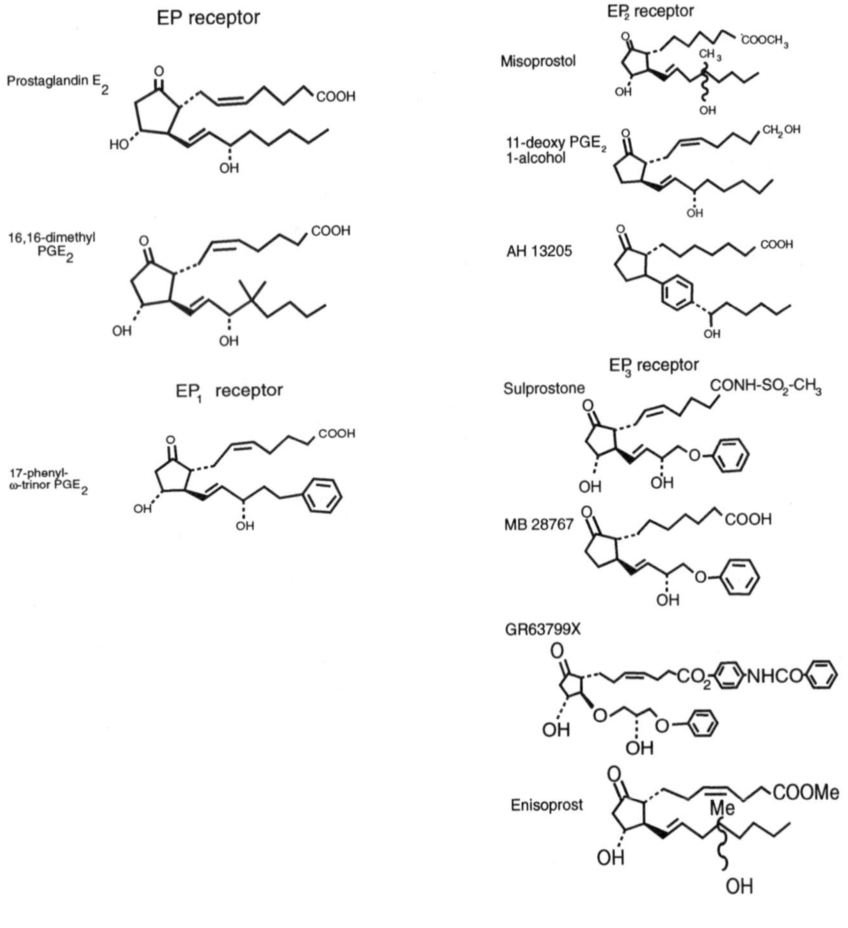

EP receptor

Prostaglandin E_2

16,16-dimethyl PGE_2

EP_1 receptor

17-phenyl-ω-trinor PGE_2

EP_2 receptor

Misoprostol

11-deoxy PGE_2 1-alcohol

AH 13205

EP_3 receptor

Sulprostone

MB 28767

GR63799X

Enisoprost

B

EP1 receptor antagonist

SC 19220

AH 6809

DP receptor antagonist

BW686C

TP receptor antagonist

SQ 29548

I-SAP

OH-LTR receptor antagonist

8-[(4-phenyl-2-quinolyl) oxy]octanoic acid

SC -41930

LY223982

CYS-LTR1 receptor antagonist

FPL 55712

ICI 198,615

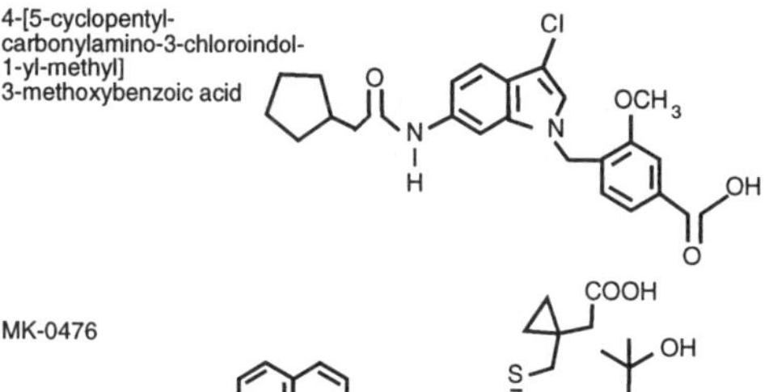

MK-0476

CYS-LTR2 receptor antagonist

BAY u9773

C

FIG. 5-2. A: Chemical structures of eicosanoid receptor agonists; **B:** Chemical structures of EP receptor agonists; **C:** Chemical structures of eicosanoid receptor antagonists.

TABLE 5-3. *EP receptor subtypes*

Receptor	Relative agonist potency	Antagonists
EP_1	DME > PGE_2 > Sulprostone > 11-Deoxy PGE_1	AH6809 SC19220
EP_2	Butaprost > PGE_2 > 11-Deoxy > PGE_1 DME >> Sulprostone	 None
EP_3	Sulprostone > DME > PGE_2 > 11-Deoxy PGE_1	None
EP_4	PGE_2 (presently no selective agonist is available; other PGs are extremely weak at this receptor)	AH23848B AH22921

postsynaptic EP_3 receptors in the ocular tissues are yet to be described.

FP RECEPTORS

Pharmacological studies in experimental animals and in humans have shown that $PGF_{2\alpha}$ reduces intraocular pressure, suggesting that FP receptors in the anterior uvea are mediating this effect (28–32). The reduction of the intraocular pressure by this agonist is thought to be the result of an increase of the uveoscleral outflow, indicating that FP receptors in the ciliary muscles are responsible for the outflow effect of $PGF_{2\alpha}$. The intact ciliary muscles of humans stimulated by FP receptor agonists formed inositol phosphates (25). Immunohistochemical studies with antibodies raised against FP receptor proteins demonstrated the expression of FP receptors in human ciliary muscles (33). Further studies at the molecular level are needed to localize FP receptors in the ocular tissues and to confirm that it is expressed in the ciliary muscle. Prostaglandin $F_{2\alpha}$ lowers intraocular pressure in the cat. Functional studies in the ciliary muscles of cats suggest that the ocular hypotensive effective of $PGF2_{2\alpha}$ probably is mediated by DP or other PG receptors but not by FP receptors (34,35).

DP, IP, AND TP RECEPTORS

These receptors have been demonstrated in a wide variety of tissues of animals and humans; DP receptors have been identified in the platelets, vascular smooth muscles, and brain and probably exist as a single receptor population. The DP receptor, however, was recently cloned; receptor protein from COS cells transfected with cDNA of DP receptors is coupled to adenylyl cyclase and the phosphoinositidase pathway (36). These observations suggest that DP receptors may have subtypes.

Both IP and TP receptors are expected to be present in the vascular endothelial cells and platelets because they are linked intimately to the pathophysiology of these two tissues (37). In fact, these receptors are expressed in these tissues and are of high affinity and density. The IP receptors are expressed in all vascular endothelia, including arterial smooth muscles. There is no evidence as yet for the existence of IP receptor subtypes. Platelets, vascular endothelium, spleen, and thymus express TP receptors. Whether TP receptors are of a single population or have subtypes remains controversial (38–41). In the absence of clear evidence for the existence of subtypes, for the time being, TP receptors can be considered a single class of receptors; however, in primary cultures of human ciliary muscle, cells express TP receptors.

In the ocular tissues, DP receptors are present in the intact iris-ciliary body and ciliary muscles of the anterior uvea of different animal species, as demonstrated by functional and transduction studies (23,42,43). The DP receptor agonist BW 245c and its antagonist BW 868c are highly selective and are extremely useful for studying DP receptors (44). Pharmacological studies showed that DP receptor stimulation causes a reduction of intraocular pressure in experimental animals.

As yet, IP and TP receptors have not been studied at the molecular level in ocular tissues; therefore, their distribution and localization in ocular tissues are not yet known. Pharmacological studies with the IP receptor agonist iloprost in rabbits suggest the presence of these receptors in the anterior uvea (45). As yet, TP receptors have not been studied in the anterior segment of the eye, with the exception of ciliary muscle cells, as mentioned. Pharmacological studies in the retinal tissues, however, suggest the presence of the TP receptors, as evidenced by the reduction of the retinal lesions in experimental autoimmune uveitis (46,47) by TP antagonist or PG synthase inhibitors.

LEUKOTRIENE RECEPTORS

Leukotriene receptors have been studied more extensively and are better characterized than the prostanoid receptors because of the availability of highly specific leukotriene receptor antagonists. In leukocytes, particularly in neutrophils, LTB_4 receptors are predominant, whereas cysteinyl-LT receptors are present in a variety of tissues, including vascular and nonvascular smooth muscles (18,48). The LTB_4 receptors have been reported to exist in high- and low-affinity forms in human neutrophils. Splictz et al. (49), however, using a photoaffinity labeling technique, demonstrated that these receptors consist of a single population.

In the ocular tissues, pharmacological studies with LTB_4 and cysteinyl LTs have shown that these agonists are chemotactic for polymorphonuclear leukocytes and eosinophils (7,8). These studies, however, do not suggest that the receptors mediating the above responses are in the ocular tissues, because the responses could have resulted from stimulation of the receptors present in the leukocytes. Cysteinyl leukotrienes cause conjunctival edema as well as eosinophil infiltration (11) in guinea pigs, suggesting the expression of LT receptors in the conjunctiva. To date, studies have not been performed to identify LT receptors in the ocular tissues by ligand-binding assays or by measuring second messengers.

In recent years, a number of highly selective antagonists of LTB_4 receptors (OH-LTR) and cysteinyl leukotriene receptors (CYS-LTR) have been synthesized. Figure 5-2C illustrates the structure of some of the antagonists of LT receptors. These antagonists have been evaluated mainly for their activity in the models of chemotaxis, chemokinesis, contractions of bronchial smooth muscles, and lung parenchyma and in animal models of human diseases. Clinically, it remains to be seen how useful these antagonists would be in diseases involving leukocytes and in allergy and asthma.

EICOSANOID RECEPTORS AND SIGNAL TRANSDUCTION

The biological responses to eicosanoids are the final event in a series of biochemical reactions initiated by receptor–ligand interaction. Receptors are coupled to adenylyl cyclase or phosphoinositidase C via guanine nucleotide binding protein (G proteins). Stimulation of PG and LT receptors leads to the activation of adenylyl cyclase or phosphoinositidase C and subsequent generation of second messengers, cyclic AMP, 1,2-diacylgycerol (DAG), and 1,4,5 inositol triphosphate (IP_3). The formation of one or more of these second messengers depends on the nature of specific receptors. Cyclic AMP activates protein kinase A (PKA), DAG activates protein kinase C (PKC), and IP_3 elevates intracellular Ca^{++}. The activated protein kinases and intracellular Ca^{++} phosphorylate various proteins; the phosphorylated proteins elicit specific cellular responses. The eicosanoid receptor signaling pathways are shown in a simplified manner in Figures 5-3 and 5-4. The receptor transduction pathways in general are highly complex because of multiple isoforms of stimulatory (G_s) and inhibitory (G_i) G proteins, adenylyl cyclase, and phosphoinositidase C. This field is under intense investigation. The specificity of the receptor-initiated cellular signaling pathway lies with the particular isoforms G proteins and enzymes. Studies at the level of second-messenger generation are useful for classifying receptors in intact tissues or

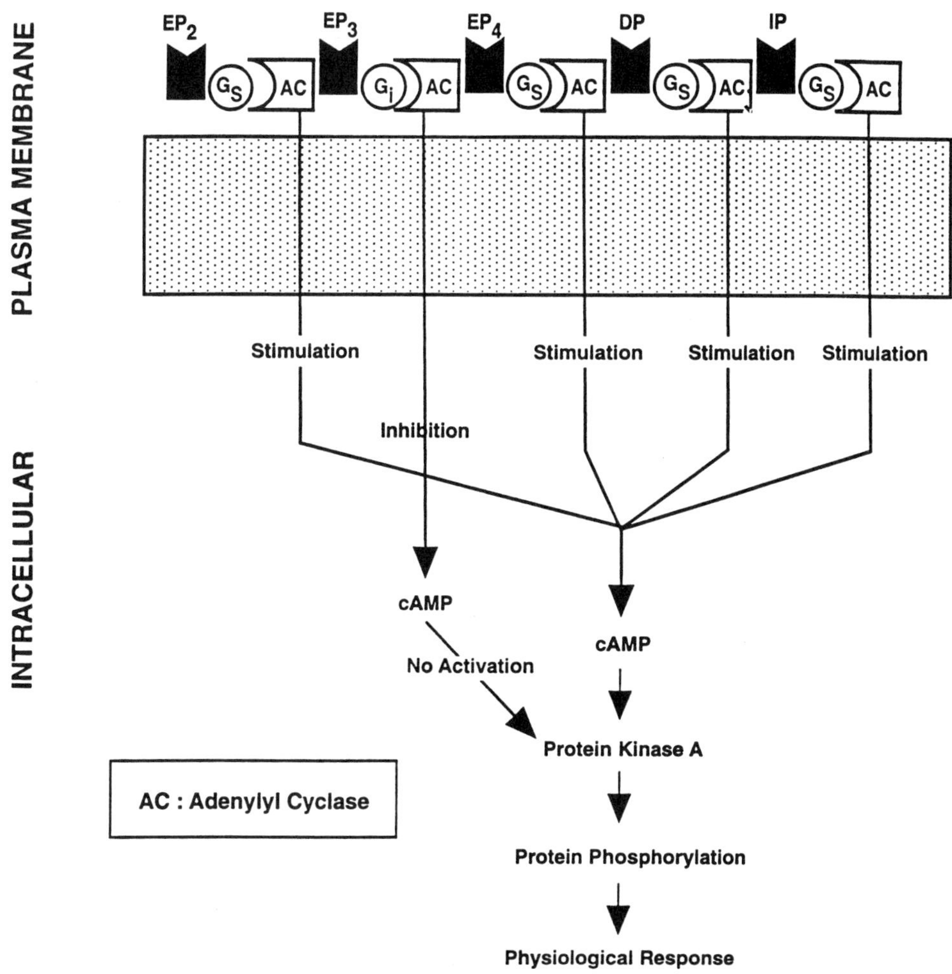

FIG. 5-3. Eicosanoid receptor signal transduction pathways.

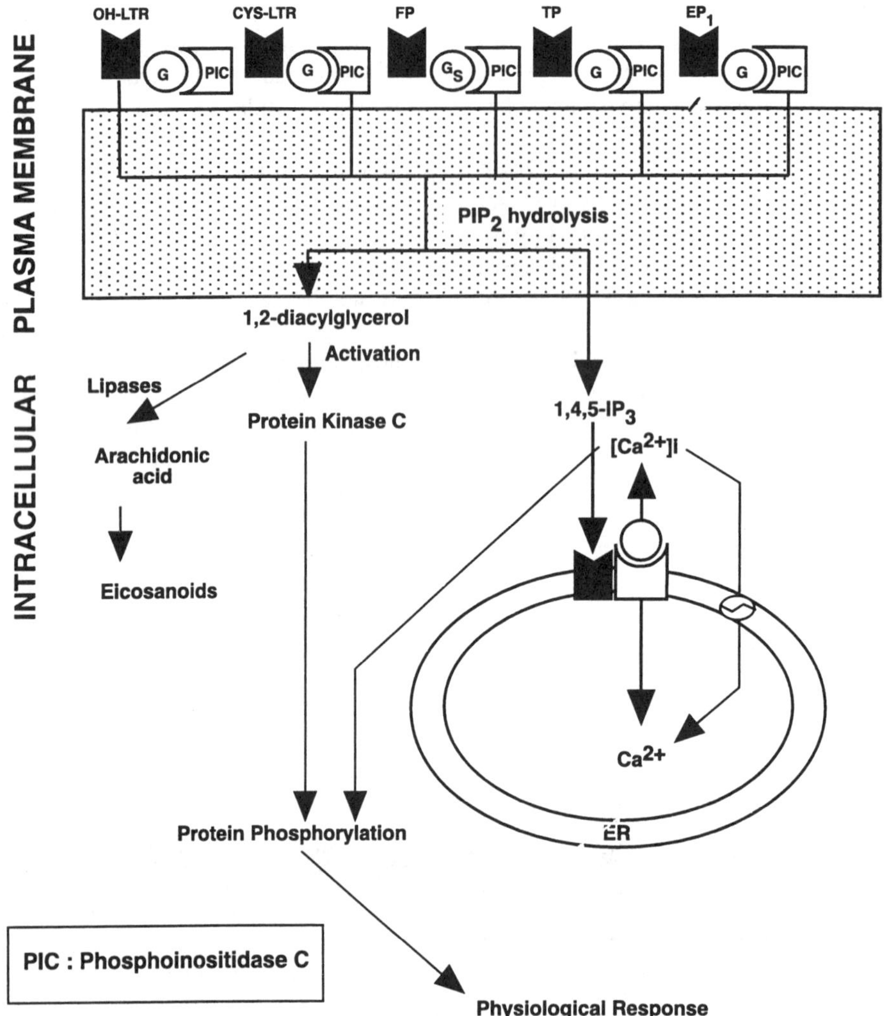

FIG. 5-4. Eicosanoid receptor signal transduction.

cultured cells and are complementary to ligand-binding and functional assays. Interested readers should consult the excellent review by Nishizuka on this subject (50,51).

In vivo, it is most likely that under some physiological and pathological conditions, neurotransmitters, hormones, and autacoids are released simultaneously. Although they act on their own receptors, it is possible that interactions at the level of protein kinases and second messengers occur. Such interactions may cause amplification or reduction of the responses to one of the endogenous mediators by upregulating or downregulating the receptors. It is hoped that an intervention at one or more of these transduction processes will provide novel therapeutic agents for the treatment of ocular and nonocular diseases.

MOLECULAR BIOLOGY OF EICOSANOID RECEPTORS

Characterization of receptors at the molecular level is of great importance because it helps us to understand the nature of receptor–ligand interaction, cellular distribution, and localization and development of novel therapeutic agents.

The characterization of receptors at the molecular level is of particular importance where the receptor density is low. For studies at the molecular level, receptor gene cloning is a prerequisite. Once the receptor gene is cloned and the nucleotide and amino acid sequences are deduced, all the aspects of receptor studies can be pursued. Among the eicosanoid receptors, cDNA of TP receptors was cloned first (52,53). Then followed a rapid succession of cloning of cDNA of EP_1, EP_2, EP_3, IP and FP receptors and their expression in different cells (54–58). Only a few studies have addressed the distribution and localization of these receptors in ocular and nonocular tissues using the respective cDNA receptor probe. Messenger RNA for TP receptors is highly expressed in the spleen, thymus, and lungs (53) and that for FP receptors is expressed abundantly in corpus luteum (58). In the ocular tissues, FP receptors have been demonstrated in the ciliary muscles of humans (33). Further studies are needed to confirm whether FP receptors are expressed in the ciliary muscle cells.

TRENDS OF FUTURE RESEARCH

Molecular biology of prostanoid receptors is still in its infancy. A great deal of work at the molecular level is necessary in the extraocular and ocular tissues at the cellular levels to localize the eicosanoid receptors. Future studies should aim at isolating and purifying the receptor proteins using cDNA transfection of appropriate cells, generation of receptor antibodies, and immunocytochemical and pharmacological studies. To establish the precise functional relevance of different eicosanoid receptors, pharmacological studies are an absolute necessity. Although molecular probes are useful, highly selective agonists and antagonists are essential for receptor-mediated functional studies. As mentioned, except for DP, TP, and LT receptors, highly selective agonists and antagonists for other prostanoid receptors are not available at present and are necessary for a complete understanding of the role of eicosanoids in health and diseases.

ACKNOWLEDGMENTS

Preparation of this communication was supported by NIH grant EY-O6918, the Kentucky Lions Eye Foundation, and an unrestricted grant from Research to Prevent Blindness, Inc. I thank Sandra Neuman, Joyce Ray, and Marilyn McLendon for secretarial assistance.

REFERENCES

1. Bhattacherjee P. The role of arachidonate metabolites in ocular inflammation. In: Bito L, Stjernschantz J, eds. *The Ocular Effects of Prostaglandins and Other Eicosanoids.* New York: Alan R Liss, 1989;211–227.
2. Bito L, Camras CB, Gum GG, Resul B. The ocular hypotensive effects and side effects of Prostaglandins on the eyes of experimental animals. In: Bito L, Stjernschantz J, eds. *The Ocular Effects of Prostaglandins and Other Eicosanoids.* New York: Alan R Liss, 1989;349–368.
3. Bhattacherjee P, Paterson CA. Inflammatory mediators in models of immunogenic and non-immunogenic inflammation of the anterior segment of the eye. In: Bazan N, ed. *Lipid Mediators in Eye Inflammation.* Basel, Switzerland: Karger Publishing, 1990;65–82.
4. Desantis LL, Sallee VL. Comparison of the effects of prostaglandins and their esters on blood-aqueous barrier integrity and intraocular pressure in rabbits. In: Bito L, Stjernschantz J, eds. *The Ocular Effects of Prostaglandins and Other Eicosanoids.* New York: Alan R Liss, 1989;379–386.
5. Alm A, Villumsen J. Effects of topically applied $PGF_{2\alpha}$ and its isopropylester on normal and glaucomatous human eyes. In: Bito L, Stjernschantz J, eds. *The Ocular Effects of Prostaglandins and Other Eicosanoids.* New York: Alan R Liss, 1989;447–458.
6. Camras CB, Schumer RA, Marsk A, Lustgurten JS, Serle JB, Stjernschantz J, eds. *Intraocular pressure reduction with PhXA34, a new prostaglandin analogue, in patients with ocular hypertension. Arch Ophthalmol* 1992;110:1733–1738.
7. Bhattacherjee P, Hammond B, Salmon JA, Eakins KE. Chemotactic response to some arachidonic acid lipoxygenase products in the rabbit eye. *Eur J Pharmacol* 1981;73:21–28.
8. Spada CS, Woodward DF, Hawley SB, Nieves AL. Leukotrienes cause eosinophil emigration into conjunctival tissue. *Prostaglandins* 1986;31:795–809.
9. Spada CS, Woodward DF, Hawley SB, Nieves AL, Williams LS, Feldman BJ. Synergistic effects of LTB_4 and LTD_4 on leukocyte emigration into the guinea pig conjunctiva. *Am J Pathol* 1988;130: 354–368.
10. Bhattacherjee P, Eakins KE. Lipoxygenase products: mediation of inflammatory responses and inhibition of their formation. In: Chakrin LW, Baily DM, eds. *The Leukotrienes: Chemistry and Biology.* New York-London: Academic Press, 1984;195–214.
11. Woodward DF, Ledagard SE. Effect of LTD_4 on conjunctival vasopermeability and blood-aqueous barrier integrity. *Invest Ophthalmol Vis Sci* 1985;26:481–485.
12. Woodward DF, Nieves AL, Gary RK, et al. Studies with a potent leukotriene antagonist, S.K.XF104353, reveal that peptidoleukotriene plays a major role in mediating experimental allergic conjunctivitis. *Invest Ophthalmol Vis Sci* 1987;28(suppl):200.
13. Ninneman JL, ed. *Prostaglandins, Leukotrienes and the Immune Response.* Cambridge: Cambridge University Press, 1988.
14. Kennedy I, Coleman RA, Humphrey PPA, Levy GP, Lumley P. Studies on the characterization of prostanoid receptors: a proposed classification. *Prostaglandins* 1982;42:667–689.
15. Coleman RA, Humphrey PPA, Kennedy I, Lumley P. Prostanoids receptors—development of a working classification. *Trends Pharmacol Sci* 1984;5:303–307.
16. Coleman RA. Prostanoid and leukotriene receptors: a progress report from the IUPHAR working parties on the classification and nomenclature [Abstracts]. *Proceedings of the 9th International Conference on Prostaglandins and Related Compounds.* Fondazione Giovanni Lorenzini, Milan, Italy, 1994; 30.
17. Coleman RA, Kennedy I, Humphrey PPA, Bunce K, Lumley P. Prostanoids and their receptors. In: Hansch C, Sammes PG, Taylor JB, eds. *Comprehensive Medicinal Chemistry.* New York-Oxford: Pergamon Press, 1990;3:693–714.
18. Kingsbury W, Daines R, Gleason J. Leukotriene receptors. In: Hansch C, Sammes PG, Taylor JB, eds. *Comprehensive Medicinal Chemistry.* New York-Oxford: Pergamon Press, 1990;3:763–796.
19. Coleman RA, Kennedy I, Sheldrick RLG, Tolowinska IV. Further evidence for the existence of three subtypes of PGE_2 sensitive (EP) receptors. *Br J Pharmacol* 1990;91:407.
20. Coleman RA, Grix SP, Head SA, Louttit JB, Lallett A, Sheldrick RLG. A novel inhibitory prostanoid receptor in pilet saphenous vein. *Prostaglandins* 1994;47:151–168.
21. Eglen RM, Whiting RL. The action of prostanoid receptor agonists and antagonists on smooth muscle and platelets. *Br J Pharmacol* 1988;94:591–601.
22. Jumblatt M, Paterson CA. PGE_2 effects on corneal endothelial cyclic AMP synthesis and cell shape are mediated by a receptor of EP_2 subtype. *Invest Ophthalmol Vis Sci* 1991;32:360–365.
23. Bhattacherjee PB, Rhodes L, Paterson CA. Prostaglandin receptors coupled to adenylyl cyclase in the iris-ciliary body of rabbits, cats and cows. *Exp Eye Res* 1993;56:327–333.
24. Jumblatt M, Neltner AA, Coca-Prados M, Paterson CA. EP_2-receptor stimulated cyclic AMP synthesis in cultured human non-pigmented ciliary epithelium. *Exp Eye Res* 1994;58:563–566.
25. Bhattacherjee P, Liu L, Eta E, Paterson CA. Expression of prostanoid receptors in ocular tissues and cultured cells [Abstract]. *Proceedings of the 9th International Conference on Prostaglandins and Related Compounds.* Fondazione Giovanni Lorenzia, Milan, Italy, 1994;133.
26. Liu L, Eta E, Kahler A, Bhattacherjee P, Paterson CA. Prostaglandin receptors and transduction pathways in ODM2 and 3T3 cells. *Invest Ophthalmol Vis Sci* 1994;35:1986.
27. Ohia S, Jumblatt J. Prejunctional inhibitory effects of prostanoids on sympathetic neurotransmission in the rabbit iris-ciliary body. *J Pharmacol Exp Ther* 1990;255:11–16.
28. Camras CB, Bito LZ. Reduction of intraocular pressure in normal and glaucomatous primate (*Aotus trivirgatus*) eyes by topically applied $PGF_{2\alpha}$. *Curr Eye Res* 1981;1:205.
29. Lee Ping-yu, Podos SM, Severin C. Effect of $PGF_{2\alpha}$ on aqueous humor dynamics of rabbit, cat and monkey. *Invest Ophthalmol Vis Sci* 1984;25:1087–1093.
30. Crawford KS, Kaufman PL. Dose-related effects of $PGF_{2\alpha}$ isopropylester on intraocular pressure, refraction, and pupil diameter in monkeys. *Invest Ophthalmol Vis Sci* 1991;32:510–519.
31. Villumsen J, Alm A. PhxA-34 A prostaglandin $F_{2\alpha}$ analogue: effect on intraocular pressure in patients with ocular hypertension. *Br J Ophthalmol* 1992;76:214–217.
32. Hothelma Y, Mishima HK. Clinical efficacy of PhxA-34 PhxA-41, two novel prostaglandin $F_{2\alpha}$ isopropylester analogues for glaucoma treatment. *Jpn J Ophthalmol* 1993;37:259–269.

33. Lake S, Ocklind A, Krook K, Stjernschantz J. A molecular biological approach to prostaglandin receptors in the eye [Abstract]. *Proceedings of the 9th International Conference on Prostaglandins and Related Compounds.* Fondazione Giovanni Lorenzini, Milan, Italy, 1994;10.
34. Woodward DF, Burke JA, Williams LS, et al. Prostaglandin $F_{2\alpha}$ receptor stimulation. *Invest Ophthalmol Vis Sci* 1989;30:1838–1842.
35. Goh Y, Hotehama Y, Mishima H. Characterization of ciliary muscle relaxation induced by various agents in cats. *Invest Ophthalmol Vis Sci* 1995;36:1188–1192.
36. Boie Y, Sawyer N, Slipetz DM, et al. Molecular cloning and characterization of the human DP prostanoid receptor. *FASEB J* 1995;39: A1373.
37. Halushka PV, Mais DE, Mayeux PR, Morinelli TA. Thromboxane, prostaglandin and leukotriene receptors. *Annu Rev Pharmacol Toxicol* 1989;10:213–239.
38. Lefer AM, Smith EF, Araki H, et al. Dissociation of vasoconstrictor and platelet aggregatory activities of thromboxane by carbocyclic TxA_2, a stable analog of TxA_2. *Proc Nat Acad Sci USA* 1980;77: 1706–1710.
39. Mais DE, Burch RM, Saussy DL, Kochel PJ, Halushka PV. Binding of thromboxane A_2/Prostaglandin H_2 receptor antagonist to washed human platelets. *J Pharmacol Exp Ther* 1985;235:729–734.
40. Tymkewycz PM, Jones RL, Wilson NH, Marr CG. Heterogeneity of thromboxane A_2(TP-) receptors: evidence from antagonist but not agonist potency measurements. *Br J Pharmacol* 1991;102:607–614.
41. Ogletree ML, Allen GT. Interspecies differences in thromboxane receptors: Studies with Tx receptor antagonists in rat and guinea pig smooth muscles. *J Pharmacol Exp Ther* 1992;260:789–794.
42. Goh Y, Nakajima M, Azuma I, Hayaishi O. Effects of prostaglandin D2 and its analogue on intraocular pressure in rabbits. *Jpn J Ophthalmol* 1995;32:471–480.
43. Chen J, Woodward DF. Prostanoid-induced relaxation of precontracted cat ciliary muscle is mediated by EP_2 and DP receptors. *Invest Ophthalmol Vis Sci* 1992;33:3195–3201.
44. Giles H, Leff P, Bolofo ML, Kelly MG, Robertson AD. The classification of prostaglandin DP-receptors in platelets and vasculature using BW A868C, a novel, selective and potent competitive antagonist. *Br J Pharmacol* 1989;96:291–300.
45. Hoyng PFJ, Groeneboer MC. The effects of prostacyclin and its stable analogue on intraocular pressure. In: Bito LZ, Stjernschantz J, eds. *The Ocular Effects of Prostanoids and Other Eicosanoids.* New York: Alan R Liss, 1989;369–378.
46. Jaramillo A, Bhattacherjee P, Sonnenfeld G, Paterson CA. Modulation of immune responses by cyclooxygenase inhibitors during intraocular inflammation. *Curr Eye Res* 1992;11:571–579.
47. Lopez JS, Lio, Caspi RR, Nussenblatt B, Kador P, Chan CC. Use of oral CGS 13080 to suppress the development of experimental autoimmune uveitis in the Lewis rats. *Invest Ophthalmol Vis Sci* 1992; 33(suppl):933.
48. Piper PJ. Biological actions of leukotrienes. In: Chakrin LW, Bailey DM, eds. *The Leukotrienes: Chemistry and Biology.* New York-London: Academic Press, 1984;215–230.
49. Splictz DM, Scoggan KA, Nicholson DW, Metters KM. Photoaffinity labeling and radiation inactivation of the leukotriene B4 receptor in human myeloid cells [Abstract]. *Proceedings of the 8th International Conference on Prostaglandins and Related Compounds,* Montreal, Canada. 1992;255.
50. Nishizuka Y. Turnover of inositol phospholipids and signal transduction. *Science* 1984;225:1385–1369.
51. Nishizuka Y. The molecular heterogeneity of protein kinase C and its implication for cellular regulation. *Nature* 1988;334:661–665.
52. Hirata M, Hayaishi Y, Ushikobi F, Yokota Y, Kageyama R, Nakanishi S, Narumiya S. Cloning and expression of cDNA for human thromboxane A2 receptor. *Nature* 1991;359:617–620.
53. Namba T, Sugimoto Y, Hiara M, et al. Mouse thromboxane A_2 receptor: cDNA cloning, expression and Northern blot analysis. *Biochem Biophys Res Comm* 1992;184:1197–1203.
54. Sugimoto Y, Namba T, Honda A, et al. Cloning and expression of a cDNA for mouse prostaglandin E receptor EP_2 subtype. *J Biol Chem* 1992; 257:6463–6466.
55. Honda A, Sugimoto Y, Namba T, et al. Cloning and expression of a cDNA for mouse prostaglandin E receptor EP_2 subtype. *J Biol Chem* 1993; 268:7759–7762.
56. Watabe P, Sugimoto Y, Honda A, et al. Cloning and expression of cDNA for a mouse EP_1 subtype of prostaglandin E receptor. *J Biol Chem* 1193; 268:20175–20178.
57. Abramovitch M, Boie Y, Nguyen T, et al. Cloning and expression of a cDNA for the human prostanoid FP receptor. *J Biol Chem* 1994; 269:2632– 2636.
58. Sugimoto Y, Hasumota K, Namba T, et al. Cloning and expression of a cDNA for mouse $PGF_{2\alpha}$ receptor. *J Biol Chem* 1994;269: 1356–1360.

Textbook of Ocular Pharmacology,
edited by T.J. Zimmerman, et al.
Lippincott–Raven Publishers, Philadelphia © 1997.

CHAPTER 6

Steroids in Ocular Therapy

Prasad S. Kulkarni

The adrenal corticoids (*steroids*) are classified in two groups: one, corticosteroids, with 21 carbons, the other, androgens, with 19 carbons. Both classes of steroids are synthesized in the adrenal cortex. Cholesterol is an intermediate in the biosynthesis of corticosteroids, used in large part from the exogenous source. Cholesterol is enzymatically metabolized into 21-carbon corticosteroids and 19-carbon androgens by a series of steps with oxidases containing P-450 NADPH pathways and oxygen (Figure 6-1). For more details, the reader is referred to physiology or biochemistry textbooks.

PHYSIOLOGY

The physiological significance of the adrenal gland began to be appreciated when Addison, in 1855, described a clinical syndrome resulting from a destructive disease of the adrenal gland (1). Consequently, Brown-Séquard (1856), in his pioneering work with experimental animals, showed that adrenal glands have an important physiological role when adrenalectomy resulted in death in these animals (2). This work provided strong and conclusive evidence for Addison's hypothesis (1) that the adrenal glands are essential to life. Despite this evidence, however, many physiologists did not support Brown-Séquard's findings because of the difficulty in removing all adrenal tissues in the rats. Furthermore, considerable confusion arose among physiologists over the function of the adrenal glands when a number of scientists demonstrated that the adrenal glands are responsible for maintaining fluid and electrolyte balance. Whereas others attributed adrenal glands as being involved in the regulation of glucose metabolism and detoxification of lethal hormonal substances circulating in the blood, the renal loss of sodium and fluids was convincingly demonstrated by Harrop and Associates (1933) (3) and by Loebs and co-workers (1933) (4) in suprarenal insufficiency in dogs and in Addison's disease.

Cori and Cori, in 1927, demonstrated that a deficiency in carbohydrate metabolism was present in adrenalectomized rodents (5) and that hypoglycemia can be corrected by adrenalcortical extracts (6). During fasting, synthesis of glucose and glycogen was increased, and it was derived from tissue protein (7). These studies supported the concept that there are two types of adrenal cortical hormones: (a) *mineralocorticoids,* which are responsible for fluid and electrolyte balance; and (b) *glucocorticoids,* which are involved in the regulation of carbohydrate metabolism. The use of adrenocortical extracts to correct deficiencies in adrenalectomized animals led to the isolation and identification of the chemical nature of the biologically active substances in these extracts (8–10). In 1943 Reichstein and Shoppee crystallized and elucidated the structures of 28 steroids from the adrenal cortex (11). Five of these compounds (cortisol, corticosterone, 11-dehydrocorticosterone, desoxy, and 11-desoxy-corticosterone) were demonstrated to be biologically active. Deming and Luetscher in 1950 isolated mineralocorticoids from urine, and further identification and purification of mineralocorticoids from adrenal cortex was done by Tait and co-workers in 1952 (12). The prototypical hormone was named *aldosterone* by Simpson et al. in 1954 (13).

Meanwhile, other physiologists showed that cell extracts of the anterior pituitary had stimulating effects on the adrenal cortex of hypophysectomized animals (14–16). Further, chemical characterization of these extracts led to the isolation of the hormone adrenocorticotropic hormone (ACTH), which acted selectively to affect chemical and morphological changes of the adrenal cortex (17–19). The structure of ACTH was established by Bell and co-workers (1956) (20).

Effective clinical use of corticosteroids has become possible because of their isolation, elucidation of their

P. S. Kulkarni: Department of Ophthalmology and Visual Sciences, University of Louisville School of Medicine, Louisville, Kentucky 40292.

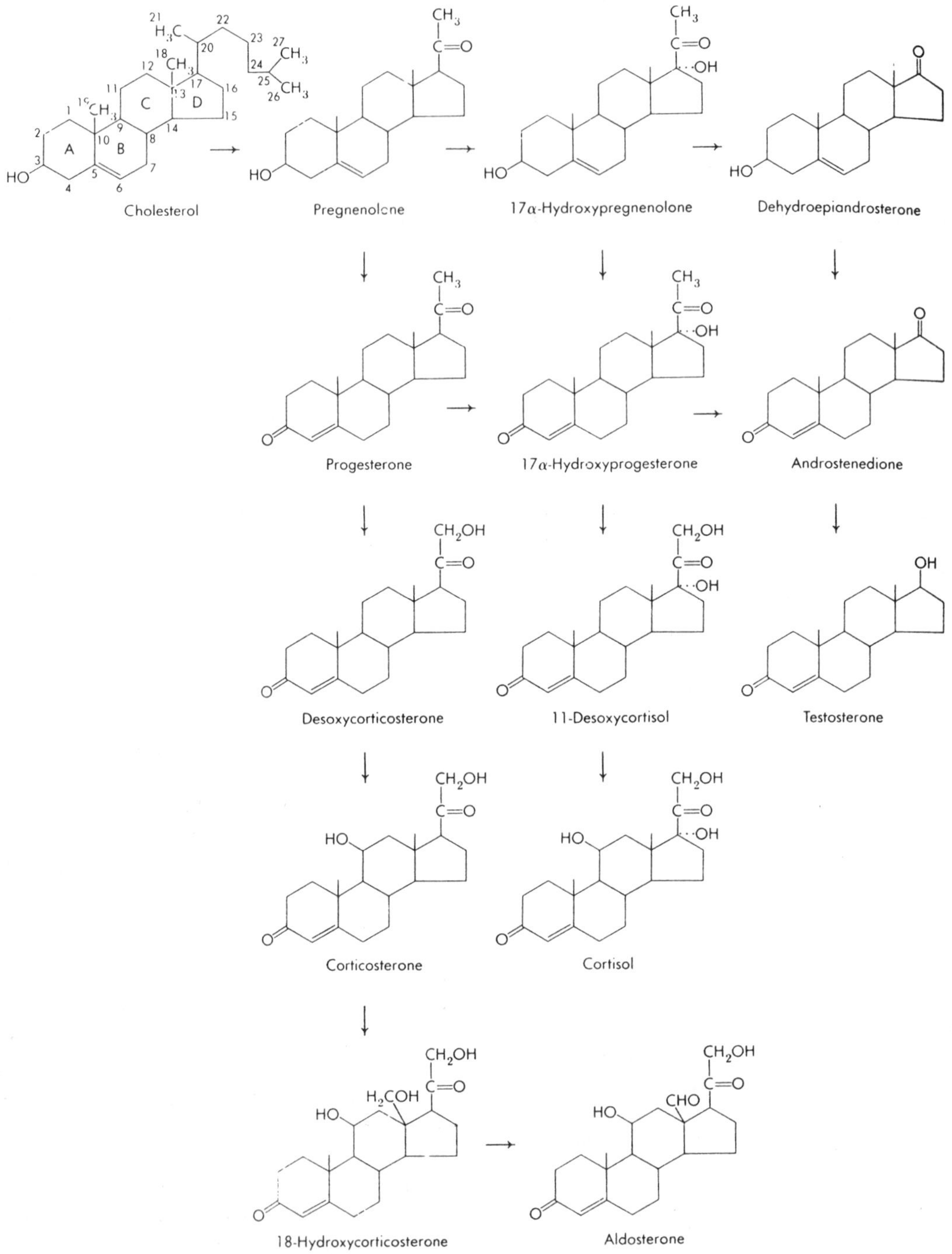

FIG. 6-1. Principal pathways for biosynthesis of adrenocorticosteroids and adrenal androgens. (Reproduced with permission from Goodman and Gilman. In: Haynes R.C., and Murad F. (eds): The Pharmacological Basis of Therapeutics, p. 472, 6th ed. MacMillan Publishing Co. Inc., NY, 1980.)

chemical structure, and their economical synthesis. Structure–activity relationship studies with various synthetic corticosteroids have led to the development of potent antiinflammatory compounds; however, their unwanted side effects are still a problem in the treatment of diseases, including in ophthalmic applications.

STRUCTURE–ACTIVITY RELATIONSHIP STUDIES OF STEROIDS

Cortisone was the first corticosteroid to be used for its antiinflammatory activity. Structural modification cortisone led to the development of more potent antiinflammatory steroids and also improved the route of administration. Changes in chemical structure not only altered the antiinflammatory activities but also altered absorption, protein binding, the rate of metabolic transformation, the rate of excretion, and the effectiveness of the molecule at its site of action. Modifications of the pregnane molecules led to the improved antiinflammatory index (Figure 6-2).

FIG. 6-2. Structure–activity relationship of adrenocorticosteroids. The molecular sites of alteration are shown in bold lines and letters. **Ring A:** The 4,5 double bond and the 3-ketone are both necessary for typical adrenocorticosteroid activity. Introduction of a 1,2 double bond, as in prednisone or prednisolone, enhances the antiinflammatory activity. **Ring B:** 6_α substitution increases antiinflammatory potency. 6_α methylprednisolone has slightly greater potency, while fluorination in the 9_α position enhances all biological activities of the cortisol. **Ring C:** The presence of an oxygen at C-11 position is important for antiinflammatory action. **Ring D:** C-16-methylation or hydrooxidation has little effect in altering antiinflammatory activities. Fluorine substitution at either C-6 or C-9 position in ring B, together with the hydroxylation or methylation of C-16 in ring D, enhances the potency of all presently used antiinflammatory steroids.

STEROIDS IN OPHTHALMOLOGY

Because ACTH and cortisone were beneficial in rheumatoid arthritis, these agents were used in the treatment of its ocular complications. Olson et al. (21) reported that patients with iridocyclitis dramatically recovered within 24 hours after steroid treatment. These patients were resistant to any other antiinflammatory therapy. For the prevention of anterior segment inflammation, cortisone was used topically for the first time in the 1950s, which led to the development of other potent corticosteroids to be used topically in ophthalmic clinical practice (21–23). This development was also important because systemic use of steroids caused significant and severe side effects.

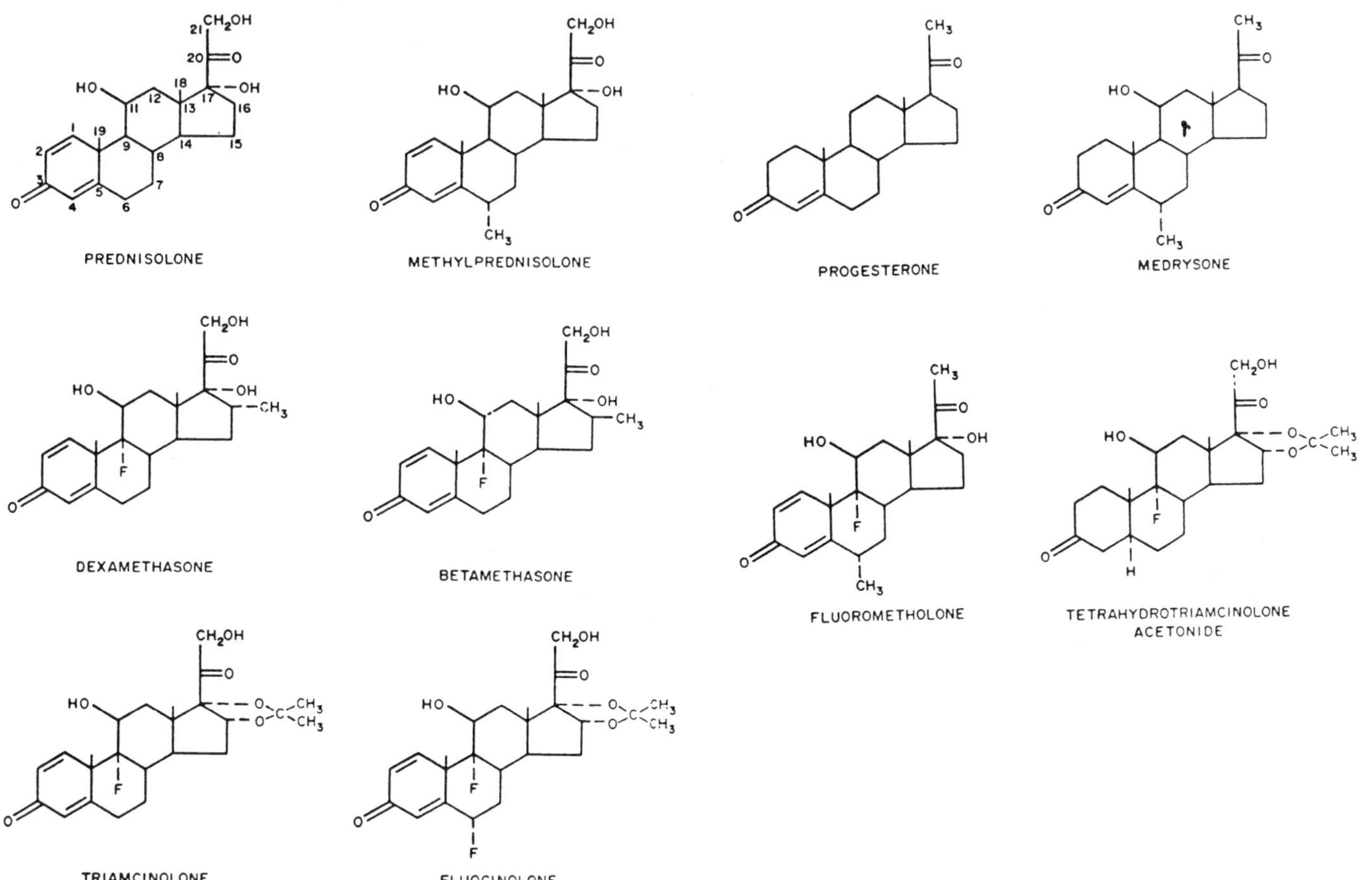

FIG. 6-3. Chemical structures of some of the newer ophthalmic steroids, medrysone and fluorometholone, compared with progesterone and tetrahydrotriamcinolone acetonide. (From Polansky and Weinreb, ref 36, with permission.)

TABLE 6-1. *Systemic glucocorticoid preparations (28)*

Commonly used name	Estimated potency relative to cortisol	
	Glucocorticoid	Mineralocorticoid
Short-acting (half-life < 12 h)		
Hydrocortisone	1	1
Cortisone	0.8	0.8
Intermediate-acting (half-life 12–36 h)		
Prednisone	4	0.25
Prednisolone	4	0.25
Methylprednisolone	5	±
Triamcinolone	5	±
Long-acting (half-life > 48 hr)		
Paramethasone	10	±
β-Methasone	25	±
Dexamethasone	30–40	±

From Williams et al., ref 28.

Concomitantly with the use of steroidal therapy in the treatment of ocular inflammatory diseases, it was also demonstrated that steroids can inhibit wound healing and corneal neovascularization (24,25). Corticosteroids were found to prevent corneal transplant rejection and postoperative inflammation and effectively to prevent inflammatory responses in uveitis and other ocular diseases (26,27); however, prolonged corticosteroid therapy has resulted in ocular hypertension, leading to glaucoma, cataract formation, delay in wound healing, and immunogenic infections caused by immunosuppression.

The three different subtypes of the commercially available corticosteroids are the short-acting, intermediate-acting, and long-acting agent preparations, based on their estimated duration of hypothalamic-pituitary suppression (28). Relative potencies of these steroids were estimated by observing the therapeutic efficacy over long periods after oral administration (29). Synthetic steroidal preparations and their chemical structures are shown in Figure 6-3. Table 6-1 shows that systemic dosage of dexamethasone has the highest glucocorticoid therapeutic efficacy. Efficacies of prednisone and cortisone after oral administrations were similar to the efficacies of prednisolone or hydrocortisone, respectively, probably because hydrocortisone and prednisolone are rapidly metabolized by the liver. Table 6-1 also lists the relative mineralocorticoid activities of hydrocortisone, cortisone, prednisone, and prednisolone. Hydrocortisone and cortisone are equally active in their glucocorticoidal and mineralocorticoidal activities. The duration of action and potency is extremely important in the treatment of various diseases, especially for the long-acting drugs, like dexamethasone (DEXA).

Table 6-2 compares the various physiological effects of the costeroids. The relative potencies of synthetic costo-

TABLE 6-2. *Comparative effects of corticosteroids (36)*

	Cortisone	Hydrocortisone	Prednisone	Prednisolone	Methylprednisolone	Triamcinolone	Dexamethasone
Equivalent daily dose (mg)	75	60	15	15	12	12	3
Edema, sodium retention	++++	+++	+	++	+	0	+
Hypertension	++	+	+	++	+	+	+
Weakness or potassium depletion	+++	++	+	+	+	++	+
Peptic ulcer	++	+	+++	+++	++	+++	++
Increased appetite and weight gain	++	++	++	++	+	–	++++
Mental stimulation	+++	+	++	++	+	0 to –	++++
Hirsutism	++	++	++	++	++	++++	+
Skin effects	+	+	+	+	+	++++	+
Adrenal atrophy	+++	+++	+++	+++	+++	+++	+++
Topical effect	+	+++	+	+++	++	+++	++
Infections	++	++	++	++	++	++	++
Diabetes	++	++	+++	++++	+++	++	+
Osteoporosis	+++	++	+++	+++	+++	+++	++

From Polanski and Weinreb, ref 36.

costeroids, like dexamethasone (DEXA), prednisolone (PDN), betamethasone (BM), hydrocortisone (HC), and fluorocortisone (FC), were found to be in a descending order: PDN < BM < DEXA < HC < FC.

Corticosteroids, like dexamethasone, prednisolone, fluoromethalone, and betamethasone, are potent antiinflammatory agents in ocular diseases, such as experimental uveitis and corneal injury in a transplant model (26,27). Indeed, corticosteroids are the most potent agents in controlling chronic inflammatory diseases. Significant investigations have explored the mechanism of the antiinflammatory action of steroids, largely through the application of molecular biological techniques. These studies may provide a new approach to developing more selective antiinflammatory drugs in the future.

MECHANISM OF STEROIDAL ANTIINFLAMMATORY ACTION OF MOLECULAR LEVELS

Receptors

Corticosteroids exert their effects by binding to a cytoplasmic glucocorticoid receptor within target cells (Fig. 6-4). These receptors are members of a supergene family, which includes cytosolic receptors for corticosteroids, progesterone, estrogen, thyroid hormone, retinoic acid, and vitamin D (30).

The cDNA coding for glucocorticoid receptors from human and other species has been cloned. The primary structure of the receptors consists of 800 amino acid residues. Although there is only a single class of glucocorticoid receptors, there are several steroid-binding domains on these receptors on the C-terminal. The DNA binding domain, in the center (80 amino acids reside) of the molecule, is folded into two zinc fingers, coordinated by a zinc molecule bound to four cysteine residues. There is an *N*-terminal domain (Tau 1) that is involved in transcriptional *trans*-activation of genes once binding to DNA occurs. This region may also be involved in binding to other transcription factors. In the human glucocorticoid receptor, there is another *trans*-acting domain (Tau 2) adjacent to the steroid binding domain. This region is also important for nuclear translocation of the receptor (see Fig. 6-4). The steroid receptor is phosphorylated at the serine amino acid on the C-terminal, but the relationship between this phosphorylation and steroidal action is yet to be elucidated.

Glucocorticoid receptors are present in every cell; however, their numbers may vary according to cell types. The inactive glucocorticoid receptor is bound to a large protein complex (= 300 kDa) that includes two subunits of the heat-shock protein 90 (hsp 90) that binds to the C-terminal end of the receptor. There is also evidence that other proteins may be associated with this complex, including immunophilin and various inhibitory proteins. The hsp facilitates the proper folding of the receptor into its optimal conformation for binding and acts as a molecular chaperone to prevent the unoccupied corticoid receptor from migrating to the nucleus. Once the corticosteroid binds to the receptor, hsp 90 dissociates and allows the rapid nuclear localization of the activated receptor-steroid complex and its binding to DNA (Figure 6-5).

Receptor Expression and Its Regulation

Corticosteroid receptor expression may be regulated by several factors at the transcriptional, translational, or the posttranslational levels (30). Downregulation of these receptors in circulating monocytes and lymphocytes occurs after steroidal therapy, but its importance in chronic steroid therapy is still unknown. A marked reduction in steroid receptor population occurs in the human lung after exposure to steroids in vitro (30). Studies with transgenic mice that express antisense steroid receptor mRNA, resulting in lower glucocorticoid receptors levels, have demonstrated that even halving steroid receptor expression causes various abnormalities, including an increase in circulating cortisol and body fat (30).

Effects on Gene Transcription

Steroids regulate gene transcription of certain target genes to elucidate their effects. It is estimated that the number of steroid-responsive genes per cell is between 10 and 100. Within the nucleus, steroid receptors form a dimer

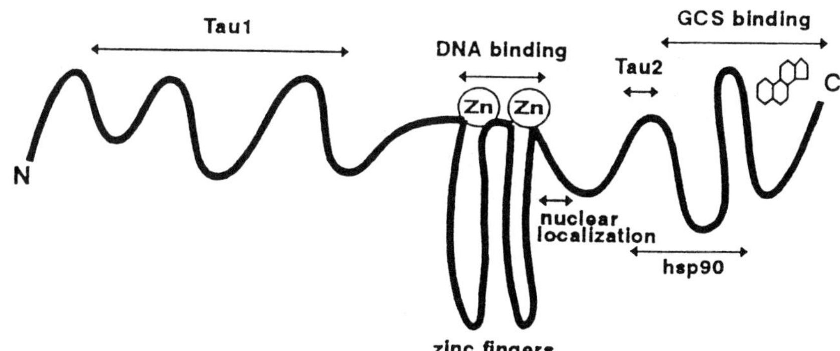

FIG. 6-4. Domains of the glucocorticoid receptor. (From Barnes and Adcock, ref 30, with permission.)

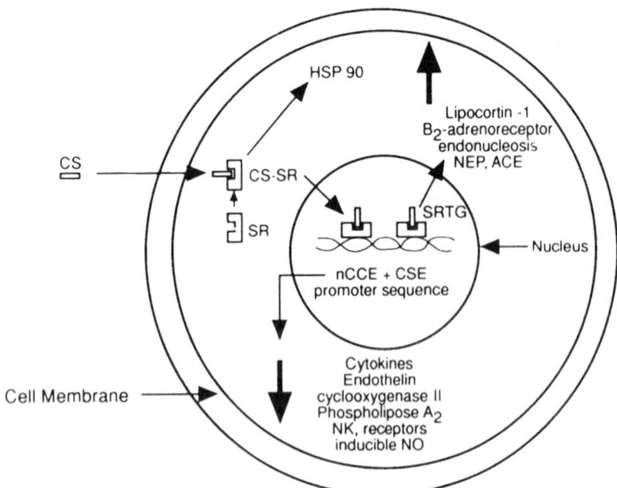

FIG. 6-5. Effects of corticosteroid on gene transcription. Corticosteroid (CS) binds to cystolic steroid receptors (SR), which are associated with two protein molecules of a 90 KDa heat shock protein (hsp90). The CS-SR complex translocates to the nucleus and binds to corticosteroid elements (CRE and NCRE) in the promoter sequences of target genes, resulting in increased or decreased transcription NCSE negative elements SRTG–steroid receptor target genes. (Reproduced from *Trends in Pharmacological Sciences*, with permission.)

that binds to DNA at consensus sites termed *glucocorticoid response elements* (SRTG), which are located in the promoter region of steroid-responsive target genes (see Fig. 6-5). This binding changes the rate of transcription, resulting in either induction or repression of the gene. The consensus sequence of SRTG binding is the palindromic 15-base-pair sequence GGTACAnnn TGTTCT, whereas for repression of transcription, the negative SRTG has a more variable sequence (ATYACnnTnTGATCn). Crystallographic studies indicate that the zinc-finger binding to DNA occurs within the major groove of DNA, with each finger interacting with half of the palindrome (30).

The number of SRTGs and their position relative to the transcriptional start site may be important determinants of the magnitude of the transcriptional response to steroids (31). Other transcriptional factors binding in the vicinity of SRTG may influence steroid inducibility. The relative abundance of various transcription factors also may contribute to the steroid responsiveness of a particular cell type. Steroid receptor–DNA interaction changes DNA I sensitivity, suggesting that there may be a change in the configuration of DNA or chromatin that will expose previously masked areas, resulting in increased binding of other transcription factors and the formation of a more stable transcription initiation complex.

The mechanisms involved in gene repression are less well understood. Glucocorticoid receptors may form complexes with activating transcription factors in the nucleus to inhibit their effect. Thus, steroids may have an inhibitory effect on the transcription of genes that do not have a negative SRTG in their promoter sequence.

Steroid receptors also may inhibit protein synthesis by reducing the stability of mRNA. This may be achieved via enhanced transcription of specific ribonucleases that break down m-RNA containing constitutive sequence(s) in the untranslated 3-region, thus shortening mRNA turnover time (30).

Corticosteroids may be effective in controlling inflammation by inhibiting several aspects of the inflammatory process through increasing or decreasing gene transcription. Glucocorticoid receptors interact directly with other transcription factors, which may be important for their antiinflammatory activities. For example, steroids are potent inhibitors of collagenase gene transcription, induced by tumor necrosis factor (TNF) or phorbol esters, which activate AP-1; and AP-1 forms a protein-protein complex with activated corticoid receptors within the nucleus, which causes mutual repression of DNA binding and thereby reduces steroid responsiveness. On the other hand, steroids may inhibit the effects of those cytokines that produce their effects on genes transcription via activation of AP-1, thus increasing AP-1 binding to DNA (30).

Corticosteroid Receptor Interaction with Transcription Factors

There is evidence that high concentrations of β-adrenoreceptor agonists can activate the transcription factor (CREB) that binds to the cAMP responsive element (CRE) on genes. These agonists increase CRE binding in the human lung in vitro and in a hepatoma cell line while reducing SRTG binding (30). These observations suggest a protein–protein interaction between CREB and glucocorticoid receptors within the nucleus. This interaction would mean that high concentration of β-adrenoreceptor agonists may interfere with the antiinflammatory actions of steroids.

Inflammatory Chemical Mediators

The antiinflammatory effects of steroids may be explained by their ability to inhibit the synthesis and release of proinflammatory chemical mediators, such as eicosanoids, platelet-activating factor (PAF), cytokines, TNF, tachykinins, nitric oxide, and others. Dexamethasone increases the synthesis of lipocortin, a 37-kDa protein that has an inhibitory effect on phospholipase A_2 (PLA_2), and therefore inhibits the release of arachidonic acid (AA), a substrate for proinflammatory leukotrienes (LTs) and prostanoids (PGs). Arachidonic acid is converted into LTs by the 5-lipoxygenase pathways and into PGs and PAF by cyclooxygenases (Cox I and Cox II) pathways. Steroids induce the synthesis of lipocortin in rat and human leukocytes (30). Recombinant lipocortin-1 has acute antiinflammatory properties, and it inhibits the release of eicosanoids from lungs; however, it is now known that lipocortin-1 is rather nonspecific, and there are doubts about the ability of steroids to induce lipocortin-1 synthesis in some cells (30).

It is possible that steroids may have a direct inhibitory action on the transcription of enzymes involved in eicosanoid synthesis. For example, corticosteroids inhibit gene transcription of a cytosolic form of PLA_2 induced by cytokines. Also, they inhibit the gene expression of cytokine-induced Cox-II in monocytes (30). Whether steroids also modulate 5-lipoxygenase expression has not been established. Although dexamethasone inhibited PG formation in ocular tissues (iris-ciliary body), it did not inhibit the synthesis of LTB_4 (a potent chemotactic factor), suggesting that steroids inhibited only the Cox II expression in rabbit uveal tissues (26,27). Steroids may also modulate or inhibit the effects of inflammatory mediators (e.g., LTB_4 and PAF), induce the expression of c-*fos* and c-*jun,* and activate AP-1 binding in inflammatory cells.

Steroids also reduce neurogenic inflammation, probably by their effects on the metabolism of mediators. Bradykinin is degraded by several enzymes, including angiotensin-converting enzyme and neural endopeptidase (NEP), both of which may be induced by steroids (30). Neural endopeptidase may also be important in degrading tachykinins, released from sensory nerves, and increased expression of NEP may therefore reduce neurogenic inflammation.

Steroids are potent antiinflammatory substances because they also inhibit cytokines, which play a vital role in chronic ocular inflammations (27). Steroids inhibit the transcription of cytokines that are vital to chronic inflammation, such as interleukin-1 (IL-1), TNF_{α}, granulocyte macrophage–colony-stimulating factor (GM-CSF), IL-2, IL-3, IL-4, IL-5, IL-6, and IL-8 (30). Cytokine genes are sensitive to steroid receptors. Inhibition is via interaction of the receptors with negative GRE, resulting in repression of gene action.

Steroids block not only the synthesis of cytokines but also their action. Steroids may inhibit synthesis of IL-1 receptors and inhibit activation of AP-1 and NF_kB (transcription factors) by $TNF_{2\alpha}$. Furthermore, activation of AP-1 leads to stimulation of T-lymphocytes, which can be inhibited by steroids.

Recently it was demonstrated that nitric oxide is a potent mediator of inflammation. Endotoxin (LPS) and cytokines induce nitrous oxide gene expression, which can be prevented by dexamethasone.

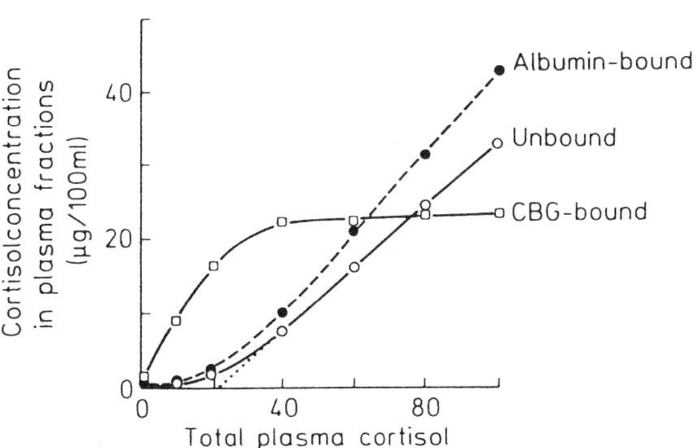

FIG. 6-6. Distribution of cortisol in plasma. (From Ballard, ref 31, with permission.)

Some patients are resistant to steroids. These patients have no abnormality with either the steroid receptors or the ability of binding with receptors and nuclear translocation (30). Therefore, the mechanism of steroid resistance has not yet been elucidated.

ABSORPTION AND DISTRIBUTION

On systemic administration, cortisol in plasma is either bound to plasma proteins, for example, albumin and corticosteroid binding globulin (CBG), or unbound as a free steroid. Ballard in 1979 (31) observed that after systemic administration of cortisol (5–25 μg), most of it binds to CBG, and over the range of 25 μg (25–80 μg) CBG binding was saturated. At this point, albumin became a steroid binding protein. Interestingly, albumin–steroid binding was not saturated even up to 100 μg of total plasma concentration. After saturation of CBG-steroid binding, about 50% of plasma cortisol was bound to albumin and the remaining was free (Figure 6-6). Only this free form of the cortisol was available for its biological action. Many synthetic compounds have lower affinity to CBG than cortisol and thus are more potent than cortisol (31). The amount of free plasma steroid may also be determined by the amount of steroid metabolized in the blood and the amount transferred into the tissues and further metabolized.

After topical application of several synthetic steroidal preparations like dexamethasone phosphate, prednisolone phosphate, prednisolone acetate, and fluoromethalone,

TABLE 6-3. *Corneal permeability (mean ± SEM) of tritiated labeled steroids*

Steroid preparation	Epithelium intact ($nM\ cm^{-2}\ h^{-1}$)	W/O epithelium ($nM\ cm^{-2}\ h^{-1}$)
Dexamethasone phosphate	7·1 ± 0·6	32·4 ± 1·8
Prednisolone phosphate	12·1 ± 0·5	37·7 ± 2·6
Prednisolone acetate	14·3 ± 1·1	11·5 ± 1·2
Fluoromethalone	15·4 ± 2·2	14·4 ± 3·3

From Hull et al., ref 32.

Hull et al. in 1974 (32) observed that the prednisolone and fluoromethalone preparations penetrated the cornea with intact epithelium cells or layer better than dexamethasone; however, penetration of the phosphate preparations through the denuded corneal epithelium was far superior than the other drugs (Table 6-3).

METABOLISM

Figure 6-7 represents the major metabolic pathways of corticosteroids. Pathways 1 and 2 are located in the liver and consist of the conjugation of the A ring to glucuronides or glucuronate, achieved by the reduction of C-4-5 double bond and hydroxylation (i.e., C-3 keto group followed by conjugation at the hydroxyl position, together with the hydroxylation, at the C-2 position). These glucuronider are excreted in the urine. Pathways 3, 4, and 5 are located in the liver and also in peripheral tissues. Pathway 3 is conversion of the C-11-hydroxyl group to a keto group; pathway 4 is the reduction of a carbonyl group at C-20 to isomeric alcohols. Pathway 5 is a hydroxylation at the C-6 position. All these compounds are excreted mainly through urine. Prednisolone is excreted either unchanged or with its side chain degraded (33). Dexamethasone and triamcinolone are more resistant to degradation than prednisolone and are excreted primarily unchanged (34,35).

Numerous studies have investigated the metabolism of steroids within the eye. For example, ocular steroid effects were observed following topical cortisone treatment, which could be due to conversion of cortisone to the active 11-hydroxy product, hydrocortisone. The presence of 11-β-hydroxylase activity in the cornea, and possibly in other ocular tissues, is indicated because cortisone and prednisolone are very active topically (37). The presence of phosphatase activity in the cornea is also equally important because the cornea can convert a less active phosphate derivative of corticosteroids to more active alcohol forms. There are other degradative pathways present in the cornea, for example, enzymatic systems that attack at the C-20 keto and C-6-B positions of progesterone (38,39). It is important to understand the metabolic and biological activities of the metabolites because corticosteroids can be biotransformed into either active or inactive compounds. These studies are helpful in determining the potency and therapeutic index of a given compound.

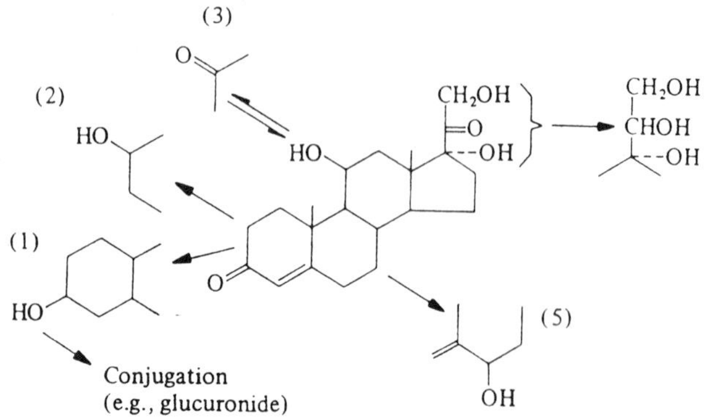

(3)
(2)
HO
CH_2OH
=O
HO
--OH
CH_2OH
CHOH
--OH
(1)
O
HO
(5)
Conjugation
(e.g., glucuronide)
OH

FIG. 6-7. Major metabolic fates of cortisol: (*1*) reduction of the 4–5 double bond, hydroxylation of the 3-keto group, with subsequent conjugation at the hydroxyl position; (*2*) hydroxylation at the 2-position; (*3*) conversion of the 11-hydroxyl to an 11-keto group; (*4*) reduction of carbonyl group at C-20 to isomeric alcohols; and (*5*) hydroxylation at the 6-position. (From Cope, ref 33, with permission.)

ROUTES OF ADMINISTRATION AND DOSAGE

Topical Application

The route of administration of corticosteroid depends on the site of involvement. Topical use will be important and effective for the anterior segment of the eye, mainly the cornea, conjunctiva, sclera, anterior chamber, lens, and uvea. This type of application is relatively easy, "patient friendly," and inexpensive. Effective ocular concentrations of the drugs will be higher than through systemic routes, with fewer complications, and almost an absence of systemic side effects. In posterior segment diseases like optic neuritis, chorioretinitis, and posterior scleritis, however, topical administration will be significantly less effective than the systemic route. In such cases, intramuscular, intravenous injections, or oral administrations are preferred. Oral administration will be most useful and preferred by most patients. Plasma corticosteroid concentrations reach peak plasma level within 1 hour after oral administration; therefore, intravenous injections are not recommended unless a rapid-loading dose is indicated. Four to 8 hours after an oral dose, plasma levels return to normal. Therefore, the one-dose regimen can be divided into equal amounts to be taken every 4 to 6 hours.

Dosage will vary with the severity and type of disease. Also, the potency of the preparation, penetration, binding affinities, and degradation will affect the efficacy. For most topical purposes, a 0.5% preparation of prednisolone, cortisone, and hydrocortisone is adequate; but for treating more severe diseases, 2.5% suspensions may be desirable. A better effect can be achieved by increased frequency than by increasing concentrations of the drug. In severe conditions, hourly instillations are used to obtain some response; then frequency is tapered off. Chronic allergic conditions, like vernal conjunctivitis, may require long-term treatment with a high concentration of steroids. Then careful monitoring is needed to detect and control severe side effects. Additionally, a possibility of relapse exists if the therapy is prematurely ceased, especially in iritis. On the other hand, in acute and less severe disease, highly potent steroids may not be required and a steroid-like fluo-

TABLE 6-4. *Ophthalmic corticosteroid preparations*

Generic name	Trade name	Concentration (%)
Hydrocortisone		
Solution	Optef drops	0.2
Acetate ointment	Hydrocortone Acetate	1.5
Acetate suspension	Hydrocortone Acetate	2.5
Prednisolone		
Phosphate ointment	Hydeltrasol	0.25
Phosphate solution	Metreton	0.5
Phosphate solution	Hydeltrasol	0.5
Sodium phosphate solution	Ak-Pred	0.125/1.0
Sodium phosphate solution	B-H Prednisolone	0.125/1.0
Sodium phosphate solution	Inflamase/Inflamase Forte	0.12/1.0
Acetate suspension	Predulose	0.25
Acetate suspension	Ak-Tate	1.0
Acetate suspension	Econopred/Econopred Plus	0.125/1.0
Acetate suspension	Pred Mild/Pred Forte	0.12/1.0
Dexamethasone		
Suspension	Maxidex	0.1
Phosphate ointment	Decadron	0.05
Phosphate solution	Decadron	0.1
Phosphate ointment	Ak-Dex	0.05
Phosphate solution	Ak-Dex	0.1
Progesterone-like compounds		
Fluorometholone ointment	FML	0.1
Fluorometholone suspension	FML/FML Forte	0.1/0.25
Medrysone	HMS	1.0

romethalone (which is metabolized in cornea) may be useful. Usually, hydrocortisone preparations are effective in the treatment of surface inflammation. The list of corticosteroid preparations and their chemical use, as well as their therapeutic treatment of ocular diseases, is given in Tables 6-4 and 6-5, respectively.

Systemic Therapy

Systemic therapy, mainly oral, has proved effective for the treatment of inflammatory disease of the posterior segment of the eye. High-dose prednisolone (80–180 mg/day) or prednisone (60–80 mg/day) with short-term administration is potentially valuable in the treatment of severe inflammation and immunogenic diseases. Orally administered steroids are also useful in the treatment of ophthalmic complications of connective tissue disorders, such as sarcoidosis. It is possible to avoid the toxic effects of steroids by short-term treatment. If the lesion progresses, doses should be increased until improvement occurs, after which the dosing regimen should be lowered in gradual steps guided by clinical and laboratory findings. In severe cases, therapy may be required for months before it can be stopped. If a reduction in dosage is followed by exacerbation of the inflammation, therapy must be restored to the initial dosage and continued until the inflammation subsides.

TABLE 6-5. *Ocular conditions reported to respond to corticosteroids*

Allergic blepharitis and conjunctivitis
Mucocutaneous conjunctival lesions
Chemical burn of the cornea and conjunctiva
Phlyctenular conjunctivitis and keratitis
Irritant conjunctivitis
Contact dermatitis of the conjunctiva and eyelid
Vernal conjunctivitis
Ocular pemphigoid
Acne rosacea keratitis
Viral ocular diseases
Herpes simplex (diskiform stage)
Herpes zoster
Adenovirus
Infiltrative corneal disease
Interstitial keratitis
Superficial punctate keratitis
Marginal corneal ulcers
Immune graft reaction
Scleritis and episcleritis
Iritis, iridocyclitis
Sympathetic ophthalmia
Posterior uveitis
Retinal vasculitis
Optic neuritis
Juvenile xanthogranuloma
Pseudotumor of the orbit
Progressive thyroid exophthalmopathy
Temporal arteritis

The dosage of steroids and the terms of treatment depend on the type of disease as well as the individual response and the patient's general state of health. A once-a-day, usually morning dose increases patient compliance. (See Section V on uveitis, this volume, for more details.)

Alternate-day Therapy

To avoid any toxic effect of steroids, such as suppression of the secretion of adrenal and other endocrine glands, growth alterations, immunosuppression, and osteoporosis, an alternate-day therapy has been advocated, especially in pediatric patients. In such cases, the total 2-day therapy dose can be given in one day, skipping the next; however, precautions must be taken to avoid exacerbation of the inflammatory condition.

Periocular Injection

Periocular injection sites depend on the nature of the disease. For example, subconjunctival injection is used for the treatment of corneal diseases, whereas anterior sub-Tenon's injections are for iritis or iridocyclitis. Posterior sub-Tenon's injection is indicated for equatorial or mid-zone "intermediate" posterior uveitis. Again, dosage depends on the severity and location of the disease. Although efficacious, these routes are underused in the clinical setting. Intravitreal injections are also an important route and a way to prevent and treat vitritis and retinitis. Triamcinolone acetonide remains in the eye longer than dexamethasone after intravitreal injections and thus was more effective in reducing the incidence of retinal detachment in an experimental model (40). The effectiveness of this route of administration in other conditions remains questionable, however.

THERAPY

Indications

Corticosteroids are potent antiinflammatory drugs and usually are more efficacious than the available nonsteroidal antiinflammatory agents. Their greater potency is probably due to their multifunctional actions. Steroids, as already discussed, inhibit cyclooxygenase activity (Cox II), phospholipase activity, synthesis, and the release of cytokines, platelet activating factor, and adhesion molecules. Steroids have these effects on virtually every cell and every tissue and even act at the molecular level through their ability to inhibit inducible enzymes and receptor synthesis regulation. Nonsteroidal antiinflammatory agents (like aspirin) are more specific and thus inhibit the release of one or two inflammatory mediators. Although steroids abolish the whole cascade of potent chemical mediators of inflammation, they also inhibit certain growth factors and β-adrenergic receptors. Although steroidal treatment is beneficial in almost all types of inflammation, their continued long-term use can be dangerous because of their side effects.

Designing Soft Drugs

A novel approach to the design of safer ophthalmic drugs with fewer side effects and a high therapeutic index has developed a new class of agents: "soft" drugs. This approach is based on the retrometabolic design technique. Among various soft-drug classes, the "inactive" metabolite and soft analogues are the most useful designs for safe and selective ophthalmic drugs. In the first case, the design process starts with a known, predicted inactive metabolite of the drug, which then is structurally modified in the chemical activation stage to the "soft" drug, which is isoteric or isoelectronic with the drug to produce activity at the target receptors similar to that of the original compound. The "soft" drug is subject to predictable metabolism, leading in one step to the starting inactive metabolite. As this deactivation takes place everywhere in the body, the desired activities are produced exclusively at the target site at or near the place of application. Successful use of this general concept led to "soft" beta blockers as safe antiglaucoma agents, "soft" anticholinergics as short-acting mydriatics, and "soft" corticosteroids as safe antiinflammatory drugs (41).

Because corticosteroids have severe side effects, the use of soft steroids in the treatment of chronic ocular inflammation is highly desirable. It is reported that a successful application of the "inactive metabolite approach" to develop a locally potent but systemically safe "soft corticosteroid" was achieved. This effort was based on the acidic inactive metabolites formed after metabolic degradation of the 17-β-hydroxyketone side chain, which in the case of hydrocortisone *17* is the corresponding cortienic acid *18*. Appropriate substitution of 17 α-OH and 17β-COOH groups led to some highly potent corticosteroids, which however showed side effects after topical, subcutaneous, or oral administration. Of more than 120 of the soft steroids, 19 have been tested, with varying R_1 and R_2 functions as well as other ring substituents, like R_3, X, Y, and Δ(41) (Figure 6-8). Many of these soft steroids show good activities (Tables 6-6 and 6-7.)

The use of steroids in various allergic and inflammatory conditions is listed in Table 6-5. Steroids are also used to reduce conjunctival and corneal scarring from chemical and thermal injuries.

The effects of various steroidal preparations are essentially similar, differing only in the concentrations required to achieve satisfactory suppression of inflammation. Steroids are also given in combination with cytotoxic an-

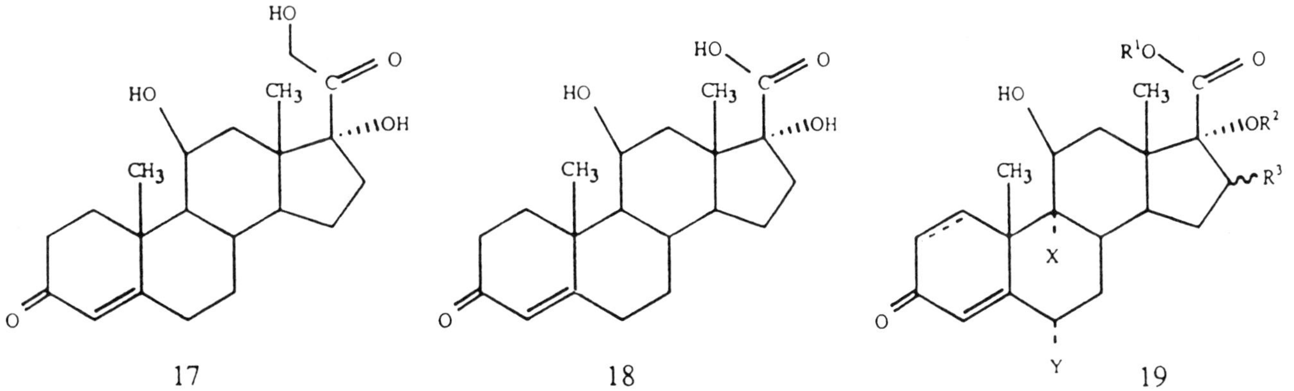

17 18 19

FIG. 6-8. Metabolites of "Soft Steroids."

tibiotics and cytonics, such as azathioprine. This approach avoids the steroidal side effects and achieves better control with a lower dosage (41).

Corticosteroid therapy has not proved beneficial in diseases like senile macular degeneration, cataracts, keratoconjunctivitis sicca, and corneal dystrophy, as well as in old inactive chorioretinitis (36). Band keratopathy, traumatic corneal scars, or old scars are not affected by these drugs. Corticosteroids can be used with antibiotics to treat infections and reduce undesirable healing sequelae. It is more important to remember that there is a possibility of relapse and pronounced inflammatory response if steroidal therapy is discontinued or dosage levels are lowered. Additionally, delay in wound healing is possible.

Complications

The side effects of prolonged use of corticosteroids are listed in Table 6-8, and significant ocular complications are discussed in the following sections.

Glaucoma

One of the primary side effects of long-term use of steroids is an increase in intraocular pressure (IOP) (42). McLean, in 1950, reported that corticosteroid therapy might increase IOP. Francois in 1964 reported a "cortisone glaucoma" case history (43). Local cortisone therapy was

TABLE 6-6. *Therapeutic indices of representative "soft steroids"* 19 *as compared to reference steroids*

Compound[a]	ED_{50}[b]	Relative potency[c]	TED_{40}[d]	Relative potency	Therapeutic index
19a					
$R_1=CH_2Cl$; $R_4=CH(CH_3)_2$ $R_3=H$; X=H(360–623)	460	1 (23.9–41.9)	31.0	1/24	24
19b					
$R_1=CH_2Cl$; $R_4=CH(CH_3)_2$ $R_3=H$; X=H; ▲	119 (60–202)	4	16.2 (11.2–23.2)	1/12	48
19c					
$R_1=CH_2Cl$; $R_4=CH_3$ X=F; ▲; $R_3=\alpha$-CH_3	2.38 (1.60–3.78)	202	46.0 (36.0–62.1)	1/36	7270
20					
Hydrocortisone-17-butyrate	4.80 (313–892)	1	1.3 (1.1–1.5)	1	1
21					
Betamethasone-17-valerate	100	5	0.3 (0.24–0.36)	4	1

[a] $R_2=CO_2R_4$ (17α-carbonates).
[b] Anti-inflammatory activity in the cotton pellet granuloma test (grams per pellet).
[c] The ratio of the relative potency for ED_{50} to the relative toxicity TED_{40}; hydrocortisone 17-butyrate *(20)* was chosen arbitrarily as the standard: all values = 1.
[d] Thymus inhibition effect subcutaneously (mg/kg).
ED_{50}, median effective dose; TED, threshold toxicity.

TABLE 6-7. *Human vasoconstrictor activity[a] of selected "soft steroids" and reference compounds*

	Compound structure[c]						Vasoconstrictor activity[b] 2 h			4 h		
Compound	R_1	R_4	R_3	X	Y	▲[1]	0.1%	0.01%	0.001%	0.1%	0.01%	0.001%
19a	CH_2Cl	$CH(CH_3)_2$	H	H	H	-	1.8	1.3	0.1	1.7	1.1	0.3
19d	CH_2Cl	C_2H_5	β-CH_3	F	H	+	1.8	1.6	0.4	1.6	1.5	0.7
19e	CH_2Cl	C_3H_5	H	H	H	-	2.4	2.1	0.6	2.1	1.8	0.6
19f	CH_2Cl	CH_3	H	H	H	+	1.7	1.6	1.0	2.1	2.0	1.4
19g	CH_2F	C_2H_5	α-CH_3	F	H	+	2.3	2.1	0.7	2.4	2.4	1.0
19h	CH_2F	n-C_3H_7	α-CH_3	F	H	+	2.2	2.0	0.7	2.4	2.1	0.8
19i	CH_2Cl	i-C_3H_7	α-CH_3	F	H	+	1.6	1.0	0.4	2.4	1.6	0.8
19j	CH_2Cl	C_2H_6	α-CH_3	H	F	+	2.4	1.8	0.5	2.8	2.4	0.7
22	Clobetasol propionate						2.4			2.7		
21	Betamethasone valerate						2.3	1.9	0.8	2.6	2.4	1.1

[a]Occlusion time of 4 h.
[b]Reading 2 and 4 h after removal of occlusion; scale: 0.3; average of six volunteers.
[c]R_4=CO_2R_2 (17α-carbonates).

In vivo studies demonstrated that LE penetrates the eye and is metabolized readily to the corresponding inactive cortienic acid derivative (30). The lack of intraocular pressure-elevating side effects, together with good pharmacological activity, was also demonstrated in humans. It is evident that the soft steroids offer significant advantages over the conventional steroids, particularly for local/topical use.

applied for 3 years in a patient with vernal conjunctivitis who developed significant visual field loss and elevated IOP. The IOP returned to normal when this therapy was discontinued. A number of reports in the last decade have shown that long-term therapy with steroids may cause glaucoma (36). Although steroids induce glaucoma in some patients, it is not clear whether and why "nonresponders" to the antiinflammatory effects of steroids develop increased IOP from steroid therapy. Some investigators (44,45) attribute this steroid-responsiveness phenomenon to genetic properties; however, the precise genetic relationship between the IOP response to steroids and primary open-angle glaucoma is not clear. Unfortunately, no animal glaucoma model exists to investigate the role and mechanism of steroids in developing primary open-angle glaucoma.

TABLE 6-8. *Toxicity of prolonged corticosteroid treatment*

Acute adrenal insufficiency
Glaucoma
Hypokalemic alkalosis
Immunosuppression
Increased susceptibility to infections like tuberculosis fungal infections and HIV
Myopathy
Nervousness, insomnia, mood changes, psychosis
Osteoporosis
Peptic ulceration and prolonged bleeding
Posterior subcapsular cataracts
Retardation of wound healing and growth
Suppression of pituitary - adrenal axis function

Cataract

Posterior subcapsular cataract (PSC) formation was reported by Oglesby et al. in 1961 as a complication of long-term, high-dosage systemic corticosteroid therapy (46). This report evaluated 72 patients receiving corticosteroid therapy and 23 control patients with rheumatoid arthritis. During the first year, PSC did not develop but PSC appeared within one to three years in 42% of those treated and in 58% of patients treated for four years or longer. After the first report by Black et al. in 1960 (47), numerous studies and clinical cases demonstrated the risks of developing significant PSC with prolonged therapy (6 months or longer) with high doses ($\geq$10 mg) of corticosteroids (48–51).

Steroid-induced PSC may be reversible, especially in younger patients (52,53). It is not yet understood, however, whether PSC was induced by direct steroid action or in association with inflammation and other complex chemical mediators. Recent developments in research using experimental cataract models have begun to shed some light on steroid-induced PSC. Specific glucocorticoid receptors have been identified in lens epithelium (50). Becker and Cotlier in 1965 reported that steroids can alter transport mechanisms in lens tissue, and Tamada et al. in 1980 demonstrated that these drugs in high doses affect phospholipid metabolism in experimental animals (54,55). An enzymatic degradation of cortisol in lens was also demonstrated (56,57). The direct relationship between high-dose steroidal therapy and cataractogenesis in experimental animal models is rather complex. In some experiments in rats, rabbits, and chickens, high steroidal doses administered systemically did not cause cataracts (58); topically applied steroids given three times daily for 6 months caused anterior subcapsular opacities in 50% of the cortisone-treated, in 35% of the hydrocortisone-treated, and in 20% of prednisolone-treated rabbits (58). Cataracts were present in one-third of mouse fetuses on the 18th day of gestation after maternal subcutaneous injection of 1 mg of hydrocortisone acetate on the ninth or tenth day of gestation. Like steroid-induced glaucoma, there is no direct evidence indicating that steroids directly cause PSC. Inflammatory disease (i.e., various chemical mediators), the aging process, and other complex factors may also play a role in this process. Again, it is not clear why some patients were prone to develop PSC after steroid therapy.

CONCLUSION

Corticosteroids are the best, and often the only, choice of treatment for various inflammatory diseases. The greater potency of these drugs compared with other classes of compounds can be explained from recent developments in steroid research. Steroids have multiple actions. They inhibit the synthesis, release, and action of several potent chemical mediators after inflammatory stimuli; thus, steroids may cause dangerous side effects, probably through actions of a similar nature. In the future, it is essential to isolate and identify the relationship between different chemical mediators and inflammatory responses. Further studies will be helpful in the design and development of specific drugs that are likely to give beneficial effects without severe steroid side effects.

ACKNOWLEDGMENTS

Preparation of this communication was supported by an unrestricted grant from Research to Prevent Blindness, Inc., from the Kentucky Lions Eye Foundation, Louisville, Kentucky. I thank Ms. Sandy Neuman for secretarial assistance.

REFERENCES

1. Addison T. *On the Constitutional and Local Effect of Disease of the Suprarenal Capsules.* London: Samuel Highley, 1855.
2. Brown-Sequard CE. Recherches experimentales sur a physiologie et la pathologie des capsules surrenales. *CR Acad Sci [D](Paris)* 1856;43:422–425.
3. Harrop GA, Soffer LJ, Ellsworth R, Trescher JH. Studies on the suprarenal cortex. III. Plasma electrolytes and electrolyte excretion during suprarenal insufficiency in the dog. *J Exp Med* 1933; 58:17–38.
4. Loeb RF, Atchley DW, Benedict EM, Leland J. Electrolyte balance studies in adrenalectomized dogs with particular reference to the excretion of sodium. *J Exp Med* 1933;57:775–792.
5. Cori CF, Cori GT. The fate of sugar in the animal body. VII. The carbohydrate metabolism of adrenalectomized rats and mice. *J Biol Chem* 1927;74:473–474.
6. Britton SW, Silvette H. Some effects of cortico-adrenal extract and other substances on adrenalectomized animals. *Am J Physiol* 1931; 99:15–32.
7. Long CNH, Katzin B, Fry EG. Adrenal cortex and carbohydrate metabolism. *Endocrinology* 1940;26:309–344.
8. Swingle WW, Pfiffner JJ. Experiments with an active extract of the suprarenal cortex. *Anat Rec* 1930;44:225–226.
9. Swingle WW, Pfiffner JJ. An aqueous extract of the suprarenal cortex which maintains the life of bilaterally adrenalectomized cats. *Science* 1930;71:321–322.
10. Hartman EF, Brownell KA, Hartman WE. A further study of the hormone of the adrenal cortex. *Am J Physiol* 1930;95:670–680.
11. Reichstin T, Shoppee CW. The hormones of the adrenal cortex. *Vitam Horm* 1943;1:346–413.
12. Tait JF, Simpson SA, Grundy HM. The effect of adrenal extract on mineral metabolism. *Lancet* 1952;1:122–124.
13. Simpson SA, Tait JF, Wettstein A, Neher R, Euw JV, Schindler O, Reichstein T. Konstitution des aldosterones des nuen mineralocorticoids. *Experientia* 1954;10:132–133.
14. Collip JB, Anderson EM, Thompson DL. The adrenotropic hormone of the anterior pituitary lobe. *Lancet* 1933;2:347–348.
15. Evans HM. Present position of our knowledge of anterior pituitary function. *JAMA* 1933;101:425–432.
16. Houssay BA, Biosotti A, Mazzoco P, Sammartino R. Accion del extracto antero-hipofisaro sobre las glandulas adrenales. *Rev Soc Argent Biol* 1933;9:262–268.
17. Li CH, Evans HM, Simpson ME. Adrenocorticotropic hormone. *J Biol Chem* 1943;149:413–424.
18. Sayer G, White A, Long CNH. Preparation and properties of pituitary adrenotropic hormone. *J Biol Chem* 1943;149:425–436.
19. Astwood EB, Raben MS, Payne RW. Chemistry of corticotrophin. *Recent Prog Horm Res* 1957;7:1–57.
20. Bell PH, Howard KS, Shepherd RG, Finn BM, Mesisenhelder. Studies with corticotropin II. Pepsin degradation of β-corticotropin. *J Am Chem Soc* 1956;78:5059–5066.
21. Olson JA, Steffenson EH, Smith RW, Margulis RR, Whitney EL. Use of adrenocorticotropic hormone and cortisone in ocular disease. *Arch Ophthalmol* 1950;45:274–300.
22. Woods AC. Clinical and experimental observation on the use of ACTH and cortisone in ocular inflammatory disease. *Am J Ophthalmol* 1950;333:1325–1349.
23. Gordon DM, McLean JM. Effects of pituitary adrenocorticotropic hormone (ACTH) therapy in ophthalmologic conditions. *JAMA* 1950;142:1271–1276.
24. Meyers FH, Jawetz E, Goldfein A. The adrenocortical steroids. In: Meyers FH, Jawetz E, Goldfein A, eds. *Review of Medical Pharmacology.* Los Altos, CA: Lange, 1950;353–370.
25. Ashton N, Cook C. Effects of cortisone on healing of corneal wounds. *Br J Ophthalmol* 1951;35:708–717.
26. Ohia E, Kulkarni PS. Corticosteroids and immunosuppressive agents in rabbit heterolamellar corneal transplant model. *Agents Actions Suppl* 1991;16:164–168.
27. Ohia EK, Mancino M, Kulkarni PS. Effects of steroids and immunosuppressive drugs on endotoxin-uveitis in rabbits. *J Ocular Pharmacol* 1992;8:295–307.
28. Williams GH, Dluhy RG, Thorn GW. Diseases of the adrenal cortex. In: Isselbacher KJ, Adams RD, Braunwald E, Peterdorf RG, Wilson JD, eds. *Harrison's principles of internal medicine,* 9th ed. New York: McGraw-Hill, 1980;1734–1750.
29. Dluhy RG, Newmark SR, Lauler DO, Thorn GW. Pharmacology and chemistry of adrenal glucocorticoids. In: Azarnoff D, ed. *Steroid Therapy.* Philadelphia: WB Saunders, 1975;1–21.
30. Barnes PJ, Adcock I. Anti-inflammatory actions of steroids: molecular mechanisms. *Trends Pharmacol Sci* 1993;172:436–441.
31. Ballard PL. Delivery and transport of glucocorticoids to target cells. In: Baxter JD, Rousseau GG, eds. *Glucocorticoid Hormone Action.* Berlin: Springer, 1979;25–30.
32. Hull DS, Hine JE, Edelhauser HF, Hyndiuk RA. Permeability of the isolated rabbit cornea to corticosteroids. *Invest Ophthalmol Vis Sci* 1974;13:457–459.
33. Cope CL. Metabolic breakdown. In: Cope CL, ed. *Adrenal Steroids and Disease,* 2nd ed. Philadelphia: Lippincott, 1972;80.
34. Vrmeulen A. The metabolism of 4-14 C prednisolone. *J Endocrinol* 1959;18:278–291.

35. Florini JR, Smith LL, Buyske DA. Metabolic fate of a synthetic corticosteroid (triamcinolone) in the dog. *J Biol Chem* 1961;236:1038–1042.
36. Polanski JR, Weinreb RN. Anti-inflammatory agents steroids as anti-inflammatory agents. In: Sears ML, ed. *Pharmacology of the Eye.* Berlin: Springer-Verlag, 1984;459–538.
37. Sugar J, Burde RM, Sugar A, Waltman SR, Kripalani KJ, Weliky I, Becker B. Tetrahydrotriamcinolone and triamcinolone I. Ocular penetration. *Invest Ophthalmol Vis Sci* 1972;11:890–893.
38. Garzon P, Delgado-Partida P, Gallegos AJ. Progesterone metabolism by human cornea. *J Steroid Biochem* 1976;7:377–379.
39. Gallegos AJ, Delgado-Partida P, Garzon P. The presence of 6-steroid hydroxylase in human cornea. *J Steroid Biochem* 1979;7:135–137.
40. Tano Y, Chandler D, Machemer R. Treatment of intraocular proliferation with intravitreal injection of triamicinolone acetonide. *Am J Ophthalmol* 1980;90:810–816.
41. Bodor N. Designing softer ophthalmic drugs by soft drug approaches. *J Ocul Pharmacol Ther* 1994;10:3–15.
42. McLean JM. Clinical and experimental observation on the use of ACTH and cortisone in ocular inflammatory disease. *Trans Am Ophthalmol Soc* 1950;48:259.
43. Francois J. Cortisone et tension oculaire. *Am Oculistique* 1954;187: 805–876.
44. Becker B. Intraocular pressure response to topical corticosteroids. *Invest Ophthalmol Vis Sci* 1965;4:198–205.
45. Armaly MF. Statistical attributes of the steroid hypertensive response in the clinically normal eye. *Invest Ophthalmol Vis Sci* 1965;71:636–644.
46. Oglesby RB, Black RL, von Sallman L, Bunim JJ. Cataract in rheumatoid arthritis patients treated with corticosteroids. *Arch Ophthalmol* 1961;66:519–523.
47. Black RL, Oglesby RB, von Sallman L, Bunim JJ. Posterior subcapsular cataracts induced by corticosteroids in patients with rheumatoid arthritis. *JAMA* 1960;174:150–171.
48. Spaeth GL, von Sallman L. Corticosteroids and cataracts. In: Schwartz B, ed. *Corticosteroids and the Eye.* Boston: Little Brown, 1966;915.
49. Yablonski ME, Burde RM, Kolker AE, Becker B. Cataract induced by topical dexamethasone in diabetics. *Arch Ophthalmol* 1978;96:474–476.
50. Southern AL, Gordon GG, Yeh HS, Dunn MW, Weinstein BI. Receptors for glucocorticoids in the lens epithelium of the calf. *Science* 1977;200:1177–1178.
51. Donshik PC, Cavanaugh HD, Boruchoff SA, Dohlman CH. Posterior subcapsular cataract induced by corticosteroids following keratoplasty for keratoconus. *Ann Ophthalmol* 1981;13:29–32.
52. Forman AR, Loreto JA, Tina LV. Reversibility of corticosteroid-associated cataracts in children with the nephrotic syndrome. *Am J Ophthalmol* 1977;84:75–78.
53. Rookin AR, Lampert SI, Jaeger EA, McGeady SJ, Mansmann HC. Posterior subcapsular cataracts in steroid-requiring asthmatic children. *Allergy* 1979;63:383–386.
54. Becker B, Cotlier E. Topical corticosteroids and galactose cataracts. *Invest Ophthalmol Vis Sci* 1965;4:806–814.
55. Tamada Y, Miyashita H, Ono S. Studies on phospholipid metabolism of rabbit lens with special reference to long-term topical administration of steroid. *Jpn J Ophthalmol* 1980;24:289–296.
56. Ono S, Hirano H, Obara K. Degradation of the side chain of cortisol by lens homogenate. *Tohoku J Exp Med* 1971;104:171–174.
57. Southern AL, Altman K, Vittek J, Boniuk V, Gordon GG. Steroid metabolism in ocular tissues of the rabbit. *Invest Ophthalmol Vis Sci* 1976;15:222–228.
58. Bettman JW, Fund WE, Webster RG, Noyes PP, Vincent NJ. Cataractogenic effect of corticosteroids on animals. *Am J Ophthalmol* 1967; 63:841–844.

Textbook of Ocular Pharmacology,
edited by T.J. Zimmerman, et al.
Lippincott–Raven Publishers, Philadelphia © 1997.

CHAPTER 7

Adrenergic Pharmacology of the Anterior Segment

David E. Potter and Gary D. Novack

Adrenergic regulation of ocular function has been studied intensely because of the ability of the sympathoadrenal (*sympathetic* nervous) system to influence aqueous humor dynamics, pupil diameter, and ocular blood flow. Adrenergic drugs affecting function of beta (β)- and alpha $(\alpha)_2$-adrenoceptors have proved useful clinically in lowering the elevated intraocular pressure that often accompanies primary open-angle glaucoma. Likewise, drugs affecting α_1-adrenoceptors have found their primary use in modifying iris function. Although most attention has focused on the action of adrenergic drugs at postjunctional (*effector*) sites in the eye, some agents modify activity at prejunctional (*neuronal*) sites as well. Studies on the role(s) of adrenoceptors in altering circadian rhythm of intraocular pressure and the advent of the clinical use of α_2-agonists in treating glaucoma have demonstrated the need to enhance the understanding of the modulation of ocular function by adrenoceptors in the central nervous system. More recently, the increased understanding of the molecular biology of adrenoceptors and their signal transduction pathways has provided new tools for evaluating adrenoceptor regulation and responsiveness in the eye. This chapter provides an overview of the basic pharmacodynamics of adrenergic drugs in the anterior segment of the eye, recent advances in this area, and avenues for future research.

PHYSIOLOGICAL ASPECTS OF SYMPATHOADRENAL FUNCTION

Because all phases of the physiologic disposition of catecholamines can be affected by drugs, a brief review of biosynthesis, storage, and release and metabolism is described below.

Biosynthesis of Catecholamines

Several enzymatic steps are involved in the biosynthesis of norepinephrine from tyrosine, with an additional step (*methylation*) in the adrenal medulla for the synthesis of epinephrine. As shown in Fig. 7-1 (step 1), the rate-limiting step in catecholamine synthesis involves the conversion of tyrosine to dopa and is carried out by tyrosine hydroxylase. The activity of this enzyme provides critical control of catecholamine biosynthesis in that it is subject to inhibition by the end product. This biosynthetic step is important pharmacologically because it can be inhibited by certain agents (such as ***a-methyl-p-tyrosine***) that cause a significant decrease in norepinephrine biosynthesis. Inhibition of tyrosine hydroxylase or of enzymes that degrade catecholamines (monoamine oxidase, MAO) can force synthesis toward alternate pathways, resulting in the synthesis of other "substitute transmitter" amines, such as octopamine. Recently, it was suggested that octopamine may be an endogenous ligand for beta (β_3)-adrenoceptors (1).

In mammals, norepinephrine is the major catecholamine biosynthesized in fetal life, being secreted by the organ of Zuckerkandl and by paraganglia. In the neonatal period and afterwards, epinephrine production by the adrenal medulla increases gradually and is secreted along with norepinephrine, the principal biogenic amine of sympathetic neurons.

Storage and Release of Catecholamines

The catecholamine neurotransmitters, norepinephrine and, to a lesser extent, dopamine, are stored in dense-core vesicles located within the highly branched nerve termi-

D. E. Potter: Department of Pharmacology/Toxicology, Morehouse School of Medicine, Atlanta, Georgia 30310.
G. D. Novack: Pharmacologic Development, Inc., San Rafael, California 94903.

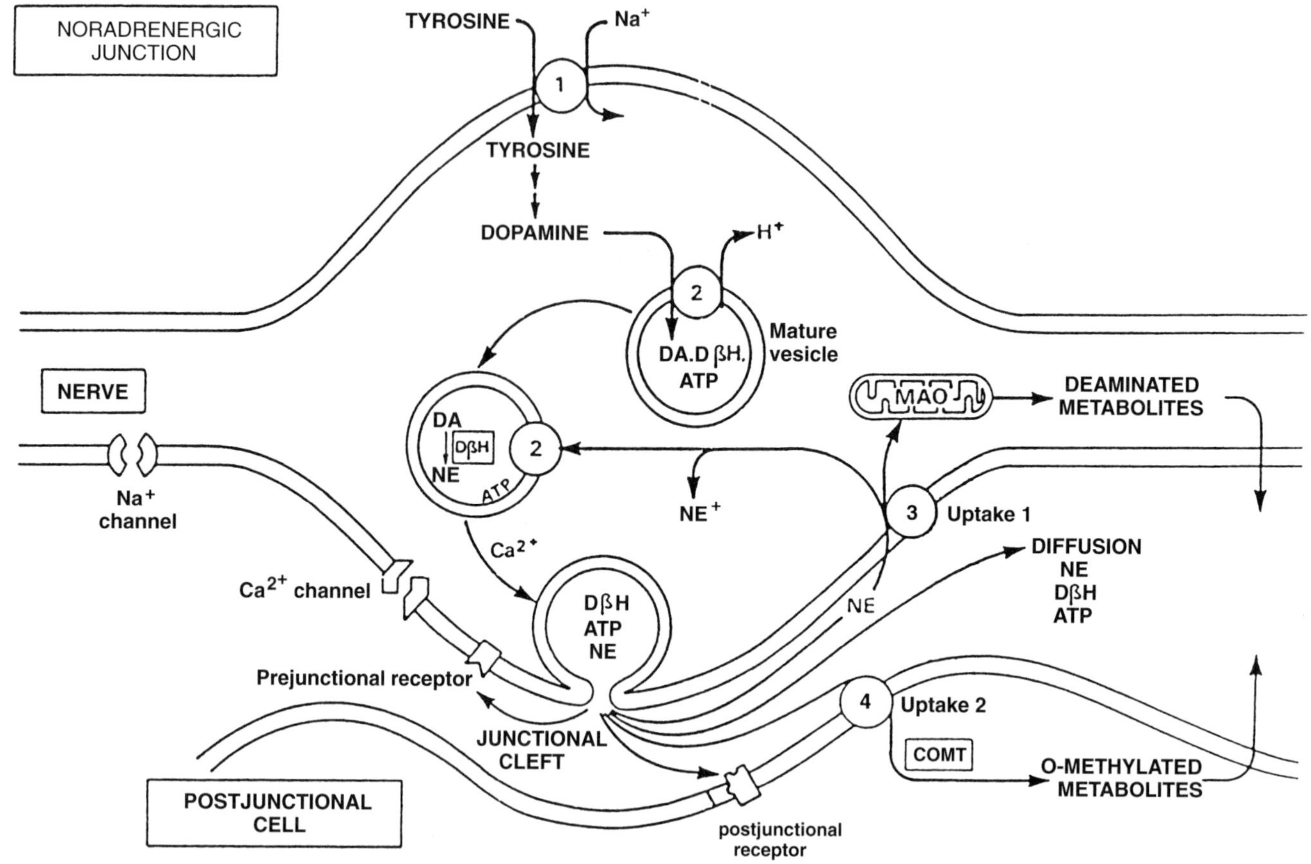

FIG. 7-1. Schematic diagram of the neuroeffector junction of the peripheral sympathetic nervous system. The nerves terminate in complex networks with varicosities or enlargements that form synaptic junctions with effector cells. Some of the processes occurring in the noradrenergic varicosity are analogous to those in cholinergic terminals, e.g., new vesicle formation in the varicosity. Tyrosine is transported into the noradrenergic varicosity by carrier (*1*) that is linked to sodium uptake. Tyrosine is hydroxylated to dopa and then decarboxylated to form dopamine (*DA*) in the cytoplasm. Dopamine is transported into the vesicle by a carrier mechanism (*2*) that can be blocked by reserpine. The same carrier transports norepinephrine (*NE*) and several other amines into these granules. Dopamine is converted to norepinephrine through the catalytic action of dopamine-β-hydroxylase (*DβH*). ATP is also present in high concentration in the vesicle. Release of transmitter occurs when an action potential is conducted to the varicosity by the action of voltage-sensitive sodium channels. Depolarization of the varicosity membrane opens voltage-sensitive calcium channels and results in an increase in intracellular calcium. The elevated calcium facilitates exocytotic fusion of vesicles with the surface membrane and expulsion of norepinephrine, ATP, and some of the dopamine-β-hydroxylase. Release is blocked by drugs such as guanethidine and bretylium. Norepinephrine reaching either pre- or postjunctional receptors modifies the function of the corresponding cells. Norepinephrine also diffuses out of the cleft, or it may be transported into the cytoplasm of the varicosity (uptake 1 [*3*], blocked by cocaine, tricyclic antidepressants) or into the postjunctional cell (uptake 2 [*4*]). The nonvesicular norepinephrine, shown schematically as *NE**, can be released by tyramine and a variety of the other indirectly acting adrenergic agonists.

nals. In the adrenal medulla, catecholamines (epinephrine, norepinephrine) are stored in chromaffin granules, which contain catecholamines complexed to adenosine triphosphate (ATP), dopamine β-hydroxylase, and at least eight species of proteins known as *chromogranins.* Neuropeptides, including neuropeptide Y and enkephalin, are synthesized, stored, and coreleased with norepinephrine and epinephrine. The storage of catecholamines in vesicles or chromaffin granules serves two purposes: (a) sequestration in an inactivated state and (b) protection from degradative enzymes (MAO) located in the mitochondria. Certain drugs (e.g., guanethidine and reserpine) can interfere with the storage of catecholamines (Fig. 7-1, step 2) and therefore have been tried in treating glaucoma, the rationale for catecholamine depletion being the production of supersensitivity at the postjunctional adrenoceptors.

The discharge of catecholamines from sympathetic nerve endings and chromaffin cells of the adrenal medulla following nerve stimulation is Ca^{2+} dependent and occurs by the process of *exocytosis.* The release of catecholamines occurs at lower frequencies of nerve stimulation, whereas higher frequencies are required for the corelease of neuropeptides. The exocytotic release of catecholamines by the action potential requires Ca^{2+} and an intact microtubular system. Release of norepinephrine from sympathetic neurons can be evoked not only by reflexively generated neuronal activity but also by indirectly acting sympathomimetic amines (tyramine, ephedrine, and amphetamine), ganglionic stimulants (e.g., nicotine), and α_2-adrenoceptor antagonists (e.g., rauwolscine). Drugs that have a negative influence on norepinephrine release include agents that alter biosynthesis (α-methyl tyrosine), storage (reserpine), and release (guanethidine) and those that activate prejunctional receptors: α_2 (clonidine), DA_2 (bromocriptine), muscarinic (carbachol), opioidergic (bremazocine), or adenosinergic (N_6-cyclohexyladenosine).

Termination of Catecholamine Activity

Several mechanisms are responsible for the termination of catecholamine action (Fig. 7-1, steps 3 and 4), including: (a) *reuptake* by the nerve terminals (Uptake-1); (b) uptake by postjunctional (*nonneuronal*) cells (Uptake-2); (c) *metabolism by enzymes,* 0-methylation extracellularly (catechol-0-methyl transferase, COMT) or oxidative deamination intracellularly (MAO); and (d) *physical removal* from the site of action by diffusion. The predominant mechanism for inactivation of endogenous catecholamine neurotransmitters is *reuptake,* however. The existence of an uptake process for catecholamines in sympathetic nerve terminals is of considerable importance in understanding the mechanism of certain drugs (e.g., cocaine, imipramine) that interact with adrenergic neurons in the peripheral nervous system and in the brain.

Both MAO-A and MAO-B have been identified in the iris-ciliary body and superior cervical ganglion of the rabbit (2). Inhibition of COMT has been reported to potentiate the pupillary and intraocular pressure (IOP) effects of topical epinephrine (3). Overall, blacks have significantly higher COMT activity than whites (4). Preliminary data suggest that Asians may also have higher COMT activity than whites. It is not clear whether these purported differences in COMT among genetically diverse groups account for alterations in the disposition of topically applied catecholamines.

The principal metabolites of catecholamine degradation by MAO and COMT are homovanillic acid for dopamine and vanillylmandelic acid for norepinephrine and epinephrine. Drugs that alter physiological reuptake can influence the relative amounts of the catecholamine available to adrenoceptors and also can result in changes in the quantities of metabolites that are formed.

Regulation of Catecholamine Turnover

Catecholamines are in a constant state of flux (*turnover*); they are continuously synthesized, released, reuptaken, and metabolized. Under normal circumstances, the tissue and fluid levels of catecholamines remain at a fairly steady level; however, both rapid and slow mechanisms exist for altering the rate of catecholamine turnover. A rapid regulatory mechanism for controlling sympathetic nerve activity involves a negative feedback receptor mechanism located prejunctionally. With neuronal firing, the concentration of norepinephrine becomes elevated in the neuroeffector junction, and the prejunctional α_2-adrenergic receptor (*autoreceptor*) is stimulated, which in turn inhibits further release of norepinephrine from nerves (Fig. 7-2). The co-release of opioid peptides and adenosine from sympathetic nerves may also help to limit the release of norepinephrine at higher frequencies of stimulation.

Tyrosine hydroxylase activity is markedly influenced by the rate of neuronal firing. With rapidly firing nerves, the activity of tyrosine hydroxylase increases. When nerve

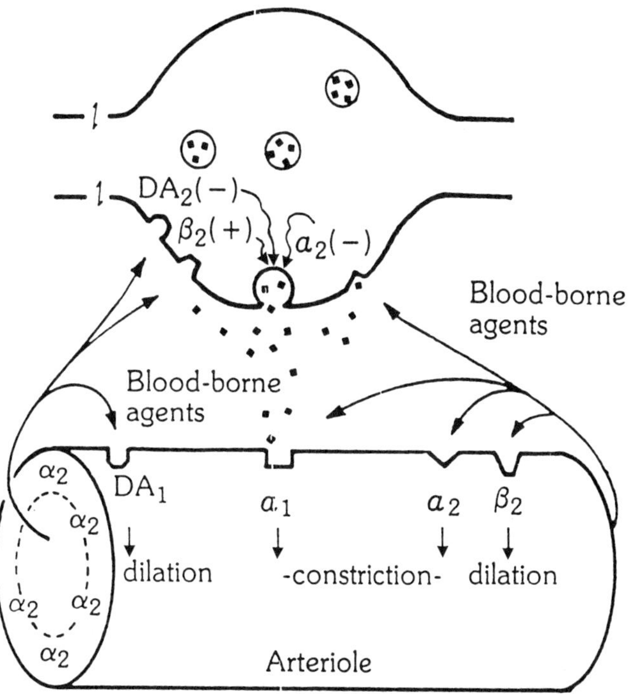

FIG. 7-2. The location of adrenoceptors at a noradrenergic neuroeffector junction. Blood-borne agents are indicated by long solid lines. Prejunctional modulation of neuronal function by blood-borne agents and norepinephrine is indicated by wavy lines within the noradrenergic nerve ending. Stimulation of α_2 and DA_2 adrenoceptors inhibits norepinephrine release, whereas stimulation of β_2 adrenoceptors enhances the release of norepinephrine. Postjunctional DA_1, α_2, and β_2 adrenoceptors are considered to be noninnervated, whereas α_1 and β_1 are innervated receptors. At the present time, dopamine receptors are considered to be of pharmacologic rather than physiologic significance.

activity is protracted, the level of cytoplasmic catecholamines becomes elevated, and tyrosine hydroxylase activity is suppressed by negative feedback. A slower control mechanism of catecholamine turnover involves the synthesis of tyrosine hydroxylase. For example, certain drugs and conditions involving stress can increase the firing of sympathetic nerves, which results in the de novo synthesis of tyrosine hydroxylase; this regulatory process is relatively slow in onset and is usually manifested only after many hours of nerve activity.

Characterization of Endogenous Catecholamines

Norepinephrine: A Neural Transmitter

Norepinephrine is active on α- (α_1, α_2) and β- (β_1, β_3) adrenoceptors. Release of norepinephrine from sympathetic nerve endings in the arterioles is one of the principal means of altering peripheral vascular resistance and thus changing systemic blood pressure and regional blood flow to various parts of the eye. It is important to note that the control of peripheral resistance in arterioles and capacitance in veins is largely a function of the sympathetic nervous system; this is principally an *α-adrenoreceptor function* in most vascular beds, including those serving the choroid of the eye. A sympathetically induced increase in pupil diameter can be produced by neurally released norepinephrine, by circulating epinephrine released from the adrenal medulla, or by topically administered drugs: directly acting (e.g., phenylephrine), and indirectly acting (e.g., hydroxyamphetamine) α_1-agonists, α_2 receptor antagonists (e.g., yohimbine), and reuptake inhibitors (e.g., cocaine). In contrast, α_1-antagonists (e.g., thymoxamine) can be used under certain circumstances to reduce pupil diameter. Thus, norepinephrine plays an important role in regulating ocular blood flow, aqueous humor formation, and iris function. In addition, norepinephrine is also found in the retina, where it serves a neurotransmitter role.

Dopamine: A Neural Transmitter

Dopamine is the immediate precursor of norepinephrine and therefore is found in the peripheral sympathoadrenal system (sympathetic nerves, ganglionic interneurons, adrenal glands) and in specific regions of the brain. Moreover, dopamine exerts important neurotransmitter functions in the retina. Systemically, the effects of dopamine differ from those of norepinephrine in that dopamine exerts dose-related vasodilation in the renal and mesenteric vascular beds. This response is selectively inhibited by antagonists (SCH23390) that are specific vascular dopaminergic (DA_1) receptors. Under special circumstances, dopamine can interact with prejunctional (DA_2, α_2) receptors on sympathetic nerve endings, resulting in an inhibition of norepinephrine release; however, this effect generally requires the presence of a neuronal (uptake-1) inhibitor to prevent dopamine's entry into nerves. Part of dopamine's action on adrenoceptors (β_1, α_1, α_2) is mediated indirectly, being produced by release of norepinephrine. Therefore, dopamine's pharmacological effects can be quite nonselective and are highly dose dependent.

Dopamine administered topically to animals produces a biphasic response in intraocular pressure. Synthetic DA_2 agonists (e.g., bromocriptine), given topically or orally, have been reported to lower intraocular pressure in laboratory animals and humans (5–7). In contrast, DA_1 receptor agonists (e.g., fenoldopam) given intravenously elevate IOP in human subjects (8), and this procedure has been proposed as a diagnostic test for glaucoma. Dopamine agonists have been demonstrated to prevent the development of myopia in laboratory animal models.

Epinephrine: A Neurohormone

Epinephrine is synthesized and released from chromaffin cells in the adrenal medulla into the circulation, thereby functioning primarily as a circulating neurohormone; however, it is synthesized by neurons in the brain and retina of various species, and any state of stress (e.g., pain, cold, hypotension, hypoxia, hypoglycemia, anxiety) triggers the release of epinephrine from the adrenal gland. The primary effect of epinephrine on cardiovascular and metabolic organs is to prepare the subject for an immediate increased level of physical activity, the "fight or flight" phenomenon. It is also important to recognize that the tissue effects of epinephrine are the combined result of interactions with α- (α_1, α_2) and β- (β_1, β_2, β_3) adrenoceptors and therefore augment the actions of neurally released norepinephrine. In times of physical activity, epinephrine shunts blood away from the skin and viscera (α_1-adrenergic effect augmented by norepinephrine) toward skeletal muscle (β_2 adrenergic effect), where it is needed, that is, constricting some vascular beds while dilating others. The actions of epinephrine are often complex but predictable if the predominant adrenoceptor population within an organ system and the dose administered are considered. For example, epinephrine tends to have greater activity on β-receptors at *low doses* and can decrease peripheral resistance principally by dilating arterioles in skeletal muscle while increasing heart rate and contractility. At *intermediate* and *high doses,* epinephrine activates both α- and β-adrenoceptors.

For a number of years, epinephrine has been used in the chronic therapy of open-angle glaucoma and in the diagnosis of Horner's syndrome. Epinephrine, like norepinephrine, acts on α-adrenoceptors on the radial muscle of the iris to produce mydriasis. The acute use of α_1-agonists in subthreshold doses in suspected Horner's patients is based on the concept of denervation supersensitivity. The chronic effect of topically administered epinephrine in lowering

IOP in glaucoma is believed to be due to an enhanced outflow of aqueous humor that involves β-adrenoceptors (9); however, some of the effects on aqueous flow could be the product of interactions with α_2-adrenergic receptors. Thus, the specific details of the cellular action of epinephrine on inflow and outflow mechanisms are understood incompletely. For example, in the outflow tract, the peak elevation of tissue cyclic adenosine monophosphate (cAMP) levels occurs much earlier (i.e., by hour) than the late-onset increase in outflow facility (10), and this asynchrony raises the possibility that other signal transduction pathways are involved in the actions of epinephrine.

SITE OF ACTION: ADRENOCEPTORS

Approaches to Adrenoceptor Classification

Three basic approaches have been used to characterize adrenoceptors: (a) functional indices, such as agonist potencies and inhibition of agonist action by antagonists (11); (b) affinity of the receptor for a drug as determined by competitive binding with a radioactively labeled ligand; and (c) molecular cloning of adrenoceptor cDNAs or genes. Recently, genetic analysis has provided additional molecular description and subtyping of adrenoceptors (12).

Historically, the classification of adrenoceptors by the use of rank-order potencies of agonists was remarkably successful, but, retrospectively, this method is now recognized to present problems because of (a) multiple events involved in the agonist-adrenoceptor interaction (binding and activation of receptors coupled to a variety of G proteins); (b) the use of naturally occurring catecholamines or other agonists that are inherently nonselective, thereby affecting multiple receptor subtypes simultaneously that may be inhibitory or stimulatory; and (c) the existence, in most tissues, of "spare receptors," which means that only a small number of receptors need to be occupied to produce a maximal response.

In contrast, the classification of adrenoceptors with antagonists is more reliable because (a) the agents are usually specific for a receptor class (α or β) if not selective for an adrenoceptor subtype (α_1, α_2, β_1, β_2); (b) the attainment of equilibrium is readily achievable with antagonists because of dependence on only one parameter of the ligand-receptor interaction (i.e., affinity), and therefore the kinetics of the interaction follow the law of mass action; and (c) an affinity constant (pA_2) for an antagonist can be calculated readily and will show reasonable consistency among a variety of tissues.

Ideally, both functional and radioligand binding assays should be used to classify receptor subtypes. Without evidence of functional (i.e., biochemical or physiological) indices, radioligand studies merely identify binding sites. Nevertheless, radioligands can be used in two paradigms to aid in defining receptor subtypes. In one type of assay, a ligand that is highly selective for a receptor subtype is used. In another scheme, a nonselective antagonist can be used to label a general class of receptors, and another ligand that has high selectivity for a particular receptor subtype can be used in a competitive fashion. In both types of binding assays, pharmacokinetic issues can be avoided by using isolated membranes instead of tissues.

In binding studies, agonists are of more limited use in classifying receptors in that the condition of the binding site with which the agonist associates is the high-affinity state. On the other hand, the agonist radioligand may reflect activity at a receptor population that is of greater biological significance. Nevertheless, antagonists continue to be the preferred ligands for binding studies.

Delineation of Adrenoceptor Subtypes

Much of the early work with adrenoceptors for catecholamines was carried out by using functional studies. As originally defined by Ahlquist (11), the *adrenoceptor* was a specific site on postjunctional effector cells, usually smooth muscle, heart, and glands, that allowed the cell to detect and respond to catecholamines and related compounds. In early studies, adrenoceptors were described in terms of the *effector response* to drug application, that is, a measured biochemical or biophysical change initiated by the drug. The distinction between two different populations of adrenergic receptors can be characterized in one of two ways: (a) by differences in agonist activity within a given organ or (b) by suppression of agonist activity with antagonist drugs that compete in a *selective* manner for receptor occupation in an organ. With the implementation of techniques in molecular biology, adrenoceptors can be isolated and their structures determined. Localization of adrenoceptors can be accomplished by many techniques, including autoradiography, selective antibodies, molecular probes, and novel fluorescent antagonists.

Because the terms *excitatory* and *inhibitory* did not always properly describe the adrenergic receptors, the arbitrary terms *alpha* (α) and *beta* (β) were chosen by Ahlquist (11). Thus, to classify an adrenergic drug, one must be prepared to identify the effector system and the receptor classes (e.g., α or β) that are operative within the effector system. In addition to α and β adrenergic receptors, there are also *dopaminergic* (DA) receptors in certain organs, that is, specific sites in effector systems (renal vasculature, nerve endings) that respond more specifically to dopamine than to epinephrine or norepinephrine. Moreover, there are subpopulations of α, DA, and β receptors. For example, increases in myocardial contractility, heart rate, and automaticity are mediated predominantly by β_1-adrenoceptor activation, whereas vasodilation and lactate production in skeletal muscle, bronchial smooth-muscle relaxation, and uterine relaxation are mediated by β_2 receptors. In white and brown adipose tissue, the β_3-adrenoceptor mediates

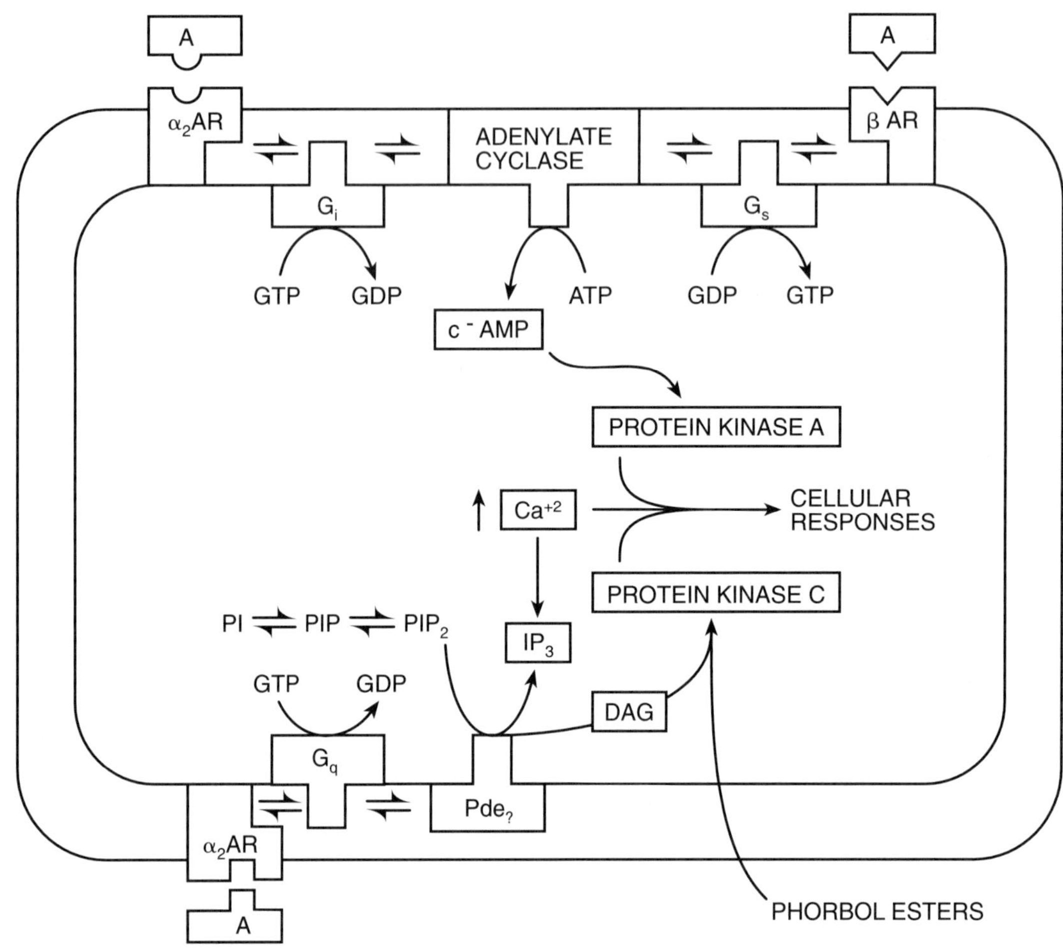

FIG. 7-3. Adenylate cyclase activity.

lipolysis and thermogenesis, respectively. The β_3-adrenoceptors appear to be more resistant to desensitization than other β-receptor subtypes. Postjunctional α_2 and β_2 adrenoceptors are activated more strongly in some tissues by the neurohormone epinephrine than by the neurotransmitter norepinephrine and sometimes are referred to as *extrasynaptic (hormonal) adrenoceptors.*

About 20 years after the adrenoceptor concept was established by Ahlquist (11), it became apparent that the major adrenoceptor classes (α and β) contained subtypes.

Based on a rank-order potency of a series of structurally related β-adrenoceptor agonists in organ experiments, it was suggested at this time that at least two subclasses of β-receptors existed: β_1 and β_2 (13). Subsequently, Langer (14), along with Berthelsen and Pettinger (15), proposed the existence of two functionally distinct α subtypes: α_1 and α_2. Beta-adrenoceptor characterization in tissues of the anterior segment of the eye has been accomplished by techniques such as ligand binding studies (16) and autoradiography (19) as well as by analysis of biochemical parameters, for example, adenylate cyclase activity (17,18) (Figure 7-3). These studies have shown adrenoceptor localization in extraocular muscles, conjunctiva, cornea, lens, iris, trabeculum, and ciliary body. The predominant receptor demonstrated in the anterior segment by these studies has been the β_2-adrenoceptor. Molecular studies indicate the existence of at least three subtypes of β-adrenoceptors in various tissues: β_1, β_2 and β_3. The ligands that have been used to classify and characterize β-adrenoceptors are shown in Table 7-1.

In the 1970s, it became apparent that α-adrenoceptors were not only at postjunctional (effector organ) sites but also could be found on autonomic nerve endings (20). Subsequent studies (15,21,22) have provided additional evidence for the subdivision of α-adrenoceptors on anatomical and functional grounds. Pharmacologically, subtypes of α-adrenoceptors could be distinguished based on their affinities for the antagonists prazosin (α_1) or yohimbine (α_2) (23). Subtypes have been shown to vary in number not only from organ to organ but also among organs from various species (24).

Current evidence suggests that α_1-adrenoceptors are heterogeneous (25). Discrete subtypes were suggested initially based on differing potency of the antagonists prazosin and phenoxybenzamine from in vitro functional studies (26,27). The α-adrenoceptors were shown to have high affinity for radiolabelled ligands such as [^{3}H] prazosin and [^{3}H] WB4101. The α_1-subtypes have also been demonstrated based on inactivation by chloroethylclonidine, with α_{1A}-receptors being insensitive and α_{1B} inactivated. Currently, α_{1A}, α_{1B}, α_{1C}, and α_{1D} adrenoceptors have been defined by pharmacological and recombinant techniques (28). Norepinephrine and epinephrine activate all known α_1-adrenoceptor subtypes. Table 7-1 illustrates the drugs typically used to subclassify α_1-adrenoceptor subtypes. Thus far, no comprehensive, systematic study has been performed to identify α_1- and α_2-adrenoceptor subtypes in various structures of the eye.

Stimulation of α_1-adrenoceptors, which are coupled to G_q proteins, activates phospholipase C, promoting the formation of inositol phosphate (IP) and the release of diacylglycerol (DAG) (29). Inositol triphosphate (IP_3) produces intracellular release of Ca^{2+}, whereas DAG activates protein kinase C (see Fig. 7-3). Some α_1-adrenoceptors influence Ca^{2+} influx into cells via a dihydropyridine-sensitive Ca^{2+} channel (30). The predominant ocular sites where α_1-adrenoceptors have relevance are in the radial muscle of the iris, lacrimal gland, and choroidal blood vessels.

Alpha-2 adrenoceptors have been classified by demonstrating a higher affinity for certain antagonists (rauwolscine, idazoxan) and agonists (clonidine, brimonidine) but a lower affinity for the α_1-adrenoceptor antagonist prazosin (31,32). Subsequently, radioligand binding evidence has been presented for the subclassification of α_2-adrenoceptors α_{2A}, α_{2B}, α_{2C}, and α_{2D}. The partial agonist oxymetazoline and the antagonist BRL44408 can bind relatively selectively to α_{2A}-adrenoceptors. The antagonist prazosin and ARC239 have a high affinity for α_{2B}-adrenoceptors, whereas BAM-1303 has high affinity for α_{2C}. Newer α_2-ligands, [^{3}H]MK-912 and RX821002 (2-methoxy idazoxan), bind to the α_{2D} sites with greater affinity than does rauwolscine.

The endogenous catecholamines norepinephrine and epinephrine seem to display no significant selectivity among the known α_2-adrenoceptor subtypes. Likewise, all subtypes can be inhibited by rauwolscine. In many tissues, including the eye, α_2-adrenoceptors are believed to be coupled to certain enzymes and ion channels through a G_i protein. A second-messenger pathway that appears to be influenced by most α_2-adrenoceptor subtypes is adenylate cyclase, which coupled to an inhibitory-G protein, Gi_2; this pathway, when activated by α_2 agonists, suppresses cAMP generation and the subsequent activation of protein kinase A (see Fig. 7-3). In the ciliary process, stimulation of α_2-adrenoceptors inhibits stimulated levels of cAMP (33), and, if basal activity is high, it may be inhibited as well. Certain α_2-adrenoceptor-mediated responses in the eye are modified by treatment with pertussis toxin, suggesting involvement of a G_i protein (34,35). In addition, α_2-adrenoceptors can be linked to other signal transduction pathways, including K^+ and Ca^{2+} channels, phospholipases C and A_2, as well as the Na^+/H^+exchange system (36).

Because α_2-adrenoceptors are located at both prejunctional (*neuronal*) and postjunctional (*effector organ*) sites in ocular tissues, there are problems differentiating between the prejunctional and the postjunctional actions of drugs in vivo. Interestingly, SKF104078 and SKF104856 produce antagonism of certain postjunctional responses without inhibition of prejunctional (neuronal) α_2-receptors (37). Thus far, subtypes of α_2-adrenoceptors in the anterior segment of the eyes of various species have not been fully characterized at prejunctional and postjunctional sites, although there is preliminary evidence that α_{2A} is the predominant subtype in the ciliary process of the rabbit.

Activation of α_2-adrenoceptors results in depression of aqueous humor flow; for this reason, α_2 agonists (e.g., apraclonidine) have been used in the therapy for glaucoma. Various compounds containing an imidazoline or guanidinium moiety not only interact with α_2-adrenoceptors but also may combine with sites referred to as *imidazoline binding sites.* Radioligand binding and photoaffinity labelling studies indicate that imidazoline binding sites rep-

TABLE 7-1. *The human adrenergic receptors*

	β			α_1[b]			α_2[b]		
	$\beta1$	$\beta2$	$\beta3$	α_{1A}	α_{1B}	α_{1C} (bovine)	α_{2A}	α_{2B}	α_{2C}
Pharmacology									
Potent agonist	Iso > bucindolol, norepi	Clenbuterol, epi ≥ iso	Isoproterenol > norepi, bucindolol	Phenylephrine	Phenylephrine	Phenylephrine	Norepi, epi	Norepi, epi	Norepi, epi
Selective agonist	Xamoterol	Procaterol	CL316,243				Oxymetazoline		
Selective antagonist	CGP20712A	ICI 118551	Bupranolol[c]	5-Methyl urapidil, Prazosin	Prazosin	Prazosin	BRL44408	ARC 239(100)	Prazosin
Mechanism of action	↑ cAMP	↑ cAMP		Ca^{2+} channel	IP_3/DG	IP_3/DG	↓ cAMP, K^+ channel ↑, Ca^{2+} channel ↓	↓ cAMP, Ca^{2+} channel	↓ cAMP
Gene									
Chromosome no.	10	5	8	5	5	8	10	2	4
Existence of introns	No	No	Yes		Yes	Yes	No	No	
Protein structure									
Length	477	413	408	515	517	466	450	451	461
Glycosylation sites (N-terminal)	2	2	2	2	4	3	2	0	2
Phosphorylation sites	PKA, βARK	PKA, βARK	0		PKA	PKA	PKA, βARK		
Prototypic tissue	Heart	Lung	Fat	Artery (renal; rat)	Heart		Platelet, brain		Spleen

From Strosberg, ref 51.

[a]Previous reports mention the existence of additional α_1 (α_{1D}) and α_2 (α_{2D}) subtypes.

[b]Bupranolol is the best β_3 antagonist identified so far, but it is not selective for this subtype.

Epi, epinephrine; norepi, norepinephrine; IP_3, phosphatidyl inositol triphosphate; DG, diacyl glycerol; PKA, protein kinase A; βARK, β-adrenergic receptor kinase (sites predicted on the basis of consensus target sequences). Blanks indicate that no definitive conclusion can be proposed.

resent a heterogeneous group referred to as I_1 and I_2 sites. Significant numbers of I_1 sites are located in the rostroventrolateral medulla of the brain and chromaffin cells of a variety of species. Functional studies in animals suggest that the IOP lowering effect of α_2-agonists (e.g., moxonidiine, brimonidine) may be due, in part, to actions on I_1 sites.

In 1971 Kebabian and Greengard (38) defined two dopamine receptors (D_1 and D_2) based on pharmacological and biochemical criteria: D_1 (DA_1) receptors, which are coupled to a G_s protein, activate adenylate cyclase when stimulated, whereas D_2 (DA_2) receptors are linked to a G_i protein, which causes inhibition of adenylate cyclase activity when activated (39). Subsequently, radioligand binding, functional studies, and receptor cloning have suggested the existence of at least three additional dopaminergic receptors, bringing the total of dopamine receptor subtypes found in the brain to five. Most of the work involving characterization of dopamine receptors has been performed in brain tissues, although dopamine and dopamine receptors have been known for some time to have a significant role in neurotransmission in the retina (40) and are thought to have a prominent role in regulating blood flow to the kidney. Dopamine is the most prominent catecholamine in the retina and is found in relatively high concentrations in amacrine cells of the inner plexiform layer.

Based on the significant role of dopamine and dopamine receptors in the retina, it is not surprising that a similar system might exist in the anterior segment. Limited functional, biochemical, and autoradiographic studies suggest that both DA_1 (41,42) and DA_2 (6) receptors are present in the anterior segment of the eyes of laboratory animals as well as in normal humans and those with glaucoma (43,44). The DA_2 agonists (e.g., pergolide, lergotrile, ciangoline, Ha117, and apomorphine) have been shown to lower IOP in animals. Although it has been assumed that DA_1 and DA_2 receptors in the anterior segment may use pathways similar to those of α- and β-adrenoceptors, the signal transduction pathways coupled to dopamine receptors in the anterior segment of the eye have not been delineated. As alluded to previously, DA_1-receptor effects often are mediated by the adenylate cyclase-cAMP system, where stimulation elevates cAMP levels (45). In the ciliary body of some, but not all, species, DA_1 receptors are positively linked to adenylate cyclase (46). Dopamine receptors, which are present in the nonpigmented ciliary epithelium, are reported to be linked to the activation of an intracellular phosphoprotein, DARPP-32 (47). In contrast, DA_2 receptors are negatively linked to cAMP and ion channels (Ca^{2+}, K^+) through G proteins in the brain and other tissues.

Ligands that are relatively selective for DA_1 receptors include agonists, such as fenoldopam, and antagonists, such as SCH-23390. Relatively selective agonists for DA_2 receptors include bromocriptine, pergolide, and lergotrile, whereas antagonists include sulpiride, remoxipride, and domperidone. In the rabbit iris-ciliary body, DA_2 receptors do not appear to be negatively coupled to adenylate cyclase at postjunctional sites. A functional association of the DA_2 receptor with inhibition of norepinephrine release has been demonstrated in the cat nictitating membrane (48) and rabbit iris-ciliary body (49).

Molecular Aspects of Adrenoceptors: Structure, Function, and Regulation

As demonstrated by a variety of investigations, receptors residing in cell membranes can be classified broadly as (a) receptors that are linked to guanine nucleotide binding (G) proteins, (b) receptors that function as ion channels, and (c) receptors that possess enzyme activity (e.g., tyrosine kinase). Adrenoceptors, through interactions with agonists and their association with G proteins,initiate cellular responses mediated by effector enzymes (e.g., adenylate cyclase, phospholipase C) and ion channels (e.g., Ca^{2+} and K^+ channels) (Fig. 7-3, Table 7-2).

TABLE 7-2. *Probable G protein and effector linkages of adrenoceptors and dopaminoceptors*

Receptor type	G protein[a]	Effectors
α_1	G_q family members(s)	Phospholipase C_β (stimulation) Phospholipase A_2 (stimulation) ? Voltage-sensitive Ca^{2+} channels (stimulation) ? Others
α_2	G_i family members (in particular G_{i2})	Adenylyl cyclase (inhibition) K^+ channels (stimulation) Voltage-sensitive Ca^{2+} channels (inhibition) ? Others
β	G_s	Adenylyl cyclase (stimulation) Voltage-sensitive Ca^{2+} channels (stimulation) ? Na channel (inhibition) ? Others
D_1	G_s	Adenylyl cyclase (inhibition) ? Others
D_2	G_i family members	Adenylyl cyclase (inhibition) Ca^{2+} channels (inhibition) K^+ channels (stimulation) ? Others

[a]These reflect preferred G protein linkages rather than absolute specificities.

As indicated, genomic or cDNA clones have been obtained for numerous adrenoceptors and include three types of α_1 (α_{1A}, α_{1B}, α_{1C}), four types of α_2 (α_{2A}, α_{2B}, α_{2C}, α_{2D}), and three types of β (β_1, β_2, β_3). Biochemical and immunological studies have shown that adrenoceptors are glycoproteins with seven domains that span the cellular membrane (Fig. 7-4). The amino terminus of the adrenoceptor and portions of the spanning domains are extracellular, whereas the carboxyl terminus and remaining portions of the spanning domains are intracellular. Specific amino acids within the extracellular membrane spanning domains serve as ligand binding sites for the amino and hydroxyl groups of the catecholamine structure and for specific moities of subtype specific ligands (50). The most important residue of the adrenoceptor is purported to be aspartate in the transmembrane domain at position 3.1, which is highly conserved in all adrenoceptors known at this time (51).

Adrenoceptors within the membrane form complexes with heterotrimeric G proteins that consist of α, β, and γ subunits. Receptors have a higher affinity for agonists when complexed with their G protein. On occupation of a β-adrenoceptor by an agonist, the Gsα-guanosine triphosphate (GTP) complex dissociates from the receptor and from the β- and γ-subunits, thereby activating adenylate cyclase. In contrast, adrenoceptor antagonists combine with both high- and low-affinity states of the receptor.

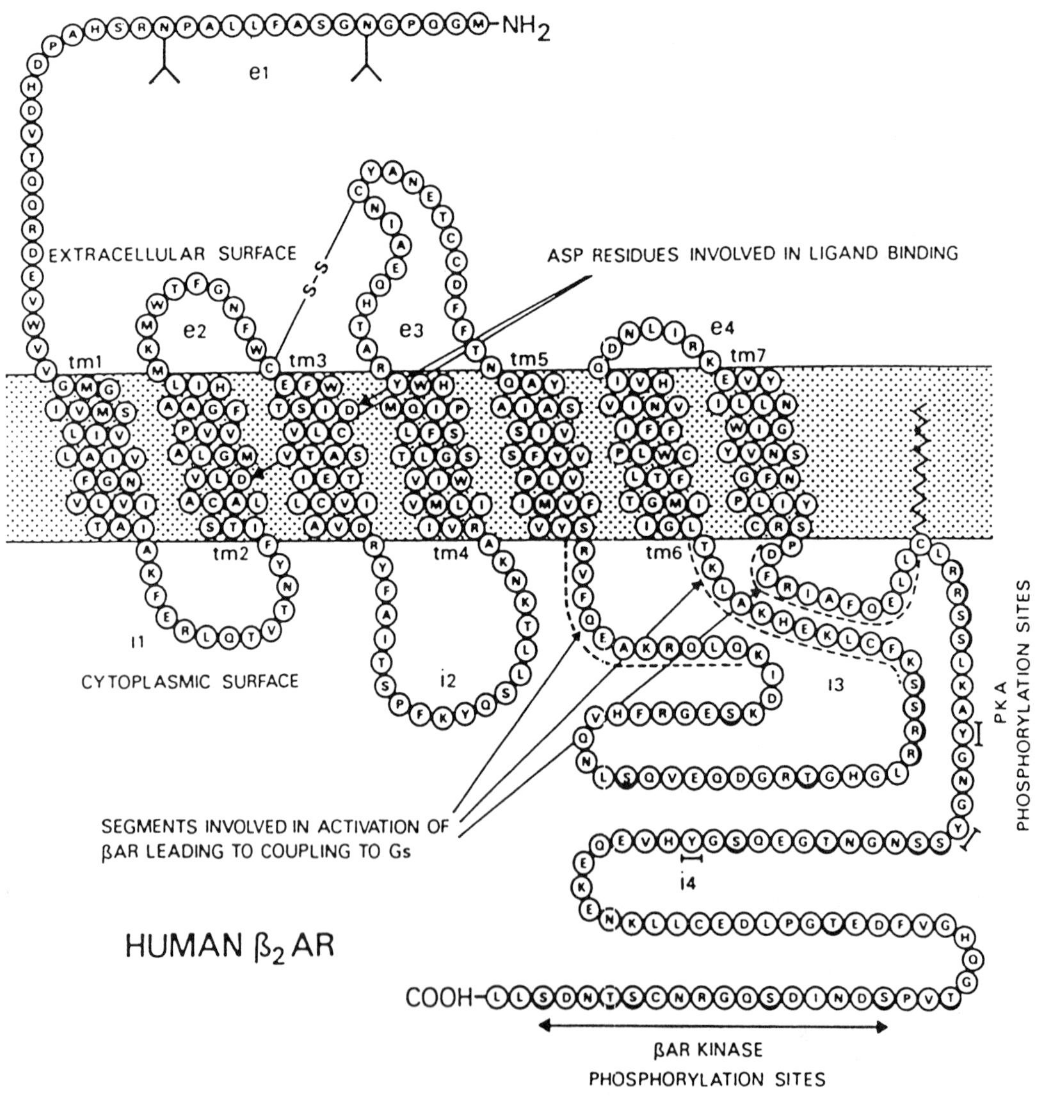

FIG. 7-4. Prototypic model of the human, β_2-adrenergic receptor. The single polypeptide chain is arranged according to the model for rhodopsin. The disulfide bond, essential for activity, linking Cys^{106} and Cys^{184} is represented by -S-S-. The two *N*-glycosylation sites in the amino-terminal portion of the protein are indicated by ⅄. The palmitoylated Cys^{341} residue in the N-terminus of the i4 loop is indicated by ⋀⋀⋀. Potential Ser and Thr phosphorylation sites are underlined. The three Tyr residues found in the i4 of β_2-, but not in β_1- or β_3AR, are indicated by ⊢⊣ (modified from Kobilka et al. [1987]).

Several types of G proteins have been characterized: G_s, G_i proteins (Gi_1, Gi_2, Gi_3) G_o, G_{OLF}, and G_t. The G_s proteins are generally associated with β-adrenoceptors and the activation of adenylate cyclase and Ca^{2+} channels (see Table 7-2). The G_i proteins are often coupled to α_2-adrenoceptors or dopamine (DA_2) receptors or both and inhibit adenylate cyclase activity but activate K^+ channels and phospholipase C and A_2. The G_o proteins are believed to modulate activity of voltage-sensitive Ca^{2+} channels and phospholipase C. G_{OLF} is thought to mediate signal transduction by olfactory receptors in the nasal epithelium, whereas G_t proteins, also known as *transducins,* mediate signal transduction by opsins in the retina.

All β-adrenoceptors (e.g., β_1, β_2, β_3) readily activate G_s (see Table 7-2). Activation of phospholipase C results from stimulation of α_1-adrenoceptors. The ability of the α_2-adrenoceptor to inhibit adenylate cyclase but to stimulate phospholipase C may be due to involvement of more than one type of G protein or the ability of the same G protein subunit to interact with more than one effector system. For example, distinct G proteins are believed to couple α_2-adrenoceptors to potassium (G_i) or to calcium (G_o) channels.

In the ciliary body of the rabbit eye, pertussis toxin will disrupt the usual inhibition of adenylate cyclase by α_2-agonists (34,35). Thus far, the signal transduction mechanisms for dopamine receptors in the anterior segment have received limited attention. In some species, DA_1-receptor activation appears to be coupled to a Gs protein in the ciliary process (46), but no effect on adenylate cyclase has been demonstrated postjunctionally for DA_2 receptors.

The coexistence of several subtypes of α- and β-adrenoceptors in the same cell suggests that regulatory systems for the various receptors must exist at the level of the gene. For example, β_3-specific mRNA may exert a more profound influence in newborns than in adults, but this effect may be related to increased thermogenesis in the newborn, hence the need for greater numbers of brown adipocytes. Evidence indicates that, through positive glucocorticoid-responsive elements, β_2-adrenoceptors can be upregulated, whereas β_1- and β_3-adrenoceptors are suppressed (52). Transcription of β-adrenoceptors also can be regulated by cAMP-responsive elements. Thus, adrenoceptors can be regulated by a variety of means.

Evidence suggests that β_2-adrenoceptors can exist in multiple forms or variants. These polymorphisms may be associated with various disease states and may explain the variability in response to agonists in patients with complex multifactorial diseases, including glaucoma. Thus, the functional consequences of β_2-adrenoceptor polymorphism may account for alterations in the severity of the disease or the response of the disease to drug therapy.

Exposing cells acutely or chronically to catecholamines or other receptor-specific agonists can promote receptor desensitization. *Desensitization* is characterized by a diminishing response despite the continuing presence of an agonist. The process of desensitization can occur rapidly (i.e., within seconds to minutes). Multiple mechanisms are involved in this diminished response, including phosphorylation of the receptor, receptor sequestration, or internalization and catabolism (i.e., downregulation) (Fig. 7-5). Although all adrenoceptors may be subject to desensitization, the mechanisms described for β-adrenoceptors may not be identical to those for α-adrenoceptors.

Adrenoceptor activity can be regulated postsynthetically by phosphorylation involving protein kinase A (PKA) or β-adrenoceptor kinase (β-ARK) (see Figs 7-4 and 7-5). Agonist-induced phosphorylation by PKA can lead to downregulation of receptor mRNA (53). Phosphorylation of β-receptors by an enzyme functionally related to rhodopsin kinase, β-ARK, was thought to be specific, but it is known currently that β-ARK can phosphorylate other receptors, for example, α_{2A}, muscarinic (M_2), and rhodopsin. In contrast to PKA, β-ARK phosphorylates only agonist-occupied receptors (54). In the presence of high agonist concentrations, both kinases can be activated, and their effects are additive (55). The finding that mRNA for β-ARK is highest in tissues amply innervated by sympathetic nerves is consistent with the hypothesis that β-ARK may be important in regulating neural transmission (56). β-ARK-induced phosphorylation does not interfere directly with the activation of G_s, but rather a cytosolic protein, arrestin, disrupts the process (57). The β-arrestins are proteins that bind phosphorylated G-protein-coupled receptors, thereby causing desensitization through an uncoupling of the signal transduction process.

Following exposure to an agonist, receptors can be functionally removed from the plasma membrane by two identifiable processes: sequestration and downregulation. *Sequestration,* that is, the reversible removal of functional receptors from the plasma membrane, is a relatively rapid process that occurs in a matter of minutes. In contrast, downregulation generally occurs more slowly (e.g., after hours of exposure to agonist) because this process involves translocation of the receptor from the membrane to the cytosol and an irreversible loss of receptors by a process that is incompletely understood. In general, exposure to an agonist for several hours is necessary for downregulation (degradation) of receptors to occur, and the event may proceed for a relatively long period (i.e., up to 24 hours). The earliest phase (i.e., the first 4 hours) of downregulation requires PKA-mediated phosphorylation of receptors. The later phase (4–24 hours) does not require phosphorylation but is believed to be due to more rapid degradation of β-adrenoceptor mRNA, which reduces new synthesis of receptors.

Other adrenoceptors can be desensitized by mechanisms similar to those described for β_2-adrenoceptors. For example, β-ARK can phosphorylate α_2-adrenoceptors (58) in an agonist-dependent manner. Protein kinase C is believed to be involved in modulating adrenoceptors linked to phospholipase C, such as α_1 and β_2 adrenoceptors. As with β-adrenoceptors, the relatively rapid process of desensitiza-

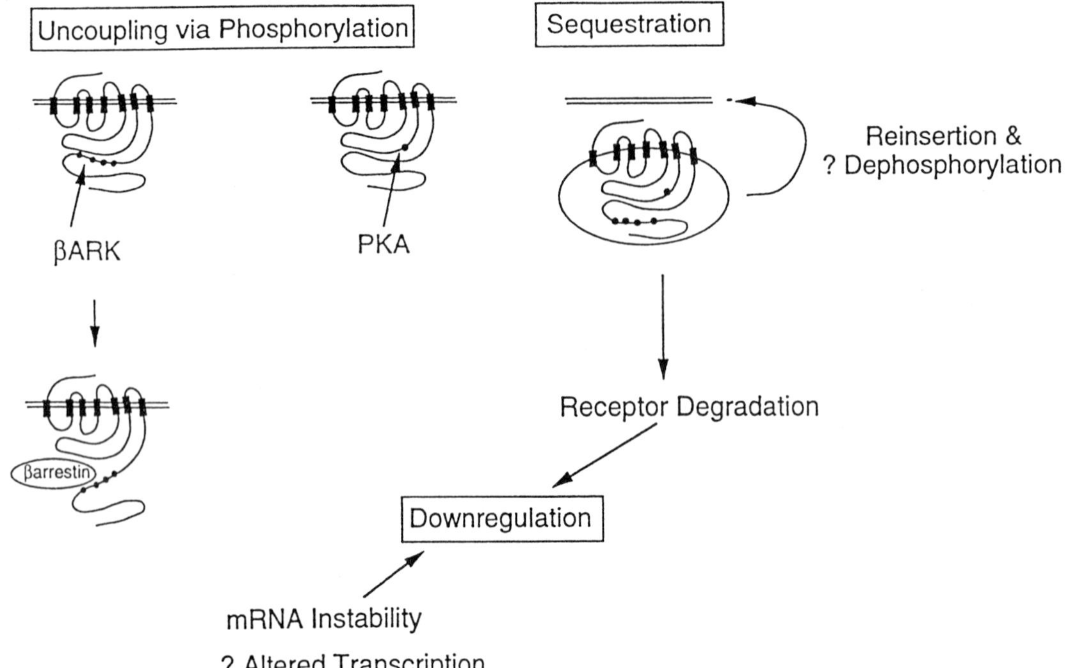

FIG. 7-5. Mechanisms of agonist-promoted desensitization of the β_2-adrenergic receptor. PKA, protein kinase A; βARK, β-adrenergic receptor kinase.

tion of D_1 receptor-stimulated adenylate cyclase is promoted by full agonists and is accompanied by an increase in receptor phosphorylation.

The α_2-adrenoceptors serve as a good example of progress that has been made at the molecular level in defining adrenoceptor subtypes. The α_2-adrenoceptors are the products of three genes located on human chromosomes 2, 4, and 10. These receptors are designated α_2C2, α_2C4, and α_2C10. Evidence suggests that expression of different α_2-subtypes are tissue specific. Thus far, oxymetazoline has been the most useful drug for discriminating among the three cloned α_2-adrenoceptors in radioligand binding assays. Further description of the physiological roles of these α_2-adrenoceptor subtypes will depend on more highly subtype-selective agonists and antagonists. Variables creating difficulty in defining the role(s) of α_2-adrenoceptor subtypes in the eye in vivo include: (a) the involvement of α_2-receptors throughout the sympathoadrenal system, making it difficult to distinguish central from peripheral effects; (b) the lipid solubility of the drug being studied, which changes disposition in tissues and ultimately the clearance of the drug; (c) the potential metabolism of the parent compound to other biologically active agents that may be more or less selective; (d) the probability of different cells within a tissue that might express different receptor subtypes. Molecular approaches that could be used to characterize α_2-adrenoceptor subtypes in the eye could include in situ hybridization with oligonucleotide probes, highly selective radioligands, or subtype-specific antibodies. Two general challenges that remain in defining the roles of adrenoceptors in the eye are (a) characterization of the cellular responses following stimulation of each receptor subtype and (b) determination of the role each subtype plays in the normal and pathophysiological processes.

ANTERIOR SEGMENT FUNCTION: ADRENERGIC PHARMACOLOGY

Functional Aspects

Aqueous Inflow/Outflow: Ciliary Process/Outflow Tract

Aqueous humor provides critical circulatory functions for all avascular tissue in the anterior segment of the eye. Avascular tissues are supplied with metabolic substrates, and waste products are evacuated through the process of aqueous humor flow. Fluid is formed in the posterior chamber by the bilayered epithelium of ciliary processes at a rate of about 2.5 μl per minute in humans (59) and somewhat higher in rabbits. Aqueous formation occurs via three physiological mechanisms: diffusion, ultrafiltration, and active secretion. The predominant process, secretion, is an active, energy-requiring process located in the nonpigmented epithelium. The two other processes involved in the formation of aqueous humor are passive (i.e., more dependent on blood flow and pressure within arterioles in the ciliary body). The bulk (~80%) of aqueous humor formation is the result of active cellular secretion by the inner nonpigmented ciliary epithelium, which contains processes such as ion transport and carbonic anhydrase activity (60). The effects of adrenergic agonists on transport processes can influence the rate of aqueous formation, but sympathetic innervation is not considered essential for formation of aqueous humor (see Fig.7-5). Therefore, although catecholamines may modulate aqueous humor dynamics, studies with Horner's syndrome patients suggest that the role of catecholamines is not obligatory (61).

Aqueous humor flows through the pupil between the posterior iris and the lens, enters the anterior chamber, and exits into the outflow system at the peripheral angle of the anterior chamber. The bulk of aqueous humor outflow occurs primarily by way of the "conventional" drainage route, that is, at the iridocorneal angle of the anterior chamber, through the trabecular meshwork, Schlemm's canal, intrascleral collector channels, aqueous veins, and the episcleral venous plexus. Although sympathetic innervation of the ciliary body has been demonstrated, innervation of the outflow tract is highly variable across the species, with monkey and human trabecular meshwork showing modest innervation that decreases with age. The "unconventional" outflow pathway consists of the passage of fluid between muscle fiber bundles of the ciliary muscle into scleral blood vessels (i.e., the uveoscleral route). This pathway accounts for IOP-independent aqueous humor outflow. The exact role of the sympathoadrenal system and adrenoceptors in modulating outflow through the uveoscleral tract is not fully appreciated at this time; however, the relative amount of aqueous flowing through the uveoscleral route assumes greater importance in patients with primary open-angle glaucoma, in whom the trabecular outflow tract is dysfunctional, and this makes the uveoscleral route a promising site for facilitating outflow by drug therapy. Most of the resistance within the conventional outflow tract is believed to reside in the outer trabecular meshwork or the inner wall of Schlemm's canal. Glycosaminoglycans, which consist mainly of hyaluronic acid and the sulfated glycans (chondroitin-4-sulfate and dermatan sulfate), coat the meshwork, thereby contributing to outflow resistance. The potential biochemical effects of adrenergic drugs on the production of glycoproteins and other functions within the outflow tract require further definition.

Intraocular Pressure

The principal determinants of IOP are aqueous inflow, resistance to outflow, and episcleral venous pressure. Adrenergic and dopaminergic drugs can lower IOP through influences on aqueous formation in the ciliary epithelium or alteration of aqueous humor outflow at the level of the trabecular meshwork, Schlemm's canal, ciliary smooth-muscle cells, episcleral vessels, or intrascleral plexus (Fig. 7-6). The precise site(s) and mechanism(s) of action of adrenergic drugs are under continuing investigation.

The various modes by which adrenoceptors and dopaminoceptors could potentially modify IOP are by (a) altering the rate of secretion of aqueous humor by the ciliary epithelium, (b) changing the rate of ultrafiltration in the ciliary process secondary to changes in hydrostatic pressure gradient across the arterioles in the ciliary body, (c) modifying the outflow resistance either directly at the conventional outflow tract or indirectly by altering resistance in the episcleral veins, or (d) changing fluid flow through the uveoscleral pathway. Although blood flow through the anterior uveal vasculature is reduced by either

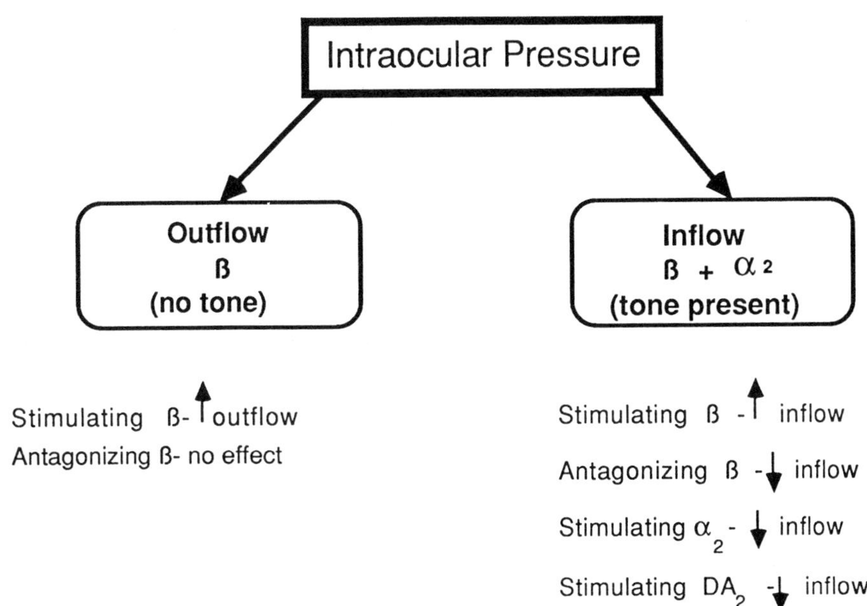

FIG. 7-6. Proposed model for the action of adrenergic and dopaminergic drugs on aqueous humor dynamics (modified from Thomas and Epstein, 1981).

electrical stimulation of the cervical sympathetic nerves or topical application α-adrenoceptor agonists, this blood flow-related mechanism does not appear to be the primary mechanism by which aqueous formation is reduced by catecholamines and other adrenoceptor agonists.

Although adrenergic mechanisms influence aqueous humor dynamics, the response is not uniform from one species to the other (62). These differences may be due in part to the fact that sympathetic nerves in various species can release a variety of neuropeptides and purines (63). There also may be differences in distribution of adrenoceptor subtypes among various species. Considerable information on adrenergic regulation of IOP has been derived largely from studies of epinephrine, a nonselective catecholamine with both α- and β-agonist properties. The effects of epinephrine are time-related, however, and undoubtedly involve multiple mechanisms and sites of action (64).

In normal human eyes, the short-term effects of relatively high doses of epinephrine and prodrugs of epinephrine (e.g., dipivefrin) include a lowering of IOP, an increase of tonographically measured outflow facility, and an increase in the rate of loss of fluorescein from the anterior chamber. Acutely, epinephrine can evoke increases in aqueous production in human subjects, and the ability of timolol to reduce aqueous humor flow is assumed to be attributable to inhibition of β_2-adrenoceptors. With more chronic use, epinephrine treatment consistently increases the outflow of aqueous humor in humans. In normal subjects and glaucoma patients, epinephrine has been reported either to increase or to decrease aqueous humor formation as well as to increase outflow facility. Therefore, the observed net effect following chronic administration of epinephrine could be due in part to an initial stimulation followed by differential downregulation of β-adrenoceptor subtypes. Little detailed information is available regarding the dynamic status of other adrenoceptors in eye tissues after chronic administration of adrenergically active drugs, such as epinephrine and timolol.

At the cellular level, effects of epinephrine on IOP are presumed to be exerted in part via β-adrenoceptors through cAMP-dependent mechanisms. The facility-enhancing effect in the outflow tract is assumed to be a cAMP-mediated event. In summary, the net effect of chronic therapy with epinephrine in glaucomatous subjects is a decrease in IOP resulting from enhancement of outflow facility.

The β-adrenoceptor antagonists (timolol, metipranolol, levobunolol, betaxolol, carteolol) are among the most widely used agents for the therapy of open-angle glaucoma, either alone or in combination with other drugs. These agents are presumed to lower IOP primarily by inhibiting aqueous humor secretion. Because topical therapy with full antagonists (e.g., timolol) can cause problems in patients predisposed to asthma and congestive heart failure, β-adrenoceptor antagonists with intrinsic sympathomimetic (agonist) activity (e.g., carteolol) have been introduced.

Dopamine, like other nonselective adrenergic agonists (epinephrine, norepinephrine), elicits a biphasic effect on IOP in rabbits following topical instillation (5). This is not surprising because dopamine acts, in part, through indirect mechanisms involving norepinephrine release. Within the first hour after instillation of dopamine to the eyes of a rabbit, a modest elevation in IOP is noted, followed for the next several hours by a decrease in IOP. The initial hypertensive effect is presumed to be due to an α-adrenoceptor-mediated stimulation of extraocular muscles. The hypotensive and hypertensive effects of topical dopamine involve a direct action on dopamine (DA_1/DA_2) receptors or release of norepinephrine. Because haloperidol can inhibit the ocular hypotensive effect of dopamine, this effect was presumed to involve dopamine receptors.

Dopamine 1 (D_1 centrally; DA_1 in the periphery) receptors usually are linked positively to adenylate cyclase, and, as a result, stimulation causes an increase in cAMP generation. In contrast, D_2 (DA_2) receptors are either negatively linked to adenylate cyclase or to ion channels, such as those for K^+ or Ca^{2+}. Peripheral DA_1 (vascular) receptors subserve vasodilation in renal, mesenteric, coronary, and cerebral vascular beds as well as in inhibition of aldosterone secretion. Relatively selective DA_1 agonists can elevate cAMP levels in the ciliary bodies of the human and bovine but not the rabbit. The DA_1 receptor agonists (e.g., ibopamine) can raise IOP in glaucomatous subjects and thus may be useful clinically as a provocative test. In contrast to DA_1 receptors, demonstration of DA_2 receptors in the rabbit ciliary body, as shown by radioligand binding and autoradiography (42), has not been accomplished; however, functional evidence suggests that activation of DA_2 (neuronal) receptors causes inhibition of norepinephrine release from sympathetic nerve endings in the iris-ciliary body (66) and lowering of IOP. Additional work has demonstrated that a phosphoprotein related to D_1 receptors, DARPP-32, is localized to nonpigmented ciliary epithelial cells (47). Unfortunately, no clearly defined role for DARPP-32 in aqueous humor dynamics has been identified thus far.

The DA_2 agonists are included in at least six chemical classes: (a) phenylethylamine, (b) aminotetralin, (c) aporphine, (d) benzazepine, (e) ergoline, and (f) benzhydroquinoline. Topical and, in some cases, oral administration of relatively selective DA_2 agonists (e.g., bromocriptine) can lower the IOP in animals as well as in normal persons and glaucoma patients. Relatively selective DA_2 antagonists, such as domperidone, metoclopramide, and sulpiride, can antagonize the ocular hypotensive effects of DA_2 agonists (67). Although administration of metoclopramide abolished the ocular hypotensive response to bromocriptine and stimulated prolactin secretion, there was no effect on basal IOP, suggesting that under normal circumstances ocular hydrodynamics in humans is not under continuous tonic dopaminergic (DA_2) control (68). In rabbits, the major effect of DA_2-agonists on aqueous dynamics is suppression of aqueous humor formation, presumably through an inhibitory effect on norepinephrine release (69).

In summary, stimulation of β-adrenoceptors can mediate increases in outflow, whereas activation of α_2- and DA_2-receptors or antagonism of β-adrenoceptors can mediate decreases in inflow. The site of action for the outflow effects of β-adrenoceptors is probably within the conventional (trabecular) outflow tract. One site of action for the β-antagonists and α_2-agonist-induced reduction in inflow is probably at the level of the nonpigmented epithelium (postjunctional site). In addition, the effect of DA_2 and α_2-agonists probably involves inhibition of norepinephrine release from sympathetic nerves (prejunctional site) within the ciliary process. Another potential site of action for α_2-agonists is in the central nervous system.

Ocular Blood Flow

Alm and Bill (70) proposed that the role of the sympathetic nerves relative to ocular blood flow is to protect the eye from overperfusion. Stimulation of the cervical sympathetic chain causes marked uveal vasoconstriction in all species studied (71–73). In most species, including the cat, α_1-adrenoceptors are probably the predominant receptor involved in causing vasoconstriction (74). Current evidence supporting this view indicates that uveal vessels respond more readily to norepinephrine (α_1, α_2) than to isoproterenol (β_2). Thus, choroidal vessels in most species appear to have limited numbers of β_2-receptors relative to α-adrenoceptors; the possible exception is the pig. Topical epinephrine, which stimulates α- and β-adrenoceptors, reduces anterior uveal blood flow for as long as 6 hours in the monkey. In another study, BHT 920, an α_2/DA_2 agonist, reduced choroidal blood flow in rabbits, suggesting that α_2-adrenoceptors are present in choroidal arterioles of this species (75).

The Lacrimal Gland

Direct stimulation of sympathetic nerves enhanced fluid secretion in the lacrimal gland of the rabbit (76). In vivo, the lacrimal gland of the rabbit responded to norepinephrine with increased release of fluid and protein (77); however, possible direct effects of catecholamines on the lacrimal gland function in vivo have been difficult to differentiate from indirect (vascular) effects. In the rat, the acinar cells of the lacrimal gland contain α-adrenoceptors, which, when activated, mediate an increase in membrane permeability to potassium. Lacrimal fluid flow in the rabbit appears to be regulated through α_1-adrenoceptors and β-adrenoceptors (78). Evidence suggests that protein secretion in the lacrimal gland also may depend on β-adrenergic-receptor stimulation. The α- and β-adrenergic responses in cultured acini are not as strong as in incubated tissue slices and may be due to perturbed postreceptor events (79). Interestingly, catecholamine concentrations in lacrimal fluid are lower than normal in glaucoma patients (80).

The Cornea

Beta-adrenoceptors have been localized in the rabbit cornea, as shown by ligand binding methods (81), and stimulation decreases collagenase production in the cornea (82). The β-adrenoceptors in the corneal epithelium are involved in secretion and mitotic activity. In the corneal endothelium, adrenergic agonists also enhance chloride transport, stimulate adenylate cyclase, and therefore activate cAMP-dependent protein kinase (83). Repetitive topical application of epinephrine decreases the density of β-adrenoceptors; as a result, the associated increase in cAMP production and chloride transport diminishes. The presence of α_2-adrenoceptors has been demonstrated by immunofluorescent labelling in human and rabbit corneal epithelium. Chloride flux is inhibited by α_2-agonists in the frog epithelium; however, the regulatory significance of these receptors has not been fully explored in the mammalian cornea.

The Lens

The lens is bathed by aqueous humor that contains varying concentrations of catecholamines. The lens will respond to β-adrenergic receptor stimulation with increased cAMP production, but isoproterenol, a nonselective β-agonist, is more potent than salbutamol, a relatively selective β_2-agonist (84). Dopamine, at a similar concentration, is relatively inactive. Propranolol treatment inhibits the effects of isoproterenol on cAMP production. During lens growth, catecholamines appear to act synergistically with chalones, proteins evidently capable of specifically inhibiting mitosis of lens epithelium (85). Beta-adrenoceptors are also present in the lens epithelium, and stimulation of these receptors suppresses mitotic activity. The functional significance of adrenoceptors in lens tissue is not fully understood.

The Iris

The radial (dilator) muscle of the iris contains extensive sympathetic innervation, and this tissue has been studied to a considerable extent to understand better signal transduction in the eye. The primary adrenoceptor in the radial muscle is the α_1-adrenoceptor, which, when stimulated, results in mydriasis (86). The iris sphincter is innervated to a lesser extent by sympathetic neurons, which form a plexus at the pupillary margin. The existence of sympathetic innervation of the sphincter has been demonstrated in a variety of species, including the rat, cat, and guinea pig. Beta-adrenoceptor stimulation will cause relaxation of the circular (sphincter) muscle in certain species, thereby causing mydriasis. Clearly, there are biochemical and functional interactions among adrenoceptors and other receptors in the iris that involve changes in second messengers, such as IP_3, CA^{2+}, and cAMP (87).

Further Definition of Drugs Affecting Ocular Adrenergic Function

Drugs that alter ocular function by modifying actions of the sympathetic nervous system can do so at multiple sites by a variety of mechanisms (88). For example, sites of action include the CNS, autonomic ganglia, postganglionic nerve endings, and effector organs. Predominant mechanisms in the CNS that may influence ocular function involve α_2 and possibly I_1 (imidazoline) receptors (89). Imidazoline (I_1) receptors are located at two principal sites, the stimulation of which can result in decreased sympathetic activity: the rostral ventrolateral medulla and adrenomedullary chromaffin cells. In contrast, α_2-adrenoceptors in the CNS appear to be located predominantly in or near the nucleus tractus solitarius.

In specific regions of the CNS, evidence exists for a novel α_2-like receptor that mediates the ocular action of certain clonidine-like compounds. Work suggests that imidazoline (clonidine-like) compounds can interact with more sites in the brainstem than can be accounted for by rauwolscine (α_2)-binding studies (90). These sites of action in the medullary region may explain the considerable contralateral effect that is observed in response to topical unilateral administration of clonidine-like drugs (brimonidine, moxonidine, rilminidine, oxymetazoline) (89). Thus, of all the drugs that can affect the function of the sympathoadrenal system, it would appear that there are more sites and mechanisms of action associated with α_2/I_1 agonists than with any other known group of drugs.

An array of drug actions can occur at peripheral postganglionic nerve endings in the eye, where agents can modify the synthesis, storage, release, reuptake, and biotransformation of norepinephrine. Although many agents have been tested, the most applicable mechanism employed to date at sympathetic nerve endings has been with agents that provoke release through an action on mobile stores of norepinephrine (e.g., hydroxyamphetamine) or inhibit release by an action on prejunctional receptors (e.g., apraclonidine). In particular, clonidine-like drugs have several potential sites by which ocular function can be modified: central (presynaptic or postsynaptic) and peripheral (prejunctional or postjunctional).

Although not classically included among the adrenoceptor-reactive compounds, dopamine can stimulate a broad range of receptors as the result of direct (i.e., postjunctional) effects on dopamine (DA_1, DA_2) receptors and indirect (i.e., prejunctional) effects mediated by the release of norepinephrine (β_1,α_1/α_2) from sympathetic nerve endings. Although special conditions are required to allow the expression of DA_2-receptor activation by dopamine (i.e., the uptake of dopamine into sympathetic neurons must be inhibited), synthetic dopamine (DA_2) receptor agonists (e.g., bromocriptine, BHT 920, Ha 117) that are not substrates for neuronal uptake are effective inhibitors of norepinephrine release from sympathetic nerve terminals (91).

At the postjunctional adrenoceptors, stimulation and inhibition of both classes of $\alpha(\alpha_1/\alpha_2)$ and $\beta(\beta_1/\beta_2)$ adrenoceptors have proved therapeutically useful. Epinephrine is the primary example of an agonist that will stimulate a wide variety of adrenoceptor subtypes (α_1/α_2,β_1/β_2) in a dose-dependent fashion. Epinephrine stimulates β_1/β_2-adrenoceptors at lower concentrations and β-adrenoceptors plus α_1/α_2 adrenoceptors at higher concentrations; these complex actions have hindered a clear definition of the primary mechanism of action of epinephrine.

Beta-adrenoceptor antagonists are among the preferred topical medical therapies for open-angle glaucoma. In addition to timolol (Timoptic), four other β-receptor antagonists are available: betaxolol (Betoptic), levobunolol (Betagan), metipranolol (OptiPranolol), and carteolol (Ocupress) (91). Betaxolol has the theoretical advantage of being relatively selective for β_1-adrenoceptors. Levobunolol has pharmacodynamically active metabolites (e.g., dihydrolevobunolol) that extend the pharmacological half-life. Carteolol is unique among the currently used β-adrenoceptor antagonists in that it has intrinsic sympathomimetic activity (93). Both betaxolol and carteolol are purported to have less tendency to antagonize β_2-adrenoceptors, which should decrease the probability of untoward systemic side effects (e.g., bronchospasm). It remains to be shown, however, whether these pharmacodynamic properties will prove to be of significant clinical value. All these β-adrenoceptor antagonists lower IOP by about 20% to 30% in patients with glaucoma or ocular hypertension.

FUTURE DIRECTIONS

Two basic approaches have been used to improve the medical therapy for glaucoma: (a) the pharmacokinetic approach (i.e., improving drug delivery by physical or chemical means) and (b) the pharmacodynamic approach (i.e., enhancing the receptor selectivity of drugs, thereby improving efficacy in the eye). Recent definition of adrenoceptor subtypes at the molecular level should, in fact, facilitate the development of subtype-selective agonists and antagonists. These types of advances could serve to improve the efficacy of therapeutic agents while reducing adverse systemic effects of topically applied drugs.

Because β-adrenoceptor antagonists and α_2-adrenoceptor agonists may have less systemic and ocular efficacy in some populations (e.g., in blacks) than in others (e.g., whites), it is important to determine whether ethnic differences in responsiveness are due to (a) insensitivity or polymorphism at the receptor level, (b) unusual linkages at postreceptor (e.g., signal transduction) sites, or (c) differences in pharmacokinetics (e.g., binding to darker-pigmented irides).

If IOP continues to serve as the principal surrogate endpoint for the medical therapy for glaucoma, it might be advantageous to try rational combinations of drugs in the therapy of glaucoma in a manner similar to that used in the treatment of essential hypertension. For example, a combination of agents that act to suppress aqueous humor formation along with agents that enhance outflow by way of the trabecular and uveoscleral routes may offer greater efficacy. For maximal effectiveness, it may be necessary to administer these agents in accordance with known changes in the circadian rhythm of neurotransmitter release and receptor activities.

In the future, it should become possible to manipulate cellular responses beyond the receptor, that is, at the level of signal transduction. Because several isozymes of phosphodiesterase exist, drugs that inhibit different types III, IV, and V phosphodiesterase (e.g., rolipram, zaprinast, and cilostamide) could be used to augment responses to agonists that are mediated by cAMP and cGMP. Also, it may be possible in the future to develop specific, directly acting inhibitors and activators of the intracellular enzymes (e.g., protein kinase A, C, and G).

REFERENCES

1. Galitzky J, Carpene C, Lafontan M, Berlan M. Specific stimulation of adipose tissue adrenergic beta 3 receptors by octopamine. *CR Acad Sci III* 1993;316:519–523.
2. Bausher LP. Identification of A and B forms of monoamine oxidase in the iris-ciliary body, superior cervical ganglion and pineal gland of albino rabbits. *Invest Ophthalmol Vis Sci* 1976;15:529–537.
3. Bausher LP, Sears ML. Potentiation of the effects of topical epinephrine on the pupil and intraocular pressure in the sympathetically denervated rabbit eye by a catechol-o-methyltransferase inhibitor. *Invest Ophthalmol Vis Sci* 1976;15:854–857.
4. McLeod HL, Fang L, Luo X, Scott EP, Evans WE. Ethnic differences in erythrocyte catechol-o-methyltransferase activity in black and white Americans. *J Pharmacol Exp Ther* 1994;270:26–29.
5. Shannon RP, Mead A, Sears ML. The effects of dopamine on the intraocular pressure and pupil of the rabbit eye. *Invest Ophthalmol Vis Sci* 1976;15:371–380.
6. Potter DE, Burke JA. Effects of ergoline derivatives on intraocular pressure and iris function in rabbits and monkeys. *Curr Eye Res* 1982;2:281–288.
7. Mekki QA, Hassan SM, Turner P. Bromocriptine lowers intraocular pressure without affecting blood pressure. *Lancet* 1983;1:1250–1251.
8. Karnezis TA, Murphy MB, Weber RR, Nelson KS, Tripathi BJ, Tripathi RC. Effects of selective dopamine-1 activation on intraocular pressure in man. *Exp Eye Res* 1988;47:689–697.
9. Sears ML. Autonomic nervous system: Adrenergic agonists. In: Sears ML, ed. *Handbook of Experimental Pharmacology.* Berlin: Springer-Verlag, 1984;69:193–247.
10. Erickson-Lamy KA, Nathanson JA. Epinephrine increases facility of outflow and cyclic AMP content in the human eye in vitro. *Invest Ophthalmol Vis Sci* 1992;33:2672–2678.
11. Ahlquist RP. A study of adrenotropic receptors. *Am J Physiol* 1948;153:586–600.
12. Caron MG, Kobilka BK, Frielle T, et al. Adrenergic receptors: molecular and regulatory properties revealed by cloning of their genes. In: Melchiorre C, Giannella M, eds. *Recent Advances in Receptor Chemistry.* Amsterdam: Elsevier, 1988;63–75.
13. Lands AM, Arnold A, McAuliff JP, Lunduena FP, Brown RG. Differentiation of receptor systems activated by sympathomimetic amines. *Nature* 1967;214:597–598.
14. Langer SZ. Presynaptic regulation of catecholamine release. *Biochem Pharmacol* 1974;23:1793–1800.
15. Berthelsen S, Pettinger WA. A functional basis for classification of alpha-adrenergic receptors. *Life Sci* 1977;21:595–606.
16. Wax MB, Molinoff PB. Distribution and properties of β-adrenergic receptors in human iris-ciliary body. *Invest Ophthalmol Vis Sci* 1987; 28:420–430.
17. Cepelik J, Cernohorsky M. The effects of adrenergic agonists and antagonists on adenylate cyclase in albino rabbit ciliary processes. *Exp Eye Res* 1981;32:291–299.
18. Nathanson JA. Adrenergic regulation of intraocular pressure: identification of β-adrenergic stimulated adenylate cyclase in ciliary process epithelium. *Proc Natl Acad Sci USA* 1980;77:7420–7424.
19. Elena P-P, Kosina-Boix M, Moulin G, Lapalus P. Autoradiographic localization of beta-adrenergic receptors in rabbit eye. *Invest Ophthalmol Vis Sci* 1987;28:1436–1441.
20. Starke K. Presynaptic of noradrenaline release by presynaptic receptor system. *Rev Physiol Biochem Pharmacol* 1977;77:1–124.
21. Ruffolo RR Jr. Mode of action and structure-activity relationships among imidazoline-like α-adrenoceptor agonists. In: Melchiorre C, Giannella M, eds. *Recent Advances in Receptor Chemistry.* Amsterdam: Elsevier Science Publishers, 1988;77–106.
22. Ruffolo RR Jr, Nichols AJ, Stadel JM, Hieble JP. Pharmacologic and therapeutic applications of α_2-adrenoceptor subtypes. *Annu Rev Pharmacol Toxicol* 1993;32:243–279.
23. Starke K. Alpha adrenoceptor subclassification. *Rev Physiol Biochem Pharmacol* 1981;88:199–236.
24. Oriowo MA, Hieble JP, Ruffolo RR. Evidence for heterogeneity of prejunctional alpha-2-adrenoceptors. *Pharmacology* 1991;43:1–13.
25. Morrow AL, Creese I. Characterization of α_1-adrenergic receptor subtypes in rat brain: a re-evaluation of ^{3}H-WB4101 and ^{3}H-prazosin binding. *Mol Pharmacol* 1986;29:321–330.
26. Coates J, Jahn U, Weetman DF. The existence of a new subtypes of α-adrenoceptor is revealed by SGD100/75 and phenoxybenzamine. *Br J Pharmacol* 1982;75:549–552.
27. Medgett IC, Langer SZ. Heterogeneity of smooth muscle alpha adrenoceptors in the rat tail artery in vitro. *J Pharmacol Exp Ther* 1984;229:823–830.
28. Bylund DB, Eikenberg DL, Hieble JP, et al. IV International Union of Pharmacology Nomenclature of Adrenoceptors. *Pharmacol Rev* 1994; 46:121–142.
29. Insel PA. Adrenergic receptors, G proteins and cell regulation: implications for aging research. *Exp Gerontol* 1993;28:341–348.
30. Lomasney JW, Cottechia S, Lefkowitz RJ, Caron M. Molecular biology of α-adrenergic receptors: implications for receptor classification and for structure function relationships. *Biochim Biophys Acta* 1991; 1095:127–139.
31. Bylund DB. Heterogeneity of α_2-adrenergic receptors. *Pharmacol Biochem Behav* 1985;22:835–843.
32. Nahorski SR, Barnette DB, Cheung Y-D. Alpha-adrenergic receptor effector coupling: affinity states or heterogeneity of the alpha-2 adrenergic receptor? *Clin Sci* 1985;68(suppl 10):395–342s.
33. Mittag TW, Tormay A. Drug responses of adenylate cyclase complex in iris-ciliary body determined by adenine labeling. *Invest Ophthalmol Vis Sci* 1985;26:396–399.
34. Hynie S, Cepelik J. Effects of pertussis toxin on intraocular pressure and adenylate cyclase activity of ciliary processes in rabbits. *Gen Physiol Biophys* 1993;12:141–153.
35. Ogidigben M, Chu T-C, Potter DE. Alpha-2 adrenoceptor mediated changes in aqueous dynamics: effects of pertussis toxin. *Exp Eye Res* 1994;58:729–736.
36. Limbird LE. Receptors linked to inhibition of adenylate cyclase: additional signalling mechanisms. *FASEB J* 1988;2:2686–2695.
37. Crosson CE, Heath AR, DeVries GW, Potter DE. Pharmacological evidence for heterogeneity of ocular α_2 adrenoceptors. *Curr Eye Res* 1992;11:963–970.
38. Kebabian JW, Greengard P. Dopamine-sensitive adenylyl cyclase;

possible role in synaptic transmission. *Science* 1971;174:1346–1349.
39. Onali P, Olianas MC, Gessa GL. Characterization of dopamine receptors mediating inhibition of adenylate cyclase activity in rat striatum. *Mol Pharmacol* 1985;28:138–145.
40. Haggendal J, Malmfors T. Evidence of dopamine containing neurones in the retina of the rabbit. *Acta Physiol Scand* 1963;59:295–299.
41. Lograno MD, Daniele E, Govoni S. Biochemical and functional evidence for the presence of dopamine D_1 receptors in the bovine ciliary body. *Exp Eye Res* 1990;51:495–501.
42. Elena PP, Denis P, Kosina-Boix M, Lapalus P. Dopamine receptors in rabbit and rat eye: characterization and localization of DA_1 and DA_2 binding sites. *Curr Eye Res* 1989;8:75–83.
43. Mekki QA, Warrington SJ, Turner P. Bromocriptine eyedrops lower intraocular pressure without affecting prolactin levels. *Lancet* 1984;1: 287–288.
44. Lustig A. Verstärkt Bromocriptin die Wirkung augeninnendruksenkender Mittel? *Dtsch Med Wochenschr* 1983;108:1656–1657.
45. Kebabian JW, Calne DB. Multiple receptors for dopamine. *Nature* 1979;227:93–96.
46. DeVries GW, Mobasser A, Wheeler LA. Stimulation of endogenous cyclic AMP levels in ciliary body by SKF82526, a novel dopamine receptor agonist. *Curr Eye Res* 1986;5:449–455.
47. Stone RA, Laties AM, Hemmings HC, Ouimet CC, Greengard P. DARPP-32 in ciliary epithelium of the eye: a neurotransmitter-regulated phosphoprotein of brain localized to secretory cells. *J Histochem Cytochem* 1986;34:1465–1468.
48. Enero MA, Langer SZ. Inhibition by dopamine of ^{3}H-noradrenaline release elicited by nerve stimulation in the isolated cat's nictitating membrane. *Naunyn Schmiedebergs Arch Pharmacol* 1975;289: 179–203.
49. Potter DE, Ogidigben MJ, Heath AR. Ocular actions of an octahydrobenzo[f]quinoline: Ha117. *Eur J Pharmacol* 1993;236:61–68.
50. Kobilka B. Adrenergic receptors as models for G protein-coupled receptors. *Annu Rev Neurosci* 1992;15:87–114.
51. Strosberg AD. Structure, function and regulation of adrenergic receptors. *Protein Sci* 1992;2:1198–1209.
52. Feve B, Baude B, Krief S, Strosberg AD, Pairault J, Emiorine LJ. Dexamethasone down-regulates β_3-adrenergic receptors in 3T3-F442A adipocytes. *J Biol Chem* 1992;267:15909–15915.
53. Bouvier M, Collins S, O'Dowd BF, Campbell PT, DeBlasi A, Kobilka BK, McGregor C, et al. Two distinct pathways for cAMP-mediated down-regulation of the β_2-adrenergic receptor. *J Biol Chem* 1989; 264:16786–16792.
54. Benovic JL, Major F Jr, Staniszewski C, Lefkowitz RJ, Caron MG. Purification and characterization of the β-adrenergic receptor kinase. *J Biol Chem* 1987;262:9026–9032.
55. Hausdorff WP, Bouvier M, O'Dowd BF, Irons GP, Caron MG, Lefkowitz RJ. Phosphorylation sites on two domains of the human β_2-adrenergic receptor are involved in distinct pathways of receptors desensitization. *J Biol Chem* 1989;265:12657–12665.
56. Benovic JL, DeBlasi A, Stone WC, Caron WG, Lefkowitz RJ. β-adrenergic receptor kinase: primary structure delineates a multigene family. *Science* 1989;246:235–246.
57. Lohse MJ, Benovic JC, Codina J, Caron MG, Lefkowitz RJ. β-Adrenergic receptor function. *Science* 1990;248:1547–1550.
58. Benovic JL, Regan JW, Matsui H, et al. Agonist-dependent phosphorylation of the α_2-adrenergic receptor by the β-adrenergic receptor kinase. *J Biol Chem* 1987;262:17251–17253.
59. Brubaker RF, Nagataki S, Townsend DJ, Burns RR, Higgins RG, Wentworth W. The effect of age on aqueous humor formation in man. *Ophthalmology* 1981;88:283–288.
60. Cole DF. Secretion of aqueous humor. *Exp Eye Res* 1977;25(suppl): 161–176.
61. Wentworth WO, Brubaker RF. Aqueous humor dynamics in a series of patients with third neuron Horner's syndrome. *Am J Ophthalmol* 1981;92:407–415.
62. Potter DE. Adrenergic pharmacology of aqueous humor dynamics. *Pharmacol Rev* 1981;33:133–153.
63. Burnstock G. Cotransmitters of catecholamines. *J Auton Pharmacol* 1994;14:5–6.
64. Neufeld AH. The mechanisms of action of adrenergic drugs in the eye. In: Drance SM, Neufeld AH, eds. *Glaucoma: Applied Pharmacology in Medical Treatment.* New York: Grune & Stratton, 1984; 277–302.
65. Caccavelli L, Cussac D, Pellegrini I, Audinot V, Jaquet P, Enjalbert A. D_2 Dopaminergic receptors: normal and abnormal transduction mechanisms. *Horm Res* 1992;38:78–83.
66. Ogidigben M, Chu T-C, Potter DE. Ocular hypotensive action of a dopaminergic (DA_2) agonist, 2, 10, 11 trihydroxy-N-n-propylnoraporphine. *J Pharmacol Exp Ther* 1993;267:822–827.
67. Al-Sereiti MR, Quik RFP, Hedges A, Turner P. Antagonism by domperidone of the ocular hypotensive effect of pergolide. *Eur J Clin Pharmacol* 1990;38:461–463.
68. Mekki QA, Turner P. Stimulation of dopamine receptors (type 2) lowers human intraocular pressure. *Br J Ophthalmol* 1985;69:909–910.
69. Potter DE. Do dopamine and dopamine receptors have roles in modulating function in the anterior segment: the evidence. *Progress in Retinal Eye Research* 1995;15:103–111.
70. Alm A, Bill A. Ocular circulation. In: Moses RA, Hart WM, eds. *Adler's Physiology of the Eye.* St. Louis: CV Mosley, 1987;183–203.
71. Adler FH, Landis EM, Jackson CL. The tonic effect of the sympathetic on the ocular blood vessels. *Arch Ophthalmol* 1924;53:239–253.
72. Alm A, Bill A. The effect of stimulation of the cervical sympathetic chain on retinal oxygen tension and on uveal, retinal and cerebral blood flow in cats. *Acta Physiol Scand* 1973;88:84–94.
73. Alm A. The effect of sympathetic stimulation on blood flow through the uvea, retina, and optic nerve in monkeys (*Macaca iru*). *Exp Eye Res* 1971;25:19–24.
74. Koss MC, Gherezghiher T. Adrenoceptor subtypes involved in neurally evoked sympathetic vasoconstriction in the anterior choroid of cats. *Exp Eye Res* 1993;57:441–447.
75. Thörig L, Bill A. Effects of B-HT920 in the eye and on regional blood flows in anesthetized and conscious rabbits. *Curr Eye Res* 1986; 5:565–573.
76. Tankrisanavincont V. Stimulation of lacrimal secretion by sympathetic nerve impulses in the rabbit. *Life Sci* 1984;34:2365–2371.
77. Botelho SY, Goldstein AM, Martinez EV. Norepinephrine-responsive beta-adrenergic receptors in rabbit lacrimal gland. *Am J Physiol* 1973;224:1119–1122.
78. Bromberg BB. Autonomic control of lacrimal protein secretion. *Invest Ophthalmol Vis Sci* 1981;20:110–116.
79. Meneray MA, Fields TY, Bromberg BB, Moses RL. Morphology and physiologic responsiveness of cultured rabbit lacrimal acini. *Invest Ophthalmol Vis Sci* 1994;35:4144–4158.
80. Zubareva TV, Kiseleva ZM. Catecholamine content of the lacrimal fluid of healthy people and glaucoma patients. *Ophthalmologica* 1977;175:339–344.
81. Butterfield LC, Neufeld AH. Cyclic nucleotides and mitosis in the rabbit cornea following superior cervical ganglionectomy. *Exp Eye Res* 1977;25:427–433.
82. Walkenbach RJ, LeGrand RD. Adenylate cyclase activity in bovine and human corneal endothelium. *Invest Ophthalmol Vis Sci* 1982;22: 120–124.
83. Neufeld AH, Zawistowski KA, Page ED, Bromberg BB. Influences on the density of beta-adrenergic receptors in the cornea and iris-ciliary body of the rabbit. *Invest Ophthalmol Vis Sci* 1978;17:1069–1075.
84. Osborne NN. Agonist-induced stimulation of cAMP in the lens: presence of functional β-receptors. *Exp Eye Res* 1991;52:105–106.
85. Grimes P, vonSallman L. Possible cyclic adenosine monophosphate mediation in isoproterenol-induced suppression of cell division in rat lens epithelium. *Invest Ophthalmol Vis Sci* 1972;11:231–235.
86. Koss MC, Gherezghiher T. Pharmacological characterization of alpha-adrenoceptors involved in nictitating membrane and pupillary responses to sympathetic nerve stimulation in cats. *Naunyn Schmiedebergs Arch Pharmacol* 1988;337:18–23.
87. Abdel-Latif AA. Calcium-mobilizing receptors, polyphosphoinositides, generation of second messengers and contraction in the mammalian iris smooth muscle; historical perspectives and current status. *Life Sci* 1989;45:757–786.
88. Potter DE, Rowland JR. Adrenergic drugs and intraocular pressure. *Gen Pharmacol* 1981;12:1–13.
89. Campbell WR, Potter DE. Centrally mediated ocular hypotension:

potential role for imidazoline receptors. *Ann NY Acad Sci* 1995; 763:463–485.
90. Boyajian CL, Leslie FM. Pharmacological evidence for α_2-heterogeneity: differential binding properties of [^{3}H] idazoxan in rat brain. *J Pharmacol Exp Ther* 1987;241:1092–1098.
91. Potter DE, Crosson CD, Heath AR, Ogidigben MJ. Alpha-2 and DA-2 agonists as antiglaucoma agents: comparative pharmacology and clinical potential. *J Ocul Pharmacol Ther* 1990;6:251–257.
92. Frishman WH, Fuksbrunner MS, Tannenbaum M. Topical ophthalmic β-adrenergic blockade for the treatment of glaucoma and ocular hypertension. *J Clin Pharmacol* 1994;34:795–803.
93. Chrisp P, Sorkin EM. Ocular carteolol: a review of its pharmacological properties and therapeutic use in glaucoma and hypertension. *Drugs Aging* 1992;2:58–77.

Textbook of Ocular Pharmacology,
edited by T.J. Zimmerman, et al.
Lippincott–Raven Publishers, Philadelphia © 1997.

CHAPTER 8

Immunosuppressive Therapy for Uveitis

Margaret K. L. Cheung and James T. Rosenbaum

The major immunosuppressive medications are divided into the antimetabolites, the alkylators, and the noncytotoxic immunosuppressive medications, such as cyclosporine. The major indication for use of these medications in ophthalmology is for noninfectious, nonmalignant causes of uveitis that have proven refractory to systemic corticosteroids (1). In general, immunosuppressive medications are reserved for patients whose vision interferes with the activities of daily living. Candidates for immunosuppressive therapy should have active, bilateral disease with visual acuity in the better eye usually ≤20/40. An infection or a specific contraindication to a medication should preclude its use. Other ophthalmic diseases that occasionally require systemic immunosuppression include scleritis, ocular cicatricial pemphigoid, corneal melt, and orbital pseudotumor.

Usually, the goal of immunosuppressive therapy is to ameliorate rather than to eliminate inflammation. Patients and physicians must carefully weigh the risk-to-benefit ratio in making a decision to try specific medications. Use of each of the immunosuppressive medications entails a certain degree of risk and cost. Often, the onset of benefit from these medications is delayed such that an adequate trial may require 3 months on the medication before concluding that it is ineffective.

Unless the pace of inflammation is extremely rapid, we prefer to use immunosuppressive medications in a stepwise fashion. Antimetabolite therapy is usually well tolerated, unlikely to predispose to an infection at recommended doses, and relatively inexpensive by immunosuppression standards. Although no study has compared directly the efficacy of azathioprine or methotrexate in the treatment of uveitis with either cyclosporine or an alkylating drug, we consider these medications to be safer but also somewhat less likely to be effective than the comparable alkylators or cyclosporine. If antimetabolite therapy is ineffective or not tolerated, the patient and physician must consider therapy with either an alkylating drug or cyclosporine. The use of cyclosporine is supported by many more clinical trials than the use of an alkylator; however, cyclosporine therapy is expensive; it fails to induce permanent resolution of disease in most instances, and it frequently is complicated by hypertension, renal toxicity, or malaise. On the other hand, therapy with an alkylating drug frequently is complicated by sterility, increased risk of infection, and increased risk of malignancy. These relative considerations must be weighed carefully in counseling a patient about selection of one of these medications. Individual patients may elect to accept visual disability rather than undertake the risks of medication. Because the medicines can be used in a progressive fashion, a therapeutic trial of one can be followed by a therapeutic trial of an alternate medicine after a brief respite from therapy. Corticosteroids generally potentiate the immunosuppressive benefit from any of these medications. The desire to reduce corticosteroid therapy is frequently used as an appropriate indication for immunosuppressive therapy.

In addition to approved forms of immunosuppression, a variety of experimental pharmaceuticals are currently being studied for their potential use in the therapy for inflammatory diseases. These medications include inhibitors of cytokine synthesis or function, monoclonal antibodies directed against T-lymphocytes or their subsets, and inhibitors of adhesion molecules that allow the homing of leukocytes to specific sites of inflammation. An animal study of uveitis has reported encouraging benefit from lipocortin topically (2). Lipocortin is a protein that is induced by corticosteroids and that interferes with the metabolism of arachidonic acid. Leumedins may act as functional inhibitors of adhesion molecules and have had reported success in two animal models for uveitis (3,4). Approaches to induce immune tolerance, for example, by oral administration of antigen, are undergoing active clini-

M. K. L. Cheung: Department of Ophthalmology, St. Francis Medical Center, and John A. Burns School of Medicine, University of Hawaii, Honolulu, Hawaii 96822.
J. T. Rosenbaum: Casey Eye Institute, Portland, Oregon 97201.

cal trial (5). Future therapy may also be able to target very specific T-cell receptors such that only a very discrete subset of the immune system is altered by therapy. It is likely that future generations will regard immunosuppression in the 1990s as a crude and relatively toxic approach to reducing immune-mediated disease.

AZATHIOPRINE (AZA)

History and Source

Azathioprine (AZA), a cytotoxic drug developed initially for cancer treatment, was adapted for therapy for rheumatoid arthritis and other systemic autoimmune diseases because of its immunosuppressive activity (6–8). It became one of the first immunosuppressive agents to be used to treat autoimmune uveitis (9,10). Favorable results were noted in the treatment of steroid-resistant uveitis (11).

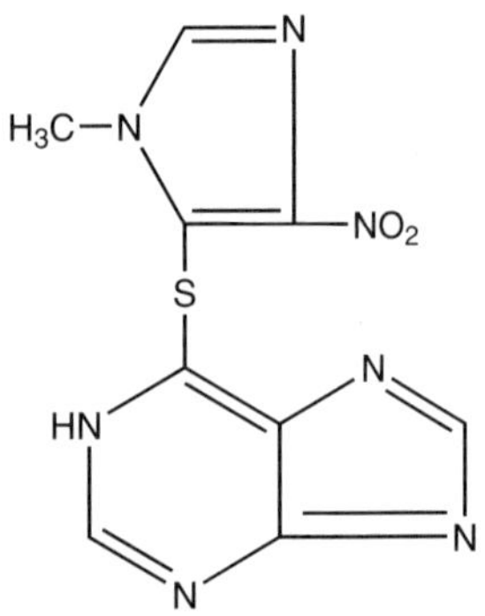

Official Drug Name and Chemistry: Azathioprine (Imuran)

Chemically, AZA is 6-[(1-methyl-4-nitroimidazol-5-yl)thio]purine, a purine analog. It is an imidazolyl derivative of 6-mercaptopurine(6-MP), and is a pale yellow powder, odorless, insoluble in water but soluble in alcohol. It hydrolyzes in alkaline solutions and remains stable in neutral or acidic solutions and converts to 6-MP in the presence of sulfhydryl compounds (oxidizing agents), such as cysteine, glutathione, and hydrogen sulfide (12).

Pharmacology

Azathioprine is a purine antagonist antimetabolite. It is a prodrug of 6-MP. Many of its biological effects are similar to those of the parent compound, 6-MP. Following absorption, it is rapidly metabolized to 6-MP and to other active metabolites: 6-thioinosinic acid and 6-thioguanylic acid (12,13). These metabolites incorporate into nucleotides and generate false codes, affecting the synthesis of nucleic acids and proteins. It also interferes with cellular metabolism by inhibiting the formation and function of coenzymes.

Clinical Pharmacology

The mechanism by which AZA exerts its immunosuppressive effects has not been determined. It inhibits cell-mediated immunity and T-cell-dependent antibody production in animal models (14). This suppression is temporally dependent on the time when the antigen is presented. Therefore, the therapeutic efficacy of AZA varies considerably with the time when therapy is initiated. It works best when administered before an antigen challenge (15). In humans, AZA suppresses the induction of delayed hypersensitivity reactions but does not prevent delayed hypersensitivity to already primed antigens. The immunosuppressive effects are dose dependent; AZA is slow acting, and its effects may persist even after the drug is discontinued.

Pharmaceutics

Oral administration of AZA is in 50-mg scored tablets; the unit dose pack is 100 tablets. Parenterally, AZA is administered in a dose of 100 mg (as the sodium salt) in a 20-ml vial for intravenous (i.v.) injection. It should be stored at 15°to 25°C (59°to 77°F) in a dry place and protected from light. The manufacturer is Burroughs Wellcome.

Pharmacokinetics, Concentration-effect Relationship and Metabolism

Orally, AZA is well absorbed. After oral administration, it is rapidly metabolized to 6-MP (7,12,13). The serum concentrations are low, usually <μg/ml. The drug serum levels have little therapeutic predictive value; only 30% of AZA and 6-MP are bound to serum proteins. The magnitude and duration of the clinical effects correlate, rather, with the tissue levels of thiopurine nucleotide. Both AZA and 6-MP are rapidly eliminated from the blood and are oxidized or methylated in erythrocytes and the liver to inactive metabolites that are excreted in the urine. Although the dose is reduced in patients with poor renal function, creatinine clearance is probably not an important parameter to monitor. Azathioprine is degraded by xanthine oxidase to its inactive form. Therefore, concomitant use of allopurinol, an inhibitor of xanthine oxidase, delays inactivation, and only 25% of the standard dose should be given (7,16).

Therapeutic Use

Azathioprine is effective in the management of a wide variety of autoimmune diseases. It is particularly successful in the treatment of rheumatoid arthritis (6–8); however, its use in juvenile rheumatoid arthritis is limited, and its safety in children has not been well established. This drug can be useful in achieving a corticosteroid-sparing effect in other autoimmune diseases, such as systemic lupus erythematosus (9), Wegener's granulomatosis (9,17,18), pars planitis (10), Vogt-Kayanagi-Harada syndrome (9,10), and, despite some conflicting results (9), with sympathetic ophthalmia (19). In the treatment of Behçet's disease, several studies have reported favorable results with the use of AZA (20–22), although some less successful outcomes also have been reported (23,24). In a randomized, double-blind study by Yazici et al., AZA at a daily dose of 2.5 mg/kg was effective in controlling the progression as well as the ocular manifestation of Behçet's disease (22). It can prevent the development and recurrence of new ocular manifestations in the disease.

For the anterior segment, AZA is effective in prolonging corneal graft survival in high-risk cases (25–27). It serves as a steroid-sparing agent for the control of scleritis and scleritis associated with relapsing polychondritis (28). Furthermore, it is an effective adjunctive agent, although not the first line of therapy in controlling the inflammation associated with cicatricial pemphigoid (29). For the treatment of iritis or iridocyclitis, however, a double-blind study showed that AZA is no more effective than placebo (30).

For ocular diseases, the recommended starting daily dose is 1 mg/kg. After 12 weeks, the daily dose can be slowly increased to a maximum of 2.5 mg/kg; however, higher doses produce a greater likelihood of neutropenia and frequently do not improve efficacy. The dose should be reduced by 75% if allopurinol is used concomitantly.

Side Effects and Toxicity

At a daily dosage level of 1 to 2 mg/kg, minimal complications of AZA are seen when used in the treatment of ocular diseases. Similar to most antimetabolites, AZA is myelotoxic (31), which may result in severe leukopenia, macrocytic anemia, or thrombocytopenia. The hematologic toxicities are dose dependent. A prompt reduction in dosage or temporary withdrawal of the drug may be necessary. Hematologic suppression may be acute or delayed; however, if an acute leukopenia occurs within a week of therapy, it is most likely an idiosyncratic reaction. Patients on AZA are recommended to have complete blood counts and platelet levels checked weekly during the first month, twice monthly for the second and third months of treatment, and monthly thereafter.

Gastrointestinal side effects can be serious; nausea and vomiting are common. Symptoms of gastrointestinal toxicity most often develop within the first several weeks of treatment (32–34). The incidence of gastric disturbance can be reduced by administering the drug in divided doses or after meals. Although rare, an acute hypersensitivity pancreatitis may present with vomiting and abdominal pain. Hepatotoxicity is manifested by an elevation of serum alkaline phosphatase, bilirubin, and serum transaminases. Although hepatic toxicity is uncommon, hepatic venoocclusion has been reported in some transplant patients and in one patient with panuveitis (35,36). Periodic measurement of serum transaminases, alkaline phosphatase, and bilirubin should be performed. If hepatic venoocclusive disease is documented, AZA should be permanently withdrawn.

Serious infection is an important concern for patients receiving chronic immunosuppression. Azathioprine causes a total lymphocytopenia of both T and B cells and reduces the synthesis of gamma globulin. It is also mutagenic in animals and humans and may increase the patient's risk of neoplasia. Some data have shown an increased incidence of lymphoproliferative disease in rheumatoid arthritis patients receiving AZA (37–39).

High-risk Groups

Pregnancy

Azathioprine and its metabolites cross the placenta (40,41). It is a teratogenic agent and can cause harm to the fetus when administered to a pregnant woman, and its use should be avoided in pregnant patients. Women of childbearing age should be informed of the risks and advised against pregnancy.

Nursing Mothers

Nursing mothers are not recommended to take AZA because of the low levels of drug present in breast milk (42); AZA has carcinogenic potential.

Pediatric Use

The safety and efficacy of AZA in children have not been established.

Patients with Impaired Renal or Hepatic Function

It is necessary to reduce the dosage of the drug or discontinue it in the presence of liver disease or unexplained abdominal pain.

Drug Interactions

The concomitant use of allopurinol and AZA can result in an overdose of AZA (7,16). Elevated levels of AZA are due to a decrease in the degradation of mercaptopurine by xanthine oxidase, an enzymatic reaction that is inhibited by allopurinol. A reduction of the normal AZA dosage by 65% to 75% is recommended for patients receiving allopurinol. When used with angiotensin-converting enzyme inhibitors, severe leukopenia has been known to be induced (43).

The combination of AZA with low-dose prednisone produced enhanced immunosuppressive effects and gave better results than either one used individually in the management of some uveitis patients (44). Another combination therapy of AZA, cyclosporine, and prednisone has been used for the suppression of organ rejection in some centers (45), but this regimen caused a high incidence of malignancies and infectious complications. For immune-mediated diseases, it is reserved for patients who do not respond adequately to less toxic therapy (46).

Major Clinical Trials

Several studies have reported favorable results with AZA in the treatment of Behçet's disease. In a double-masked, randomized controlled study, at a daily dose of 2.5 mg/kg, AZA decreased the incidence and recurrence of ocular involvement of Behçet's disease (22).

CYCLOPHOSPHAMIDE

History and Source

Cyclophosphamide (CTX) was synthesized in 1958 during an effort to develop a more selective antineoplastic agent (47). It is a derivative of nitrogen mustard with some similar chemical properties and has been used either alone or in combination with other chemotherapeutic agents in the treatment of numerous myeloproliferative disorders or solid malignancies (48). Furthermore, CTX is immunosuppressive and effective in controlling the immune reactivity of various disorders, namely, polyarteritis nodosa, Wegener's granulomatosis, and glomerulonephritis associated with systemic lupus erythematosus.

Official Drug Name and Chemistry: Cyclophosphamide (Cytoxan, Neosar)

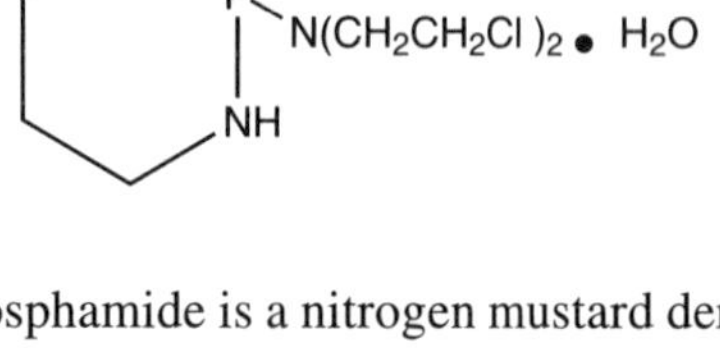

O, P, O, $N(CH_2CH_2Cl)_2 \bullet H_2O$, NH

Cyclophosphamide is a nitrogen mustard derivative with a molecular formula of $C_7H_{15}Cl_2N_2O_2P \cdot H_2O$ and a molecular weight of 279 (47). The chemical name is 2[bis(2-choroethyl)amino]tetrahydro-2H-1,3,2-oxazaphosphorine 2-oxide monohydrate. It is a white crystalline powder that is soluble in water, saline, or ethanol.

Pharmacology

Cyclophosphamide is an alkylating agent. It is metabolized by the mixed-function microsomal oxidase system in the liver to various active metabolites that interfere with the growth of rapidly proliferating malignant cells. Alkylation, the mechanism through which CTX induces cross-linking of cellular DNA (49), occurs when covalent bonds are formed between the electrophilic moieties of the metabolites and the nucleophilic substances of the DNA molecule. Cyclophosphamide acts on the 7-nitrogen atom of the nucleotide, guanine, leading to the formation of guanine–thymidine linkages, which subsequently results in DNA miscoding and disruption of nucleic acid function and protein synthesis.

Clinical Pharmacology

CTX was shown to have a marked suppressive effect on the humoral immune system in particular (50,51); however, several recent studies demonstrated that CTX affected the cellular immune system as well (52,53). Differences in the immunomodulating effect appear to be dose related. At lower dosage levels, CTX affects T-suppressor cells primarily and consequently leads to an enhanced response in cellular immunity, such as the delayed-type hypersensitivity and cytotoxicity (53); however, CTX suppresses both T-suppressor and T-helper cells at higher doses, which results in an inhibition of delayed hypersensitivity and T-cell-mediated humoral responses leading to a decrease in B-cell functions.

Pharmaceutics

Oral preparations are in 25-mg or 50-mg tablets, anhydrous. Parenteral preparations are 100 mg, 200 mg, 500 mg, 1 g, or 2 g of CTX (anhydrous). The potency of the drug is estimated by its anhydrous form. The parenteral form is commercially available as a mixture of CTX with sodium chloride or a sterile, lyophilized mixture with mannitol.

Storage at or below 77°F (25°C) is recommended. The tablets should be stored in tight containers. For the parenteral form, the preparation is stable for 24 hours at room temperature or 6 days when refrigerated at 2°to 8°C following reconstitution with bacteriostatic water. When reconstituted with sterile water, it should be used within 6 hours. Manufacturers are Bristol-Myers Oncology, Elkins-Sinn, and Adria.

Pharmacokinetics, Concentration-effect Relationship, and Metabolism

Orally, CTX is well absorbed and has a bioavailability >75% (54). It is completely metabolized within 24 hours by the liver microsomal enzymes, cytochrome-P450 to different active phosphoramide mustard, and inactive 4-keto CTX metabolites (55). No single metabolite has been demonstrated to be responsible for either the therapeutic or the toxic effects, except for acrolein, which causes hemorrhagic cystitis, a side effect that can be minimized by adequate hydration (56,57). The binding of unchanged drug to plasma protein is low, yet some of the metabolites bind >60%. It is primarily eliminated in the form of metabolites with only 5% to 25% of the dose excreted in the urine as unchanged drug. The pharmacokinetics of orally and intravenously administered CTX are similar. After an i.v. dose, the plasma concentration of the metabolites reaches a peak in 2 to 3 hours. The half-life varies between 3 and 12 hours.

Therapeutic Use

Cyclophosphamide has been established as the drug of choice for Wegener's granulomatosis, which otherwise has a grave prognosis. The work of Fauci and colleagues showed that CTX alone or in combination with corticosteroids can markedly improve patient survival (58,59). Furthermore, it also controls their ocular manifestations, especially necrotizing scleritis. In addition to Wegener's granulomatosis, CTX has been useful in managing necrotizing scleritis associated with rheumatoid arthritis (60) or relapsing polychronditis not responsive to other immunosuppressants (61).

Favorable results have been obtained with CTX controlling the inflammatory activity of ocular cicatricial pemphigoid (62) because CTX slows conjunctival shrinkage in these patients. In a randomized double-masked clinical trial conducted by Foster et al., combination therapy with prednisone was more effective than prednisone alone in suppressing the inflammation of ocular cicatricial pemphigoid (63).

Cyclophosphamide has been reported to be efficacious in treating sympathetic ophthalmia (64), Mooren's ulcers (65), ocular and systemic manifestations of polyarteritis nodosa (66), orbital vasculitis (67), and various peripheral uveitis (68). It is also the drug of choice for active lupus nephritis and is effective for various other forms of systemic vasculitides (58). In the treatment of Behçet's disease, CTX is a more effective immunosuppressant than systemic steroids (69,70).

The recommended daily oral doses of CTX in the treatment of ocular diseases is 1–2 mg/kg (65). Oral CTX is recommended to be taken before meals because the presence of phosphatase in food assists with activation of the drug. Intravenous CTX given monthly is an alternative to daily oral CTX. Intravenous delivery allows minimization of the total amount of medication and shortens greatly the duration of neutropenia. The risks of infection and bladder toxicity are reduced. Transient nausea is, of course, more frequent. The danger of bladder toxicity can be reduced further with the concomitant use of Mesna. Intravenous CTX (500 mg/M^2 monthly) plus prednisone is effective for lupus nephritis. The dose is escalated monthly based on tolerance and the nadir leukocyte count. The treatment of uveitis with i.v. CTX has been disappointing (71). Some patients respond to daily oral CTX even after failing i.v. CTX.

Side Effects and Toxicity

Cyclophosphamide is myelosuppressive and causes leukopenia, thrombocytopenia, and anemia (72). Leukopenia is dose dependent; leukopenia of <2,000 cells/mm^3 commonly occurs from an initial loading dose and occurs less frequently when maintained at a lower dose. Recovery from leukopenia usually begins 17 to 28 days after therapy is discontinued. Complete blood cell counts with white cell differentials and platelet levels should be performed before starting therapy and then weekly until the dosage, disease activity, and hematologic parameters stabilize; after that, a biweekly monitoring is appropriate.

Cyclophosphamide may markedly suppress immune responses and can lead to susceptibility to infection (72). The amount of neutropenia is particularly important in resistance to infections. Treatment should be discontinued or dosage reduced in patients who have developed viral, bacterial, or fungal infection.

Cyclophosphamide may cause sterility in both sexes because it interferes with oogenesis and spermatogenesis (73). The development of sterility appears to depend on the dose of CTX, the duration of therapy, and the state of gonadal function at the time of treatment. The azospermia or oligospermia in male patients is associated with increased gonadotropin. These patients have normal testosterone levels, and their sexual potency and libido are unimpaired. Prepubescent boys treated with CTX develop secondary sexual characteristics normally, although they may have oligospermia and some degree of testicular atrophy. Similarly, prepubescent girls treated with CTX develop secondary sex characteristics. In postpubertal females, amenorrhea is induced because of the decrease in estrogen levels and increased gonadotropin secretions. Affected patients generally resume regular menses when treatment is discontinued. Although the CTX-induced azospermia may reverse, reversibility may not occur until several years after therapy is discontinued. Gonadal dysfunction occurs in about 60% of patients after 6 months of therapy, regardless of the mode of delivery.

Hemorrhagic cystitis develops in up to 20% of patients on long-term therapy (56). Fibrosis of the urinary bladder can be extensive, even without accompanying cystitis. The bladder injury is thought to be due to CTX metabolites, especially acrolein excreted into the urine (57). This risk can be minimized by having the patient take the medicine in the morning and use adequate hydration. Patients who have developed hemorrhagic cystitis or microscopic hematuria are at an increased risk of developing bladder carcinoma. Discontinuation of the drug may be necessary in cases of hemorrhagic cystitis. Urinalysis is recommended before therapy, every 7 to 14 days initially, and then every 2 to 4 weeks once the disease and dose have been stable for 2 or 3 months.

Neoplasia, particularly myeloproliferative, lymphoproliferative, and cutaneous types, have developed in some patients treated with CTX either used alone or in association with other antineoplastic drugs (74). The risk increases with the duration of therapy, the cumulative dose (over 50 g), and the history of previous exposure to other cytotoxic agents. In rheumatoid arthritis patients, the risk of secondary neoplasia is increased tenfold compared with the normal population. The possibility of CTX-induced malignancy should be considered in any benefit-to-risk ratio. Administration of CTX for longer than 2 years is not recommended. An annual physical examination is important.

Alopecia is a common side effect; however, hair grows back after cessation of the drug (75). Anorexia, abdominal discomfort, nausea, and vomiting may occur with CTX treatment. There are other reports of hemorrhagic colitis, oral mucosal ulceration, and jaundice. At doses >50 mg/kg, the syndrome of inappropriate secretion of antidiuretic hormone has been reported in conjunction with CTX use (76). A few cases of elevated intraocular pressure (IOP) have been reported, and about 50% of patients complain of dry eyes. Cardiac toxicity has been observed only in some patients receiving high doses of CTX ranging from 120 to 270 mg/kg adjusted over a few days.

High-risk Groups

Cyclophosphamide is a highly toxic drug with a low therapeutic index. When treating with CTX, special attention should be given to patients with any history of leukopenia, thrombocytopenia, tumor infiltration to bone marrow, adrenalectomy, previous therapy with radiation or cytotoxic agents, and impaired hepatic or renal function. These patients are the most likely to develop deleterious side effects from using CTX.

Pregnancy

Cyclophosphamide can be harmful to the fetus when administered to pregnant women. If this drug is used during pregnancy, or if the patient becomes pregnant while taking this drug, the patient should be apprised of the potential hazard to the fetus. Women of childbearing age should be advised to avoid becoming pregnant.

Nursing Mothers

Cyclophosphamide is excreted in breast milk and causes leukopenia in breast-fed infants. Taking into account the importance of the drug to the mother, a decision should be made whether to discontinue nursing or to discontinue the drug because of the potential for serious adverse reactions and tumorigenicity.

Drug Interactions

Concomitant administration of phenobarbital and other drugs that potentiate hepatic enzyme metabolism shortens the half-life of CTX, and adjustment of dosage is necessary. Cyclophosphamide inhibits cholinesterase activity and potentiates the effect of succinylcholine chloride. If a patient has been treated with CTX within 10 days of general anesthesia, the anesthesiologist should be informed. Concomitant administration of allopurinol increases the risk of leukopenia by an unknown mechanism.

Major Clinical Trials

No major clinical trials have been reported to date.

METHOTREXATE (MTX)

History and Source

Methotrexate (MTX) was first introduced in 1958 as an antineoplastic agent for the treatment of leukemias (77). Its inhibitory action on the immune system has made it an efficacious drug in treatment of psoriasis, an indication that was approved by the Food and Drug Administration (FDA) in 1971 (78). Favorable results have also been shown in treatment of other nonmalignant autoimmune conditions, such as rheumatoid arthritis and uveitis.

Official Drug Name and Chemistry: Methotrexate (Rheumatrex)

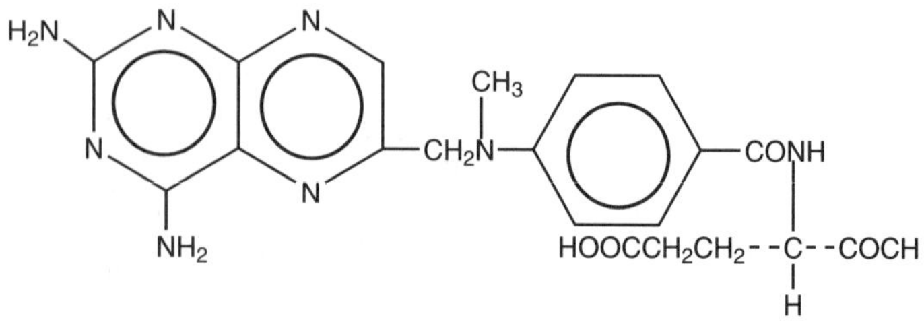

H_2N N N N CH_3 CH_2N CONH N NH_2 $HOOCCH_2CH_2$--C--COCH H

Chemically, MTX is a N-{4-{[(2,4-diamino-6-pteridinyl)-methyl]methylamino}benzoyl}-L-glutamic acid, a folic acid analogue (77). It differs from the parent compound by the substitution of an amino group instead of a hydroxyl group in the pteridine nucleus and the addition of a methyl group on the amino nitrogen between the pteroyl and benzoyl groups. It is an orange-brown, crystalline powder (79), a weak acid, and insoluble in water or alcohol. The commercial oral and parenteral preparation is a yellow powder, a sodium salt that is water soluble.

Pharmacology

As a folate analogue, MTX acts on the enzyme dihydrofolate reductase (DHFR), which catalyzes the reduction of folate to tetrahydrofolate (80). Inhibition of this enzymatic reaction decreases the amount of tetrahydrofolate, a one-carbon group carrier in the purine nucleotide and thymidylate synthesis, which interferes with DNA synthesis and cellular replication. Because the affinity of DHFR for MTX exceeds that of folic acid or dihydrofolic acid, the effect of MTX cannot be blocked even by an enormous amount of folic acid when given simultaneously. Instead, folinic acid (Leucovorin), a coenzyme of the DHFR enzymatic process, can be given to protect normal tissues from the effects of MTX when a high dosage of the drug is used (81).

Clinical Pharmacology

Methotrexate has profound effects on rapidly proliferating tissues, such as malignant cells, bone marrow, and lining of the gastrointestinal tract (82). Because the cellular proliferation in malignant tissues is greater than that in most normal tissues, MTX impairs malignant growth without irreversible damage to normal tissues. It affects the function of T and B cells and acts mostly against the humoral response, with only some activity against cellular immunity (83). Although the mechanism by which MTX affects the immune system is unclear, some studies have shown that it inhibits the multiplication of lymphocytes (84). Some studies reported that MTX affects cellular responses in the spleen and suppresses interleukin (IL)-2 production (85), but these results were not confirmed. Recent experimental studies indicate that MTX increases the level of adenosine, which has multiple anti-inflammatory effects (86). The antiinflammatory effects via adenosine may be independent of immunosuppression or antiproliferative effects. Adenosine may play a role in attenuating the effects of platelet-activating factor, which mediates the leukocyte-endothelial cell adhesion (87).

Pharmaceutics

The oral dose is in 2.5-mg tablets, in a unit dose pack of 100, or in a packaging system, called Rheumatrex (Lederle), which is designed for weekly dosing schedules of 5 mg, 7.5 mg, 12.5 mg and 15 mg.

Parenterally, MTX is in 20 mg, 50 mg, 100 mg, 250 mg, and 1 g doses (MTX sodium parenteral, Lederle; Folex, Adria). It should be stored at room temperature, 15°to 30°C (59°to 86°F), and protected from light. Manufacturers are Lederle Laboratories Division, Adria, Astra, Cetus, and Lyphomed.

Pharmacokinetics, Concentration-effect Relationship, and Metabolism

The oral absorption of MTX varies. Up to 35% of orally administered MTX may be metabolized by the intestinal flora before absorption (88). The percentage of absorption decreases as the dose increases as a result of the saturation of absorption transport at a higher dosage. Parenterally, MTX is completely absorbed (89). After an intramuscular injection, peak serum levels occur in 30 to 60 minutes. About 50% of MTX binds to serum protein, which can be displaced by various medications, such as sulfonamides, salicylates, tetracyclines, chloramphenicol, and phenytoin (79). The drug is distributed in various tissues, with the highest concentrations in the kidney, gallbladder, spleen, liver, and skin. Small amounts of MTX polyglutamate deposit in the tissue for extended periods and remain functional. The primary route of elimination is through the kidney. Depending on the dosage and route of administration, a large percentage of the drug is excreted unchanged in the urine. The half-life of MTX is approximately 3 to 10 hours. At a higher dosage, the half-life may extend from 8 to 15 hours.

Therapeutic Use

When given intravenously, MTX is effective in treating necrotizing scleritis associated with rheumatoid arthritis (90) or relapsing polychondritis (91), steroid refractory cyclitis, and sympathetic ophthalmia (92–95). Low-dose MTX therapy (12.5–15 mg/week) can be effective in controlling some chronic steroid-resistant ocular inflammatory diseases, such as chronic uveitis-vitritis, orbital myositis, idiopathic orbital inflammation, retinal vasculitis, and scleritis (96,97). It is also the drug of choice (7.5–15 mg/week) of many rheumatologists in treating patients with rheumatoid arthritis who have failed nonsteroidal antiinflammatory drugs, sulfasalazine, or antimalarials. It is also efficacious for other inflammatory disorders, such as psoriasis (98), inflammatory bowel disease (99), and recalcitrant juvenile rheumatoid arthritis (100).

The recommended dose is 10 to 25 mg/week. It is usually 4 weeks before the clinical effects are noticed. Although most patients prefer to take MTX orally, it also can be given safely intramuscularly or subcutaneously. For some patients, parenteral administration is better tolerated, particularly because it causes less nausea. Occasionally, the efficacy of MTX is improved by parenteral administration.

Side Effects and Toxicity

Hepatotoxicity is a serious side effect (101–103). Cirrhosis and hepatic fibrosis appear to be related to the total dose of MTX received. Cirrhosis is less likely if the patient does not have predisposing factors to liver disease, such as advanced age, diabetes mellitus, gross obesity, recent or active hepatitis, heavy alcohol use, or any significant liver abnormality. To monitor the liver conditions, it is recommended that a liver function test be done every 1.5 to 2 months; some authorities recommend a liver biopsy after a cumulative dose of 1.5 g. Because of the morbidity of liver biopsy and the safety of MTX, if liver function tests are persistently normal, we recommend liver biopsy only for patients predisposed to hepatic disease or who have liver function test abnormalities on several occasions. Guidelines for monitoring hepatotoxicity during methotrexate therapy for rheumatoid arthritis have been reviewed (104,105).

At any dose, MTX can cause interstitial pneumonitis, which may lead to pulmonary fibrosis (106). It may also cause an acute hypersensitivity reaction in the lungs, which improves promptly once the drug is discontinued. When restarted at a lower dosage (<8–25 mg/week), recurrences occur in about 10% of the patients. It is necessary to obtain a chest radiograph when patients develop cough or dyspnea. When there is pulmonary involvement, MTX should be discontinued.

Gastrointestinal distress, oral ulceration, and diarrhea are common complications that usually improve by reducing the dosage (106,107). Other side effects reported in association with MTX use are leukopenia, thrombocytopenia, anemia, weight loss, alopecia, increased risk of fungal infections, teratogenicity, and CNS effects, such as dysphoria and memory loss (79).

Although ocular side effects are relatively uncommon, transient aggravation of seborrheic blepharitis, photophobia, and tearing have been reported (108). It has not been necessary to discontinue the therapy because these symptoms will eventually resolve.

High-risk Groups

Pregnancy

Methotrexate is teratogenic and can cause fetal death when administered to a pregnant woman (79). Women of childbearing age should not be started on MTX until pregnancy is excluded and should be advised of the serious risk to the fetus. Pregnancy should be avoided if either partner is receiving MTX. After discontinuation of the medication, the recommended waiting period is 3 months in male patients and one ovulatory cycle in female patients before attempting conception.

Nursing Mothers

Small amounts of MTX appear in breast milk. It is contraindicated in nursing mothers because of the serious adverse effects on infants. The decision to continue with breast-feeding or to discontinue the drug depends on the risk-to-benefit ratio of the drug to the nursing mother.

Pediatric Use

Except for cancer chemotherapy, the safety and effectiveness in children have not been completely established for autoimmune diseases.

Compromised Patients

Patients with impaired hepatic or pulmonary function are at an increased risk of developing deleterious consequences.

Drug Interactions

Because 50% of methotrexate is bound to plasma proteins, certain drugs, such as sulfonamides, salicylates, tetracycline, and chloramphenicol, can displace MTX from its binding and increase the drug level (88). The coadministration of these drugs can increase the level of MTX markedly. Adjustments of dosage are particularly important. Drugs that affect the renal tubular functions, such as nonsteroidal antiinflammatory drugs, probenecid, and salicylates, can increase serious side effects by prolonging the half-life of MTX in circulation. Oral antibiotics (e.g., tetracycline, chloramphenicol, and other nonabsorbable drugs) decrease the intestinal absorption of MTX. They inhibit the bowel flora, which leads to a decreased metabolism of the drug by the bacteria.

Vitamins that contain folic acid, on the other hand, may decrease the response to MTX, whereas therapeutic and toxic effects of MTX may be potentiated in patients with folate deficiency. A particularly effective combination therapy of cyclosporin A-steroid-MTX was reported to give a total, lasting remission in 32 patients whose uveitis had failed high doses of corticosteroids and other immunosuppressive agents (109).

Major Clinical Trials

To date, no major clinical trials have been reported.

CHLORAMBUCIL (LEUKERAN)

History and Source

Chlorambucil (CRB) is a derivative of nitrogen mustard, synthesized in 1953 as a selective antineoplastic agent (110). It was used in the treatment of various neoplastic diseases, such as chronic lymphocytic leukemia, malignant lymphomas, and Hodgkin's disease (111,112). Reports of successful results in the treatment of Behçet's disease made CRB an added therapeutic agent for autoimmune and rheumatological diseases (113).

Official Drug Name and Chemistry: Chlorambucil (Leukeran)

$(ClCH_2CH_2)_2N$—[benzene ring]—$CH_2CH_2CH_2COOH$

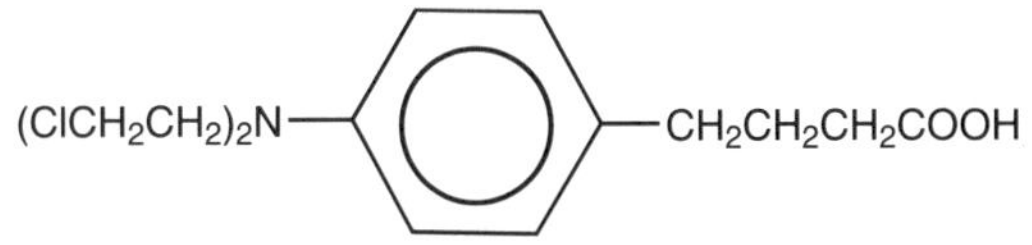

The chemical formula of CRB is 4-[bis(2-chlorethyl)amino]benzenebutanoic acid, a derivative of nitrogen mustard (110). The drug is a creamy white, granular powder. It hydrolyzes in water and has a pKa of 5.8.

Pharmacology

Both CRB and its major metabolite, phenylacetic acid mustard, are bifunctional alkylating agents with in vivo antitumor activity of CRB (114). They interfere with the DNA replication and transcription of RNA, disrupting the functions of nucleic acids (115). Although the mechanism is unclear, CRB possesses some immunosuppressive activity and causes lymphocytic suppression.

Clinical Pharmacology

It is the slowest-acting nitrogen mustard derivative. It shares many properties with CTX.

Pharmaceutics

This drug comes in 2-mg tablets that should be stored in a tight container and protected from light. The storage temperature is recommended to be between 15°and 30°C. The expiration date is 1 year after the date of manufacture. The manufacturer is Burroughs Wellcome.

Pharmacokinetics, Concentration-effect Relationship, and Metabolism

Orally administered CRB is rapidly absorbed (116). It is extensively metabolized in the liver, mainly to phenylacetic acid mustard, which is also active pharmacologically. Phenylacetic acid mustard is formed by β-oxidation of the butyric acid side chain of CRB (117). Both CRB and phenylacetic acid mustard undergo spontaneous degradation, forming monohydroxy and dihydroxy derivatives. They are almost completely metabolized, and only a small amount is excreted in the urine. Although the distribution of CRB in humans has not been fully characterized, 99% of the drug binds extensively to plasma proteins, especially albumin (118). After a single oral dose of CRB, the concentration of the drug peaks within 1 hour, and that of phenylacetic acid mustard occurs in 2 to 4 hours. The half-life of CRB and phenylacetic acid mustard is 1.5 and 2.5 hours, respectively.

Therapeutic Use

The successful results of CRB in the treatment or Behçet's disease led many ophthalmologists and rheumatologists to recommend CRB as the drug of choice for the disease (113,119–126). Many reports, except that of Tabbara et al. (121), demonstrated the efficacy of CRB in the management and long-term control of the disease.

There are also other favorable reports of CRB in the treatment of other autoimmune diseases, namely, Wegener's granulomatosis, polyarteritis nodosa (128), rheumatoid arthritis (129), and sympathetic ophthalmia (130,131). Chlorambucil is an effective drug in patients who are refractory to steroids and for whom other immunosuppressive modalities have failed. Favorable results also were reported in treatment of ocular inflammation associated with juvenile rheumatoid arthritis (121,132).

Two dosing schedules were recommended. The starting oral dose recommended by Godfrey is 2 mg daily with an increment of 2 mg/day each week until a favorable response is achieved or a maximum dose of 10 to 12 mg/day reached (121). Chlorambucil is a slow-acting agent, and typically the response is not noted until 3 to 4 weeks after initiation of therapy. If no response is observed at this dosage and no adverse effects are noted, the dosage can be increased up to as much as 22 mg/day. Foster, on the other hand, recommends a starting daily dose of 0.1 mg/kg (133). The dosage is then adjusted every 3 weeks according to the clinical response and tolerance of the patient. The maximum daily dose is 18 mg. Safe use of the drug is emphasized, with special attention to its effects on bone marrow suppression, of which the extent increases exponentially at daily doses >10 mg.

Side Effects and Toxicity

The most common side effect is bone marrow suppression. Most patients develop neutropenia during treatment, with the maximum effect noted 14 to 28 days after the start of the therapy (114,134). The suppression of bone marrow is dose related and usually occurs in patients who have received a total dosage of 6.5 mg/kg or more in one course of therapy (111). This risk increases exponentially once the daily doses go above 10 mg, when severe leukopenia can occur abruptly. Cumulative marrow toxicity also occurs. It is necessary to monitor carefully the hematologic parameters. Thrombocytopenia can be the first sign of bone marrow suppression. The dose should be decreased when the leukocyte count falls below normal value and discontinued if the depression is severe. Although bone marrow suppression occurs frequently, it is usually reversible if CRB is withdrawn early enough. The lymphocyte count usually returns to normal levels rapidly with completion of drug therapy; however, irreversible bone marrow suppression also has been reported.

This drug is the slowest acting and perhaps the least toxic of the presently available nitrogen mustard derivatives; however, CRB should be used with caution because of its carcinogenic properties (135–137). Neoplasia, mostly leukemias, have been reported after prolonged use. Although it is difficult to define the amount of cumulative dose to induce neoplasia, the risks appear to increase with a cumulative dose of 1 g or more.

Both reversible and permanent sterility has occurred as a result of CRB treatment. Azospermia was reported in males as an uncommon complication when the daily dose was <0.2 mg/kg or treatment was for <6 weeks (138). Recovery of spermatogenesis is possible within 3 years after discontinuation of therapy if the total cumulative dose is <400 mg, although irreversible azospermia may occur in some. Amenorrhea, ovary fibrosis, and follicle depletion are reported in female patients receiving CRB treatment (139,140). These changes can lead to permanent sterility. This adverse effect makes us especially reluctant to recommend an alkylating agent for pediatric patients.

In patients receiving high doses of CRB, there may be an increased risk of developing seizures (141,142). Neurological toxicity ranging from agitated behavior and ataxia to multiple grand mal seizures has also reported. Other reported complications include hypersensitivity, pulmonary fibrosis, and gastrointestinal upset (134,143).

High-risk Groups

Pregnancy

Chlorambucil crosses the placenta and can cause fetal harm when administered to a pregnant woman (144). Urogenital malformation has been reported in offspring whose mothers had received CRB during the first trimester. If this drug is used during pregnancy or if the patient becomes pregnant while taking this drug, the patient should be apprised of the potential hazard to the fetus.

Nursing Mothers

It is not known whether this drug is excreted in human milk. Because of CRB's carcinogenic properties and the potential for serious adverse reactions in nursing infants, caution should be taken in giving it to nursing mothers. It may be better to avoid its use while nursing.

Pediatric Use

The safety and effectiveness in children have not been established.

Drug Interactions

There are no known interactions with drugs. Combined use of CRB with other immunosuppressive medications will lead to greater risk of opportunistic infection.

Major Clinical Trials

To date, no major clinical trials have been reported.

DAPSONE

History and Source

Dapsone was synthesized in 1908 and was used as an antibiotic agent against streptococcal infections (145). With the development of newer antibiotics of less toxicity, other uses of dapsone were explored. It was found to be effective against chloroquine-resistant *Plasmodium falciparum* and also a good adjunctive medication for prophylaxis against other malarial infections (146). Dapsone is the drug of choice for treatment of leprosy (147). For the treatment of various bullous dermatologic diseases, especially dermatitis herpetiformis and bullous pemphigoid, good therapeutic results were noted (148,149). In another dermatological mucosal disease, ocular cicatricial pemphigoid of grave prognosis, dapsone was also effective in controlling the inflammatory processes (150,151).

Official Drug Name and Chemistry: Dapsone

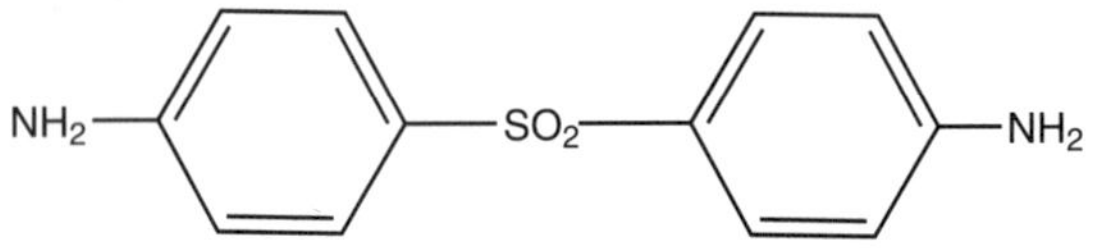

NH_2 — SO_2 — NH_2

Dapsone is a 4-4′diaminodiphenylsulfone. It is a white, odorless crystalline powder, practically insoluble in water or vegetable oils (145).

Pharmacology

Dapsone appears particularly effective for diseases that are thought to be mediated by immune complexes and polymorphonuclear leukocytes (PMNLs). The mechanisms through which dapsone downregulates immune responses may be explained by its ability to interfere with myeloperoxidase-H_2O_2-halide-mediated cytotoxic actions of PMNLs (152–154), as well as its ability to inhibit the release of lysosomal enzymes (155). Chemotaxis of PMNLs occurs in Arthus's reaction following the fixation of antigen–antibody complexes and complement activation; dapsone prevents tissue damage in this reaction by inhibition of the lysosomal enzyme release by PMNLs (156).

Pharmaceutics

Scored tablets are in 25- and 50-mg tablets. The manufacturer is Jacobus Pharmaceutical Co., Inc. (Princeton, NJ, USA). Tablets should be stored at room temperature (59°–86°F) and protected from light.

Pharmacokinetics, Concentration-effect Relationship and Metabolism

The oral absorption of dapsone is slow but complete (157). Peak plasma levels are reached in 1 to 3 hours; about 50% of the drug is bound to plasma protein (158). The drug is acetylated in the liver, and about 80% is excreted in the urine in the form of water-soluble metabolites (159).

Therapeutic Use

Dapsone is effective in controlling the systemic and ocular inflammatory activity of cicatricial pemphigoid (150,151). Foster et al. reported good responses with dapsone in 70% of his 130 patients with ocular cicatricial pemphigoid and recommended it as the drug of choice for this disease (160–162). According to this study, dapsone works best if the disease has moderate inflammatory activity and slow progression and if the patient has a normal red blood cell level of glucose-6-phosphate dehydrogenase (G-6PD). Other successful results have been reported in the treatment of systemic relapsing polychondritis (163–165) and its associated scleritis (166).

A recommended starting regimen is 25 mg, twice a day for one week (160). The dosage then can be adjusted or increased according to the therapeutic response, hematocrit, and drug tolerance of the patient. In most patients, the dosage is adjusted to maintain the hematocrit at 30% or above. A response to the treatment is usually evident within 4 weeks of therapy.

Side Effects and Toxicity

Hemolytic anemia is the most common side effect (145). The reduced form of glutathione is essential in protecting the red blood cells from hemolysis. Not only do G-6PD deficient patients lack the enzyme to keep the intracellular glutathione in its reduced form but the oxidation of glutathione by dapsone causes even more hemolysis to occur (167). Hemolytic anemia is dose dependent and is certainly present if the daily dose is at 200 to 300 mg (168). A mild reduction in hematocrit is frequent and can be acceptable. In normal persons, anemia usually is not observed until the third or fourth week of therapy. Because G-6PD-deficient persons have severe hemolysis earlier and at a lower dosage level, G-6PD levels must be determined before therapy.

Dapsone, being a sulfone, can precipitate cutaneous hypersensitivity reactions. The drug sensitization can lead to serious complications, such as toxic erythema, erythema multiforme, or toxic epidermal necrolysis (169). Dapsone should be discontinued immediately once a patient presents with hypersensitivity reaction.

There are also other side effects, including an infectious mononucleosis-like syndrome, methemoglobinemia, gastrointestinal upset, blurred vision, reversible peripheral neuropathy, and psychosis (145,152,169). These symptoms are encountered less commonly. Recently, dapsone-induced neutropenia has been reported in patients treated for ocular cicatricial pemphigoid. This side effect did not appear to be dose dependent, and leukocyte monitoring was recommended (170).

High-risk Groups

Pregnancy

There is no animal or controlled human study regarding the adverse effect of dapsone in pregnancy. Clinical experiences, however, have shown an absence of harmful effects of the drug even when given to pregnant women during all three trimesters.

Nursing Mothers

Dapsone is excreted in the breast milk and can cause hemolysis in neonates. Nursing mothers required to be on dapsone should not breast-feed their infants.

Pediatric Use

Dapsone does not affect the growth and development of a child. It can be administered to children but in smaller doses.

Drug Interactions

Rifampin accelerates the clearance rate of dapsone in the plasma and lowers the drug levels by 7 to 10 times (171). On the other hand, pyrimethamine, a folic acid antagonist, lowers the drug levels by increasing the incidence of hemolysis (2). It is necessary to adjust the dosage of dapsone in patients who are taking these drugs simultaneously.

Major Clinical Trials

To date, no major clinical trials have been reported.

RAPAMYCIN (RAPA)

History and Source

Rapamycin (RAPA) is extracted from the fermentation broth of *Streptomyces hygroscopicus,* a fungus found in the soil sample from Easter Island (Rapa Nui) (172,173). It was initially tested as an antifungal agent and was found to be very effective against the *Candida* species, especially *Candida albicans* (174); however, the immunosuppressive effects were so significant that it has subsequently become an important new immunosuppressive agent (175). In various animal models of the heart, kidney, pancreas, and small bowel transplantation, RAPA prolongs the survival rate of allografts (176,177). Further research studies have also demonstrated the potency of RAPA in preventing the occurrence of noninfectious autoimmune diseases (178,179). This drug is not approved by the U.S. FDA; it is investigational at the time of this writing. Its potential value in the treatment of uveitis is untested.

Official Drug Name and Chemistry: Rapamycin (RAPA)

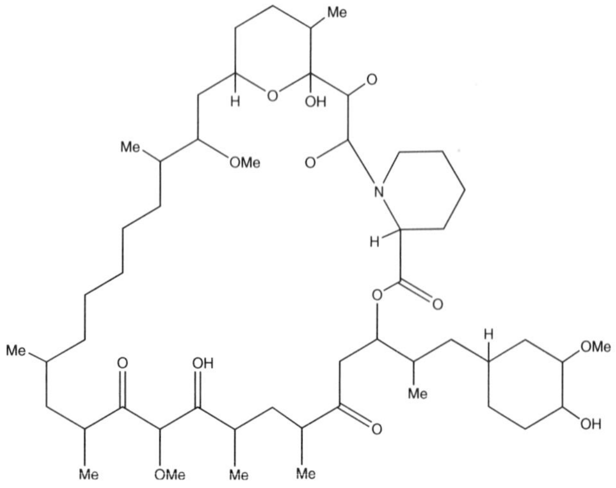

Me
H O OH O
Me OMe O
N
H
O O
Me H OMe
O OH
Me O
OH
Me OMe Me Me

Rapamycin is a colorless, crystalline solid (172). Structurally, it has some resemblance to FK 506. The molecular formula is $C_{56}H_{89}NO_{14}$, and the molecular weight is 999. It melts at 183°to 185°C. It is soluble in alcohol and insoluble in water.

Pharmacology

Quite different from the mechanisms of CSA and FK506, which inhibit the transcription of T-cell IL-2 and IL-4 genes, RAPA operates by inhibiting the transduction signal of growth factors, leading to immunosuppression of lymphocytes (180–182). It also interferes with the activation of the kinase cascade induced by IL-2. Rapamycin inhibits the proliferation of T cells by its action on IL-4 and IL-6. Compared with CSA and FK 506, the B cells are least affected by RAPA, an important attribute in the prolonged treatment of autoimmune diseases (183).

Pharmacokinetics, Concentration-effect Relationship, and Metabolism

Studies on the pharmacokinetics and the metabolism of the drug are under way.

Therapeutic Use

Rapamycin has been shown to be an effective immunosuppressant in various animal models of organ transplant and autoimmune diseases. A recent study on a rat corneal allograft model showed that RAPA not only prolonged survival but significantly inhibited neovascularization of corneal grafts (184). At present, a clinical study is being conducted to evaluate the use of this medication in humans and its efficacy in the treatment of psoriasis. The manufacturer is Wyeth-Ayerst Research, Philadelphia.

Side Effects and Toxicity

In contrast to CSA and FK 506, RAPA has low renal toxicity. Weight loss has been reported during the first week of treatment but usually stabilizes over the course of the treatment. All the studies so far have shown limited side effects (179).

Drug Interactions

Synergistic effects have been observed when RAPA was coadministered with steroids and cyclosporine in animal models (185). Refer to the drug interaction section on FK 506 for information about RAPA administered with this drug.

Major Clinical Trials

A major clinical trial is being conducted in patients with psoriasis to evaluate the therapeutic value of RAPA in humans.

FK 506

History and Source

FK 506 was isolated from the fermentation broth of *Streptomyces tsukubaensis,* a fungus that was first found in a soil sample obtained from Tsukuka, Japan, in 1984 (186). It has potent immunosuppressive activity with a mechanism of action similar to that of cyclosporine, which impairs T-cell functions (187). FK 506 was studied extensively in transplantation models in rats and primates and was more efficacious than cyclosporine A (CSA) in prolonging allograft survival (188,189). Studies were also conducted in various experimental autoimmune uveitis models with results suggesting the effectiveness of FK 506 in treating various immunologically mediated ocular diseases (190,191).

Official Drug Name and Chemistry: FK 506

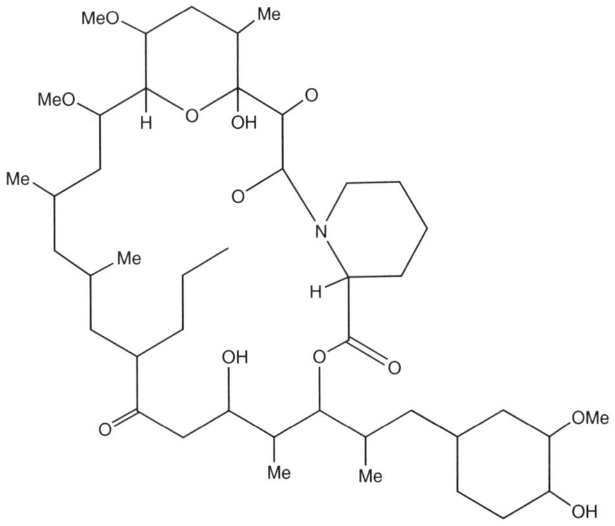

FK 506 is a colorless powder with a molecular formula of $C_{44}H_{69}NO_{12}\cdot H_2O$. The anhydrous molecular weight is 804. It is a neutral macrolide and is highly lipophilic in nature. It is soluble in alcohol and moderately soluble in polyethylene glycol and olive oil but insoluble in water.

Pharmacology

Although FK 506 is structurally different from CSA, the pharmacological mechanisms of the two compounds are very similar. Both CSA and FK 506 function as prodrugs. Each binds to a separate cytoplasmic receptor, immunophilin (immunosuppressant binding protein), forming a complex that acts on protein phosphatase, calcineurin, to exert immunosuppressive effects (192–194). FK 506 binds to an immunophilin named FK-binding protein (FKBP). Similar to the mechanisms of CSA, FK 506 inhibits genes that encode IL-2, IL-3, IL-4, interferon-gamma, tumor necrosis factor-alpha, granulocyte-colony stimulating factor, and *c-myc* that are responsible for the early activation of T cells (195). FK 506, furthermore, suppresses the mixed lymphocyte reactions, the production of T-cell-mediated soluble factors, and the expression of IL-2 receptors. In addition to its effects on T cells, FK 506 acts on B cells indirectly through its action on T-helper cells. By reducing the recruitment of T-helper cells, FK 506 decreases the numbers of infiltrating B cells in a humoral response (196).

Clinical Pharmacology

FK 506 inhibits T-cell functions and appears to be 10 to 100 times more effective than CSA (188,189). In experimental autoimmune uveoretinitis animal models, FK 506 inhibits the expression of IL-2 receptors on T cells and also that of the major histocompatibility complex (MHC) class II antigens on ocular resident cells (197). It prolongs the recruitment time of the T-suppressor/cytotoxic cells in an inflammatory response. An important advantage of FK 506 in the treatment of uveitis is that it suppresses ongoing inflammatory processes. It acts on the effector limb of an immune process, even when development of the event is at an advanced stage (198).

Pharmaceutics

Dosages of 0.05, 0.1, and 0.2 mg/kg twice a day were used in the clinical trial of FK 506 for treatment of uveitis in Japan (199). It was recommended that the trough level of FK 506 in the whole blood be maintained at below 20 ng/ml. The manufacturer of FK 506 is Fujisawa Pharmaceutical Co. (Osaka, Japan).

Pharmacokinetics, Concentration-effect Relationship, and Metabolism

After an oral intake, FK 506 is absorbed rapidly into the gastrointestinal tract (200). The serum level peaks in 2 to 3 hours and decreases to baseline in 8 to 10 hours. The oral bioavailability of FK 506 averages approximately 27% because of the low aqueous solubility of FK 506 in the gastric fluids. With i.v. administration, the peak plasma concentration occurs at 0.5 to 4 hours. FK 506 binds extensively to red blood cells. It is possible that intracellular contents of RBCs may contain large amounts of FKBP. In plasma, FK 506 binds primarily to α-1-acidic glycoprotein, which is in contrast to CSA, which associates with lipoproteins. At equilibrium, FK 506 distributes in the heart, lung, spleen, kidney, and pancreas (201). FK 506 has not been detected in the cerebrospinal fluid of patients with neurotoxicity, even though it was thought to be related to the therapy (200).

FK 506 is primarily eliminated by metabolism. It undergoes demethylation and hydroxylation. Most of the metabolites are excreted in the bile. Less than 5% of the drug is excreted unchanged or as its conjugates in the bile. The half-life is based on the plasma concentration of the drug and ranges between 3.5 and 40.5 hours.

Therapeutic Use

In humans, FK 506 (0.15 mg/kg/day) prolongs allograft survival in patients undergoing liver transplantation (202) and was recently approved by the FDA for this indication. This new immunosuppressive agent has potential efficacy in treatment of other autoimmune diseases, such as uveitis, in humans. The multicenter study in Japan showed that FK 506 is effective in treating some patients with steroid-resistant Behçet's disease (199). When tested in various animal models, FK 506 was effective as therapy for corneal allograft rejection, endotoxin-induced uveitis, and experimental autoimmune uveoretinitis (190,191,203,204).

Side Effects and Toxicity

The side effects of FK 506 are very similar to that of CSA except the incidence of hypertension occurs at a different frequency (205). Similar to CSA, nephrotoxicity is a serious side effect. FK 506 causes renal damage. Pathologic studies revealed morphological changes in the juxtaglomerular cells of the renal vasculature in animals treated at a high dosage level (206). Focal medial necrosis of the renal arterioles and changes in the proximal tubules also were observed. Renal biopsy specimens obtained from human subjects, however, showed primarily tubular changes, especially the proximal tubules (207). Based on the clinical trial study in Japan, renal impairment was noted in patients receiving 0.2 mg/kg of FK 506 (199). Patients with renal dysfunction are particularly vulnerable. It is imperative to obtain a baseline renal function test before treatment and to monitor patients at regular intervals. At high doses, FK 506 affects the synthesis of insulin and the response to glucose challenge in vitro (208). Similar observations also were observed in animal and human studies (209). FK 506 inhibits insulin secretion from the islet cells; however, both metabolic and histologic studies failed to reveal any significant toxic effects on the islet cells. This effect is dose dependent and is observed when the serum level is significantly higher than the therapeutic levels, which affects glucose metabolism and leads to hyperglycemia in some patients; however, FK 506 causes degenerative changes in the pancreatic exocrine cells and can lead to decreased secretion of various digestive enzymes (210).

Liver toxicity has been reported in animals treated with FK 506 (206). Some patients had significantly elevated serum titers of lactate dehydrogenase and aspartate aminotransferase when treated with higher doses of FK 506. Similarly, pathologic studies also revealed diffuse multiple granulomas in the livers of some animals treated with FK 506 (191).

A disconcerting side effect of FK 506 is its involvement of the CNS (206). There have been reports of patients developing seizures, confusion, dysarthria, and even coma. These CNS effects, however, do not appear to be dose related. FK 506 was not detected in the cerebrospinal fluid of patients who suffered CNS effects (200).

Other reported side effects include hyperkalemia, chest discomfort, tremor, and weight loss (206). The change in weight is probably due to anorexia, lethargy, and diarrhea that patients experience while on the medication. An increase in blood urea nitrogen (BUN) without an associated rise in serum creatinine is more likely a result of dehydration from anorexia and diarrhea (211). Although there is a significant decrease in the hematocrit early in treatment, it usually normalizes by the third week of therapy. Intervention may not be needed, but close monitoring is necessary.

High-risk Groups

Pregnancy

It is unclear whether FK 506 is teratogenic. The concentration of FK 506 in placental tissue has been found higher than that of the plasma, suggesting a potential transfer to the fetus (206). Until more detailed studies are done, it is best to refrain from administering this medication to pregnant women.

Patients with Liver Dysfunction

The concentrations of FK 506 are higher in patients with liver dysfunction. The decrease in metabolism results in a longer half-life and a lower clearance rate, a condition that can further potentiate the side effects of the drug, even when given at a lower dosage level.

Pediatric Use

Pediatric patients tolerate FK 506 better than adults (212,213). Although they absorb FK 506 as well as adults, on average pediatric patients require twice the dosages given to an adult to maintain a similar therapeutic level. This requirement may simply be due to the higher clearance rate of FK 506 in the pediatric group.

Drug Interactions

Synergistic immunosuppressive responses as well as increased nephrotoxicity were observed in patients receiving both CSA and FK 506 (214). Based on the studies done on dogs, the synergistic response of the two drugs is accounted for by the increase in oral bioavailability of FK 506 through some unknown mechanisms (215).

Drugs that affect liver metabolism, enzyme inhibitors, or inducers, also will affect the metabolism of FK 506 and its plasma concentration (216). The concentration of FK 506 increases when it is coadministered with enzyme inhibitors, such as clotrimazole, ketoconazole, erythromycin, fluconazole, diltiazam, and cimetidine.

Because FK 506 and RAPA are inhibitory to each other's action, both may act on a common receptor-binding protein (217). An excess of one drug can revert the other drug's mediated inhibition of IL-2 production. Laboratory findings suggest that FK 506 interferes with the antigen-receptor-induced signals and that rapamycin affects the IL-2-induced signals.

Major Clinical Trials

The results of the Japanese multicenter clinical open trial showed that FK 506 was efficacious in the treatment of refractory uveitis patients (199); 80% of the patients maintained or improved their visual acuity with FK 506 treatment. Currently in Japan, another clinical trial of FK 506 is under way in treating patients with severe uveitis of noninfectious etiology. The role of FK 506 in treating uveitis or other autoimmune disease is currently experimental; its use in treating uveitis should be reserved for well-designed clinical trials.

CYCLOSPORIN(E) (CSA)

History and Source

Cyclosporin (CSA) is an important drug for the treatment of uveitis. It was isolated from the fungus *Tolypocladium inflatum Gams* as an antifungal agent in 1970 (218). During the course of the research, it was found to have a potent immunosuppressive activity against T cells (219). This property made it a vital drug for the management of allograft rejections. Because a wide spectrum of uveitic diseases are T-cell mediated, Nussenblatt and colleagues pioneered in using CSA for the treatment of uveitis (220,221). It is effective and useful for a variety of ocular autoimmune inflammatory diseases, especially in cases where steroids or other immunosuppressants have failed.

Official Drug Name and Chemistry: Cyclosporin A, Cyclosporine, USP (Sandimmune)

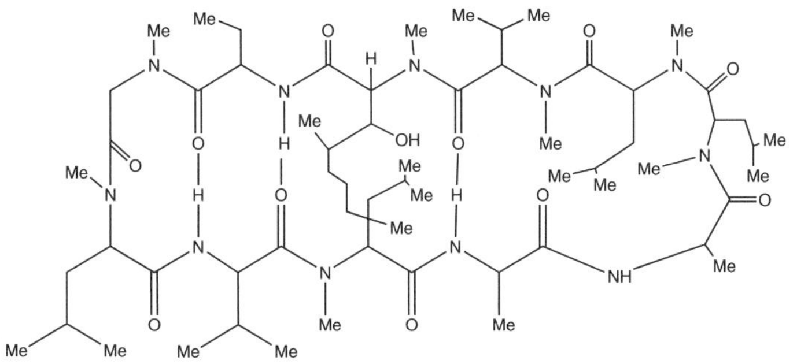

The chemical formula is (R-(R*,R*-(E)))-cyclic(L-alanyl-*D*-alanyl-*N*-methyl-L-leucyl-*N*-methyl-L-leucyl-*N*-methyl-L-valyl-3-hydroxy-*N*,4-dimethyl-L-2-amino-6 octenoyl -L-α-amino-butyryl-*N*-methylglycyl-*N*-methyl-L-leucyl-L-valyl-*N*-methyl-L-leucyl). This drug is a powdery white crystalline compound; it is a neutral, lipophilic, cyclic polypeptide consisting of 11 amino acids; and it has a molecular weight of 1,203 g (218). The drug is fairly soluble in lipids and organic solvents but practically insoluble in aqueous. For clinical applications, CSA is dissolved in castor oil or olive oil with ethanol.

Pharmacology

The precise mechanisms of the immunosuppressive activity of CSA are still not fully understood, but it is known that CSA affects T-cell activation at different cellular levels. It becomes activated when it binds to endogenous intracellular receptors (immunophilins), named cyclophilin (222). The CSA-cyclophilin complexes then act through a calcium-dependent cytoplasmic pathway via a protein phosphatase, calcineurin (223), which inhibits activation cascade of immune reactions by suppressing mRNA transcription of the necessary lymphokines (224,225). The production of IL-2, an activator of T cells, particularly T-helper cells, is markedly reduced by the inhibition of CSA on the synthesis of the α- and β-chains of IL-2 receptor. The drug interferes with the recognition of T-lymphocyte surface receptors to DR antigens on antigen-presenting cells, thus inhibiting the activation of T cells (226,227); however, CSA does not affect the responsiveness of antigen-primed T cells (228).

Clinical Pharmacology

Because CSA acts predominantly on T cells, it is a potent immunosuppressant for cell-mediated immunity (219,221). Clinically, it is an extremely effective drug in suppressing allograft rejections in various organ transplants (i.e., heart, kidney, pancreas, liver, bone marrow, and lung). Furthermore, it suppresses graft-versus-host disease, delayed hypersensitivity, and autoimmune diseases. Some studies showed that CSA also may inhibit humoral responses to some extent. The mechanisms of CSA involve mostly the inhibition of lymphocytic proliferation and functions by suppressing the production of various lymphokines. Cyclosporine is important for treating noninfectious sight-threatening inflammatory eye diseases, particularly in patients who have failed other therapies.

Pharmaceutics

Sandimmune (cyclosporine) oral solution, USP, is supplied in 50-ml bottles containing 100 mg/ml of cyclosporine. Each milliliter contains 100 mg of cyclosporine dissolved in olive oil with 12.5% ethanol by volume and peglicol 5 oleate. The drug must be diluted further with milk, chocolate milk, or orange juice before oral administration. It also comes in gelatine capsules, 25 and 100 mg, and Neoral is available in a micropulverized oral version.

For parenteral administration, Sandimmune i.v. is supplied at a concentration of 50 mg/ml dissolved in castor oil with 32.9% ethanol by volume.

The drug is recommended for storage at a temperature below 66°F (30°C). It should not be refrigerated. Once opened, the contents must be used within 2 months. The manufacturer is Sandoz Pharmaceuticals.

Pharmacokinetics, Concentration-effect Relationship, and Metabolism

The oral absorption of cyclosporine from the small intestine is incomplete and highly variable, ranging between 4% and 60%, with an average of 30% absorption of the agent (229). Absorption is affected by biliary diversion and gastrointestinal motility. The peak drug levels occur approximately 4 to 5 hours after ingestion; 90% of the CSA in circulation is associated with lipoproteins. The distribution volume appears to correlate with the levels of cytoplasmic binding proteins, through which the drug may be retained for months even after discontinuation of the therapy. The median half-life is 6.4 to 8.7 hours. The drug is concentrated in lipid-containing tissues, with the liver being the major depot, followed by the pancreas, fat, breast, blood, heart, lung, kidney, and neural and muscular tissues. It is metabolized on first pass through the liver by the cytochrome P-450 microsomal enzyme system (230) and is excreted primarily through the bile and intestines; only 6% is excreted by the kidney. The clearance rate in children is 45% higher than in adults (231), whereas in the elderly and patients with hepatic impairment, the drug clearance is slower.

The ocular bioavailability of CSA depends on the integrity of the blood–ocular barrier. In experimental animals, systemic or topically administered CSA does not penetrate through noninflamed intact ocular tissues, such as the corneal epithelium or the vascular endothelium (232). In the eyes of patients with chronic flare, however, the concentration in the aqueous humor is about 40% of the plasma concentration, indicating good intraocular penetration of the drug (233). When either the corneal or conjunctival epithelium is damaged, high levels of CSA are detected in the aqueous humor.

Therapeutic Use

Generally, CSA is used when other forms of therapy have failed, particularly in treating bilateral sight-threatening uveitis in patients who are refractory or unable to tolerate systemic steroids and cytotoxic agents. It is an especially effective treatment for ocular complications of Behçet's disease (234), but nephrotoxicity is noted at the high dosage used. There are conflicting results regarding the efficacy of lower dose of CSA in the treatment of Behçet's disease (235,236). A double-blind study by Masuda et al. showed that CSA as the sole therapeutic agent was more effective than colchicine (237). When used at 5 mg/kg/day, mixed results were obtained with some success in three of ten patients; in five patients therapy failed (238).

In a randomized short-term study, CSA as a sole agent was effective in 46% of the uveitic patients (239). It was efficacious for birdshot retinochoroidopathy, pars planitis, sarcoidosis, Vogt-Koyanagi-Harada syndrome, and sympathetic ophthalmia (231,240,241). Favorable results with low-dose CSA were reported in the management of birdshot retinochoroidopathy, granulomatous optic neuropathy, and orbitopathy (242,243). Towler showed effectiveness in 97% of patients with posterior uveitis (19). A combination of low-dose CSA and systemic steroids was effective with a significant reduction of side effects (244). Therapy with azathioprine, CSA, and prednisone was proposed for treatment of serpiginous choroiditis (245). Cyclosporine was also efficacious in stopping corneal melts associated with Wegener's granulomatosis (246).

We recommend an initial dose of 2.5 to 5 mg/kg/day with the drug delivered in divided doses every 12 hours. In patients with a 30% drop in the glomerular filtration rate (GFR) or a sustained increase in the creatinine and the BUN levels, we recommend a dosage reduction. In pediatric use, the same dose and dosing regimen may be used as in adults. In several studies, children have required and tolerated higher doses than adults (231). Cyclosporine is also available in capsule form. Dosage adjustment is more accurate but less convenient with the oral solution. There is a new micropulverized oral version, Neoral, which supposedly provides more consistent bioavailability. Periocular administration has proved not to be particularly efficacious.

Two percent topical CSA is efficacious in delaying corneal rejection in high-risk corneal grafts (247,248). It had a success rate of 89% when used postoperatively and a success rate of 91% when the medication was begun 2 days before surgery. Ben Ezra showed in a double-blind study that topical CSA was effective in treating severe vernal keratoconjunctivitis (249). Favorable results have also been reported for the treatment of ligneous conjunctivitis (250) and corneal ulceration associated with rheumatoid arthritis with or without scleral melts (251).

Little has been published about the optimal topical dosage with CSA. In most animal studies, a 1 to 2% solution was given five times/day. In human studies, a 2% solution was administered with a frequency ranging from four times a day to every 2 hours. The preparation of topical cyclosporine requires evaporation of the alcohol from the oral solution before dilution with olive oil.

Side Effects and Toxicity

Nephrotoxicity is the most serious side effect of systemic cyclosporine use (252). The severity of renal dysfunction is dependent on the dosage used, the duration of the therapy, and the individual's underlying renal status. Most early nephrotoxicity is probably physiologic and can be reversed by lowering the dosage; however, progressive morphologic changes in the kidney, as characterized by interstitial fibrosis and tubular atrophy, occur with long-term therapy (253). Signs of nephrotoxicity include increased serum creatinine and BUN, elevated blood pressure, reduced creatinine clearance, and reduced GFR. A 30% rise in BUN/creatinine or a 30% drop in GFR should prompt a reduction in the dose of cyclosporine. It is recommended, therefore, to have blood pressure, serum creatinine, and BUN levels checked at every visit. A 24-hour creatinine clearance every 3 to 6 months, and glomerular filtration rate every year or following a significant drop in the 24-hour creatinine clearance should be obtained.

A common side effect is hypertension (254), but it is usually not severe. The effect can be reversed by decreasing the dosage or by using antihypertensive medications. Because cyclosporine may cause hyperkalemia, potassium-sparing diuretics should be avoided. Calcium antagonists can be effective, but they interfere with the metabolism of cyclosporine, and dosage adjustment may be required (255). The only exception is nifedipine.

Hepatotoxicity is dose dependent and can be reversible (252). It occurs mostly in transplant patients and less commonly in uveitis patients. Longer dosing intervals may be required in the presence of elevated serum levels of bilirubin or alanine aminotransferase, and liver function tests should be monitored every 6 to 12 months.

Increased susceptibility to infection may occur from oversuppression of the immune system. Other complications include gingival hyperplasia, which occurs in 25% of the patients and is exacerbated by poor oral hygiene (256). Hirsutism can be distressing to female or pediatric patients. Paresthesia, temperature hypersensitivity, nausea, and vomiting are common. Elevation of the serum cholesterol levels probably is due to increased low-density lipoprotein levels (257).

Cyclosporine has not been found to be mutagenic or genotoxic, but there is an increased associated risk of developing lymphomas and other malignancies, particularly those of the skin (258). The incidence is higher than in the normal, healthy population but similar to that in patients receiving other immunosuppressive therapies. This increased risk probably is related more to the intensity and duration of immunosuppression than the use of CSA.

Many adverse changes reported with cyclosporine were seen at 10 mg/kg/day (252). These changes were not noted when a lower dose was used. The long-term use of CSA at a minimal dose of 0.75 to 2 mg/kg/day, when closely monitored, stabilized or improved vision in 76% of patients with uveitis who had follow-up for a median of 7 years (259). The only significant side effect was hypertension. None of the patients developed renal failure, and the serum creatinine level was only minimally elevated. Creatinine clearance, serum minerals, and cholesterol were minimally affected.

The only side effect of topical CSA is related to allergic reactions to the vehicle, causing redness, itching, tearing, and burning of the eye. No other ocular side effects have been reported.

High-risk Groups

Pregnancy

When given at 2 to 5 times the human dose, CSA has been shown to be embryotoxic and fetotoxic in rats and rabbits (260); however, within the well-tolerated dose range, the oral solution has proved to be without any embryolethal or teratogenic effects. Well-controlled studies in pregnant women have not been done. It should be used during pregnancy only if the potential benefit justifies the potential risks to the fetus. Data based on pregnant women taking cyclosporine throughout gestation showed premature birth, low birth weight, and other complicated disorders, such as preeclampsia, eclampsia, premature labor, abruptio placentae, oligohydramnios, and fetoplacental dysfunction.

Nursing Mothers

Because CSA is excreted in human milk (260), nursing should be avoided.

Pediatric Use

Although there is no well-controlled study done in children and long-term follow-up data are unavailable, patients as young as 6 months of age have received the drug with no unusual adverse effects (231).

Drug Interactions

Cyclosporine is primarily metabolized in the liver by cytochrome P-450. Co-administration of drugs that affect the cytochrome P-450 will decrease the hepatic metabolism and increase the circulating cyclosporine levels (261). Drugs that induce cytochrome P-450 enzymes will increase the hepatic metabolism and decrease the circulating CSA levels. Adjustment of dosage is necessary when these drugs are used concomitantly.

The following drugs increase CSA levels: erythromycin, oral contraceptives, androgens, methylprednisolone, calcium channel blockers except nifedipine, ketoconazole, fluconazole, traconazole, bromocriptine, metoclopramide, and danazol. The following drugs decrease cyclosporine levels: rifampin, phenobarbital, phenytoin, and carbamazepine.

Renal function should be monitored carefully when CSA is used with other nephrotoxic drugs (262), such as nonsteroidal antiinflammatory drugs, gentamicin, tobramycin, vancomycin, cimetidine, ranitidine, diclofenac, amphotericin B, ketoconazole, melphalan, trimethoprim with sulfamethoxazole, and azapropazan.

Ketoconazole is a potent inhibitor of cytochrome P-450 (263). When coadministered with ketoconazole, the required dose of CSA can be reduced by more than 30%. A combination therapy of low-dose CSA (<2 mg/kg/day) and systemic steroids has been shown effective and has significantly reduced the incidence of side effects. Furthermore, triple therapy with azathioprine and prednisone has been extremely effective in selected patients.

Clinical Trials

Two clinical studies of topical CSA for indications such as vernal conjunctivitis, keratoconjunctivitis sicca, and corneal transplantation are in progress.

RETINAL S-ANTIGEN

History and Source

S-antigen was first isolated and purified from bovine retinal extract in 1977 by Wacker and associates (264). It is a soluble protein located in the photoreceptor cell layer of the retina and is an autoantigen responsible for autoimmune reactions against the retina (265).

Official Drug Name and Chemistry

Retinal S-antigen is found in retinal photoreceptors and also in cells of the pineal gland (264). There are 403 to 405 amino acids. The calculated molecular weight from the amino acid sequences is 45 kDa. Amino acid sequencing of bovine (266), human (267), and murine (268) S-antigens were deduced from cDNA. There is 81% identity between bovine and human sequence. Uveitogenic sites are present along several short amino acid sequences (269), showing that an intact molecule is not necessary to induce uveitis.

Therapeutic Use

Oral tolerance is a state of specific immunologic unresponsiveness toward an antigen administered orally. This natural means of inducing immunosuppression has long been recognized (270). Various animal models of experimental autoimmune disease were studied to investigate the effectiveness of this method as a possible immunotherapy as well as the mechanisms. Some of these disease models are multiple sclerosis, rheumatoid arthritis, and diabetes type 1 (271). The results of these studies have shown that oral tolerance is induced with oral immunization of the respective antigens and that the disease process is ameliorated. Although the mechanism of oral tolerance is unclear, studies have shown that the immunosuppressive activity is mediated through both the cellular and humoral aspects of the immune system.

Side Effects and Toxicity

Until now, no side effect or toxicity has been reported.

Major Clinical Trials

Favorable results have been reported in a double-blind pilot trial of oral tolerance to myelin basic proteins in multiple sclerosis (272) as well as oral tolerization to type II collagen in rheumatoid arthritis (273).

A randomized, masked clinical trial is currently under way at the National Eye Institute to evaluate the effectiveness of oral administration of ocular antigens to induce tolerance in patients with various uveitis diseases.

LEUMEDINS

History and Source

NPC 15669 is a synthetic peptide that possesses antiinflammatory activities by inhibiting the recruitment of neutrophils and lymphocytes (274). It belongs to a new class of antiinflammatory agents termed leumedins.

Official Drug Name and Chemistry: NPC 15669

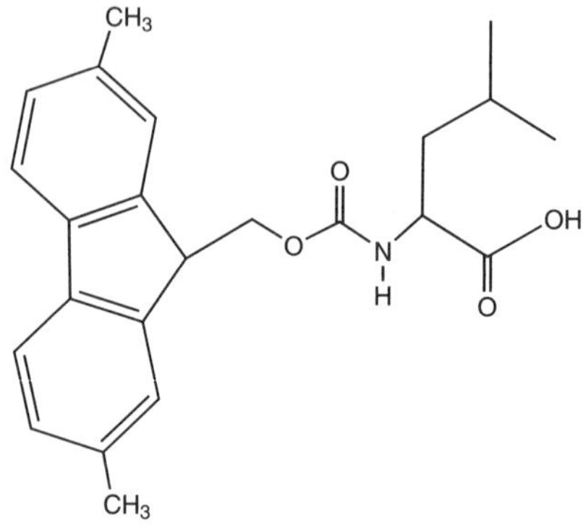

CH_3 O OH O N H O CH_3

NPC 15669 is *N*-carboxy-L-leucine,N-{(2,7-dimethylfluoren-9-yl)methyl}ester (274). It is a nonpeptide with a low molecular weight of 381.5. When prepared as sodium salt, it is readily soluble in water. The agent requires storage at 4°C and must be prepared fresh daily.

Pharmacology

NPC 15669 acts predominantly on neutrophils. It not only inhibits the recruitment of neutrophils into inflammatory lesions but also prevents the degranulation of these cells (275). Because NPC 15669 downregulates the expression of CD 11b/CD18 (MAC-1) on neutrophils, it blocks the adherence of neutrophils to vascular endothelium (276). NPC 15669 does not block metabolic enzymes or chemoattractant receptors for leukotriene B4, platelet-activating factor, complement 5a and f-met-leu-phe. It also does not inhibit the respiratory burst or phagocytosis of neutrophils and macrophages. Moreover, the agent also has some actions on lymphocytes. NPC 15669 effectively blocks two T-cell-mediated models of oxazolone dermatitis and adjuvant arthritis through its inhibitory action on the activation and recruitment of T cells (277).

Pharmacokinetics, Concentration-effect Relationship, and Metabolism

After intraperitoneal administration of NPC 15669 in a rat model, the plasma concentration of the drug rose rapidly with a peak level between 30 minutes and 1 hour (277). The agent appeared to distribute in total body water. The half-life was estimated to approximately 2 hours.

Therapeutic Use

The drug is effective in preventing septic shock (278). In two ocular inflammatory disease models, endotoxin-induced uveitis and experimental autoimmune uveoretinitis, NPC 15669 was effective in abrogating the inflammatory process (279,280).

Side Effects and Toxicity

Weight loss was noted in 50% of the animals studied. Hemolysis is a serious complication. The manufacturing company has been working to synthesize another compound with similar antiinflammatory properties as NPC 15669 and yet eliminate this untoward hemolytic side effect.

REFERENCES

1. Rosenbaum JT. Immunosuppressive therapy of uveitis. *Ophthalmological Clinics of North America* 1993;6:167–175.
2. Chan CC, Miele NM, Cordella-Miele L, et al. Effects of antiflammins on endotoxin-induced uveitis in rats. *Arch Ophthalmol* 1991;109:275.
3. Cheung MK, Dastgheib K, Chan CC, et al. Inhibition of polymorphonuclear leukocyte recruitment by NPC 15669 prevents endotoxin-induced uveitis. 1994. *Proceedings of the Meetings of the Association for Research in Vision and Ophthalmology.*
4. Cheung MK, Dastgheib K, Chan CC, et al. Prevention of uveitis by NPC 15669, an inhibitor of polymorphonuclear leukocyte recruitment in animal models. 1994. *Proceedings of the Sixth International Symposium of the Immunology and Immunopathology of the Eye.*
5. Grejerson DS, Obritsch WF, Donoso LA, et al. Oral tolerance in experimental autoimmune uveoretinitis. *J Immunol* 1993;151:5751–5761.
6. Elion GB, Callahan S, Bieber S, Hitchings GH, Rundles RW. A summary of investigations with 6[(1-methyl-4-nitro-5-imidazolyl)-thio] purine. *Cancer Chemother Rep* 1961;14:93–98.
7. Gilman AG, Goodman LS, Rall TW, Murad F. In: *The Pharmacological Basis of Therapeutics.* New York: Macmillan Publishing Company, 1985.
8. Davis JD, Muss HB, Turner RA. Cytotoxic agents in the treatment of rheumatoid arthritis. *South Med J* 1978;71:58–64.
9. Newell FW, Krill AE. Treatment of uveitis with azathioprine (Imuran). *Trans Ophthalmol Soc UK* 1967;87:499–511.
10. Newell FW, Krill AE, Thomson A. The treatment of uveitis with six-mercaptopurine. *Am J Ophthalmol* 1966;61:1250–1255.
11. Corley CC, Lessner SE, Larsen WE. Azatheioprine therapy of "autoimmune" diseases. *Am J Med* 1966;41:404–412.
12. Elion GB. Biochemistry and pharmacology of purine analogs. *Fed Proc* 1967;26:898–904.
13. Elion GB, Hitchings GH. Metabolic basis for the actions of analogs of purines and pyrimidines. *Adv Chemother* 1965;2:91–177.
14. McIntosh J, Hansen P, Ziegler J. Defective immune and phagocytic functions in uraemia and renal transplantation. *Int Arch Allergy Immunol* 1976;15:544–549.
15. McGeown M. Immunosuppression for kidney transplantation. *Lancet* 1973;2:310–312.
16. Elion GB, Callahan S, Rundles RW, Hitchings GH. Relationship between metabolic fates and anti-tumor activities of thiopurines. *Cancer Res* 1963;23:1207–1217.
17. Koyama T, Matsuo N, Watanabe Y. Wegener's granulomatosis with destructive ocular manifestations. *Am J Ophthalmol* 1984;98:736–740.
18. Bouroncle BA, Smith EJ, Cuppage FE. Treatment of Wegener's granulomatosis with Imuran. *Am J Med* 1967;42:314–318.
19. Moore CE. Sympathetic ophthalmia treated with azathioprine. *Br J Ophthalmol* 1968;52:688–690.
20. Bietti GB, Cerulli L, Pivetti-Pezzi P. Behçet's disease and immunosuppressive treatment. *Mod Probl Ophthalmol* 1976;16:314–323.
21. Aoki K, Sugiura S. Immunosuppressive treatment of Behçet's disease. *Mod Probl Ophthalmol* 1976;16:309–313.
22. Yazici H, Pazarli H, Barnes CG, et al. A controlled trial of azathioprine in Behçet's syndrome. *N Engl J Med* 1990;322:281–285.
23. Baer JC, Foster CS, Raizman MB. Ocular Behçet's syndrome: clinical presentation and visual outcome in 26 patients. *Ophthalmology* 1989;96(suppl):128 (abst).
24. Martenet AC. Resultats de l'immunodepression par cytostatiques en ophthalmologie. *Ophthalmologica (Basel)* 1976;172:106–115.
25. Leibowitz HM, Elliott JH. Chemotherapeutic immunosuppression of the corneal graft rejection. I. Systemic antimetabolites. *Arch Ophthalmol* 1966;75:826–835.
26. Leibowitz HM, Elliott JH. Chemotherapeutic immunosuppression of the corneal graft rejection. II. Combined systemic antimetabolites and topical corticosteroid therapy. *Arch Ophthalmol* 1966;76:826–835.
27. Polack FM. Effect of azathioprine (Imuran) on corneal graft rejection. *Am J Ophthalmol* 1967;64:233–244.
28. Watson PG. The nature and the treatment of scleral inflammation. *Trans Ophthalmol Soc UK* 1982;102:257–281.
29. Tauber J, Sainz de la Maza M, Foster CS. Systemic chemotherapy for ocular cicatricial pemphigoid. *Ophthalmology* 1988;95:146.
30. Mathews JD, Crawford BA, Bignell JL, Mackay IR. Azathioprine in active iridocyclitis, a double blind controlled trial. *Br J Ophthalmol* 1969;53:327–330.

31. Burchenal JH. The treatment of leukemias. *Bull NY Acad Med* 1954;30:429–447.
32. Assini JF, Hamilton R, Strosberg JM. Adverse reactions to azathioprine mimicking gastroenteritis. *J Rheumatol* 1986;13:1117–1118.
33. Cochrane D, Adamson AR, Halsey JP. Adverse reactions to azathioprine mimicking gastroenteritis. *J Rheumatol* 1987;14:1075.
34. Cox J, Daneshmend JK, Hawkey CJ. Devastating diarrhoea caused by azathioprine: management difficulty in inflammatory bowel disease. *Gut* 1988;29:686–688.
35. Katzka DA, Saul SH, Jorkasky D. Azathioprine and hepatic venocclusive disease in renal transplant patients. *Gastroenterology* 1986;90: 446–454.
36. Weitz H, Gokel JM, Loeschke K. Veno-occlusive disease of the liver in patients receiving immunosuppressive therapy. *Virchows Arch* 1982;395:245–246.
37. Hoover R, Fraumeni JF. Drug-induced cancer. *Cancer* 1981;47: 1071–1080.
38. Silman AJ, Petrie J, Hazlman B. Lymphoproliferative cancer and other malignancy in patients with rheumatoid arthritis treated with azathioprine: a 20-year follow-up study. *Ann Rheum Dis* 1988;47: 988–992.
39. Hoover R, Fraumeni JF Jr. Risks of cancer in renal transplant recipients. *Lancet* 1973;2:55–57.
40. Tagatz GE, Simmons RL. Pregnancy after renal transplantation. *Ann Intern Med* 1975;82:113–114.
41. Saarikoski S, Seppälä M. Immunosuppression during pregnancy: transmission of azathioprine and its metabolites from the mother to the fetus. *Am J Obstet Gynecol* 1973;115:110–116.
42. Coulam CB, Moyer TP, Jiang NS. Breast-feeding after renal transplantation. *Transplant Proc* 1982;14:605–609.
43. Kirchertz EJ, Grone HJ, Rieger J. Successful low dose captopril rechallenge following drug-induced leucopenia. *Lancet* 1981;1234: 1362–1363.
44. Andrasch RH, Profsky B, Burns RP. Immunosuppressive therapy for severe chronic uveitis. *Arch Ophthalmol* 1978;96:247–251.
45. Lorber MI, Flechner SM, Van Buren CT. Cyclosporine toxicity: the effect of combined therapy using cyclosporin, azathioprine, and prednisone. *Am J Kidney Dis* 1987;9:476–484.
46. Hooper PI, Kaplan HJ. Triple agent immunosuppression in serpiginous choroiditis. *Ophthalmology* 1991;98:944–952.
47. Calabresi P, Welch AD. Chemotherapy of neoplastic diseases. *Ann Rev Med* 1962;13:147–202.
48. Coggins PR, Randin RG, Eisman SM. Clinical pharmacology and preliminary evaluation of cyclophosphamide. *Cancer Chemother Rep* 1959;3:9–11.
49. Colvin M, Chabner BA. Alkylating agents. In: Chabner BA, Collins JM, eds. *Cancer Chemotherapy: Principles and Practice.* Philadelphia: JB Lippincott, 1990;276–313.
50. Lerman SP, Weidanz WP. The effect of cyclophosphamide on the ontogeny of the humoral immune response in chickens. *J Immunol* 1970;105:614–619.
51. Stockman GD, Heim LR, South MA, Trentin JJ. Differential effects of cyclophosphamide on the B and T cell compartments of adult mice. *J Immunol* 1973;110:277–282.
52. Shand FL, Liew FY. Differential sensitivity to cyclophosphamide of helper T cells for humoral responses and suppressor T cells for delayed-type hypersensitivity. *Eur J Immunol* 1980;10:480–483.
53. Legrange PH, Maekaness GB, Miller TE. Potentiation of T-cell mediated immunity by selective suppression of antibody formation with cyclophosphamide. *J Exp Med* 1974;139:1529.
54. Brock N. Pharmacologic characterization of cyclophosphamide and cyclophosphamide metabolites. *Cancer Chemother Rep* 1967;51: 315–325.
55. Brock N. Oxazaphosphorine cytostatics: past-present-future: Seventh Cain Memorial Award Lecture. *Cancer Res* 1989;49:1–7.
56. deVries CR, Freiha FS. Hemorrhagic cystitis: a review. *J Urol* 1990;143:1–9.
57. Spiers ASD. Haemorrhagic cystitis and cyclophosphamide. *Lancet* 1963;1:1282–1283.
58. Fauci AS, Haynes BF, Katz P. The spectrum of vasculitis, clinical, pathologic, immunologic, and therapeutic considerations. *Ann Intern Med* 1978;89:660–676.
59. Fauci AS, Haynes BF, Katz P, et al. Wegener's granulomatosis: prospective clinical and therapeutic experience with 85 patients for 21 years. *Ann Intern Med* 1983;98:76–85.
60. Fosdick WM, Parsons JL, Hill DF. Long term cyclophosphamide therapy in rheumatoid arthritis. *Arthritis Rheum* 1968;9:151–161.
61. Hoang-Xuan T, Foster CS, Rice BA. Scleritis in relapsing polychondritis: response to therapy. *Ophthalmology* 1990;97:892–898.
62. Mondino BJ, Brown SI. Immunosuppressive therapy in ocular cicatricial pemphigoid. *Am J Ophthalmol* 1983;96:453–459.
63. Foster CS. Cicatricial pemphigoid. *Trans Am Ophthalmol Soc* 1986;84:527–663.
64. Martenet AC. Resultats de l'immunodepression par cytostatiques en ophthalmologie. *Ophthalmologica* 1976;172:106–115.
65. Brown SI, Mondino BJ. Therapy of Mooren's ulcer. *Am J Ophthalmol* 1984;98:1–6.
66. Fauci AS, Doppman JL, Wolff SM. Cyclophosphamide-induced remissions in advanced polyarteritis nodosa. *Am J Med* 1978;64: 890–894.
67. Garrity JA, Kennerdell JS, Johnson BL, Ellis LD. Cyclophosphamide in the treatment of orbital vasculitis. *Am J Ophthalmol* 1986; 102: 97–103.
68. Buckley CE, Gills JP. Cyclophosphamide therapy of peripheral uveitis. *Arch Intern Med* 1969;124:29–35.
69. Gills JP, Buckley CE. Cyclophosphamide therapy of Behçet's disease. *Ann Ophthalmol* 1970;2:399–405.
70. Oniki S, Kurakazu K, Kawata K. Immunosuppressive treatment of Behçet's disease with cyclophosphamide. *Jpn J Ophthalmol* 1976; 20:32–40.
71. Rosenbaum JT. Treatment of severe refractory uveitis with intravenous cyclophosphamide. *J Rheumatol* 1994;21:123–125.
72. Gershwin ME, Goetz EJ, Steinberg AD. Cyclophosphamide: use in practice. *Ann Intern Med* 1974;80:531–540.
73. Fairley KF, Barrie JU, Johnson W. Sterility and testicular atrophy related to cyclophosphamide therapy. *Lancet* 1972;1:568–569.
74. Baker GL. Malignancy following treatment of rheumatoid arthritis with cyclophosphamide: long-term case-control follow-up study. *Am J Med* 1987;83:1–9.
75. DeFronzo RA, Braine H, Colvin OM. Water intoxication in man after cyclophosphamide therapy: time course and relation to drug activation. *Ann Intern Med* 1973;78:861–869.
76. Claube S, Kury G, Murphy ML. Teratogenic effects of cyclophosphamide in rats. *Cancer Chemother Rep* 1967;51:363–376.
77. Huennekens FM. The methotrexate story: a paradigm for development of cancer chemotherapeutic agents. *Adv Enzyme Regul* 1994; 34:397–419.
78. Nirenberg DW. Methotrexate therapy for psoriasis. *JAMA* 1988; 260:3003.
79. *Drug Evaluation Annual 1993.* Chicago, IL: American Medical Association, 1993;1990–1991.
80. Peters LJ, Olsen NJ. Mechanisms of action of methotrexate. *Bull Rheum Dis* 1991;41:5–8.
81. Borsi JD, Sagen E, Romslo I, et al. Rescue after intermediate and high-dose methotrexate: background; rationale, and current practice. *Pediatr Hematol Oncol* 1990;7:347–363.
82. Olsen EA. The pharmacology of methotrexate. *J Am Acad Dermatol* 1991;25:306–318.
83. Hitchings GH, Elion RB. Chemical suppression of the immune response. *Pharmacol Rev* 1963;15:365.
84. Segal R, Yaron M, Tartakovsky B. Methotrexate: mechanism of action in rheumatoid arthritis. *Semin Arthritis Rheum* 1990;20:190–200.
85. Gilman AG, Goodman LS, Rall TW, Murad F. *The Pharmacological Basis of Therapeutics.* New York: Macmillan Publishing Company, 1985;x–x.
86. Cronstein BN, Naime D, Ostad E. The antiinflammatory mechanism of methotrexate: increased adenosine release at inflamed sites diminishes leukocyte accumulation in an in vivo model of inflammation. *J Clin Invest* 1993;92:2675–2682.
87. Asako H, Wolf RE, Granger DN. Leukocyte adherence in rat mesenteric venules: effects of adenosine and methotrexate. *Gastroenterology* 1993;104:31–37.
88. Grosflam J, Weinblatt ME. Methotrexate: mechanism of action, pharmacokinetics, clinical indications, and toxicity. *Curr Opin Rheumatol* 1991;3:363–368.

89. Werkheiser W. The biochemical, cellular, and pharmacologic action and effects of the folic acid antagonists. *Cancer Res* 1963;23: 1277–1285.
90. Kremer JM, Lee JK. Long-term prospective study of the use of methotrexate in rheumatoid arthritis. *Arthritis Rheum* 1988;31:577–584.
91. Hoang-Xuan T, Foster CS, Rice BA. Scleritis in relapsing polychondritis: response to therapy. *Ophthalmology* 1990;97:892–898.
92. Wong VG, Hersh EM. Methotrexate in the therapy of cyclitis. *Trans Am Acad Ophthalmol Otolaryngol* 1965;69:279–293.
93. Wong VG, Hersh EM, McMaster PR. Treatment of a presumed case of sympathetic ophthalmia with methotrexate. *Arch Ophthalmol* 1966;76:66–76.
94. Wong VG. Methotrexate treatment of uveal disease. *Am J Med Sci* 1966;251:239–241.
95. Lazar M, Weiner MJ, Leopold IH. Treatment of uveitis with methotrexate. *Am J Ophthalmol* 1969;67:383–387.
96. Shah SS, Careen CY, Schmitt MA, et al. Low-dose methotrexate therapy for ocular inflammatory disease. *Ophthalmology* 1992;99: 1419–1423.
97. Holz FG, Krastel H, Breitbart A, et al. Low-dose methotrexate treatment in noninfectious uveitis resistant to corticosteroids. *Ger J Ophthalmol* 1992;1:142–144.
98. Tung JP, Maibach HI. The practical use of methotrexate in psoriasis. *Drugs* 1990;40:697–712.
99. Kozarek RA. Methotrexate induces clinical and histologic remission in patients with refractory inflammatory bowel disease. *Ann Intern Med* 1989;110:353–356.
100. Giannini EH, Cassidy JT. Methotrexate in juvenile rheumatoid arthritis. Do the benefits outweigh the risks? *Drug Saf* 1993;9:325–329.
101. Dahl MGC, Gregory MM, Scheuer PJ. Methotrexate hepatotoxicity in psoriasis-comparison of different dose regimens. *Br Med J* 1972;1:654–656.
102. Weinstein GD, Cox JW, Suringa DW, et al. Evaluation of possible chronic hepatotoxicity from methotrexate for psoriasis. *Arch Dermatol* 1970;102:613–618.
103. Weinstein G, Roenigk H, Maibach H, et al. Psoriasis-liver methotrexate interactions. *Arch Dermatol* 1973;108:36–42.
104. Petrazzuoli M, Roth MJ, Grin Jorgensen C, et al. Monitoring patients taking methotrexate for hepatotoxicity. Does the standard of care match published guidelines? *J Am Acad Dermatol* 1994; 31:969–977.
105. Kremer JM, Alarcon GS, Lightfoot RW, et al. Methotrexate for rheumatoid arthritis: suggested guidelines for monitoring liver toxicity. *Arthritis Rheum* 1994;37:316–328.
106. Goodman TA, Polisson RP. Methotrexate: adverse reactions and major toxicities. *Rheum Dis Clin North Am* 1994;20:513–528.
107. Decker JL. Toxicity of immunosuppressive drugs in man. *Arthritis Rheum* 1973;16:89–91.
108. Fraunfelder FT, Meyer SM. Ocular toxicity of antineoplastic agents. *Ophthalmology* 1983;90:1–3.
109. Pascalis L, Pia G, Aresu G, et al. Combined cyclosporin A-steroid-MTX treatment in endogenous non-infectious uveitis. *J Autoimmun* 1993;6:467–480.
110. Everett JL, Roberts JJ, Ross WC. Aryl-2-halogenoalkylamines. Part XII. Some carboxylic derivatives of NN-Di-2-chloroethylaniline. *J Chem Soc* 1953;3:2386–2392.
111. Galton DA, Israels LG, Nabarro JD, et al. Clinical trials of *p*-(DI-2-chloroethylamino)-phenylbutyric acid (CB 1348) in malignant lymphoma. *Br Med J* 1955;2:1172–1176.
112. Sawitsky A, Raj KR, Glidewell O, et al. Comparison of daily versus intermittent chlorambucil and prednisone therapy in the treatment of patients with chronic lymphocytic leukemia. *Blood* 1977;50: 1049–1059.
113. Mamo JG, Azzam SA. Treatment of Behçet's disease with chlorambucil. *Arch Ophthalmol* 1970;84:446–450.
114. *Drug Evaluation Annual 1993.* Chicago: American Medical Association, 1993;1966–1967.
115. Stevenson AC, Patel C. Effects of chlorambucil on human chromosomes. *Mutat Res* 1973;18:333–351.
116. Alberts DS, Chang SY, Chen HS, et al. Pharmacokinetics and metabolism of chlorambucil in man. *Cancer Treat Rev* 1979;6 (suppl):9–17.
117. McLean A, Woods RL, Catovsky D, et al. Pharmacokinetics and metabolism of chlorambucil in patients with malignant disease. *Cancer Treat Rev* 1979;6(suppl):33–42.
118. Ehrsson H, Lonroth U, Wallin I, et al. Degradation of chlorambucil in aqueous solution: influence of human albumin binding. *J Pharm Pharmacol* 1981;33:313–315.
119. BenEzra D, Cohen E. Treatment and visual prognosis in Behçet's disease. *Br J Ophthalmol* 1986;70:589–592.
120. Bietti GB, Cerulli L, Pivetti-Pezzi P. Behçet's disease and immunosuppressive treatment. *Mod Probl Ophthalmol* 1976;16:314–23.
121. Godfrey WA, Epstein WV, O'Connor GR, et al. The use of chlorambucil in intractable idiopathic uveitis. *Am J Ophthalmol* 1974;78: 415–28.
122. Nozik RA, Godfrey WA, Epstein WV, et al. Immunosuppressive treatment of uveitis. *Mod Probl Ophthalmol (Basel)* 1976;16: 305–308.
123. O'Duffy JD, Robertson DM, Goldstein NP. Chlorambucil in the treatment of uveitis and meningoencephalitis of Behçet's disease. *Am J Med* 1984;76:75–84.
124. Pezzi PP, Gasparri V, De Liso P, et al. Prognosis in Behçet's disease. *Ann Ophthalmol* 1985;17:20–25.
125. Elliott JH, Ballinger WH. Behçet's Syndrome: treatment with chlorambucil. *Trans Am Ophthalmol Soc* 1984;82:264–281.
126. Smulders SM, Oosterhuis JA. Treatment of Behçet's disease with chlorambucil. *Ophthalmologica (Basel)* 1975;171:347–352.
127. Tabbara KF. Chlorambucil in Behçet's disease, a reappraisal. *Ophthalmology* 1983;90:906–908.
128. Rossert J, Druet P. Immunosuppresseurs chimiques et maladies autoimmune. *Ann Biol Clin* 1991;49:327–337.
129. Sterling LP. Rheumatoid arthritis: current concepts and management, part 2. *Am Pharm NS* 1990;30:49–54.
130. Yang CS, Liu JH. Chlorambucil therapy in sympathetic ophthalmia. *Am J Ophthalmol* 1995;119:482–488.
131. Jennings T, Tessler HH. Twenty cases of sympathetic ophthalmia. *Br J Ophthalmol* 1989;73:140–145.
132. Kanski JJ. Anterior uveitis in juvenile rheumatoid arthritis. *Arch Ophthalmol* 1977;95:1794–1797.
133. Hermady R, Tauber J, Foster CS. Immunosuppressive drugs in immune and inflammatory ocular disease. *Surv Ophthalmol* 1991;35:369–385.
134. Moore GE, Bross ID, Ausman R, et al. Effects of chlorambucil in 374 patients with advanced cancer: Eastern Clinical Drug Evaluation Program. *Cancer Chemother Rep* 1968;52:661–666.
135. Cameron S. Chlorambucil and leukemia. *N Engl J Med* 1977;296:1065.
136. Zarrabi MH, Grunwald HW, Rosner F. Chronic lymphocytic leukemia terminating in acute leukemia. *Arch Intern Med* 1977;137:1059–1064.
137. Steigbigel RT, Kim H, Potolsky A, Schrier SL. Acute myeloproliferative disorder following long-term chlorambucil therapy. *Arch Intern Med* 1974;134:728–731.
138. Callis L, Nieto J, Vila A, Rende J. Chlorambucil treatment in minimal lesion nephrotic syndrome: a reappraisal of its gonadal toxicity. *J Pediatr* 1980;97:653–656.
139. Bur GE. Ovarian lesions due to cytostatic agents during the treatment of Hodgkin's disease. *Surg Gynecol Obstet* 1972;134: 826–828.
140. Sobrinho LG, Levine RA, DeConti RC. Amenorrhea in patients with Hodgkin's disease treated with antineoplastic agents. *Am J Obstet Gynecol* 1971;109:135–139.
141. LaDelfa I, Bayer N, Myers R, et al. Chlorambucil-induced myoclonic seizures in an adult. *J Clin Oncol* 1985;3:1691–1692.
142. Naysmith A, Robson RH. Focal fits during chlorambucil therapy. *Postgrad Med J* 1979;55:806–807.
143. Knisley RE, Settipane GA, Albala MM. Unusual reaction to chlorambucil in a patient with chronic lymphocytic leukemia. *Arch Dermatol* 1971;104:77–79.
144. Shotton D, Monie IW. Possible teratogenic effect of chlorambucil on a human fetus. *JAMA* 1963;186:74–75.
145. DeGowin RL. A review of therapeutic and hemolytic effects of dapsone. *Arch Intern Med* 1967;120:242–248.
146. Lucas AO, Hendrickse RG, Okubadejo OA, Richards WH, Neal RA, Kofie BA. The suppression of malarial parasitaemia by pyri-

methamine in combination with dapsone or sulphormethoxine. *Trans R Soc Trop Med Hyg* 1969;63:216–229.
147. Lowe J, Smith M. The chemotherapy of leprosy in Nigeria. *Int J Lepr Other Mycobact Dis* 1949;17:181–195.
148. Wolf M. Dermatitis herpetiform: response to diaminodiphenylsulfone. *Arch Dermatol* 1960;82:1020–1021.
149. Cornbleet T. Sulfoxone sodium for dermatitis herpetiformis. *Arch Dermatol* 1951;64:684–687.
150. Person JR, Rogers RS. Bullous pemphigoid responding to sulfapyridine and the sulfones. *Arch Dermatol* 1977;113:610–615.
151. Rogers RS, Seehafer JR, Perry HO. Treatment of cicatricial (benign mucous membrane) pemphigoid with dapsone. *J Am Acad Dermatol* 1982;6:215–223.
152. Lang PG. Solfones and sulfonamides in dermatology today. *J Am Acad Dermatol* 1979;1:479–492.
153. Stendahl O, Molin L, Dahlgren C. The inhibition of polymorphonuclear leukocyte cytotoxicity by dapsone, a possible mechanism in the treatment of dermatitis herepetiformis. *J Clin Invest* 1978;62:214–220.
154. Lehrer RI. Inhibition by sulfonamides of the candicidal activity of human neutrophils. *J Clin Invest* 1971;50:2498–2505.
155. Mier PD, van der Hank JMA. Inhibition of lysosomal enzymes by dapsone. *Br J Dermatol* 1975;93:471–472.
156. Barranco VP. Inhibition of lysosomal enzymes by dapsone. *Arch Dermatol* 1974;110:563–566.
157. Shepard CC, Ellard GA, Levy L, et al. Experimental chemotherapy of leprosy. *Bull WHO* 1976;53:425–433.
158. Riley RW, Levy L. Characteristics of the binding of dapsone and monoacetyldapsone by serum albumin. *Proc Soc Exp Biol Med* 1973;142:1168–1170.
159. Shepard CC, Ellard GA, Levy L, et al. The sensitivity to dapsone of *Mycobacterium leprae* from patients with and without previous treatment. *Am J Trop Med Hyg* 1969;18:258–263.
160. Foster CS. Cicatricial pemphigoid. *Trans Am Ophthalmol Soc* 1986;84:527–663.
161. Foster CS, Wilson SA, Ekins MB. Immunosuppressive therapy for progressive ocular cicatricial pemphigoid. *Ophthalmology* 89:340–353.
162. Tauber J, Sainz de la Maza M, Foster CS. Systemic chemotherapy for ocular cicatricial pemphigoid. *Ophthalmology* 1988;95(suppl): 146 (abst).
163. Barranco VP, Minor DB, Solomon H. Treatment of relapsing polychondritis with dapsone. *Arch Dermatol* 1976;112:1286–1288.
164. Martin J, Roenig HH, Lynch W, Tingwald FR. Relapsing chondritis treated with dapsone. *Arch Dermatol* 1976;112:1272–1274.
165. Ridgway HB, Hansotia PL, Schorr WF. Relapsing polychondritis, unusual neurological findings and therapeutic efficacy of dapsone. *Arch Dermatol* 1979;115:43–45.
166. Hoang-Xuan T, Foster CS, Rice BA. Scleritis in relapsing polychondritis: response to therapy. *Ophthalmology* 1990;97:892–898.
167. Desforges JF, Thayer WW, Dawson JP. Hemolytic anemia induced by sulfoxone therapy with investigation into the mechanism of its production. *Am J Med* 1959;27:132–136.
168. Pengally CDR. Dapsone-induced haemolysis. *Br Med J* 1963 2:662–664.
169. Rapoport AM, Guss SB. Dapsone-induced peripheral neuropathy. *Arch Neurol* 1972;27:184–186.
170. Raizman MB, Fay AM, Weiss JS. Dapsone-induced neutropenia in patients treated for ocular cicatricial pemphigoid. *Ophthalmology* 1994;101:1805–1807.
171. Peters JH, Murray JF, Gordon FR, Jacobson RR. Metabolic-bacteriologic relationships in the chemotherapy of lepromatous patients with dapsone or dapsone-rifampin. *Int J Lepr Other Mycobact Dis* 1978;46:115–116.
172. Vezina C, Kudelski A, Sehgal SN. Rapamycin (AY-22,989), a new antifungal antibiotic. I. Taxonomy of the producing streptomycete and isolation of the active principle. *J Antibiotics* 1975;28:721–726.
173. Sehgal SR, Baker H, Vezina C. Rapamycin (AY-22,989), a new antifungal antibiotic. II. Fermentation, isolation and characterization. *J Antibiotics* 1975;28:727–732.
174. Martel RR, Klicius J, Galet S. Inhibition of the immune response by Rapamycin, a new fungal antibiotic. *Can J Physiol Pharmacol* 1977;55:48–51.
175. Eng CP, Gullo-Brown J, Chang JY, Sehgal SH. Inhibition of skin graft rejection in mice by Rapamycin: a novel immunosuppressive macrolide. *Transplant Proc* 1991;23:868–869.
176. Stepkowski SM, Chen H, Daloze P, et al. Rapamycin, a potent immunosuppressive drug for vascularized heart, kidney and small bowel transplantation in the rat. *Transplantation* 1991;51:22–26.
177. Chen HF, Wu JP, Luo HY, Daloze PM. Reversal of ongoing rejection of allografts by Rapamycin. *Transplant Proc* 1991;23:2241–2242.
178. Peng B, Li Q, Luyo D, et al. Treatment of allergic conjunctivitis in murine model. In: Nussenblatt RB, Whitcup SM, Caspi RR, Gery I, eds. *Ocular Immunology.* Amsterdam: Elsevier, 1994;249–252.
179. Roberge FG, Xu D, Chan CC, et al. Treatment of autoimmune uveoretinitis in the rat with rapamycin, an inhibitor of lymphocyte growth factor signal transduction. *Curr Eye Res* 1993;12:197–203.
180. Dumont FJ, Staruch MJ, Koprak SL, et al. Distinct mechanisms of suppression of murine T-cell activation by the related macrolides FK-506 and rapamycin. *J Immunol* 1990;144:251–258.
181. Bierer BE, Mattila PS, Standaert RF, et al. Two distinct signal transmission pathways in T-lymphocytes are inhibited by complexes formed between an immunophilin and either FK506 or rapamycin. *Proc Natl Acad Sci USA* 1990;87:9231–9235.
182. Henderson DJ, Naya I, Bundick RV, et al. Comparison of the effects of FK-506, cyclosporin A and rapamycin on IL-2 production. *Immunology* 1991;73:316–321.
183. Kawashima H, Fujino Y, Mochizuki M. Effects of a new immunosuppressive agent, FK 506, on experimental autoimmune uveoretinitis ni rats. *Invest Ophthalmol Vis Sci* 1988;29:1265–1271.
184. Olsen TW, Benegas NM, Joplin AC, et al. Rapamycin inhibits corneal allograft rejection and neovascularization. *Arch Ophthalmol* 1994;112:1471–1475.
185. Martin DF, DeBarge LR, Nussenblatt RB, et al. Synergistic effect of rabamycin and cyclosporin A in the treatment of experimental autoimmune uveoretinitis. *J Immunol* 1995;154:922–927.
186. Goto T, Kino T, Hatanaka H, et al. F.K. 506: historical perspectives. *Transplant Proc* 1991;23:2713–2717.
187. Starzl T, Abu-elmagd K, Tzakis A, et al. Selected topics on FK 506, with special references to rescue of extrahepaticwhole organ grafts, transplantation of "forbidden organs," side effects, mechanisms, and practical pharmacokinetics. *Transplant Proc* 1991;23:914–919.
188. Todo S, Fung JI, Demetris AJ, et al. Early trials with FK 506 as primary treatment in liver transplantation. *Transplant Proc* 1990;22: 13–16.
189. Inamura N, Nakahara K, Kino T, et al. Prolongation of skin allograft survival in rats by a novel immunosuppressive agent, FK 506. *Transplantation* 1988;45:206.
190. Kawashima H, Fujino Y, Mochizuki M. Effects of a new immunosuppressive agent, FK 506, on experimental autoimmune uveoretinitis in rats. *Invest Ophthalmol Vis Sci* 1988;29:1265–1271.
191. Fujino Y, Chan CC, deSmet M, et al. FK 506 treatment of experimental autoimmune uveoretinitis in primates. *Transpl Proc* 1991;23:3335–3338.
192. Siekierka JJ, Hunt SH, Poe M. *Nature* 1989;341:755.
193. Bierer BE, Schreiber SL, Burakoff SJ. The effect of the immunosuppressant FK 506 on alternate pathways of T cell activation. *Eur J Immunol* 1991;21:439–445.
194. Schreiber SL, Liu J, Albers MW, et al. Immunophilin-ligand complexes as probes of intracellular signaling pathways. *Transpl Proc* 1991;23:2839–2844.
195. Tocci MJ, Matkovich DA, Collier KA, et al. The immunosuppressant FK 506 selectively inhibits expression of early T cell activation genes. *J Immunol* 1989;143:718–726.
196. Stevens C, Lempert N, Freed BM. The effects of immunosuppressive agents on in vitro production of human immunoglobulins. *Transplantation* 1991;51:1240–1244.
197. Ming N, Chan CC, Nussenblatt RB, et al. FR900506 (FK 506) and 15-deoxyspergualin (15-DSG) modulate the kinetics of infiltrating cells in eyes with experimental autoimmune uveoretinitis. *Autoimmunity* 1990;8:43–51.
198. Kawashima H, Mochizuki M. *Exp Eye Res* 1990;51:565.
199. Mochizuki M, Masuda K, Sakane T, et al. A multicenter clinical open trial of FK 506 in refractory uveitis, including Behçet's disease. *Transplant Proc* 1991;23:3343.

200. Venkataramanan R, Jain A, Warty VS, et al. Pharmacokinetics of FK 506 in transplant patients. *Transplant Proc* 1991;23:2736–2740.
201. Venkataramanan R, Jain A, Cadoff E, et al. Pharmacokinetics of FK 506: Preclinical and clinical studies. *Transplant Proc* 1990; 22:52–56.
202. Fung J, Abu-Elmagd K, Jain A, et al. A randomized trial of primary liver transplantation under immunosuppression with FK 506 vs cyclosporine. *Transplant Proc* 1991;23:2977–2983.
203. Hikita N, Lopez JS, de Smet MD, et al. Use of topical FK 506 in the corneal graft rejection model in Lewis rats. The Association for Research in Vision and Ophthalmology Meeting, 1993.
204. Hikita N, Chan CC, Whitcup SM, et al. Effect of topical FK 506 on endotoxin-induced uveitis in Lewis rats. *Curr Eye Res* 1995;14: 209–214.
205. Fung J, Alessian M, Abu-Elmagd K, et al. Adverse effects associated with the use of FK 506. *Transplant Proc* 1991;23:3105–3108.
206. Yamada K, Sugisaki Y, Akimoto M, et al. Short term FK 506-induced morphological changes in rat kidneys. *Transplant Proc* 23: 3130–3132.
207. Japanese FK 506 Study Group. Clinicopathological evaluation of kidney transplants in patients given a fixed dose of FK 506. *Transplant Proc* 1991;23:311–315.
208. Rilo HL, Zeng Y, Alejandro R, et al. Effect of FK 506 on function of human islets of Langerhans. *Transplant Proc* 1991;23:3164–3165.
209. Tse WJ, Tai J, Cheung S. In vitro effects of FK 506 on human and rat islets. *Transplant Proc* 1990;49:1172–1174.
210. Doi R, Tangoku K, Inoue K, et al. Mechanisms by which FK 506 affects exocrine pancreas in rats. *Transplant Proc* 1991;23:3161–3163.
211. Sumpio BE, Phan S. Nephrotoxic potential of FK 506. *Transplant Proc* 1991;23:1789–1790.
212. Tzakis AG, Fung JJ, Toda S, et al. Use of FK 506 in pediatric patients. *Transplant Proc* 1991;23:924–927.
213. Jain AB, Fung JJ, Tzakis AG, et al. Comparative study of cyclosporine and FK 506 dosage requirements in adult and pediatric orthotopic liver transplant patients. *Transplant Proc* 1991;23:2763–2766.
214. Christains U, Braum F, Sattler M, et al. Interactions of FK 506 and cyclosporine metabolism. *Transplant Proc* 1991;23:2794–2796.
215. Wu YM, Venkataramanan R, Suzuki M, et al. Interaction between FK 506 and cyclosporine in dogs. *Transplant Proc* 1991;23: 2797–2799.
216. Pichard L, Fabre I, Domergue J, et al. Effect of FK 506 on human hepatic cytochromes P-450: interaction with cyclosporine A. *Transplant Proc* 1991;23:2791–2793.
217. Bierer BE, Mattila S, Standaert RF, et al. Two distinct signal transmission pathways in T-lymphocytes are inhibited by complexes formed between an immunophilin, either FK 506 or rapamycin. *Proc Natl Acad Sci USA* 1990;87:9231–9235.
218. Borel JF. The history of cyclosporin A and its significance. In: White DJG, ed. *Cyclosporin A*. New York: Elsevier Biomedical Press, 1982;5–17.
219. Borel JF, Feurer C, Magnee C, Stahelin H. Effects of the new antilymphocytic peptide cyclosporin A in animals. *Immunology* 1977;32:1017–1025.
220. Nussenblatt RB, Palestine AG, Chan CC. Cyclosporine A therapy in the treatment of intraocular inflammatory disease resistant to systemic corticosteroids and cytotoxic agents. *Am J Ophthalmol* 1983;96:275–282.
221. Nussenblatt RB, Palestine AG. Cyclosporine: immunology, pharmacology and therapeutic uses. *Surv Ophthalmol* 1986;31:159–169.
222. Haitt WN, Harding MW, Handschumacher RE. Calmodulin, cyclophilin, and cyclosporin A. *Science* 1986;233:987–989.
223. Schreiber SL, Crabtree GR. The mechanism of action of cyclosporin A and FK 506. *Immunology Today* 1992;13:136–142.
224. Reem GH, Cook LA, Palladino MA. Cyclosporine inhibits interleukin-2 and interferon gamma synthesis by human thymocytes. *Transplant Proc* 1983;15:2387–2389.
225. Abb J, Abb H. Effect of cyclosporine on human leukocytes interferon production: selective inhibition of IFN-gamma synthesis. *Transplant Proc* 1983;15(suppl):2380–2382.
226. Borel JF, Lafferty KJ. Cyclosporin: speculation about its mechanism of action. *Transplant Proc* 1983;15:1881–1885.
227. Palacios R, Moller G. Cyclosporin A blocks receptors for HLA-DR antigens on T-cells. *Nature* 1981;290:792–794.
228. Kupiec-Weglinski JW, Filho MA, Strom TB, et al. Sparing of suppressor cells: a critical action of cyclosporine. *Transplantation* 1984;38:97–101.
229. Wood AJ, Maurer G, Neiderberger W, et al. Cyclosporine: pharmacokinetics, metabolism, and drug interactions. *Transplant Proc* 1983;15:2409–2414.
230. Freed BM, Rosano RG, Lempert N. In vitro immunosuppressive properties of cyclosporine metabolites. *Arthritis Rheum* 1987;25: 235–256.
231. Palestine AG, Nussenblatt RB, Chan CC. Cyclosporine therapy of uveitis in children. In: Saari KM, ed. *Uveitis Update*. Netherlands: Elsevier Science Publishers B.V. 1984;499–503.
232. Vine W, Bowers LD. Cyclosporine: structure, pharmacokinetics, and therapeutic drug monitoring. *Crit Rev Clin Lab Sci* 1987;25:275–311.
233. Palestine AG, Nussenblatt RB, Chan CC. Cyclosporine penetration into the anterior chamber and cerebrospinal fluid. *Am J Ophthalmol* 1985;99:210–211.
234. Nussenblatt RB, Palestine AG, Chan CC, et al. Effectiveness of cyclosporine therapy for Behçet's disease. *Arthritis Rheum* 1985;28: 671–679.
235. Binder AI, Graham EM. Sanders MD, et al. Cyclosporine in the treatment of severe Behçet's uveitis. *Br J Rheumatol* 1987;26: 285–291.
236. Towler HMA, Cliffe AM, Whiting PH, et al. Low dose cyclosporin A therapy in chronic posterior uveitis. *Eye* 1989;3:282–287.
237. Masuda K, Nakajima A, Urayama A, et al. Double masked trial of cyclosporin versus colchicine and long term open study of cyclosporin in Behçet's disease. *Lancet* 1989;1:1093–1096.
238. Bear JC, Foster CS, Raizman MB. Ocular Behçet's syndrome: clinical presentation and visual outcome in 26 patients. *Ophthalmology* 1989;96:128.
239. Nussenblatt RB, Palestine AG, Chan CC, et al. Randomized, double-masked study of cyclosporine compared to prednisolone in the treatment of endogenous uveitis. *Am J Ophthalmol* 1991;112: 138–146.
240. Le Hoang P, Girard B, Le Minh H, et al. Cyclosporine in the treatment of Birdshot retinochoroidopathy. *Transplant Proc* 1988; 20(suppl):128–130.
241. Nussenblatt RB, Palestine AG, Chan CC. Cyclosporin A therapy in the treatment of intraocular inflammatory disease resistant to systemic corticosteroids and cytotoxic agents. *Am J Ophthalmol* 1983;96:275–282.
242. Vitale AT, Rodriquez A, Foster CS. Low-dose cyclosporine therapy in the treatment of birdshot retinochoroidopathy. *Ophthalmology* 1994;101:822–831.
243. Bielory L, Frohman LP. Low-dose cyclosporine therapy of granulomatous optic neuropathy and orbitopathy. *Ophthalmology* 1991; 98:1732–1736.
244. Towler HM, Whiting PH, Forrester JV. Combination low dose cyclosporin A and steroid therapy in chronic intraocular inflammation. *Eye* 1990;4:514–520.
245. Hooper PL, Kaplan HJ. Triple agent immunosuppression in serpiginous choroiditis. *Ophthalmology* 1991;98:944–952.
246. Kruit PJ, Van Bale A, Stilma JS. Cyclosporin A treatment in two cases of corneal peripheral melting syndromes. *Doc Ophthalmol* 1985;59:33–39.
247. Goichot-Bonnat L, De Beauregard C, Saragoussi JJ, et al. usage de la cyclosporine A collyre dans la prevention dy rejet de greffe de cornee chez l'homme. *J Fr Ophthalmol* 1987;10:207–211.
248. Belin MW, Bouchard CS, Frantz S, et al. Topical cyclosporine in high-risk corneal transplants. *Ophthalmology* 1989;96:1144–1150.
249. Ben Ezra D, Pe'er J, Brodsky M, Cohen E. Cyclosporine eyedrops for the treatment of severe vernal keratoconjunctivitis. *Am J Ophthalmol* 1986;101:278–282.
250. Holland EJ, Chan CC, Kuwabara T, et al. Immunohistochemical findings and results of treatment with cyclosporine in ligneous conjunctivitis. *Am J Ophthalmol* 1983;107:160–166.
251. Wiebking J, Mehlfeld T. Topical treatment of corneal ulcers and scleromalacias with cyclosporin A. *Fortschr Ophthalmol* 1986; 83:345–347.

252. Kahan BD, Flechner SM, Lorber MI, et al. Complications of cyclosporin therapy. *World J Surg* 1986;10:348–360.
253. Bennett WM, Pulliam JP. Cyclosporine nephrotoxicity. *Ann Intern Med* 1983;99:851–854.
254. Feutren G. The optimal use of cyclosporin A in autoimmune diseases. *J Autoimmun* 1992;5:183–195.
255. Feutren G, Abeywickrama K, Friend D, et al. Renal function and blood pressure in psoriatic patients treated with cyclosporin A. *Br J Dermatol* 1990;122:57–69.
256. Wysocki GP, Gretzinger HA, Laupacis A, et al. Fibrous hyperplasia of the gingiva: a side effect of cyclosporin A therapy. *Oral Surg* 1983;55:274–278.
257. Ballantyne CM, Podet EJ, Patsch WP, et al. Effects of cyclosporine therapy on plasma lipoprotein levels. *JAMA* 1989;262:53–56.
258. Cockburn I. Assessment of the risks of malignancy and lymphomas developing in patients using Sandimmune. *Transplant Proc* 1987; 19:1804–1807.
259. Callanan DG, Cheung MK, Martin DF, et al. Outcome of uveitis patients treated with long term cyclosporine. The Association for Research in Vision and Ophthalmology Meeting, 1994.
260. Hamilton DV, Evans DB, Thiru S. Toxicity of cyclosporin A in organ grafting. In: White DJG, ed. *Cyclosporin A.* New York: Elsevier Biomedical Press, 1982;393–411.
261. Beveridge T. Pharmacokinetics and metabolism of cyclosporine A. In: White DJG, ed. *Cyclosporin A.* New York: Elsevier Biomedical Press, 1982;35–44.
262. Harris KP, Jenkins D, Wall J. Nonsteroidal antiinflammatory drugs and cyclosporine: a potentially serious adverse interaction. *Transplantation* 1988;46:598–599.
263. de Smet MD, Rubin BJ, Whitcup SM, et al. Combined use of cyclosporine and ketoconazole in the treatment of endogenous uveitis. *Am J Ophthalmol* 1992;113:687–690.
264. Wacker WB, Donoso LA, Kalsow CM, et al. Experimental allergic uveitis. Isolation, characterization and localization of a soluble uveitopathogenic antigen from bovine retina. *J Immunol* 1977; 119:1949–1958.
265. Faure JP. Autoimmunity and the retina. *Curr Top Eye Res* 1980;2:215–302.
266. Shinohara T, Dietzschold B, Craft CM, et al. Primary and secondary structure of bovine retinal S-antigen (48-kDa protein). *Proc Natl Acad Sci USA* 1987;84:6975–6979.
267. Yamaki K, Tsuda M, Shinohara T. The sequence of human retinal S-antigen reveals similarities with alpha-transducin. *FEBS Lett* 1988;234:39–43.
268. Tsuda M, Syed M, Bugra K. Structural analysis of mouse S-antigen. *Gene* 1988;73:11–20.
269. Gregerson DS, Obritsch WF, Fling SP. S-antigen-specific rat T cell lines recognize peptide fragments of S-antigen and mediate experimental autoimmune uveoretinitis and pinealitis. *J Immunol* 1986; 136:2875–2882.
270. Friedman A, Al-Sabbagh A, Santos LM, et al. Oral tolerance: a biologically relevant pathway to generate peripheral tolerance against external and self-antigens. *Chem Immunol* 1994;58:259–290.
271. Sosroseno W. A review of the mechanisms of oral tolerance and immunotherapy. *J R Soc Med* 1995;88:14–17.
272. Weiner HL, Mackin GA, Matsui M, et al. Double-blind pilot trial of oral tolerization with myelin antigens in multiple sclerosis. *Science* 1993;259:1321–1324.
273. Trentham DE, Dynesius-Trengtham RA, Orav EJ, et al. Effects of oral administration of type II collagen on rheumatoid arthritis. *Science* 1993;261:1727–1730.
274. Burch RM, Weitzberg M, Blok N, et al. *N*-(fluorenyl-9-methoxycarbonyl) amino acids, a class of antiinflammatory agents with a different mechanism of action. *Proc Natl Acad Sci USA* 1991;88: 355–359.
275. Pou S, Surichamorn W, Cao GL, et al. The effect of NPC 15669, an inhibitor of neutrophil recruitment, and neutrophil-mediated inflammation, on neutrophil function, in vitro. In preparation.
276. Bator JM, Weitzberg M, Burch RM. *N*-[9H-(2,7-Dimethylfluorenyl-9-methoxy)carbonyl]-L-leucine, NPC 15669, prevents neutrophil adherence to endothelium and inhibits CD 11b/CD 18 upregulation. *Immunopharmacology* 1992;23:139–149.
277. Burch RM, Connor JR, Bator JM, et al. NPC 15669 inhibits the reversed arthus reaction in rats by blocking neutrophil recruitment. *J Pharmacol Exp Therapeutics* 1992;263:933–937.
278. Noronha-Blob L, Lowe VC, Weitzberg M, et al. NPC 15669 enhances survival and reverses leukopenia in endotoxin-treated mice. *Eur J Pharmacol* 1991;199:387–388.
279. Cheung MK, Dastgheib K, Chan CC, et al. Inhibition of polymorphonuclear leukocyte recruitment by NPC 15669 prevents endotoxin-induced uveitis. The Association for Research in Vision and Ophthalmology Meeting, 1994.
280. Cheung MK, Dastgheib K, Chan CC, et al. Prevention of uveitis by NPC 15669, an inhibitor of polymorphonuclear leukocyte recruitment in animal models. Proceedings of the Sixth International Symposium of the Immunology and Immunopathology of the Eye, 1994.

Textbook of Ocular Pharmacology,
edited by T.J. Zimmerman, et al.
Lippincott–Raven Publishers, Philadelphia © 1997.

CHAPTER 9

Ocular Pharmacokinetics

Ronald D. Schoenwald

BACKGROUND

The kinetic processes, collectively referred to as *pharmacokinetics,* are defined by the study of the movement of drugs into, within, and out of the body. Specifically, these processes, called absorption, distribution, and elimination, are consecutive; that is, drugs are first absorbed, then distributed, then eliminated by either metabolism or excretion out of the body. These latter four processes are best known by the abbreviation ADME (i.e., by the first letter of each process: *a*bsorption, *d*istribution, *m*etabolism, and *e*xcretion). In general, the study of pharmacokinetic processes and the factors that influence them is fundamental in determining the appropriate dosing regimen for a particular patient and is likewise critically important to the design of new therapeutic agents.

Because we are considering the eye as a separate entity, the well-known definitions for ADME must be modified from those that were developed for systemically administered drugs. *Absorption* is defined as the process by which a drug enters the aqueous humor. The *rate* and *extent* of absorption (defined as *bioavailability*) refer to how quickly and extensively the administered dose enters aqueous humor. Both the rate and extent of absorption are determined by the physicochemical behavior of the drug and the permeability factors of the barrier membrane. They are also influenced significantly by the precorneal factors competing with absorption (i.e., tearing, blinking, drainage, and uptake into the lids).

Distribution to a peripheral compartment refers to the process by which a drug is transferred from aqueous humor to the surrounding tissues and is affected by flow dynamics, partitioning, and binding. In the eye, the conjunctiva, cornea, lens, iris-ciliary body, choroid, and vitreous are specific tissues that may be associated with the peripheral compartment. If a significant rate-determining step for drug distribution separates the aqueous humor from any of these tissues, a peripheral compartment becomes an integral part of the pharmacokinetic model (Fig. 9-1). Tissues representing the peripheral compartment must also be reversibly connected to the central compartment, but if redistribution into aqueous humor is slow or nonexistent, these tissues can act as a sink or reservoir for the drug. Ideally, drug distribution to the active site should be significant, or the pharmacological response may not be optimal. Also, if distribution is variable, the response likewise will vary.

Drugs are eliminated from the eye by bulk flow mechanisms, metabolism, or passage across the blood-ocular barriers. The latter mechanism may be an active process and, to this extent, is analogous to the process of excretion for systemically administered drugs.

To quantitate each process and to calculate dosage regimens, pharmacokinetics has been defined most effectively by "compartmentalizing" the system it attempts to describe. The term *kinetically homogeneous,* often used to describe a compartment, refers to groups of tissues that behave the same kinetically, even though these tissues may be quite different anatomically or physiologically. In practice, this means that when drug concentration in kinetically homogeneous tissues is plotted over time, the drug's half-life remains the same. It is important to understand, however, that the various tissues in a compartment may have significantly higher or lower drug concentrations over time, depending on the extent of partitioning and binding of drug to that particular tissue.

Without actually determining the profile for each tissue over time, one cannot be certain which tissues actually reside in the central or peripheral compartments. One exception is the aqueous humor, which is always assigned to the central compartment. A clear distinction between the central and peripheral compartment comes from how rapidly a drug enters and leaves the tissues bathed by aqueous humor. If distribution is relatively rapid (i.e., a distribution half-life of 15–20 minutes or less), then the tissue is as-

R. D. Schoenwald: Division of Pharmaceutics, College of Pharmacy, The University of Iowa, Iowa City, Iowa 52242.

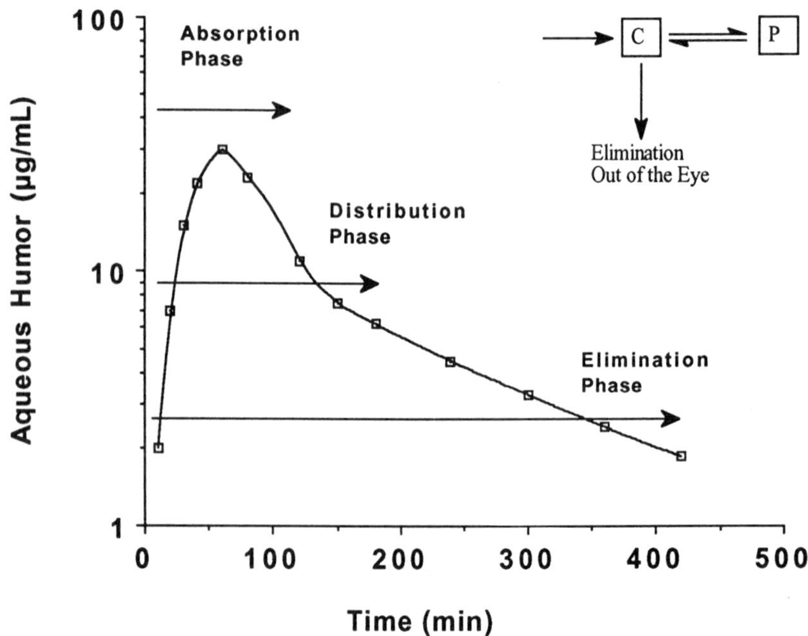

FIG. 9-1. Semilogarithmic plot of an ocular drug showing the curve segments representative of absorption, distribution, and elimination and a typical two-compartment pharmacokinetic model. C, central; P, peripheral compartments.

signed to the central compartment, whereas if drug distribution to a particular tissue is relatively slow, the tissue is assigned to a peripheral compartment.

Figure 9-1 gives a profile of aqueous humor concentration of drug over time and shows the two-compartment model that best describes the data. The rate-determining steps between the central and peripheral compartments as well as absorption and elimination from the eye are represented by arrows. In contrast, a one-compartment model assigns all the tissues of the eye to a single compartment. One should realize that distribution to the tissues residing in a one-compartment model may be just as extensive as distribution to tissues assigned to the peripheral compartment of a two-compartment model. The major difference is that the rate of distribution to tissues in the one-compartment model is considered quite rapid; therefore, rate-determining barriers do not exist for the particular drug. Although a one-compartment model may be an oversimplification of a complex kinetic process, in practice it is usually justified because drug concentrations in tissues of importance over time may be predicted adequately from equations that represent the model.

PHARMACOKINETIC PROCESSES IN THE EYE

The eye is one of the few organs that can be considered pharmacokinetically separate from the body. This separation is possible because of two main factors: (a) absorption occurs directly into the eye before reaching systemic circulation and (b) because elimination occurs directly into the body, which can be considered a large reservoir that can dilute drug concentration below a therapeutic threshold.

Although the application of pharmacokinetic models has been immensely useful in developing optimal dosing regimens for systemic drugs, this has not occurred for ophthalmic drugs. One reason is that meaningful pharmacokinetic studies cannot be conducted routinely in the human eye because tissues or fluids cannot be sampled without risking severe injury or pain. Pharmacokinetic parameters, such as the fraction absorbed, absorption rate constant, volume of distribution, and ocular clearance, cannot be determined easily in the human eye. Unfortunately, the anatomy and physiology of the eyes of various animal species are not similar enough to human eyes in anatomy and physiology to estimate pharmacokinetic parameters of importance (Table 9-1). Nevertheless, the ophthalmic literature contains the results of many animal studies and, to a much lesser extent, human studies in which surgical patients have consented to participate in the pharmacokinetic evaluation of drugs. Despite the inability of ophthalmologists to optimize individual dosing regimens for patients, the results of human ocular studies have been indispensable to both the design and delivery of ophthalmic drugs.

Absorption

Rate and Extent of Ocular Absorption

The rate and extent of absorption of drugs applied topically to the eye are exceptionally difficult to measure experimentally (1), but experimental results clearly indicate that competition from noncorneal absorption (i.e., lids and adnexa) and, particularly, drainage are responsible for suppressing the absorption of drugs into the eye (2–5). To ex-

TABLE 9-1. *Anatomical and physiological differences in the New Zealand rabbit and human eye pertinent to ophthalmic pharmacokinetics*

Pharmacokinetic factor	Human eye	Rabbit eye
Tear volume	7.0–30.0 μl	7.5 μl[a]
Tear turnover rate	0.5–2.2 μL/min	0.6–0.8 μl/min
Spontaneous blinking rate[b]	15 ×/min	4–5 times/min
Nictitating membrane[c]	Absent	Present
pH of tears	7.14–7.82	[d]
Milliosmolarity of tears	305 mOsm/L	[d]
Corneal thickness	0.52 mm	0.40 mm
Corneal diameter	15 mm	12 mm
Ratio of surface area (conj/cornea)	17.2	8.6–9.6
Aqueous humor volume	310 μl	[d]
Aqueous humor turnover rate	1.53 μl/min	[d]

[a]Approximate, depending on blinking rate and conjunctival sac volume.
[b]Occurs during normal waking hours without external stimuli.
[c]Significance of nictitating membrane is small relative to overall loss rate from precorneal area.
[d]Approximately same measurement as human eye.

acerbate the problem, tear secretion promotes the dilution of the instilled dose, and blinking facilitates its removal. The biggest factor is the drainage rate, which is about 100 times more rapid than the absorption rate. Because of these precorneal factors, it is not surprising to find that drugs reside in the conjunctival sac for only about 3 to 5 minutes; therefore, a relatively small fraction of the instilled dose actually penetrates the cornea (2–4).

For drugs applied topically to the eye, the extent of absorption is quite poor compared with systemic routes of administration, such as oral, rectal, and intramuscular (i.m.) administration. The extent of absorption is measured by taking the ratio of the total amount of drug that has entered the eye divided by the instilled dose. For ophthalmic drugs, this ranges from 1% to 7% (1,5,6), whereas systemic drugs are usually >75%. Improvement in the extent of absorption can come from either better retention at the site of absorption induced by the dosage form (e.g., Ocusert) or from improved penetrability from the use of a lipophilic modification of the drug (e.g., prodrugs, such as dipivefrin).

Corneal Membrane Barriers

Although the human cornea consists of five layers, only three layers provide significant barrier resistance to absorption into the aqueous humor: the epithelium, which for most drugs provides the highest resistance to penetration; the stroma; and the endothelium. Bowman's membrane and Descemet's membrane are important anatomically but are not significant rate-determining barriers.

The outer epithelium is cellular, consisting of superficial layers of flat, tightly fitting squamous cells with underlying columnar cells. Drugs penetrate this outer layer either by partitioning through the cells (*intracellular*) or passing between the cells (*paracellular* or *intercellular*) by diffusing through the interstitial aqueous media. Because of the lipophilic nature of the epithelium as well as its low porosity and high tortuosity, most drugs penetrate the cornea via the intracellular route. The paracellular route predominates for hydrophilic drugs or ions of small molecular weight (<350 MW), whereas the intracellular route predominates for lipophilic drugs (based on an octanol/buffer, pH 7.6 partitioning system where $\log p < 0$ or $\log p > 0$ represents hydrophilic or lipophilic drugs, respectively).

For barrier purposes, the stroma, with its 78% water content, can be considered an aqueous environment, interspersed geometrically with collagen fibrils, imparting a high porosity and a low tortuosity so that drugs diffuse through the stroma with relatively minor resistance at diffusional rates about a fourth that of an aqueous system (7,8). Differences in partitioning behavior have little, if any, effect on stromal penetration. Theoretically, the cube root of the molecular weight is the most important factor; however, ophthalmic drugs have a relatively narrow molecular weight range, and stromal penetration therefore is nearly the same for all therapeutic agents. Although the endothelium is cellular, it is only one cell thick and does not provide significant resistance to the penetration of ophthalmic drugs (9).

When the intact cornea is considered, drug penetration depends primarily on the partitioning behavior of the therapeutic agent as well as the collective effect of each individual membrane. Fig. 9-2 summarizes the relationship between the log of the permeability coefficient (cm/s $\times 10^{-6}$) calculated for an analog series of beta-blocking agents and the log of their respective partition coefficients (octanol/buffer, pH 7.65). The permeability coefficients for each analog were determined from penetration measurements made across various layers of excised rabbit corneas (9). As mentioned previously and shown in Figure 9-2, stromal permeability is independent of a drug's partition-

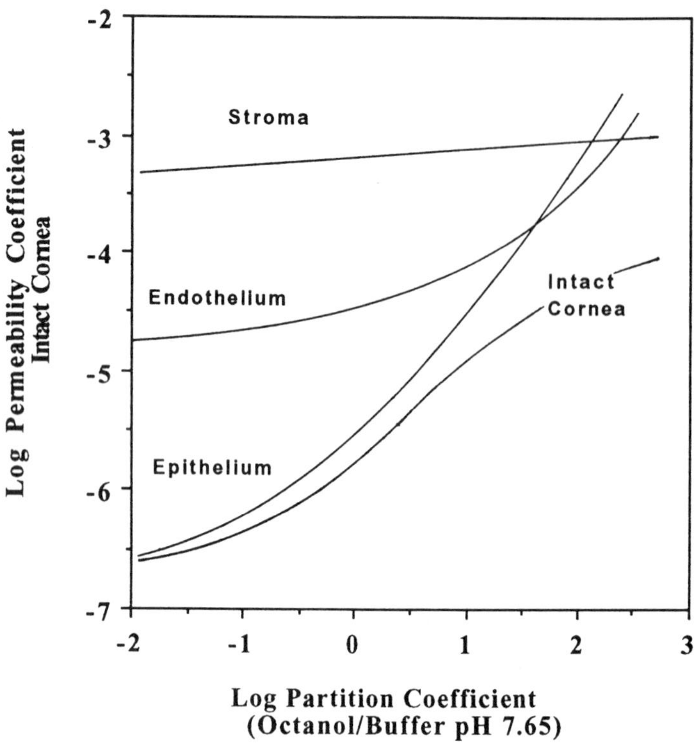

FIG. 9-2. Relationship between log corneal permeability coefficient and the log octanol/buffer (pH 7.65) partition coefficient for each membrane barrier of the cornea.

ing behavior, whereas both epithelial and endothelial permeability are linearly dependent on partitioning. The intact cornea shows a linear relationship for drugs with intermediate partitioning behavior, but for extremely hydrophilic or lipophilic drugs a plateau region is evident in the plot. The upper plateau region occurs because the very lipophilic drugs penetrate the epithelium readily but penetrate the aqueouslike stroma more slowly, eventually becoming rate determining. The lower plateau region is the rate-determining region for hydrophilic drugs that penetrate the epithelium slowly or not at all; therefore, the paracellular pathway predominates.

Based on the use of log octanol/buffer (pH 7.65) as a reference system, examples of very hydrophilic drugs are tobramycin, phenylephrine, sulfacetamide, gentamycin, prednisolone sodium phosphate, dexamethasone sodium phosphate, carbachol, cromolyn, fluorescein, and idoxuridine. Few very lipophilic drugs are commercially available; these are the acetate esters of dexamethasone and prednisolone. The large majority of drugs of ophthalmic interest have partitioning behavior that ranges between the two extremes.

Conjunctiva/Scleral Route of Entry

The corneal route has always been assumed to be the major route of entry into the eye; however, recent evidence suggests that penetration across the conjunctiva and sclera may also contribute significantly to penetration into the anterior chamber. In a series of studies of various designs (10–16), results have shown that the outer layer of the sclera provides much less barrier resistance to hydrophilic drugs than does the epithelium of the cornea. The sclera also contains arterial vessels that lead to the uvea and retina and could explain drug entry into the eye by this route. Another explanation is that drugs, once absorbed into the conjunctiva, diffuse laterally into the sclera of the cornea and then directly enters the aqueous humor (7).

Although less plausible than vessel uptake or lateral diffusion into corneal stroma, drug entry into the eye could occur by first penetrating the conjunctiva, proceeding through the sclera, ciliary muscle, ciliary processes, and finally by diffusing into the anterior chamber. If drug enters the anterior chamber by corneal penetration, it becomes diluted by aqueous humor and must diffuse against the flow rate. Further, adjacent tissues compete for aqueous humor concentrations of drug. Therefore, if the iris/ciliary body is the active site, it seems reasonable to assume that the conjunctiva/scleral pathway is more likely to yield higher drug concentrations than from absorption by the corneal pathway. At present, more research must be conducted to determine the precise conjunctiva/scleral route, the critical factors, and the signficance of this pathway to drug absorption into the eye.

Routes of Administration

Usually, preference is given to topical instillation of ophthalmic drugs because this route of administration is noninvasive, simple for the patient to use, and most often nontoxic to the body. Bacterial corneal ulcers or other eye infections that threaten vision and require immediate therapy often are treated by the simultaneous administration of topical and subconjunctival routes of administration. Although the choice of a dosage form can influence the rate or the extent to which a drug penetrates the eye, an alternate route of administration may be more effective. Systemic routes, however, such as oral or parenteral routes, may not produce high enough concentrations of drug in the eye because of resistance to entry from blood-ocular barriers, metabolism of drug to an inactive species, or significant uptake into another organ or tissue.

The selection of a periocular or intraocular route of administration depends on the inability of the drug to penetrate the cornea and on the location of the target site. In general, lids and lid margins are best treated with ointments, whereas the conjunctiva, limbus, cornea, and anterior chamber are treated most effectively by instillation of solutions or suspensions or, if unresponsive, by subconjunctival injection (17). Table 9-2 summarizes the results from measurement of aqueous humor concentrations of various aminoglycosides, cephaloridine, carbenicillin, or Chloromycetin (chloroamphenicol) after subconjunctival injection to patients undergoing elective surgeries (11–23). Whereas none of these antibiotics reach significant intraocular concentrations following topical instillation, subconjunctival injections maintain therapeutically effective concentrations in the aqueous humor for many hours (see Table 9-2). In general, hydrophilic drugs are more effective when given by the subconjunctival route because absorption occurs from the reservoir of drugs at the conjunctival depot, which is not subject to precorneal factors responsible for their loss of drugs when instilled topically. Also, a drug given by this route of administration is not required to penetrate the conjunctival epithelium, a significant rate-determining barrier for water-soluble drugs. The conjunctival route of administration often provides therapeutically effective drug levels for 8 to 12 hours after a single injection.

Application of a drug using drug-soaked soft contact lenses has been studied as an alternative approach to sustaining the levels of water-soluble antibiotics in the eye (24). In a comparison study using 466 patients undergoing cataract surgery, chloramphenicol sodium succinate, gentamicin, or carbenicillin was given by either subcutaneous injection or by drug-soaked soft contact lenses. The subcutaneous route of administration provided a longer duration of drug concentration in the aqueous humor but much lower peak concentrations than drug-soaked contact lenses (18).

Because of the risk of retinal damage and loss of vision, intravitreal injection is not considered a desirable method for reaching therapeutic drug concentrations in the vitreous, particularly with the use of steroids in the treatment of endophthalmitis. With the recent increase in retinitis due to infection by either bacterial endophthalmitis or cytomegalovirus in HIV patients, however, intravitreal injection is being used more often (25,26). Previous work established that the penetration of antibiotics into the vitreous from topical, subconjunctival, or systemic routes of administration is nearly always inadequate in treating bacterial endophthalmitis. Although toxicity to the retina remains a concern, intravitreal injection of certain antibiotics (ciprofloxacin, ceftriaxone, tobramycin, and other aminoglycosides) or antivirals (ganciclovir, acyclovir, and foscarnet) is considered the most effective route of administration (27).

Iontophoresis has been used occasionally in the human eye in an attempt to enhance the penetration of a charged molecule without resorting to intraocular injection (28,29). Also, in the human eye, the iontophoresis of fluorescein has been used to determine accurately the rate of aqueous

TABLE 9-2. *Mean aqueous humor concentrations of various antibiotics after subconjunctival injection to human eyes*

Antibiotic	Dose (mg)	Pk aqueous Concentration (μg/ml)[a]	Duration (h) above MIC	Reference
Gentamycin	20	14.6 (60)	12	18
Gentamycin	20	14.9 (60)	18	19
Gentamycin	5	4.0 (120)	10	20
	10	6.5 (120)	16	20
	20	15.0 (120)	16	20
Gentamycin	20	14.6 (60)	12	18
Tobramycin	20	22.4 (120)	20	18
Tobramycin	10	16.5 (120)	8	21
Sisomicin	20	16.4 (78)	20	22
Sisomicin	20	19.0 (60)	18	19
Cephaloridine	100	30.8 (60)	12	19
Chloramphenicol sodium succinate	50	16.2 (60)	8	18
Carbenicillin	50	80.5 (30)	4	18
Netilmicin	12.5	36.0 (120)	7–9	23
	25	85.6 (105)	9	23

[a]Peak concentration and corresponding time (min).

humor flow. A recent review (30), however, indicated that most iontophoresis studies over the past 20 years have been in animals. The method involves application of a small current (about 2 mA) to the eye by means of an anode or cathode attached to an eyecup. The current, applied for a few minutes, establishes an electrical gradient across the cornea or sclera. The difference in charge on each side of the membrane promotes the passage of drug and identically charged ions across the tissue barrier. With both corneal and transcleral iontophoresis, tissue burns may occur. Nevertheless, this latter route of administration may have much less risk of damage to the retina than intravitreal injection. For charged water-soluble drugs, particularly antibiotics, the method may be applicable for use in bacterial endophthalmitis (31,32).

In general, treatment of conjunctiva, lids, cornea, or anterior chamber is most often achieved from topical application of drugs; however, subconjunctival injection may be necessary for poorly absorbed drugs in reaching anterior chamber tissues. If high vitreal concentrations are necessary, intravitreal injection or systemic routes of administration should be considered. In cases of optic nerve or macular inflammations, sub-Tenon's or retrobulbar injections have been used. Despite the advantage of emergency management of acute disorders, alternatives to direct injections into the eye are being studied because of their disadvantages (e.g., inconvenience, expense, patient apprehension, and intraocular tissue damage).

DISTRIBUTION

Although precorneal and corneal factors discourage absorption, tissues in the anterior and posterior chambers are bathed continuously by circulating aqueous humor. Therefore, peripheral issues are readily available for distribution, provided drug properties, such as partitioning and binding, are optimal. Factors that reduce the opportunity for distribution to an active site are binding to melanin in the iris and the ciliary body, binding to protein in the aqueous humor, and rapid elimination of drug as a result of turnover of aqueous humor. Binding of drug to an inactive site can act as a biological reservoir, releasing drug slowly over time but producing relatively low therapeutic concentrations. For example, the binding of catecholamines and atropine to melanin is responsible for a delayed onset and a reduced but prolonged response in darker-eyed persons (33). Melanin binding is also responsible for a reduced effect of timolol in persons with darker irides (34).

For medication administered systemically, the volume of distribution (V_{ss}) measured at plasma steady-state concentrations of drugs is used to assess the relative extent of drug distribution to tissues and extravascular fluids. Theoretically, V_{ss} can be estimated from the amount of drugs in the body at steady state divided by the steady-state drug concentration and is a function of partitioning and binding within tissues and extravascular fluids. In addition, competition between these tissue factors and the binding of drug to plasma or blood components determines the extent to which a drug will distribute.

In the eye, V_{ss} is experimentally difficult to measure but has been estimated for a few drugs administered to the rabbit eye. Some examples of drugs used clinically but measured in rabbit eyes are pilocarpine (0.58 ml), clonidine (0.53 ml), phenylephrine (0.42 ml), flubiprofen (0.62), and levobunolol (1.65) (6). These values are not much greater than the aqueous humor volume of 0.31 ml but indicate distribution of drug to tissues bathed by aqueous humor. As more V_{ss} values become available, a better understanding of drug distribution within the eye will emerge. Although tissues within animal eyes are often removed and measured for drug concentration over time, not much is known about the binding and partitioning properties of various ocular tissues relative to drugs.

Cornea

Although the cornea is a complex barrier to drug entry into the eye, more than any other tissue, it is capable of accumulating drug. Accumulation is possible because the cornea is large, readily accessible to drugs, and has layers with widely varying partitioning properties. Pilocarpine and particularly the nonsteroidal antiinflammatory drugs (i.e., flurbiprofen and suprofen) accumulate in the cornea. Increased delivery of water-soluble drugs (e.g., prednisolone sodium phosphate, gentamicin, tobramycin, and the cephalosporins) can be accomplished by soaking a contact lens or collagen shield in a concentrated solution and then placing the lens on the cornea to improve ocular retention and thereby increase corneal uptake and anterior chamber concentrations.

Iris

The iris tissue is highly vascular and porous, possesses a large surface area, and is thus able to equilibrate rapidly with drugs in aqueous humor. In animal studies, when drugs are instilled topically, peak concentration in the iris often is reached before it occurs in the aqueous humor. This phenomenon can occur only if drug is absorbed from the anterior ciliary arteries embedded in the episclera, which also supply the iris (and ciliary body). If drugs enter the iris from the anterior chamber, the porous nature of the anterior surface of the stroma permits a rapid uptake of drugs. The sphincter and dilator muscles are the target sites for miotics and mydriatics. The former is located in the pupillary zone of the posterior stroma, and the latter is a smooth sheet of muscle located between the stroma and the pigmented epithelium. Because of its anatomical location and porosity, diffusion into the iris musculature most likely occurs from the anterior surface. A pigmented epithelial layer is located on the posterior side of the iris, which would be more resistant to drug uptake. For highly lipophilic drugs that can penetrate the epithelium layer, however, it is possible that this tissue can act as a reservoir for drugs.

In ocular pharmacokinetic studies, the iris and ciliary body often are removed and treated as a kinetically homogeneous tissue and measured for drug concentration over time. The resulting data may be misleading because drugs may actually accumulate in one portion of the tissue only but are reported as though the tissue were homogeneous (i.e., mass/unit weight of tissue). Although it is difficult to separate surgically the ciliary body from iris tissue in the rabbit eye, knowledge that many different receptors reside in one tissue or the other makes it increasingly important to know the exact location of drugs distribution of new drug agents. Information that drug distributes to the active site in high concentrations, as opposed to accumulation in a reservoir site, is critical in deciding whether a pharmacokinetic process is responsible for the success or failure of a new test agent. This knowledge helps to determine a direction in designing a more active therapeutic agent.

Ciliary Body

In contrast to the iris, the ciliary body contains a significant barrier to penetration: the pigmented and nonpigmented epithelial layers. Nevertheless, the ciliary body is the target tissue for many active topical drugs reported to lower intraocular pressure (IOP) in experimental animal eyes. Muscarinic, dopaminergic, serotonergic, α_1, α_2, and β-adrenergic receptors all have been identified in the ciliary body. In addition, forskolin, cannabinoid, prostaglandin, carbonic anhydrase inhibitors (CAIs), and xanthine derivatives all have lowered IOP in the animal eye and require high concentrations in the ciliary body for these agents to function.

Inhibition of carbonic anhydrase isoenzymes (II–IV) is the mechanism by which the CAIs lower IOP. In order for IOP to decline by this mechanism, a number of rather stringent requirements must be met. First, carbonic anhydrase (CA), which is located in the nonpigmented layer of the ciliary body, must be inhibited by +99%. Second, the large turnover of CA requires that a relatively high concentration of CAI must be present at the active site for a significant time for the IOP to fall for an acceptable time interval. Because the enzyme is located intracellularly, the CAI must be sufficiently lipophilic to enter the nonpigmented cell. Besides the requirement for distribution to the active site, a lipophilic CAI was initially considered essential to achieving adequate bioavailability into the eye; however, as development of the new antiglaucoma agent progressed, it became apparent that the most active topical CAIs were not the most lipophilic and also were not the most rapid in penetrating the cornea (35–39). Evidence suggested that scleral penetration was occurring for the most effective CAIs and, along with high potency, produced the best clinical candidates. Not surprisingly, a number of studies (40–43) were conducted to develop a topically active CAI. Merck scientists were the most successful and clinically tested two agents (44–47), MK-927 (sezolamide) and MK-507 (dorzolomide). In vitro studies showed that dorzolamide was the most potent of the CAIs intended for topical application and was at least 20 times more potent in inhibiting CA II than acetazolamide. Dorzolamide is converted to a metabolite that inhibits CA II less than the parent drug, but it also inhibits CA I. Dorzolamide (Trusopf, Merck) is considered the most active in glaucoma patients and possesses less ocular stinging and longer duration than sezolamide (48).

Lens

Drug distribution within the lens has not been well studied; however, whenever drug concentration in eye tissues has been measured over time and the lens has been included, a lack of accumulation is usually evident. Because the lens is bathed continuously by aqueous humor, one might first expect that accumulation should occur readily. The apparent lack of accumulation is likely a result of the structure of the lens. The lens, like the iris-ciliary body, is often incorrectly treated as a kinetically homogeneous tissue. The outer lens capsule consists of an elastic collagen-like material that theoretically should not provide much resistance to drug penetration. The primary barrier to entry into the lens is a single layer of epithelial cells lying just below the anterior lens capsule, which is absent on the posterior side of the lens. Internal to the epithelial layer are densely packed lens fibers and the nucleus, which consists of hard condensed cellular material. The nucleus possesses high tortuosity and low porosity. With age, old fibers are not disposed of but become compressed centrally to form a larger, less elastic nucleus. Consequently, hydrophilic drugs are not expected to penetrate the various layers of the lens, particularly with the rapid turnover of aqueous humor and with age.

The structure of the lens suggests that the epithelium is an initial barrier for uptake. Once drugs enter the lens, the most significant rate-determining step to accumulation is diffusion through the lens fibers. This phenomenon was successfully identified in vitro for the uptake and accumulation of timolol using excised rabbit lens. The model then was fit mathematically in vivo to concentration-time data for timolol (25 μl of 0.65%) given topically to rabbits (49).

When accumulation does occur, cataract formation becomes a concern. Because of the long time required for a cataract to develop, it becomes difficult to identify a causative agent. Nevertheless, chronic use of chlorpromazine, eosin, or sulfonamides is considered potentially responsible for the formation of cataracts (50).

Fluorescein, a water-soluble dye, diffuses laterally within the outermost layers of the lens more rapidly than it diffuses within the lens. A more lipophilic dye, rhodamine B, penetrated the lens more effectively during the same exposure time (51). If drugs are continuously available to the lens through chronic administration of either high or frequent dosing, it may have the capacity to accumulate significant levels of drugs. In an example using perfloxacin (52), a fluroquinolone antibiotic proposed for use in treating endophthalmic bacterial infections, 400 mg of drugs was infused over 1 hour to 20 patients undergoing cataract extraction. Plasma, aqueous humor, and lens concentrations were measured at 2, 6, 12, and 24 hours after the initiation of drug infusion. In plasma, the elimination half-life was 12.6 (±3.1) hours; however, at 24 hours, drug concentrations in aqueous humor had not reached distribution equilibrium, whereas the lens showed successively higher levels of drugs at each time interval. If the lens absorbs enough drug relative to the drug concentration in aqueous humor, and if this process occurs slowly, slow redistribution from the lens may inadvertantly lead to an overestimation of the half-life for drugs eliminated from aqueous humor. With the present interest in aldose reductase inhibitors preventing monsaccharide-induced lens degeneration in diabetic patients (53–55), more studies will focus on the role of the lens in influencing ocular pharmacokinetics and lead to a more precise model for lens pharmacokinetics.

Vitreous Cavity Gradient

For drugs to reach adequate levels in the retina, choroid, or optic nerve following topical application, drugs must first distribute from the aqueous to the vitreous humor. Although the vitreous is a circulating fluid that constitutes about 80% of the volume of the eye, drugs topically applied to the eye does not enter the vitreous in significant concentrations. Two main factors explain the relative lack of penetration into the vitreous cavity. One factor is that the available space between the ciliary processes and the lens is small, and drugs must diffuse against an aqueous humor gradient. Another factor is the relatively slow diffusion of drugs in vitreous. Molecular charge, lipophilicity, and even molecular size have little effect on the diffusion of drugs of ocular interest. Drug diffusion depends on molecular movement through an aqueous environment and, although it is not restricted by the presence of collagen in the vitreous (0.01%), drug diffusion is too slow to allow significant vitreous accumulation to occur. If high vitreal drug concentrations are critical to therapy, then either subconjunctival, iontophoretic, intravitreal, or systemic parenteral routes of administration must be considered.

ELIMINATION

Once drugs are absorbed into the anterior chamber, they are eliminated mostly by aqueous humor turnover, which is 1.5% per minute of the anterior chamber volume. When expressed as a half-life, aqueous turnover is 46.2 minutes, or 0.77 hours (7). Therefore, if drugs are eliminated from the eye with a half-life of approximately 0.77 hours, their elimination can be explained by aqueous turnover. Table 9-3 gives values determined for the rabbit eye from various ocular routes of administration and shows that most of the drugs of ophthalmic interest range from 0.6 to 3.0 hours. Certainly, extrapolation to human ocular pharmacokinetics must be done with great caution because metabolic pathways, volume of aqueous or vitreous humor, and other physiological factors vary significantly between rabbit and human eyes. Unfortunately, and for good reason, the half-lives of ophthalmic drugs have not been extensively determined. It is imperative in calculating an aqueous humor half-life of a drug that the latter portion of the concentration-time curve is clearly linear. As mentioned, slow redistribution of drugs from the lens may result in an overestimation of the half-life that may not be obvious if calculated from two to three time intervals or calculated from data with significant variability in the latter portion of the elimination phase.

For drugs with a half-life >0.77 hours, strong tissue binding is likely responsible for the longer half-life. If the half-life is <0.77 hours, metabolism and uptake by blood vessels in the anterior uvea or iris are likely pathways for elimination of drugs in addition to aqueous turnover. Many of the drugs in Table 9-3 with short half-lives act on receptors located in the iris-ciliary body. It is conceivable that their short half-lives may be a result of greater access to, and thus removal by, blood vessels located in this region of the eye.

For systemic drugs, the half-life is important in predicting both the time and extent of *accumulation,* defined as the ratio of the minimum concentration at steady state at the end of a dosing interval (C_{minSS}) to the concentration at the end of the first interval ($C_{min(1)}$). Accumulation can likewise be defined for drug administration to the eye. Ideally, C_{minSS} represents drug concentrations within the therapeutic range. In theory, C_{minSS} is reached after 5 elimination half-lives (96.8%), assuming a fixed dose and a fixed dosing interval are maintained. C_{minSS} can be calculated from the following equation:

$$C_{minSS} = \frac{C_{min(1)}}{1 - e^{-K\tau}}$$

where, K represents the elimination rate constant and τ is the time of the dosing interval. C_{minSS} is a relatively easy value to predict for systemically adminstered drugs but less clear for ocular drugs. At present, K is not well established for various ophthalmic patient populations, and $C_{min(1)}$ is not easily measured because of the inability to sample eye tissues without causing injury.

Blood-ocular Barriers

The blood-ocular barriers consist of the blood-aqueous barrier and the blood-retinal barrier. Anatomically, the

TABLE 9-3. *Aqueous humor half-lives[a] of drugs administered to the rabbit eye by topical, intracameral, or subconjunctival routes of administration*

Drug	Half-life (min)	Reference
Dapiprazole	348	56
Imirestat	285	57
6-Mercaptopurine	276	58
Falintolol	180	59
Fusidic acid	168	60
Prostaglandin $F_{2\alpha}$ methyl ester	162	61
Suprofen	156	62
Histamine	132	63
Cimetidine	132	63
Forskolin	128	64
Ketorolac tromethamine	126	65
Prednisolone sodium phosphate	123	66
Benzolamide	120	67
Ceftazidime	120	68
L-alphamethyldopa[b]	108	69
Diclofenac	102	70
Flurbiprofen	102	71
2-(4-Hydroxyethoxyphenyl) acetic acid	100	72
Oxacillin	96.3	73
Fluorometholone acetate	90	74
Cefamandole	90	75
Thiamphenicol	87	76
Amikacin	85.2	77
Phenylephrine	84	78
D-alphamethyldopa[b]	84	69
Acyclovir	77	79
Timolol	72	80
	50.4	81
Chloramphenicol	61.8	77
Lincomycin	72	82
6 Amino-2-benzothiazolesulfon amide	69	83
Dexamethasone	68.5	84
D-timolol	66.6	85
Acetbutolol	66	81
Dacarbazine	64.1	86
2-(4-Hydroxyethoxyphenyl)proprionic acid	60.3	72
Cefsulodin	60	87
Fluorouracil	60	88
	46.2	89
Dihydrolevobunolol	58.8	90
N-methylacetazolamide	58.8	91
6-hydroxyethoxy-2-benzothiazole-sulfonamide	58.2	38
6-acetamido-2-benzothiazolesul-fonamide	55.8	83
Prednisolone acetate	51.0	66
	90.8	92
Saperconazole	47.7	93
Tobramycin	45.	74
	40.4	94
	70.7	94
Pilocarpine	43.2	95
Trifluoromethazolamide	46.8	67
Methazolamide	34.8	67
Cefotaxime	34.2	96
Bufuralol	30.	81
Levobunolol	40.2	90
Ethoxzolamide	37.8	38
	13.8	67
Pyrilamine	36.6	63
Clonidine	29.4	97
Acetazolamide	21.	91
1,3-Bis(2-chloroethyl)-1,1-nitrosurea (BCNU)	20.4	98
Ibuprofen	18.8	83
2-benzothiazolesulfonamide	17.4	38
Ibufenac	16.8	72

[a]Concentrations from the last two to four time intervals were used in calculating $t_{1/2}$ values.
[b]A small dose dependency was observed (statistically n.s.); i.v. dose = 10 mg/kg.

blood-aqueous barrier is bordered by the ciliary nonpigmented epithelium and the endothelium of the iridial vessels. The blood-retinal barrier comprises the pigmented epithelium of the retina and the endothelial cells of the retinal capillaries. The cells of these various layers possess "tight junctions" and therefore resist penetration by hydrophilic drugs. For example, fluorescein is relatively impermeable to intact blood-ocular barriers and is used as a basis for testing the degree of barrier damage (i.e., fluorescein angiophraphy and vitreous fluorophtometry) (99,100). Certain drugs and endogeneous substances, either because of their lipophilicity or because of active transport (e.g., glucose and amino acids), can readily penetrate the blood-ocular barrier.

A breakdown of these barriers can occur either as a result of certain disease states, by surgical intervention, or from the use of toxic agents (100–103). Although no research has been published relating drug elimination and the breakdown of the blood-ocular barriers, it is logical to anticipate that half-lives may be decreased, and either smaller doses or more frequent dosing regimens might be required for these patients.

Metabolism

Metabolic pathways in the eye have not been extensively studied. The exception is corneal esterases, which are important in the conversion of dipivefrin to epinephrine, the former a lipophilic dipivalyl ester of epinephrine. When applied to the eye as dipivefrin HCl, approximately tenfold to 17-fold as much epinephrine is absorbed across the cornea compared with equal doses of epinephrine salts. Esterases exist in relatively high concentrations in anterior segment tissues of the rabbit eye, particularly the iris-ciliary body, which contains about twice as much esterase as the corneal epithelium (104,105). Acetyl-, butyryl- and carboxyl-esterases have been identified in albino and pigmented rabbit eyes, suggesting that esterases differ slightly with respect to the substrate (106). In general, the corneal epithelium and endothelium, the iris-ciliary body, and the retina are the tissues most likely to contain enzyme systems capable of metabolizing drugs. Because drugs do not appreciably reach the retina from topical application, retinal enzymes are less important to ophthalmic drug metabolism unless drugs are given by systemic or periocular routes of administration.

In designing new drugs for the eye, one attractive course of action is to develop a lipophilic prodrug that is absorbed rapidly across the cornea and then converted into the active drug species before reaching the target tissue. This approach has been attempted many times, as exemplified by the following list of drugs for which prodrugs have been studied: phenylephrine (107,108), timolol (109), pilocarpine (110), idoxuridine (111), and prostaglandin $F_{2\alpha}$ (112). Mostly, ocular prodrugs have not been commercially successful, which can be attributed to one of a number of factors. Lipophilic prodrugs are often relatively insoluble and difficult to manufacture as sterile, homogeneous suspensions and also may be unstable to an extent that an adequate shelf life is not possible. Further, as a general rule, ocular absorption in animal models must be fivefold to tenfold greater than an equal dose of the parent drug in order for clinical efficacy to be significantly improved.

Although the eye is not a primary drug-metabolizing organ, identification of metabolites of ocular drugs is important because of the potential of finding new drugs. Also, identification of phenotypes that might exist for enzyme systems could possibly explain variability in therapeutic efficacy. The enzyme systems that have been identified from the study of animal eyes are *N*-acetyltransferase (113), ketone reductase (114), catechol-O-methyltransferase, monamine oxidase, steroid 6-betahydroxylase, oxidoreductase, lysosomal enzymes, aminopetidases, glucuronide and sulfate transferase, and glutathione-conjugating enzymes (36, 115).

Recently, Bodar and co-workers (116–118) applied a knowledge of metabolic pathways to alter a drug's elimination profile. These new drug entities are referred to as *soft drugs* and are designed to improve therapy. For example, a soft analog of atropine has shown a much-reduced duration of action compared with atropine and had no effect on the fellow eye (119). A potent, short-acting mydriatic would be advantageous for use in ophthalmoscopy or other ocular procedures. In another example using rabbits (120), an adamantylethyl ester of metoprolol showed a prolonged and greater reduction of IOP and also a reduced potential to cause bradycardia compared with timolol.

PHARMACOKINETICS OF SELECTED OCULAR DRUGS

Fluoroquinolone Antibacterial Agents

The fluoroquinolone derivatives are new antibacterial agents with a wide spectrum of activity against both gram-positive and gram-negative bacteria. When given orally or parenterally, their distribution into eye tissues is less than adequate. Based on ratios of peak concentrations of aqueous humor to serum, measurements of 16% to 22% were obtained in volunteer surgical subjects for ciprofloxacin, perfloxacin, ofloxacin, or norfloxacin (121) given as single doses. Peak concentrations in aqueous humor varied from 0.22 to 1.48 μg/ml and were considered for the most part below the minimum inhibitory concentrations (MIC_{90s}: 0.5–4 μg/ml for most organisms). In one study (122), an approximation of the aqueous humor half-life was estimated as 1.9 hours for ciprofloxacin following 200 mg i.v. administration to 25 patients undergoing cataract surgery. Levels ranged from 0.1 to 0.2 μg/ml from 3 through 7 hours before declining rapidly. Topical application of these agents has proved efficacious for the treatment of external eye infections.

Studies in rabbits (123,124) in which either 0.3% norfloxacin (Chibroxin, Merck) or 0.3% ciprofloxacin (Ciloxan, Alcon) was given topically indicated that corneal and conjunctival drug concentrations were well above the MIC_{90}s for relevant organisms but below the MIC_{90}s in aqueous humor, iris, lens, vitreous, or retina/choroid. In a carefully conducted pharmacokinetic study using rabbits (125), fleroxacin was administered both intravenously (10 mg/kg) and intravitreally (100 μg), followed by frequent monitoring of drug concentrations in serum, aqueous, and vitreous humors over 5 hours. The half-lives were not significantly different and ranged from 2.34 to 3.88 hours. The relatively short half-life for these agents suggests that frequent systemic or periocular administration is required to maintain therapeutic concentrations if the drug is used to treat intraocular infections. When used topically for conjunctival or corneal infections, however, these agents also must be instilled frequently because of precorneal factors (e.g., drainage and blinking) that do not permit drugs to remain in the conjunctival sac for more than 5 to 10 minutes at the longest.

Prostaglandin F2α Isopropyl Ester

Topical application of prostaglandin $F_{2\alpha}$ isopropyl ester (PhXA34) has been studied for its potential use in glaucoma patients. Studies in the human eye suggest that it significantly lowers IOP by increasing the "nonconventional" outflow facility and may only require a single topical daily dose; however, ocular irritation and conjunctival hyperemia are side effects that have been noted even with lower doses (10 μg daily to the eye). Fluorophotometery measurements showed a 10 to 20% increase in the total amount of fluorescein during the first 2 hours, indicating a disruption of the blood-aqueous barrier. An attempt was made to use a 1,15-diester to separate the lowering of IOP from the unwanted side effects, but it was not successful (112).

PhXA34 was designed to penetrate the cornea rapidly and therefore increase the amount of drug reaching the anterior chamber. In vitro incubation of PhXA34 with isolated pig corneas (126,127) indicated that butyrylcholinesterase, but not acethycholinesterase or carbonic anhydrase (a nonspecific esterase), was responsible for enzymatic hydrolysis of the prodrug to the active species, prostaglandin F2α. It was also determined that conversion to the active drug was occurring mainly in the corneal epithelium. PhXA41 (latanoprost) is a more active isomer (R-epimer) of PhXA34 and also lowers IOP to a greater extent on an equimolar basis. Both isomers are long acting, and although conjunctival hyperemia occurs in a significant number of patients, a single daily dose effectively lowers IOP for both isomers.

Cyclosporine

Cyclosporine is an effective immunosuppressive agent in kidney, liver, bone marrow, pancreas, and heart transplant patients. It has also been used to inhibit the rejection of corneal grafts and in the treatment of uveitis. Cyclosporine is a highly lipophilic cyclic polypeptide with a large molecular weight (MW 1200). When dosed topically to the human eye in a concentration of 2% in olive oil, very little drug reaches the anterior chamber. Patients with severe uveitis who took cyclosporine orally (5 mg/kg/day) had significant levels of cyclosporine in both aqueous and vitrous humor. Patients without intraocular inflammation or with mild uveitis did not have detectable levels of drug in the aqueous humor (128). The absorption of cyclosporine after oral administration is slow, incomplete ($\approx$30%), and quite variable so that a relatively wide range of tissue levels can be expected. It is extensively metabolized to 15 metabolites in most subjects with a half-life range of 10 to 27 hours (average, 19 hours).

Animal studies (129–131) indicate that disruption of the blood-ocular barriers is necessary for drugs to reach intraocular tissues following oral ingestion. Also, topical instillation produces significant levels in both the cornea and conjunctiva but not within the eye. Topical administration of 2% cyclosporine in a petrolatum ointment appears to have a role in preventing graft rejection, especially in high-risk patients.

Ganciclovir

Ganciclovir is currently the drug of choice for treatment of cytomegalovirus (CMV) retinitis in patients with AIDS, although about a third of patients taking the drug intravenously must discontinue therapy because of systemic side effects (e.g., neutropenia). Intravitreal injection (200–400 μg) significantly reduces these side effects but requires at least weekly injections. The intravitreal half-life of ganciclovir in one patient was estimated as 13.3 hours (132).

To circumvent the problems associated with systemic and intravitreal administration of ganciclovir, a surgically implantable device was designed for slow release of drugs over a 4- to 5-month period (133). Because of the drug's relatively long vitreal half-life and high water solubility, it can be designed as a sustained release implant using a diffusional polymer barrier to control the release rate and to obviate the need for frequent intravitreal injections. Studies in rabbits indicated that sustainable vitreous concentrations of drugs above the ID_{50} for CMV (0.2–2.6 μg/ml) can be maintained in the human eye (134). The implant was tested in eight patients with AIDS and associated CMV (135). Results indicated that the surgically implanted intravitreal device (13 eyes) effectively released ganciclovir above the ID_{50} for 4 to 5 months. All eyes with the implanted device showed resolution of the CMV retinitis, which suggests that treatment by this approach is feasible. An implanted device, along with a reduced parenteral dose of ganciclovir, may prove to be more effective.

Imirestat, An Aldose Reductase Inhibitor

Aldose reductase is present in ocular tissues, particularly the lens. Inhibition of this enzyme blocks the sorbitol accumulation as a result of excess glucose, which contributes to the formation of cataracts, a complication of diabetes. Aldose reductase is also involved in other diabetic complications, namely, retinopathy and neuropathy. The ocular pharmacokinetics of imirestat (ALO1576), a hydantoin derivative of 2,7-difluorofluorenone, was studied extensively in the rabbit eye by Brazzell and co-workers (55,57,136, 137). When given systemically to rats or rabbits, the drug accumulated in tissues that contain high concentrations of aldose reductase (i.e., eye, testis, adrenal, and kidney).

The pharmacokinetics of imirestat following topical dosing to the rabbit eye (0.05% suspension) showed rapid absorption into the cornea and extensive distribution into the lens, with relatively high residual concentrations remaining in the cornea over time. Slow elimination was observed from the cornea and lens, probably a consequence of the high affinity of drug for aldose reductase in these tissues. The half-life of drug in the lens was 140 minutes. It persisted at detectable levels in aqueous and vitreous humor for 12 and 72 hours, respectively. Drugs increased in the lens with an increase in dose. The cortex showed a consistently higher drug concentration than the nucleus, and on multiple dosing (0.05% twice daily for 6 weeks), the nucleus levels increased proportionately, whereas the cortex levels remained nearly the same, suggesting, as expected, that the two lens tissues have different kinetic behaviors (57).

Because aldose reductase apparently plays a role in retinopathy and neuropathy as well as in the formation of cataracts, clinical application of these agents is likely to reflect the need for systemic treatment. Other potent aldose reductase inhibitors are being studied in human subjects but are designed for systemic administration (53,54).

5-Fluorouracil

5-Fluorouracil (5FU) inhibits cellular proliferation and is proposed for use extraocularly in high-risk glaucoma patients undergoing filtering surgery and also intraocularly to accompany retinal detachment complicated by proliferative vitreoretinopathy (138,139). Although both topical drops and intravitreal injections produce therapeutic drug concentrations, the drug's toxicity to the cornea or retina eliminates both routes of administration from consideration. A subconjunctival injection also produces therapeutic drug levels but assumes the risk of hemorrhage, scarring, ocular penetration, and infection (89). Given systemically, 5FU is rapidly eliminated from the body (half-life = 8–20 min), mostly by metabolism; so little of the drug is available for distribution to eye tissues (140). Therefore, recent scientific studies focused on determining the lowest dose necessary for therapeutic success, identifying potentially less toxic but active metabolites or developing ocular drug-delivery approaches (141).

In an attempt to demonstrate the applicability of delivering 5FU from liposomes, rabbits were given liposome-encapsulated 5FU containing 10.6 mg of the drug by either subconjunctival or intravitreal injections and compared with similar treatments of drugs dissolved in a phosphate buffer (142). Over 8 hours, drug concentrations from the liposome-encapsulated injections produced approximately twofold higher drug levels than from drug dissolved in phosphate buffer. Maximum concentrations for 5FU reached 64.8 μg/m; versus 29.4 μg/ml for each formulation, respectively; however, in another rabbit study in which 5 and 10 mg of liposome-encapsulated 5FU was given, peak concentrations in the aqueous humor were only 6.2 and 12.0 μg/ml but sustained these concentrations relatively well from 0.5 through 8 hours.

Evidence suggests that reduced toxicity occurs from drugs encapsulated in liposomes (143); so, if lower concentrations can be delivered over extended periods, the use of liposomes may prove beneficial. Given the drug's narrow therapeutic window, the successful use of 5FU (or a less toxic metabolite) in the eye likely depends on delivering it to the site of action at a sustainable rate, just above its median infective dose (ID_{50}) for cellular proliferation.

Pilocarpine

The ocular pharmacokinetics of pilocarpine has been studied extensively, mostly in the rabbit eye, and has led to a better understanding of ocular ADME processes in general. Various modeling approaches have been applied to explain the ocular absorption and disposition of the drug following topical dosing, including physiologic (98,144) and classical pharmacokinetic methods (145–149). From this work, critical bioavailability factors have been identified: the precorneal factors, such as drainage, blinking, and noncorneal absorption into and away from the eye. One of the most significant findings is that the drainage rate is so large compared with corneal absorption (i.e., about 100-fold) that little of the instilled dose is actually absorbed into the eye and that the time to peak, regardless of the drug administered, is relatively fixed between 20 and 60 minutes. The study of pilocarpine pharmacokinetics has also led to a clearer understanding of retention of an instilled viscous dose at the absorption site from the use of cellulosic polymers or polyvinyl alcohol. As a result, optimal bioavailability is attained if drugs are instilled at least 3 to 5 minutes apart or if they are formulated as a combination product.

Pilocarpine penetrates the cornea at moderate rates compared with other ocular drugs, which is indicative of its intermediate lipophilicity. Various studies agree that about 1% to 2% of the instilled dose is absorbed (146,147) and that its elimination half-life from aqueous humor closely approximates the half-life for aqueous turnover (i.e., 43.2 minutes). Pilocarpine binds to melanin, which potentially acts as a reservoir for drug accumulation in the iris. As with other drugs instilled topically into the eye, little of the absorbed dose diffuses into the vitreous (<5%). The drug is metabolized rapidly once it reaches the bloodstream; therefore, systemic uptake and subsequent cholinergic activity (i.e., muscarinic) are of minor concern from its topical use. Stinging and burning upon instillation are common side effects but typical of amine drugs used in the eye.

Timolol and Other Beta-Blocking Agents

Timolol is a potent nonselective beta-blocking agent that penetrates the cornea moderately well, which is predicted by its intermediate lipophilic behavior; however, its concentration in the rabbit eye is much higher than estimated from either its corneal permeability or partition coefficient (9,81,109), suggesting an additional route of entry, perhaps the conjunctiva/scleral pathway. Studies in rabbits (150) in which 20 μl of 0.5% timolol was administered topically in single and multiple doses (twice daily for 6 days) to both pigmented and albino rabbits showed that treated and untreated pigmented eyes resulted in a concentration profile of iris>ciliary body≥cornea>choroid and retina>>aqueous humor. The albino rabbit showed a much lower concentration profile in which cornea>>iris≈ciliary body≈aqueous humor. The tissue profiles indicate that differences were due to melanin binding and tend to support the hypothesis of a significant scleral pathway into the anterior chamber. The half-life for elimination of timolol from the rabbit aqueous humor is reported to be 50 min (81), which is nearly equal to aqueous humor turnover (half-life = 42.7 min). In the human eye, there is a slight elevation of aqueous protein after topical application of timolol, but this is not a drug effect on the blood-aqueous barrier but rather a consequence of a decrease in aqueous humor production (151).

Both cardiovascular and respiratory side effects have been associated with the topical use of timolol and have led to the development of levobunolol, betaxolol, and metipranolol. Only betaxolol is a relatively selective beta-blocking agent and should have fewer side effects. Although drug-receptor specificity is an important factor in the design of a drug devoid of systemic side effects, another approach has been to design lipophilic prodrugs of timolol that penetrate the cornea more readily and allow a twofold reduction in administered dose (109). Stereochemical specificity from the use of D-timolol has produced a nearly equipotent antiglaucoma agent with fewer cardiovascular side effects (152). In the rabbit eye, its half-life of 66 minutes in aqueous humor is similar to L-timolol (85).

Levobunolol is a potent nonselective beta-blocking agent with physicochemical and permeability properties similar to timolol (90). The ocular pharmacokinetics of levobunolol have been well studied in the rabbit eye by Tang-Liu and co-workers (90,153). Its ocular bioavailability is about 7.5%; however, about two-thirds that amount is represented by the equipotent metabolite dihydrolevobunolol (DHB), which is formed mostly in the cornea, presumably the epithelium, but also in the iris-ciliary body. After distribution equilibrium, DHB is the major component found in the cornea, aqueous humor, and iris-ciliary body (153). The half-lives for elimination of parent drug and DHB from aqueous humor are 40 and 59 minutes, respectively.

Phenylephrine

Phenylephrine HCl is a potent α_1-adrenergic agonist with little or no β-receptor stimulation. It is used in ophthalmology in concentrations of 2.5 and 10% for pupillary dilatation in surgery as well as ophthalmoscopic examination. The drug is polar and penetrates the cornea so poorly that it must be administered in a high concentration to exert its effect. At 10% the commercial product is hypertonic and therefore quite uncomfortable upon instillation. After topical application of 10% phenylephrine, a sufficient amount is systemically absorbed to increase blood pressure by 10 to 40 mm Hg in both healthy and hypertensive patients. In susceptible patients, severe transient hypertension, subarachnoid hemorrhage, ventricular arrhythmia, and possible myocardial infarction have been reported (154). The drug is metabolized extensively if given systemically; when its disposition is followed in the eye of either rabbits (78), monkeys (108), or humans (155), it rapidly falls below detection within 30 to 60 minutes, partly due to metabolism and partly to distribution to the active site. In 30 patients undergoing vitreoretinal surgery (155), administration of 2.5% drops to the eye of either viscous or nonviscous aqueous solutions showed little difference in the drug's plasma profile.

These observations prompted the development of phenylephrine oxazolidine, a lipophilic prodrug of phenylephrine. It is highly lipophilic and promotes rapid absorption of the drug into the anterior chamber so that in either rabbits (78) or monkeys (108), 1% of the prodrug was equipotent to 10% of the parent drug. In clinical trials (107) in which healthy subjects received either 1% of the prodrug, 10% phenylephrine HCl, or vehicle, a pupillary diameter of 8.8 mm was achieved in 30 minutes in those receiving the prodrug compared with 6.5 mm obtained at 30 minutes with 10% phenylephrine.

Gentamicin and Tobramycin

Both gentamicin and tobramycin are large molecular-weight, very polar, broad-spectrum aminoglycosides, which, because of their efficacy against *Pseudomonas aeruginosa,* are particularly useful in the treatment of ocular infections. In vitro studies indicate that tobramycin has a slightly lower MIC against *P. aeruginosa.* The epithelium of the cornea is the primary barrier that resists their entry into the anterior chamber after topical application of either drug. When given systemically, plasma concentrations are monitored frequently because of these drugs' narrow therapeutic window. Although nephrotoxicity is of concern when given systemically, concentrations instilled topically do not provide systemic levels of drugs that are significant. Nevertheless, the lack of penetration of aminoglycosides into the anterior chamber from topical dosing has prompted clinicians to give the drug parenterally.

In a study in which 22 patients underwent penetrating keratoplasty, patients were given either gentamicin 13.6 mg/ml topically per minute for three doses 5 to 70 minutes before surgery or a dose of 1 mg/kg intramuscularly 1 to 1.5 hours before surgery (156). In patients receiving the topical dose, drug levels in the cornea ranged from 2.6 to 56 μg/g, which is above the MIC (1–2 μg/ml for *P. aeruginosa*), whereas aqueous humor levels ranged from nondetectable to 1 μg/ml. The patients receiving parenteral drug averaged 6.1 μg/g and 0.4 μg/ml in the cornea and aqueous humor, respectively, with considerably less variability. Although the topical route is preferred, significant penetration into the anterior chamber is not feasible with conventional drop therapy. A number of animal and human studies involving inflamed eyes have shown that for either gentamicin (many manufacturers) or tobramycin (Tobrex, Alcon) fortified preparations and greater frequency of administration produce high levels of drugs in the cornea and adnexa but not within the eye. Consequently, topical administration of either drug is indicated for external eye infections, whereas systemic or periocular routes of administration must be used for intraocular infections.

It is often debated whether continuous infusion or intermittent administration gives better tissue levels of gentamicin. Barza et al. (157) tested each method of administration based on the intraocular distribution of gentamicin in rabbits with bacterial endophthalmitis. The rabbits were treated with the same dose over 12 hours either by continuous infusion or i.m. injection every 3 hours. From the infusion, steady-state serum levels measured about 7 μg/ml, whereas the repeated i.m. injection produced peaks and troughs of 11.4 and 1.6 μg/ml. Areas under the serum-concentration curves were similar for each route of administration. Mean vitreous humor levels at the end of treatment were 2.8 and 2.6 μg/ml for continuous versus intermittent administrations, respectively.

For bacterial endophthalmitis, intravitreal drug administration is the preferred method of administration. Once injected, it requires about 8 hours to produce a uniform concentration throughout the vitreous of an infected cat eye. Infected eyes yielded an elimination half-life of 12.6 hours, whereas normal eyes have much shorter vitreal half-lives, most likely because of an intact blood-vitreous barrier.

Although frequent topical instillation of either tobramycin or gentimycin eyedrops are effective means of treating external eye infections, the use of liposome-encapsulated subconjunctival injection or drug-soaked collagen shields were tested in rabbit eyes to improve compliance (158–160). The use of drug-soaked collagen shields showed no benefit to therapy, but the use of liposome encapsulation did show a prolonged effect from the subconjunctival depot for both gentamicin (161) and tobramycin (162). Also, intravitreal injection of liposome-encapsulated gentamicin in the normal rabbit eye showed a twofold increase in available drug compared with the same dose given without encapsulation (163).

Iontophoresis also appears to be an effective means of delivering either drug into the eye. For example, the transcorneal iontophoresis of tobramycin (25 mg/ml for 10 min at 0.8 mAmps) generated high concentrations of 103.2, 20.7, and 5.9 μg/ml for 8 hours in the normal rabbit eye for epithelium, stroma, and aqueous humor, respectively. This treatment, although effective in delivering therapeutic levels of drugs over an extended period compared with fortified drop therapy, also produced epithelial edema. Transcorneal iontophoresis has produced therapeutic levels of gentamicin into the vitreous of aphakic rabbit eyes of 6.2 μg/ml after 24 hours but not into the vitreous humor of normal rabbit eyes (164).

Steroidal and Nonsteroidal Antiinflammatory Agents

Corticosteroids used in the eye can be classified into two types: those that are lipophilic, relatively insoluble, and formulated as suspensions; and those that are very polar, water soluble, and formulated as viscous solutions. The former are indicated for intraocular inflammations of the uveal tract because they effectively penetrate the cornea, whereas the latter are used for external eye inflammations and do not appreciably penetrate the cornea. Prednisolone acetate and dexamethasone acetate penetrate the cornea rapidly and are also the most lipophilic steroids. Although they are potent antiinflammatory agents, their effectiveness is also a consequence of their optimal corneal penetration.

During the decade of the 1970s, Leibowitz and co-workers (165–169) indirectly determined the ocular pharmacokinetics of many commercially available corticosteroids by measuring the ability of steroids to suppress a chemically induced corneal inflammation and also directly by measuring their concentrations in various eye tissues after topically administering radiolabelled steroids. These researchers devised an inflammatory response in the rabbit eye from an intracorneal injection of 0.03 ml of clove oil. To quantify this phenomenon, they injected radiolabeled thymidine intravenously before the inflammatory response induced by the clove oil. During inflammation, large numbers of inflammatory cells, mostly radiolabelled polymorphonuclear leukocytes (PMN), migrated to the site. To suppress the migration of PMNs to the site of inflammation, various steroids were given topically in repeated doses (standard protocol). Antiinflammatory activity was measured by counting radioactivity in corneas before, during, and after treatment. Table 9-4 summarizes their results for a few commercially available steroids. The results show that the percent of suppression of each steroid depends in part on its antiinflammatory potency, the concentration that applied, and corneal permeability, which in turn depends on lipophilicity. Clearly, the water-soluble steroids, dexamethasone sodium phosphate and methylprednisolone sodium succinate, are the least effective in suppressing corneal inflammation in this model, mostly because of their high water solubility and hence their inability to penetrate across corneal barriers.

Although corticosteroids effectively suppress external and anterior-chamber eye inflammations, they also may induce glaucoma and enhance actively replicating herpes simplex virus in susceptible persons. Consequently, the ocular use of nonsteroidal antiinflammatory agents (NSAIDs) has been investigated. Recently, flurbiprofen (Ocufen, Allergan) and suprofen (Profenal, Alcon) have been marketed, and others are also likely to become available for patient use.

The ocular pharmacokinetics of flurbiprofen, an arylacetic acid NSAID, was studied thoroughly by Tang-Liu et al. (170). Topical application of suspended flurbiprofen to the normal rabbit eye indicated that 7% to 10% of the applied dose (75 and 150 μg) was absorbed into the eye, whereas systemic bioavailability from the ophthalmic dose

TABLE 9-4. *Suppression of radiolabeled polymorphonuclear leucocytes (PMN) in the inflamed cornea following topical and subjunctival administration*[a]

Drug and dosage form	Suppression (%)[b]
Topical treatment[c]	
Prednisolone acetate, 1% suspension (Econopred Plus)	52.1 ± 3.8
Dexamethasone, 0.5% suspension (Maxidex)	38.9 ± 2.6
Fluorometholone, 0.1% suspension (FML)	30.8 ± 5.0
Dexamethosone sodium phosphate, 1.0% solution	27.6 ± 2.0
Dexamethasone sodium phosphate, 0.1% solution (Decadron)	18.7 ± 1.9
Suprofen 1.0 solution (profenal)[d]	16.9 ± 4.7
Dexamethasone sodium phosphate, 0.05% ointment (Decadron)	12.3 ± 2.9
Saline 0.9%	7.3 ± 2.9
Suprofen vehicle	9.6 ± 4.1
Subconjunctival treatment[d]	
Prednisolone acetate, 100 mg/ml suspension (Durapred)	24.3 ± 3.8
Prednisolone acetate, 25 mg/ml suspension (Durapred)	14.8 ± 2.0
Methylprednisolone sodium succinate, 40 mg/ml solution (Solu-Medrol)	29.9 ± 4.5
Saline 0.9%	0.9 ± 1.4

From Leibowitz et al., ref 92; Leibowitz and Kupferman, refs 165 and 169.

[a]Inflammatory activity produced by 0.03 ml of clove oil injected into stroma of rabbit cornea.

[b]Mean ± standard deviation from 12 eyes.

[c]Topical treatment: 0.05 ml every 1 h for 6 h beginning 24 h after induction of inflammation, then lapse of 18 h, then 0.05 ml every 1 h for 7 h.

[d]Topical treatment: same as footnote "c" above, except suprofen was administered 24 h before induction of inflammation.

[e]Subconjunctival treatment: two injections of 0.5 ml 5 h apart, beginning 24 hours after induction of inflammation, then lapse of 18 h, then two additional injections of 0.5 ml 6 h apart.

was 74%. Once absorbed into the eye, an ocular distribution half-life of 15 minutes indicated rapid uptake by anterior chamber tissues. The drug is highly bound to serum proteins (99%) and also presumably highly bound to proteins in aqueous humor. An aqueous humor elimination half-life of 93 minutes was measured, which is somewhat longer than elimination by aqueous turnover (i.e., 42.7 minutes). In either normal or aphakic rabbit eyes following the instillation of 50 μl of 0.03% of a radiolabeled drug, flurbiprofen showed no difference in tissue levels. The ratio of drug levels for cornea/aqueous humor at time intervals between 0.5 and 6 hours varied from tenfold to 30-fold, suggesting either poor corneal permeability or the existence of a corneal binding site. The latter may be more likely because conjunctival levels, which have equal access to the instilled drug, were only a tenth the concentration of the cornea. In this particular study, the aqueous humor elimination half-life measured 2 hours.

Leibowitz et al. (62) studied both the bioavailability as well as the corneal antiinflammatory effect of topical suprofen in rabbit eyes and showed that it possesses pharmacokinetic behavior similar to that of flurbiprofen. The ratio of drug in cornea/aqueous humor was 15- to 25-fold at distribution equilibrium, and the aqueous humor half-life was 2.6 hours. The antiinflammatory activity of suprofen depended on the time of treatment. When drug treatment was begun either immediatedly after the induction of inflammation or 24 hours later, the antiinflammatory activity was low; however, when treatment was begun 48 hours before clove oil injection and continued on the day of injection and 2 days thereafter, a significant decrease in PMNs was measured. Although corneal levels of drug were high, the percent of suppression of PMN migration was not dramatic and suggests either that the inflammatory rabbit model described above does not adequately measure the drug's activity or that NSAIDs are inferior to corticosteroids in antiinflammatory activity. Clinical studies suggest the latter; in fact, their approval for use in the human eye has been limited thus far to inflammations associated with intraoperative miosis. Nevertheless, the topical use of NSAIDs does not pose the safety risk that has been experienced with the topical use of corticosteroids. The most frequent adverse effect reported with the use of NSAIDs has been the initial discomfort experienced upon instillation, which may be related to their surfactantlike physicochemical properties (72).

SYSTEMIC ABSORPTION OF OCULAR DRUGS

As mentioned previously, when drugs are instilled topically, only a small percentage of the dose is actually absorbed into the eye (i.e., 1–7%). The remainder of the drug in contact with conjunctival and nasolacrimal mucosa can be systemically absorbed, leading to the possibility of an unwanted side effect. Nevertheless, because of the small dose administered and the likelihood of rapid dilution by the large blood reservoir, the risk of systemic side effects from topical administration is minimal with many ocular drugs. The ideal conditions for a systemic drug effect depend on factors such as high potency and a rapid rate of systemic absorption. In particular, the larger the volume of the instilled drop, the faster the drainage rate and the greater the potential for rapid systemic absorption (3,171). When absorption is rapid, the peak serum concentration is high. The extent of absorption may be a less critical factor, particularly if the drug enters the systemic pool slowly. Reduction of systemic absorption may be promoted either by enhancing corneal absorption or by retarding drainage of the instilled drug, accomplished from the use of vehicles that extend ocular contact (e.g., viscous solutions or semisolids), from the preparation of lipophilic prodrugs (e.g., phenylephrine oxazolidine or dipivephrine), from the use of nasolacrimal occlusion, or from the use of microdrops of 10 μl or less (1,5–8).

In a recent review by Salminen (172), a summary of drugs known to produce significant serum levels following topical administration are timolol, levbunolol, atropine, cyclopentolate, scopolamine, phenylephrine, and betamethasone. Systemic absorption occurs partly from the vascularized conjunctiva/scleral pathway and partly from the large nasal mucosa. When the puncta are occluded, systemic absorption is variable with regard to serum levels of drugs and may be due to preferential absorption from the conjunctiva/scleral pathway once nasolacrimal drainage is prevented.

CONCLUSION

The knowledge necessary to understand the pharmacokinetics of human ocular drugs has advanced in recent years, but it has not evolved to a level comparable to that of systemic drugs. The precorneal physiological factors and corneal absorption are better known than distribution within the eye, particularly the lens and vitreal kinetics. Currently, pharmacokinetic measurements in the human eye can be made only in patients undergoing eye surgery, severely limiting the application of ADME to designing optimal dosing regimens. Individualized dosing regimens for ocular drugs remain a goal until noninvasive techniques can be developed as has been done for fluorescein.

A knowledge of ocular pharmacokinetic behavior is also important to the development of new drug entities. For many years, ocular drugs were screened from drugs originally intended for systemic use. The recent clinical trials of dorzolamide, prostaglandin $F_{2\alpha}$ isopropyl ester, and imirestat indicate that in the future more new agents will be developed specifically for the eye. Least is known regarding the metabolic pathways of ocular drugs. Such knowledge would be useful in providing leads to new drug entities and also in suggesting alternate dosing regimens in which variability or genetic phenotype behavior is identified.

REFERENCES

1. Schoenwald RD. Ocular drug delivery pharmacokinetic considerations. *Clin Pharmacokinet* 1990;19:255–269.
2. Chrai SS, Patton TF, Mehta A, Robinson JR. Lacrimal and instilled fluid dynamics in rabbit eyes. *J Pharm Sci* 1973;62:1112–1121.
3. Chrai SS, Makoid MC, Eriksen SP, Robinson JR. Drop size and initial dosing frequency problems of topically applied ophthalmic drugs. *J Pharm Sci* 1974;63:333–338.
4. Mackoid MC, Sieg JW, Robinson JR. Corneal drug absorption: an illustration of parallel first-order absorption and rapid loss of drug from absorption depot. *J Pharm Sci* 1976;65:150–152.
5. Lee VH, Robinson JR. Review: topical ocular drug delivery: recent developments and future challenges. *J Ocul Pharmacol* 1986;2: 67–108.
6. Schoenwald RD. Ocular pharmacokinetics/pharmacodynamics. In: Mitra AK, ed. *Ophthalmic Drug Delivery Systems.* New York: Marcel Dekker, 1993;83–110.
7. Maurice DM. Ocular pharmacokinetics. In: Sears ML, ed. *Pharmacology of the Eye.* New York: Springer-Verlag, 1984;19–116.
8. Schoenwald RD. Pharmacokinetics in ocular delivery. In: Edman P, ed. *Biopharmaceutics of Ocular Drug Delivery.* Boca Raton, FL: CRC Press, 1993;159–191.
9. Huang HS, Schoenwald RD, Lach JL. Corneal penetration behavior of beta-blocking agents II: assessment of barrier contributions. *J Pharm Sci* 1983;72:1272–1279.
10. Doane MG, Jensen AD, Dohlman CH. Penetration routes of topically applied eye medications. *Am J Ophthalmol* 1978;85:383–386.
11. Ahmed I, Patton TF. Importance of the noncorneal absorption route in topical ophthalmic drug delivery. *Invest Ophthalmol Vis Sci* 1985;26:584–587.
12. Edelhauser HF, Maren TH. Permeability of human cornea and sclera to sulfonamide carbonic anhydrase inhibitors. *Arch Ophthalmol* 1988;106:1110–1114.
13. Chien DS, Honsy JJ, Gluchowski C, Tang-Liu DDS. Corneal and conjunctival/scleral penetration of p-aminoclonidine, AGN 190342, and clonidine in rabbit eyes. *Curr Eye Res* 1990;9:1051–1059.
14. Weng W, Sasaki H, Chien DS, Lee VHL. Lipophilicity influence on conjunctival drug penetrtion in the pigmented rabbit: a comparison with corneal penetration. *Curr Eye Res* 1991;10:571–579.
15. Lee DY, Schoenwald RD, Barfknecht CF. Biopharmaceutical explanation for the topical activity of 6-hydroxyethoxy-2-benzothiazole-sulfonamide in the rabbit eye. *J Ocul Pharmacol* 1992;8:247–265.
16. Pech B, Chetoni P, Saettone MF, Duval O, Benoit JP. Preliminary evaluation of a series of amphiphilic timolol prodrugs: possible evidence for transscleral absorption. *J Ocul Pharmacol* 1993;9:141–150.
17. McCloskey RV. Topical antimicrobial agents and antibiotics for the eye. *Med Clin North Am* 1988;72:717–722.
18. Jain MR. Drug delivery through soft contact lenses. *Br J Ophthalmol* 1988;72:150–154.
19. Jain MR, Goyal M, Jain V. Ocular penetration of subconjunctivally injected gentamicin, sisomicin and cephaloridine. *Jpn J Ophthalmol* 1988;32:392–400.
20. Van Rooyen MMB, Coetzee JF, Du Toit DF, Van Jaarsveld, PP. Intra-ocular concentration-time relationships of subconjunctivally administered gentamicin. *S Afr Med J* 1991;80:236–239.
21. Gorden TB, Cunningham RD. Tobramycin levels in aqueous humour after subconjunctival injection in humans. *Am J Ophthalmol* 1982;93:107–110.
22. Desai S, Desai R, Bhatt V, Sharma R. Aqueous kinetics of sisomicin sulphate. *Eye* 1992;6:469–472.
23. Orr WM, Jackson WB, Colden K. Intraocular penetration of netilmicin. *Can J Ophthalmol* 1985;20:171–175.
24. Marmion VJ, Jain MR. Role of soft contact lenses and delivery of drugs. *Trans Ophthalmol Soc UK* 1976;96:319–321.
25. Jabs DA, Enger C, Bartlett JG. Cytomegalovirus retinitis and acquired immunodeficiency syndrome. *Arch Ophthalmol* 1989;107: 75–80.
26. Ashton P, Brown JD, Pearson PA, et al. Intravitreal ganciclovir pharmacokinetics in rabbits and man. *J Ocul Pharmacol* 1992;8: 343–347.
27. Schulman JA, Peyman GA. Intracameral, intravitreal, and retinal drug delivery. In: Mitra AK, ed. *Ophthalmic Drug Delivery Systems.* New York: Marcel Dekker, 1993;383–425.
28. Hughes L, Maurice DM. A fresh look at iontophoresis. *Arch Ophthalmol* 1984;102:1825–1829.
29. Yoshizumi MO, Cohen D, Verbukh I, Leinwand M, Kim J, Lee DA. Experimental transscleral iontophoresis of ciprofloxacin. *J Ocul Pharmacol* 1991;7:163–167.
30. Hill JM, O'Callaghan RJ, Hobden J. Ocular iontophoresis. In: Mitra AK, ed. *Ophthalmic Drug Delivery Systems.* New York: Marcel Dekker, 1993;331–354.
31. Yoshizumi MO, Cohen D, Verbukh I, Leinwand M, Kim J, Lee DA. Experimental transscleral iontophoresis of ciprofloxacin. *J Ocul Pharmacol* 1991;7:163–167.
32. Kwon BS, Gangarosa LP, Burch KD, deBack J, Hill JM. Induction of ocular herpes simplex virus shedding by iontophoresis of epinephrine into rabbit cornea. *Invest Ophthalmol Vis Sci* 1981;21: 442–449.
33. Havener WH. Autonomic drugs. In: *Ocular Pharmacology,* 5th ed. St. Louis: Mosby, 1983;264–269.
34. Katz IM, Berger ET. Effects of iris pigmentation on response of ocular pressure to timolol. *Surv Ophthalmol* 1979;23:395–398.
35. Grove J, Gautheron P, Plazonnet B, Sugrue MF. Ocular distribution studies of the topical anhydrase inhibitors L-643,799 and L-650,719 and related alkyl prodrugs. *J Ocular Pharmacol* 1988;4:279–290.
36. Plazonnet B, Grove J, Durr M, Mazuel C, Quint M, Rozier A. Pharmacokinetics and biopharmaceutical aspects of some anti-glaucoma drugs. In: Saettone MF, Bucci M, Speiser P, eds. *Ophthalmic Drug Delivery,* vol 11, Fidia Research Series. Berlin: Liviana Press, Springer-Verlag, 1987;117–139.
37. Eller MG, Schoenwald RD, Dixson JA, Segarra T, Barfknecht. Topical carbonic anhydrase inhibitors III: optimization model for corneal penetration of ethoxzolamide analogues. *J Pharm Sci* 1985;74:155–160.
38. Eller MG, Schoenwald RD, Dixson JA, Segarra T, Barfknecht CF. Topical carbonic anhydrase inhibitors IV: relationship between excised corneal permeability and pharmacokinetic factors. *J Pharm Sci* 1985;74:525–529.
39. Brechue W, Maren TH. pH and drug ionization affects ocular pressure lowering of topical carbonic anhydrase inhibitors. *Invest Ophthalmol Vis Sci* 1993;34:2581–2587.
40. Lewis RA, Schoenwald RD, Eller MG, Barfknecht CF, Phelps CD. Ethoxzolamide analog gel: a topical carbonic anhydrase inhibitor. *Arch Ophthalmol* 1984;102:1821–1824.
41. Maren TH, Jankowska L, Sanyal G, Edelhauser HF. The transcorneal permeability of sulfonamide carbonic anhydrase inhibitors and their effect on aqueous humor secretion. *Exp Eye Res* 1983;36:457–479.
42. Lewis RA, Schoenwald RD, Barfknecht CF, Phelps CD. Aminozolamide gel: a trial of a topical carbonic ahydrase inhibitor in ocular hypertension. *Arch Ophthalmol* 1986;104:842–844.
43. Sugrue MF, Gautheron P, Schmitt C, Viader MP, Conquet P, Smith RL, Share NN, Stone CA. On the pharmacology of L-645,151: a topically effective ocular hypotensive carbonic anhydrase inhibitor. *J Pharmacol Exp Ther* 1985;232:534–540.
44. Serle JB, Lustgarten JS, Lippa EA, Camras CB, Panebianco DL, Podos SM. MK-927, a topical carbonic anhydrase inhibitor. *Arch Ophthalmol* 1990; 108:838–841.
45. Serle JB, Lustgarten J, Lippa EA, Camras CB, Framm L, Payne JE, Deasy D, Podos SM. Six week safety study of 2% MK-927 administered twice daily to ocular hypertensive volunteers. *J Ocul Pharmacol* 1992;8:1–9.
46. Wang RF, Serle JB, Podos SM, Sugrue MF. The ocular hypotensive effect of the topical carbonic anhydrase inhibitor L-671,152 in glaucomatous monkeys. *Arch Ophthalmol* 1990;108:511–513.
47. Bron A, Lippa EA, Gunning F, et al. Multiple-dose efficacy comparison of the two topical carbonic anhydrase inhibitors sezolamide and MK-927. *Arch Ophthalmol* 1991;109:50–53.

48. Lippa EA, Carlson LE, Ehinger B, et al. Dose Response and duration of action of dorzolamide, a topical carbonic anhydrase inhibitor. *Arch Ophthalmol* 1992;102:495–499.
49. Ahmed I, Francoeur ML, Thombre AG, Patton TF. The kinetics of timolol in the rabbit lens: implications for ocular drug delivery. *Pharm Res* 1989;6:772–778.
50. Zigman S. Photobiology of lens. In: Maisel H, ed. *Ocular Lens.* New York: Marcel Dekker, 1985;301.
51. Maurice D. Kinetics of topically applied ophthalmic drugs. In: Saettone MF, Bucci M, Speiser P, eds. *Ophthalmic Drug Delivery,* vol 11, Fidia Research Series. Berlin: Liviana Press, Springer-Verlag, 1987;19–26.
52. Salvanet A, Fisch A, Lafaix C, Montay G, Dubayle P, Forestier F, Haroche G. Perfloxacin concentrations in human aqueous humor and lens. *J Antimicrob Chemother* 1986;18:199–201.
53. Crabbe MJ, Petchey M, Burgess SEP, Cheng H. The penetration of sorbinil, an aldose reductase inhibitor, into lens, aqueous humour and erythrocyttes of patients undergoing cataract extraction. *Exp Eye Res* 1985;40:95–99.
54. Park YH, Mayer PR, Barker R, et al. Comparison of the pharmacokinetics and pharmacodynamics of the aldose reductase inhibitors, AL03152 (RS), AL03802 (R), and AL03803 (S). *Pharm Res* 1993; 10:593–597.
55. Chien JY, Banfield CR, Brazzell RK, Mayer, Slattery JT. Saturable tissue binding and imirestat pharmacokinetics in rats. *Pharm Res* 1992;9:469–473.
56. Valeri P, Palmery M, Severini G, Piccinelli D, Catanese B. Ocular pharmcokinetics of dapiprazole. *Pharmacol Res Commun* 1986; 18:1093–1105.
57. Brazzell RK, Wooldridge CB, Hackett RB, McCue BA. Pharmacokinetics of the aldose reductase inhibitor imirestat following topical ocular administration. *Pharm Res* 1990;7:192–198.
58. Gudauskas G, Kumi C, Dedhar C, Bussanich N, Rootman J. Ocular pharmacokinetics of subconjunctivally versus intravenously administered 6-mercaptopurine. *Can J Ophthalmol* 1985;20:110–113.
59. Andermann G, Guggenbuhl P, de Burlet G, Himber J. Pharmacokinetics of falintolol II. absorption, distribution and elimination from tissues and organs following ocular administration and intravenous injection of falintolol in albino rabbits. *Methods Find Exp Clin Pharmacol* 1989;11:747–754.
60. Taylor PB, Burd EM, Tabbara K. Corneal and intraocular penetration of topical and subconjunctival fusidic acid. *Br J Ophthalmol* 1987;71:598–601.
61. Bito LZ, Baroody RA. The ocular pharmacokinetics of eicosanoids and their derivatives. I. comparison of ocular eicosanoid penetration and distribution following the topical application of $PGF_{2\alpha}$, $PGF_{2\alpha}$-1-methyl ester, and $PGF_{2\alpha}$-1-isopropyl ester. *Exp Eye Res* 1987;44: 217–226.
62. Leibowitz HM, Ryan WJ, Kupferman A, DeSantis L. Bioavailability and corneal anti-inflammatory effect of topical suprofen. *Invest Ophthalmol Vis Sci* 1986;27:628–631.
63. Hui HW, Zeleznick L, Robinson JR. Ocular disposition of topically applied histamine, cimetidine and pyrilamine in the albino rabbit. *Curr Eye Res* 1984;3:321–330.
64. Matsumoto S, Yamashita T, Araie M, Kametani S, Hosokawa T, Takase M. The ocular penetration of topical forskolin and its effects on intraocular pressure, aqueous flow rate and cyclin amp level in the rabbit eye. *Jpn J Ophthalmol* 1990;34:428–435.
65. Ling TL, Combs DL. Ocular bioavailability and tissue distrubition of [^{14}C] ketorolac tromethamine in rabbits. *J Pharm Sci* 1987; 76:289–294.
66. Schoenwald RD, Boltralik JJ. A bioavailability comparison in rabbits of two steroids formulated as high-viscosity gels and reference aqueous preparations. *Invest Ophthalmol Vis Sci* 1979;18:61–66.
67. Maren TH, Jankowska L. Ocular pharmacology of sulfonamides: the cornea as barrier and depot. *Curr Eye Res* 1985;4:399–408.
68. Walstad RA, Hellum KB, Blika S, et al. Pharmacokinetics and tissue penetration of ceftazidime: studies on lymph, aqueous humor, skin blister, cerebrospinal and pleural fluid. *J Antimicrob Chemother* 1983;12(suppl A):275–282.
69. Auclair E, Laude D, Wainer IW, Chaouloff F, Elghozi JL. Comparative pharmacokinetics of D- and L-alphamethyldopa in plasma, aqueous humor, and cerebrospinal fluid in rabbits. *Fundam Clin Pharmacol* 1988;2:283–287.
70. Agata M, Tanaka M, Nakajima A, Fujii A, Kuboyama N, Tamura T, Araie M. Ocular penetration of topical diclofenac sodium, a nonsteroidal anti-inflammatory drug, in rabbit eye. *Nippon Ganka Gakkai Zasshi* 1984;88:991–996.
71. Anderson JA, Chen CC, Vita JB, Shackleton M. Disposition of topical flurbiprofen in normal and aphakic rabbit eyes. *Arch Ophthalmol* 1982;100:642–645.
72. Rao CS, Schoenwald RD, Barfknecht CF, Laban SL. Biopharmaceutical evaluation of ibufenac, ibuprofen, and their hydroxyethoxy analogs in the rabbit eye. *J Pharmacokinet Biopharm* 1992;20:357–387.
73. Barza M, Kane A, Baum J. Ocular penetration of subconjunctival oxacillin, methicillin and cefazolin in rabbits with staphylococcal endophthalmitis. *J Infect Dis* 1982;145:899–903.
74. Schoenwald RD, Harris RG, Turner D, Knowles W, Chien DS. Ophthalmic bioequivalence of steroid/antibiotic combination formulations. *Biopharm Drug Dispos* 1987;8:527–548.
75. Barza M, Kane A, Baum JL. Intraocular levels of cefamandole compared with cefazolin after subconjunctival injection in rabbits. *Invest Ophthalmol Vis Sci* 1979;18:250–255.
76. Aldana I, Fos D, Gonzalez P. Ocular pharmacokinetics of thiamphenicol in rabbits. *Arzneimittelforschung* 1992;42:1236–1239.
77. Mayers M, Rush D, Madu A, Motyl M, Miller MH. Pharmacokinetics of amikacin and chloramphenicol in the aqueious humor of rabbits. *Antimicrob Agents Chemother* 1991;35:1791–1798.
78. Schoenwald RD, Chien DS. Ocular absorption and disposition of phenylephrine and phenylephrine oxazolidine. *Biopharm Drug Dispos* 1988;9:527–538.
79. Kitagawa K, Fukuda M, Sasaki K. Intraocular penetration of topically administered acyclovir. *Lens Eye Toxicol Res* 1989;6:365–373.
80. Huupponen R, Kaila T, Salminen L, Urtti A. The pharmacokinetics of oclarly applied timolol in rabbits. *Acta Ophthalmol* 1987;65: 63–66.
81. Huang HS, Schoenwald RD, Lach JL. Corneal penetration behavior of β-blocking agents III: In vitro-in vivo correlations. *J Pharm Sci* 1983;72:1279–1281.
82. Kleinberg J, Dea FJ, Anderson JA, Leopold IH. Intraocular penetration of topically applied lincomycin hydrochloride in rabbits. *Arch Ophthalmol* 1979;97:933–936.
83. Putnam ML, Schoenwald RD, Duffel MW, Barfknecht CF, Segarra TM, Campbell DA. Ocular disposition of aminozolamide in the rabbit eye. *Invest Ophthalmol Vis Sci* 1987;28:1373–1382.
84. Hwang DG, Stern WH, Hwang PH, MacGowan-Smith LA. Collagen shield enhancement of topical dexamethasone penetration. *Arch Ophthalmol* 1989;107:1375–1380.
85. Zhao F, Ji XC, Zheng YZ. Effects of D-timolol on intraocular pressure (IOP), beta blocking activity, and the dynamic changes of drug concentrations in aqueous humor. *J Ocul Pharmacol* 1989;5:271–279.
86. Kalsi GS, Hulbert KB, Silver KB, Rootman J. Ocular pharmacokinetics of dacarbazine following subconjunctival versus intravenous administration in the rabbit. *Can J Ophthalmol* 1991;26:247–251.
87. Mester U, Krasemann C, Werner H. Cefsulodine concentrations in rabbit eyes after intravenous and subconjunctival administration. *Ophthalmol Res* 1982;14:129–134.
88. Rootman J, Ostry A, Gudauskas G. Pharmcokinetics and metabolism of 5-fluorouracil following subconjunctival versus Intravenous administration. *Can J Ophthalmol* 1984;19:187–191.
89. Fantes FE, Heuer DK, Parrish RK, Sossi N, Gressel MG. Topical fluorouracil. *Arch Ophthalmol* 1985;103:953–955.
90. Tang-Liu DDS, Liu S, Neff J, Sandri R. Disposition of levobunolol after an ophthalmic dose to rabbits. *J Pharm Sci* 1987;76:780–783.
91. Eng IS. *N*-Methylacetazolamide ocular disposition and enzyme kinetics. Iowa City, Iowa: Ph.D. Thesis, University of Iowa College of Pharmacy, 1986.
92. Leibowitz HM, Berrospi AR, Kupferman A, Restropo GV, Galvis V, Alvarez JA. Penetration of topically administered prednisolone acetate into the human aqueous humor. *Am J Ophthalmol* 1977;402–406.
93. O'Day DM, Head S, Robinson RD, Williams TE, Wolff R. Ocular pharmacokinetics of saperconazole in rabbits. *Arch Ophthalmol* 1992;110:550–554.
94. Gilbert ML, Wihelmus KR, Osato MS. Comparative bioavailability and efficacy of fortified topical tobramycin. *Invest Ophthalmol Vis Sci* 1987;881–885.

95. Sieg JW, Robinson JR. Mechanistic studies on transcorneal permeation of pilocarpine. *J Pharm Sci* 1976;65:1816–1822.
96. Virgo JF, Rafart J, Concheiro A, Martinez R, Cordido M. Ocular penetration and pharmacokinetics of cefotaxmine: an experimental study. *Curr Eye Res* 1988;1149–1154.
97. Chiang CH, Schoenwald RD. Ocular pharmacokinetic models of clonidine-^{3}H hydrochloride. *J Pharmacokin Biopharm* 1986;14: 175–211.
98. Lee VHL, Robinson JR. Mechanistic and quantitative evaluation of precorneal pilocarpine disposition in albino rabbits. *J Pharm Sci* 1979;68:673–684.
99. Marmor MF. Barriers to fluorescein and protein movement. *Jpn J Ophthalmol* 1985;29:131–138.
100. Miyake K. Fluorophotometric evaluation of the blood-ocular barrier function following cataract surgery and intraocular lens implantation. *J Cataract Refract Surg* 1988;14:560–568.
101. Araie M, Surgiura Y, Minota K. Akazawa K. Effects of the encircling procedure on the aqueous flow rate in retinal detachment eyes: a fluorometric study. *Br J Ophthalmol* 1987;71:510–515.
102. Grimes PA. Carboxyfluorescein transfer across the blood-retinal barrier evaluated by quantitative fluorescence microscopy: comparison with fluorescein. *Exp Eye Res* 1988;46:769–783.
103. Yoshida A, Ishiko S, Kojima M, Ogasawara H. Permeability of the blood-ocular barrier in adolescent and adult diabetic patients. *Br J Ophthalmol* 1993;77:158–161.
104. Lee VHL, Chang SC, Oshiro CM, Smith RE. Ocular esterase composition in albino and pigmented rabbits: possible implications in ocular prodrug design and evaluation. *Curr Eye Res* 1985;4:1117–1125.
105. Lee VHL. Esterase activities in adult rabbit eyes. *J Pharm Sci* 1983;72:239–244.
106. Lee VHL, Smith RE. Effect of substrate concentration, product concentration, and peptides on the in vitro hydrolysis of model ester prodrugs by corneal esterases. *J Ocul Pharmacol Ther* 1985;1:269– 278.
107. Miller-Meeks MJ, Farrell TA, Munden PM, Folk JC, Rao C, Schoenwald RD. Phenylephrine prodrug: report of clinical trials. *Ophthalmology* 1991;98:222–226.
108. Schoenwald RD, Folk JC, Kumar V, Piper JG. *In Vivo* comparison of phenylephrine and phenylephrine oxazoldine instilled in the monkey eye. *J Ocul Pharmacol Ther* 1987:3:333–339.
109. Chang SC, Bundgaard H, Burr A, Lee VHL. Improved corneal penetration of timolol by prodrugs as a means to reduce systemic drug load. *Invest Ophthalmol Vis Sci* 1987;28:487–491.
110. Bundgaard H, Falch E, Larsen C, Mosher GL, Mikkelson T. Pilocarpine prodrugs II. Synthesis, stability, bioconversion, and physicochemical properties of sequentially labile pilocarpine acid diesters. *J Pharm Sci* 1986;75:775–778.
111. Narukar MM, Mitra AK. Prodrugs of 5 iodo-2′-deoxyuridine for enhanced ocular transport. *Pharm Res* 1989;6:887–891.
112. Alm A, Villumsen J. PhXA34, a new potent ocular hypotensive drug: A study on dose-response relationship and on aqueous humor dynamics in healthy volunteers. *Arch Ophthalmol* 1991;109:1564–1568.
113. Campbell DA, Schoenwald RD, Duffel MW, Barfknecht CF. Characterization of arylamine acetyltransferase in the rabbit eye. *Invest Opthalmol Vis Sci* 1991;32:2190–2200.
114. Lee VHL, Chien DS, Sasaki H. Ocular ketone reductase distribution and its role in the metabolism of ocularly applied levobunolol in the pigmented rabbit. *J Pharmacol Exp Ther* 1988;246:871–878.
115. Sichi H, Nerbert DW. Drug metabolism in ocular tissues. In: Gram TE, ed. *Extrahepatic Metabolism of Drugs and Other Foreign Compounds.* New York: S.P. Medical and Scientific Books, 1980;333– 363.
116. Kumar GN, Hammer RH, Wu WM, Bodor NS. Soft drugs 15: mydriatic activity and transcorneal penetration of phenylsuccinic soft analogs of methscopolamine as short acting mydriatics. *Curr Eye Res* 1993;12:501–506.
117. Hammer RH, Wu W, Sastry JS, Bodor N. Short acting soft mydriatics. *Curr Eye Res* 1991;10:565–570.
118. Bodor N, Varga M. Effect of a novel soft steroid on the wound healing of rabbit cornea. *Exp Eye Res* 1990;50:183–187.
119. Bodor N, Prokai L. Site- and stereospecific ocular drug delivery by sequential enzymatic bioactivation. *Pharm Res* 1990;7:723–725.
120. Bodor N, El-Koussi A, Kano M, Khalifa MM. Soft drugs. 7. soft β-blockers for systemic and ophthalmic use. *J Med Chem* 1988;31: 1651–1656.
121. Barza M. Use of Quinolones for treatment of ear and eye infections. *Eur J Clin Microbiol Infect Dis* 1991;10:296–303.
122. Athanasios ST, Gartaganis SP, Chrysanthopoulos CJ, Beermann D, Papachristou C, Bassaris HP. Aqueous humor penetration of ciprofloxacin in the human eye. *Arch Ophthalmol* 1988;108:404–405.
123. Bron AM, Péchinot A, Garcher C, Guyonnet G, Kazmierczak A. Ocular penetration of topically applied norfloxacin 0.3% in the rabbits and in humans. *J Ocul Pharmacol* 1992;8:241–246.
124. Marchese AL, Slana VS, Holmes EW, Jay WM. Toxicity and pharmacokinetics of ciprofloxacin. *J Ocul Pharmacol* 1993;9:69–76.
125. Miller MH, Madu A, Samathanam G, Rush D, Madu CN, Mathisson K, Mayers M. Fleroxacin pharmacokinetics in aqueous and vitreous humors determined by using complete concentration-time data from individual rabbits. *Antimicrob Agents Chemother* 1992;36:32–38.
126. Camber O, Edman P, Olsson LI. Permeability of prostaglandin $R_{2\alpha}$ and prostaglandin $F_{2\alpha}$ esters across cornea in vitro. *Int J Pharm* 1986;29:259–266.
127. Camber O, Edman P. Factors influencing the corneal permeability of prostaglandin $F_{2\alpha}$ and its isopropyl ester in vitro. *Int J Pharm* 1987; 37:27–32.
128. BenEzra D, Mftzir G, de Courten C, Timonen P. Ocular penetration of cyclosporin A. III: the human eye. *Br J Ophthalmol* 1990;74: 350–352.
129. Newton C, Gebhardt BM, Kaufman HE. Topically applied cyclosporine in azone prolongs corneal allograft survival. *Invest Ophthalmol Vis Sci* 1988;29:208–215.
130. Gregory CR, Hietala SK, Pedersen NC, Gregory TA, Floyd-Hawkins KA, Patz JD. Cyclosporine pharmacokinetics in cats following topical ocular administration. *Transplantation* 1989;47:516–519.
131. BenEzra D, Maftzir G. Ocular penetration of cyclosporin A: the rabbit eye. *Invest Ophthalmol Vis Sci* 1990;31:1362–1366.
132. Henry K, Cantrill H, Fletcher C, Chinnock BJ, Balfour HH. Use of intravitreal ganciclovir (dihydroxy propoxymethyl guanine) for cytomegalovirus retinitis in a patient with AIDS. *Am J Ophthalmol* 1987;103:17–23.
133. Smith TJ, Pearson PA, Blandford DL, et al. Intravitreal sustained-release ganciclovir. *Arch Ophthalmol* 1992;110:255–258.
134. Faulds d, Heel RC. Ganciclovir: a review of its antiviral activity, pharmacokinetic properties and therapeutic efficacy in cytomegalovirus infections. *Drugs* 1990;39:597–638.
135. Sanborn GE, Anand R, Torti RE, et al. Sustained-release ganciclovir therapy for treatment of cytomegalovirus retinitis. *Arch Ophthalmol* 1992;110:188–195.
136. Vaidyanathan G, Jay M, Vera RK, PR Mayer, Brazzell RK. Scintigraphic evaluation of the ocular disposition of ^{18}F-Imirestat in rabbits. *Pharm Res* 1990;7:1198–1200.
137. Brazzell RK, Mayer PR, Dobbs R, McNamara PJ, Teng R, Slattery JT. Dose-dependent pharmacokinetics of the aldose reductase inhibitor imirestat in man. *Pharm Res* 1991;8:112–118.
138. Smith TJ, Maurin MB, Milosovich SM, Hussain AA. Polyvinyl alcohol membrane permeability characteristics of 5-fluorouracil. *J Ocul Pharmacol* 1988;4:147–152.
139. Wong VKW, Shapourifar-Tehrani S, Kitada S, Choo PH, Lee DA. Inhibition of rabbit ocular fibroblast proliferation by 5-fluorouracil and cytosine arabinoside. *J Ocul Pharmacol* 1991;7:27–39.
140. Smyth RJ, Moore JJ, Shapourifar-Tehrani S, Lee DA. The effects of 5-fluorouridine, 5-fluorodeoxyuridine, and 5-fluorodeoxyuridine monophosphate on rabbit tenon's capsule fibroblasts in vitro. *J Ocul Pharmacol* 1991;7:329–338.
141. Simmons ST, Sherwood MB, Nichols DA, Penne RB, Sery T, Spaeth GL. Pharmacokinetics of a 5-fluorouracil liposomal delivery system. *Br J Ophthalmol* 1988;72:688–691.
142. Fishman P, Peyman GA, Hendricks R, Hui SL. Liposome-encapsulated 3H-5FU in rabbits. *Int Ophthalmol* 1989;13:361–365.
143. Tremblay C, Barza M, Szoka F, Lahav F, Baum J. Reduced toxicity of liposome-associated amphtericin B injected intravitreally in rabbits. *Invest Ophthalmol Vis Sci* 1985;26:711–718.
144. Miller SC, Himmelstein KJ, Patton TF. A physiologically based pharmacokinetic model for the intraocular distribution of pilocarpine in rabbits. *J Pharmacokinet Biopharm* 1981;9:653–657.
145. Makoid MC, Robinson JR. Pharmacokinetics of topically applied pilocarpine in the albino rabbit eye. *J Pharm Sci* 1979;68:435–443.

146. Patton TF, Robinson JR. Quantitative Precorneal Disposition of topically applied pilocarpine nitrate in rabbit eyes. *J Pharm Sci* 1976; 65:1295–1301.
147. Conrad JM, Robinson JR. Aqueous chamber drug distribution volume measurement in rabbits. *J Pharm Sci* 1977;66:219–224.
148. Lee VHL, Robinson JR. Disposition of pilocarpine in the pigmented rabbit eye. *Int J Pharm* 1982;11:155–165.
149. Himmelstein KJ, Guvenir I, Patton TF. Preliminary pharmacokinetic model of pilocarpine uptake and distribution in the eye. *J Pharm Sci* 1978;67:603–606.
150. Salminen L, Urtti A. Disposition of ophthalmic timolol in treated and untreated rabbit eyes: a multiple and single dose study. *Exp Eye Res* 1984;38: 203–206.
151. Stur M, Grabner G, Huber-Spitzy, Schreiner J, Haddad R. Effect of timolol on aqueous humor protein concentration in the human eye. *Arch Ophthalmol* 1986;104:899–900.
152. Chiou GCY. Development of D-timolol for the treatment of glaucoma and ocular hypertension. *J Ocul Pharmacol* 1990;6:67–74.
153. Tang-Liu DDS, Shackleton M, Richman JB. Ocular metabolism of levobunolol. *J Ocul Pharmacol* 1988;4:269–278.
154. Fraunfelder FT, Meyer SM. Possible cardiovascular effects secondary to topical ophthalmic 2.5% phenylephrine. *Am J Ophthalmol* 1985;99:362–363.
155. Kumar V, Schoenwald RD, Barcellos WA, Chien DS, Folk JC, Weingeist TA. Aqueous vs viscous phenylephrine I. systemic absorption and cardiovascular effects. *Arch Ophthalmol* 1986;104: 1189–1191.
156. Insler MS, Helm CJ, George WJ. Topical vs systemic gentamicin penetration into the human cornea and aqueous humor. *Arch Ophthalmol* 1987;105:922–924.
157. Barza M, Kane A, Baum J. Comparison of the effects and intermittent systemic adminstration on the penetration of gentamicin into infected rabbit eyes. *J Infect Dis* 1983;147:144–148.
158. Lee VHL. Review: new directions in the optimization of ocular drug delivery. *J Ocul Pharmacol* 1990;6:157–164.
159. Assil KK, Zarnegar SR, Fouraker BD, Schanzlin DJ. Efficacy of tobramycin-soaked collagen schields vs tobramycin eyedrop loading dose for sustained treatment of experimental *Pseudomonas aeruginosa*-induced keratitis in rabbits. *Am J Ophthalmol* 1992;113:418–423.
160. Chen CC, Takruri H, Duzman E. Enhancement of the ocular bioavailability of topical tobramycin with use of a collagen shield. *J Cataract Refract Surg* 1993;19:242–245.
161. Barza M, Baum J, Szoka F. Pharmacokinetics of subconjunctival liposome-encapsulated gentamicin in normal rabbit eyes. *Invest Ophthalmol Vis Sci* 1984;25:486–490.
162. Assil KK, Frucht-Perry J, Ziegler E, Schanzlin DJ, Schneiderman T, Weinreb RN. Tobramycin liposomes: single subconjunctival therapy of pseudomonal keratitis. *Invest Ophthalmol Vis Sci* 1991;32: 3216–3220.
163. Fishman PH, Peyman GA, Lesar T. Intravitreal liposome-encapsulated gentamycin in a rabbit model: prolonged therapeutic levels. *Invest Ophthalmol Vis Sci* 1986;27:1103–1106.
164. Fishman PH, Jay WM, Rissing JP, Hill JM, Shockley RK. Iotophoresis of gentamycin into aphakic rabbit eyes. *Invest Ophthalmol Vis Sci* 1984;25:343–345.
165. Leibowitz HM, Lass JH, Kupferman A. Quantitation of inflammation in the cornea. *Invest Ophthalmol Vis Sci* 1974;92:427–430.
166. Leibowitz HM, Kupferman A. Pharmacology of topically applied dexamethasone. *Trans Acad Ophth Otol* 1974;78:856–861.
167. Cox WV, Kupferman A, Leibowitz HM. Topically applied steroids in corneal disease I: The role of inflammation in stromal absorption of dexamethasone. *Arch Ophthalmol* 1972;88:308–313.
168. Kupferman A, Leibowitz HW. Therapeutic effectiveness of fluorometholone in inflammatory keratitis. *Arch Ophthalmol* 1975;93: 1011–1014.
169. Leibowitz HW, Kupferman A. Periocular injection of corticosteroids: an experimental evaluation of its role in the treatment of corneal inflammation. *Arch Ophthalmol* 1977;95:311–314.
170. Tang-Liu DDS, Liu SS, Weinkam RJ. Ocular and systemic bioavailability of ophthalmic flurbiprofen. *J Pharmacokin Biopharm* 1984; 12:611–626.
171. Chrai SS, Patton TF, Mehta A, Robinson JR. Lacrimal and instilled fluid dynamics in rabbit eyes. *J Pharm Sci* 1973;62:1112–1121.
172. Salminen L. Review: systemic absorption of topically applied ocular drugs in humans. *J Ocul Pharmacol* 1990;6:243–249.

Textbook of Ocular Pharmacology,
edited by T.J. Zimmerman, et al.
Lippincott–Raven Publishers, Philadelphia © 1997.

CHAPTER 10

Basic Considerations of Ocular Drug-Delivery Systems

Amir Bar-Ilan and Ron Neumann

Drugs topically applied to the eye are subjected to the normal (or *pathological*) physiology of the conjunctival sac, which in turn regulates the rate of clearance (*drainage*) of drugs from the sac into the nasal cavity. Most drugs penetrate the eye through the cornea, protected by a complex tear-washing mechanism that easily washes away most compounds in a few minutes. The rate of the secretion and clearance of tears determines variable contact time for any given drug with the ocular surface. Radioactive tracers applied to the eyes are readily washed by the tears, with elimination of approximately two thirds of the radioactive signal within the first 2 minutes (1). The drug volume is readily cleared to the nasal cavity, where systemic absorption takes place. It follows that, despite variable intraocular penetration, systemic absorption may be effective, and nearly all drug dosages applied to the eye are absorbed systemically, leading sometimes (e.g., timolol, atropine, epinephrine) to substantial systemic drug effects.

DRUGS AS CHEMICAL COMPOUNDS

Commonly used drugs are chemical compounds with distinct physicochemical properties that largely control their penetration into active sites within the eye. High molecular weight and size may limit efficient corneal penetration. Ionic/nonionic partition and acid/base balance in solution, as well as the solubility constant and the "octanol/water partition coefficient," all determine the drug dissolution rate in distinct solvents and, hence, the effective drug concentration in solution. As detailed in the sections to follow, the physicochemical properties of the preparation (*formulation*) control corneal contact time and thus may largely affect bioavailability.

A. Bar-Ilan and R. Neumann: Pharmos Limited, Kiryat Weizmann, Rehovot, Israel.

Tear Film Physiology and Corneal Contact Time

The conjunctival sac and external epithelium are washed constantly by a basic tear secretion averaging 1.2 μl per minute. The total volume of fluids held by the conjunctival sac is approximately 10 μl (~20% the amount delivered by a typical eyedropper) (2). Ocular irritation, however, induces a reflex secretion of tears that may increase tear secretion up to 400 μl per minute (3) and may easily wash out the irritating compound (i.e., the drug). In addition, pathological conditions that disrupt the normal tear physiology (e.g., dry eyes, external inflammation with excessive tearing, eyelid malpositioning, and others) may exert a major effect on topical ocular drug delivery.

The corneal surface is densely innervated with sensory nerve fibers, causing extreme sensitivity to any change in the composition of the tear solution bathing the cornea. Eyedrops may easily destroy the delicate interactions between the corneal surface and the tear film, resulting in corneal irritation in mild cases and toxic epitheliopathies in severe cases. Among the basic parameters to be considered are osmolality (266 mOsm/kg to 445 mOsm/kg are acceptable to the eye) and pH. Basic pH is especially irritating to the ocular surface. Buffer capacity is also important because tears can neutralize a wide range of pH levels with low buffer capacity. Thus, pH in some pilocarpine commercial solutions may be as low as 3.5 to 4.0 without producing excessive irritation. The mere instillation of a drop of fluid may induce some reflex tearing, and high levels of viscosity may cause an especially unpleasant sensation. Moreover, the chemical compound itself (the active drug) may induce either lacrimation (e.g., with pilocarpine and antazoline) or reduced tear flow (e.g., with timolol and anaesthetics). Generally, the more irritating a chemical compound, the more difficult it is to extend its corneal contact time. (More details are found in the section entitled Ophthalmic Aqueous Solutions.)

The Barriers

The cornea is composed of a complex network of barriers comprising distinct layers of fluid and tissues that confront any molecule that "dares" to cross. A drug molecule dissolved in the tear film may be washed easily from the corneal surface. As soon as the compound penetrates the corneal epithelium, however, the probability of intraocular penetration becomes much higher. It follows that rapid movement of chemical compounds from the tear film to the corneal epithelium is essential for efficient ocular drug delivery.

The tear film is composed of approximately 10 μl of lipophilic, aqueous, and mucin layers totalling up to 7 μm thick. The molecular trip through the tear film involves crossing through hydrophobic and hydrophilic environments. Moreover, in the mucin layer, a significant fraction of the drug molecules may bind to "carrier" proteins, allowing only the "free," unbound molecules to cross into the epithelium.

Once in the corneal matrix, the drug should cross distinct layers of corneal tissue, constituting a variety of barriers. The external corneal epithelium, composed of five to seven layers of a nonkeratinized squamous epithelium with an external net of tight junctions, allows only selective penetration of compounds. Because of the high concentration of lipophilic membranes, nonpolar molecules (as well as nonpolar molecular moieties) have easier access into the epithelium. On the other hand, the hydrophilic corneal stroma has a low cellular content and may easily be crossed by polar molecules. The *endothelium* is a cellular monolayer that allows much better penetration of hydrophilic compounds compared with the epithelium. A profound description of the implications of this complex structure on pharmacokinetics can be found in Chapter 9. It has been estimated that under optimal conditions only 1% to 10% of the total drug applied directly onto the cornea is absorbed into the eye (4).

GOALS OF THE OCULAR DRUG-DELIVERY SYSTEM

The self-explanatory goal of the ocular drug-delivery system (DDS) is extended corneal contact time, resulting in increased drug penetration and a higher intraocular level. Nevertheless, sometimes the goals of a DDS may be more subtle, that is, reduced irritation leading to increased corneal contact time on one hand and increased patient compliance on the other hand. In other instances, aqueous levels may suffice but only with such dosages that induce systemic side effects. An efficient DDS may enable reduced dosages, thus bypassing significant systemic side effects without compromising the ocular therapeutic effect. Another use of an "unorthodox" delivery system may be reduced anterior chamber penetration for drugs needed for external ocular indications with potential intraocular adverse effects, such as topical steroids. Any system that can reduce the penetration of a topical corticosteroid to the anterior chamber without compromising drug presence on the ocular surfaces would allow safer administration of the drug for external indications, such as allergic conjunctivitis. Similarly, minimizing systemic absorption of topically administered ophthalmic drugs is sometimes a major goal of ocular DDS.

The definition of optimal drug delivery differs with the drug involved. For example, pilocarpine exerts its intraocular pressure (IOP)-lowering effect with minimal side effects (miosis and increased accommodation) when introduced continuously to the anterior chamber in constant lower levels. It follows that for pilocarpine the best mode of delivery should abolish the initial high peak of intraocular penetration, thereby avoiding unpleasant ocular side effects without compromising the desired therapeutic effect. For other medications, an initial high peak of intraocular drug concentration may be advantageous in reaching higher therapeutic levels (i.e., antibiotics and steroids). In the following sections, we review the delivery aspects of ophthalmic aqueous solutions, suspensions, ointments, inserts, collagen shields, liposomes, emulsions, and gels.

OPHTHALMIC AQUEOUS SOLUTIONS

Ophthalmic solutions are sterile solutions, essentially free from foreign particles, suitably compounded and packaged for instillation into the eye (5). Aqueous solutions are the most commonly used ocular DDS and are the least expensive to formulate compared with other types of DDS. All the ingredients are completely dissolved; so there is only minimal interference with vision. The major drawback of aqueous solutions is their relatively short contact time with the drug-absorbing surfaces, namely, the cornea, conjunctiva, and sclera.

In addition to the active drug, ophthalmic solutions contain other ingredients, or *excipients,* that are added to control various characteristics of the formulation, such as the tonicity, buffering and pH, viscosity, sterility, and antimicrobial preservation. Although these added ingredients are listed as "inactive additives," they can affect (i.e., enhance or reduce) the permeability of the drug across the ocular surface barriers and thus significantly alter the therapeutic effectiveness of a given drug (the *active* ingredient). Because the effects of different additives are interrelated, the final product's composition usually reflects a compromise between contradictory requirements rather than the optimized condition for each individual property.

pH and Buffering

The pH of an ophthalmic solution can play an important role in determining the therapeutic effectiveness of a drug.

Most ophthalmic drugs, being weak acids or bases, are present in solutions as both the nonionized (*nondissociated*) and the ionized (*dissociated*) species. It is generally accepted that the nonionized species (being more lipid soluble) diffuses across cellular barriers at a higher rate than the ionized (less lipid-soluble) species (6). The degree of ionization of a drug in solution is determined by its pK and the solution's pH. Thus, a pH that favors a higher proportion of the nonionized species should result in a higher transcorneal permeability, as is well illustrated by the findings of Mitra and Mickelson (7), who showed that the permeability of pilocarpine across isolated cornea, which was 4.72×10^6 cm/s^{-1} at pH 4.67 (99% of the pilocarpine in the ionized form), increased by almost twofold to 8.85×10^6 cm/s^{-1} at pH 7.40 when 84% of the drug was in the nonionized form. Similar changes, that is, twofold to threefold increases in transcorneal permeability concomitant with 2 to 2.5 pH unit changes (5–7.5, 6.2–8.4, etc.), were reported for various carbonic anhydrase inhibitors (8). Similarly, alterations in the pH of solutions of the carbonic anhydrase inhibitor MK-927 from pH-7 (11% ionized) to pH-4.8 (91% ionized) or pH-9.1 (86% ionized), increased the IOP-lowering activity of the drug in rabbits by fivefold to sixfold, respectively (9).

Tonicity

To avoid irritation, ophthalmic formulations intended for topical instillation should be approximately isotonic with tears (10). Normal human tears are considered isotonic, or slightly hypertonic to plasma, that is, about 300 mOsmol/kg or 0.90 to 1.01 NaCl equivalents. Significant interindividual and intraindividual variability has been reported for the tonicity of normal human tears, ranging between 260 and 440 mOsmol (11–13).

Various studies have shown that the eye can tolerate a considerable range of tonicity before any pain or discomfort is detected (14,15). Also, increased tonicity of topically applied solutions (above that of the body fluids) resulted in their immediate dilution by osmosis in the eye (16). Thus, the tonicity of an ophthalmic solution may range from 0.2% to 2.0% in NaCl equivalents or 220 to 640 mOsM without exceeding the safety range. Most ophthalmic drugs listed in the *Physician's Desk Reference* (PDR) 22 (17) do not exceed 5% of an active compound, and even with additional tonicity resulting from adjustments in pH, preservatives, and surfactants they are within this range of tonicity. Only a few ophthalmic solutions (i.e., pilocarpine 8% and 10%; phenylephrine 10%; sulfacetamide 10%, 15%, and 30%) have an osmolarity of 700 to 1,000 mOsM and would cause a strong burning-stinging sensation upon instillation.

In one class of ophthalmic drugs, hypertonic ophthalmic solutions, which are used for temporary relief of corneal edema, the hypertonic factor (5% NaCl) is listed as the active ingredient. It is reasonable to believe that a similar effect would occur during treatment with other hypertonic (high drug concentration) ophthalmic formulations.

Viscosity

Increasing the viscosity of topically applied ocular formulations is expected to reduce drainage, increase the residence time in the conjunctival sac, and thus lead to an enhanced intraocular penetration and this therapeutic effect. Substances like methylcellulose (MC), hydroxypropylmethylcellulose (HPMC), hydroxypropylcellulose (HPC), hydroxyethylcellulose (HEC), and polyvinyl alcohol (PVA), listed in the *U.S. Pharmacopeia* (USP) 23 (5) as viscosity-increasing agents, are frequently added to ophthalmic liquid formulations.

The use of MC for improving contact with the ocular surface was reported some 50 years ago by Swan (18). Linn and Jones (19) showed that an increase in the drainage time of topically applied fluorescein solution is directly related to the concentration of added HPMC in human subjects. A solution containing 0.25% HPMC increases drainage time by 1.5-fold and a 1% solution of HPMC by 3.5-fold compared with an aqueous solution. Although a 2.5% solution of HPMC increased drainage time by 4.5-fold, it caused irritation, which made it unsuitable for routine clinical use. Mueller and Deardorff (20) reported that although a 0.25% homatropine hydrobromide solution failed to produce a cycloplegic or mydriatic response in human subjects, the addition of 1% MC 4,000 centipoise (cps) to this solution reduced accommodation by 80% and led to significant pupillary dilation. Later, Chrai and Robinson (21) showed that increasing the viscosity of a pilocarpine solution over the range of 1 to 100 cps (achieved by increasing the added concentration of MC) resulted in a significant reduction in the drainage rate constant (by tenfold) and an increase in aqueous humor pilocarpine concentration (by twofold). Patton and Robinson (22) reported that most of the improvement in ocular drug delivery was observed over the viscosity range of 1 to 15 cps and suggested that the optimal viscosity should be 12 to 15 cps. The use of formulations with higher viscosity causes ocular surface irritation, resulting in reflex blinking and lacrimation and increased drainage of the applied formulation.

Saettone et al. (23) compared the effects of different polymers, including HPC and PVA, added to an aqueous solution of 0.2% tropicamide, on the mydriatic responses of albino rabbits and human subjects. All test solutions were isoviscous (73 cps). They found that the PVA-containing solution had the highest activity: a 3.7-fold increase compared with the aqueous solution and a twofold increase over the other polymers. The author suggested that the surface-spreading effect of PVA, which did not characterize the other polymer solutions tested, was responsible for the observed advantage of PVA. An important finding was that the advantage of the PVA-tropicamide formulation was observed in the human subjects but not in the albino rabbit. The lower blinking and tear production rates of the rabbit compared with humans could contribute to the discrepancy and highlights the importance of clinical testing in defining the actual advantages of modifications in ocular DDS.

Preservatives

Ophthalmic solutions packaged in multiple-dose containers must contain a suitable substance, or mixture of substances, to prevent the growth of or to destroy microorganisms accidentally introduced when the container is opened during use (USP 23) (5). Quaternary ammonium compounds (benzalkonium chloride), organic mercurials (thimerosal), parahydroxy benzoates, chlorobutanol, and aromatic alcohols are used as preservatives in ophthalmic preparations.

Banzalkonium chloride (BAk), the most commonly used preservative in ophthalmic preparations, was demonstrated repeatedly to enhance corneal permeability of various drugs. A 50- to 80-fold increase in the permeability of carbaminochline chloride caused by 0.02% BAk was reported by O'Brien and Swan (24). A 10- to 18-fold increase in inulin permeability was attained by 0.01% and 0.02% BAk, respectively (25). This preservative was also reported to increase the permeability of pilocarpine (26) and fluorescein (27,28).

In rabbits, preservatives used in ophthalmic solutions (BAk and others) are toxic to the ocular surface following topical application as well as to retinal functions following intravitreal administration (29–34). The clinical significance of the toxic effects and the enhanced ocular penetration attributed to preservatives are not completely clear, however. Most of these studies used rabbits as experimental subjects, and rabbits are more susceptible to ocular surface drainage (28) and permeability changes (35) than humans.

OPHTHALMIC SUSPENSIONS

Ophthalmic suspensions are sterile preparations in which relatively water-insoluble drugs are delivered in the form of solid particles dispersed in a liquid vehicle. They are sometimes commercially identified by the "forte" suffix. Because the small drug particles tend to remain in the cul-de-sac longer than an aqueous solution, drug delivery from a suspension is characterized by two consecutive phases: the first, rapid delivery of the dissolved drug; the second, slower, more prolonged delivery resulting from dissolution of the retained particles. Thus, in order for a suspension to attain a higher bioavailability than that of a saturated solution, it must have a rapid, significant rate of dissolution in the tear film (36).

Ocular bioavailability from topically applied suspension is correlated with particle size (37): (a) the area accessible for drug dissolution, and hence the dissolution rate, is related to particle size; (b) larger particles can lead to increased ocular irritation with enhanced tearing and drug loss by drainage. Use of the drug in a micronized form with a particle size $<10\ \mu m$ should minimize ocular discomfort and irritation (38). Formulation factors that affect the ocular bioavailability of topically instilled ophthalmic solution (i.e., pH and buffering, tonicity, viscosity) would also influence the bioavailability from ophthalmic suspensions.

Because precipitation is the major problem with ophthalmic suspensions, they must be resuspended before use to obtain an accurate dose. The degree of resuspension of commercially available formulations varies considerably among patients and formulations (39).

OPHTHALMIC OINTMENTS

Ointments are a popular, frequently prescribed ocular DDS. Fifty-eight ophthalmic ointments are listed in the USP 23 (5) compared with 59 ophthalmic solutions and 29 ophthalmic suspensions. The ointment bases commonly used in ophthalmic preparations are usually those that permit the incorporation of aqueous solutions and the formation of a water-in-oil emulsion (e.g., white hydrophilic petrolatum and anhydrous liquid lanolin). The addition of mineral oil to the petrolatum base lowers the melting point of the base, allowing the ointment to become a liquid at eye temperature, with improved spreading and mixing with the tear film and reduced effect on vision. Hydrophilic drugs are dispersed in the ointment as fine, solid particles, similar to aqueous suspensions, whereas lipid-soluble drugs are dissolved in the ointment base. Like ophthalmic solutions and suspensions, ophthalmic ointments must contain preservatives to prevent the growth of microorganisms introduced accidentally during routine use. The effects related to inactive ingredients (e.g., preservatives, pH, tonicity), described earlier for ophthalmic solutions, are pertinent to ophthalmic ointments and should be controlled accordingly.

Similar to ophthalmic solutions, some ophthalmic ointments contain a high drug concentration, exceeding tears' tonicity, and thus would cause stinging, burning, and reflex tearing upon instillation. A hypertonic ointment (5% NaCl formulated in white petrolatum, mineral oil, and lanolin) is available for temporary relief of corneal edema.

The major advantage of ointments as an ocular DDS is their tendency to serve as a drug depot, made possible by their extended retention in the conjunctival sac (i.e., increased ocular contact time), resulting in enhanced and sustained corneal absorption (40,41). This enhanced effect is related to the lipid-aqueous differential solubility of the drug. The bioavailability of a water-soluble drug like pilocarpine resulted in a fourfold increase when a 0.01 *M* ointment was compared with a 0.01 *M* solution. On the other hand, the bioavailability of the lipid-soluble drug, fluorometholone, formulated as an ointment, increased by more than eightfold compared with that observed following treatment with a saturated solution of fluorometholone (42).

On the other hand, Riegelman (43) pointed out that the solubility of most drugs in commercial petrolatum ointments is very low. Therefore, most of the drug is present within the ointment as solid microcrystals and must diffuse through the petrolatum to reach the surface. Thus, under conditions of low tear turnover (i.e., during sleep), the drug may reach the tear film at a rate lower than necessary to achieve therapeutic levels, as was the case for various preparations of 5 mg/g of neomycin ointment. Thus, ointment may not be always advantageous to solutions and suspensions.

The major disadvantages of ophthalmic ointments are an annoying blurring of vision following instillation; difficulties in properly applying an exact dose of the drug compared with applying a solution or a suspension; an initial delay in drug delivery; and sensitivity to ambient temperatures (under cold-weather conditions petrolatum-based ointments are difficult to extrude from the ointment tube, and the formulation exhibits a poor ocular drug release rate). Water-containing bases tend to separate into two phases. Elevated temperatures also can enhance melting and nonhomogeneity within the ointment tube.

STRIPS

Paper strips impregnated with fluorescein are used for diagnostic purposes by staining the anterior segment of the eye. The sterile paper strips are impregnated with a sufficient amount of the drug and then released by the tears on contact with the bulbar conjunctiva. Direct contact of the paper with the eye can be avoided by leaching the drug from the paper strip with the aid of sterile water or sodium chloride solution. Like many other ocular DDS, these paper strips contain, in addition to the active ingredient, a preservative, surface-acting agent, and buffering agents.

OCULAR INSERTS

Hydrogel Contact Lenses

Hydrogel contact lenses can absorb water up to 80% of their weight; thus, when soaked in a drug solution and placed over the cornea, they can greatly extend the contact time of the drug solution with the ocular surface and hence increase drug penetration. Waltman and Kaufman (44) showed that placing a contact lens presoaked with fluorescein over the cornea resulted in increased fluorescein levels in the anterior chamber of rabbits (by fourfold) and humans (by eightfold) compared with levels observed following frequent topical instillation of fluorescein solution.

Similar findings were later reported for various ophthalmic drugs, including idoxuridine, polymyxine B, phenylephrine (45), chloramphenicol and tetracycline (46), pilocarpine (47,48), prednisolone (49), and carbonic anhydrase inhibitors (50). Despite the demonstrated improved ocular drug delivery by this system, it did not gain widespread use and is restricted to a few clinical examples.

Membrane-bound Devices

The first marketed device to achieve the goal of a zero-order delivery kinetics was the Ocusert. The drug, pilocarpine, bound to olginic acid and present as a free base, is contained in a reservoir formed by two thin, transparent ethylene-vinyl-acetate (EVA) membranes. An annular ring of EVA, made opaque by impregnation with titanium dioxide, aids in visualization and handling of the insert. The hydrophobic polymer impedes the permeation of water into the device, and the drug delivery rate is determined by the coefficient of diffusion and the concentration gradient. The elliptical device, measuring 13.4 by 5.7 mm, 0.3 mm thick, delivers 20 μg/h (Pilo-20) or 40 μg/h (Pilo-40); the higher delivery rate is achieved by the addition of a flux enhancer (di(2-ethylhexyl)phtalate) to the reservoir. The initial clinical studies with Ocusert (51,52) showed that the 20 μg/h device, delivering 500 μg/day, was effective in maintaining IOP as a standard drop treatment delivering 4 mg/day (an eightfold reduction in the daily dose). The device could be used in combination with other antiglaucoma drugs, for example, epinephrine (53,54). The major advantage of this ocular DDS is the maintenance of therapeutic effectiveness using a smaller amount of drug concomitant with a lower incidence of induced miosis and myopia and reduction in visual acuity (53).

Ocusert therapy is more expensive than standard ophthalmic solution therapy. Patients must check that the device has not been lost and that it is in position in the lower cul-de-sac, that is, has not migrated around the eye. The device must be removed and replaced once a week. Excessive foreign body sensation can sometimes preclude its use. Cases of sudden leakage of the drug have been reported (51).

COLLAGEN SHIELDS

Collagen shields were originally developed by Fyodorov (55) for use as a corneal bandage after radial keratotomy, keratorefractive procedures, and corneal abrasion. The commercially available collagen shields (Bio-Cor, Bausch and Lomb, Pharmaceuticals, Tampa, FL, U.S.A.) are biodegradable contact-lens-shaped clear films made of porcine scleral collagen. They dissolve over 12 to 72 hours, depending on the degree of collagen cross-linking induced by ultraviolet irradiation during production of the device. Collagen shields are indicated for relief of discomfort and to promote corneal epithelial wound healing.

Because corneal shields have a water content >60%, they can be used as a depot for ophthalmic drug delivery. Drugs can be coalesced into the collagen matrix during production, absorbed during rehydration of the device before ocular application, or added topically over a shield already installed in the eye. Animal studies have demonstrated repeatedly that corneal shields can deliver various drugs to the cornea, aqueous humor, or vitreous better than multiple-drop treatments, including tobramycin (56,57), gentamycin, vancomycin (58–60), dexamethasone (61), prednisolone acetate (62), cyclosporine A (63), and amphotericin B (64).

Studies in animal disease models (*Pseudomonas keratitis,* anterior chamber fibrin, and corneal allograft rejection) also showed that the efficacy of collagen shields is superior to that of drop treatments of tobramycin (57), cyclosporine A (65), heparin (66), and tissue plasminogen activator (67). Some studies, however, reported comparable or even lower efficacy for the collagen shield compared with drops of tobramycin (68), amphotericin B (69), and gentamycin (70,71).

Only a limited number of clinical studies using collagen shields as ocular DDS have been published. Reidy et al. (72) found better delivery of fluorescein to aqueous humor by collagen shields in human subjects compared with delivery by a soft contact lens or frequent drop application. Poland and Kaufman (73) tested collagen shields rehydrated in 4% tobramycin in an uncontrolled series of 60 patients with epithelial defects. In general, patients tolerated the collagen shield well (58 of 60 patients), and the impression was that epithelial defects healed faster and provided better prophylaxis against infection than conventional methods. Improved reepithelization, protection, and lubrication were reported by Aquavella et al. (74) in a series of 122 postsurgical patients (67 with penetrating keratoplasty and 55 with cataract extraction) treated with tobramycin- or gentamycin-soaked collagen shields in combination with pilocarpine, dexamethasone, or flurbiprofen. Renard et al. (75) reported reduced subconjunctinal hemorrhage and postoperative inflammation in patients after cataract surgery who were treated with dexamethasone and gentamycin delivered by collagen shields compared with patients treated with subconjunctival injections. These findings indicate that ocular drug delivery by collagen shields can be beneficial in promoting epithelial healing and prophylaxis against ocular infection. Further clinical testing is needed to determine which drugs and indications would benefit from the use of collagen shield as an ocular DDS.

LIPOSOMES

Liposomes are microscopic (0.01–10 μm) structures consisting of spheres (*vesicles*) of lipid bilayers separated by water or an aqueous buffer compartment. Liposomal preparations can be composed of either (a) a single bilayer lipid membrane surrounding an aqueous droplet, classified as small unilamellar vesicles (SUR) if <100 nm or as large unilammellar vesicles (LUV) if >100 nm; or (b) a series of concentric-compartment multilamellar vesicles (MLV) (76,77). The lipids most commonly used in the preparation of lipsomes include glycerol-containing phospholipids like phosphatidylcholine (Lecitin), phosphatidylethanolamine (Cephalin), phosphatidylserine, and phosphatidylglycerol. Steroid cholesterol and its derivatives are often included as components of liposomal membranes to improve the stability of the membrane in the presence of biological fluids. The addition of substances like glycolipids, organic acids, bases, membrane proteins, and synthetic polymers alters liposomal characteristics, such as size, charge, bilayer rigidity/fluidity, and drug-loading capacity (entrapment efficiency).

Liposomes initially were conceived as a DDS for the i.v. route. The major advantage ascribed to liposomal formulation was the ability to circumvent cell membrane permeability barriers by cell membrane-liposome interactions (adsorption, fusion, and endocytosis) (78). It was postulated that liposomes could protect the delivered drug from metabolic and immune attacks, reduce drug toxicity, and enhance the therapeutic effects.

Liposomes are used in cosmetics and dermatologicals. The first parenterally applied formulation was an amphotericin-liposomal formulation for the treatment of disseminated fungal infections (Ambisome), launched in 1990.

The first reports of liposome-based ocular DDS were by Smolin et al. (79), who showed an improvement in the treatment of herpetic keratitis in rabbits by using an idoxuridine-liposome preparation; by Schaeffer et al. (80,81), who reported a twofold increase in the corneal flux of penicillin G, indoxole, and carbachol; and by Singh and Mezei (82), who found increased ocular tissue levels of triamcinolone acetonide, in rabbits, following topical application of a liposomal formulation. Ahmed and Patton (83) found that although topical treatment with an inulin-liposome formulation did not yield increased aqueous humor inulin levels, iris-ciliary body inulin levels were significantly higher than those obtained following administration of inulin in aqueous solution. These findings may be due to a higher drug influx across the conjunctiva. Multivesicular liposomes were used successfully for sustained delivery of antimetabolites (cytarabine, 5-fluorouridine 5-monophosphate) in rabbits and owl monkeys after periocular and intravitreal administration (84–87).

Some studies failed to demonstrate elevated aqueous humor drug levels delivered by liposome-formulated drugs, like epinephrine, inulin, and pilocarpine (88,89). Singh and Mezei (90) found that ocular drug levels, following topical treatment with liposome-dihydrostreptomycin sulfate formulation, were lower than those following treatment with the drug in solution. Taniguchi et al. (91) found that topical treatment with liposomal preparations of dexamethasone and dexamethasone palmitate yielded lower drug levels than those obtained with suspensions of these drugs.

The improved ocular bioavailability reported for some drug-liposomal formulations can be attributed to an increased ocular residence time. Fitzgerald et al. (92) found in rabbits a slower drainage rate of liposomal preparations for the ocular surface compared with the drainage rate of solutions. Positively charged liposomes were retained longer than negatively charged or neutral liposomes or the suspending buffer. These findings correspond well with those of Schaeffer and Krohn (80), who showed that the binding affinities of liposomes to the cornea are greatest for positively charged liposomes, less for negatively charged liposomes, and least for neutral liposomes.

The findings obtained so far from in vitro and animal studies clearly demonstrate the potential of liposomes as ocular DDS. Studies of the efficacy and long-term safety in humans as well as product development are needed to determine the prospect of liposomes as a successful ocular DDS.

EMULSIONS

Emulsions are traditionally defined as two-phase systems in which one liquid is dispersed throughout another liquid in the form of small droplets. Emulsifying agents (*surfactants*) are added to stabilize the emulsion and prevent coalescence of the dispersed drops. All emulsions require an antimicrobial agent because the aqueous phase favors the growth of microorganisms (5).

As a DDS, emulsions offer some advantages: the ability to deliver lipid-soluble drugs in a liquid aqueouslike form, enhanced bioavailability, protection of drugs susceptible to oxidation or hydrolysis, and patient acceptability in cases where the free drug is irritating or has an objectionable taste or texture. Nevertheless, there is a general reluctance on the part of the pharmaceutical industry to develop liquid dispension systems, as they are considered the most complex of the various pharmaceutical dosage forms, and their formulation is still at an experimental level (93–95).

Emulsions are commonly used in ophthalmology in the form of ointments, as mentioned earlier, but only rarely have emulsions been tested or used in the form of liquid eyedrops. Some earlier studies on oil-in-water emulsions reported them to be too irritating (96). A major contributing factor was the ionic surfactants used to stabilize the emulsion.

Interest in emulsions as an ophthalmic DDC was renewed with the development of the specialized submicron emulsion (SME) (97), which is characterized by the droplet size of the oily phase in the range of 0.1 to 0.3 μm, smaller than those of the classic macroemulsion but generally larger than those of a classic microemulsion (94,95). Nonionic (nonirritating) surfactants are used to stabilize the emulsion. Animal studies demonstrated improved performance of some ophthalmic drugs formulated in SME. Improvements over aqueous, commercially available solutions and suspensions were evident in both bioavailability, increased aqueous humor drug levels of indomethacin (98), effectiveness (a 30% increase in IOP lowering activity of timolol and betaxolol) (99), and a reduction in ocular irritation (stinging-burning, conjuctival redness, iris hyperemia, and corneal fluorescein staining) (98,99).

Increased ocular retention time (100) of fluorescently labeled SME (both lipid and aqueous phases) can explain the improved bioavailability. The mechanism behind the reduced irritation is currently unknown. Reduced irritation for both hydrophilic and hydrophobic drugs suggests that the irritation is not merely a result of drug entrapment within the emulsion vesicles. The SME formulation also allowed safe and effective delivery of the very lipophylic compound HU-211 (a nonpsychotropic, synthetic cannabinoid) by both the topical (eyedrops) and parenteral (i.v.) routes in rabbits (101,102). After the findings in rabbits, some SME formulations were also tested in human subjects with promising results. Pilocarpine-SME (2%) twice daily was as effective as a 2% pilocarpine solution four times a day in lowering IOP in ocular hypertensive patients, with no major side effects (103,104). Adaprolol maleate, a novel soft β-blocking agent, formulated in SME was safe, comfortable, and effective in lowering IOP in normotensive subjects (105) as well as in ocular hypertensive patients (106).

GELS

Gels are single or multiphase semisolid systems. In two-phase gels, the gel mass consists of a network of small, discrete particles suspended in a liquid. In single-phase gels, the macromolecules are distributed uniformly throughout a liquid, and there are no apparent boundaries between the dispersed macromolecules and the liquid. Gels can be termed as inorganic or organic, depending on the nature of the colloidal, dispersed phase. The type of solvent used determines whether the gel is a *hydrogel* (water-based) or an *organogel* (nonaqueous solvent). *Xerogels* are solid gels with low solvent concentration; when a solvent is introduced, xerogels swell to gel matrix.

A variety of gel-forming compounds have been used in the manufacture of gels: (a) natural gums, which are typically anionic, branched-chain polysacharides (alginates, carrageenan, pectin, xanthan gum); (b) carbomer, a group of acrylic polymers cross-linked with polyalkenyl ether (carbopol 934p), that form gels at concentrations as low as 0.5%, and whose viscosity can be lowered by the addition of ions; (c) cellulose derivatives; (d) polyethylenes; (e) Colloidally dispersed solids (1,107,108). Many gels can be degraded by microorganisms requiring the inclusion of a preservative. Gels are used as delivery systems for oral administration, topical-dermal application, i.m. injections of long-acting drugs, and a wide variety of cosmetic products.

Polymer-based aqueous gels have been tested and developed as delivery systems for a variety of ophthalmic drugs, including hydroxypropylcellulose (HPC), HEC, ethylhydroxyethylcellulose (EHEC), pluronic acid, carbopol, polyacrylamide (PAA), and polyvinylalcohol (PVP).

PILOPLEX

Piloplex is a dispersed system containing a polymeric pilocarpine salt. The polymer constituent is a copolymer of lauryl methacrylate and acrylic acid, and pilocarpine is in the form of an amine salt with the carboxylic groups. Tests in rabbits showed that the duration of hypotensive effects of a single drop of piloplex is equipotent to 2 drops of pilocarpine given at 6-hour intervals. In a preliminary clinical study, piloplex produced a prolonged therapeutic effect in open-angle glaucoma patients (109,110).

Pilopine HS Gel

A carbopol 940 gel (cross-linked polymer of acrylic acid) was developed by Alcon as a delivery system for once-a-day pilocarpine. In rabbits, pilopine showed higher efficacy than commercially available pilocarpine solutions, although this effect was not seen in squirrel monkeys (111). Clinical studies showed that this formulation can be used as a once-a-day pilocarpine treatment for the control of IOP (112–114).

In Situ Gel-forming Systems

In these systems, ophthalmic eyedrops undergo gelation on contact with the ocular surface; they combine the advantages of dispensing an aqueous solution with the increased retention time of high viscosity formulations. Gelation can be triggered by changes in external factors (e.g., temperature, pH, or ionic composition).

Ion-activated Gelation

Gelrite (developed at Merck Sharp and Dohme (MSD)-Chibret) is a polysaccharide, low-acetyl gellan gum that forms clear gels in the presence of monovalent or bivalent ions. The concentration of sodium ions in tears is sufficient to cause gelation in the conjuctival sac, even when a low concentration of the polymer (0.6%) is used. This gel was reported to increase bioavailability about twofold over aqueous solutions of both timolol maleate and pilocarpine in rabbits (115,116).

pH-Activated Gelation

These specially selected systems are composed of a large amount of an anionic polymer in the form of nanodispersion, which has a very low viscosity at pH ≤5. On contact with the tear film, with a normal pH of 7.2 to 7.4, the particles agglomerate, coacervate, and assume a gel form. The gelation process is due to swelling of the particles from neutralization of the acid groups on the polymer chain and the absorption of water. Testing such a system in rabbits showed that for a 2% pilocarpine in a cellulose acetate, phthalate latex (CAP), the amount of drug retained on the ocular surface was 3.8 times more than that of a 2% pilocarpine solution (117). Measurements of aqueous humor kinetics of pilocarpine in rabbits showed that a CAP-pilocarpine formulation increased ocular bioavailability by about twofold (118).

Temperature-sensitive Gels

Miller and Donovan (119) used a 25% poloxamer 407 gel that exhibits reverse thermal gelation; that is, its viscosity increases with the increase in temperature, from that of ambient temperature (~25°C) to that of the ocular surface (~32–34°C). Incorporation of pilocarpine nitrate into this gel led to a twofold increase in the miotic response (area under the pupil diameter/time curve) compared with an aqueous solution of pilocarpine.

Harsh and Gehrke (120) developed a temperature-sensitive hydrogel based on cross-linking cellulose ethers like hydroxycellulose. These gels swell as the temperature rises and thus would release the solvent, which can be a drug solution. Because cellulose ethers are Food and Drug Administration (FDA)-approved for food and drug use, they offer an advantage over many synthetic gels that are based on polymers or monomers shown to be carcinogenic or teratogenic. The advantages of such gels as an ocular DDS are yet to be proved. Lindel and Egnstrom (121) reported that the in vitro release of timolol maleate from a thermogelling DDS based on ethylhydroxyethyl cellulose (EHEC) is similar to that for the Gelrite-timolol delivery system described by Rozier et al. (115).

Another approach to in situ gelation was presented by Joshi et al. (122), who used a formulation containing a combination of polymers responding simultaneously to two gelating factors (i.e., pH and temperature). An aqueous solution containing a combination of 0.3% carbopol, a polyacrylic acid polymer that gelates when the pH is raised over its pk of 5.5, and a 1.5% methylcellulose that gelates when the temperature is raised above 30°C was reported to form a gel under simulated physiological conditions, thus reducing the total polymer content of the delivery system (123). Thus, many varieties of gels potentially can be used as an ocular DDS. Future development efforts would demonstrate which ones are best suited for clinical use.

The ocular DDS mentioned here represent a variety of techniques aimed at extending ocular contact time. Additionally, attempts have been made to overcome another major obstacle, the structural barriers at the ocular surface that impede the intraocular penetration of drugs, especially ionized (charged) molecules.

IONTOPHORESIS

Iontophoresis is a process of moving a charged molecule (*ion*) by an electric current across a barrier. Iontophoresis has been used in medicine to improve the penetration of various drugs into the body (e.g., glucocorticosteroids for the treatment of arthritis or local anesthesia of oral mucosa or the middle ear) (124–126). Iontophoresis was reported to be used in ophthalmology since the turn of the century (127) for the treatment of a wide variety of diseases using various ions and drugs. These earlier clinical reports, as well as the experimental animal studies of Von Sallman, were reviewed by Karbowski (128), Smith (129), and Erlanger (130).

Sarraf and Lee (131) summarized and reviewed the experimental work done between 1987 and 1994, mostly in rabbits, investigating transcorneal and transscleral iontophoresis of various antibiotics, antiviral, antimetabolite, and steroid drugs. These studies generally showed that intraocular drug levels obtained following iontophoresis are significantly higher than those found after multiple drop treatments or intravitreal injections.

Animal studies also showed that drug delivery by iontophoresis may be accompanied by toxic tissue-damaging effects. Transcorneal iontophoresis resulted in some corneal epithelial or endothelial damage; the severity of damage was related to the current density, duration of application, and the drug being used (132–136). Local retinal and choroidal lesions were also reported in some animal studies following transcleral iontophoresis of various drugs (137–139). Current density and duration of application affected the size and severity of the lesions.

Although these animal studies demonstrated that iontophoresis can greatly improve drug delivery into the eye, randomized, controlled clinical trials have not been done. The fact that multiple-drop therapy with antibiotics proved relatively successful with few complications and that relatively successful management of endophthalmitis can be achieved with a single intravitreal injection probably curtailed part of the incentive to develop a safe and effective transcorneal/transcleral antibiotic iontophoresis.

Future studies of drugs with high iontophoresis conductivity, representing additional classes of ophthalmic drugs (e.g., anticancer, antifungal, antiviral, cytokines, or peptide hormones) may lead to the development of a safe and efficient iontophoresis ocular drug delivery.

Ion Pairing

Ion *pairing* is a coulombic association between large organic ions of opposite charge. As a pair, they do not have a net charge; so the ion pair is more lipophilic than its respective constituent ions. The increased lipophilicity should result in enhanced permeability of the ion pair compared with the permeability of the individual ions. Ion pairs, like salicylate and 1-dodecylazacyclo heptane-2-one (Azone) or physostigmine-salicylate, improve transport across artificial membranes or isolated human skin (140,141). Improved transcorneal permeability of the anti-inflammatory drug cromoglycate was obtained by ion pairing with a quarternary ammonium compound (142,143). This enhanced permeability could be due in part to the adverse effects of quarternary ammonium compounds (like benzalkonium chloride; see section on preservatives) on the structural integrity of the corneal epithelium. Improved permeability across isolated rabbit cornea was also reported for some carbonic anhydrase inhibitors ion-paired with quarternary ammonium, phosphonium and arsonium salts (144). The full potential of ion pairing as a means of improving ocular drug delivery would be better appreciated only after additional demonstrations of the efficacy and safety of this DDS.

REFERENCES

1. Sorensen B, Jensen FT. Tear flow in normal human eyes: determination by mean of radioisotope and gamma camera. *Acta Ophthalmol Scand Suppl* 1979;57:564–581.
2. Peduzzi M, Debbia A, Monzani A. Ocular anatomy and physiology: its relevance to transcorneal drug absorption and to vehicle effects. In: Saettone MF, Bucci M, Speiser P, eds. *Ophthalmic Drug Delivery,* Fidia Research Series, vol 11. Liviana Press and Springer Verlag, 1987;1–6.
3. Van Ootegham MM. Factors influencing the retention of ophthalmic solutions on the eye surface. In: Saettone MF, Bucci M, Speiser P, eds. *Ophthalmic Drug Delivery,* Fidia Research Series, vol 11. Liviana Press and Springer Verlag, 1987;7–18.
4. Schoenwald RD. The control of drug bioavailability from ophthalmic dosage forms. In: Smolen VF, Ball VA, eds. *Controlled Drug Bioavailability,* vol 3: *Bioavailability Control by Drug Delivery System Design.* New York: John Wiley & Sons, 1985;257–306.
5. *U.S. Pharmacopeia (USP) 23 1995.* Rockville, Maryland: United States Pharmacopeial Convention, 1994;1945–1946.
6. Benet LZ, Mitchell JR, Sheiner HB. Pharmacokinetics: the dynamics of drug absorption, distribution and elimination. In: *Goodman and Gilman's The Pharmacological Basis of Therapeutics,* 8th ed. New York: Pergamon Press, 1945–46;3–32.
7. Mitra AK, Mickelson TJ. Mechanisms of transcorneal permeation of pilocarpine. *J Pharm Sci* 1988;77:771–775.
8. Jankowska LM, Bar-Ilan A, Maren TH. The relations between ionic and non-ionic diffusion of sulfonamides across the rabbit cornea. *Invest Ophthalmol Vis Sci* 1986;27:29–37.
9. Brechue WF, Maren TH. pH and drug ionization affects ocular pressure lowering of topical carbonic anhydrase inhibitors. *Invest Ophthalmol Vis Sci* 1993;34:2581–2587.

10. Siegel FP. Tonicity, osmoticity, osmolality and osmolarity. In: Gennaro AR, ed. *Remington's Pharmaceutical Sciences,* 18th ed. Easton, Pennsylvania: Mack Publishing Co., 1990;1481–1498.
11. Scheile HG, Albert DM. *Textbook of Ophthalmology,* 9th ed. Philadelphia: WB Saunders, 1977;122–124.
12. Terry JE, Hill RM. Human tear osmotic pressure. *Arch Ophthalmol* 1978;96:120–122.
13. Benjamin WJ, Hill RM. Human tears: osmotic characteristics. *Invest Ophthalmol Vis Sci* 1983;24:1624–1626.
14. Krogh A, Lung CG, Pedersen-Bjergard K. The osmotic concentration of human lacrymal fluid. *Acta Physiol Scand* 1945;10:88–90.
15. Fenton AH. Solutions of sulfacetamide sodium. *Pharm J* 1951;166: 6–8.
16. Maurice DM. The tonicity of an eye drop and its dilution by tears. *Exp Eye Res* 1971;11:30–33.
17. *Physician's Desk Reference for Ophthalmology,* 22nd ed. Montvale, NJ: Medical Economics Data Production Co., 1994;1–22, 103–106, 201–323.
18. Swan KC. Use of methylcellulose in ophthalmology. *Arch Ophthalmol* 1945;33:378–380.
19. Linn ML, Jones JT. Rate of lacrimal excretion of ophthalmic vehicles. *Am J Ophthalmol* 1968;65:76–78.
20. Mueller WH, Deardruff DL. Ophthalmic vehicles: the effect of methylcellulose on the penetration of homatotropin hydrobromide through the cornea. *J Am Pharm A Sci* 1956;48:334.
21. Chrai SS, Robinson JR. Ocular evaluation of methylcellulose vehicle in Albino rabbits. *J Pharm Sci* 1974;63:1218–1223.
22. Patton TF, Robinson JR. Ocular evaluation of polyvinyl alcohol vehicle in rabbits. *J Pharm Sci* 1975;64:1312–1316.
23. Saetone MF, Giannaccini B, Ravecca S, La Marca F, Tota G. Polymer effects on ocular bioavailability: the influence of different liquid vehicles on the mydriatic response of tropicamide in humans and rabbits. *Int J Pharm* 1984;20:187–202.
24. O'Brien CS, Swan KC. Carbaminocholine chloride in the treatment of glaucoma simplex. *AMA Arch Ophthalmol* 1942;27:255–269.
25. Keller N, Moore DM, Carper D, Longwell A. Increased corneal permeability induced by the dual effects of transient tear film acidification and exposure to benzalkonium chloride. *Exp Eye Res* 1980; 30:203–210.
26. Green K, Downs SJ. Ocular penetration of pilocarpine in rabbits. *Arch Ophthalmol* 1978;931:1165–1168.
27. Green K, Tonjum AM. Influence of various agents on corneal permeability. *Am J Ophthalmol* 1971;72:897–905.
28. Burstein NL. Preservative alteration of corneal permeability in humans and rabbits. *Invest Ophthalmol Vis Sci* 1984;25:1453–1457.
29. Swan KG. Reactivity of the ocular tissues to wetting agents. *Am J Ophthalmol* 1944;27:1118–1122.
30. Dormans JAMA, Van Logten MJ. The effects of ophthalmic preservatives on corneal epithelium of the rabbit: a scanning electron microscopical study. *Toxicol Appl Pharmacol* 1982;62:251–261.
31. Pfister RR, Burstein NL. The effects of ophthalmic drugs, vehicles, and preservatives on corneal epithelium: a scanning electron microscope study. *Invest Ophthalmol* 1976;15:246–259.
32. Gasset A, Ishi Y, Kaufman H. Cytotoxicity of ophthalmic preservatives. *Am J Ophthalmol* 1974;78:98–105.
33. Mietz H, Niessen U, Kreiglstein GK. The effect of preservatives and antiglaucomatous medication on the histopathology of the conjunctiva. *Graefes Arch Clin Exp Ophthalmol* 1994;232:561–565.
34. Loewenstein A, Zemel E, Lazar M, Perlman I. The effects of depomedrol preservative on the rabbit visual system. *Invest Ophthalmol Vis Sci* 1991;32:3053–3060.
35. Buehler EV, Newman EA. A comparison of eye irritation in monkeys and rabbits. *Toxicol Appl Pharmacol* 1964;6:701–710.
36. Sieg JW, Robinson JR. Vehicle effects of ocular drug bioavailability: I. Evaluation of fluorometholone. *J Pharm Sci* 1975;64: 931–936.
37. Schoenwald RP, Stewart P. Effect of particle size on ophthalmic bioavailability of dexamethasone suspensions in rabbits. *J Pharm Sci* 1980;69:391–394.
38. Sieg JW, Robinson JR. Vehicle effects of ocular bioavailability: II. Evaluation of pilocarpine. *J Pharm Sci* 1977;66:1222–1228.
39. Apt Z, Henrick A, Silverman LM. Patient compliance with use of topical ophthalmic corticosteroid suspension. *Am J Ophthalmol* 1979; 87:210–214.
40. Harberger RE, Hanna C, Bond CM. Effects of drug vehicles on ocular contact time. *Arch Ophthalmol* 1975;92:42–47.
41. Harberger RE, Hanna C, Goodart R. Effects of drug vehicles on ocular uptake of tetracycline. *Am J Ophthalmol* 1975;80:133–138.
42. Sieg JW, Robinson JR. Vehicle effects on ocular drug bioavailability. III. Shear facilitated pilocarpine release from ointments. *J Pharm Sci* 1979;68:724–728.
43. Riegelman S. Pharmacokinetic factors affecting epidermal penetration and percutaneous absorption. *Clin Pharmacol Ther* 1974;16: 873–883.
44. Waltman SR, Kaufman HE. Use of hydrophilic contact lenses to increase ocular penetration of topical drugs. *Invest Ophthalmol* 1970;9:250–255.
45. Kaufman HE, Uotila MH, Gasset AR, Wood TO, Ellison ED. The medical uses of soft contact lenses. *Am Acad Ophthalmol Otolaryngol* 1970;75:361–366.
46. Praus R, Brettschneider I, Krejcl L, Kalodowa D. Hydrophilic contact lenses as a new therapeutic approach for the topical use of chloramphenicol and tetracycline. *Ophthalmologica* 1972;165:62–70.
47. Podos SM, Becker B, Asseff C, Hartstein J. Pilocarpine therapy with soft contact lenses. *Am J Ophthalmol* 1972;73:336–341.
48. Hillman JS. Management of acute glaucoma with pilocarpine-soaked hydrophilic lens. *Br J Ophthalmol* 1974;58:674–679.
49. Hull DS, Edelhauser HF, Hyndiuk RA. Ocular penetration of prednisolone and the hydrophilic contact lens. *Arch Ophthalmol* 1974;92: 413–416.
50. Friedman Z, Allen RC, Raph SM. Topical actazolamide and methazolamide delivered by contact lenses. *Arch Ophthalmol* 1985;103: 963– 966.
51. Armaly MD, Rao KR. The effect of pilocarpine Ocusert with different release rates on ocular pressure. *Invest Ophthalmol* 1973;12: 491–496.
52. Worthen DM, Zimmerman TJ, Wind CA. An evaluation of the pilocarpine Ocusert. *Invest Ophthalmol* 1974;13:296–299.
53. Macoul KL, Pavan-Langston D. Pilocarpine Ocusert® system for sustained control of ocular hypertension. *Arch Ophthalmol* 1975;93: 587–590.
54. Lee PF, Shen YT, Eberle M. The long-acting Ocusert pilocarpine system in the management of glaucoma. *Invest Ophthalmol* 1975;14: 43–46.
55. Fyodorov SN, Moroz ZI, Kramskaya ZI, Bagrov SN, Amstislavskaya TS, Zolotarevsky AV. Complex medical treatment of endothelial epithelial corneal distrophy with the use of therapeutic collagen bandages. *Vestn Oftalmol* 1985;101:33–36.
56. O'Brien TP, Sawusch MR, Dick JD, Hamburg TR, Gottsch JD. Use of collagen corneal shields versus soft contact lenses to enhance penetration of topical tobramycin. *J Cataract Refract Surg* 1988;14: 505–507.
57. Sawusch MR, O'Brien TP, Dick JD, Gottsch JD. Use of collagen corneal shields in treatment of bacterial keratitis. *Am J Ophthalmol* 1988;106:279–281.
58. Phinney RB, Schwartz SP, Lee DA, Mondino BJ. Collagen-shield delivery of gentamicin and vancomycin. *Arch Ophthalmol* 1988; 106:1599–1604.
59. Fong-Qi L, Viola RS, Del Cerro M, Aquavella JV. Noncross-linked collagen discs and cross-linked collagen shields in the delivery of gentamicin to rabbit's eyes. *Invest Ophthalmol Vis Sci* 1992; 33:2194– 2198.
60. Baziuk N, Gremillion CM, Peyman GA, Cho HK. Collagen shield and intraocular drug delivery: concentration of gentamicin in the aqueous and vitreous of a rabbit eye after lensection and vitrectomy. *Int Ophthalmol* 1992;16:101–107.
61. Hwang DG, Stern WH, Hwang PH, McGowan-Smith LA. Collagen shield enhancement of topical dexamethasone penetration. *Arch Ophthalmol* 1989;107:1375–1380.
62. Sawusch MR, O'Brien TP, Undegraff BS. Collagen corneal shields enhance penetration of topical prednisolone acetate. *J Cataract Refract Surg* 1989;15:625–628.
63. Reidy JJ, Gebhardt BM, Kaufman HE. The collagen shield: a new vehicle for delivery of cyclosporin A to the eye. *Cornea* 1990; 9:196–199.
64. Schwartz SD, Harrison SA, Engtrom RE, Bawdon RE, Lee DA, Mondino BJ. Collagen shield delivery of amphotericin B. *Am J Ophthalmol* 1990;109:701–704.

65. Chen YF, Gebhardt BM, Reidy JJ, Kaufman HE. Cyclosporine-containing collagen shields suppress corneal allograft rejection. *Am J Ophthalmol* 1990;109:132–137.
66. Murray TG, Stern WH, Chin DH, McGowan-Smith EA. Collagen shield heparin delivery for prevention of postoperative fibrin. *Arch Ophthalmol* 1990;108:104–106.
67. Murray TG, Jaffe GJ, Mckay BS, Han DP, Burke JM, Abrams GW. Collagen shield delivery of tissue plasminogen activator: functional and pharmacokinetic studies of anterior segment delivery. *Refract Corneal Surg* 1992;8:44–48.
68. Hobden JA, Reidy JJ, O'Callaghan RJ, Hill JM, Insler MS, Rootman DS. Treatment of experimental pseudomonas keratitis using collagen shields containing tobramycin. *Arch Ophthalmol* 1988; 106:1605–1607.
69. Pleyer U, Legmann A, Mondino BJ, Lee DA. Use of collagen shields containing amphotericin B in the treatment of experimental *Candida albicans*-induced keratomycosis in rabbits. *Am J Ophthalmol* 1992;113:303–307.
70. Sibliger J, Stern GA. Evaluation of corneal collagen shields as a drug delivery device for the treatment of experimental pseudomonas keratitis. *Ophthalmology* 1992;99:889–892.
71. Brockman EB, Tarantino PA, Hobden JA. Keratotomy model of pseudomonas keratitis: gentamicin chemotherapy. *Refract Corneal Surg* 1992;8:39–43.
72. Reidy JJ, Limberg M, Kaufman HE. Delivery of fluorescein to the anterior chamber using the corneal collagen shield. *Ophthalmology* 1990;97:1201–1203.
73. Poland DE, Kaufman HE. Clinical uses of collagen shields. *J Cataract Refract Surg* 1988;14:489–491.
74. Aquavella JV, Musco PS, Ueda S, Lo Cascio JS. Therapeutic application of a collagen bandage lens: a preliminary report. *CLAO J* 1988; 14:47–50.
75. Renard GY, Bennani N, Lutaj P, Richard C, Trinquand C. Comparative study of a corneal collagen shield and a subconjuctival injection at the end of cataract surgery. *J Cataract Refract Surg* 1993;19: 48–51.
76. Weiner N, Martin F, Riaz M. Liposomes as a drug delivery system. *Drug Dev Indust Pharm* 1989;15:1523–1554.
77. Lee VHL, Urrea PT, Smith RE, Schanzlin DJ. Ocular drug bioavailability for topically applied liposomes. *Surv Ophthalmol* 1985;29: 335–348.
78. Pagano RE, Weinstein JN. Interactions of liposomes with mammalian cells. *Annu Rev Biopsy Bioeng* 1978;7:435–468.
79. Smolin G, Okumoto M, Feiler S, Condon D. Idoxuridine-liposome therapy for herpes simplex keratitis. *Am J Ophthalmol* 1981;91: 220– 225.
80. Schaeffer HE, Krohn DL. Liposomes in topical drug delivery. *Invest Ophthalmol Vis Sci* 1982;22:220–227.
81. Schaeffer HE, Brietfeller JM, Krohn DL. Lecitin-mediated attachment of liposomes to cornea: influence on transcorneal drug flux. *Invest Ophthalmol Vis Sci* 1983;23:530–533.
82. Singh K, Mezei M. Liposomal ophthalmic drug delivery system. I. Triamenilone acetonide. *Int J Pharm* 1993;16:339–344.
83. Ahmed I, Patton TF. Selective intraocular delivery of liposome encapsulated inulin via the non-corneal absorption route. *Int J Pharm* 1986;34:163–167.
84. Assil KK, Weinreb RN. Multivesicular liposomes sustain release of the antimetabolite cytarabine in the eye. *Arch Ophthalmol* 1987; 105:400–403.
85. Assil KK, Lane J, Weinreb R. Sustained release of the antimetabolite 5-fluorduridine-5-monophosphate by multivesicular liposomes. *Ophthalmic Surg Lasers* 1988;19:408–413.
86. Assil KK, Hartzer M, Weinreb RN, Neharayan M, Ward T, Blumenkranz M. Liposome suppression of proliferative vitreoretinopathy. *Invest Ophthalmol Vis Sci* 1991;32:2891–2897.
87. Skuta G, Assil K, Parish R, Folberg R, Weinreb RN. Filtering surgery in owl monkey treated with the antimetabolite 5-fluorovridine-5-monophosphate entrapped in multivesicular Hiposomes. *Am J Ophthalmol* 1987;103:714–716.
88. Stratford RE, Yang DC, Redell MA, Lee VHL. Effects of topically applied liposomes on disposition of epinephrine and inulin in the albino rabbit eye. *Int J Pharm* 1983;13:263–272.
89. Benita S, Plenecassegne JA, Cave G, Drovin D, Dong PLH, Sincholle D. Pilocarpine hydrochloride liposomes characterization in vitro and preliminary evaluation in-vivo in rabbit exe. *J Microencapsul* 1984; 1:203–216.
90. Singh KK, Mezei M. Liposomal ophthalmic drug delivery system II. Dihydrostreptomycin sulphate. *Int J Pharm* 1984;19:263–266.
91. Taniguchi K, Itakura K, Yamazawa N, Morisaki K, Hayashi S, Yamada Y. Efficacy of a liposome preparation of anti-inflammatory steroid as an ocular drug delivery system. *J Pharmacobiol Dyn* 1988;11:39–116.
92. Fitzgerald P, Hadgrraft J, Wilson CG. A gamma scintigraphic evaluation of the precorneal residence of liposomal formulations in the rabbit. *J Pharm Pharmacol* 1987;39:487–490.
93. Idson B. Pharmaceutical emulsion. In: Lieberman HA, Rieger MM, Banker GS, eds. *Pharmaceutical Dosage Forms—Disperse Systems,* vol 1. New York: Marcel Dekker, 1988;199–243.
94. Rosoff M. Specialized pharmaceutical emulsions. In: Liebgerman HA, Rieger MM, Banker GS, eds. *Pharmaceutical Dosage Forms–Disperse Systems,* vol 1. New York: Marcel Dekker, 1988;245–283.
95. Block LH. Emulsions and microemulsions. In Liebgerman HA, Rieger MM, Bank GS, eds. *Pharmaceutical Dosage Forms—Disperse Systems,* vol 2. New York: Marcel Dekker, 1988;335–378.
96. Stenbeck-Gjertz A, Ostholm I. Ointments for ophthalmic use. *Acta Ophthalmol* 1954;32:405–423.
97. Aviv H, Friedman D, Bar-Ilan A, Vered M. Submicron Emulsion as Ocular Drug Delivery Vehicles. Patient PCT/vs93/00044; I.P. Number W094/05298; 1994;1–27.
98. Bar-Ilan A, Baru H, Beilin M, Friedman D, Amselem S, Neumann R. Extended activity and increased bioavailability of indomethacin formulated in submicron emulsion, compared to commercially available formulation. *Reg Immunol* 1996;6:166–168.
99. Bar-Ilan A, Aviv H, Friedman D, Vered M, Belkin M, Amselem S, Baru H, Beilin M, Wellner E, Wolf Y, Schwartz J, Neumann R. Improved performance of ocular drugs formulated in submicron emulsions. *Invest Ophthalmol Vis Sci* 1993;34:1488.
100. Beilin M, Bar-Ilan A, Amselem S, Schwartz J, Yogev A, Neumann R. Ocular retention time of submicron emulsion (SME) and the miotic response to pilocarpine delivered in SME. *Invest Ophthalmol Vis Sci* 1995;36:S166;805.
101. Beilin M, Aviv H, Friedman D, Vered M, Belkin M, Neumann R, Amselem S, Schwarz J, Bar-Ilan A. HU-211, a novel synthetic nonpsychotrophic cannabinoid with ocular hypotensive activity. *Invest Ophthalmol Vis Sci* 1993;34:925.
102. Beilin M, Bar-Ilan A, Belkin M, Howes JF, Neumann R. Mechanistic studies on the IOP lowering effect of systemic HU-211, a nonpsychotropic cannabinoid. *Invest Ophthalmol Vis Sci* 1994; 35:1400.
103. Melamed S, Kurtz S, Greenbaum A, Vered M, Garty N. Effect of pilocarpine in sub-micron emulsion on intraocular pressure in healthy volunteers. *Invest Ophthalmol Vis Sci* 1993;34:926.
104. Garty N, Lusky M, Zalish M, Rachmiel R, Greenbaum A, Desatnik H, Neumann R, Howes JF, Melamed S. Pilocarpine in submicron emulsion formulation for treatment of ocular hypertension: a phase II clinical trials. *Invest Ophthalmol Vis Sci* 1994;35:2175.
105. Melamed S, Kurtz S, Greenbaum A, Howes JF, Neumann R, Garty N. Adaprolol maleate in submicron emulsion—a novel soft β-blocking agent is safe and effective in human studies. *Invest Ophthalmol Vis Sci* 1994;35:1387.
106. Garty N, Melamed S, Ticho U, Zalish M, Howes JF, Rachmiel R, Greenbaum A, Neumann R. Adaprolol: a site active β-blocker for the treatment of glaucoma: a two week clinical trial. *Invest Ophthalmol Vis Sci* 1995;36:5736.
107. Zatz JL, Kushla GP. Gels. In: Lieberman HA, Ringer MM, Bankers GS, eds. *Pharmaceutical Dosage Forms: Dispersed Systems,* vol II. New York: Marcel Dekker, 1989;495–510.
108. Peppas NA, Khare AR. Preparation, structure and diffusional behavior of hydrogels in controlled release. *Adv Drug Del Rev* 1993;11:1–35.
109. Ticho U, Blumenthal M, Zonis S, Gal A, Blank I, Mazor ZW. A clinical trial with piloplex—a new long-acting pilocarpine compound preliminary report. *Ann Ophthalmol* 1979;11:555–561.
110. Mazor Z, Kasan R, Kain N, Ladkani D, Ross M, Weiner B. Glaubid (piloplex 3,4)-a long-acting, anti-glaucoma medication. In: Ticho V, David R, eds. *Recent Advances in Glaucoma.* New York: Elsevier Science Publishers B.V. 1984;225–229.

111. Cheeks L, Green K, Stone RP, Riedhammer T. Comparative effects of Pilocarpine in different vehicles on pupil diameter in albino rabbit and squirrel monkeys. *Curr Eye Res* 1989;8:1251–1258.
112. Goldberg I, Ashborne F, Kass M. Efficacy and patient acceptance of pilocarpine gel. *Am J Ophthalmol* 1979;88:843–846.
113. Marck WF, Stewart RM, Mandell II, Bruce LA. Duration of effect of pilocarpine gel. *Arch Ophthalmol* 1982;100:1270–1271.
114. Samples JR. Pilocarpine gel. *Ophthalmol Clin North Am* 1989;2: 109–111.
115. Roziere A, Mazuel C, Grove J, Plazonnet B. GTelrite: a novel, ion-activated, in-situ gelling polymer for ophthalmic vehicles: effect on bioavailability of Timolol. *Int J Pharm* 1989;57:163–168.
116. Chastaing C, Rozier A, Plazonnet B, Grove J. Gelrite enhances the ocular penetration of pilocarpine in the pigmented rabbit. *Invest Ophthalmol Vis Sci* 1995;36:5159;680.
117. Gurny R, Boye T, Ibrahim H. Ocular therapy with nanoparticulate systems for controlled drug delivery. *J Contr Rel* 1985;2:353–361.
118. Ibrahim H, Gurny R, Buri P, Grove J, Rozier A, Plazonnet B. Ocular bioavailability of pilocarpine from phase transition latex system triggered by pH. *Eur J Drug Metab Pharmacokinet* 1990;15(Suppl): 7;206.
119. Miller SC, Donovan MD. Effect of poloxamer 407 gel on the motic activity of pilocarpine nitrate in rabbits. *Int J Pharm* 1982;12: 147–152.
120. Harsh DC, Gehrke SH. Controlling the swelling characteristics of temperature-sensitive cellulose ether hydrogels. *J Contr Rel* 1991; 17:175–185.
121. Lindel K, Engstrom S. In vitro release of timolol maleate from an in-situ gelling polymer system. *Int J Pharm* 1993;95:219–228.
122. Joshi A, Ding S, Himmelstein KJ. Patent application US 91/04101 (Publication Wo 91/19481).
123. Kumar S, Haglund BO, Himmelstein KJ. In situ-forming gels of ophthalmic drug delivery. *J Ocul Pharmacol Ther* 1994;19:47–56.
124. Murray W. Lavine LS, Seifter E. The Iontophoresis of C21 Esterified Glucocorticoids. *J Am Phys Ther Assoc* 1963;43:579–581.
125. Gangarosa LP. Iontophoresis for surface local anesthesia. *J Am Dent Assoc* 1974;88:125–128.
126. Comeau M, Brummett R, Vernon J. Local anesthesia of the ear by Iontophoresis. *Arch Otolaryngol* 1973;98:114–120.
127. Wirtz R. Die Iontophoresis in Der Augenheilkunde. *Klin Monatsbl Augenheilkd* 1908;46:543–579.
128. Karbowski M. Iontophoresis in ophthalmology. *Ophthalmolica* 1939;97:166–202.
129. Smith VL. Iontophoresis in ophthalmology. *Am J Ophthalmol* 1951;34:698–704.
130. Erlanger G. Iontophoresis, a scientific and practical tool in ophthalmology. *Ophthalmologica* 1954;128:232–246.
131. Sarraf D, Lee DA. The role of iontophoresis in ocular drug delivery. *J Ocular Pharmacol Ther* 1994;10:69–81.
132. Hill FM, Park NH, Gangarosa LP, Hull DS, Tugle CL, Bowman K, Green K. Iontophoresis of vidarabine monophosphate into rabbit eye. *Invest Ophthalmol Vis Sci* 1978;17:473–476.
133. Hughes L, Maurice DM. A fresh look at Iontophoresis. *Arch Ophthalmol* 1984;102:1825–1829.
134. Rootman DS, Jantzen JA, Gonzalez JR, Fischer MJ, Beuerman R, Hill JM. Pharmacokinetics and safety of transcorneal Ionthophoresis of Tobramycin in the rabbit. *Invest Ophthalmol Vis Sci* 1988; 29:1397–1401.
135. Choi TB, Lee DA. Transscleral and transcorneal iontophoresis of vancomycin in rabbit eyes. *J Ocular Pharmacol Ther* 1988;4: 153–264.
136. Grossman RE, Chu DF, Lee DA. Regional ocular gentamycin levels after transcorneal and transscleral Iontophoresis. *Invest Ophthalmol Vis Sci* 1990;31:909–916.
137. Maurice DM. Iontophoresis of fluorescein into the posterior segment of the rabbit eye. *Ophthalmology* 1986;93:128–132.
138. Barza M, Peckman C, Baum J. Transscleral iontophoresis of cephazolin, ticarcillin, and gentamicin in the rabbit. *Ophthalmology* 1986;93:133–139.
139. Lam TT, Fu J, Tso MOM. A histopathologic study of retinal lesions inflicated by transscleral iontophoresis. *Graefes Arch Clin Exp Ophthalmol* 1991;229:389–394.
140. Hadgraft J, Walters KA, Wotton PK. Facilitated transport of sodium salicylate across artificial lipid membrane by Azone. *J Pharm Pharmacol* 1985;37:725–727.
141. Pardo A, Shiri Y, Cohen S. Kinetics of transdermal penetration of an organic ion pair: physostigmine salicylate. *J Pharm Sci* 1992;81: 990–995.
142. Tomlinson E, Davis SS, Dlejnik D, Wilson CG. Altered ocular absorption and disposition of sodium cromoglycate upon ion-pairing and complex coaccervate formation with dodecylbenzyl dimethyl amonium chloride. *J Pharm Pharmacol* 1981;31:749–753.
143. Davis SS, Tomlinson E, Wilson CG. The effect of ion-association on the transcorneal transport of drugs. *Br J Pharmacol* 1989;64:444–445.
144. Conroy CW, Buck RH. Influence on ion pairing salts on the transcorneal permeability of ionized sulfonamides. *J Ocular Pharmacol* 1992;8:233–240.

Textbook of Ocular Pharmacology,
edited by T.J. Zimmerman, et al.
Lippincott–Raven Publishers, Philadelphia © 1997.

CHAPTER 11

Development of New Drugs for Ophthalmology

Gary D. Novack

Although great progress has been made in the diagnosis and treatment of a large number of ocular disorders, there is still a great need for innovative therapies. Ideas for these therapies may come from basic scientists, clinical scientists, practitioners, internists, and other more systemically oriented physicians. The development of these ideas into therapies requires scientific assessment, clinical evaluation of efficacy and safety, review by regulatory agencies, and adoption by third-party payers. In this chapter, various aspects of these processes are discussed.

FINANCIAL AND TIME PERSPECTIVES

The financial requirements for the adoption of a novel therapeutic agent are immense. The exact assignment of costs is an accounting nightmare. For example, when does research in an area of basic science (e.g., how the immune system distinguishes self from foreign) become assignable to a given drug (e.g., evaluating Drug A as a suppressor of the inflammatory response) (1). The task of estimating these costs was undertaken by DiMasi and colleagues. Working with confidential data supplied by pharmaceutical firms for all medical specialties, they calculated an average time of 12 years and $114 million to develop a drug from initial chemical synthesis to approval for marketing (Fig. 11-1) (2). Factoring in the opportunity cost at a 9% interest rate yields an average cost estimate of $231 million. Both these figures are presented in 1987 U.S. dollars (3).

Many drugs used in ophthalmology were developed originally for the treatment of systemic disease, and their ophthalmic utility was found subsequently. Frequently, ophthalmic pharmaceutical companies have licensed the ophthalmic rights to another firm's systemic drug, which tends to decrease risk, costs, and time. Examples include ofloxacin, flurbiprofen, levobunolol, metipranolol, and fluorometholone. Systemic development of these drugs probably was near the estimate provided by DiMasi et al. (3), but the incremental cost of ophthalmic development was probably much less. More importantly, the U.S. Food and Drug Administration (FDA)'s review of ophthalmic compounds (Table 11-1) tends to be shorter than that of systemic drugs. As we explore more drugs targeted for ophthalmology as first indications rather than secondary indications, costs of development are no longer incremental but approach the large sums discussed for systemic drugs. Examples of these approaches for ophthalmic indications first, rather than later, include dorzolamide (MK-507) and latanoprost.

Given the requirement for a major outlay of funds over a long time, drug development typically is undertaken in a capitalistic framework. Heretofore predominantly the domain of large, established firms, in the past decade, we have seen a large increase in the entry of smaller, entrepreneurial firms with private funding sources. In a few cases, development has been sponsored by academic or government institutions. More typical in that case is that an academic center may conduct an initial clinical study, which in turn stimulates the interest of an industrial firm with the resources to commit to the longer-term development. In the 1990s, academic centers are finding competition for government-sponsored grants increasing and the per capita reimbursement for clinical procedures decreasing. Thus, industrial-sponsored research in either basic or clinical areas is increasingly attractive as a source of funding. Additional development alternatives being considered are joint ventures between academia and industry or between two industrial firms sharing the risks and benefits of research.

G. D. Novack: Pharma•Logic Development, Inc., San Rafael, California 94903.

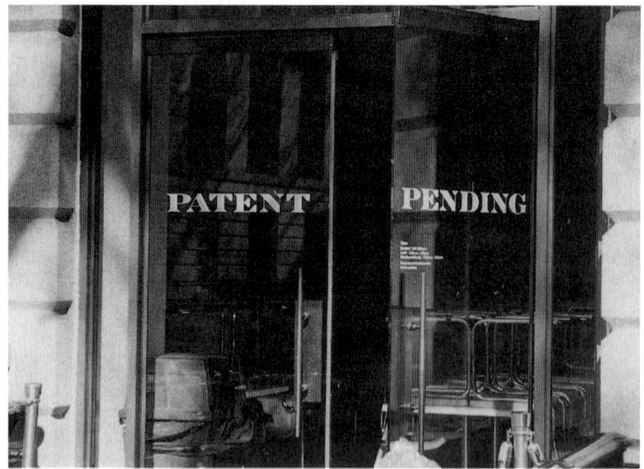

FIG. 11-1. Photograph of Old U.S. Patent Office, Washington, D.C.

PATENTS

An inherent assumption in the investment in research and development (R & D) by a pharmaceutical firm in a compound is a proprietary patent position. In other words, when a product is approved, the firm desires a period in which only it can market the product. In a sense, a patent is a limited, government-approved monopoly. The life of a U.S. patent traditionally has been 17 years. With implementation of the North American Free Trade Agreement, some interpret that this will be extended to 20 years. Also under discussion is a change in the U.S. system from "first to invent" to "first to file." The duration of patent life varies in other countries. Patents typically are applied for in the preclinical stage of development. Given review time by the patent office (see Fig. 11-1) and the time to develop and gain approval for the drug, the period of marketing protection is usually 10 years.

A *composition of matter* patent is awarded to the inventor who first patents a unique chemical entity. Inventors who later discover an application of this compound not claimed or "not obvious to one trained in the art" may obtain a *use* patent. Inventions of novel ophthalmic formulations (e.g., extended-duration vehicles) tend to be in this latter category. A composition of matter patent is preferred, as it typically provides the inventor a stronger proprietary position. In addition, use patents, which are issued in the United States, are not generally valid in countries such as Japan, Germany, and the U.K.

In the United States, the *Waxman-Hatch Act* of the 1980s provides some extension to the patent life of a product based on the time required for development and regulatory review. On the other hand, this same act makes it much easier for firms to market generic forms of the drug once the patent expires. Together, this means that "ethical" pharmaceutical firms (in contrast to generic firms) need to redevelop their business totally every 10 years. An example of the duration of proprietary protection is levobunolol, approved for marketing in the United States in 1982. The period of proprietary protection for the innovator firm ended in 1993, and generic forms of levobunolol were first marketed in 1994. The development period for a new drug is also approximately 10 years, which means it will be a decade before any revenue is realized for a compound being synthesized today, which in turn will generate significant revenue only for another decade before its proprietary protection expires. Thus, long-term strategic planning is an essential component for any major pharmaceutical firm. A corollary of this environment is that many of the employees who research a product may no longer be in their present positions when that product is marketed or when it reaches full market potential.

Whereas investors in pharmaceutical firms may have an opportunity for profit, there is also great risk. Approximately 99.9% of compounds synthesized do not become revenue-producing products for the company as a result of inadequate efficacy, unacceptable toxicity, or other reasons. The key in the scientific method of drug development is to ask the decisive question (experiment) as early as possible, before resources are expended unnecessarily. For example, if the goal is to develop a longer-acting pilocarpine, the duration of ocular hypotensive action of the new agent relative to conventional pilocarpine is the most important experiment. If a more comfortable antiinflammatory agent is the goal, an early experiment should be a comparison of the new agent to a currently marketed one. Another area of risk is product liability. One need only consider the lawsuits regarding birth defects from Bendectin (doxylamine and pyridoxine), immune disorders from breast implants, and psychoses from Halcion (triazolam) to realize the potential for substantial losses related to product use.

THE PHARMACEUTICAL INDUSTRY

The pharmaceutical industry is a major sector of the U.S. economy, with approximately 500,000 employees and 100 billion dollars per year in revenue, representing 3% of the total sales of Fortune 500 companies (4). Given the intense capital investment, extensive development times, shortening product life cycles, and publicity of many pharmaceutical firms, the financial world follows the financial performance of these firms closely. This increased scrutiny includes careful review of research results presented at scientific meetings, such as efficacy and safety results of major clinical trials. In one extreme case, a stockbroker changed his buy/sell recommendation of a given stock based on the selection of the data as a poster rather than an oral paper at a major meeting.

As startup companies recruit personnel required to research and develop compounds, their expenses increase. The use of funds per unit time is called the *cash burn rate*. This rate is particularly critical in small firms that have no

TABLE 11-1. *NDA review times for selected ophthalmic products*

Drug	Sponsor	Initial	Approval date	Interval (mo)	Indication	NCE
Antazoline/ Naphazoline (Vasocon-A)	IOLAB	26 February 1982	30 April 1990	98	Conjunctivitis	No
Apraclonidine (Iopidine)	Alcon	1 October 1987[a]	31 December 1987	3	Glaucoma	Yes
Caretolol HCl (Optipress)	BW	20 April 1989	23 May 1990	13	Glaucoma	No
Ciprofloxacin (Ciloxan)	Alcon	20 July 1989	31 December 1990	18	Infection	No
Diclofenac (Voltaren)	Ciba	18 December 1989	28 March 1991	16	Inflammation	No
Disodium cromoglycate (Opticrom)	Fisons	17 March 1981	3 October 1984	42	Allergic conjunctivitis	No
Dorzolamide (Trusopt)	Merck	17 December 1993	20 December 1994	12	Glaucoma	Yes
Fluorometholone acetate (Omnitrol)	Alcon	21 July 1983	11 February 1986	31	Inflammation	Yes
Fluorometholone/ sulfacetamide (FML-S)	Allergan	16 September 1985	29 September 1989	48	Inflammation	No
Foscarnet (intravenous, Foscavir)[b]	Astra	18 November 1990	27 August 1991	10	CMV retinitis	Yes
Ganciclovir (intravenous; Cytovene)[b]	Syntex	25 December 1985	23 June 1989	43	CMV retinitis	Yes
Ganciclovir (intravitreal, Vitrasert)	Chiron	28 June 1995	4 March 1996	9	CMV retinitis	No
Ketorolac (Accular)	Syntex	27 May 1987	9 November 1992	66	Allergic conjunctivitis	No
Levobunolol (generic)	Bausch and Lomb	30 December 1992	24 June 1994	7	Glaucoma	No (ANDA)
Levocabastine (Livostin)	IOLAB	10 October 1991	10 November 1993	25	Allergy	Yes
Metipranolol (Optipranolol)	Bausch and Lomb	19 October 1988	29 December 1989	14	Glaucoma	Yes
Norfloxacin (Chibroxin)	Merck	31 August 1987	17 June 1991	47	Infection	No
Pilocarpine Gel (Pilopine)	Alcon	19 May 1982	17 March 1983	10	Glaucoma	No
Rimexolone (Vexol)	Alcon	31 May 1994	30 December 1994	7	Inflammation	Yes
Timolol gel (Timoptic-XE)	Merck	20 January 1993	4 November 1993	10	Glaucoma	No
Timolol hemihydrate (Betimol)	Leiras	17 February 1994	31 March 1995	13	Glaucoma	Yes (new salt)
Tobramycin/ fluorometholone acetate (Tobrasone)	Alcon	31 December 86	21 July 1989	31	Inflammation	No

From FDA Approved Drug Products (through December 1995) and Summary Bases of Approval (SBA) obtained through Freedom of Information Action.

Submission dates are as stated on the SBA cover letter. These are dates assigned by the FDA and may differ from the date actually submitted by the sponsor.

[a]Estimate.

[b]The primary reviewing division for Cytovene and Foscavir was the Anti-Virals Division.

NCE, new chemical entity (A Yes indicates that this molecule was not previously approved by any route for any indication by the FDA); BW, Burroughs Wellcome; CMV, cytomegalovirus

product revenue as yet. For many such firms, at projected cash burn rates, cash reserves will last 2 years or less, which means that additional funding is needed. These potential investors typically want to know how much progress the company has made in its R & D plan. Thus, there is always a push for frequent and rapid communication with the results of experiments, particularly clinical efficacy trials. Contrast this need for rapid communication to the investment community with the typical time frame of a clinical study. When a study is completed and the results are analyzed, a clinical scientist typically would submit an abstract for presentation at a meeting with a 6-month lead time. In that interval, a manuscript might be submitted for publication. Given review time and publication lag, such a publication might appear within a year. This long lead time, as well as copyright standards, may be at odds with the communication needs of the financial side of the firm (5,6).

A firm typically has many possible research ideas that could be developed. Because resources are rarely sufficient to develop all candidates fully, a selection process must occur. The factors typically considered include the project cost and time for development, the chance of success, the projected expenses, projected revenues, and patent life. The product needs of the medical community in coming years must also be assessed. Focused discussions with opinion leaders in the specialty can occur or current sales trends be projected; however, in the long run, these are only estimates, and, in the end, intuition is an equally important attribute used in selecting candidates for further development.

Optimization of company resources in the simultaneous development of several products is a field called *project management.* In this ever-increasingly sophisticated area, specialists determine the tasks, their absolute timing (stability data on a formulation will be available 6 months after start), their interrelationship (e.g., task A must occur 3 months before task B but 6 weeks after task C), and their cost. The concepts of "as late as possible" or "as soon as possible" must also be considered. Air travel across the United States provides a useful analogy (Fig. 11-2). Assume that one must travel from the west coast to a relatively small town in the southeast, which would require three planes: from city A to city B, city B to city C, and finally, city C to city D. Bad weather at city B frequently delays the arrival of the flight from city A; however, it also delays the departure of the second flight from city B to city C. The bad weather at city B rarely affects plane schedules

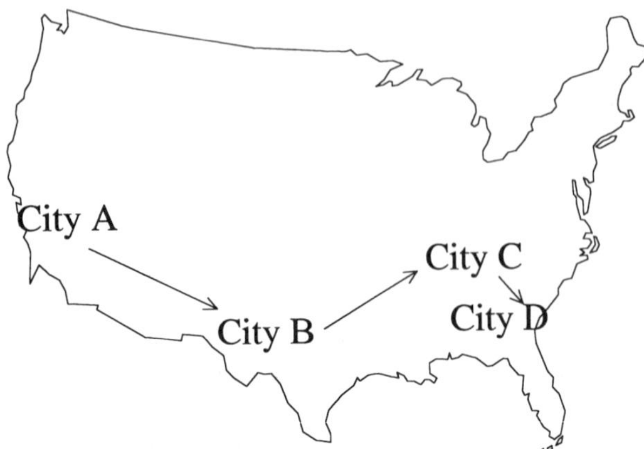

FIG. 11-2. Theoretical cross-country plane flight with multiple connections used in analogy to project management.

at city C. Thus, one might frequently arrive late in city C, with no delay in the scheduled departure of the flight from city C to city D. If that interflight interval, scheduled at 50 minutes, is still 20 minutes, one can generally make that third flight. If that interval is only 10 minutes, the third flight is missed and the passenger would have to wait 2 hours for the next one. Thus, the first two flights could be up to 30 minutes late with no impact on the final arrival time in city D, but if the second flight is 45 minutes late, one would be 2 hours late. In the same way, project managers assess whether a delay of X months in a given task will delay the overall project by X months, $3X$ months, or not at all.

IMPACT OF U.S. HEALTH CARE REFORM AND THIRD-PARTY PAYERS

As the proportion of the U.S. gross national product spent on health care remains significant, the government and third-party payers (e.g., health care insurance firms) will be concerned with costs. Although physicians and pharmaceuticals represent only about a fourth of U.S. health care expenses, the nature of their billing and compensation makes them obvious targets for cost reduction. To date, the American Medical Association and the Pharmaceutical Research and Manufacturers Association have been visible participants in health care system reform.

It seems likely that this reform will focus on utilization issues; that is, the cost of a given therapeutic intervention is to be judged on the total cost of using the health care system by this patient. In one scenario, a given drug may be less expensive than another, but if it requires an additional four office visits to adjust dosing adequately, in the long run it may be more expensive to the health-care provider. If the provider is a health-maintenance organization, the therapy with a lower overall cost may be selected. In a situation where a private practitioner is compensated on a capitation basis, any additional expense "comes out of pocket." Another example is the cost of medical versus surgical therapy for a chronic condition. A given surgical procedure may be more expensive than a year's worth of medical therapy. If the patient is expected to live for an additional 20 years, however, the surgical procedure might be less expensive in the long run. Today, we see hospitals competing with each other for technological advances, such as the $3 million gamma knife (7). In the future, we may see a greater financial analysis of the need for expensive technologies that provide incremental benefit to only a few.

It will be increasingly difficult to recoup development expenses with a product of only marginal improvement on existing therapies. One would project that the managed care environment would be slow to adopt new therapies that do not provide a substantial benefit. Adoption is even less likely if these newer products are more expensive. Conceptually, the pharmaceutical firm could set the selling price of such products at less than the existing therapies, although to do so would be difficult. These newer agents may be more expensive to produce (e.g., biotechnology products versus simple botanical extracts). More importantly, the substantial costs of research and development must be recouped. If this investment of time, money, and risk is not rewarded within the period of proprietary protection, a business is less likely to make the investment in the first place.

SEQUENTIAL NATURE OF RESEARCH AND DEVELOPMENT PROCESS

Discovery and development of drugs are parts of a sequential process, as displayed in Fig. 11-3 (2). A novel therapeutic agent frequently begins as a theoretical modification of a physiological process. Examples include the antagonism of the chronotropic effects of catecholamines (propranolol) (8) or antagonism of carbonic anhydrase in the ciliary body (acetazolamide) (9). In such cases, the body's own agonist or enzyme substrate is the chemical starting point for a series of analogs. So, for example, the first compounds synthesized as potential antagonists of epinephrine were analogs of epinephrine. In the same schema, the first compounds synthesized as antagonists at H_2-histamine receptors were analogs of histamine.

Preclinical Pharmacology

The various chemical analogs are screened for activity in in vitro and in vivo pharmacological and biochemical models for this disease. The biological model need not be an exact model *of* the disease, merely a model *for* the disease. That is, the model's sensitivity and specificity with respect to existing clinical therapies are more important than whether the animal disease actually looks like the human disease (10). For example, β-adrenoceptor antagonists, although not so effective as ocular hypotensive agents in normal rabbits, can antagonize the ocular hypotensive effects of isoproterenol. This action of the β-

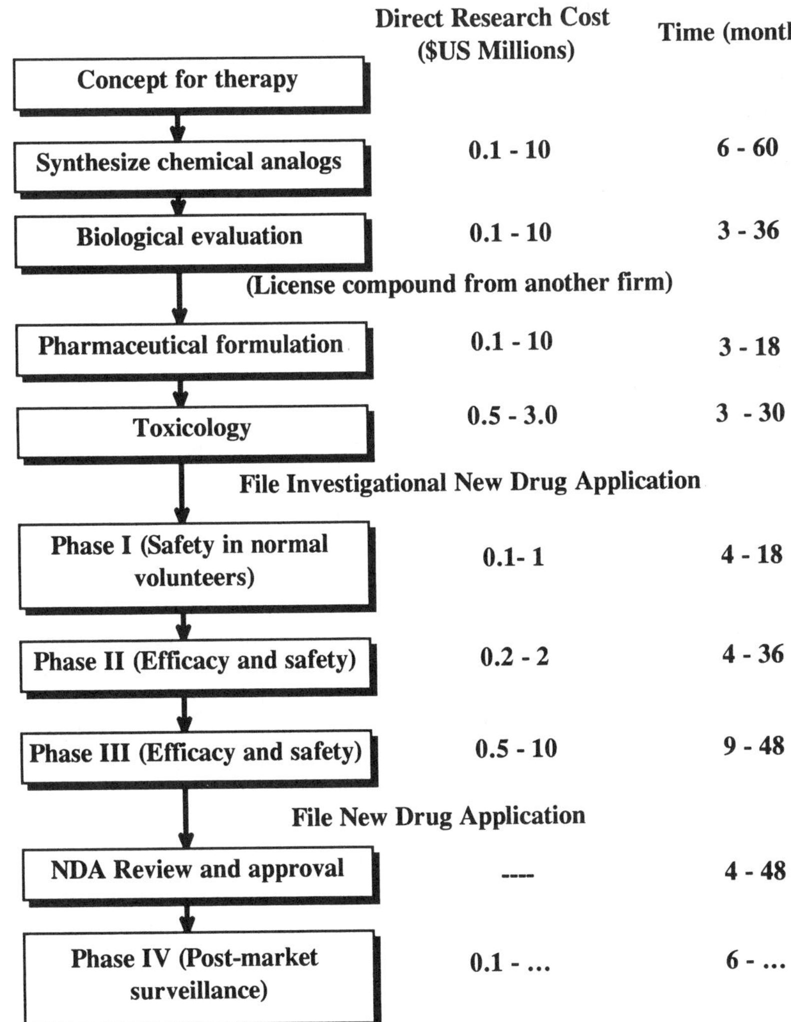

FIG. 11-3. The drug development process. Timing and direct research cost are provided based on the author's experience. Additional developmental costs, not displayed, may include chemistry and manufacturing expenses, capital equipment and facilities, administrative and management time, insurance, and the cost of funds. IND, Investigational New Drug Application; NDA, New Drug Application. (From Novack, ref. 2, with permission.)

adrenoceptor antagonist, which is actually a hypertensive effect, can be used to evaluate new agents for intraocular β-adrenoceptor blockade in a relatively inexpensive model (11).

In many research laboratories today, chemists use three-dimensional computer modeling programs to evaluate the interaction of potential molecules with the putative active site. Such "rational drug development" means that fewer compounds need to be synthesized and evaluated. Unfortunately, these techniques are still being refined, and one still needs to synthesize many molecules, a large proportion of which do not have the desired biological activity.

Combination Products

In addition to novel chemicals synthesized for ophthalmic use and compounds previously used systemically, there is a third route for novel product development: combination products. These products take two agents and combine them in one bottle. Examples include the combination of a corticosteroid and an antibiotic (e.g., Tobradex, Pred-G), two antiglaucoma agents (e.g., PE, TimPilo), and two or more antibiotics (e.g., Polytrim). Whereas formulation, toxicology, and clinical work are still substantially involved in these products, they are typically less risky than development of novel chemical entities. Of course, from a marketing perspective, they are also less rewarding and often involve merely the switch from one of the firm's older products to another, newer one ("cannibalization").

Pharmaceutics (Formulation)

The next step is *pharmaceutical formulation,* which begins with an evaluation of the molecule's stability and solubility, that is, how one can best put the drug into a vehicle (e.g., water, oil, gel) in which it will be comfortable for the patient, consistent in its delivery, and stable on the drugstore shelf for a long time. An ideal drug candidate has the requisite balance of hydrophilicity and lipophilicity to enable it to cross the corneal barrier readily. The most preferred delivery system for ophthalmic agents is an aqueous eyedrop. A drug may be insoluble in water, necessitating a micronized suspension (e.g., corticosteroids). Thus, pharmaceutical scientists are challenged to develop aqueous formulations in which the drug remains stable for a product shelf life of at least 2 years at room temperature. Multidose containers require protection against microbial contamination; thus, a preservative that is compatible with the drug and not irritating to the eye must be added. The pH and buffering of the formulation must not lead to discomfort nor the viscosity interfere with instillation or visual clarity. Some drugs are inherently discomforting, and acceptance can be provided only by decreasing the concentration of the active molecule in the final formulation.

Toxicology

The next step in drug development is toxicology. Also known as safety evaluation, this step involves exposing several species of animals to increasingly larger doses and durations of treatment with the test compound. This continuum begins with *acute* (one dose up to several instillations per day), continues with *subacute* (up to 1 month), and finally *chronic* studies (6 to 12 months). These studies evaluate any changes in animal health or behavior as well as extensive gross and microscopic pathology. Acute and subacute studies are generally required before testing the novel drug in humans. The commitment of resources for chronic studies is generally not made until there are some positive data from the short-term human trials. Drugs intended for chronic use also may require in vitro evaluation of their mutagenicity and in vivo evaluation of their potential for eliciting birth defects (teratogenicity) and cancer (carcinogenicity).

Investigational New Drug Application

At this point, the company evaluates the biological evidence for activity, its potency for efficacy relative to its potency for toxicity, and the suitability of the compound for acceptable formulations. If these criteria are met and there is still a large projected therapeutic need for this type of compound, the firm proposes clinical evaluation. A regulatory submission is required in most countries to administer an investigational drug to humans. In the United States, this regulatory submission is called an Investigational New Drug (IND) application. This submission includes reports from the biology, toxicology, and pharmaceutics studies; the proposed clinical plan and indication for use; and the chemistry and pharmaceutics to demonstrate a stable, known product. In practice, a firm generally confers with the FDA before this point ("pre-IND Application" meeting) to ensure that the early development plan will provide sufficient data and be of limited risk to volunteers and patients. Over the past 15 years, responsibility for FDA review of ophthalmic drugs have resided with the Division of Anti-Infective Drugs, the Division of Medical Imaging, Surgical and Dental Drug Products, the Division of Topical Drugs, and, as of early 1996, the Division of Analgesic, Anti-inflammatory, and Ophthalmic Drug Products. Technically, the IND Application is a notification to the FDA that, if no word to the contrary is heard, the company will begin the proposed clinical studies in approximately 30 days. The filing of an IND application and its status are confidential unless released by the firm. Therefore, it is not possible to state accurately the number of drugs under active clinical investigation for ophthalmological indications or their developmental status. In other countries, the IND process may be either longer or shorter than in the United States. For example, the review period in Spain is

4 months; in England and Germany, essentially only local institutional review board (IRB) approval is required for evaluation in normal volunteers.

Clinical Phases

Clinical research studies are divided into four major phases: Phases I through IV. *Phase I* studies are intended primarily to evaluate the safety and pharmacokinetics of the new drug in normal volunteers, starting with low doses for brief periods (e.g., one drop) and continuing to more extended concentrations, frequencies, and durations. The objective is to monitor the safety of the product while slowly increasing the exposure (dose, frequency, and duration) to the volunteer. The comfort of the formulation is often assessed at this time (12–14). Several potential products have been found unacceptable at this stage, either because of discomfort caused by a novel vehicle or by a combination of two agents that were comfortable given separately but not together. In America today, it is important to know the systemic exposure of ocularly instilled drugs. It is during Phase I that many firms choose to evaluate plasma levels of the topically applied drugs (15). Only about a third of all drugs entering Phase I evaluation make it to Phase III evaluation (3). A drug clears Phase I evaluations with negative data, that is, the absence of significant ocular or systemic toxicity at intended therapeutic doses. The patent position on the proprietary nature of the new drug may not be clear at this time. For these reasons, few Phase I studies are submitted for publication. Because toxicology studies on the drug's potential teratogenicity are generally not complete at this time, use by women of child-bearing potential in these studies is restricted.

Phase II studies also employ dosage escalation regimens similar to those in Phase I but in patients with the intended disease rather than in normal volunteers. Phase II studies include dose-response, time-response evaluations (16,17). Early Phase II studies are generally placebo controlled, as absolute efficacy is the first question (18,19). If enhanced efficacy or safety over existing therapy is a sine qua non for the putative product, then Phase II studies may incorporate active controls. It is only after the completion of a Phase II trial that the pharmaceutical company gets human efficacy data for its compound. The interval from demonstration of efficacy in animal models until receiving results from Phase II studies may be up to several years and may cost several million dollars. When one hears of early reports of efficacy in the literature or at meetings, it is generally a pilot Phase II study. Examples of ophthalmic drugs for which further development was stopped after Phase II include metoprolol (too short-acting) (20) and diacetyl-nadolol (blepharoconjunctivitis) (21).

Once efficacy in patients has been demonstrated many ethical, financial, scientific, and political pressures remain to proceed rapidly toward the next step: Phase III trials; however, investigation as to the selection of the appropriate concentration and frequency of use should be a key segment of Phase II investigations. Many clinical pharmacologists in industry, government, and academia feel that hastening Phase III trials results in failure to optimize the dose. With oral therapy in systemic medicine, one can modify dosing by taking two pills rather than one pill or by scoring a pill in half. In ophthalmology, one cannot realistically modify dose by instilling a second drop or by giving half a drop. Many of our marketed drugs are available only in one or two concentrations; so doses can be modified only by modifying frequency of use. If only one concentration is to be selected for further development, one generally errs on the side of a higher concentration to maximize efficacy rather than to risk a lower concentration, for which there might be greater potential safety. This tendency to select dosing that represents the "plateau" phase of the dose-response curve is probably reasonable for drugs with large therapeutic indices (e.g., antibiotics) but probably worthy of further exploration for drugs with narrower therapeutic indices (e.g., autonomic drugs and corticosteroids).

Phase III studies are extended trials (up to one year of dosing per patient) in large patient populations (generally in the hundreds) with the concentration, formulation, and dosing regimens as intended for use in patients when the product is marketed (22–25). Both safety and efficacy are measured in Phase III. For most drugs, at least two Phase III trials are required to provide substantive evidence of efficacy and safety. As with all clinical trials, the cost of Phase III trials includes the physician's time for examining and treating the patient, laboratory tests, in-patient stays, the study medications, and study management and data handling. As one must conduct at least two Phase III trials, and they must include large numbers of patients for long treatment periods, this is the most expensive phase of drug development, with costs ranging from hundreds of thousands to millions of dollars. The logistics of administering these large studies will often exceed the ability of the pharmaceutical company's staff; so independent private research organizations are sometimes employed to assist in the trial management. An example of an ophthalmic drug rejected after Phase III trials is oral sorbinil, intended for diabetic retinopathy, because of inadequate efficacy (26).

Biostatistical Issues

An important definition in comparative trials of efficacy and safety is the *clinically significant difference.* Any measurement in a patient is confounded by inherent variability among patients, the pathological condition, drug manufacture, compliance, and the measurement error of any device employed. One must define what change, if observed consistently, would constitute a meaningful difference. Both the firm that designs the studies and the FDA reviewers must agree on the dividing line for differences as being clinically meaningful or not. For the recently approved ophthalmic quinolone antibiotics, a clinically significant difference was a 20% difference in cure rates between the quinolone and the standard therapy (tobramycin or gentamycin). This approval required approximately 80 to 100 evaluable patients per treatment group. Given that only 42% of patients who entered with clinical bacterial infections met the rigorous culture requirements (24), approximately 450 patients per trial or 900 Phase III patients were required. For a recently approved topical antiinflammatory drug, a clinically significant difference was 0.5 to 1.0 grades in anterior chamber cells (0–3 scale), requiring about 100 patients per group per study (27).

In the mid-1980s, published papers on antiglaucoma therapies assumed a clinically significant difference in ocular hypotensive therapies of approximately 4 mm Hg (28). In other words, if the two drugs are declared equivalent in the trial, the difference in ocular hypotensive efficacy between them would be, at most, 4 mm Hg. From today's perspective, that was too liberal, as several agents were found to be equivalent to timolol within 4 mm Hg but not within 2 mm Hg. For recently approved novel ocular hypotensive agents, a clinically significant difference was judged to be 2 mm Hg (12), which required about 30 to 50 patients per group per trial. Should an even more rigorous standard, such as a 1 mm Hg difference, be set? This standard is most likely too rigorous, as most clinicians would judge two agents that differed by only 1 mm Hg in their ocular hypotensive efficacy to be similar. If this more rigorous standard were selected, the sample size (and therefore costs and time) would have to be doubled to reach this standard. Thus, it is probably an inappropriate use of resources to detect a difference smaller than clinically relevant. Even with relatively large Phase III trials (e.g., 1,000 patients), only relatively frequent adverse events (that is, incidence of $\geq$1% or greater) are expected to be detected, and differences in safety between agents are extremely difficult to detect.

In designing a Phase III trial, one must project what the standards for regulatory review and clinical utility will be several years in the future. For example, antiglaucoma drugs have been approved to date on the basis of their ocular hypotensive efficacy. It is generally accepted that increased intraocular pressure (IOP) carries with it an increased risk of further progressive loss of visual field (29,30). Also monitored in studies for approved drugs were visual field (either by manual Goldmann or automated threshold techniques) and cup-disk ratio (by direct ophthalmoscopy). There is a large body of peer-reviewed literature on the influence of accepted glaucoma therapies on these measures. We know what the standard therapies do to these measures and how to interpret statistically significant differences vis-à-vis their clinical relevance (31). There are a host of developing methodologies for the measurement of ocular pathology, including novel visual field tests (32,33), stereoacuity (34), retinal nerve fiber layer photographs (35,36), and measures of color function (34, 37,38). In the future, these measures of visual function may become standards of care in evaluating the effect of glaucoma therapy; however, such tests are not fully validated as to their ability to measure the efficacy of glaucoma therapy. Validation would come from controlled clinical trials as well as clinical experience in how meaningful such measures are in diagnosis and therapeutic management. One would hesitate to risk the time and resources of a Phase III trial using investigational measurement systems to evaluate investigational agents.

Another decision in study design is the crossover versus parallel comparison. In a *crossover study,* each patient receives each treatment in a separate period. In a *parallel study,* patients are randomized to receive only one of the treatments. Crossover studies require fewer patients than parallel studies and have the inherent appeal of using each patient as their own control; however, all patients must complete all periods, there can be no unequal carryover of treatment effect from one period to the next, and the disease must remain stable (39). With β-adrenoceptor antagonists having effects for at least 2 weeks (40), it is unlikely that a crossover trial is the preferred method for evaluating these types of agents.

Patients generally underdose both in number and in interval between doses (41,42), which tends to underestimate both the efficacy and toxicity of a drug and complicate the evaluation of a novel therapy. One would like to be able to separate the actions of the drug per se from the actions of the drug plus its method of use. Ideally, one would have an objective measure of compliance and then correlate the lack of efficacy or adverse events to underdosing or overdosing. Such devices are available for oral medications. In evaluation of an antiepileptic therapy, it was clear that cases of apparent inadequate efficacy (seizures) were correlated with inadequate compliance and thus most likely not related to the drug (43). One would not want to discontinue development of a drug for inadequate efficacy when it was really just a case of inadequate compliance. Whereas there are devices that have been used to monitor compliance with oral medication regimens (44), none is currently available for ophthalmic medication.

All clinical evaluations should be conducted by an independent investigator in studies designed to minimize bias. Where possible, this involves masking the study medications and the use of positive and negative controls (45). For example, when evaluating the mydriatic potential of a new drug, one should attempt to include both a mydriatic (i.e., cyclopentolate) as a positive control and the vehicle of the new drug as a negative control. If it is difficult to mask the investigator from the treatment (i.e., laser or surgical procedures), an independent observer may be employed to make critical measurements (46). Any proprietary relationship of the clinical investigator with the product being evaluated should be disclosed.

Good Clinical Practices

Clinical researchers and regulatory agencies are developing a series of guidelines for the conductance of clinical trials. These guidelines, called Good Clinical Practices (GCP), dictate a clear written record of the clinical trial. The wide range of GCP covers protocols, patient informed consent, IRB review, patient exposure to the drug, analysis, and reporting. For example, it is important to document clearly the version and date of a protocol, and any changes need to be documented and signed by the sponsor and, in most cases, the IRB. In another example, clinical data need to be entered into a computer in an organized, auditable format and reviewed against the source data (e.g., computer printout needs to be checked against a case report form and then, in some cases, against patient records). A major underlying idea of GCP is that after a study is complete, an independent individual could go back and confirm exactly what was done, how it was done, and who did it.

It may seem that such efforts toward "paperwork" are unwarranted, but these studies involve major commitments of time, money, and patients. Moreover, regulatory approval and health care system decisions are based on them. In one instance, there was some question about the traceability of data in a large study sponsored by the National Cancer Institute. After the trial was completed and published and had influenced the choice of various surgical therapies for breast cancer, there were some questions about the entry and analysis of patient data (47).

The American, European, and Japanese standards for GCP differ today, but through the International Conference on Harmonization, a universal worldwide standard is being developed. Among the issues being addressed are the complexities of informed consent. Fully informed consent requires a number of key elements, including a description of the study, its benefits and risks, the total number of subjects being recruited, and the right of the subject to withdraw from the study at any time. The role of informed consent in the development of new therapies was evidenced by a 1994 FDA decision to put a hold on further studies of an investigational device. The device enabled an emergency worker to both compress and decompress the chest during cardiopulmonary resuscitation (48). This situation was resolved through a "community informed consent," but such issues will continue to arise in sight-threatening and life-threatening diseases with new, relatively untested therapies.

Orphan Drugs and Ethics Issues

The U.S. Congress passed the *Orphan Drug Act* in 1983 to provide incentives for development of drugs for rare diseases. The incentives of the orphan drug act include (a) tax credits for human clinical research undertaken by a sponsor to generate data required for approval; and (b) exclusive U.S. marketing rights for 7 years after marketing approval. A pending bill may limit this exclusivity to 4 years with the potential for a 3-year extension (49). Generally, a *rare* disease is defined as one with fewer than 200,000 affected Americans. Amendments to the act in subsequent years deleted the requirement that designations be allowed only for drugs for which no U.S. patent was issued. These amendments also clarified that the orphan indication could be filed anytime before the filing of a New Drug Application (NDA) or Product License Application (PLA; the equivalent of an NDA for a biological product). Also, orphan designations can be requested for antibiotics but not for devices or medical foods (50).

The Congress intended that the FDA assist firms that obtain orphan drug indications. Contrary to perception, there is no explicit requirement that the FDA lower the requirements for product approval for drugs with orphan designation. As orphan drugs, however, the available patient population is by definition low. Thus, the clinical development plans generally employed are unique. Open-label protocols for compassionate use of the drug while it is in development are typically allowed. The firm is required to present documentation of the incidence of the targeted disease as well as a rationale for the proposed use of the drug in treating the disease and some manufacturing information.

The orphan designation is given based on the disease and the drug but not the formulation. Thus, exclusivity, as granted by the FDA, could allow more than one firm to market the same drug as long as the indication is different (Table 11-2, Situation 1); the inverse may be also allowed. More than one firm could market for the same indication if the drugs were different (Table 11-2, Situation 2). It is in this definition of what a different drug is that interesting situations could develop. Oculinum/Botox has been approved, and, based on its orphan designation, it received exclusive marketing rights in the U.S. for 7 years. Thus, additional botulinum toxin products may be barred from receiving marketing approval for the same disease unless they are determined to be a drug different from Oculinum/Botox.

Differences in formulation (e.g., suspension versus solution) are typically not considered different enough to be a

TABLE 11-2. *Theoretical application of the orphan drug designation*

Drug	Indication	Firm
Situation 1: Multiple indications for the same drug		
1	1	1
1	2	2
1	3	3
Situation 2: Multiple drugs for the same indication		
1	1	1
2	1	2
3	1	3

different drug; however, the former director of the FDA Center for Biologics Evaluation and Research stated, "... if the second drug [with a different formulation or stabilizing proteins] were shown to be clinically superior, this could provide a basis for granting it orphan drug status" (51). The "hair-splitting" tactics in this arena are evident (Table 11-3). Porton obtained an orphan designation for "essential blepharospasm" for serotype A several years after Allergan obtained a designation for "blepharospasm associated with dystonia in adults." For example, whereas Allergan has exclusivity for serotype A in cervical dystonia, Athena was granted the same indication for serotype B. Also, BioPure (now Associated Synapse Biologics) was able to obtain a designation for serotype A for a rather narrow use (even in orphan designation terms): eyelid closure problems after facial nerve damage. Additional examples of orphan designations within ophthalmology include vernal conjunctivitis (lodoxamide) and treatment of refractory glaucoma as an adjunct to externoglaucoma surgery (mitomycin-c). At this time, such orphan drug incentives do not exist in Europe or Japan, although they are being discussed.

Treatment for life-threatening illnesses, such as AIDS, generates significant discussion regarding the ethics of drug development. One would question whether a full preclinical package of pharmacology, toxicology, and pharmaceutics would be required to evaluate the clinical efficacy of a treatment of such a disease. On the one hand, some would argue that if the patient is already terminally ill, any potential therapy should be made available, even if there is some toxicity. On the other hand, some argue that certain basic information is required. An interim case is the possibility of a drug that allowed the patient to worsen to a near-death state but prevented the final event that precipitated death. It would actually be unethical to allow widespread use of such an agent, as it would prolong the suffering of a patient with no benefit. A further posit is an investigational agent that would decrease the bioavailability of a concomitant medication that has already proved effective. In this way, the investigational agent, which itself is of unproved efficacy, actually could harm the patient in attenuating the efficacy of an existing medication. To my knowledge, neither of these situations exists. On the positive side, an agent developed in the 1940s to prolong the time course of penicillin, probenecid, prolongs the time course of selected antiviral compounds. Although of limited clinical benefit for other reasons, this example points out a rationale for early pharmacokinetic evaluation of compounds, even in life-threatening diseases (47, 52,53).

TABLE 11-3. *U.S. orphan drug designations for botulinum toxins*[a]

Type	Firm/brand	Indication	Designated	Date marketed
A	Allergan (Oculinum/ Botox)	Blepharospasm associated with dystonia in adults (≥12 yr)	22 March 1984	29 December 1989
A	Allergan (Oculinum/ Botox)	Strabismus associated with dystonia in adults (≥ 12 yr)	22 March 1984	29 December 1989
A	Allergan (Oculinum/ Botox)	Cervical dystonia	20 August 1986	
A	Porton (Dysport)	Essential blepharospasm	23 March 1989	
A	Allergan (Oculinum Botox)	Dynamic muscle contracture in pediatric cerebral palsy patients	6 December 1991	
A	Associated Synapse Biologics	Synkinetic closure of the eyelid associated with VII cranial nerve aberrant regeneration	15 September 1992	
B	Athena (BotB)	Cervical dystonia	16 January 1992	
F	Porton (Dysport)	Essential blepharospasm	3 December 1991	
F	Porton (Dysport)	Cervical dystonia	24 October 1991	

Source: Food and Drug Administration (FDA)-approved drug products (through December 1993) and Summary Bases of Approval (SBA) obtained through *Freedom of Information Action.*

[a]The California Department of Health (Berkeley) also has an orphan indication for a botulinum toxin antibody (botulism immune globulin) for the treatment of infant botulism (i.e., food poisoning).

New Drug Application

If the agent proves effective, relatively safe, and has the intended characteristics (i.e., safer than current therapy or greater efficacy or longer duration of action), the firm decides to request marketing approval from the FDA. This request, called a New Drug Application (NDA) in America, is a large submission (up to 150 volumes) requiring the integration of the extensive clinical program (which may involve millions of pieces of data). Each piece of clinical data must have been checked from its source (generally a case report form) through its various electronic manipulations. At least several months are involved in the equality check of these data and the subsequent rigorous statistical analysis. The NDA must include the toxicology, chemistry, manufacturing, and controls data. The firm must have demonstrated that the product can be manufactured at a site that meets rigorous demands of quality control and repeatability.

As mentioned, many drugs have already been approved for systemic use before submission of the NDA for the ophthalmic indication (e.g., norfloxacin). This systemic experience provides a larger knowledge base for the FDA in their review of the possible risks associated with the drug. The review of NDA for all specialties by the FDA ranges from 1 to 3 years (54). There are examples of short review times in ophthalmology (e.g., apraclonidine was reviewed in less than 3 months), but the review time for most recently approved ophthalmic drugs falls into the published range noted previously. The review is generally an interactive process in which the FDA may ask for clarification, reanalysis, additional studies, or revisions to the proposed indications. After approval of the NDA, the company may sell the drug as prescribed by physicians.

Not all drugs and their indications used by ophthalmologists have approved NDA at the FDA. Drugs introduced before 1962 (e.g., pilocarpine, epinephrine, or oral fluorescein) are not "approved," but their use is acceptable in standard practice. Still other drugs are approved for one indication but prescribed for another. For example, at this time, no topical nonsteroidal antiinflammatory drug is approved in the United States for the treatment of cystoid macular edema. These agents may be prescribed for this indication by an ophthalmologist, but a firm may not promote its drug for this unapproved claim. The FDA has taken a strong line against promotion for unapproved indications (55). Although such promotion is not generally allowed in the United States, a physician is generally allowed to use approved medications for unapproved, or "off-label," use.

On the Market

Phase IV studies are conducted either during the review period or after approval. These may be for extended indications (56) (i.e., additional dosage regimens or diseases) or extended human experience for safety evaluation in larger patient populations in more "real-world" use (i.e., postmarket surveillance) (57–59). In this phase, one may further evaluate the utility of one agent when used in combination with another marketed product. For example, the NDA for levobunolol was for the 0.5% strength for once and twice daily use, with both placebo- and timolol-controlled studies. During the approximately 2-year review period, and in the subsequent years, Phase IV studies were conducted on the 0.25% strength, both once and twice daily, on the use of levobunolol for elevations in IOP after laser or cataract surgery and compared with other marketed agents, such as betaxolol and metipranolol (60–64). Supplements to the NDA have so far resulted in approval for 0.25% levobunolol, twice daily.

As noted, good long-range planning is required to keep useful therapeutic agents that are adopted by physicians and payers alike. In considering this factor, the firm needs to understand clearly the difference between *features* and *benefits*. As an example, an analogy to automobiles is provided. The American family has demanded that minivans have built-in holders for cups. In an effort to better the competition, one manufacturer has included the feature of a special holder for a garage door opener. To the driver who lives in a house in the suburbs with an automatic garage door, this probably will be a benefit, but this feature would be of no consequence, and thus will not be a benefit, to a driver who has no garage. In the same way, features of a drug (e.g., multiplicity of target enzyme inhibitors) may or may not be a benefit in terms of differential therapeutic efficacy. In the managed health-care scenario, the features of a novel drug must result in a benefit to the health-care system over older, generally less costly medications.

Additional Regulatory Issues

In addition to GCP, there are other guidelines, including *Good Laboratory Practices* (GLP), which apply to certain pharmacology studies and most toxicology studies, and *Good Manufacturing Practices* (GMP). Similar in concept to GCP, these guidelines require clear, consistent, auditable documentation. In particular, GMP requires traceability of all constituents of a product (actives, excipients, preservatives), as well as reproducibility.

SUMMARY

In summary, many of our novel therapies in ophthalmology will come from the development of compounds as sponsored by private pharmaceutical firms. This process is lengthy, challenging, and requires rigorous controls in scientific methodology, interpretation, and quality control. An overview of the drug development process was given, with emphasis on the clinical investigation for ophthalmic drugs. With the synergistic cooperation of basic and clinical scientists, clinical investigators, and our colleagues in pharmaceutics and regulatory affairs, we can continue to provide novel therapies to patients.

REFERENCES

1. Vagelos PR. Are prescription drug prices high? *Science* 1991;252: 1080–1084.
2. Novack GD. The development of new drugs for ophthalmology. *Am J Ophthalmol* 1992;114:357–364.
3. DiMasi JA, Hansen RW, Grabowski HG, Lasagna L. Cost of innovation in the pharmaceutical industry. *J Health Econ* 1991;10:107–142.
4. Anonymous. The Fortune 500 ranked within industries. *Fortune* 1994;129:257–276.
5. Steiner J. Problems in clinical development for the start-up company. *Appl Clin Trials* 1994;3:41–46.
6. Werth B. *The Billion Dollar Molecule: One Company's Quest for the Perfect Drug.* New York: Simon and Schuster, 1994.
7. Anders G. High-Tech Health: hospitals rush to buy a $3 million device few patients can use. *Wall Street Journal* 1994 Apr 20.
8. Black J. Drugs from emasculated hormones: the principle of syntopic antagonism. *Science* 1989;245:486–493.
9. Kupfer C, Gaasterland D, Ross K. Studies of aqueous humor dynamics in man. V. Effects of acetazolamide and isoproterenol in young and old normal volunteers. *Invest Ophthalmol* 1976;15:349–355.
10. Novack GD, Zwolshen JM. Predictive value of muscle relaxant models in rats and cats. *J Pharmacol Methods* 1983;10:175–183.
11. Woodward DF, Chen J, Padillo E, Ruiz G. Pharmacological characterization of b-adrenoceptor subtype involvement in the ocular hypotensive response to β-adrenergic stimulation. *Exp Eye Res* 1986; 43:61–75.
12. Novack GD, Lue JC, Duzman E. Power estimates for glaucoma trials. *Clin Pharmacol Ther* 1987;41:208(abst).
13. Weisweiler PS, Barnett PS, Chen KS, Kelley EP, Novack GD. Comparative comfort of flurbiprofen solution and indomethacin suspension eyedrops. *J Clin Res Drug Dev* 1988;2:233–239.
14. Scoville B, Kreiglstein GK, Then E, Yokoyama S, Yokoyama T. Measuring drug-induced eye irritation: a simple new clinical assay. *J Clin Pharmacol* 1985;25:210–218.
15. Novack GD, Tang-Liu D, Glavinos EP, Liu S, Shen D. Plasma levels following topical administration of levobunolol. *Ophthalmologica* 1987;194:194–200.
16. Repass R, Eto CY, Lee PH, Sinclair I. An evaluation of the duration of action and safety of PilaSite in ocular hypertensive patients. *Invest Ophthalmol Vis Sci* 1991;32(suppl):946(abst).
17. Vogel R, Shedden A, Kulaga S, Laurence JK, Neafus R, Study Group for Timolol-in-Gelrite. The ocular hypotensive effect of once daily administration of timolol-in-Gelrite (TG) vs. timolol solution (TS). *Invest Ophthalmol Visual Sci* 1991;32(suppl):946(abst).
18. Bensinger R, Keates E, Gofman J, Novack GD, Duzman E. Levobunolol: a three month efficacy study in the treatment of glaucoma and ocular hypertension. *Arch Ophthalmol* 1985;103:375–378.
19. Feghali JG, Kaufman PL. Decreased intraocular pressure in the hypertensive human eye with betaxolol, a beta-1-adrenergic antagonist. *Am J Ophthalmol* 1985;100:777–782.
20. Ros FE, Dake CL, Nagelkerke NJD, Greve EL. Metoprolol eye drops in the treatment of glaucoma: A double-blind single-dose trial of a beta-1-adrenergic blocking drug. *Graefes Arch Klin Exp Ophthalmol* 1978;206:247–254.
21. Duzman E, Rosen N, Lazar M. Di-acetyl nadolol: 3-month ocular hypotensive effect in glaucomatous eyes. *Br J Ophthalmol* 1983;67: 668–673.
22. Caldwell DR, Hartwich-Young R, Drake M. Efficacy and safety evaluation of lodoxamide 0.1% ophthalmic solution versus cromolyn sodium 4% ophthalmic solution in patients with vernal keratoconjunctivitis (VKC). *Invest Ophthalmol Vis Sci* 1991;32(suppl): 736(abst).
23. Levobunolol Study Group. Levobunolol: a four-year study of efficacy and safety in glaucoma treatment. *Ophthalmology* 1989;96:642–645.
24. Leibowitz HM. Antibacterial effectiveness of ciprofloxacin 0.3% ophthalmic solution in the treatment of bacterial conjunctivitis. *Am J Ophthalmol* 1991;112(suppl):29S–33S.
25. Brown RH, Stewart RH, Lynch MG, et al. ALO 2145 reduces the intraocular pressure elevation after anterior segment laser surgery. *Ophthalmology* 1988;95:378–384.
26. The Sorbinil Retinopathy Trial Research Group. A randomized trial of sorbinil, an aldose reductase inhibitor, in diabetic retinopathy. *Arch Ophthalmol* 1990;108:1234–1244.
27. Vickers FF, McGuigan LJB, Ford C, et al. The effect of diclofenac sodium ophthalmic on the treatment of postoperative inflammation. *Invest Ophthalmol Vis Sci* 1991;32(suppl):793 (abst).
28. Allen RC, Cagle GD, Bruce LA. Controlled clinical evaluations of betaxolol (0.5%) ophthalmic solution intraocular pressure and adjunctive therapy. *Program and Abstracts of the Glaucoma Society Meeting.* Turin: *XXV International Congress on Ophthalmology.* 1986;1–20.
29. Sommer A. Intraocular pressure and glaucoma. *Am J Ophthalmol* 1989;107:186–188.
30. David R, Zangwill L, Stone D, Yassur Y. Epidemiology of intraocular pressure in a population screened for glaucoma. *Br J Ophthalmol* 1987;71:766–771.
31. Werner EB, Petrig B, Krupin T, Bishop KI. Variability of automated visual fields in clinically stable glaucoma patients. *Invest Ophthalmol Vis Sci* 1989;30:1083–1089.
32. Lachenmayr BJ, Drance SM, Douglas GR, Mikelberg FS. Light-sense, flicker and resolution perimetry in glaucoma: a comparative study. *Graefes Arch Klin Exp Ophthalmol* 1991;229:246–251.
33. House P, Schulzer M, Drance S, Douglas G. Characteristics of the normal central visual field measured with resolution perimetry. *Graefes Arch Klin Exp Ophthalmol* 1991;229:8–12.
34. Bassi CJ, Galanis JC. Binocular visual impairment in glaucoma. *Ophthalmology* 1991;98:1406–1411.
35. Sommer A, Katz J, Quigley HA, et al. Clinically detectable nerve fiber atrophy precedes the onset of glaucomatous field loss. *Arch Ophthalmol* 1991;109:77–83.
36. Sommer A, Quigley HA, Robin AL, Miller NR, Katz J, Arkell S. Evaluation of nerve fiber layer assessment. *Arch Ophthalmol* 1984; 102:1766–1771.
37. Yu TC, Falcao-Reis F, Spileers W, Arden GB. Peripheral color contrast: a new screening test for preglaucomatous visual loss. *Invest Ophthalmol Vis Sci* 1991;32:2779–2789.
38. Motolko M, Drance SM, Douglas GR. The early psychophysical disturbances in chronic open-angle glaucoma: a study of visual functions with asymmetric disc cupping. *Arch Ophthalmol* 1982;100:1632–1634.
39. Fleiss JL. *The Design and Analysis of Clinical Experiments.* New York: John Wiley and Sons, 1986, pp. 263–290.
40. Schlecht LP, Brubaker RF. The effects of withdrawal of timolol in chronically treated glaucoma patients. *Ophthalmology* 1988;95:1212–1216.
41. Kass MA, Meltzer DW, Gordon M, Cooper D, Goldberg J. Compliance with topical pilocarpine treatment. *Am J Ophthalmol* 1986; 101:515–523.
42. Kass MA, Gordon M, Morley RE, Meltzer DW, Goldberg JJ. Compliance with topical timolol treatment. *Am J Ophthalmol* 1987;103: 188–193.
43. Cramer JA, Mattson RH, Prevey ML, Scheyer RD, Ouellette VL. How often is medication taken as prescribed? A novel assessment technique. *JAMA* 1989;261:3273–3277.
44. Engstrom FW, Urquhart J. Electronic monitoring of medication compliance in depressed outpatients. *Clin Pharmacol Ther* 1989;45: 159.
45. Smith EB. Effect of investigator bias on clinical trials. *Arch Dermatol* 1989;125:216–218.
46. The Glaucoma Laser Trial Research Group. The Glaucoma Laser Trial (GLT). 2. Results of argon laser trabeculoplasty versus topical medicine. *Ophthalmology* 1990;97:1403–1413.
47. Petty BG, Kornhauser DM, Lietman PS. Zidovudine with probenecid: a warning [Letter]. *Lancet* 1990;335:1044–1045.
48. Winslow R. FDA halts test on device that shows promise for victims of cardiac arrest. *Wall Street Journal* 1994 11 May.
49. Anonymous. 'Orphan drug' overhaul approved by Senate panel. *Wall Street Journal* 1994 12 May.

50. Haffner ME. Orphan products: origins, progress, and prospects. *Annu Rev Pharmacol Toxicol* 1991;31:603–620.
51. Halpern JL, Habig WH. An overview of some issues in the licensing of botulinum toxins. In: DasGupta BR (ed). *Botulinum and Tetanus Neurotoxins: Neurotransmission and Biomedical Aspects.* New York: Plenum Press, 1993;661–669.
52. Kornhauser DM, Petty BG, Hendrix CW, et al. Probenecid and zidovudine metabolism. *Lancet* 1989;2:473–475.
53. Laskin OL, de Miranda P, King DH, et al. Effects of probenecid on the pharmacokinetics and elimination of acyclovir in humans. *Antimicrob Agents Chemother* 1982;21:804–807.
54. DiMasi JA, Bryant NR, Lasagna L. New drug development in the United States from 1963 to 1990. *Clin Pharmacol Ther* 1991;50:471–486.
55. Novack GD. Failure of controlled trial data to reach the literature [Letter]. *Clin Pharmacol Ther* 1993;53:43–46.
56. Spivey RN, Lasagna L, Trimble AG. New indications for already-approved drugs: time trends for the new drug application review phase. *Clin Pharmacol Ther* 1987;41:368–370.
57. Novack GD, Eto CY, Lue JC, Branin M. A post-marketing evaluation of levobunolol, a topical ophthalmic drug. *J Clin Res Drug Dev* 1987;1:197–203.
58. Novack GD, Kelley EP, Lue JC. A multicenter evaluation of levobunolol (VISTAGAN) in Germany. *Ophthalmologica* 1988;197: 90–96.
59. Schnarr K-D. Vergleichende multizentrische untersuchung von carteolol-augentropfen mit anderen betablockern bei 768 patienten unter alltagsbedingungen. *Klin Monatsbl Augenheilkol* 1988;192:167–176.
60. Long DA, Johns GE, Mullen RA, et al. Levobunolol and betaxolol: a double-masked controlled comparison of efficacy and safety in patients with elevated intraocular pressure. *Ophthalmology* 1988;95: 735–741.
61. Silverstone DE, Novack GD, Kelley EP, Chen KS. Prophylactic treatment of intraocular pressure elevations after Neodymium:YAG laser posterior capsulotomies and extracapsular cataract extractions with levobunolol. *Ophthalmology* 1988;95:713–718.
62. Silverstone D, Zimmerman T, Choplin N, et al. Evaluation of once-daily levobunolol 0.25% and timolol 0.25% for increased intraocular pressure. *Am J Ophthalmol* 1991;112:56–60.
63. Krieglstein GK, Novack GD, Voepel E, et al. Levobunolol and metipranolol: comparative ocular hypotensive efficacy, safety and comfort. *Br J Ophthalmol* 1987;71:250–253.
64. Ober M, Scharrer A, Novack GD, Lue JC. Die lokale subjektive Verträglich keit von Levobunolol und Metipranolol in einer Doppelblink-Vergliechsstudie bie Patienten mit erhohtem intraokularem druck. *Ophthalmologica* 1986;192:159–164.

Textbook of Ocular Pharmacology,
edited by T.J. Zimmerman, et al.
Lippincott–Raven Publishers, Philadelphia © 1997.

CHAPTER 12

Ethical Issues in Ophthalmic Research

Mark P. Nasisse

The massive volume of literature generated over the past 20 years that addresses the use of animals in scientific research attests to the level of maturity this issue has achieved within the academic community. This is not to say that controversy no longer exists. There are still those who argue that there is no defensible basis for using animals as experimental subjects (1,2), whereas others persist in their belief that the value of research to humans supersedes concern for the welfare of the animals involved (3,4). It does mean that an equilibrium, however unstable, has been reached between those with diametrically opposed perspectives on the issue. The days of debating whether animal welfare should be considered when designing experimental studies have been permanently supplanted by institutional and governmental policies and procedures intended to ensure that animal welfare issues are seriously balanced with scientific merit. This issue undoubtedly is still evolving, and only time will determine where the pendulum will stop and the extent to which animal welfare concerns become balanced by societal needs for information produced by animal research. It is not the intention of this chapter to debate either side of the issue but to summarize contemporary practices and to highlight issues of particular relevance to ophthalmic research as perceived from the perspective of a veterinarian engaged in ophthalmic research.

HISTORICAL BACKGROUND

Evidence of the use of animals in scientific research can be found at least as far back as A.D. 129, when the use of pigs in medical experimentation was recorded by the Greek physician Galen. The use of animals in medical research became more common during the 1800s and reached commonplace status in the academic community by 1900 (5). Although concern for animal welfare had been expressed for centuries, it was not until 1824 that the Society for the Prevention of Cruelty to Animals was founded in Britain to ensure that guidelines for the protection of farm animals were observed. It was in the second half of the nineteenth century, however, that concern for animal welfare in Britain extended to animals used for research. The enactment of the *Cruelty to Animals Act of 1876* finally required some oversight of experiments that might cause pain to vertebrates.

The first United States animal protection legislation, the *Twenty-Eight Hour Law,* was passed in 1873 and regulated the number of hours that livestock could be confined for transport. It was not until the passing of the *Laboratory Animal Welfare Act of 1966* (PL 89–544), however, that protection was extended to nonfarm animals. Aimed specifically at the welfare of pet dogs and cats, this legislation set forth guidelines for the licensure of individuals and organizations that bought or sold animals for laboratory use as well as guidelines for animals' care. The legislation did not, however, specifically address the welfare of the dog or cat while in the possession of the research institution. The *Laboratory Animal Welfare Act* became the *Animal Welfare Act* (AWA) (PL 91–579) in 1970 when it was broadened to cover other species of animals as well as to the care of the animals while in the research facility. The AWA was further amended in 1976 (PL 94–279) to include recommendations that expanded species coverage and addressed the transport of animals and animal fighting.

Two pieces of legislation passed in 1985 significantly impacted the care and use of animals in research. The first of these, the *Health Research Extension Act* (6) (PL 99–158), also referred to as the *NIH Reauthorization Act,* stipulated that research facilities establish animal care and use committees to review the care and treatment of animals and required that applicants for National Institutes of Health (NIH) funds file assurances certifying that the investigator and the institution adhere to NIH guidelines. The second was an amendment to the AWA entitled the

M. P. Nasisse: College of Veterinary Medicine, University of Missouri, Columbia, Missouri 65211.

Improved Standards for Laboratory Animals Act (PL 99–198), which addressed the need for the psychological well-being of nonhuman primates and exercise for dogs. This amendment to the AWA also required that an information service be established at the National Agricultural Library to disseminate information that would minimize the unnecessary duplication of animal experiments, provide information on alternatives to animals, and provide information on humane practices of animal use for individuals involved in animal research. They also stipulate that investigators consider alternatives to animal use and consult a veterinarian before beginning any experiment that could cause pain.

OVERSIGHT OF ANIMAL RESEARCH

Policies of the NIH and the Public Health Service (PHS)

Since 1971 institutions doing research funded by the NIH that involves any live vertebrate animal have been required to have their use, care, and treatment of animals evaluated, either by acquiring accreditation from the professional laboratory animal accreditation organization, the American Association for Accreditation of Laboratory Care (AAALAC), or by being overseen by an internal committee that includes a veterinarian and complies with NIH guidelines. This policy was replaced by the first *Public Health Service Policy* in 1973, which was revised in 1979 and again in 1985 and 1986. The current *Public Health Service Policy on Humane Care and Use of Laboratory Animals* (7) incorporates the changes in the Public Health Service Act and was mandated for PHS-funded institutions by the *Health Research Extension Act of 1985.* The current policy adopts the *Guide for the Care and Use of Laboratory Animals* (8), the details of which are summarized subsequently, and applies to all intramurally or extramurally funded PHS research. The policy also mandates that institutions have an animal use and care committee and specifies procedures for reviewing and submitting proposals, as well as for reporting research conducted with PHS funds. The PHS policy also endorses the *U.S. Government Principles for the Utilization and Care of Vertebrate Animals Used in Testing, Research and Training,* developed by the Interagency Research Animal Committee, which summarizes the principles by which animal research is to be conducted. A detailed description of the operating procedures of these agencies can be found in several authoritative references on the subject of animal use in research (9–11).

Guide for the Care and Use of Laboratory Animals

The *Guide for the Care and Use of Laboratory Animals* (8) is the most thorough description of animal care policies in the United States that addresses the ethical treatment of animals in laboratory research environments. Originally published in 1963 as the *Guide for Laboratory Animal Facilities and Care,* it has been revised many times, most recently in 1985. The guide is prepared by the Committee on Care and Use of Laboratory Animals of the Institute of Laboratory Animal Resources Commission on Life Sciences, National Research Council, which consists of 14 members of diverse backgrounds of expertise in laboratory animal care. This detailed document describes specific policies for monitoring all aspects of animal care, including facilities, personnel, and guidelines on acceptable experiments (i.e., experimental design, use of hazardous agents, and surgical procedures).

Position of the American Veterinary Medical Association (AVMA)

In recognition of its incumbent responsibility to provide leadership on animal welfare issues, the AVMA executive board established a special joint committee in 1980 to study contemporary welfare issues of importance to the veterinary profession and to develop position statements on animal welfare. The results of these efforts are detailed in the AVMA publication, *Animal Welfare; Positions and Recommendations and Background Information* (12), which was most recently revised in 1989. The guidelines were produced in view of the stated recognition that "veterinarians have certain ethical, philosophical, and moral values that must be considered." By "recognizing the central and essential role of animals in research experimentation and testing for continued improvement in the health and welfare of all animals including man," the AVMA in essence endorses animal experimentation. The AVMA does, however, "encourage the refinement of animal experimentation and more development of non-animal alternatives in research." The AVMA further endorses the policies defined in the *Guide for the Care and Use of Laboratory Animals* and concludes that current laws and regulations governing the use of animals, if properly enforced and implemented, are adequate to ensure humane care and treatment of laboratory animals.

In May 1987, the AVMA established a panel to organize a Colloquium on Recognition and Alleviation of Animal Pain and Distress, the results of which were subsequently published (13). The focus of this colloquium was a wide variety of topics relating to animal pain, ranging from its physiologic basis to its identification and management. In addition to providing a unique insight into the perspective of veterinarians regarding the issue of animal pain, the panel provided a series of recommendations in its concluding remarks that included the need for scientific investigators to reexamine their research designs to determine whether they will induce unintended pain or distress and to minimize those aspects of the design when they cannot be avoided.

GUIDELINES FOR THE USE OF ANIMALS IN OPHTHALMIC RESEARCH

There are no specific detailed regulations or guidelines that address ophthalmic research involving animals, nor is this issue specifically addressed by the *Guide for the Care and Use of Laboratory Animals.* Instead, ophthalmic research proposals must be evaluated on a case-by-case basis by animal-use committees. The Association for Research in Vision and Ophthalmology (ARVO) has attempted to provide leadership on this issue and has produced a document detailing its own guidelines (14). The ARVO document emphasizes that animals must not be subjected to avoidable stress or discomfort and recommends that the "investigator's first concern be to avoid the use of animals whenever possible." In accordance with conventional animal use committee guidelines, these require that distress be limited by careful experimental design incorporating the use of analgesics or anesthesia or both. They further support the careful justification of animal use, including the species and number to be involved. In a 1993 supplement to this document, ARVO highlights the importance of considering the potential effects of research on the animal's vision and points out that in the view of the PHS (8), any survival procedure that has the potential for producing a visual disability sufficient to disrupt an animal's normal daily activity should be considered a *major* survival procedure, requiring appropriate justification. Attention is also called to the PHS guide's recommendation that animals not be subjected to multiple major survival surgical procedures unless they are related components of a particular project. One implication to ophthalmic research is that bilateral ocular surgery not be performed unless special justification is provided.

Oversight of Ophthalmic Research Involving Animals

The sponsoring institution bears the ultimate responsibility for seeing that research involving animals adheres to existing federal guidelines and regulations. Failure to comply with these guidelines can lead to revocation of permits for research animal use by the U.S. Department of Agriculture (USDA) and suspension of institution-wide funding by the PHS. As prescribed by the PHS *Policy on Humane Care and Use of Laboratory Animals,* Institutional Animal Care and Use Committees (IACUC) form the focal point of institutional oversight. The IACUC is required to comprise at least five members, including one laboratory animal veterinarian who is responsible for the animal program of the institution, a practicing scientist with experience in animal research, a nonscientist, and one member who is unaffiliated with the institution. The animal program of the institution is required to be evaluated by the IACUC at least every 6 months to ensure its compliance with federal guidelines. Probably the most important IACUC function relative to animal welfare is its responsibility for reviewing and approving all animal research proposals by its constituent members before the initiation of the project. Approval by the IACUC is required for disbursement of PHS funds. Although most institutions generally discharge these duties admirably, inherent limitations exist within the system. First, the difficulty of this task is made enormous by the fact that whereas federal guidelines for the use of animals are explicit in their intent, they leave it to the IACUC to develop its own specific procedures and policies to ensure that the general guidelines are met. The committee is left the unenviable task of balancing scientific merit with animal welfare when deciding on the disposition of proposals for animal use. It is easy to appreciate that consistency in animal project review between institutions might be difficult to achieve. The ability of IACUCs to administer their duties effectively is further complicated by the limited level of expertise that committee members may have regarding the specifics of a proposal. This problem is particularly present in proposals of ophthalmic research, where peculiarities in ocular sensory innervation and the difficulty of maintaining ocular surface analgesia make assessing the merits of certain proposals difficult. It is intended that adjunct committee members with specific expertise in the area of question be consulted to contribute to the review.

SPECIFIC ISSUES IN ANIMAL OPHTHALMIC RESEARCH

Appropriateness of Animal Species

One of the most justifiable criticisms of animal research is that applicability of the results to the human disease to which it is intending to contribute is often difficult to determine. This is particularly true in ophthalmology, where substantial anatomic, physiologic, and naturally occurring disease differences exist between humans and animals. With the exception of certain primates, there is no animal species whose normal ocular features are similar to those of humans. As a comparative ophthalmologist, I have often provided advice on the appropriateness of the intended animal species for comparative research. I have been impressed that investigators are at times unaware of major anatomic and physiologic differences between animal species that might preclude or diminish their usefulness as models. Examples of this include the intention of using dogs, which have no macula, to study the mechanisms of macular disease and using rabbits, which have the bulk of their secretory epithelium located on iridal processes rather than ciliary processes, to study the pressure-lowering effects of transscleral cyclodestructive surgery. As is the case for justifying the number of animals to be used, it is incumbent on the investigator to justify to the IACUC that data produced from the intended species will be applicable. Veterinary ophthalmologists are uniquely qualified to contribute to this aspect of project planning.

Appropriateness of Animal Number

It is not only ethically appropriate to consider welfare issues when determining the number of animals to be used in a scientific study, but it is mandated by the U.S. Food and Drug Administration (FDA) that the research and testing derive the maximum amount of scientific information from the minimum number of animals (15). Obviously, the fewest animals should be used that will produce valid scientific data. It is the responsibility of the investigator to justify in the IACUC application the number of animals to be used and the responsibility of the IACUC to see that the justification is valid. There are surprisingly few guidelines, however, that provide advice on how exactly this is to be done. The complexity of the issues surrounding the justification of animal numbers for the IACUC has been addressed elsewhere (Weigler, B. J., manuscript in review). The problem of assessing animal numbers is particularly difficult in ophthalmic research because investigators tend to use both eyes of an animal, presumably for the purpose of reducing study costs. In many situations, however, it is difficult to argue that data from the different eyes of a single animal represent truly independent events. Suggestions currently being considered by the authors' IACUC to ensure that careful consideration has been given to the appropriate animal number include reviewing the investigator's attention to detail in study design, and redesigning IACUC applications to make it easier to determine the extent to which the investigator has considered all possible alternative models and study designs for the proposed project (including consultation with the appropriate biostatistician and informing investigators of available sources of statistical expertise). Because the IACUC must walk the fine line between impeding and facilitating research, its role in oversight of this issue will undoubtedly evolve slowly.

Control of Pain

Despite the numerous works published in recent years that address the phenomena of pain, its physiologic basis, and optimum ways to detect it, pain remains poorly understood, particularly in animals (16,17). Because the cornea is the most richly innervated structure in the body, however, issues of pain recognition and control are particularly relevant to ophthalmic research. Pain can be classified as either *neuropathic,* occurring secondary to sensory nerve system dysfunction, or *nociceptive,* representing the neural response to the application of noxious stimulation (18,19). Nociceptive pain is mediated by A-delta and C fiber nerve types, both of which are found in the cornea (20,21). Discomfort caused by corneal stimulation is the most severe form of ocular pain and is aggravated indirectly through intraocular mechanisms such as miosis, ciliary spasm, and blood ocular barrier disruption. Although considered less intense than corneal pain, intraocular stimulation resulting from elevated intraocular pressure or uveal inflammation can result in substantial discomfort.

Because pain can be anticipated as the result of any study in which direct stimulation to either the globe's surface or intraocular structures is anticipated, some form of analgesia is routinely indicated in ophthalmic research. In the event of uncertainty about whether the proposed study might induce discomfort, general guidelines are available for the recognition of pain and distress in animals (22,23). Because of the eyes' unique sensitivity and conspicuous nature, monitoring for discomfort is much less complex than for other organ systems. Having treated a wide variety of domestic animal species with naturally occurring ocular disease for the past 14 years, there is little question in my mind that overt squinting (*blepharospasm*) represents a reliable indicator of moderate to severe discomfort.

Finding ways to suppress experimentally induced ocular discomfort adequately remains a significant problem. Although numerous guidelines have been provided for the selection of analgesic agents for both mammalian and nonmammalian species (24–27), unique features of the eye and of ophthalmic research make their effective application less than predictable. Because of the cornea's rich innervation, systemically administered analgesics are unlikely to be entirely effective at controlling extreme corneal pain. The limited toxic effects and duration of topical analgesics limit their effectiveness for controlling corneal discomfort to only the shortest procedures. The antimicrobial effects of topically applied anesthetics also preclude their use in studies addressing microbial pathogenesis or drug efficacy. In many situations, therefore, the benefits to be gained by the research must be weighed carefully against the discomfort to be anticipated. Conflicts also arise when contemplating control of the discomfort caused by intraocular pain, as many analgesics also have immunomodulating effects that may be incompatible with the objectives of the research. It is clear from reading the most contemporary guidelines that although a conscientious effort has been made, we are a long way from having a comprehensive set of guidelines for managing pain resulting from ocular research in animals.

Alternatives to Using Mammals in Ophthalmic Research

The increasing awareness of ethical as well as practical and economic limitations of animal research has stimulated a concerted search for alternatives. Nonmammalian research models have been developed using everything from protozoa and insects to amphibians, fish, and reptiles (28). The simplistic generalization that pain is a less significant issue in nonmammalian species is no longer tenable, however, as the anatomic and physiologic basis of nociception has been clearly demonstrated in nonmammalian vertebrates (29,30). Nonetheless, nonmammalian research models do provide much less politically sensitive systems with which we can work. Except for a few very basic areas, however, the application of nonmammalian systems to human-oriented ophthalmic research is seriously hampered by substantial anatomic and physiologic differences, the specifics of which can easily be identified by consulting a comparative ophthalmologist or a variety of comparative texts (31–33).

Undoubtedly, the political and regulatory pressure to identify in vitro alternatives to animal research will continue to increase. The USDA *Improved Standards for Laboratory Animals Act* and PHS laws currently require that the investigator consider alternatives to animal use, and guidance in identifying alternatives is available from the Animal Welfare Information Center of the National Agricultural Library (Beltsville, Maryland).

ACKNOWLEDGMENT

I gratefully acknowledge the assistance of Dr. Benjamin Weigler in preparing this chapter.

REFERENCES

1. Regan T. Cruelty, kindness, and unnecessary suffering. *Philosophy* 1988;55:532–541.
2. Regan T. Animal rights, human wrongs. *Environmental Ethics* 1980;2:99–120.
3. Frey RG. Interests and animal rights. *Philosophical Quarterly* 1977; 27:254–259.
4. Frey RG. *Interests and Rights: The Case Against the Animals.* Oxford: Clarendon Press, 1980.
5. McGrew RE. *Encyclopedia of Medical History.* New York: McGraw-Hill, 1985.
6. *Health Research Extension Act of 1985,* Public Law 99–158, Section 495, 1985.
7. U.S. Department of Health and Human Services, Public Health Service, National Institutes of Health. *Public Health Service Policy on Human Care and use of Laboratory Animals,* 1986.
8. Committee on Care and Use of Laboratory Animals of the Institute of Laboratory Animal Resources. *Guide for the Care and Use of Laboratory Animals.* Bethesda, Maryland: U.S. Department of Health and Human Services, Public Health Service, National Institutes of Health, 1985, NIH Publication No. 85–23.
9. Rollin BE, Kesel ML, eds. *The Experimental Animal in Biomedical Research,* vol I, *A Survey of Scientific and Ethical Issues for Investigators.* Boca Raton, Florida: CRC Press, 1990.
10. *Use of Laboratory Animals in Biomedical and Behavioral Research.* Washington: National Academy Press, 1988.
11. Tyckoson DA, ed. Oryx Science Bibliographies, vol 9, *Animal Experimentation and Animal Rights.* Phoenix: Oryx Press, 1987.
12. Animal Welfare Committee, American Veterinary Medical Association, Chicago, Illinois. *Animal Welfare; Positions, Recommendations, and Background Information,* 1989.
13. AVMA Colloquium on Recognition and Alleviation of Animal Pain and Distress. *J Am Vet Med Assoc* 1989;191:1186–1196.
14. The Association for Research in Vision and Ophthalmology, Animals in Research Committee. *Handbook for the Use of Animals in Biomedical Research,* vol 2., 1993.
15. United States Department of Health and Human Services, Food and Drug Administration. *Good Laboratory Practice Regulations:* Final Rule, 21 CFR, Part 58, 1987.
16. Kitchell RL. Problems defining pain and peripheral mechanisms of pain. *J Am Vet Med Assoc* 1987;191:1195–1199.
17. Moberg GP. Problems defining stress and distress in animals. *J Am Vet Med Assoc* 1987;191:1207–1211.
18. Tanelian DL, Brunson DB. Anatomy and physiology of pain with special reference to ophthalmology. *Invest Ophthalmol Vis Sci* 1994;35: 759–763.
19. Burgess PR, Perl ER. Cutaneous mechanoreceptors and nociceptors. In: Iggo A, ed. *Handbook of Sensory Physiology,* vol 2. *Somatosensory System.* Berlin: Springer-Verlag, 1973;29–78.
20. Rozsa AJ, Beuerman RW. Density and organization of free nerve endings in the corneal epithelium of the rabbit. *Pain* 1982;14: 105–120.
21. Marfurt CF, Kingsley RE, Echtenkamp SE. Sensory and sympathetic innervation of the mammalian cornea: a retrograde tracing study. *Invest Ophthalmol Vis Sci* 1989;30:461–472.
22. Morton DB, Griffiths PHM. Guidelines on the recognition of pain, distress and discomfort in experimental animals and a hypothesis for assessment. *Vet Rec* 1985;116:431–436.
23. Spinelli JS, Harkowitz H. Clinical recognition and anticipation of situations likely to induce suffering in animals. *J Am Vet Med Assoc* 1987;191:12–18.
24. Benson GJ, Thurmon JC. Species difference as a consideration in alleviation of animal pain and distress. *J Am Vet Med Assoc* 1987; 191:1227–1230.
25. Jenkins W. Pharmacologic aspects of analgesic drugs in animals: an overview. *J Am Vet Med Assoc* 1987;191:1231–1240.
26. Daunt DA. Pain and analgesia in mammals. *Invest Ophthalmol Vis Sci* 1994;35:763–774.
27. Stoskopf MK. Pain and analgesia in birds, reptiles, amphibians and, fish. *Invest Ophthalmol Vis Sci* 1994;35:775–780.
28. Woodhead AD, ed. *Nonmammalian Animal Models for Biomedical Research.* Boca Raton, Florida: CRC Press, 1989.
29. Spray DC. Pain and temperature receptors of anurans. In: Llinbas R, Precht W, eds. *Frog Neurobiology.* Berlin: Springer-Verlag, 1976; 607–628.
30. Szolcsanyi J, Sann H, Pierau FK. Nociception in pigeons is not impaired by capsaicin. *Pain* 1986;27:289–293.
31. Davson H, Graham LT, ed. *The Eye,* vol 5, *Comparative Physiology.* New York: Academic Press, 1974.
32. Duke-Elder. *System of Ophthalmology,* vol 1, *The Eye in Evolution.* St. Louis: CV Mosby, 1958.
33. Gelatt KN. *Veterinary Ophthalmology (2nd Ed).* Philadelphia: Lea & Febiger, 1991.

Textbook of Ocular Pharmacology,
edited by T.J. Zimmerman, et al.
Lippincott–Raven Publishers, Philadelphia © 1997.

CHAPTER 13

The Ophthalmologist as Clinical Investigator

Gary D. Novack

The development of new therapeutic agents for the treatment of ophthalmic diseases as well as expansion of our knowledge about existing therapeutics requires research at both the basic and clinical levels. As part of the clinical research, ophthalmologists are frequently called on to serve as clinical investigators. This chapter is oriented toward the ophthalmologist who is considering participating as a clinical investigator and covers the practical, scientific, ethical, and legal aspects of this role.

Most opportunities to serve as a clinical investigator arise from clinical studies sponsored by the private sector. Thus, the orientation of this chapter is for the ophthalmologist approached by a pharmaceutical firm. In addition, it is assumed that studies would be conducted in the United States.

THE PHARMACEUTICAL INDUSTRY

Given that most opportunities for sponsored research involve a relationship with a pharmaceutical firm, it is useful for the clinician to have some information about this industry. The pharmaceutical industry is a major sector of the U.S. economy, with approximately 500,000 employees and 100 billion dollars per year in revenue, representing 3% of the total sales of Fortune 500 companies (1). As with any industry, the primary goals of a pharmaceutical firm are to increase its market valuation (i.e., stock price) and to make a profit. What is somewhat unique about this industry is the long time lines required from concept until marketing. The research and development (R & D) process for a new drug may exceed 10 years, with additional years required for regulatory approval. The cost of this product development may be several hundred million dollars (2). Given a 17-year patent life in America, a pharmaceutical firm essentially must reinvent its product line every decade. The U.S. orphan drug law provides special tax allowances for pharmaceutical products for small populations (typically fewer than 200,000 cases per year) (3). As of late 1994, however, the United States was unique in having such a law enacted. Furthermore, a firm still needs to have revenues to take advantage of tax credits; that is, in the long-term, most firms cannot afford to develop, produce, and sell a product at a substantial loss.

Clinical studies conducted on a new drug are intended to identify its potency, efficacy, and relative safety profile. There are three preapproval stages of clinical studies (Phases I, II and III) and a postapproval phase (Phase IV). To gain product approval by the Food and Drug Administration (FDA), the large Phase III, multicenter, controlled trials must provide substantial evidence of efficacy and safety. Protocols presented to an ophthalmologist may range from early Phase I studies, typically of short duration and low dose and in normal patients, to long-term Phase III studies, to studies on additional indications or more real-world concomitant therapy situations (Phase IV). Given the increasing costs and timing for pharmaceutical development as well as harmonization of international regulatory requirements, there is a tendency toward a worldwide approach to drug development. After signing a confidentiality agreement, the ophthalmologist typically is provided several documents by the pharmaceutical firm, including the clinical investigator brochure (CIB) and protocol.

BEFORE THE STUDY

Clinical Investigator Brochure

The sponsor is obligated to provide the clinical investigator with adequate information about the drug to make an educated judgment about potential benefits and risks in exposing patients to this investigational agent. This information typically is included in the CIB. Key sections of the

G. D. Novack: Pharma•Logic Development, Inc., San Rafael, California 94903.

CIB are outlined in Table 13-1 and include the following sections.

Description of Product and Formulation

This section includes the chemical description and structure of the drug. The formulation of the product for clinical use (e.g., capsule, solution) and any excipients used (fillers, preservatives) are described. The dosage form also (solution, suspension, erodible implant, etc.) needs to be described here. Both the drug substance (i.e., raw chemicals) and the drug product (i.e., product as delivered for clinical use) should be well characterized and reproducibly manufactured. For clinical studies, the sponsor is obligated to manufacture the product in a consistent, documented, controlled environment. Further, the product must be demonstrated, primarily by chemical tests, to be stable in its packaging; that is, the concentration of the active product as well as the preservative must remain within tight limits (typically 10%) of the stated amount for the shelf life. Although straightforward in concept, these requirements, embodied in *Good Manufacturing Practices* (GMP) regulations, are constantly upgraded. For many projects currently in development, preparation of GMP supplies is the rate-limiting step. Products of biological origin (e.g., potent proteins), which can be assayed only by biological rather than by chemical means, present special challenges in manufacturing and control.

Pharmacology

The pharmacology of a compound should be assessed in several in vitro and in vivo models of drug action. Depending on the molecule and its novelty, this assessment may include a wide range of systemic and ocular models. The range of tests should include a measure of the drug's intended efficacy (e.g., a selective agonist of a given subtype of a receptor) as well as unintended effects (e.g., other related subtypes of this receptor) and general physiological models. Drugs given to the eye frequently enter the systemic circulation and thus can be presented to various organ systems. It is therefore important that both the systemic and ocular pharmacology of a compound be assessed. Receptors in the eye may differ from those in other organ systems in their selectivity for receptor subtypes and stereoisomers.

TABLE 13-1. *Contents of a clinical investigator's brochure*

Description of product and formulation
Pharmacology
Absorption, distribution, metabolism and excretion
Toxicology
Previous systemic clinical experience
Previous ophthalmic experience
Draft labeling

Absorption, Distribution, Metabolism, and Excretion

This quartet of characteristics, known as ADME, describes how a drug moves from its site of application to its site of action and how it is removed from the body (See Chapter 9). Some drugs are extremely unstable and must be applied near the site of action and at frequent intervals. Other drugs are stable and long lasting. Drugs are generally foreign compounds to the body (*xenobiotics*). Functional chemical groups on a molecule may be recognizable to the body's endogenous chemicals; thus, drugs may be metabolized by a host of biological pathways.

A general rule for ophthalmic solutions applied as eyedrops is that approximately 2% to 5% of the instilled amount enters the eye. Using the rough estimate of approximately 100 μl of aqueous humor, with a flow rate of approximately 2 μl per minute, once distributed into the aqueous humor, drugs tend to be removed at this physiological rate, which represents a half-life of 1 to 2 hours.

Toxicology

Before a novel compound is administered to humans, its mammalian toxicity should be assessed at exaggerated doses and frequencies. These tests are a series of increasingly larger doses and longer durations of treatment. The battery of tests employed should include both systemic and ocular administration and evaluation of both ocular and extraocular tissues. In the early stages of clinical evaluation, the preclinical exposure should always exceed the clinical exposure. For a one-drop clinical study, animal evaluations probably should include a minimum dosing period of several days. For a 2-week clinical study, animal evaluations probably should include a minimum dosing period of a month. If the compound is intended for use in women of childbearing potential, its potential for teratogenicity and mutagenicity should be evaluated, and if intended for chronic use for a long-term disease, its carcinogenicity should be assessed.

Previous Systemic Clinical Experience

Many ophthalmic compounds were first evaluated for a systemic disease. The sponsor has an obligation to inform the investigator about any systemic clinical experience with the compound. These reports should include the doses, routes and frequency of administration, duration of treatment, efficacy, toxicity, and pharmacokinetics. The level of detail in these reports depends on the amount of experience. For a compound new to the eye but with an established systemic profile and relatively few clinical studies, the level of detail should be great. In contrast, for a well-known compound already approved for systemic use, the level of detail can be less. The perspective of this section should be global, including information on the experience and marketing status of the compound throughout the world.

Previous Ophthalmic Experience

Similar to systemic experience, the sponsor has an obligation to inform the investigator about any ophthalmic clinical experience with the compound. Special attention should be given to safety, both subjective (e.g., comfort) and objective (e.g., biomicroscopy). As with systemic application, these reports should include the doses, routes and frequency of administration, duration of treatment, efficacy, toxicity, and pharmacokinetics.

Draft Labeling

This draft label includes the same sections as an approved label. In addition to some of the sections already noted for the CIB, this section includes indications, contraindications, warnings, precautions, and treatment for overdoses. Examples of indications include allergic conjunctivitis, postsurgical inflammation, or prophylaxis of glaucomatous visual field loss.

Protocol

Overview

The clinical protocol represents the *methods* section, or the recipe for the clinical study. It is the essence of the "contract" between the sponsor and the clinician performing the study. In order for the data to be scientifically, ethically, and legally valid, the investigator must follow a set pattern of drug administration and data recording, especially in multicenter studies, where many independent clinicians are cooperating. The restrictions on drug exposure in the protocol are most likely present for a reason, and to exceed them might put a patient in jeopardy. Further, regulatory restrictions demand that the investigator administer the investigational agent only in the manner stated in the protocol. A protocol may be presented in draft form, allowing the investigator to provide input before it is finalized. Alternatively, a protocol also may be presented after it is finalized and approved by the firm's internal review committee as well as selected IRBs. A clinician who does not believe he or she can follow the protocol should not become an investigator.

Throughout the protocol and the study, the overriding elements of written informed consent and benefit-to-risk ratio need to be considered. The consent form, typically provided by the sponsor, but also typically requiring modification for each governing IRB, should clearly outline in readable terms the rationale for the study, the number of patients anticipated in the study, the potential benefits and risks, compensation or inducement for participation (financial and nonfinancial), as well as the option of the patient to withdraw without prejudice at any time. Key sections of a protocol are outlined in Table 13-2 and include the following.

Synopsis, Personnel, and Facilities

The synopsis should present in 1 or 2 pages the critical elements of patient qualifications and number, investigational drug exposure, examination methods required, and clinical phase (i.e., I, II, III, or IV). The responsible individuals at the sponsor and investigational site should be listed here, including telephone and facsimile numbers.

Introduction and Objectives

This section is similar to the introduction of a published paper and should include background of the disease and the investigational drug, leading to the rationale for and the explicit objectives of the present study.

Study Design and Patient Population

This section should clearly state the method of assignment to treatment group (e.g., randomized, unequal), masking (e.g., open, single-masked, double-masked), and

TABLE 13-2. *Contents of a clinical protocol*

Overview
Clinical phase
Personnel and facilities
Synopsis
Background and rationale
Study objective
Study design
Study population
Number
Inclusion criteria
Exclusion criteria
Materials and methods
Study medications and regimen
Warnings, precautions, and contraindications
Concomitant medications
Washout
Clinical assessment/examination procedures
Study flowchart
Subject entry procedure
Study endpoints
Adverse experience considerations
Statistical considerations
Consent form

treatment sequence (e.g., parallel, crossover, paired comparison). The population section should include the projected number of patients to be enrolled, the disease qualifications (e.g., adult-onset, insulin-dependent stable diabetes), other requirements for inclusion, and characteristics that would exclude a patient from participation.

Materials

The investigational product and any comparative marketed product should be clearly described. The concentration of the active ingredient and any preservatives is required. The excipients must be listed, although their exact concentration may be considered proprietary and therefore not disclosed. Whereas "approved" labeling for the investigational product generally does not exist, warnings, precautions, and contraindications should be presented. Labeling for the marketed product should be included. Any special requirements as to concomitant medications should be presented.

Examinations and Schedule

This section describes the step-by-step procedure for enrolling, treating, and monitoring patients. Typically, there is an explicit visit schedule, which may include a period of washout from existing medications. Certain procedures may be very exacting, for example, visual acuity according to the Early Treatment of Diabetic Retinopathy Study method (4) or visual fields by a certain program on a certain machine. A flowchart of examinations and visits should be presented.

Adverse Experience Considerations

The FDA and other regulatory authorities have strict guidelines regarding the reporting of adverse experiences. Because of the occurrence of deaths in a National Institutes of Health study of a potential hepatitis treatment, these regulations are expected to become even more rigorous. Stated broadly, the investigator is required to report immediately to the sponsor any death or any serious or unexpected adverse event, whether or not it is thought to be related to the treatment. More explicit wording, together with 24-hour emergency telephone numbers, is provided in this section.

Statistical Considerations

A biostatistician should be consulted in the protocol preparation stage rather than merely after the study is complete and data are ready to be analyzed. There are many areas where the preparer of a protocol and the biostatistician can work together. The results of this collaboration should be apparent in the protocol and should include identification of the measurements as primary efficacy measures (e.g., intraocular pressure reduction for a glaucoma drug or reduction in cell and flare for an antiinflammatory drug), secondary efficacy measures, or safety measures. The design of forms on which clinical data are recorded (*case report forms*) is critical to the success of the trial as is the time required for key punching the data and its analysis. Experienced clinical trialists can provide substantial input on how to optimize these forms. If any form of automated data entry is considered (e.g., visual field data, output from an office computer system, or data from a centralized clinical laboratory), this is the time to plan for it.

The power of a given study to detect a clinically significant difference is critical in judging the relevance of a study. The power calculation should be clearly identified in a protocol, and it is essential to state the clinically significant difference (e.g., 2 mm Hg for a glaucoma study or one grade in inflammation or comfort), the presumed standard deviation of that measurement, the sample size per group, and the alpha level (generally $p = 0.05$, two-tailed). The critical minimum for biostatistical power is typically 80% (5,6).

References and Appendices

An investigator can request a copy of any "data on file" references (e.g., toxicology, previous clinical studies). Although these should be summarized in the CIB, additional information may be required. The sponsor may elect to send the investigator a summary first, as some of these internal documents comprise more than 500 pages. The appendices typically include statements regarding investigator and sponsor obligations, specialized measurement techniques, and human subject information.

Compensation

Compensation to the investigator is one of the issues that must be resolved before study start. A good "rule of thumb" is to add the normal costs of the procedures for a patient who completes the study as planned and then add 20% of that amount for administrative costs and overhead. Direct expenses (e.g., laboratory fees, patient transportation fees, express fees) are normally passed through at cost. Other issues involve compensation for patients who are discontinued or terminated from further study participation, bonus payments for meeting enrollment deadlines, expenses for fellows and residents to present the research at key meetings, and any other consulting role for the clinical investigator.

Investigator Decisions

If to an ophthalmologist and a clinical investigator the protocol has appeal, then the investigator needs to consider the additional issues (Table 13-3).

Patients

A potential investigator should ask, "Do I have the patients?" Carefully review the inclusion and exclusion criteria for the study. Consider also the implicit assumption that these patients return for frequent follow-up, which generally requires that they live nearby, and they must be mobile. Consider also patients who are "snowbirds" who migrate to warmer climates during winter months.

Whereas there is no hard and fast rule, typically only 20% to 40% of apparently eligible patients will qualify and desire to participate in the study. Most studies require a minimum of 20 patients or more to be enrolled at each site within 3 to 6 months, which means that an investigator may have to plan to locate 100 patients to complete enrollment.

Aside from the actual pharmacology of the investigational drug, the rate of patient enrollment is usually the major rate-limiting step of most clinical studies and is also the most variable. Thus, it is utmost in the mind of a clinical manager and the sponsor in selecting a site. Of potential investigators who have an office computer system, some routinely request an electronic search of the patient database for patients with the required disease within a restricted zip code. This information plus a demonstrated track record are important factors in selecting a clinical site.

Expertise

Does the study require any special expertise? Is the investigator sufficiently experienced and trained in this special procedure (e.g., phacoemulsification, photorefractive keratectomy)? One should develop expertise in the procedure before conducting a study of an investigational treatment in the procedure. In addition, are residents and fellows allowed to participate in this study as surgeons, examiners, or both?

TABLE 13-3. *Selected considerations of an ophthalmologist in deciding to serve as a clinical investigator*

Sufficient patients?
Professional expertise?
Staff skills?
Sufficient physician and staff time available?
Any specialized equipment or facilities required?
Ethics of this trial?

Staff

Does the investigator have the necessary staff to complete this task? Study patients require more staff interaction than standard clinical patients. The staff must be trained to anticipate this need as well as specific questions about the concepts of randomization, masking, frequent follow-up, and the need to report any symptoms immediately. If there are any special examination procedures (e.g., Goldmann Visual Fields or fluorophotometry), does the investigator have staff with the proper training or who can be trained to perform these tasks?

Equipment

Does the investigator have all the equipment required to conduct the study? Some studies may require a given piece of capital equipment, and the sponsor may not always be in a position to purchase it for the site (e.g., specific perimeter, laser-flare meter). With standard clinical practice, it may be acceptable to send patients to a local university setting for some procedures (e.g., fundus photography), but this practice may not be an acceptable solution for study patients, especially if the procedure is required frequently.

Time

Clinical studies take substantial time from the principal investigator, fellows, residents, and office staff. Clinical examinations and their documentation tend to be significantly longer for investigational studies than for standard practice. A rough estimate is 20% to 30% more "chair time" than for a standard patient. In addition, the prestudy and poststudy administrative issues could require substantial time. Although there are certainly benefits and recognition for participating in a clinical trial, it is paramount that the potential investigator make a realistic assessment of the time available vis-à-vis the time required for such a commitment.

Ethics

As already noted, there are several formal ethical reviews that occur before an investigational clinical study begins. The investigator must realize that an investigational compound of unknown efficacy and safety is being put in a patient's eye. In most cases, this patient is otherwise "normal" and receiving some therapy for the disease. Although the new compound may hold promise as providing greater efficacy or a better safety profile, it is still investigational. A synonym for *investigational* is *experimental.* Whereas there may be a good deal of excitement at the sponsoring firm regarding a new chemical entity, the clinical investigator bears an ethical burden to decide whether it is appropriate to expose humans to this new agent. A physician has the right to remain skeptical about any claims and to question, in a professional manner, the adequacy of the supporting pharmacology and toxicology.

When questioned by a potential investigator about whether it is "safe" to test this new drug, it is advisable that each investigator question his or her own ethical stance on the planned investigation. These questions might include the following: "Do I truly feel that the risk to my patients is outweighed by the potential benefits of this trial?" When this trial is completed and the information released by the firm, "How would I feel if my participation in this trial became known?"

There is a wide range of risk in clinical studies. Some studies (typically Phase IV) of relatively low risk may involve evaluation of an approved product for a new indication (e.g., a drug approved for open-angle glaucoma in narrow-angle glaucoma) or a reformulation (e.g., removal of a preservative or excipient). Other studies of much higher risk may be a compound never evaluated previously in human eyes, a compound with significant ocular or systemic toxicity (e.g., an antimetabolite), or a compound evaluated in very ill patients (e.g., opportunistic cytomegalovirus retinitis). Clinicians new to investigational studies may wish to develop their expertise first by selecting a study of lower risk.

CONDUCTING THE STUDY

The major tasks involved in actually conducting the study relate to recruiting patients, conducting the appropriate examinations, and exposing patients to the investigational treatment. These tasks usually are fully described in the protocol.

The investigator needs to be hyperalert to the possibility for untoward or unusual reactions. As Goethe said, "Was man nicht weiss, seight man nicht" ("What man does not know, man does not see"). Although one cannot know what the unexpected is, one can heighten the senses to increase the potential to detect it. As Pasteur said, "Science favors the prepared mind."

The sponsor typically will send a *clinical monitor* (also known as a *clinical research associate*) to visit the site frequently. The role of this monitor is to review pedantically all the data for completeness and potential adverse experiences. There is an increasing trend to "document the documents," and "source data" for the case report forms may be required (e.g., visual fields, laboratory reports, and the initial observations of the investigator as noted in the patient's chart). These case report forms are essentially legal documents, and thus the sponsor must review seemingly minute aspects of the forms for completeness. The investigator may also interact with other members of the sponsor's firm, including the *study coordinator* (sometimes known as a *manager, director,* or *project leader*) as well as more senior members of the firm (e.g., executive directors, vice presidents).

The investigational drug provided by the sponsor must be kept in a restricted access environment and used only in patients entered in the study consistent with the protocol. It is a serious violation for an investigator to use an investigational drug outside the approved protocol.

GOOD CLINICAL PRACTICES

Clinical researchers and regulatory agencies are developing a series of guidelines for the conductance of clinical trials. These guidelines, called *Good Clinical Practices* (GCP), dictate a clear written record of the clinical trial. The wide range of GCP covers protocols, patient informed consent, IRB review, patient exposure to the drug, analysis, and reporting. For example, it is essential to document clearly the version and date of a protocol, and any changes need to be documented and signed by the sponsor and, in most cases, the IRB. In another example, clinical data need to be entered into a computer in an organized, auditable format and reviewed against the source data (e.g., the computer printout should be checked against a case report form and then, in some cases, against patient records). A major underlying idea of GCP is that after a study is complete, an independent individual could go back and confirm exactly what was done, how it was done, and who did it. It may seem that such efforts toward "paperwork" are unwarranted, but these studies involve major commitments of time, money, and patients. Moreover, regulatory approval and health-care system decisions are based on them. In one instance, there was some question about the traceability of data in a large study sponsored by the National Cancer Institute. After the trial was completed and published and had influenced the choice of various surgical therapies for breast cancer, there was some question about the entry and analysis of patient data.

The American, European, and Japanese standards for GCP differ today, but through the International Conference on Harmonization, a universal worldwide standard is being developed. Among the issues being addressed are the complexities of informed consent. Fully informed consent requires a number of key elements, including a description of the study, its benefits and risks, the total number of subjects being recruited, and the right of the subject to withdraw from the study at any time. The role of informed consent in the development of new therapies was evidenced by a recent FDA decision to stop further studies on an investigational device that enables an emergency worker to both compress and decompress the chest during cardiopulmonary resuscitation. Issues concerning attainment of informed consent from an unconscious patient in cardiac arrest led to the cessation, at least for now, of further investigations (7).

As with any practice, GCPs are a combination of statutes, regulations, and generally understood practices. The reference text for U.S. regulations is the *Code of Federal Regulations* (CFR). These volumes are updated annually, and interim revisions are published as part of the *Federal Register,* attainable from any federal Government Printing Office. Some of the regulations concerning the FDA and clinical use of investigational drugs are found in CFR Parts 1 to 100 and Parts 300 to 500. More specifically, obligations of sponsors and clinical investigators may be found in CFR (subpart D), Parts 312.50 to 312.70. Potential investigators should be aware that this is a mechanism for disqualifying investigators. One certainly does not want to conduct studies in any unacceptable way and thus be included on the FDA's "blacklist" of prohibited investigators.

After completion of the study, multiple audits may be conducted at the clinical investigator's site. Auditors may be the same clinical monitors with whom the clinical investigator interacts during the study, different ones from the sponsor, or an independent group of auditors. The presence of auditors generally has nothing to do with any wrongdoing on the clinician's part; rather, it is part of the checks and balances system of any pharmaceutical organization. Further, these persons are trying to detect any potential problems before audit by the FDA or other regulatory agencies. The FDA typically audits clinical sites from at least one of the two Phase III trials submitted in a New Drug Application.

AFTER THE STUDY

Patents

An inherent assumption in the R & D investment by a pharmaceutical firm in a compound is a proprietary patent position. In other words, when a product is approved, the firm desires a period in which only it can market the product. In a sense, a patent is a limited, government-approved monopoly. At present, the life of a U.S patent is 17 years, but the duration of patent life varies in other countries. Typically, patents are applied for in the preclinical stage of development. Given review time by the patent office and the time to develop and gain approval for the drug, the period of marketing protection is usually ten years.

Most clinical studies are viewed as "work for hire." In this regard, the clinical investigator is similar to an employee or a contractor in that the compensation received for the work includes payment for any inventions found in the process of completing the work. All rights thus remain with the sponsor. Most confidentiality agreements ask that the investigator disclose from the start any prior inventions that might conflict or present a priority position. Confidentiality agreements also typically cover not just the period before the study start and the period of study conductance but also the poststudy period until the information has been publicly released.

Publications

Most sponsors would like the results of their clinical studies to be published in peer-reviewed journals; however, such publications usually occur after preparation of the complete final clinical report, which typically comprises 60 pages of text plus hundreds of pages of supporting tables, figures, and individual patient listings. There is good reason for this prioritization. The business of the company depends on regulatory approvals, which depend on regulatory filings, which require the complete report, not just a manuscript or article of the study. Thus, the preparation of such reports receives preference over manuscripts. In addition, good compliance and audit trail dictate that the manuscript should agree with the data submitted to regulatory authorities. The simplest, most straightforward way to ensure such agreement is to prepare the larger report first and then to prepare the manuscript as a reduced report. If there is a serious discrepancy between the publication and the report, some regulatory authorities will not allow the publication to be used in the promotion of the product.

To investigators accustomed to conducting single-site studies, where a fellow uncodes the study a few days after completion and the manuscript is prepared within the next few months, this process will seem interminable, especially for multicenter trials; however, it is important to realize that for a complete report to be prepared, every site must finish with all patients. The data must be checked at each site, a database prepared and repeatedly checked to ensure that it represents the hard copy case report form, a formal analysis of all study variables performed, and a final clinical report prepared. The time frame is more like that typically seen with a National Eye Institute multicenter extramural project rather than the small fellow's project. Such patience is usually worthwhile, as the data and analysis behind the manuscript have a good deal of assuredness. Further, when questions arise in the preparation or review of a manuscript, the detailed data are usually readily available without additional effort. The investigator as well as clinical research personnel at the sponsoring firm must realize that, given review time and publication lag, such a publication might not appear until a year or more after completion of the study. This long lead time as well as copyright standards may be at odds with the communication needs of the financial side of the firm (8,9).

IMPACT OF THE CHANGING HEALTH-CARE SYSTEM

Several changes in the health-care system, especially in the United States, have affected the business aspects of clinical research. Market pressures in the United States are decreasing the physician reimbursement per procedure as well as increasing the competitive environment for patient populations. In this environment, private specialists may find that they must associate with larger firms who have the patients (e.g., health maintenance organizations). For more and more ophthalmologists, clinical studies represent a way to perform quality medical practice and receive reasonable compensation. This trend probably will continue as long as there are clinical studies to perform and ophthalmologists with sufficient, qualified study patients. In fact, some anticipate that the per patient reimbursement for clinical trials actually may decrease as the number of ophthalmologists competing for such studies increases.

The recent trend in ophthalmic drug approvals in the United States has been for an increasingly larger study patient population. This trend is related to several factors, including the desire for higher power on efficacy measures in equivalency studies, evaluation of drugs with incremental (as contrasted with dramatic) improvement over existing therapy, and a desire to detect low-incidence adverse events preapproval rather than postapproval. These factors, some generated by the FDA and some by the sponsor, have tended to increase the demand for clinical study patients. Given the reasonable assumption that the number of compounds being studied remains constant or increases, one would predict an increase in the requirement for clinical patients overall.

Changes in the health-care environment also put pressures on pharmaceutical firms. The distribution of market share within a given product area will probably dramatically sharpen. Whereas previously a firm with the third most popular drug in a given area (e.g., corticosteroids) might still enjoy a reasonable market share, it is more likely that the first and second drugs in any category will take more and more of the market. Thus, a company needs either to develop a highly demanded drug (e.g., timolol in the late 1970s) or accept a much lower reimbursement rate for a "me-too" drug. Demands of third-party payers for demonstration of a real clinical benefit or lower utilization cost to the provider will probably result in a host of Phase IV "quality of life" studies. Firms that wish to participate in the higher level of product sales probably will continue to increase their investment in this type of clinical trial. Other firms may feel that this sizable investment in time and money may not be worthwhile, and they will move to the "lower" end of the reimbursement continuum. In the arena of the 1970s and 1980s, when the physician's choice of a medication was paramount, having a strong relationship with the prescribing physician was very important to pharmaceutical firms. In the late 1990s, when physician choice is more numerically weighed against cost by pharmacists and financial personnel, a decrease in the investment of pharmaceutical firms in support of the physician (e.g., continuing medical education courses, resident's rounds) has been seen; however, overall, the demand for clinical patients probably will increase.

SUMMARY

There are many scientific, regulatory, and ethical considerations for an ophthalmologist who participates in a clinical research study. This chapter notes many of the factors to consider in deciding whether to participate as a clinical investigator, which should be viewed as a long-term commitment to a relationship with the pharmaceutical firm, the compound, and the study patients.

ACKNOWLEDGMENTS

I acknowledge the hours of patient training from colleagues, including Alan L. Robin, M.D., William C. Stewart, M.D., Daniel Mufson, Ph.D., and Maggie Reents Timms.

REFERENCES

1. Anonymous. The Fortune 500 ranked within industries. *Fortune* 1994; 129:257–276.
2. DiMasi JA, Hansen RW, Grabowski HG, Lasagna L. Cost of innovation in the pharmaceutical industry. *J Health Econ* 1991;10:107–142.
3. Haffner ME. Orphan products: origins, progress, and prospects. *Annu Rev Pharmacol Toxicol* 1991;31:603–620.
4. Ferris FL, Sperduto RD. Standardized illumination for visual acuity testing in clinical research. *Am J Ophthalmol* 1982;94:97–98.
5. Novack GD. Ophthalmic beta-blockers since timolol. *Surv Ophthalmol* 1987;31:307–327.
6. Novack GD, Lue JC, Duzman E. Power estimates for glaucoma trials. *Clin Pharmacol Ther* 1987;41:208(abst).
7. Winslow R. FDA halts test on device that shows promise for victims of cardiac arrest. *Wall Street Journal* 1994;11 May.
8. Steiner J. Problems in clinical development for the start-up company. *Applied Clinical Trials* 1994;3:41–46.
9. Werth B. *The Billion Dollar Molecule: One Company's Quest for the Perfect Drug.* New York: Simon and Schuster, 1994.

Textbook of Ocular Pharmacology,
edited by T.J. Zimmerman, et al.
Lippincott–Raven Publishers, Philadelphia © 1997.

CHAPTER 14

Introduction to Toxicology

Harrell E. Hurst

Toxicology is the basic science involving the study of undesirable effects of matter and energy on living systems. To date, most of the research effort and published information in this field concern the detrimental effects of chemicals on living systems. As chemical and drug exposures currently represent the overwhelming majority of actual human exposures and issues of safety are extremely important in public opinion, the essence of toxicological science focuses on understanding interactions between exogenous chemicals and the internal chemical milieu of living systems.

Early efforts in toxicology were descriptive in nature and provided observational details regarding chemical poisonings. A brief historical perspective will illustrate development of toxicological knowledge. Anecdotal accounts dating from antiquity, such as the poisoning of Socrates with hemlock (coniine), today seem to represent the essence of legend rather than science. Poisoning was a black art during Roman times and was used for surreptitious advantage. The use of poison to eliminate enemies or to elevate one's status was epidemic to the extent that Sulla issued *Lex Cornelia,* which became the first legal proclamation against poisoning, in about 80 B.C. Toxicological knowledge remained in a similar state throughout the Middle Ages.

The writings of Paracelsus (1493–1541) provided the basis for toxicological science. This key figure of the Renaissance articulated the concept of *dose,* which is taken for granted today. His key observation stated that all substances are poisons; the right dose differentiates a *remedy* from a *poison.* This idea effectively replaced the philosophy of magic that had dictated power to that time. Additionally, Paracelsus generated ideas that initiated the practices of experimentation and examination of responses to chemicals. His concepts of differentiation between desirable and toxic effects, with emphasis on dose as a determinant, began the construct of *selective toxicity,* which is fundamental in medicine today.

The Spanish physician Orfila (1787–1853) served as court physician to Louis XVIII of France and lectured at the University of Paris. His book of 1815 regarding mineral, vegetable, and animal poisons can be viewed as the first toxicology text. He was the first to use autopsy material and chemical analysis systematically as legal proof; thus began the field of forensic toxicology. One might say that he began to elevate toxicology to an *analytical science* from its former *descriptive* origins. Others continued this tradition of learned study. Magendie (1783–1855), a physiologist and physician, studied actions of emetine, strychnine, and curare. Bernard (1813–1878), a student of Magendie, continued these efforts and, notably, observed the action of carbon monoxide in combination with hemoglobin.

As understanding of functional mechanisms of physiological systems developed, toxicologists began to provide hypotheses based on these mechanisms. Scottish physicians at the University of Edinburgh played important roles in toxicology and ophthalmology. Here the well-known actions of atropine and other belladonna alkaloids were studied. Christison (1797–1882), a former student of Orfila, studied the actions of the recently described Calabar bean (the seed of *Physostigma venenosum*), which had been used in a concoction for tribal justice in West Africa. Pharmacological experiments by Fraser (1863) revealed the miotic action of extracts of the bean; in the same year, Robertson (1837–1909) realized the antagonism between the active principal (later named physostigmine, or eserine) and atropine. Shortly thereafter (1877), Laquere suggested that this drug, the first methylcarbamate anticholinesterase, would be effective in the therapy for glaucoma.

This trend continues today as advances in biological and clinical sciences increase our understanding of physiological mechanisms. As knowledge of molecular biology de-

H. E. Hurst: Department of Pharmacology and Toxicology, University of Louisville School of Medicine, Louisville, Kentucky 40292.

velops, so do research efforts toward detailed explanation of the undesirable interactions between exogenous chemicals and mechanisms of normal function in living organisms. Formulated mechanistic hypotheses of therapeutic effects or chemically mediated diseases provide necessary elements for systematic attempts toward strategic prevention or intervention.

Otherwise, only serendipity provides such insight. This text necessarily is limited in scope to ocular pharmacology and thus provides focus on the eye as the major physiological system of interest. This chapter attempts to give a summary toxicological approach and, in so doing, will reach beyond the oculus for perspective. The intent is to provide information that may prove useful in the discovery of causal relationships between chemical exposures that may result in adverse consequences to living systems and, ultimately, to ourselves.

CLASSIFICATION OF TOXIC AGENTS

Traditional classification of toxic agents provides a means to organize or catalog toxic interactions to assess this information readily as needed. Some general means for classification of toxic agents are chemical functionality, chemical use or source, types of adverse effect, biological system affected, biochemical mechanism of the effect, and potential for toxicity. Choice of a classification system depends on the purpose for which the classification system will be used; that is, the classification system should serve as an index by which the chemistry or toxic effect can be accessed for future study.

Chemical group classification is particularly useful in toxicological studies of structure-activity relationships. As specific chemical functional groups most often provide the basis for receptor-mediated drug effects, so do specific chemical moieties cause receptor-based toxic effects. The drug-receptor interaction often is related to students as a "lock-and-key" analogy. A corresponding analogy for toxic chemicals might consider a toxicant a "monkey wrench in the cogs" of the exquisite biochemical, physiological machine that is the human body. The chemical group classification provides systematic order to the wrenches: their types, sizes, and material from which they are constructed.

Classifications by *chemical use* or *source* might be more appropriate for commercial or regulatory purposes. Such a system provides the advantage of focus on the use of the chemical. The hazards of toxic agents are derived, directly or indirectly, from the manner in which chemicals are used. Perhaps the most substantial impact in diminishing the hazards of chemicals arises from associating specific risks with the various ways chemicals are handled or used. An obvious example is the beneficial impact made by child-resistant drug container caps on the incidence of accidental poisoning.

Similarly, the affected *biological system* or *biochemical mechanism* could be advantageous as classification schemes for physiologists, biologists, or biochemists. This approach assists scientists whose focus is a specific physiologic system for study. Suffice it to say that individuals can construct organizational elements advantageously for the purpose at hand.

CHARACTERIZATION OF EXPOSURE

Characterization of exposure gives insight into the manner in which a chemical gains access to the body. Critical determinants governing systemic presentation of toxicant and, usually, the toxic consequences are the amount or *dose* of chemical, the specific *route* by which it enters the physiological system, the *duration,* and *frequency* of exposure(s). Obviously, the dose of chemical determines the mass of substance available for potential for systemic poisoning. The effects of dosage depend on the potential disruptive effects that the chemical can cause at the molecular level of the living system. Collectively, these undesirable, detrimental actions, or *toxicity,* should be considered a property of the chemical as it interacts with a given living system. As different species have evolved or adapted with defense mechanisms against certain toxic chemicals, characterization of the specific chemical-species interaction offers a more reliable basis for understanding toxicity. The primary objectives of toxicology as a science currently are characterization of the nature and extent of such toxic effects, determination of the dosage required for the expression of toxicity, and, ultimately, prevention of such exposures.

Additional objectives of toxicology include elucidation of less obvious interactions among dose, exposure route, duration, and dosage frequency, which result in unexpected increases or decreases in typical toxic effects. If an adverse action follows from exposure of the protein, lipid, or ionic material of the living system to chemicals, the magnitude of toxic effect most commonly is a function of the dose $\times$ time product. The consequence of repeated doses depends on the reversibility of the toxicity or the time required for such repair.

If the action of a toxic chemical on tissue is reversible or repairable and the insult occurs infrequently, the physiologic system can maintain homeostasis. In contrast, with toxic effects that are not truly reversible or that are repaired only slowly, damage will accumulate with repeated presentation of the noxious, tissue-damaging material. The effect of dosage generally is additive toxicity if the frequency of toxic material presentation is more rapid than the processes of repair. This view may be an oversimplification, however, when genetic material or other critical or irreplaceable sites of toxicity are involved.

Characterization of toxic effects with repeated chemical exposure often reveals undiscovered toxic effects. The anticoagulant drug and rodenticide warfarin increases both vitamin K-dependent prothrombin time and capillary fragility. The combination of these effects causes repeated small doses to be much more toxic than a large single dose. Careful observation noted the combined effects of lengthened clotting time and damage to capillary walls, which result in lethal hemorrhage. Likewise, knowledge of the mechanism of action provided the critical information that vitamin K was antidotal through reversal of the clotting inhibition.

Similarly, comparison of toxicity following different routes of toxicant entry can illustrate critical steps in the poisoning process. If a chemical is more toxic given orally than parenterally, one might suspect that a metabolite of the chemical formed in the liver immediately following absorption was the active toxic principal. Conversely, a lower oral toxicity might lead to the hypothesis that the first-pass effect of the liver was defending the system by detoxifying a substantial portion of the chemical. This type of observed differential toxicity is significant in industrial settings, which often include parenteral exposure through inhalation or dermal contact.

MECHANISMS OF TOXICITY

The actions of a toxicant can be characterized by the nature and degree of selectivity of effect. The actions range from very specific interaction with tissue, which may induce a subtle change in protein conformation, to a gross tissue injury, which destroys the intricate chemical superstructure of cells. An example of a specific, selective toxic effect involves formation of a receptor-ligand complex. In this instance, the three-dimensional shape of the toxicant, here referred to as the *ligand,* conforms to a complex surface of the receptor. The interaction produces an undesired effect on the normal function of the receptor, often disabling its normal role. Many instances of this type of toxic action exist. A classic example is the interaction of carbon monoxide, which binds to hemoglobin with affinity some 200 times greater than that of oxygen. This displacement of oxygen can occur in an atmosphere of as little as 0.1% carbon monoxide, leading to inadequate oxygenation and potential death by asphyxia.

A characteristic of receptor-ligand interactions is *reversibility.* As the complex is held together by ionic forces, hydrophobic or hydrogen bonding, the complex can dissociate into the two components, resulting in return of normal function. In mild cases of carbon monoxide exposure, such as occurs with cigarette smoking, reversal of the toxic process occurs on termination of exposure as oxygen diffuses in and replaces carbon monoxide. Alternatively, if a physiologic ligand can be presented to compete with the toxic moiety, the reversibility can be accelerated in some instances. This is, in part, the basis for treatment of carbon monoxide poisoning in which oxygen is given in concentration or pressure greater than that in the normal atmosphere. This type of intervention requires an understanding of the nature and extent of the poisoning. Discovery of the nature of such a process is the ideal of the toxicological scientist, as this knowledge may provide a new approach in treatment of such poisoning. Mechanisms of reversibility are varied; in simplest terms, these mechanisms involve dissociation of pharmacological agents or replacement with the physiological ligand, as previously discussed. Alternatively, recovery of function may require synthetic tissue repair, which requires considerably longer for recovery of function and provides little opportunity for therapeutic intervention.

Toxic effects on excitable membranes also present a high degree of selectivity. This category includes compounds and ions that alter normal functions of nerve tissue. The special properties of nerve membranes, which include the maintenance of neurotransmitter packaging and differing ion concentrations on either side of the membranes, are targets of numerous toxicants. Agents that bind to active transport systems or disrupt critical structures effectively disrupt these essential structures. Generally, receptor-ligand-type interactions at nerve membranes are reversible, and treatment of such toxicity is supportive. That is, the patient is assisted in overcoming the functional deficit caused by the toxicant until toxicant removal by metabolism and excretion is sufficient for approach to normal function. In contrast, toxic agents that cause nerve-cell death may not be reversible, particularly if toxicity involves a specific, critical neural tract. A dramatic example is the severe type of parkinsonism induced by 1-methyl-4-phenyl-1,2,5,6-tetrahydropyridine (MPTP). This experimental compound causes selective destruction of dopaminergic neuronal cells of the substantia nigra, leading to loss of willful muscle control; MPTP contamination of improperly synthesized meperidine caused catatonic reactions in numerous illicit drug users. This "case of the frozen addicts" was solved mechanistically in a model series of investigations during the 1980s (Singer et al., 1987).

Macromolecular binding is a mechanism by which many reactive materials disrupt normal function. A distinguishing feature in this category is formation of one or more covalent bond(s) between the toxicant and the biological macromolecule. It is likely that such interaction occurs frequently, often without toxicity, as many reactive materials are produced by oxidative metabolism. If the macromolecule is sufficiently redundant or without critical function, such binding is without overt toxicity. Examples include the formation of adducts at various sites on hemoglobin by reactive metabolites of exogenous compounds or from lipid peroxidation. On the other hand, if the macromolecule has critical function, such binding may result in disease. An example is unrepaired genetic damage produced by genotoxic or mutagenic materials. The result of such toxic binding may be cancer, although many of the drugs used to treat cancer work through similar mechanisms. Such chemotherapeutic agents derive their cell-killing action through covalent binding to macromolecules of rapidly dividing cells. Toxic side effects of such therapy are common problems. The alkylating agent busulfan has caused subcapsular lens opacities during treatment of chronic myeloid leukemia and experimental cataracts in rodents chronically fed this drug.

Selective cell loss is a fascinating type of toxicity that occurs when particular toxins exhibit lethal affinity with a particular cell type, as in the previously mentioned loss of dopaminergic neurons in the substantia nigra caused by MPTP. These poisons often result in dramatic toxicity in which a particular function is lost without apparent damage to other systems. Another example is the selective loss of optic nerve ganglion cells after poisoning with methanol. This toxicity, which can result in blindness, is a consequence of the formation of oxidative metabolites of methanol (formaldehyde and formic acid). Evidence for metabolic involvement in this toxicity is the antidotal action of ethanol, which is preferentially oxidized while methanol is removed by other mechanisms. Infusions containing ethanol prevent the metabolic formation of the toxic metabolite(s) and, thereby, the threat of permanent blindness.

Gross tissue injury is a nonspecific destruction of all cells in a selected area. This toxicity generally is associated with physical damage, as opposed to selective molecular events. This mechanism is quite common in cases of alkali or acid burns by splash or other eye contact, where extreme pH conditions result in chemical degradation of the chemical matrix of tissue. The best approach to this type of problem is prevention through transparent eye protection. Lacking that, rapid removal of the offending agent, as by rapid flushing with water at an emergency eyewash station, can be critical in the prevention of serious, persistent damage. In such a serious accident, rapid action is paramount to successful recovery.

DOSE-RESPONSE RELATIONSHIPS

As mentioned earlier, the relationship of dose to the toxic response is the cornerstone of toxicological science. In all scientific discussions of dose-response relationships, certain assumptions are implicit but require examination, as all too often perceived toxic episodes are associated with products or environmental contaminants without scientific evidence. The fundamental assumption is that a toxic response is due to some chemical with which the physiologic system has come in contact. For appropriate scientific documentation or study, the toxic response must be measurable, directly or indirectly. Additionally, a site of action must exist for the toxic chemical, and the response must be a function of the concentration of the chemical at the site. Lastly, the concentration at the site must be related to the dose of the chemical. These essential assumptions are necessary elements to establish a cause-effect relationship. Those who associate an undesirable event without acceptable evidence that these assumptions are valid are no more scientific in approach than those earlier humans who associated magical properties with toxic events.

Dose-response functions vary according to the nature of the mechanism of toxicity. *Irreversible* toxic effects generally are additive over time, less any tissue repair that occurs during intervals between exposures to the toxic agent. The outcome of this mechanism is highly dependent on the frequency and duration of dosage compared with the time required for repair of damage. Thus, if exposures are of such frequency and duration that homeostatic repair mechanisms cannot undo the damage, tissue destruction is inevitable. With this general mechanism, quality of repair may be an issue as well. If the repair does not exhibit the full capacity of the original tissue, a deficit in function will remain. For example, a caustic burn destroys tissue, which is replaced by scar tissue. If the scar is not as elastic or as transparent, depending on the normal function of the tissue involved, loss of physiological function will impair the quality of life of the organism.

With *reversible* toxic effects, the outcome is more complex. Consideration must be given to the nature and function of the involved physiological system, the extent of reversible inhibition, and the kinetics of reversibility. Impairment of a highly vital system for a sufficient time can result in death, even though the effect is reversible. A classic example of such a system is the reversible binding of carbon monoxide to hemoglobin. As the affinity of hemoglobin for this gas is some 200 times that of oxygen, a small fractional percentage of carbon monoxide in the atmosphere (0.1% versus 20% for oxygen for about 50% binding) can result in lethal interruption of the vital oxygen-carrying function of the red cells. On the other hand, the reversibility of the effect provides opportunity for significant therapeutic intervention. With this example, removal of a poisoned patient from the source of carbon monoxide to fresh air provides relief from the toxicity. The therapeutic effects can be hastened significantly, if necessary, through the use of increased exposure to oxygen beyond that naturally present in the atmosphere. The essential determinant for successful detoxication is adequate reversal of lost function before other consequential, irreversible damage occurs.

Less vital systems can suffer more extensive reversible inhibition without lethal effect or even obvious toxicity. Many possible examples of pharmacological effects exist without overt toxicity from functional redundancy in physiologic systems or adaptive changes at various levels of physiologic function; however, many of these cause undesirable change in the overall quality of life. For example, drug dependency may not result in direct or overt toxicity but if continued over time may have substantial negative effects. Such drug effects, although technically reversible at the cellular level, cause changes at higher levels of physiologic integration. Taken to the extreme, such reversible effects can produce withdrawal syndromes resulting from adaptive cellular effects in the nervous system and can lead to certain behaviors that can be lethal.

Dose-response curves of the previously discussed effects differ. The irreversible toxic response can be considered a series of step functions with increasing loss of function between exposures. If such effects occur without repair, the loss of capacity with repeated dose can be represented by the cumulative total of these step functions. As such toxicity is additive in nature, the dose-response curves often may be plotted on an arithmetic axis. The toxic effect will rise in proportion to increases in dosage according to the specific injury caused by the dosage.

More reversible effects give a cumulative effect that is dependent on the extent of repair or the continuing presence of toxicant. Toxicity requiring the continuing presence of chemical, a so-called receptor-mediated effect, generally follows the laws of mass action. That is, the toxicity is dependent on the continuing presence of the toxicant at some site of action. Therefore, removal of molecules from that site by diffusion to other sites, metabolic detoxification, or excretion diminishes the toxic effect with time.

Individuals in most samples of populations exhibit differences in sensitivity to a toxic effect, resulting in a distribution of responses across dosage that ranges from obvious effects at lower doses in sensitive individuals ultimately to those in more resistant persons at higher levels. The statistical nature of this sensitivity distribution sometimes is represented by a normal, bell-shaped curve of frequency of effect versus dose. Alternatively, the cumulative mortality is plotted as dose is increased, which is the traditional *sigmoid curve.* Often the dose axis is scaled according to the logarithm of dose. Logarithms are used because responses often vary quickly with small changes in low doses, with lesser increases at higher doses. Another transform, used to linearize dose-response curves, involves the probability of effect based on the normal or other evident distribution. This scaling of the response axis into probit units uses standard deviations of response as the fundamental units. The median response is set arbitrarily at a probit unit of 5, and standard deviations of the experimental sample responses range in either direction. With probit units, responses rarely range beyond the extremes of probit values 2 through 8, as these units encompass >99% of the represented population.

Comparisons of dose-response values among different chemicals exhibiting a similar toxic effect often are useful for risk evaluation or selection of the least toxic drug. The dose producing the median toxic response is a common means of such evaluation and is useful for drugs with identical specificity and therapeutic and toxic effects. Such parallel therapeutic response between two drugs is unusual. In this case, the relative potency can be determined by the ratio of the median responses. The most frequently considered example in toxicology is the LD_{50}, or median lethal dose.

Other side effects or differing responses, such as dose increase, often mar convenient comparisons of therapeutic response versus dosage. Many apparently similar drugs exhibit different slopes in their respective dose-response curves. It is possible for two such curves to have similar doses, which produce the median effect, but widely different responses at extremes of dosage. Therefore, besides the dose giving the median response, the slope of the curve

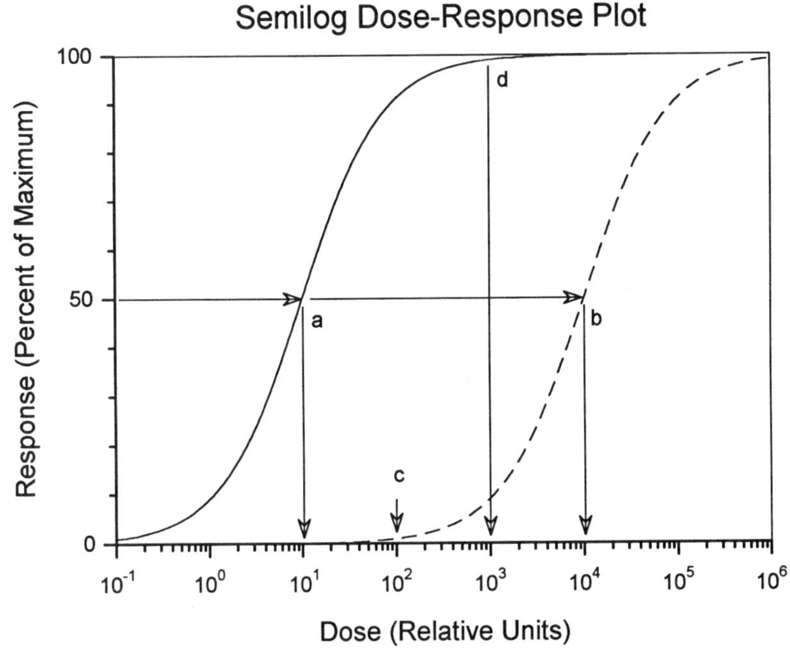

FIG. 14-1. Theoretical semilog dose-response curves for therapeutic response (solid line) and lethal response (dashes) as functions of dosage. Vertical arrows indicate (**a**) the median (50%) effective dose, (**b**) median lethal dose, and, similarly, doses producing (**c**) 1% lethal and (**d**) 99% effective therapeutic responses.

must be considered. Several indices are derived from dose-response curves so that such information can be included in comparisons. The safety of drugs is sometimes compared by the *margin of safety,* or the margin between therapeutic (ED) and lethal doses (LD). This concept is illustrated in Figure 14-1, where the *therapeutic response* of a population may be considered as the solid curve (left), and the *lethal response* is represented as the dashed curve (right). Please note that this example uses curves with similar slopes and that overlap exists between points (c) and (d). A conservative estimate of the margin of safety is determined in this case as the ratio $LD_{1\%}/ED_{99\%}$, or dose values (c/d). This estimate of margin of safety indicates that dosage required for achieving therapeutic effect in the most refractory individuals of the population (the highest effective doses) can be lethal to the most sensitive individuals (lowest lethal doses), as this ratio is <1.0.

Another more common measure, although less protective, is the *therapeutic index,* which is derived from the ratio of the median lethal and therapeutic doses, or $LD_{50\%}/ED_{50\%}$. In the example, this ratio is determined using the dose value (b/a), which gives a therapeutic index of 10^3. Note the contrast between this value based on median response compared with the previous estimate of margin of safety. In real cases, the measures of relative safety are related directly to the spacing between and the slopes of the dose–response curves, which depend on the mechanism(s) of therapeutic and toxic effects.

Another comparative term used in toxicology is the *chronicity index,* a measure of accumulation of chemical or its toxic effects, which is estimated for a chemical by dividing the single-dose LD_{50} by the 90-day LD_{50}. Theoretically, if no toxicant accumulation or residual effect occurs, the chronicity index would be 1.0; if a residual toxicant remained without tolerance or if irreversible effects occurred, this number would be higher.

INTERACTIONS OF TOXICANTS

Rarely, if ever, in practice, are people exposed to single chemicals because of the widespread distribution of environmental chemicals in water, air, and dietary components. Therefore, it is important to understand the nature of chemical interactions. It is also true, however, that people are not often exposed acutely to health-threatening doses of such toxicants, despite the fear frequently expressed in the general concern for environmental chemical exposure. Analysis of multiple chemical exposures and the mechanisms of resultant toxicity has yielded an understanding of the ways in which chemicals jointly interact with a living system. The effects of such interactions of chemicals can lead to decreases or increases in the express toxicity compared with the effects of each chemical alone.

Antagonism is a term applied when one chemical moderates, or lessens, the toxicity of another. This effect results when one or both of the chemicals interfere with the toxic action of the other. A number of possible mechanisms can cause this effect. Changes in the absorption, distribution, metabolism, or elimination of either chemical and interruptions of specific toxic events occur as a result of the presence of the chemical(s) at some critical cellular or molecular site(s). Antidotal drugs are exploited therapeutically for precisely this reason. Many of these, such as the narcotic antagonist naloxone, derive their efficacy from specific antagonism of the active binding site at the receptors. Others, such as chelating agents used in metal element poisoning, hasten the reduction of toxic concentrations through increased rates of toxicant elimination.

Conversely, toxic agents can increase toxicity when combined. For chemicals and drugs with similar modes of action, or that make similar critical biochemical systems active, *additive effects* are the most commonly observed type of interaction. This term refers to the instance when the combined toxic effect can be considered the sum of the toxic effects that occur when each chemical is given separately. A distinctly different term, *synergism,* describes the situation when two chemicals combined produce a more toxic effect than the sum of their individual doses. In this instance, both chemicals have similar toxic effects, and, in some manner, each chemical promotes the toxic combined action, thereby magnifying the overall effect. Another term, *potentiation,* is used to describe an interaction in which one chemical is without apparent effect alone but, when combined with a known toxicant, produces a much greater toxic action than the toxicant alone. The latter effect is akin to the opposite of antagonism. Often, characterization of these interactions depends on knowledge of the mechanisms of toxicity.

SAFETY TESTING

One of the major roles for toxicologists is *testing* of commercial products. The purpose of this important function is premarket discovery of hazardous conditions that might result from the projected use of chemicals. This objective supports the important task of discovery of chemicals or product forms that can be used for commercial purposes without adverse effect. Elucidation of toxic mechanisms is a secondary objective for critical chemicals to which some exposure is unavoidable or for products of sufficiently important use to justify the cost of such research.

The toxicological testing paradigm initially involves short-term *acute tests,* which usually require one dosage or exposure for a few hours. One variation of this test type involves testing for acute lethality. The usual measure is the *median lethal dose,* or LD_{50}, which is the dose sufficient to kill 50% of exposed animals. In such a study, another, more useful objective is to determine roughly the exposure range to which animals may be exposed without overt toxicity. Experimental observations made in acute testing are simple and relate to overall toxic effects and the range of exposures that cause these effects. Other acute tests of interest include dermal and inhalation toxicity, dermal and eye irritation, as well as skin sensitization.

If the results of the acute test are deemed successful by the appropriate criteria to continue the testing paradigm, a second stage of testing is invoked. This phase, termed *subacute* or *subchronic testing,* involves repeated dosing. Subchronic testing may involve exposure for up to 10% of the test animal species' lifetime, usually about 90 days for rodents. Three dosage levels are chosen, which ideally cause no overt effects at the low level and not more than 10% fatalities at the high level. During this time, tests of increasing sophistication are employed, including clinical chemistry panels. Observations made during acute testing are examined in greater depth, with more refined tests designed to probe previously noted toxic events. An important objective at this point is to find a level of treatment at which no apparent ill effects are noted. This level is termed the *no observable effect level.* Another goal is estimation of a dose that suppresses weight gain by about 10%; this dosage is called the *maximum tolerable dose.* These critical doses will be used in design of chronic tests. For chemicals being developed for use as drugs, acute and subchronic testing must be completed before an Investigational New Drug application is done.

The last phase of testing, assuming successful outcomes of previous efforts, involves treatment in the range of exposure conditions previously determined to cause none to moderate toxic effects. This phase, termed *chronic testing,* is continued over the lifetime of the rodent. The number of animals used should allow for premature loss during testing. Chronic testing involves extensive, detailed observation, complete biochemical parameters, and extensive pathological study of animals killed for necropsy. The objective is to develop a whole profile of exposure effects along with dose-response and time-response toxicological data. A wide spectrum of other tests may be involved in this phase, depending on the potential use of the chemical. Detailed examination of these is beyond the scope of this chapter, but such testing may include testing for carcinogenesis and for developmental and reproductive toxicity. Rodents, including mice and rats, account for most of the routine animal models used in safety testing. These species are used for reasons of convenience and cost and because humans usually do not have these animals as pets. Other species are used occasionally for specific physiological features, including monkeys as surrogate primates. Other important animal models include the guinea pig (testing for skin sensitization) and the rabbit (acute dermal and eye irritation testing).

The eye irritation test, conducted in rabbits, has drawn criticism from the public, who bemoan the use of rabbits for eye-irritation testing. Such testing is known formally as the *Draize test,* after the author of a published testing procedure. Advantages of using rabbits in such in vivo tests include ease of handling, large surface area of the eyeball, inexpensive cost, a large background literature for comparison, and requirement by certain regulatory protocols. Disadvantages include the presence of a nicitating membrane, which may clear the surface of chemical. Additionally, the tearing mechanism for removal of a chemical is less effective in the rabbit than in the human. Also different are the blink reflex, the pH, and the buffering capacity of the aqueous humor as well as the thickness and histology of the cornea.

Alternatives to the Draize test have been proposed and are gaining some measure of acceptance. These alternatives involve quantitative in vivo estimates of irritation at threshold levels below frank irritation scoring. Another approach involves in vitro cytotoxicity assays based on corneal epithelial cells, Chinese hamster ovary cells, lung fibroblasts, and canine renal cells. Ocular preparations exposed in vitro include enucleated rabbit eye, isolated bovine cornea, or lens in culture. Hen's egg chorioallantoic membrane is a nonocular preparation that has been used as a predictor for eye irritation. Each of these test methods has a scoring system that correlates to some degree with the classic Draize test for eye irritation. As use of these systems increases, acceptance will increase in suitable systems as a result of decreased cost and greater acceptability to humanitarian concerns.

RISK ASSESSMENT

Currently, considerable money and resources are spent on efforts devoted to assessment of risk from real and perceived chemical exposures. Most such efforts originate from regulatory mandates, such as those issued by the Environmental Protection Agency, or conflicts between commercial or government objectives and local public opinion. Lack of understanding of essential toxicological mechanisms represents a fundamental problem that leaves many such efforts flawed and scientifically unsatisfactory; that is, risk estimates tend to be ad hoc without general applicability or are derived from "pseudo"-science that is subject to public debate and scientific revision.

Two approaches to the use of toxicological data in policy determination may help to illustrate the dilemma of hazard prevention. One technique that has been in use for many years involves safety factors. With this approach, scientists have taken dosage or exposure data derived from toxicological animal experiments and arbitrarily divided animal doses by factors of 10 to 1,000, depending on the severity and type of toxicity. The rationale was that lack of understanding of mechanisms or actual target-tissue exposure made it better to err on the conservative side. Safety factors can be increased, if necessary, to protect more sensitive individuals as the need becomes apparent; however, the use of safety factors is not founded on fundamental mechanistic understanding. Additionally, this approach is subject to criticism, as it relies on subjective judgment, and regulatory officials are increasingly reticent to use it in our litigious and political society.

Another approach relies on scientific techniques for extrapolation, but the data used are incomplete for definition of the appropriate mathematical function for such extrapolation. As a result, default assumptions are used which are not necessarily mechanistically derived. These techniques rely on more sophisticated statistical manipulations than the safety factor approach, but their scientific enhancement seems to serve more to baffle the uninformed than to support judgment with appropriate mechanistic data for extrapolation. In this approach, safety factors are implicit as statistical confidence limits.

Much argument surrounds the idea of a dosage threshold for biological effects. At this time, the term hardly can be discussed intelligently, as two pervasive, conflicting views exist, each of which is adamantly defended without definitive data on either part. On the one hand, many optimistic toxicologists view the homeostatic biological organism with considerable reserve detoxication capacity. The capacity to overcome toxic insult represents a threshold, and the task of hazard prevention in this view is to define and protect limits of homeostasis. The other view is that perhaps as little as one molecule suitably targeted can cause disease. Our understanding of the detailed mechanisms of life and the fate of large numbers of the diverse molecules to which current life is exposed, is limited. Therefore, unwarranted exposure must be prevented at all cost.

Some recent innovative approaches offer some hope of additional insight for future use. An increased understanding of molecular biology is beginning to detail the mechanisms of control of cellular replication and homeostasis. Confluence of formerly separate biological disciplines, such as biochemistry and immunology, serves to reinforce resources that may bc applied to toxicological problems. Use of computer techniques, such as biological and pharmacokinetic simulations, offers new ways to pose dynamic, rather than static, hypotheses. Noninvasive imaging of tissues and organs graphically depicts disease states in ways to which we formerly were blind. New surgical techniques offer means of remediation of maladies for which suffering was once inevitable. Now the daunting task of toxicological science is to define the appropriate use of such tools and to provide an integrated means of information focus and exchange for true risk assessment and prevention.

REFERENCES

Amdur MO, Doull J, Klaassen CD, eds. *Casaret and Doull's Toxicology: The Basic Science of Poisons,* 4th ed. New York: Pergamon Press, 1991;

Ballantyne B, Marrs T, Turner P, eds. *General and Applied Toxicology.* New York: Stockton Press, 1993;567–593.

Hodgson E, Levi PE, eds. *Introduction to Biochemical Toxicology,* 2nd ed. Norwalk, Connecticut: Appleton & Lange, 1994;

Singer TP, et al. Biochemistry of the neurotoxic action of MPTP: or how a faulty batch of "designer drug" led to Parkinsonism in drug abuse. *Trends Biochem Sci* 1987;12:266–270.

Textbook of Ocular Pharmacology,
edited by T.J. Zimmerman, et al.
Lippincott–Raven Publishers, Philadelphia © 1997.

CHAPTER 15

Effect of Disease on Drug Disposition

Bruce A. Mueller and Steven R. Abel

A patient's response to drug therapy relies on pharmacodynamics and pharmacokinetics. These terms can be easily defined. *Pharmacodynamics* refers to the biological response of the patient to the drug (what the drug does to the patient). *Pharmacokinetics* refers to the disposition of the drug once administered to the patient (what the patient does to the drug). Optimal pharmacotherapy cannot occur without a working knowledge of both concepts. As clinicians, we prescribe and administer drug therapies with the purpose of achieving a particular pharmacodynamic effect, usually to treat or prevent a particular disease state. If the desired pharmacodynamic response does not occur, we change the dosing regimen or use a different drug to achieve the desired effect. Frequently, the lack of therapeutic response or the presence of a toxic reaction from a drug derives from pharmacokinetic considerations. Drug absorption, distribution to the site of action, metabolism, and elimination from the body all must be considered before initiating pharmacotherapy. All these pharmacokinetic factors can be altered by a patient's concomitant disease states. Although most ocular treatments are topical, certain diseases of the eye (e.g., uveitis, endophthalmitis, and glaucoma) are treated systemically. These aspects, together with the implications of systemic absorption of topical medications, need special attention. This chapter explores the effects of disorders of the hepatic, renal, cardiopulmonary, central nervous system, and gastrointestinal tract on pharmacokinetics.

DISORDERS OF THE LIVER

Liver disease, whether from hepatitis, cirrhosis, or drug-induced hepatotoxicity, is a common cause of morbidity and mortality worldwide. Unlike renal disease, in which one can estimate the renal function of a patient using urine output and creatinine clearance, hepatic function is more difficult to quantify. The diversity of tasks performed by the liver means that clinicians must monitor more than a single laboratory test to assess liver function. Generally, by the time a patient notices symptoms of liver failure, serious damage has already occurred. From absorption to elimination, the liver performs many functions that control the pharmacokinetic disposition of drugs in patients. Developing empiric dosing recommendations for patients is difficult because all these physiologic changes must be evaluated (1).

Oral drug absorption from the gastrointestinal tract can increase significantly in patients with liver failure because of a reduced *first-pass effect,* that is, the metabolism of drug as it crosses the gastrointestinal membrane and travels through the liver for the first time. Drugs that have a much smaller parenteral dose compared with their oral dose usually are affected by the first-pass phenomenon. Higher oral doses of these drugs are required to account for the hepatic metabolism that occurs during first pass. Table 15-1 lists drugs that exhibit significant first-pass effects and compares their usual oral and parenteral doses for patients with normal liver and renal function. For example, the recommended oral versus parenteral antiarrhythmic doses of propranolol differ by a factor of ten. Another antiarrhythmic, lidocaine, is not listed in Table 15-1 because it cannot be given orally for antiarrhythmic qualities. The first-pass effect of lidocaine is so profound that little drug reaches the systemic circulation and the heart tissue to exert an antiarrhythmic effect. In patients with liver disease, hepatic extraction of drugs is reduced, therefore increasing the oral bioavailability of highly extracted drugs. Table 15-1 also lists the increase in bioavailability seen in patients with advanced liver disease as a result of the reduced first-pass effect.

To assume that the reduction in hepatic drug clearance in liver disease is due solely to reductions in overall hepatic enzymatic activity or functional hepatic mass is too sim-

B. A. Mueller and S. R. Abel: Department of Pharmacy Practice, School of Pharmacy and Pharmacal Sciences, Purdue University, West Lafayette, Indiana 46202.

TABLE 15-1. *Oral versus parenteral dosing consequences of first-pass effect on selected drugs and subsequent increase in oral bioavailability in liver disease*

Drug	Usual oral dose[a] (mg)	Usual i.v. dose[a] (mg)	Increase in oral bioavailability in liver disease (%)
Meperidine	100–150	50–100	40–80
Nifedipine	10–20	Not marketed	77
Pentazocine	50–100	30–60	250–400
Propranolol	10–30	0.5–3	40–60
Verapamil	40–80	5–10	60–240

[a]Usual doses in patients with normal renal and hepatic function.

plistic. Although these factors may occur, the fibrotic changes in the liver induced by cirrhosis also result in an increased portal blood pressure, which leads to shunting of blood through extrahepatic circuits and away from the metabolizing cells of the liver. The clearance of drugs that are rapidly metabolized by the liver (*high-extraction drugs*) is dependent on the hepatic blood flow rate. The shunting of blood away from the metabolic enzymes of the liver yields a decreased clearance of these drugs. Examples of high-extraction agents appear in Table 15-1.

It is more difficult to predict changes of hepatic clearance in drugs that are poorly extracted by the liver (*low-extraction drugs*). Some of these drugs, like tolbutamide, lorazepam, and oxazepam, actually have increased clearances in patients with liver disease compared with those with normal livers. Warfarin's clearance is unchanged in liver disease, whereas other low-extraction drugs, like theophylline and diazepam, have substantial diminutions in hepatic clearance in patients with liver disease. As a result, generalizations about the dosing of low-extraction drugs in liver failure should not be made. Clinicians may use this information to select certain drugs from a pharmacologic class for patients with liver disease; for example, oxazepam or lorazepam probably should be considered the benzodiazepines of choice in liver disease compared with diazepam.

The unpredictability of hepatic drug clearance in liver disease arises because drug metabolism is an extremely heterogeneous process. Many different enzymatic pathways are used in drug metabolism, and each is affected differently by liver disease. Often many different pathways are used as a drug is metabolized into active and inactive metabolites. Metabolic pathways can be classified into phase I and phase II reactions. *Phase I* reactions are oxidation, reduction, and hydrolysis and are profoundly affected by liver disease. *Phase II* reactions involve coupling between the drug and an endogenous substrate. Examples of phase II reactions include conjugation with amino acids, sulfate, glucuronic acid (glucuronidation), and the process of acetylation. Generally, phase II processes, like glucuronidation, are preserved in liver disease compared with phase I reactions. This finding explains why the clearances of lorazepam and oxazepam are unchanged or slightly elevated in liver disease, whereas another benzodiazepine, diazepam, has a decreased clearance. Diazepam is metabolized into active metabolites through phase I reactions. These hydroxylated active metabolites also may be metabolized by other phase I reactions until finally pharmacologic inactivation and elimination occur. This metabolic process is substantially delayed in patients with impaired liver function. Other benzodiazepines, including chlordiazepoxide, chlorazepate, and flurazepam, also undergo phase I metabolism to form active metabolites that accumulate in liver failure. Lorazepam and oxazepam metabolites are not pharmacologically active, which is another reason why they should be used preferentially in liver disease patients who require benzodiazepine therapy.

Wide variability in hepatic metabolism exists even among normal subjects. Genetic factors play a significant role in drug metabolism. Polymorphism of acetylation has been recognized for decades. Patients who are slow acetylators of isoniazid, an antituberculosis agent, are at increased risk of isoniazid-induced neurotoxicity (2). As shown in this example, "fast" or "slow" acetylator status alters the biotransformation rate of drugs to active, inactive, and sometimes toxic metabolites. Fast acetylators metabolize isoniazid rapidly to acetylhydrazine, which then may be converted to a toxic metabolite that causes isoniazid-induced hepatitis (3). Acetylation status also can affect the efficacy of isoniazid therapy in patients with tuberculosis. Fast acetylators receiving once weekly isoniazid have a poorer antituberculosis response rate than slow acetylators (4). Other drugs metabolized by acetylation that can be influenced by a patient's genetically determined acetylator status appear in Table 15-2. Note that sulfonamides used to treat glaucoma, are affected by acetylator status.

An individual's acetylator status is either fast or slow (no intermediate acetylator status exists) based on one's acetylator phenotype. Slow acetylation is an autosomal, homozygous recessive condition, whereas fast acetylators are either heterozygous or homozygous dominant. Because this is a genetic trait, significant ethnic differences exist in acetylator status. For example, slow acetylator status occurs in 42 to 51% of black Americans, 52 to 58% of white Americans, 10% of Japanese Americans, 5 to 6% of Canadian Eskimos, and 13% of Mainland Chinese (5).

TABLE 15-2. *Selected drugs metabolized by acetylation*

Acebutolol
Aminoglutethamide
Caffeine
Clonazepam
Dapsone
Hydralazine
Isoniazid
Procainamide
Sulfonamides

More recently, it was learned that other metabolic pathways are genetically determined. The cytochrome P450 isoenzyme system is a group of many different metabolizing enzymes involved in the oxidation of several clinically important drugs. Each isoenzyme differs slightly in its amino acid sequencing. Considerable research is under way to identify not only each isoenzyme but also which drugs are affected by the altered metabolism. Like acetylation, hepatic drug oxidation is a polymorphic process. Whether an individual is an extensive metabolizer or a poor metabolizer of a particular drug is genetically predetermined. The metabolizer status of one P450 isoenzyme may be different from another P450 isoenzyme in the same patient. Metabolizer status is determined using pharmacologic probes with model drugs known to be specific for a particular P450 isoenzyme. Currently, metabolizer status is primarily a research issue; however, therapeutic and toxic responses to many pharmaceuticals probably depend on the individual's own metabolizer status. Table 15-3 lists selected drugs known to undergo polymorphic metabolism, among which is the ocular hypotensive agent timolol.

Drug binding to plasma proteins is altered considerably in liver disease. Drugs bind to two primary plasma proteins: albumin and α-1 acid glycoprotein. The production of both proteins is reduced in liver disease, resulting in a subsequent reduction in protein binding. Consequently, an increase in the pharmacologically active, unbound fraction of drug will occur. Furthermore, drug affinity for α-1 acid glycoprotein is reduced in cirrhosis, suggesting that the protein is morphologically or qualitatively different from that in healthy subjects (6). Reduced protein binding in liver failure also results in a corresponding increased apparent volume of distribution for drugs that are normally highly protein bound.

The decreased production of plasma proteins in liver failure results in a reduction of intravascular oncotic pressure that leads to edema and ascites. The presence of ascites will increase the distribution volume of water-soluble drugs, like the aminoglycosides. Gentamicin and tobramycin distribution volumes are significantly higher in patients with ascites compared with healthy subjects (7,8). An increased distribution volume will require a larger loading dose to achieve a therapeutic serum concentration. The larger volume also may lead to a longer half-life as the drugs

TABLE 15-3. *Selected drugs that undergo polymorphic metabolism in man by different cytochrome P450 isoenzymes*[a]

CNS depressants	Antiarrhythmic agents
Alcohol	Alprenolol
Amobarbital	Encanide
Codeine	Flecanide
Hexobarbital	**Lidocaine**
Antidepressants	Metoprolol
Amitriptyline	Nifedipine
Clomipramine	Propafenone
Desipramine	Propranolol
Imipramine	Quinidine
Nortriptyline	**Timolol**
Antipsychotics	Miscellaneous
Perphenazine	4-Hydroxyamphetamine
Thioridazine	**Cyclosporin A**
Benzodiazepines	**Dextromethorphan**
Diazepam	**Erythromycin**
Midazolam	Mephenytoin
Triazolam	

[a]Drugs in bold print are used directly or indirectly in ophthalmology.

leach out of the ascites into the intravascular space to be eliminated by the liver and kidneys.

DISORDERS OF THE KIDNEYS

Kidney failure is a final manifestation of common diseases like hypertension, diabetes mellitus, and systemic lupus erythematosus. Advances in renal replacement therapies over the past two decades have improved the prognosis of patients with end-stage renal disease (ESRD). More than 100,000 Americans receive maintenance dialysis therapy to treat their ESRD. Another 10,000 per year receive kidney transplants. Renal insufficiency that has not yet progressed to renal failure affects millions more. Obviously, kidney disease alters the clearance of drugs eliminated by the kidneys; however, renal disease may significantly change all other pharmacokinetic parameters as well.

The oral bioavailability of most drugs has not been researched extensively in patients with renal disease. More attention is usually focused on changes in drug elimination and volume of distribution. Nonetheless, a significant reduction in the oral bioavailability of furosemide has been reported (9). This reduction in oral bioavailability is important because furosemide is a loop diuretic commonly used to treat patients with acute renal failure or chronic renal insufficiency. Higher doses of oral furosemide are required to yield the same effect as lower parenteral doses; however, the oral bioavailability of most drugs is not reduced by ESRD. Indeed, bioavailability may increase for certain drugs because of reductions in hepatic metabolism that occur in patients with ESRD (10). As described in the liver disease section of this chapter, diminished hepatic metabolism results in a lower first-pass effect; therefore, more drug absorbed from the gastrointestinal tract is available to the systemic circulation. D-propoxyphene is one example of a drug that may have a greater oral bioavailability in ESRD because of a reduced first-pass effect (11).

Drug interactions account for the most common change in oral bioavailability in patients with renal disease. In nearly every patient with ESRD, calcium- or aluminum-containing antacids are administered with meals to reduce dietary phosphate absorption. A nonabsorbable aluminum or calcium phosphate salt is formed from the antacid and dietary phosphate. These phosphate-binding antacids also affect the absorption of many medications. Table 15-4 lists the effects of antacids on the oral bioavailability of commonly used drugs. Many of the absorption interactions have important clinical consequences. Concomitant antacids might interfere with the absorption of steroid treatment of uveitis, necessitating an increased steroid dose or a staggering of administration times of these agents.

End-stage renal disease greatly affects the distribution of drugs within the body. Intuitively, it would seem that this change would be due to fluid overload in patients with anuria or oliguria, but most of the important changes in drug distribution volume in ESRD come from the reduction in circulating plasma protein concentrations. Drugs that are normally highly bound to plasma proteins have a higher unbound fraction in patients with ESRD. Two major consequences arise when a drug has a higher unbound fraction than normal. First, the volume of distribution of the drug increases (12). The second consequence is more clinically significant. Only drug that is unbound can exert pharmacologic activity. Consequently, the "therapeutic" total drug concentration may differ in patients with ESRD because they may have a higher unbound drug concentration as a result of their reduced plasma protein levels.

Phenytoin is a drug that exemplifies this change in its total serum concentration therapeutic range because of decreased plasma protein binding. Phenytoin has a high affinity for albumin and is 90% protein bound. In healthy patients with normal renal function and plasma protein concentrations, the usual therapeutic total serum concentration is 10 to 20 mg/L. It follows that the therapeutic unbound concentration would be 10% of this value, or 1 to 2 mg/L. Hypoalbuminemia results in a reduction in phenytoin binding sites and a subsequent increased unbound (and pharmacologically active) fraction of phenytoin. Furthermore, uremic by-products that are not removed by dialysis therapies also have a high binding affinity for albumin. These by-products preferentially bind to albumin and displace phenytoin from binding to albumin. Renal failure patients may have a twofold to threefold increased unbound fraction at any given total serum concentration. The increased unbound fraction of phenytoin is a function of the patient's serum albumin concentration and degree of renal failure. Where possible, free (*unbound*) drug serum concentrations rather than total concentrations should be monitored to assess efficacy and to evaluate toxicity in these patients more accurately. Special calculations to estimate free drug concentrations have been developed to help the clinician in instances where free drug assays are unavailable (13).

The protein binding of other drugs can be altered in patients with ESRD (14) or acute renal failure (15). Generally, these alterations occur in acidic drugs that, like phenytoin, have a high affinity for albumin. Table 15-5 lists examples of commonly used drugs that have altered protein binding in uremia. Many drugs used to treat ocular diseases are also highly protein bound, including certain beta blockers, sulfonamides, cyclosporin, ceftriaxone, and local anesthetic agents. The pharmacokinetic monitoring of drugs that are highly protein bound and have a narrow therapeutic index may be difficult in these patients. Reduc-

TABLE 15-4. *Drug absorption effects of antacids*

Decreased absorption	Increased absorption
Atenolol	Levodopa
Captopril	Triazolam
Cefaclor	
Cefpodoxime	
Chlordiazepoxide	
Cimetidine	
Ciprofloxacin	
Dexamethasone	
Diazepam	
Dicumarol	
Digoxin	
Indomethacin	
Iron Salts	
Isoniazid	
Ketoconazole	
Nitrofurantoin	
Norfloxacin	
Ofloxacin	
Penicillamine	
Phenytoin	
Prednisone	
Ranitidine	
Tetracycline	
Valproic acid	

[a]Drugs in bold print are used directly or indirectly in ophthalmology.

TABLE 15-5. *Clinically important drugs that show decreased binding in uremic patients*

Chloramphenicol
Diazepam
Furosemide
Pentobarbital
Phenytoin
Salicylate
Thiopental
Valproic acid
Warfarin

tions in protein binding must be considered when attempting to titrate the dosing of these agents to a desired therapeutic effect.

Another common kidney disease that alters drug protein binding is *nephrotic syndrome,* which is characterized by proteinuria, hypoalbuminemia, and edema. Each of these factors can alter pharmacodynamics or pharmacokinetics. Furosemide, a diuretic that exerts its action at the loop of Henle, is normally >90% protein bound. In nephrotic syndrome, furosemide activity is inhibited because of binding to the abnormally high concentrations of protein in the urine (16). Urinary furosemide becomes protein bound and cannot exert its effect in the tubules, leading to a condition of diuretic resistance. The subsequent hypoalbuminemia of nephrotic syndrome results in an increased unbound, pharmacologically active fraction of highly protein bound drugs. The increased unbound and pharmacologically active drug may lead to drug toxicity in these patients (17). Finally, the massive edema seen in some patients may increase the volume of distribution of water-soluble drugs, like the aminoglycoside antibiotics.

Kidney disease can have clinically important effects on drug metabolism. Practitioners do not always appreciate the metabolic functions of the kidney (10). An example of a drug that is actively metabolized by the kidneys is the broad-spectrum antibiotic imipenem. Imipenem is rapidly degraded by tubular dihydropeptidases. The renal metabolism of imipenem is so efficient that therapeutic urine concentrations of imipenem are not achieved when imipenem is given as monotherapy. Therefore cilastatin, a dihydropeptidase inhibitor, has been added to the commercially available product yielding high, efficacious urinary imipenem concentrations for the treatment of urinary tract infections. Many other drugs actively metabolized by the kidneys may have clearance alterations in renal disease. Table 15-6 lists substances metabolized by the kidneys.

Worsening renal function is associated with derangements in the hepatic metabolism of many drugs. The mechanism(s) that slow the metabolic pathways responsible for this nonrenal clearance, for example, reduction (18) and ester hydrolysis (19), have not been studied extensively, but it appears that retained uremic byproducts are responsible for the reduced enzymatic activity. Table 15-7 illustrates how nonrenal clearance rates of certain drugs differ in patients with normal renal function and in those with ESRD.

TABLE 15-6. *Substances partially metabolized by kidneys*

Acetaminophen
Calcitonin
Cephalothin
Growth hormone
Imipenem
Insulin
Isoproterenol
Meperidine
Morphine
Salicylate
Sulindac

Of interest are the nonrenal clearance parameters of drugs in patients with acute renal failure (ARF). Little research has examined whether nonrenal clearance in ARF approximates normal values or values obtained in ESRD patients. The calculated doses of the drugs listed in Table 15-7 would differ substantially, depending on the assumed nonrenal clearance. Our research indicates that the nonrenal clearance of vancomycin and imipenem is preserved in early ARF (20,21). With vancomycin, hepatic clearances decline with time until they approach the values observed in patients with ESRD. Therefore, the dosing of drugs listed in Table 15-7 may need to be substantially higher in patients with early ARF compared with patients with ESRD.

A final impact of kidney disease on drug metabolism and patient response to drug therapy pertains to retained active metabolites. Hepatic metabolism of drugs often constitutes the formation of active metabolites eliminated by the kidney. In renal disease, these metabolites are retained and are not always removed by dialysis therapies. The retained active metabolites can be responsible for therapeutic and toxic consequences. For example, morphine has two major metabolites, morphine-3 glucuronide and morphine-6 glucuronide. Morphine-6 glucuronide is pharmacologically active as an analgesic and usually is eliminated by the kidneys. In ESRD, morphine-6 glucuronide accumulates, maintaining pharmacologically active serum concentrations for days after a morphine dose (24). The retention of morphine-6 glucuronide accounts for an apparent increased sensitivity to morphine in ESRD patients.

In the case of morphine in ESRD, the active metabolite has pharmacologic properties similar to those of the parent drug. Some retained active metabolites have effects that differ from the parent compound. Normeperidine is a metabolite of meperidine that accumulates in patients with renal failure and is not removed efficiently by dialysis therapies. Unlike meperidine, normeperidine has central nervous system (CNS) excitatory activity that may promote seizure activity (25). Another opiate, propoxyphene, has a renally eliminated active metabolite, norpropoxyphene, which is cardiotoxic (26). Norpropoxyphene accumulates in ESRD and is negligibly removed by dialysis. Normeperidine and norpropoxyphene are salient examples of active, toxic metabolite accumulation that complicates pharmacotherapy in patients with ESRD.

Retained drug metabolites in renal failure can also invalidate certain drug assay methodologies, causing the spurious appearance of a change in a patient's pharmacokinetics. Vancomycin's main metabolite, crystalline degradation product (CDP), is retained in ESRD and is not removed by dialysis. Although CDP is pharmacologically inactive, the most commonly used vancomycin assay, the polyclonal fluorescence polarization immunoassay, reports CDP as vancomycin (27).

TABLE 15-7. *Nonrenal clearance of drugs in patients with normal renal function and chronic renal failure*

Drug	Normal renal function (ml/min/70 kg)	Chronic renal failure (ml/min/70 kg)	Decline in nonrenal clearance (%)
Acyclovir	65	29	55
Aztreonam	40	27	33
Cefotaxime	217	130	40
Imipenem	128	54	56
Isoniazid			
Fast acetylators	311	262	16
Slow acetylators	106	56	47
Procainamide	257	102	60
Vancomycin	40	6	85

From Gibson, ref 10; Matzke et al., ref 22; and Kim et al., ref 23.

If the clinician does not account for CDP accumulation over time, it can appear that the patient's vancomycin clearance continues to slow throughout the course of vancomycin therapy. Clinicians acting on these false laboratory results might unwittingly reduce the vancomycin dose and inadequately treat a serious bacterial infection.

The most important and most obvious pharmacokinetic change that occurs in kidney disease is the decline in the renal elimination of drugs. By the time a patient needs dialysis therapy, no clinically important renal drug clearance remains. The challenge for the clinician is to assess the pharmacokinetic changes caused by dialysis therapies. The two predominant maintenance dialytic therapies are hemodialysis and continuous ambulatory peritoneal dialysis (CAPD). The drug-clearance properties of these two modalities differ. Hemodialysis is much more efficient in removing "dialyzable" drugs than CAPD, as it is accomplished in short "bursts" of clearance usually lasting 3 to 4 hours thrice weekly. On the other hand, CAPD is a slow process that results in gradual, nonstop clearance. Dosing recommendations for drugs derived from hemodialysis studies cannot be applied to patients receiving CAPD and vice versa because of these clearance differences; however, not all drugs are removed by dialysis. Table 15-8 lists factors that increase dialysis drug clearance.

Many recommendations for hemodialysis drug dosing have been published (28), most of which derive from early dialysis studies that used old hemodialysis membranes and machines. New, "high-flux" hemodialysis membranes remove drugs with larger molecular weights more efficiently than the membranes used in early studies. Pharmacokinetic monitoring for drugs like vancomycin (29) and the aminoglycosides is probably a better method for adjusting doses than relying on older published dosing guidelines in patients receiving high-flux hemodialysis (30).

TABLE 15-8. *Factors that may increase drug clearance by dialysis*

Dialysis-specific factors	Drug-specific factors
Large dialysis membrane	Smaller molecular weight (<500 Da)
Increased duration of dialysis	Nonprotein bound
Increased amounts of dialysate	Small volume of distribution
Higher blood flow rates	Water soluble
Larger dialyzer pore size	Electrical charge
High-flux membrane composition	

In the acute-care setting, newer renal replacement therapies like continuous arteriovenous hemofiltration (CAVH) and continuous venovenous hemofiltration (CVVH) are used to treat renal failure (31). Hemofiltration does not use a dialysate and therefore removes drugs differently than the dialysis therapies. The convective clearance of hemofiltration results in the removal of all nonprotein bound drug that has a molecular weight small enough (<5,000–10,000 daltons) to pass through the hemofilter membrane. These hemofiltration therapies impact the pharmacokinetic dosing in two manners. First, large amounts of extracellular fluid can be removed from edematous patients, thereby changing drug distribution volume. Second, most drugs are removed at least partially by hemofiltration, resulting in the necessity of calculating hemofiltration drug loss (32). The hemofiltration-induced drug clearance values must be added to nonhemofiltration drug doses to appropriately dose patients receiving these therapies (20,21).

DISORDERS OF THE CARDIOPULMONARY SYSTEM

Cardiovascular disease remains the primary cause of morbidity and mortality in the United States. Despite the high prevalence of cardiovascular disease, the effects of cardiovascular diseases on pharmacokinetics generally are not considered by clinicians to be as important as disorders of the renal or hepatic systems. Of the most common cardiovascular complications, congestive heart failure (CHF) alters pharmacokinetics to the greatest extent. The significant reduction in cardiac output associated with CHF significantly reduces hepatic, renal, and gastrointestinal-tract blood flow. The biotransformation rates of high-extraction drugs like lidocaine are extremely sensitive to changes in liver blood flow secondary to CHF. Lidocaine clearance in adults with CHF is only 60 to 65% of the clearance of normal subjects without CHF (33). Similarly, theophylline, a low-extraction drug, has a reduced clearance in CHF (34,35).

Reductions in renal blood flow secondary to CHF may decrease glomerular filtration rate and the clearance of drugs eliminated by the kidneys. The reduction in renal blood flow induced by CHF also leads to fluid retention. Volume overload, in theory, may result in changes in the volume of distribution of certain agents that are water soluble.

Reduced blood flow to the gastrointestinal tract in patients with CHF has been identified as an important factor affecting the bioavailability of various drugs. Furosemide absorption in patients with CHF is extremely variable compared with that in healthy controls (36). The potential for reduced oral bioavailability of certain drugs in CHF patients may be offset somewhat by a reduction in the renal and hepatic metabolism and elimination also induced by CHF. The area under the blood concentration versus time curve (AUC) is a measure of absolute bioavailability. The AUC of a drug depends on the extent of absorption and the rate of metabolism and elimination. In patients with CHF, clinicians must examine all these factors before determining the optimal dosing.

Myocardial infarction can also affect pharmacokinetics, independent of the reduction in cardiac output commonly seen in this clinical situation. Alpha-1 acid glycoprotein is an acute-phase reactant protein that increases in concentration when the body is under stress. Concentrations of α-1 acid glycoprotein increase by 50% within 36 to 48 hours after an acute myocardial infarction (37). Drugs that normally bind to α-acid glycoprotein will have more protein with which to bind following a myocardial infarction. Lidocaine is highly bound to α-1 acid glycoprotein and is commonly used in patients with myocardial infarction. The clinical significance of increased α-1 acid glycoprotein concentrations following myocardial infarction is that higher total lidocaine concentrations must be achieved to yield a therapeutic unbound lidocaine concentration. Unbound lidocaine concentrations are not measured by most clinical laboratories; therefore, an increased "therapeutic" range of total drug must be used by the clinician to account for this increase in protein binding. Other drugs that are highly bound to α-1 acid glycoproteins that might be used in patients with myocardial infarction include alprenolol, dipyridamole, disopyramide, propranolol, and quinidine.

Although the lungs do not contribute to the metabolism of most drugs, patients with pulmonary disease often have an altered pharmacokinetic profile. Patients with severe pulmonary disease requiring mechanical ventilation have special pharmacokinetic changes secondary to the ventilator. Positive end-expiratory pressure (PEEP) reduces cardiac output, glomerular filtration rate, and hepatic blood flow (38). Although never studied directly, reductions in liver blood flow secondary to PEEP should reduce the hepatic clearance of the high extraction drugs like lidocaine, propranolol, and verapamil. A diminished glomerular filtration rate should reduce the clearance of drugs that are primarily removed by filtration or tubular secretion. Examples of these types of drugs include the aminoglycosides, digoxin, some penicillins, and furosemide (38).

Clinicians who treat patients with cystic fibrosis (CF) know that drug-dosing regimens must be adjusted considerably because of the unusual pharmacokinetic parameters found in these patients. Patients with CF often require theophylline and antibiotic therapies for the treatment of their disease. Interestingly, the pharmacokinetics of these drugs differ significantly in CF patients compared with age- and sex-matched normal controls. The reasons for the differences are not well described. Patients with CF may have altered drug absorption as a result of alterations in pancreatic secretions, altered bile acid turnover, or lengthened gastrointestinal transit time. Renal blood flow and glomerular filtration rate are probably not different from matched controls, but tubular secretion of drugs may differ in patients with CF (39).

Frequent bacterial bronchial infections in CF patients lead to many courses of aminoglycoside therapy; however, aminoglycoside clearance in CF patients is substantially greater than in healthy control patients. Curiously, the primary route of aminoglycoside elimination is renal clearance, which does not differ in patients with CF compared with normals. The precise mechanism for the difference in aminoglycoside clearance is not known (40). The distribution volume of gentamicin and tobramycin appears to be larger in CF patients compared with normal subjects, but when corrected for lean body mass, the differences disappear (41). Patients with CF are usually smaller and have less adiposity, thereby appearing to have a larger distribution volume based on liters per kilogram (L/kg).

Theophylline clearances are twice as fast in patients with CF compared with control patients (42). The volume of distribution of theophylline is significantly larger in CF as well. The effect of these two factors combined means that loading and maintenance theophylline doses must be larger to "fill" the larger distribution volume and to offset the more rapid clearance of the drug. More frequent dosing

TABLE 15-9. *Drugs with an increased clearance in cystic fibrosis patients compared with normal volunteers*

Amikacin
Aztreonam
Ceftazidime
Ciprofloxacin
Dicloxacillin
Gentamicin
Imipenem
Methicillin
Netilmicin
Ofloxacin
Piperacillin
Theophylline
Ticarcillin
Tobramycin
Trimethoprim

of nonsustained release formulations is also needed to maintain a therapeutic serum concentration because of the rapid theophylline clearance. Table 15-9 lists other commonly used drugs that have an increased clearance in CF patients. For all these agents, an increased volume of distribution and clearance results in the necessity of higher doses to achieve therapeutic serum concentrations.

DISORDERS OF THE CENTRAL NERVOUS SYSTEM

Even diseases of the CNS can affect pharmacokinetic parameters. The blood–brain barrier (BBB) generally inhibits the passage of most drugs from the blood into the cerebrospinal fluid. In the patient with meningitis, however, the meninges become inflamed, and the integrity of the BBB is compromised. Serendipitously, many antibiotics used to treat meningitis can cross the BBB when the meninges are inflamed, allowing for the administration of intravenous drugs to treat this CNS infection. Examples of drugs that achieve only therapeutic CNS concentrations in the presence of inflamed meninges include imipenem, ciprofloxacin, and many penicillins and cephalosporins (43).

Epilepsy is another disease of the CNS associated with pharmacokinetic changes. Increases in α-1 acid glycoprotein blood concentrations have been observed after seizures. Lidocaine, which binds preferentially to α-1 acid glycoprotein, will have a reduced unbound fraction and potentially a reduced therapeutic effect postictally (44). The primary pharmacokinetic change observed in patients with seizure disorders arises from the antiseizure medications themselves. The drugs used to treat seizures are notorious for inducing drug interactions in other antiseizure medications as well as many drugs dependent on hepatic metabolism. Carbamazepine even induces its own hepatic metabolism, resulting in a faster clearance after 3 to 4 weeks of therapy. Newer antiepilepsy agents also are susceptible to drug interactions.

DISORDERS OF THE GASTROINTESTINAL TRACT AND OF NUTRITION

Alterations in drug absorption from an orally administered dosage form are the most obvious way that diseases of the gastrointestinal tract can affect pharmacokinetics. "Short-gut" syndrome is a real phenomenon that arises in patients who have undergone extensive surgery to remove portions of their gastrointestinal tract. Without much of their gastrointestinal tract, only a limited amount of nutrients and drugs can be absorbed. Further, certain gastrointestinal diseases, like Crohn's disease and ulcerative colitis, can reduce the rate and extent of drug absorption (45). Overcoming the drug bioavailability problems in these types of patients may involve administering higher doses at more frequent intervals. Therapeutic drug monitoring may be necessary to ensure that therapeutic serum concentrations are achieved. In severe cases, oral drugs cannot be used because of the limited absorption caused by short-gut syndrome.

The pharmacokinetic effects of gastrointestinal disease go beyond oral drug absorption, however. The food that we eat can affect how the body absorbs and metabolizes drugs. Cyclosporin A, an agent used to treat uveitis, has changing absorption and metabolic patterns based on the food that is ingested simultaneously. The oral bioavailability of cyclosporin A increases significantly in the presence of a high-fat meal in healthy subjects (46). Total cyclosporin A clearance and volume of distribution also increase when the drug is administered with a high-fat meal. The exact mechanism for these findings is unknown. Lower doses of cyclosporin A may be necessary when the drug is administered with food. Clinically important drug-nutrient interactions appear in Table 15-10.

The malnourished patient will handle drugs differently from the well-nourished patient. Drugs that are water soluble will appear to have a higher volume of distribution on a total body weight basis (L/kg). Correcting for lean body mass should normalize this finding. The malnourished patient may have an increased sensitivity to drugs that are highly protein bound. The malnourished patient will have lower concentrations of plasma proteins like albumin and α-1 acid glycoprotein. Highly protein-bound drugs will have a higher unbound concentration in these patients and therefore will have more drug that is pharmacologically active.

In contrast to the malnourished patient, the obese patient has many more factors that complicate pharmacotherapy. Doubling the drug dose in a patient who is twice as large as other patients is probably not an appropriate response because of the many pharmacokinetic differences between obese patients and their leaner counterparts. Obese patients not only have an increase in their adipose tissue mass but also their lean body mass. Consequently, the distribution volume of fat-soluble drugs will be larger in obese patients. Water-soluble drugs will have a slightly larger total distribution volume because of the increased lean body mass, but on a L/kg basis, the volume of distribution will tend to be smaller than that of patients of ideal weight. Glomerular filtration rates in obesity tend to be higher than in patients of normal weight, which complicates the dosing of aminoglycoside antibiotics that are water soluble and eliminated by the kidneys. The absolute volume of distribution of aminoglycosides increases in obesity but is actually decreased on a L/kg basis. A correction factor for determining the aminoglycoside volume of distribution and subsequent loading dose has been suggested (47). Similar corrections have been useful in the dosing of other drugs (48); however, correction factors for additional drugs need to be developed. Aminoglycoside loading dose (corrected for obesity) = (desired peak serum concentration) (0.26 L/kg)[IBW + (0.4 $\times$ (TBW − IBW)], where IBW = ideal

TABLE 15-10. *Drug nutrient interactions*

Drug	Nutrient	Interaction
Acetaminophen	Brussels sprouts and cabbage	Increased acetaminophen clearance
Cyclosporin A	High-fat meal	Increased cyclosporin A absorption
Fluoroquinolone antibiotics	Calcium, magnesium, iron	Reduced fluoroquinolone absorption
Ciprofloxacin		
Ofloxacin		
Norfloxacin		
Phenytoin	Enteral feeding products	Reduced phenytoin absorption
Tetracycline	Calcium, magnesium, iron	Reduced tetracycline absorption
Theophylline	Charbroiled meats	Increased theophylline clearance
	High-carbohydrate, low-protein meals	Reduced theophylline clearance
	Low-carbohydrate, high-protein meals	Increased theophylline clearance
Warfarin	Vitamin K-rich foods	Reduced anticoagulant effect of warfarin

body weight and TBW = total body weight. Protein-binding alterations occur in the obese patient. Serum concentrations of α-1 acid glycoprotein are elevated in the obese, thereby providing more binding sites for drugs like propranolol (49). This reduction in unbound propranolol in the obese patient may result in reduced pharmacological effect of the drug.

Drug metabolism via phase II pathways (e.g., glucuronidation and sulfation) is increased in the obese patient. Acetaminophen is metabolized primarily by these phase II routes. Acetaminophen clearance is about 50% faster in obese patients than in normal weight controls (50). Generally, drugs metabolized by phase I pathways (e.g., oxidation, reduction) have slightly increased or no change in clearance in the obese. Theophylline undergoes phase I metabolism and is a representative example. The clearance of theophylline in obese patients is not markedly different from that in normal subjects. Consequently, published studies have suggested conflicting dosing recommendations of whether one should dose based on ideal body weight or total body weight (51,52). Like many disease states discussed in this chapter, dosing must be adjusted based on serum concentrations.

SUMMARY

Pharmacodynamics is the result of complex interactions between patients and drugs. Desired and undesired consequences of pharmacotherapy often are grounded in pharmacokinetics. Disease states profoundly influence pharmacokinetics and ultimately therapeutic outcomes. When a patient does not respond to drug therapy as expected, the diseases themselves should be considered as a possible explanation. Therapeutic drug monitoring is essential for many agents to ensure a positive pharmacotherapeutic outcome in patients with disease states that alter pharmacokinetic parameters.

REFERENCES

1. Bass NM, Williams RL. Guide to drug dosage in hepatic disease. *Clin Pharmacokinet* 1988;15:396–420.
2. Hughes HB, Biehl JP, Jones AP, Schmidt LH. Metabolism of isoniazid in man as related to the occurrence of peripheral isoniazid neuritis. *American Review of Tuberculosis* 1954;70:266–273.
3. Mitchell JR, Thorgeirsson UP, Black M, et al. Increased incidence of isoniazid hepatitis in rapid acetylators—possible relation to hydrazine metabolites. *Clin Pharmacol Ther* 1975;18:70–79.
4. Ellard GA, Gammon PT. Acetylator phenotyping of tuberculosis patients using matrix isoniazid or sulphadimidine and its prognostic significance for treatment with several intermittent isoniazid-containing regimens. *Br J Clin Pharmacol* 1977;4:5–14.
5. Wood AJJ, Zhou HH. Ethnic differences in drug disposition and responsiveness. *Clin Pharmacokinet* 1991;20:350–373.
6. Aguirre C, Calvo R, Rodriguez-Sasiain JM. Serum protein binding of penbutolol in patients with hepatic cirrhosis. *Int J Clin Pharmacol Ther* 1988;26:566–569.
7. Gill MA, Kern JW. Altered gentamicin distribution in ascitic patients. *Am J Hospital Pharmacy* 1979;36:1704–1706.
8. Sampliner R, Perrier D, Powell R, Finley P. Influence of ascites on tobramycin pharmacokinetics. *J Clin Pharmacol* 1984;24:43–46.
9. Anonymous. Furosemide. In: McEvoy GK, ed. *AHFS Drug Information 94.* Bethesda, MD: American Society of Hospital Pharmacists, Inc., 1994;1709–1713.
10. Gibson TP. Renal disease and drug metabolism: an overview. *Am J Kidney Dis* 1986;8:7–17.
11. Gibson TP, Giacomini KM, Briggs WA, Whitman W, Levy G. Propoxyphene and norpropoxyphene plasma concentrations in the anephric patient. *Clin Pharmacol Ther* 1980;27:665–670.
12. Oie S, Tozer TN. Effect of altered plasma protein binding on apparent volume of distribution. *J Pharm Sci* 1979;68:1203–1205.
13. Winter ME, Tozer TN. Phenytoin. In: Evans WE, Schentag JJ, Jusko WJ, eds. *Applied Pharmacokinetics,* 2nd ed. Spokane, Washington: Applied Therapeutics, Inc. 1986;493–539.

14. Reidenberg MM. The binding of drugs to plasma proteins from patients with poor renal function. *Clin Pharmacokinet* 1976;1:121–125.
15. Belpaire FM, Bogaert MG, Mussche MM. Influence of acute renal failure on the protein binding of drugs in animals and man. *Eur J Clin Pharmacol* 1977;11:27–32.
16. Voelker JR, Jameson DM, Brater DC. In vitro evidence that urine composition affects the fraction of active furosemide in the nephrotic syndrome. *J Pharmacol Exp Ther* 1989;250:772–778.
17. Bridgeman JG, Rosen SM, Thorp JM. Complication during clofibrate treatment of nephrotic-syndrome hyperlipoproteinemia. *Lancet* 1972; 2:506.
18. Reidenberg MM. The biotransformation of drugs in renal failure. *Am J Med* 1977;62:482–485.
19. Reidenberg MM, James M, Dring LG. The rate of procaine hydrolysis in serum of normal subjects and diseased patients. *Clin Pharmacol Ther* 1972;13:279–284.
20. Macias WL, Mueller BA, Scarim SK. Vancomycin pharmacokinetics in acute renal failure: preservation of non-renal clearance. *Clin Pharmacol Ther* 1991;50:688–694.
21. Mueller BA, Scarim SK, Macias WL. Comparison of imipenem pharmacokinetics in patients with acute or chronic renal failure treated with continuous hemofiltration. *Am J Kidney Dis* 1993;21: 172–179.
22. Matzke GR, McGory RW, Halstenson CE, et al. Pharmacokinetics of vancomycin in patients with varying degrees of renal function. *Antimicrob Agent Chemother* 1984;25:433–437.
23. Kim YG, Shin JG, Shin SG, et al. Decreased acetylation of isoniazid in chronic renal failure. *Clin Pharmacol Ther* 1993;54:612–620.
24. Osborne R, Joel S, Grebenik K, Threw D, Levin M. The pharmacokinetics of morphine and morphine glucuronides in kidney failure. *Clin Pharmacol Ther* 1993;54:158–167.
25. Szeto HH, Inturrisi CE, Houde R, et al. Accumulation of normeperidine, an active metabolite of meperidine, in patients with renal failure or cancer. *Ann Intern Med* 1977;86:738–741.
26. Giacomini KM, Gibson TP, Levy G. Effect of hemodialysis on propoxyphene and norpropoxyphene concentrations in blood of anephric patients. *Clin Pharmacol Ther* 1980;27:508–514.
27. Perino LM, Mueller BA. Accuracy of vancomycin serum concentrations in patients with renal failure. *Ann Pharmacother* 1993;27:892–893.
28. Bennett WM, Aronoff GR, Golper TA, Morrison G, Singer I, Brater DC. *Drug Prescribing in Renal Failure,* 2nd ed. Philadelphia: American College of Physicians, 1991.
29. Pollard T, Lampasona V, Akkerman S, et al. Vancomycin redistribution: dosing recommendations following high-flux hemodialysis. *Kidney Int* 1994;45:232–237.
30. Matzke GR. Pharmacotherapeutic consequences of recent advances in hemodialysis therapy. *Ann Pharmacother* 1994;28:512–514.
31. Macias WL, Mueller BA, Scarim SK, Robinson M, Rudy DW. Continuous venovenous hemofiltration: an alternative to continuous arteriovenous hemofiltration and hemodiafiltration in acute renal failure. *Am J Kidney Dis* 1991;18:451–458.
32. Bickley SK. Drug dosing during continuous arteriovenous hemofiltration. *Clin Pharm* 1988;7:198–206.
33. Thomson PD, Melmon KL, Richardson JA, et al. Lidocaine pharmacokinetics in advanced heart failure, liver disease, and renal failure in humans. *Ann Intern Med* 1973;78:499–508.
34. Jusko WJ, Gardner MJ, Mangione A, Schentag JJ, Koup JR, Vance JW. Factors affecting theophylline clearances: age, tobacco, marijuana, cirrhosis, congestive heart failure, obesity, oral contraceptives, benzodiazepines, barbiturates, and ethanol. *J Pharm Sci* 1979;68: 1358–1366.
35. Vicuna N, McNay JL, Ludden TM, Schwertner H. Impaired theophylline clearance in patients with cor pulmonale. *Br J Clin Pharmacol* 1979;7:33–37.
36. Greither A, Goldman S, Edelen JS, Cohn K, Benet LZ. Erratic and incomplete absorption of furosemide in congestive heart failure. *Am J Cardiol* 1976;37:139 (abst).
37. Routledge PA, Stargel W, Wagner GS, Shand DG. Increased alpha-1-acid glycoprotein and lidocaine disposition in myocardial infarction. *Ann Intern Med* 1980;93:701–704.
38. Perkins MW, Dasta JF, DeHaven B. Physiologic implications of mechanical ventilation of pharmacokinetics. *DICP* 1989;23:316–323.
39. Wang JP, Unadkat JD, Al-Habet SMH, et al. Disposition of drugs in cystic fibrosis. IV. Mechanisms for enhanced renal clearance of ticarcillin. *Clin Pharmacol Ther* 1993;54:293–302.
40. de Groot R, Smith AL. Antibiotic pharmacokinetics in cystic fibrosis. *Clin Pharmacokinet* 1987;13:228–253.
41. Levy J, Smith AL, Koup JR, Williams-Warren J, Ramsey B. Disposition of tobramycin in patients with cystic fibrosis: a prospective controlled study. *J Pediatr* 1984;105:117–124.
42. Isles A, Spino M, Tabachnik E, Levison H, Thiessen J, MacLeod S. Theophylline disposition in cystic fibrosis. *Am Rev Respir Dis* 1983; 127:417–421.
43. Zabinski RA, Vance-Bryan K, Rotschafer JC. Central nervous system infections. In: DiPiro JT, Talbert RL, Hayes PE, Yee GC, Matzke GR, Posey LM, eds. *Pharmacotherapy: A Pathophysiologic Approach,* 2nd ed. New York: Elsevier Science Publishing, 1992;1524–1542.
44. Routledge PA, Stargel WW, Finn AL, Barchowsky A, Shand DG. Lignocaine disposition in blood in epilepsy. *Br J Clin Pharmacol* 1981;12:663–666.
45. Gubbins PO, Bertch KE. Drug absorption in gastrointestinal disease and surgery. *Clin Pharmacokinet* 1991;21:431–447.
46. Gupta SK, Manfro RC, Tomlanovich SJ, Gambertoglio JG, Garovoy MR, Benet LZ. Effect of food on the pharmacokinetics of cyclosporin in healthy subjects following oral and intravenous administration. *J Clin Pharmacol* 1990;30:643–653.
47. Blouin RA, Chandler MHH. Special pharmacokinetic considerations in the obese. In: Evans WE, Schentzg JJ, Jusko WJ, eds. *Applied Pharmacokinetics,* 3rd ed. Vancouver, Washington: Applied Therapeutics, 1992;11.1–11.20.
48. Allard S, Kinzig M, Boivin G, Sörgel F, LeBel M. Intravenous ciprofloxacin disposition in obesity. *Clin Pharmacol Ther* 1993;54: 368–373.
49. Bendedek IH, Blouin RA, McNamara PJ. Serum protein binding and the role of increased $alpha_1$-acid glycoprotein in moderately obese patients. *Br J Clin Pharmacol* 1984;18:941–946.
50. Abernethy DR, Divoll M, Greenblatt DJ, et al. Obesity, sex, and acetaminophen disposition. *Clin Pharmacol Ther* 1982;31:783–790.
51. Gal P, Jusko WJ, Yurchak AM, Franklin BA. Theophylline disposition in obesity. *Clin Pharmacol Ther* 1978;23:438–444.
52. Blouin RA, Elgert JF, Bauer LA. Theophylline clearance; effect of marked obesity. *Clin Pharmacol Ther* 1980;28:619–623.

Textbook of Ocular Pharmacology,
edited by T.J. Zimmerman, et al.
Lippincott–Raven Publishers, Philadelphia © 1997.

CHAPTER 16

Effect of Age on Drug Disposition

William F. Buss, Steven R. Abel, and Bruce A. Mueller

As the title suggests, age influences not only the sites into which a drug distributes and its rate of removal from the body but also the pharmacologic and adverse effects seen in a given patient. The study of maturational changes in drug absorption, distribution, metabolism, and elimination is called *developmental pharmacology.* Children have been referred to as the *therapeutic orphans* of drug therapy because most drugs marketed in the United States do not have Food and Drug Administration (FDA)-approved labeling for pediatric use (1,2). This situation should not be surprising considering the lack of financial incentive to develop a drug for a population that will use only small amounts of it, the ethical and technical difficulties of conducting clinical trials in pediatric patients, and the growing elderly population in the United States.

As with pediatric patients, deficiencies exist in our knowledge of the effect of aging on drug disposition in the elderly patient. Historically, dosage regimens have been developed based largely on pharmacokinetic data generated from studies involving healthy young adults. Application of these data in the design of dosage regimens for elderly patients may result in excessive dosage and untoward effects. Several factors complicate the design and interpretation of age-related studies: the definition of age (chronological versus biological), the health status of the patient (chronic or acute illness versus good health), the acute or chronic nature of therapy, nutritional status, and the environment, to name a few (3). It is anticipated that by the year 2,000, elderly patients will constitute 40% of the U.S. population (4). About 50% of marketed drugs will be used to treat elderly patients, who use about twice as many prescription drugs as the general population (5,6). These difficulties in identifying and applying pharmacokinetic and pharmacodynamic studies to treatment are complicated by the fact that the incidence of adverse drug reactions increases with age (7). Adverse drug reactions are responsible for as many as 10% of hospital admissions for elderly patients. The incidence of adverse reactions appears to increase exponentially with the number of drugs administered (7).

This chapter provides an overview of the effects of age on drug disposition in the pediatric and elderly patient. For purposes of this discussion, a *neonate* is aged <1 month, a *preterm* neonate is born at <36 weeks' gestation; an infant is aged 1 to 12 months, a *child* is aged 1 to 10 years, an *adolescent* is aged 10 to 15 years, and *elderly* patients are aged >65 years.

W. F. Buss: Department of Pharmacy, Indiana University Medical Center, Indianapolis, Indiana 46202.

S. R. Abel and B. A. Mueller, Department of Pharmacy Practice, School of Pharmacy and Pharmacal Sciences, Purdue University, West Lafayette, Indiana 46202.

ABSORPTION

Gastrointestinal Tract

A number of factors contribute to the rate and extent of drug absorption from the gastrointestinal tract (Table 16-1). The desire to ensure adequate drug delivery to the site of action makes the oral route the least desirable method of drug administration during the immediate postnatal period. The pH of the gastrointestinal tract markedly affects drug absorption. Drugs are best absorbed in an un-ionized lipophilic form. Most medications are weak bases, and an alkaline pH such as in the small intestine favors their absorption because they are in an un-ionized form in this environment. The same alkaline conditions would greatly reduce the absorption of acidic medications because they would be ionized and less lipophilic.

Gastric pH in the term infant is usually between 6 and 8 at birth and decreases to between 1.5 and 3.0 within a few hours (8,9). Secretion of gastric acid postnatally in the term infant appears to follow a biphasic pattern with the highest acid concentrations within the first 10 days of life and the lowest between days 10 and 30 (10). The premature

TABLE 16-1. *Factors influencing drug absorption*

Gastric and intestinal pH	Degree of ionization (pKa)
GI motility	Local GI enzyme activity
Lipid solubility	Regional blood flow
GI flora	Rate of dissolution of drug product
Area of absorptive surface	Bile salt pool

GI, gastrointestinal.

infant has a state of relative achlorhydria, which gradually resolves such that basal gastric acid output is comparable to that in older infants by 4 weeks of age (11). Gastric pH correlates with postnatal age and decreases to adult values in all children by 3 years of age (12).

The incidence of achlorhydria increases in men and women from age 20 to about age 79 (13). Basal and histamine-stimulated peak gastric acid secretion declines with age (14). The influence of decreased gastric acidity on drug absorption in the elderly has not been evaluated adequately. Age-related reductions in gastric fluid acidity could adversely affect the dissolution of basic drugs (3). Increases in gastric pH may influence the efficiency of drug absorption. Drugs that are unstable in acidic media (e.g., penicillin, erythromycin) may degrade to a lesser extent in the gastric fluids of elderly patients, resulting in a greater percentage of drug absorbed (3). Gastric emptying time and intestinal motility are also major factors in oral drug absorption. Gastric emptying time during the neonatal period is prolonged (up to 6–8 hours) compared with that of an adult and is extremely delayed during the immediate postnatal period (up to 24 hours) (15). Rates of emptying are slower with lesser gestational and postnatal ages, ingestion of formula versus breast milk, and increasing caloric content of feedings (8,15). Gastric emptying time approaches adult values by 6 to 8 months of life (16). Prolongation of intestinal transit time has also been noted in 3- to 5-day-old term infants (17).

Gastrointestinal muscle tone and motor activity are believed to be reduced in the elderly as a result of atrophic conditions (3). These differences with age may also be influenced by diet and laxative use. Clinical studies evaluating gastric emptying in young and elderly subjects have not clearly established a difference with age (3).

Drug absorption also may be altered by the relatively low duodenal concentrations of amylase and lipase, which persist until 4 months of age (18) and may result in reduced absorption of drugs such as chloramphenicol and the benzodiazepines. The neonatal bile acid pool is diminished as well in term infants (approximately 50% of adult values) and in premature neonates (to 33–50% of term infant values), partially because of a reduction in bile acid synthesis and ineffective bile acid reabsorption (19). Within the first few months of life, bile salt metabolism matures and the infant becomes able to absorb dietary fat (20). The production and secretion of digestive enzymes may decrease with advancing age; however, sufficient amounts appear to be available for digestive purposes in elderly patients (21).

Under normal conditions, blood flow to the gastrointestinal tract appears to allow for rapid drug absorption (3). Although it is likely that gastrointestinal blood perfusion is diminished in the elderly, leading to a reduced rate of absorption, there appears to be little influence on the extent of absorption (3). Age-related reductions in portal blood flow have been associated with reduced first-pass hepatic metabolism. The systemic oral bioavailability of drugs such as levodopa and propranolol is greater in elderly patients as a result of this reduction in first-pass hepatic metabolism (22,23). Table 16-2 summarizes the net effect of these factors on overall drug absorption. The net effect of all of these alterations in gastrointestinal status is that most orally administered drugs are adequately absorbed, but the time to peak concentration may be delayed significantly, and the peak levels may be blunted by the slow absorption phase. In the case of theophylline, it may take up to 4 hours after oral dosing in infants for peak levels to be reached. Practically speaking, rarely are these factors of sufficient magnitude to preclude oral drug administration in the infant who is tolerating oral feedings; however, they have been responsible for therapeutic failures of oral phenytoin and indomethacin and probably contributed to the increased toxicity seen with early use of chloramphenicol (24–26). The rate of drug absorption may be decreased in elderly patients, but the extent of absorption is similar to young adults.

Skin

The skin is the body's largest organ, and it plays a vital role in preventing excessive loss of fluids and serving as a barrier to external substances. Percutaneous drug absorption in newborns, especially in premature infants, is much greater than in adults. Several factors account for this increase in absorption. First, the ratio of surface area to body weight is higher in neonates; so the same application/M^2

TABLE 16-2. *Net effect of alterations in gastrointestinal tract*

Factor	Effect
↑ Gastric pH	↓ Absorption of acidic drugs (phenytoin, phenobarbital) ↑ Absorption of basic drugs (penicillin, ampicillin)
↓ Gastric emptying	↑ Time to reach peak drug level
↓ Lipase activity	↓ Absorption of fat-soluble drugs
↓ Bile acids	↓ Absorption of fats and fat-soluble drugs (vitamin E)
↓ Gastric blood flow	↓ Rate of absorption; little influence on extent of absorption

will result in a greater amount of drug absorbed per kilogram of body weight. Second, the epidermis is immature at <34 weeks' gestation and causes increased insensible water losses. Third, in the most immature neonate, there is little or no stratum corneum present and little keratinization, resulting in increased permeability to substances applied to the skin.

The premature infant's epidermis matures rapidly after birth and resembles a full-term infant's skin by 2 to 3 weeks of age (27). Failure to consider these alterations in skin permeability have led to a number of therapeutic misadventures, including methemoglobinemia and death from absorption of aniline diaper dyes, acute encephalopathy from topical hexachlorophene, hemorrhagic necrosis of the skin from topical alcohol use, and hypothyroidism associated with the topical use of povidone (27). Evans and colleagues took advantage of the increased drug permeability of neonatal skin by administering topical theophylline gel and were able to achieve therapeutic levels for up to 72 hours following application and to maintain these levels in a few patients even as late as 3 weeks of age. Absorption decreased as the infants' age increased so that beyond 3 weeks of age, therapeutic serum concentrations could no longer be maintained (28). In the elderly, little attention has been focused on absorption from routes of administration other than oral. Although one might expect altered barrier function of the skin of elderly patients, there is little qualitative information about the efficacy of transdermal absorption through aged skin (3). With increased use of transdermal drug-delivery systems (estrogen, nicotine, nitroglycerin), further study in the elderly is warranted.

AGE-RELATED CHANGES IN DRUG DISTRIBUTION

Drugs distribute throughout the body. Following an initial bolus dose of medication, the apparent volume in which the drug distributes can be calculated using the following equation:

$$\text{volume of distribution } (V_d) = \text{dose given/concentration observed}$$

or

$$V_d \text{ (in liters)} = \text{dose (in mg)/concentration (in mg/L)}$$

This V_d is a theoretical value that describes the volume necessary to account for the total amount of drug in the body if it were present throughout the body at the same concentration found in the plasma. Drugs that preferentially distribute into fat, myocardial tissue, or the central nervous system will have a $V_d > 1$ L/kg (i.e., digoxin, diazepam). Obviously, it would be physically impossible for one to obtain >1 L/kg of fluid from a person. Practically speaking, an apparent $V_d > 1$ L/kg indicates that the drug distributes into places other than total body water. Volumes of distribution <1 L/kg are found with drugs that remain primarily in the intracellular and extracellular fluid, such as the aminoglycoside antibiotics and vancomycin. These drugs have the most marked increases in V_d when comparing neonates and adults.

Total body water (TBW) and extracellular fluid constitute a greater percentage of an infant's body weight compared with adult values (Table 16-3). It is primarily these increases in body fluid that explain the larger volumes of distribution observed in the neonate compared with the adult for those drugs that distribute primarily into body water (water-soluble drugs). The TBW rapidly decreases during the first year of life and reaches adult values by about 12 years of age (29). Further declines in TBW are seen in the elderly (30). Other factors that affect drug distribution are plasma protein binding and the presence of adipose tissue. Protein binding is reduced in the neonate by a combination of decreased overall plasma protein concentrations, reduced binding affinity of these proteins, increased concentrations of substances that compete for binding sites (bilirubin and fatty acids), and acidosis if present (31). The net effect is that for any given total drug concentration reported, there is a greater percentage of "free" drug. A larger percentage of free drug means that more drug is available to be distributed throughout the body, leading to an increase in V_d. It is the free drug that exerts both the beneficial and adverse pharmacologic effects. For this reason, neonates may experience beneficial pharmacologic effects as well as adverse effects at lower total drug concentrations than in adults. Total protein and serum albumin concentrations increase to adult values by the age of 1 year (31).

Albumin concentrations are reduced by about 10 to 20% in elderly patients compared with younger adults (32). The elderly may also exhibit an alteration in protein binding that is independent of the reduction in albumin concentration. This alteration in binding implies the involvement of other factors, such as drug displacement from binding sites by drug metabolites or endogenous compounds whose concentrations increase due to renal impairment (3). In contrast, α-1-acid glycoprotein concentrations increase with age, which may result in increased binding of basic drugs (33).

TABLE 16-3. *Body water expressed as a percentage of body weight*

Age	TBW (%)	ECF (%)
Premature neonate	87	57
Full-term neonate	75	45
Infant, 3 months old	73	33
Child, 1 year old	59	28
Adult	55	26
Elderly	50	17

From Friss-Hansen, ref 29; Shock et al., ref 30, with permission.

ECF, extracellular fluid; TBW, total body weight.

TABLE 16-4. *Plasma protein binding and volume of distribution*

Drug	% Bound		V_d (L/kg)	
	Neonate	Adult	Neonate	Adult
Diazepam	82–85	94–98	1.4–1.8	2.2–2.6
Digoxin	14–26	23–40	4.9–10.2	5.2–7.4
Gentamycin			0.4	0.2
Phenobarbital	10–30	58	0.8	0.6
Phenytoin	75–84	89–92	1.2–1.4	0.6–0.7
Theophylline	36	56	0.8	0.45

From Roberts, ref 35; Morselli, ref 36; McEvoy et al., ref 37, with permission.

Adipose tissue is decreased in the neonate as well; the premature infant is virtually fat free, and the term newborn has approximately 16% body fat. In boys, body fat continues to increase during normal development until 10 years of age and then decreases up to age 17. In girls, body fat continues to increase, most rapidly at puberty, so that girls have about twice as much fat as boys at puberty (34). The relative lack of adipose tissue in neonates and infants results in a lower volume of distribution for fat-soluble drugs compared with adults. Because fat represents a higher percentage of body weight in the elderly, fat-soluble agents such as cyclosporine, digoxin, or the benzodiazepines may have a larger volume of distribution than in younger patients. Table 16-4 summarizes the differences in volumes of distribution and protein binding for some common medications.

RENAL FUNCTION

Renal function is the sum of glomerular filtration, tubular secretion, and tubular reabsorption. Renal elimination of medications in the newborn infant is decreased because of a number of factors. The kidneys of the neonate receive only 5 to 6% of the total cardiac output, compared with 15 to 20% in the adult, meaning that neonatal kidneys have less drug presented to them per unit of time and therefore less opportunity to eliminate the medication. Figure 16-1 shows the time frame of renal organ development and the ability to eliminate drugs that are cleared by glomerular filtration.

Premature infants have a decreased number of glomeruli at birth. All glomeruli are generally present by 35 weeks' gestational age. Although term neonates have the same number of nephrons as an adult, they have only 20 to 40% of the renal function of older children or adults. The glomerular filtration rate (GFR) is decreased in premature neonates <34 weeks' gestation. Marked maturation in renal function occurs at 34 to 36 weeks' gestational age, and an improvement in renal function also occurs over the first week of life regardless of gestational age (Figure 16-2).

In term neonates, the GFR doubles from 10 to 20 ml/min/m^2 during the first 2 weeks of life. The GFR is directly proportional to gestational age after 34 weeks' gestation. Overall renal function matures by 6 to 8 months of age (39–41). Table 16-5 shows the effect of age on the GFR. This table demonstrates that the GFR reaches adult values by 3 years of age and declines in the elderly.

Tubular function is also immature at birth, with tubular secretion only 20 to 30% of adult values. The decrease in tubular secretion affects primarily weak acids, such as the penicillins, sulfa drugs, and cephalosporins. Secretion reaches adult values by 30 weeks' postnatal age (45). Reductions in passive tubular reabsorptive capacity resolve with increasing gestational age.

The kidneys decrease in size after the third decade of life; the average kidney of a person aged 70 to 80 years weighs about 20% less than one from a young adult. Progressive reduction in glomerular surface area also occurs with advanced age, with an average prevalence of 12% sclerotic glomeruli by age 80. Total renal blood flow declines by about 10% per decade after young adulthood. GFR also declines after age 40 at a yearly rate of about 0.8 ml/min divided by 1.73 times the body surface area (46).

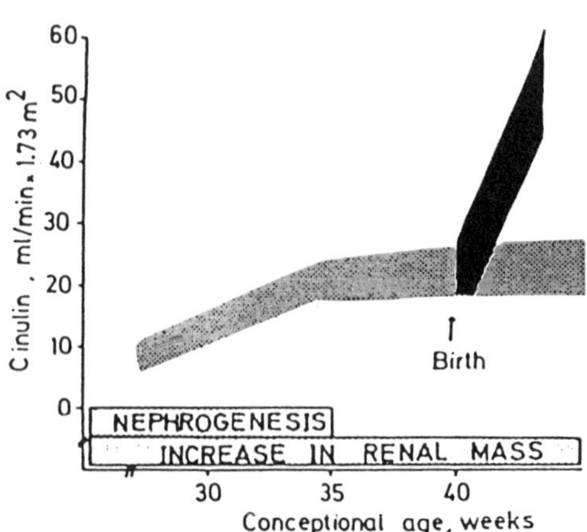

FIG. 16-1. Time course of renal tissue and functional development. (From ref. 38, with permission.)

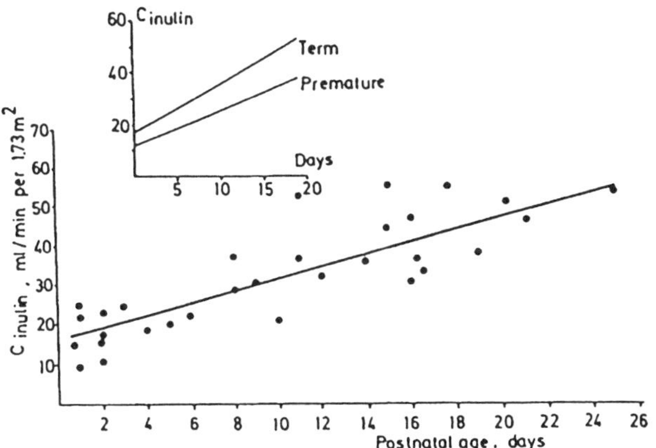

FIG. 16-2. Postnatal development of renal function (inulin clearance). (From ref. 38, with permission.)

Decreased cortical perfusion rate, atrophy affecting the renal cortex more than the medulla, and vascular lesions of small arteries resulting in a decrease in filtration pressure in a large number of glomeruli all may contribute to the reduction in GFR seen in elderly patients (47). Tubular function, including reabsorption, also declines with age (3). Clinically, elderly patients may be described as having mild renal insufficiency. Creatinine clearance decreases by 30 to 40% at an average age of 80 years (3). "Normal" serum creatinine values may be misleading because there is an age-related reduction in muscle mass. The Cockroft-Gault equation is used to estimate creatinine clearance in adult patients with stable serum creatinine values (48):

$$\text{Creatinine clearance (CrCl)} = (140 - \text{age}) \times \text{weight (kg)}/72 \times \text{serum creatinine}$$

This value is multiplied by the factor of 0.85 for women, reflecting their smaller muscle mass. This equation facilitates the estimation of creatinine clearance for the purpose of calculating drug dosages in the elderly patient. Because renal function declines with age, drug doses may need to be reduced or dosage intervals extended. One comprehensive reference to assist with drug dosing is *Drug Prescribing in Renal Failure* (49).

TABLE 16-5. *Relationship of age to glomerular filtration rate (GFR)*

Age	GFR (ml/min/1.73 m^2)
Term infant	38.5
2 mo	70.2
6 mo	111
12–19 mo	118
3 yr to adult	127
>75 yr	50

From Boreus, ref 42; Friedman et al., ref 43; Hadj-Aissa et al., ref 44, with permission.

MATURATION OF HEPATIC METABOLISM WITH INCREASING AGE

No significant alterations in hepatic blood flow in the neonate have been documented. The liver undergoes anatomic and physiologic changes with advancing age. Liver blood flow decreases at a rate of 0.5% to 1.5% per year after age 25 (3), representing a 40% to 45% reduction in flow in a 65-year-old compared with that in a young adult (3). Lidocaine hepatic metabolism is governed by the blood flow to the liver (6). Its rate of clearance is a good indicator of liver metabolism. A significant correlation between lidocaine clearance and age has been identified (50). As age increases, lidocaine elimination decreases. In the elderly, the first-pass effect is also reduced secondary to decreased liver blood flow (6). The liver is responsible for transforming drugs from their original less water-soluble form into a more water-soluble form that is more easily eliminated from the body. It accomplishes these transformations using enzyme systems and reactions that can be classified into two categories: phase I and phase II. For many drugs, a combination of both phase I and II reactions result in drug elimination. Phase I reactions include oxidation, reduction, hydrolysis, and hydroxylation. These reactions make a drug more polar and less lipophilic. In general, phase I reactions proceed at a diminished rate for the first 2 to 3 weeks of life and then dramatically increase. The cytochrome P450 mixed-function oxidase system components are present in term newborns but in lower concentrations. Metabolic activity of the P450 system in full-term neonates is 50 to 70% of adult values. Premature neonates, however, have a virtually absent oxidative metabolic capacity (caffeine, diazepam, phenobarbital, and phenytoin). *N*-demethylation (diazepam, meperidine, theophylline, and caffeine) and hydroxylation (phenobarbital) rates are greatly depressed in the newborn as well, whereas dealkylation and methylation reactions are less impaired (45). Figure 16-3 illustrates the differences between metabolic pathways used in the neonate and adult for theophylline metabolism. Note that because of the immaturity of the demethylation pathways, the neonate uses the methylation path to form caffeine, an active metabolite that is not formed in adults.

Increasing age results in marked maturation of these hepatic metabolic systems; therefore, the clearance of carbamazepine, phenytoin, procainamide, quinidine, and theophylline in children exceeds adult values (52). Figure 16-4 shows the increases in theophylline clearance from birth to childhood, followed by a reduction in clearance in the adult years.

Most studies indicate an age-related decline in phase I metabolism occurring primarily in late adulthood. The elimination of diazepam, chlordiazepoxide, alprazolam, theophylline, propranolol, and nortriptyline appears to be reduced in the elderly (53,54). Other studies have suggested no change in the elimination of diazepam, labetolol,

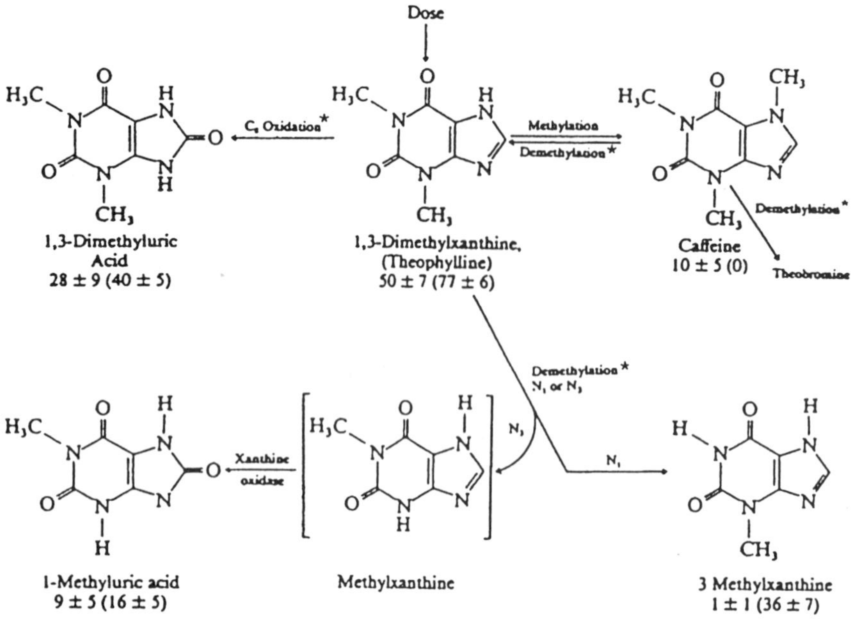

Dose

1,3-Dimethyluric Acid
28 ± 9 (40 ± 5)

C_8 Oxidation*

1,3-Dimethylxanthine, (Theophylline)
50 ± 7 (77 ± 6)

Methylation

Demethylation*

Caffeine
10 ± 5 (0)

Demethylation*

Theobromine

Demethylation* N_1 or N_3

N_3

N_1

Xanthine oxidase

1-Methyluric acid
9 ± 5 (16 ± 5)

Methylxanthine

3 Methylxanthine
1 ± 1 (36 ± 7)

FIG. 16-3. Metabolism of theophylline in the neonate and the adult. The values beneath each compound show the percentage of administered theophylline excreted in the urine and metabolites. Values in parentheses are for adults. Asterisks identify pathways catalyzed by the cytochrome P450 oxidases. (From ref. 51, with permission.)

lidocaine, phenytoin, theophylline, tolbutamide, and warfarin in older versus younger patients (55). No consensus has been reached to confirm the reduction in the rate of phase I metabolism in the elderly.

Phase II reactions include glucuronidation, sulfation, acetylation, methylation, and glycine and amino acid conjugation. These reactions add a water-soluble component to the drug molecule, which changes its characteristics so that it becomes less lipophilic. Glucuronidation is decreased in newborns (chloramphenicol, steroids, bilirubin, benzodiazepines, and morphine) and reaches adult values between the third and fourth year of life (45). In 1959, the decreased capacity of the neonate to glucuronidate chloramphenicol was reported to result in accumulation of drug, causing the "gray baby syndrome" of circulatory collapse, cyanosis, and death (56).

Acetylation is also decreased in newborns (sulfonamides). Premature neonates exhibit a lower metabolic rate of acetylation compared with term infants. Both rates are lower than those seen in adults. Sulfate and glycine conjugation capabilities in the newborn are approximately equal to adult values. Sulfation is the pathway relied on for acetaminophen elimination in the neonate, as glucuronidative capacity is limited. Esterase activity is diminished at birth (lower in premature than term infants) but normalizes during the first year of life. In general, an increase in the over-

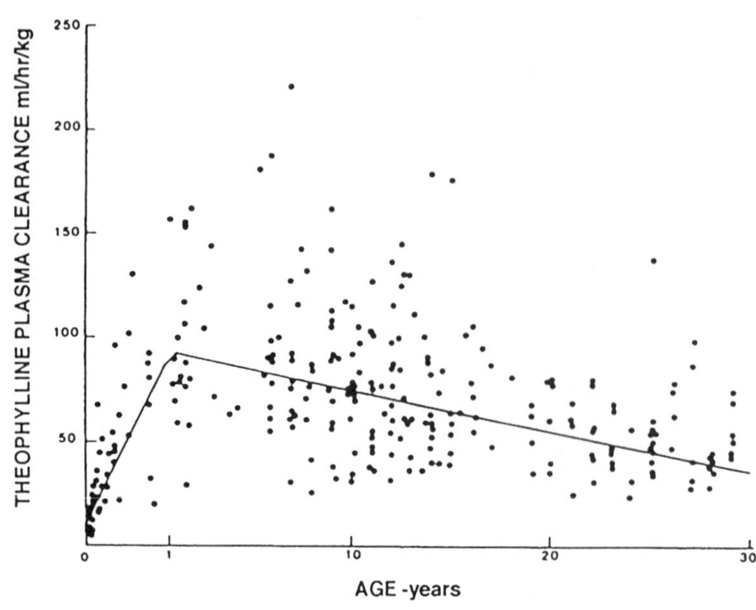

FIG. 16-4. Changes in theophylline plasma clearance with increasing age. (From ref. 52, with permission.)

TABLE 16-6. *Mechanisms used to eliminate some common drugs*

Hepatic, phase I	
Oxidation	Acetaminophen, caffeine, cimetidine, codeine, diazepam, hydralazine, morphine, phenobarbital, phenytoin, propranolol
Reduction	Chloral hydrate, chloramphenicol
Hydrolysis	Acetylsalicylic acid, indomethacin
N-demethylation	Caffeine, diazepam, phenobarbital, phenytoin
Hepatic, phase II	
Glucuronidation	Acetaminophen, chloramphenicol, morphine, steroids
Sulfation	Acetaminophen
Acetylation	Sulfonamides, procainamide
Methylation	Dopamine, dobutamine, theophylline
Amino acid conjugation	Salicylic acid
Renal	
Glomerular filtration	Aminoglycosides, digoxin, vancomycin
Tubular secretion	Cephalosporins, digoxin, furosemide, ethacrynic acid, penicillin, thiazides, tolazoline
Tubular reabsorption	Aminoglycosides, caffeine

From Polin and Fox, refs 59 and 60.

all hepatic metabolic rate occurs after the first 2 weeks of life (57).

The effect of aging on phase II conjugation reactions appears to be less pronounced in adults. Aging appears to have little effect on the metabolism of isoniazid, rifampin, valproic acid, salicylate, indomethacin, lorazepam, oxazepam, or temazepam (53). Except for lorazepam, these observations are of doubtful significance (3,53,54,58). Although most data concerning the benzodiazepines suggest that elimination by conjugation is affected little by aging, considerable variation exists with respect to other drug classes (53). There is evidence that glucuronidation, sulfation, and glycine conjugation are variably affected by aging (53). Like phase I metabolism, phase II metabolism may be reduced in the elderly.

Because of the limited capabilities of the neonatal hepatic enzyme system, saturation of these enzymes may play an important role in drug clearance in this population.

TABLE 16-7. *Half-lives ($T_{1/2}$) of drugs in the neonate and adult*

Drug	Serum $T_{1/2}$ (h) Neonate	Adult
Phase I (P-450)		
Phenytoin sodium	17–60	21–29
Theophylline	12–58	6–12.8
Caffeine	40–230	3.5–5.2
Meperidine	6	3
Phenobarbital	40–500	53–118
Phase II (conjugation)		
Morphine	7	2–3
Acetaminophen	3.5	2
Renal elimination		
Aminoglycoside	3.7–16	1.5–4
Penicillin	1.1–6.2	2

Reductions in metabolic capacity can result in accumulation of the parent drug as well as active metabolites, which may contribute greatly to the therapeutic and toxic effects. Enzyme induction may also be important (anticonvulsants, glucocorticoids) in drug elimination in the neonate. Conflicting data exist regarding the relationship between age and induction of hepatic metabolism. It does not appear that induction occurs more frequently in the elderly. As with induction, inhibition of drug metabolism such as that seen with cimetidine has not been shown to be altered with increasing age (53).

Table 16-6 summarizes the metabolic and renal pathways that are used to eliminate some common medications, and Table 16-7 summarizes the differences in neonatal and adult half-lives that result from the immaturity of these drug-elimination systems. The reduced ability of the neonate to metabolize some medications results in prolongation of drug effects, especially for drugs with active metabolites, such as chloral hydrate, diazepam, meperidine, propranolol, and theophylline.

SUMMARY

Age may influence various aspects of drug disposition in pediatric and elderly patients. The potential impact on drug disposition should be considered in determining appropriate drug-therapy regimens in these patient populations.

REFERENCES

1. Shirkey H. Editorial comment: therapeutic orphans. *J Pediatr* 1968;72:119–120.
2. American Academy of Pediatrics. Guidelines for the ethical conduct of studies to evaluate drugs in pediatric populations. *Pediatrics* 1977; 60:91–101.

3. Mayersohn MB. Special pharmacokinetic considerations in the elderly. In: *Applied Pharmacokinetics. Principles of Therapeutic Drug Monitoring,* 3rd ed. Vancouver: Applied Therapeutics, Inc., 1992;9-1–9-43.
4. Ouslander JG. Drug therapy in the elderly. *Ann Intern Med* 1981;95:711–722.
5. Massoud N. Pharmacokinetic considerations in geriatric patients. In: *Pharmacokinetics: Basis for Drug Treatment.* New York: Raven Press, 1984;283–310.
6. Yuen GJ. Altered pharmacokinetics in the elderly. *Clin Geriatr Med* 1990;6:257–267.
7. Cadieux RJ. Drug interactions in the elderly: how multiple drug use increases risk exponentially. *Postgrad Med* 1989;86:179–185.
8. Grand RJ, Watkins JB, Torti FM. Development of the human gastrointestinal tract: a review. *Gastroenterology* 1976;70:790–810.
9. Avery GB, Randolph JG, Weaver T. Gastric acidity in the first days of life. *Pediatrics* 1966;37:1005–1007.
10. Agunod M, Yomaguchi N, Lopez R, Luhby AL, Glass GBJ. Correlative study of hydrochloric acid, pepsin and intrinsic factor secretion in newborns and infants. *Am J Dig Dis* 1969;14:400–414.
11. Hyman PE, Feldman EJ, Ament ME, Byrne WJ, Euler AR. Effect of external feeding on the maintenance of gastric acid secretory function. *Gastroenterology* 1983;84:341–345.
12. Deren JS. Development of structure and function of the fetal and newborn stomach. *Am J Clin Nutr* 1971;24:144–159.
13. Vanzant FR, Alvarez WC, Eusterman GB, Dunn HL, Berkson J. The normal range of gastric acidity from youth to old age. *Arch Intern Med* 1932;49:345–359.
14. Baron JH. Studies of basal and peak acid output with an augmented histamine test. *Gut* 1963;4:136–144.
15. Cavell B. Gastric emptying in preterm infants. *Acta Pediatr Scand* 1979;68:725–730.
16. Heimann G. Enteral absorption and bioavailability in children in relation to age. *Eur J Clin Pharmacol* 1980;18:43–50.
17. Rubaltelli FF, Largajolli G. Effect of light exposure on gut transit time in jaundiced newborns. *Acta Pediatr Scand* 1973;62:146–148.
18. Lebenthal L, Lee PC, Heitlinger LA. Impact of development of the gastrointestinal tract on infant feeding. *J Pediatr* 1983;102:1–9.
19. Watkins JB, Ingall D, Szczepanek P, et al. Bile salt metabolism in the newborn: measurement of pool size and synthesis by stable isotope technique. *N Engl J Med* 1973;288:431–434.
20. Heubi JE, Balistreri WF, Suchy FJ. Bile salt metabolism in the first year of life. *J Lab Clin Med* 1982;100:127–136.
21. Sklar M. Gastrointestinal diseases in the aged. In: *Clinical Aspects of Aging.* Baltimore: Williams and Wilkins, 1978;173–181.
22. Robertson DRC, Wood ND, Everest H, Monks K, Waller DG, Renwick AG, et al. The effect of age on the pharmacokinetics of levodopa administered alone and in the presence of carbidopa. *Br J Clin Pharmacol* 1989;28:61–69.
23. Castleden CM, George CF. The effect of aging on the hepatic clearance of propranolol. *Br J Clin Pharmacol* 1979;7:49–54.
24. Painter MJ, Pippenger C, MacDonald H. Phenobarbital and diphenylhydantoin levels in neonates with seizures. *J Pediatr* 1978;92: 315–319.
25. Evans M, Bhat R, Vidyasagar D, Patel M, Hastreiter A. A comparison of oral and intravenous indomethacin dispositions in the premature infant with patent ductus arteriosus. *Pediatr Pharmacol* 1981;1:251–258.
26. Lischner H, Seligman SJ, Krammer A. An outbreak of neonatal deaths among term infants associated with administration of chloramphenicol. *J Pediatr* 1961;59:21–34.
27. Rutter N. Percutaneous drug absorption in the newborn: hazards and uses. *Clin Perinatol* 1987;14:911–930.
28. Evans NJ, Rutter N, Hadgraft J. Percutaneous administration of theophylline in preterm neonates. *J Pediatr* 1985;107:307–311.
29. Friss-Hansen B. Body water compartments in children: changes during growth and related changes in body composition. *Pediatrics* 1961;28:169–181.
30. Shock NW, Watkin DM, Yiengst MJ, Norris AH, Gaffney GW, Gregerman RI, et al. Age differences in the water content of the body as related to basal oxygen consumption in males. *J Gerontol* 1963; 18:1–8.
31. Friss-Hansen B. Body composition during growth. *Pediatrics* 1971; 47:264–274.
32. Wallace SM, Whiting B. Factors affecting drug binding in plasma of elderly patients. *Br J Clin Pharmacol* 1976;3:327–330.
33. Verbeek RK, Wallace SM, Lowewen GR. Reduced elimination of ketoprofen in the elderly is not necessarily due to impaired glucuronidation. *Br J Clin Pharmacol* 1984;17:783–784.
34. Widdowson EM. Changes in body proportions and composition during growth. In: Davies JA, Dobbing J, eds. *Scientific Foundations of Pediatrics.* London: Heinemann Medical Books Ltd., 1974;153–163.21.
35. Roberts RJ. Pharmacologic principles in therapeutics in infants. In: *Drug Therapy in Infants. Pharmacologic Principles and Clinical Experience.* Philadelphia: WB Saunders, 1984;3–12.
36. Morselli PL. Clinical pharmacokinetics in neonates. *Clin Pharmacokinet* 1976;1:81–98.
37. Anonymous. Respiratory smooth muscle relaxants. In: McEvoy GK, Litvak K, Welsh OH, eds. *AHFS Drug Information 93.* Maryland: ASHP, 1993.
38. Guignard JP. Drugs and the neonatal kidney. *Dev Pharmacol Ther* 1982;4(suppl):19–27.
39. Guignard JP. Glomerular filtration rate in the first three weeks of life. *J Pediatr* 1975;87:268–272.
40. Leake RD, Trygstad CW, Oh W. Inulin clearance in the newborn infant. Relationship to gestational and postnatal age. *Pediatr Res* 1976;10:759–762.
41. Arant BS. Developmental patterns of renal functional maturation compared in the human neonate. *J Pediatr* 1978;92:705–712.
42. Boreus LO. Principles of pediatric pharmacology. In: *Monographs in Clinical Pharmacology.* New York: Churchill Livingstone, 1982;118.
43. Friedman JR, Norman DC, Yoshikawa TT. Correlation of estimated renal function parameters versus 24-hour creatinine clearance in ambulatory elderly. *J Am Geriatr Soc* 1989;37:145–149.
44. Hadj-Aissa A, Dumarest C, Maire P, Pozet N. Renal function in the elderly. *Nephron* 1990;54:364–365.
45. Assael BM. Pharmacokinetics and drug distribution during postnatal development. *Pharmacol Ther* 1982;18:159–197.
46. Meyer RB, Hirsch BE. Renal function and the care of the elderly. *Compr Ther* 1990;16:30–37.
47. Hollenberg NK, Adams DF, Solomon HS, Rashid A, Abrams HL, Merrill JP. Senescence and the renal vasculature in normal man. *Circ Res* 1974;34:309–316.
48. Cockroft DW, Gault MH. Prediction of creatinine clearance from serum creatinine. *Nephron* 1976;15:31–41.
49. Bennett WM, Aronoff GR, Golper TA, Morrison G, Singer I, Brater DC. *Drug Prescribing in Renal Failure,* 3rd ed. Philadelphia: American College of Physicians, 1994.
50. Cusson J, Nattel S, Matthews RT, Talajic M, Lawand S. Age-dependent lidocaine disposition in patients with acute myocardial infarction. *Clin Pharmacol Ther* 1985;37:381–386.
51. Takieddine FN, Tserng KY, King KC, Kalhan SC. Postnatal development of theophylline metabolism in preterm infants. *Semin Perinatol* 1981;5:351–355.
52. Milsap RL, Hill MR, Szefler SJ. Special pharmacokinetic considerations in children. In: Evans WE, Schentag JJ, Jusko WJ, eds. *Applied Pharmacokinetics: Principles of Therapeutic Drug Monitoring.* Vancouver: Applied Therapeutics, Inc., 1992;1–25.
53. Durnas C, Loi Cm, Cusack BJ. Hepatic drug metabolism and aging. *Clin Pharmacokinet* 1990;19:359–389.
54. Greenblatt DJ, Sellers EM, Shader RI. Drug disposition in old age. *N Engl J Med* 1982;306:1081–1088.
55. Loi CM, Vestal RE. Drug metabolism in the elderly. *Pharmacol Ther* 1988;36:131–149.
56. Sutherland JM. Fatal cardiovascular collapse of infants receiving large amounts of chloramphenicol. *Am J Dis Child* 1959;97:761–767.
57. Stewart CF, Hampton EM. Effect of maturation on drug disposition in pediatric patients. *Clin Pharm* 1987;6:548–564.
58. Greenblatt DJ, Allen MD, Locniskar A, Marmatz JC, Shader RI. Lorazepam kinetics in the elderly. *Clin Pharmacol Ther* 1979;26:103.
59. Polin RA, Fox WW. Basic pharmacologic principles. In: *Fetal and Neonatal Physiology.* Philadelphia: WB Saunders, 1992;107–119.
60. Polin RA, Fox WW. Physiologic differences of clinical significance. In: *Fetal and Neonatal Physiology.* Philadelphia: WB Saunders, 1992;169–177.
61. Roberts RJ. Pharmacologic principles in therapeutics in infants. In: *Drug Therapy in Infants. Pharmacologic Principles and Clinical Experience.* Philadelphia: WB Saunders, 1984;37–138.

Textbook of Ocular Pharmacology,
edited by T.J. Zimmerman, et al.
Lippincott–Raven Publishers, Philadelphia © 1997.

CHAPTER 17

Effect of Pregnancy on Drug Disposition

Helen Y. How and Joseph A. Spinnato

In prescribing drugs during pregnancy, two major factors should be considered. The first is that as a result of physiologic changes, the pregnant woman manifests altered drug handling. Hence, for the benefit of the mother, it is necessary to ensure that an effective dose is administered. Second, the fetus is an additional, discrete, and sensitive target organ on which certain drug effects may be irreversible and inapparent for several months or years; therefore, one should be aware of the potential teratogenic effects of available drugs. In general, ocular drugs are usually applied locally in the form of eyedrops; the effect on the fetus is therefore nil and at most minimal.

PREGNANCY-ASSOCIATED MATERNAL PHYSIOLOGIC CHANGES

Drug Absorption

From the Gastrointestinal Tract

Both the tone and the motility of the maternal gastrointestinal tract may be reduced as a consequence of physical displacement by the enlarging uterus and progesterone effect (1). Gastric emptying is slowed from a nonpregnancy average of 50 minutes to between 80 and 130 minutes (2), which may cause stagnation of drugs in the stomach and delayed attainment of peak drug concentrations. A 40% reduction in acid secretion, combined with increased production of alkaline mucus, can affect gastric pH and, consequently, the degree of ionization and solubility of drugs (3). A reduction of 30% to 50% in transit time through the small bowel may lead to increased metabolism of drugs in the gut wall (3,4) or, conversely, may allow a more complete absorption with increased bioavailability (5,6).

From the Lungs

As pregnancy progresses, increases occur in respiratory minute volume of up to 50% and in cardiac output of about 40%. These increases lead to a more rapid absorption and clearance of highly lipid-soluble anesthetic agents and bronchodilator aerosols (7).

From the Skin, Mucous Membranes, and Other Sites

Skin perfusion is increased up to fourfold in pregnancy (8). Increased blood flow to mucous membranes also occurs (7). These changes may improve the absorption of drugs administered by these routes. Conversely, blood flow to the legs is reduced late in pregnancy (9), and absorption of an intramuscular (i.m.) injection from this site may be delayed (10).

Drug Distribution

Plasma volume increases progressively from 6 to 8 weeks' gestation and reaches a maximal volume of 4,700 to 5,200 ml at 32 weeks, an increase of 45% (1,200 to 1,600 ml) above nonpregnant values (11). The net result is an increased volume of distribution for drugs, leading to decreased maternal serum concentration.

Serum concentration of albumin, the principal drug-binding protein, decreases progressively from a mean of 4.3 g/dl in the nonpregnant state to a mean of 3.0 g/dl (12). This change, along with altered binding to α-1 acid glycoprotein (13), an increase in fatty acids and lipids, and hormonal changes, may lead to an increase in the unbound drug fraction (6).

H. Y. How: Department of Obstetrics and Gynecology, University of Cincinnati, Cincinnati, Ohio 45267.

J. A. Spinnato: Department of Obstetrics and Gynecology, Division of Maternal-Fetal Medicine, University of Louisville School of Medicine, Louisville, Kentucky 40292.

Drug Elimination

The glomerular filtration rate (GFR) begins to increase by as early as 6 weeks' gestation, with a peak of 50% over nonpregnant values by the end of the first trimester (14), resulting in an increased drug clearance and the potential for subtherapeutic drug concentrations. Increased progesterone-activated hepatic metabolism leads to an increased rate of biotransformation to either active or inactive metabolites (15). The changes affecting drug distribution and elimination imply a need for a larger loading dose or a decreased dosing interval.

EFFECTS OF THE FETOPLACENTAL UNIT

The amount of drug reaching the fetus by passive diffusion depends on several factors: the molecular weight of the drug (higher-molecular-weight agents, i.e., >1,000, do not cross the placenta well); the lipid solubility (lipophilic agents cross the placenta more easily); the degree of ionization (only nonionized drugs cross the placenta rapidly); and the extent of plasma protein binding (only unbound drugs cross the placenta) (16).

Drug transfer is greater during late gestation as a result of the following factors (17):

1. Increased free drug available for transport
2. Uteroplacental blood flow (500 ml/min)
3. Increased placental surface area
4. Decreased thickness of the semipermeable lipid membranes (2 μm at term) between the placental capillaries
5. Greater physical disruption of placental membranes
6. More acidic fetal circulation to "trap" basic drugs

The placenta contains several enzymes that are capable of metabolizing drugs by oxidation, reduction, hydrolysis, or conjugation (18). Fetal tissues also metabolize drugs, although in most cases this contributes little to maternal drug concentrations, and the fetus relies largely on the maternal system for the clearance of drugs (19).

Drug Effects on the Fetus

Drugs and environmental chemicals currently are believed to account for 2% to 3% of malformations (20). The effect of a teratogen depends on (21) the following:

1. Specificity of the agent. Some agents are obviously more teratogenic than others. For example, thalidomide produces phocomelia in primates but not in rodents; cortisol is a teratogen in rodents but not in humans.
2. The dose reaching the developing fetus. At a low dose, there is no effect. At an intermediate dose, a pattern of organ-specific malformations can result. At a high dose, the embryo may be killed, causing the organ-specific teratogenic action to go unrecognized.
3. Stage of embryonic development. The embryo is relatively resistant to teratogenic insults during the first 2 weeks in humans. The presumed explanation is that early embryonic cells have not differentiated irrevocably. If one cell is destroyed, a surviving cell may be able to assume that function. The susceptibility to teratogens is maximal during organogenesis, between embryonic weeks 3 and 8; however, differentiation occurs later in the brain and gonads. Table 17-1 (22) lists the time when major organ systems develop.
4. The genotype of the mother and the fetus. Species differences in teratogenic effect abound in the literature and illustrate the difficulty in applying animal research to predict either the safety or adverse effects on human pregnancy.

To address the issues surrounding the use of drugs in pregnancy, the Food and Drug Administration (FDA) promulgated the labeling of drugs and drug products as to their effect on the fetus into the following categories (23):

Category A: controlled studies in women fail to demonstrate a risk to the fetus in the first trimester; the potential of fetal anomalies is low.

Category B: Reproductive studies in animals demonstrate no risk to the fetus, but no controlled studies in pregnant women exist, or animal studies have shown an adverse effect that was unconfirmed in controlled studies in pregnant women in the first trimester.

TABLE 17-1. *Development of fetal organ systems*

Embryonic age (wk from conception)	Embryonic development
1	Period of dividing zygote, implantation; embryo relatively resistant to teratogenic effects except embryocides
2–3	Craniofacial development; musculoskeletal and neural tube formation and differentiation
4	Limb buds; cardiovascular system enlarges
5	Limb buds segment; nose, eyes, ears become prominent
	Urinary system and gonadal differentiation
6	Formation of fingers and toes; heart septation
7–8	Maxilla fused; palate closed; eyelids formed
9–10	External and internal genitalia differentiate; most other major organ systems formed; embryo relatively resistant to teratogens
11	Genitourinary system complete

Category C: Animal studies have revealed adverse effects on the fetus, and there are no available controlled studies in pregnant women or in animals. These agents should be used only if the potential benefit justifies the potential risk to the fetus.

Category D: Positive evidence of fetal risk in humans exists, but the benefits from use in pregnant women may be acceptable in spite of the risk, such as a life-threatening situation for which a safer agent cannot be used or is ineffective.

Category X: Studies in animals or humans demonstrate fetal abnormalities, and the risk of using this drug during pregnancy clearly outweighs any possible benefits.

It is clinically useful to categorize drugs in one of four general categories: drugs with known teratogenic effects, drugs with probable teratogenic effects, drugs without known teratogenic effects at customary dosage levels, and drugs with potential adverse effects on the neonate (Tables 17-2, 17-3, 17-4 and 17-5) (21).

Topical application is the most common route of administration for ophthalmic drugs. To minimize systemic absorption, the rule of thumb is compression of the lacrimal sac for 3 to 5 minutes following instillation of drops, which retards the passage of drops via the nasolacrimal duct into areas of potential absorption such as the nasal and pharyngeal mucosa, thereby reducing systemic absorption (24).

TABLE 17-2. *Drugs with known teratogenic effects*

Drugs	Fetal effects
Anti-acne	
Isotretenoin (Accutane)	Microcephaly, cardiac defects and CNS lesions
Antibiotics	
Streptomycin	Ototoxicity (long duration of maternal therapy)
Tetracycline	Stained deciduous teeth (if exposed during the month 5 of fetal life to 7 to 8 yr of age)
Anticonvulsants	
Trimethadione, phenytoin	Facial dysmorphogenesis, mild mental retardation, growth restriction
Valproic acid	1–2% Neural tube defect
Anticoagulants	Nasal hypoplasia, epiphyseal stippling, optic atrophy, microcephaly, mental retardation
Coumadin and congeners	
Alcohol	Fetal alcohol syndrome: growth restriction, mild mental retardation, increase in anomalies
Angiotensin-converting enzymes	Fetal hypotension leading to fetal and neonatal death, pulmonary hypoplasia, neonatal anuria, growth restriction, skull hypoplasia
Folic acid antagonists	
(methotrexate, aminopterin)	Abortion, craniofacial dysmorphism, growth restriction, bone maldevelopment
Hormones	
Diethylstilbestrol and congeners	Vaginal adenosis, carcinogenesis, uterine anomalies, epididymal anomalies
Androgens	Masculinization of female fetus
Expectorants	
Inorganic iodides (≥12 mg/day)	Fetal goiter, neonatal deaths secondary to respiratory obstruction
Antidepressants	
Lithium	Ebstein's anomaly and other heart and great-vessel defects
Methyl mercury (contaminated fish)	Central nervous system damage, growth restriction
Thalidomide	Phocomelia

TABLE 17-3. *Drugs with probable teratogenic effects*

Drugs	Fetal effect
Alkylating agents	Increased abortion, anomalies
Aminoglycosides (kanamycin, gentamycin, neomycin)	Ototoxicity
Methimazole	Ulcerlike midline scalp defect
Nicotine	Growth retardation
Sulfonylureas	Increased anomalies
Benzodiazepines	Facial clefts

Occasionally, oral or parenteral administration of drugs may be necessary to achieve adequate therapeutic levels of drug in ocular tissue. It would be beyond the scope of this chapter to cover the pregnancy pharmacokinetics of all classes of drugs; so we have singled out some of the more commonly used ocular drugs not mentioned in Tables 17-2 through 17-5 for detailed discussion. For a detailed discussion of the different drugs used during pregnancy and lactation, see *Drugs in Pregnancy and Lactation,* 4th edition by Briggs et al. (25).

ANTIALLERGY AGENTS

Decongestants

Ephedrine/Pseudoephedrine

Ephedrine and ephedrine-like drugs are teratogenic in some animal species, but human teratogenicity has not been suspected (26). An association in the first trimester was found between the drugs as a whole and minor malformations, such as congenital dislocation of the hip, inguinal or umbilical hernia, and clubfoot (27). Breast-fed infants of mothers consuming long-acting preparations of these drugs exhibit transient irritability, excessive crying, and disturbed sleeping patterns (28). These drugs are risk category C.

TABLE 17-4. *Drugs without known teratogenic effects in humans at customary dosages*

Analgesics	Antituberculosis
Acetaminophen	Isoniazid
Narcotics	Ethambutol
Salicylates	Para-aminosalicylic acid
	Rifampicin
Antibiotics	Corticosteroids
Penicillin	
Cephalosporin	General anesthesia (short time exposure)
Sulfonamides	
Antiemetics	Heparin
Bendectin	
Promethazine	Phenobarbitol
Meclizine	

TABLE 17-5. *Drugs with potential adverse effects on the neonate*

Drugs	Potential adverse effects
Alcohol	Intoxication, hypotonia, delayed mental and motor development
Azathioprine	Decreased immunologic competence
Amphetamines	Irritable, poor feeding
Anesthetics	
General	Depression
Anticonvulsant	Bleeding, withdrawal
Benzodiazepines	Depression, floppy infant
Chloramphenicol	Gray syndrome
Caffeine	Jitteriness
Cigarette smoking	Intrauterine growth retardation
Hexamethonium	Paralytic ileus
Magnesium sulfate	Hypermagnesemia, respiratory depression
Napthalene	Hemolysis (G6PD deficiency)
Narcotic	Depression, withdrawal
Nitrofurantoin	Hemolysis (G6PD deficiency)
Propranolol	Hypoglycemia, bradycardia
Quinine	Thrombocytopenia
Reserpine	Nasal congestion
Salicylates	Platelet dysfunction
"Street" drugs	Withdrawal
Terbutaline	Tachycardia, hypothermia, hypocalcemia, hypoglycemia and hyperglycemia
Thiazides	Thrombocytopenia and electrolyte imbalance

Epinephrine/Phenylephrine/Phenylpropanolamine

In addition to what is already mentioned, these drugs are predominantly or in part α-adrenergic stimulants; theoretically, a large dose given intravenously could cause constriction of uterine blood vessels and could cause reduced blood flow, thereby producing fetal hypoxia (bradycardia) (29). These drugs are risk category C.

Antihistaminics

Antazoline Phosphate

No data are available concerning fetal risk and breastfeeding. This drug is risk category C.

Chlorpheniramine/Diphenhydramine/Pyrilamine Maleate/Tripelennamine/Triprolidine

There is no increase in minor and major malformations in fetuses exposed to these drugs. Generalized tremulousness and diarrhea as a result of diphenhydramine withdrawal was reported in a newborn infant whose mother had taken 150 mg/day during pregnancy (30). These drugs (diphenhydramine, triprolidine) are excreted into human breast milk in low concentrations. These drugs are risk category B (chlorpheniramine, tripelennamine) and risk category C (diphenhydramine, pyrilamine maleate, triprolidine) (31).

Lodoxamine Tromethamine

There are no available data of this drug in human pregnancy and lactation.

CYCLOPLEGICS (ANTICHOLINERGICS)

Atropine, Homatropine, Scopolamine

The Collaborative Perinatal Project reported no increased association of malformations with the use of these anticholinergic drugs individually anytime during pregnancy (32). When the group of parasympatholytics were taken as a whole, however, a possible association with minor malformations, like clubfoot and inguinal hernia, was found (33). Anticholinergics readily cross the placenta (32,34). When scopolamine is administered to the mother at term, fetal effects include tachycardia, decreased heart-rate variability, and decreased heart-rate deceleration. It has not been adequately documented whether measurable amounts are excreted into breast milk or, if excretion does occur, whether the nursing infant is affected (35). Although neonates are particularly sensitive to anticholinergic agents, no adverse effects have been reported in nursing infants whose mothers were taking these drugs, and the American Academy of Pediatrics considers these agents to be compatible with breast-feeding (36). These drugs are risk category C.

ANTIMICROBIAL AGENTS

Aminoglycosides (Gentamycin, Tobramycin, Kanamycin, Streptomycin)

These drugs rapidly cross the placenta into the fetal circulation and amniotic fluid (37). No congenital defects have been reported with their use. Ototoxicity has not been reported following in utero exposure to gentamycin or tobramycin; however, eighth cranial nerve toxicity in the fetus is well known following exposure to kanamycin and streptomycin and may occur with gentamycin (38). Data on the excretion of gentamycin into breast milk are lacking. Insignificant amounts of tobramycin are excreted into the breast milk. These drugs are risk category C.

Bacitracin

Congenital defects have not been reported in association with use of bacitracin. One study listed first-trimester exposure in 18 patients. The route of administration was not specified, and no association with malformations was found (39). Data on breast-feeding are not available. These drugs are risk category C.

Cephalosporin

The use of cephalothin, cefoperazone, ceftizoxime, ceftriaxone, and cephalexin has not been reported to be associated with congenital defects or toxicity in the newborn. These drugs can cross the placenta and distribute in fetal tissue. Most cephalosporins are excreted into breast milk in low concentrations. These drugs are risk category B.

Nalidixic Acid

No reports linking the use of nalidixic acid with congenital defects can be found. Nalidixic acid is excreted into breast milk in low concentration. Hemolytic anemia was reported in one infant with glucose-6-phosphate dehydrogenase deficiency whose mother was taking 1 g four times per day (40). Insignificant amounts of nalidixic acid are excreted into the breast milk (41). The drug is risk category B.

Fluoroquinolones (Norfloxacin/Ciprofloxacin)

These drugs were found to be embryotoxic, fetotoxic, and teratogenic (permanent cartilage lesions) when used in high dosages in animal studies. Norfloxacin and ciprofloxacin are excreted into breast milk in low concentrations; however, because of the unknown neonatal effect, the manufacturer does not recommend its use in breast-feeding mothers. These drugs are risk category C (31).

Sulfonamides

The sulfonamides readily cross the placenta to the fetus during all stages of gestation. Equilibrium with maternal blood is usually established after 2 to 3 hours, with fetal levels averaging 70% to 90% of maternal levels. Sulfonamides compete with bilirubin for binding to plasma albumin. Several authors have related severe jaundice in the newborn to maternal sulfonamide ingestion at term (42–44); however, a study of 94 infants exposed to sulfadiazine in utero for maternal prophylaxis of rheumatic fever failed to show an increase in prematurity, hyperbilirubinemia, or kernicterus (45). Our experience with the use of sulfonamides at term has been consistent with that of the latter study. The Collaborative Perinatal Project concluded that, taken in sum, sulfonamides do not appear to pose a significant teratogenic risk. Sulfonamides are excreted into breast milk in low concentrations. Milk : plasma ratios during therapy ranged between 0.06 and 0.5. This drug is risk category B.

ANTIVIRAL AGENTS

Acyclovir

This drug readily crosses the placenta to the fetus (46). After an intravenous (i.v.) dose, fetal cord acyclovir levels were higher than those in maternal serum with ratios of 1.4 and 1.25 reported (47,48). Topically, acyclovir may produce low levels of the drug in maternal serum, urine, and vaginal secretions (49). No adverse fetal effects attributable to acyclovir have been reported (50). The theoretical milk : plasma ratio is 0.15; however, ratios of 0.16 to 4.1 have been reported (51). This finding may be due to active or facilitated processes. The American Academy of Pediatrics considers acyclovir to be compatible with breastfeeding (36). This drug is risk category C.

Vidarabine

This drug has not been studied in human pregnancy. It is a potent teratogen in some species of animals after topical and i.m. administration (52,53). Daily instillations of a 10% solution into the vagina of pregnant rats in late gestation had no effect on the offspring (53). No reports involving the use of vidarabine in lactating women have been located. This drug is risk category C.

Idoxuridine

This drug has not been studied in human pregnancy and lactation. The drug is teratogenic in some species of animals after injection and ophthalmic use (54,55). This drug is risk category C.

ANTIINFLAMMATORY AGENTS

Corticosteroids

Dexamethasone

The congenital defects have been reported with the use of dexamethasone. It has been used widely in obstetrics for preterm labor to enhance fetal pulmonary maturation (56,57). Dexamethasone crosses the placenta to the fetus (58,59) and is partially metabolized (54%) by the placenta to its inactive 11-ketosteroid derivative. Leukocytosis has been observed in infants with in utero exposure to dexamethasone (60,61). Long-term follow-up of these children has not shown any adverse effects (62,63). There are no available data about this drug in human lactation. This drug is risk category C.

Prednisone/Prednisolone

Prednisolone is the biologically active form of prednisone. The placenta can oxidize prednisolone to inactive prednisone or less-active cortisone. Human studies have shown that these corticosteroids have little, if any, effect on the developing fetus (64,65). At 80 mg/day, the nursing infant would ingest <0.1% of the dose, which corresponds to <10% of the infant's endogenous cortisol production (66). This drug is risk category B.

Nonsteroidal Antiinflammatory Agents

There are no published reports linking the use of nonsteroidal antiinflammatory agents (diclofenac sodium, flurbiprofen sodium, ketorolac, tromethamine, and suprofen) with congenital defects. Theoretically, these drugs are prostaglandin synthetase inhibitors and could cause constriction of the ductus arteriosus in utero (67). Persistent pulmonary hypertension of the newborn should also be considered (67). Ophthalmic nonsteroidals probably should be avoided during late pregnancy. These drugs are risk category B (diclofenac) and risk category C (flurbiprofen, ketorolac, suprofen). During the third trimester, these drugs are considered risk category D. These drugs do not enter human milk in significant quantities (68).

CYTOTOXIC AGENTS

Azathioprine (Imuran)

Most investigators have found azathioprine to be relatively safe in pregnancy (50,69–71). It readily crosses the placenta, and trace amounts of its active metabolite, 6-mercaptopurine, have been found in fetal blood. Intrauterine growth restriction and immunosuppression of the newborn have been associated with in utero exposure (72,73). Azathioprine has been reported to interfere with the effectiveness of intrauterine contraceptive devices (74,75); hence, additional or other methods of contraception should be considered in sexually active women. No data are available on the effect of this drug in human lactation. This drug is risk category D.

Cyclophosphamide (Cytoxan)

Multiple congenital anomalies have been associated with in utero first-trimester exposure of cyclophosphamide (76). Data indicate that intrauterine growth retardation and neonatal immunosuppression may occur with in utero exposure of this drug at any time during the pregnancy (77,78). Cyclophosphamide is excreted into breast milk (79). Except for the neutropenia and a brief episode of diarrhea (80), no other adverse effects have been observed in infants. The American Academy of Pediatrics considers cyclophosphamide to be contraindicated during breast-feeding because of the reported case of neutropenia and because of the potential adverse effects relating to immune suppression, growth, and carcinogenesis (36). This drug is risk category D.

Fluorouracil

There is limited experience with fluorouracil during pregnancy. Topical use of the drug has not been associated with adverse fetal effects. Animal studies showed that fluorouracil crosses the placenta, and maternal doses of >40 mg/kg resulted in abortion of all embryos. Teratogenic dosages in animals that are one to three times the maximum recommended human therapeutic dose have been associated with malformations such as cleft palate, skeletal defects, and deformed appendages (paws and tails) (31). There are no data available on the effects of this drug in human lactation. This drug is risk category D.

Mitomycin C

Safety for use during pregnancy has not been established. Animal studies have demonstrated a relative fetal exposure of 6.4% following maternal dosing (81). Teratogenic effect includes skeletal abnormalities, specifically that of the vertebrae and ribs (82), as well as neural tube defects (83). No data are available on breast-feeding. This drug is risk category C.

Cyclosporin A

Oral cyclosporin A in a daily dose of 1 to 10 mg/kg was used successfully in the treatment of Graves' ophthalmopathy and uveitis (31). Cyclosporin crosses the placenta readily, and the cord blood : maternal plasma ratio at delivery was 0.63 (84). The manufacturer in 1987 had knowledge of 34 pregnancies involving the use of cyclosporin (A. Poploski and D. A. Colasante, Sandoz Pharmaceuticals, personal communication, 1987). These pregnancies resulted in 27 live births, six abortions (two spontaneous, three elective, and one for anencephaly). Cyclosporin is embryotoxic and fetoxic in rats and rabbits when given in doses of two to five times the human dose (31). Based on relatively small numbers, cyclosporin has not been found to be a human teratogen. Cyclosporin is excreted into human breast milk. At a dose of 450 mg/day, milk levels on postpartum days 2, 3, and 4 were 101 ng/ml, 109 ng/ml, and 263 ng/ml, respectively (85). The American Academy of Pediatrics considers cyclosporin to be contraindicated during breast-feeding because of the potential for immune suppression and neutropenia, possible intrauterine growth restriction, and possible association with carcinogenesis (86). This drug is risk category C.

ANTIGLAUCOMA AGENTS

Beta-adrenergic Blocking Agents

Timolol Maleate

Its use in pregnancy has been reported. Newborns exposed in utero to timolol should be observed closely during the first 24 to 48 hours after birth for effects of persistent beta blockade (e.g., bradycardia and hypoglycemia). High maternal timolol levels in milk (5.6 ng/ml) and plasma (0.93 mg/ml) were noted approximately 1.5 hours after a dose of 0.5% timolol maleate ophthalmic drops. A milk sample taken 12 hours after the last dose contained 0.5 ng/ml of timolol maleate. Assuming that the infant nursed every 4 hours and received 75 ml at each feeding, the daily dose would be below that expected to produce cardiac effects in the infant. The American Academy of Pediatrics considers timolol to be compatible with breast-feeding (36). This drug is risk category C.

Betaxolol

No data describing the use of betaxolol in human pregnancy exist. In oral studies in rats, there is evidence of skeletal and visceral anomalies at doses 600 times the maximum recommended human dose, whereas in rabbits, there is an increase in postimplantation loss at doses 54 times the recommended human dose (87). Betaxolol is excreted into human milk in quantities sufficient to produce beta-blockage in a nursing infant (88). These infants should be closely observed for hypotension, bradycardia, and other signs and symptoms of beta-blockage. This drug is risk category C.

Levobunolol

Fetotoxicity was observed in rabbits at doses 200 and 700 times the dose for glaucoma. It is not known whether levobunolol is excreted in breast milk. This drug is risk category C (31).

Metipranolol

During organogenesis, an oral dose of 50 mg/kg has been associated with increased fetal resorption, fetal death, and delayed development in rabbits. It is not known whether metipranolol is excreted in breast milk. This drug is risk category C (31).

Carteolol

Increased resorptions and decreased fetal weights occurred in rabbits and rats at maternal doses of 1,052 and 5,264 times the maximum human dose, respectively. A dose-related increase in wavy ribs was noted in the developing rat fetus when pregnant rats received doses of 212 times the maximum human dose. Carteolol is excreted in the breast milk of animals. Caution is advised when administering this drug to a nursing mother. This drug is risk category C (31).

Miotics (Cholinergics)

Carbachol/Demacarium/Echothiophate/Isoflurophate

No reports of their use in pregnancy can be found. As quaternary ammonium compounds, these drugs are ionized at physiologic pH, and transplacental passage in significant amounts would not be expected (75). There are no available data about the effects of these drugs in human lactation. These drugs are risk category C.

Physostigmine

Congenital defects associated with physostigmine use have not been reported. Physostigmine is an anticholinesterase agent that does not contain a quaternary ammonium element; hence it is expected to cross the placenta (88). The transplacental passage of anti-acetylcholine receptor immunoglobulin G antibodies leads to transient muscular weakness in about 20% of newborns of mothers with myasthenia gravis (89–91). The onset of characteristic weakness in the infant may be delayed as long as 48 hours by coincident acquisition by the infant of anticholinesterase drugs given to the mother. There are no data available about the effects of this drug in human lactation. This drug is risk category C.

Pilocarpine

No reports of its use in pregnancy and lactation have been located. This drug is risk category C.

Sympathomimetics (Dipivefrin HCL)

There are no available data on the effect of this drug in human pregnancy and lactation. This drug is risk category B (31).

Carbonic Anhydrase Inhibitors

Acetazolamide

Except for a single case of a neonatal teratoma in a mother who received 750 mg daily for glaucoma during the first and second trimester (92), there are no reports linking the use of acetazolamide with congenital defects. The Collaborative Perinatal Project monitored 50,282 mother-child pairs, 12 of which had first trimester exposure to acetazolamide. For use anytime during pregnancy, 1,024 exposures were recorded. No evidence was found to suggest a relationship to major or minor malformations (33). The milk : plasma ratio 1 hour after a dose was 0.25. This drug is risk category C.

Methazolamide

No reports describing the use of methazolamide in human pregnancy and lactation exist. This drug is risk category C.

Dorzolamide

Studies in rabbits at oral dose of higher than 2.5 mg/kg/day (31 times the recommended human ophthalmic dose) revealed malformations of the vertebral bodies. It is not known whether dorzolamide is excreted in breast milk. This drug is risk category C (31).

Osmotic-Diuretic

Mannitol

Mannitol is an osmotic diuretic. No reports of its use in pregnancy following intravenous administration have been located. There are no available data on the effects of these drugs in human lactation. This drug is risk category C.

Glycerol 50%

No data on its use in human pregnancy and lactation exist. This drug is risk category C (31).

Isosorbide

No data are available of its use in human pregnancy and lactation. This drug is risk category C (25).

GENERAL AND LOCAL ANESTHESIA

It is beyond the scope of this chapter to discuss in detail the possible effects of the use of each general and local anesthetic during pregnancy; however, the following are recommendations for anesthetic management during pregnancy (93):

1. Elective surgery should be deferred until after delivery when the physiologic changes of pregnancy have returned to normal. Women of reproductive age scheduled for elective surgery should be screened carefully for the possibility of pregnancy.
2. Urgent surgery—that is, operations that are essential but can be delayed without increasing the risk of permanent disability—should be deferred until the second or third trimester. At present, no anesthetic drug has been proved to be teratogenic in humans; however, it is prudent to minimize fetal exposure to drugs during the vulnerable first trimester.
3. Emergency surgery during the first trimester is ideally performed under regional block.
4. If pharmacologic premedication is necessary, barbiturates are preferable to minor tranquilizers such as diazepam or meprobamate. Glycopyrrolate does not cross the placenta and is preferred over atropine and scopolamine.
5. If a general anesthetic is necessary, adequate oxygenation and avoidance of hyperventilation are mandatory. Pregnant patients are at increased risk of aspiration, and the usual safeguards to prevent aspiration pneumonitis should be performed.
6. Aortocaval compression during the second and third trimesters may be prevented by a left lateral tilt position.
7. Ideally, continuous fetal heart rate monitoring during surgery should be employed after week 16 of gestation, which may produce an indication of abnormalities in maternal ventilation or uterine perfusion.
8. Abortion following surgery is not common unless uterine manipulation was done intraoperatively. Uterine activity should be monitored continuously with an external tocodynamometer during the postoperative period to detect the onset of preterm labor. Tocolytic agents, instituted early, may prevent preterm delivery.

DRUGS AND BREAST MILK

Most drugs taken by a lactating mother are excreted in her milk, but usually the amount will be too small to affect the baby (94). Principles of drug transfer across the placenta also apply to the transfer of drugs into the breast tissue; for example, the breast milk pH ranges from 6.8 to 7.3, which is lower than plasma and interstitial fluid. Weak bases are more unionized in the higher pH of the plasma and pass readily into the more acidic milk where they become ionized and "trapped," creating a higher concentration in milk than in plasma. Weak acids, such as sulfonamides and benzyl penicillin, have an equal or lower concentration in milk than in plasma (95); however, even if milk concentrations are low, the total daily dose received in 500 to 1,000 ml of milk may approach an effective dose for a 3 to 4 kg baby, especially in premature babies, because of slower drug excretion. If a potentially harmful drug is prescribed, it is sometimes possible to minimize the amount reaching the baby by avoiding feeding at times when milk levels are highest, usually between 30 minutes and 2 hours after oral dosing. Thus, in general, if a drug is used therapeutically in the neonatal period, there is no need to be concerned about its use in breast-feeding women (95).

TABLE 17-6. *Effects of radiation*

Dose (rads)	Effects
<5	No increased incidence of congenital malformation and growth restriction
>10	May have low-risk tumorigenic or genetic hazards
>50	Growth restriction, microcephaly, mental retardation
>100	Microcephaly/hydrocephaly; mental retardation; growth restriction; congenital malformation of the eyes, ears, limbs and genitalia. Radiation sickness.
450	Fifty percent of exposed persons die; survivors may be predisposed to malignancy

DIAGNOSTIC RADIATION AND PREGNANCY

Medical personnel are often asked by patients how much radiation they are receiving or how dangerous the radiation is that they receive in routine radiologic studies. Tables 17-6 and 17-7 summarize the dose effects of radiation and the adverse outcomes that may occur following maternal high-dose ionizing radiation (97). So, for example, a lateral skull roentgenogram will expose the patient's gonad and the fetus to <0.5 mrad of radiation, and this dose becomes negligible if the patient wears a lead apron (Tables 17-6 and 17-7).

TABLE 17-7. Adverse pregnancy outcomes with a radiation dose of >250 rads

Gestational age at exposure (wk)	Outcome
0–3	Spontaneous abortion or normal
4–11	Microcephaly, mental retardation, microphthalmia, cataracts, growth restriction
12–16	Mental retardation and/or growth restriction
17–19	Same but less severe than at 12–16 weeks
>20	As seen with postnatal exposure: hair loss, skin lesions, bone marrow suppression

REFERENCES

1. Krauer B, Krauer F. Drug kinetics in pregnancy. *Clin Pharmacokinet* 1977;2:167–181.
2. Davison JS, Davison MC, Hay DM. Gastric emptying time in late pregnancy and labour. *J Obstet Gynaecol Br Commonw* 1970;77: 37–41.
3. Parker WA. Effects of pregnancy on pharmacokinetics. In: Benet LZ, et al. eds. *Pharmacokinetic Basis for Drug Treatment.* New York: Raven Press, 1984;251.
4. Dahl SG, Strandjard RE. Pharmacokinetics of chlorpromazine after single and chronic dosage. *Clin Pharmacol Ther* 1977;21:437–448.
5. Eadie MJ, Lander CM, Tyrer JH. Plasma drug level monitoring in pregnancy. *Clin Pharmacokinet* 1977;2:427–436.
6. Welling PG. Effects of gastrointestinal disease on drug absorption. In: Benet LZ, et al, eds. *Pharmacokinetic Basis for Drug Treatment.* New York: Raven Press, 1984;30.
7. Krauer B, Krauer F, Hytten FE. Pregnancy and its effect on drug handling: the influence of physiological changes in pregnancy. In: Lind T, Singer A, eds. *Current Reviews in Obstetrics and Gynecology.* Edinburgh: Churchill Livingstone, 1984;19–50.
8. Katz M, Sokal MM. Skin perfusion in pregnancy. *Am J Obstet Gynecol* 1980;137:30–33.
9. Hytten FE, Leitch I. *The Physiology of Human Pregnancy,* 2nd ed. Oxford: Blackwell, 1964;1–86.
10. Krauer B. In: Eskes TKAB, Finster M, eds. *Drug Therapy During Pregnancy.* London: Butterworths, 1985;9–31.
11. Pritchard JA. Changes in the blood volume during pregnancy and delivery. *Anesthesiology* 1965;26:393.
12. Mendenhall NW. Serum protein concentrations in pregnancy. I. Concentrations in maternal serum. *Am J Obstet Gynecol* 1970;106: 388–399.
13. Herngren L, Ehrnebo M, Boreus LO. Drug binding to plasma proteins during human pregnancy and in the perinatal period. *Dev Pharmacol Ther* 1983;6:110–124.
14. Davison JM, Dunlop W. Changes in renal hemodynamics and tubular function induced by normal human pregnancy. *Semin Nephrol* 1984; 4:198.
15. Fever G. Action of pregnancy and various progesterones on hepatic microsomal activities. *Drug Metab Rev* 1979;9:147–169.
16. Mirkin BL, Singh S. Placental transfer of pharmacologically active molecules. In: Mirkin BL, ed. *Perinatal Pharmacology and Therapeutics.* New York: Academic, 1976;1–30.
17. Juchau MR, Dyer DC. Pharmacology of the placenta. *Pediatr Clin North Am* 1972;19:65.
18. Juchau MR. Drug biotransformation in the placenta. *Pharmacol Ther* 1980;8:501–524.
19. Juchau MR, Chao ST, Omiecinski CJ. Drug metabolism by the human fetus. *Clin Pharmacokinet* 1980;5:320–339.
20. Wilson JG. Environmental effects on development-teratology. In: Assali NS, ed. *Pathophysiology of Gestation.* II. New York: Academic Press, 1972;288.
21. Simpson JL, Golbus MS. Principles of teratology. In: Simpson JL, Golbus MS, eds. *Genetics in Obstetrics and Gynecology.* Philadelphia: WB Saunders, 1992;241–274.
22. Moore KL, Persaud TVN. *The Developing Human: Clinically Oriented Embryology,* 5th ed. Philadelphia: WB Saunders, 1993.
23. Food and Drug Administration: *Federal Register* 1980;44:37,434–37,487.
24. Bartlett JD. Dosage forms and routes of administration. In: Bartlett JD, Ghormley NR, Jaenus SD, Rowsey JJ, Zimmerman TJ, eds. *Ophthalmic Drug Facts.* St. Louis: Wolters Kluwer Co., 1993.
25. Briggs GG, Freeman RK, Yaffe SJ, eds. *Drugs in Pregnancy and Lactation,* 4th ed. Baltimore: Williams & Wilkins, 1994.
26. Shepard TH. *Catalog of Teratogenic Agents,* 4th ed. Baltimore: Johns Hopkins University Press, 1983;177–178.
27. Heinonen OP, Slone D, Shapiro S. *Birth Defects and Drugs in Pregnancy.* Littleton: Publishing Sciences Group, 1977;355, 491.
28. Mortimer EA Jr. Drug toxicity from breast milk? *Pediatrics* 1977; 60:780–781.
29. Entmann SS, Moise KJ. Anaphylaxis in pregnancy. *South Med J* 1984;77:402.
30. Parkin DE. Probable Benadryl withdrawal manifestations in a newborn infant. *J Pediatr* 1974;85:580.
31. Olin BR, ed. *Drug Facts and Comparisons.* St. Louis: JB Lippincott, 1996.
32. Nishimura H, Tanimura T. *Clinical Aspects of the Teratogenicity of Drugs.* Amsterdam: Excerpta Medica, 1976;233.
33. Heinonen OP, Slone D, Shapiro S. *Birth Defects and Drugs in Pregnancy.* Littleton: Publishing Sciences Group, 1977;350, 493.
34. Kanto J, Virtanen R, Iisalo E, Maenpaa K, Liukko P. Placental transfer and pharmacokinetics of atropine after a single maternal intravenous and intramuscular administration. *Acta Anaesthesiol Scand* 1981;25:85–88.
35. Stewart JJ. Gastrointestinal drugs. In: Wilson JT, ed. *Drugs in Breast Milk.* Balgowlah, Australia: ADIS Press, 1981;65–71.
36. Committee on Drugs, American Academy of Pediatrics. Transfer of drugs and other chemicals into human milk. *Pediatrics* 1989;84: 924–936.
37. Daubenfeld O, Modde H, Hirsch H. Transfer of gentamicin to the foetus and the amniotic fluid during a steady state in the mother. *Arch Gynecol* 1974;217:233–240.
38. Nishimura H, Tanimura T. *Clinical Aspects of the Teratogenicity of Drugs.* Amsterdam: Excerpta Medica, 1976;129–131.
39. Heinonen OP, Slone D, Shapiro S. *Birth Defects and Drugs in Pregnancy.* Littleton: Publishing Sciences Group, 1977;297, 301.
40. Belton EM, Jones RV. Hemolytic anemia due to nalidixic acid. *Lancet* 1965;2:691.
41. Wilson JT. Milk/plasma ratios and contraindicated drugs. In: Wilson JT, ed. *Drugs in Breast Milk.* Balgowlah, Australia: ADIS Press, 1981;78–79.
42. Heckel GP. Chemotherapy during pregnancy: danger of fetal injury from sulfanilamide and its derivatives. *JAMA* 1941;117:1314–1316.
43. Lucey JP, Driscoll TJ Jr. Hazard to newborn infants of administration of long-acting sulfonamides to pregnant women. *Pediatrics* 1959;24: 489–499.
44. Kanto HI, Sutherland DA, Leonard JT, Kamholz FH, Fry ND, White WL. Effect on bilirubin metabolism in the newborn of sulfisoxazole administration to the mother. *Obstet Gynecol* 1961;17:494–500.
45. Baskin CG, Law S, Wenger NK. Sulfadiazine rheumatic fever prophylaxis during pregnancy: does it increase the risk of kernicterus in the newborn? *Cardiology* 1980;65:222–225.
46. Haddad J, Simeoni U, Messer J, Willard D. Transplacental passage of acyclovir. *J Pediatr* 1987;110:164.
47. Landsberger EJ, Hager WD, Grossman JH III. Successful management of varicella pneumonia complicating pregnancy: a report of three cases. *J Reprod Med* 1986;31:311–314.
48. Utley K, Bromberger P, Wagner L, Schneider H. Management of primary herpes in pregnancy complicated by ruptured membranes and extreme prematurity: case report. *Obstet Gynecol* 1987;69:471–473.
49. Zovirax. Product information. Burroughs-Wellcome, 1985.
50. Key TC, Resnik R, Dittrich HC, Reisner LS. Successful pregnancy after cardiac transplantation. *Am J Obstet Gynecol* 1989;160:367–371.
51. Lau RJ, Emery MG, Galinsky RE. Unexpected accumulation of acyclovir in breast milk with estimation of infant exposure. *Obstet Gynecol* 1987;69:468–471.
52. Pavan-Langston D, Buchanan RA, Alford CA Jr, eds. *Adenine Arabinoside: An Antiviral Agent.* New York: Raven Press, 1975;153.
53. Schardein JL, Hertz DL, Petretre JA, Fitzgerald JE, Kutz SM. The effect of vidarabine on the development of the offspring of rats, rabbits and monkeys. *Teratology* 1977;15:213–242.
54. Nishimura H, Tanimura T. *Clinical Aspects of the Teratogenicity of Drugs.* Amsterdam: Excerpta Medica, 1976;148:258–259.
55. Itoi M, Gefter JW, Kaneko N, Ishii Y, Ramer RM, Gasset AR. Teratogenicities of ophthalmic drugs. I. Antiviral ophthalmic drugs. *Arch Ophthalmol* 1975;93:46–51.
56. Caspi E, Schreyer P, Weinraub Z, Lifshitz Y, Goldberg M. Dexamethasone for prevention of respiratory distress syndrome: multiple perinatal factors. *Obstet Gynecol* 1981;57:41–47.
57. Bishop EH. Acceleration of fetal pulmonary maturity. *Obstet Gynecol* 1981;58(suppl):48S–51S.
58. Osathanondh R, Tulchinsky D, Kamali H, Fencl MdeM, Taeusch HW Jr. Dexamethasone levels in treated pregnant women and newborn infants. *J Pediatr* 1977;90:617–620.

59. Levitz M, Jansen V, Dancis J. The transfer and metabolism of corticosteroids in the perfused human placenta. *Am J Obstet Gynecol* 1978;132:363–366.
60. Otero L, Conlon C, Reynolds P, Duval-Arnould B, Golden SM. Neonatal leukocytosis associated with prenatal administration of dexamethasone. *Pediatrics* 1981;68:778–780.
61. Anday EK, Harris MC. Leukemoid reaction associated with antenatal dexamethasone administration. *J Pediatr* 1982;101:614–616.
62. Wong YC, Beardsmore CS, Silverman M. Antenatal dexamethasone and subsequent lung growth. *Arch Dis Child* 1982;57:536–538.
63. Collaborative Group on Antenatal Steroid Therapy. Effects of antenatal dexamethasone administration in the infant: long-term follow-up. *J Pediatr* 1984;104:259–267.
64. Warrell DW, Taylor R. Outcome for the foetus of mothers receiving prednisolone during pregnancy. *Lancet* 1968;1:117–118.
65. Walsh SD, Clark FR. Pregnancy in patients on long-term corticosteroid therapy. *Scott Med J* 1967;12:302–306.
66. Ost L, Wettrell G, Bjorkhem I, Rane A. Prednisolone excretion in human milk. *J Pediatr* 1985;106:1008–1011.
67. Levin DL. Effects of inhibition of prostaglandin synthesis on fetal-development, oxygenation, and the fetal circulation. *Semin Perinatol* 1980;4:35–44.
68. Townsend RJ, Benedetti TJ, Erickson S, Cengiz C, Gillespie WR, Gschwend J, Albert KS. Excretion of ibuprofen into breast milk. *Am J Obstet Gynecol* 1984;149:184–186.
69. Sharon E, Jones J, Diamond H, Kaplan D. Pregnancy and azathioprine in systemic lupus erythematosus. *Am J Obstet Gynecol* 1974; 118:25–27.
70. Erkman J, Blythe JG. Azathioprine therapy complicated by pregnancy. *Obstet Gynecol* 1972;40:708–709.
71. Price HV, Salaman JR, Laurence KM, Langmaid H. Immunosuppressive drugs and the foetus. *Transplantation* 1976;21:294–298.
72. Scott JR. Fetal growth retardation associated with maternal administration of immunosuppressive drugs. *Am J Obstet Gynecol* 1977;128: 668–676.
73. Cote CJ, Meuwissen HJ, Pickering RJ. Effects on the neonate of prednisone and azathioprine administered to the mother during pregnancy. *J Pediatr* 1974;85:324–328.
74. Davison JM, Lindheimer MD. Pregnancy in renal transplant recipients. *J Reprod Med* 1982;27:613–621.
75. Kossoy LR, Herbert CM III, Wentz AC. Management of heart transplant recipients: guidelines for the obstetrician-gynecologist. *Am J Obstet Gynecol* 1988;159:490–499.
76. Kirshon B, Wasserstrum N, Willis R, Herman GE, McCabe ERB. Teratogenic effects of first-trimester cyclophosphamide therapy. *Obstet Gynecol* 1988;72:462–464.
77. Pizzuto J, Aviles A, Noriega L, Niz J, Morales M, Romero F. Treatment of acute leukemia during pregnancy: presentation of nine cases. *Cancer Treat Rep* 1980;64:679–683.
78. Nicholson HO. Cytotoxic drugs in pregnancy: review of reported cases. *J Obstet Gynaecol Br Commonw* 1968;75:307–312.
79. Wiernik PH, Duncan HJ. Cyclophosphamide in human milk. *Lancet* 1971;1:912.
80. Amato D, Niblett JS. Neutropenia from cyclophosphamide in breast milk. *Med J Aust* 1977;1:383–384.
81. Boike GM, Deppe G, Young JD, Gove NL, Bottoms SF, Malone JM Jr, et al. Chemotherapy in a pregnant rat model. 1. Mitomycin-C: pregnancy-specific kinetics and placental transfer. *Gynecol Oncol* 1989;34:187–190.
82. Gregg BC, Snow MHL. Axial abnormalities following disturbed growth in Mitomycin C-treated mouse embryos. *J Embryol Exp Morphol* 1983;73:135–149.
83. Seller MJ, Perkins KJ. Effect of Mitomycin C on neural tube defects of the curly-tail mouse. *Teratology* 1986;33:305–309.
84. Pawliger DF, McClean FW, Noyes WD. Normal fetus after cytosine arabinoside therapy. *Ann Intern Med* 1971;74:1012.
85. Lewis GJ, Lamont CAR, Lee HA, Slapak M. Successful pregnancy in a renal transplant recipient taking cyclosporin A. *Br Med J* 1983;286: 603.
86. Committee on Drugs, American Academy of Pediatrics. Transfer of drugs and other chemicals into human milk. *Pediatrics* 1994;93:137–150.
87. Kerlone. Product information. G D Searle & Co., 1993.
88. Taylor P. Anticholinesterase agents. In: Gilman AG, Goodman LS, Gilman A, eds. *The Pharmacological Basis of Therapeutics,* 6th ed. New York: MacMillan, 1980;100–119.
89. McNall PG, Jafarnia MR. Management of myasthenia gravis in the obstetrical patient. *Am J Obstet Gynecol* 1965;92:518–525.
90. Blackhall MI, Buckley GA, Roberts DV, Roberts JB, Thomas BH, Wilson A. Drug-induced neonatal myasthenia. *J Obstet Gynaecol Br Commonw* 1969;76:157–162.
91. Plauche WG. Myasthenia gravis in pregnancy: an update. *Am J Obstet Gynecol* 1979;135:691–697.
92. Worsham GF, Beckman EN, Mitchell EH. Sacrococcygeal teratoma in a neonate: association with maternal use of acetazolamide. *JAMA* 1978;240:251–252.
93. Levinson G, Shnider SM. Anesthesia for surgery during pregnancy: In: Shnider SM, Levinson G, eds. *Anesthesia for Obstetrics.* Baltimore: Williams & Wilkins, 1987;201–202.
94. Beeley L. Drugs and breast feeding. *Clin Obstet Gynecol* 1988;23: 247–251.
95. Lien EJ, Kuwahara J, Koda RT. Diffusion of drugs into prostatic fluid and milk. *Drug Intell Clin Pharm* 1974;8:470.
96. Brent RL. The effects of embryonic and fetal exposure to x-ray, microwaves, and ultrasound. *Clin Perinatol* 1986;13:615.
97. Dekaban AS. Abnormalities in children exposed to x-radiation during various stages of gestation: tentative timetable of radiation injury to the human fetus. Part I. *J Nucl Med* 1968;9:471.

SECTION II

Glaucoma

Section Editors: Karanjit S. Kooner, Robert D. Fechtner, and Thom J. Zimmerman

OVERVIEW

The world of glaucoma therapy has been rapidly changing. During the preparation of this textbook, we saw the introduction of the first topical carbonic anhydrase inhibitor (CAI), dorzolamide. More recently, the first drug in a new class, latanoprost, a topical prostaglandin analogue was introduced. With the availability of several beta blockers, the alpha-2 agonists, and the parasympathetic drugs, clinicians now enjoy an ever-widening choice of IOP-lowering drugs for their patients with glaucoma. The introduction of these new agents may present the first real challenge to the topical beta blockers which have been the first line in glaucoma therapy for nearly 20 years. As our understanding of the glaucomas deepens, we may find therapies directed at factors other than intraocular pressure play an increasingly important role. Blood flow and neuroprotection are two such areas of active investigation that may result in novel glaucoma therapies in the future.

The section on glaucoma therapy covers all the drugs currently available in the United States to treat this disease. Each author has extensive experience in the use of the respective drugs. Chapters are arranged to offer continuous flow of thought for the reader. Each subsection is self-explanatory: glaucoma classification (Fechtner and Kooner), parasympathetic drugs (Kaufman and Gabelt), sympathetic drugs: epinephrine and dipivefrin (Fang and Kass), alpha-2 agonists (Juzych, Robin, and Novack), alpha-adrenergic antagonists (Kooner), and beta-adrenergic antagonists (Juzych and Zimmerman). Next come chapters on the oral carbonic anhydrase inhibitors (Piper), the new topical carbonic anhydrase inhibitors (Sharir), hyperosmotic agents (Singh and Krupin), antifibrosis agents (Henderson and Nardin), and prostaglandins (Camras, Bito, and Toris). The next two chapters look into future drug development areas: namely, the neuroprotective agents (Abbasoglu and Kooner) and the approach to medical trabeculocanulotomy (Allingham). This section ends with a thought-provoking, provocative, and often-alternative view concerning glaucoma and its management (Bito).

Textbook of Ocular Pharmacology,
edited by T.J. Zimmerman, et al.
Lippincott–Raven Publishers, Philadelphia © 1997.

CHAPTER 18

Definitions and Classification of Glaucoma

Robert D. Fechtner and Karanjit S. Kooner

DEFINITION OF GLAUCOMA

The term glaucoma refers to a syndrome of retinal ganglion cell loss often manifested as excavation of the optic nerve head with corresponding visual functional defects. The etiologies of the optic nerve damage are not well understood and may be multifactorial. Several mechanisms have been invoked to explain this syndrome, and each may play a role in some cases (see Chapter 31 by Bito, this volume; Fechtner, ref. 1). Historically, glaucoma has been defined based on elevated intraocular pressure (IOP). It is now appreciated that while elevated IOP is a prominent risk factor, there are many with the syndrome of glaucoma without elevated IOP (normal tension glaucoma) and many with elevated IOP without damage (ocular hypertension). Other mechanisms such as microvascular abnormalities, genetic predisposition, and excitotoxin injury have been suggested as contributing to glaucomatous optic neuropathy. The definition of the syndrome will doubtless undergo further evolution as our understanding of the pathophysiologic and genetic basis of these injuries evolves.

CLASSIFICATION OF GLAUCOMA

Classifying the glaucomas helps distinguish the known differences in clinical presentation, pathophysiology, and therapeutic approach. These classifications are useful as they can help guide diagnostic and therapeutic interventions. The major glaucoma textbooks contain long lists classifying the glaucomas by various criteria (Shields, ref. 2; Hoskins, ref. 3.)

A few important distinctions can be drawn from such classifications. One important distinction is the anatomic classification of glaucomas as open-angle and angle-closure. The angle-closure glaucomas include conditions in which there is anatomic obstruction of the trabecular meshwork outflow pathway. This anatomic distinction has important implications for the clinician.

The glaucomas are often separated into categories of primary and secondary. The primary glaucomas have no known association with other ocular or systemic disease. The secondary glaucomas have an identifiable ocular or systemic abnormality associated with the glaucoma. Primary open-angle glaucoma is the most common of the glaucomas. It accounts for about 70 percent of glaucoma in the United States. The secondary open-angle glaucomas are characterized by an anatomically open angle and an identifiable associated condition such as pigment dispersion, pseudoexfoliation, or elevated episcleral venous pressure. Primary angle closure with pupillary block is a condition in which aqueous trapped behind the iris pushes the iris forward to occlude the trabecular meshwork. Neovascular glaucoma, in which a fibrovascular membrane grows across the angle occluding outflow, is a secondary angle closure.

Developmental glaucoma is a general term that refers to glaucoma present at birth or presenting during childhood generally related to a developmental abnormality of ocular structures.

Any classification of the glaucomas will be somewhat arbitrary. Classifying a poorly understood condition may limit our readiness to accept new theories. Nevertheless, a classification can help in diagnosis and treatment. The reader can find further information in any major glaucoma textbook.

TREATMENT OF THE GLAUCOMAS

Although recent evidence strongly suggests that factors other than elevated intraocular pressure are important in the pathogenesis of glaucoma, lowering IOP has remained the mainstay of glaucoma therapy. Medical therapy is generally directed at decreasing aqueous production or in-

R. D. Fechtner and K. S. Kooner: Department of Ophthalmology, Southwestern Medical School, Dallas, Texas 75235.

creasing aqueous outflow. There do not yet exist proven therapies for treating glaucoma through alteration of the circulation or neuroprotection. These are currently areas of active research (see Chapter 28 by Abbasoglu).

The surgical therapy of glaucoma is directed toward improving existing pathways or providing an alternate pathway for aqueous outflow. Laser trabeculoplasty aims to improve trabecular outflow. The many glaucoma filtering procedures create a fistula to allow aqueous to enter the subconjunctival space. Angle closure resulting from pupillary block can often be relieved with laser iridotomy.

Proper glaucoma management consists of accurate diagnosis with appropriate combinations of medical and/or surgical therapies. As our appreciation of the multifactorial nature of this syndrome has increased, new therapeutic approaches are being explored. Investigations into the genetic and molecular basis of these syndromes will likely provide further insights. As we grow better able to distinguish between the underlying pathophysiology resulting in optic nerve damage in an individual, we are likely to use more targeted therapies.

REFERENCES

1. Fechtner RD, Weinreb RN. Mechanisms of optic nerve damage in primary open angle glaucoma. *Surv Ophthalmol* 1994;39:23–42.
2. Shields MB. Classification of the glaucomas. In: *Textbook of Glaucoma,* 3rd ed. Baltimore: Williams & Wilkins, 1992;167–171.
3. Hoskins HD, Kass M. Introduction and classification of the glaucomas. In: *Becker-Shaffer's Diagnosis and Therapy of the Glaucomas,* 6th ed. St. Louis: The C. V. Mosby Company, 1989;2–9.

Textbook of Ocular Pharmacology,
edited by T.J. Zimmerman, et al.
Lippincott–Raven Publishers, Philadelphia © 1997.

CHAPTER 19

Direct, Indirect, and Dual-Action Parasympathetic Drugs

Paul L. Kaufman and B'Ann True Gabelt

Cholinergic drugs mimic the effects of acetylcholine (ACh), which is a transmitter at postganglionic parasympathetic junctions as well as at other autonomic, somatic, and central synapses. Acetylcholine is synthesized by the enzyme choline acetyltransferase and produces its effects by binding to cholinergic receptors at the effector site (1).

Acetylcholine, released from vesicles in nerve terminals, then is hydrolyzed within a few milliseconds by acetylcholinesterase (AChE). This rapid destruction of ACh permits the cholinergic receptors to repolarize in preparation for the next stimulation. Cholinergic drugs act either directly by stimulating cholinergic receptors or indirectly by inhibiting the enzyme cholinesterase, thereby protecting endogenous ACh (1).

Cholinergic drugs have been used in glaucoma therapy for more than a century (1–3). They have a minimal effect on aqueous humor formation and episcleral venous pressure (4). Rather, their effect on intraocular pressure (IOP) is the result of various actions on aqueous humor outflow, which have been thought consequent to agonist-induced, muscarinic receptor-mediated contraction of the ciliary muscle.

The modified Goldmann equation can be used to describe the hydraulics of aqueous humor dynamics as follows (5):

$$F = C_{trab}(\mathrm{IOP} - P_e) + U$$

where F is the aqueous humor flow, C_{trab} is the facility of outflow from the anterior chamber via the trabecular meshwork and Schlemm's canal, P_e is the episcleral venous pressure (the pressure against which fluid leaving the anterior chamber via the trabecular-canalicular route must drain), and U is the uveoscleral outflow. If we rearrange the equation to isolate IOP,[1] it is apparent that for a modality (e.g., a drug) to lower IOP, it must either decrease F or P_e or increase C_{trab} or U (5). The effect of cholinergic agents on IOP is thought to be mainly through their effect on trabecular outflow facility (C_{trab}).

Uveoscleral Flow

There are two ways in which ciliary muscle contraction can affect aqueous outflow. Because there is no epithelial or endothelial barrier separating the spaces between the trabecular lamellae from those between the ciliary muscle bundles, in the absence of cholinergic stimulation, aqueous humor is free to flow down a pressure gradient from the former to the latter, thence into the suprachoroidal space, through the sclera, and into the orbit (Figure 19-1) (4). This posterior unconventional or uveoscleral route can account for nearly one third of aqueous drainage in normal young monkeys (6) and humans (7) but probably less in older primates (8). Ciliary muscle contraction obliterates the intermuscular spaces (Fig. 19-2) (9,10), obstructing uveoscleral outflow (11).

Outflow Facility

There is an intimate anatomic relationship of the anterior tendons of the ciliary muscle bundles with the scleral spur, peripheral cornea, trabecular meshwork, and inner wall of Schlemm's canal (12,13). One function of some of these tendons is to anchor the muscle to the spur and the cornea.

P. L. Kaufman and B. T. Gabelt: Department of Ophthalmology and Visual Sciences, University of Wisconsin, Madison, Wisconsin 45219.

[1] $\mathrm{IOP} = \dfrac{F - U}{C_{trab}} + P_e$

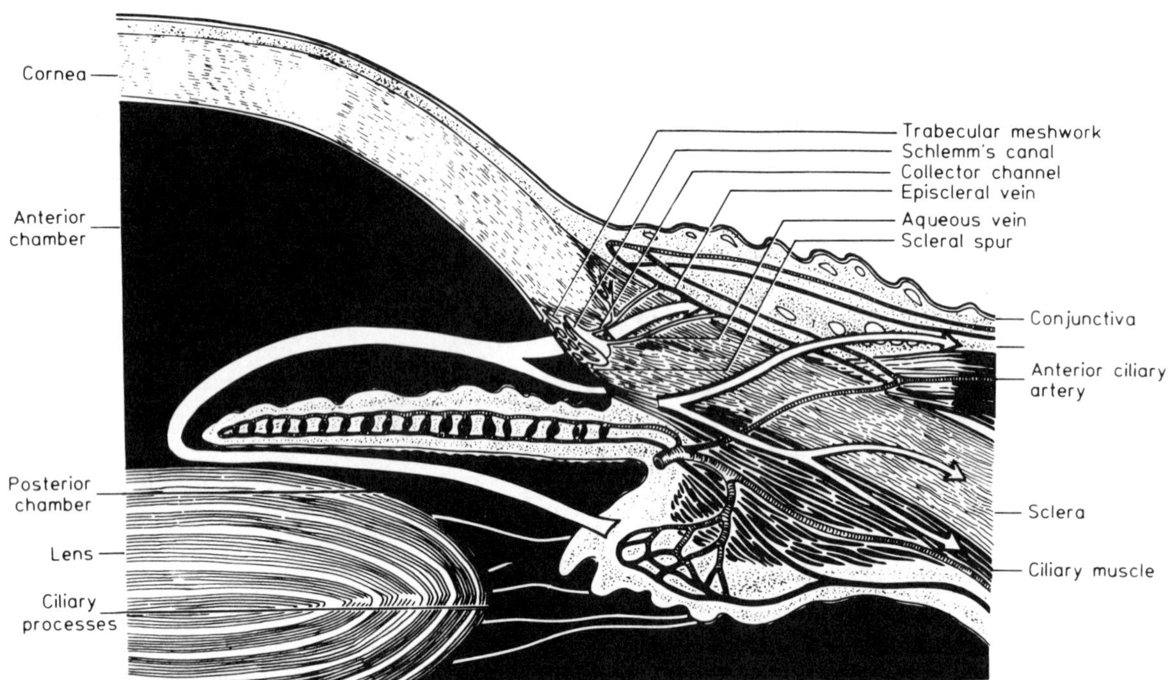

FIG. 19-1. Schematic representation of the primate anterior ocular segment. Arrows indicate aqueous humor flow pathways. Aqueous humor is formed by the ciliary processes, enters the posterior chamber, flows through the pupil into the anterior chamber, and exits at the chamber angle via the trabecular and uveoscleral routes. (From ref. 4, with permission.)

Other tendons splay out and intermingle with the elastic network within the mesh, ultimately inserting onto specialized regions on the surface of the inner wall endothelial cells via connecting fibrils. Muscle contraction results in an unfolding of the meshwork and widening of the canal, facilitating aqueous outflow from the anterior chamber through the mesh into the canal lumen and thence into the venous collector channels and the general venous circulation (4,14). Facilitation of outflow via the conventional route more than compensates for the obstruction of the uveoscleral route; thus, the net effect of ciliary muscle contraction is to decrease IOP (15).

Cholinomimetic drug effects on IOP have been presumed to be due to these biomechanical consequences of ciliary muscle contraction, with little or no effect due to iris sphincter constriction (16), except in angle closure (e.g., pupillary block, plateau iris), where sphincter contraction pulls the iris root away from the trabecular meshwork. Total removal of the iris from the monkey eye does not alter the facility response to pilocarpine, indicating that neither miosis nor even the presence of the iris is necessary for the response (17). The pilocarpine effect on outflow facility is abolished if the anterior tendons of the ciliary muscle are severed (Fig. 19-3) (18), indicating the necessity of the muscle-meshwork attachment and the absence of a facility-relevant effect directly on the trabecular or Schlemm's canal cells; however, other cholinomimetics were never tested in this system. Pilocarpine is only a partial agonist (19,20) and is atypical in other ways, which may be relevant in light of evidence that cultured trabecular meshwork cells produce second messengers in response to physiologic concentrations of carbachol (21,22) but only to pilocarpine concentrations that are several orders of magnitude higher (21). Detection of smooth-muscle actin and myosin in the collector channel and outer wall region of Schlemm's canal and, to a lesser extent, within the trabecular meshwork itself (23–25) suggests that these cells may be capable of contracting and thus contributing to the regulation of aqueous outflow (23,24); however, muscarinic receptors in the trabecular meshwork seem not to be coupled to outflow facility changes in the human eye in vitro (26). There have been no studies investigating possible cholinomimetic effects on the biosynthesis or degradation of the connective tissue matrix between the ciliary muscle bundles.

Accommodation

Another major consequence of ciliary muscle contraction is accommodation, causing near rather than distant objects to be in focus. Accommodative myopia produced by cholinomimetic antiglaucoma drugs is a major drawback to their use, especially in younger patients; however, there

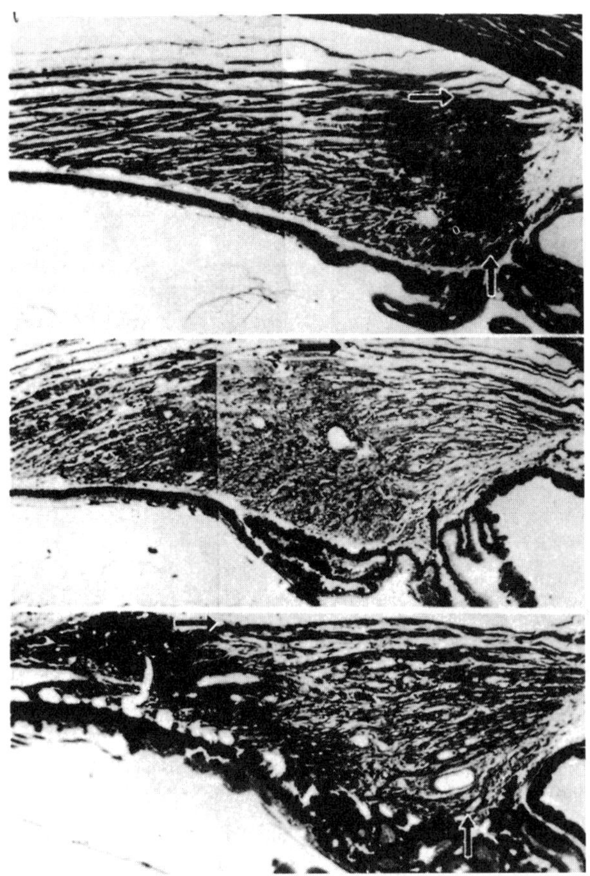

FIG. 19-2. Effect of pilocarpine and atropine on intramuscular spaces within the ciliary muscle of the vervet monkey. Top, intracameral heavy pilocarpine solution: crowding of muscle bundles within the anterior part of the longitudinal muscle. Zone of localized contraction indicated by arrows. Middle, intramuscular pilocarpine followed by intracameral heavy atropine solution (atropine was allowed to act for 3 min); loose arrangement of anterior longitudinal muscle bundles. Arrows indicate boundary between zone of localized relaxation and other contracted parts of muscle. Bottom, same protocol as middle, but atropine was allowed to act for 10 min. The zone of loosely arranged muscle bundles reaches far toward the posterior region. Only the posterior extremity of the muscle appears intensely contracted. Arrows indicate boundary between contracted and relaxed muscle portions (Heidenhain's Azan stain, ×63). (From ref. 9, with permission.)

may be some regionalization of the accommodative and outflow functions within the ciliary muscle, as evidenced by recent anatomic and physiologic studies (27). Muscle-fiber bundles appear to be grouped in three major orientations, and it is likely that the directional force exerted by each group is different (Fig. 19-4) (28). Studies are now in progress to characterize more fully such regionalization. If the accommodative and outflow functions are mediated by different subtypes of muscarinic acetylcholine receptors, it may be possible to employ subtype-specific agonists to maximize contraction mediating the outflow effect while minimizing contraction mediating the accommodative effect.

Miosis

A similar strategy might be useful in minimizing the pupillary constriction produced by the action of cholinomimetic drugs on the iris sphincter muscle. The latter continues to be a serious drawback to the use of cholinomimetic agents in elderly patients with incipient cataracts, in whom the induced miosis can significantly compromise visual acuity (29).

Evidence for Response Separation

There are three distinct morphologic regions of the primate ciliary muscle: an outer longitudinal portion, an inner apical circular portion, and an intermediate obliquely oriented reticular region. In relaxed versus cholinergic agonist-contracted muscle, the appearance, relative sagittal section area, and topographic interrelationship of the three regions differ (see Fig. 19-4) (28,30).

The meridional tips of the ciliary muscle resemble fast fibers of striated muscle by virtue of their histochemical differences from the bulk of the muscle (31). Stronger staining for myosin adenosine triphosphatase (ATPase) and lactate dehydrogenase can be demonstrated in the tips, whereas the rest of the muscle stains more strongly for succinic dehydrogenase, NADH-tetazoliumreductase, and lipids. Fewer paranuclear mitochondria and more myofibrils are also found in the tips.

Aceclidine, a potent muscarinic agonist used in Europe to treat glaucoma (32–36), causes considerable miosis, but the IOP decrease is associated with minimal accommodation and anterior chamber shallowing (34–39). Increased tonographic outflow facility is most frequently associated with the reduced IOP (32–35), although at least one author attributed the decrease of IOP to reduced aqueous humor production (33). The intracameral dose of aceclidine or pilocarpine required to double perfusion outflow facility in monkeys induces markedly different levels of accommodation: ~2 diopters with aceclidine, ~20 diopters with pilocarpine (40).

Following parasympathetic denervation of the ciliary muscle in the same monkey species by surgical ciliary ganglionectomy, the accommodative response to topical eserine and electrical stimulation of the midbrain Edinger-Westphal nucleus were lost, whereas the response to topical or systemic pilocarpine became supersensitive despite a marked decrease in the number of muscarinic receptors, estimated from ^{3}H-quinuclidinyl benzilate (QNB) binding sites in the ciliary muscle (41). Denervation was confirmed biochemically by the absence of choline acetyltransferase activity in the muscle (42) and histologically by

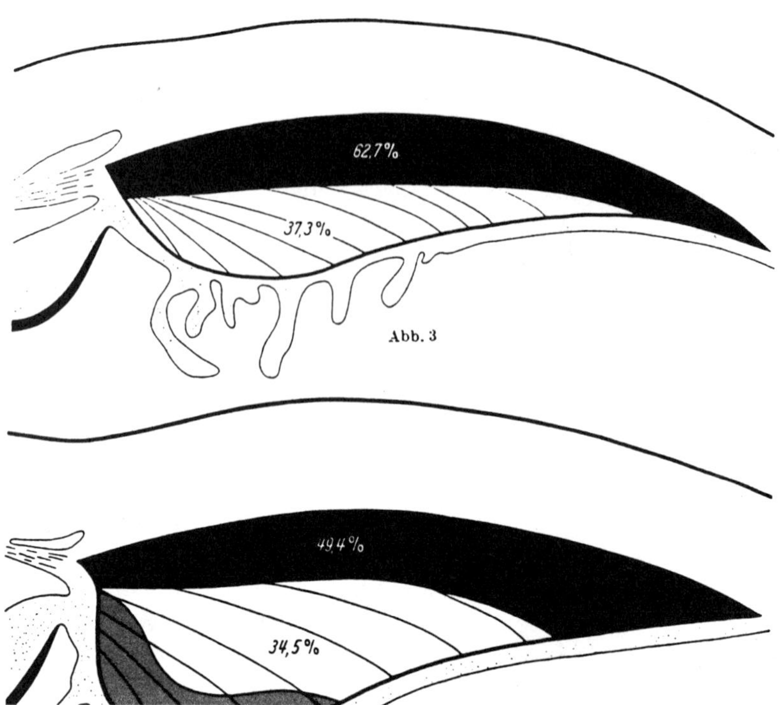

FIG. 19-3. Outflow facility and facility responses to intravenous and intracameral pilocarpine (PILO) hydrochloride (i.v. PILO, a.c. PILO) before and after unilateral ciliary muscle disinsertion in a typical bilaterally iridectomized cynomolgus monkey. Intramuscular atropine sulfate (i.m. ATR) was given before each perfusion to minimize systemic effects of intravenous pilocarpine. Note the absence of facility increase following i.v. and a.c. PILO in the iridectomized and disinserted eye (solid circles), as opposed to the large facility increases in the opposite iridectomized-only eye (open circles). (From ref. 18, with permission.)

examination of the excised surgical specimen and absence of parasympathetic nerves within the ciliary muscle (43). Subsequent reinnervation was evidenced by the reappearance of choline acetyltransferase activity in the muscle (42); by the return to normal of accommodative responses to eserine (44), central electrical stimulation (43), and pilocarpine (41); and the reappearance of parasympathetic nerves (31). The number of QNB binding sites in the ciliary muscle also returned to normal; the affinity for the ligand was unchanged throughout (41). Interestingly, in these putatively normally reinnervated eyes, IOP and resting perfusion outflow facility were normal, as was the facility response to intracameral eserine, but there was virtually no facility response to intracameral pilocarpine (Fig. 19-5) (45).

In monkeys, topical or intracameral pilocarpine induces a greater facility response per diopter of accommodation than does systemic pilocarpine (46), and in humans topical pilocarpine increases facility more per diopter of accommodation than does voluntary near focus (47). In summary, these findings indicate that under some circumstances the outflow facility and accommodative responses of the ciliary muscle to cholinergic agonists may have different pharmacologic profiles, perhaps mediated by different muscarinic receptor subtypes.

Subsensitivity to cholinergic stimulation induced by topical echothiophate in the owl monkey iris and ciliary muscle also suggests the existence of muscarinic subtypes. Pilocarpine, which induced miosis and a decrease in IOP before echothiophate treatment, produced an increase in IOP and only partial miosis after 16 days of echothiophate treatment. The existence of two receptor populations was postulated to explain this finding, one for which pilocarpine is selective and is abolished by echothiophate treatment and another that mediates the effects of ACh (48). Subsensitivity in the ciliary muscle of cynomolgus monkeys produced by treatment with carbachol or pilocarpine could not be accounted for by the small reduction in the number of available QNB binding sites, suggesting that a subpopulation of receptors may be involved in mediating the accommodative response to pilocarpine (19).

Finally, agonists other than pilocarpine might act via mechanisms different from ciliary muscle contraction to increase outflow facility. For example, the eserine-induced facility increase in eyes that had reinnervated following ciliary ganglionectomy could have been mediated by a mechanism other than cholinesterase inhibition (45). Earlier studies demonstrated eserine to be still capable of increasing outflow facility in monkey eyes after complete

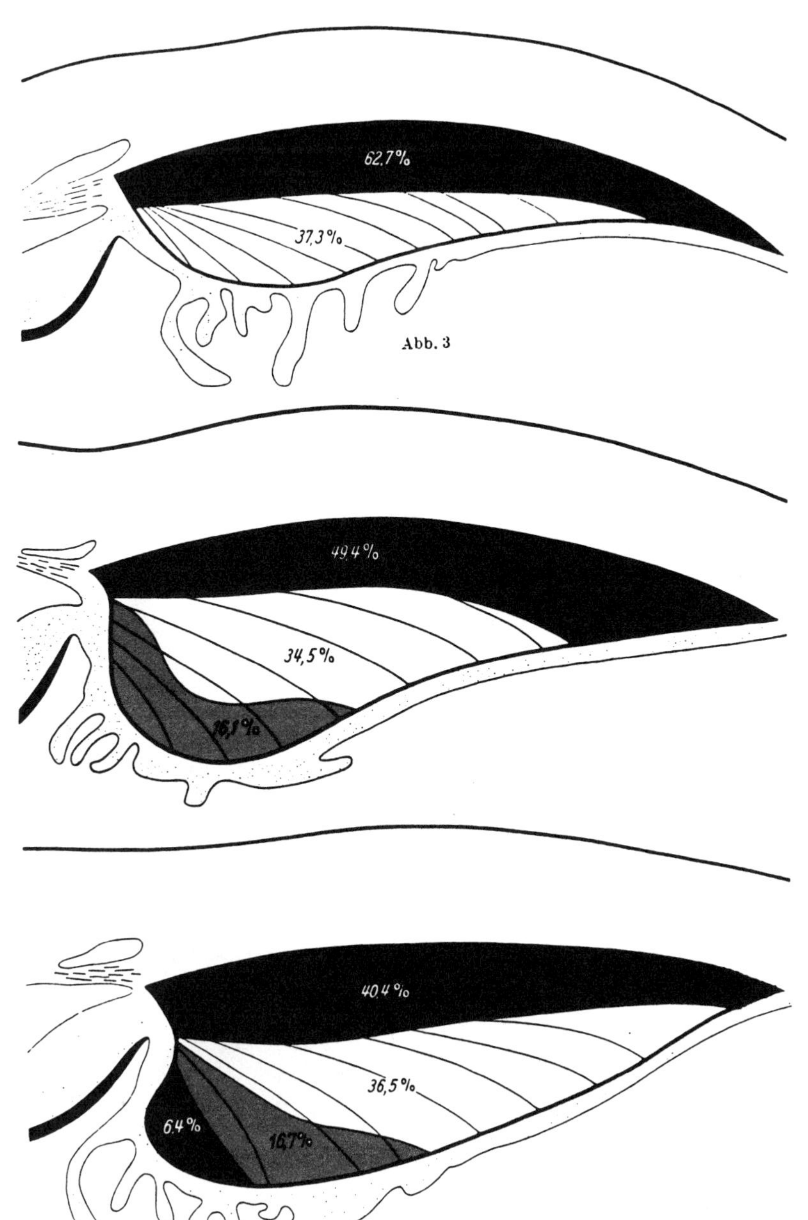

FIG. 19-4. Results of morphometric analysis of the ciliary muscle of vervet monkeys during relaxation (top) and during moderate (middle) and strong (bottom) contraction induced by pilocarpine. Area of longitudinal (black), reticular (white), reticular plus circular (gray), and purely circular (6.4% black in bottom only) muscle portions as percent of the entire muscle area. (Modified from ref. 28.)

ganglionic blockade by hexamethonium (49). Recently, eserine has been shown to interact directly with the nicotinic ACh receptor (50). These findings suggest that eserine may have stimulated neurotransmitter release from noncholinergic nerves in the ciliary muscle (e.g., VIP) (51) or from adrenergic, parasympathetic, or sensory fibers in the trabecular meshwork (52,53). Eserine, therefore, may increase outflow facility in the normal eye by both the expected ACh-mediated ciliary muscle contraction mechanism (due to AChE activity) as well as through a direct, as yet to be determined, mechanism perhaps involving innervation of the trabecular meshwork. The direct mechanism may be detected only when the cholinesterase-mediated mechanism is no longer operative (e.g., parasympathetic denervation, damage to the ciliary muscle, ciliary muscle disinsertion) (18,54).

Muscarinic Receptors

Drugs used in glaucoma therapy alter cellular functions in the eye by direct interaction either with receptors or with certain specific enzymes. Although no current therapeutic agent is known to interact directly with ion channels of cells, channels are probably important effectors of responses initiated by glaucoma drugs acting via receptors.

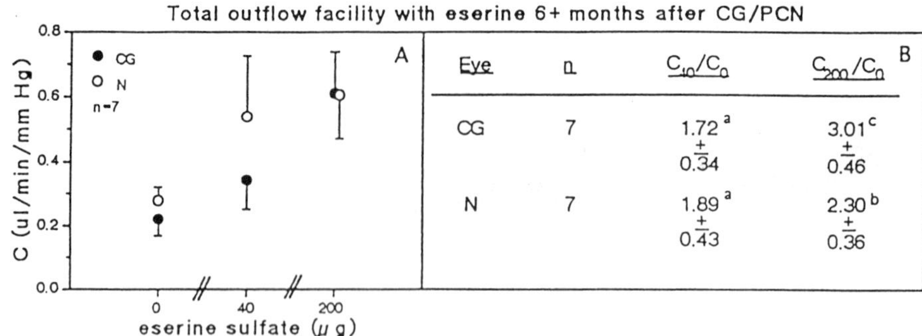

Eye	n	C_{40}/C_0	C_{200}/C_0
CG	7	1.72[a] ± 0.34	3.01[c] ± 0.46
N	7	1.89[a] ± 0.43	2.30[b] ± 0.36

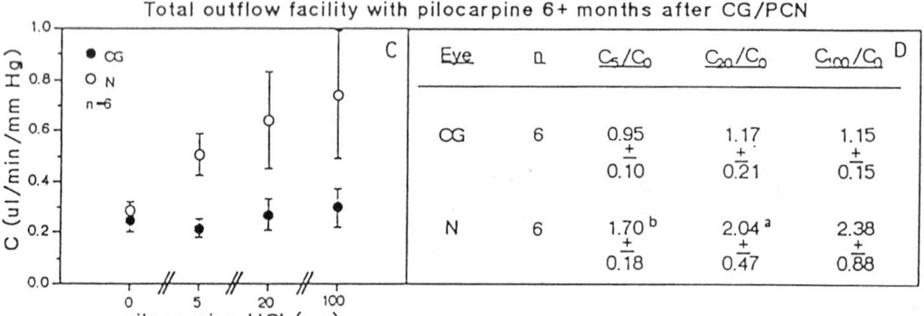

Eye	n	C_5/C_0	C_{20}/C_0	C_{100}/C_0
CG	6	0.95 ± 0.10	1.17 ± 0.21	1.15 ± 0.15
N	6	1.70[b] ± 0.18	2.04[a] ± 0.47	2.38 ± 0.88

FIG. 19-5. Total outflow facility (C_0, μl/min/mm Hg) was measured in several monkeys by two-level constant pressure perfusion approximately 1 month and 6 or more months after unilateral ciliary ganglionectomy (CG)/posterior ciliary neurectomy (PCN). **A,B:** At 6 or more months after CG/PCN, baseline facility was determined, after which successive doses of eserine sulfate were given, and facility was measured for 45 min following each dose; subscripts indicate dose in micrograms (B). **C,D:** At 1 to 2 months after the eserine experiments, a similar protocol employing pilocarpine HCl was conducted. When calculating the postdrug/baseline facility ratios, the measured postdrug facilities were adjusted downward by 15% to compensate for the facility increase induced by perfusion itself. Data are mean ±SEM facility for *n* paired eyes. Ratio significantly different from 1.0 by the two-tailed paired *t* test: $^a p < 0.10$, $^b p < 0.02$, $^c p < 0.005$. (Modified from ref. 45.)

Application of molecular biology techniques has led to the discovery of at least five subtypes of muscarinic acetylcholine receptors (AChR-M_1–M_5) identified from their mRNA sequences (55,56). Autoradiography conducted on the primate iris, ciliary muscle, trabecular meshwork, and collector channels using probes for the various muscarinic receptor subtypes has provided information as to the predominate subtypes present as well as their distributions (57–60). The physiological or pharmacological significance of these subtypes remains uncertain, but their presence offers promise for future development of more selective drugs targeted to specific subtypes of receptors expressed on specific cell types.

Knowledge of the biochemical events of signal transduction initiated by receptor activation is rapidly expanding. The general pattern for signal transduction can be described as follows (29): Interaction of the primary signal molecule (the *first messenger*) with its specific receptor triggers a cascade of one or more amplification steps involving small intermediate signal molecules (*second* and *third messengers*), culminating in the regulation of a specific effector protein at the end of the first stage of the signal pathway. The active effector protein(s) (usually an enzyme such as a kinase) may directly mediate the cellular response (for example, regulate the closing of ion channels by protein phosphorylation); activate additional regulatory proteins that act by further protein-protein interactions; or generate the second, third, and even a fourth messenger. Several components of a signal transduction cascade, including small molecule messengers, effector proteins, or regulatory proteins can contribute to the overall final cellular response(s). Most of our present knowledge involves the biochemical steps from receptor to effector protein (*enzyme*). Much less is known about the specific events from the effector protein to the final cellular response, but specific protein phosphorylation and dephosphorylation seem to be a major mechanism.

Signal transduction initiated by AChR-M receptor binding often mediates contractile responses of many cells. Contractile responses involve the second messengers inositol triphosphate (IP_3), IP_4, and diacylglycerol (DAG), third messengers $[Ca^{2+}]_i$ or its complex with calmodulin (CAM), and the effector enzymes protein kinase C and Ca^{2+}/CAM-activated kinase enzymes. In smooth muscle and other cells, calcium ion can be released from internal stores. There are at least two types of internal stores: one in which a large calcium release is triggered by a small increase in internal [Ca^{2+}] (this store is characterized by the release of its calcium by caffeine) and a second type of internal calcium store where IP_3 induces the release of calcium. The proportion of these two types of internal stores varies widely from one type of smooth muscle to another and has not been characterized in iris or ciliary muscle cells. This signal pathway also can trigger the entry of calcium from outside the cell via Ca^{2+} channels. In some cells, IP_3 or IP_4 seems to be a direct regulator of such channels, but usually they are more regulated via the second-messenger DAG, which activates protein kinase C. These mechanisms to control intracellular Ca^{2+} ions are clearly important in the contractile responses of vascular, ciliary, and iris muscle cells (e.g., responses to pilocarpine or epinephrine) and perhaps also for contractile elements in the trabecular outflow apparatus.

The reduction in iris responses may be possible by targeting cholinomimetic drugs. Some muscarinic antagonist drugs are partially selective for mydriasis as compared with cycloplegia (e.g., tropicamide), suggesting a difference in receptors on the two muscles. Although the dominant contractile control of the pupil is via mAChR, a second cholinergic component causing iris dilator relaxation has been reported (61), suggesting that when cholinergic miosis occurs, sphincter muscle contraction and dilator fiber relaxation work together. In some other primate sphincter muscles, cholinergic relaxation occurs by opening a K^+ channel, possibly via a different subtype of MAChR than that mediating muscle contractions (29). One could postulate a decreased miotic effect for a cholinergic agonist that does not cause iris dilator fibers to relax, although cholinergic relaxation has not been specifically shown for primate iris dilator muscles. Several lines of evidence suggest that the muscarinic receptors of the mammalian iris sphincter are predominantly of the M_3 subtype. The M_3 muscarinic receptor subtype antagonist 4-DAMP is a more potent inhibitor of ^{3}H-QNB binding and carbachol-induced PI hydrolysis than are PZ (M1) and AF-DX 116 (M_2) in cat and human iris sphincter cells (62,63). When oligonucleotide probes specific for four mAChR subtypes were hybridized to mRNA from bovine iris sphincter, the predominant binding was to the m_3 probe with minor amounts of m_2 detected (64).

In cultured human trabecular meshwork cells, approximately 20,000 muscarinic receptors per cell have been detected by binding of the nonsubtype-specific muscarinic receptor antagonist QNB (65). 4-DAMP inhibition of carbachol stimulated Ca^{2+} mobilization suggests these receptors are predominantly of the M_3 subtype (65).

The mAChRs have been detected in rabbit and cynomolgus monkey nonpigmented ciliary epithelial cells (66,67). Human nonpigmented ciliary epithelial cells transfected by SV40 produced inositol phosphatides in response to carbachol stimulation, which was inhibited by 4-DAMP, indicating the presence of M_3 receptors (68,69). Northern blot hybridization has shown that bovine ciliary processes contain predominantly the m_3 subtype, minor amounts of m_2, and trace amounts of m_4 (64). Localization of the m_3 subtype in the ciliary epithelium was demonstrated in postmortem human tissue (70). There is no evidence to date that cholinergic mechanisms play a major role in the volumetric rate of aqueous production in the living primate eye (45,71). It is possible that muscarinic receptors on the ciliary processes mediate the transport of anions (72) and amino acids (73,74) or modulate the effects of other modulators of aqueous production (e.g., decrease cAMP levels that were increased by catecholamines, vasoactive intestinal polypeptide (VIP), or forskolin) (75), although these mechanisms have yet to be investigated.

The m_3 receptor mRNA has been found in cultured human ciliary muscle cells and in postmortem tissues (59,60). The M_3-like mAChR subtype is found in cultured human ciliary muscle cells and may be involved in carbachol-induced activation of phosphoinositide metabolism (63). Functional assays have shown that an M_3-like muscarinic receptor mediates the muscarinic agonist activation of phospholipase C and increases in intracellular calcium concentration (76), causing contraction (77).

Ciliary muscle is a rich source of mAChRs (19). Evidence for the presence of the M_3 subtype in cat and human ciliary muscle cells was shown by competitive inhibition of QNB binding (78), inositol phospholipid hydrolysis (78), or agonist-induced muscle contraction (62) with PZ, AF-DX 116, and 4-DAMP. [^{3}H]-4-DAMP binding sites and m_3 mRNA were localized in postmortem human ciliary muscle tissue (70). Autoradiographic studies in human eyes with the M_2 agonist [^{3}H] oxotremorine also suggest that M_2 receptors may be localized to the longitudinal portion of the ciliary muscle (57). In vivo, in normally innervated rhesus monkeys, M_3 is the muscarinic receptor subtype predominantly involved in the facility, accommodative, and miotic responses to pilocarpine (79) and aceclidine (80), suggesting no basis for selective stimulation of outflow facility without the other two undesirable side effects. There was also no apparent dissociation of responses to carbachol, aceclidine, or oxotremorine in the longitudinal and circular vectors of the rhesus ciliary muscle in vitro (81). The responses to each drug in each vector were mediated by the M_3 muscarinic receptor subtype. Although our knowledge is still far from complete, at present we must view all cholinomimetic effects on aqueous humor dynamics as consequent to the mechanical effects of ciliary muscle contraction, mediated by the M_3 muscarinic receptor subtype.

Directly Acting Muscarinic Agonists

Directly acting muscarinic agonists can elicit numerous ocular responses, including reduction in intraocular pressure; stimulation of the iris sphincter, producing miosis;

and stimulation of the ciliary muscle, increasing outflow facility, decreasing uveoscleral outflow, and producing accommodation. Muscarine, pilocarpine, aceclidine (3-acetoxyquinuclidine), arecoline, and acetyl B-methylcholine (methacholine) are examples of directly acting muscarinic drugs. Carbachol (carbamylcholine) is both a directly acting muscarinic agonist and a directly acting nicotinic agonist, in addition to having indirect agonist activities (i.e., it is a cholinesterase inhibitor). Aceclidine is also slightly cholinesterase resistant and has weak AChE activity (82).

The intrinsic muscarinic activity of pilocarpine is less than that of ACh and carbachol (83,84); however, primarily pharmacokinetic factors play a role in determining clinical efficacy (82). Hydrolysis by tissue esterases may prevent drugs such as ACh and acetyl B-methylcholine from reaching the desired site of action. Tertiary amines can penetrate the corneal epithelium more readily than the positively charged quaternary amines because of their better lipid solubility. The proportions of nonionized drug can be dependent on the pH of eyedrops and tears. Topical anesthetics and surfactants also aid penetration. Prolonged drug delivery may be accomplished through the use of continuous release membranes (Ocusert) (85–88), polymer emulsions (89–92), or gels (93,94).

Carbachol and pilocarpine, topically active cholinergic agonists in common clinical use, have somewhat different characteristics (29). Carbamylcholine (carbachol), the methylcarbamyl ester of choline, is permanently positively charged (quaternary ammonium group) and must be used at high concentrations (up to 3%) to penetrate the cornea effectively. Carbachol has a dual action: Directly at the receptors, it is as effective as ACh; indirectly, due to its carbamyl group, it is also a weak suicide substrate for AChE.

Pilocarpine acts only on mAChR (29). It effectively penetrates the cornea in its uncharged form, but because it is only a partial agonist (i.e., the maximal response is less than can be obtained with a full agonist like carbamylcholine) (95–100), it must be administered in about the same concentration as carbachol to be therapeutically effective. Unlike most other antiglaucoma medications, directly acting cholinomimetics such as pilocarpine and carbachol virtually never cause systemic side effects, because the systemic levels achieved after their topical administration are just too low (3). Attempts have been made to minimize side effects by specialized drug formulations, delivery systems, targeted administration times, or, in the case of miosis, by concurrent administration of phenylephrine to stimulate the iris dilator muscle (1,2). Thus far, these efforts have met with only limited success, although the work continues.

Indirectly Acting Cholinergic Agents

This group of drugs (physostigmine, demecarium, echothiophate, isoflurophate) all block cholinesterase (AChE), thus preventing metabolic inactivation of ACh released from parasympathetic nerve endings (29). None of these drugs has any affinity for mACh receptors but act instead by either carbamylating or phosphorylating the AChE. The terminal half-life ($T_{1/2}$) for the carbamyl enzyme is hours, days for the phosphoryl enzyme. Thus, these drugs are suicide substrates of AChE, and some of their effects can last for days or weeks.

When AChE is blocked by such a suicide substrate, the local concentration of endogenously released ACh and its time of action are increased, thus increasing and prolonging the endogenous cholinergic response (*tone*). Drugs that compete with ACh can alter the response to these indirect agonists. Thus, pilocarpine, which has less intrinsic muscarinic activity than ACh, can diminish the miosis and hypotension of a maximally effective dose of physostigmine or DFP (101).

The use of cholinesterase (ChE) inhibitors to treat glaucoma is declining because of their substantial adverse ocular effects (Table 19-1) (29) and ocular toxicities (82). Additionally, their use must be discontinued 3 weeks before induction of general anesthesia (increased risk of prolonged apnea if succinylcholine is used as a muscle relaxant) and before ophthalmic surgery (increased risk of postoperative inflammation and hemorrhage). Monkey eyes treated for 5 or more months with topical echothiophate had elevated IOP associated with histologic evidence of damage to the aqueous humor outflow system (102).

The most widely used phosphorylating ChE inhibitor has been echothiophate. In addition to glaucoma, ChE inhibitors have been used to correct accommodative esotropia by stimulating accommodation peripherally without stimulating convergence centrally (82). Dilute concentrations of physostigmine have been used with variable success to reduce the mydriasis and improve the accommodation in eyes with Adie's syndrome (103).

Cholinergic Sensitivity

There is no advantage in administering two miotic drugs in combination because no greater reduction in IOP is achieved than the appropriate concentration of either agent alone (104,105). Some glaucoma patients may become refractory to the IOP-lowering effects of pilocarpine during long-term therapy, even with higher doses. Topical treatment of the monkey eye with echothiophate drops, sustained-release pilocarpine delivery systems, or a single dose of carbachol under a contact lens causes decreased accommodative and aqueous outflow responsiveness to cholinergic agonists, attributed to agonist-induced cholinergic subsensitivity in the ciliary muscle. Discontinuation of agonist treatment restores function (95,106–108), even after permanent anatomic abnormalities in the ciliary muscle and trabecular meshwork have been produced (102,109).

The mechanism underlying the observed subsensitization and recovery is unclear; however, several studies

TABLE 19-1. Cholinomimetics[a]

Drug	Delivery/duration/ frequency	Side effects	
		Ocular	Systemic
Directly acting *imitate acetylcholine (ACh)*			
Pilocarpine	Eyedrops[b] 0.5–10% sol 4% usually maximal Gel (Pilopine HS) 4% pilocarpine in gel applied q.h.s. 24-h effect? Ocusert 20 μg/h, 40 μg/h constant release rate 7-day duration equivalent to 1–2%, 3–4% drops	Ciliary and conjunctival congestion Ocular and periocular pain Accommodative myopia Pupillary constriction (decreased acuity with lens changes) Iris cysts (with ChE inhibitors; prevented by phenylephrine) Increased pupillary block: angle closure (stronger miotics) Iritis (especially anti-cholinesterases) Posterior synechiae (even without overt iritis)	Nausea Vomiting Diarrhea Bradycardia Salivation Sweating CNS (depression, delusions) Apnea (anticholin-esterases, if succinylcholine used during general anesthesia)
Carbachol	0.75–3% sol'n q. 6 or 8 h	Retinal detachment (especially with strong miotics in aphakes) Lacrimal canalicular	
Aceclidine (Glaucostat)	0.5–4% sol'n	stenosis (especially anticholinesterase) Allergic conjunctivitis and dermatitis (unusual) Irritaive conjunctivitis and follicular hypertrophy (eserine)	
Indirectly acting-anticholinesterases *bind acetylcholinesterase*		Cataracts (anticholinesterases) Decreased ocular rigidity (anticholinesterases)	
Echothiophate (Phospholine iodide, Echodide)	0.03–0.25% q 12 or 24 h		
Demecarium (Humorsol, Tosmilen)	0.125–0.25% solution q 12 or 24 h		

Modified from Kaufman and Mittag, ref 29

[a]Additive to all other currently available antiglaucoma drugs

[b]Timpilo drops combine 2% or 4% pilocarpine and 0.5% timolol; administer twice daily; available only in Europe.

suggest that responsiveness may be mediated in part by muscarinic receptor content of the relevant smooth muscle. Diminished sensitivity of the mammalian iris sphincter to cholinergic agonists, induced by continuous illumination or topical cholinesterase inhibitors, is accompanied by parallel decreases in binding of the muscarinic antagonist QNB. Similarly, increased sensitivity following continuous darkness or parasympathetic denervation is accompanied by increased QNB binding (110–114). Thus, cholinergic sensitivity of the iris sphincter muscle apparently varies inversely with local ACh concentration (110,113), the negative feedback putatively mediated by downregulation and upregulation of muscarinic receptors without a change in the rate of receptor degradation (113,114).

Subsensitivity of the accommodative response to cholinergic agonists was observed in monkeys treated with a single dose of carbachol administered under a corneal contact lens or a few days of pilocarpine released continuously into the conjunctival sac from a membrane delivery system, accompanied by a 23% decrease in the number of ciliary muscle binding sites (B_{max}) for n-methylscopolamine (NMS, another nonsubtype-specific muscarinic receptor antagonist), with no change in affinity (19). An approximate 25% decrease in monkey ciliary muscle-binding sites for QNB occurred after either a single topical dose of pilocarpine or up to 7 months of twice-daily topical pilocarpine administration (20). Monkeys receiving twice-daily topical treatment with echothiophate demonstrated a far more profound loss of accommodative responsiveness to pilocarpine and a greater loss (~65%) of ciliary muscle QNB binding sites, with no change in affinity, whether the treatment duration was 2 weeks or 7 months. Discontinuation of echothiophate treatment resulted in a return of functional accommodative sensitivity and a parallel increase in the number of QNB binding sites, with both actually overshooting the contralateral normal control values (20,115).

These and other data collectively indicate that in the monkey ciliary muscle, cholinergic agonist-induced subsensitivity is rapid in onset and is accompanied by decreased numbers of muscarinic receptors. The decreases in physiologic responsiveness and muscarinic receptor number in these studies are more pronounced with echothiophate than with pilocarpine or carbachol (20). Factors possibly contributing to the differences might be that (a) the concentration of endogenous ACh achieved at the postjunctional membrane by maximal cholinesterase inhibition is higher than the concentrations of pilocarpine or carbachol achieved by topical agonist administration; (b) the local agonist concentration may be elevated continuously by irreversible cholinesterase inhibition, but only intermittently by topical pilocarpine or carbachol eye drops and (c) ACh may have a greater effect on physiological and receptor regulatory mechanisms in primate ciliary muscle than do pilocarpine or carbachol, perhaps because ACh is a more complete agonist (95–100) or because of the presence of physiologically relevant receptor subpopulations more sensitive to it (19,48,110). Thus, the parallel between the degree of induced subsensitivity and decreased muscarinic receptor content is consistent with (but does not definitely prove) regulation of functional cholinergic sensitivity of the ciliary muscle by its receptor content (110, 113–115).

Other data suggest that coupling of these parameters does not occur under all conditions. Subsensitivity of accommodative responses to threshold doses of pilocarpine, carbachol, and bethanechol in normosensitive and carbachol-desensitized monkey eyes was thought not to be related to the reduced ciliary muscle muscarinic receptor content (19,116). Supersensitivity of the accommodative response to pilocarpine following parasympathetic denervation of the monkey ciliary muscle by surgical ciliary ganglionectomy (41) or panretinal photocoagulation (117, 118) was associated with decreased rather than increased ciliary-muscle QNB binding (Table 19-2) without altered affinity (41,117,118). Both functional sensitivity and receptor content gradually returned to normal (41,117,118), concurrent with reinnervation by other criteria such as the return of choline acetyltransferase activity and the reappearance of nerves containing agranular synaptic vesicles in the ciliary muscle (reviewed in refs 44 and 117). Cholinergic denervation supersensitivity also has been associated with unchanged or decreased overall numbers of muscarinic receptors in the cat iris (119), rat sympathetic ganglion (120), and rat parotid (121), again suggesting that nonreceptor mechanisms can contribute to ciliary muscle cholinergic agonist sensitivity.

Denervation supersensitivity in cholinergic systems may be postjunctional and involve nonspecific (122,123) or specific (124) mechanisms. Nonspecific supersensitivity could be due to altered permeability to K^+ (125) or Ba^{++} (126), altered Ca^{++} usage (127), and alterations in cyclic nucleotide levels (128). Increased responsiveness without any change in muscarinic receptor content could result from both prejunctional and nonspecific postjunctional mechanisms. A prejunctional mechanism related to decreased ChE activity (123) cannot explain these findings because the supersensitivity could be elicited by the non-

TABLE 19-2. *Ciliary muscle muscarinic receptor concentration (B_{max}) after ciliary ganglionectomy (CG)*[a]

Time p̄ CG	no. of monkeys	B_{max} D	N	D/N
1 wk	2	1606 ± 102	4084 ± 264	0.39 ± 0.0
3–6 wk	8	834 ± 245	1602 ± 210	0.46 ± 0.10
2–3 yr	3	1083 ± 112	1126 ± 181	0.99 ± 0.11

Modified from Erickson-Lamy et al., ref 41.

[a]Data are mean ± SEM fmol/mg ciliary muscle protein for cynomolgus monkeys, each contributing one previously denervated (D) and one normal control (N) eye.

choline ester, pilocarpine, and AChE activity was increased in supersensitive ciliary muscles (42).

The mechanism underlying the efficacy of cholinomimetics in glaucoma therapy has been considered to be the most straightforward of all the drug classes used; however, our knowledge about cholinergic mechanisms and ciliary neuromuscular physiology in relation to glaucoma pathophysiology and therapy continues to grow and could lead to significant new clinical benefits. The agents currently or imminently available for clinical use, along with their dosages and side effects, are shown in Table 19-1 (29).

DRUG OUTLINE (refs 129–136; see below)

Pilocarpine

History and Source

Pilocarpine is a chief alkaloid produced from the leaflets of South American shrubs of the genus *Pilocarpus* (*P. microphyllus*). The first experiments were performed in 1874 by Brazilian physician Coutinhou. The alkaloid was isolated in 1875. Shortly thereafter, the actions on the pupil and sweat and salivary glands were described by Weber. Pilocarpine was introduced for glaucoma therapy in 1877.

Official Drug Name and Chemistry

Pilocarpine, (3S-cis)-3-Ethyldihydro-4-[(1-methyl-1H-imidazol-5-yl)methyl]-2(3H)-furanone, $C_{11}H_{16}N_2O_2$, is sold under the following brand names: Adsorbocarine, Akarpine, l-Pilocarpine, Isopto Carpine, Minims Pilocarpine, Miocarpine, OcuCarpine, Ocusert-Pilo, Pilagan, Pilocar, Pilokair, Pilopine-HS, Piloptic, Pilostat, P.V. Carpine Liquifilm, Spectro-Pilo, Spersacarpine, Storzine, and Pilagan. Its chemical structure is as follows:

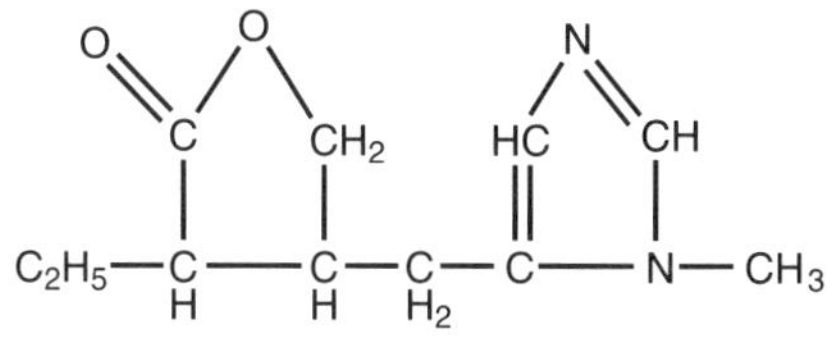

```
  O     O                    N
   \\  / \                  / \\
     C     CH2           HC     CH
     |      |            ||     |
C2H5—C——————C——C——C——————N—CH3
     H      H  H2
```

Pharmacology

This cholinomimetic alkaloid acts by direct stimulation of muscarinic cholinergic receptors. Pilocarpine duplicates the muscarinic effect of ACh but not its nicotinic effects; hence, it will stimulate smooth muscle and secretory glands but has no effect on striated muscle. It will cause lacrimation, salivation, sweating, vomiting, and diarrhea, but these effects are virtually unheard of following proper topical ocular dosing.

Clinical Pharmacology

Pilocarpine produces miosis through contraction of the iris sphincter muscle, which pulls the iris root away from the trabecular meshwork in angle-closure glaucoma and allows aqueous humor to exit the eye, thereby lowering the IOP. It also causes ciliary muscle contraction, resulting in accommodation and increased tension on and opening of the trabecular meshwork spaces, facilitating aqueous humor outflow and lowering IOP in open-angle glaucoma.

Pharmaceutics

Pilocarpine hydrochloride solutions usually contain methylcellulose or a similar polymer and range in concentrations from 0.25% to 10%. Pilocarpine nitrate solutions range from 1% to 4%. The usual vehicles for pilocarpine are hydroxypropyl methylcellulose and polyvinyl alcohol. Benzalkonium chloride and sodium EDTA are added to prevent microbial growth.

Pilocarpine can be sealed within a multilayered polymeric membrane envelope to form the Ocusert delivery system. Two forms are manufactured that release the drug continuously into the tear film at either 20 μg/h or 40 μg/h for 7 days. Pilocarpine is also formulated in a high-viscosity gel. A single dose of 4% pilocarpine gel applied at bedtime is approximately equal in effect to 4% pilocarpine eyedrops applied four times daily.

Pilocarpine polymer is an aqueous emulsion consisting of a polymeric material to which pilocarpine base is chemically bound. The drug is released over a period of hours as the polymer is hydrolyzed.

When maintained in a buffered, slightly acid solution, pilocarpine is indefinitely stable, retaining full activity at 6 months. Its effectiveness is maintained across a broad temperature range.

Pharmacokinetics, Concentration-effect Relationship, and Metabolism

Pilocarpine penetrates the cornea well and produces a low incidence of allergic reactions. Animal studies indicate that the cornea absorbs pilocarpine rapidly and then releases it slowly to the aqueous humor.

The onset of miosis with a 1% solution is 10 to 30 minutes. The maximum reduction in IOP occurs by 1.5 to 2 hours with the membrane delivery system and within 75 minutes with a solution, depending on its strength. The duration of action for miosis is about 4 to 8 hours following administration with a solution. The reduction in IOP lasts for 7 days with the membrane delivery system and 4 to 14 hours with a solution, depending on the strength used. In light-eyed persons, 2% solution is at the top of the dose-response curve for lowering IOP. In brown-eyed white patients, 4% solution may be required for maximum effect, whereas extremely dark-eyed individuals (blacks, Hispanics, Asians) may require an 8 to 10% solution. These differences relate to binding of the drug by pigment within the eye, making it unavailable to the relevant muscarinic receptors. In light-eyed persons, the higher concentrations have been used to extend the duration of action, thereby reducing the frequency of administration to twice daily.

Pilocarpine is inactivated by tissues of the anterior segment of the eye, partly by reversible binding of the drug to tissues, but also by appreciable enzymatic hydrolysis to the primary metabolite, pilocarpic acid. Human serum contains a heat-labile component capable of inactivating pilocarpine. Incubation of 500 mg of pilocarpine with 0.5 ml of human serum at 37°C for 1 hour will inactivate 40% of the pilocarpine. The amount of pilocarpine-hydrolyzing enzyme is not changed by prolonged pilocarpine use by glaucoma patients. The mean elimination half-life is 0.76 hours following 5 mg three times per day for 2 days.

Resistance to the IOP lowering effect may occur after prolonged use. Responsiveness may be restored by substituting another miotic for a short time and then resuming treatment with pilocarpine.

Therapeutic Use

Pilocarpine is used in the chronic treatment of glaucoma; it is generally administered as a 0.5% to 4.0% aqueous solution four times per day. It is the standard cholinergic agent for treatment of open-angle glaucoma. During episodes of acute primary angle-closure glaucoma with pupillary block, 1% or 2% pilocarpine is administered two or three times over a 30-minute period to produce miosis, pulling the peripheral iris away from the trabecular meshwork, thereby allowing aqueous humor to leave the eye. The miotic action of pilocarpine is also occasionally used to overcome the mydriasis produced by anticholinergics. Alternated with mydriatics, pilocarpine is employed to break adhesions between the iris and the lens. Pilocarpine also has been used in the treatment of Adie's syndrome.

Side Effects and Toxicity

Transient symptoms of stinging and burning may occur. Conjunctival vascular congestion and true allergy may occur but are unusual. Recent evidence suggests that prolonged use of topical antiglaucoma drug therapy, including pilocarpine, may alter the conjunctival tissues so as to make subsequent glaucoma filtration surgery more likely to fail. Intraocular vascular congestion may occur in and aggravate uveitic conditions. Ciliary spasm, temporal or supraorbital headache, and induced myopia may occur, all consequent to drug-induced contraction of the ciliary muscle; these occur most commonly in younger, prepresbyopic patients. Reduced visual acuity in poor illumination is frequently experienced by older persons and those with lens opacities, consequent to miosis reducing the amount of light reaching the retina through an already partially opaque lens. Young persons with clear lenses are rarely bothered by the miosis. A few cases of retinal detachment have been attributed to pilocarpine in certain susceptible individuals. Some evidence suggests that long-term use of pilocarpine may accelerate the development of lens opacities, but this is not proven conclusively. Intense miosis and cyclotonia produced at the higher doses may, respectively, increase pupillary block or induce ciliary block sufficiently to induce angle-closure glaucoma in susceptible persons.

Systemic toxicity following appropriate topical ocular administration is extremely rare (135). Theoretically, sensitive persons may develop sweating and gastrointestinal overactivity following suggested dosage and administration, but this is much more likely to occur with inappropriate dosing or in children (because of their lower body weight). Overdosage can produce sweating, salivation, nausea, tremors, slowing of the pulse, and a decrease in blood pressure. In moderate overdosage, spontaneous recovery is to be expected and is aided by intravenous fluids to compensate for dehydration. For severe poisoning, atropine is the pharmacologic antagonist to pilocarpine.

High-risk Groups

This drug is not recommended under conditions where pupillary constriction and intraocular vascular congestion are undesirable, such as in acute iritis. It should not be given to patients with a history of or predisposition to retinal detachment, a proven sensitivity to pilocarpine, severe asthma or bronchial obstruction, or acute infectious conjunctivitis or keratitis (for membrane delivery dosage form). Caution should be exercised in administering this drug to children because of their lower body weight and greater likelihood of accidental systemic overdosage.

Drug Interactions

In combination with beta-adrenergic antagonists, carbonic anhydrase inhibitors, alpha- or beta-adrenergic agonists, or hyperosmotic agents, pilocarpine may be used to control IOP. Its therapeutic additivity with the recently released prostaglandin $F_{2\alpha}$ analog latanoprost remains to be definitively determined. Pilocarpine-induced contraction of the ciliary muscle may interfere with $PGF_{2\alpha}$'s enhancement of uveoscleral outflow (137–139).

Concurrent local use of anticholinergic drugs will interfere with the antiglaucoma action of pilocarpine; appropriate doses of systemic anticholinergics usually will not interfere because of insufficient ocular drug levels.

Major Clinical Trials

To date, no major clinical trials have been reported. This compound was already in use before clinical trials were standardized; however, numerous smaller studies have documented pilocarpine's safety, efficacy, and mode of action.

Carbachol

History and Source

Carbachol is the carbamyl ester of choline and was synthesized in the early 1930s.

Official Drug Name and Chemistry

Carbamyl choline chloride, 2-[(Aminocarbonyl)oxy]-N,N,N-trimethylethanaminium chloride $NH_2COOCH_2CH_2N(CH_3)_3CL$, is sold under the brand names Isopto Carbachol and Miostat. Its chemical structure is as follows:

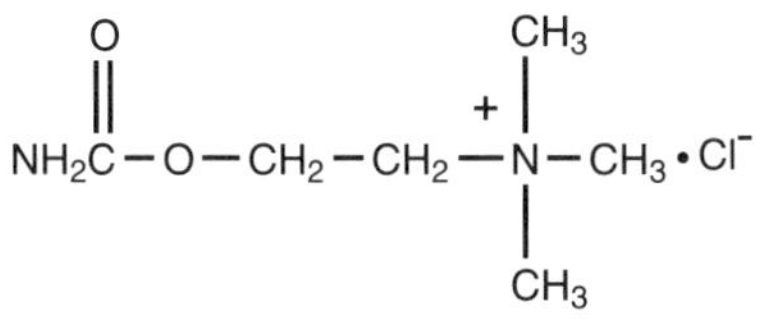

$$NH_2\overset{\overset{\large O}{\|}}{C}-O-CH_2-CH_2-\overset{+}{\underset{\underset{\large CH_3}{|}}{\overset{\overset{\large CH_3}{|}}{N}}}-CH_3 \cdot Cl^-$$

Pharmacology

Carbachol has direct parasympathomimetic action as well as an indirect mechanism of action by inhibition of AChE (132).

Clinical Pharmacology

Carbachol's clinical pharmacology is the same as for pilocarpine.

Pharmaceutics

Isopto Carbachol (0.75, 1.5, 2.25, 3.0%) solution is administered as eyedrops every 8 hours for therapy of open-angle glaucoma. Miostat (0.01%) solution is administered by intraocular injection to induce rapid miosis during eye surgery and to prevent postoperative elevation of eye pressure. It should be stored at 46° to 80°F (8°–27°C).

Pharmacokinetics, Concentration-effect Relationship, and Metabolism

Carbachol is not destroyed by cholinesterase; therefore, its action is not increased by anticholinesterase drugs. It is stable in solution and is not lipid soluble at any pH; hence, it penetrates the intact corneal epithelium poorly. To be clinically useful, carbachol must be dispensed in combination with a wetting agent, such as 0.03% benzalkonium chloride, which increases corneal penetration. A 1.5% solution of carbachol used three times daily has been reported to be more effective than a 2% solution of pilocarpine given four times daily in the control of IOP in chronic simple glaucoma. When administered as a solution, the onset of miosis is within 10 to 20 minutes. The maximum reduction in IOP occurs within 4 hours and then lasts about 8 hours. Miosis lasts 4 to 8 hours.

When used intracamerally, carbachol (Miostat, 0.01%) is an intensely powerful miotic. It is 100 times more potent and longer lasting than ACh and 200 times more potent than pilocarpine. Maximal miosis is achieved within 5 minutes and lasts about 24 hours.

Therapeutic Use

The 0.75 to 3.0% solution is used three times daily to control IOP in open-angle glaucoma. The 0.01% solution (0.5 ml) is given intracamerally at the conclusion of cataract surgery to prevent postsurgical IOP elevation or to produce miosis during ocular surgery.

Side Effects and Toxicity

These are the same as for pilocarpine.

High-risk Groups

In general, these are the same as for pilocarpine; however, because carbachol is a more complete agonist than pilocarpine, systemic effects, although still extremely rare, are more likely to occur. Its use is contraindicated in acute iritis, and caution should be used in the presence of corneal abrasion to avoid excessive penetration, which can produce systemic toxicity. Caution should also be exercised when used in patients with acute cardiac failure, bronchial asthma, active peptic ulcer, hyperthyroidism, gastrointestinal spasm, urinary tract obstruction, Parkinson's disease, recent myocardial infarct, systemic hypertension, or hypotension (133).

Drug Interactions

These are the same as for pilocarpine. Additionally, the miotic effect of intraocularly administered carbachol may be reduced if topical flurbiprofen is administered preoperatively.

Major Clinical Trials

Many smaller studies have attested to carbachol's safety and efficacy, although no major clinical trials have been conducted.

Echothiophate

History and Source

Eserine was isolated from the Calabar bean (also called the Esére nut), which was brought to England in 1840 from West Africa. The first use of a cholinesterase inhibitor for glaucoma therapy was with the introduction of the alkaloid eserine (physostigmine) in 1877 by Laqueur.

The first account of the synthesis of a highly potent compound of the organophosphorus anticholinesterase type was published by Clermont in 1854. Schrader in 1952 defined the structural requirements for insecticidal activity. A widely used insecticide of this class was parathion. Compounds of greater toxicity were synthesized for chemical warfare during World War II. In the 1950s, carbamate derivatives were found to have a high degree of selective toxicity against insects and to be potent anticholinesterase agents.

Several cholinesterase inhibitors have been used medicinally for ocular diagnostic and therapeutic purposes, including edrophonium (Tensilon, ultra-short-acting, used in the diagnosis of myasthenia gravis), neostigmine, diisopropylfluorophosphate (isofluorophate, DFP), demecarium, and echothiophate.

Official Drug Name and Chemistry

Echothiophate iodide, 2-[(Diethoxyphosphinyl)-thio]-N,N,N-trimethylethanaminium iodide; 2-mercaptoethyl) trimethylammonium iodide O,O-diethyl phosphorothioate $C_9H_{23}INO_3PS$, has the following chemical structure:

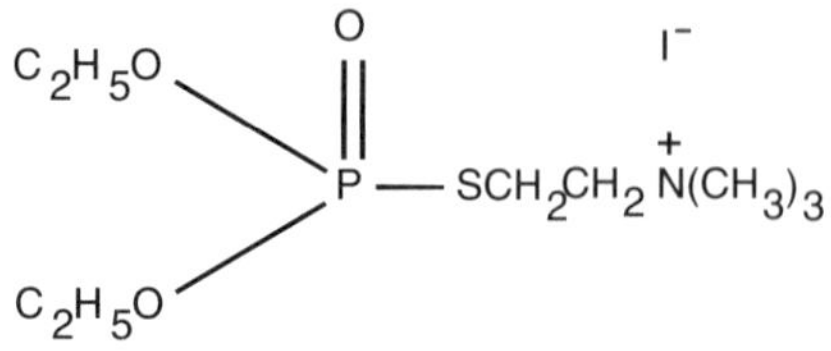

$$(C_2H_5O)_2P(=O)-SCH_2CH_2\overset{+}{N}(CH_3)_3 \quad I^-$$

Other cholinesterase inhibitors that have been or are still available for clinical ocular use include eserine, neostigmine, isofluorophate, and demecarium. Echothiophate is by far the one most commonly used and is discussed as the paradigm for this drug class.

Pharmacology

This indirect-acting parasympathomimetic agent is classified as a cholinesterase inhibitor or anticholinesterase. Cholinesterase inhibitors prolong the effect of ACh, the physiologic muscarinic neurotransmitter released at the neuroeffector junction of parasympathetic postganglion nerves, by inactivating the cholinesterase enzymes that break it down.

Clinical Pharmacology

Echothiophate inactivates pseudocholinesterase and incompletely inactivates AChE, enhancing and prolonging the effects of ACh endogenously released from parasympathetic nerve endings. In the eye, this has the same consequences as direct stimulation of the muscarinic receptors of the iris sphincter and ciliary muscle (miosis, accommodation, facilitation of aqueous humor outflow, and consequent decrease in IOP).

Pharmaceutics

Phospholine iodide (0.03%, 0.06%, 0.125%, 0.25%) remains indefinitely stable when dry; it must be kept in tightly sealed containers because the powdered form is hygroscopic. Assay of refrigerated aqueous solutions show a drop to 90% of the original potency within 4 weeks. At room temperature, this drop is to 83% of the original potency within 4 weeks and to 76% in 8 weeks. Benzalkonium is incompatible; so chlorobutanol is used instead as a preservative.

Echothiophate is marketed as a powder accompanied by a separately packaged diluent; the two are mixed for clinical use. The 0.125% solution is the most commonly employed strength for treatment of open-angle glaucoma and accommodative esotropia. In many instances, a 0.06% solution gives satisfactory therapeutic results and causes less irritation.

Pharmacokinetics, Concentration-effect Relationship, and Metabolism

Dose-response analysis of echothiophate with respect to IOP and outflow facility indicates that little additional pharmacologic response is obtained by increasing the drug concentration to more than 0.06%. A 0.03% concentration of echothiophate iodide has an effect similar to 1% to 2% pilocarpine. Echothiophate has a duration of action significantly longer than pilocarpine, with a maximal effect in 4 to 6 hours and a substantial effect maintained after 24 hours.

The onset of miosis is less than 1 hour; IOP reduction occurs within 4 hours. Maximum miosis occurs within

2 hours, maximum IOP reduction within 24 hours. Miosis and IOP reduction can last for several weeks but usually lasts at least 24 to 48 hours.

Therapeutic Use

Because of its toxicity, echothiophate should be reserved for use in patients with open-angle glaucoma that is not satisfactorily controlled with short-acting miotics and other agents: primary open-angle or nonuveitic secondary open angle glaucoma, angle-closure glaucoma after iridectomy, and accommodative esotropia (enhanced the cyclotonic effect of parasympathetic neuronal input to the ciliary muscle necessitates less input to achieve accommodation, stimulating less accommodation-linked convergence).

Side Effects and Toxicity

Side effects may include corneal toxicity; conjunctival and intraocular vascular congestion; fibrinous iritis, especially in predisposed individuals or following intraocular surgery; retinal detachment in predisposed individuals; lacrimal canalicular stenosis; and formation of posterior synechiae, iris cysts, and, most importantly, cataracts. Pupillary constriction and ciliary muscle contraction will produce the same symptoms as described for pilocarpine but to a more pronounced degree.

Systemic toxic effects caused by echothiophate include diarrhea, nausea, abdominal cramps, general fatigue and weakness, hypotension, and bradycardia. Topical echothiophate reduces blood cholinesterase activity, making patients more susceptible to prolonged paralysis following depolarizing muscle relaxants such as succinylchyoline and procaine. Frequency of dosage is an important factor in systemic toxicity. Pure echothiophate powder should never be applied directly to the eye, as serious systemic poisoning will result.

High-risk Groups

The risk-benefit should be considered when the following medical problems exist: bronchial asthma (systemic absorption of medication may precipitate an attack), bradycardia and hypotension, Down's syndrome (echothiophate may cause hyperactivity), epilepsy, gastrointestinal disturbances, narrow anterior chamber angle glaucoma associated with iridocyclitis (medication may aggravate the inflammatory process and lead to the development of posterior synechiae), hypertension, hyperthyroidism, iritis, myasthenia gravis, myocardial infarction, parkinsonism, peptic ulcer, retinal detachment or predisposition thereto (may result from intense drug induced cyclotonia), intraocular surgery (may be complicated by severe uveitis), urinary tract obstruction, active or quiescent uveitis, and marked vagotonia.

Drug Interactions

Use of ophthalmic physostigmine before echothiophate use may partially block the effects of the latter medication and shorten the duration of action. Concurrent use of echothiophate with ester-derived local mucosal or parenteral anesthetics may inhibit the metabolism of these anesthetics, leading to prolonged anesthetic effect and increased risk of toxicity. Concurrent local use of anticholinergics may antagonize the antiglaucoma and miotic actions of echothiophate. Exposure of patients using echothiophate to carbamate or organophosphate-type insecticides or pesticides may increase the possibility of systemic effects resulting from absorption of the insecticide or pesticide through the respiratory tract or skin. Inhibition of cholinesterase activity by echothiophate reduces or slows cocaine metabolism thereby increasing and/or prolonging cocaine's effects and increasing the risk of toxicity.

Caution is recommended in administering edrophonium to patients with symptoms of myasthenic weakness who are also using echothiophate; symptoms of cholinergic crisis (overdosage) may be similar to those occurring with myasthenic crisis (underdosage), and the patient's condition may be worsened by use of edrophonium.

Echothiophate may decrease plasma concentrations or activity of pseudocholinesterase, the enzyme that metabolizes succinylcholine, thereby enhancing the neuromuscular blockade of succinylcholine when it is used concurrently; cardiovascular collapse may occur; in addition, increased or prolonged respiratory depression or paralysis may occur; the effects of this interaction may persist for weeks or months after echothiophate is discontinued.

Major Clinical Trials

In general, the efficacy, safety, and toxicity of this drug have been adequately documented by smaller studies; however, no major clinical trials have been done.

ACKNOWLEDGMENTS

This work was supported by USPHS National Institutes of Health grant EY02698 and Research to Prevent Blindness.

REFERENCES

1. Hoskins HD, Kass MA. Cholinergic drugs. In: Hoskins HD, Kass MA, eds. *Becker-Shaffer's Diagnosis and Therapy of the Glaucomas.* St. Louis: CV Mosby, 1989;420–434.
2. Nardin GF, Zimmerman TJ, Zaita AH, Felts K. Ocular cholinergic agents. In: Ritch R, Shields MB, Krupin TH, eds. *The Glaucomas.* St. Louis: CV Mosby, 1989;515–521.

3. Leopold IH. The use and side effects of cholinergic agents in the management of intraocular pressure. In: Drance SM, Neufeld AH, eds. *Glaucoma: Applied Pharmacology in Medical Treatment.* Orlando: Grune and Stratton, 1984;357–393.
4. Kaufman PL, Wiedman T, Robinson JR. Cholinergics. In: Sears ML, ed. *Handbook of Experimental Pharmacology.* Berlin: Springer-Verlag, 1984;149–191.
5. Kaufman PL. Aqueous humor dynamics. In: Duane TD, ed. *Clinical Ophthalmology.* Philadelphia: Harper & Row, 1985;1–24.
6. Bill A. Aqueous humor dynamics in monkeys (Macaca inus and Cercopithecus ethiops). *Exp Eye Res* 1971;11:195–206.
7. Townsend DJ, Brubaker RF. Immediate effect of epinephrine on aqueous formation in the normal human eye as measured by fluorophotometry. *Invest Ophthalmol Vis Sci* 1980;19:256–266.
8. Bill A, Phillips I. Uveoscleral drainage of aqueous humor in human eyes. *Exp Eye Res* 1971;21:275–281.
9. Bárány EH, Rohen JW. Localized contraction and relaxation within the ciliary muscle of the vervet monkey (*Cercopithecus ethiops*). In: Rohen JW, ed. *The Structure of the Eye, Second Symposium.* Stuttgart: FK Schattauer Verlag, 1965;287–311.
10. Rohen JW, Lütjen E, Bárány E. The relation between the ciliary muscle and the trabecular meshwork and its importance for the effect of miotics on aqueous outflow resistance. *Albrecht von Graefes Arch Clin Exp Ophthalmol* 1967;172:23–47.
11. Bill A. Effects of atropine and pilocarpine on aqueous humor dynamics in cynomolgus monkeys (*Macaca inus*). *Exp Eye Res* 1967;6:120–125.
12. Rohen JW, Futa R, Lütjen-Drecoll E. The fine structure of the cribriform meshwork in normal and glaucomatous eyes as seen in tangential sections. *Invest Ophthalmol Vis Sci* 1981;21:574–585.
13. Lütjen-Drecoll E, Futa R, Rohen JW. Ultrahistochemical studies on tangential sections of the trabecular meshwork in normal and glaucomatous eyes. *Invest Ophthalmol Vis Sci* 1981;21:563–573.
14. Bárány EH. The immediate effect on outflow resistance of intravenous pilocarpine in the vervet monkey. *Invest Ophthalmol* 1967; 6:373–380.
15. Hart WM. Intraocular pressure. In: Hart WM, ed. *Adler's Physiology of the Eye.* St. Louis: Mosby, 1992;248–267.
16. Kaufman PL. Total iridectomy does not alter outflow facility responses to cyclic AMP in cynomolgus monkeys. *Exp Eye Res* 1986; 43:441–447.
17. Kaufman PL. Aqueous humor dynamics following total iridectomy in the cynomolgus monkey. *Invest Ophthalmol Vis Sci* 1979;18:870–875.
18. Kaufman PL, Bárány EH. Loss of acute pilocarpine effect on outflow facility following surgical disinsertion and retrodisplacement of the ciliary muscle from the scleral spur in the cynomolgus monkey. *Invest Ophthalmol* 1976;15:793–807.
19. Bárány E, Berrie CP, Birdsall NJM, Burgen ASV, Hulme EC. The binding properties of the muscarinic receptors of the cynomolgus monkey ciliary body and the response to the induction of agonist subsensitivity. *Br J Pharmacol* 1982;77:731–739.
20. Erickson-Lamy KA, Polansky JR, Kaufman PL, Zlock DM. Cholinergic drugs alter ciliary muscle response and receptor content. *Invest Ophthalmol Vis Sci* 1987;28:375–383.
21. Ruiz G, WoldeMussie E. Signal transduction in cultured bovine and human trabecular meshwork cells by several agents. *FASEB J* 1988;2(suppl):A614.
22. Friedman Z, Bloom E, Crook RB, Polansky JR. Inositol phosphate formation and prostaglandin production in cultured human trabecular meshwork (HTM) cells. *Invest Ophthalmol Vis Sci* 1990;31 (suppl):247.
23. de Kater AW, Spurr-Michaud SJ, Gipson IK. Localization of smooth muscle myosin-containing cells in the aqueous outflow pathway. *Invest Ophthalmol Vis Sci* 1990;31:347–353.
24. de Kater AW, Shahsafaei A, Epstein DL. Localization of smooth muscle and nonmuscle actin isoforms in the human aqueous outflow pathways. *Invest Ophthalmol Vis Sci* 1992;33:424–429.
25. Flügel C, Tamm E, Lütjen-Drecoll E, Stefani FH. Age-related loss of α-smooth muscle actin in normal and glaucomatous human trabecular meshwork of different age groups. *J Glaucoma* 1992;1: 165–173.
26. Schroeder A, Erickson K. Cholinergic agonists do not increase trabecular outflow facility in the human eye. *Invest Ophthalmol Vis Sci* 1994;34(suppl):2054.
27. Kaufman PL, Gabelt BT. Cholinergic mechanisms and aqueous humor dynamics. In: Drance SM, Van Buskirk EM, Neufeld AH, eds. *Pharmacology of Glaucoma.* Baltimore: Williams & Wilkins, 1992; 64–92.
28. Lütjen E. Histometrische Untersuchungen über den Ziliarmuskel der Primaten. *Albrecht von Graefes Arch Clin Exp Ophthalmol* 1966; 171:121–133.
29. Kaufman PL, Mittag TW. Medical therapy of glaucoma. In: Kaufman PL, Mittag TW, eds. *Textbook of Ophthalmology Series.* London: Mosby-Year Book Europe Ltd, 1994;9.7–9.30.
30. Rohen JW. The evolution of the primate eye in relation to the problem of glaucoma. In: Lutjen-Drecoll E, ed. *Basic Aspects of Glaucoma Research.* Stuttgart: Schattauer, 1982;3–33.
31. Flügel C, Bárány EH, Lütjen-Drecoll E. Histochemical differences within the ciliary muscle and its function in accommodation. *Exp Eye Res* 1990;50:219–226.
32. Étienne R, Barut C, Gonzalès-Bouchon J. Un nouvel hypotenseur oculaire: l'acéclidine. *Ann Oculist* 1967;200:287–292.
33. Lieberman TW. Keopold IH. The use of aceclidine in the treatment of glaucoma: its effect on intraocular pressure and facility of aqueous outflow as compared to that of pilocarpine. *Am J Ophthalmol* 1967;64:405–415.
34. Demailly PH. Place de l'acéclidine dans le traitement du glaucome chronique simple à angle ouvert. *Arch Ophthalmol* 1968;28: 735–744.
35. Romano JH. Double-blind crossover comparison of aceclidine and pilocarpine in open-angle glaucoma. *Br J Ophthalmol* 1970;54:510–521.
36. Drance SM, Fairclough M, Schulzer M. Dose response of human intraocular pressure to aceclidine. *Arch Ophthalmol* 1972;88:394–396.
37. Fechner PU, Teichman KD, Weyrauch W. Accommodative effects of aceclidine in the treatment of glaucoma. *Am J Ophthalmol* 1975;79:104–106.
38. Keren G, Treister G. Effect of aceclidine (+) isomer and pilocarpine on the intraocular pressure decrease and the miosis in glaucomatous eyes: effect on accommodation in normal eyes of young subjects. *Ophthalmologica* 1980;180:181–187.
39. François J, Goes F. Ultrasonographic comparative study of the effect of pilocarpine and aceclidine on the eye components. *Ophthalmologica* 1974;168:299–307.
40. Erickson-Lamy K, Schroeder A. Dissociation between the effect of aceclidine on outflow facility and accommodation. *Exp Eye Res* 1990;50:143–147.
41. Erickson-Lamy KA, Kaufman PL, Polansky JR. Dissociation of cholinergic supersensitivity from receptor number in ciliary muscle. *Invest Ophthalmol Vis Sci* 1988;29:600–605.
42. Erickson-Lamy KA, Johnson CD, True-Gabelt B, Kaufman PL. Ciliary muscle choline acetyltransferase and acetylcholinesterase after ciliary ganglionectomy. *Exp Eye Res* 1990;51:295–299.
43. Erickson-Lamy KA, Kaufman PL. Reinnervation of primate ciliary muscle following ciliary ganglionectomy. *Invest Ophthalmol Vis Sci* 1987;28:927–933.
44. Kaufman PL, Erickson-Lamy KA, Rohen JW, Polansky Jr. The ciliary muscle and nerves after ciliary ganglionectomy. In: Krieglstein GK, eds. *Glaucoma Update IV. Proceedings of the Symposium of the Glaucoma Society of the International Congress of Ophthalmology in Bali.* Springer-Verlag, 1991;36–51.
45. Erickson-Lamy KA, Kaufman PL. Effect of cholinergic drugs on outflow facility after ciliary ganglionectomy. *Invest Ophthalmol Vis Sci* 1988;29:491–494.
46. Bárány EH. Dissociation of accommodation effects from outflow effects of pilocarpine. In: Paterson G, Miller SJH, Paterson GH, eds. *Drug Mechanisms in Glaucoma.* London: Churchill Ltd, 1966;275–282.
47. Croft MA, Oyen MJ, Gange SJ, Fisher MR, Kaufman PL. Aging effects on accommodation and outflow facility responses to pilocarpine in humans. *Arch Ophthalmol* 1996;114:586–592.
48. Bito LZ. Paradoxical ocular hypertensive effect of pilocarpine on echothiophate iodide-treated primate eyes. *Invest Ophthalmol Vis Sci* 1980;19:371–377.

49. Bárány EH. Action of eserine, hexamethonium, and atropine on outflow resistance of monkey eyes indicating that eserine releases acetylcholine besides protecting it. *Doc Ophthalmol* 1966;20:150–156.
50. Cohen S, Sololovsky M. Complexity apparent in muscarinic mechanisms. *Trends Pharmacol Sci* 1987;8:41–44.
51. Stone RA. Vasoactive intestinal polypeptide and the ocular innervation. *Invest Ophthalmol Vis Sci* 1986;27:951–957.
52. Nomura T, Smelser GK. The identification of adrenergic and cholinergic nerve endings in the trabecular meshwork. *Invest Ophthalmol* 1974;13:525–532.
53. Ruskell GL. The source of nerve fibres of the trabeculae and adjacent structures in monkey eyes. *Exp Eye Res* 1976;23:449–459.
54. Kaufman PL, Bárány EH. Residual pilocarpine effects on outflow facility after ciliary muscle disinsertion in the cynomolgus monkey. *Invest Ophthalmol* 1976;15:558–561.
55. Bonner TI. New subtypes of muscarinic acetylcholine receptors. In: Levine RR, Birdsall JJM, eds. *Subtypes of muscarinic receptors IV. Trends Pharmacol Sci.* Cambridge, United Kingdom: Elsevier Trends Journals, 1989;11–15.
56. Goyal RK. Muscarinic receptor subtypes: physiology and clinical implications. *N Engl J Med* 1989;15:1022–1028.
57. Gupta N, McAllister R, Drance SM, Rootman J, Cynader MS. Muscarinic receptor M1 and M2 subtypes in the human eye: QNB, pirenzipine, oxotremorine, and AFDX-116 in vitro autoradiography. *Br J Ophthalmol* 1994;78:555–559.
58. Honkanen RE, Howard EF, Abdel-Latif AA. M3 muscarinic receptor subtype predominates in the bovine iris sphincter muscle and ciliary processes. *Invest Ophthalmol Vis Sci* 1990;31:590–593.
59. Erickson-Lamy KA, Chen MC, Hernandez MR. Expression of muscarinic receptor mRNA in cultured ciliary muscle cells. *Invest Ophthalmol Vis Sci* 1991;32(suppl):833.
60. Zhang X, Hernandez MR, Cheng MC, Erickson-Lamy KA. Further characterization of muscarinic receptor subtype mRNA in the human ciliary muscle. *Invest Ophthalmol Vis Sci* 1992;33(suppl):1200.
61. Suzuki R, Oso T, Kobayashi S. Cholinergic inhibitory response in the bovine iris dilator muscle. *Invest Ophthalmol Vis Sci* 1983;24:760–765.
62. Chen J, WoldeMussie E. Similarities of muscarinic receptor subtypes in smooth muscles of cat iris sphincter, ciliary and guinea-pig ilium. *FASEB J* 1988;2:A788.
63. WoldeMussie E, Feldmann B, Chen J. Characterization of muscarinic receptors in cultured human iris sphincter and ciliary smooth muscle cells. *Exp Eye Res* 1993;56:385–392.
64. Honkanen RE, Howard EF, Abdel-Latif AA. M3 muscarinic receptor subtype predominates in the bovine iris sphincter smooth muscle and ciliary processes. *Invest Ophthalmol Vis Sci* 1990;31:590–593.
65. WoldeMussie E, Ruiz G, Feldmann B. Muscarinic receptor subtype involved in signalling mechanisms in cultured human trabecular meshwork cells. *Invest Ophthalmol Vis Sci* 1990;31(suppl):338.
66. Polansky JR, Zlock D, Brasier A, Bloom E. Adrenergic and cholinergic receptors in isolated nonpigmented ciliary epithelial cells. *Curr Eye Res* 1985;4:517–522.
67. Mallorga P, Babilon RW, Buisson S, Sugrue MF. Muscarinic receptors in the albino rabbit ciliary process. *Exp Eye Res* 1989;48:509–522.
68. Wax MB, Coca-Prados M. Receptor-mediated phosphoinositide hydrolysis in human ocular ciliary epithelial cells. *Invest Ophthalmol Vis Sci* 1989;30:1675–1679.
69. Wheeler LA, Moore A, Coca-Prados M, Sachs G. Cholinergic stimulation of the non-pigmented cell of ciliary epithelium. *Invest Ophthalmol Vis Sci* 1990;31(suppl):248.
70. Gupta N, Drance SM, McAllister R, Prasad S, Rootman J, Cynader MS. Localization of M3 muscarinic receptor subtype and mRNA in the human eye. *Ophthalmic Res* 1994;26:207–213.
71. Nagataki S, Brubaker RF. The effect of pilocarpine on aqueous humor formation in humans. *Arch Ophthalmol* 1982;100:818–821.
72. Bito LZ, Davson H, Snider N. The effects of autonomic drugs on mitosis and DNA synthesis in the lens epithelium and on the composition of the aqueous humor. *Exp Eye Res* 1965;4:54–61.
73. Wålinder P-E, Bill A. Aqueous flow and entry of cycloleucine into the aqueous humor of vervet monkeys (*Cercopithecus ethiops*). *Invest Ophthalmol* 1969;8:434–445.
74. Wålinder P-E, Bill A. Influence of intraocular pressure and some drugs on aqueous flow and entry of cycloleucine into the aqueous humor of vervet monkeys (*Cercopithecus ethiops*). *Invest Ophthalmol* 1969;8:446–458.
75. Jumblatt JE, North GT, Hackmiller RC. Muscarinic cholinergic inhibition of adenylate cyclase in the rabbit iris-ciliary body and ciliary epithelium. *Invest Ophthalmol Vis Sci* 1990;31:1103–1108.
76. Matsumoto S, Yorio T, DeSantis L, Pang I-H. Muscarinic effects on cellular functions in cultured human ciliary muscle cells. *Invest Ophthalmol Vis Sci* 1994;35:3732–3738.
77. Pang I-H, Shade D, Tamm E, DeSantis L. Single-cell contraction assay for human ciliary muscle cells: Effect of carbachol. *Invest Ophthalmol Vis Sci* 1993;34:1876–1879.
78. WoldeMussie E, Feldmann B. Characterization of muscarinic receptors in human ciliary and iris smooth muscle cells by ligand binding and biochemical response studies. *FASEB J* 1988;2:A364.
79. Gabelt BT, Kaufman PL. Inhibition of outflow facility, accommodative, and miotic responses to pilocarpine in rhesus monkeys by muscarinic receptor subtype antagonists. *J Pharmacol Exp Ther* 1992;263:1133–1139.
80. Gabelt BT, Kaufman PL. Inhibition of aceclidine-stimulated outflow facility, accommodation and miosis by muscarinic receptor subtype antagonists in rhesus monkeys. *Exp Eye Res* 1994;58:623–630.
81. Poyer JF, Gabelt BT, Kaufman PL. The effect of muscarinic agonists and selective receptor subtype antagonists on the contractile response of the isolated rhesus monkeys ciliary muscle. *Exp Eye Res* 1994;59:729–736.
82. Mindel JS. Cholinergic pharmacology. In: Tasman W, Jaeger EA, eds. *Duane's Biomedical Foundations of Ophthalmology.* Philadelphia: JB Lippincott Company, 1989;1–59.
83. Rossum JMV, Cornelissen MJWJ, de Groot CTP, Hurkmans JATM. A new view on an old drug: pilocarpine. *Experientia* 1960;16:373–375.
84. Furchgott RF, Bursztyn P. Comparison of dissociation constants and of relative efficacies of selected agonists acting on parasympathetic receptors. *Ann NY Acad Sci* 1967;144:882–899.
85. Armaly MF, Rao KR. The effect of pilocarpine Ocusert with different release rates on ocular pressure. *Invest Ophthalmol* 1973;12:491–496.
86. Lee P, Shen Y, Eberle M. The long-acting Ocusert-pilocarpine system in the management of glaucoma. *Invest Ophthalmol* 1975;14:43–46.
87. Quigley HA, Pollack IP, Harbin TS Jr. Pilocarpine ocuserts: long-term clinical trials and selected pharmacodynamics. *Arch Ophthalmol* 1975;93:771–775.
88. Worthen DM, Zimmerman TJ, Wind CA. An evaluation of the pilocarpine Ocusert. *Invest Ophthalmol* 1974;13:296–299.
89. Mazor Z, Ticho U, Rehany U, Rose L. Piloplex, a new long-acting pilocarpine polymer salt. B: Comparative study of the visual effects of pilocarpine and Piloplex eye drops. *Br J Ophthalmol* 1979;63:48–51.
90. Ticho U, Blumenthal M, Zonis S, Gal A, Blank I, Mazor AW. A clinical trial with Piloplex—a new long-acting pilocarpine compound: preliminary report. *Ann Ophthalmol* 1979;11:555–561.
91. Ticho U, Blumenthal M, Zonis S, Gal A, Blank I, Mazor ZW. Piloplex, a new long-acting pilocarpine polymer salt. A. Long-term study. *Br J Ophthalmol* 1979;63:45–47.
92. Klein HZ, Lugo M, Shields MB, Leon J, Duzman E. A dose-response study of piloplex for duration of action. *Am J Ophthalmol* 1985;99:23–26.
93. Goldberg I, Ashburn FS, Kass MA, Becker B. Efficacy and patient acceptance of pilocarpine gel. *Am J Ophthalmol* 1979;88:843–846.
94. Magder H, Bayaner D. The use of a longer acting pilocarpine in the management of chronic simple glaucoma. *Can J Ophthalmol* 1974;9:285–288.
95. Kaufman PL, Bárány EH. Subsensitivity to pilocarpine in primate ciliary muscle following topical anticholinesterase treatment. *Invest Ophthalmol* 1975;14:302–306.
96. Zacharias J, Guerrero S. Effects of cholinergic drugs and 4-aminopyridine on cat ciliary muscle contractility. *Invest Ophthalmol Vis Sci* 1985;26:1309–1313.
97. Lommatzsch P. Über Versuche mit Pilokarpin am isolierten Ciliarmuskel und Sphincter iridis. *Graefes Arch Clin Exp Ophthalmol* 1963;165:487–494.

98. Takagi K, Takayanagi I, Shih CK. A new view on the site of action of pilocarpine and arecoline in the isolated guinea pig ileum. *Chem Pharm Bull (Tokyo)* 1967;15:1744–1748.
99. Barlow RB. *Introduction to Chemical Pharmacology.* London: Methuen, 1964.
100. Goldstein A, Aronow L, Kalman SM. *Principles of Drug Action: The Basis of Pharmacology.* New York: John Wiley & Sons, 1974.
101. Swan KC, Gehrsitz L. Competitive action of miotics on the iris sphincter. *Arch Ophthalmol* 1951;46:477–481.
102. Lütjen-Drecoll E, Kaufman P. Biomechanics of echothiophate-induced anatomic changes in monkey aqueous outflow system. *Graefes Arch Clin Exp Ophthalmol* 1986;224:564–575.
103. Wirtschafter JD, Herman WK. Low concentration eserine therapy for the tonic pupil (Adie) syndrome. *Ophthalmology* 1980;87:1037–1043.
104. Kini MM, Dahl AA, Roberts CR, Lehwalder LW, Grant WM. Echothiophate, pilocarpine, and open-angle glaucoma. *Arch Ophthalmol* 1973;89:190–192.
105. Kronfeld PC. The efficacy of combinations of ocular hypotensive drugs: a tonographic approach. *Arch Ophthalmol* 1967;78:140–146.
106. Kaufman PL, Bárány EH. Subsensitivity to pilocarpine of the aqueous outflow system in monkey eyes after topical anticholinesterase treatment. *Am J Ophthalmol* 1976;82:883–891.
107. Bárány E. Pilocarpine-induced subsensitivity to carbachol and pilocarpine of ciliary muscle in vervet and cynomolgus monkeys. *Acta Ophthalmol* 1977;55:141–163.
108. Kaufman PL. Anticholinesterase-induced cholinergic subsensitivity in primate accommodative mechanism. *Am J Ophthalmol* 1978;85: 622–631.
109. Lütjen-Drecoll E, Kaufman PL. Echothiophate-induced structural alterations in the anterior chamber angle of the cynomolgus monkey. *Invest Ophthalmol Vis Sci* 1979;18:918–929.
110. Bito LZ, Dawson MJ, Petrinovic L. Cholinergic sensitivity: normal variability as a function of stimulus background. *Science* 1971;172: 583–585.
111. Bito LZ, Hyslop A, Hyndman J. Antiparasympathomimetic effects of cholinesterase inhibitor treatment. *J Pharmacol Exp Ther* 1967; 157:159–169.
112. Bito LZ, Banks N. Effects of chronic cholinesterase inhibitor treatment. I. The pharmacological and physiological behavior of the anti-ChE-treated (*Macaca mulatta*) iris. *Arch Ophthalmol* 1969;82: 681–686.
113. Bito LZ, Dawson MJ. The site and mechanism of the control of cholinergic sensitivity. *J Pharmacol Exp Ther* 1970;175:673–684.
114. Claesson H. Bárány E. Time course of light-induced changes in pilocarpine sensitivity of rat iris. *Acta Physiol Scand* 1978;102:394–398.
115. Croft MA, Kaufman PL, Erickson-Lamy KA, Polansky JR. Accommodation and ciliary muscle muscarinic receptors after echothiophate. *Invest Ophthalmol Vis Sci* 1991;32:3288–3297.
116. Bárány EH. Muscarinic subsensitivity without receptor change in monkey ciliary muscle. *Br J Pharmacol* 1985;84:193–198.
117. Kaufman PL. Parasympathetic denervation of the ciliary muscle following retinal photocoagulation. *Trans Am Ophthalmol Soc* 1990; 88:513–553.
118. Kaufman PL, Rohen JW, Gabelt BT, Eichhorn M, Wallow IHL, Polansky JR. Parasympathetic denervation of the ciliary muscle following panretinal photocoagulation. *Curr Eye Res* 1991;10:437–455.
119. Sachs DI, Kloog Y, Korczyn AD, Heron DS, Sokolovsky M. Denervation, supersensitivity, and muscarinic receptors in the cat iris. *Biochem Pharmacol* 1979;28:1513–1518.
120. Burt DR. Muscarinic receptor binding in rat sympathetic ganglion is unaffected by denervation. *Brain Res* 1978;143:573–579.
121. Talamo BR, Adler OC, Burt DR. Parasympathetic denervation decreases muscarinic receptor binding in rat parotid. *Life Sci* 1979;24: 1573–1580.
122. Emmelin N. Supersensitivity following "pharmacological denervation." *Pharmacol Rev* 1961;13:17–37.
123. Westfall DP, McPhillips JJ, Foley DJ. Inhibition of cholinesterase activity after postganglionic denervation of the rat vas deferens: evidence for prejunctional supersensitivity to acetylcholine. *J Pharmacol Exp Ther* 1974;189:493–498.
124. Hata F, Takeyasu K, Morikawa YL R, Ishida H, Yoshida H. Specific changes in the cholinergic system in guinea pig vas deferens after denervation. *J Pharmacol Exp Ther* 1980;215:716–722.
125. Fleming WW. A comparative study of supersensitivity to norepinephrine and acetylcholine produced by denervation, decentralization and reserpine. *J Pharmacol Exp Ther* 1963;141:173–179.
126. Morrison JM, Fleming WW. The nonspecific supersensitivity of the cat nictitating membrane. *Pharmacologist* 1967;9:234(abstr).
127. Carrier OJ, Jurevics HA. The role of calcium in "nonspecific" supersensitivity of vascular muscle. *J Pharmacol Exp Ther* 1973;184: 81–94.
128. Westfall DP. Nonspecific supersensitivity of the guinea pig vas deferens produced by decentralization and reserpine treatment. *Br J Pharmacol* 1970;39:110–120.
129. Hoskins HD, Kass MA. Cholinergic drugs. In: Hoskins HD, Kass MA, eds. *Becker-Shaffer's Diagnosis and therapy of the glaucomas,* 6th ed. St. Louis: CV Mosby, 1989;420–434.
130. Taylor P. Cholinergic agonists. In: Goodman Gilman A, Rall TW, Nies AS, Taylor P, eds. *The Pharmacological Basis of Therapeutics,* 8th ed. New York: McGraw-Hill, 1990;122–130.
131. Taylor P. Anticholinesterase agents. In: Goodman Gilman A, Rall TW, Nies AS, Taylor P, eds. *The Pharmacological Basis of Therapeutics,* 8th ed. New York: McGraw-Hill, 1990;131–149.
132. Weisbecker CA, Fraunfelder FT, Gold AA, Naidoff M, Tippermann R, eds. *Physician's Desk Reference for Ophthalmology,* 23rd ed. Montvale, NJ: Medical Economics Data Production Company, 1995;354.
133. Autonomic drugs. In: Mauger TF, Craig EL, eds. *Havener's Ocular Pharmacology,* 6th ed. St. Louis: CV Mosby, 1994;53–171.
134. *Drug Information for the Health Care Professional,* 15th ed. vol 1. Rockville, Maryland: The United States Pharmacopeial Convention, 1995;3279.
135. Abel SR, ed. Micromedix computerized clinical information system (R) drug information. Staff DE, ed. Vol 83. Denver: Micromedix, 1995.
136. Maurice DM, Mishima S. Ocular pharmacokinetics. In: Sears ML, ed. *Pharmacology of the Eye.* Berlin: Springer-Verlag, 1984;19–116.
137. Crawford K, Kaufman PL. Pilocarpine antagonizes $PGE_{2\alpha}$-induced ocular hypotension: Evidence for enhancement of uveoscleral outflow by $PGF_{2\alpha}$. *Arch Ophthalmol* 1987;105:1112–1116.
138. Nilsson SFE, Samuelsson M, Bill A, Stjernschantz J. Increased uveoscleral outflow as a possible mechanism of ocular hypotension caused by prostaglandin $F_{2\alpha}$-1-isopropylester in the cynomolgus monkey. *Exp Eye Res* 1989;48:707–716.
139. Gabelt BT, Kaufman PL. Prostaglandin $F_{2\alpha}$ increases uveoscleral outflow in the cynomolgus monkey. *Exp Eye Res* 1989;49:389–402.

Textbook of Ocular Pharmacology,
edited by T.J. Zimmerman, et al.
Lippincott–Raven Publishers, Philadelphia © 1997.

CHAPTER 20

Epinephrine and Dipivefrin

Ervin N. Fang and Michael A. Kass

History and Source

At the turn of the nineteenth century, Oliver and Schaffer first synthesized epinephrine. By 1900 Erdmann began to employ subconjunctival injections of epinephrine for his glaucoma patients (26). In 1923 Hamburger administered topical epinephrine to lower intraocular pressure (IOP). The use of epinephrine waned, however, because it was unstable in solution and had the potential to aggravate or precipitate angle-closure glaucoma. With the addition of stabilizing antioxidants and the advent of gonioscopy for the correct classification of the glaucomas, epinephrine compounds regained their place in the management of elevated intraocular pressure.

Official Name and Chemistry

Epinephrine

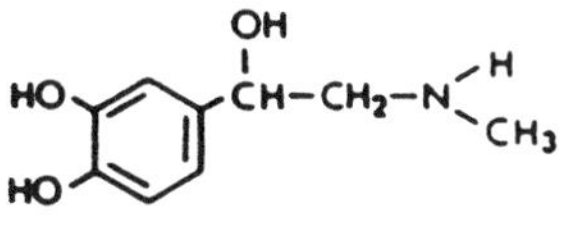

Dipivefrin (Propine)

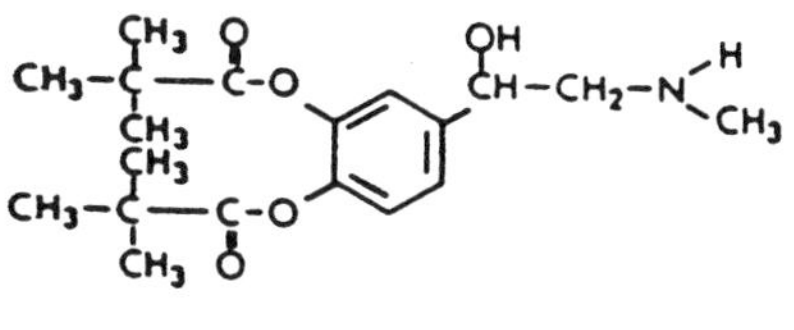

Pharmacology

Epinephrine ($C9H_{13}NO_3$) is a directly acting sympathomimetic agent. It is 1,2-benzenediol,4-[1-hydroxy-2-(methylamino)ethyl],(R)-(-)-3,4-dihydroxy-α-[(methylamino) methyl]benzyl alcohol. It mediates reduction of intraocular pressure through stimulation of alpha (α) and beta (β)-adrenergic receptors. The prodrug form of epinephrine is dipivefrin, which must be biochemically transformed to its active state. Esterase enzymes in the cornea cleave the two pivalic acid side chains on dipivefrin, liberating epinephrine.

E. N. Fang and M. A. Kass: Department of Ophthalmology and Visual Sciences, Washington University School of Medicine, St. Louis, Missouri 63110.

Clinical Pharmacology

Epinephrine

Epinephrine is an endogenous neurohumor, synthesized by the adrenal medulla and carried by the circulation to local effector sites. It is metabolized primarily by the enzymes, monoamine oxidase, and catechol-O-methyltransferase. A small fraction of epinephrine is removed by active uptake into tissues.

Despite its long use in the treatment of open-angle glaucoma, the effects of epinephrine on aqueous humor dynamics and its mechanism of IOP reduction are still controversial. The most widely accepted theory is that epinephrine lowers IOP by its effects on conventional and unconventional outflow channels of the eye. Epinephrine enhances conventional outflow in human as well as animal eyes through a β_2-receptor-mediated mechanism. Epinephrine stimulates β_2-receptors, which, in turn, activate adenyl cyclase and increase production of cyclic adenosine monophosphate (cAMP) (81,83). This mechanism lowers IOP by reducing outflow resistance in the conventional outflow channels (83,96,99). Epinephrine also improves uveoscleral outflow in human and primate eyes (98). Recent studies have suggested that this phenomenon may occur through a complex mechanism involving prostaglandin production (4,19,76) and cAMP.

Acute administration of epinephrine increases IOP and aqueous humor formation. This phenomenon may be mediated by β-receptors because timolol, a β-adrenergic antagonist, can block this increase in aqueous production (39), but thymoxamine, an α-adrenergic antagonist, does not

(65). This effect on aqueous production seems to diminish with chronic administration of epinephrine.

Dipivefrin

Dipivalyl epinephrine (DPE) is a lipophilic prodrug derivative of epinephrine, with two pivalic acid groups added (122). It has limited sympathomimetic activity. It is propanoic acid, 2,2-dimethyl-,4-[1-hydroxy-2-(methyl-amino) ethyl]-1,2-phenylene ester, hydrochloride, (±)-(±)-3,4-dihydroxy-α-[(methylamino)methyl]benzyl alcohol 3,4-dipivalate hydrochloride. After entering the corneal stroma, corneal esterases cleave off the two pivalic acid side chains (16,41), thereby liberating epinephrine. This hydrolytic conversion increases dipivefrin's lipid solubility to 600 times that of its original compound and its ocular penetration to 17 times that of epinephrine alone (70,122).

Pharmaceutics (Table 20-1)

Epinephrine

Epinephrine is commercially manufactured for topical use as a concentration of its salt rather than available free base. There are three preparations available: bitartrate, borate, and hydrochloride. These salt preparations are relevant when considering doses, as a 2% bivalent salt solution of epinephrine bitartrate is equivalent to that of 1.1% epinephrine base. All three preparations appear to be equally effective in reducing IOP (25).

Borate solutions ($C_9H_{12}BNO_4$), which are available in 0.5 and 1% concentrations, are better tolerated because of their more neutral pH (7.4). Hydrochloride solutions ($C_9H_{13}NO_3$), which are available and stable in 0.5, 1, and 2% concentrations, cause more discomfort because of a more acidic pH (3.5). Bitartrate preparations ($C_9H_{13}NO_3\ C_4H_6O_6$) are stable at 2% concentrations but also cause irritation because of their low pH.

Commercial preparations of epinephrine eyedrops must contain preservatives as well as antioxidants because once epinephrine solutions become oxidized, they are notably less effective and also more irritating. Patients should be warned to discard discolored solutions or those that appear muddy.

Epinephrine is usually instilled every 12 hours. The utilization of epinephrine-pilocarpine combinations may require four-times-a-day dosing to be effective, but this dosage represents an overdose of the epinephrine component in order to dose pilocarpine adequately.

Dipivefrin

Dipivefrin comes in a single concentration of 0.1% and is usually well tolerated. Administered twice daily, dipivefrin 0.1% is roughly equivalent in its ocular hypotensive effect to 1% to 2% epinephrine (18,22,41,58).

PHARMACOKINETICS, CONCENTRATION-EFFECT RELATIONSHIP, AND METABOLISM

Epinephrine

Following topical epinephrine administration, IOP diminishes within 1 hour, reaching a minimum in 1 to 4 hours. Intraocular pressure returns to baseline in 12 to 24 hours. Although the IOP of some patients can be controlled by once-daily dosing, this should be confirmed by an IOP check 24 to 26 hours after the last dose.

Epinephrine has been tested in a polymeric matrix, which releases the drug osmotically at a rate of 1 to 4 μg of epinephrine base per hour over 12 hours (17). This drug-delivery system provides good control of IOP while delivering less medication to the patient than standard eyedrop preparations.

Epinephrine's effectiveness in lowering IOP is directly proportional to its concentration. The concentrations of most commercial preparations of epinephrine (free-base or active form) range from 0.5% to 2%. Although most studies have shown efficacy in the concentration rate of 0.5 to 1%, doses as low as 0.06% and as high as 2% can effectively reduce IOP. We recommend that clinicians initiate therapy at lower concentrations, increasing only as needed.

The pharmacologic action of circulating epinephrine is terminated by the liver and other tissues through various

TABLE 20-1. *Pharmaceutics of epinephrine preparations and dipivefrin*

Generic name	Brand name	Concentration (%)	Dose
Dipivefrin HCl	Propine	0.1	Q12–24h
Epinephrine bitartrate	Epitrate	2	Q12–24h
Epinephrine borate	Epinal	0.5, 1	Q12–24h
	Eppy/N	0.5, 1, 2	Q12–24h
Epinephrine HCl	Epinephrine	0.25	Q12–24h
	Epifrin	0.5, 1, 2	Q12–24h
	Glaucon	1, 2	Q12–24h
Pilocarpine/epinephrine	E-Pilo$_{n\%}$	$P_{1\%}E_{1\%}$–$P_{6\%}E_{1\%}$	Q6h

enzymatic reactions involving catechol-O-methyltransferase and monoamine oxidase. Remaining active drug is also taken up and metabolized by sympathetic nerve terminals. Metanephrine and 3-methoxy,4-hydroxymandelic acid (vanillylmandelic acid) are inactive metabolites of epinephrine, and they are excreted by the kidney.

Dipivefrin

Following topical administration of dipivefrin, IOP declines in 30 to 60 minutes and attains its lowest level in 1 to 4 hours. It returns to baseline in 12 to 24 hours. Because dipivefrin produces its ocular hypotensive effect by biotransformation to epinephrine, there is no added benefit to concurrent administration of epinephrine preparations with dipivefrin. The metabolites of dipivefrin include 3-monopivalic acid, 4-monopivalic acid, and dipivalyl mandelic acid; however, their biochemical activity is still unclear (73).

Therapeutic Use

Epinephrine and Dipivefrin

Epinephrine is widely employed for the management and treatment of open-angle glaucoma. It can also be helpful in the treatment of patients with secondary glaucoma as well as patients with angle-closure glaucoma who have patent iridectomies.

Because many patients can receive maximal benefit from lower drug concentrations (34,91), epinephrine therapy should be initiated with a low concentration and increased as needed for IOP reduction. In addition, some of the side effects of epinephrine are dose related. Initial epinephrine treatment should begin with a monocular trial, as only 70% of patients with open-angle glaucoma will respond with a substantial IOP reduction. Because epinephrine has a slight effect on the intraocular pressure of the contralateral, untreated eye, it is unlikely to confound the results of a monocular trial. Patients and family physicians should be made aware that topical epinephrine preparations can produce blood levels sufficient to induce systemic side effects. Patients should be instructed to instill only one drop of medication per eye and educated on the use of nasolacrimal duct occlusion (or gentle eyelid closure) to lessen systemic absorption.

It is well known that angle-closure glaucoma can be precipitated or aggravated by topical epinephrine. Therefore, all patients must undergo careful gonioscopic examination before and soon after initiating epinephrine therapy. Mydriasis after epinephrine is more marked with concurrent β-adrenergic antagonist treatment and can occur despite concomitant miotic therapy. While the epinephrine-induced pupillary dilation can prove beneficial for patients with media opacities (22), others may describe diminution of vision due to the loss of the pinhole effect.

Side Effects and Toxicity

Epinephrine and Dipivefrin

Ocular Side Effects

At least 50% of glaucoma patients on chronic epinephrine therapy become intolerant to the drug (13). Most of these adverse reactions are external in nature, including hyperemia, irritation, tearing, and hypersensitivity blepharoconjunctivitis. Other ocular side effects are included in Table 20-2.

TABLE 20-2. *Signs and symptoms of side effects*

Symptoms	Ocular signs
Burning	Lid and conjunctiva
Stinging	Hyperemia
Tearing	Blepharoconjunctivitis
Blurred/distorted vision	Skin Blanching
Photophobia	Adrenochrome deposits
Headache	Madarosis
Browache	Ocular pemphigoid
Palpitations	Lacrimal system
Nervousness	Punctal stenosis
Faintness	Epidermalized puncta
Tremor	Lacrimal stones
	Cornea
	Epithelial toxicity
	Edema
	Erosion from tarsal adrenochrome deposit
	"Black cornea" from diffuse adrenochrome
	Soft contact lens and prosthesis staining
	? herpetic reactivation
	Uveal tract
	Mydriasis
	Angle closure
	Iridocyclitis
	Retina
	Macular edema
	? Central retinal vein occlusion
	Systemic signs
	Tachyarrhythmia
	Premature ventricular contractions
	Pallor
	Systemic hypertension
	Bronchospasm
	Cerebrovascular accident
	Myocardial infarction
	Death

Epinephrine-induced conjunctival hyperemia results from an initial vasoconstriction followed by a rebound vasodilation. Because of the α-adrenergic mediated vasoconstriction, some patients erroneously believe that the topical epinephrine may actually relieve their hyperemia, and they thereby commence a cycle of misguided overuse. Many people associate the appearance of red eyes with heavy alcohol consumption.

Tearing and burning are other common complaints related to the acidic pH of some preparations. These symptoms may be relieved by switching to dipivefrin or an epinephrine borate preparation.

Topical epinephrine produces *hypersensitivity blepharoconjunctivitis* in 10% to 15% of patients. These patients present with lid erythema, lichenification, conjunctival chemosis, vascular engorgement, and follicular conjunctivitis. Patients may also present with asymptomatic follicular conjunctival hypertrophy. Mild iridocyclitis and subepithelial corneal infiltrates also have been found in this syndrome (6). Symptoms can occur acutely or after several years of use. Some patients who develop epinephrine-related hypersensitivity blepharoconjunctivitis can tolerate dipivefrin without similar symptoms (124). Other patients can continue epinephrine treatment only if a weak topical corticosteroid, such as 1% medrysone (hydroxymesterone, HMS), is concurrently administered. Long-term use of medrysone is unlikely to raise IOP.

Adrenochrome deposits are a type of black melanin pigment formed by the oxidation and polymerization of epinephrine. These deposits are usually asymptomatic and often found in the lower conjunctival cul-de-sac (20,24,116), encapsulated by squamous epithelium. They generally do not produce symptoms. Adrenochrome deposits of the upper tarsal conjunctiva, however, typically have a branching or "staghorn" appearance and can cause corneal epithelial abrasions (20,93,116). Adrenochrome material also can be deposited in the corneal epithelium, especially if the IOP is elevated and bullous keratopathy is present (23,30,36,42, 57,66,69,95). A diffuse plaque of adrenochrome covering the cornea can simulate a malignant melanoma (105). Adrenochrome deposits can also be found in the lacrimal sac (9), nasolacrimal ducts (106), senile scleral plaque (105), corneal transplants, and prosthetic eyes (30). They occasionally may be mistaken for a foreign body. Adrenochrome deposits are found more frequently in patients using old and discolored epinephrine solutions.

Mydriasis is a well-known, usually benign result of epinephrine therapy. Mydriasis can precipitate or aggravate an angle-closure attack in predisposed eyes. Epinephrine is contraindicated in glaucoma patients with narrow or occludable angles until a patent iridectomy is present.

Macular edema after topical epinephrine therapy occurs in approximately 10 to 20% of aphakic eyes (51,68,71,90, 95,112). Visual acuity is usually reduced to the range of 20/25 to 20/200, and the reduction can occur months to years after institution of epinephrine therapy. Fortunately, this condition seems to be reversible if the drug is discontinued, but resolution may take months. If vision begins to diminish and epinephrine treatment is not discontinued, chronic structural injury to the retina can permanently decrease visual acuity. Fluorescein angiographic findings of leakage are similar to aphakic cystoid macular edema. Theories regarding epinephrine-induced macular edema in aphakic eyes include vasospasm, increased prostaglandin synthesis, sensitization of the retina to the effects of ultraviolet radiation, or alteration of macular blood flow (77).

Epinephrine should *not* be the first line of therapy for treating glaucoma in aphakic eyes. If epinephrine is necessary, the aphakic patient should check his or her vision at home daily. Any diminution in vision requires a thorough examination to determine whether epinephrine treatment should be discontinued. Unfortunately, this condition is underrecognized, and the reduction in vision is often misdiagnosed. An intact posterior capsule may provide a mechanical barrier to posterior migration of epinephrine and its possible effects on retinal and choroidal circulation (54,56).

Halos and blurred vision have been reported with epinephrine therapy by patients who have corneal haze and edema despite good IOP control. The symptoms and corneal findings disappear when the drug is discontinued. Intracameral injections of high concentrations of epinephrine (e.g., 1 : 1,000 dilution) are toxic to the corneal endothelium (40). There was one report of reduced corneal endothelial cell density in a small series of patients receiving topical unilateral epinephrine treatment (117). Their findings, however, were not confirmed in a larger series of patients treated with a variety of antiglaucoma drugs (52).

Headache and brow ache occur infrequently in patients receiving topical epinephrine but may be severe.

Staining of soft contact lenses can occur in patients instilling epinephrine while their lenses are in place (72,107). The lens discoloration can be removed by soaking the lenses in 3% hydrogen peroxide for 5 hours (72). Dipivefrin does not produce stains and can be used freely in contact lens patients (84).

Less common side effects of topical epinephrine include photophobia, madarosis (45), and epidermalization of the lacrimal puncta (97). There are a few reports of ocular cicatricial pemphigoid associated with epinephrine administration, but no direct cause-and-effect relationship has been established (31,59). One case report of central retinal vein occlusion has been described after a single use of dipivefrin (33), but it was thought to be a coincidental finding in a patient with uncontrolled glaucoma. Some researchers have postulated that an epinephrine-induced vasoconstriction may compromise optic nerve perfusion. Herschler suggested that this effect is worse with unilateral treatment because the fellow untreated eye does not have a lowered IOP to offset any decrease in perfusion. Further studies of the effects of topical and systemic epinephrine on human optic-nerve blood flow are required to resolve this issue. In rabbits, epinephrine administered intramuscularly or by iontophoresis can activate latent herpes simplex virus (61,62); however, there is no evidence that topical epinephrine treatment activates herpetic disease in humans.

Systemic Side Effects

A small subset of patients experience systemic side effects, including palpitations, hypertension, and premature ventricular contractions. It is important to note that one drop of a 2% epinephrine solution contains 1 mg of epinephrine, which is in the upper limit of systemic usage (i.e., 0.5–1.0 mg of 1 : 1000 intravenously repeated every 3–5 minutes). Some investigators have postulated that primary open-angle glaucoma patients are more sensitive to the effects of epinephrine in the eye (in specific) and in the body (in general), which makes them more susceptible to develop systemic side effects (12,92). One study showed that 69% of the patients with primary open-angle glaucoma treated with epinephrine developed premature ventricular contractions as noted on tonography as compared with 19% of patients with secondary glaucoma (12).

There are a number of ways to reduce or limit the side effects associated with topical epinephrine therapy. The side effects from systemic absorption can be reduced by employing the lowest concentration of the drug possible, instilling only one drop to each eye, and applying punctal occlusion or gentle eyelid closure. Periorbital and adnexal side effects can be reduced by using a different salt solution or a concomitant mild topical corticosteroid, such as medrysone.

Another approach to reducing epinephrine-related side effects is to prescribe dipivefrin. Dipivefrin is stable in solution and produces a lower incidence of external side effects than standard epinephrine solutions. In some patients, however, it can also cause significant external ocular reactions (118), including giant follicular bulbar conjunctivitis (67). Whereas some patients who develop hypersensitivity blepharoconjunctivitis related to epinephrine treatment can tolerate long-term dipivefrin treatment (124), others demonstrate cross-reactivity (108). Both dipivefrin and epinephrine can produce macular edema in aphakic eyes or angle closure glaucoma in predisposed eyes.

Epinephrine treatment is contraindicated in a number of medical conditions, including severe hypertension, cardiac disease, and thyrotoxicosis (7). All in all, because of the lower concentration of drug administered, dipivefrin produces fewer systemic side effects than epinephrine and is a better choice for patients with substantial cardiovascular disease.

High-risk Groups

The safety of topical epinephrine treatment in children and pregnant women has not been fully tested. Topical epinephrine instillation can result in systemic adsorption; therefore, epinephrine can cross the placenta as well as enter breast milk. Epinephrine does not cross the blood–brain barrier. Reproductive animal studies with dipivefrin have shown no untoward effects; however, no well-controlled human studies exist. Because administration of the prodrug, dipivefrin, produces lower blood levels of epinephrine, it is probably the preferred drug when treatment with an epinephrine compound is required in these special situations.

Drug Interactions

Beta-Blockers

Epinephrine stimulates β-adrenergic receptors, whereas β-adrenergic antagonists inhibit these receptors. Some clinical reports have revealed additive effects of timolol and epinephrine or dipivefrin on IOP reduction (47,85, 104); however, most studies have shown that adding epinephrine or dipivefrin to a regimen that includes a nonselective beta-blocker produces a 1 to 3 mm Hg reduction in IOP (47,49,87) in a minority of patients (1,11). Thus, it is recommended that epinephrine be added in a one-eyed trial. The minimal benefit of this combined regimen is attributed to the fact that β-blockers inhibit epinephrine's effects on the ocular outflow channels.

Recent reports have found that epinephrine or dipivefrin are additive in their effects on IOP when combined with betaxolol, a relatively selective β_1-antagonist (2,3). This finding supports the idea that epinephrine's mechanism of action is through stimulation of β_2-adrenergic receptors, as it is not counteracted by betaxolol's β_1 selective blockade. The effect of combined betaxolol and epinephrine treatment on IOP is equivalent to timolol alone.

Miotics

The ocular hypotensive effects of epinephrine and the miotics are additive. Commercial pilocarpine-epinephrine combinations are available and useful in the treatment of selected glaucoma patients. In human eyes, dipivefrin can be used effectively in conjunction with the cholinesterase inhibitor echothiophate iodide (74).

Carbonic Anhydrase Inhibitors

The ocular hypotensive effects of epinephrine and the carbonic anhydrase inhibitors are also additive. Moreover, the combination of epinephrine, a miotic, and a carbonic anhydrase inhibitor is more effective than any two agents alone.

Other Agents

Patients treated with drugs that block the uptake of epinephrine and norepinephrine (e.g., reserpine) or that inhibit monoamine oxidase (e.g., phenylzine, tranylcypromine) or catechol-*O*-methyltransferase are at greater risk of developing systemic side effects with epinephrine therapy. These combinations should be avoided.

Major Clinical Studies

No major clinical studies have been conducted to date.

REFERENCES

1. Abramovsky I, Mindel JS. Dipivefrin and echothiophate contraindications to combined use. *Arch Ophthalmol* 1979;97:1937.
2. Albrecht DC, LeBlanc RP, Cruz AM, Lamping KA, Siegel LI, Stern KL, Kelley EP, Stoecker JF. A double-masked comparison of betaxolol and dipivefrin for the treatment of increased intraocular pressure. *Am J Ophthalmol* 1993;116:307.
3. Allen RC, Epstein DL. Additive effect of betaxolol and epinephrine in primary open-angle glaucoma. *Arch Ophthalmol* 1986;104:1178.
4. Anderson L, Wilson WS. Inhibition by indomethacin of the increased facility of outflow induced by adrenaline. *Exp Eye Res* 1990;50:119.
5. Araie M, Takase M. Effects of various drugs on aqueous humor dynamics in man. *Jpn J Ophthalmol* 1981;25:91.
6. Aronson SB, Yamomoto EA. Ocular hypersensitivity to epinephrine. *Invest Ophthalmol* 1966;5:75.
7. Ballin N, Becker B, Goldman M. Systemic effects of epinephrine applied topically to the eye. *Invest Ophthalmol* 1966;5:125.
8. Ballintine EJ, Garner LL. Improvement of the coefficient of outflow in glaucomatous eyes prolonged local treatment with epinephrine. *Arch Ophthalmol* 1961;66:314.
9. Barishak R, Romano A, Stein R. Obstruction of lacrimal sac caused by topical epinephrine. *Ophthalmologica* 1969;159:373.
10. Bealka N, Schwartz B. Enhanced ocular hypotensive response to epinephrine with prior dexamethasone treatment. *Arch Ophthalmol* 1991;109:346.
11. Becker B, Ley AP. Epinephrine and acetazolamide in the therapy of the glaucomas. *Am J Ophthalmol* 1958;45:639.
12. Becker B, Montgomery SW, Kass MA, Shin DH. Increased ocular and systemic responsiveness to epinephrine in primary open-angle glaucoma. *Arch Ophthalmol* 1977;95:789.
13. Becker B, Morton WR. Topical epinephrine in glaucoma suspects. *Am J Ophthalmol* 1966;62:272.
14. Becker B, Pettit TH, Gay AJ. Topical epinephrine therapy of glaucoma. *Arch Ophthalmol* 1961;66:219.
15. Becker B, Shin DH. Response to topical epinephrine: a practical prognostic test in patients with ocular hypertension. *Arch Ophthalmol* 1976;94:2057.
16. Bigger JF. Dipivefrin and glaucoma. *Perspect Ophthalmol* 1980; 4:85.
17. Birss SA, Longwell A, Heckbert S, Keller N. Ocular hypotensive efficacy of topical epinephrine in normotensive and hypertensive rabbits continuous drug delivery vs. eyedrops. *Ann Ophthalmol* 1978; 10:1045.
18. Bischoff P. Clinical studies conducted with a new epinephrine derivative for the treatment of glaucoma (dipivalyl epinephrine). *Klin Monatsbl Augenheilkd* 1978;172:565.
19. Camras CB, Feldman SG, Podos SM, Christensen RE, Gardner SK, Fazio DT. Inhibition of the epinephrine-induced reduction of intraocular pressure by systemic indomethacin in humans. *Am J Ophthalmol* 1985;100:169.
20. Cashwell LF, Shields MB, Reed JW. Adrenochrome pigmentation. *Arch Ophthalmol* 1977;95:514.
21. Cass E, Kadar D, Stein HA. Hazards of phenylephrine topical medication in persons taking propranolol. *Can Med Assoc J* 1979;120: 126.
22. Chin NB, Gold AA, Breinin G. Iris cysts and miotics. *Arch Ophthalmol* 1964;71:611.
23. Cleasby G, Donaldson DD. Epinephrine pigmentation of the cornea. *Arch Ophthalmol* 1967;78:74.
24. Corwin ME, Spencer WJ. Conjunctival melanin depositions: a side effect of topical epinephrine therapy. *Arch Ophthalmol* 1963;69:73.
25. Criswick VG, Drance SM. Comparative study of four different epinephrine salts on intraocular pressure. *Arch Ophthalmol* 1966;75: 768.
26. Darier A. De l'extrait de capsule surrenales en therapeutique oculaire. *Lab Clin Ophthalmol* 1900;6:141.
27. Drance SM, Saheb NE, Schulzer M. Response to topical epinephrine in chronic open-angle glaucoma. *Arch Ophthalmol* 1978;96: 1001.
28. Eakins KE, Eakins HMT. Adrenergic mechanisms and the outflow of aqueous humor from the rabbit eye. *J Pharmacol Exp Ther* 1964; 144:60.
29. Ferry AP, Zimerman LE. Black cornea: a complication of topical use of epinephrine. *Am J Ophthalmol* 1964;58:205.
30. Ferry JF. Black prosthesis. *Am J Ophthalmol* 1967;64:162.
31. Fiore PM, Jacobs IH, Goldberg DB. Drug-induced pemphigoid: a spectrum of diseases. *Arch Ophthalmol* 1987;105:1660.
32. Flach AJ, Kramer SG. Supersensitivity to topical epinephrine after long term epinephrine therapy. *Arch Ophthalmol* 1980;98:482.
33. Fledelius HC. Central vein thrombosis and topical dipivalyl epinephrine. *Ophthalmologica* 1990;68:491.
34. Garner LL, Johnstone WW, Ballintine EJ, Carroll ME. Effect of 2% levo rotary epinephrine on the intraocular pressure of the glaucomatous eye. *Arch Ophthalmol* 1959;62:230.
35. Goldberg I, Ashburn FS Jr, Palmberg PF, et al. Timolol and epinephrine: a clinical study of ocular interactions. *Arch Ophthalmol* 1980; 98:484.
36. Green WR, Kaufer GI, Dubroff S. Black cornea: a complication of topical use of epinephrine. *Ophthalmologica* 1967;154:88.
37. Harrison R, Kaufmann CS. Clonidine: effects of a topically administered solution on intraocular pressure and blood pressure in open-angle glaucoma. *Arch Ophthalmol* 1980;95:1368.
38. Hayasaka S, Sears M. Effects of epinephrine indomethacin, acetylsalicylic acid, dexamethasone, and cyclic AMP on the in vitro activity of lysosomal hyaluronadase from the rabbit iris. *Invest Ophthalmol Vis Sci* 1978;17:1109.
39. Higgins RG, Brubaker RF. Acute effect of epinephrine on aqueous humor formation in the timolol-treated normal eye as measured by fluorophotometry. *Invest Ophthalmol Vis Sci* 1980;19:420.
40. Hull DS, Chemotti T, Edelhauser HF, Van Horn DL, Hyndiuk RA. Effect of epinephrine on the corneal endothelium. *Am J Ophthalmol* 1975;79:245.
41. Kaback MB, Podos SM, Harbin TS Jr, Mandell A, Becker B. The effects of dipivalyl epinephrine on the eye. *Am J Ophthalmol* 1976;81: 768.
42. Kaiser PK, Pineda R, Albert DM, Shore JW. "Black cornea" after long term epinephrine use. *Arch Ophthalmol* 1992;110:1273.
43. Kass MA, Mandell AL, Goldberg I, Paine M, Becker B. Dipivefrin and epinephrine treatment of elevated intraocular pressure: a comparative study. *Arch Ophthalmol* 1979;97:1865.
44. Kass MA, Reid RW, Neufeld AH, Bauscher LP, Sears ML. The effect of *d*-isoproterenol on intraocular pressure of the rabbit, monkey, and man. *Invest Ophthalmol* 1976;15:113.
45. Kass MA, Stamper RL, Becker B. Madarosis in chronic epinephrine therapy. *Arch Ophthalmol* 1972;88:429.
46. Kaufman PL, Barany EN. Adrenergic drug effects on aqueous outflow following ciliary muscle displacement in the cynomolgus monkey. *Invest Ophthalmol Vis Sci* 1981;20:644.
47. Keates EC, Stone RA. Safety and effectiveness of concomitant administration of dipivefrin and timolol maleate. *Am J Ophthalmol* 1981;91:243.
48. Keates EU. Evaluation of timolol maleate combination therapy in chronic open-angle glaucoma. *Am J Ophthalmol* 1979;88:565.
49. Knupp JA, Shields MB, Mandell AI, et al. Combined timolol and epinephrine therapy for open angle glaucoma. *Surv Ophthal* 1983; 28(suppl):280.

50. Kohn AN, Moss AP, Hargett NA, Ritch R, Smith H Jr, Podos SM. Clinical comparison of dipivalyl epinephrine and epinephrine in the treatment of glaucoma. *Am J Ophthalmol* 1979;85:196.
51. Kolker AE, Becker B. Epinephrine maculopathy. *Arch Ophthalmol* 1968;79:552.
52. Korey M, Gieser D, Kass MA, Waltman SR, Gordon M, Becker B. Central corneal endothelial cell density and central corneal thickness in ocular hypertension and primary open-angle glaucoma. *Am J Ophthalmol* 1982;94:610.
53. Korey MS, Hodapp E, Kass MA, et al. Timolol and epinephrine. Long term evaluation of con-current administration. *Arch Ophthalmol* 1982;100:742.
54. Kramer SG. Bilateral epinephrine uptake in drops to one eye. *Invest Ophthalmol* 1977;16(ARVO Suppl):125.
55. Kramer SG. Considerations on epinephrine therapy in glaucoma. *Ann Ophthalmol* 1978;10:1077.
56. Kramer SG. Aphakic eyes. *Trans Am Ophthalmol Soc* 1980;78:947.
57. Krejci L, Harrison R. Corneal pigment deposits from topically administered epinephrine experimental production. *Arch Ophthalmol* 1969;82:836.
58. Krieglstein GK, Leydhecker W. The dose-response relationships of dipvalyl epinephrine in open-angle glaucoma. *Graefes Arch Clin Exp Ophthalmol* 1978;205:141.
59. Krimensen EB, Norn MS. Benign mucous membrane pemphigoid. 1. Secretion of mucus and tears. *Acta Ophthal* 1974;52:266.
60. Kupfer C, Gaasterland D, Ross K. Studies of aqueous humor dynamics in man. II. Measurements in young normal subjects using acetazolamide and lepinephrine. *Invest Ophthalmol* 1971;10: 523.
61. Kwon BS, Gangarosa LP, Burch KD, deBack J, Hill JM. Induction of ocular herpes simplex virus shedding by iontophoresis of epinephrine into rabbit cornea. *Invest Ophthalmol Vis Sci* 1981;21:442.
62. Laibson PR, Kibreck S. Reactivation of herpetic keratitis by epinephrine in rabbit. *Arch Ophthalmol* 1966;75:254.
63. Langham ME, Diggs E. Beta-adrenergic responses in the eyes of rabbits, primates and man. *Exp Eye Res* 1974;19:281.
64. Langham ME, Krieglstein GK. Biphasic intraocular response of conscious rabbits to epinephrine. *Invest Ophthalmol* 1976;15:119.
65. Lee DA, Brubaker RF, Nagataki S. Acute effects of thymoxamine on aqueous humor formation in the epinephrine treated normal eye as measured by flurophotometry. *Invest Ophthalmol Vis Sci* 1983; 24:165.
66. Levine RA. Ocular pigmentation due to topical epinephrine: review and case report. *Ophthalmol Dig* 1973;34.
67. Liesegang TJ. Bulbar conjunctival follicles associated with dipivefrin therapy. *Ophthalmology* 1985;92:228.
68. Mackool RJ, Muldoon T, Fortier A, Nilsen D. Epinephrine-induced cystoid macular edema in aphakic eyes. *Arch Ophthalmol* 1977; 95:791.
69. Madge GE, Geeraets WJ, Guerry DP III. Black cornea secondary to topical epinephrine. *Am J Ophthalmol* 1971;71:402.
70. Mandell AL, Stentz F, Kitabchi AE. Dipivalyl epinephrine: a new pro-drug in the treatment of glaucoma. *Ophthalmology* 1978;85: 268.
71. Michaels RG, Maumenee AE. Cystoid macular edema associated with topical applied epinephrine in aphakic eyes. *Am J Ophthalmol* 1975;80:379.
72. Miller D, Brooks SM, Mobilia E. Adrenochrome staining of soft contact lenses. *Ann Ophthalmol* 1976;8:65.
73. Mindel JS. Who, what, where, when and how. *Ann Ophthalmol* 1982;14:10.
74. Mindel JS, Yablonski ME, Tavitian HO, Podos SM, Orellana J. Dipivefrin and echothiophate: efficacy of combined use in humans. *Arch Ophthalmol* 1981;99:1583.
75. Mishima H, Bausher L, Sears M, Cochu M, Ono H, Gregory D. Fine structured studies of ciliary processes after treatment with cholera toxin or its B subunit. *Graefes Arch Clin Exp Ophthalmol* 1982;219: 272.
76. Miyake K, Miyake Y, Kuratomi R. Long-term effects of topically applied epinephrine on the blood-ocular barrier in humans. *Arch Ophthalmol* 1984;105:1360.
77. Miyake K, Shirasawa E, Hikita M, Miyake Y, Kuratomi R. Synthesis of prostaglandin E in rabbit eyes with topical epinephrine. *Invest Ophthalmol Vis Sci* 1988;29:332.
78. Miyake K, Shirasawa E, Hikita M. Active transport system of prostaglandins: Clinical implications and considerations. *J Cataract Refract Surg* 1992;18:100.
79. Nagataki S. Effects of adrenergic drugs on aqueous humor dynamics in man. *Acta Soc Ophthalmol Jpn* 1977;81:1795.
80. Nagataki S, Brubaker RF. Early effect of epinephrine on aqueous formation in the normal human eye. *Ophthalmology* 1981;88:278.
81. Neufeld AH, Jampol LM, Sears ML. Cyclic-AMP in the aqueous humor: the effects of adrenergic agents. *Exp Eye Res* 1972;14: 242.
82. Neufeld AH, Page ED. In vitro determination of the ability of drugs to bind to adrenergic receptors. *Invest Ophthalmol Vis Sci* 1979;16: 1118.
83. Neufeld AH, Sears ML. Adenosine 3′-5′-monophosphate analogue increases the outflow facility of the primate eye. *Invest Ophthalmol Vis Sci* 1975;14:688.
84. Newton MJ, Nesburn AB. Lack of hydrophilic lens discoloration in patients using dipivalyl epinephrine for glaucoma. *Am J Ophthalmol* 1979;87:193.
85. Nielsen NV, Eriksen JS. Timolol in maintenance treatment of ocular hypertension and glaucoma. *Acta Ophthal* 1979;57:1070.
86. Norm MS. Pemphigoid related to epinephrine treatment. *Am J Ophthalmol* 1977;83:138.
87. Ober M, Scharrer A. The effect of timolol and dipivalyl-epinephrine in the treatment of the elevated intraocular pressure. *Graefe's Arch Clin Exp Ophthalmol* 1980;213:273.
88. Ohrstrom A, Kattstrom O. Interaction of timolol and adrenaline. *Br J Ophthal* 1981;65:53.
89. Ohrstrom A, Pandolfi M. Regulations of intraocular pressure and pupil size by beta-blockers and epinephrine. *Arch Ophthal* 1980;98: 2182.
90. Ostbaum SA, Galin MA, Poole TA. Topical epinephrine and cystoid macular edema. *Ann Ophthalmol* 1976;8:455.
91. Ostbaum SA, Kolker AE, Phelps CD. Low-dose epinephrine. *Arch Ophthalmol* 1974;92:1181.
92. Palmberg PF, Hajak S, Cooper D, Becker B. Increased cellular responsiveness to epinephrine in primary open-angle glaucoma. *Arch Ophthalmol* 1977;95:855.
93. Pardos GJ, Krachmer JJ, Mannis MJ. Persistent corneal erosion secondary to tarsal adrenochrome deposit. *Am J Ophthalmol* 1980;90: 870.
94. Potter DE, Rowland JM. Adrenergic drugs and intraocular pressure: effects of selective beta-adrenergic agonists. *Exp Eye Res* 1978;27: 615.
95. Reinecke RD, Kuwabara T. Corneal deposits secondary to topical epinephrine. *Arch Ophthalmol* 1963;70:170.
96. Robinson JC, Kaufman PL. Effects and interactions of epinephrine, norepinephrine, timolol, and betaxolol on outflow facility in the cynomolgus monkey. *Am J Ophthal* 1990;109:189.
97. Romano A, Barishak R, Stein R. Obstruction of lacrimal puncta caused by topical epinephrine. *Ophthalmologica* 1973;166:301.
98. Schenker HE, Yablonski ME, Podos SM, Kinder L. Fluorophotometric study of epinephrine and timolol in human subjects. *Arch Ophthal* 1981;99:1212.
99. Sears M, Caprioli J, Kondo K, Bauscher L. A mechanism for the control of aqueous humor formation. In: Drance SM, Neufeld AH, eds. *Glaucoma: Applied Pharmacology in Medical Treatment.* New York: Grune and Stratton, 1984;303–324.
100. Sears ML, Mead A. A major pathway for the regulation of intraocular pressure. *Int Ophthalmol* 1983;6:201.
101. Sears ML, Neufeld AH. Adrenergic modulation of the outflow of aqueous humor. *Invest Ophthalmol* 1975;14:83.
102. Shenker HI, Yablonski ME, Podos SM, Linder L. Fluorophotometric study of epinephrine and timolol in human subjects. *Arch Ophthalmol* 1981;99:1212.
103. Shin DH, Tsai CS, Parrow KA, Bsee CK, Wan JY, Shi DX. Intraocular pressure-dependent retinal vascular changes in adult chronic open-angle glaucoma patients. *Ophthalmology* 1991;98:1087.
104. Smith RJ, Nagasubramanian S, Watkins R, Poinoosawmy D. Addition of timolol maleate to routine medical therapy: a clinical trial. *Br J Ophthalmol* 1980;64:779.
105. Soong HK, McKenney MJ, Wolter JR. Adrenochrome staining of senile plaque resembling malignant melanoma. *Am J Ophthalmol* 1986;101:380.

106. Spaeth GL. Nasolacrimal duct obstruction caused by topical epinephrine. *Arch Ophthalmol* 1967;77:355.
107. Sugar J. Adrenochrome pigmentation of hydrophilic lenses. *Arch Ophthalmol* 1974;91:11.
108. Theodore JA, Leibowitz HM. External ocular toxicity of dipivalyl epinephrine. *Am J Ophthalmol* 1979;88:1013.
109. Thomas JV, Epstein DL. Study of the additive effect of timolol and epinephrine in lowering intraocular pressure. *Br J Ophthalmol* 1981;65:596.
110. Thomas JV, Epstein DL. Timolol and epinephrine in primary open angle glaucoma: transient additive effect. *Arch Ophthalmol* 1981; 99:91.
111. Thomas JV, Epstein DL. Transient additive effect of timolol and epinephrine in primary open angle glaucoma. *Arch Ophthalmol* 1981; 99:91.
112. Thomas JV, Gragoudas ES, Blaire NP, Lapus JV. Correlation of epinephrine use and macular edema in aphakic glaucomatous eyes. *Arch Ophthalmol* 1978;96:625.
113. Townsend DJ, Brubaker RF. Immediate effect of epinephrine on aqueous formation in the normal human eye as measured by fluorophotometry. *Invest Ophthalmol Vis Sci* 1980;19:256.
114. Tripathi BJ, Tripathi RC. Effect of epinephrine in vitro on the morphology, phagocytosis, and mitotic activity of human trabecular endothelium. *Exp Eye Res* 1984;39:731.
115. Ueno K. The effect of beta and alpha adrenergic drugs on the ciliary body of the rabbit eye: an electron microscopic study. *Folia Ophthalmol Jpn* 1976;27:1012.
116. Veirs ER, McGrew JC. Ocular complications from topical epinephrine therapy of glaucoma. *EENT Monthly* 1963;42:46.
117. Waltman SR, Yarian D, Hart W Jr, Becker B. Corneal endothelial changes with long-term topical epinephrine therapy. *Arch Ophthalmol* 1977;95:1357.
118. Wandel T, Spinak M. Toxicity of dipivalyl epinephrine. *Ophthalmology* 1981;88:259.
119. Weekers R, Delmarcelle Y, Gustin J. Treatment of ocular hypertension by adrenalin and diverse sympathomimetic amines. *Am J Ophthalmol* 1955;40:666.
120. Weekers R, Prijot E, Gustin J. Measure de la resistance a l'ecoulement de l'humeur aqueuse au moyen du tonometre electronique. 6. Mode d'action de l'adrenaline dans le glaucome chronique. *Ophthalmologica* 1954;128:312.
121. Weekers R, Prijot E, Gustin J. Recent advances and future prospects in the medical treatment of ocular hypertension. *Br J Ophthalmol* 1954;38:742.
122. Wei CP, Anderson JA, Leopold I. Ocular absorption and metabolism of topically applied epinephrine and a dipivalyl ester of epinephrine. *Invest Ophthalmol Vis Sci* 1978;17:315.
123. Wilke K. Early effects of epinephrine and pilocarpine on the intraocular pressure and the episcleral venous pressure in the normal human eye. *Acta Ophthalmol (Scand)* 1974;52:231.
124. Yablonski ME, Shin DH, Kolker AE, Kass MA, Becker B. Dipivefrin use in patients with intolerance to topically applied epinephrine. *Arch Ophthalmol* 1977;95:215.

Textbook of Ocular Pharmacology,
edited by T.J. Zimmerman, et al.
Lippincott–Raven Publishers, Philadelphia © 1997.

CHAPTER 21

Alpha-2 Agonists in Glaucoma Therapy

Mark S. Juzych, Alan L. Robin, and Gary D. Novack

In 1948 Ahlquist first recognized the distinct physiological actions of two classes of adrenergic receptors: alpha (α)-receptors and beta (β)-receptors (1). Over the next 20 years, α- and β-receptors were further subclassified. Scientists classified α-receptors into α_1- and α_2-receptors primarily on the basis of their physiological function and anatomical location within the synaptic cleft, either presynaptic or postsynaptic. With the increasing sophistication of receptor localization in recent years, α_2-adrenoceptors have been further subdivided into at least four subtypes. The α_2 receptors are found predominantly presynaptically but also may be found postsynaptically. Interestingly, these receptors were also discovered on platelets and smooth-muscle cells (2). In the eye, α_2-receptors are the predominant receptor in the iris and ciliary body (3). Stimulation of these receptors causes a number of different physiological responses, depending on the tissue: lowering of blood pressure, lowering of intraocular pressure (IOP), platelet aggregation, sedation, growth hormone release, water and electrolyte reabsorption in the intestines, inhibition of insulin release, lipolysis, and renin release (4,5).

Recognizing the potential to lower IOP by manipulating adrenergic receptors, ocular pharmacologists developed various pharmaceuticals with applications in the treatment of glaucoma. It was discovered that aqueous humor production can be decreased by blocking β-adrenergic receptors with an antagonist (6). Stimulation of both α- and β-adrenergic receptors with an agonist also lowers IOP through other mechanisms of action. For many years, epinephrine, which is both an α- and β-agonist, was the only agonist, or sympathomimetic drug, used in the treatment of glaucoma. In recent years, a new class of sympathomimetic drugs, α_2-adrenoceptor agonists, has been introduced for glaucoma management.

M. S. Juzych: Department of Ophthalmology, Kresge Eye Institute, Wayne State University, Detroit, Michigan 48201.

A. L. Robin: Johns Hopkins University and University of Maryland Schools of Medicine, Baltimore, Maryland 21209.

G. D. Novack: PharmaLogic Development, Inc., San Rafael, California 94903.

CLONIDINE

Clonidine was the first relatively selective α_2-agonist with clinical application in ophthalmology. Chemically, it is classified as an imidazoline. In the 1960s, it was evaluated as a nasal decongestant because of its ability to cause vasoconstriction of the nasal mucosa. In clinical trials, however, clonidine caused orthostatic hypotension and a significant decrease in mean resting blood pressure. After observing this cardiovascular effect, researchers began developing clonidine for the treatment of essential hypertension. Oral clonidine (Catapress) has been available as an antihypertensive medication for more than a decade.

The mechanism of action for the decrease in blood pressure is mediated through the central nervous system (CNS). After being systemically absorbed, clonidine, a lipophilic drug, readily passes through the blood–brain barrier and stimulates presynaptic α_2-receptors in the brainstem. These receptors in the vasomotor center then inhibit central sympathetic activity, resulting in peripheral vasodilatation, and consequently produce systemic hypotension.

In 1966 it was noted that administration of intravenous clonidine caused a decrease in IOP (7). A few years later, it was reported that topical clonidine resulted in the same effect (7). Since then, topical clonidine 0.25% and 0.5% has been found to lower IOP effectively (8–10). In the original studies, in which only a single drop of clonidine was applied, there was no significant change in blood pressure. When given repeatedly for 1 week, however, it markedly lowered systemic blood pressure (8,9).

In addition to its cardiovascular side effects, concern arose over the possibility that clonidine caused a decrease in blood flow to the optic nerve. In part, this concern was caused by a small number of articles involving animal studies. Heilmann demonstrated that a decrease in ophthalmic artery pressure could occur in eyes with elevated IOP that received topical clonidine 0.05% and 0.25% (11). In retrospect, although historically excellent articles, these studies were limited in their generalization by their design. Additionally, other investigators found no change in ophthalmic artery pressure in normal volunteers receiving clonidine 0.25% (12). Nevertheless, topical clonidine hydrochloride (Isoglaucon) 0.125%, 0.25%, and 0.5% has been available in Europe in a three-times-daily dosing regimen. The 0.125 solution appears to be safer than the other higher concentrations. Concern over the systemic side effects of topical clonidine has led to the development of other α_2-agonists, specifically apraclonidine and brimonidine, which would decrease IOP without influencing blood pressure.

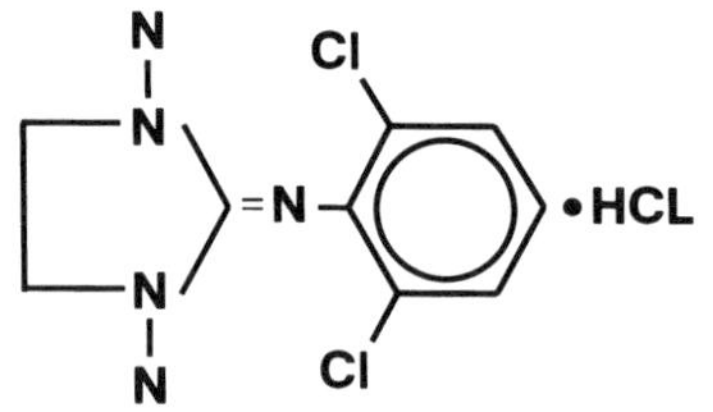

APRACLONIDINE

The official drug name is apraclonidine hydrochloride; the trade name, Iopidine; and the trivial names, aplonidine hydrochloride, ALO 2145. Apraclonidine's chemical name is 2-[(4-amino-2,6 dichlorophenyl) imino]imididazoline monohydrochloride, and the molecular formula is $C_9H_{11}Cl_3N_4$. Its molecular weight is 281.6.

Apraclonidine comes in two strengths. Apraclonidine 0.5% is supplied in 5 and 10 ml, and apraclonidine 1% is supplied in 0.1 ml in a plastic dispensor, packaged two per foil pouch.

Pharmacology

Apraclonidine hydrochloride is a relatively selective α_2-adrenergic agonist. It is an imidazoline derivative that differs from clonidine (Fig. 21-1) by the addition of an amide group (-NH_2) at the C_4 (paraposition) of the benzene ring (Fig. 21-2). This amide group results in a highly ionized molecule at physiological pH (96.4% versus clonidine 71.5%) with a PKa of 9.2. The increased polarity of apraclonidine limits its penetration through the blood–brain barrier, theoretically decreasing unwanted CNS side effects. In contrast to clonidine, whose lipophilicity facilitates penetration through the cornea, apraclonidine's polarity slows penetration through the cornea and decreases its bioavailability to the ciliary body. Research has suggested that, although corneal penetration is the major pathway for apraclonidine into the aqueous humor, the primary route of delivery of apraclonidine to the ciliary body is through the conjunctiva and sclera. This route of delivery accounted for 65% of intraocular absorption in rabbits (13). The significance is that it is the ciliary body that may be the major target tissue for the drug; this is yet to be confirmed in other studies.

Apraclonidine is an effective ocular hypotensive agent. Within 1 hour of drop instillation, IOP decreases significantly, lasting for at least 12 hours. The maximal effect is observed between 3 and 5 hours after dosing. At peak effect, apraclonidine 1% lowers IOP by 30% to 40% compared with baseline and at trough 20 to 30% (14,15). In dose-response studies comparing 0.125%, 0.25%, 0.5%, and 1.0%, either 0.25% or 0.5% appear to be at the top of the dose-response curve for the reduction of IOP (16,17). Recently, it was also suggested that uveoscleral outflow may account for some of the decrease in IOP.

N Cl N =N •HCL N N Cl

FIG. 21-1. Structural formula of clonidine.

Mechanism of Action

Apraclonidine primarily lowers IOP by decreasing the production of aqueous humor without altering aqueous outflow as measured by tonography (14,18–20). Using fluorophotometry, Gharagozolo demonstrated a reduction in aqueous flow by 35% in normal volunteers at 4 hours, which corresponds to the maximal effect seen clinically (19).

The principal site of action of apraclonidine is probably at the sympathetic nerve-ciliary body junction; however, the complete cellular mechanism is not yet fully understood. Normally, an action potential arrives at an adrenergic synapse, causing the release of norepinephrine from synaptic vesicles into the synaptic cleft. Norepinephrine then diffuses across the synapse to bind with the postsynaptic receptors (21,22). At the ciliary body, these postsynaptic receptors are predominantly β_2-adrenoceptors, which are coupled to G_S proteins that stimulate adenylate cyclase (23). As a result, cyclic adenosine monophosphate (cAMP) levels are increased, stimulating formation of aqueous humor.

It is believed that the reduction in aqueous humor production by apraclonidine is mediated through α_2 receptors. The α_2-receptors are located on the presynaptic sympa-

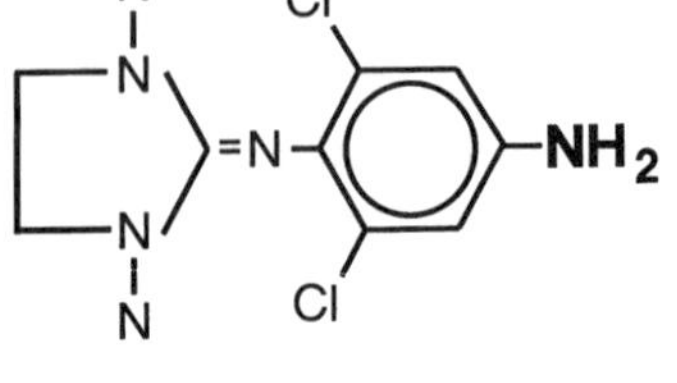

N Cl N =N NH_2 N N Cl

FIG. 21-2. Structural formula of apraclonidine.

thetic nerve terminal, where they modulate neurotransmitter release. They are also located postjunctionally in the ciliary body, where they can inhibit cellular response to neurotransmitters. It appears that α_2-agonists, such as clonidine, apraclonidine, and brimonidine, may bind to both presynaptic and postsynaptic receptors. Activation of presynaptic α_2 receptors inhibits neurotransmitter release when the sympathetic nerve is stimulated. This activation decreases the amount of norepinephrine that is released and was destined for postsynaptic β-receptors on the ciliary epithelium (22). The net effect is a decrease in aqueous humor production.

Activation of the postsynaptic ciliary body α_2-receptor, which is coupled to a G_i protein, reduces production of intracellular cAMP by suppressing the activity of adenylate cyclase (23). This reduced accumulation of intracellular cAMP also decreases aqueous humor production. In addition to decreasing cAMP by stimulating G_i protein, the activated postsynaptic α_2-receptor has also been discovered to stimulate the Ca^{++}-dependent protein kinase C pathway. Regardless of the initiating event, it appears that the final common pathway of the postsynaptic-mediated cascade is an inhibition of chloride secretion. Although the process is poorly understood, the decreased secretion affects the cell's ability to respond to the binding of a neurotransmitter to its postsynaptic β-receptor (24,25).

A new receptor, the imidazoline-preferring receptor, has been localized (26). This receptor is distinct from the α_2 receptor and can be further subclassified to I_1 and I_2; however, many α_2 agonists bind not only to both presynaptic and postsynaptic α_2 receptors but also to the various subclasses of imidazoline receptors. Currently, it is not known which of these receptors is responsible for mediating the lowering of IOP in response to the α_2-agonist.

Although it is unlikely, apraclonidine may also lower IOP by affecting ocular blood flow. Although apraclonidine is predominantly an α_2-agonist, at higher concentrations, it can also stimulate α_1-adrenoceptors. Stimulation of α_1-receptors causes vasoconstriction by contraction of smooth muscle in blood vessels. The vasoconstriction then may reduce the blood flow to the ciliary body and decrease production of the aqueous humor (27). Jin et al., however, found that lofexidine, an α_2-agonist, also lowers IOP but does not decrease blood flow to the ciliary body (28).

Another proposed mechanism by which apraclonidine lowers IOP is a decrease in episcleral venous pressure. Kriegelstein et al. found a significant decrease in episcleral venous pressure, up to a maximum decrease of 4 mm Hg, in subjects treated with clonidine (12). As further indirect evidence, in one study >50% of normal volunteers taking apraclonidine 0.5% had an IOP below the normal mean episcleral venous pressure of 10 mm Hg (16). The reduction in episcleral venous pressure is possibly linked to reduced blood flow to the limbal area. Limbal blood flow is known to be reduced with clonidine (29,30).

Previously, it was postulated that the decrease in IOP may have been mediated through the release of endogenous prostaglandins (31,32); however, this early work in animals was not supported in human clinical trials, where it was shown that pretreatment with flurbiprofen, a prostaglandin inhibitor, did not blunt the decrease of aqueous humor (33–35). Flurbiprofen is a weak prostaglandin inhibitor and only inhibits cyclooxygenase, however.

Side Effects

Systemic

Although rare, the most common nonocular side effects of apraclonidine are a sensation of dry mouth or dry nose or both; these effects are not unexpected considering that clonidine was first introduced as a nasal decongestant, probably as a result of the direct absorption of apraclonidine through the nasolacrimal system, which causes vasoconstriction of the nasal and oral mucosa. The symptoms appear to be dose related and decrease in severity over time. They appear in about 20% of patients using apraclonidine 0.5% and in only 5% of patients using 0.25% and 0.125% (17). Although no studies have evaluated it, these symptoms may be minimized by nasolacrimal occlusion or forced eyelid closure.

As mentioned previously, one of the advantages of apraclonidine is the reduction of centrally mediated side effects because of its reduced ability to cross the blood–brain barrier. Mild sedation is a frequent complaint of persons using systemic clonidine. In contrast, in a dose-response study of apraclonidine 0.125%, 0.25%, and 0.5%, the occurrence of fatigue in patients ranged from 0% to 10% (17); however, in double-masked studies, the frequency of fatigue was not any greater compared with placebo (14,16).

Either topical beta-blockers or clonidine can produce systemic hypotension and bradycardia, whereas apraclonidine has minimal adverse cardiovascular side effects. It apparently does not effect either the mean resting heart rate or mean arterial blood pressure (15,17,36,37). Additionally, apraclonidine has minimal effect on exercise-induced heart rate in normal healthy volunteers (38), whereas topical 0.5% timolol significantly decreases exercise-induced heart rate (39); however, there has been a case report of a patient experiencing chest tightness and near syncope after instillation of apraclonidine before argon laser iridotomy (40). Apraclonidine has now been available for 3 years. There have been no reports linking it conclusively to any commonly observed adverse systemic side effects. This is an extremely safe drug outside of topical allergy.

Ocular Side Effects

The most common ocular side effects of apraclonidine include conjunctival blanching, lid retraction, and mydriasis. These effects are suggestive of α_1-adrenoceptor stimulation. Conjunctival blanching occurs most commonly and is found in 85% of patients (14).

Eyelid retraction occurred in at least 50% of normal volunteers and is most noticeable with unilateral therapy because of the asymmetry (14). It begins within minutes and is maximal 3 to 5 hours after instillation of a drop. The mean interpalpebral fissure increased 1.4 mm (17). It is believed that the lid retraction is probably due to an increased sympathetic stimulation of α_1-adrenoceptors in the Müller muscle.

A small amount of mydriasis, a mean of 0.4 mm in 45% of treated eyes, occurs with apraclonidine use. It is more noticeable with unilateral treatment and is not dose related. The apraclonidine-induced mydriasis is less than that associated with dipivefrin. The mydriasis is not sufficient to cause pupillary block in an eye with occludable angles (41,42).

The most troublesome side effect of chronic use of apraclonidine appears to be an allergic-type (to toxic) blepharoconjunctivitis and dermatitis, similar to that seen with epinephrine and dipivefrin (43). The periorbital region of an affected patient becomes erythematous and edematous with the skin becoming scaly. Symptoms have been reported within 9 hours of starting apraclonidine therapy (14), but typically the reaction occurs weeks or months after initiation. The typical patient presents complaining of red, itchy eyes after being placed on chronic apraclonidine therapy. The follicular conjunctivitis clears 3 to 5 days after cessation of the medication without the need of additional treatment. The percentage of persons developing the allergy varies, averaging about 20% and increasing to nearly 50% with longer use. In one 3-month study, there was a higher incidence of ocular allergy with apraclonidine 0.5% (36%) than with apraclonidine 0.25% (9%) (44). With a twice-daily rather than a three-times-daily dosing schedule, the number of patients developing the allergy decreased to 9% (45). Thus, decreasing the concentration and dosing schedule decreases the frequency of ocular allergy.

With the increasing use of apraclonidine, one potential side effect that has been of particular interest and debate is apraclonidine's effect on ocular hemodynamics. Ralli and Bill and Heilman showed that clonidine reduces blood flow to both the anterior and posterior segments of monkey and cat eyes (29,30). Similar to clonidine, investigators have shown apraclonidine's vasoconstrictive activity on the anterior segment of the eye, including the conjunctiva, ciliary body, and iris (46–48). One particular study found that apraclonidine 1% decreases conjunctival oxygen tension (48). Additionally, the technique of microvascular corrosion casting suggests that apraclonidine 1% produces vasoconstriction of the uveal precapillary sphincters (27). In contrast to clonidine, however, there are no definitive data supporting the vasoconstrictive effect of apraclonidine on the posterior segment of the eye (the retina, choroid, and the optic nerve) (46,49–51). For example, acute administration of topical and intravenous apraclonidine did not affect retinal or optic-nerve blood flow measured by laser Doppler flowmetry (51).

Therapeutic Use

Anterior Segment Laser Surgery

Apraclonidine was first approved in 1987 by the U.S. Food and Drug Administration (FDA) to prevent acute rises in IOP after argon and neodymium-yttrium aluminum garnet (Nd:YAG) laser procedures of the anterior segment. Postoperative IOP elevation of greater than 10 mm Hg following 360-degree argon laser trabeculoplasty (ALT) occurs in up to 50% of patients (52,53). Apraclonidine has been shown to lower IOP and decrease the incidence of IOP spikes after ALT (42,54). The dosing regimen consisted of apraclonidine 1% instilled, both 1 hour before and then immediately after the laser procedure. In one double-masked, placebo-controlled study, none of the apraclonidine-treated eyes had a pressure spike >10 mm Hg, compared with 17.6% in the placebo-treated group (54). In another study of 260 eyes randomized to apraclonidine 1%, acetazolamide 250 mg, dipivefrin 0.1%, pilocarpine 4%, and timolol 0.5%, only 3% of the apraclonidine-treated eyes developed a IOP spike >5 mm Hg after 360-degree ALT compared with a third of the patients in each of the other treatment groups (55).

In addition to ALT, apraclonidine also decreases the incidence of IOP spikes following other anterior-segment laser procedures: Q-switched Nd:YAG capsulotomy (56,57) and argon (41) and Nd:YAG iridotomy (58); however, it is important to remind physicians that apraclonidine does not blunt all IOP spikes (59).

Chronic Medical Therapy

Apraclonidine has been evaluated in several studies as a primary ocular hypotensive agent. The first of these studies compared 0.25%, 0.5%, and 1% in a dose-response study lasting 8 days (17). The first long-term study compared apraclonidine 0.25% and 0.5% three times a day with timolol 0.5% twice a day in a 3-month double-blind study (44). All three treatment groups exhibited similar IOP lowering; however, over the 90-day study period, 36% of patients on 0.5% apraclonidine and 9% of patients on 0.25% apraclonidine developed an ocular allergy and were withdrawn from the study. In contrast, none of the timolol-treated patients developed an allergy. The risk of allergy, therefore, makes apraclonidine desirable as a first-line agent only in situations in which patients are unable to tolerate other glaucoma medications.

Another possible role for apraclonidine is as a second-line adjunctive agent. Apraclonidine is effective in further lowering IOP in patients taking β-blockers, in both short-

and long-term studies (37,60,61); however, the number of patients in these studies was small. In a well-designed 3-month study, Stewart and co-workers demonstrated that apraclonidine 0.5% twice daily can significantly lower IOP when added to timolol 0.5% (45). With the twice-daily dosing, only 9% of patients developed an allergy requiring withdrawal from the study. Thus, it appears that apraclonidine can be a good second-line medication.

In October 1993, apraclonidine 0.5% three times a day was approved by the FDA as a short-term adjunctive in patients on maximally tolerated medication. A number of preliminary studies demonstrated varying effectiveness of adding apraclonidine to glaucoma patients on maximally tolerated medication (62,63). These studies were limited by design and sample size. In a large double-masked, multicenter, parallel study, apraclonidine 0.5% three times a day given to glaucoma patients on maximally tolerated medication definitively lowered IOP compared with vehicle. At 90 days' follow-up, 61% of patients on apraclonidine avoided surgery, compared with 33.9% in the control group (64). In this study, an insignificant IOP-lowering effect was seen in eyes already on two aqueous humor suppressants; however, the numbers are minimal.

In the only known randomized, double-masked study comparing clonidine and apraclonidine, eyes treated with apraclonidine 1% had a mean IOP decrease of 34%, compared with 22% in the clonidine 0.125% group (65). In the apraclonidine group, there was no change in blood pressure and pulse, whereas in the clonidine group there was no change in pulse but a significant decrease in blood pressure. As expected, the apraclonidine-treated eyes exhibited lid retraction, conjunctival blanching, and mydriasis, which were not noted with clonidine. Interestingly, the clonidine group showed a contralateral IOP-lowering effect, which the apraclonidine group did not. This contralateral effect may be mediated through the CNS, which is accessible to clonidine but not to apraclonidine (66,67).

Intraocular Surgery

Some studies suggest the use of apraclonidine to decrease postoperative IOP spikes after intraocular surgery, but the results are inconclusive. In a study of extracapsular cataract extraction, Fry demonstrated that carbachol was the most effective agent, whereas apraclonidine was ineffective given at the end of surgical procedure (68). In another study in which apraclonidine 1% was instilled 1 hour preoperatively, apraclonidine decreased the incidence of IOP elevation (69). It is believed that preoperative apraclonidine may stabilize the vascular or epithelial structures of the ciliary body such that it responds poorly to mediators released in response to surgery. Thus, postoperative instillation of apraclonidine is ineffective because surgical trauma has already occurred with its release of inflammatory mediators. Furthermore, apraclonidine 1% used immediately before and after cataract extraction by phacoemulsification with intraocular lens implantation was shown to blunt IOP spikes. A decrease in aqueous flare was seen in patients receiving the apraclonidine treatment compared with those receiving a vehicle as a control (70). In a randomized double-blind study of extracapsular cataract extraction combined with trabeculectomy, apraclonidine 1% instilled preoperatively and postoperatively was more effective than placebo control in decreasing postoperative IOP elevations (71), but it did not totally eliminate IOP spikes. At 24 hours after surgery, 20% placebo eyes and 2% (one patient) apraclonidine-treated eyes had IOPs >40 mm Hg.

Other possible applications that have been proposed include use in vitreoretinal surgery (72) to decrease IOP elevation following cycloplegia in glaucoma patients (73) and upper-lid retraction for ptosis (74).

BRIMONIDINE

The official drug name is brimonidine tartrate; the trade name, Alphagan; trivial names, AGN 190342-LF, UK-14,304, and SK&F 190342; and chemical name, 5-bromo-6-[imidazolin-2-ylamino]-quinoxaline tartrate.

Pharmacology

Brimonidine tartrate is another relatively selective α_2-agonist, recently approved by the FDA. Structurally, it is similar to clonidine (Fig. 21-3); like clonidine, but in contrast to apraclonidine, brimonidine is a lipophilic drug (50% unionized at pH of 7.5 versus 1.7% for apraclonidine and 22% for clonidine) (13). Because of brimonidine's high lipophilicity, its major route of ocular penetration is through the cornea. In lower-order animals, it also should be more receptive to α_2-receptors than either clonidine or apraclonidine.

Brimonidine's efficacy and safety appear to be similar to apraclonidine's. Brimonidine lowers IOP in normotensive and ocular hypertensive monkeys, rabbits, and cats over a dose range of 0.001% to 1.0% (75). Like apraclonidine, it decreases aqueous humor production, up to 67%, without altering outflow (76). Twice daily administration for 5 days to glaucomatous monkey eyes reduced IOP up to 49%, with the IOP lowering lasting at least 18 hours (76). This is the rationale for brimonidine's twice-a-day dosing sched-

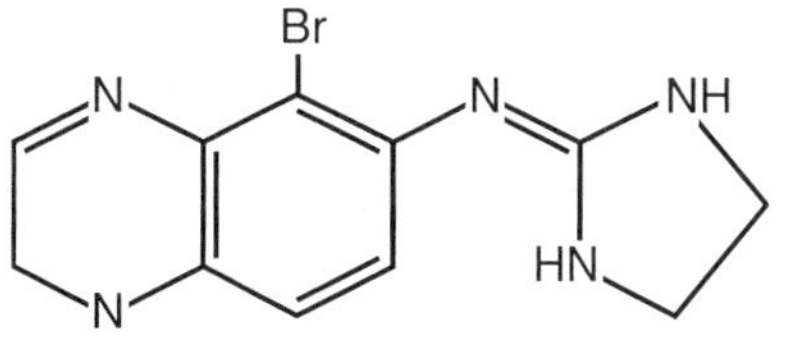

FIG. 21-3. Structural formula of brimonidine.

ule. However, it is labeled for TID use. Brimonidine appears to have a contralateral effect. Unilateral topical application significantly reduced IOP in the contralateral eye in monkeys, and this effect is believed to be mediated through the CNS.

Therapeutic Use

The first clinical trials with brimonidine in humans evaluated the efficacy of brimonidine in the prevention of acute IOP increases after trabeculoplasty. Brimonidine 0.5%, like apraclonidine, is effective in decreasing IOP elevations after argon laser trabeculoplasty (77,78). In a vehicle-controlled, double-masked multicenter study, brimonidine 0.5% was effective whether used before 360-degree ALT, after the procedure, or both before and following the trabeculoplasty. A drop, both before and after, was more effective than just one single drop; however, this difference was not apparently statistically significant enough for the FDA to grant approval of one-drop therapy. From this study, it appears that a single dose given before or after the laser procedure suffices to prevent postoperative pressure spikes (77).

In a 1-month dose-response study, brimonidine in concentrations of 0.08, 0.2, and 0.5%, in a twice-daily dosing regimen, lowered IOP in open-angle glaucoma and ocular hypertensive patients (79). The maximum IOP decrease ranged between 20% and 30%. This study concluded that brimonidine 0.2% appears to be the most effective dose because it was not only at the top of the dose response curve but also had the fewest systemic and local side effects. The 0.5% concentration was associated with problems with systemic hypotension and CNS effect. In a preliminary study, brimonidine, like apraclonidine, effectively lowered IOP in glaucoma patients on maximally tolerated medical therapy (80).

Side Effects

The most frequent side effects reported with brimonidine are dry mouth, conjunctival blanching, and fatigue or drowsiness. These side effects appear to be dose related. The dry mouth and conjunctival blanching are α_1-receptor-mediated side effects similar to those experienced with apraclonidine. Chronic use of apraclonidine is associated with an allergic follicular conjunctivitis. In chronic, 1-year studies, the allergic rate is about 10%. This allergy appears to be different from that associated with apraclonidine. It occurs later than in eyes with apraclonidine allergy.

Brimonidine, like clonidine, is a highly lipophilic drug possessing the ability to pass through the blood–brain barrier and causes central nervous side effects. Complaints of fatigue and drowsiness, both centrally mediated symptoms, appear to be higher with brimonidine, ranging from 4% to 29%, compared with apraclonidine, a less lipophilic drug. Another potential concern with brimonidine is the systemic hypotension that was noted with topical clonidine. Nordlund and co-workers demonstrated the cardiopulmonary safety of single-dose brimonidine 0.2% in young, healthy males (81). In this study, there were no significant changes in heart rate, and the cardiovascular effects were limited to a slight reduction in systolic blood pressure during recovery from exercise. In the study evaluating brimonidine during laser trabeculoplasty, brimonidine 0.5% had minimal effects and systolic and diastolic blood pressure (77); however, in the 1-month dose-response study, brimonidine did significantly lower blood pressure, but clinical adverse effects were not seen (79). With multiple dosing, it appears that brimonidine causes less hypotension than clonidine but greater than that observed with apraclonidine.

REFERENCES

1. Alhquist RP. A study of adenotropic receptors. *Am J Physiol* 1948;153:586–599.
2. Hoffmann BB, Lefkowitz RJ. Alpha-adrenergic receptor subtypes. *N Engl J Med* 1980;302:1390–1396.
3. Matsuo T, Cynader MS. Localization of alpha-2 adrenergic receptors in the eye. *Ophthalmic Res* 1992;24:213–219.
4. Alabaster V, Davey M. Effects of the sympathetic nervous system and catecholamines. *J Cardiovasc Pharmacol* 1984;3:365–376.
5. McGrath JC. Evidence for more than one type of postjunctional alpha adrenoreceptor. *Biochem Pharmacol* 1982;31:467–475.
6. Zimmerman TJ, Kaufman HE. Timolol, a beta-adrenergic blocking agent for the treatment of glaucoma. *Arch Ophthalmol* 1977;95: 601–604.
7. Hasslinger R. Catapres: a new drug lowering intraocular pressure. *Klin Montasbl Augenheilkd* 1969;154:95–105.
8. Hodapp E, Kolker AE, Kass MA, Goldberg I, Becker B, Gordon M. The effect of topical clonidine on intraocular pressure. *Arch Ophthalmol* 1981;99:1208–1211.
9. Harrison R, Kaufmann CS. Clonidine: effects of a topically administered solution on intraocular pressure and blood pressure in open-angle glaucoma. *Arch Ophthalmol* 1977;95:1368–1373.
10. Heilmann K. Clonidine in glaucoma therapy—inferences for therapy and obvious problems. *Buch Augenarzt* 1974;63:56–59.
11. Heilmann K. Studies on the effect of Catapress on intraocular pressure. *Klin Montasbl Augenheilkd* 1972;161:425–430.
12. Kriegelstein GK, Langham ME, Leydhecker W. The peripheral and central neural actions of clonidine in normal and glaucomatous eyes. *Invest Ophthalmol Vis Sci* 1978;17:149–158.
13. Chien DS, Homsy JJ, Gluchowski C, Tang-Liu DD. Corneal and conjunctival/scleral penetration of p-aminoclonidine, AGN 190342, and clonidine in rabbit eyes. *Curr Eye Res* 1990;9:1051–1059.
14. Robin AL. Short-term effects of unilateral 1% apraclonidine therapy. *Arch Ophthalmol* 1988;106:912–915.
15. Abrams DA, Robin AL, Pollack IP, DeFaller JM, DeSantis L. The safety and efficacy of topical 1% ALO 2145 (*p*-Aminoclonidine hydrochloride) in normal volunteers. *Arch Ophthalmol* 1987;105:1205–1207.
16. Abrams DA, Robin AL, Crandall AS, et al. A limited comparison of apraclonidine's dose response in subjects with normal or increased intraocular pressure. *Am J Ophthalmol* 1989;108:230–237.
17. Jampel HD, Robin AL, Quigley HA, Pollack IP. Apraclonidine: a one-week dose-response study. *Arch Ophthalmol* 1988;106:1069–1073.
18. Lee DA, Topper JE, Brubaker RF. Effect of clonidine on aqueous humor flow in normal human eyes. *Exp Eye Res* 1984;38:239–246.
19. Gharagozloo NZ, Relf SJ, Brubaker RF. Aqueous flow is reduced by the alpha-2 adrenergic agonist, apraclonidine hydrochloride (ALO 2145). *Ophthalmology* 1988;95:1217–1220.

20. Kaufman PL, Gabelt B. Alpha-adrenergic agonist effects on aqueous humor dynamics. *J Glaucoma* 1995;4(suppl):S8–S14.
21. Leopold IH, Potter DE, Duzman E, Novack GD. Pharmacology of ocular catecholamines. In: Tasman W, Jaeger EA, eds. *Biomedical Foundations of Ophthalmology.* Philadelphia: Harper and Row, 1988; 1–34.
22. Langer SZ. Presynaptic receptors and the regulation of transmitter release in the peripheral and central nervous system. Sixth Gaddum Memorial Lecture. *Br J Pharmacol* 1977;60:481–497.
23. Kobilka BK, Kobilka TS, Daniel K, Regan JW, Caron MG, Lefkowitz RJ. Chimeric α2-, β2-adrenergic receptors: delineation of domains involved in effector coupling and ligand binding specificity. *Science* 1989;240:1310–1316.
24. Marshall WS, Bryson SE, Garg D. Alpha 2-adrenergic inhibition of Cl-transport by opercular epithelium is mediated by intracellular Ca2+. *Proc Natl Acad Sci U S A* 1993;90:5504–5508.
25. Warhurst G, Turnberg LA, Higgs NB, Tonge AJG, Fogg KE. Multiple G-protein-dependent pathways mediate the antisecretory effects of somatostatin and clonidine in the HT29-19A colonic cell line. *J Clin Invest* 1993;92:603–611.
26. Lehmann J, Koenig-Berard E, Vitou P. The imidazoline preferring receptor. *Life Sci* 1989;14:1690–1715.
27. Van Buskirk EM, Bacon DR, Fahrenbach WH. Ciliary vasoconstriction after topical adrenergic drugs. *Am J Ophthalmol* 1990;109:511–517.
28. Jin V, Verstappen A, Elko E, Cammarata P, Yorio T. Effect of lofexidine, an alpha 2-adrenoceptor agonist, on ocular blood flow and ion transport of rabbit iris-ciliary body. *J Ocul Pharmacol* 1992;8:23–33.
29. Ralli R. Clonidine effect on the intraocular pressure and eye circulation. *Acta Ophthalmologica* 1975;125:37.
30. Bill A, Heilman K. Ocular effects of clonidine in cats and monkeys (*Macaca irus*). *Exp Eye Res* 1978;21:481–488.
31. Camras CB, Podos SM, Rosenthal JS, Lee PY, Severin CH. Multiple dosing of prostaglandin F2 alpha or epinephrine on cynomolgus monkey eyes. I. Aqueous humor dynamics. *Invest Ophthalmol Vis Sci* 1987;28:463–469.
32. Camras CB, Bhuyan KC, Podos SM, Bhuyan DK, Master RW. Multiple dosing of prostaglandin F2 alpha or epinephrine on cynomolgus monkey eyes. II. Slit-lamp biomicroscopy, aqueous humor analysis, and fluorescein angiography. *Invest Ophthalmol Vis Sci* 1987;28: 921–926.
33. Siegel MJ, Camras CB, Lustgarten JS, Podos SM. Effect of flurbiprofen on the reduction of intraocular pressure after administration of 1% apraclonidine in patients with glaucoma. *Arch Ophthalmol* 1992;110: 598–599.
34. McCannel C, Koskela T, Brubaker RF. Topical flurbiprofen pretreatment does not block apraclonidine's effect on aqueous flow in humans. *Arch Ophthalmol* 1991;109:810–811.
35. Sulewski ME, Robin AL, Cummings HL, Arkin LM. Effects of topical flurbiprofen on the intraocular pressure lowering effects of apraclonidine and timolol. *Arch Ophthalmol* 1991;109:807–809.
36. Hernandez Y, Hernandez H, Cervantes R, et al. Cardiovascular effects of topical glaucoma therapies in normal subjects. *J Toxicol Cutaneous Ocul Toxicol* 1983;2:99–106.
37. Morrison JC, Robin AL. Adjunctive glaucoma therapy: a comparison of apraclonidine to dipivefrin when added to timolol maleate. *Ophthalmology* 1989;96:3–7.
38. Robin AL, Coleman AL. Apraclonidine hydrochloride: an evaluation of plasma concentrations, and a comparison of its intraocular pressure lowering and cardiovascular effects to timolol maleate. *Trans Am Ophthalmol Soc* 1990;88:149–162.
39. Doyle WJ, Weber PA, Meeks RH. Effect of topical timolol maleate on exercise performance. *Arch Ophthalmol* 1984;102:1517–1518.
40. King MH, Richards DW. Near syncope and chest tightness after administration of apraclonidine before argon laser iridotomy. *Am J Ophthalmol* 1990;110:308–309.
41. Robin AL, Pollack IP, DeFaller JM. Effects of topical ALO 2145 (*p*-aminoclonidine hydrochloride) on the acute intraocular pressure rise after argon laser iridotomy. *Arch Ophthalmol* 1987;105:1208–1211.
42. Brown RH, Stewart RH, Lynch MG, et al. ALO 2145 reduces the intraocular pressure elevation after anterior segment laser surgery. *Ophthalmology* 1988;95:378–384.
43. Wilkerson M, Lewis RA, Shields MB. Follicular conjunctivitis associated with apraclonidine. *Am J Ophthalmol* 1991;111:105–106.
44. Nagasubramanian S, Hitchings RA, Demailly P, et al. Comparison of apraclonidine and timolol in chronic open-angle glaucoma. *Ophthalmology* 1993;100:1318–1323.
45. Stewart WC, Ritch R, Shin DH, et al. The efficacy of apraclonidine as an adjunct to timolol therapy. *Arch Ophthalmol* 1995;113:287–292.
46. Chandler ML, DeSantis L. Studies of *p*-amino clonidine as a potential antiglaucoma agent. *Invest Ophthalmol Vis Sci* 1985;26(suppl): 227.
47. Fahrenbach WH, Bacon DR, Van Buskirk EM. Vasoactive drug effects on the uveal vasculature of the rabbit: a corrosion casting study. *Invest Ophthalmol Vis Sci* 1989;30(suppl):100.
48. Serdahl CL, Galustian J, Lewis RA. The effects of apraclonidine on conjunctival oxygen tension. *Arch Ophthalmol* 1989;107:1777–1779.
49. Harris A, Caldemeyer KS, Mansberger SL, Martin BJ. Alpha-adrenergic agonists' effects on ocular hemodynamics. *J Glaucoma* 1995;4 (suppl):S19–S23.
50. Cioffi GA, Orgul S, Bacon DR, Van Buskirk EM. Acute vasomotor effects in the anterior optic nerve of topical apraclonidine hydrochloride. *J Glaucoma* 1995;4(suppl):S15–S18.
51. Barnes GE, Riva CE, Chandler ML, DeSantis L. Retinal and optic nerve head flow responses to apraclonidine in anesthetized cats. *Invest Ophthalmol Vis Sci* 1993;34(suppl):1394.
52. Krupin T, Kolker AE, Kass MA, et al. Intraocular pressure the day of argon laser trabeculoplasty in primary open-angle glaucoma. *Ophthalmology* 1984;91:361–365.
53. Hotchkiss ML, Robin AL, Pollack IP, et al. Non-steroidal anti-inflammatory agents after argon laser trabeculoplasty. *Ophthalmology* 1984;91:969–976.
54. Robin AL, Pollack IP, House B, Enger C. Effects of ALO 2145 on intraocular pressure following argon laser trabeculoplasty. *Arch Ophthalmol* 1987;105:646–650.
55. Robin AL. Argon laser trabeculoplasty medical therapy to prevent the intraocular pressure rise associated with argon laser trabeculoplasty. *Ophthalmic Surg Lasers* 1991;22:31–37.
56. Pollack IP, Brown RH, Crandall AS, Robin AL, Stewart RH, White GL. Prevention of the rise in intraocular pressure following neodymium:YAG posterior capsulotomy using topical 1% apraclonidine. *Arch Ophthalmol* 1988;106:754–757.
57. Silverstone DE, Brint SF, Olander KW, et al. Prophylactic use of apraclonidine for intraocular pressure increase after Nd:YAG capsulotomies. *Am J Ophthalmol* 1992;113:401–405.
58. Kitazawa Y, Taniguchi T, Sugiyama K. Use of apraclonidine to reduce acute intraocular pressure rise following Q-switched Nd:YAG laser iridotomy. *Ophthalmic Surg Lasers* 1989;20:49–52.
59. Nesher R, Kolker AE. Delayed increased intraocular pressure after Nd:YAG laser posterior capsulotomy in a patient treated with apraclonidine. *Am J Ophthalmol* 1990;110:94–95.
60. Yaldo MK, Shin DH, Parrow KA, Lee SH, Lee SY. Additive effect of 1% apraclonidine hydrochloride to nonselective β-blockers. *Ophthalmology* 1991;98:1075–1078.
61. Blasini M, Shields MB. Apraclonidine hydrochloride as an adjunct to timolol maleate therapy. *J Glaucoma* 1992;1:148–152.
62. Lish AJ, Camras CB, Podos SM. Effect of apraclonidine on intraocular pressure in glaucoma patients receiving maximally tolerated medications. *J Glaucom* 1992;1:19–22.
63. Cardakli UF, Smythe BA, Eisele JR, Kaufman PL, Perkins TW. Effect of chronic apraclonidine treatment on intraocular pressure in advanced glaucoma. *J Glaucoma* 1993;2:271–278.
64. Robin AL, Ritch R, Shin DH, Smythe B, Mundorf T, Lehmann RP. The short-term efficacy of apraclonidine hydrochloride when maximum tolerated medical therapy fails to control intraocular pressure. *Am J Ophthalmol* 1995;120:423–432.
65. Yuksel N, Guler C, Caglar Y, Elibol O. Apraclonidine and clonidine: a comparison of efficacy and side effects in normal and ocular hypertensive volunteers. *Int Ophthalmol* 1992;16:337–342.
66. Liu JH, Neufeld AH. Study of central regulation of intraocular pressure using ventriculocisternal perfusion. *Invest Ophthalmol Vis Sci* 1985;26:136–143.
67. Innemee HC, Van Zwieten PA. The central ocular hypotensive effect of clonidine. *Graefes Arch Clin Exp Ophthalmol* 1979;210:93–102.
68. Fry LL. Comparison of the postoperative intraocular pressure with Betagan, Betoptic, Timoptic, Iopidine, Diamox, Pilopine Gel, and Miostat. *J Cataract Refract Surg* 1992;18:14–19.

69. Wiles SB, MacKenzie D, Ide CH. Control of intraocular pressure with apraclonidine hydrochloride after cataract extraction. *Am J Ophthalmol* 1991;111:184–188.
70. Araie M, Ishi K. Effects of apraclonidine on intraocular pressure and blood-aqueous barrier permeability after phacoemulsification and intraocular lens implantation. *Am J Ophthalmol* 1993;116:67–71.
71. Robin AL. Effect of topical apraclonidine on the frequency of intraocular pressure elevations after combined extracapsular cataract extraction and trabeculectomy. *Ophthalmology* 1993;100:628–633.
72. Pulido JS, Sneed SR, Blodi CF. Apraclonidine hydrochloride in vitreoretinal surgery. *Arch Ophthalmol* 1989;107:316–317.
73. Hill RA, Minckler DS, Lee M, Heuer DK, Baerveldt G, Martone JF. Apraclonidine prophylaxis for postcycloplegic intraocular pressure spikes. *Ophthalmology* 1991;98:1083–1086.
74. Munden PM, Kardon RH, Denson CE, Carter KD. Palpebral fissure responses to topical adrenergic drugs. *Am J Ophthalmol* 1991;111: 706–710.
75. Burke JA, Potter DE. Ocular effects of a relatively selective α-2 agonist (UK-14, 304-18) in cats, rabbits, and monkeys. *Eye Res* 1986;5: 665–676.
76. Serle JB, Steidl S, Wang R-F, Mittag TW, Podos SM. Selective α-2 adrenergic agonists B-HT920 and UK14304-18: effects on aqueous humor dynamics in monkeys. *Arch Ophthalmol* 1991;109:1158–1162.
77. Barnebey HS, Robin AL, Zimmerman TJ, et al. Efficacy of brimonidine in decreasing elevations in intraocular pressure after laser trabeculoplasty. *Ophthalmology* 1993;100:1083–1088.
78. David R, Spaeth GL, Clevenger CE, et al. Brimonidine in the prevention of intraocular pressure elevation following argon laser trabeculoplasty. *Arch Ophthalmol* 1993;111:1387–1390.
79. Derick RJ, Walters TR, Robin AL, et al. Brimonidine tartrate: A one-month dose response study. *Invest Ophthalmol Vis Sci* 1993;34 (suppl):1138.
80. Serle JB, Podos SM, Abundo GP, et al. The effect of brimonidine tartrate in glaucoma patients on maximal medical therapy. *Invest Ophthalmol Vis Sci* 1993;34(suppl):1137.
81. Nordlund JR, Pasquale LR, Robin AL, Rudikoff MT. The cardiovascular, pulmonary, and ocular hypotensive effects of brimonidine tartrate 0.2%. *Arch Ophthalmol* 1995;113:77–83.

Textbook of Ocular Pharmacology,
edited by T.J. Zimmerman, et al.
Lippincott–Raven Publishers, Philadelphia © 1997.

CHAPTER 22

Thymoxamine (Alpha-Adrenergic Antagonist)

Karanjit S. Kooner

ALPHA-ADRENERGIC BLOCKING AGENTS

Currently there are two alpha (α)-receptor blocking agents with some ophthalmic therapeutic roles. In the United States, thymoxamine hydrochloride is still investigational, and dapiprazole hydrochloride was introduced in 1991 to reverse mydriasis. The former drug was originally synthesized by Greef and Schumann in 1953 (1). Many other α-adrenergic blocking drugs are known but have not been introduced in ophthalmology because of ocular side effects.

THYMOXAMINE HYDROCHLORIDE

Chemical Structure

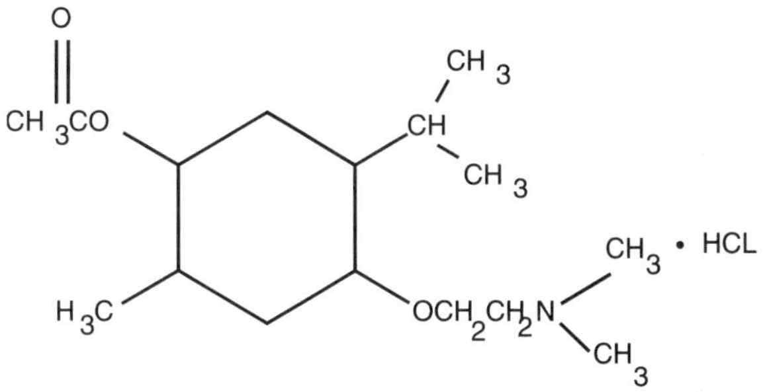

O
CH_3CO
CH_3
CH
CH_3
CH_3 • HCL
H_3C
OCH_2CH_2N
CH_3

Thymoxamine (Moxisylyte) hydrochloride is 4-[2-(dimethylamino) ethoxy]-5-isopropyl -2- methylphenyl acetate hydrochloride. It is a white to colorless crystalline powder with no odor, but it has a bitter taste (2). The drug has a molecular weight of 315.8, and the molecular formula is $C_{16}H_{25}No_2$.HCl.

K. S. Kooner: Department of Ophthalmology, Southwestern Medical School, Dallas, Texas 75235.

Pharmacology

Thymoxamine is an α-adrenergic blocking agent that is primarily used topically to reverse phenylephrine-induced mydriasis. Topical thymoxamine solution competes with norepinephrine and other adrenergic agonists at the postjunctional α_1-adrenoceptors (3,4). Miosis is produced by blockade of α-receptors in the dilator muscle of the iris, which facilitates parasympathetic dominance via the iris sphincter muscle. The drug has no effect on intraocular pressure (IOP), facility of outflow of aqueous humor, or rate of aqueous humor formation (5). There is also no effect on ciliary muscle or depth of anterior chamber, as may occur with cholinergic drugs. The minimal effective concentration for induction of miosis is 0.01%; the maximum effective concentration is 1.3% (4).

Thymoxamine effectively reverses the mydriatic effects of sympathomimetic amines, including phenylephrine, ephedrine, and hydroxyamphetamine (6–9). The reversal of mydriasis produced by anticholinergic drugs like tropicamide and homatropine is incomplete.

Clinical Pharmacology

To reverse phenylephrine-induced mydriasis, the usual effective dose is one drop of a 0.1% ophthalmic solution. In patients with darkly pigmented irides, it is necessary either to repeat the 0.1% concentration or to use a higher concentration of 0.5% (8–10). More local adverse effects, like stinging or burning, occur with the use of a higher concentration.

The role of thymoxamine in the treatment of acute-angle closure glaucoma is ambiguous. Some studies have shown effective resolution of acute angle-closure glaucoma attacks with the use of one drop of 0.5% thymoxamine ophthalmic solution in the involved eye every minute for 5 minutes, followed by instillation of one drop every

15 minutes for up to 3 hours (11). Other investigators have reported that treatment with thymoxamine alone is ineffective (12).

Thymoxamine also has been used to differentiate angle-closure glaucoma from open-angle glaucoma with narrow angles (12). In this thymoxamine test, two drops of 0.5% thymoxamine hydrochloride are applied, 2 minutes apart to the eye(s) to be studied. After an hour, gonioscopy is repeated. Thymoxamine-induced miosis helps to establish a diagnosis of open-angle glaucoma with functionally noncontributory narrow angles by causing the angles to open up without any effect on IOP. In patients with long-standing angle-closure glaucoma, thymoxamine-induced miosis may cause no or little change in the angle or IOP; however, if the patient has acute or subacute angle-closure glaucoma or combined mechanism glaucoma, the angle may open with some reduction of IOP.

Pharmaceutics

Thymoxamine ophthalmic solution is currently investigational in the United States, with IOLAB Pharmaceuticals acting as sponsor. The drug is supplied as a sterile solution for topical ophthalmic application in a concentration of 1 mg/ml. The solution should be protected from light. The pH of a 0.5% thymoxamine hydrochloride solution in water is 4.5 to 5.5. The drug is soluble in water, alcohol, and chloroform and it is insoluble in ether.

Pharmacokinetics, Concentration-effect Relationships, and Metabolism

There are no studies investigating the pharmacokinetics of thymoxamine following ocular instillation. Following oral doses, thymoxamine is rapidly and completely metabolized to *N*-monomethyldeacetyl thymoxamine. Peak serum concentrations of these metabolites occur 1 hour after oral absorption of the drug. After instillation of one drop of 0.5% thymoxamine, the half-life effect on pupillary miosis is 10 hours.

In the normal human eye, miosis is evident almost immediately after instillation of one drop of thymoxamine 0.5% ophthalmic solution, with peak miotic effects noticed at 1 hour (4). After instillation of 0.1% thymoxamine ophthalmic solution in patients with mydriasis induced by phenylephrine, pupillary diameter generally returns to baseline in 1 to 1.5 hours in eyes with light irides. In patients with dark irides, it may take 2 to 4 hours or longer (9,10).

When 0.5% thymoxamine was used in subjects with phenylephrine-induced mydriasis, there was no difference in the rapidity of pupillary constriction between eyes with light or brown irides (8,13). With the 0.5% concentration, Saheb et al. (8) reported that pupils constricted to their original size in approximately 20 minutes.

After instillation of 0.1% thymoxamine ophthalmic solution for reversal of mydriasis by ophthalmic phenylephrine 2.5%, pupillary diameter continued to decrease from 3 hours postinstillation until the end of observation at 8 hours postinstillation (9). The duration of pupillary constriction with thymoxamine exceeded the effect of phenylephrine. No patients in this study experienced a rebound pupillary dilation after effective reversal of phenylephrine mydriasis with thymoxamine. The miotic effect of thymoxamine 0.5% may persist for 24 hours.

Metabolism

Thymoxamine is rapidly hydrolyzed to deacetylthymoxamine following oral absorption. This process appears to be complete. Deacetylthymoxamine is further demethylated to *N*-monomethyldeacetyl thymoxamine, and both metabolites are subsequently metabolized to sulfate and glucuronide derivatives (14). There are no studies investigating the metabolism of thymoxamine in the eye following topical use. The plasma half-life of active metabolites of thymoxamine is approximately 1 to 1.5 hours.

Clinical Uses

Parasympatholytic-induced Mydriasis

Topical thymoxamine has been used to reverse mydriasis induced by topical parasympatholytic agents such as tropicamide and homatropine. With a 0.1% or 0.2% solution of thymoxamine, the reversal is incomplete (6). For a complete reversal, a higher concentration of 0.5% is required.

Phenylephrine-induced Mydriasis

Topical thymoxamine effectively reverses mydriasis produced by phenylephrine during routine ocular examinations (5,10,13). Unlike pilocarpine, thymoxamine does not increase pupillary block secondary to iris sphincter constriction and has no effect on the depth of the anterior chamber. In eyes with mydriasis caused by 2.5% phenylephrine, the usual effective dose for pupillary reversal is one drop of 0.1% thymoxamine in each eye, repeated 5 minutes thereafter. In patients with dark irides, the miotic response to thymoxamine 0.1% solution is slower and less complete compared with light irides. Some patients with dark brown irides may not respond at all to 0.1% thymoxamine. In patients with light irides, the pupillary diameter generally returns to baseline 1 to 1.5 hours after instillation of 0.1% thymoxamine. Similarly, in phenylephrine-induced mydriasis in dark irides, return to baseline occurs in 2 to 4 hours or longer. In studies using 0.5% thymoxamine, no difference in pupillary constriction between eyes with light and brown irides was observed (8,13). In darkly pigmented irides, a concentration >0.1% may have to be used, or the instillation of 0.1% concentration may need to be repeated. A higher concentration of thymoxamine is associated with a higher incidence of local adverse effects.

Saheb et al. (8) compared thymoxamine 0.5% with pilocarpine 2% in reversing mydriasis induced by 10% phenylephrine in 19 patients. The subjects were either normal or had ocular hypertension. One drop each of thymoxamine or pilocarpine was instilled approximately 1 hour after the application of phenylephrine. Both agents induced effective miosis, and the onsets of action were similar. The half-lives for onsets of action were 12 minutes and 10 minutes for thymoxamine and pilocarpine, respectively. Pilocarpine constricted the pupil to its normal baseline size in 10 minutes, compared with 19 minutes by thymoxamine. The maximal miotic effect was also greater with pilocarpine, but the half-life for disappearance of pupillary constriction was significantly longer with thymoxamine at 12 hours compared with only 5 hours for pilocarpine.

Lid Retraction

Thymoxamine 0.5% ophthalmic solution has been reported to be effective in treating eyelid retraction primarily in patients with thyroid ophthalmopathy (2,15). Significant decreases in palpebral fissures, up to 75%, were observed.

Glaucoma

Some studies reported successful breaking of acute attacks of angle-closure glaucoma in a majority of patients (2,11). One drop of 0.5% thymoxamine solution was instilled into the involved eye every minute for 5 minutes, followed by instillation of one drop every 15 minutes for up to 3 hours. Other studies, however, report that thymoxamine alone was ineffective in treating angle-closure glaucoma (2).

Another promising use of thymoxamine may be in pigmentary dispersion syndrome or pigmentary glaucoma (2). The constant mechanical rubbing between the anterior ciliary zonules and the peripheral iris results in pigment dispersion in the anterior chamber. Over time, this pigment may raise IOP. Drugs such as thymoxamine might be ideal in this situation. The miosis without ciliary muscle contraction may stretch the iris and lift it away from the lens' surface.

Side Effects and Toxicity

The most common adverse effects observed with thymoxamine ophthalmic solution are burning, stinging, and blurring of vision (2,5,7,9,10). With the 0.1% concentration, these local effects occurred in 20% to 50% of subjects but were usually mild and short-lived, subsiding within several minutes (5,9,10). In one study, the incidence of local adverse effects were similar in placebo and thymoxamine-treated eyes (10).

The incidence and severity of local effects are greater with higher concentrations of thymoxamine 0.5% or 1.0% (2,9,10). Transient ptosis is also observed with 0.5% and 1.0% thymoxamine ophthalmic solution (2,7,13). This complication is rare with the lower concentration of 0.1% thymoxamine. Blepharoptosis has also been reported during oral therapy with thymoxamine (16). Ptosis improved following *discontinuation* of the drug, but the patient was not rechallenged. A definite cause-effect relationship could not be established in this case.

Transient conjunctival hyperemia was reported to occur with 0.5% thymoxamine ophthalmic solution (2). Chemosis has been observed with 5.0% concentrations of thymoxamine but is rare with 0.5% solution (2). It has not been reported with 0.1% solution.

Vertigo in association with tinnitus was reported in one patient treated with 0.1% thymoxamine solution for reversal of phenylephrine-induced mydriasis (10). This patient had a history of severe motion sickness, and it was unclear whether symptoms were drug related.

Green et al. investigated the effects of 0.02% and 0.2% thymoxamine on the isolated rabbit corneal endothelium and measured the corneal swelling rate by using specular microscopy (17). The 0.02% concentration produced a swelling rate of 10.3 μm/hour compared with 34.1 μm/hour by the 0.2% concentration ($p < 0.05$). They recommended against using thymoxamine at a concentration greater than 0.02% for future intracameral use. In a large randomized clinical trial involving 171 eyes of patients undergoing extracapsular cataract extraction with or without posterior chamber intraocular lens implantation, Grehn (18) compared the efficacy of 1.0% acetylcholine with a mixture of 0.01% thymoxamine and 0.5% acetylcholine injected intracamerally after intraocular lens insertion. The mixture of thymoxamine 0.01% and acetylcholine 0.5% produced twice as much pupillary constriction as acetylcholine 1% alone. Postoperative slit-lamp examination revealed no toxic reaction to thymoxamine.

Contraindications

Thymoxamine is contraindicated in patients with previous episodes of hypersensitivity to thymoxamine.

Precautions

Caution must be exercised when using thymoxamine in patients with angina pectoris, a history of recent myocardial infarction, or diabetes mellitus. It should be avoided during pregnancy and in nursing mothers.

DAPIPRAZOLE HYDROCHLORIDE

Chemical Structure

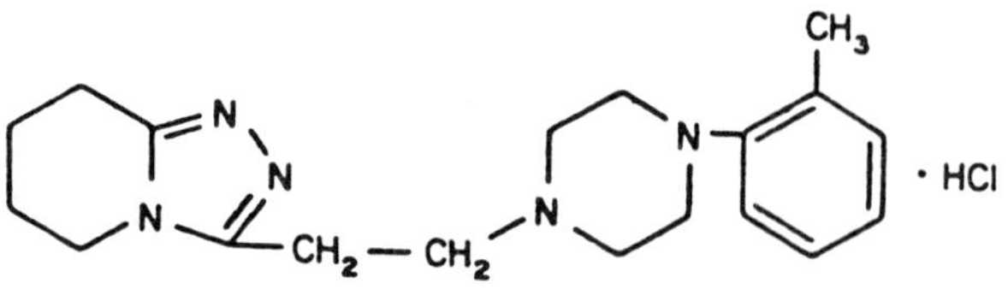

Dapiprazole hydrochloride (Rev-Eyes) is 5, 6, 7, 8 -tetrahydro-3-[2-(4-0, tolyl-1-piperazinyl) ethyl]-S-triazolo [4,3-a] pyridine hydrochloride. The empirical formula is $C_{19}H_{27}N_5HCl$ with a molecular weight of 361.93. Dapiprazole is a sterile, white, lyophilized powder-soluble in water.

Pharmacology

Dapiprazole is a selective α-adrenergic blocking agent, exerting effects primarily on α_1 adrenoceptors (19). It induces miosis secondarily by relaxation of smooth dilator muscle of the iris. The nature of miosis produced by dapiprazole suggests a minimal role in inducing pupillary block glaucoma compared with cholinergic agents (20). The drug also partially reverses cycloplegia induced with parasympatholytic agents, such as tropicamide. Dapiprazole has no significant effect on the ciliary muscle contraction, but it may partially increase accommodative amplitude, therefore relieving the symptoms of paralysis of accommodation (20). There is no effect on IOP or the thickness of the lens or any significant change in the anterior chamber depth (21).

Clinical Pharmacology

The main clinical use of dapiprazole is in reversing mydriasis produced by adrenergic drugs (e.g., phenylephrine) and, to a lesser degree, by parasympatholytic drugs (e.g., tropicamide).

To produce the reversal of mydriasis, two drops of 0.5% dapiprazole solution are instilled into the lower conjunctival cul-de-sac at the end of an ophthalmic examination, followed by another set of two drops 5 minutes later. The rate of pupillary constriction depends on the eye color. In persons with brown irides, the rate of pupillary constriction may be slightly slower than in individuals with blue or green irides. The final pupil size, however, is independent of eye color. Dapiprazole does not significantly alter IOP in normotensive eyes or in eyes with elevated IOP.

Pharmaceutics

Dapiprazole is a clear, colorless, slightly viscous solution for topical application. Each milliliter, after reconstitution, contains 5 mg of dapiprazole hydrochloride as the active ingredient. The reconstituted solution has a pH of approximately 6.6 and an osmolarity of approximately 415 mOsm. The inactive ingredients include mannitol (2%) sodium chloride, hydroxypropyl methylcellulose (0.4%), edentate sodium (0.01%), sodium phosphate dibasic, sodium phosphate monobasic, water for injection, and benzalkonium chloride (0.01%) as a preservative. To reconstitute dapiprazole ophthalmic solution, aseptic technique should be used. The aluminum seals are torn off, followed by removal of the rubber plugs from both the drug (25 mg) and diluent vials (5 ml). The diluent is then poured into the drug vial, the dropper assembly is attached to the drug vial, and the solution is shaken for several minutes to ensure complete drug dissolution. After reconstitution, dapiprazole ophthalmic solution should be stored at room temperature, 15° to 30° C (59 to 86° F), and is stable for 21 days. Any solution that is not clear and colorless should be discarded.

Pharmacokinetics, Concentration-effect Relationship, and Metabolism

Dapiprazole is well absorbed after topical application to the conjunctival cul-de-sac. The antimydriatic effect of dapiprazole usually occurs within 1 hour of administration. Reversal of mydriasis induced by either 2.5% phenylephrine, 1% tropicamide, or the combination of the two drugs develops 30 minutes to 2 hours after application. Eye color influences the rate of dapiprazole-induced papillary constriction. In patients with brown eyes the rate of constriction may be slower than in patients with blue or green eyes, but the eye color does not effect the final pupil size. The miotic effect of dapiprazole lasts about 6 hours.

Therapeutic Uses

Reversing Phenylephrine-induced Mydriasis

Dapiprazole effectively reverses phenylephrine-produced mydriasis. Bonomi et al. (22) administered 10% phenylephrine topically to healthy volunteers between the ages of 24 and 68 years, followed by dapiprazole 0.125%, 0.25%, or 0.5% or saline 30 minutes later. The baseline pupil size in these subjects was approximately 4.5 mm before instillation of phenylephrine, increasing to 5.5 to 7 mm at the time of dapiprazole administration. Thirty minutes after instillation of 0.25% and 0.5% dapiprazole, the mean pupillary diameter was about 5 mm compared with 7.5 mm with saline. One hour after dapiprazole, the mean pupil size was approximately 4.5 and 5 mm in the 0.25% and 0.5% groups, respectively, compared with 7 mm with saline. Two hours after dapiprazole, the mean pupil size was approximately 4.5 mm in the 0.25% and 0.5% groups, compared with 6.5 mm with saline. Although these values were statistically significant with 0.25% and 0.5% dapiprazole (p <0.001), the difference was not significant with 0.125% concentration (p <.05).

Allinson et al. (23) evaluated the efficacy of dapiprazole in reversing mydriasis induced by tropicamide 1% and phenylephrine 2.5% in 50 normal subjects. Twenty-six men and 24 women were tested. Eye color was brown in 18 patients and blue or green in the remainder of the subjects. Pregnant or nursing mothers were excluded from trials, as were persons with narrow anterior-chamber angles or a previous history of intraocular surgery. All patients received one drop of tropicamide 1% followed by one drop of 2.5% phenylephrine. After examination for maximal mydriasis, two drops of dapiprazole 0.5% were placed into one eye followed 5 minutes later by two additional drops. The contralateral eye served as a control. The mean premydriatic pupil size was 3.7 mm. After mydriatics, the mean pupillary diameter was approximately 9 mm. At 30 minutes after instillation of dapiprazole, there was a significant (p = 0.001) difference in pupillary diameter between treated and untreated eyes. Fifty-two percent of the treated eyes achieved premydriatic diameter at 2 hours compared with none for untreated eyes. The mean pupillary diameter in the untreated eye at 2 hours was greater than 8 mm, whereas in the treated eyes it was 4.5 mm. In all subjects, pupils completely returned to normal after 24 hours.

The effect of dapiprazole on amplitude of accommodation was tested by Nyman and Reich (20) in a single-mask fashion. They measured accommodative amplitudes in 48 age-matched subjects through a 3-mm artificial pupil. For dilation, 0.5% tropicamide was used, followed by random instillation of 0.5% dapiprazole in one eye and a placebo drop in the other eye. The effect of dapiprazole on amplitude of accommodation was significant (p < 0.001). The authors concluded that the effect on pupil size had no relation to dapiprazole's effect in accelerating the return of accommodation.

Reversal of Mydriasis During Intraocular Surgery

A miotic pupil after placement of a posterior chamber intraocular lens may help to avoid iris capture and lens decentration. Prosdocimo and DeMarco (24) evaluated the efficacy of buffered 0.1% dapiprazole injected intracamerally in 40 patients during extracapsular cataract extraction with posterior chamber lens implantation. Preoperatively, the pupils were dilated with 10% phenylephrine, 0.5% tropicamide, and 0.1% cyclopentolate. The infusion fluid also contained a 1 : 500,000 diluted solution of phenylephrine. After lens implantation and aspiration of viscoelastic substance, each eye randomly received either 0.2 ml of 0.1% dapiprazole or 0.2 ml of balanced salt solution. The pupillary diameters were measured with calipers at 1, 2, or 3 minutes after injection. Dapiprazole reversed mydriasis in all eyes independent of eye color. Balanced salt solution had no effect on pupillary diameter. The study found no untoward reaction or any significant effect on endothelial cells, IOP, or inflammatory responses between the two series.

In a double-blind study involving 120 patients undergoing extracapsular cataract extraction with posterior chamber intraocular lens, Ponte et al. (25) found significant reversal of mydriasis by intraocular 0.25% dapiprazole. The effect of the drug was observed within minutes of injection with maximal response in 2 hours, and the action persisted for 8 hours. The investigators detected no toxic effect of the drug during the 4-month follow-up period.

Glaucoma

Based on the pharmacologic action of dapiprazole, there is a potential use of the drug in the prevention and treatment of narrow-angle glaucoma and pigmentary glaucoma. In the latter condition, miosis without ciliary muscle constriction would decrease iris-zonule contact while avoiding symptoms of ciliary spasm seen with drugs like pilocarpine. Dapiprazole has no effect on ciliary body, anterior chamber depth, or IOP.

Precautions

Dapiprazole ophthalmic solution is not currently recommended to be used more frequently than once a week. Miosis induced by dapiprazole may cause difficulty in dark adaptation and may reduce field of vision. It should be used with caution when driving at night or when other activities in poor illumination are anticipated. The drug is classified as Food and Drug Administration (FDA) Pregnancy Category B by the manufacturer (21). There are no adequate well-controlled studies in pregnant women. The safety and effectiveness of the use of this drug in children or nursing mothers have not been established.

Contraindications

Dapiprazole is contraindicated in patients with a history of hypersensitivity to any component of the formulation. It should also be avoided in patients with acute intraocular inflammation.

Side Effects and Toxicity

Dapiprazole has been reported to produce transient conjunctival injection in 80% of patients (23). Almost 50% also report blurring on instillation; ptosis, lid erythema or edema, chemosis, aching, punctate keratitis, corneal edema, brow ache, photophobia, and headaches occur in 10% to 40%. Other less-frequent findings are dry eyes, tearing, or blurred vision. There are no reports of precipitation of angle-closure glaucoma.

Although mutagenicity and impairment of fertility tests with dapiprazole have been negative, the drug was shown to increase the incidence of hepatic tumors in male rats given 300 mg/kg/day orally (80,000 times the human doses) for 104 weeks (21). This was not observed in male and female rats at doses of 30 and 100 mg/kg/day or female rats at doses of 300 mg/kg/day. The clinical significance of this finding is unknown. Reproduction studies with dapiprazole in rats and rabbits at doses up to 128,000 (rat) and 27,000 (rabbit) times the human ophthalmic dose have revealed no evidence of impaired fertility or harm to the fetus.

Using a specular microscope, Cheeks et al. tested dapiprazole's effect on isolated rabbit corneal endothelium (26). They found no toxicity using concentrations up to 125 μg/ml. When concentrations of 250 μg/ml to 1000 μg/ml were used, corneal swelling rates of 17.1 μm/hour to 23.2 μm/hour were noted. The study showed no evidence of toxic effect on the cornea at levels used for topical application.

REFERENCES

1. Greef K, Schumann HJ. Zur Pharmakologie des Sympathicolyticums 6-acetoxy thymoxyaethyldimethylamin. *Arzneimittelforschung* 1953; 3:341–345.
2. Wand M, Grant M. Thymoxamine hydrochloride: an alpha-adrenergic blocker. *Surv Ophthalmol* 1980;25:75–84.
3. Drew GM. Effects of alpha-adrenoceptor agonists and antagonists on pre and post synaptically located alpha-adrenoceptors. *Eur J Pharmacol* 1976;36:313–320.
4. Lee DA, Rimele TJ, Brubaker RF, Nagataki S, VanHoutte PM. Effect of thymoxamine on the human pupil. *Exp Eye Res* 1983;36:655–662.
5. Relf SJ, Gharagozloo NZ, Skuta GL, Alward WLM, Anderson DR. Brubaker RF. Thymoxamine reverse phenylephrine-induced mydriasis. *Am J Ophthalmol* 1988;106:251–255.
6. Mayer GL, Stewart-Jones JH, Turner P. Influence of alpha-adrenoceptor blockade with thymoxamine on changes in pupil diameter and accommodation produced by tropicamide and ephedrine. *Curr Med Res Opin* 1977;4:660–663.
7. McKinna H, Steward-Jones JH, Edgar DF, Turner P. Reversal of tropicamide-induced mydriasis by thymoxamine eye drops. *Curr Med Res Opin* 1988;11:1–3.
8. Saheb NE, Lorenzetti D, East D, Salpeter Carlton S. Thymoxamine versus pilocarpine in the reversal of phenylephrine induced mydriasis. *Can J Ophthalmol* 1982;17:266–267.
9. Wright MM, Skuta GL, Drake MV, Chang LF, Rabbani R, Musch DC, Teikari J. Time course of thymoxamine reversal of phenylephrine induced mydriasis. *Arch Ophthalmol* 1990;108:1729–1732.
10. Diehl DLC, Robin AL, Wand M. The influence of iris pigmentation on the miotic effect of thymoxamine. *Am J Ophthalmol* 1991;111: 351–355.
11. Halasa AH, Rutkowski PC. Thymoxamine therapy for angle closure glaucoma. *Arch Ophthalmol* 1973;90:177–179.
12. Wand M, Grant MW. Thymoxamine test: differentiating angle-closure glaucoma from open-angle glaucoma with narrow angles. *Arch Ophthalmol* 1978;96:1009–1011.
13. Mapstone R. Safe mydriasis. *Br J Ophthalmol* 1970;54:690–692.
14. Jones NS, Lewis LD. Ergotamine-induced peripheral ischaemia reversed by oral thymoxamine hydrochloride. *Hum Toxicol* 1986;5: 61–62.
15. Dixon RS, Anderson RL, Hatt MV. The use of thymoxamine in eyelid retraction. *Arch Ophthalmol* 1979;97:2147–2150.
16. Chitkara DK, Hudson JM. Blepharoptosis caused by systemic thymoxamine. *Am J Ophthalmol* 1991;111:524–525.
17. Green K, Chapman JM, Cheeks L, Hull DS. Effects of thymoxamine on corneal endothelium. *Lens Eye Toxicol Res* 1991;8:1–8.
18. Grehn F. Intraocular thymoxamine for miosis during surgery. *Am J Ophthalmol* 1987;103:709–711.
19. Nencini P, Valeri P, Morrone LA. Dapiprazole, a selective alpha 1 adrenoceptor antagonist, inhibits diuresis but not polydipsia produced by amphetamine in rats. *Brain Res Bull* 1990;25:765–767.
20. Nyman N, Reich L. The effect of dapiprazole on accommodative amplitude in eyes dilated with 0.5% tropicamide. *J Am Optom Assoc* 1993;64:625–628.
21. Product Information: Rev-Eyes (R), dapiprazole. St. Louis: Storz Ophthalmics, Inc., 1992.
22. Bonomi L, Marchini G, DeFeo G, Piccinelli D, Bettini A. On the reversal of diagnostic mydriasis with dapiprazole. *Curr Ther Res* 1985;38:945–952.
23. Allinson RW, Gerber DS, Bieber S, Hodes BL. Reversal of mydriasis by dapiprazole. *Ann Ophthalmol* 1990;22:131–138.
24. Prosdocimo G, DeMarco D. Intraocular dapiprazole to reverse mydriasis during extracapsular cataract extraction. *Am J Ophthalmol* 1988;105:321–322.
25. Ponte F, Cillino S, Faranda F, Casanova F, Cucci F. Intraocular dapiprazole for the reversal of mydriasis after extracapsular cataract extraction with intraocular lens implantation. *J Cataract Refract Surgery* 1991;17:780–784.
26. Cheeks L, Chapman JM, Green K. Corneal endothelial toxicity of dapiprazole hydrochloride. *Lens Eye Toxicol Res* 1992;9:79–84.

Textbook of Ocular Pharmacology,
edited by T.J. Zimmerman, et al.
Lippincott–Raven Publishers, Philadelphia © 1997.

CHAPTER 23

Beta-blockers

Mark S. Juzych and Thom J. Zimmerman

Historical Perspective

The concept of adrenoreceptors dates to 1948, when Ahlquist concluded that there were two distinct types of adrenergic receptors in the autonomic nervous system which he classified as α and β (1). Ten years later, β-adrenoreceptor antagonists, β-blockers, were discovered, which initiated the development of pharmaceutical agents that affected specifically this subpopulation of receptors and their physiological responses (2). Since then, this class of drug has been used for a variety of clinical indications. Thus, the development of β-blockers represents one of the major pharmacotherapeutic advances in medicine. The first β-blocker synthesized with widespread application in medicine was propranolol, which is used for the management of systemic hypertension, cardiac arrhythmias, and angina. In 1967 it was observed that intravenous propranolol not only lowered blood pressure in hypertensive patients but also lowered their intraocular pressure (IOP) (3,4). The same effect was also noted when the medication was administered orally (5,6) and topically (7–9). A number of oral β-blockers used for cardiovascular disease then were evaluated for ocular hypotensive efficacy, notably atenolol, pindolol, and bupranolol.

Adverse side effects limited the ocular use of the early β-blockers. Propranolol, which possesses membrane-stabilizing activity, caused significant corneal anesthesia (8). Practolol, another systemic β-blocker, induced an immunologically mediated oculomucocutaneous syndrome, including eczematous rash, keratoconjunctivitis sicca (dry eye), subconjunctival scarring, and corneal ulceration (10,11). Thus, research efforts focused on the development of β-blockers possessing the ocular hypotensive effect without the undesirable side effects and led to the development of timolol, which revolutionized the treatment of glaucoma. Since timolol's introduction in 1978, a number of other topical β-blockers have been developed. Together, they have become the most commonly used medical therapeutic agents in the treatment of glaucoma.

M. S. Juzych: Kresge Eye Institute, Detroit, Michigan 48201.
T. J. Zimmerman: Department of Ophthalmology and Visual Sciences, University of Louisville School of Medicine, Louisville, Kentucky 40292.

General Pharmacology

Beta adrenoreceptors are not homogenous but can be subcategorized into two distinct classes on the basis of their differential binding and physiological responses to various agents. β_1-receptors are mainly found in the heart, and β_2-receptors in bronchial muscle, peripheral blood vessels, and uterus. Stimulating β_1-receptors increases heart rate, A-V conduction, and cardiac contractility, whereas stimulating β_2-receptors causes dilatation of bronchi and peripheral blood vessels. This classification has allowed for the development of specific agonists and antagonists that are relatively selective for either the β_1- or β_2-receptors. Agonists interact and elicit a response, and antagonists interact and block the agonists' action. Recently, a third β-receptor was identified in the mammalian body and denoted as β_3. Most of the commonly used β-antagonists possess a relatively low affinity to β_3-receptors. These β-receptors are involved in lipolysis and may be responsible for the metabolic and lipid effects of β-blockers.

The β-adrenergic antagonists, β-blockers, are competitive inhibitors of catecholamines, such as norepinephrine, which bind to β-adrenoreceptors. Individual β-blockers can be classified further as *selective* or *nonselective,* depending on their ability to bind to β_1- and β_2-receptors. Nonselective blocking agents inhibit both β_1 and β_2 adrenoreceptors, whereas selective blocking agents primarily inhibit either β_1- or β_2-adrenoreceptors. It is important to note that all selective β-blockers, applied at high enough concentrations, will also block the other β-adrenoreceptors. The term *cardioselectivity* refers to β-blockers that relatively selectively block β_1-receptors (cardiovascular) and have less effect on the β_2-receptors (respiratory system).

Mechanism of Action

Beta-blockers lower IOP by reducing the formation of aqueous humor by the ciliary body, up to 50% (12,13), without affecting aqueous outflow (14). Although the exact mechanism by which β-blockers lower IOP is not fully understood, it is most commonly attributed to the adrenergic receptor blockade of the aqueous inflow apparatus, the ciliary epithelium and ciliary body blood vessels. Of the β-adrenoreceptors populating the ciliary body stroma and epithelium and the ciliary blood vessels, β_2 receptors predominate (75–90%) (15). Aqueous humor is produced by the ciliary body through a combination of ultrafiltration of blood and active secretion by the ciliary epithelium. It is therefore speculated that at the cellular level, β-blockers either affect active transport at the nonpigmented ciliary epithelium or alter ultrafiltration of blood in the ciliary body.

To understand the cellular process requires a basic working knowledge of β-receptor pharmacology. When a catecholamine binds to the β-receptor, it induces a change in the receptor. The receptor-agonist complex then activates a regulatory protein (G protein). In general, both β_1- and β_2-receptors activate a stimulatory G protein, called G_S protein, which stimulates the membrane-bound enzyme adenylyl cyclase. This enzyme is responsible for converting adenosine triphosphate (ATP) to cyclic adenosine monophosphate (cAMP). Once adenylyl cyclase is activated, there is an accelerated rate of production and accumulation of intracellular cAMP, which acts as a "second messenger" coupling activation of receptors to a physiological or biochemical response. In the β-adrenergic cascade, cAMP activates a protein kinase, which phosphorylates proteins (enzymes or ion channels) through a series of poorly understood intermediate steps leading to secretion of aqueous humor from the ciliary processes.

By classic β-adrenergic blockade, a β-receptor antagonist binds to a β-receptor, preventing binding of the agonist, a catecholamine, causing the level of cAMP to decrease and leading to a reduction in the production of aqueous humor. In fact, this was shown to be true for timolol and other β-blockers. After topical instillation, these drugs bound to β-receptors and blocked the synthesis of cAMP in the ciliary body. Further, β_1-blockers were shown to be much less *potent* in decreasing cAMP synthesis than β_2-antagonists.

The association between ciliary epithelium, β-blockade, and reduction in aqueous humor production is still somewhat unclear. One study found no relationship between reduction of cAMP by β-blockers and the ability of β blockers to lower IOP (16). One hypothesis postulates that β-blockers reduce aqueous formation by directly blocking the tonic adrenergic stimulation of the secretory ciliary epithelium by endogenous epinephrine. Under steady-state conditions, β-receptors of the ciliary processes are stimulated continuously by circulating catecholamines to produce aqueous humor. The β-blockers are theorized to interfere with this β-adrenergic stimulation of the ciliary processes that promote the normal production of aqueous humor (17).

A number of observations do not support a simple β-antagonist receptor hypothesis. It has been noted that drugs that increase the cAMP level in the cell, such as cholera toxin (18) and forskolin (18), also lower IOP. This finding contrasts with the hypothesis that a decrease in cAMP, not an increase in cAMP, is responsible for lowering IOP. Other evidence for an alternative mechanism of action of β-blockers is that the dextroisomer of timolol, which has a low affinity for the β-receptors, is equally as effective in decreasing aqueous humor flow as the clinically used levoisomer (19).

As mentioned, stromal ultrafiltration is the second component of aqueous formation, and an alternative hypothesis suggests that aqueous humor production may be affected by a decrease in ocular blood flow (20). It is hypothesized that β-blockade is exerted on vascular smooth muscle of the ciliary body, preventing vasodilatation and promoting vasoconstriction in ciliary arterioles. The resultant decrease in capillary perfusion reduces ultrafiltration. Thus, the decreased blood flow in the ciliary body would indirectly decrease production of aqueous humor and thereby lower IOP. In their study, Watanabe and Chiou found that IOP reduction was related to decreased ciliary body blood flow and not to inhibition of active processes in the ciliary epithelium; however, decreased blood flow was related to decreased dopamine. Furthermore, it was shown that haloperidol, a dopamine blocking agent, also significantly reduces IOP (20).

In summary, the relationship between β-receptors and ocular hypotension is not well characterized. It may be that it is independent of β-blocker interaction with β-adrenergic receptors of the ciliary processes. Further research is needed to elucidate this mechanism of action.

INDIVIDUAL β-BLOCKERS

Currently in the United States there are five topical β-blockers approved for lowering IOP in the treatment of glaucoma and ocular hypertension: betaxolol, carteolol, levobunolol, metipranolol, and timolol. A detailed description of each of these β-blockers follows. Figure 23-1 shows the chemical structures of the β blocker. Tables 23-1 and 23-2 summarize the salient similarities and differences between the individual drugs in their pharmacological activity and pharmaceutics.

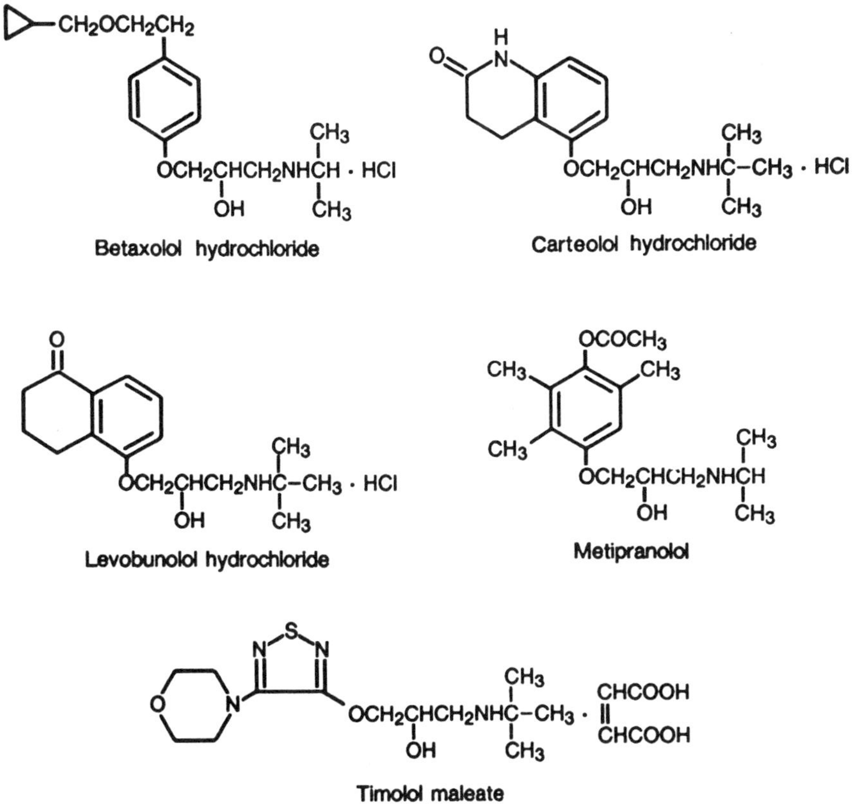

Betaxolol hydrochloride

Carteolol hydrochloride

Levobunolol hydrochloride

Metipranolol

Timolol maleate

FIG. 23-1. Chemical structure of β-blockers.

TIMOLOL

One form of timolol has the official drug name of timolol maleate (trade names, Timoptic and Timoptic XE), and its chemical name, (s)-1-[(1,1-dimethylethyl)-amino]-3-[[4-(4-morphoninyl)-1,2,5 thiadiazol-3-yl]-oxy]-2-propanol, (2) butenedioate. The molecular formula is $C_{13}H_{24}O_3N_4S{\cdot}C_4H_4O_4$, and the molecular weight is 432.5. The second form of timolol has the official drug name timolol hemihydrate (trade name, Betimol), and the chemical name is (s)-1-[(1,1-dimethylethyl)-amino]-3-[[4-(4-morphoninyl)-1,2,5 thiadiazol-3-yl]-oxy]-2-propanol. The molecular formula is $C_{13}H_{24}O_3N_4S$ and the molecular weight is 650.9.

Clinical Pharmacology

In 1978 timolol maleate was the first topical β-blocker approved by the U.S. Food and Drug Administration (FDA), an important turning point in glaucoma therapy, because

TABLE 23-1. *Properties of beta-blockers*

Property	Betaxolol	Carteolol	Levobunolol	Metipranolol	Timolol
Relative beta blockade potency (propranolol = 1)	1.0	10.0	14.6	1.8	4.7
Serum half-life (h)	12–20	3–7	6	2	3–5
Cardioselectivity (β_1-blockade)	++	0	0	0	0
Intrinsic sympathomimetic activity	0	++	0	0	0
Local anesthetic effect (membrane stabilizing activity)	0	0	0	0	0
Ocular discomfort (stinging, burning)	+++[a]	±	++	+	++
Heart rate decrease	±	+	++	++	++
Bronchoconstriction	±	+	++	++	++
Dyslipidemia	?	0	?	?	+
Ocular perfusion	±	±	?	?	±

[a]Betaxolol 0.25% suspension (Betoptic S) has similar ocular discomfort as timolol (++).

TABLE 23-2. *Beta-blockers and their trade names, ingredients, and other properties*

Generic preparations	Brand name (manufacturer)	Concentrations (%)	Supplied bottles (ml)	Preservative	Vehicle ingredients	Adjusted pH
Betaxolol	Betoptic (Alcon)	0.5	2.5, 5, 10, 15	Benzalkonium chloride 0.01%	Edetate disodium NaCl Purified water	HCl/NaOH 5.5–8.0
	Betoptic S (Alcon)	0.25	2.5, 5, 10, 15	Benzalkonium chloride 0.01%	Mannitol Poly (Styrene-Divynyl Benzene) sulfonic acid Carbomer 934P Edetate disodium Purified water	HCl/NaOH 5.5–8.0
Carteolol	Ocupress (Otsuka)	1.0	5, 10	Benzalkonium chloride 0.005%	Monobasic sodium phosphate Dibasic sodium phosphate NaCL Water for injection	NaOH 6.2–7.5
Levobunolol	Betagan (Allergan) Generic (Schein) (Bausch and Lomb)	0.25 0.5	5, 10, 15	Benzalkonium chloride 0.004%	Polyvinyl alcohol Edetate disodium Sodium metabisulfite Monobasic potassium phosphate NaCl Purified water	HCl/NaOH 7.2
Metipranolol	OptiPranolol (Baush and Lomb)	0.3	5, 10	Benzalkonium chloride 0.004%	Glycerol Edetate disodium Povidone NaCl Purified water	HCl/NaOH 6.0(?)
Timolol	Timoptic (Merck Sharp and Dohme)	0.25 0.5	2.5, 5, 10, 15	Benzalkonium chloride 0.01%	Monobasic sodium phosphate Dibasic sodium phosphate Water for injection	NaOH 6.5–7.5
	Timoptic XE (Merck Sharp and Dohme)	0.25 0.5	2.5, 5, 10, 15	Benzalkonium bromide 0.01%	GELRITE, gellan gum Tromethamine Mannitol Purified water	
	Betimol (CIBA Vision) Generic	0.25 0.5	2.5, 5, 10, 15	Benzalkonium bromide 0.01%	Monosodium phosphate dihydrate Disodium phosphate dihydrate Water for injection	NaOH 6.5–7.5

before the introduction of timolol, the only pharmaceutics that were available for the treatment of glaucoma were sympathomimetics (epinephrine), parasympathomimetics (pilocarpine and phospholine iodide), and oral carbonic anhydrase inhibitors. These latter medications were not well tolerated because of their side-effects profile. In early trials, timolol was shown to be more effective in lowering IOP than pilocarpine (21) and epinephrine (22). Timolol rapidly replaced these drugs as the first-line therapy for glaucoma, and now β-blockers are the most widely prescribed glaucoma medications. Because of its unique position in history (the first topical β-blocker), timolol maleate has become the gold standard to which not only all other β-blockers are compared in terms of efficacy and toxicity, but also new non-β-blocker glaucoma medications.

Timolol maleate (Merck and Co., Inc., West Point, PA, U.S.A.) is a lipophilic, nonselective β-adrenergic blocker with a pKa of 9.0. It lacks intrinsic sympathomimetic activity and the ability to act as a partial agonist and also lacks membrane-stabilizing property (local anesthetic activity). Timolol maleate is effective in lowering IOP in normal eyes (23), ocular hypertensive eyes (24), and glaucoma patients (25). Topically applied timolol maleate in concentrations of 0.1 to 1.5% was shown to be efficacious, with the optimal therapeutic dose being 0.25% or 0.5% (24,26); however, even concentrations as low as 0.008% have a noticeable, although minimal, effect on lowering IOP (27). Topical timolol maleate not only reduces IOP in the eye receiving the medication, but it also produces a significant reduction in pressure in the contralateral, untreated eye (24,25). This effect is speculated to be due to systemic absorption.

The onset of significant IOP reduction is seen 20 to 30 minutes after instillation, with the maximum decrease seen after 2 hours (26). Duration of action with timolol maleate 0.25% and 0.5% was approximately 24 hours, with maximal decrease in IOP for at least 12 hours after topical application. Although the recommended dosing for timolol is twice-daily administration, several studies have shown that once-daily administration with either 0.25% or 0.5% may be equally efficacious (28,29). A reduction of aqueous humor inflow by timolol maleate has been shown to be effective only during waking hours, when it is presumed that there is greater endogenous adrenergic stimulation of aqueous production (17). During sleep, aqueous humor inflow is decreased by approximately half.

As mentioned, the duration of action of topically administered β-blockers is between 12 and 24 hours; however, the half-life of topically administered timolol is approximately 1.5 hours (30). The difference in the prolonged effect may be explained by the significant binding of β-blockers to melanin pigment. The β-blockers have an affinity for pigment and bind to ocular melanin easily (31). Topically applied timolol maleate is five times higher in concentration in the iris-ciliary body of pigmented rabbits compared with that in albino rabbits, leaving less medication available to exert its pharmacological action. The melanin is near the site of pharmacological action, however, and does not inactivate the drug, thus acting as a drug depot and allowing for "slow release" of the β-blocker, increasing the medication duration of action. Additionally, the melanin competitively inhibits timolol. The net effect is that highly pigmented (brown) eyes may need a higher concentration than eyes with less pigment (blue eyes), thereby explaining the decreased hypotensive effect seen in patients with heavily pigmented eyes compared with lightly pigmented eyes (32).

In some patients, the ocular hypotensive effect of timolol maleate may be reduced with continued use. This reduction occurs in two phases: *short-term escape* and *long-term drift* (33). Most patients will have a dramatic reduction in IOP immediately after instillation of timolol maleate; however, after several weeks of continued administration, a number of patients lose IOP control, or short-term escape (34). In these patients, the IOP does not return to pretreatment levels but stabilizes at a 25% decrease from pretreatment IOP. One possible explanation is drug-induced receptor upregulation, in which the number of β-receptors in the iris and ciliary body significantly increase during this same period (35). Over a period of months and years, in some patients who were initially controlled, timolol's ocular hypotensive efficacy will be reduced. This phenomenon has been termed long-term drift (36). Brubaker showed that aqueous flow was higher in most patients at 1 year compared with 1 week after starting therapy (37). With both these phenomena, there is a great deal of individual variation.

The "washout" period for timolol maleate is up to 4 weeks after the cessation of chronic timolol therapy (38). The IOP does not elevate significantly for 14 days after discontinuing long-term timolol, and aqueous flow does not return to normal for 2 to 6 weeks (38).

Timolol maleate has a long history of success as a single-therapy agent in the reduction of IOP; however, almost 50% of glaucomatous eyes require more than one drug to lower IOP to the desirable target level. A number of studies have shown the additive effect of additional antiglaucoma medications to timolol maleate; however, the relationship of timolol maleate with epinephrine or dipivefrin is somewhat controversial. Epinephrine compounds enhance aqueous outflow facility when added to a β-blocker. There have been conflicting findings, with some studies showing an additive effect (39,40) and others showing no effect (41,42). In general, the addition of epinephrine agents slightly decreases the IOP an additional 1 to 3 mm Hg; however, there is a wide variability in efficacy from patient to patient, with some studies claiming no additive effect in 50% of patients (43).

As of September 1993, timolol maleate became available in an anionic heteropolysaccaride gellan gum (Gelrite) administered once a day (Timoptic XE 0.25% and 0.5%). This novel ophthalmic vehicle, purified from *P. elodea* cell wall, gels on contact with the monovalent and divalent cations in the tear film, especially the sodium in tears (44). The gel formulation increases the viscosity of the drug, allowing increased bioavailability. Thus, timolol is in contact with the ocular surface longer, allowing more drug penetration. The ocular hypotensive effect is similar for timolol maleate solution twice daily and timolol XE once daily (45,46). One of the theoretical advantages of Timoptic XE is that less timolol maleate is administered over a 24-hour period, which decreases the amount available for systemic absorption and theoretically decreases systemic side effects; however, there is a significant incidence of transient blurred vision, lasting 30 seconds to 5 minutes, in patients taking Timoptic-XE.

In 1995, Betimol, timolol hemihydrate (CIA Vision, Atlanta, Georgia) was approved for use in the United States. Pharmacologically, the only difference between timolol maleate and timolol hemihydrate is the substitution of the hemihydrate for the maleate anion. Unpublished multicenter double-masked studies report that the two drugs have similar IOP-lowering effect and side-effect safety profiles.

Pharmaceutics and Therapeutic Use

Commercially available timolol maleate and timolol hemihydrate 0.25% and 0.5% concentrations contain the L (levo)-isomer, which yields a higher affinity for adrenergic receptors. The 0.25% and 0.5% concentrations are also available as an ophthalmic gel. They are supplied in 2.5-, 5-, 10-, and 15-ml bottles.

The recommended dosing of timolol maleate and timolol hemihydrate 0.25% and 0.5% ophthalmic solutions is one drop twice daily. For Timoptic XE, the gel-forming preparation, the recommended dosing is one drop once a day. In patients with an inadequately controlled IOP, other antiglaucoma medications, such as pilocarpine or carbonic anhydrase inhibitors, may be used in combination with timolol to lower the IOP further. The clinical indication for timolol is for the lowering of IOP, which may be useful in the treatment of ocular hypertension and a variety of glaucomas.

Pharmacokinetics

There is little information concerning the pharmacokinetics of topical timolol in humans because of the difficulty in obtaining samples. Thus, most of our knowledge comes either from animal models or in humans from orally or intravenously administered timolol. In single-dose studies in rabbits, peak levels of topical timolol occur in aqueous humor and blood 30 minutes after administration of 0.5% timolol, with a half-life of 1.5 hours (30). Oral timolol is widely distributed, with an elimination half-life of 2 to 5 hours. Systematically absorbed timolol is biotransformed in the liver into inactive metabolites, which then are excreted primarily in the urine, with 20% of the drug eliminated unchanged (47). The concentration of drug at the ciliary body may be an important consideration for β-blocker pharmacokinetics. Unfortunately, to date, definitive studies developing this relationship are lacking.

Side Effects

Although timolol has been shown to be a relatively safe drug over its long history of clinical use, some ocular and systemic side effects have been reported.

Ocular Effects

Ocular toxicity is a rare occurrence with timolol. The most common adverse effect is stinging or burning on ocular instillation. This local irritation may manifest itself as conjunctival hyperemia. Other reported subjective side effects include itching, photophobia, blurring of vision, and foreign-body sensation. Objective side effects include keratitis, ptosis, superficial punctate keratopathy, corneal anesthesia, and allergic blepharoconjunctivitis (48,49). Timolol may also decrease tear production, resulting in a mild dry eye (50). Ocular cicatricial pemphigoid has been reported in patients receiving topical timolol (51). Chronic timolol therapy was shown to decrease goblet cell density, which alters mucus production (52). This finding may explain the pathogenesis of timolol-induced pemphigoid. Additionally, studies have shown that nonselective β-blockers inhibit corneal reepithelization more than β_1-antagonists (53).

Systemic Effects

Although topical agents are used for their local effects on the eye, there is significant systemic absorption, which may lead to serious systemic consequences. The ocular doses administered are much lower than those administered orally. The amount of timolol in four drops of 0.5% ophthalmic solution is only about 1 mg. In contrast, the oral dose of timolol maleate for treatment of systemic hypertension is 20 to 60 mg per day. Thus, plasma levels of the drug after ophthalmic administration are below those of cardiovascular therapeutic doses but are still high enough to cause systemic adverse effects (54).

The conjunctival cul-de-sac can hold approximately 7 to 11 μl of volume; however, the size of most eyedrops ranges from 30 to 80 μl. Thus, the medication is lost within a few minutes of drop instillation, with most lost within the first 15 seconds, either by running down the patient's cheek or by passing through the nasolacrimal drainage system. A small amount of topically administered drug is absorbed into the systemic circulation through the conjunctival capillaries, but the vast majority, approximately 80%, is absorbed by draining through the puncta into the lacrimal system and nasal cavity, where it is absorbed by the mucosal vasculature (55).

This type of absorption is significant because the absorbed drug enters the systemic circulation, avoiding the first-pass hepatic metabolism, which is quite relevant for β-blockers. Oral β-blockers undergo extensive first-pass hepatic metabolism, with 90% of the drug inactivated, so that relatively little drug reaches the systemic circulation. In this respect, topical administration is akin to intravenous administration of the drug because systemically absorbed timolol bypasses hepatic metabolism. By avoiding first-pass metabolism, higher drug plasma levels relative to their starting dose are achieved, which may explain the systemic side effects of topical β-blockers despite low dosages.

Systemic absorption can be reduced by occluding the lacrimal puncta or by eyelid closure. Nasolacrimal occlusion is performed by gentle pressure over the nasal corner of the eye from the fingertips before and for 2 minutes after instillation of the eyedrop. This maneuver reduces the plasma drug level by 60% (56).

In its premarketing clinical studies, timolol showed a high therapeutic index with few systemic effects; however, increased experience with timolol has revealed a number of systemic effects. In general, systemic adverse events with timolol have been reported more frequently and are more serious than the ocular side effects. The systemic adverse events that β-blocking cause can be divided into four broad categories: cardiovascular, pulmonary, central nervous system (CNS), and metabolic effects.

Cardiovascular Effects

Cardiovascular side effects are caused by *blocking* the β_1-receptors. This blockage interferes with normal sympathetic stimulation, which is important in cardiac function. Blocking the β_1-receptors may lower heart rate and blood pressure, decrease myocardial contractility, and slow cardiac conduction. In most healthy patients, these effects are of little consequence, but in patients with already compromised myocardial function, these effects may precipitate congestive heart failure, arrhythmias, severe bradycardia, heart block, or death (57). Other potential cardiovascular effects include syncope, palpitations, angina, and myocardial infarction. In one study, cardiac arrhythmias (55%) were the most common timolol-associated cardiovascular adverse event (58). Timolol significantly decreased heart rate and oxygen consumption in young, healthy volunteers during exercise (59). Caution must be used when prescribing timolol to patients with a compromised cardiovascular system.

Pulmonary Effects

Among the most important adverse events of timolol are bronchospasm-related respiratory events. β_2-adrenergic tone is important for maintaining open airways. Blocking the β_2-receptors may cause contraction of the smooth muscle in the pulmonary bronchi, leading to bronchospasm and airway obstruction. This fact is especially important in patients with preexisting asthma and chronic obstructive pulmonary disease. The most common reported complaints in patients with a history of pulmonary disease are wheezing, dyspnea, and cough (58,60,61). Respiratory depression and death from status asthmaticus have been reported in patients with history of reactive airway disease and on timolol (62).

Central Nervous System Effects

Adrenergic neurotransmission plays an important role in many CNS activities, best exemplified by antidepressants, which enhance central adrenergic activity by increasing the availability of neurotransmitter at synaptic junctions. It has been postulated that β-blockers may cause CNS effects by blocking seratonin receptors in the CNS. Although numerous reports have linked oral β-blockers with the development of central nervous system symptoms (63), few cases have been reported with ophthalmic use of β-blockers (64,65).

Timolol is a lipophilic drug with low-protein binding, which allows it to penetrate the blood–brain barrier easily. It has been reported to cause a number of CNS effects, including light-headedness, weakness, fatigue, memory loss, depression, anxiety, confusion, weakness, emotional lability, sleep disturbances, memory loss, and drowsiness (48, 66). Additionally, timolol can cause sexual dysfunction by decreasing libido and causing impotence (67).

Metabolic Effects

Oral β-blockers are known to affect different metabolic processes. In diabetic patients, β-blockers may mask the signs and symptoms of acute hypoglycemia and not allow proper physiological response to low blood-glucose levels.

Increasing interest in ophthalmology has developed regarding the effect of topical β-blockers on lipid metabolism. The triglyceride levels increased 12% and high-density lipoproteins decreased 9% in normal volunteers taking topical timolol, which theoretically could increase the risk of coronary heart disease (68). Further studies are needed to correlate these observations to other patient populations (e.g., older glaucoma patients).

BETAXOLOL

Betaxolol's official drug name is betaxolol hydrochloride; its trade names, Betoptic and Betoptic S; and its chemical name, (±)-1-[p-[2-(Cyclopropylmethoxy) ethyl] phenoxy]-3-(isopropylamino)-2-propanol hydrochloride. Its molecular formula is $C_{18}H_{29}NO_3 \cdot HCl$, and it has a molecular weight of 343.9.

Clinical Pharmacology

Betaxolol hydrochloride (Alcon Laboratories, Fort Worth, TX, U.S.A.) is a relatively cardioselective β_1-adrenergic blocking drug and was the second topical β-blocker approved for ophthalmic use, in 1985. It is a phenoxypropanolamine and lacks local anesthetic activity (membrane stabilizing) and partial agonist (intrinsic sympathomimetic) activity. In guinea pigs, betaxolol was 200 times more potent in atrial tissue than in tracheal tissue (69). As the concentration of betaxolol increases, however, β_2-receptors in the trachea are also blocked, and selectivity is relative, not absolute.

Betaxolol is effective in lowering IOP. It significantly reduces IOP compared with placebo (70–73). In ocular hypertensives and glaucoma patients, betaxolol and timolol reduce IOP by 20% to 30% from baseline, with most studies showing betaxolol to have slightly less pressure-lowering efficacy difference (<2 mm Hg) (74–76). This difference is also observed when betaxolol is compared with other β-blockers (77). Physiologically, betaxolol reduces aqueous humor flow but less than other β-blockers (78).

Non-β-blocker glaucoma medications have been shown to be additive to betaxolol. The combined use of betaxolol with pilocarpine or a carbonic anhydrase inhibitor results in a lower IOP (79). A study by Allen found a significant additional reduction by adding epinephrine to betaxolol therapy, but not when it was added to timolol therapy (80). The mechanism of additional IOP lowering may be the stimulation of β_2-receptors by epinephrine increasing aqueous outflow. Betaxolol produces less β_2-blockade than timolol, which would not prohibit possible β_2-receptor-mediated increase in outflow produced by epinephrine. Further research is needed to clarify the mechanism by which this is mediated.

A newer ophthalmic delivery vehicle for betaxolol was introduced in 1991. In this formulation, betaxolol 0.25% is suspended in 5-μm beads consisting of a sterile polymeric resin, allowing slower, more gradual release of medication. Betaxolol 0.25% suspension (Betoptic S) has the same IOP-lowering effect and safety profile as the 0.5% solution but with lower prevalence of ocular discomfort (81).

Because ocular perfusion may play a role in the development of optic nerve damage in glaucoma, there has been increasing interest in the effects of β-blockers on ocular blood flow (82). In a recent study by Messmer (82), the visual fields in glaucoma patients taking betaxolol, with 48-month follow-up, were slightly better compared with patients taking timolol, even though the IOP was slightly higher in the betaxolol group (83). In a second independent visual field study, Collington-Brach found similar results comparing betaxolol and timolol (84). It is theorized that this paradox may be explained by betaxolol's lesser effect on the blood flow to the optic nerve; however, these studies had small sample size, and larger clinical trials are necessary to confirm these observations.

Pharmaceutics and Therapeutic Use

The commercially available product is a racemic mixture containing both inactive dextro isomer and active levo isomer. It is available in 0.5% solution supplied in 2.5-, 5-, 10-, and 15-ml bottles. Betoptic S is supplied as a suspension of betaxolol 0.25% in 2.5-, 5-, 10-, and 15-ml bottles. Betaxolol may be used alone or in combination with other glaucoma medications, such as a miotic or a carbonic anhydrase inhibitor. The recommended dose is one drop twice daily for both concentrations of betaxolol.

The indication for use is the same as for all β-blockers: reducing IOP in ocular hypertensive and glaucoma patients to prevent damage to the optic nerve. The potential advantage of betaxolol over other β-blockers is the relative lack of β_2 blockade, which may be beneficial in patients with a history of respiratory problems.

Pharmacokinetics

Pharmacokinetic studies in humans are limited to data for oral and intravenous betaxolol. Betaxolol is very lipid soluble with a pKa of 9.4. It has a large volume of distribution and rapidly disperses throughout the body. It binds to plasma proteins fairly well (50%) and has a longer elimination half-life (14 to 22) than most other β-blockers. Intravenous and oral betaxolol are metabolized into mainly inactive metabolites by liver microsomal enzymes, which are excreted in the urine; some unchanged drug (15%) is also excreted in the urine (85).

Side Effects

The most common ocular adverse effect with betaxolol solution is transient discomfort (i.e., burning and stinging), which may occur in up to 25% of patients (74,76). It is believed that the discomfort of betaxolol is attributable to its molecular structure and is not a local anesthetic effect. The incidence of ocular adverse events is higher than reported for timolol (74,86). There appears to be a significant difference in ocular tolerability between betaxolol solution and the newer betaxolol suspension. Only 13% patients taking betaxolol suspension complained of burning and stinging versus 37% for the 0.5% betaxolol solution (81).

Patients with a history of reactive airway disease are at particular risk of pulmonary problems from β-blockers. The major advantage of betaxolol is the relatively selective $\beta 1$-adrenergic blockade, which should minimize $\beta 2$-mediated bronchoconstriction and airflow problems. A number of clinical studies have shown that glaucoma patients with respiratory diseases tolerate betaxolol well (87–90). Patients on betaxolol had minimal changes in forced expiratory volume in 1 second (FEV_1), vital capacity, and forced expiratory flow compared with those on timolol and levobunolol (89,91). Although formal clinical trials have shown a relative lack of adverse pulmonary effects, $\beta 1$ selectivity is not absolute, and betaxolol has some $\beta 2$-blocking properties. In rabbits, the concentration of betaxolol after topical instillation was high enough to block both $\beta 1$- and $\beta 2$-receptors. Several reports have associated betaxolol with nonfatal respiratory distress in elderly and asthmatic patients (92,93). Thus, a careful history and assessment of risk benefit must still be performed even when considering betaxolol for clinical use.

Oral or intravenous betaxolol decreases heart rate, blood pressure, and exercise-induced tachycardia; however, in the original clinical trials with topical betaxolol, changes in cardiovascular parameters were not observed. There was also no evidence of cardiovascular blockade during exercise seen with betaxolol as measured by blood pressure and heart rate (94). In clinical practice, where medications are prescribed less selectively, adverse cardiovascular effects have been documented from usage of topical betaxolol. These include congestive heart failure (95), bradycardia, sinus arrest (96), and cardiac arrhythmias (97).

It has been suggested that betaxolol produces fewer CNS side effects than timolol (66,98,99). A likely explanation is betaxolol's high volume of distribution, which allows minimal penetration of the drug into the CNS. It is important to remember, however, that, as with pulmonary side effects, this is not absolute, but relative, and betaxolol has been reported to cause severe clinical depression (65).

CARTEOLOL

Carteolol's official drug name is carteolol hydrochloride; its trade name, Ocupress; and its chemical name, (±)-5-[3-[(1,1-dimethylethyl)amino]-2-hydroxypropoxyl] -3,4-dihydro-2 (1H)-quinolinone monohydrochloride. The molecular formula is $C_{16}H_{24}N_2O_3 \cdot HCl$ and molecular weight, 328.8.

Clinical Pharmacology

Carteolol hydrochloride (Otsuka Pharmaceuticals, Rockville, MD, U.S.A.) is a hydrophilic, relatively potent, nonselective β_1- and β_2-antagonist developed in Japan. It was approved for use in the United States in 1992. Carteolol, along with other β-blockers, possesses little or no local anesthetic activity. It is distinguished from other β-blockers by its partial agonist activity, termed *intrinsic sympathomimetic activity* (ISA). The β-blocking drugs with ISA, in addition to preventing access of endogenous circulating catecholamines to the receptor, also cause an early slight activation of the receptor. Compared with complete agonists, partial agonists produce a reduced pharmacological response. The partial agonist activity of carteolol appears to be attributable to its main metabolite, 8-hydroxy-carteolol. This metabolite is also a potent IOP-lowering agent, which may be responsible for prolonging the duration of IOP lowering of carteolol. Theoretically, ISA has the potential clinical value of producing fewer unwarranted side effects, such as bronchoconstriction, bradycardia (by slight cardiac stimulation), and vasoconstriction, compared with other β-blockers without ISA; however, this claim with topical carteolol remains controversial.

Carteolol hydrochloride effectively reduces normal and elevated IOP; there is no difference in efficacy of carteolol 1% and 2% (100,101). In studies of healthy volunteers, a single dose of carteolol 1% or 2% reduced IOP by 14% to 38% (102,103). A significant reduction in IOP is observed within 1 hour of instillation of carteolol 1%, with peak effect occurring 4 hours after eyedrop instillation. The reduction in IOP persists for 24 to 48 hours, but significant IOP reduction is seen only up to 12 hours (102,103). In a 2-week crossover study in patients with elevated IOP, carteolol 2% lowered IOP by 2 mm Hg more than placebo (104). In one study, 1% or 2% carteolol reduced mean IOP in patients with elevated baseline IOP by a mean of 8.7 mm Hg, a reduction of 32% from pretreatment values for up to 14 months.

Carteolol appears to be as effective as other β-blockers in reducing IOP. In studies comparing timolol and carteolol, no difference was found in efficacy of the two drugs (101,105,106). In a 4-week, double-masked study of 97 ocular hypertensives, no significant difference was found between carteolol 1% and timolol 0.25% (107).

Pharmaceutics and Therapeutic Use

Carteolol is available in the 1% solution in 5- and 10-ml bottles. The recommended dosing is one drop of the 1% solution twice daily. If the IOP is not controlled adequately, concomitant therapy with other antiglaucoma medications may be instituted. As with all β-blockers, carteolol is used to lower IOP for the treatment of glaucoma or ocular hypertension.

Pharmacokinetics

There are few studies published on the pharmacokinetics of ocular carteolol. Most of our knowledge is derived from studies with oral and intravenous carteolol. The drug is widely and rapidly distributed in the body, and the degree of protein binding is small (15%). In healthy volunteers, between 63% and 87% of the drug is excreted unchanged in the urine, with its major metabolite 8-hydroxy-carteolol constituting 4 to 10%. The elimination half-life of carteolol is 5 to 7 hours (108).

Side Effects

In general, nonselective adrenergic blocking agents can reduce cardiac function and increase airway resistance in bronchi and bronchioles, which may lead to problems in already medically compromised patients. The intrinsic sympathomimetic activity of carteolol, with its partial β-agonist activity, may help to reduce these systemic side effects. Although a few preliminary studies with topical carteolol are encouraging, these clinical advantages need to be confirmed in formal clinical trials. The evidence supporting this claim is certainly not absolute, with some studies showing no increased protection from adverse systemic effects (101,109–111). In general, topical carteolol's influence on cardiovascular function has been demonstrated to reduce heart rate and blood pressure, similar to that observed for other β-blockers without ISA. Interestingly, in two separate studies, carteolol reduced heart rate for subjects with a baseline heart rate >70 beats per minute but not in patients with a heart rate <70 beats per minute (105, 112). Compared with timolol 0.5%, less ocular irritation has been seen with carteolol 1% and 2% (113).

Carteolol is a hydrophilic molecule and thus is limited in its penetration. This is best illustrated by the fact that a 1% concentration is needed to achieve IOP lowering compared with 0.25% or 0.5% concentration of timolol, a lipophilic drug. On the other hand, carteolol's hydrophilicity may be an advantage in reducing systemic side effects. Carteolol's poor penetration of membranes may decrease its systemic absorption in the nasolacrimal system and also limit penetration of the blood–brain barrier. Theoretically, less drug would be available to produce systemic side effects (114).

Topical nonselective β-blockers have been associated with the alteration of blood lipid profile, an increase in triglycerides (12%), and reduction of high-density lipoprotein (HDL) cholesterol (8%) (68). In preliminary studies, carteolol, possibly because of its partial agonist activity, was shown to have less effect on lipid parameters (105, 115). In an 8-week study on healthy volunteers, timolol was associated with a 7.4% statistically significant decrease in HDL, whereas carteolol was associated with a smaller decrease in HDL (3.4%) (115).

LEVOBUNOLOL

Levobunolol's official drug name is levobunolol hydrochloride; its trade name, Betagan; and its chemical name, (-)-5[3-*tert*-butylamino)-2-hydroxypropoxy]-3,4-dihydro-1(2H)naphthalenone, hydrochloride. Its molecular formula is $C_{17}H_{26}O_3N_1Cl_1$ and its molecular weight is 327.9.

Clinical Pharmacology

Levobunolol hydrochloride (Allergan Pharmaceuticals, Irvine, CA, U.S.A.) is a lipophilic propranolol derivative with nonselective β_1 and β_2-blocking ability, which was approved for use in late 1985. It is also now available in generic form (Bausch and Lomb, Tampa, FL, U.S.A.; Schein Pharmaceutical, Florham Park, N.J., U.S.A.). It has a pKa of 9.4 and its pharmacokinetics are similar to timolol. Levobunolol does not have significant local anesthetic activity and lacks intrinsic sympathomimetic activity. The levoisomer of levobunolol is 60 times more potent in its β-blocking activity than its dextroisomer (116). Thus, the commercially available product of levobunolol contains only the levoisomer.

Levobunolol was effective in decreasing IOP in normal volunteers as well as in persons with elevated IOP. Initial studies demonstrated that 0.3% and 0.6% concentrations reduced IOP significantly for up to 4 hours, and 1% and 2% concentrations reduced IOP for 12 hours (117,118). Intraocular pressure reduction occurs within 1 hour after instillation of levobunolol; the maximum effect, a reduction of 30%, was seen at 2 to 6 hours (119). In long-term and short-term studies, levobunolol has been shown to be equivalent to timolol and other β-blockers in its ability to lower IOP (118,120–122).

A significant decrease in IOP can be maintained for up to 24 hours following single dosing of levobunolol. Thus, in selected patients, levobunolol may be effective in lowering IOP when it is administered in once-daily dosage (123–125). Levobunolol is metabolized to dihydrobunolol, which also has β-blocking ability, which may account for the prolonged efficacy of levobunolol. A 3-month clinical trial compared once-a-day administration of 0.5% levobunolol, 1% levobunolol, and 0.5% timolol in 92 patients (123). The study found that the overall decrease in intraocular pressure was significantly greater for the levobunolol group (0.5% levobunolol 7 mm Hg and 1% levobunolol 6.5 mm Hg) than for the timolol group (4.5 mm Hg). The probability of IOP control over the study period was 83% for 0.5% levobunolol, 86% for 1% levobunolol, and 72% for 0.5% timolol. Although there appears to be a difference, it did not achieve statistical significance.

Few studies have examined the additive effect of antiglaucoma medications to levobunolol; however, one would expect effects similar to those reported for the nonselective β-blockers. One study found that the combination of levobunolol and dipivefrin had the same efficacy as timolol plus dipivefrin (126). The additive effect of pilocarpine to levobunolol is similar to the combined effect of pilocarpine and timolol (127).

Pharmaceutics and Therapeutic Use

Levobunolol hydrochloride is available commercially in 0.25% and 0.5% concentrations in 5-, 10-, and 15-ml bottles. The usual dosing is one drop twice daily in the affected eye; however, current data suggest that once-daily dosage of levobunolol may be tried first in selected patients before increasing to the typical twice-daily schedule. If the IOP is not controlled, combination therapy with other glaucoma medications may be used to achieve the target IOP. Levobunolol hydrochloride is indicated for ocular hypertension and glaucoma, for which lowering of IOP may be beneficial.

Pharmacokinetics

As with all other β-blockers, scarce information is available regarding ocular levobunolol in humans. In animal experiments, peak aqueous humor levels were obtained 30 minutes after administration of racemic bunolol. The half-life of the drug was 60 to 90 minutes. With oral or intravenous administration, levobunolol is metabolized to dihydrolevobunolol, a potent pressure-lowering metabolite, which may explain the prolonged effect of topical levobunolol. The half-life of systemically administered levobunolol is 6 to 7 hours (128).

Side Effects

Levobunolol can produce a number of potential ocular and systemic adverse side effects similar to those of other nonselective β-blockers. These effects are summarized in detail in the section on timolol maleate. As expected, more side effects are observed with the 1% solution, available only as an investigational concentration, compared with the 0.5% solution (129). A recent study by Lewis illustrated reduced heart rates and systolic blood pressure during exercise in patients treated with 0.25% levobunolol as compared to 0.25% betaxolol suspension (130). In general, the cardiovascular effect of β-adrenergic blockade reduces cardiac output, which may be hazardous in patients with preexisting myocardial dysfunction and may lead to cardiac failure. Beta-blockade also increases airway resistance in the bronchi and bronchioles from unopposed parasympathetic activity. In persons with asthma or other pulmonary problems, this effect can be dangerous.

METIPRANOLOL

Metipranolol's official drug name is metipranolol; its trade name, Optipranolol; and its chemical name, (±)-1-(4-Hydroxyl-2,3,5-trimethylphenoxyl)-3-(isopropylamino)-2-propanol-4-acetate. The molecular formula is $C_{17}H_{27}NO_4$, and its molecular weight is 309.4.

Clinical Pharmacology

Metipranolol (Bausch and Lomb, Tampa, FL, U.S.A.), introduced in the United States in 1991, is a nonselective β_1- and β_2-adrenergic receptor blocking agent, as are timolol and levobunolol. It lacks intrinsic sympathomimetic activity or membrane-stabilizing effect.

The efficacy of metipranolol in lowering IOP has been reported in a number of studies. Metipranolol begins to act within 30 minutes, with a maximum effect (30% decrease from baseline) at 2 hours. After a single dose, IOP remains lower than baseline for at least 24 hours (131). Metipranolol, like levobunolol, has a biologically active metabolite, des-acetyl metipranolol, which may explain the prolonged duration of action (132). There was no difference in IOP-lowering when using 0.1%, 0.3%, and 0.6% solutions (133). In a 6-week, double-masked study, metipranolol 0.3% reduced IOP by 21% from baseline, and 0.6% metipranolol reduced it by 31% (134). The efficacy of metipranolol is comparable to the currently used ocular β-blockers. Studies have shown that metipranolol lowers IOP comparably to timolol (135–137) and levobunolol (138).

Pharmaceutics and Therapeutic Use

Metipranolol has been available in Europe for more than a decade in a range of concentrations. In the United States, it is available only as a 0.3% solution in 5- and 10-ml bottles. The recommended dose is one drop twice daily. Metipranolol may be used as a single-drug therapy or in conjunction with other glaucoma medications when IOP is not adequately controlled. As with all the β-blockers discussed herein, metipranolol is indicated to lower IOP in ocular hypertensives and glaucoma patients.

Pharmacokinetics

Pharmacokinetic data for topically administered metipranolol are not available in humans. Oral and intravenous metipranolol rapidly undergo acetylation in plasma to an active metabolite, desacetyl metipranolol. The absolute bioavailability is 50%, and 70% of the drug is bound to plasma proteins; the half-life is 2.5 to 4 hours. It has been reported that metipranolol does not undergo first-pass hepatic metabolism (139).

Side Effects

Metipranolol has generally been well tolerated, although patients have complained of transient stinging, particularly with the first few doses. Other ocular adverse side effects attributed to metipranolol (burning, photophobia, punctate keratopathy, ocular foreign body sensation, and blurred vision) are similar to those of timolol and other β-blockers. Metipranolol is less tolerated than other β-blockers because of stinging and burning on instillation (135,137).

Patients on metipranolol may develop a wide range of adverse clinical effects (respiratory, cardiovascular, and CNS) from systemic absorption similar to those of other nonselective β-blockers.

Since 1991 in England, a number of patients treated with metipranolol 0.3% and 0.6% developed granulomatous uveitis (140–142). Although the exact pathogenesis was not determined, this problem was believed to be related to the manufacturing process in England. Since then, the United Kingdom has withdrawn the 0.1%, 0.3%, and 0.6% strengths of metipranolol from clinical use. There has been an isolated report in the United States of uveitis associated with metipranolol (143).

GENERAL CONSIDERATIONS

The following section summarizes current thought and makes some general statements regarding β-blockers.

Clinical Pharmacology

For glaucoma therapy to be most efficacious, the most important principle to remember is that, regardless of the type of medication prescribed, it is imperative for success that patients be provided with instructions for proper administration of these drugs. Topical β-blockers are the most widely used treatment for glaucoma. To date, comparative trials in patients with elevated IOP demonstrated that carteolol, levobunolol, metipranolol, and timolol have a similar degree and maintenance of IOP-lowering (20–30%). Betaxolol appears to have slightly less IOP-lowering efficacy.

Approximately 50% of glaucoma patients on a β-blocker require additional glaucoma medications to control their IOP adequately. Combination therapies with all the β-blockers have similar efficacy. The additivity of epinephrine compounds to β-blockers is variable: Some studies suggest that additivity is greater with betaxolol than with timolol. At best, there is mean reduction of IOP of 1 to 2 mm Hg, with a small proportion of patients showing a greater reduction of IOP pressure and a significant percent showing no change in IOP.

Side Effects

The nature of side effects from medications used to treat glaucoma may be overlooked easily when evaluating patients. Ophthalmologists may not routinely question patients about their symptoms, and patients often do not think these problems are related to the use of their eyedrops. Thus, it is important to remember that topical β-blockers have systemic absorption and therefore have the potential to lead to significant cardiovascular, respiratory, and CNS side effects. These problems are rarely encountered with well patients, but the possibility increases in sick patients, particularly in those with cardiovascular and pulmonary disease. Specifically, topical β-blockers are contraindicated in patients with reactive airway disease (asthma and chronic obstructive pulmonary disease), greater than first-degree heart block, overt heart failure, and symptomatic sinus bradycardia. Thus, as with any form of treatment, medical or surgical, the ratio of risk to benefits must be weighed in consultation with the patient.

A wide variety of systemic side effects have been reported with the use of topical β-blockers. Beta-blockers produce their cardiopulmonary side effects by nonspecific blockade of both β_1- and β_2-receptors. Betaxolol, which is a cardioselective β-blocker, has the advantage of causing less systemic β_2-blockade. Although betaxolol does not entirely prevent systemic side effects, the incidence of pulmonary side effects with betaxolol is significantly less than that reported with nonselective beta blockers. As with all β-blockers, however, caution must be exercised.

Clinical trials have not definitively evaluated the differential effect of the β-blockers on the CNS. The lipid solubility of a β-blocker allows the drug to pass through the blood–brain barrier into the CNS. It is unclear, however, whether drugs that are less lipid soluble, such as carteolol, cause fewer adverse reactions in the CNS. Preliminary evidence suggests that selective β-blockers may offer an advantage over nonselective β-blockers in terms of lessening CNS effects.

As with all eyedrops, methods to minimize systemic absorption should be considered. Nasolacrimal occlusion before and 2 minutes after drop application is a simple technique to reduce systemic absorption of eyedrops and to ensure maximum ocular absorption. This technique may be expected to reduce the plasma levels of the drugs and concomitantly reduce systemic side effects.

Ocular adverse reactions are relatively uncommon with topical β-blockers. There are some variations in ocular side effects, but in general the side effects of the different β-blockers are similar. The variations in ocular side effects may reflect the different vehicles used, pHs, and concentrations of the drugs.

REFERENCES

1. Ahlquist RP. A study of the adrenotropic receptors. *Am J Physiol* 1948;153:586–600.
2. Powell CE, Slater IH. Blocking of inhibitory adrenergic receptors by a dichloro analog of isoproterenol. *J Pharmacol Exp Ther* 1958; 122:480–488.
3. Phillips CI, Howitt G, Rowlands DJ. Propranolol as ocular hypotensive agent. *Br J Ophthalmol* 1967;51:222–526.
4. Takats I, Szilvassy I, Kerek A. Intraocular pressure and circulation of aqueous humor in rabbit eyes following intravenous administration of propranolol (Inderal). *Graefes Arch Clin Exp Ophthalmol* 1972;185:331–342.
5. Pandolfi M, Ohrstrom A. Treatment of ocular hypertension with oral beta-adrenergic blocking agents. *Acta Ophthalmol* 1974;52:464–467.
6. Ohrstrom A, Pandolfi M. Long-term treatment of glaucoma with systemic propranolol. *Am J Ophthalmol* 1978;86:340–344.
7. Bucci MG, Missiroli A, Giraldi JP, Virno M. Local administration of propranolol in the treatment of glaucoma. *Boli Oculist* 1968;47: 51–80.
8. Musini A, Fabbri B, Bergamaschi M, Mandelli V, Shanks RG. Comparison of the effect of propranolol, lignocaine, and other drugs on normal and raised intraocular pressure in man. *Am J Ophthalmol* 1971;72:773–781.
9. Merte HJ, Merkle W. Long-term treatment of glaucoma with propanolol ophthalmic solution. *Klin Monatsbl Augenheilkd* 1980; 177:437–442.
10. Rahi AHS, Chapman CM, Garner A, Wright P. Pathology of practolol-induced ocular toxicity. *Br J Ophthalmol* 1976;60:312–323.
11. Skegg DCG, Doll R. Frequency of eye complaints and rashes among patients receiving practolol and propranolol. *Lancet* 1977;2:475–478.
12. Yablonski ME, Zimmerman TJ, Waltman SR, Becker B. A fluorophotometric study of the effect of topical timolol on aqueous humor dynamics. *Exp Eye Res* 1978;27:135–142.
13. Neufeld AH, Bartels SP, Liu JH. Laboratory and clinical studies on the mechanism of action of timolol. *Ophthalmology* 1983;28:286–290.
14. Zimmerman TJ, Harbin R, Pett M, Kaufman HE. Timolol and facility of outflow. *Invest Ophthalmol Vis Sci* 1977;16:623–624.
15. Nathanson JA. Human ciliary process adrenergic receptor: pharmacological characterization. *Invest Ophthalmol Vis Sci* 1981;21: 798–804.
16. Schmitt C, Lotti VJ, DeDouarec JC. Beta-adrenergic blockers: lack of relationship between antagonism of isoproterenol and lowering of intraocular pressure in rabbits. In: Sear ML, ed. *New Directions in Ophthalmic Research.* New Haven: Yale University Press, 1983; 147–162.
17. Topper JE, Brubaker RF. Effects of timolol, epinephrine, and acetazolamide on aqueous flow during sleep. *Invest Ophthalmol Vis Sci* 1985;26:1315–1319.

18. Caprioli JC, Sears M, Bausher L, Gregory D, Mead A. Forskolin lowers intraocular pressure by reducing aqueous outflow. *Invest Ophthalmol Vis Sci* 1984;25:268–277.
19. Keates EV, Stone R. The effect of d-timolol on intraocular pressure in patients with ocular hypertension. *Am J Ophthalmol* 1984;98: 73–78.
20. Watanabe K, Chiou GCY. Mechanism of action of timolol to lower the intraocular pressure in rabbits. *Ophthalmic Res* 1983;15:160–167.
21. Boger WP, Steinert RF, Puliafito CA, Pavan-Langston D. Clinical trial comparing timolol ophthalmic solution to pilocarpine in open-angle glaucoma. *Am J Ophthalmol* 1978;86:8–18.
22. Sonntag JR, Brindley GO, Shields MB, Arafat NT, Phelps CD. Timolol and epinephrine: comparison of efficacy and side effects. *Arch Ophthalmol* 1979;97:273–277.
23. Katz IM, Hubbard WA, Getson AJ, Gould AL. Intraocular pressure decrease in normal volunteers following timolol ophthalmic solution. *Invest Ophthalmol Vis Sci* 1976;15:489–492.
24. Zimmerman TJ, Kass MA, Yablonski ME, Becker B. Timolol maleate: efficacy and safety. *Arch Ophthalmol* 1979;97:656–658.
25. Zimmerman TJ, Kaufman HE. Timolol: a beta-adrenergic blocking agent for the treatment of glaucoma. *Arch Ophthalmol* 1977;95: 601–604.
26. Zimmerman TJ, Kaufman HE. Timolol: dose response and duration of action. *Arch Ophthalmol* 1977;95:605–607.
27. Mottow-Lippa LS, Lippa EA, Naiidoff MA, Clementi R, Bjornsson T, Jones K. 0.008% timolol ophthalmic solution: a minimal effect dose in a normal volunteer model. *Arch Ophthalmol* 1990;108:61–64.
28. Soll DB. Evaluation of timolol in chronic open angle glaucoma: once a day vs twice a week. *Arch Ophthalmol* 1990;98:2178–2181.
29. Letchinger SL, Frohlichstein D, Gieser DK, et al. Can the concentration of timolol or the frequency of its administration be reduced? *Ophthalmology* 1993;100:1259–1262.
30. Schmitt CJ, Lotti VJ, LeDouarec JC. Penetration of timolol into the rabbit eye: Measurement after ocular instillation and intravenous injection. *Arch Ophthalmol* 1980;98:547–551.
31. Aula P, Kaila T, Huupponen R, et al. Timolol binding to bovine ocular melanin in vitro. *J Ocul Pharmacol Ther* 1988;4:29–36.
32. Katz IM, Berger ET. Effects of iris pigmentation on response of ocular pressure to timolol. *Surv Ophthalmol* 1979;23:395–398.
33. Boger WI. Short-term "escape" and longterm "drift". The dissipation effects of the beta adrenergic blocking agents. *Surv Ophthalmol* 1983;28:235–242.
34. Boger WP, Puliafito CA, Steinert RF, Langston DP. Long-term experience with timolol ophthalmic solution in patients with open-angle glaucoma. *Ophthalmology* 1978;85:259–267.
35. Neufeld AH, Zawistowski KA, Page ED, Bromberg BB. Influences on the density of beta adrenergic receptors in the cornea and iris-ciliary body of the rabbit. *Invest Ophthalmol Vis Sci* 1978;17:1069–1075.
36. Steinert RF, Thomas JV, Boger WP. Long-term drift and continued efficacy after multiyear timolol therapy. *Arch Ophthalmol* 1981;99: 100–103.
37. Brubaker RF, Nagataki S, Bourne WM. Effect of chronically administered timolol on aqueous humor flow in patients with glaucoma. *Ophthalmology* 1982;89:280–283.
38. Schlect LP, Brubaker RF. The effect of withdrawal of timolol in chronically treated glaucoma patients. *Ophthalmology* 1988;95: 1215–1216.
39. Cyrlin M, Thomas JV, Epstein DL. Additive effects of epinephrine to timolol therapy in primary open angle glaucoma. *Arch Ophthalmol* 1982;100:414–418.
40. Goldberg I, Ashburn FS, Palmberg PF. Timolol and epinephrine: a clinical study of intraocular interactions. *Arch Ophthalmol* 1980;98: 484–486.
41. Korey MS, Hodapp E, Kass MA, et al. Timolol and epinephrine: long-term evaluation of concurrent administration. *Arch Ophthalmol* 1982;100:742–745.
42. Moss AP, Ritch R, Hargett NA. A comparison of the effects of timolol and epinephrine on intraocular pressure. *Am J Ophthalmol* 1978; 86:489–491.
43. Alexander DW, Berson F, Epstein DL. A clinical trial of timolol and epinephrine in the treatment of primary open-angle glaucoma. *Ophthalmology* 1988;95:247–251.
44. Greaves JL, Wilson CG, Rozier A, Grove J, Iazonnet B. Scintigraphic assessment of an ophthalmic gelling vehicle in man and rabbit. *Curr Eye Res* 1990;9:415–420.
45. Timoptic-XE Study Group. Multiclinic, double-masked study of 0.5% Timoptic-XE once daily versus 0.5% Timoptic twice daily. *Ophthalmology* 1993;100(suppl):111.
46. Laurence J, Holder D, Vogel R, et al. A double-masked, placebo-controlled evaluation of timolol in gel vehicle. *J Glaucoma* 1993;2:177–181.
47. Vermeij P, el Sherbini-Shepers M, van Zweiten PA. The disposition of timolol in man. *J Pharm Pharmacol* 1978;30:53–55.
48. McMahon CD, Shaffer RN, Hoskin HD, Hetherington J. Adverse effects experienced by patients taking timolol. *Am J Ophthalmol* 1979;88:736–738.
49. Van Buskirk EM. Corneal anesthesia after timolol maleate therapy. *Am J Ophthalmol* 1979;88:739–743.
50. Bonomi L, Zavarise G, Noya E. Effects of timolol maleate on tear flow in human eyes. *Graefes Arch Clin Exp Ophthalmol* 1980;213: 19–22.
51. Fiore PM, Jacobs IH, Goldberg DB. Drug-induced pemphigoid: a spectrum of disease. *Arch Ophthalmol* 1987;105:1660–1663.
52. Herreras JM, Pastor JC, Calonge M, Asensio VM. Ocular surface alteration after long-term treatment with an antiglaucomatous drug. *Ophthalmology* 1992;99:1082–1088.
53. Liu GS, Trope GE, Basu PK. Beta adrenoreceptors and regenerating corneal epithelium. *J Ocul Pharmacol Ther* 1990;6:101–112.
54. Alvan G, Calissendorf B, Slideman P, Widmark K, Widmark G. Absorption of ocular Timolol. *Clin Pharmokinet* 1980;5:95–100.
55. Shell JW. Pharmacokinetics of topically applied ophthalmic drugs. *Surv Ophthalmol* 1982;26:207–218.
56. Zimmerman TJ, Kooner KS, Kandarakris AS, et al. Improving the therapeutic index of topically applied ocular drugs. *Arch Ophthalmol* 1984;102:551–553.
57. Van Buskirk EM. Adverse reactions from timolol administration. *Ophthalmology* 1988;87:447–450.
58. Nelson WL, Fraunfelder FT, Sills JM, et al. Adverse respiratory and cardiovascular events attributed to timolol ophthalmic solutions 1978–1985. *Am J Ophthalmol* 1986;102:606–611.
59. Doyle WJ, Weber PA, Meeks RH. Effects of timolol maleate on exercise performance. *Arch Ophthalmol* 1984;102:517–518.
60. Jones FL, Ekberg NL. Exacerbation of asthma by timolol. *N Engl J Med* 1979;301:270.
61. Schoene RB, Martin TR, Charan NB, French CL. Timolol-induced bronchospasms in asthmatic bronchitis. *JAMA* 1981;245:1460–1461.
62. Van Buskirk EM, Fraunfelder FT. Ocular beta-blockers and systemic effects. *Am J Ophthalmol* 1984;98:623–624.
63. Petire WM, Maffucci RJ, Woosley RL. Propranolol and depression. *Am J Psychiatry* 1982;139:92–94.
64. Nolan BT. Acute suicidal depression associated with use of timolol [Letter]. *JAMA* 1982;247:1567.
65. Orlando RG. Clinical depression associated with betaxolol. *Am J Ophthalmol* 1986;102:275.
66. Duch S, Duch C, Pasto L, Ferrer P. Changes in depressive status associated with topical beta-blockers. *Int Ophthalmol* 1992;16:331–335.
67. Fraunfelder FT. Sexual dysfunction secondary to topical ophthalmic timolol. *JAMA* 1985;253:3092–3093.
68. Coleman AL, Diehl DLC, Jampel HD, Bachorik PS, Quigley HA. Topical timolol decreases plasma high-density lipoprotein cholesterol level. *Arch Ophthalmol* 1990;108:1260–1263.
69. Cavero I, Lefevero-Borg F, Manoury P, et al. In vitro and in vivo pharmacologic evaluation of betaxolol, a new potent, selective $\beta 1$ adrenoreceptor antagonist. In: Morseli PL, ed. *Betaxolol and Other $\beta 1$-Adrenoreceptor Antagonists.* Laboratories d'edites et de recherches synthelabo. New York: Raven Press, 1983;31–42.
70. Feghali JG, Kaufman PL. Decreased intraocular pressure in the hypertensive human eye with betaxolol, beta1-adrenergic antagonist. *Am J Ophthalmol* 1985;100:777–782.
71. Caldwell DR, Salisbury CR, Guzek JP. Effects of topical betaxolol in ocular hypertensive patients. *Arch Ophthalmol* 1984;102:539–540.
72. Berrospi AR, Leibowitz HM. A new beta-adrenergic blocking agent for the treatment of glaucoma. *Arch Ophthalmol* 1982;200:943–946.

73. Radius RL. Use of betaxolol in the reduction of elevated intraocular pressure. *Arch Ophthalmol* 1983;101:898–900.
74. Berry DP, Van Buskirk EM, Shields MB. Betaxolol and timolol. A comparison of efficacy and side effects. *Arch Ophthalmol* 1984;102: 42–45.
75. Stewart RH, Kimbrough RL, Ward RL. Betaxolol vs timolol. A six month double blind comparison. *Arch Ophthalmol* 1986;104:46–48.
76. Feghali JG, Kaufman PL, Radius RL, et al. A comparison of betaxolol and timolol in open angle glaucoma and hypertension. *Acta Ophthalmol* 1988;66:180–186.
77. Long DA, Johns GE, Mullen RS, et al. Levobunolol and betaxolol. A double masked controlled comparison of efficacy and safety in patients with elevated intraocular pressure. *Ophthalmology* 1988; 95:735–738.
78. Gaul GR, Will NJ, Brubaker RF. Comparison of a noncardioselective beta-adrenoreceptor and a cardioselective blocker in reducing aqueous flow in humans. *Arch Ophthalmol* 1989;107:1308–1340.
79. Smith JP, Weeks RH, Newland EF, et al. Betaxolol and acetazolamide. Combined ocular hypotensive effect. *Arch Ophthalmol* 1984;102:1794–1795.
80. Allen RC, Epstein DL. Additive effects of epinephrine to betaxolol and timolol, in primary open-angle glaucoma. *Arch Ophthalmol* 1986;104:1178–1184.
81. Weinreb RN, Caldwell DR, Goode SM, et al. A double masked three month comparison between 0.25% betaxolol suspension and 0.5% betaxolol ophthalmic solution. *Am J Ophthalmol* 1990;110:189–192.
82. Messmer C, Flammer J, Stumpfig D. Influence of betaxolol and timolol on the visual fields of patients with glaucoma. *Am J Ophthalmol* 1991;112:678–681.
83. Kaiser HJ, Flammer J, Stumpfig D, Hendrickson P. Long-term visual field follow-up of glaucoma patients treated with beta-blockers. *Surv Ophthalmol* 1994;38(suppl):156–160.
84. Collignon-Brach J. Long-term effect of topical beta-blockers on intraocular pressure and visual field sensitivity in ocular hypertension and chronic open-angle glaucoma. *Surv Ophthalmol* 1994;38 (suppl):149–155.
85. Beresford R, Heel RC. Betaxolol. A review of its pharmacodynamics and pharmacokinetic properties, and therapeutic efficacy in hypertension. *Drugs* 1986;31:6–28.
86. Allen RC, Hertzmark E, Walker AM, Epstein DL. A double masked comparison of betaxolol vs timolol in the treatment of open-angle glaucoma. *Am J Ophthalmol* 1986;101:534–535.
87. Brooks AMV, Burdon JG, Gillies WE. The significance of reactions to betaxolol reported by patients. *Aust N Z J Ophthalmol* 1989;17: 353–355.
88. Ofner S, Smith TJ. Betaxolol in chronic obstructive pulmonary disease. *J Ocul Pharmacol* 1987;3:171–176.
89. Schoene RB, Abuan T, Ward RL, Beasley CH. Effects of topical betaxolol, timolol, and placebo on pulmonary function in asthmatic bronchitis. *Am J Ophthalmol* 1984;97:86–92.
90. Weinreb RB, Van Buskirk EM, Cherniack R, Drake MM. Long-term betaxolol therapy in glaucoma patients with pulmonary disease. *Am J Ophthalmol* 1988;106:162–167.
91. Dunn TL, Gerber MJ, Shen AS, et al. The effect of topical ophthalmic instillation of timolol and betaxolol on lung function in asthmatic subjects. *Am Rev Respir Dis* 1986;133:264–268.
92. Rohalt PC. Betaxolol and restrictive airway disease: case report. *Arch Ophthalmol* 1987;102:1072.
93. Harris LS, Greenstein SH, Bloom AF. Respiratory difficulties with betaxolol. *Am J Ophthalmol* 1986;201:274–275.
94. Atkins JM, Pugh BR, Timewell RM. Cardiovascular effects of topical beta-blockers during exercise. *Am J Ophthalmol* 1985;99:173–175.
95. Ball S. Congestive heart failure from betaxolol. *Arch Ophthalmol* 1987;105:320.
96. Zabel RW, MacDonald IM. Sinus arrest associated with betaxolol ophthalmic drops. *Am J Ophthalmol* 1987;104:431.
97. Nelson WL, Kuritsky N. Early post-marketing surveillance of betaxolol ophthalmic drops. *Am J Ophthalmol* 1987;103:592.
98. Cohn JB. A comparative study of the central nervous system effects of betaxolol versus timolol. *Arch Ophthalmol* 1989;107:633–634.
99. Lynch MG, Whitson JT, Brown RH, Nguyen H, Drake MM. Topical beta-blocker therapy and central nervous system side effects: a preliminary study comparing betaxolol and timolol. *Arch Ophthalmol* 1988;106:908–911.
100. Duff GR. A double masked cross-over study comparing the effects of carteolol 1% and 2% on intraocular pressure. *Acta Ophthalmol* 1987;65:618–621.
101. Stewart WC, Shields MB, Allen RC, Lewis RA, Cohen JS, et al. A 3 month comparison of 1% and 2% carteolol and 0.5% timolol in open-angle glaucoma. *Graefes Arch Clin Exp Ophthalmol* 1991; 229:258–261.
102. Araie M, Takase M. Effects of S-696 and carteolol, new beta-adrenergic blockers, and flurbiprofen on the human's eye: a fluorophotometric study. *Graefes Arch Clin Exp Ophthalmol* 1985;222:259–262.
103. Negishi C, Kanai A, Nakajima A, Funahashi M, Kitazawa Y. Ocular effects of beta-blocking agent carteolol on healthy volunteers and glaucoma patients. *Jpn J Ophthal* 1981;25:464–476.
104. Duff GR, Graham PA. A double cross-over trial comparing the effect of topical carteolol and placebo on intraocular pressure. *Br J Ophthalmol* 1988;72:27–28.
105. Kitazawa Y. Multicenter double-blind comparison of carteolol and timolol in primary open-angle glaucoma and ocular hypertension. *Advances in Therapy* 1993;10:95–131.
106. Tsuchisaka H, Kin K, Matsumoto S, Ishiwata T, et al. Multi-institutional evaluation of timolol and carteolol for glaucomas. *Ganka Rhinsho Iho* 1991;85:1136–1140.
107. Scoville B, Muller B, White BG, Kriegelstein GK. A double-masked comparison of carteolol and timolol in ocular hypertension. *Am J Ophthalmol* 1988;105:150–154.
108. Chrisp P, Sorkin EM. Ocular carteolol. A review of its pharmacological properties, and therapeutic use in glaucoma and ocular hypertension. *Drugs Aging* 1992;2:58–77.
109. Brazier DJ, Smith SE. Ocular and cardiovascular response to topical carteolol 2% and timolol 0.5% in healthy volunteers. *Br J Ophthalmol* 1988;72:101–103.
110. Hugues FC, Le Jeunne C, Munera Y. Systemic effects of topical antiglaucomatous drugs. *Glaucoma* 1992;14:100–104.
111. Le jeune CI. Cardiovascular effects of beta-blocker eyedrops (timolol, carteolol, metipranolol, betaxolol) in elderly patients. *Therapie* 1988;6:489–492.
112. Flury H, Tournoux A, Martenet AC. Vertaglichkeit und pharmakologische Wirksamkeit von antiglaukomatosen Augentropfen. *Klin Monatsbl Augenheilkd* 1986;188:573–575.
113. Scoville B, Kriegelstein GK, Then E, Yokoyama S, Yokoyama T. Measuring drug-induced eye irritation: a simple new clinical assay. *J Clin Pharmacol* 1985;25:210–218.
114. Zimmerman TJ. Topical ophthalmic beta blockers: a comparative review. *J Ocul Pharmacol Ther* 1993;9:373–384.
115. Freedman SF, Freedman NJ, Shields MB, et al. Effects of ocular carteolol and timolol on plasma high density lipoprotein cholesterol level. *Am J Ophthalmol* 1993;116:600–611.
116. Woodward DF, Novack GD, Williams LS, Nieves AL, Potter DE. Dihydrolevobunolol is a potent ocular beta-adrenoreceptor antagonist. *J Ocul Pharmacol* 1987;3:11–15.
117. Partamian LC, Kass MA, Gordon M. A dose response study of the effect of levobunolol on ocular hypertension. *Am J Ophthalmol* 1983;95:229–232.
118. Berson FG, Cohen HB, Foerster RJ, et al. Levobunolol compared with timolol for the long term control of elevated intraocular pressure. *Arch Ophthalmol* 1985;103:379–382.
119. Duzman E, Ober M, Scharr A, et al. A clinical evaluation of the effects of topically applied levobunolol and timolol on increased intraocular pressure. *Am J Ophthalmol* 1982;94:318–327.
120. The Levobunolol Study Group. Levobunolol: a four year study of efficacy and safety in glaucoma treatment. *Ophthalmology* 1989; 96:642–645.
121. Cinotti A, Cinotti D, Grant W, et al. Levobunolol compared with timolol for the long-term control of elevated intraocular pressure. *Am J Ophthalmol* 1985;99:11–17.
122. Geyer O, Lazar M, Novack G, et al. Levobunolol compared with timolol for the control of elevated intraocular pressure. *Ann Ophthalmol* 1986;18:289–292.
123. Wandel T, Fishman D, Novack GD, et al. Ocular hypotensive efficacy of 0.25% levobunolol instilled once daily. *Ophthalmology* 1988;95:252–255.

124. Rakofsky SI, Melamed S, Cohen JS, et al. A comparison of the ocular hypotensive efficacy of once-daily and twice-daily levonolol treatment. *Ophthalmology* 1989;96:8–11.
125. Derick RJ, Robin AL, Tielsch J, et al. Once daily versus twice daily levobunolol (0.5%) therapy. *Ophthalmology* 1992;99:424–429.
126. Allen R, Long D, Robin A, et al. Efficacy and safety of levobunolol compared with timolol in combination with dipivefrin in glaucoma. *Invest Ophthalmol Vis Sci* 1986;27:181.
127. David R, Ober M, Masi R, et al. Treatment of elevated intraocular pressure with concurrent levobunolol and pilocarpine. *Can J Ophthalmol* 1987;22:208–211.
128. Lesar TS. Comparison of ophthalmic β-blocking agents. *Clinical Pharmacy* 1987;6:451–463.
129. The Levobunolol Study Group. Levobunolol, a beta-adrenoreceptor antagonist effective in the long-term treatment of glaucoma. *Ophthalmology* 1985;92:1271–1276.
130. Lewis SE. Controlled comparison of the cardiovascular effects of levobunolol 0.25% ophthalmic solution and betaxolol 0.25% ophthalmic suspension. *J Glaucoma* 1994;3:308–314.
131. Dausch D, Brewitt H, Edelhoff R. Metipranolol eye drops: clinical suitability in the treatment of chronic open angle glaucoma. In: Merte HJ, ed. *Metipranolol.* New York: Springer-Verlag Wien, 1983; 132–147.
132. Pentikainen PJ, Neuvonen PJ, Penttila A. Assessment of beta-blocking activity of trimepranol in man. *Int J Clin Pharmacol Ther* 1978;16:279–284.
133. Hickey-Dwyer M, Campbell SH, Harding S. Double-masked three-period crossover investigation of metipranolol in control of raised intraocular pressure. *J Ocul Pharmacol* 1991;7:277–283.
134. Serle JB, Lustgarten JS, Podos SM. A clinical trial of metipranolol, a noncardioselective beta-adrenergic antagonist, in ocular hypertension. *Am J Ophthalmol* 1991;112:302–307.
135. Mills KB, Wright G. A blind randomised cross-over trial comparing metipranolol 0.3% with timolol 0.25% in open-angle glaucoma: a pilot study. *Br J Ophthalmol* 1986;70:39–42.
136. Merte HJ, Stryz JR, Mertz M. Comparative studies on initial pressure reduction using metipranolol 0.3% and timolol 0.25% in eyes with open-angle glaucoma. *Klin Monatsbl Augenheikd* 1983;182: 286–289.
137. Mertz M. Results of a 6 weeks' multicenter double-blind trial: Metipranolol vs timolol. In: Merte HJ, ed. *Metipranolol: Pharmacology of Beta-blocking Agents and Use of Metipranolol in Ophthalmology.* New York: Springer-Verlag, 1984;93–105.
138. Kriegelstein GK, Novack GD, Voepel E, et al. Levobunolol and metipranolol: comparative ocular hypotensive efficacy, safety, and comfort. *Br J Ophthalmol* 1987;71:250–253.
139. Battershill PE, Sorkiin EM. Ocular metipranolol: a preliminary review of its pharmacodynamic and pharmacokinetic properties, and therapeutic efficacy in glaucoma and ocular hypertension. *Drugs* 1988;36:601–615.
140. Kinshuck D. Glauline (metipranolol) induced uveitis and increase in intraocular pressure. *Br J Ophthalmol* 1991;75:575.
141. Akingbehin T, Villada JR. Metipranolol-associated granulomatous anterior uveitis. *Br J Ophthalmol* 1991;75:519–523.
142. Akingbehin T, Villada JR, Walley T. Metipranolol-induced adverse reactions: I. The rechallenge study. *Eye* 1992;6:277–279.
143. Schultz JS, Hoenig JA, Charles H. Possible bilateral anterior uveitis secondary to metipranolol (OptiPranolol) therapy. *Arch Ophthalmol* 1993;111:1606–1607.

Textbook of Ocular Pharmacology,
edited by T.J. Zimmerman, et al.
Lippincott–Raven Publishers, Philadelphia © 1997.

CHAPTER 24

Oral Carbonic Anhydrase Inhibitors

Jeffrey G. Piper

ACETAZOLAMIDE (DIAMOX)

History and Source

Acetazolamide, a synthetic sulfonamide without antimicrobial properties, was initially described as a diuretic agent by Miller and associates in 1950 (1). Its initial use in the therapy for glaucoma was based on a theory of aqueous production proposed by Friedenwald in 1949 (2). This theory, combined with the report by Wistrand of carbonic anhydrase in the aqueous-producing structures of the eye (3), prompted Becker to investigate acetazolamide as a pressure-lowering agent in humans (4). The use of acetazolamide has since become widespread, with an estimated 250,000 patients receiving the drug annually (5).

Chemistry

Acetazolamide (trade name, Diamox) has the chemical name N-(5-sulfamoyl, 1,3,4-thiadiazole-2yl)-acetamide and chemical formula $C_4H_6N_4O_3S_2$. Its molecular weight is 222.24, and it has a PKa of 7.4. Its appearance is white to faintly yellow; it is an odorless, crystalline powder. Its solubility in water is slight.

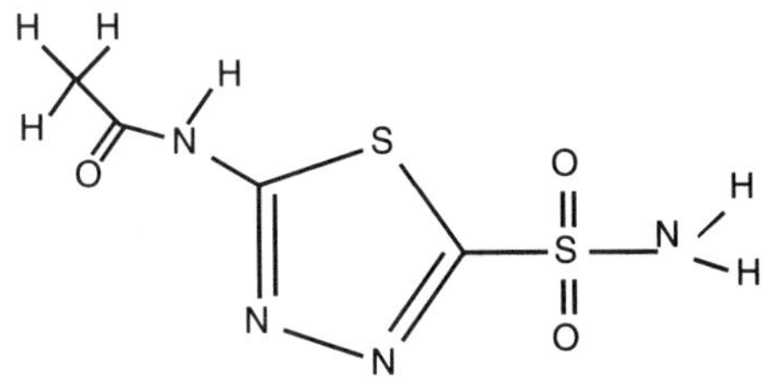

Acetazolamide

J. G. Piper: Department of Ophthalmology, University of Texas Southwestern Medical Center, Dallas, Texas 75235.

Pharmacology

Acetazolamide inhibits the enzyme carbonic anhydrase, which catalyzes the reversible hydration of carbon dioxide to form carbonic acid. A subsequent spontaneous disassociation of carbonic acid to hydrogen and bicarbonate ions is not under enzymatic control. Acetazolamide acts to reduce intraocular pressure by inhibiting isoenzyme II in the ciliary processes of the eye (6). Carbonic anhydrase is also found in multiple other tissues of the body, including the renal cortex, pancreas, and gastric mucosa (7,8).

Clinical Pharmacology

Mechanism

Acetazolamide acts to decrease intraocular pressure by reducing aqueous production. Support for this comes from multiple studies, including tonography (9), the transport of fluorescein (10), dilution of intraocular substances (11), and direct observation of the ciliary processes (12).

Acetazolamide acts locally at the ciliary processes to reduce aqueous production. Isolated ciliary processes respond to directly administered acetazolamide (12). Once problems with limited penetration are overcome, topically administered acetazolamide will produce local pressure effects (13). Furthermore, intracarotid injection of acetazolamide produces only ipsilateral pressure reduction (14).

The effect of acetazolamide is mediated by its action on carbonic anhydrase. Zimmerman and colleagues demonstrated an acetazolamide-induced reduction in bicarbonate transport into the posterior chamber (15). Others have also shown altered CO_2 turnover in response to acetazolamide (16). These chemicals represent the substrate of carbonic anhydrase, which is found in significant quantity in the ciliary processes. Additionally, patients with autosomal recessive deficiency of carbonic anhydrase failed to respond to acetazolamide (17).

Alternate hypotheses about the mechanism of action have failed to find wide support. Although a small group of postoperative patients appeared to have an increased facility of outflow with acetazolamide therapy (18), this effect has not been generally demonstrated (9,19). The pressure-lowering effect of acetazolamide was shown to be unrelated to its diuretic action by Becker's studies of nephrectomized rabbits (9).

Based on the observation that intraocular pressure is often reduced in systemic acidotic states, Bietti and others proposed that acetazolamide acts via metabolic acidosis rather than directly on ocular carbonic anhydrase (20). Other authors emphasize the countervailing finding that concomitant bicarbonate administration does not prevent a pressure effect (21) and report that the rapidity of acetazolamide's action suggests a direct effect (9).

Dose-response Relation

Zimmerman and others demonstrated a maximum 50% reduction of bicarbonate transfer following acetazolamide administration (15). This finding is reflected in the reduced aqueous production of a similar magnitude (19). At least 99% of carbonic anhydrase must be inhibited before a pressure effect is demonstrated (22). A concentration of 10.5 *M* acetazolamide will block carbonic anhydrase staining in the ciliary processes (23). The serum concentration found in clinical doses ranges from 4 to 30 μg/ml (24).

Friedland and colleagues studied patients with ocular hypertension and demonstrated linear relations between dose and peak plasma level as well as plasma level and percentage of carbonic anhydrase inhibition. Short-term pressure response was found to plateau with doses >63 mg. The maximum pressure effect was a 30 to 35% reduction of pretreatment levels (~9 mm Hg) (24).

Lichter's group found pressure reductions of a similar degree but emphasized that maximum response and speed of onset increased with doses up to 500 mg. They also reported an increased response in patients who had been pretreated with acetazolamide (25).

Nonocular Effects

Acetazolamide acts in the red blood cells and kidneys to induce metabolic acidosis. Some authors suggest that this effect may contribute to the pressure-lowering effects of the agent (20), whereas others attribute the malaise often associated with chronic carbonic anhydrase inhibitor use to this acidosis (26). Urinary citrate excretion is reduced in acetazolamide therapy, which may account for the occurrence of renal stones in patients receiving the drug (27,28). Conversely, renal excretion of potassium is increased in acetazolamide treatment. Therefore, patients taking other potassium-wasting diuretics may be at increased risk for hypokalemia (26).

Pharmaceutics

Tablets

Acetazolamide tablets are available in two forms. The 125-mg oral tablets are white, round, and beveled. They bear the marks "Diamox" and "125" on the obverse and are scored in half with the marks "LL" and "D1" on the reverse. The 250-mg oral tablets are white and of similar shape but bear the marks "Diamox," "acetazolamide," and "250" on the obverse, with quarter scores, "LL," and "D2" on the reverse.

The tablets contain the inactive ingredients cornstarch, dibasic calcium phosphate, magnesium stearate, Povidone, and sodium starch glycolate. According to the manufacturer, they should be stored at 15° to 30°C. Generic forms of the medication are equally effective in reducing intraocular pressure (29).

Sustained-release Capsules

An oral sustained-release form of acetazolamide is available under the brand name Diamox Sequels. These are 500-mg orange capsules bearing the marks "Diamox" and "D3" on each capsule. They contain the inactive ingredients beeswax, Benzoin gum, cornstarch, ethylcellulose, FD & C, blue no. 1, FD & C yellow no. 6, gelatin, glycerin, magnesium stearate, methylparaben, mineral oil, monoglycerides and diglycerides, propylene glycol, propylparaben, silica, sucrose talc, terpene, resin, and vanillin. The manufacturer recommends storage at 15 to 30°C.

Parenteral

Diamox is available for intravenous injection as a lyophilized powder of acetazolamide sodium. Each vial contains the equivalent of 500 mg of acetazolamide and, according to the manufacturer, should be stored at 15° to 30°C.

Pharmacokinetics

Acetazolamide is absorbed completely following oral administration (30). Peak plasma levels occur 1 hour after ingestion and are linearly related to dose (24). A 500-mg dose produces a peak level of 30 μg/ml. Maximum pressure reduction occurs 2 to 6 hours after an oral dose (24, 25), and the effect persists beyond 7 hours.

The sustained-release capsule produces peak plasma levels in 3 to 4 hours (31). Serum levels remain above 10 μg/ml for 10 hours, and the pressure effect lasts 6 to 18 hours (32). Approximately 90% of acetazolamide is protein bound in plasma. At physiological pH, about 50% of acetazolamide is in the active, nonionized form (33).

The principal route of excretion is via active secretion of the unaltered drug by the renal tubules (34). Plasma drug levels can be determined by high-performance liquid chromatography (HPLC), but most practitioners adjust the dose based on pressure response and side effects (36).

Therapeutic Use

Indications

Acetazolamide is useful in the treatment of primary and secondary open-angle glaucoma and chronic angle-closure glaucoma. Because of its side-effect profile, it is usually reserved for use in patients who have not had an adequate response to topical agents or are intolerant to them. The effect of acetazolamide in combination with topical agents is additive (37–39). It is useful in short-term management of infantile, neovascular, and angle-closure glaucoma but should not be used as a substitute for definitive surgical management of these conditions.

Contraindications

Acetazolamide produces metabolic acidosis (20) and may potentiate acid-base imbalance in patients with preexisting acidosis. Because of its transient diuretic effect, acetazolamide should be used with caution in combination with other diuretic agents causing potassium wasting (26). Extra caution should be used in clinical situations where adequate potassium levels are particularly important, such as digitalis glycoside therapy.

A combination of acetazolamide and high-doses of aspirin increases the risk for salicylate toxicity and metabolic acidosis (40). Acetazolamide is structurally related to sulfa antibiotics and is known to cause sulfa-type allergic reactions (41). The incidence of cross reactivity may, however, be low (42).

Acetazolamide-induced acidosis and hemoconcentration may predispose patients with hemoglobinopathies to sickling of red blood cells. Therefore, sickle-cell patients with glaucoma secondary to hyphema should receive topical pressure-lowering agents in preference to carbonic anhydrase inhibitors (42). Acetazolamide should not be used as chronic therapy for neovascular and angle-closure glaucoma to the exclusion of definitive therapy. In angle-closure states, pressure reduction caused by carbonic anhydrase inhibitors may reduce pressure temporarily, allowing subsequent permanent synechiae of the angle to ensue.

Method of Use

The usual dosages of acetazolamide for chronic glaucoma therapy in adults is 250 mg to 1,000 mg daily, typically delivered in four divided doses. Clinicians should consider beginning therapy with a low dose, gradually increasing dosage until an adequate therapeutic effect is achieved. To do so may improve patient acceptance of medication (36). Sustained-release preparations (Diamox Sequels 500 mg orally, twice daily) are better tolerated over the long term than equivalent dosages in tablet form (42).

Elderly patients are less tolerant to carbonic anhydrase inhibitors (42). Initial dosages should be reduced. Consideration should be given to using methazolamide in preference to acetazolamide in elderly patients (36).

There is a body of clinical experience with acetazolamide administered to children. The usual pediatric dose of acetazolamide is 5 mg to 10 mg/kg four to six times a day (43). The safety and efficacy of acetazolamide therapy in children are unproven.

In the acute setting, a 500-mg oral dose of acetazolamide causes a more rapid decrease in intraocular pressure than lower doses (25). Intravenous administration of acetazolamide causes a pressure fall within minutes (9).

Some authors suggest periodic monitoring of blood counts because of the potential for severe hematologic abnormalities in chronic acetazolamide therapy (44). Other authors point out that the cost of screening blood counts per case detected would be extremely high and that early detection may not influence the outcome of hematologic side effects (45). Most practitioners, including specialists in the field of glaucoma, do not monitor blood counts routinely (46).

Adverse Reactions

Life-threatening reactions (e.g., marrow suppression and aplastic anemia) occasionally are attributed to acetazolamide (44). In addition, sulfa-type allergic reactions, including anaphylactic shock, have been reported (41).

Potassium depletion is of concern in patients concurrently receiving other diuretic agents (26). Metabolic acidosis is a consistent finding in acetazolamide use (20), and this drug may produce severe effects in patients with other acid-base disturbances. Renal stones occur at the rate of 2.4% of patients per year among patients on acetazolamide therapy (47). Previous stone formation on carbonic anhydrase inhibitors is a significant predictor of future nephrolithiasis (47).

Less severe but still significant reactions from acetazolamide are quite common. Only 26% of patients were able to tolerate acetazolamide over a 6-week period. This rate rose to 58% with Diamox Sequels (42). Epstein and Grant reported a symptom complex of malaise, weight loss, depression, anorexia, and loss of libido in almost half of patients on carbonic anhydrase inhibitor therapy (26). Other reported side effects include paresthesias (36), metallic taste to carbonated beverages (48), gastrointestinal disturbances (36), and hirsutism (49). Transient myopia caused by ciliary body swelling also can occur (50).

Overdosage

Despite the frequent occurrence of side effects, acetazolamide has relatively little additional toxicity, even at very high doses. If overdose were to occur, gastric lavage and supportive therapy are recommended.

HIGH-RISK GROUPS

Children

In neonates and children, dosage should be reduced to approximately 5 to 10 mg/kg four times a day (43). The metabolic acidosis induced by acetazolamide can cause feeding problems in children. Long-term studies of the safety of acetazolamide in children are lacking.

Pregnant and Nursing Women

Although acetazolamide has been used without ill effects in late pregnancy (51), it is known to produce forelimb deformities in the offspring of rodents (52). Therefore, acetazolamide use during pregnancy should be avoided when possible. Low concentrations of Diamox have been detected in human breast milk (53). Therefore, women requiring acetazolamide should not breast-feed.

Elderly Patients

Elderly patients have a higher incidence of side effects from carbonic anhydrase inhibitors and are less able to tolerate therapy (54). Reduced initial dosage is recommended, and consideration should be given to using methazolamide rather than acetazolamide (36).

Drug Interactions

The combination of acetazolamide and high doses of aspirin can lead to severe acidosis and salicylate toxicity (40). Diflunisal raises the serum levels of acetazolamide and enhances the pressure-reducing effect (55); however, the safety of this combination has not been determined (55).

Acetazolamide in combination with topical glaucoma agents has an additive effect (37–39). The potential exists for acetazolamide to potentiate potassium depletion caused by other diuretics (26).

DICHLORPHENAMIDE (DARANIDE)

History and Source

After its introduction, acetazolamide gained widespread use as an antiglaucoma agent. It was recognized early, however, that the agent was associated with side effects for many patients (56). The search for a clinically effective carbonic anhydrase inhibitor with fewer toxic side effects led to the investigation of dichlorphenamide (57). It was hoped that the higher potency of this agent compared with other carbonic anhydrase inhibitors and its consequent reduced dosage would allow for better tolerance of therapy (57). Unfortunately, this has not proved to be the case (42).

Chemistry

Dichlorphenamide (trade name, Daranide) has the chemical name 4,5-dichloro-benzenedisulfonamide, and its chemical formula is $C_6H_6Cl_2N_2O_4S_2$. Its molecular weight is 305.16 and its PKa 8.3. It has extremely slight solubility in water. Its appearance is that of a white crystalline powder.

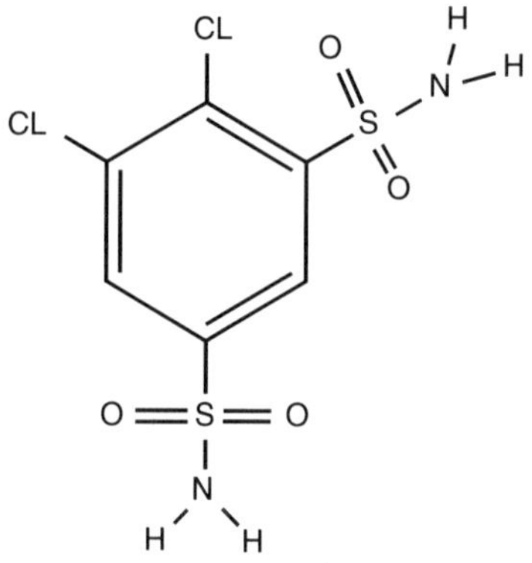

Dichlorphenamide

Pharmacology and Clinical Pharmacology

Dichlorphenamide (Daranide) is a carbonic anhydrase inhibitor with effects similar to those of acetazolamide. The concentration of drug required to inhibit 50% of carbonic anhydrase activity is 30 times higher for acetazolamide than for dichlorphenamide. Despite this higher potency, dichlorphenamide has not been found more clinically efficacious than acetazolamide.

Intraocular pressure is reduced following administration of dichlorphenamide (57,58). This effect can be observed in both normal and glaucomatous subjects (57). As with other carbonic anhydrase inhibitors, the pressure reduction results from decreased aqueous production (57). Aqueous flow is reduced by approximately 39% after a 300-mg dose (57).

Clinical reduction of pressure begins within 30 minutes of a 200-mg oral dose (57). The maximum pressure reduction occurs in approximately 2 hours and persists for 6 hours (57). The average pressure reduction in glaucoma with a single 200-mg dose is 6.8 mm Hg (57). A sensitive assay for drug levels in serum has been described (42).

Pharmaceutics

Daranide is available as oral tablets containing 50 mg of dichlorphenamide. The tablets are yellow and round. They are scored and bear the mark "MSD 49." The inactive ingredients are D & C yellow no. 10, lactose, magnesium stearate, and starch. There are no special storage requirements.

Therapeutic Use

Indications

Dichlorphenamide is indicated for the control of intraocular pressure in open-angle glaucoma. It is also indicated for the short-term treatment of angle-closure glaucomas preoperatively or as adjunct therapy after surgical intervention. Substitution of agents within the carbonic anhydrase inhibitor class can reduce side effects in some patients (36). Therefore, dichlorphenamide may be tolerated in a minority of patients who are unable to tolerate the other carbonic anhydrase inhibitors (36,59).

Contraindications

Dichlorphenamide has a persistent chloruretic effect (60). The resulting persistent diuresis may contribute to potassium depletion. The agent is therefore contraindicated in patients with hypokalemia. Dichlorphenamide should be used with caution in patients using other potassium-depleting drugs, such as thiazides and adrenal steroids.

Hyperkalemic metabolic acidosis has been reported in one patient with aldosterone deficiency (61). The combination of high-dose aspirin and dichlorphenamide carries the potential risk of severe metabolic acidosis and salicylate toxicity (40). Methazolamide may be preferable in patients taking salicylates (40). Patients with chronic obstructive pulmonary disease are less able to compensate for metabolic acidosis associated with the carbonic anhydrase inhibitors.

There is the potential for cross-reactivity among sulfa drugs; therefore, alternate therapies should be considered in patients with sulfa allergy. Because of the shared properties of carbonic anhydrase inhibitors, dichlorphenamide should be considered contraindicated in cirrhosis and nephrolithiasis. Angle-closure and neovascular glaucoma should not be treated with dichlorphenamide to the exclusion of definitive therapy.

Method of Use

The usual dose of dichlorphenamide is 25 to 50 mg orally, one to four times a day. The manufacturer suggests a priming dose of 100–200 mg. Patient tolerance of carbonic anhydrase inhibitors may, however, be enhanced by low initial doses (36). Dosage should be adjusted according to patient tolerance and clinical response. Consideration should be given to periodic monitoring of electrolytes, especially in those at increased risk for hypokalemia or acidosis.

Adverse Reactions

The common side effects for the other carbonic anhydrase inhibitors also have been reported in dichlorphenamide therapy. Among these are paresthesias, loss of appetite, dizziness, malaise, depression, and confusion (57,59). Compared with the other carbonic anhydrase inhibitors, dichlorphenamide was particularly associated with anorexia and confusion (42).

Patient tolerance for dichlorphenamide is lower than for the other available carbonic anhydrase inhibitors (42). Only 21% of glaucoma patients can tolerate Daranide beyond 6 weeks of therapy.

Metabolic disturbances, including hypokalemia and hyperkalemia and acidosis have been reported with dichlorphenamide (61). Rare hematologic reactions have been reported in association with all the carbonic anhydrase inhibitors, including dichlorphenamide (44). The clinician should be alert to the possibility of aplastic anemia, agranulocytosis, and other reactions.

High-risk Groups

Children

The safety and efficacy of dichlorphenamide in children have not been established. Acetazolamide should be considered in children who require a carbonic anhydrase inhibitor.

Pregnant or Nursing Women

Dichlorphenamide causes forelimb abnormalities in the offspring of rodents when administered during pregnancy (62). It should not be used during pregnancy unless the benefits clearly outweigh the potential risks. It is not known whether dichlorphenamide is excreted in breast milk.

Elderly Patients

Elderly patients have an increased incidence of intolerance to acetazolamide but not to methazolamide (36). In the absence of agent-specific data regarding dichlorphenamide, extra caution should be used when administered to elderly patients.

Drug Interactions

The combination of dichlorphenamide and aspirin may lead to salicylate toxicity and severe metabolic acidosis (40). The combination of dichlorphenamide and other potassium-depleting agents may lead to significant hypokalemia (26).

METHAZOLAMIDE (NEPTAZANE)

History and Source

Sisson and colleagues described a new carbonic anhydrase inhibitor, methazolamide, in 1956 (63). Hoping to find a clinically effective agent with fewer side effects than acetazolamide, Becker reported on the use of methazolamide in 1960 (64). The drug has proved somewhat less effective, but better tolerated, than the other carbonic anhydrase inhibitors (64).

Chemistry

The chemical name of methazolamide (trade name, Neptazane) is N-[5-(aminosulfamoyl)-3-methyl-1,3,4-thiadiazol-2(3H)-ylidine]-acetamide, and its molecular weight is 236.26 and its PKa 7.2. It has the appearance of a white crystalline powder, and its solubility in water is slight.

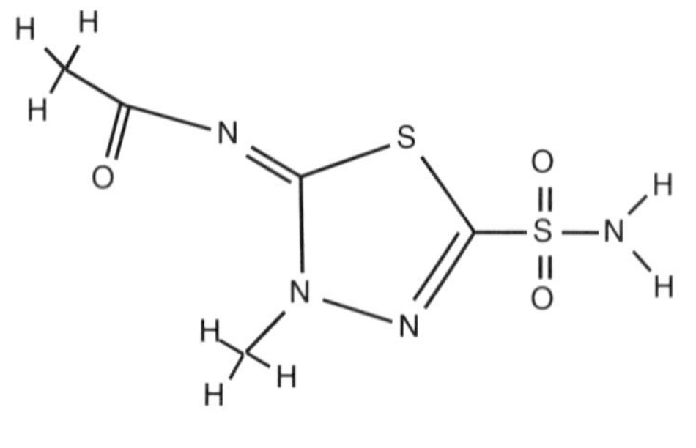

Methazolamide

Pharmacology and Clinical Pharmacology

Methazolamide is a carbonic anhydrase inhibitor with somewhat greater activity, in vitro, than acetazolamide (63). The in vivo effect is enhanced by a high proportion of unbound drug and greater tissue penetration (64,65).

As with the other carbonic anhydrase inhibitors, methazolamide acts to decrease aqueous production. Most patients treated with methazolamide will have >40% reduction in aqueous flow (64).

The serum concentration of methazolamide is linearly related to dose, and peak plasma levels occur 2 to 3 hours after oral administration (66,67). The peak serum concentration following a 100-mg dose is approximately 17 μg/ ml (66). The half-life of methazolamide in blood is significantly longer than that of acetazolamide. Significant plasma levels persist beyond 9 to 14 hours (66,67).

Reported pressure reduction with methazolamide ranges from 2.5 mm Hg, with a 25-mg twice-daily dose, to 5.6 mm Hg, with a 100-mg three-times-daily dose (66,67).

Approximately one quarter of methazolamide is excreted unchanged in the urine (65). The metabolic disposition of the remaining portion is unknown.

Pharmaceutics

Methazolamide is available in 25-mg and 50-mg tablets both in brand name (Neptazane, MZM) and generic preparations. The 25-mg tablets are square and white. The obverse is marked N, and the reverse is marked N2. The 50-mg tablets are round, white, and scored in half, marked "LL" on the obverse and "N" and "1" on the reverse.

The inactive ingredients are Acacia, alginic acid, cornstarch, dibasic calcium phosphate, gelatin, and magnesium stearate. Neptazane should be stored at 15° to 30°C.

Therapeutic Use

Indications

Methazolamide is indicated for the reduction of intraocular pressure in open-angle glaucoma. It may also be useful as adjunct therapy in the management of neovascular and angle-closure glaucoma. At low doses, methazolamide is better tolerated than the other carbonic anhydrase inhibitors (67). It may prove useful in patients who cannot tolerate acetazolamide, particularly the elderly (36,67).

Contraindications

Methazolamide produces less metabolic disturbance than the other carbonic anhydrase inhibitors. With low-dose therapy, few changes in acid-base balance or serum electrolytes are noted (67). Nonetheless, caution should be used when employing methazolamide in patients at risk for metabolic acidosis or hypokalemia.

Patients with angle-closure glaucoma should not receive methazolamide in place of surgical intervention. Permanent synechial closure of the angle could result.

Sulfa-type allergic reactions to methazolamide have been reported (64). Patients with a history of sulfa allergy have the potential for cross-reactivity with methazolamide (42).

Method of Use

The usual dose of methazolamide is 25 to 50 mg orally two or three times per day. Low initial doses may be desirable, especially in elderly patients (36,67). Dosage should be titrated to the desired clinical effect while minimizing adverse reactions. Diamox sequels may be preferable to increased doses of Neptazane for patients who do not adequately respond to methazolamide 50 mg twice a day (67).

Adverse Reactions

Severe hematologic reactions, including aplastic anemia, have been reported in association with methazolamide use (68). The clinician should be alert to the signs and symptoms of platelet or leucocyte deficiency.

In contrast to the other carbonic anhydrase inhibitors, low-dose methazolamide appears to cause relatively few metabolic disturbances (67). Nephrolithiasis has occurred in patients using methazolamide (69), but it appears to be uncommon (65).

Many less severe side effects commonly associated with other carbonic anhydrase inhibitors are also caused by methazolamide. These side effects include nausea, anorexia, paresthesias, malaise, and fatigue (64,67). Malaise and fatigue are particularly associated with methazolamide (64).

Compared with other carbonic anhydrase inhibitors, overall tolerance of methazolamide is high. Moderate-dose methazolamide (50 mg four times daily) is second only to Diamox Sequels in terms of patient tolerance (42). Low-dose methazolamide (25–50 mg twice daily) actually may be the most well-tolerated therapy (67).

High-risk Groups

Children

The safety and efficacy of methazolamide in children have not been established.

Pregnant and Nursing Women

Methazolamide causes forelimb deformities in the offspring of rodents (70). The risk of teratogenicity should be considered when making therapeutic judgments in pregnant women. It is not known whether methazolamide is secreted in breast milk. Women should not breast-feed while using methazolamide.

Elderly Patients

Methazolamide appears to be equally well tolerated in elderly and younger adults (36). It may therefore be the preferred carbonic anhydrase inhibitor in elderly patients (36).

Drug Interactions

High-dose aspirin combined with carbonic anhydrase inhibitors may cause severe metabolic disturbances (40). Therefore, caution should be used when combining methazolamide and salicylates. Low-dose methazolamide itself does not appear to cause hypokalemia (67), but carbonic anhydrase inhibitors may enhance the potassium-depleting effects of other drugs (26).

CLINICAL TRIALS

The early introduction date of the carbonic anhydrase inhibitors as well as the limited therapeutic alternatives at that time account for the relatively small number of clinical trials that have been conducted. Most existing studies use acetazolamide as the standard and compare newer agents with it.

Timolol Versus Acetazolamide

Kass and colleagues compared the pressure effects of Timolol and Acetazolamide in a 1982 study (38). Thirty-eight patients with ocular hypertension were randomized into two groups following a 30-day washout of pressure-lowering medications. After baseline pressure measurements, half received acetazolamide 500 mg, every 12 hours, in a time-released preparation. The other group received timolol 0.5% every 12 hours. The intraocular pressure was measured at 4 weeks for the timolol group and at 1 week for the acetazolamide group.

Measurement of outflow pressure (intraocular pressure minus episcleral venous pressure) showed a 36% reduction for the timolol group and a 48.6% reduction for the acetazolamide group. The authors did not draw a conclusion regarding the statistical significance of this difference. Analysis of the presented data, however, indicates a statistically significant superiority of acetazolamide.

A similar comparison of betaxolol and acetazolamide by Smith et al. confirmed the superiority of acetazolamide to beta blockers in terms of pressure reduction (71). Each of these studies was designed principally to determine the additive effects of beta-blockers and carbonic anhydrase inhibitors. Therefore, the trials provide a less-detailed comparison than one might wish.

Epinephrine Versus Acetazolamide

Becker and Ley compared the effectiveness of acetazolamide, 250 mg every 6 hours, and epinephrine, 4.5% at bedtime, in the eyes of 23 patients (39). All patients were concurrently receiving pilocarpine of unspecified dosage for chronic glaucoma.

Acetazolamide caused an average reduction of 13.0 mm Hg in intraocular pressure. The pressure decrease in the epinephrine group averaged 13.4 mm Hg. This demonstrates a roughly equal effectiveness of the two agents, but the effects in patients not receiving pilocarpine may vary.

Acetazolamide Versus Methazolamide

In a well-controlled, randomized study, Lichter and others compared the effect of two formulations of acetazolamide with methazolamide (25). The 19 glaucoma patients studied were all uncontrolled by epinephrine and pilocarpine therapy. Therapy with these agents was continued during the trial. Dosage of the carbonic anhydrase inhibitors ranged up to 500 mg for acetazolamide, 1,000 mg for sustained-release acetazolamide, and 100 mg for methazolamide.

Maximum mean pressure reduction for acetazolamide was 9.9 mm Hg. The greatest mean pressure reduction for sustained-release acetazolamide was 7.2 mm Hg; the maximum reduction for methazolamide was 8.5 mm Hg.

In a rare comparison of long-term clinical success, Becker compared acetazolamide and methazolamide over 2 years (64). Success was defined as pressure reduction to <30 mm Hg (alternately <24 mm Hg), with no progressive visual field loss or intolerable side effects.

The success rate was 31% for methazolamide and 46% for acetazolamide (15% and 31%, respectively, with the lower pressure criterion). Although this study sets a pressure target that may not be appropriate for all patients and reports few of the controls common in more recent studies, it does give an indication about the overall usefulness of the two agents in glaucoma therapy.

Tolerance of Side Effects

Lichter and colleagues compared the three available carbonic anhydrase inhibitors in terms of patient tolerance (42). Nineteen patients with uncontrolled glaucoma completed a randomized crossover study including placebo.

The highest tolerance was to sustained-release acetazolamide 500 mg twice daily (58% tolerance beyond 6 weeks). The least tolerated of the three agents was dichlorphenamide 50 mg four times daily (21% tolerance beyond 6 weeks). Tolerance to methazolamide (47% beyond 6 weeks) was inferior only to Diamox Sequels. The dose of methazolamide studied (50 mg four times daily) was higher than the dose that often is clinically used. Others have reported that lower-dose therapy is even better tolerated than Diamox Sequels (67).

REFERENCES

1. Miller WH, Dessert AN, Roblin RO Jr. Heterocyclic sulfonamide as carbonic anhydrase inhibitors. *J Am Chem Soc* 1950;72:4893–4896.
2. Friedenwald JS. The formation of the intraocular fluid. *Am J Ophthalmol* 1949;32:9–27.
3. Wistrand PJ. Carbonic anhydrase in the anterior uvea of the rabbit. *Acta Physiol Scand* 1951;24:144–148.
4. Becker B. Decrease in intraocular pressure in man by a carbonic anhydrase inhibitor, Diamox. *Am J Ophthalmol* 1954;37:13–15.
5. Zimran A, Beutler E. Can the risk of acetazolamide-induced aplastic anemia be decreased by periodic monitoring of blood cell counts? *Am J Ophthalmol* 1987;104:654–658.
6. Dobbs PC, Epstein DL, Anderson P. Identification of isoenzyme C as the principal carbonic anhydrase in human ciliary processes. *J Invest Ophthalmol Vis Sci* 1979;18:867–870.
7. Janowitz HD, Colcher H, Hollander F. Inhibition of gastric secretion of acid in dogs by carbonic anhydrase inhibitor 2 - acetylamine - 1,3,4, thiadiazole - 5 - sulfonamide. *Am J Physiol* 1953;171:325–330.
8. Birnbaum D, Hollander F. Inhibition of pancreatic secretion by the carbonic anhydrase inhibitor 2 - acetylamine - 1,3,4, thiadiazole - 5 - sulfonamide, Diamox. *Am J Physiol* 1953;174:191–195.
9. Becker B. The mechanism of the fall in intraocular pressure induced by the carbonic anhydrase inhibitor, Diamox. *Am J Ophthalmol* 1955; 39:177–182.
10. Linner E, Friedenwald JS. The appearance time of fluoroscein as an index of aqueous flow. *Am J Ophthalmol* 1957;44:225–229.
11. Oppelt WW. Measurement of aqueous humor formation rates by posterior-anterior chamber perfusion with inulin: normal values and the effect of carbonic anhydrase inhibition. *Invest Ophthalmol* 1967;6: 76–83.
12. Berggren L. Direct observation of secretory pumping in vitro of the rabbit eye ciliary processes: influence of ion mileu and carbonic anhydrase inhibition. *Invest Ophthalmol* 1964;3:266–272.
13. Friedman Z, Allen RC, Raph SM. Topical acetazolamide and methazolamide delivered by contact lenses. *Arch Ophthalmol* 1985;103: 963–966.
14. Wistrand PJ. Local action of the carbonic anhydrase inhibitor acetazolamide on the intraocular pressure in cats. *Acta Pharmacol Toxicol* 1957;14:27–37.
15. Zimmerman TJ, Garg LC, Vogh BP, Maren TH. The effect of acetazolamide on the movements of anions into the posterior chamber of the dog eye. *J Pharmacol Exp Ther* 1976;196:510–516.
16. Kinsey VE, Reddy DVN. Turnover of carbon dioxide in the aqueous humor and the effect thereon of acetazolamide. *Arch Ophthalmol* 1959;62:78–83.
17. Krupin T, Sly WS, Whyte MP, Dodgson SJ. Failure of acetazolamide to decrease intraocular pressure in patients with carbonic anhydrase II deficiency. *Am J Ophthalmol* 1985;99:396–399.
18. Galin MA, Harris L. Acetazolamide and outflow facility. *Arch Ophthalmol* 1966;76:493–497.
19. Becker B, Constant MA. Experimental tonography: the effect of the carbonic anhydrase inhibitor acetazolamide on aqueous flow. *Arch Ophthalmol* 1955;54:321–329.
20. Bietti G, Virno M, Pecon-Geraldi J, Pellegrino N. Acetazolamide, metabolic acidosis and intraocular pressure. *Am J Ophthalmol* 1975; 80:360–369.
21. Benedikt O, Zirm M, Harmoncourt K. Die Beziehungen zwischen metabolischer azidose und intraokularem druck nach carboanhydrasehemmung mit acetazolamid. *Graefes Arch Clin Exp Ophthalmol* 1974;190:247–255.
22. Friedenwald JS. Current studies on acetazolamide (Diamox) and aqueous humor flow. *Am J Ophthalmol* 1955;40:139–146.
23. Barany EH. A pharmacologist looks at medical treatment in glaucoma—in retrospect and prospect. *Ophthalmology* 1979;86:80–94.
24. Friedland BR, Mallonnee J, Anderson DR. Short-term dose response characteristics of acetazolamide in man. *Arch Ophthalmol* 1977;95: 1809–1812.

25. Lichter PR, Musch DC, Medzihradsky F, Standardi CL. Intraocular pressure effects of carbonic anhydrase inhibitors in primary open-angle glaucoma. *Am J Ophthalmol* 1989;107:11–17.
26. Epstein DL, Grant WM. Carbonic anhydrase inhibitor side effects: serum chemical analysis. *Arch Ophthalmol* 1977;95:1378–1382.
27. Constant MA, Becker B. The effect of carbonic anhydrase inhibitors on urinary excretion of citrate by humans. *Am J Ophthalmol* 1960;49: 929–934.
28. Shah A, Constant MA, Becker B. Urinary excretion of citrate in humans following administration of acetazolamide (Diamox). *Arch Ophthalmol* 1958;59:536–540.
29. Ellis PP, Price PK, Kelmenson R, Rendi MA. Effectiveness of generic acetazolamide. *Arch Ophthalmol* 1982;100:1920–1922.
30. Maren TH, Mayer E, Wadsworth BD. Carbonic anhydrase inhibitors I. The pharmacology of Diamox, 2 - acetylamino - 1,3,4, - thiadiazole - 5 - sulfonamide. *Bull Johns Hopkins Hosp* 1954;95:199–243.
31. Bayne WF, Rogers G, Crisologo N. Assay for acetazolamide in plasma. *J Pharm Sci* 1975;64:402–404.
32. Garner L, Franklin E, Ferwerda JR. Advantages of sustained-release therapy with acetazolamide in glaucoma. *Am J Ophthalmol* 1963;55: 323–327.
33. Maren TH. Carbonic anhydrase: chemistry, physiology, and inhibition. *Physiol Rev* 1967;47:595–781.
34. Maren TH, Robinson B. The pharmacology of acetazolamide as related to cerebrospinal fluid and the treatment of hydrocephalus. *Bull Johns Hopkins Hosp* 1960;106:1–24.
35. Chambers DM, White MH, Korstenlauder HB. Efficient extraction and reversed phase high performance liquid chromatography ultraviolet quantitation of acetazolamide in serum. *J Chromatogr* 1981;225: 231–235.
36. Lichter PR. Reducing side effects of carbonic anhydrase inhibitors. *Ophthalmology* 1981;88:266–269.
37. Dailey RA, Brubaker RF, Bourne WM. The effects of timolol maleate and acetazolamide on the rate of aqueous formation in normal human subjects. *Am J Ophthalmol* 1982;93:232–237.
38. Kass MA, Korey M, Gordon M, Becker B. Timolol and acetazolamide: a study of concurrent administration. *Arch Ophthalmol* 1982; 100:941–942.
39. Becker B, Ley AP. Epinephrine and acetazolamide in the therapy of the chronic glaucomas. *Am J Ophthalmol* 1958;45:639–643.
40. Anderson CJ, Kaufman PL, Sturm RJ. Toxicity of combined therapy with carbonic anhydrase inhibitors and aspirin. *Am J Ophthalmol* 1978;86:516–519.
41. Perlata J, Abelairas J, Fernandez-Guardiola J. Anaphylactic shock and death after intake of acetazolamide. *Am J Ophthalmol* 1992;114: 367.
42. Lichter PR, Newman LP, Wheeler NC, Beall OV. Patient tolerance to carbonic anhydrase inhibitors. *Am J Ophthalmol* 1978;85:495–502.
43. Kolker AE, Hetherington J Jr. Becker-Shaffer's diagnosis and therapy of the glaucomas. St. Louis: CV Mosby Co., 1976;314–322.
44. Fraunfelder FT, Meyer SM, Bagby GC Jr, Dries MW. Hematologic reactions to carbonic anhydrase inhibitors. *Am J Ophthalmol* 1985; 100:79–81.
45. Johnson T, Kass MA. Hematologic reaction to carbonic anhydrase inhibitors. *Am J Ophthalmol* 1986;101:128–129.
46. Mogk LG, Cyrlin MN. Blood dyscrasia and carbonic anhydrase inhibitors. *Ophthalmology* 1988;95:768–771.
47. Kass MA, Kolker AE, Gordon M, Goldberg I, et al. Acetazolamide and urolithiasis. *Ophthalmology* 1981;88:261–265.
48. Graber M, Kelleher S. Side effects of acetazolamide: the champagne blues [letter]. *Am J Med* 1988;84:979–980.
49. Weiss IS. Hirsutism after chronic administration of acetazolamide. *Am J Ophthalmol* 1974;78:327–328.
50. Galin MA, Baras I, Zweifach P. Diamox-induced myopia. *Am J Ophthalmol* 1962;54:237–240.
51. Heinonen OP, Sloan D, Shapiro S. Birth defects and drugs in pregnancy. Littleon, MA: Publishing Sciences Group, Inc., 1977;494–495.
52. Layton WM, Hallesy DM. Deformity of forelimb in rats: association with high doses of acetazolamide. *Science* 1965;149:306–308.
53. Soderman P, Hartvig P, Fagerlund C. Acetazolamide excretion into human breast milk. *Br J Clin Pharmacol* 1984;17:599–600.
54. Shrader CE, Thomas JV, Simmons RJ. Relationship of patient age and tolerance to carbonic anhydrase inhibitors. *Am J Ophthalmol* 1983; 96:730–733.
55. Yablonski ME, Maren TH, Hayashi M, Naveh N, Potash SD, Pessah N. Enhancement of ocular hypotensive effect of acetazolamide by diflunisal. *Am J Ophthalmol* 1988;106:332–336.
56. Becker B, Middleton WH. Long-term acetazolamide (Diamox) administration in therapy of glaucomas. *Arch Ophthalmol* 1955;54: 187–192.
57. Gonzales-Jiminez E, Leopold IH. The effect of dichlorphenamide on the intraocular pressure of humans. *Arch Ophthalmol* 1958;60: 427–436.
58. Bleckmann H. Die wirkung von Dichlorphenamid bei der behandlung des akuten glaukomanfalls. *Graefes Arch Clin Exp Ophthalmol* 1976; 201:69–77.
59. Henry MM, Lee PF. Clinical comparison of dichlorphenamide, chlorothiazide and sulocarbilate with acetazolamide in control of glaucoma. *Am J Ophthalmol* 1959;47:199–202.
60. Beyer KH, Baer JE. Physiological basis for the action of newer diuretic agents. *Pharmacol Rev* 1961;13:517–562.
61. Wakabayashi Y. Hyperkalemia induced by carbonic anhydrase inhibitor. *Br J Ophthal* 1991;75:176–177.
62. Hallesy DW, Layton WM Jr. Forelimb deformity of offspring of rats given dichlorphenamide during pregnancy. *Proc Soc Exp Biol Med* 1967;126:6–12.
63. Sisson GM, Maren TH. Pharmacology of 5-acetylimino-4-methyl-Δ-1,3,4-thiadiazoline-2-sulfonamide: a new carbonic anhydrase inhibitor with reference to its penetration into central nervous system and eyes. *Fed Proc* 1956;15:484.
64. Becker B. Use of methazolamide in the therapy of glaucoma. *Am J Ophthalmol* 1960;49:1307–1311.
65. Maren TH, Maywood JR, Chapman SK, Zimmerman TJ. The pharmacology of methazolamide in relation to the treatment of glaucoma. *Invest Ophthalmol* 1977;16:730–742.
66. Dahlen K, Epstein DL, Grant WM, Hutchinson BT, Prien EL, Krall JM. A repeated dose-response study of Methazolamide in glaucoma. *Arch Ophthalmol* 1978;96:2214–2218.
67. Stone RA, Zimmerman TJ, Shin DH, Becker B, Kass MA. Low-dose methazolamide and intraocular pressure. *Am J Ophthalmol* 1977;83: 674–679.
68. Thomas RP, Riley MW. Acetazolamide and ocular tension: notes concerning the mechanism of action. *Am J Ophthalmol* 1965;60: 241–246.
69. Shields MB, Simmons RJ. Urinary calculas during methazolamide therapy. *Am J Ophthalmol* 1976;81:622–624.
70. Maren TH. Teratology and carbonic anhydrase inhibition. *Arch Ophthalmol* 1971;85:1–2.
71. Smith JP, Weeks RH, Newland EF, Ward RL. Betaxolol and acetazolamide combined ocular hypotensive effect. *Arch Ophthalmol* 1984; 102:1794–1795.

Textbook of Ocular Pharmacology,
edited by T.J. Zimmerman, et al.
Lippincott–Raven Publishers, Philadelphia © 1997.

CHAPTER 25

Topical Carbonic Anhydrase Inhibitors

Mordechai Sharir

DORZOLAMIDE HYDROCHLORIDE (TRUSOPT)

History and Source

Carbonic anhydrase [(CA); carbonate hydrolyase; E.C. 4.2.1.1] is a metalloenzyme that catalyzes the reversible hydration of CO_2 and the dehydration of carbonic acid. Of the identified human isoenzymes of CA, it is isoenzyme II (CA-II), abundant in the ciliary epithelium, that plays an important role in the production and secretion of aqueous humor into the posterior chamber of the eye.

Although systemic carbonic anhydrase inhibitors (sCAI) can suppress aqueous production by up to 60% and effectively reduce intraocular pressure (IOP), their use has been associated with a variety of systemic side effects that can decrease patient compliance by up to 50% (1). Therefore, a topical carbonic anhydrase inhibitor (TCAI) that would provide effective ocular hypotension with a minimum of adverse effects would be highly desirable. Numerous previous attempts to develop such a tCAI failed as a result of instability or poor transcorneal movement (2–9). Various difficulties in achieving the goal of developing a tCAI were extensively reviewed by Maren (10), among which were the prerequisite of inhibiting >99.9% of the ciliary CA before gaining a significant reduction in the IOP. It was determined that acetazolamide would be topically effective only in extreme conditions because of its poor lipid solubility (6,7). Based on the concept of improving lipid solubility without losing water solubility and efficacy, a trifluoro derivative of methazolamide was developed. Although efficacious, its chemical instability precluded further investigations (5).

M. Sharir: Department of Ophthalmology, The Edith Wolfson Hospital, Holon, Israel; Department of Ophthalmology and Visual Sciences, Department of Microbiology and Immunology, University of Louisville School of Medicine, Louisville, Kentucky 40292.

Experimental use of 6-hydroxyethoxzolamide, an ethoxzolamide analogue, in a gel vehicle, as a tCAI enhanced its corneal permeability and prolonged its action (9,11), but a multidose study of another analogue (6-amino-benzothiazole-sulfonamide [aminozolamide]) was precluded by a high incidence of bulbar injection and follicular conjunctivitis (12). In a 2% solution, MK-927 (not available commercially), another ethoxzolamide analogue developed by Merck Research Laboratories, was effective in reducing the IOP in normal volunteers and in patients with primary open-angle glaucoma (13–17, 18). MK-927 was well tolerated, and a dose-response study demonstrated dose-dependent IOP-lowering in glaucoma patients as well as in glaucoma suspects (16). The S-enantiomer of MK-927, sezolamide (also not available commercially), was even more efficacious against CA-II than MK-927.

Of the novel class of ethoxzolamides titled thienothiopyrans, dorzolamide possessed the highest potency. In humans, dorzolamide demonstrated good tolerance and efficacy.

Chemistry

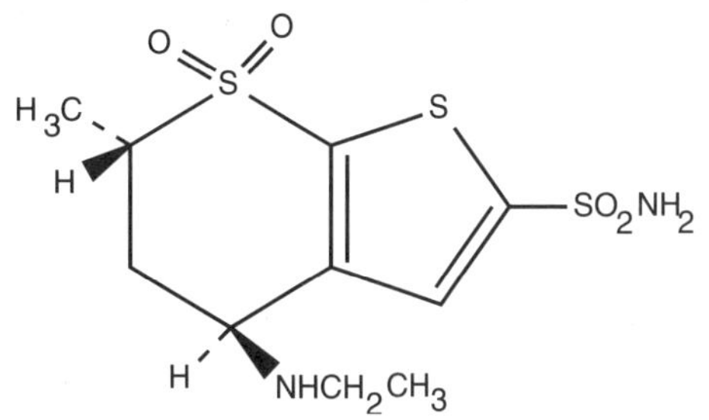

O O S H₃C H S SO₂NH₂ H NHCH₂CH₃

Dorzolamide hydrochloride (Trusopt) is supplied as a sterile, isotonic, buffered, slightly viscous aqueous solution, with a pH of 5.6. Its chemical name is (4S-trans)-4-(ethylamino)-5,6-dihydro-6-methyl-4H-thieno [2,3-b]thiopyran-2-sulfonamide 7,7-dioxide monohydrochloride and its chemical formula is $C_{10}H_{16}N_2O_4S_3$*HCl. Dorzolamide hydrochloride has a molecular weight of 360.9. Its appearance is white to off-white crystalline powder; it is soluble in water and slightly soluble in methanol and ethanol.

Pharmacology

Mechanism of Action

Dorzolamide inhibits the enzyme carbonic anhydrase (CA), which catalyzes the reversible hydration of CO_2. Dorzolamide is specifically effective against CA-II, found primarily in red blood cells, but also in the ciliary processes. Inhibition of CA decreases aqueous humor production and secretion, presumably by slowing the formation of bicarbonate ions, with subsequent reduction in sodium and fluid transport. The pharmacodynamic result is a reduction in the IOP. Topical dorzolamide reduces elevated IOP, a major risk factor in the pathogenesis of glaucomatous visual-field loss and optic nerve damage.

Dose-response Relation

In a randomly allocated placebo-controlled study in ocular hypertensive patients, dorzolamide at three different concentrations (0.7%, 1.4%, and 2%) effectively lowered the IOP when given twice a day for 5 days and three times a day for an additional 7 days (peak effect of 21% reduction in IOP 2 hours after dosing), with 2.0% concentration producing a slightly greater IOP lowering effect at day 12 at the twice-daily regimen (17). Dorzolamide at 3.0% concentration, given three times a day, did not lower the IOP any further (18). In a Phase III dose-response study in 333 primary open-angle glaucoma patients, dorzolamide at 2.0% concentration showed numerical but not statistical advantage over the 0.7% concentration, but both were significantly different from either 0.2% or placebo. Half of the patients were controlled successfully on monotherapy with dorzolamide 2.0% three times a day for one year. Therefore, the 2.0% concentration was chosen for the final product because it achieves the maximum IOP-lowering effect (19).

Pharmaceutics

Dorzolamide HCl 2% ophthalmic is a colorless, slightly viscous solution supplied in OCUMETER, a white, opaque, plastic ophthalmic dispenser in either a 5- or 10-ml dropper.

Pharmacokinetics

Following chronic topical application, dorzolamide reaches the systemic circulation and binds to erythrocytic CA-II. A steady state is reached within 4 weeks. The parent drug is metabolized via *N*-desethylation. The metabolite retains some CAI activity, with more affinity to erythrocytic CA-I. About 95% of CA-II activity and about 88% of total CA activity in the erythrocyte is inhibited by the drug and its metabolite.

Dorzolamide is about 33% bound to plasma proteins. Plasma concentrations of dorzolamide and its metabolite are generally below the assay limit (15 nM). Dorzolamide and *N*-desethyl-dorzolamide are excreted unchanged in the urine. After termination of therapy, the washout period is nonlinear, characterized by an initial rapid decline, followed by a slow decay over several months (19).

Therapeutic Use

Indications

Dorzolamide is indicated in the treatment of elevated IOP in patients with open-angle glaucoma and in patients in whom glaucoma is suspected. Like sCAI, dorzolamide should be useful in short-term management of neovascular, juvenile, traumatic, and angle-closure glaucoma.

Dorzolamide is additive to beta-adrenoreceptor antagonists. In one study, an additional decrease of 6.3 mm Hg (or 34%) in IOP was noticed in patients receiving 2% dorzolamide three times daily when 0.5% timolol maleate twice daily was added (19).

Contraindications

Dorzolamide is contraindicated in patients who are hypersensitive to any of the components of the medication.

Method of Use

The dose is one drop three times daily in the affected eye. Dorzolamide can be used concomitantly with other topical ocular hypotensive agents. If polytherapy is indicated, the medications should be instilled at least 10 minutes apart.

Dorzolamide, which is absorbed systemically following topical application, has not been associated with any of the major side effects reported after long-term therapy with sCAI. Chronic treatment with dorzolamide is generally well tolerated, with no change in pupillary diameter, no acid-base and electrolyte disturbances, or alterations in blood pressure or heart rate. Nevertheless, dorzolamide is a sulfonamide, and some rare fatalities have occurred from sulfonamides including Stevens-Johnson syndrome, fulminant hepatic necrosis, toxic epidermal necrosis, and aplastic anemia. Therefore, regardless of the route of administration, the danger of hypersensitization is not avoided.

Adverse Reactions

Based on reports of 1,108 patients receiving dorzolamide, the most frequently reported symptoms and adverse experiences were transient burning, stinging, and discomfort (33%), and bitter taste (26%). Ocular allergy and superficial punctate keratitis occurred in one-tenth of the patients. Blurred vision, dryness, tearing and photophobia were encountered in 1 to 5%. Headaches, nausea, fatigue, skin rashes, urolithiasis and iridocyclitis were reported infrequently.

In only 5% of patients were the adverse effects so severe that termination of treatment was warranted. The most frequent causes for discontinuation with dorzolamide were local lid edema and conjunctivitis, which resolved when therapy was stopped (19).

Overdosage

Significant lethality was reported in female rats after a single oral dose of approximately 2 g/kg dorzolamide hydrochloride. Human data are not available as yet, but, theoretically, acid-base disturbances and changes in serum potassium levels must be monitored in cases of overdose.

Carcinogenesis/Mutagenesis, Impairment of Fertility

Urinary bladder papillomas were seen in Sprague-Dawley rats that received orally 250 times the recommended human ocular dose but not in lower doses or in mice given oral dose or about 900 times the human recommended ocular dose. It should be mentioned that rats are especially susceptible to developing papillomas in response to foreign bodies, sodium salts, and compounds causing crystalluria. Ames test, alkaline elution assay, in vitro chromosomal aberration assay, and in vivo mouse cytogenetic assay were all negative as markers for potential mutagenicity. There was no noticeable change in reproductive ability in rats receiving >150 times the recommended human ophthalmic dose (19).

High-risk Groups

Children

No data are available as regards efficacy and safety in the pediatric age.

Pregnancy/Nursing Mothers

No adequate, well-controlled studies have been done on the use of dorzolamide in pregnant women. It should be used during pregnancy only if the potential benefit justifies the potential risks to the fetus. Species sensitivity was encountered in developmental toxicity studies. In rabbits receiving oral dorzolamide in more than 30 times the recommended dose revealed vertebral body malformations and decreased body-weight gain secondary to metabolic acidosis, but none were reported with half that dose. There were no fetal malformations in rats receiving orally 125 times the recommended daily dose (19). It is not known whether dorzolamide is excreted in human milk.

A slight delay in postnatal development of vaginal canalization, eye opening, and incisor eruption together with a 5% decrease in weight gain were reported in lactating rats receiving 94 times the recommended human ocular dose. Because of the lack of sufficient data, a clinical decision about therapy with dorzolamide in the nursing mother should take into account the risk-to-benefit ratio.

Elderly Patients

Elderly patients are more sensitive to medications as a result of changes in absorption, metabolism, and elimination that occur with age (see Chapter 16, *this volume*). Forty-four percent of the patients enrolled in clinical studies with dorzolamide hydrochloride were aged ≥65 years, and 10% were aged at least 75 years old. No overall differences in effectiveness or safety were observed between the older and younger age groups.

Drug Interactions

The potential of toxicity when any CAI is used in combination with high-dose salicylates or diuretics should be remembered, although no alterations in acid-base balance or electrolytes was reported with dorzolamide hydrochloride (20).

REFERENCES

1. American Medical Association. Drugs used for glaucoma. In: *Drug Evaluation Annual 1991.* Chicago: AMA, 1991;1811–1829.
2. Grant WM, Trotter RR. Diamox (acetazolamide) in treatment of glaucoma. *Arch Ophthalmol* 1954;51:735–739.
3. Foss RH. Local application of Diamox: an experimental study of its effect on the intraocular pressure. *Am J Ophthalmol* 1955;39:336– 339.
4. Green H, Leopold IH. Effects of locally administered diamox. *Am J Ophthalmol* 1955;40:137–139.
5. Maren TH, Jankowska L, Sanyal G, et al. The transcorneal permeability of sulfonamide carbonic anhydrase inhibitors and their effect on aqueous humor secretion. *Exp Eye Res* 1983;36:457–479.
6. Flach AJ, Peterson JS, Seligmann KA. Local ocular hypotensive effect of topically applied acetazolamide. *Am J Ophthalmol* 1984;98: 66–72.
7. Friedman Z, Allen RC, Raph SM. Topical acetazolamide and methazolamide delivered by contact lenses. *Arch Ophthalmol* 1985;103: 963–967.
8. Sugrue MF, Gantheron P, Schmitt C, et al. On the pharmacology of L-645,151: a topically effective ocular hypotensive carbonic anhydrase inhibitor. *J Pharmacol Exp Ther* 1985;232:534–540.

9. Lewis RA, Schoenwald RD, Eller MG, et al. Ethoxzolamide analogue gel: a topical carbonic anhydrase inhibitor. *Arch Ophthalmol* 1984;102: 1821–1824.
10. Maren TH. HCO_3^- formation in aqueous humor: mechanism and relation to the treatment of glaucoma. *Invest Ophthalmol* 1974;13:479–484.
11. Lewis RA, Schoenwald RD, Barfknecht CF, et al. Aminozolamide gel: a trial of a topical carbonic anhydrase inhibitor in ocular hypertension. *Arch Ophthalmol* 1986;104:842–844.
12. Kalina PH, et al. 6-amino-2-benzothiazole sulfonamide: the effect of a topical carbonic anhydrase inhibitor on aqueous humor formation in the normal human eye. *Ophthalmology* 1988;95:772–777.
13. Higginbotham EJ, Kass MA, Lippa EA, et al. MK-927: A topical carbonic anhydrase inhibitor: dose response and duration of action. *Arch Ophthalmol* 1990;108:65–68.
14. Lippa EA, von-Denffar HA, Hofmann HM, et al. Local tolerance and activity of MK-927, a novel topical carbonic anhydrase inhibitor. *Arch Ophthalmol* 1988;106:1694–1696.
15. Bron AM, Lippa EA, Hofmann HM, et al. MK-927: a topically effective carbonic anhydrase inhibitor in patients. *Arch Opthalmol* 1989; 107:1143–1146.
16. Lippa EA, Schuman JS, Higginbotham EJ, et al. MK-507 versus sezolamide: Comparative efficacy of two topically active carbonic anhydrase inhibitors. *Ophthalmology* 1991;98:308–313.
17. Lippa EA. Dose response and duration of action of dorzolamide, a topical carbonic anhydrase inhibitor. *Arch Ophthalmol* 1992;110: 495–499.
18. McMahon CD, et al. IOP lowering activity of the topical CAI MK-507 at 3%. *Invest Ophthalmol Vis Sci* 1991;32:989.
19. Manufacturer's information. Trusopt product monograph, 1995.
20. Anderson CJ, Kaufman PL, Sturm RJ. Toxicity of combined therapy with carbonic anhydrase inhibitors and aspirin. *Am J Ophthalmol* 1978;86:516.

Textbook of Ocular Pharmacology,
edited by T.J. Zimmerman, et al.
Lippincott–Raven Publishers, Philadelphia © 1997.

CHAPTER 26

Hyperosmotic Agents

Kuldev Singh and Theodore Krupin

Hyperosmotic agents are a class of compounds that are administered systemically to lower intraocular pressure (IOP) acutely (Table 26-1). They are effective in lowering IOP during attacks of acute angle-closure glaucoma as well as conditions of marked IOP elevation with secondary glaucoma. Hyperosmotics also can be used to reduce vitreous volume and decrease IOP before intraocular surgery. Hyperosmotic drugs, although diverse in their organic characteristics, have similar mechanisms of action and side effects.

Historical Background

Cantonnet recommended the use of an oral mixture of sodium chloride and lactose (4-0-B-D-galactopyranosyl-D-glucose) in the treatment of glaucoma in 1904 (1). Hertel, in 1914, described the use of concentrated intravenous saline to lower IOP transiently (2). Studies of other intravenous agents followed, including glucose and sucrose, which were limited by their systemic side effects. In the late 1950s, intravenous urea was noted by Javid to reduce both intracranial and the intraocular pressure (3). Galin et al. were the first to use urea to treat glaucoma (4,5). Urea was compared with sucrose and found to be a better osmotic agent. Intravenous urea was associated with fewer systemic side effects than previously used hyperosmotic agents and thus became the drug of choice among this class of compounds. Its poor penetration of the blood–aqueous barrier allowed a prolonged period of effect. Mannitol (D-mannitol) was subsequently shown to be an effective IOP-lowering agent when administered systemically by Weiss et al. in 1962 (6). Weiss also cautioned against the use of hyperosmotics in patients with cardiocirculatory insufficiency. Glycerol (1,2,3-propanetriol) and isosorbide (1,4,3,6-dianhydro-D-glucitol) were introduced as oral hyperosmotic agents in the mid-1960s by Virno et al. (7) and Becker et al., (8), respectively.

Pharmacology

The principal mechanism by which hyperosmotic agents lower IOP is thought to be reduction of vitreous volume. The rise in serum osmolality following the administration of a hyperosmotic agent causes a net movement of intraocular water (primarily from the vitreous) into intraocular vessels (retinal and uveal). With time, the osmolality gradient between the serum and vitreous decreases, and thus the flow of water out of the eye diminishes. The duration of the IOP-lowering effect is dependent on the permeability of the blood–ocular barrier and the size of the hyperosmotic molecule. With clearing of the compound from the systemic circulation, there may be a relative reversal of the osmotic gradient and a subsequent rebound rise in IOP. Rabbit studies have shown a 2.7% to 3.9% reduction in the vitreous body weight following hyperosmotic agent administration (9). When the results are extrapolated to the human eye, with a vitreous volume of approximately 4 ml, the effect may reduce vitreous volume by about 0.015 ml, which is about 10% the volume of the anterior chamber. This reduction in vitreous volume not only reduces IOP but may deepen the anterior chamber by allowing a posterior movement of the iris–lens diaphragm. This is particularly useful in certain cases of angle-closure glaucoma.

An alternative theory that osmotic agents lower IOP through receptors in the brain has been proposed. This theory is supported by the observation that small intravenous doses of hyperosmotic agents lower IOP in normal rabbit eyes but not those with optic nerve lesions or transected optic nerves (10–13). Phenobarbital prevents the IOP-lowering effect of oral isosorbide or intravenous urea in rabbits with intact optic nerves (14). The mechanism by which the

K. Singh: Department of Ophthalmology, Stanford University Medical Center, Stanford, California 94305.
T. Krupin: Department of Ophthalmology, Northwestern University Medical School, Chicago, Illinois 60611.

TABLE 26-1. *Hyperosmotic agents*

Agent	Brand names	Chemical structure	Molecular weight	Dosage (g/kg)	Distribution	Ocular penetration
Oral agents						
Glycerol	Glyrol Osmoglyn	CH_2 OH H-C-OH CH_2OH	92	1–1.5	Extracellular	Poor
Isosorbide	Ismotic	$C_6H_{10}O_4$	146	1–1.5	Total body water	Good
Alcohol		H H_3C-C-OH H	46	0.4–1.0	Total body water	Good
Intravenous agents						
Mannitol	Osmitrol	CH_2OH HO-C-H HO-C-H HO-C-H HO-C-H CH_2OH	182	1–1.5	Extracellular	Very poor
Urea	Ureaphil	O H_2N-C-NH_2	60	0.6–2.1	Total body water	Good

Modified from Shields, ref 26, and Feitl and Krupin, ref 48.

central nervous system may affect IOP through the optic nerve when exposed to hyperosmotics is not well understood. An alternative explanation may be that the secondary reduction in the number and caliber of vessels near the inner retinal surface often associated with optic atrophy may decrease the amount of fluid that can be removed from the eye with hyperosmotic use (15). The effectiveness of individual hyperosmotic agents is proportional to the extent of the induced blood–ocular osmotic gradient. Likewise, the duration of this effectiveness is directly related to the duration of this osmotic gradient. The following factors influence the osmotic gradient:

1. Dosage: Small molecules increase osmolality greater than large molecules per unit of weight. Thus, low-molecular weight compounds, such as urea, increase plasma osmolality to a greater extent than high-molecular-weight compounds.
2. Rate of administration: A faster rate of administration allows a larger osmotic gradient to be established than with slower delivery. Intravenous administration is advantageous when oral absorption is delayed.
3. Rate of ocular penetrance: Poor ocular penetrance allows the blood–ocular gradient to persist longer and thus increase the IOP-lowering effect. Drugs and ocular conditions (e.g., inflammation) that alter the blood–ocular barrier decrease the effect of hyperosmotics.
4. Systemic clearance of the drug: The rapidity of drug metabolism and clearance is inversely proportional to the duration of action.
5. Oral ingestion of fluids: Ingestion of fluids after hyperosmotic use decreases serum osmolality and thus hinders the IOP-lowering effect.
6. Distribution of drug in body fluids: Substances that remain predominately in the extracellular space (e.g., mannitol) allow a greater osmotic effect than drugs that pass intracellularly and are distributed in total body water (e.g., urea).

A rebound increase in IOP can occur after administration of a hyperosmotic agent. With the passage of time, a variable amount of the hyperosmotic agent enters the eye, and the compound is cleared from the systemic circulation. This action creates a reverse osmotic gradient with a dehydrated vitreous pulling fluid from the serum and resulting in elevation of IOP. This effect is transient.

ORAL AGENTS

Oral administration of hyperosmotic agents is less effective with slower onset of action than intravenous administration (16). This decreased effect is due to variable gastrointestinal absorption with oral agents. These differences are not large and can be partially compensated by adjusting dosage. Patients with nausea and vomiting generally tolerate oral agents poorly. The presence of cardiac disease makes oral drugs preferable, as they are less likely to result in cardiac overload than intravenous hyperosmotic agents.

Glycerol (Glyrol, Osmoglyn)

Glycerol ($C_3H_8O_3$) is administered most commonly as a liquid with a dosage of 1 to 1.5 g/kg (2–3 cc/kg) of body weight of a 50% solution (16,17). Glyrol, a 75% solution, is also available. Often a 100% solution of glycerol is diluted with an equal volume of juice.

The ocular hypotensive effect begins 10 minutes after ingestion, with a peak effect at about 30 to 60 minutes (7,18). The effect lasts for approximately 5 hours, after which the dose can be repeated, as the drug penetrates the eye poorly and largely remains in the extracellular space. Glycerol is absorbed rapidly from the gastrointestinal tract and metabolized in the liver. Its metabolism produces 4.32 kilocalories per gram (7,19).

Glycerol has an intense, sweet taste that may induce nausea and vomiting, especially in patients with angle-closure glaucoma, who often have nausea on presentation. Adding lemon juice and serving over ice may make the medication more palatable. An antiemetic can be used before administering glycerol.

The presence of diabetes mellitus is a relative contraindication to the use of oral glycerol as a hyperosmotic agent. High caloric content combined with osmotic diuresis and dehydration may lead to hyperglycemia and hyperosmolar nonketotic coma in some patients, especially with repeated dosage (20).

Isosorbide (Ismotic)

Isosorbide ($C_6H_{10}O_4$), like glycerol, is a hyperosmotic agent that can be given orally. Its main advantage over glycerol is that it has fewer side effects (21–25). Isosorbide is rapidly absorbed from the gastrointestinal tract and excreted unmetabolized in the urine. Because it is not metabolized, isosorbide does not provide calories and is relatively safer for diabetics than glycerol. It is also less likely to cause nausea and vomiting but is associated more often with diarrhea than glycerol (19,20). The usual dosage of isosorbide is 1.5 g/kg (3 cc/kg) of body weight administered as a 45% (0.45 mg/ml) solution (22,25). The peak ocular hypotensive effect occurs in 1 to 3 hours and lasts 3 to 5 hours (26). As with glycerol, the dose can be repeated. Isosorbide may be confused with the similarly named antiangina vasodilating drug isosorbide dinitrate (Isordil) (27). Isosorbide has no antiangina properties.

Ethyl Alcohol (Ethanol)

Ethyl alcohol (C_2H_6O) can be used as a hyperosmotic agent to decrease IOP acutely. The hyperosmotic effect is achieved both by an increased serum osmolality and the inhibition of antidiuretic hormone, with a resultant hypotonic diuresis that prolongs the osmotic gradient.

Dosages of 1 to 2 ml/kg of 40% to 50% solution may adequately lower IOP but the effect is very brief, as alcohol rapidly penetrates the eye. Side effects, including acute alcohol intoxication, nausea, and vomiting, limit the use of ethyl alcohol as a hyperosmotic agent. In addition, ethyl alcohol produces a profound hypotonic diuresis, which increases serum osmolality (28). Like glycerol, ethyl alcohol is metabolized and may present a caloric problem, especially in diabetic patients. Because of its side effects and relatively short duration of effect, ethyl alcohol is rarely used as a hyperosmotic agent when glycerol or isosorbide are available.

Other Oral Agents

Other oral agents that have been used effectively as hyperosmotics in lowering IOP include glycine (29), sodium lactate (30), propylene glycol (1,2-propanediol), calcium chloride, and ascorbic acid (L-ascorbic acid) (31).

INTRAVENOUS AGENTS

Intravenous agents have a greater ocular hypotensive effect than oral agents. They also act more rapidly because the gastrointestinal system is bypassed. Intravenous drugs are often administered when oral agents are insufficient or when nausea and vomiting preclude their use.

Mannitol

Mannitol ($C_6H_{14}O_6$) is currently the most commonly used intravenous hyperosmotic agent. It is effective and relatively safer than urea (10–15 cc/kg). The recommended dosage is 1 to 1.5 g/kg of body weight of a 10% or 20% (5–8 cc/kg) solution at a delivery rate of 3 to 5 ml per minute (32,33). Significantly lower doses may be nearly as effective. The onset of action is at 10 to 30 minutes, with a peak effect at about 40 to 60 minutes (6,21,33,34). The duration of action is 2 to 6 hours (26). The rate of dosage is important, and the drug dosage may be titrated to the desired IOP reduction. Mannitol is not effective as an oral agent.

Mannitol is not metabolized and thus is not contraindicated in diabetic patients. It is excreted in urine (33). Mannitol penetrates the eye poorly and thus is especially effective in the presence of ocular inflammation, when the blood–ocular barrier has been disrupted (5). The drug is confined to extracellular water. One of the major advantages of mannitol over urea is the absence of tissue necrosis if the solution extravasates during administration.

Side effects are rare with mannitol use. Because the drug has limited solubility, a larger volume of administration is necessary. Patients with cardiac and renal disease should be monitored closely and perhaps treated with lower doses (35). It has been recommended that the 20% solution of mannitol be warmed before administration to dissolve crystals. A blood filter should be used in the intravenous line.

Urea (Urevert, Ureaphil)

Urea (CH_4N_2O) is a less frequently used hyperosmotic agent than mannitol. The usual dosage is 2 to 7 ml/kg of body weight of a 30% solution. It has an onset of action of 15 to 30 minutes, with maximum effect in 60 minutes and duration of action of 4 to 6 hours (36–39). Urea is generally considered less effective than mannitol because it diffuses throughout body fluids and has relatively greater ocular penetration. The ocular penetration may make urea ineffective with ocular inflammation as well as cause a rebound increase in IOP after administration (40). Urea is excreted in the urine unmetabolized. Unlike mannitol, urea does not have a long shelf life and may decompose to ammonia. This instability in solution makes it necessary to use only fresh solutions. Urea also has the disadvantage of causing local thrombophlebitis and skin necrosis if it extravasates during administration (39).

Other Intravenous Drugs

Intravenously administered 30% glycerol has been used as a hyperosmotic agent, but the side effect of hematorrhea limits its clinical usefulness. Intravenous mixtures of 20% ascorbic acid and 30% glycerol or 15% sorbitol (D-glucitol) and 30% glycerol similarly reduce IOP without significant side effects (41,42).

Clinical Use

Angle-Closure Glaucoma

Perhaps the most common use of hyperosmotic agents in ophthalmology is in the presence of acute angle-closure glaucoma. Although topical beta-blockers and oral carbonic anhydrase inhibitors will decrease aqueous humor production in such attacks, topical miotics are often not effective in an eye with a very high IOP and iris ischemia. Oral glycerol or isosorbide can help decrease IOP acutely. This decrease in IOP may allow concurrently administered pilocarpine to more produce miosis and break the angle-closure attack. Alternatively, the transient reduction in IOP may allow adequate corneal clearing to make laser iridotomy easier and safer. If nausea and vomiting accompany the angle-closure attack, intravenous mannitol is preferable to the use of oral agents.

Secondary Glaucoma

With many of the secondary glaucomas, hyperosmotic agents allow temporary reduction in IOP, which may be adequate therapy for self-limited processes, such as traumatic hyphema with secondary elevation of IOP. In other situations, the use of hyperosmotics may delay the need for surgical intervention. Hyperosmotics also may be used preoperatively in eyes with extremely high IOP in an effort to minimize the extent of intraoperative decompression.

Ciliary Block Glaucoma

In conjunction with oral carbonic anhydrase inhibitors, topical beta-blockers, and cycloplegics (such as atropine), hyperosmotics play an important role in the medical treatment of ciliary block glaucoma. Hyperosmotic agents dehydrate the vitreous body and reduce posterior vitreous pressure (43,44). Oral glycerol or intravenous mannitol can be given once or twice a day. If prolonged use is necessary, isosorbide is preferred over glycerol to prevent the administration of a large caloric load.

Preoperative Preparation

There are instances when a soft eye is desired prior to surgery. Dehydration of the vitreous body before corneal or retinal detachment and other types of surgery can be achieved with hyperosmotics. A few ophthalmologists advocate the routine use of hyperosmotics before cataract surgery in an effort to decrease the occurrence of vitreous loss.

Other Considerations

Long-term use of hyperosmotics is generally not as safe as short-term use. Electrolytes should be followed closely with long-term use, as dehydration can occur.

Oral glycerol and intravenous mannitol are associated with lesser ocular penetration than isosorbide and urea and are thus preferable in eyes with inflammatory glaucomas where there is a disruption of the blood–ocular barrier. With marked ocular inflammation, all hyperosmotics may be ineffective, as the osmotic gradient rapidly equilibrates.

Side Effects

All hyperosmotic agents have the potential to cause serious and even fatal side effects (Table 26-2) (45). The magnitude of these effects is related to the specific agent as well as the mode of delivery. Intravenous agents are associated more commonly with severe systemic side effects than oral agents. Elderly patients with cardiac, renal, or hepatic disease are at increased risk for severe side effects (46).

Headache, nausea, vomiting, and diuresis are among the most common side effects. Nausea and vomiting are encountered more frequently with the oral agents, possibly because of the intensely sweet taste of some agents. Vomiting often results in loss of the medication and the necessity to use an intravenous agent. Nausea and headache make

TABLE 26-2. *Side effects*

General constitutional
Nausea
Vomiting
Fever
Chills
Confusion
Disorientation
Thirst
Genitourinary
Diuresis
Urinary retention
Hyperosmosis
Renal insufficiency
Central nervous system
Headache
Syncope
Light headedness
Vertigo
Subdural hemorrhage
Others
Pulmonary edema
Congestive heart failure
Hypersensitivity

patients irritable during surgery. Antiemetics are sometimes helpful. Diuresis is a greater problem with intravenous than oral agents. An indwelling catheter may sometimes be required intraoperatively after hyperosmotic administration. Urinary retention can follow the intense diuresis, especially in men with prostatic hypertrophy (19).

Patients with renal failure cannot adequately excrete hyperosmotic agents, such as mannitol, and thus the dose must be adjusted appropriately to prevent a prolonged hyperosmotic state (47). Cerebrospinal fluid acidosis and neurologic deterioration are side effects of a prolonged hyperosmotic state (47). Total mannitol dosage should be limited to <50 mg in patients with renal failure (48). Post-hyperosmotic administration renal function should be monitored carefully in these patients with attention to *osmolality gap* (the difference between measured and calculated osmolality), electrolytes, and urine output (48). Extracorporeal hemodialysis is necessary to remove mannitol quickly (half-life, 6 hours) from the extracellular space and to correct electrolyte abnormalities once toxicity is determined. Peritoneal dialysis (half-life, 21 hours) is relatively slower in removing mannitol (47). Mannitol-induced renal failure has also been described in previously normal patients (49). The mechanism of this renal failure is uncertain, but it may be a directly nephrotoxic effect or secondary to mannitol's effect on the renal vasculature. Treatment of this condition is similar to that of other forms of renal failure. Pulmonary edema and congestive heart failure are known complications of hyperosmotic use and are more common with drugs that are restricted to extracellular water (47,50). Cellular dehydration is another side effect that may result in mental status changes, including disorientation and agitation. These effects are secondary to cerebral dehydration. Hypokalemia may exacerbate the symptoms. Subdural hemorrhage, which is potentially life threatening, may occur following dehydration and retraction of the brain surface from the dura and tearing of the bridging veins between the sagittal sinus and the brain surface (45).

Hypersensitivity reactions following mannitol use are rare but have been described (51,52). Respiratory distress, cyanosis, and hives are some of the manifestations. When such a reaction is encountered, mannitol infusion should be halted and supportive treatment with epinephrine, diphenhydramine, and corticosteroids initiated.

REFERENCES

1. Cantonnet A. Essai de traitment du glaucome par les substances osmotiques. *Arch Ophthalmol (Paris)* 1904;24:1.
2. Hertel E. Experimentelle Untersuchungen Ueber die Abhangigkeit des Argendrucks von der Blutbeschaffenheit. *Graefes Arch Clin Exp Ophthalmol* 1914;88:197.
3. Javid M. Urea: new use of an old agent. Reduction of intracranial and intraocular pressure. *Surg Clin North Am* 1958;38:907.
4. Galin MA, Aizawa F, McLean LM. A comparison of intraocular pressure reduction following urea and sucrose administration. *Arch Ophthalmol* 1960;63:281.
5. Galin MA, Davidson R, Schachter N. Ophthalmological use of osmotic therapy. *Am J Ophthalmol* 1966;62:629.
6. Weiss DI, Shaffer RN, Wise BL. Mannitol infusion to reduce intraocular pressure. *Arch Ophthalmol* 1962;68:341.
7. Virno M, Cantore P, Bietti C, Bucci MG. Oral glycerol in ophthalmology: a valuable new method for the reduction of intraocular pressure. *Am J Ophthalmol* 1963;55:1133.
8. Becker B, Kolker AE, Krupin T. Isosorbide, an oral hyperosmotic agent. *Arch Ophthalmol* 1967;78:147.
9. Robbins R, Galin MA. Effect of osmotic agents on the vitreous body. *Arch Ophthalmol* 1969;82:694.
10. Podos SM, Krupin T, Becker B. Effect of small-dose hyperosmotic injections on intraocular pressure of small animals and man when optic nerves are transected and intact. *Am J Ophthalmol* 1971;71:898.
11. Riise D, Simonsen SE. Intraocular pressure in unilateral optic nerve lesion. *Acta Ophthalmol* 1969;47:750.
12. Krupin T, Podos SM, Becker B. Effect of optic nerve transection on osmotic alterations of intraocular pressure. *Am J Ophthalmol* 1970; 70:214.
13. Krupin T, Podos SM, Lehman RAW, Becker B. Effects of optic nerve transection on intraocular pressure in monkeys. *Arch Ophthalmol* 1970;84:668.
14. Podos SM, Krupin T, Becker B. Mechanism of intraocular pressure response after optic nerve transection. *Am J Ophthalmol* 1971;72:79.
15. Serafano DM, Brubaker RF. Intraocular pressure after optic nerve transection. *Invest Ophthalmol Vis Sci* 1978;17:68.
16. Havener WH. *Ocular Pharmacology,* 4th ed. St. Louis: CV Mosby, 1978;440.
17. Krupin T, Kolker AE, Becker B. A comparison of isosorbide and glycerol for cataract surgery. *Am J Ophthalmol* 1970;69:737.
18. Drance SM. Effect of oral glycerol on intraocular pressure in normal and glaucomatous eyes. *Arch Ophthalmol* 1964;72:491.
19. Hoskins H, Kass M. *Becker-Shaffer's Diagnosis and Therapy of the Glaucomas.* Baltimore: Mosby, 1989;485–491.
20. Oakley DE, Ellis PP. Glycerol and hyperosmolar nonketotic coma. *Am J Ophthalmol* 1976;81:469.
21. Barry KG, Khoury AH, Brooks MH. Mannitol and isosorbide: sequential effects on intraocular pressure, serum osmolality, sodium, and solids in normal subjects. *Arch Ophthalmol* 1969;81:695.
22. Wisznia KI, Lazar M, Leopold IH. Oral isosorbide and intraocular pressure. *Am J Ophthalmol* 1970;70:630.
23. Wood TO, Waltman SR, West C, Kaufman HE. Effect of isosorbide on intraocular pressure after penetrating keratoplasty. *Am J Ophthalmol* 1973;75:221.

24. Mehra KS, Singh R, Char JN, Rajyashree K. Lowering of intraocular tension: effects of isosorbide and glycerin. *Arch Ophthalmol* 1971;85: 167.
25. Mehra KS, Singh R. Lowering of intraocular pressure by isosorbide: effects of different doses of drug. *Arch Ophthalmol* 1971;86:623.
26. Shields MB. *Textbook of Glaucoma,* 3rd ed. Baltimore: Williams and Wilkins, 1992;512.
27. Buckley EG, Shields MB. Isosorbide and isosorbide dinitrate. *Am J Ophthalmol* 1980;89:457.
28. Becker B, Kolker AE, Krupin T. Hyperosmotic agents. In: Leopold IM: *Symposium on Ocular Therapy,* vol 3. St. Louis: CV Mosby Company, 1968;41–43.
29. Fox SL, Kranta JC Jr. The use of glycine in the reduction of intraocular pressure. *EENT Monthly* 1972;51:469.
30. Chiang TS, Stocks A, Jones C, Thomas RP. The ocular hypotensive effect of sodium lactate in rabbits. *Arch Ophthalmol* 1971;86:566.
31. Bietti G. Recent experimental, clinical, and therapeutic research on the problem of intraocular pressure and glaucoma. XXV Francis I Proctor Memorial Lecture. *Am J Ophthalmol* 1972;73:475.
32. O'Keefe M, Nabil M. The use of mannitol in intraocular surgery. *Ophthalmic Surg* 1983;14:55.
33. Smith EW, Drance SM. Reduction of human intraocular pressure with intravenous mannitol. *Arch Ophthalmol* 1962;68:734.
34. Adams RE, Kirschner RJ, Leopold IH. Ocular hypotensive effect of intravenously administered mannitol: a preliminary report. *Arch Ophthalmol* 1963;69:55.
35. Grabie MT, Gipstein RM, Adams DA, Hepner GW. Contraindications for mannitol in aphakic glaucoma. *Am J Ophthalmol* 1981;91:265.
36. Davis MD, Duehr PA, Javid M. The clinical use of urea for reduction of intraocular pressure. *Arch Ophthalmol* 1961;65:526.
37. Galin MA, Aizawa F, McLean JM. Urea as an osmotic ocular hypotensive agent in glaucoma. *Arch Ophthalmol* 1959;62:347.
38. Javid M, Settlage P. Effect of urea on cerebrospinal fluid pressure in human subjects: preliminary report. *JAMA* 1956;160:943.
39. Tarter RC, Linn JG Jr. A clinical study of the use of intravenous urea in glaucoma. *Am J Ophthalmol* 1961;52:323.
40. Galin MA, Davidson R. Hypotensive effect of urea in inflamed and noninflamed eye. *Arch Ophthalmol* 1962;68:633.
41. Virno M, Bucci MG, Pecori-Giraldi J, Cantore G. Intravenous glycerol-vitamin C (sodium salt) as osmotic agents to reduce intraocular pressure. *Am J Ophthalmol* 1966;62:824.
42. Bartkowska-Orlowska M, Orlowski WJ, Warchaloska D, Masiakowski J, Wojnerowicz-Pawlakowej E, Piskorz-Sobcynskiej M. Effect of osmotic agents on intraocular pressure. II. Intravenous administration of glycerol and glycerol with sortibol under experimental conditions. *Klin Oczna* 1973;43:371.
43. Chandler PA, Simmons RJ, Grant WM. Malignant glaucoma: medical and surgical treatment. *Am J Ophthalmol* 1968;66:495.
44. Dickens CJ, Shaffer RN. The medical treatment of ciliary block glaucoma after extracapsular cataract extraction. *Am J Ophthalmol* 1987; 103:237.
45. Marshall S, Hinman F. Subdural hematoma following administration of urea for diagnosis of hypertension. *JAMA* 1962;182:813.
46. D'Alena P, Ferguson W. Adverse effects after glycerol orally and mannitol parenterally. *Arch Ophthalmol* 1966;75:201.
47. Borges MF, Mochs J, Kjellstrand CM. Mannitol intoxication in patients with renal failure. *Arch Intern Med* 1982;142:63.
48. Feitl ME, Krupin T. Hyperosmotic agents. In: Ritch R, Shields MB, Krupin T. *The Glaucomas,* vol 1. St. Louis: Mosby, 1989;551–555.
49. Whelan TV, Bacon ME, Madden M, Patel TG, Handy R. Acute renal failure associated with mannitol intoxication. *Arch Intern Med* 1984; 144:2053.
50. Almog Y, Geyer O, Laser M. Pulmonary edema as a complication of oral glycerol administration. *Ann Ophthalmol* 1986;18:38.
51. Spaeth GL, Spaeth EB, Spaeth PG, Lucier AC. Anaphylactic reaction to mannitol. *Arch Ophthalmol* 1967;78:583.
52. McNeill IY. Hypersensitivity reaction to mannitol. *Drug Intell Clin Pharm* 1985;19:552.

Textbook of Ocular Pharmacology,
edited by T.J. Zimmerman, et al.
Lippincott–Raven Publishers, Philadelphia © 1997.

CHAPTER 27

Antifibrosis Agents: Pharmacologic Inhibition of Wound Healing

Bruce C. Henderson and George F. Nardin

RATIONALE FOR MODULATION OF WOUND HEALING

The response of the body to injury is to initiate a complex process of wound healing, resulting in the formation of fibrous or fibrovascular tissue, in which collagen is a major component. The manifestation of this process is the formation of a scar, usually a desirable endpoint. In certain clinical situations, however, such as glaucoma filtration surgery (GFS), the goal is to achieve incomplete healing of the surgical wound. In other situations, such as pterygium removal, the primary disease process involves aberrant fibrovascular proliferation, and the goal is to eliminate the offending tissue and prevent its recurrence by interrupting the "healing" process. Therefore, there has been longstanding interest in manipulating this process by pharmacologic means to achieve a desired therapeutic goal.

Wound Healing

Healing Sequence

Tissue healing commences with initial ocular injury and damage to vasculature, leading to release of blood and plasma proteins. The subsequent release of local hormonal factors, such as prostaglandin, serotonin, and histamine, results in even greater vascular leakage (1,2). Plasma fibrinogen is transformed in the extravascular tissue to fibrin and a clot forms, trapping red blood cells, platelets, and fibronectin (3). Chemotactic factors enhance the orderly movement into the wound of neutrophils, followed by macrophages and then fibroblasts (4).

Fibroblasts are attracted by platelet-derived growth factor, macrophage-released factors, fibronectin, and tissue hormones, such as serotonin and prostaglandin (5,6). Originating from blood mesenchymal cells and adjacent tissues, fibroblasts appear on the third day after injury and are the dominant cellular component by the fifth day (Fig. 27-1). Procollagen secreted by fibroblasts is transformed into tropocollagen and then to collagen fibrils, which cross-link to form mature collagen (7).

The fibroblastic phase of wound healing is accompanied by neovascular proliferation to form granulation tissue. Contraction of the wound along with epithelialization completes the wound closure. Remodeling of the wound continues for a year or longer and is accompanied by a gradual decrease in fibroblasts and vessels (5). Variations in the degree and intensity of this scarring process can have clinical significance. For example, increased density and thickness of fibrous tissue have been noted in animal and human eyes with failed GFS compared with eyes in which results were successful (8,9). Different phases of the sequence can be more or less exuberant. Early bleb failure after GFS has demonstrated a hypercellular appearance, whereas late failure has been associated with thicker hypocellular collagen disposition (10).

Opportunities for Inhibition

Inhibition of scarring can occur at various stages of the sequence by both physical and pharmacologic means (Fig. 27-2). Decreased size of the operative site and careful hemostasis (to avoid both excessive fibrin and thermal tissue injury) serve to lessen the scope of initial injury and subsequent fibrosis-stimulating inflammation. Avoidance of other sources of inflammation, such as a simultaneous sur-

B. C. Henderson: Department of Ophthalmology, Louisiana State University Medical School in Shreveport, Shreveport, Louisiana 71104.
G. F. Nardin: Private practice, Kailua, Hawaii 96734.

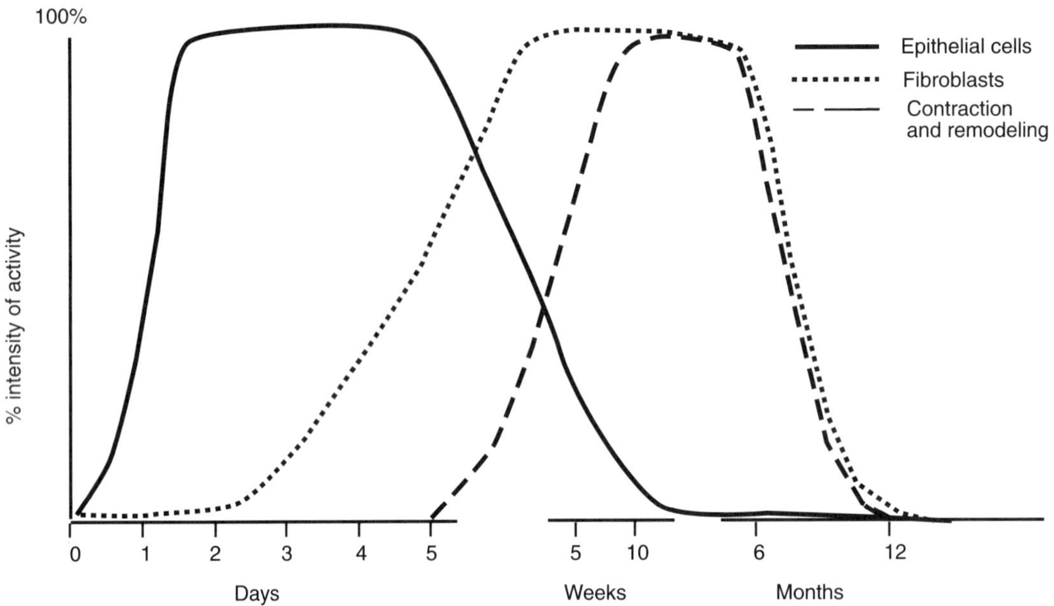

FIG. 27-1. Chronologic activity of wound healing components in glaucoma filtration surgery. (From Costa et al., ref 4, with permission.)

gical procedure, has the same effect; however, the risk must be assessed in light of the total clinical picture, as with combined cataract and glaucoma procedures. The effect of human aqueous humor on wound healing is unclear, with various studies demonstrating both inhibition and stimulation of some healing sequence phases (5). Certainly, as with other fistulae, the physical flow of aqueous through a sclerostomy serves to prolong or prevent its closure.

Many of the drugs studied and used for modulation of wound healing are antimetabolites interfering at the cellular level with the cell-replication cycle of fibroblasts, which are the chief architects of the healing wound (Fig. 27-3). The particular phases of the replication cycle inhibited are specific for each substance. The clinical applications of these agents in ophthalmology are discussed in the remainder of this chapter.

USE OF ANTIFIBROSIS AGENTS IN GLAUCOMA FILTRATION SURGERY

The goal of GFS is to lower intraocular pressure (IOP) by creating a new drainage system for the aqueous humor to leave the anterior chamber and eventually to find its way into the venous return to the heart or into the tears, thus bypassing the conventional outflow pathway. Ideally, this is accomplished without great risk of infection, severe hypotony, or derangement of the optical system. In broadest terms, GFS includes techniques of guarded (trabeculectomy) or unguarded (trephination and posterior lip sclerectomy) limbal drainage to the subconjunctival space and tube shunting to subconjunctival and intraorbital spaces. The desired outcomes of these procedures can be thwarted by proliferation of scar tissue; use of drugs to inhibit such proliferation has increased in recent years. Some, such as corticosteroids, are used routinely, whereas other agents are often reserved for eyes with poor prognosis as a result of increased scarring. Characteristics of patients with increased risk for scarring include young age, black race, previous unsuccessful GFS, aphakia and pseudophakia, neovascular glaucoma, uveitic glaucoma, iridocorneal endothelial syndrome, previous prolonged topical glaucoma therapy, or other forms of conjunctival scarring, such as alkali burns or pseudopemphigoid (11–18).

Antiinflammatory Drugs

Corticosteroids

The structures and properties of corticosteroids and nonsteroidal antiinflammatory drugs (NSAIDs) are discussed in depth elsewhere (Chapter 61) in this text. The beneficial effects of *topical* corticosteroids in the prevention of bleb scarring after GFS, first noted by Sugar, was confirmed by Starita et al. at 1 and 5 years postoperatively (19–21). No additional benefit was derived from the addition of *systemic* steroids; however, they are sometimes used postoperatively in the presence of post-GFS suprachoroidal effusions to discourage vascular permeability. *Subconjunctival* injection of steroids is frequently employed at operation's end to begin treatment,

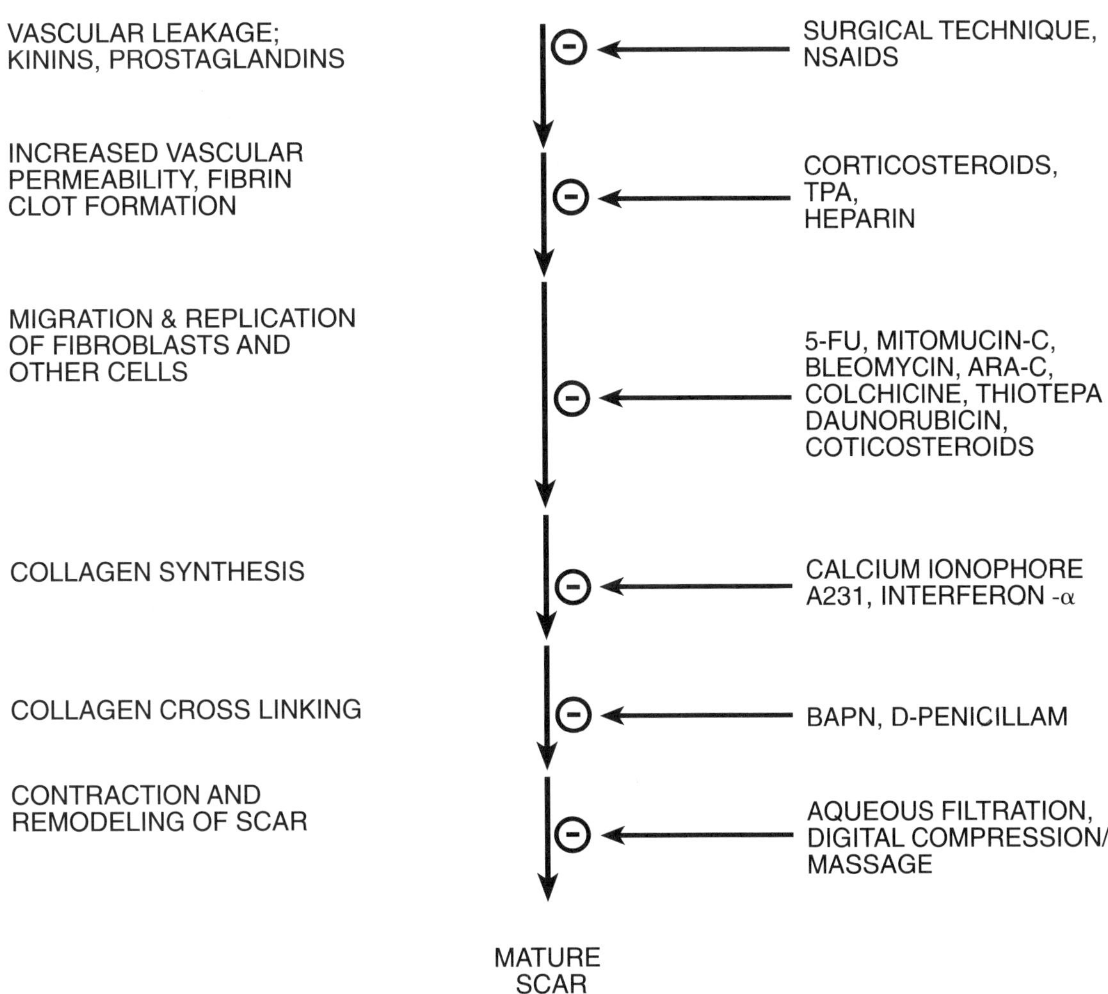

FIG. 27-2. Sequence of wound-healing process with opportunities for inhibition by drugs or other modalities.

followed by moderate to high-dose topical therapy tapering over several weeks. Reports on the use of *preoperative* topical, systemic, and subconjunctival corticosteroids appear to be inconclusive or preliminary.

The presumed mechanism of the antifibrosis activity of corticosteroids in GFS—the inhibition of the inflammatory response—is mediated via blockage of the lipo-oxygenase and cyclooxygenase pathways by direct inhibition of phospholipase A2. This results in decreased capillary permeability, chemotaxis inhibition, and suppression of fibrin deposition (22). Decreased fibroblast proliferation occurs at higher concentrations while a stimulatory effect may be seen at lower concentrations (23).

Nonsteroidal Antiinflammatory Drugs

The NSAIDs, including inhibitors of both lipooxygenase and cyclooxygenase pathways, have demonstrated suppression of human ocular fibroblast proliferation (24); however, in clinical trials, use of topical postoperative flurbiprofen 0.03% after GFS resulted in a higher rate of encapsulated blebs and higher final IOP (25).

Antineoplastic Agents

Many of the pharmacologic agents that hinder the scarring process do so via antimetabolic activity, typically inter-

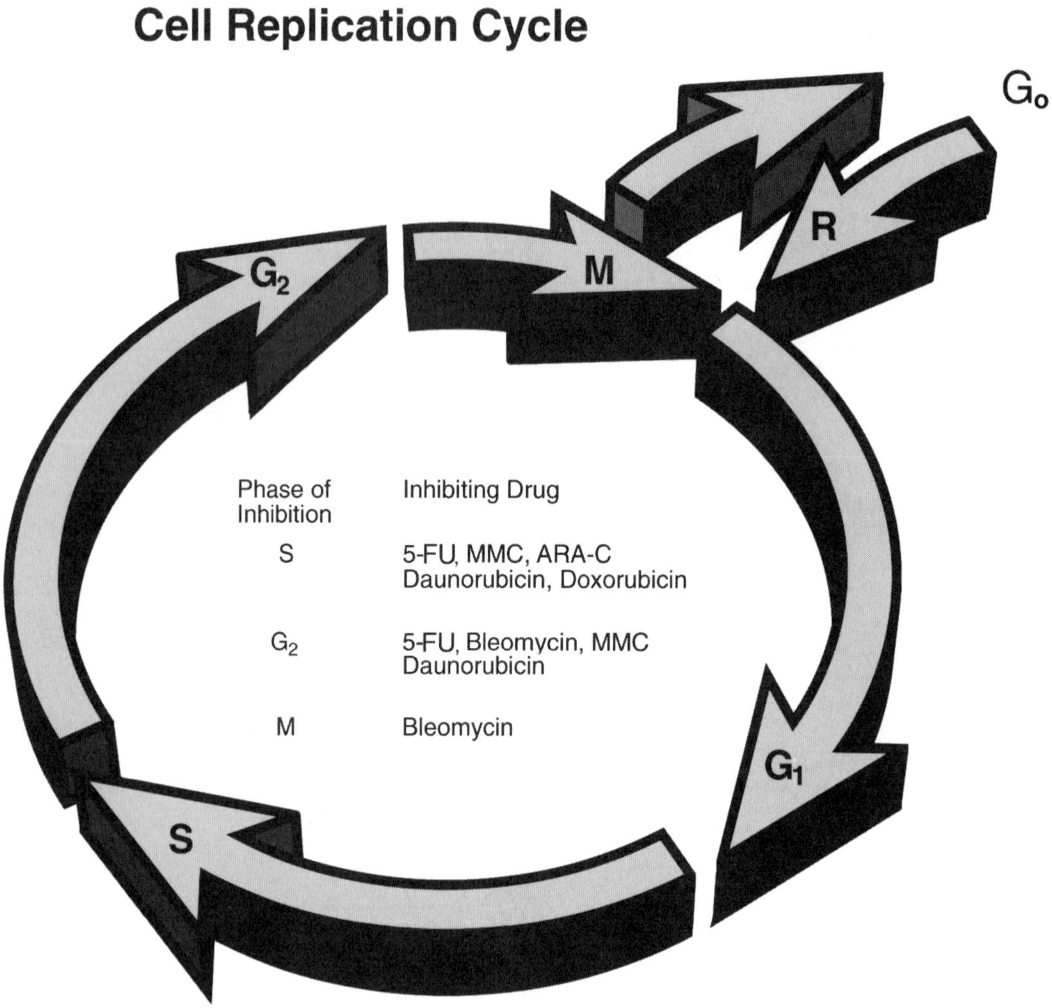

Cell Replication Cycle

Phase of Inhibition	Inhibiting Drug
S	5-FU, MMC, ARA-C Daunorubicin, Doxorubicin
G_2	5-FU, Bleomycin, MMC Daunorubicin
M	Bleomycin

FIG. 27-3. Inhibition of cell replication by various agents. G_0, resting phase; G_1, pre-DNA synthesis; S, DNA synthesis; G_2, RNA synthesis; M, mitosis; R, recruitment phase.

fering with one or more phases of the cell replication cycle of fibroblasts (see Fig. 27-3). Most are antineoplastic antibiotics derived from *Streptomyces* organisms. Only two drugs, 5-fluorouracil (5-FU) and mitomycin C (MMC), have been used extensively in GFS, although many others have been studied or may eventually see clinical application.

5-Fluorouracil

History

5-Fluororidine (5-FUR) and 5-FU are pyrimidine nucleotide analogs. Like other pyrimidine analogs, they owe their antineoplastic activity to small structural dissimilarities from endogenous pyrimidines. They require metabolic conversion to nucleotides to exert cytotoxicity (26). Simultaneous catabolism, on the other hand, can inactivate these drugs. Variations in these opposing activities among different cell types helps to explain the increased toxicity to actively proliferating cells seen with drugs such as 5-FU.

First synthesized by Duschinsky et al. in 1957, 5-FU has seen a flurry of clinical investigation and use in GFS since the first reported human pilot study by Heuer and co-workers in 1984 (27). It is a fluorinated pyrimidine with a molecular weight of 130.08, which undergoes intracellular conversion to the active deoxynucleotide, 5-fluoro-2′-deoxyuridine 5′-monophosphate (FdUMP). The conversion of deoxyuridylic acid to thymidylic acid is hampered by the action of FdUMP on thymidylate synthetase, thus impeding DNA synthesis (26). FdUMP also is incorporated directly into DNA molecules after conversion by intracellular kinases to a triphosphate. Such DNA, with fluorouracil substituted for thymine, may be more unstable than native DNA. It also interferes with RNA processing and function after its conversion to the ribonucleotide, fluorouridine monophosphate (FUMP), which is incorporated into the RNA molecule. Thus, three mechanisms may be involved in the antimetabolic activity of 5-FU, although it is primarily due to competitive inhibition of thymidylate synthetase in the S-phase of the cell-replication cycle.

Therapeutic Use

Primarily, 5-FU has been employed in the chemotherapeutic management of metastatic carcinomas of the breast and gastrointestinal tract, and it has also been used parenterally for treatment of hepatomas and carcinomas of the ovary, cervix, bladder, prostate, and pancreas (28). It is used topically to treat actinic keratoses and superficial basal cell carcinomas.

In GFS, 5-FU has been used mostly in the form of postoperative subconjunctival injections. Different concentrations may be used. The usual single dose is 5 mg and can be accomplished by using 0.1 ml of the undiluted form at 50 mg/ml (Adrucil, Adria Laboratories or Fluorouracil, Roche). Alternatively, it may be diluted with nonpreserved saline under a laminar flow hood to 10 mg/ml and then given as a 0.5-ml injection. Either is performed 90 to 180 degrees away from the bleb using a tuberculin syringe with a 30-gauge needle directed tangentially to the globe, bevel away from the sclera. This step is preceded by topical anesthetic on a cotton-tipped applicator, often with 2% to 4% lidocaine, although proparacaine also works well (29). Avoidance of conjunctival vessels minimizes bleeding.

Subconjunctival diffusion to the wound site may occur, although much of the effect occurs as a result of leakage back through the needle track into the tear film. Whereas this leakage is intended, the rapid release of undiluted drug into the tear film may encourage epithelial toxicity. To decrease the leakage when using a larger bolus of 0.5 ml, one may use tamponade of the needle track with a moist cotton-tipped swab, light massage with the swab to move the bolus away from the track, and irrigation of residual undiluted 5-FU from the conjunctiva and eyelids with saline (30). A smaller 0.1-ml bolus (also with 5 mg of drug) can be deposited well away from the track by advancing the needle cautiously for some distance under the conjunctiva. These techniques may result in a more gradual release of 5-FU into the tear film, hopefully lessening corneal epithelial toxicity.

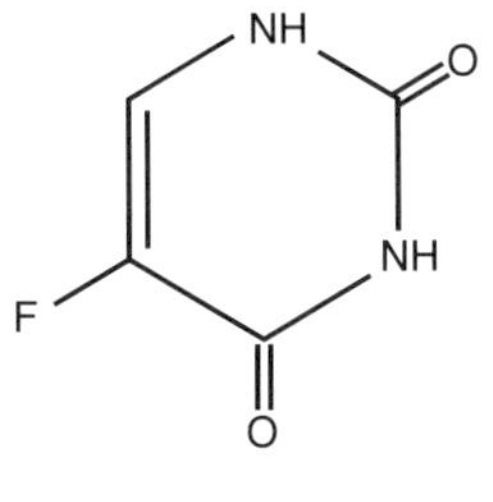

5-Fluorouracil

Both the frequency and duration of postoperative subconjunctival 5-FU can be varied considerably. Initially, the regimen employed required 5 mg twice daily for 7 days postoperatively followed by once daily for 7 more days (27). Lower total dosage employed in other studies, ranging from 13 mg to 87 mg, has achieved similar success with fewer complications (30). The dosage can be adjusted based on clinical judgment, response to therapy, development of complications, and occasionally on a patient's access to care.

Another reported method of 5-FU application in GFS is the intraoperative *implantation* of a purified collagen sponge containing 100 μg of 5-FU in the quadrant of surgery (31), which results in a slow release of the agent over time with less epithelial exposure. Undiluted 5-FU (50 mg/ml) has also been used *intraoperatively* using drug-soaked cellulose sponges placed under and over the scleral flap and subconjunctivally for a 5-minute period followed by copious balanced salt irrigation (32). Supplementary 5-FU injections can still be used postoperatively.

Toxicity of 5-FU

Toxicity is inherent with antimetabolic drugs, and adverse toxic side effects are not surprising. Systemic absorption of 5-FU in the course of adjunctive use in GFS is extremely small because of the minuscule dosages employed subconjunctivally: on the order of 1% to 3% of the amount used intravenously for antitumor therapy. The absorbed drug undergoes hepatic catabolism and elimination by respiration as carbon dioxide or by renal excretion as one of several metabolites and as free drug (33). The low quantities administered explain the virtual absence of systemic toxicity from 5-FU in local ocular applications. Side effects seen with high-dose intravenous therapy, such as bone marrow suppression, nausea, stomatitis, and alopecia, have not been reported with human ocular use (although one case of bone marrow aplasia occurred in primate studies with a closely related compound) (34,35). Its risk in pregnancy is unclear, however, and it is classified in U.S. Food and Drug Administration (FDA) pregnancy category D. It has, in high concentrations, demonstrated mutagenic activity in murine bone-marrow cells and has shown teratogenicity in mice, rats, and hamsters but not in monkeys.

Toxicity from ocular 5-FU administration is related to its effect on rapidly dividing epithelial cells of the cornea and conjunctiva. The Flouorouracil Filtering Surgery Study (FFSS) group reported nearly universal occurrence of punctate corneal epitheliopathy (98%) and conjunctival epithelial defects along with a significant incidence of corneal epithelial defects (64%), some of long duration (36). The same epithelial toxicity is believed to be responsible for the high incidence of conjunctival wound leaks observed after the use of 5-FU in GFS, with a reported incidence of 5% to 37% (5). Other corneal complications include filamentary keratitis, keratinized corneal plaques, infectious corneal ulcers, and striate melanokeratosis, the latter resulting from centripetal migration of pigment-laden stem cells from the limbus (37–39).

During parenteral use, 5-FU's presence in the tear layer is associated with ocular complications, including punctal-canalicular stenosis and cicatricial ectropion due to lower-eyelid dermatitis (40–42). Contact dermatitis and increased pigmentation of periocular skin have been seen with periocular use of topical 5-FU for skin lesions (43). These effects are potentially relevant to current ophthalmic use because of the high levels of 5-FU seen in the tear layer after subconjunctival injection. Use of 5-FU has been associated with a higher incidence of thin blebs. Complications typical of thin cystic blebs, such as late bleb leaks, late endophthalmitis, and hypotony maculopathy, have been reported to occur with increased frequency with 5-FU use (36, 44,45). Although corneal endothelial toxicity has been shown in vitro at high concentrations, it has not been reported in clinical trials (46). Other complications of hypotony, such as prolonged choroidal effusion and persistent shallow chambers, can be expected to occur at a somewhat increased rate with antimetabolite use in GFS.

Prevention of complications from 5-FU use in GFS begins with patient selection. Use of 5-FU should be avoided or only with caution in patients with known corneal diseases that might encourage corneal toxicity, such as bullous keratopathy, severe dry-eye syndrome, preexisting corneal epithelial defect, recurrent erosion syndrome, corneal melting syndrome, preexisting dellen, and conditions with decreased limbal stem cells, such as Stevens-Johnson syndrome, pemphigoid, pseudopemphigoid, and old alkali burns.

Epithelial defects and wound leaks appear to be dose related, and the use of lesser total dosages or the adjustment of dosage by clinical response has lessened toxicity while maintaining the increased success of GFS seen in problem eyes using 5-FU (37,47). Methods to decrease concentrated free drug in the tear film after injection were described previously. *Careful closure of the conjunctival wound* is critical to the prevention of early postoperative wound leaks, which then are prolonged by antimetabolite exposure. Some authors believe that fornix-based conjunctival flaps are inappropriate in this setting. The use of a small taper-point needle (to prevent needle track leaks) on 8-0 to 10-0 suture material of various types and a running horizontal mattress closure (which everts both wound edges) results in the near absence of significant early bleb wound leaks. The running horizontal mattress closure, taking suture bites in both Tenon's capsule and conjunctiva, eliminates the need for a two-layer closure in the prevention of bleb leaks.

Some authors advocate avoidance of antimetabolites with primary filtration in young and myopic patients because of an increased incidence of hypotony maculopathy, whereas others recommend precautionary techniques to avoid hypotony in such higher-risk patients (48). Larger scleral trabeculectomy flaps, sutured more tightly, help in this regard, still leaving the option of selective laser suturolysis. A more anterior placement of the sclerostomy during guarded filtration, described by Palmberg, can create a *partial corneal valve effect* (as seen with self-sealing cataract wounds), thereby giving an additional site of resistance to outflow independent of conjunctival or episcleral scarring (49).

Clinical Trials

After initial success in prolonging bleb formation in owl monkeys, human clinical studies were undertaken (27,50). Multiple studies have confirmed the increased success rates for GFS in poor-prognosis eyes when using postoperative 5-FU. Such eyes include those with neovascular, congenital, inflammatory, and pseudophakia or aphakic glaucomas as well as those with previous filtration surgery and in the black population (14,36,37,51–54). No clear benefit has been shown in glaucoma associated with iridocorneal endothelial syndrome and epithelial downgrowth (17,55). The FFSS confirmed that 5-FU decreased the failure rate to 49% at 3 years postoperatively for GFS in poor prognosis eyes compared with a 74% failure rate in control eyes (51).

Lower postoperative pressures, higher success rates, and fewer required postoperative glaucoma medications are seen after GFS for uncomplicated glaucomas when 5-FU is used; however, adverse side effects are increased compared with control eyes (56–58). The results have been mixed with 5-FU used as an adjunct to combined cataract/glaucoma surgery, although one might expect a benefit in larger randomized trials (59,60). 5-FU may reduce the incidence of encapsulated blebs and may enhance needling revision of failing filter blebs (61,62).

Intraoperative application of 5-FU appears to increase success rates in GFS and allow decreased postoperative injections of 5-FU with decreased surface toxicity. Other alternative methods of delivering 5-FU, such as bioerodable polymeric disks, collagen implants, and liposomal encapsulation, have not been extensively studied in humans (31,65,66).

Mitomycin C

History

Wakaki and colleagues in 1958 isolated MMC, a naturally occurring antibiotic-antineoplastic compound (molecular weight 334.33), from the organism *Streptomyces caespitosus* (67). Because of its toxicity, it has not been found useful for antimicrobial therapy. After enzyme activation in tissue, it functions as an alkylating agent, cross-linking DNA. Although it is cell-cycle phase nonspecific, MMC is most active in the G and S phases of cell division (68).

Therapeutic Use

Mitomycin C has been used intravenously in the treatment of malignant neoplasms of the stomach, pancreas, bladder, colon, rectum, lung, cervix, and breast. Bladder instillation has been used to prevent tumor recurrence, and intraarterial treatment has been tried for hepatic tumors. The drug is broken down in the liver and excreted in urine, 10% unchanged, with a half-life of 5 to 15 minutes.

In GFS, mitomycin is used to prevent replication of fibroblasts. Based on animal and human studies, subconjunctival fibroblast proliferation is inhibited in a manner that is dependent on both drug concentration and time of exposure (69,70). Potency is as much as 100 times greater than 5-FU. Fibroblasts migration and attachment are unaffected at usually employed dosages (71). The effectiveness of single-dose administration, which is commonly used, may be due to the ability of MMC to impede future replication even of cells not synthesizing DNA at the time of exposure. The marked hypovascularity of blebs after MMC exposure presumably stems from toxicity to vascular endothelium and may contribute to a decrease in scarring. In addition to enhanced filtration, some have hypothesized additional IOP lowering as a result of hyposecretion of aqueous caused by toxicity to ciliary body (72,73); however, the observed suppression of aqueous production appears transient in animal studies, even with exposure much greater than usual (74). Additionally, most patients with persistent hypotony respond to bleb revisions with a significant pressure elevation, indicating overfiltration as having a major contribution to the pressure decrease (73).

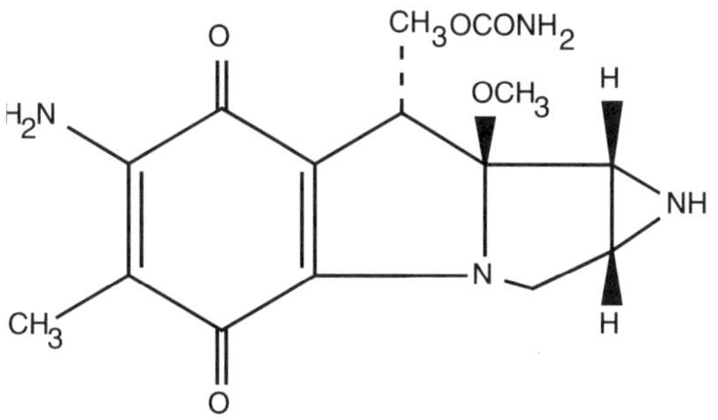

O
CH_3OCONH_2
OCH_3
H
H_2N
NH
N
CH_3
H
O

Mitomycin C (MMC)

Mitomycin requires special handling procedures, with mixing under a hood and filtration through a 5-μm filter. It should be mixed for ophthalmic use by a pharmacist in sterile water to a concentration between 0.1 mg and 0.5 mg/ml, stable for 7 days at room temperature or 14 days refrigerated (75). If nonpreserved, it should be used within 24 hours. It should be properly labeled, with handling and disposal precautions used by all personnel.

Currently MMC is used for GFS almost exclusively in the form of transient intraoperative topical application. Typically, a soaked sponge vehicle containing a solution of MMC is placed on the scleral bed after conjunctival dissection, either before or after the trabeculectomy scleral flap has been fashioned, but *before any entry into the eye.* The conjunctival/Tenon's flap is then draped over the sponge, thus exposing the episcleral layer and undersurface of Tenon's capsule to the solution for a measured period. Some surgeons also place a piece of sponge beneath the flap. Care is taken to avoid full contact with the free wound margin of the conjunctival flap, which might encourage postoperative wound leaks.

Sponge removal is followed by irrigation of the field with saline or balanced salt solution to prevent drug entry into the eye through subsequent incisions. Should inadvertent chamber entry occur during flap dissection, the dissection should be stopped and the chamber overfilled with viscoelastic. Then cautious separate application to the underside of the conjunctival flap and to episclera adjacent to the scleral flap can be performed, taking care to dry any free solution collecting near the entry site. We have encountered no complications with this technique in isolated cases. The procedure is otherwise unaltered, except for methods employed to avoid hypotony.

Practices vary considerably in this type of application of MMC with respect to sponge type, concentration of solution, and exposure time. A recent informal survey by IOP, Inc., of 48 ophthalmologists experienced in MMC use indicated that they used the drug in almost 80% of all filtering procedures. Mean concentration used was 0.34 mg/ml, and mean application time was 3.1 minutes. Many surgeons used variations either in concentration or in application time based on the clinical situation. Most used modified cellulose surgical spear sponges (either whole or in pieces), although Gelfoam was also used. The area of application varied among surgeons and with the clinical outcome desired.

Toxicity of MMC

As with 5-FU, the current clinical ophthalmic use of mitomycin yields minimal systemic exposure to the drug. No systemic complication resulting from ocular therapy has been reported. Because of its teratogenicity in animals, however, it should be avoided during pregnancy. Carcinogenicity in rats leaves some concern about future sequelae of local tissue application; the brevity of exposure and the technique employed should give some reassurance with regard to surrounding tissues.

The potential for *corneal endothelial* toxicity has been demonstrated, but the concentration used properly in the clinical setting results in insufficient aqueous concentrations to cause such damage (76–78). The saline irrigation after exposure lowers resulting aqueous concentrations even more (79). Topical use of MMC after pterygium surgery and associated complications are discussed later in this chapter. The scleral thinning and necrosis seen occasionally with topical use have not been reported with MMC use in GFS as described.

One of the major advantages of MMC over 5-FU in glaucoma surgery is the much decreased incidence of *corneal epithelial toxicity.* Punctate epitheliopathy may occur with MMC, but it is much less frequent and less severe than with 5-FU (5,80). In fact, no major corneal complications have been reported with MMC use in GFS except for one incidence of necrotizing keratitis occurring greater than 6 months posttrabeculectomy in the third corneal graft of a patient suffering from an old alkali burn (81). There is some evidence that the lack of corneal toxicity observed is due mainly to the method of administration, as MMC is more toxic to corneal epithelium than 5-FU (82). *Conjunctival epithelial* defects are sometimes seen over an area of intense exposure (i.e., high concentration and long duration; R. K. Parrish II, personal communication).

Most problems encountered with MMC in glaucoma surgery simply stem from its desired antiproliferative effect. Conjunctival *wound leak* may occur more frequently, but wide variation in incidence suggests that meticulous closure may be the key to prevention (5,80,83). The persistent antiproliferative effect on the fibroblasts, along with vascular toxicity, probably accounts for the thin avascular blebs frequently seen and the ability to achieve successful laser suturolysis much later postoperatively than is possible without mitomycin (84). Differences in long-term complications related to altered bleb characteristics, such as late bleb leaks and infection, have not been firmly established relative to surgery without MMC.

Hypotony maculopathy is characterized by decreased visual acuity, macular retinal and choroidal folds, vascular tortuosity, and sometimes disc edema. It is a known complication of filtration surgery in which prolonged hypotony occurs, usually <5 mm Hg (85). Such hypotony occurs more frequently after mitomycin filter procedures and is more likely with longer exposure time; it may be more common with primary than with repeat operations (86). An associated peculiar marked reversal of disc cupping frequently occurs (even without nerve fiber layer edema); the cup usually will reenlarge upon elevation of pressures to normal or higher levels, whereas visual fields remain unimproved throughout. Surgical techniques, as described with 5-FU, may decrease the incidence of this problem (49). Treatment modalities for hypotony maculopathy include autologous blood injection into the bleb, cryotherapy of the bleb, and topical application of trichloroacetic acid (48,87,88). Significant improvement usually occurs with early reversal of hypotony. Other complications of hypotony, such as shallow anterior chamber and cataract, may be more frequent with MMC use (5) (Fig. 27-4).

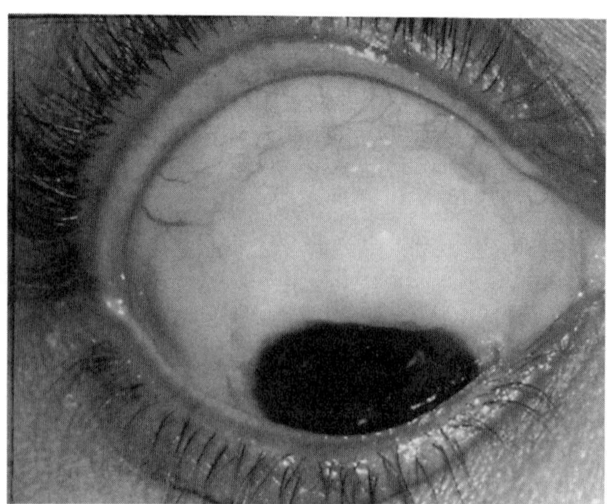

FIG. 27-4. Pale avascular bleb seen typically after mitomycin C filtration surgery.

Clinical Trials

Chen first described adjunctive use of mitomycin in glaucoma surgery, reporting enhanced success (89,90); however, the expanded use by glaucomatologists did not occur until Palmer reported an excellent success rate in eyes with a high risk for failure with GFS. His technique, derived from that described by Chen, is essentially the same used by most surgeons today. Eyes selected included those with neovascular, aphakic, low-tension, or secondary glaucomas and those with previous surgery. Using strict criteria for failure (target pressures), 28 of 33 eyes were deemed successful (84%), with only three requiring medication. Four of the five failures had IOP decreased by 25% to 82% (91).

Kitazawa and co-workers confirmed this beneficial effect and demonstrated a greater success rate with MMC than 5-FU in a controlled study (80). Eyes treated with MMC had lower pressures, required fewer medications, and had fewer corneal complications. Other studies confirmed these advantages over 5-FU in both animal models and humans (83,92,93). Anterior chamber reaction was less with MMC than with 5-FU (94).

Use of mitomycin in primary trabeculectomies is open to debate. High success rates have been shown but with some significant complications (95). The answer may be in restricting its use in primary filters to eyes needing a very low IOP or by decreasing the exposure significantly below that currently practiced (96). Salutary effects on bleb survival and pressure control seem apparent in the setting of combined cataract and trabeculectomy procedures. Two controlled studies, reported to the American Academy of Ophthalmology in late 1994, yielded conflicting results on this issue (97,98). As an adjunct to glaucoma tube-shunt surgery, MMC has been suggested, whereas some believe that the better risk-to-benefit profile of mitomycin trabeculectomies may preclude the use of shunts in many cases (99,100).

Other developments regarding MMC include suturing techniques allowing fornix-based conjunctival flaps, although early postoperative wound leaks are still significant (101). Given by subconjunctival injection before a laser sclerostomy procedure, MMC has been studied in animals with some success; however, the use of an irreversible antimetabolite in a procedure already limited by its full-thickness nature and associated complications should be viewed with skepticism, when more control is possible through surgical technique or withholding of medication (as with 5-FU) (102). An alternate method of administration of MMC by an implanted crosslinked poly (HEMA) device shows promise in high-risk glaucoma surgery (103). The ability of MMC to lower IOP by subconjunctival injection alone, seen in animals and a small human study, may be related to ciliary body toxicity; further study is anticipated (104,105).

Other Antineoplastic Agents

Antibiotics

Bleomycin, daunorubicin, doxorubicin, and mithramycin are all antineoplastic antibodies isolated from *Streptomyces,* as is MMC. Each demonstrated inhibition of fibroblasts in tissue culture or animal model (23,72,106,107).

Bleomycin inhibits cell replication primarily in the G_2 (premitosis) phase of cell division but also has some activity in the M, G_1, and early S phases. A ferrous iron-bleomycin complex intercalates between DNA base pairs, splitting DNA strands, thus inhibiting DNA, RNA, and protein synthesis (108). It is used to treat testicular tumors, malignant lymphomas, and squamous cell carcinomas. Bleomycin bound in a collagen polymer sponge implanted at the time of filtration surgery has shown increased bleb survival in rabbits and humans in limited studies (109,110).

Daunorubicin and doxorubicin, both anthracycline antibiotics, are not cell-cycle specific but are most toxic to cells in the S phase of the cell-replication cycle via combination with DNA (108). Daunorubicin, discussed later in this chapter, is used systemically in the treatment of acute leukemias and markedly increased bleb survival in GFS on rabbits, exhibiting some corneal toxicity, particularly with higher dosage (111).

Pyrimidine Analogs

Pyrimidine analogs, including cytosine arabinoside (Ara-C), trifluorothymidine, 5-fluoroorotate, and metabolites of 5-FU have shown promise for use in GFS by their antiproliferative actions. Arabinoside C acts selectively in the S phase of the cell cycle, completely inhibiting DNA polymerase and thus impeding DNA synthesis (112). This antileukemia agent has demonstrated more potent inhibition of fibroblast proliferation than 5-FU (113). In a bioerodible polymer, Ara-C caused significant prolongation of bleb survival after GFS in rabbits (114). One drawback may be its corneal epithelial toxicity (115). Trifluorothymidine inhibits fibroblast proliferation in tissue culture and possibly enhances GFS in humans (116,117). 5-Fluoroorotate proved beneficial in promoting bleb formation in a primate model (118). Lee et al. observed that fluorouridine (5-FUR), FUMP, 5-fluorodeoxyuridine (FudR), and FdUMP all had greater potency than 5-FU for inhibiting proliferation of human Tenon's capsule fibroblasts (119).

Alkaloids

Some alkaloids derived from natural plants have inhibited rabbit or human fibroblast in vitro. Those that have been studied are vincristine, vinblastine, and taxol (120, 121).

Other Antifibrosis Agents for Glaucoma Surgery

There has been great interest in impeding not only cellular proliferation but also collagen synthesis and maturation in an attempt to reduce scar formation. Interferon-α, calcium ionophore A23187, β-aminoproprionitrile, (BAPN), and D-penicillamine (DPA) have been studied.

Interferon-α inhibits not only collagen production but also fibroblast proliferation and chemotaxis in vitro (122–124). Gillies and co-workers have observed a possibly beneficial effect in a human GFS study (125) using postoperative subconjunctival injections of 200,000 IU in 0.2 ml N saline two to three times weekly for up to 3 weeks. Less corneal toxicity was observed than with 5-FU. Calcium ionophore A23187 also inhibits collagen synthesis in human episcleral fibroblast cell cultures and has been suggested as an adjunct to GFS (125).

Both DPA and BAPN inhibit collagen fibril cross-linking after synthesis, decreasing tensile strength of scar tissue; DPA, a chelating agent and a degradation product of penicillin, has been studied in animal models for GFS with only modest results (127), and BAPN, an alkaloid from the sweet pea *Lathyrus odoratus,* inhibits lysl oxidase, the enzyme active in cross-linking of tropocollagen fibrils. Used in 10 to 20% topical ointment in human GFS on high-risk patients, a 74% success rate was observed at a 6-month mean follow-up, with some corneal and dermal toxicity (128).

Inhibitors of fibrin deposition in the earliest phases of wound healing may prove beneficial in GFS. Tissue plasminogen activator (TPA) is an enzyme that converts plasminogen to plasimin, which is fibrinolytic. Some evidence from animal studies suggests that TPA may enhance GFS (130,179). Heparin may be helpful in the same way; it also shows some inhibition of proliferation in human scleral fibroblasts with frequent exposure (131).

OTHER USES OF ANTIFIBROSIS AGENTS

Strabismus

An uncommon but well-recognized complication of strabismus surgery is the postoperative development of a hypertrophic scar over an operated extraocular muscle, particularly the medial rectus muscle. Despite its rarity, this complication can be cosmetically quite disfiguring. Once this scarring occurs, the rate of recurrence with excision and application of topical corticosteroid drops has been estimated to be as high as 33%. At the time of this publication, only limited data are available on the use of antimetabolites in the management of this problem.

Mitomycin-C

Urban and Kaufman have described the application of topical MMC eyedrops in a concentration of 0.4 mg/ml and 0.2 mg/ml applied four times daily for 7 to 10 days following surgical excision of the scar to prevent recurrence (132). With a follow-up of 16 to 20 weeks, these investigators found a recurrence rate of one in four, with the single recurrence described as being only partial (Fig. 27-5).

No scleromalacia or other complications known to occur with topical MMC administration were found in this small study. Longer follow-up (2–3 years) has demonstrated no recurrence in the original three patients who were considered successes at the time. In the 2-year follow-up of the fourth patient, who showed partial recurrence, the recurring scar had undergone spontaneous regression. To date, no serious complications have arisen from the use of mitomycin in these patients (personal communication, Lawrence M. Kaufman).

Corneal Vascularization and Pterygium

Thiotepa

Triethylene thiophosphoramide (Thoitepa) was first investigated for ophthalmic use in the management of corneal vascularization and recurrent pterygia. Thiotepa is a synthetic antimitotic agent chemically and pharmacologically similar to the nitrogen mustards used in chemical warfare in the early part of the twentieth century. It is a polyfunctional alkylating agent that is most effective in inhibiting tissue growth in rapidly growing normal and neoplastic tissue (133,134). Its suspected mode of action is the release of ethylenamine radicals and their effect on actively dividing cells. The inhibition of vascular neogenesis seems to be due to the inhibition of capillary endothelial cell proliferation.

Originally, thiotepa came under investigation for use in the inhibition of corneal scarring and vascularization following alkali burns (135). Lavergne and Colman found that the administration of thiotepa drops inhibited the progression of corneal vascularization in the alkali-burned rabbit cornea by impeding the replication of capillary endothelial cells (136). Initial results seemed promising, but further studies in animal models and in humans failed to show any permanent inhibition of corneal vascularization with the use of thiotepa. Furthermore, corneal thinning and ulceration occurred occasionally with its use. As a result, thiotepa has never gained popularity in the management of corneal vascularization.

Antimetabolites have found their most common clinical use in the management of *recurrent pterygia.* Because β irradiation using Strontium^{90} had previously been shown to be effective in the management of recurrent pterygia, investigators were interested in finding some type of radiomimetic drug that might be as useful but with fewer un-

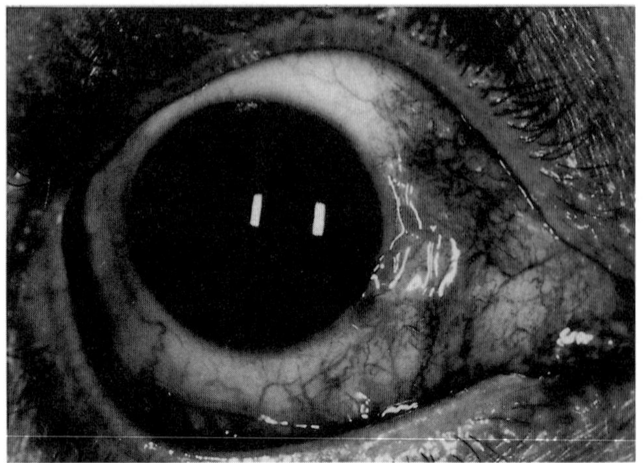

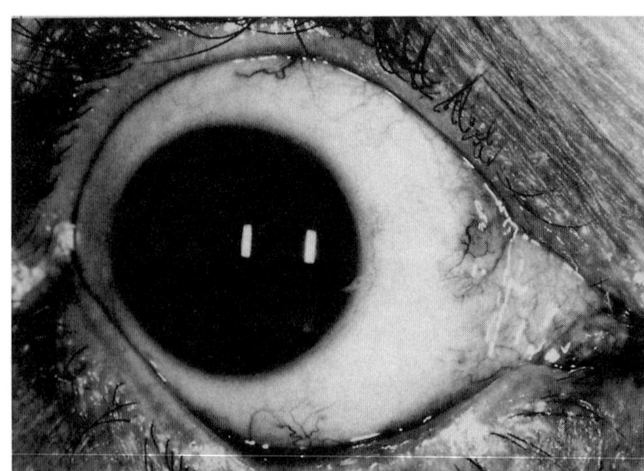

FIG. 27-5. Preoperative (left) and postoperative (right) appearance in excision of hypertrophic scar after strabismus surgery (courtesy of L.M. Kaufman).

desirable side effects and complications of irradiation. Such treatment might be simpler and less expensive, thus the choice of thiotepa. Meacham pioneered its use in the prevention of recurrence of pterygia in humans in 1962. He initially applied it in topical form in a solution of 15 mg in 30 ml of Ringer's solution (1 : 2,000) applied every 3 hours while awake. Treatment was begun 2 or 3 days after pterygium excision and was continued for 6 weeks. He found a nearly tenfold decrease (from 30% to 3.3%) in the rate of recurrence with this regimen of thiotepa therapy administered four times a day for 1 to 2 weeks (137,138).

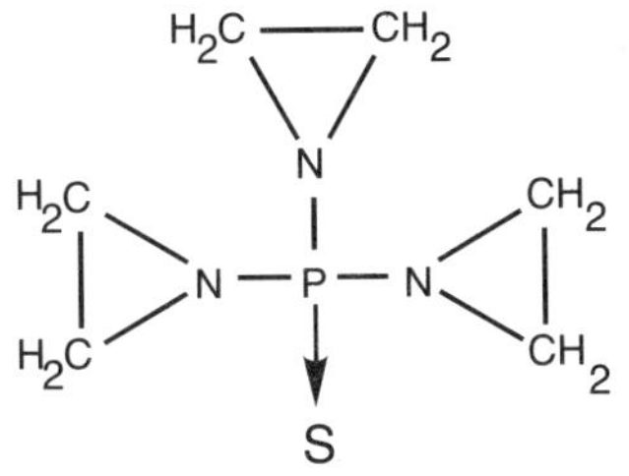

Triethylene thiophosphoramide (Thio-tepa)

Initially, concentrations of 1 : 500 and 1 : 1,000 were used, but the postoperative management of pterygium recurrence using topical thiotepa appeared to be just as effective and less likely to cause irritation using low concentrations, such as 1 : 2,000. Used in this manner, it caused little irritation and appeared to prevent recurrences over a follow-up period of 1 to 3 years; however, when the higher concentration of 1 : 100 in oil was used, significant eye irritation and occasional stenosis or obstruction of the nasolacrimal duct occurred (139). Over time, other side effects were noted to arise with repeated topical application of thiotepa (140): allergic contact dermatitis, rare cases of depigmentation of the eyelids and eyelashes, and occasional keratitis and corneal edema. In some cases of skin depigmentation, the depigmentation process continued for several months after discontinuation of the thiotepa treatment.

As yet, no consensus has been agreed on as to the single best way to manage the problem of recurrence after pterygium excision. Thiotepa administration, β-irradiation using Strontium^{90}, and conjunctival autograft placement all have significantly reduced the rate of recurrence (141). Adjunctive β-irradiation therapy appears to offer nearly the same recurrence rate (10.9%) as the use of thiotepa (8%) (142). Cataract formation, corneal melt, scleral melt, and keratitis sicca have limited the use of β-irradiation, and reports of occasional skin depigmentation and recommendations against its use in darkly pigmented people have prevented thiotepa from being used as widely as irradiation in preventing recurrence (143). With the success of autograft placement and the use of MMC, the use of both β-irradiation and thiotepa has been on the decline in the United States. Elsewhere in the world, all three modalities are still commonly employed.

Mitomycin-C

Kunimoto and Mori first reported the successful use of MMC in the management of pterygium recurrence in 1963 (144). In 1988, Singh et al. reported the results of a large study in which MMC was used to prevent the recurrence of pterygia (145). They originally used topical MMC at concentrations of 1.0 mg/ml and 0.4 mg/ml to treat both primary and recurrent pterygia. In the course of their study, it became apparent that the use of the 1.0 mg/ml concentration was greater than necessary, was accompanied by a higher rate of complication, and therefore was discontinued. Compared with the group treated by surgical excision alone, in which recurrence occurred in 16 of 18 cases (88.9%), the groups treated by surgical excision followed by the topical administration of MMC had one recurrence in 44 cases (2.3%). The MMC drops were administered four times daily for 2 weeks. Mild to moderate conjunctival injection was observed in the mitomycin-treated groups, and conjunctival epithelial defects persisted for up to 4 weeks postoperatively in this group as well. Complete healing of the conjunctiva was noted in the placebo-treated group within the first 2 weeks of surgery. In the course of the study, many patients treated with the higher dosage of MMC complained of a much longer period (up to 3 months) of ocular pain, photophobia, lacrimation, and foreign-body sensation after the drops were discontinued. Hayasaka et al. found that the use of MMC at a dosage of 2.0 mg/ml twice daily for 5 days resulted in a very low recurrence rate as well (146,147). Frucht-Pery and Ilsar found that with twice-daily administration for 5 days of 0.1 mg/ml MMC the recurrence rate was 8%, and with 0.2 mg/ml the recurrence rate was 4% (148). Of 50 patients treated with one of these two dosages, only two experienced complications. One patient had an 8-week delay in conjunctival reepithelialization, and one patient experienced degenerative calcification of the conjunctiva 18 months after surgery. Both complications occurred in patients receiving the higher dosage. The use of topical MMC has been accompanied by a number of rare but serious complications, including scleral ulceration, necrotizing scleritis, corneal perforation, uveitis, cataract formation, infection, glaucoma, and scleral calcification (149–151).

Pingyangmycinum (Bleomycin A5)

In China, pingyangmycinum, a naturally occurring compound produced by *Streptomyces pingyanggensis* n. spp. was shown to be effective in preventing the recurrence of pterygium following surgical excision (152). Pingyangmycinum, identical to bleomycin A5, is a cytotoxic compound that, like all bleomycins, derives its activity from the ability to incise and fragment DNA molecules. This naturally occurring antibiotic antimetabolite is under study in some preliminary work in China to inhibit the recurrence of pterygium formation. Although scarce, the data suggest that postoperative treatment of pterygia with bleomycin A5 may significantly reduce the rate of pterygium recurrence.

Posterior Capsule Opacification

Despite improved intraocular lens design, improved cortical removal, and careful capsule polishing at the time of surgery (which carries some risk), posterior capsule opacification following cataract surgery continues to be a problem. It is known to occur in 30% to 50% of all cataract patients within 4 to 5 years after cataract surgery (153,154). Surviving lens epithelial cells, remaining adherent to the equatorial lens capsule after cataract surgery, multiply and spread across the posterior capsule. The resulting distortion and opacification of the lens capsule cause diminished contrast sensitivity and visual acuity. If severe enough, this problem can limit the patient's ability to function.

Before the early 1980s, the management of capsular opacification involved surgical discission of the posterior capsule either at the slit lamp or in the operating room under sterile operating room conditions. With the advent of the neodymium-yttrium aluminum garnet (Nd:YAG) laser, handling this problem became much simpler and safer. Despite this advance, opening the capsule with the Nd:YAG carries with it certain complications and considerable expense. Damage to the intraocular lens, retinal detachment, and retinal breaks all occur with greater frequency in patients undergoing capsular discission with conventional surgery and with the Nd:YAG laser (155–157). Because of the inherent risks associated with opening the posterior capsule as well as the added cost, there continues to be strong interest in primary prevention of capsular opacification through the use of pharmacologic agents. Two chemotherapeutic agents in particular have been investigated.

Daunorubicin

Power and co-workers examined the effects of daunorubicin in cultured human and bovine lens epithelial cells by applying four different concentrations of daunorubicin to cultured human lens cells for 10 minutes and then observing cell viability for 5 days. Application of 2.2 μg/ml for 10 minutes resulted in a 50% reduction in the number of cells compared with a control group receiving no daunorubicin (158). Exposure to higher concentrations left few viable cells. Because short exposure times completely inhibit cell proliferation, a single intraoperative infusion might be useful in inhibiting capsular opacification. Other investigators have found no corneal damage with the use of intraocular concentrations as high as 7.5 μg/ml for 10 minutes (159,160).

Colchicine

Colchicine, derived from *Colchicum autumnale* (autumn crocus, meadow saffron), is a potent antimitotic agent used in the treatment of gouty arthritis since the mid-eighteenth century. The antiinflammatory effects of colchicine are fairly specific for gout, but its effects on the inhibition of mitosis have rendered it a useful tool in the study of cell division.

Colchicine arrests mitosis at metaphase and can arrest cell division both in vitro and in vivo in plants and in animals. High concentrations of this agent are capable of preventing cells from entering mitosis at all and can lead to cell death. Cells undergoing the highest rate of cell division are affected the earliest. Administered systemically, colchicine has a wide variety of other effects. It can inhibit release of histamine from mast cells and insulin from pancreatic islets. It can lower body temperature, increase sensitivity to central nervous system depressants, and can induce hypertension by central vasomotor stimulation (161).

Colchicine has been investigated experimentally for use in the prevention of posterior capsule opacification following cataract surgery. Legler and co-workers studied the effects of applying three different concentrations of the drug on the rate of posterior capsule opacification after endocapsular cataract extraction in rabbits (162). Using a polymer matrix wafer to achieve sustained drug delivery, colchicine was applied to 34 eyes following cataract extraction. All three concentrations of colchicine resulted in a significantly lower rate of posterior capsule opacification than found in untreated control eyes. Higher concentrations appeared to offer no improvement over lower ones, suggesting that even the lowest dosage used in this study was adequate for the desired effect. Side effects included anterior chamber reaction and corneal and retinal complications.

Retinopathy of Prematurity

Retinopathy of prematurity (ROP) is a disease of premature underweight infants in which low birth weight, short gestation period, and high arterial oxygen tension are all significant risk factors for the development of fibrovascular damage to retina. The fibrovascular process seen in this disease may either regress and cause little or no harm to the retina, or it may progress to extremely severe stages that lead to total retinal detachment and blindness. Since the earliest descriptions of this disease, therapeutic measures have been controversial and not fully satisfactory. The overall incidence of ROP in all premature infants is about 16%, whereas in high-risk infants with a birth weight <1,300 g or <31 weeks' gestation, the incidence of ROP ranges from 44% to 59% (163,164). Cryotherapy and laser therapy have met with success in the management of this condition, but the medical management of ROP continues to be an active area of investigation (165–167).

D-Penicillamine

In 1976 Lakatos published the results of a study of DPA used in treating hemolytic disease of the newborn (168). High doses of DPA (300 mg/kg) were administered in four equal doses daily for 2 to 5 days beginning in the first 24 hours of life. In a separate retrospective study of 195 infants, 109 treated with DPA and 86 untreated (otherwise evenly matched for age, gestational age, and neonatal factors associated with oxygen administration), Lakatos observed 11 cases of ROP (169). One case occurred among the 109 infants treated with DPA, and the other ten occurred among the 86 untreated infants. Since 1980 DPA has been used to treat both hyperbilirubinemia and ROP in premature infants. It is a noncytotoxic chelating agent that is known to have disease-suppressing properties in rheumatoid arthritis; its primary uses have been in the management of Wilson's disease, lead poisoning, and cystinuria because of its chelating action and in rheumatoid arthritis where its mechanism of action is unknown.

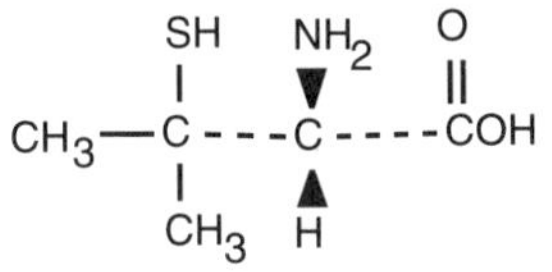

```
         SH    NH2    O
         |     ▼      ||
CH3—C - - - C - - - - COH
         |     ▲
        CH3    H
```

D-penicillamine

Unlike cytotoxic immunosuppressants, DPA lowers IgM rheumatoid factor, but it does not appear to lower absolute levels of serum immunoglobulins. It also seems to suppress T-cell (but not B-cell) activity and is known to interfere with collagen cross-linking, cleaving the bonds when newly formed. Its mechanism of action in ROP is unknown, but the therapeutic effect may lie in its ability to inhibit collagen synthesis or possibly through its activity as an antioxidant.

Proliferative Vitreoretinopathy

Proliferative vitreoretinopathy (PVR) continues to plague the vitreoretinal surgeon as the most common cause of failure in retinal detachment surgery. Surgical procedures for its management are complex and expensive, require extensive instrumentation, and have achieved widely variable levels of success in the past. Surgical fluid-gas exchange techniques have improved the success rate of retinal reattachment surgery in recent years. Nonetheless, interest has continued in understanding the pathophysiology of PVR and pharmacologic methods to manage it.

Proliferative vitreoretinopathy and other cicatricial disorders of the vitreous are characterized by the rapid proliferation of cells on the surface of the retina and in the collagen matrix of the vitreous gel. The subsequent contraction of the resulting fibrous membrane leads to the clinical pathology of PVR. Early attempts at pharmacologic management of this disorder were aimed at inhibiting the proliferative phase of the disease using 5-FU, 5-FUR (a ribonucleotide metabolite of 5-fluorouracil), and daunomycin (170–172).

5-Fluorouracil and 5-Fluorouridine

Both 5-FU and 5-FUR, a more potent inhibitor of ocular cell proliferation than 5-FU, have been studied as possible therapeutic agents in the prevention of proliferative vitreoretinopathy. Numerous investigators have demonstrated the ability of 5-FU and 5-FUR to inhibit the proliferation of fibroblasts in cell culture (171,173–175). Leon and co-workers examined the effects of 5-Fu and 5-FUR on protein synthesis in retinal ganglion cells in laboratory animals and found a significant reduction in protein synthesis (22%) with daily intravitreal injections of 0.1 mg of 5-FUR and a notable inhibition of protein synthesis after intravitreal injections of 2.5 mg of 5-FU (176). Accompanying these effects were a marked decrease in incorporation of newly synthesized protein into retinal photoreceptors. Additionally, there was nearly a 50% inhibition of axonal transport in retinal ganglion cells. Other investigators also reported significant retinal toxicity with the use of small doses of 5-FU. Binder and Kulnig found after intravitreal injection of fibroblasts into rabbits that 5-FU (1 or 5 mg) caused damage to the retina as shown by degranulation of the retinal pigment epithelium and migration of cells towards the vitreous (177). The higher of the two concentrations appeared to cause more damage. More importantly, they found no significant reduction in detachment rate with the use of these concentrations of 5-FU. More recent investigation in animals suggests that 5-FU reduces the rate of tractional retinal detachment from 90% (control group with PVR) to 32% in the 5-FU-treated group. Although both 5-FU and 5-FUR appear to be effective in reducing vitreous scarring and subsequent tractional retinal detachment, 5-FUR may be much more potent and efficacious (178). Use of a biodegradable intravitreal implant for sustained release of 5-FU in the prevention of experimental PVR in rabbits shows promise and may be useful with other agents (179).

Daunorubicin

In the early 1980s, investigators began to look for other antiproliferative drugs for use in the management of PVR. Kirmani et al. and Santana et al. observed that experimentally induced PVR in rabbits was effectively inhibited clinically and microscopically by the use of intravitreal daunorubicin (180,181). At the dosage of 10 nmol injected per eye, they noted no electroretinogram changes that suggested drug-induced retinal toxicity. Subsequent investigations showed that daunorubicin is capable of completely inhibiting retinal pigment epithelial cells and fibroblasts at a concentration of 7.5 μg/ml with an exposure time of 10 minutes (182), which offers the advantage of a brief exposure time compared with the use of fluoropyrimidines, which require repeated exposure or several hours of constant exposure.

Using this dosage and an infusion of the drug into the eye over a 10-minute period, Wiedemann and co-workers treated 15 humans with advanced posttraumatic PVR (183). Successful anatomic reattachment was achieved in 14 of the 15 patients. Visual acuity improved postoperatively in all 14 patients with reattachment. Importantly, the investigators noted no toxic effects on the optic nerve, retina, lens, or cornea. More recent work, in which daunomycin has been incorporated into liposomes (20 μg daunomycin liposomes) and placed in the vitreous cavity, has shown that lower dosages may enhance activity and lower toxicity (184). Administration of daunomycin in divided dosages has been more efficacious than a single administration but may offer no reduction in retinal toxicity (185). Concerns over ocular toxicity, in particular the morphologic and functional damage it causes to the retina, have limited its use in this disease entity (186).

CONCLUSION

Certainly, the *science* of controlled wound healing modulation is in its infancy. Numerous agents with promise have been identified for application to that end, but only a few have been tested thoroughly. The search will continue for inexpensive, controllable agents that are minimally toxic and have predictable actions. Nevertheless, we have already entered a new era in which selective pharmacologic suppression of the scarring process will pave the way to desired clinical outcomes.

The difficulties and complications encountered in harnessing these often-toxic substances to do our bidding should not be dismissed; but neither can we ignore the substantial advantages they already present in the treatment of some diseases. We must weigh the risks and benefits of these imperfect tools as we treat our patients. Such is the *art* of medicine.

REFERENCES

1. Peacock EE Jr. Biological and pharmacological control of scar tissue. In: Peacock EE Jr, ed. *Wound Repair.* Philadelphia, PA: WB Saunders, 1984;491–492.
2. Skuta GL, Parrish RK II. Wound healing in glaucoma filtering surgery. *Surv Ophthalmol* 1989;20:350–357.
3. Jampel HD, Morrison J, Vocci M, Quigley H. Identification of fibrin/fibrinogen in glaucoma filtration surgery wounds. *Ophthalmic Surg* 1988;19:576–579.
4. Tahery MM, Lee DA. Review: pharmacologic control of wound healing in glaucoma filtration surgery. *J Ocul Pharmacol* 1989; 5:155–179.
5. Costa VP, Spaeth GL, Eiferman RA, Orego-Nania S. Wound healing modulation in glaucoma filtration surgery. *Ophthalmic Surg* 1993; 24:152–170.
6. Knighton DR, Hunt TK, Thakral KK, et al. Role of platelets and fibrin in the healing sequence: an in vivo study of angiogenesis and collagen synthesis. *Ann Surg* 1982;196:379.
7. White A, Handler P, Smith EL. *Principles of Biochemistry.* New York: McGraw-Hill, 1978;1139–1141.
8. Desjardins DC, Parrish RK, Folberg R, Nevarez J, Heuer DK, Gressel MG. Wound healing after fitting surgery in owl monkeys. *Arch Ophthalmol* 1986;104:1835–1839.
9. Addicks EM, Quigley HA, Green WR, Rolina AL. Histologic characteristics of filtering blebs in glaucomatous eyes. *Arch Ophthalmol* 1983;101:795–798.
10. Hitchings RA, Grierson I. Clinico pathological correlation in eyes with failed fistulizing surgery. *Transaction of the Ophthalmic Society of the United Kingdom* 1983;103:84–88.
11. Gressel MG, Heuer DK, Parrish RK II. Trabeculectomy in young patients. *Ophthalmology* 1984;91:1242–1246.
12. Freedman J, Shen E, Ahrens M. Trabeculectomy in a black American glaucoma population. *Br J Ophthalmol* 1976;60:573–574.
13. Inaba Z. Long-term results of trabeculectomy in the Japanese: an analysis of life-table method. *Jpn J Ophthalmol* 1982;26:361–373.
14. Heuer DK, Gressel MG, Parrish RK II. Trabeculectomy in aphakic eyes. *Ophthalmology* 1984;91:1045–1051.
15. Allen RC, Bellows AR, Hutchinson BT, Murphy SD. Filtration surgery in the treatment of neovascular glaucoma. *Ophthalmology* 1982;89:1181–1189.
16. Epstein DL. Glaucoma due to intraocular inflammation. In Epstein DL, ed. *Chandler and Grant's Glaucoma,* 3rd ed. Philadelphia: Lea and Feiberger, 1986;362.
17. Wright MM, Grajewski AL, Cristol SM, Parrish RK II. 5-Fluorouracil after trabeculectomy and iridocorneal endothelial syndrome. *Ophthalmology* 1991;98:314–316.
18. Broadway DC, Grierson I, O'Brien C, Hitchings RA. Adverse effects of topical antiglaucoma medication. II. The outcome of filtration surgery. *Arch Ophthalmol* 1994;112:1446–1454.
19. Sugar HS. Clinical effect of corticosteroids on filtering blebs; a case report. *Am J Ophthalmol* 1965;59:854–860.
20. Starita RJ, Fellman RL, Spaeth GL. Short and long-term effects of postoperative corticosteroids on trabeculectomy. *Ophthalmology* 1985;92:938–946.
21. Roth SM, Spaeth GL, Starita RJ, Birbillis EM, Steinmann WL. Effects of postoperative corticosteroids on trabeculectomy and the clinical course of glaucoma. The five year follow up study. *Ophthalmic Surg* 1991;22:724–729.
22. Havener WH. Cortisteroid therapy. In: Havener WH, ed. *Ocular Pharmacology.* St. Louis: CV Mosby, 1983;437–442.
23. Blumenkranz MS, Clafin A, Hajek AS. Selection of therapeutic agents for intraocular proliferative disease, cell culture evaluation. *Arch Ophthalmol* 1984;102:598–604.
24. Nguyen K, Kitoda S, Shapourifar-Tehrani S, Lee DA. The effect of steroids and nonsteroidal antiinflammatory agents on proliferation of human ocular fibroblasts. *Invest Ophthalmol Vis Sci* 1991;32 (suppl):1121.
25. Cantor LB, Boeglin RJ, Kramer DM, Phillips CA. The effect of topical flurbiprofen on trabeculectomy. *Invest Ophthalmol Vis Sci* 1991;32(suppl):1121.
26. Bennett DR, ed. *Drug Evaluation Annual.* American Medical Association, 1995;2132–2133.
27. Heuer DK, Parrish RK II, Gressel MG, et al. 5-fluorouracil and glaucoma filtering surgery II. A pilot study. *Ophthalmology* 1984; 91:384–394.
28. Goodman L, Gilman A. *The Pharmacologic Basis of Therapeutics.* New York: Permagon Press, 1990;1227–1232.
29. Rader JE, Parrish RK II. Update on antimetabolites in glaucoma surgery. *Ophthalmology Clinics of North America* 1991;4,4:861.
30. Henderson BC. 5-Fluorouracil: ophthalmic use. *Ophthalmology Clinics of North America* 1989;2:131–139.
31. Herschler J. Long-term results of trabeculectomy with collagen sponge implant containing low dose antimetabolite. *Ophthalmology* 1992;99:666–671.
32. Smith FM, Sherwood MB, Doyle JW, Khaw PT. Results of intraoperative 5-fluorouracil supplementation on trabeculectomy for open-angle glaucoma. *Am J Ophthalmol* 1992;114:737–741.
33. Precup AV, ed. *Drug Information for the Health Care Professional.* Taunton, Mass: Rand McNally, 1995;1355–1357.

34. Chabner BA, Myers CE, Oliverio VT. Clinical pharmacology and anticancer drugs. *Semin Oncol* 1977;4:165.
35. Skuta GL, Assil K, Parrish RK II, et al. Filtering surgery in owl monkeys treated with the antimetabolite 5-fluorouridine 5-mono phosphate entrapped in multivesicular liposomes. *Am J Ophthalmol* 1987;103:714–716.
36. The Fluorouracil Filtering Study Group. Fluorouracil filtering surgery study one-year follow-up. *Am J Ophthalmol* 1989;108:627–635.
37. Weinreb RN. Adjusting the dose of 5-fluorouracil after filtration surgery to minimize side effects. *Ophthalmology* 1987;94:564.
38. Knapp A, Heuer DK, Stern GA, Driebe WT. Serious corneal complications of glaucoma filtration surgery with 5-fluorouracil. *Am J Ophthalmol* 1987;103:183–187.
39. Peterson MR, Skuta GL, Phelan MJ, et al. Striate melanokeratosis following trabeculectomy with 5-fluorouracil. *Arch Ophthalmol* 1990;108:1216.
40. Christophidis N, Vajda FJE, Lucas I, et al. Ocular side effects with 5-fluorouracil. *Aust N Z J Med* 1979;9:143.
41. Caravella LP, Burns JA, Zangmeister M. Punctal-canalicular stenosis related to systemic fluorouracil therapy. *Arch Ophthalmol* 1981; 99:284–286.
42. Straus DJ, Mausolf FA, Ellerby RA, et al. Cicatricial ectropion secondary to 5-fluorouracil therapy. *Med Pediatr Oncol* 1977;3:15–19.
43. Fraunfelder FT, Meyer SM. Ocular toxicity of antineoplastic agents. *Ophthalmology* 1983;90:1–3.
44. Wolner B, Liebmann JM, Sassani JW, et al. Late bleb-related endophthalmitis after trabeculectomy with adjunctive 5-fluorouracil. *Ophthalmology* 1991;98:1053–1060.
45. Lotfield K, Ball SF. 5-fluorouracil in primary trabeculectomy: a randomized trial. *Invest Ophthalmol Vis Sci* 1991;32(suppl):745.
46. Mannis MJ, Sweet EH, Lewis RA. The effect of fluorouracil on corneal endothelium. *Arch Ophthalmol* 1988;106:816–817.
47. Krug JH Jr, Melamed S. Adjunctive use of delayed and adjustable low dose 5-fluorouracil in refractory glaucoma. *Am J Ophthalmol* 1990;109:412.
48. Stamper RL, McMenemy MG, Lieberman MF. Hypotonus maculopathy after trabeculectomy with subconjunctival 5-fluorouracil. *Am J Ophthalmol* 1992;114:544–553.
49. Boyd BF. The use of mitomycin. *Highlights of Ophthalmology* 1993;21:58.
50. Gressel MG, Parrish RK II, Folberg R. 5-fluorouracil and glaucoma filtering surgery. I. an animal model. *Ophthalmology* 1984; 91:378.
51. The Fluorouracil Filtering Surgery Study Group. Three-year follow-up of the fluorouracil filtering surgery study. *Am J Ophthalmol* 1993;115:82–92.
52. Whiteside-Michel J, Liebmann JM, Ritch R. Initial 5-fluorouracil in young patients. *Ophthalmology* 1992;99:7.
53. Zalish M, Leiba H, Oliver M. Subconjunctival injection of 5-fluorouracil following trabeculectomy for congenital and infantile glaucoma. *Ophthalmic Surg* 1992;23:203–205.
54. Egbert PR, Williams AS, Singh K, Dazie P, Egbert TB. A prospective trial of intraoperative fluorouracil during trabeculectomy in a black population. *Am J Ophthalmol* 1993;116:612–616.
55. Loane ME, Weinreb RN. Glaucoma secondary to epithelial downgrowth and 5-fluorouracil. *Ophthalmic Surg* 1990;21:704–706.
56. Liebmann JM, Ritch R, Marmor M, Nunez J, Wolner B. Initial 5-fluorouracil trabeculectomy in uncomplicated glaucoma. *Ophthalmology* 1991;98:1036–1041.
57. Wilson RP, Steinmann WC. Use of trabeculectomy with postoperative 5-fluorouracil in patients requiring extremely low intraocular pressure levels to limit further glaucoma progression. *Ophthalmology* 1991;98:1047–1052.
58. Goldenfeld M, Krupin T, Ruderman J, et al. 5-fluorouracil in initial trabeculectomy. *Ophthalmology* 1994;101:1024–1029.
59. Hurvitz LM. 5-FU-supplemented phacomulsification, posterior chamber intraocular lens implantation, and trabeculectomy. *Ophthalmic Surg* 1993;24:674–676.
60. Wong PC, Ruderman JM, Krupin T, et al. 5-fluorouracil after primary combined filtration surgery. *Am J Ophthalmol* 1994;117: 149–154.
61. Younghyun O, Katz LJ, Spaeth GL, Wilson RP. Risk factors for the development of encapsulated filtering blebs. *Ophthalmology* 1994; 101:629–632.
62. Shin DH, Juzych MS, Khatana AK, Swendris RP, Parrow KA. Needling revision of failed filtering blebs with adjunctive 5-fluorouracil. *Ophthalmic Surg* 1993;24:242–244.
63. Dietze PJ, Feldman RM, Gross RL. Intraoperative application of 5-fluorouracil during trabeculectomy. *Ophthalmic Surg* 1992;23: 662–665.
64. Williams RD, Sakamoto MJ, Pastor SA, Hoskins HD. Intraoperative sponge 5-fluorouracil application decreases the number of postoperative injections. *Invest Ophthalmol Vis Sci* 1992;33(suppl):1393.
65. Lee DA, Flores RA, Anderson PJ, et al. Glaucoma filtration surgery in rabbits using bioerodible polymers and 5-fluorouracil. *Ophthalmology* 1987;18:187–190.
66. Winter DF, Jones NA, Simmons ST, et al. A histologic analysis of 5-fluorouracil liposomal delivery system following subconjunctival injection in rabbits. *Invest Ophthalmol Vis Sci* 1987;(suppl):271.
67. Wakaki S, Marumo H, Tornoika K. Isolation of new fractions of antitumor mitomycins. *Antibiot Chemother* 1958;8:228–240.
68. Precup AV, ed. *Drug Information for the Health Care Professional.* Taunton, Mass: Rand McNally, 1995;1889–1891.
69. Jampel HC. Effect of brief exposure to mitomycin C on viability and proliferation of cultured human Tenon's capsule fibroblasts. *Ophthalmology* 1992;99:1471–1476.
70. Yamamoto T, Varani J, Soong HK, Lichter PR. Effects of 5-fluorouracil and mitomycin C on cultured rabbit subconjunctival fibroblasts. *Ophthalmology* 1990;97:1202–1210.
71. Lee DA, Lee TC, Cortes AE, Kitada S. Effects of mithramycin, mitomycin, daunorubicin and bleomycin on human subconjunctival fibroblast attachment and proliferation. *Invest Ophthalmol Vis Sci* 1990;31:2136–2144.
72. Meitz H, Addicks K, Diestelhorst M, Krieglstem G. Extraocular application of mitomycin C in a rabbit model: cytotoxic effects on the ciliary body and epithelium. *Ophthalmic Surg* 1994;25:240–244.
73. Nuyts RMMA, Felten PC, Pels E, et al. Histopathologic effects of mitomycin C after trabeculectomy in human glaucomatous eyes with persistent hypotony. *Am J Ophthalmol* 1994;188:225–237.
74. Kee C, Pelzek C, Kaufman P. Mitomycin C suppresses aqueous humor flow in cynomolgus monkeys. *Arch Ophthalmol* 1995;113: 239–242.
75. *Physicians Desk Reference 1995.* Montvale, NJ: Medical Economics Data Production Company, 1995;671–672.
76. Derich RJ, Pasquale L, Quigley HA, Jampel H. Potential toxicity of mitomycin C. *Arch Ophthalmol* 1991;109:1635.
77. Nuyts RMMA, Pels E, Greve EL. The effects of 5-fluorouracil and mitomycin C on the corneal endothelium. *Curr Eye Res* 1992; 11:565–570.
78. Sarraf D, Eezzuduemhoi D, Cheng Q, Wilson R, Lee D. Aqueous and vitreous concentration of mitomycin C by topical administration after glaucoma filtration surgery in rabbits. *Ophthalmology* 1993;100:1574–1579.
79. Prata JA, Minckler DS, Koda RT. Effects of external irrigation on mitomycin C concentration in rabbit aqueous and vitreous humor. *J Glaucoma* 1995;4:32–35.
80. Kitazawa Y, Kawase K, Matsushita H, Minobe M. Trabeculectomy with mitomycin—a comparative study with fluorouracil. *Arch Ophthal* 1991;32(suppl):1122.
81. Oram O, Gross R, Wilhelmus K, Hoover J. Necrotizing keratitis following trabeculectomy with mitomycin. *Arch Ophthalmol* 1995; 113:19.
82. Ando H, Ido T, Kawai Y, Yamamoto T, Kitazawa Y. Inhibition of corneal epithelial wound healing: a comparative study of mitomycin C and 5-fluorouracil. *Ophthalmology* 1992;99:1809–1814.
83. Skuta GL, Beeson CC, Higginbotham EJ, et al. Intraoperative mitomycin versus postoperative 5-fluorouracil in high-risk glaucoma filtering surgery. *Ophthalmology* 1992;99:438–444.
84. Pappa KS, Derick RJ, Weber PA, et al. Late argon laser suture lysis after mitomycin C trabeculectomy. *Ophthalmology* 1993;100:1268–1271.
85. Gass JDM. Hypotony maculopathy. In: Bellows JG, ed. *Contemporary Ophthalmology: Honoring Sir Stewart Duke-Elder.* Baltimore: Williams and Wilkins, 1972;343–366.
86. Zacharia PT, Deppermann SR, Schuman JS. Ocular hypotony after trabeculectomy with mitomycin C. *Am J Ophthalmol* 1993;116: 314–326.
87. Wise JB. Treatment of chronic postfiltration hypotony by intrableb injection of autologous blood. *Arch Ophthalmol* 1993;111:827–830.

88. Costa VP, Wilson RP, Moster MR, Schmidt CM, Ganham S. Hypotony maculopathy following the use of topical mitomycin C in glaucoma filtration surgery. *Ophthalmic Surg* 1993;6:389–392.
89. Chen C-W. Enhanced intraocular pressure controlling effectiveness of trabeculectomy in local application of mitomycin C. *Transactions of the Asia Pacific Academy of Ophthalmology* 1983;9:172–177.
90. Chen C-W, Huang H-T, Shen M-M. Enhancement of IOP control effect of trabeculectomy by local application of anticancer drug. In: *ACTA XXV Concilium Ophthalmologicum (Rome)* 1986;2:1487–1491.
91. Palmer S. Mitomycin as adjunct chemotherapy with trabeculectomy. *Ophthalmology* 1991;98:317–321.
92. Sherwood MB, Khaw PT, Doyle JW, et al. Comparison of five minute intraoperative treatments with 5-fluorouracil in high risk glaucoma surgery. *Ophthalmology* 1992;99:438–444.
93. Norlund JR, Pasquale LR, Quigley HA, Jampel HD. Effectiveness of intraoperative 5-fluorouracil versus intraoperative mitomycin C in experimental rabbit glaucoma surgery. *Invest Ophthalmol Vis Sci* 1992;33(suppl):1393.
94. Kawase K, Nishimura K, Yamamoto T, Jikihava S, Kitazawa Y. Anterior Chamber reaction after mitomycin and 5-fluorouracil trabeculectomy: a comparative study. *Ophthalmic Surg* 1993;24:24–27.
95. Costa VP, Moster MR, Wilson RP, et al. Effects of topical mitomycin C on primary trabeculectomies and combined procedures. *Br J Ophthalmol* 1993;77:693–697.
96. Kitazawa Y, Suemori-Matsuchita H, Yamamoto T, Kawase K. Low dose and high dose mitomycin trabeculectomy as initial surgery in primary open angle glaucoma. *Ophthalmology* 1993;100:1624–1628.
97. Cohen JS, Greff LJ, Novack GD. A placebo controlled, double-masked evaluation of mitomycin C in combined phacoemulsification, IOL, and glaucoma filtering surgery. AAO abstracts. *Ophthalmology* 1994;(suppl):78.
98. Simone PA, Reed SY, Juzych MS. Adjunctive subconjunctival mitomycin C in glaucoma triple procedure. AAO abstracts. *Ophthalmology* 1994;(suppl):82.
99. Susanna R Jr, Nicolela MT, Takahoshi WY. Mitomycin C as adjunctive therapy with glaucoma implant surgery. *Ophthalmic Surg* 1994;25:458–462.
100. Sayyad FE, Helal M, Elsherif Z, El-Magrhaby A. Molteno implant versus trabeculectomy with adjunctive intraoperative mitomycin C in high risk glaucoma patients. *J Glaucoma* 1995;4:80–85.
101. Wise JB. Mitomycin-compatible suture technique for fornix-based conjunctival flaps in glaucoma surgery. *Arch Ophthalmol* 1993;111: 992–997.
102. Wang T-H, Hung PT, Ho T-C. THC:YAG laser sclerostomy with preoperative mitomycin C subconjunctival injection in rabbits. *J Glaucoma* 1993;2:260–265.
103. Akata RF, Onol M, Reisoglu B. Crosslinked poly (HEMA) glaucoma filtration device for controlled release of fluorouracil and mitomycin C. AAO abstracts. *Ophthalmology* 1994;(suppl):108.
104. Letchinger SL, Becker B, Wax MB. The effects of subconjunctival administration of mitomycin C on intraocular pressure (IOP) in rabbits. *Invest Ophthalmol Vis Sci* 1992;33(ARVO suppl):736.
105. Gandolfi SA, Vecchi M, Braccio L. Decrease of intraocular pressure after subconjunctival injection of mitomycin in human glaucoma. *Arch Ophthalmol* 1995;113:585.
106. Kwong EM, Litin BS, Jones MA, Herschler J. Effect of antineoplastic drugs on fibroblast proliferation in rabbit aqueous humor. *Ophthalmic Surg* 1984;15:847–851.
107. McGuigan LJB, Quigley HA, Young E, Lutty GA. Drug effects on proliferation and collagen synthesis of conjunctival fibroblasts. ARVO abstracts. *Invest Ophthalmol Vis Sci* (suppl) 1985;26:125.
108. Bennett DR, ed. *Drug Evaluation Annual.* Chicago: American Medical Association, 1995;2147–2155.
109. Kay JS, Litin BS, Jones MA, et al. Delivery of antifibroblast agents as adjuncts to filtration surgery. Part II. Delivery of 5-fluorouracil and bleomycin in a collagen implant: pilot study in the rabbit. *Ophthalmic Surg* 1986;17:796–801.
110. Herschler J. Long-term results of trabeculectomy with collagen sponge implant containing low dose antimetabolite. *Ophthalmology* 1992;99:666–671.
111. Xu Y, Yang GH, Gin WM, Chen KQ, Song XH. Effect of subconjunctival daunorubicin on glaucoma surgery in rabbits. *Ophthalmic Surg* 1993;24:382–388.
112. Bennett DR, ed. *Drug Evaluation Annual.* Chicago: American Medical Association, 1995;2130–2151.
113. Hajek AS, Parrish RK II, Mallick KS, Gressel M. In vitro inhibition of ocular cell proliferation with ara-C: blockage of the antiproliferative effect with 2′-deoxycytidine. *Invest Ophthalmol Vis Sci* 1986; 27:1010–1012.
114. Lee DA, Goodwin LT, Panek WC, Leong KW, Glasgow BJ. Effects of cytosine arabinoside-impregnated bioerodible polymers on glaucoma filtration surgery in rabbits. *J Glaucoma* 1993;2:96–100.
115. Kaufman HE, Capella JA, Maloney ED, et al. Corneal toxicity of cytosine arabinoside. *Arch Ophthalmol* 1964;72:535–540.
116. Katz LJ, Spaeth GL, Steinmann WC, Fahmi IA, Moones AA, Gross RL. Topical trifluridine use following filtering surgery: a randomized prospective trial. *Invest Ophthalmol Vis Sci* 1991;32(suppl):1121.
117. Rivera AH, Hajek AS, Fantes F, et al. Trifluorothymidine and 5-fluorouracil: antiproliferative activity in tissue culture. *Can J Ophthalmol* 1987;22:13–16.
118. Alvarado JA. The use of liposomal-encapsulated 5-fluoroorotate for glaucoma surgery: I. Animal studies. *Trans Am Ophthalmol Soc* 1989;87:487–514.
119. Lee DA, Shapourifar-Tehrani S, Stephenson TR, Kitada S. The effects of fluorinated pyrimidines FUR, FUDR, FUMP, and FDUMP on human Tenon's fibroblasts. *Invest Ophthalmol Vis Sci* 1991; 32:2599–2609.
120. Cheng O, Fukunaga S, Lee DA. The effects of vincristine and vinblastine on rabbit and human Tenon's capsule fibroblast cell lines. *Invest Ophthalmol Vis Sci* 1992;33(suppl):735.
121. Joseph JP, Grierson I, Hitchings RA. Taxol cytochalasin B and colchicine effects on fibroblasts migration and contraction: a role in glaucoma filtration surgery. *Curr Eye Res* 1989;8:203–215.
122. Jimenez SA, Freundlich B, Rosenbloom J. Selective inhibition of human diploid fibroblast collagen synthesis by interferons. *J Clin Invest* 1984;74:1112–1116.
123. Gillies MC, Su T, Sarossy M, Hollows FC. Interferon-alpha 2b inhibits proliferation of human Tenon's capsule fibroblasts. *Graefes Arch Clin Exp Ophthalmol* 1993;231:118–121.
124. Adelmann-Grill BC, Hein R, Wach F, Kreig T. Inhibition of fibroblast chemotaxis by recombinant human interferon gamma and interferon alpha. *J Cell Physiol* 1987;130:270–275.
125. Gillies MC, Goldberg I, Young S, Su T. Glaucoma filtering surgery with interferon-α-2b. *J Glaucoma* 1993;2:229–235.
126. Assil KK, Saperstein D, Weinreb RN, Chojkier M. Inhibition of collagen synthesis in human episcleral fibroblasts by calcium ionophore A23187. *J Glaucoma* 1995;4:41–44.
127. McGuigan LJB, Cook DJ, Yablonski ME. Dexamethasone, D-penicillamine and glaucoma filter surgery in rabbits. *Invest Ophthalmol Vis Sci* 1986;27:1755.
128. Moorhead LC, Smith J, Stewart R, et al. Effects of beta-aminopropionitrile after glaucoma filtration surgery: pilot human trial. *Ann Ophthalmol* 1987;19:223.
129. Fourman S, Vaid K. Effects of tissue plasminogen activator on glaucoma filter blebs in rabbits. *Ophthalmic Surg* 1989;20:663–667.
131. Del Vecchio PJ, Bizios R, Holleran LA, Judge TK, Pinto GL. Inhibition of human scleral fibroblast proliferation with heparin. *Invest Ophthalmol Vis Sci* 1998;29:1272–1276.
132. Urban RC, Kaufman LM. Mitomycin in the treatment of hypertrophic scars after strabismus surgery. *J Pediatr Ophthalmol Strabismus* 1994;31:96–98.
133. Watson GW, Turner RL. Breast cancer: a new approach to therapy. *Br Med J* 1995;5133:1315–1320.
134. Sparks SJ, Walsh ME, et al. Chemotherapy of a granulocytic chloroleukemia in the rat. *Cancer Res* 1954;14:753–757.
135. Langham M. The inhibition of corneal vascularization by triethylene thiophosphoramide. *Am J Ophthalmol* 1960;49:1111.
136. Lavergne G, Colman I. Comparative study of the action of thio-tepa and triamcinolone on corneal vascularization in rabbits. *Br J Ophthalmol* 1964;48:416.
137. Meacham C. Triethylene thiophosphoramide in the prevention of pterygium recurrence. *Am J Ophthalmol* 1962;54:751.
138. Meacham C. Prevention of recurrence of pterygium. *Eye Ear Nose Throat Monthly* 1965;44:62.
139. Cooper JC. Pterygium: prevention of recurrence by excision and post-operative thio-tepa. *Eye Ear Nose Throat Monthly* 1966;45:59–61.
140. Grant WM. *Toxicology of the Eye,* 2nd ed. Springfield, IL: Charles C Thomas Publisher, 1974.

141. Sebban A, Hirst LW. Treatment of pterygia in Queensland. *Aust N Z J Ophthalmol* 1991;19:123–127.
142. Olander K, Haik KG, Haik GM. Management of pterygia: should thio-tepa be used? *Ann Ophthalmol* 1978;10:853–862.
143. Talbot AN. Complication of beta ray treatment of pterygia. *Trans Ophthalmol Soc N Z* 1979;31:62–63.
144. Kunimoto N, Mori S. Studies on the pterygium. Part IV. A treatment of pterygium by mitomycin-C instillation. *Nippon Ganka Gakkai Zasshi* 1963;67:601–607.
145. Singh G, Wilson MR, Foster CS. Mitomycin eye drops as treatment for pterygium. *Ophthalmology* 1988;95:813–821.
146. Hayasaka S, Noda S, Yamamoto Y, Setogawa T. Postoperative instillation of low-dose mitomycin-C in the treatment of primary pterygium. *Am J Ophthalmol* 1988;106:715–718.
147. Hayasaka S, Noda S, Yamamoto Y, Setogawa T. Postoperative instillation of low-dose mitomycin-C in the treatment of recurrent pterygium. *Ophthalmic Surg* 1989;20:580–583.
148. Frucht-Pery J, Ilsar M. The use of low-dose mitomycin-C for prevention of recurrent pterygium. *Ophthalmology* 1994;101:759–762.
149. Dunn JP, Seamone CD, Ostler HB, Nicket BL, Beallo A. Development of scleral ulceration and calcification after pterygium excision and mitomycin therapy. *Am J Ophthalmol* 1991;112:343–344.
150. Fujitani A, Hayasaka S, Shibuya Y, Noda S. Corneoscleral ulceration and corneal perforation after pterygium excision and topical mitomycin-C therapy. *Ophthalmologica* 1993;207:162–164.
151. Rubinfeld RS, Pfister RR, Stein RM, et al. Serious complications of topical mitomycin-C after pterygium surgery. *Ophthalmology* 1992; 99:1647–1654.
152. Yang ZH. The curative effect of pingyangmycinum in treating pterygium. *Chung Hua Chung Liu Tsa Chih* 1993;28:663–664.
153. Lindstrom RL, Harris WS. Management of the posterior capsule following posterior chamber lens implantation. *American IntraOcular Implant Society Journal* 1980;6:255–258.
154. Nishi O. Incidence of posterior capsule opacification in eyes with and without implantation of posterior chamber intraocular lenses. *J Cataract Refract Surg* 1986;12:519–522.
155. American Academy of Ophthalmology. Nd:YAG photodisrupters. *Ophthalmology Nove* 1993;100:1736–1742.
156. Javitt JC, Tielsch JM, Canner JK, Kolb MM, Sommer A, Steinberg EP. National outcomes of cataract extraction: increased risk of retinal complications associated with Nd:YAG laser capsulotomy. The Cataract Patient Outcomes Research Team. *Ophthalmology* 1992; 99:1487–1497.
157. Rickman-Barger L, Florine CW, Larson RS, Lindstrom RL. Retinal detachment after neodymium:YAG laser posterior capsulotomy. *Am J Ophthalmol* 1989;107:531–536.
158. Power WJ, Neylan D, Collum LM. Daunomucin as an inhibitor of human lens epithelial cell proliferation in culture. *J Cataract Refract Surg* 1994;20:287–290.
159. Weller M, Wiedemann P, Fischbach R, Hartmann C, Heimann K. Evaluation of daunomycin toxicity on lens epithelium in vitro. *Int Ophthalmol* 1988;12:127–130.
160. Wiedemann P, Lemmen K, Schmiedl R, Heimann K. Intraocular daunorubicin for the treatment and prophylaxis of traumatic proliferative vitreoretinopathy. *Am J Ophthalmol* 1987;104:10–14.
161. *Goodman and Gilman's: The Pharmacologic Basis of Therapeutics*, 8th ed. New York: Permagon Press, 1990;674–676.
162. Legler UF, Apple DJ, Assie EI, Bluestein EC, Castenada VE, Mowbray SL. Inhibition of posterior capsule opacification: the effect of colchicine in a sustained drug delivery system. *J Cataract Refract Surg* 1993;19:462–470.
163. Tasman W. The natural history of active retinopathy of prematurity. *Ophthalmology* 1984;91:1499–1502.
164. Acheson JF, Schulenburg WE. Surveillance for retinopathy of prematurity in practice: experience from one neonatal intensive care unit. *Eye* 1991;5:80–85.
165. Cryotherapy for retinopathy of prematurity cooperative group: multicentre trial of cryotherapy for retinopathy of prematurity. 3 month outcome. *Arch Ophthalmol* 1990;108:195–204.
166. Cryotherapy for retinopathy of prematurity cooperative group: multicentre trial of cryotherapy for retinopathy of prematurity. 1 month outcome. *Arch Ophthalmol* 1990;108:1408–1416.
167. McNamara JA, Tasman W, Brown GC, Federman JL. Laser photocoagulation for stage 3+ retinopathy of prematurity. *Ophthalmology* 1991;98:576–580.
168. Lakatos L, Kover B, Oroszlan G, Verkedy Z. D-Penicillamine therapy in ABO hemolytic disease of the newborn infant. *Eur J Pediatr* 1976;123:133–137.
169. Lakatos L, Hatvani I, Oroszlan G, Karmazsin L. Prevention of retrolental fibroplasia in very low birth weight infants by D-Penicillamine. *Eur J Pediatr* 1982;138:199–200.
170. Binder S, Riss S, Skorpik C, Kulnig W. Inhibition of experimental intraocular proliferation with intravitreal 5-fluorouracil. *Graefe's Arch Clin Exp Ophthalmol* 1983;221:126–129.
171. Blumenkranz M, Ophir A, Claflin A, Hajek A. Fluorouracil for the treatment of massive periretinal proliferation. *Am J Ophthalmol* 1982;94:458–467.
172. Stern W, Guerin C, Erickson P, Lewis G, Anderson D, Fisher S. Ocular toxicity of 5-fluorouracil after vitrectomy. *Am J Ophthalmol* 1983;96:43–51.
173. Sunalp M, Wiedemann P, Sorgente N, Ryan S. Effects of cytotoxic drugs on proliferative vitreoretinopathy in the rabbit cell injection model. *Curr Eye Res* 1984;3:619–623.
174. Hartzer M, Blumenkranz M, Hajeck A, Dailey W, Cheng M, Margherio A. Selection of therapeutic agents for intraocular proliferative disease III. Effects of fluoropyrimidines on cell-mediated contraction of human fibroblasts. *Exp Eye Res* 1988;48:321–328.
175. Stern WH, Lewis GP, Erickson PA, Guerin CJ, Anderson DH, Fischer SK, O'Donnell JJ. Fluorouracil therapy for proliferative vitreoretinopathy. *Arch Ophthalmol* 1988;106:669.
176. Leon JA, Britt JM, Hopp RH, Mills RP, Milam AH. Effects of fluorouracil and fluorouridine on protein synthesis in rabbit retina. *Invest Ophthalmol and Vis Sci* 1990;31:1709–1716.
177. Binder S, Riss B, Skorpik C, Kulnig W. Inhibition of experimental intraocular proliferation with intravitreal 5-fluorouracil. *Graefes Arch Clin Exp Ophthalmol* 1983;221:126.
178. Ward T, Hartzer M, Blumenkranz M, Lin LR. A comparison of 5-fluorouridine and 5-fluorouracil in an experimental model for the treatment of vitreoretinal scarring. *Curr Eye Res* 1993;12:397–401.
179. Rubsamen P, Davis P, Hernandez E, O'Grady G, Cousins S. Prevention of experimental proliferative vitreoretinopathy with a biodegradable intravitreal implant for the sustained release of fluorouracil. *Arch Ophthalmol* 1994;112:407–413.
180. Kirmani M, Santana M, Sorgente N, Wiedemann P, Ryan SJ. Antiproliferative drugs in the treatment of experimental proliferative vitreoretinopathy. *Retina* 1983;3:269–272.
181. Santana M, Wiedemann P, Kirmani M, Minckler DS, Patterson R, Sorgente N, Ryan SJ. Daunomycin in the treatment of experimental proliferative vitreoretinopathy: retinal toxicity of intravitreal daunomycin in the rabbit. *Graefes Arch Clin Exp Ophthalmol* 1984;221:210–213.
182. Wiedemann P, Sorgente N, Bekhor C, Patterson R, Tran T, Ryan SJ. Daunomycin in the treatment of experimental proliferative vitreoretinopathy: effective doses in vitro and vivo. *Invest Ophthalmol Vis Sci* 1985;25:719–725.
183. Wiedemann P, Lemmen K, Schmiedl R, Heimann K. Intraocular daunorubicin for the treatment and prophylaxis of traumatic proliferative vitreoretinopathy. *Am J Ophthalmol* 1987;104:10–14.
184. Hui YN, Loang HC, Cai YS, Kirchhof B, Heimann K. Corticosteroids and daunomycin in the prevention of experimental proliferative vitreoretinopathy induced by macrophages. *Graefes Arch Clin Exp Ophthalmol* 1993;231:109–114.
185. Steinhorst UH, Hatchell DL, Chen EP, Machemer R. Ocular toxicity of daunomycin effects of subdivided doses on the rabbit retina after vitreous gas compression. *Graefes Arch Clin Exp Ophthalmol* 1993;231:591–594.
186. Steinhorst UH, Chen EP, Freedman SF, Machemer R, Hatchell DL. Growth inhibition of human Tenon's capsule fibroblasts and rabbit dermal fibroblasts with non-carcinogenic N-alkylated anthracyclines. *Graefes Arch Clin Exp Ophthalmol* 1994;232:347–354.

Textbook of Ocular Pharmacology,
edited by T.J. Zimmerman, et al.
Lippincott–Raven Publishers, Philadelphia © 1997.

CHAPTER 28

Prostaglandins and Prostaglandin Analogues

Carl B. Camras, Laszlo Z. Bito, and Carol B. Toris

History and Source

As is apparent from the previous chapters, the clinical management of glaucoma has been dominated in the twentieth century by drugs that mimic or inhibit the effects of the neurotransmitters, namely, acetylcholine (ACh) or norepinephrine, or the enzyme carbonic anhydrase (1). This is not surprising considering that both ACh and epinephrine were discovered in the nineteenth century. By the middle of this century, their biological effects were reported to include many biologic phenomena, and carbonic anhydrase was found to be present in the ciliary processes (95).

In contrast to the long-term history of neurotransmitters, the first prostaglandins (PGs) were extracted from seminal fluid in the 1930s. It was not until the 1950s that the structures of the E- and F-type PGs were identified. The discovery of PGs in lipidic extract of the iris was among the first indications that PGs are produced outside the reproductive system, representing a major step toward their recognition as ubiquitous local hormones (3).

Four decades ago, Ambache discovered the capacity of the iris to synthesize PGs (4) in his search for the mediator of the neurogenic ocular irritative response. When synthetic PGs became readily available at the end of the 1960s, research efforts focused on substantiation of the role of PGs in ocular pathophysiology. Consequently, the first ocular studies used large amounts of PGs delivered directly into the anterior chamber of rabbit eyes, specifically, to reproduce the signs of ocular irritation and inflammation, including a breakdown of the blood-aqueous barrier (BAB), *increased* intraocular pressure (IOP), and iridial hyperemia. In addition, PGs produced atropine-resistant miosis in some species (5,6). This early association of PGs with the signs of ocular inflammation was strengthened greatly by the claim that aspirin prevents disruption of the BAB in the rabbit eye (7), even though the actual findings showed inhibition, rather than prevention, of the disruption. Unfortunately, the resulting misconceptions greatly delayed the elucidation of the more subtle physiologic roles and the ocular therapeutic potential of PGs (8).

The assumed primary role of PGs in ocular inflammation had a beneficial effect: It stimulated research in the ability of ocular tissues to synthesize PGs. By the 1970s, it was well established that several ocular tissues could produce these local hormones from endogenous membrane phospholipids or from exogenous arachidonic acid (9). By the end of the 1970s, it was recognized that the release of arachidonic acid from membrane phospholipids, by physiologic or pathologic stimuli, resulted not only in the synthesis of the classic E and F PGs but also of other potent eicosanoids, such as prostacyclin, thromboxane, leukotrienes, and platelet-activating factor (PAF) (3,10–12). One leukotriene, LTB_4, was found to have a potent chemotactic effect in the eye, causing the accumulation of leukocytes in the anterior segment after intracameral injection in extremely small amounts. On the other hand, PGE_2 was not chemotactic, even when administered in much higher doses (13). Some key members of this eicosanoid family of mediators, also referred to as the *arachidonic acid cascade,* are shown in Fig. 28-1.

The discovery of other potent mediators, such as the neuropeptides, PAF, the interleukins, and the nitric oxide system and their roles in the inflammatory response led to the recognition by the end of the 1980s that PGs play a minor, mostly modulatory, role in ocular inflammation. It also was recognized that PGs can downregulate some aspects of the inflammatory response and can be regarded as antiinflammatory as well as proinflammatory agents (12,13). Intraocular release of neuropeptides occurred during ocular irritation, and PGs potentiated the ocular effect of substance P. These findings suggested that the adverse effects of exogenous PGs in the early studies was due, at least in

C. B. Camras and C. B. Toris: Department of Ophthalmology, University of Nebraska Medical Center, Omaha, Nebraska 68198-5540.

L. Z. Bito: Department of Ophthalmology, Research Division, Columbia University, New York, New York 10032.

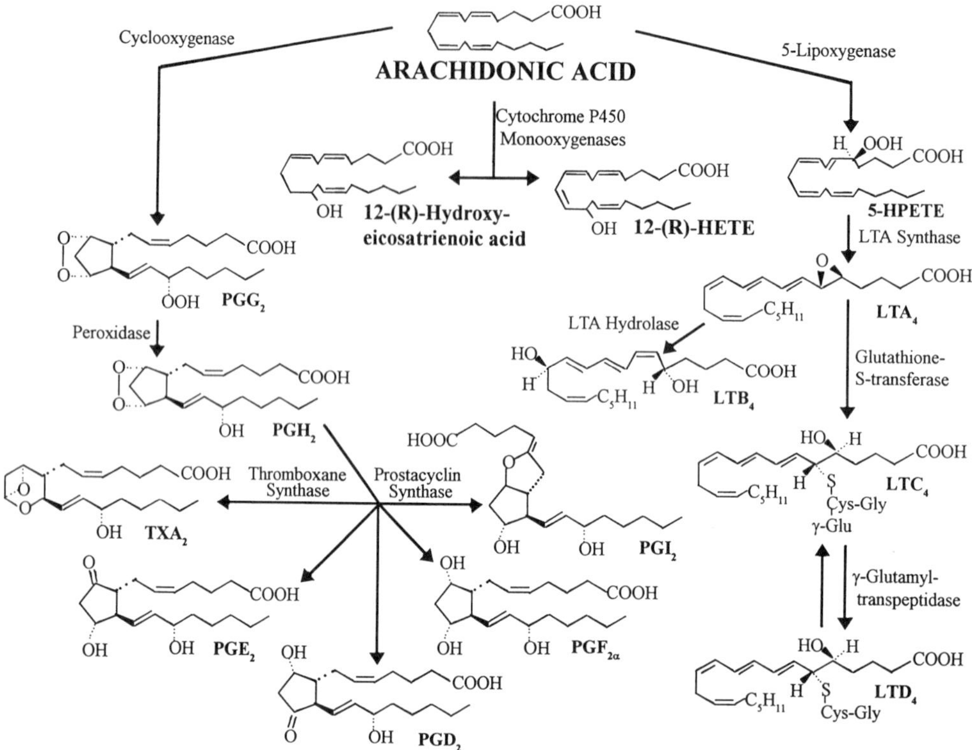

FIG. 28-1. Arachidonic acid cascade. (Modified from ref 14.)

part, to PG-induced potentiation of endogenous neuropeptides released following cannulation of the anterior chamber. These considerations required reevaluation of the concept that PGs are involved primarily with ocular irritative and inflammatory responses in species other than rabbits (1,3,11,13) and opened up an avenue toward the elucidation of the therapeutic potential of PGs.

Much of the first two decades of ocular PG research, including the initial misconceptions, was reviewed in a multiauthored monograph, *The Ocular Effects of Prostaglandins and Other Eicosanoids* (96). This book also describes the studies that first demonstrated the therapeutic potential of PGs in the management of IOP. Some more recent major contributions to our understanding of the complexity of the eicosanoid system and the role of PGs in physiologic versus pathophysiologic ocular processes also were reviewed (12,15–18). The ocular hypotensive effect and side-effect profile of several PG analogues have been established over the past decade on ocular normotensive volunteers and glaucoma patients.

Official Drug Names and Chemistry

The chemical structures of PGs and their prodrugs/analogues that have been used in clinical trials are found in Fig. 28-2.

Two analogues of PGF$_{2\alpha}$ have been approved for clinical use. The phenyl-substituted prostaglandin analogue, 13,14-dihydro-17-phenyl-18,19,20-trinor-prostaglandin F$_{2\alpha}$-isopropyl ester (latanoprost), is approved for clinical use in several countries, including the United States, Scandinavia, and the United Kingdom. It was previously denoted as PhXA41 and is being marketed under the trade name Xalatan.

The isopropyl ester prodrug form of the 20-ethyl derivative of the pulmonary metabolite of PGF$_{2\alpha}$, 20-ethyl-13,14-dihydro-15-keto-PGF$_{2\alpha}$-isopropyl ester (isopropyl unoprostone), is approved for clinical use in Japan. It was previously denoted UF-021 and is being marketed under the trade name Rescula.

Pharmacology

The main action of topical latanoprost, unoprostone, and related PGF$_{2\alpha}$ analogues is a reduction in IOP, which occurs predominantly by increasing uveoscleral outflow (reviewed in 19). The increase in uveoscleral outflow may result initially from relaxation of the ciliary muscle and later from biochemical restructuring of the components of its extracellular matrix.

Clinical Pharmacology (20)

PGF$_{2\alpha}$ Tromethamine Salt (PGF$_{2\alpha}$-TS)

In the first clinical study evaluating the effects of PGs, a single dose of 200 μg (0.5%) of PGF$_{2\alpha}$-TS (Fig. 28-2)

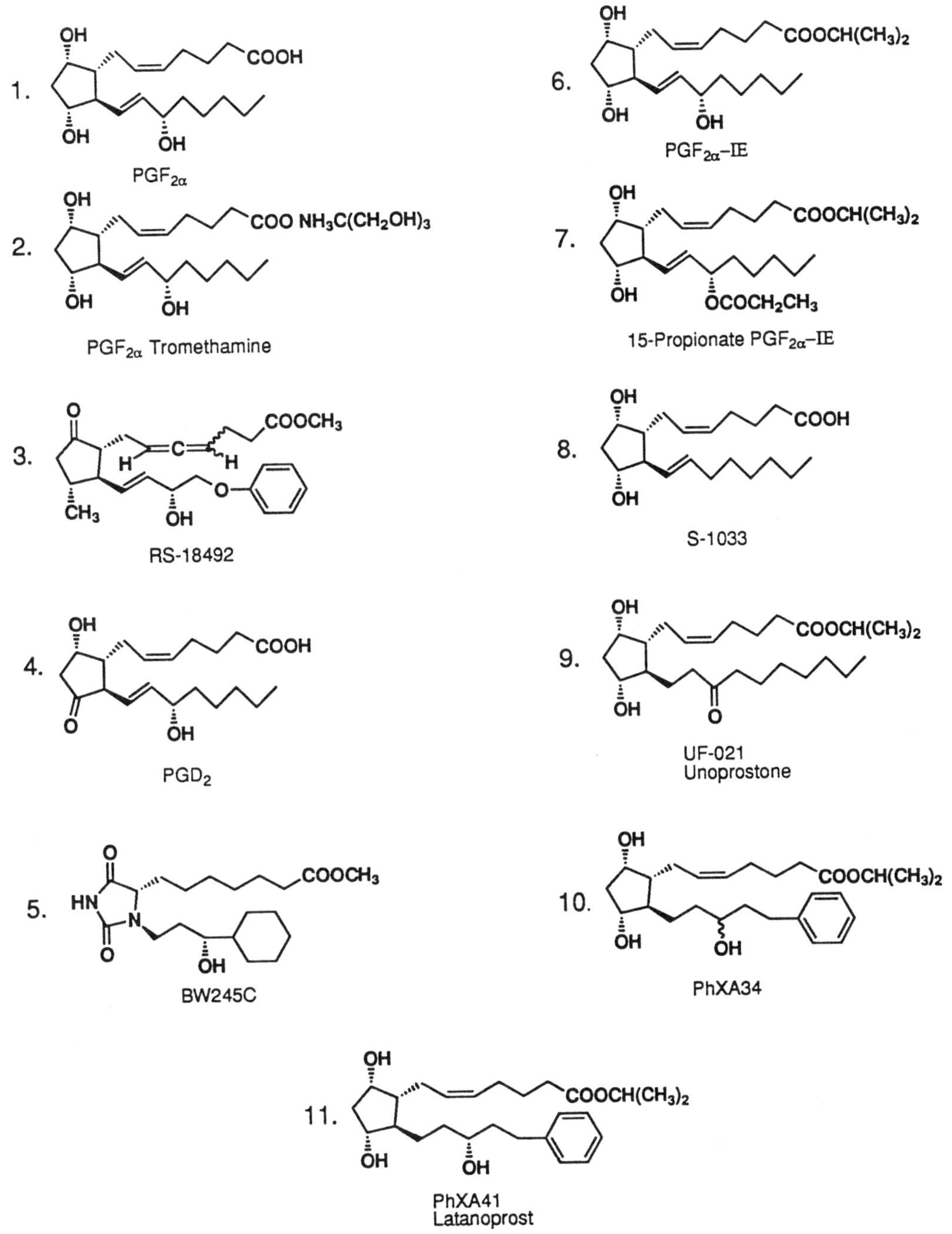

FIG. 28-2. Chemical structures of prostaglandins and their prodrugs/analogues that have been used in clinical trials. (From ref 20, with permission.)

was topically applied to one eye in each of 18 normotensive volunteers in a randomized fashion (21); PGF$_{2\alpha}$-TS significantly reduced IOP for 24 hours, with a mean reduction of as much as 3 to 4 mm Hg occurring at 7 hours. Aqueous flare, abnormal leakage of the iris after fluorescein angiography, an anterior chamber cellular response, and miosis were not observed; however, PGF$_{2\alpha}$ produced marked conjunctival hyperemia, "smarting," foreign-body sensation, and headaches in one third of patients. Although most of these side effects dissipated over the first 2 to 3 hours after application of the PG, they were severe enough for the author to conclude that the use of PGF$_{2\alpha}$-TS in clinical therapy would be limited by its external irritative effects (21).

A double-masked, randomized, parallel group study comparing three concentrations of $PGF_{2\alpha}$-TS was performed in 45 normotensive volunteers (22). A single dose of 62.5 μg (0.125%), 125 μg (0.25%), or 250 μg (0.5%) of $PGF_{2\alpha}$-TS was applied to one eye in each of 15 subjects. $PGF_{2\alpha}$-TS caused a mean reduction of IOP of as much as 2 to 3 mm Hg in each of the three groups of subjects. A peak reduction occurred at 2 to 9 hours. The duration of the hypotensive effect was 12, 21, and >24 hours for doses of 62.5, 125, and 250 μg, respectively. Confirming results of the previous study (21), $PGF_{2\alpha}$-TS caused dose-dependent conjunctival hyperemia, irritation, foreign-body sensation, headaches (50% of patients treated with the 125 or 250 μg doses), and occasional erythema of the skin of the lower lid. Pupillary diameter was not altered. Neither aqueous flare nor an anterior cellular response was observed in any eyes (22).

PGE_2 Analogue

After demonstrating an ocular hypotensive effect in rabbits (23), a single application of a PGE_2 analogue, RS 18492 (see Fig. 28-2) 0.02% was administered to one eye in each of 20 normotensive volunteers in a randomized, double-masked fashion (24). This PG analogue caused an initial mean rise in IOP of as much as 3 to 4 mm Hg, peaking at 1 to 2 hours. As an extreme, two individual patients showed rises of 13 to 20 mm Hg. Following this initial hypertensive response, mean IOP was reduced by no more than 1 to 2 mm Hg at 6 hours. Similar to the effects with the $PGF_{2\alpha}$-TS, this PGE_2 analogue caused conjunctival hyperemia, aching, tenderness, and photophobia, beginning within the first hour and lasting up to 6 hours after administration. Once again, these results were not encouraging for the development of PGs for glaucoma therapy.

PGD_2 and its Selective Analogue

Based on studies demonstrating that PGD_2 and BW245C (Fig. 28-2), an agonist selective for the DP receptor, are not only effective ocular hypotensive agents but also the best tolerated PGs in terms of the BAB and ocular surface pathology in rabbits (25–27), a dose-response study was carried out in five to nine normotensive volunteers (28). This clinical study was performed despite the demonstration of poor tolerance of BW245C in monkeys (29). Like the PGE_2 analogue, PGD_2 caused a dose-dependent initial rise in IOP of 1 to 4 mm Hg for the 5 μg (0.01%), 10 μg (0.02%), and 50 μg (0.1%) doses, peaking at 30 minutes (28). A subsequent mean reduction in IOP of no more than 1.5 to 2 mm Hg peaked at 1.5 to 2 hours after a single application. BW245C 2.5 μg (0.005%) induced an initial rise in IOP of 3 to 4 mm Hg at 30 minutes, followed by a reduction of 1 to 1.5 mm Hg at 3 hours. PGD_2 and BW245C caused conjunctival hyperemia, foreign-body sensation, itching, and burning during the first 2 hours after application. Neither aqueous flare nor an anterior chamber cellular response was observed. Similar to the PGE_2 analogue and $PGF_{2\alpha}$-TS, PGD_2 and BW-245C had a poor therapeutic index and side-effect profile.

$PGF_{2\alpha}$-1-Isopropyl Ester ($PGF_{2\alpha}$-IE)

The first improvement in therapeutic index for PGs occurred with the development of the isopropyl ester (IE) of $PGF_{2\alpha}$ (Fig. 28-2). The enhanced lipophilicity resulting from esterification of the carboxylic acid group improved corneal penetration to increase potency (30). Maintaining similar efficacy as $PGF_{2\alpha}$ at considerably lower concentrations in rabbits, cats (6,31), and monkeys (6,32,33), $PGF_{2\alpha}$-IE produced fewer external ocular side effects. Analogous to the relationship between dipivefrin and epinephrine, $PGF_{2\alpha}$-IE is a prodrug of $PGF_{2\alpha}$ and is converted to the free acid by esterases in the cornea (30).

In a dose-response study in six normotensive volunteers, single applications of $PGF_{2\alpha}$-IE produced a dose-dependent reduction of IOP at 8 to 12 hours by 1.9, 1.9, 3.3, and 5.7 mm Hg at doses of 0.1 μg (0.0004%), 0.5 μg (0.002%), 2.5 μg (0.01%), and 10 μg (0.04%), respectively (34). Only the highest doses showed a tendency toward an initial rise in IOP at 30 minutes. The reduction in IOP was maintained for 12 to 24 hours with the higher two doses. Twice-daily application of 0.5 μg (0.002%) in ten normotensive volunteers produced a 1.5 to 2.5 mm Hg reduction in IOP for the 16 days of treatment. Compared with $PGF_{2\alpha}$, $PGF_{2\alpha}$-IE reduced IOP with a lower incidence and intensity of conjunctival hyperemia, pain, foreign-body sensation, and photophobia (34).

Based on these initial favorable results in normotensive volunteers, $PGF_{2\alpha}$-IE was tested in patients with ocular hypertension or glaucoma (70,35). Doses of 0.25 μg (0.001%) or 0.5 μg (0.002%) reduced IOP by as much as 6 mm Hg (25%). A 4 to 6 mm Hg IOP reduction was maintained on the eighth day of twice-daily treatment (70,35). Although conjunctival hyperemia and irritation were noted by many patients, these side effects were reduced compared with those observed with $PGF_{2\alpha}$.

This esterified prodrug of $PGF_{2\alpha}$ provided evidence that with appropriate modification of PGs or their analogs, external ocular side effects could be reduced without sacrificing ocular hypotensive efficacy. Nevertheless, although reduced, local side effects persisted at sufficient levels that would lead to problems with medical compliance and would prevent $PGF_{2\alpha}$-IE from becoming a useful primary therapy for glaucoma.

15-Propionate-PGF$_{2\alpha}$-IE

In an effort to reduce the irritation and conjunctival hyperemia produced by PGF$_{2\alpha}$-IE, esterification at the 15 carbon position, in addition to esterification at the carboxylic acid moiety (Fig. 28-2), was tried (36). In a double-masked, dose-response, comparative study with PGF$_{2\alpha}$, 15-propionate-PGF$_{2\alpha}$-IE effectively reduced IOP in 12 normotensive volunteers but failed to offer any advantages compared with PGF$_{2\alpha}$-IE in terms of therapeutic index (36).

15-Deoxy-PGF$_{2\alpha}$ (S-1033)

S-1033 is PGF$_{2\alpha}$ without the hydroxyl group at the 15 carbon position (Fig. 28-2). It reduced IOP in rabbits, cats, dogs, and monkeys with minimal side effects (25). In the only clinical trial using this agent, a dose-dependent reduction in IOP of as much as 2 to 3 mm Hg peaked at 2 to 8 hours after a single application of 0.3% solution in six normotensive volunteers (37). The highest dose of 0.4% resulted in both an ipsilateral and contralateral reduction of IOP of 4 to 5 mm Hg at 8 hours. This contralateral effect was difficult to explain. S-1033 0.3% produced mild conjunctival hyperemia in three of the six subjects and a slight "smarting" sensation in all six patients that lasted a few minutes after a single application. Twice-daily application of S-1033 0.3% in the six normotensive volunteers reduced IOP by 2 to 3 mm Hg for the 8 days of treatment.

Isopropyl Unoprostone, a Modified PGF$_{2\alpha}$ Metabolite

Isopropyl unoprostone (UF-021; Rescula; isopropyl 20-ethyl-13,14-dihydro-15-keto-PGF$_{2\alpha}$-isopropyl ester) is the isopropyl ester prodrug form of the 20-ethyl derivative of the common pulmonary metabolite of PGF$_{2\alpha}$ (Fig. 28-2). In a dose-response study involving 8 to 11 normotensive volunteers, isopropyl unoprostone 0.03%, 0.06%, 0.09%, and 0.12% caused a dose-dependent IOP reduction, with a peak of 1 to 4 mm Hg at 1 to 2 hours after a single dose (39). Compared with all previously discussed PG analogues, isopropyl unoprostone seems best tolerated in terms of external ocular surface side effects (39). In another dose-response study involving normal volunteers treated twice daily for 2 weeks, isopropyl unoprostone 0.06% or 0.12% produced a similar dose-dependent reduction of IOP without ocular or systemic side effects (38). In 10 normotensive volunteers, isopropyl unoprostone 0.12% caused a peak reduction of IOP of 1 to 2 mm Hg at 6 hours (40). Twice-daily treatment in seven normotensive volunteers reduced IOP for 2 weeks, but no significant IOP reduction was present after 4 weeks of treatment (40). In a larger study involving 129 patients with elevated IOP, isopropyl unoprostone 0.03%, 0.06%, or 0.12%, or placebo was randomly applied twice daily for 4 weeks in these four parallel groups (41). A dose-dependent reduction in IOP of 1 to 3 mm Hg (5–15%) was produced with only mild side effects (41).

The initial investigations led to evaluation of isopropyl unoprostone in larger multicenter studies (42–44). In one Phase III trial (43,44), 114 patients with elevated IOPs were randomly assigned to twice-daily treatment with either 0.06% or 0.12% isopropyl unoprostone for 1 year. Of the 57 patients who started in each group, 31 patients (54%) completed the 0.06% treatment, and 39 patients (68%) completed the 0.12% treatment. Excluding all withdrawals, some of whom dropped out because of lack of IOP control, patients treated with 0.06% isopropyl unoprostone for 1 year exhibited a 3.4 mm Hg reduction from baseline and those treated with 0.12% exhibited a 4.5 mm Hg reduction.

In a second Phase III trial, 158 patients with elevated IOPs were treated twice daily for 12 weeks with either 0.12% isopropyl unoprostone or 0.5% timolol (42,44). Both groups exhibited a significant IOP reduction of 5 mm Hg from the baseline of 24; however, IOP was measured only 4 hours after the last dose of either drug. A comparison of the important trough values at 12 hours was not evaluated. Mild conjunctival hyperemia occurred in 4% of patients in each group. Blood pressure decreased significantly in the timolol treatment group but not in the isopropyl unoprostone treatment group. The results of these clinical trials led to governmental approval for the use of isopropyl unoprostone in glaucoma therapy in Japan.

PhXA34

PhXA34 (13,14-dihydro-15(R,S)-17-phenyl-18,19,20-trinor-PGF$_{2\alpha}$-IE) is a 17-phenyl substituted analogue of the isopropyl ester of PGF$_{2\alpha}$ (Fig. 28-2). In addition to the phenyl group at the 17th position on the carbon chain, the double bond at the C_{13-14} is reduced. The 17-phenyl substituted PGF$_{2\alpha}$ analogues were 90 times as potent as PGF$_{2\alpha}$ in an in vitro assay that measured luteolytic activity and considerably more potent in several in vivo assays (45). These analogues are selective for the FP receptor, the prostanoid receptor responsible for the IOP reduction in primates (46,47). Although not an effective ocular hypotensive agent in rabbits or cats, PhXA34 produced fewer and less severe external ocular side effects compared with other analogues (48–50). In monkeys, this PG analogue maintained ocular hypotensive efficacy (50,51).

On the basis of an improved therapeutic index found in experimental animals, PhXA34 was evaluated in clinical trials. In a dose-response study in 16 normotensive volunteers, PhXA34 1 μg (0.003%), 3 μg (0.01%), and 10 μg (0.03%) caused a dose-dependent IOP reduction by as much as 5 mm Hg, peaking at 8 to 10 hours after a single dose (52). The hypotensive effect lasted at least 24 hours after each application of the higher dose and was maintained during the 7 days of treatment. External ocular side effects were markedly reduced using this analogue compared with others (52,53). In patients with ocular hypertension or glaucoma, PhXA34 0.003% or 0.01% reduced IOP by as much as 40% on the second day of therapy (54,55); a 20 to 35% IOP reduction was maintained for 1 week (54). Adverse sensory side effects of burning, stinging, irritation, and foreign-body sensation were virtually totally eliminated. Conjunctival hyperemia was reduced significantly to a level tolerated by all patients (54,55).

Latanoprost

PhXA34 is an epimeric mixture. Because the 15S-epimer has only 10% the activity of the 15R-epimer (56), the R-epimer of PhXA34 is about twice as potent as the epimeric mixture. This R-epimer, or latanoprost (PhXA41; Xalatan; Fig. 28-2), reduced IOP by 25 to 35% in initial clinical trials evaluating dose-response relationships in normotensive volunteers and in patients with ocular hypertension or glaucoma (53,57–60). Multiple dosing once daily maintained a consistent IOP reduction over at least a 24-hour period (53,58–60). Conjunctival hyperemia was minimal, and adverse symptomatology was virtually nonexistent. These favorable initial clinical trials led to testing in international multicenter trials (61–66). A summary of these studies is found in the Major Clinical Trials section of this chapter.

Pharmaceutics

Xalatan (latanoprost) is available in a 2.5-ml dropper bottle and can be stored at room temperature after opening for at least 6 weeks. The molecular alterations in latanoprost were such that the most important pharmacokinetic attributes of $PGF_{2\alpha}$ and its agonistic potency on the FP receptor were retained (48). Thus, latanoprost effectively reduces IOP at a concentration of 0.005% and maintains this IOP reduction when applied only once a day. During the course of bilateral latanoprost treatment, the daily dose applied is about 3 μg.

Pharmacokinetics

Bioavailability. The isopropyl ester prodrug latanoprost is absorbed through the cornea and hydrolyzed to the biologically active acid form. Peak concentrations of the active agent in the aqueous humor occur at about 2 hours after topical application.

Distribution. The distribution volume in humans is 0.16 ± 0.02 L/kg. The acid form of latanoprost was measurable in the aqueous humor for at least 4 hours and in the plasma during the first hour after administration. The half-life for elimination from the anterior segment of the eye is 3 to 4 hours (98).

Rate and Route of Elimination. After both intravenous and topical administration, the active form of latanoprost from human plasma was eliminated with a half-life of 17 minutes (67). Systemic clearance is approximately 7 ml/min/kg. The free-acid form and metabolites from hepatic β-oxidation are eliminated mainly by the kidneys through an active transport process (68). After topical or intravenous dosing, the recovered amount of drug in the urine is 88% or 98%, respectively.

Routes of Metabolism. Latanoprost is hydrolyzed by esterases in the cornea to the biologically active acid. This active form is stable in the eye because it is not metabolized by intraocular tissues. The active agent reaching the systemic circulation is metabolized primarily by the liver to the 1,2-dinor and 1,2,3,4,-tetranor metabolites via fatty acid β-oxidation (Fig. 28-3).

Therapeutic Use

Latanoprost is used therapeutically to reduce IOP. It is an effective ocular hypotensive agent both in hypertensive and normotensive glaucoma when used alone or in combination with other glaucoma medications. Latanoprost is not indicated for anyone with a known hypersensitivity to latanoprost or benzalkonium chloride.

Side Effects and Toxicity

Ocular Surface

Conjunctival hyperemia was noted after the topical application of all naturally occurring PGs to rabbit, cat, or human eyes. In addition, irritation of sensory nerves was evident from the tendency of cats to keep their treated eyes closed for 1 to 20 minutes after the topical application of ocular hypotensive doses of such PGs. In general, these side effects could not be detected in monkeys. Because primates have heavily pigmented perilimbal bulbar conjunctivae, hyperemia cannot be observed. Also, monkeys do not close their eyes even when given a solution that is clearly irritating to the human eye (Bito, unpublished observation).

In clinical studies, conjunctival hyperemia and irritation of the sensory nerves, typically expressed as pain or foreign-body sensation, were observed after topical application of the naturally occurring PGs or many of their analogues. In addition, PGE_2, PGD_2, tromethamine salt of $PGF_{2\alpha}$, and some of their analogues produced headaches in some patients (21,22,24,69). The side effects of the E and D compounds were more severe than those of $PGF_{2\alpha}$.

Esterification of the carboxylic acid group of $PGF_{2\alpha}$, such as in $PGF_{2\alpha}$-IE, allowed the use of much lower concentrations to achieve comparable IOP reductions with less conjunctival hyperemic and fewer sensory side effects (34,35,70); however, these side effects could not be completely eliminated even with the esterification of a hydroxyl group of $PGF_{2\alpha}$ in addition to the carboxylic acid group (36, 71).

It became necessary to modify the PG moiety itself chemically to reduce or eliminate the side effects further.

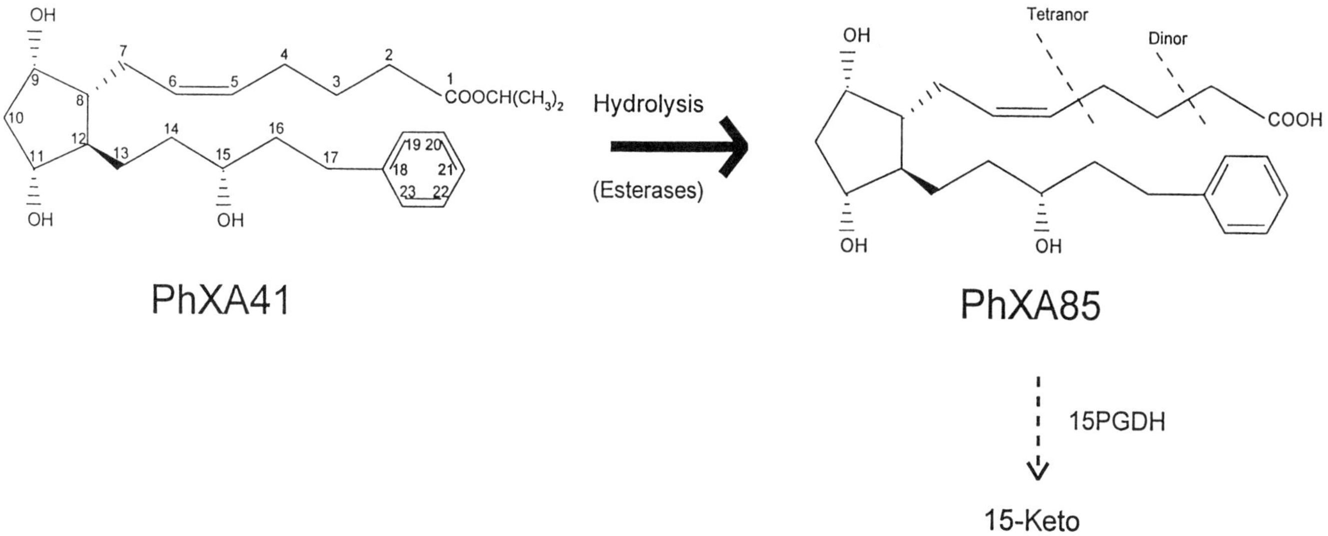

FIG. 28-3. Metabolism of latanoprost (PhXA41). Hydrolysis to the free acid (PhXA85) occurs in the eye. Fatty acid β-oxidation forming the 1,2-dinor and 1,2,3,4-tetranor metabolites occurs primarily in the liver.

Latanoprost is a $PGF_{2\alpha}$ analogue that shows very high selectivity for the FP type of PG receptor, with greatly reduced potency toward the EP, TP, DP, and IP types of receptors (47). This selectivity enabled maintenance of the ocular hypotensive potency with elimination of the adverse sensory side effects and marked reduction of the conjunctival hyperemia.

With isopropyl unoprostone, reduction of side effects was achieved by selecting the pulmonary metabolite of $PGF_{2\alpha}$, thus reducing the overall ocular potency of the analogue compared with $PGF_{2\alpha}$-IE. Whether this actually resulted in appreciable improvement of therapeutic index is difficult to conclude from the published findings. Reduced hyperemic and sensory side effects on the conjunctival and corneal surfaces of the eye were also reported following the topical application of $PGF_{2\alpha}$-IE in doses that yielded less than the maximum IOP reduction achievable with this $PGF_{2\alpha}$ prodrug. A low dose of $PGF_{2\alpha}$-IE may produce a comparable IOP reduction with similar side effects as isopropyl unoprostone.

Anterior Chamber Cells and Flare

PGs do not cause cellular invasion of the anterior chamber, such chemotactic effects were later found to be attributable to a leukotriene, LTB_4 (13). It is not surprising, therefore, that none of the clinical studies discussed in this chapter reported observing cells in the anterior chamber as a side effect of any topically applied ocular hypotensive PG or PG analogue. These clinical studies excluded most eyes with signs of uveitis. Thus, in view of current concepts that assign to PGs both proinflammatory and antiinflammatory effects (12,13), it remains to be seen whether topically applied PG analogues will enhance or minimize ocular inflammation, including the accumulation of leukocytes.

Similarly, clinically observable flare in the anterior segment, the breakdown of the BAB, was not observed in any of these clinical studies, although such breakdown of this barrier was one of the most consistent effects of higher doses of PGs in rabbit eyes (5).

Comparative studies on the ocular irritative response suggest the existence of profound species differences, including the existence of a highly sophisticated PG-mediated mechanism for the breakdown of the BAB in rabbits (98). It appears that such a mechanism evolved only in species with monitoring-type visual systems, which enable a 360-degree field of vision. Because these eyes protrude from the head and are not protected, they require a system that provides rapid delivery of plasma-borne clotting factors into the anterior chamber to stabilize the eye after inadvertent penetrating injuries. The site of BAB breakdown in rabbit eyes is primarily the iridial ciliary processes. Such processes are abundant in rabbits but absent or vestigial in primates. Because the primate eye is well protected in the orbit, it does not require the exquisitely sensitive BAB for protection against the infrequent ruptured globe. Instead, it developed a different mechanism to deliver plasma proteins into the anterior chamber (1,98). It is not surprising, therefore, that anterior chamber flare has not been reported to be a side effect of ocular hypotensive doses of PGs in human volunteers or in glaucoma patients.

Fluorophotometric methods can detect extremely small changes in the permeability of the BAB by measuring the entry of systemically administered fluorescein from the circulation into the aqueous humor, yielding a measurable value even in normal eyes. Several antiglaucoma drugs have been reported to increase the permeability of the BAB to fluorescein. Some studies using $PGF_{2\alpha}$ predrugs and analogs have reported similar small increases in fluorescein accumulation in the aqueous humor in some patients (34,52). The most sophisticated use of this technique was developed at the Mayo clinic by Brubaker and co-workers. Studies conducted on human volunteers in that laboratory revealed no significant change in BAB permeability following the topical application of ocular hypotensive doses of either $PGF_{2\alpha}$-isopropyl ester (72,99) or latanoprost (73). In one clinical study of PhXA34, a statistically significant increase in aqueous fluorescence was reported after 7 days of treatment with a high dose (52); even in this case, however, the increase was too small to suggest a breakdown of the barrier associated with clinically observable flare.

The more recently developed laser-flare meter allows the noninvasive determination of the protein concentration in the aqueous humor, even at normal levels. The first report using this instrument showed no significant change in photon count after a single administration of 0.005% latanoprost (53). More recently, the same technique was used to estimate protein concentration in the anterior chamber following 4 weeks of once-daily application of 0.005% latanoprost or twice-daily application of 0.0015% latanoprost compared with 0.5% timolol in a crossover study. Timolol, but not latanoprost, yielded a statistically significant ($p < 0.004$) increase in photon count.

Small increases in protein concentration do not necessarily imply an effect on BAB barrier permeability. In the case of timolol, it is attributable to a slower rate of aqueous humor flow, leading to somewhat greater than normal accumulation of the proteins that continually enter the anterior chamber in small amounts from the systemic circulation. On the other hand, by increasing uveoscleral outflow, latanoprost can be expected to modify the properties of the extracellular matrix of the iris root—ciliary body complex and affect the rate of normal protein entry into the anterior chamber from this region. The iris root is the major source of the proteins that enter the anterior chamber in primates (76). Thus, even if significant increases in protein concentration in the anterior chamber are found in the PG-treated eyes in the future, such increases in the 10 to 50% range should not necessarily be interpreted as an adverse effect on BAB function. True breakdown of the BAB is associated with a 10- to 20-fold (i.e., 1,000–2,000%) increase rather than a 10% to 20% increase in the protein concentration in the anterior chamber.

Similar evaluation of the effect of isopropyl unoprostone on the BAB has not been reported. Considering, however, that unoprostone is a weak FP receptor agonist and reportedly has an even lower affinity for EP receptors, this $PGF_{2\alpha}$ analogue, like latanoprost, would not be expected to lead to any cellular response in the anterior chamber and would be expected to have no physiologically or clinically significant effects on BAB permeability.

Lack of Retinal Effects

Several studies in monkeys and humans have failed to find any effect of topical $PGF_{2\alpha}$-TS or latanoprost on the retinal vasculature. In monkeys undergoing fluorescein angiography, high doses of $PGF_{2\alpha}$-TS (250 μg applied twice daily) (77) or latanoprost (10 μg/eye/day) (78) did not produce leakage of fluorescein from retinal blood vessels suggestive of cystoid macular edema in phakic or aphakic eyes treated for 2 weeks to 6 months. Furthermore, high doses of either $PGF_{2\alpha}$-TS (79) or latanoprost (80) in phakic or aphakic cynomolgus monkey eyes did not result in any pathological effects in the retina (including cystoid macular edema) or other adverse histopathologic changes in other parts of the eye as determined by light or electron microscopy after 2 weeks to 6 months of treatment. In pseudophakic patients with elevated IOP treated with latanoprost 0.006% twice daily for 4 weeks, no evidence of leakage or other drug-induced changes in the retinal vasculature was found by fluorescin angiography (81).

Iridial Pigmentation (15)

In cynomolgus monkeys, all PGs and PG analogues studied so far, including latanoprost and isopropyl unoprostone, caused increased pigmentation of the anterior surface of the iris in some eyes after several months of treatment (82). Consequently, baseline and follow-up photographs were obtained in all Phase III latanoprost studies. In some unilaterally treated patients, heterochromia became recognizable after a few months of latanoprost treatment. In general, however, an increase in iridial pigmentation in patients treated with latanoprost in both eyes became apparent only from the evaluation of the photographic record and was not noticed by the patients, their relatives, or their ophthalmologists.

The most striking changes in iridial color occurred in persons with a concentric brown color around the pupil and a light grey-green or blue color around the periphery. Latanoprost did not alter eye color in white patients with uniformly blue or brown eyes or in patients of African or Japanese descent (2). Similar changes in eye color have not been reported in patients treated with isopropyl unoprostone for several months; however, studies published to date with isopropyl unoprostone have been limited to patients in Japan with uniformly dark eyes.

Increased iridial pigmentation, or the restoration of the age-dependent loss of iridial pigmentation, which may be the cause of the observed effect, was reported for the first time in the Phase III latanoprost studies (62). Thus, the physiologic and pharmacologic parameters that may be involved, as well as the basis for the apparent assumption that iridial pigmentation is invariant past early childhood in all individuals, are examined in some detail here.

Without question, the greatest risk factor for the development of increased iridial pigmentation is the baseline eye color. Therefore, we can assume that a fundamental aspect of this effect is associated closely with the conditions that cause this type of heterogenous iridial pigmentation. Genetically determined set points of melanin accumulation in subgroups of melanocytes, as occurs in piebaldism, produces sharply demarcated light and dark iridial halves (83). We must assume, therefore, that in eyes that are most susceptible for the PG-induced darkening, the somewhat concentrically arranged brown and lightly pigmented or unpigmented areas arise because of regional or focal differences in the availability of some factor(s) in the chemical milieu of iridial melanocytes. The only such factor currently known to be required for achieving or maintaining the genetically determined level of iridial pigmentation is normal sympathetic innervation. The absence of this innervation causes hypopigmentation in clinical Horner's syndrome or in experimental animals following sympathectomy (84,86,100). Based on the known interactions between PGs and the adrenergic system (86) as well as on the demonstrated (sympathetic) innervation of the anterior border layer of the iris (84,85), our working hypothesis for the PG-induced increase in iridial pigmentation assumes two alternatives: (a) that PGs potentiate the insufficient but still existing (sympathetic) neurohumoral influences on hypopigmented melanocytes; or (b) that PGs can substitute for the lack of neuronal influences normally derived from the sympathetic innervation, which may be required for maintaining the genetically determined level of pigmentation in iridial melanocytes.

The observation that latanoprost causes increased iris pigmentation in sympathetically denervated rabbit (86) or monkey (82) eyes supports the second alternative. The hypothesis that the increased iris pigmentation reflects the ability of PGs to compensate for a sympathetic insufficiency, which leads to hypopigmentation of some iridial melanocytes, is fully testable experimentally. One such experiment has already shown that, in contrast to normal rabbits that do not show this response, the iris color darkens in sympathetically denervated hypopigmented rabbit eyes after chronic treatment with latanoprost (86). The observation that eye color is variable during childhood (87), adolescence, and even into adulthood in a subpopulation of 10 to 20% of whites (85,88) supports the concept that the melanin content of the melanocytes of the anterior border layer of the iris, which determines eye color (85,89,101,102), may be influenced by neurohumoral or hormonal mechanisms throughout life.

Not all eyes with the susceptible baseline iris color develop the PG-induced increase in iridial pigmentation; therefore, some other factor(s), such as insufficient local concentration of melanocyte-stimulating hormone (MSH) or some other mediator(s), also may be involved. Alternatively, this marked difference in PG-induced increase in iridial pigmentation, even in eyes with similar susceptible colors at baseline, may simply reflect individual differences in drug sensitivity or in ocular pharmacokinetic properties.

Systemic Side Effects

Except for the portion of eyedrops that falls on the skin of the eyelid or is blinked out of the tear film, the whole dose of a topically applied medication is systemically absorbed. On a molar basis, this amount is equivalent to about 2 μg of $PGF_{2\alpha}$, which is a small fraction of the approximately 1,000 to 2,000 μg of PGs that are normally produced, metabolized, and excreted by the body daily (90). For other therapeutic purposes, PGs also have been administered intravaginally or intravenously in milligram amounts (1). In addition, as stated in the section on pharmacokinetics, latanoprost enters the aqueous humor and the circulation in the free acid form, which is a good substrate for the PG transport system (68). Thus, latanoprost free acid and its initial metabolites, mainly β-oxidation products, are effectively excreted primarily by the kidneys into the urine. These considerations suggest that the daily doses of topically applied latanoprost are not expected to exert any systemic side effects (1), and no such systemic effects attributable to latanoprost were observed during any of the three Phase III latanoprost studies (62).

In one Phase II safety study using a placebo control, up to sevenfold the recommended daily ocular hypotensive dose of latanoprost was applied topically to the eyes of 11 asthmatic and 12 healthy volunteers. This excessive dose had no effect on pulmonary function tests, which included forced expiratory volume, peak expiratory outflow, and forced vital capacity (FVC). In addition, no difference in bronchodilator response to β-adrenergic agonists was observed in the asthmatic volunteers after either latanoprost or vehicle (91).

The topically applied PG dose that is drained through the nasolacrimal sac into the nose and is swallowed to reach the stomach would be expected to have cytoprotective, rather than harmful, effects in this organ. It is the inhibition of PG synthesis by aspirin or indomethacin that occasionally causes gastric ulceration. This effect has been shown to be prevented or minimized by the use of some PG analogues (92).

Drug Interactions

In in vitro studies, precipitation occurs when eyedrops containing thimerosal are mixed with latanoprost. To avoid this reaction, these drugs should be administered at least 5 minutes apart.

Major Clinical Trials

Four large multicenter trials have been conducted comparing latanoprost to timolol, one each in the United States (U.S.), the United Kingdom (U.K.), Scandinavia, and Japan.

Scandinavian Study (62,63)

Patients (n = 267) with elevated IOP were included in the study. Patient demographics and baseline characteristics of the eyes of each patient in this and the other two multicenter trials are listed in Table 28-1. Patients previously treated with topical β-adrenergic blockers were excluded. Eligible patients were randomized into three groups: 0.5% timolol twice daily (n = 84), 0.005% latanoprost once daily in the morning for 3 months and then in the evening for 3 months (n = 89), and 0.005% latanoprost once daily with the treatment regimen reversed (n = 94). Examinations were made at 8 AM, noon, and 4 PM on baseline day and after 3 and 6 months of treatment. Additional morning visits were made at 0.5, 1.5, and 4.5 months of treatment.

The efficacy of the two drugs was determined from the mean diurnal IOP, that is, the average of the three IOP measurements at 8 AM, noon, and 4 PM. Both drugs significantly ($p < 0.001$) reduced IOP for the entire 6-month period. Latanoprost given once a day in the morning reduced diurnal IOP by 7.8 mm Hg (31%) when given either the first 3 months or the second 3 months of treatment. This effect did not differ significantly from that of twice-daily timolol given for the first 3 months or second 3 months. When given once daily in the evening during the alternate 3-month period, the IOP reduction was even greater than both morning latanoprost and twice-daily timolol. After 6 months of treatment, 69% of patients treated with latanoprost in the evening had IOPs <17 mm Hg compared with 34% of patients treated with twice-daily timolol (Fig. 4D,E). In patients with unilateral treatment, there was no significant contralateral effect with latanoprost; however, timolol caused a slight but significant ($p < 0.01$) decrease (1.1 $\pm$0.3 mm Hg) in IOP in the contralateral eye.

Adverse subjective symptomatology, such as burning, itching, foreign-body sensation, stinging, tearing, or eye pain, occurred infrequently and at a similar rate in all groups. Compared with baseline, mild conjunctival hyperemia was noted in 31% of patients treated with latanoprost and in 16% of patients taking timolol. The average hyperemia was considered less than mild in all groups. Hyperemia reported as an ocular side effect or adverse event was 4% with latanoprost and 0% with timolol. A change in iris color was considered definite in five patients (3%) and suspect in seven patients (4%) treated with latanoprost for at least 3 months. No aqueous flare was observed in any patient.

Latanoprost had no effect on blood pressure or heart rate, whereas timolol slightly reduced heart rate by 2.7 beats/minute ($p < 0.005$) at 6 months.

U.K. (62,66)

Patients (n = 294) with the same diagnoses as in the Scandinavia study were assigned to one of two treatment groups: latanoprost 0.005% administered once daily in the evening (149 patients) and timolol 0.5% administered twice daily, morning and evening (145 patients).

Similar to the Scandinavia study, latanoprost significantly ($p < 0.0001$) reduced the diurnal IOP by 8.5 mm Hg (34%) at 6 months. Timolol reduced ($p < 0.0001$) IOP by a similar amount (8.4 mm Hg, 33%). At 3 and 4.5 months only, the IOP in latanoprost-treated eyes was significantly less than in timolol-treated eyes. The difference in IOP reduction between latanoprost and timolol was 0.4 mm Hg ($p < 0.04$) at 3 months and 0.9 mm Hg ($p < 0.001$) at 4.5 months (Fig. 28-4B).

Latanoprost caused more conjunctival hyperemia than timolol ($p < 0.001$); however, the degree of hyperemia was slight. Neither drug caused significant aqueous flare or cellular infiltration into the anterior chamber. In the la-

TABLE 28-1. *Percentage of patients exhibiting specified ocular signs and symptoms at least once during the study*

	Scandinavia		United Kingdom[a]		United States		Japan	
Signs and symptoms	Lat (n = 183)	Tim (n = 84)	Lat (n = 149)	Tim (n = 145)	Lat (n = 128)	Tim (n = 140)	Lat (n = 80)	Tim (n = 83)
Superficial punctate keratopathy	7%	2%	13%	4%	13%	18%	NR	NR
Conjunctival hyperemia	3%	0%	15%	6%	5%	3%	15%	9%
Foreign-body sensation	5%	5%	22%	8%	4%	11%	NR	NR
Blurred vision	3%	7%	11%	13%	10%	6%	1%	0%
Eye pain	1%	0%	9%	7%	2%	4%		
Eye irritation[b]	22%	25%	40%	32%	24%	45%	15%	12%
Iris color change								
Definite	3%	0%	1%	0%	1%	0%	NR	NR
Suspect	4%	0%	9%	0%	2%	0%	NR	NR

[a]Includes adverse events as well as ocular symptoms.
[b]Includes burning, stinging, itching, and tearing.
From refs 63, 64, 66, 94 with permission.
Lat, latanoprost; Tim, timolol. NR, not reported.

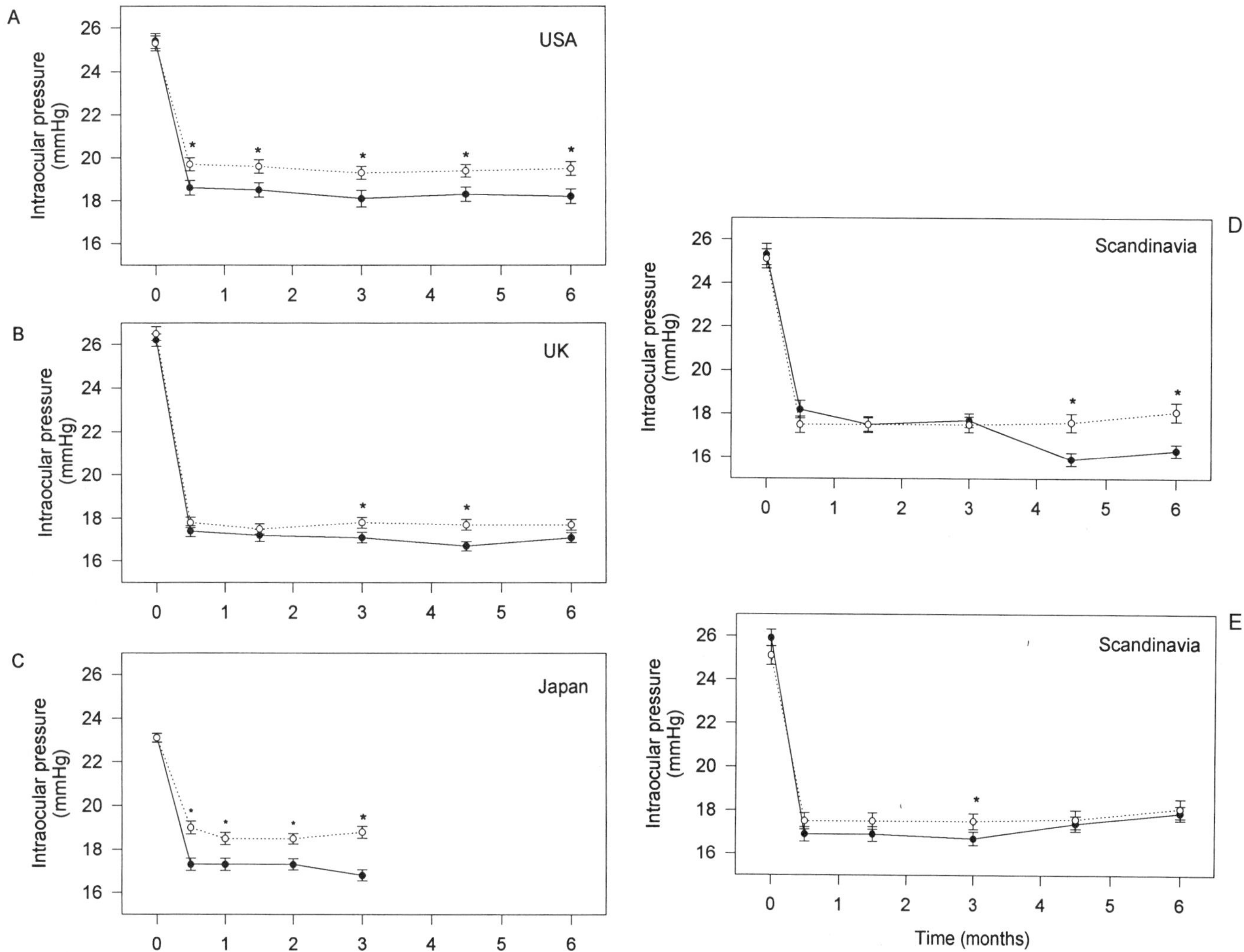

FIG. 28-4. Comparison of the effects on intraocular pressure (IOP) (measured at 8:00–9:00 AM) of latanoprost (0.005%) given once daily (solid circles) and timolol (0.5%) given twice daily (open circles) for 3 to 6 months to patients with elevated IOP. Each value is the mean IOP (±SEM) of 84 to 149 patients. **A:** Clinical trials conducted in the United States. Latanoprost significantly (p <0.001) reduced IOP more than timolol at all time points after pretreatment baseline. (Data from Camras et al., ref 64.) **B:** Clinical trials conducted in the United Kingdom. The IOPs were reduced significantly with both latanoprost and timolol and were significantly lower in the latanoprost-treated eyes compared with the timolol-treated eyes at 3 and 4.5 months. (Data from Watson et al., ref 66.) Timolol was as effective as latanoprost at the other time points. **C:** Clinical trials conducted in Japan. The IOPs were reduced significantly with both drugs. Following baseline measurements, latanoprost reduced IOP significantly more than timolol during the 3-month study. (Data from ref 94.) **D, E:** Clinical trials conducted in Scandinavia. In D, latanoprost was administered in the morning for 3 months and then treatment was switched to the evening. In E, the reverse latanoprost regimen was given. When latanoprost was given in the morning, timolol and latanoprost were equally effective in reducing IOP. When latanoprost was given in the evening, IOPs were significantly lower than when timolol was given twice daily. Asterisks indicate significant (p <0.05) differences in IOP between timolol and latanoprost treatment. (From ref 63, with permission.)

tanoprost group, a darkening of the iris color was considered definite in two patients (1%) and suspect in 13 (9%). Timolol had no effect on iris pigment in this 6-month study. Latanoprost had no effect on blood pressure and heart rate, whereas timolol significantly (p <0.02) reduced heart rate by 2 beats/minute. These effects are similar to those reported in the Scandinavia study.

U.S. Study (62,64)

Patients (n = 268) with ocular hypertension or primary open-angle glaucoma were enrolled in one of two treatment groups. The study design was similar to that of the UK trial. Compared with baseline measurements, both latanoprost and timolol caused a significant (p <0.001) and stable reduction of IOP for the 6 months of the study. In latanoprost-treated eyes, IOPs were significantly ($p < 0.001$) lower than in timolol-treated eyes at all time points. At 6 months, the mean diurnal reduction in IOP was 6.7 mm Hg (27%) with latanoprost and 4.9 mm Hg (20%) with timolol compared with baseline measurements (Fig. 28-4A).

More conjunctival hyperemia appeared in latanoprost-treated compared with timolol-treated eyes; however, the amount of hyperemia and differences between groups were slight. Fewer subjective side effects occurred in latanoprost-treated eyes than in timolol-treated eyes.

A definite change in iris color was observed in one patient in the latanoprost group (1%) and was suspected in three (2%). No pigmentation effect was observed in the timolol group.

One Year of Treatment with Latanoprost in the United States, United Kingdom, and Scandinavia (62,94)

All patients completing 6 months of treatment in the United States, United Kingdom, and Scandinavia double-masked studies were given the option of continuing on latanoprost therapy once daily in an open-label fashion for an additional 6 months. If needed, timolol 0.25% or 0.5% was added to the patient's regimen to control the IOP. Results of the first 198 patients who completed one year of therapy were evaluated to provide information on efficacy and safety for more prolonged periods.

Latanoprost significantly ($p < 0.001$) reduced diurnal IOP from a baseline of 25.3 ± 3.0 mm Hg (mean ± SD) to 17.4 ± 2.7 mm Hg (32% reduction) at 12 months with no evidence of drift. Timolol was added to the latanoprost therapy in 6% of patients. Age, gender, race, and eye color had no significant effect on the IOP reduction.

An increase in iris pigmentation was suspected or definite in 16 (8%) of the 198 patients who completed 1 year of treatment with latanoprost. Other examinations and tests were not appreciably changed a year after treatment. These tests included visual field, optic disc cupping, visual acuity, refractive error, conjunctival hyperemia, aqueous flare, anterior chamber cellular response, lens examination, blood pressure, blood tests, heart rate, and urinalysis.

Japanese Study (95)

A total of 184 patients with open-angle glaucoma or ocular hypertension were randomized to receive either 0.005% latanoprost (n = 89) once daily in the morning or 0.5% timolol maleate (n = 95) twice daily, morning and evening, for 12 weeks. The IOPs were measured at baseline and at weeks 2, 4, 8, and 12.

Latanoprost reduced the IOP at 12 weeks by 6.2 mm Hg (27%), whereas timolol reduced IOP by 4.4 mm Hg (20%). At all visits, latanoprost reduced IOP significantly ($p < 0.001$) more than timolol. An IOP reduction of 10 mm Hg or more was noted in 25% of eyes treated with latanoprost and 7% of eyes treated with timolol (Fig. 28-4C).

Mild conjunctival hyperemia was observed in 15% of patients treated with latanoprost and 9% treated with timolol. Statistical analysis of these differences was not done. In all cases, the degree of hyperemia was slight. Neither drug caused significant aqueous flare or cells in the anterior chamber. Iris color was not evaluated photographically, but the change was observed.

No serious side effects occurred in either group. There was a slight, but statistically significant ($p < 0.01$), reduction in mean heart rate of patients in the timolol group after treatment for 4 weeks or longer. Latanoprost had no effect on heart rate or blood pressure.

All the phase III studies provide clear evidence that latanoprost is a very effective ocular hypotensive agent with few side effects in patients with elevated IOP in the United States, United Kingdom, Scandinavia, and Japan.

REFERENCES

1. Bito LZ. A physiological approach to glaucoma management: the use of local hormones and the pharmacokinetics of prostaglandin esters. In: Bito L, Stjernschantz J, eds. *The Ocular Effects of Prostaglandins and Other Eiconsanoids.* New York: Alan R. Liss, 1989; 329–347.
2. Wistrand P, Stjernschantz J, Ohlsson K. The incidence and time-course of latanoprost-induced iridial pigmentation, as a function of eye color. *Surv Ophthalmol* (suppl), 1997;41(2):S129–S138.
3. Stjernschantz J, Bito LZ. The ocular effects of eicosanoids and other autacoids: Historic background and the need for a broader perspective. In: Bito L, Stjernschantz J, eds. *The Ocular Effects of Prostaglandins and Other Eiconsanoids.* New York: Alan R Liss, 1989;1–13.
4. Ambache N. Irin, a smooth-muscle contracting substance present in rabbit iris. *J Physiol* 1955;129:65P.
5. Eakins KE. Prostaglandin and non-prostaglandin mediated breakdown of the blood-aqueous barrier. *Exp Eye Res* 1977;25:483–498.
6. Bito LZ, Camras CB, Gum GG, Resul B. The ocular hypotensive effects and side effects of prostaglandins on the eyes of experimental animals. In: Bito L, Stjernschantz J, eds. *The Ocular Effects of Prostaglandins and Other Eiconsanoids.* New York: Alan R Liss, 1989; 349–368.
7. Neufeld AH, Jampol LM, Sears ML. Aspirin prevents the disruption of the blood-aqueous barrier of the rabbit eye. *Nature* 1972;238: 158–159.
8. Bito LZ. Prostaglandins: old concepts and new perspectives. *Arch Ophthalmol* 1987;105:1036–1039.
9. Kulkarni PS, Srinivasan BD. Cyclooxygenase and lipoxygenase pathways in anterior uvea and conjunctiva. In: Bito L, Stjernschantz J, eds. *The Ocular Effects of Prostaglandins and Other Eiconsanoids.* New York: Alan R Liss, 1989;39–52.
10. Bazan NG. Metabolism of arachidonic acid in the retina and retinal pigment epithelium: biological effects of oxygenated metabolites of arachidonic acid. In: Bito L, Stjernschantz J, eds. *The Ocular Effects of Prostaglandins and Other Eicosanoids.* New York: Alan R Liss, 1989;15–37.
11. Unger WG. Mediation of the ocular response to injury and irritation: Peptides versus prostaglandins. In Bito L, Stjernschantz J, eds. *The Ocular Effects of Prostaglandins and Other Eiconsanoids.* New York: Alan R Liss, 1989;293–328.
12. Bazan NG, Allan G. Signal transduction and gene expression in the eye: A contemporary view of the pro-inflammatory, anti-inflammatory, and modulatory roles of prostaglandins and other bioactive lipids. *Surv Ophthalmol* 1997 (In press)
13. Bhattacherjee P. The role of arachidonate metabolites in ocular inflammation. In: Bito L, Stjernschantz J, eds. *The Ocular Effects of*

Prostaglandins and Other Eiconsanoids. New York: Alan R Liss, 1989;211–227.

14. Brestel E, Van Dyke K. Lipid mediators of homeostasis and inflammation. In: Craig CR, Stitzel RE, eds. *Modern Pharmacology.* Boston: Little, Brown and Company, 1990;562.
15. Bito LZ. Prostaglandins: a new approach to glaucoma management with a new, intriguing side effect. *Surv Ophthalmol* 1997; (Suppl) 41(2):S1–S14.
16. Woodward DF, Regan JW, Lake S, Ocklind A. The molecular biology and ocular distribution of prostanoid receptors. *Surv Ophthalmol (Suppl)* 1997;41(2):S15–S22.
17. Schuster V. The prostaglandin transporter is widely expressed in ocular tissues. *Surv Ophthalmol* (suppl) 1997;41(2):S41–S46.
18. Masferrer J, Kulkarni P. Cyclooxygenase-2 inhibitors: A new approach to the therapy of ocular inflammation. *Surv Ophthalmol* (Suppl), 1997;41(2):S35–S40.
19. Toris CB, Yablonski ME, Camras CB, Brubaker RF. Effects of exogenous prostaglandins on aqueous humor dynamics and blood-aqueous barrier function. *Surv Ophthalmol* (suppl), 1997;41(2):S69–S76.
20. Camras CB, Alm A. Initial clinical studies with prostaglandins and their analogues. *Surv Ophthalmol* (suppl), 1997;41(2):S61–S68.
21. Giuffrè G. The effects of prostaglandin $F_{2\alpha}$ in the human eye. *Graefe's Arch Clin Exp Ophthalmol* 1985;222:139–141.
22. Lee P-Y, Shao H, Xu L, Qu C-K. The effect of prostaglandin $F_{2\alpha}$ on intraocular pressure in normotensive human subjects. *Invest Ophthalmol Vis Sci* 1988;29:1474–1477.
23. Waterbury LD, Eglen RM, Faurot GF, Cooper GF. EP_3, but not EP_2, FP, or TP prostanoid-receptor stimulation may reduce intraocular pressure. *Invest Ophthalmol Vis Sci* 1990;31:2560–2567.
24. Flach AJ, Eliason JA. Topical prostaglandin E_2 effects on normal human intraocular pressure. *J Ocular Pharm* 1988;4:13–18. [Erratum] *J Ocular Pharm* 1991;7:189.
25. Goh Y, Hirono S, Yoshimura K. Ocular hypotensive and adverse effects after topical application of prostaglandin analogue, S-1033, in animals: A comparative study with UF-021 and PhXA34. *Jpn J Ophthalmol* 1994;38:215–227.
26. Woodward DF, Hawley SB, Williams LS, et al. Studies on the ocular pharmacology of prostaglandin D_2. *Invest Ophthalmol Vis Sci* 1990; 31:138–146.
27. Woodward DF, Spada CS, Hawley SB, et al. Further studies on ocular responses to DP receptor stimulation. *Eur J Pharm* 1993;230: 327–333.
28. Nakajima M, Goh Y, Azuma I, Hayaishi O. Effects of prostaglandin D_2 and its analogue, BW245C, on intraocular pressure in humans. *Graefes Arch Clin Exp Ophthalmol* 1991;229:411–413.
29. Wang R-F, Camras CB, Lee P-Y, Podos SM. Effect of BW245C, a prostaglandin (PG) D_2-sensitive (DP) agonist, on aqueous humor dynamics after topical application in monkeys and rabbits. *Invest Ophthalmol Vis Sci* 1991;(suppl)32:990.
30. Bito LZ, Baroody RA. The ocular pharmacokinetics of eicosanoids and their derivatives. 1. Comparison of ocular eicosanoid penetration and distribution following the topical application of $PGF_{2\alpha}$, $PGF_{2\alpha}$-methyl ester, and $PGF_{2\alpha}$-1-isopropyl ester. *Exp Eye Res* 1987;44:217–226.
31. Bito LZ. Comparison of the ocular hypotensive efficacy of eicosanoids and related compounds. *Exp Eye Res* 1984;38:181–194.
32. Camras CB, Podos SM. Reduction of intraocular pressure by exogenous and endogenous prostaglandins in monkeys and humans. In: Drance SM, Van Buskirk EM, Neufeld AH, eds. *Pharmacology of Glaucoma.* Baltimore: Williams & Wilkins, 1992;175–183.
33. Wang R-F, Camras CB, Lee P-Y, et al. Effects of prostaglandins $F_{2\alpha}$, A_2, and their esters in glaucomatous monkey eyes. *Invest Ophthalmol Vis Sci* 1990;31:2466–2470.
34. Villumsen J, Alm A. Prostaglandin $F_{2\alpha}$-isopropyl ester eye drops: effects in normal human eyes. *Br J Ophthalmol* 1989;73:419–426.
35. Camras CB, Siebold EC, Lustgarten JS, et al. Maintained reduction of intraocular pressure by prostaglandin $F_{2\alpha}$-1-isopropyl ester applied in multiple doses in ocular hypertensive and glaucoma patients. *Ophthalmology* 1989;96:1329–1337.
36. Villumsen J, Alm A. Ocular effects of two different prostaglandin $F_{2\alpha}$ esters: a double masked cross-over study on normotensive eyes. *Acta Ophthalmol* 1990;68:341–343.
37. Ando Y, Matsunami C, Yamamoto T, Kitazawa Y. Ocular hypotensive effect of a new prostaglandin analogue, S-1033, in normal human volunteers. *Jpn J Ophthalmol* 1994;38:337–342.
38. Takase M, Murao M, Koyano S, Ueno R. Ocular effects of continuous topical instillations of UF-021 ophthalmic solution in healthy volunteers. *Atarashii Ganka (J Eye)* 1992;9:1055–1059.
39. Takase M, Murao M, Koyano S, et al. Ocular effects of topical instillation of UF-021 ophthalmic solution in healthy volunteers. *Nippon Ganka Gakkai Zasshi* 1992;96:1261–1267.
40. Sakurai M, Araie M, Oshika T, et al. Effects of topical application of UF-021, a novel prostaglandin derivative, on aqueous humor dynamics in normal human eyes. *Jpn J Ophthalmol* 1991;35:156–165.
41. Azuma I, Masuda K, Kitazawa Y, et al. Phase II double-masked dose-determination study of UF-021 ophthalmic solution in primary open-angle glaucoma and ocular hypertension. *Nippon Ganka Kiyo* 1992;43:1425–1431.
42. Azuma I, Masudo K, Kitazawa Y, Takase M, et al. Double-masked comparative study of UF-021 and timolol ophthalmic solutions in patients with primary open-angle glaucoma or ocular hypertension. *Jpn J Ophthalmol* 1993;37:514–525.
43. Azuma I, Masuda K, Kitazawa Y, Takase M. Long-term study of UF-021 (Rescula) ophthalmic solution in patients with primary open-angle glaucoma and ocular hypertension. *Atarasii Ganka (J Eye)* 1994;11:1435–1444.
44. Yamamoto T, Kitazawa Y, Azuma I, Masuda K. Clinical evaluation of UF-021 (Rescula; isopropyl unoprostone). *Surv Ophthalmol* (suppl), 1997 (In press)
45. Miller WL, Weeks JR, Lauderdale JW, Kirton KT. Biological activities of 17-phenyl-18,19,20-trinorprostaglandins. *Prostaglandins* 1975; 9:9–18.
46. Stjernschantz J. Prostaglandins as ocular hypotensive agents; development of an analogue for glaucoma treatment. In: Samuelsson B, et al., eds. *Advances in Prostaglandin, Thromboxane, and Leukotriene Research,* vol 23. New York: Raven Press, 1995;63–68.
47. Stjernschantz J. Selen G, Sjöquist B, Resul B. Preclinical pharmacology of latanoprost, a phenyl-substituted $PGF_{2\alpha}$ analogue. In: Samuelsson B et al., eds. *Advances in Prostaglandin, Thromboxane, and Leukotriene Research,* vol 23. New York: Raven Press, 1995; 513–518.
48. Resul B, Stjernschantz J, Selen G, Bito LZ. Structure-activity relationships and receptor profiles of some ocular hypotensive prostanoids. *Surv Ophthalmol* (Suppl), 1997; (In press)
49. Resul B, Stjernschantz J, No K, et al. Phenyl-substituted prostaglandins: potent and selective antiglaucoma agents. *J Med Chem* 1993;36:243–248.
50. Stjernschantz J, Resul B, Marsk A, et al. Phenyl substituted prostaglandin esters—effects in the eye. *Invest Ophthalmol Vis Sci* 1991; 32(suppl):1257.
51. Justin N, Wang R-F, Camras CB, et al. Effect of PhXA34, a new prostaglandin (PG) derivative, on intraocular pressure (IOP) after topical application to glaucomatous monkey eyes. *Invest Ophthalmol Vis Sci* 1991;32(suppl):947.
52. Alm A, Villumsen J. PhXA34, a new potent ocular hypotensive drug. *Arch Ophthalmol* 1991;109:1564–1568.
53. Hotehama Y, Mishima HK. Clinical efficacy of PhXA34 and PhXA41, two novel prostaglandin $F_{2\alpha}$-isopropyl ester analogues for glaucoma treatment. *Jpn J Ophthalmol* 1993;37:259–269.
54. Camras CB, Schumer RA, Marsk A, et al. Intraocular pressure reduction with PhXA34, a new prostaglandin analogue, in patients with ocular hypertension. *Arch Ophthalmol* 1992;110:1733–1738.
55. Villumsen J, Alm A. PhXA34—a prostaglandin $F_{2\alpha}$ analogue: Effect on intraocular pressure in patients with ocular hypertension. *Br J Ophthalmol* 1992;76:214–217.
56. Stjernschantz J, Resul B. Phenyl substituted prostaglandin analogs for glaucoma treatment. *Drugs of the Future* 1992;17:691–704.
57. Alm A, Villumsen J, Törnquist P, et al. Intraocular pressure-reducing effect of PhXA41 in patients with increased eye pressure: A one-month study. *Ophthalmology* 1993;100:1312–1317.
58. Hotehama Y, Mishima HK, Kitazawa Y, Masuda K. Ocular hypotensive effect of PhXA41 in patients with ocular hypertension or primary open-angle glaucoma. *Jpn J Ophthalmol* 1993;37:270–274.
59. Nagasubramanian S, Sheth GP, Hitchings RA, Stjernschantz J. Intraocular pressure-reducing effect of PhXA41 in ocular hypertension. *Ophthalmology* 1993;100:1305–1311.
60. Rácz P, Ruzsonyi MR, Nagy ZT, Bito LZ. Maintained intraocular pressure reduction with once-a-day application of a new prostaglandin $F_{2\alpha}$ analogue (PhXA41). *Arch Ophthalmol* 1993;111:657–661.
61. Alm A. Comparative phase III clinical trial of latanoprost and timo-

lol in patients with elevated intraocular pressure. In: Samuelsson B et al., eds. *Advances in Prostaglandin, Thromboxane, and Leukotriene Research,* vol 23. New York: Raven Press, 1995;527–532.

62. Alm A, Camras CB, Watson PG. Phase III latanoprost studies in Scandinavia, the United Kingdom and the United States. *Ophthalmol* (Suppl) 1997;41(2):S105–S110.
63. Alm A, Stjernschantz J, the Scandinavian Latanoprost Study Group. Effects on intraocular pressure and side effects of 0.005% latanoprost applied once daily, evening or morning: a comparison with timolol. *Ophthalmology* 1995;102:1743–1752.
64. Camras CB, the United States Latanoprost Study Group. Comparison of latanoprost and timolol in patients with ocular hypertension and glaucoma: a six-month, masked, multicenter trial in the United States. *Ophthalmology* 1996;103:138–147.
65. Camras CB, Bito LZ, Parkhede U, et al. Comparison of latanoprost and timolol in patients with ocular hypertension and glaucoma—preliminary results of the USA multicenter trial. In: Krieglstein GK, ed. *Glaucoma Update,* vol V. Heidelberg: Springer-Verlag, 1995;205–216.
66. Watson P, Stjernschantz J, the Latanoprost Study Group. A six-month, randomized, double-masked study comparing latanoprost with timolol in open-angle glaucoma and ocular hypertension. *Ophthalmology* 1996;103:126–137.
67. Sjöquist B, Byding P, Resul B, Stjernschantz J. The systemic pharmacokinetics of latanoprost in man after intravenous and topical administration. *Invest Ophthalmol Vis Sci* 1994;35(suppl):2220.
68. Bito LZ, Stjernschantz J, Resul B, et al. The ocular effects of prostaglandins and the therapeutic potential of a new $PGF_{2\alpha}$ analog, PhXA41 (latanoprost), for glaucoma management. *J Lipid Med* 1993;6:535–543.
69. Goh Y, Nakajima M, Azuma I, Hayaishi O. Effects of prostaglandin D_2 and its analogues on intraocular pressure in rabbits. *Jpn J Ophthalmol* 1988;32:471–480.
70. Villumsen J, Alm A, Söderström M. Prostaglandin $F_{2\alpha}$-isopropylester eye drops: effect on intraocular pressure in open-angle glaucoma. *Br J Ophthalmol* 1989;73:975–979.
71. Woodward DF, Chan MF, Burke JA, et al. Studies on the ocular hypotensive effects of prostaglandin $F_{2\alpha}$ ester prodrugs and receptor selective prostaglandin analogs. *J Ocul Pharmacol* 1994;10: 177–193.
72. Kerstetter Jr, Brubaker RF, Wilson SE, Kullerstrand LF. Prostaglandin $F_{2\alpha}$-1-isopropyl ester lowers intraocular pressure without decreasing aqueous humor flow. *Am J Ophthalmol* 1988;105:30–34.
73. Ziai N, Dolan JW, Kacere RD, Brubaker RF. The effects on aqueous dynamics of PhXA41, a new prostaglandin $F_{2\alpha}$ analogue, after topical application in normal and ocular hypertensive human eyes. *Arch Ophthalmol* 1993;111:1351–1358.
74. Diestelhorst M, Roters S, Krieglstein GK. The effect of latanoprost (PHXA41) on the intraocular pressure and aqueous humor protein concentration: A randomized, double masked comparison of 50 μg/ml vs 15 μg/ml with timolol 0.5% as control. *Invest Ophthalmol Vis Sci* 1995;(Suppl) 36:S823.
75. Diestelhorst M, Krieglstein GK, Lusky M, Nagasubramanian S. Dose-finding and dose-regimen studies with latanoprost, a new ocular hypotensive $PGF_{2\alpha}$ analogue. *Surv Ophthalmol* (Suppl), 1997; 41(2):S77–S82.
76. Barsotti MF, Bartels SP, Freddo TF, Kamm RD. The source of protein in the aqueous humor of the normal monkey eye. *Invest Ophthalmol Vis Sci* 1992;33:581–595.
77. Camras CB, Bhuyan KC, Podos SM, Bhuyan DK, Master RWP. Multiple dosing of prostaglandin $F_{2\alpha}$ or epinephrine on cynomolgus monkey eyes. II. Slit-lamp biomicroscopy, aqueous humor analysis and fluorescein angiography. *Invest Ophthalmol Vis Sci* 1987;28: 921–926.
78. Astin M, Gjotterberg M, Holst A, et al. Fluorescein angiographic study of the fundus in phakic and aphakic monkey eyes treated with PhXA41. *Invest Ophthalmol Vis Sci* 1992;33(suppl):1078.
79. Camras CB, Friedman AH, Rodrigues MM, et al. Multiple dosing of prostaglandin $F_{2\alpha}$ or epinephrine on cynomolgus monkey eyes. III. Histopathology. *Invest Ophthalmol Vis Sci* 1988;29:1428–1436.
80. Svedbergh B, Forsberg I. A morphological study on the effects of chronic administration of latanoprost (LP) on the ciliary muscle and trabecular meshwork in monkeys. *Invest Ophthalmol Vis Sci* 1993;34 (suppl):932.
81. Rulo A, Greve E, Hoyng P, Alm A. A study of the effect of latanoprost on the intraocular pressure and retinal vasculature in pseudophakic patients. *Invest Ophthalmol Vis Sci* 1994;(suppl)35:1483.
82. Selen G, Stjernschantz J, Resul B. Prostaglandin-induced iridial pigmentation in primates. *Surv Ophthalmol* (suppl), 1997;41(2): S125–S128.
83. Nordlund JJ. The pigmentary system: An expanded perspective. *Ann Dermatol* 1994;6:109–123.
84. Laties A. Ocular melanin and the adrenergic innervation to the eye. *Trans Am Ophthalmol Soc* 1974;72:560–605.
85. Imesch PD, Wallow IHL, Spritz RA, Albert DM. The color of the human eye: A review of morphologic correlates and some conditions that affect iridial pigmentation. *Surv Ophthalmol* (Suppl), 1997; 41(2):S117–S125.
86. Camras CB, Zhan GL, Wang YL, et al. Effect of sympathectomy (SX) and prostaglandin (PG) analog (latanoprost) treatment on iris color in pigmented rabbits. *Invest Ophthalmol Vis Sci* 1995; 36(suppl):S720.
87. Matheny AP, Dolan AB. Changes in eye colour during early childhood: Sex and genetic differences. *Ann Hum Biol* 1975;2:191–196.
88. Carino OB, Matheny AP, DeRousseau CJ, Bito LZ. Changes in iridial pigmentation past childhood through adolescence. *Invest Ophthalmol Vis Sci* 1994;35(suppl):1530.
89. Eagle RC. Iris pigmentation and pigmented lesions: an ultrastructural study. *Trans Am Ophthalmol Soc* 1988;88:581–687.
90. Nugteren DH. The determination of prostaglandin metabolites in human urine. *J Biol Chem* 1975;250:2808–2812.
91. Hedner J, Svedmyr N, Lunde H, Mandahl A. The lack of respiratory effects of the ocular hypotensive drug latanoprost in patients with moderate steroid treated asthma. *Surv Ophthalmol (suppl)* 1997; 41(2):S111–S116.
92. Campbell WB, Halushka PV. Lipid-derived autacoids: Eicosanoids and platelet-activating factor. In: Mardman JG, Limbird LE, Molinoff PB, Ruddon RW, Gilman AG, eds. *The Pharmacological Basis of Therapeutics,* 9th ed. New York: McGraw-Hill, 1996;601–616.
93. Camras CB, Alm A, Watson P, et al. Latanoprost, a prostaglandin analog, for glaucoma therapy: efficacy and safety after one year of treatment in 198 patients. *Ophthalmology* 1996;103:1916–1924.
94. Mishima HK, Kiuchi Y, Takamatsu M, et al. Circadian intraocular pressure management with latanoprost: diurnal and nocturnal intraocular pressure reduction and increased uveoscieral outflow. *Surv. Opthalmol* (Suppl) 1997:41(2).
95. Wistrand PJ. Carbonic anhydrase in the anterior uvea of the rabbit. *Acta Physiol Scand* 1951;24:144.
96. Bito L, Stjernschantz J (eds): *The Ocular Effects of Prostaglandins and Other Eicosanoids.* New York: Alan R Liss, Inc, 1989.
97. Sjoquist B, Johansson A. The ocular pharmacokinetics of latanoprost, a new antiglaucoma drug, studied by autoradiography. *Invest Ophthalmol Vis Sci* (Suppl) 1995;36:S823.
98. Bito LZ. Species differences in the responses of the eye to irritation and trauma: A hypothesis of divergence in ocular defense mechanisms, and the choice of experimental animals for eye research. *Exp Eye Res* 1984;39:807–829.
99. Brubaker RF. Fluorophotometric studies of prostaglandin effects on the human eye: The lack of association of reduced intraocular pressure with altered flow or barrier function. In: Bito L, Stjernschantz J (eds). *The Ocular Effects of Prostaglandins and Other Eiconsanoids.* New York: Alan R Liss, Inc. 1989;477–481.
100. Camras CB, Podos SM. The role of endogenous prostaglandins in clinically-used and investigational glaucoma therapy. In: Bito L, Stjernschantz J (eds). *The Ocular Effects of Prostaglandins and Other Eiconsanoids.* New York: Alan R Liss, Inc. 1989;459–475.
101. Wilkerson CL, Syed NA, Fisher MR, et al. Melaonocytes and iris color. Light microscopic findings. *Arch Ophthalmol* 1996;114: 437–442.
102. Imesch PD, Bindley CD, Khademian Z, et al. Melanocytes and iris color. Electronic microscopic findings. *Arch Ophthalmol* 1996;114: 443–447.

Textbook of Ocular Pharmacology,
edited by T.J. Zimmerman, et al.
Lippincott–Raven Publishers, Philadelphia © 1997.

CHAPTER 29

Future Role of Neuroprotective Agents in Glaucoma

Ozlem Evrem Abbasoglu and Karanjit S. Kooner

In 1989, Hoskins and Kass stressed the traditional definition of glaucoma as "a disturbance of the structural or functional integrity of the eye that can be arrested or diminished by adequate lowering of intraocular pressure (IOP)" (1). Another well-accepted definition stated that glaucoma was "a disease characterized by IOP sufficient to cause either temporary or permanent impairment of vision" (2). In both definitions, glaucoma is considered a disease condition in which high IOP is the sole reason for optic nerve damage. Considering that there are patients who show characteristic glaucomatous cupping and visual field changes with normal IOP (normal-tension glaucoma) and some with high IOP without any evidence of optic nerve damage or visual field loss (ocular hypertension), there should be several factors other than IOP that make the optic nerve susceptible to glaucomatous optic atrophy. The definition of glaucoma has been broadened in such a way to include all patients most appropriately. Only if we believe IOP is the sole causative factor in glaucoma may we define glaucoma as "a disorder in which the intraocular pressure exceeds the level that is tolerated by the optic nerve" (3).

Intraocular pressure, no doubt, is an important risk factor for the development of glaucoma. A number of studies showed the close relation between high IOP and glaucoma. In an experimental glaucoma model, high IOP was induced in one eye of monkeys, and the other eye was used as a control (4). Severe degenerative changes occurred in the eyes with higher IOP and longer duration of glaucoma. Cartwright et al. reported that in patients with normal-tension glaucoma exhibiting asymmetric IOP, glaucomatous cupping and visual field loss were greater in eyes with higher pressure (5). Other studies also showed that, in the presence of unequal IOPs, visual damage is almost always greater on the side with higher mean IOP (6). In experimental models, high IOP appears to cause obstruction of axonal transport (7).

Quigley reviewed the effect of IOP on the optic nerve (8). He considered the scleral canal a defect in the eye wall. Because of the pressure differential between the eye and the optic nerve tissue, there is an inside-out vector of force. This vector is present in all ranges of IOP. The condition that makes the nerve head more susceptible to a certain IOP is the susceptibility of the eye's connective tissues, vasculature, and neurons to these forces. His other studies showed that even in the advanced glaucomatous optic neuropathies, optic nerve head vasculature may be well preserved (9). The site of susceptibility to increased IOP was found to be at the level of lamina cribrosa of the optic nerve. Although this finding seems to oppose the vascular theory, the functional status of the vasculature was not considered.

Wide variation of clinical presentations of glaucomatous optic neuropathy shows that there are some factors other than IOP causing optic neuropathy. The Baltimore Eye Survey Group reported that half of all glaucomatous eyes had IOPs below 21 mm Hg on initial examination (10). In some patients, although IOP is decreased satisfactorily, progression of optic neuropathy can be seen (11). This finding implies that there is no cut-off point for safe IOP. Several factors may act in combination to cause optic nerve damage. There is evidence of a relation between vascular vasospasm and ocular circulation. Guthauser et al. demonstrated that visual fields of patients with ocular vasospasm may deteriorate after exposing one hand to cold water and improve after administration of nifedipine (12). Others have seen increased prevalence of peripheral vasospasm in patients with glaucoma compared with normal controls (13). Migraine headaches, which are believed to

O. E. Abbasoglu and K. S. Kooner: Department of Ophthalmology, University of Texas Southwestern Medical Center at Dallas, Dallas, Texas 75235-9057.

be due to a vasospastic disorder, are also more common in patients with normal-tension glaucoma (14).

Other well-known risk factors for glaucomatous damage are age, race, myopia, diabetes, and hypertension (3). Results of a prospective study investigating the risk factors for glaucomatous visual field defects showed that out of 26 factors only outflow facility, age, IOP, cup-to-disc ratio, and pressure change after water drinking were significant in the development of visual field changes (15). With multivariate analysis, however, their collective predictive power was quite poor, showing some other, yet unknown risk factors exist that cause glaucomatous optic neuropathy.

Recently, Brubaker discussed the well-recognized situation of patients exhibiting progressive visual-field defects long after normalization of their IOP (16). He presented several hypotheses to explain the delayed functional loss. First, a process independent of IOP may kill ganglion cells, such as the toxic effects of neurotransmitters like glutamate or inappropriate vasoconstrictive activity. Second, undetected increases of IOP may kill ganglion cells. Third, the ganglion cells may have a genetically determined hypersensitivity to IOP. Fourth, the ganglion cells may have been rendered hypersensitive to IOP by irreversible damaging effects of previously increased IOP. Finally, apoptosis was discussed as an additional possible mechanism for glaucomatous optic neuropathy.

The multifactorial analysis of the causes of glaucomatous optic neuropathy shows that decreasing IOP may not prevent the progression of glaucoma. Our treatment modalities should consider additional neuroprotection. Current understanding of neuronal death shows that, independent of the insult (ischemia, trauma, hypoglycemia, etc.), the pathophysiological changes in neuronal death have a common pathway (17). The optic nerve, being an extension of the central nervous system (CNS), may respond similarly to different insults. Many investigators are trying different approaches to make the nerves more resistant to those insults. This chapter emphasizes the common pathway for neuronal death and current implications for neuronal protection as a future approach for glaucoma therapy. Several articles have discussed neurological advances in cellular death in the CNS as pertaining to ocular diseases (18–20).

PATHOPHYSIOLOGY OF NEURONAL DEATH

Recent studies showed that many different kinds of insults to the nerves (e.g., ischemia, hypoglycemia, hereditary, and degenerative neurological diseases) cause damage by a common pathway (17,19). This final common pathway for neuronal death is mediated by the excitatory amino acids glutamate and aspartate. Glutamate and aspartate are the major excitatory amino acids in the CNS. Glutamate receptors are located on virtually all neurons in the CNS, and glutamate is capable of exciting almost all cells of the CNS (21).

Excitotoxicity refers to the clinical condition in which these amino acids excite the nerve excessively, resulting in neurotoxicity and neuronal death (19,22). Some other structurally related amino acids are capable of inducing the excitotoxic damage, like *N*-methyl D-aspartate (NMDA), homocysteate, cysteine sulfinate, and cysteate (23). In 1957 Lucas and Newhouse reported the toxic effects of L-glutamate on the inner layers of retina (24). Cytotoxicity of glutamate in the rat CNS was shown by Olney et al., the pioneers in this field (23).

NERVE INJURY

Mechanisms of excitotoxic nerve injury are reviewed by Choi (25). Following injury to the neuron in the form of ischemia, trauma, or hypoglycemia, excitatory amino acids are released into the surrounding medium (Fig. 29-1). Once glutamate is released into the medium, it activates two kinds of receptors: ionotropic and metabotropic. Ionotropic receptors are identified by their preferred agonists: NMDA, alpha-amino-3-hydroxy 5-methyl 4-isoxandepropionic acid (AMPA), and kainate (KA). Metabotropic receptors are coupled to G-regulatory protein. A few minutes after the release of glutamate, Na^+ enters into the cell primarily via AMPA receptor channels. Chloride ion and water passively diffuse into the cell following Na^+, resulting in cellular swelling. These pathophysiological events represent the *acute phase* of neuronal injury. Cellular swelling is infrequently lethal. The cell may recover, depending on the severity of the insult.

In the second phase (*delayed phase*), calcium ion enters the cell primarily via NMDA channels. Ca^{++} influx also occurs indirectly through non-NMDA receptors. Depolariza-

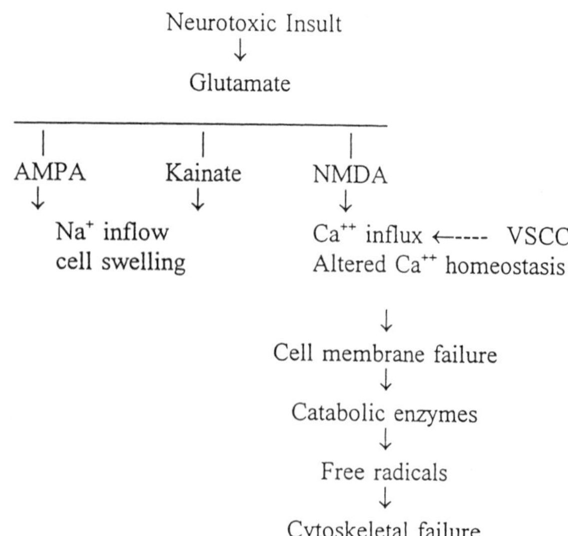

FIG. 1. Proposed neurotoxic cellular pathways (AMPA = alpha-amino-3-hydroxy 5-methyl 4-isoxandepropionic acid; NMDA = N-methyl D-asparate; VSCC = voltage sensitive Ca^{++} channels).

tion causes Ca^{++} influx through voltage-sensitive Ca^{++} channels (VSCC) or receptor-operated Ca^{++} channels. All these reactions cause altered calcium homeostasis in the cell and induce a cascade of metabolic reactions. Increased cytoplasmic calcium can activate a variety of Ca^{++}-dependent enzymes, including protein kinase C, phospholipase A2, phospholipase C, Ca/calmodulin-dependent protein kinase II, nitric oxide synthase, and various proteases and endonucleases (21). Ca^{++} activates protease and lipase, leading to the formation of free fatty acids and destruction of membrane stability. Once the enzyme phospholipase is activated, it breaks down the cell membrane, liberating phospholipase A2, which triggers arachidonic acid and free radical formation and also liberates endonuclease, which breaks the DNA genome. Increased intracellular calcium also leads to calcium accumulation in the mitochondria, thus disturbing the oxidative phosphorylation process and causing a decrease in adenosine triphosphate (ATP) synthesis. The reaction further leads to anaerobic metabolism of glucose, causing accumulation of lactose. Lactose accumulation results in cell acidosis, disturbance in metabolic functions, and decreased buffering capacity of the cell resulting in the cell death. Another action of Ca^{++} is conversion of xanthine dehydrogenase to xanthine oxidase, a rich enzymatic source of free radicals.

Murphy et al. suggested that glutamate exposure and high intracellular calcium levels decrease cysteine uptake (26). Cysteine is an important precursor for glutathione synthesis, and glutathione is important for the removal of free radicals. Once its production is decreased, free radicals accumulate in the cell, further disturbing cellular metabolic functions and increasing vulnerability to stress. Calcium increases the excitation process by further activating NMDA channels.

Glutamate also activates metabotropic receptors. Stimulation of metabotropic receptors causes activation of G protein, which in turn activates phospholipase C. Activated phospholipase C induces hydrolysis of phosphotidyl inositol 4,5-biphosphate, which liberates the dual messengers inositol 1,4,5-triphosphate (IP3) and diacylglycerol (DAG). In the presence of calcium, DAG activates protein kinase C, calmodulin, and calmodulin kinase II. Protein kinase alters the phosphorylation of proteins, which are integral parts of receptor and ion channels, which disturbs cellular function. It also induces Ca^{++}-dependent glutamate release and calcium entry through VSCCs. Also, IP3 causes Ca^{++} release from endoplasmic reticulum, further increasing intracellular calcium levels. The importance of calcium is evident from the finding that neurons containing high concentrations of calcium-binding proteins are relatively resistant to excitotoxic injury.

Glutamate is present in the nerve terminals in synaptic vesicles. It is concentrated in these vesicles by active transport (27). Upon depolarization of the nerve terminal, glutamate is released into the synaptic cleft. Glutamate generates its effects via specific glutamate receptors. Neurons and glial cells have carriers that are responsible for removal of glutamate from the synaptic cleft (28). The removal of glutamate from the nerve terminals stops glutamate's effect on neurons. Glutamate that is carried to glial cells or neurons by the carriers is recycled and again concentrated in synaptic vesicles. In normal conditions, glutamate is removed from the synaptic cleft efficiently.

Excitotoxicity occurs when nerves are stimulated excessively so that they lose their Ca^{++} homeostasis and can occur in several ways (29). Excitotoxicity may be seen when there is hypersensitivity of postsynaptic neurons to glutamate, insufficient removal of glutamate, or any abnormality at the level of glutamate receptors. Also, in some disease states, glutamate receptors show an abnormally high Ca^{++} conductance. In hypoxic and ischemic states, large increases in extracellular glutamate and marked depression of glutamate uptake system occur (30,31).

Another pathway of cellular death after exposure to excitotoxic amino acids is programmed cellular suicide, namely *apoptosis* (16). The loss of calcium homeostasis causes apoptosis (32). Apoptosis differs from necrosis in that it is an active process. The cell synthesizes new enzymes for organized condensation of its nucleus and convolution of both nuclear and plasma membranes, allowing preservation of membrane and organelle stability and enabling the cell to die without liberating its digestive enzymes, which could harm neighboring cells.

EXCITOTOXICITY AND DISEASES OF THE EYE AND GLAUCOMA

Various experimental models showed excitotoxicity to be mediated by glutamate in the CNS and also in retina. A recent study by Dreyer and Lipton was conducted to determine whether the mechanism of neuronal cell loss in glaucoma was mediated via glutamate excitotoxicity (33). Vitreous specimens from patients with open-angle glaucoma were analyzed for their amino acid levels and compared with those of normal subjects. Only glutamate concentrations were significantly higher in patients with glaucoma. The investigators concluded that glutamate-mediated excitotoxicity may play a role in retinal ganglion cell death in glaucoma.

Lucas and Newhouse were the first to demonstrate toxic effects of glutamate on the inner retinal layers, especially retinal ganglion cells, after subcutaneous injection of glutamate in rats (24). More recently, Sesma et al. explored the sensitivity of retinal ganglion cells to different subtypes of excitotoxins (34). They injected NMDA and KA intravitreally into one eye of rats and used the other eye as control. Their results showed that ganglion cell loss was significant in both NMDA- and KA-treated eyes.

Dreyer et al. suggested that larger retinal ganglion cells are more sensitive to NMDA receptor-mediated neurotoxicity both in vivo and in vitro (35). Their studies in tissue culture and intact rat eye have demonstrated that cells smaller than 10 μm were relatively unaffected by glutamate or NMDA. These agents were markedly toxic to retinal ganglion cells 10 >μm. Their observations indicate that glutamate-mediated loss is seen first in larger retinal ganglion cells, in a fashion similar to the pattern of loss seen in glaucoma (8).

Another study, by Caprioli and Kitano, investigated the effect of excitotoxic and hypoxic damage on cultured rat retinal ganglion cells (36). Their results showed that large rat retinal ganglion cells are more susceptible to excitotoxic and hypoxic damage than smaller cells. They also emphasized that this susceptibility is consistent with observations of preferential loss of larger ganglion cells in glaucoma.

This preferential susceptibility of large ganglion cells to excitotoxic injury may help to explain the pathophysiology of glaucoma. Excitotoxicity is a common final pathway for neuronal damage after different insults to the CNS. If glaucomatous optic neuropathy (either by mechanical injury or vascular insufficiency) occurs as a result of toxicity of excitatory amino acids (EAAs), drugs that modulate excitotoxicity may help to prevent optic neuropathy (18,20).

MECHANISMS OF DRUG ACTIONS FOR NEUROPROTECTION

The principal causative factor in excitotoxicity, regardless of the causative problem, is the disturbed intracellular calcium metabolism that causes neuronal death. Several drugs may potentially prevent excitotoxicity, such as Ca^{++} channel antagonists, EAA receptor antagonists, nitric oxide inhibitors, and free-radical scavengers (18,20,37) (Table 29-1).

Calcium-channel Blockers

Fleckenstein and Godfraind et al. first proposed that calcium-channel blockers become active on excitation-contraction coupling in myocardium (38,39). The same group developed verapamil, nifedipine, and diltiazem, which are widely used for coronary artery disease and systemic hypertension.

In glaucoma, calcium-channel blockers have three potential applications: for their effect on IOP (*ocular hypotension*); on vascular smooth muscles (*vasodilatation*), thereby improving optic nerve blood flow; and on intracel-

TABLE 29-1. *Drugs currently being evaluated for neuroprotection*

- Calcium-channel blockers
  - SNX-III
  - Flunarizine
  - Nimodipine
  - Nicardipine
  - Levemopamil
- Calcium chelators
  - BAPTA-AM
- EAA antagonists
  - Drugs that decrease glutamate release
    - Sodium channel blockers
      - 619C89
      - Lamotrigine
      - Riluzole
      - Lubeluzole
      - CNS 1237 (Na^{+} and Ca^{++} channels blocker)
    - Kappa opioid agonists
      - CI977
  - Drugs that block glutamate receptors
    - Acting on NMDA receptors (noncompetitive)
      - Aptiganel HCl (CNS 1102)
      - Phencyclidine
      - Ketamine
      - Dextromethorphan derivatives (Ro-01-6794/706)
      - Remacemide hydrochloride
      - Magnesium
      - Dizocilpine (MK 801)
    - Acting on NMDA receptors (competitive)
      - AP5
      - AP7
      - APV
      - d-CCPene
      - CGS 19755
    - Glycine site antagonists
      - ACEA 1021 and 1031
    - Polyamine site antagonists
      - Ifenprodil
      - Eliprodil
    - AMPA receptor antagonists
      - NBQX
      - GYKI 52466
- Nitric oxide inhibitors
  - Nitric oxide synthase inhibitor
    - Nitroarginine
  - PARS inhibitor
    - Benzamine derivatives
  - Calcineurin antagonists
    - FK 506
    - Cyclosporin A
- Oxygen radical scavengers
  - Endogenous
    - Vitamin E
    - Beta-carotene
    - Ascorbic acid
    - DHLA
  - Xanthine oxidase inhibitors
    - Allopurinol
- Others
  - Dimethylthiourea
  - 21 (lazaroids) aminosteroids (U7400GF
  - Carvedilol
  - HU-211

EAA, excitatory amino acids; CNS, central nervous system.

lular calcium metabolism (*neuroprotection*). Tsien identified five types of voltage-dependent calcium channels and named them according to their electrophysiological and pharmacological properties (40). *L-type* Ca^{++} channels (L stands for the "long-lasting" action of these channels) are activated by high voltage and are inactivated slowly so that they have long-lasting current. They are found in all excitable and in many nonexcitable cells, primarily in the heart, smooth and skeletal muscles, and some neurons. They are involved in excitation–contraction and secretion processes. *T-type* Ca^{++} channels (T stands for their "transient" action and "tiny" structure) are low-voltage-activated channels and are found primarily in heart, smooth muscles, and endocrine cells. They have spontaneous pacemaker activity. *N-type* Ca^{++} channels (N stands for "neuronal" and "non-L and non-T") are high-voltage-activated channels that show a moderate rate of inactivation. They are found only in neurons and are active in neurotransmitter release. *P-type* Ca^{++} channels (newly defined Ca^{++} channels; P stands for "Purkinje") are moderately high-voltage-activated and noninactivated type Ca^{++} channels. They are found in some CNS neurons, like cerebellar Purkinje cells. Recently, a fifth subclass of calcium channels was identified, called *Q-type* Ca^{++} channels (41). Closely related to P-type channels, they are presynaptic calcium channels and are involved in neurotransmitter release.

The use of Ca^{++} channel blockers in the treatment of normal-tension glaucoma is a new approach. There are several conflicting reports regarding the effect of Ca^{++} channel blockers on IOP, but the general tendency is toward a decrease in IOP. Experimental animal studies have shown a mild increase or no change in IOP with Ca^{++} channel blockers, whereas the application of these drugs in normal human subjects, ocular hypertensives, and primary open-angle glaucoma patients has generally shown a decrease in IOP (42). The mechanism of action of these drugs is mainly increased outflow facility (43). The other action of calcium-channel blockers that may be useful in normal-tension glaucoma is vasodilatation, which may increase blood flow to the optic nerve. In at least some patients with normal-tension glaucoma, it is believed the blood flow to the optic nerve is compromised, causing optic nerve damage (42). Netland et al. compared the visual-field progression of patients with open-angle glaucoma or normal-tension glaucoma who were using calcium-channel blockers with similar patients who were not taking such medications. They reported that the use of calcium-channel blockers was associated with a slowed progression of visual-field deterioration in normal-tension glaucoma (44).

Calcium homeostasis is vital for neural function. Currently, direct "neural" effects of calcium-channel blockers are under investigation for their presumed neuroprotective function and their role in neuronal survival by maintaining calcium homeostasis. It is generally accepted that the neuroprotective effect is due to a neuronal site of action of the drugs (37). There are several ways by which calcium-channel blockers may be neuroprotective. The first is their action on presynaptic neurons to decrease the neurotransmitter release and, second, their inhibition of calcium influx via the VSCC.

Recent evidence suggests that N-, P-, and Q-type channels all contribute to the presynaptic regulation of glutamate release in the CNS (45). SNX-111 (the cone snail peptide w-conotoxin M-VII-A) blocks neurotransmitter release by blocking N-type channels. It was effective in animal models of transient global ischemia (46) and is currently in human clinical trials for the prevention of global ischemic brain damage (41). The second mechanism is via blockade of VSCC. Nimodipine, nicardipine, flunarizine, and levemopamil are lipophilic calcium-channel blockers that can pass the blood–brain barrier. Nimodipine has both vasodilating and direct neuronal action. The neuroprotective effect was independent of its vasodilating effect by blocking calcium influx via VSCCs (47). Flunarizine, rather than blocking L-type calcium channels, reduces intracellular calcium by inhibiting its release from intracellular stores (48). In experimental studies, flunarizine reduced neuronal necrosis even when given postischemically in rats (49). Takahashi and Akaike suggest that the neuroprotective effect of flunarizine is due to blockade of T-type calcium channels (50). T-type channels are involved in EAA-mediated neurotoxicity.

Another approach to neuroprotection may be intracellular calcium chelation. Neuronal ischemic injury can be treated successfully in vivo by cell-permeant Ca^{++} chelators derived from 1,2 bis-(2-aminophenoxy) ethane-N,N,N′, N′-tetraacetic acid acetomethyl ester (BAPTA-AM) (51). Cell-permeant Ca^{++} chelators constitute a unique pharmacotherapeutic approach to cerebral ischemia that protects neurons for at least 24 hours following permanent focal neocortical ischemia. Their actions may be related to their calcium-buffering capacity or their inhibition of synaptic transmission (52).

Excitatory Amino Acid Antagonists

Excitotoxicity is the common pathway to neuronal damage in many disease conditions (18,19,25). Drugs that block EAA function have shown to be neuroprotective in many experimental models. Currently, many agents are undergoing human clinical trials worldwide.

Glutamate antagonists may act on different steps of EAA-induced excitotoxicity: those drugs that cause decreased glutamate release and drugs that block postsynaptic glutamate receptors. Drugs that decrease glutamate release are Na^{+}-channel blockers and kappa opioid agonists.

Sodium-channel Blockers

These drugs inhibit voltage-sensitive presynaptic Na^+-channels and decrease glutamate release:

The first of these drugs, 619C89 [4 amino-2-(4 methyl-1-piperazinyl)-5-(2,3,5-trichlorophenyl) pyrimidine], is one of the Na^+-channel blockers that is in Phase II clinical trial for its neuroprotective actions on stroke and brain trauma. It is manufactured by Burroughs-Wellcome. It decreases ischemia-induced presynaptic glutamate release (53). Leach and colleagues showed that glutamate-release inhibitors may provide an alternative to EAA receptor antagonists in the treatment of ischemic nerve injury. On administration to rats after permanent middle cerebral artery (MCA) occlusion, it reduces focal cerebral infarction by 60% to 70% (54). Mercer et al. administered 619C89 to healthy volunteers to evaluate pharmacokinetics and effects on vital signs. It was well tolerated, with light-headedness the most common side effect. It also decreased alpha waves in electroencephalograms in a dose-dependent manner (55).

Lamotrigine (3,5 diamino-6-[2,3-dichlorophenyl]-1,2,4 triazine), an antiepileptic drug, acts via blockade of voltage-activated sodium channels and inhibits presynaptic release of glutamate (56). In experimental studies, when lamotrigine was given 24 hours after MCA occlusion in rats, it was cerebroprotective and decreased cerebral infarct volume. Also, lamotrigine had protective effects in a gerbil model of global ischemia. It protected against neurological deficits resulting from 15 minutes of carotid artery occlusion and prevented histological damage resulting from 5 and 15 minutes of global cerebral ischemia (57).

Riluzole (2-amino-6-trifluoromethoxy-benzothiazole) is under clinical trial (Phase III) for its use in amyotrophic lateral sclerosis (ALS). Recent studies suggest that neurodegeneration in ALS could be related to an excitotoxic disorder. Riluzole represents a new pharmacological approach for the treatment of patients with ALS (58). Its neuroprotective effects have been shown in animal models. Wahl and colleagues investigated the effects of riluzole on the histological and neurobehavioral consequences of MCA occlusion in rats. Their results indicate that the drug depresses glutaminergic neurotransmission without blocking the glutamate receptors, thereby exerting antiischemic activity (59).

Lubeluzole (R 87926) is an S-enantiomer of a related benzothiazole. Its Phase II trial for ischemic stroke has shown that, given to patients with a clinical diagnosis of acute ischemic stroke, it may reduce mortality significantly (60). Its neuroprotective action is now in Phase III trial for use in stroke.

CNS 1237 (N-acenaphthyl-N `-methoxynaphthyl guanidine) is a "use-dependent" inhibitor of neurotransmitter release; it blocks glutamate release by blocking Na^+ and Ca^{++} channels with greater efficiency when there is persistent depolarization of the nerve (as in pathological conditions) rather than in transient depolarizations (as seen in normal physiological conditions). Its neuroprotective property has been demonstrated in experimental studies (61).

Kappa Opioid Agonists

CI 977 (5R)-(5 alpha, 7 alpha, 8 beta)-N-methyl-N-[7-(1 pyrrolidinyl) -1-oxaspiro[4,5]dec-8-y1]-4-benzofuranacetamide monohydrochloride is produced by Parke-Davis under the trade name Enadoline. It is being investigated for analgesia and treatment of brain trauma. The ability of the kappa opioids to attenuate hypoxia/hypoglycemia, but not NMDA- or kainate-induced toxicity, suggests that these drugs exert their neuroprotective role predominantly by a presynaptic mechanism, possibly by inhibiting ischemic-mediated glutamate release (62). Studies by Mackay et al. also showed CI 977 to be neuroprotective in a model of focal ischemia in a gyrencephalic species (63).

Postsynaptic EAA Inhibitors

The NMDA receptor is a ligand-gated ion channel. For its activation, the presence of NMDA and glycine is needed. Also, removal of Mg^{++} (a physiological inhibitor of NMDA-receptor activation) from the receptor site is needed. When the nerve is depolarized, Mg^{++} is removed from the receptor. Pharmacological action sites of postsynaptic EAA inhibitors are the glutamate recognition site, glycine recognition site, Mg^{++} site in the channel, phencyclidine blocking site, polyamine site, and redox site. Recently Muir and Lees reviewed the clinical uses of the EAA inhibitors (64). For noncompetitive drugs to act, the nerve should be depolarized and the ion channel should be open. Thus, these drugs cause a state-dependent block.

Drugs Acting on the NMDA Receptor Site

Aptiganel HCL (=CNS 1102) N-(1-naphthyl)-N'(3-ethyl phenyl)-N'methylguanidine hydrochloride) is produced under the name Cenestat by Cambridge Neuroscience. CNS 1102 is a selective ligand for the NMDA ion-channel modulatory site to which dizocilpine (MK-801) and ketamine bind. In a focal ischemia model in rats, it reduced the extent of cerebral infarction by 66% when given before ischemia and by 40% when administered up to 30 minutes after permanent MCA occlusion (65). When tried in healthy humans, CNS 1102 caused dose-dependent elevation of blood pressure accompanied by clinical evidence of vasoconstriction (66). Total cerebral blood flow is unaltered, but MCA flow velocity is increased. Symptoms of light-headedness, disorientation, paresthesia, hallucination, paranoia, and catatonia are seen with increasing dosage. Wagstaff et al. tried CNS 1102 in 15 patients with severe head injury (67). They found that mean intracranial pressure and temperature were transiently decreased during administration of the drug. It is now undergoing trial use in traumatic brain injury and stroke.

Phencyclidine (PCP) is one of the oldest drugs to be used as an anesthetic agent. It binds to its specific site within activated receptor-operated Ca^{++} channels, called the PCP-binding site. Some other drugs, like ketamine and dizocilpine (MK-801), can also bind to the phencyclidine site. All PCP-site acting drugs are lipophilic and can have high concentrations in the brain when administered systematically. They have potent neuroprotective effects both in vitro and in vivo experiments. The main problems with these drugs are the side effects: agitation, disinhibition, hallucination, and paranoid reaction (68,69). Another drawback for ketamine and dizocilpine is that they cause neuronal vacuolization, probably secondary to a drug-induced increase in metabolic activity.

Dextrorphan HCl (Ro-01-6794/706), a dextromethorphan derivative, is the o-demethylated monohydrochloride derivative of dextromethorphan, a drug that was previously used as an antitussive drug. In rabbit and rat models of focal ischemia, it reduced the extent of infarcted brain tissue (70). In vivo models of ischemic stroke suggest that the neuroprotective effects are dose dependent and increase with higher concentrations of the drug. It is currently undergoing trial for use in stroke. When tested in patients with stroke, it caused side effects such as nystagmus, nausea, agitation, hallucination, confusion, and somnolence (71).

Remacemide hydrochloride ((+1-)-2-amino-N-(1-methyl-1, 2-diphenyl-ethyl)-acetamide hydrochloride is produced by Fisons. Initially, it was used as an antiepileptic drug. Its desglycinated metabolite (FPL 12495) is more active pharmacologically. The drug is a weak noncompetitive NMDA antagonist and a moderate inhibitor of the Na^{+} channel; FPL 12495 is a moderate noncompetitive NMDA antagonist and a potent inhibitor of Na^{+} channel (64). Remacemide was neuroprotective in cats after permanent occlusion of one MCA. To evaluate its neuroprotective activity, it is undergoing trial in patients with acute ischemic stroke, coronary artery bypass, and Huntington's disease. Muir and Lees used it in patients with acute ischemic stroke and found that the drug is well tolerated (72).

Magnesium is the physiological voltage-dependent inhibitor of NMDA receptors. Under normal conditions, Mg^{++} induces a voltage-dependent block of the activated NMDA receptor-associated calcium channel. When the nerve is depolarized, this inhibition terminates and the channel opens. In experimental studies, it decreased the volume of cerebral infarct by up to 20% after MCA occlusion (73). Also, after traumatic focal ischemia, it decreases the infarct volume. It is now in Phase III trials for its action on acute stroke.

Competitive NMDA Receptor Antagonists

There are several structural analogs of L-glutamate. These drugs include 2-amino-5-phosphono-pentanoate (AP5), 2- amino-5-phosphono-heptanoate (AP7), 2- amino-5-phosphonovalerate (APV), and 4-[3-phosphonopropyl]-2-piperazinecarboxylic acid (CPP). Their most important limitation is their hydrophilicity, which prevents their diffusion across the blood–brain barrier.

d-CPPene (R)-4-(3-phosphono-2-propyl)-2-piperazinecarboxilic acid is a newer, more lipophilic drug and currently is on trial. It is produced under the name of EAA 494 by Sandoz. In a model of brain edema in rats, it was useful (74). The drug was previously administered intrathecally for pain. It is now in trial for use in seizures and brain trauma.

CGS 19755 (Selfotel) is a competitive NMDA antagonist that limits neuronal damage in animal stroke models. It is produced under the name Selfotel by Ciba Geigy. When administered to patients with acute ischemic stroke, adverse reactions like agitation, hallucination, confusion, and paranoid reaction are seen (75). It is now in Phase II clinical trials for use in stroke, brain trauma, and high risk neurosurgical prophylaxis.

Glycine Site Antagonists

Glycine is a coagonist of NMDA receptors. Its presence is required for receptor activation. ACEA 1021 and 1031 (5-nitro-6,7-dichloro, and 5-nitro-6,7-dibromo 4-dihydro-2, 3 quinoxalinedione) are two glycine site antagonists. ACEA 1021 is currently produced by ACEA. Warner et al. compared neuroprotective effects of ACEA 1011, 1021, and 1031 in rats after 90 minutes of MCA occlusion (76). They concluded that ACEA 1021 and 1031 but not ACEA 1011 reduced cerebral infarct significantly. ACEA 1021 is now in Phase I clinical trials for use in stroke and brain trauma.

Polyamine Site Antagonists

The polyamine site is present in the intracellular part of the ion channel. The drugs that are active on the polyamine site increase Ca^{++} permeability of the receptor-operated Ca^{++} channels. Ifenprodil and (SL82) eliprodil have been shown to be neuroprotective in experimental studies (64). These drugs lack phencyclidine-like psychological and cardiovascular side effects (37). Eliprodil is currently in Phase III clinical trials for its neuroprotective effects on stroke and brain trauma.

AMPA Receptor Antagonists

The AMPA receptors are much more involved in the acute phase of neuronal injury, which is manifested by cellular swelling as a result of high conductance of Na^+ and passive diffusion of water. These receptors are also permeable to calcium. The best known antagonists are the competitive 6-nitro-7-sulphamoylbenzo(f)quinoxaline-2,3-dione (NBQX) and the noncompetitive GYKI 52466. Both were neuroprotective in focal and global ischemic models (64). When NMDA and non-NMDA antagonists are both used in ischemic conditions, postischemic neuronal damage is reduced (37).

Nitric Oxide Inhibitors

Nitric oxide (NO) is a free-radical gas. In the nervous system, it acts as a neurotransmitter. It is also present in white blood cells and is involved in bactericidal and tumoricidal effects. In blood vessels, NO causes vasodilatation. It was previously known as the endothelium-derived relaxing factor because of its vasodilator effect via production of cyclic guanosine 3,5′-monophosphate (cGMP) (77). Nitric oxide was identified in some amacrine cells in the inner nuclear layer and in some ganglion cells of the retina (78) and in blood vessels of the choroid and limbus (79).

In the CNS, NO can be both neurodestructive and neuroprotective (80). The mechanism of action of NO was reviewed by Bredt and Snyder (79). Several studies showed NO to be produced in response to activation of the NMDA subtype of glutamate receptor. When glutamate activates NMDA, Ca^{++} channels open and Ca^{++} influx occurs. High levels of intracellular calcium, along with intracellular calmodulin and NADPH, stimulate the nitric oxide synthase enzyme to produce NO from arginine. Nitric oxide is not stored in synaptic vesicles but formed on demand and is released by diffusion rather than exocytosis. It activates iron at the active site of guanyl cyclase. When nitric oxide synthase (NOS) is inhibited by N^G-monomethylarginine (L-NMMA), cGMP formation is completely prevented.

Nitric oxide damages DNA and causes mutations. There are conflicting reports that neurons possessing NOS activity are actually more resistant to neuronal damage in ischemia (81). On the other hand, NO was neurotoxic in stroke models. Neurotoxicity in ischemia is mediated by glutamate through activation of NMDA receptors. Dawson et al. showed that NO mediates the glutamate toxicity in neuronal cultures (82). Normally, neurons making NO release it to elevate cGMP in adjacent neurons without toxicity. In the presence of large, toxic levels of glutamate, NOS neurons would behave like macrophages, releasing large amounts of NO to kill nearby neurons (79).

Another mechanism to explain the dual action of NO was studied by Lipton and Stamler (80). They proposed that the local redox milieu of the biological system is of critical importance for explaining actions of the nitrogen monoxide moiety. Nitric oxide can be found in different redox-related states: nitrosonium ion (NO^+), nitric oxide (NO^0), and nitroxyl ion (NO^-) containing one additional electron. The co-agonist NMDA receptors have several subunits. There is a coagonist binding site for glycine and a redox modulatory site with a thiol group. When the redox site is oxidized to the disulfide form, channel activity is downregulated, and when the site is reduced more calcium enters through NMDA channels. The chemical pathways involving distinct redox-related congeners of NO may trigger neurotoxic or neuroprotective pathways. The reaction of nitric oxide (NO^0) with superoxide can lead to neurotoxicity through formation of peroxynitrite, whereas No^0 alone does not. Reactions of NO equivalents to thiols on the NMDA receptor can lead to neuroprotection by inhibiting Ca^{++} influx. The neuroprotective effects of NO suggest that acceleration of disulfide bond formation at the NMDA receptor is important in attenuation of Ca^{++} influx and constitutes another strategy for neuroprotection such that downregulation of NMDA receptors can be achieved through sulphydryl oxidation by S-nitrosylation with NO^+donors or with NO^-donors.

Zeevalk and Nicklas showed that NO pathways are involved in EAA-stimulated cGMP formation in chick retina (83). MK-801, an NMDA blocker, can prevent NMDA-induced cGMP rise. Nowicki et al. showed that the neuroprotective effect of nitroarginine, which is an inhibitor of NOS, was greater than MK-801 in a model of stroke in mice (84).

The functions of NO were reviewed by Zhang (85). As a free radical, NO can damage DNA and cause mutations; DNA strand breaks activate polyadenosine diphosphate (ADP)-ribose synthetase (PARS). This enzyme is important for DNA repair, cellular differentiation, transformation, and gene arrangements. In turn, PARS catalyzes polyADP ribosylation of many nuclear proteins. With overstimulation of PARS in stroke or metabolic stress, NAD, which is a substrate for PARS, is depleted. The destruction of DNA overwhelms its repair and the neuron dies. Nitric oxide also inhibits ribonucleotide reductase, which is necessary for DNA synthesis and repair. So, in the presence of NO, DNA repair is delayed. The presence of DNA fragments causes prolonged activation of PARS.

In cortical cultures, NMDA neurotoxicity is blocked by PARS inhibitors. Benzamine and its derivatives (3-aminobenzamide and 4- aminobenzamide) are shown to be PARS inhibitors; benzamine is the most active of the three. The PARS inhibitors may become the new therapeutic approaches to prevent ischemic neuronal death. Another novel target for neuroprotective drugs regarding NOS activity is phosphorylation of NOS (85), which decreases its catalytic activity, and dephosphorylation causes increased NO production. FK506 is an immunosuppressant drug. It forms a complex with FK binding protein (FKBP) that in turn inhibits calcineurin, a calmodulin-dependent phosphoprotein phosphatase. It dephosphorylates phosphorylated NOS and makes it more active in NO production. The inhibition of calcineurin by the FK506/FKBP complex decreases NO production and reduces NMDA neurotoxicity.

Sharkey showed that in an in vivo model of focal cerebral ischemia, FK506 is neuroprotective (86). Another drug that inhibits calcineurin is cyclosporin A, a well-known immunosuppressive drug (85). These findings show that calcineurin can be another potential target in the search for neuroprotection.

Oxygen Radical Scavengers

A *free radical* is a molecule with one or more unpaired electrons. Oxygen free radicals are implicated in tissue injury during ischemia and reperfusion. Free radicals are constantly produced in normal cellular metabolism, such as in oxidative-reduction reactions in the electron transport chain in mitochondria for generation of ATP or in arachidonic acid metabolism (87). Endogenous defense mechanisms against these free radicals include antioxidant enzymes, like superoxide dismutase, catalase, and glutathione peroxidase, and also some free-radical scavengers, like glutathione, alpha tocopherol (vitamin E), and beta-carotene.

The production of free radicals is related to increased intracellular calcium in several ways. Increased levels of calcium activate phospholipases, leading to arachidonic acid oxidation and free radical formation (88). Also, high levels of intracellular calcium activate xanthine oxidase enzyme, which in turn produces uric acid and superoxide radical (89). Another source of calcium-induced free radical formation is activation of nitric acid synthase, which leads to nitric acid production (90). Previous studies showed that free radicals are produced in response to brain trauma and ischemia due to extensive oxidation of proteins and lipid peroxidation (91); and antioxidants have neuroprotective actions (92).

DL-6,8-dithioloctanoic acid (DHLA) has antioxidant activity against microsomal lipid peroxidation. It is a biological dithiol found in mitochondria. Prehn et al. reported that DHLA is able to protect neurons against ischemic damage in rodents (93). Experimental studies showed that other physiological free radical scavengers, like alpha-tocopherol and ascorbic acid, are neuroprotective in ischemia models in vivo (94).

Several synthetic compounds have been developed as free-radical scavengers. Dimethylthiourea (1,3-dimethyl-2-thiourea) is a hydroxyl radical scavenger. It reduces infarct size after MCA occlusion in rats without changing the cerebral blood flow (95). Allopurinol is a xanthine oxidase inhibitor. Williams et al. showed that high-dose allopurinol pretreatment protected against hypoxic-ischemic injury in rats (96). Similarly, Martz et al. found that pretreatment with dimethylthiourea and allopurinol reduced the cerebral infarct volume by 30% and 35%, respectively, in a model of continuous partial ischemia in rats (97). These compounds also significantly reduced cerebral edema and improved blood–brain barrier function.

Recent studies suggest that there may be interactions between free radicals and EAAs in the formation of ischemic neuronal damage. When free radicals are formed by stimulation of EAA, they stimulate further release of EAA, creating a vicious cycle (98). Studies by Oh and Betz indicate that pretreatment with dimethylurea or MK-801 can reduce brain edema during early stages of cerebral ischemia (98). These experiments suggest that EAAs and oxygen free radicals may damage the brain by a common pathway.

The 21-aminosteroids (lazaroids) are steroidal compounds that were developed for acute treatment of traumatic or ischemic CNS injury. Their action involves inhibition of lipid peroxidation. The glucocorticoid steroid methylprednisolone possesses significant antioxidant efficacy. When administered to animals or humans in antioxidant dosages, it improves chronic neurologic recovery after spinal cord injury. The antioxidant action of methylprednisolone is independent of the steroid's glucocorticoid receptor-mediated actions. U-74OOGF (21 aminosteroid trilazad mesylate) does not have glucocorticoid activity, but it has greater antioxidant efficacy than methylprednisolone. The compound is effective in animal models of brain and spinal cord injury and is the subject of Phase III clinical trials (99).

Carvedilol, a new antihypertensive drug, also had neuroprotective action in both in vitro and in vivo models of neuroinjury (100). It may reduce risk of cerebral ischemia and stroke by virtue of both its antihypertensive action and its antioxidative properties. HU-211 (dexanabinol) is a synthetic cannabinoid with negligible affinity to cannabinoid receptors and no psychotropic effects in animals. It was evaluated in a number of animal models, including closed head injury, optic nerve trauma, global ischemia, and focal ischemia. Dexanabinol holds a unique position among putative neuroprotective agents because it combines NMDA-blocking activity and free-radical scavenging properties in one molecule without having cannabinoid activity (101).

The understanding of glaucoma has made broad progress in the past 25 years. The more we learn about the pathophysiology of the disease, the more options we will have for treatment. Management of glaucoma has been unimodel, with pharmacological treatment limited to decreasing the IOP. Clinicians are currently unable to treat the disease at a cellular level, such as with targeted optic-nerve protection. Neuroprotective agents under investigation may have renewed hopes for some neurological diseases, including glaucomatous optic neuropathy. Clearly, obstacles must be overcome before these agents can be introduced into clinical practice. It is hoped that in the twenty-first century we will be able to treat the glaucomas with therapies aimed at the underlying mechanisms and cellular sites of injury.

ACKNOWLEDGMENT

This work was supported in part by an unrestricted grant from Research to Prevent Blindness, Inc., New York, NY.

REFERENCES

1. Hoskins HD Jr, Kass M. Introduction and classification of glaucomas. In: Hoskins HD Jr, Kass M, eds. *Becker-Shaffer's Diagnosis and Therapy of the Glaucomas,* 6th ed. St. Louis: CV Mosby, 1989;2.
2. Chandler PA, Grant WM. General considerations. In: Chandler PA, Grant WM, eds. *Glaucoma,* 3rd ed. Philadelphia: Lea & Febiger, 1986;3.
3. Van Buskirk EM, Cioffi GA. Glaucomatous optic neuropathy. *Am J Ophthalmol* 1992;113:447–452.
4. Gaasterland D, Tanishima T, Kuwabara T. Axoplasmic flow during chronic experimental glaucoma. 1. Light and electron microscopic studies of the monkey optic nerve head during development of glaucomatous cupping. *Invest Ophthalmol Vis Sci* 1978;17:838–846.
5. Cartwright MJ, Anderson DR. Correlation of asymmetric damage with asymmetric intraocular pressure in normal-tension glaucoma (low tension glaucoma). *Arch Ophthalmol* 1988;106:898–902.
6. Crichton A, Drance SM, Douglas GR, Schulzer M. Unequal intraocular pressure and its relation to asymmetric visual field defects in low tension glaucoma. *Ophthalmology* 1989;96:1312–1314.
7. Anderson DR, Hendrickson A. Effect of intraocular pressure on rapid axoplasmic transport in monkey optic nerve. *Invest Ophthalmol* 1974;13:771–783.
8. Quigley HA. The relationship of intraocular pressure. In: Drance SM, Van Buskirk EM, Neufeld AH, eds. *Pharmacology of Glaucoma.* Baltimore: Williams and Wilkins, 1992;265–272.
9. Quigley HA, Addicks EM, Green R, Maumenee AE. Optic nerve damage in human glaucoma II. The site of injury and susceptibility to damage. *Arch Ophthalmol* 1981;99:635–649.
10. Sommer A, Tielsch JM, Katz J, et al. and the Baltimore Eye Survey Research Group. Relationship between intraocular pressure and primary open angle glaucoma among white and black Americans. *Arch Ophthalmol* 1991;109:1090.
11. Werner EB, Drance SM. Progression of glaucomatous field defects despite successful filtration. *Can J Ophthalmol* 1977;12:275–280.
12. Guthauser U, Flammer J, Mahler F. The relationship between digital and ocular vasospasm. *Graefes Arch Clin Exp Ophthalmol* 1988; 226:224–226.
13. Drance SM, Douglas GR, Wijsman K, Schulzer M, Britton RJ. Response of blood flow to warm and cold in normal and low tension glaucoma patients. *Am J Ophthalmol* 1988;105:35–39.
14. Corbett JJ, Phelps CD, Eslinger P, Montaque PR. The neurological evaluation of patients with low tension glaucoma. *Invest Ophthalmol Vis Sci* 1985;26:1101.
15. Armaly MF, Krueger DE, Maunder L, et al. Biostatistical analysis of the collaborative glaucoma study. I. Summary report of the risk factors for glaucomatous visual field defects. *Arch Ophthalmol* 1980; 98:2163–2171.
16. Brubaker RF. Delayed functional loss in glaucoma. LII Edward Jackson Memorial Lecture. *Am J Ophthalmol* 1996;121:473–483.
17. Rothman SM, Olney JW. Gluthamate and pathophysiology of hypoxic-ischemic brain damage. *Ann Neurol* 1986;19:105–111.
18. Schumer RA, Podos SM. The nerve of glaucoma. *Arch Ophthalmol* 1994;112:37–44.
19. Bresnick GH. Excitotoxins: a possible mechanism for the pathogenesis of ischemic retinal damage. *Arch Ophthalmol* 1989;107:339–341.
20. Iversen LL. Pharmacological approaches to the treatment of ischemic neuronal damage. *Eye* 1991;5:193–197.
21. Greenamyre JT. The role of glutamate in neurotransmission and in neurologic disease. *Arch Neurol* 1986;43:1058–1063.
22. Olney JW. Inciting excitotoxic cytocide among central neurons. *Adv Exp Med Biol* 1986;203:631–645.
23. Olney JW, Ho OL, Rhee V. Cytotoxic effects of acidic and sulpher containing amino acids on the infant mouse central nervous system. *Exp Brain Res* 1971;14:61–76.
24. Lucas DR, Newhouse JP. The toxic effects of sodium L-glutamate on inner layers of retina. *AMA Arch Ophthalmol* 1957;58:193–204.
25. Choi DW. Excitotoxic cell death. *J Neurobiol* 1992;23:1261–1276.
26. Murphy TH, Malouf AT, Sastre A, Schnaar RL, Coyle JT. Calcium-dependent glutamate cytotoxicity in neuronal cell line. *Brain Res* 1988;444:325–332.
27. Naito S, Ueda T. Adenosine triphosphate dependent uptake of glutamate into protein I associated vesicles. *J Biol Chem* 1983;258:696–699.
28. Kanai Y, Smith CP, Heiger MA. The elusive transporters with a high affinity for glutamate. *Trends Neurosci* 1993;16:359–365.
29. Greenamyre JT, Porter RHP. Anatomy and physiology of glutamate in the CNS. *Neurology* 1994;44(suppl 8):S7–S13.
30. Hagberg H, Lehmann A, Sandberg M, et al. Ischemia induced shift of inhibitory and excitatory amino acids from intra and extracellular compartments. *J Cereb Blood Flow Metab* 1985;5:413–419.
31. Drejer J, Benveniste H, Diemer NH, et al. Cellular origin of ischemia-induced glutamate release from brain tissue in vivo and in vitro. *J Neurochem* 1985;45:145–151.
32. Duke RC, Chervenak R, Cohen JJ. Endogenous endonuclease-induced DNA fragmentation: an early event in cell-mediated cytolysis. *Proc Natl Acad Sci USA* 1983;80:6361–6365.
33. Dreyer EB, Lipton SA. A proposed role for excitatory amino acids in glaucoma visual loss. *Invest Ophthalmol Vis Sci* 1993;34 (suppl):1504.
34. Sesma MA, Price MT, Olney JW. Sensitivity of retinal ganglion cell subtypes to specific excitotoxins. *Invest Ophthalmol Vis Sci* 1991;32(suppl):1263.
35. Dreyer EB, Pan ZH, Storm S, Lipton SA. Greater sensitivity of larger retinal ganglion cells to NMDA-mediated cell death. *Neuroreport* 1994;5:629–631.
36. Caprioli J, Kitano S. Large retinal ganglion cells are more susceptible to excitotoxic and hypoxic injury than small cells. *Invest Ophthalmol Vis Sci* 1993;34(suppl):1429.
37. Peruche B, Krieglstein J. Mechanisms of drug actions against neuronal damage caused by ischemia—an overview. *Prog Neuropsychopharmacol Biol Psychiatry* 1993;17:21–70.
38. Fleckenstein A. History of calcium antagonists. *Circ Res* 1983;52 (suppl 1):3–16.
39. Godfraind T, Miller RC, Wibo M. Calcium antagonism and calcium entry blockade. *Pharmacol Rev* 1986;38:321–416.
40. Tsien RW, Lipscombe D, Madison DV, et al. Multiple types of neuronal calcium channels and their selective modulation. *TINS* 1988; 11:431–438.
41. Goldin SM, Subbarao K, Sharma R, et al. Neuroprotective use-dependent blockers of Na^{++} and Ca^{++} channels controlling presynaptic release of glutamate. *Ann NY Acad Sci* 1995;765:210–227.
42. Netland PA, Erickson KA. Calcium channel blockers in glaucoma management. *Ophthalmol Clin North Am* 1995;8:327–334.
43. Zhang X, Schroeder A, Ericson K. Influence of Verapamil and epinephrine on outflow facility and cyclic AMP in human eye. *Invest Ophthalmol Vis Sci* 1994;35(suppl):2053.
44. Netland PA, Chaturvedi N, Dreyer EB. Calcium channel blockers in the management of low tension and open angle glaucoma. *Am J Ophthalmol* 1993;115:608.
45. Luebke JI, Dunlop K, Turner TJ. Multiple calcium channel types control glutaminergic synaptic transmission in the hippocampus. *Neuron* 1993;11:895–902.
46. Valentino K, Newcomb R, Gadbois T. A selective N-type calcium channel antagonist protects against neuronal loss after global cerebral ischemia. *Proc Natl Acad Sci USA* 1993;90:7894–7897.
47. Nuglisch J, Karkoutly C, Mennel HD, Robberg C, Krieglstein J. Protective effects of nimodipine against ischemic neuronal damage in rat hippocampus without changing postischemic cerebral blood flow. *J Cereb Blood Flow Metab* 1990;10:654–659.
48. Holmes B, Brodgen RN, Heel RG, Speight TN, Avery GS. Flunarizine: a review of its pharmacological and pharmacokinetic properties and therapeutic use. *Drug* 1984;27:6–44.
49. Deshpande JK, Wieloch T. Amelioration of ischemic brain damage following postischemic treatment with flunarizine. *Neurol Res* 1985;7:27–29.
50. Takahashi K, Akaike N. Calcium antagonist effects on low-threshold (T-type) calcium current in rat isolated hippocampal CA1 pyramidal neurons. *J Pharmacol Exp Ther* 1991;256:169–175.
51. Tymianski M, Wallace MC, Uno M, et al. Successful treatment of focal ischemic stroke by intracellular calcium chelation. *J Cereb Blood Flow Metab* 1993;13(suppl 1):S638.
52. Tymianski M, Spigelman I, Zhang L, et al. Mechanism of action and persistence of neuroprotection by cell-permeant Ca^{2+} chelators. *J Cereb Blood Flow Metab* 1994;14:911–923.

53. Muir KW, Lees KR, Hamilton SJC, George CF, Hobbiger SF, Lunnon MW. A randomized, double blind, placebo controlled ascending dose tolerance study of 619C89 in acute stroke. *Ann NY Acad Sci* 1995;765:328–329.
54. Leach MJ, Swan JH, Essential D, Dopson M, Nobbs M. BW619C89, a glutamate release inhibitor, protects against focal cerebral ischemic damage. *Stroke* 1993;24:1063–1067.
55. Mercer AJ, Lamb RJ, Hussein Z, Hobbiger S, Posner J. The tolerability, pharmacokinetics and pharmacodynamics of increasing intravenous doses of 619C89, a novel compound for the acute treatment of stroke, in healthy volunteers. *Ann NY Acad Sci* 1995;765: 324–326.
56. Burstein AH. Lamotrigine. *Pharmacotherapy* 1995;15:129–143.
57. Wiard RP, Dickerson MC, Beek O, Norton R, Cooper BR. Neuroprotective properties of the novel antiepileptic lamotrigine in a gerbil model of global cerebral ischemia. *Stroke* 1995;26:466–472.
58. Couratier P, Sindou P, Esclaire F, Louvel E, Hugon J. Neuroprotective effects of riluzole in ALS CSF toxicity. *Neuroreport* 1994;5: 1012–1014.
59. Wahl F, Allix M, Plohine M, Boulu RG. Effect of riluzole on focal cerebral ischemia in rats. *Eur J Pharmacol* 1993;230:209–214.
60. Diener HC, Hacke W, Hennerici M, Radberg J, Hantson L, De Keyser J. Lubelozole in acute ischemic stroke: a double blind, placebo controlled phase II trial. Lubeluzole International Study Group. *Stroke* 1996;27:76–81.
61. Goldin SM, Subarrao K, Sharma R, et al. Neuroprotective use-dependent blockers of Na^{+} and Ca^{++} channels controlling presynaptic release of glutamate. *Ann NY Acad Sci* 1995;765:210–229.
62. Lockhart BP, Soulard P, Benicourt C, Private A, Julien JL. Distinct neuroprotective profiles for sigma ligands against N-methyl-D-aspartate (NMDA) and hypoxia-mediated neurotoxicity in neuronal culture in toxicity studies. *Brain Res* 1995;675:110–120.
63. Mackay KB, Kusumotok K, Graham DI, McCulloch J. Focal cerebral ischemia in the cat: pretreatment with a kappa-1 opioid receptor agonist, CI 977. *Brain Res* 1993;618:213–219.
64. Muir KW, Lees KR. Clinical experience with excitatory amino acid antagonist drugs. *Stroke* 1995;26:503–513.
65. Minematsu K, Fischer M, Li L, Davis MA, et al. Effects of novel NMDA antagonist on experimental stroke rapidly and quantitatively assessed by diffusion-weighed MRI. *Neurology* 1993;43:397–403.
66. Muir KW, Grosset DG, Lees KR. Clinical pharmacology of CNS 1102 in volunteers. *Ann NY Acad Sci* 1995;765:279–289.
67. Wagstaff A, Teasdale GM, Clifton G, Steward L. The cerebral hemodynamic and metabolic effects of the noncompatitive NMDA antagonist CNS 1102 in humans with severe head injury. *Ann NY Acad Sci* 1995;765:332–333.
68. Greifenstein FE, DeVault M, Yoshikate J, Gajewski JE. A study of 1-aryl cyclohexamine for anesthesia. *Anesth Analg* 1958;37:283–294.
69. Johnstone M, Evans V, Baigel S, Sernyl (CI-395) in clinical anesthesia. *Br J Anaesth* 1959;31:433–439.
70. Steinberg GK, Saleh J, Kunis D. Delayed treatment with dextromethorphan and dextrorphan reduces cerebral damage after transient focal ischemia. *Neurosci Lett* 1988;89:193–197.
71. The Dextrorphan Study Group, Hoffmann-La Roche. Safety, tolerability and pharmacokinetics of the N-methyl-D-aspartate antagonist R0-01-6794/706 in patients with acute ischemic stroke. *Ann NY Acad Sci* 1995;765:249–261.
72. Muir KW, Lees KR. Initial experience with ramacemide hydrochloride in patients with acute ischemic stroke. *Ann NY Acad Sci* 1995;765:322–333.
73. Muir KW, Lees KR. A randomized, double blind, placebo controlled pilot trial of intravenous magnesium sulfate in acute stroke. *Ann NY Acad Sci* 1995;765:315–316.
74. Demura N, Kuroda J, Tanaka K, Seno N, Kanazawa I. Effects of continual intravenous posttreatment with D-CPPene, a potent competitive N-methyl-D-aspartate receptor antagonist on rat brain edema induced by injection of triethyltin into the cerebral hemisphere. *Neurosci Lett* 1995;192:109–112.
75. Grotta J, Clark W, Coull B, et al. Safety and tolerability of glutamate antagonist CGS 19755 (selfotel) in patients with acute ischemic stroke: results of a phase IIa randomized trial. *Stroke* 1995;26: 602–605.
76. Warner DS, Martin H, Ludwig P, McAllister A, Keana JF, Weber E. In vivo models of cerebral ischemia: effects of parenterally administered NMDA receptor glycine site antagonists. *J Cereb Blood Flow Metab* 1995;15:188–196.
77. Moncada S, Higgs A. The L-arginine-nitric pathway. *N Engl J Med* 1993;329:2002–2012.
78. Bredt DS, Hwang PM, Snyder SH. Localization of nitric oxide synthase indicating a neural role for nitric oxide. *Nature* 1990;347: 768–770.
79. Bredt DS, Snyder SH. Nitric oxide, a novel neuronal messenger. *Neuron* 1992;8:3–11.
80. Lipton SA, Stamler JS. Actions of redox-related congeners of nitric oxide at the NMDA receptor. *Neuropharmacology* 1994;33:1229–1233.
81. Uemura Y, Kowall NW, Beal MF. Selective sparing of NMDPH-diaphorase-somatostatin-neuropeptide Y neurons in ischemic gerbil striatum. *Annals Neuro* 1990;27(6):620–625.
82. Dawson VL, Dawson TM, London ED, Bredt DS, Snyder SH. Nitric oxide mediates glutamate neurotoxicity in primary cortical culture. *Proc Natl Acad Sci USA* 1991;88:6368–6371.
83. Zeevalk GD, Nicklas WJ. Nitric oxide in retina: relation to excitatory amino acids and excitotoxicity. *Exp Eye Res* 1994;58:343–350.
84. Nowicki JP, Duval D, Poignet H, Scatton B. Nitric oxide mediates neuronal death after focal cerebral ischemia in the mouse. *Eur J Pharmacol* 1991;204:339–340.
85. Zhang J, Steiner JP. Poly(ADP-ribose) synthetase: novel targets for the development of neuroprotective drugs. *Neurol Res* 1995;17: 285–288.
86. Sharkey J, Butcher SP. Immunophilins mediate the neuroprotective effects of FK506 in focal cerebral ischemia. *Nature* 1994;371: 336–339.
87. Halliwell B, Gutteridge JM. *Free Radicals in Biology and Medicine.* Oxford: Clarendon Press, 1985;139–189.
88. Verity MA. Mechanisms of phospholipase A2 activation and neuronal injury. *Ann NY Acad Sci* 1993;679:110–120.
89. McCord: Oxygen-derived free radicals in postischemic injury. *N Engl J Med* 1985;312:159–163.
90. Lipton SA. A redox-based mechanism for neuroprotective and neurodestructive effects of nitric oxide and related nitroso-compounds. *Nature* 1993;364:626–632.
91. Kontos HA, Wei EP. Superoxide production in experimental brain injury. *J Neurosurg* 1986;64:803–807.
92. Clifton GL, Lyeth BG, Jenkins LW, Taft WC, Delorenzo RJ, Hayes RL. Effect of D alpha-tocopheryl succinate and polyethylene glycol on performance tests after fluid percussion brain injury. *J Neurotrauma* 1989;6:71–81.
93. Prehn JH, Karkoutly C, Nuglisch J, Peruche B, Krieglstein J. Dihydrolipoate reduces neuronal injury after cerebral ischemia. *J Cereb Blood Flow Metab* 1992;12:78–87.
94. Yamamoto M, Shima T, Sagahe T, Yamada K, Kawasaki T. A possible role of lipid peroxidation in cellular damages caused by cerebral ischemia and the protective effect of alpha tocopherol administration. *Stroke* 1983;14:977–982.
95. Martz D, Beer M, Betz A. Dimethylthiourea reduces ischemic brain edema without affecting cerebral blood flow. *J Cereb Blood Flow Metab* 1990;10:352–357.
96. Williams GD, Palmer C, Heitjan DF, Smith MB. Allopurinol preserves cerebral energy metabolism during perinatal hypoxia-ischemia: a 31P NMR study in unanesthetized immature rats. *Neurosci Lett* 1992;144:103–106.
97. Martz D, Rayos G, Schielke GP, Betz A. Allopurinol and dimethylthiourea reduce brain infarction following middle cerebral artery occlusion. *Stroke* 1989;20:488–494.
98. Oh SM, Betz LB. Interaction between free radicals and excitatory amino acids in the formation of ischemic brain edema in rats. *Stroke* 1991;22:915–921.
99. Hall ED. Lipid antioxidants in acute central nervous system injury. *Ann Emerg Med* 1993;22:1022–1027.
100. Lysko PG, Lysko KA, Yue TL, Webb CL, Gu JL, Feuerstein G. Neuroprotective effects of carvedilol, a new antihypertensive agent, in cultured rat cerebellar neurons and in gerbil global brain ischemia. *Stroke* 1992;23:1630–1636.
101. Biegon A, Joseph AB. Development of HU-211 as a neuroprotectant for ischemic brain damage. *Neurol Res* 1995;17:275–280.

Textbook of Ocular Pharmacology,
edited by T.J. Zimmerman, et al.
Lippincott–Raven Publishers, Philadelphia © 1997.

CHAPTER 30

Medical Trabeculocanulotomy

R. Rand Allingham

The term *medical trabeculocanulotomy* was first coined in the 1970s to describe an approach to the treatment of glaucoma predicated on the biochemical manipulation of trabecular meshwork structure to reduce outflow resistance and ultimately intraocular pressure (IOP) (1). Over the last two decades, investigations into a variety of agents may be bringing the realization of this goal closer to reality.

For more than 40 years, it has been known that the trabecular meshwork is the primary site of fluid-flow resistance in normal and glaucomatous human eyes (2,3). Recent investigations lend support to the concept that the primary site of fluid-flow resistance lies within the juxtacanalicular tissue in conjunction with the endothelial lining of Schlemm's canal (4,5).

The trabecular meshwork is composed of both cellular and extracellular components. The major extracellular biochemical components of the trabecular meshwork are types I and IV collagen, elastin, fibronectin, laminin, and glycosaminoglycans (GAGs). Trabecular endothelial cells are integrated around collagenous beams and within the juxtacanalicular tissue, and they line Schlemm's canal. Several broad classes of agents alter trabecular meshwork resistance, presumably by their action on specific components of the trabecular meshwork that expand existing fluid channels through the trabecular meshwork or create new ones. These agents include various degradative enzymes, such as proteases and GAG-ases, as well as agents that act primarily on the cell cytoskeleton or cellular junctions.

ENZYMATIC AGENTS

GAG-ases

The GAGs are a major component of the trabecular meshwork in both animals and humans. They richly invest the extracellular matrix of the uveal and corneoscleral beams, the juxtacanalicular tissue, and the surface of cells lining Schlemm's canal (5,6). It is likely that GAGs and other extracellular matrix components contribute to aqueous outflow resistance. This view is supported by computer analysis of the outflow pathways in human eyes performed by Ethier and co-workers, which found that the dimensions of the outflow pathways within the juxtacanalicular tissue of human eyes does not account for measured outflow resistance (7). These investigators concluded that the outflow pathways must be filled with a matrix material such as GAGs to account for this discrepancy.

In now classic investigations, Barany found that incorporating testicular hyaluronidase into mock aqueous during anterior chamber perfusions reduced the outflow resistance in enucleated animal eyes (8). More recently, the effect of intracameral chondroitinase ABC, which digests chondroitin sulfate, dermatan sulfate, and hyaluronic acid, has been examined in monkey eyes by Sawaguchi and coworkers (9). The IOP was consistently reduced in association with structural changes of the juxtacanalicular tissue. This IOP reduction persisted for up to 2 weeks. Although these injections were well tolerated in the normal monkey eye, a severe inflammatory reaction was observed in the glaucomatous monkey model. Interestingly, a similar reaction was observed by Weekers et al. using hyaluronidase in patients with glaucoma (10). It is possible that reduced aqueous humor turnover time or increased retention time of the chondroitinase in glaucomatous eyes permits a prolonged effect on anterior segment structures other than the trabecular meshwork, such as the iris and cornea.

Alpha-Chymotrypsin

Alpha (α)-chymotrypsin is a protease that has been used clinically to promote lysis of lens zonular fibers during intracapsular cataract extraction. Marked IOP elevation secondary to zonulysis and obstruction of trabecular mesh-

R. R. Allingham: Duke University Eye Center, Durham, North Carolina 27710.

work by zonular fragments has been described following this procedure. Experimental evidence supports this assertion (11); however, Bill noted that α-chymotrypsin, when perfused in the anterior chamber, produces a pronounced reduction in IOP in the monkey eye (12,13). Experimental perfusion with α-chymotrypsin has a similar effect on outflow resistance to that of chondroitinase ABC despite a different site of action (9,12). In both cases, histological changes consist of degradation of the extracellular matrix and cell–cell separation in the juxtacanalicular tissue. Additionally, α-chymotrypsin produces breaks in the inner wall endothelial lining of Schlemm's canal. It has been proposed that both α-chymotrypsin and the GAG-ases act on components of the extracellular matrix which are integral to maintaining the cell cytoskeleton, and thus cell–cell adhesion.

CYTOSKELETAL AND CELL-ADHESIVE AGENTS

Calcium Chelators

Calcium is essential to normal cell adhesion. Calcium chelators such as Na_2EDTA and EGTA bind free calcium ion. Ocular perfusion with Na_2EDTA and EGTA produces a reduction in outflow resistance which is associated with a loss of cell processes in monkey eyes (14). Na_2EDTA binds both Ca^{2+} and Mg^{2+}, whereas EGTA binds Ca^{2+} alone. The results of anterior chamber perfusion of both agents are essentially the same, indicating that Ca^{2+} is primarily responsible for the observed effects on outflow (15).

Anterior chamber perfusions combined with alpha-chymotrypsin EDTA or EGTA produces distention of the juxtacanalicular tissue and ballooning of the inner endothelial lining into the lumen of Schlemm's canal. Washout of extracellular material is also observed. As ruptures in the lining endothelial cells close, outflow resistance returns to normal despite persistent alterations in the trabecular meshwork structure. Bill and co-workers proposed that the return to normal resistance in treated eyes may be due to closure of openings through the juxtacanalicular tissue and the endothelial lining of Schlemm's canal by platelets (15).

Again, there is a remarkable similarity in the histological effect of calcium chelator perfusion on the trabecular meshwork morphology to that seen in α-chymotrypsin and chondroitinase ABC perfusion. These investigations support the important role of cell-to-cell and cell-matrix adhesion in maintaining normal aqueous outflow resistance.

Cytochalasins

Cytochalasin B is a metabolite of the fungus *Helminthosporium dematiodeum,* which disrupts actin assembly. Cytochalasin B, when administered intracamerally, produces a marked reduction in outflow resistance within 20 minutes in monkey eyes (16). This effect is unaltered in eyes in which the ciliary muscle has been surgically disinserted and renders the trabecular meshwork insensitive to pilocarpine. Therefore, the site of action appears to be the trabecular meshwork alone rather than an indirect effect exerted through contraction of the ciliary muscle. The effect of cytochalasin is reversible. Histologically, widespread damage to cells is associated with tissue disorganization with associated blood reflux into the anterior chamber. The repair of these morphological changes is rapid, occurring within hours to days (17). Cytochalasin D is about 25 times more potent than B, although the physiologic and morphologic effects are similar.

Colchicine

Colchicine is a plant alkaloid that prevents polymerization of microtubules. Colchicine reduces IOP in the rabbit model (18,19). The peak effect is noted 24 hours after administration. Tonography measurements demonstrate an increase in outflow facility after topical administration of 50 or 100 μg of colchicine (18). Despite continued application of colchicine, outflow facility returns to baseline and is associated with marked toxicity to the cornea and anterior segment. Ultimately, IOP becomes elevated, presumably due to obstruction or disorganization of the outflow pathways. Lumilcolchicine, an inactive isomer with little affinity for tubulin, has no effect on outflow facility (20). Therefore, it appears likely that it is colchicine's interaction with tubulin and the cytoskeleton that is primarily responsible for its effect on outflow facility.

ETHACRYNIC ACID AND THE SULFHYDRYL-REACTIVE AGENTS

Cellular sulfhydryl groups appear to be involved in passive fluid movement in many tissues (21). Sulfhydryl-reactive agents covalently bind to sulfhydryl groups to form a thiol adduct (Fig. 30-1).

Sulfhydryl-reactive compounds, including iodoacetamide, *N*-ethyl maleimide, and ethacrynic acid (ECA), decrease aqueous outflow resistance in enucleated calf and monkey eyes (22,23,24) (Fig. 30-2). More recently, ECA has received increasing attention as an agent potentially useful for the treatment of glaucoma. Historically it has been used systemically as a loop diuretic and is still available for such use, although it has largely been replaced by less toxic diuretics, such as furosemide (25).

Ethacrynic acid causes reversible cell-shape changes in cultured trabecular meshwork cells (26). These changes are first evident in cell culture at 2 hours by phase-contrast microscopy and are coincident with disruption of many components of the cytoskeleton including F-actin, α-actinin, vinculin, and vimentin. The first cytoskeletal component that appears to be altered is β-tubulin. Disruption of

$$CH_2{=}\underset{\underset{CH_3}{|}}{\underset{CH_2}{|}}{C}-\overset{O}{\overset{\|}{C}}-C_6H_2Cl_2-O-CH_2-COOH + RSH \rightleftharpoons$$

$$R-SCH_2-\underset{\underset{CH_3}{|}}{\underset{CH_2}{|}}{\overset{H}{\overset{|}{C}}}-\overset{O}{\overset{\|}{C}}-C_6H_2Cl_2-O-CH_2-COOH$$

FIG. 30-1. Ethacrynic acid covalently binds to sulfhydryl groups to form a thiol adduct.

microtubules is observed within 10 minutes of ECA administration; ECA has been shown to react with tubulin, thus inhibiting conversion of tubulin to microtubules. By shifting the tubulin <-> microtubule equilibrium to the left, disassembly of microtubules exceeds assembly (27).

The role of cells as a major site of outflow resistance in the trabecular meshwork is controversial. It is known that there are both transcellular and paracellular routes of aqueous egress (28,29). Additionally, the density of endothelial pores in Schlemm's canal is related to outflow resistance and is reduced in glaucomatous eyes, although the total contribution of this cell lining to total outflow resistance is relatively small (30). Alterations in the cellular morphology of the juxtacanalicular tissue in glaucomatous eyes appears to support the role of cells as a major source of outflow resistance in the trabecular meshwork (18). Ethacrynic acid causes cell separation in cell culture and increases hydraulic conductivity in a monolayer trabecular meshwork cell-culture system (26,32). It reduces outflow resistance in the calf, monkey, and human eye (29,33,34). Histologically, ECA produces cell separation in the form of breaks in the inner-wall endothelial lining of Schlemm's canal in the monkey eye (Figure 30-3); however, ECA perfused at lower concentrations in the human-eye organ culture system (0.01–0.05 mMol) reduced outflow resistance by 34–38%, but no morphologic correlate was observed (34). In these studies, ECA produced evidence of cell toxicity, including cell swelling and death at higher concentrations. Intracameral ECA can

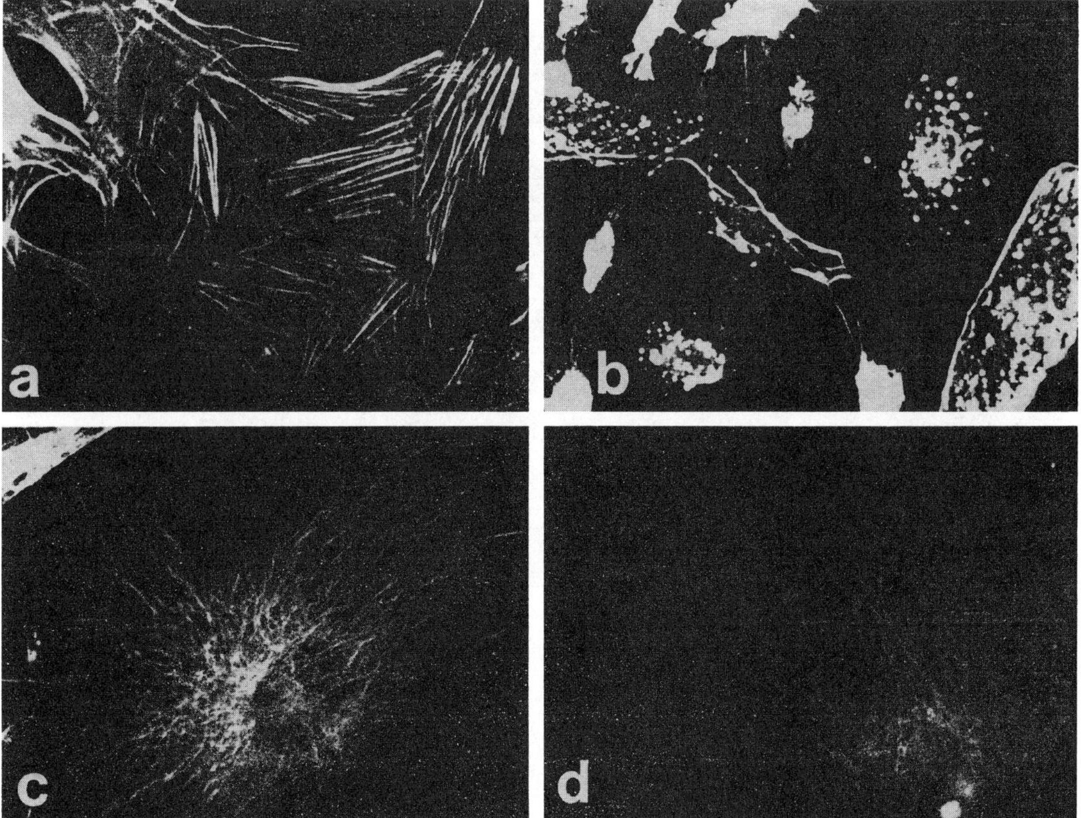

FIG. 30-2. Rhodamine phalloidin staining of filamentous actin in human trabecular meshwork cells in controls (**A**) and 2 hours after exposure to 0.2 mM of ethacrynic acid (ECA) (**B**). Immunofluorescent localization of β-tubulin in calf pulmonary artery cells in controls (**C**) and 10 minutes after exposure to 0.2 mM ECA (**D**).

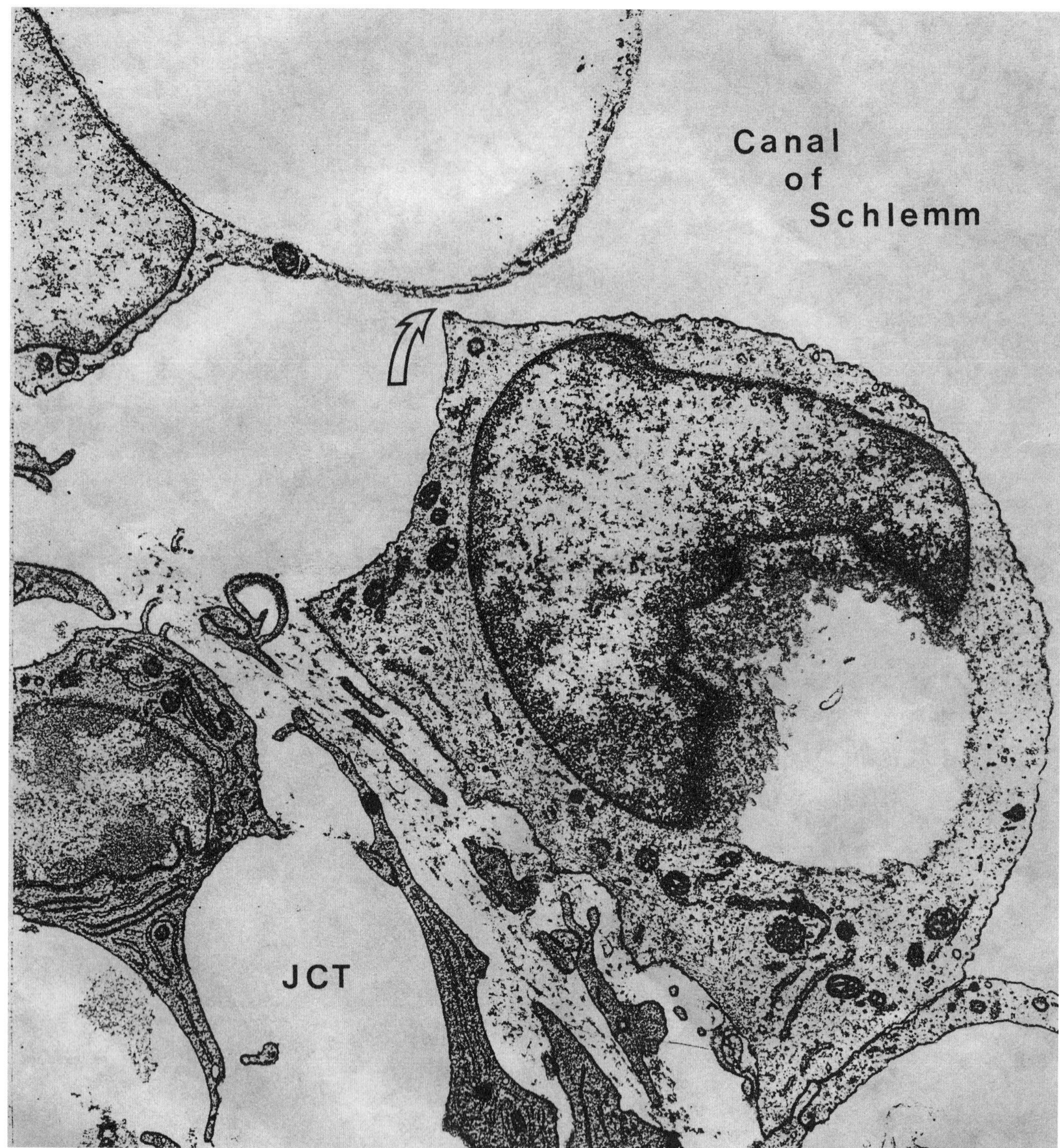

FIG. 30-3. Electron micrograph of the inner wall of Schlemm's canal and adjacent juxtacanalicular tissue in the monkey after intracameral ethacrynic acid administration. Note the focal break between inner wall endothelial cells (arrow). Original magnification, ×11,200.

produce mild-to-marked corneal edema (33). Thiol adducts of ECA may reduce the incidence of corneal toxicity (35).

To date, only one clinical study using ECA has been published (36). Intracameral ECA was administered to five patients, two with primary open-angle glaucoma, two with pseudoexfoliation glaucoma, and one with open-angle glaucoma with associated persistent hypertrophic primary vitreous. Intracameral dosage was 3.3, 6.5, and 9.8 μg, which produced an approximate anterior chamber concentration of 0.05, 0.10, and 0.15 m*M*, respectively. Intraocular pressure was reduced from 9 to 31 mm Hg. The onset of action was 3 to 24 hours following administration, and IOP reduction was sustained for 3 to 7 days. A significant reduction in IOP was noted in all patients, although the mechanism of action cannot be stated with certainty because tonography was not performed. No adverse effects were observed. Visual acuity, anterior chamber reaction, and corneal endothelial cell counts were unchanged in this limited study. No gonioscopic changes were seen. Interestingly, all three types of glaucoma appeared to respond to ECA similarly, despite presumably different pathologies.

Currently, there are no ongoing clinical studies of ECA in the management of glaucoma. A Phase II and III study examining the role of intracameral ECA for patients undergoing cataract surgery failed to demonstrate an effect of ECA on the acute, transient postoperative IOP rise commonly seen in glaucoma patients after cataract surgery (37); however, it is important to stress that ECA is a "pioneer" drug. Recent evidence suggests that sulfhydryl reactivity is not essential for an effect on aqueous outflow within this class of compounds. Nonsulfhydryl reactive agents such as indacrinone and ticrynafen, although chemically related to ECA, disrupt microtubules and increase outflow facility and may be more suitable than ECA for topical use (38). Further investigations into this class of compounds will help to clarify their mechanism of action and may help to produce new innovative treatment approaches for glaucoma patients.

SUMMARY

It is appealing to speculate on an agent or agents that can restore outflow resistance in the trabecular meshwork to normal levels, either by washing out obstructing debris or through the creation of new stable aqueous flow channels within the trabecular meshwork. It is possible that agents such as ECA may prove to be clinically useful. Ultimately, these goals may be reached through biological manipulation of the trabecular meshwork. Laser trabeculoplasty induces changes in the trabecular meshwork that result in long-term IOP reduction (39). A diffusible factor may be responsible in part for this alteration in laser-induced outflow resistance (40).

To date, the mechanism of action of these agents, whether biochemical or biological, remains largely unknown. Despite the relative simplicity of the trabecular meshwork, methods to produce long-term alterations in flow resistance remain elusive; however, it is encouraging that the diligent effort on the part of many talented investigators continues to bring us closer to realization of this important goal.

REFERENCES

1. Kaufman PL, Svedbergh B, Lütjen-Drecoll E. Medical trabeculocanalotomy in monkeys with cytochalasin B or EDTA. *Ann Ophthalmol* 1979;11:795–796.
2. Grant WM. Further studies on the facility of flow through the trabecular meshwork. *Arch Ophthalmol* 1958;60:523–533.
3. Grant WM. Experimental aqueous perfusion in enucleated human eyes. *Arch Ophthalmol* 1963;69:783–801.
4. Maepea O, Bill A. Pressures in the juxtacanalicular tissue and Schlemm's canal in monkeys. *Exp Eye Res* 1991;56:879–883.
5. Knepper PA, Farbman AI, Telser AG. Aqueous outflow pathway glycosaminoglycans. *Exp Eye Res* 1981;32:265–277.
6. Acott TS, Westcott M, Passo MS, Buskirk MV. Trabecular meshwork glycosaminoglycans in human and cynomolgus monkey eye. *Invest Ophthalmol Vis Sci* 1985;26:1320–1329.
7. Ethier CR, Kamm RD, Polaszewski BA, Johnson MC, Richardson TM. Calculations of flow resistance in the juxtacanalicular meshwork. *Invest Ophthalmol Vis Sci* 1986;27:1741–1750.
8. Barany EH. The action of different kinds of hyaluronidase on the resistance of flow through the angle of the anterior chamber. *Acta Ophthalmol Scand* 1956;34:257–290.
9. Sawaguchi S, Yue BYJT, Yeh P, Tso MOM. Effects of intracameral injection of chondroitinase ABC in vivo. *Arch Ophthalmol* 1992;110: 110–117.
10. Weekers R, Watillon M, De Rudder M. Experimental and clinical investigations into the resistance to outflow of acqueous humor in normal subjects. *Br J Ophthalmol* 1956;40:225–233.
11. Chee P, Hamasaki DI. The basis for chymotrypsin-induced glaucoma. *Arch Ophthalmol* 1971;85:103–106.
12. Bill A. Effects of Na$_2$EDTA and alpha-chymotrypsin on aqueous humor outflow conductance in monkey eyes. *Ups J Med Sci* 1980;85: 311–318.
13. Hamanaka T, Bill A. Effects of alpha-chymotrypsin on the outflow routes for aqueous humor. *Exp Eye Res* 1988;46:323–341.
14. Hamanaka T, Bill A. Morphological and functional effects of EDTA on the outflow routes of aqueous humor in monkeys. *Exp Eye Res* 1987;44:171–190.
15. Bill A, Drecoll EL, Svedbergh B. Effects of intracameral Na$_2$EDTA and EGTA on aqueous outflow routes in the monkey eye. *Invest Ophthalmol Vis Sci* 1980;19:492–504.
16. Kaufman PL, Bárány EH. Cytochalasin B reversibly increases outflow facility in the eye of the cynomolgus monkey. *Invest Ophthalmol Vis Sci* 1977;16:47–53.
17. Svedbergh B, Lütjen-Drecoll E, Ober M, Kaufman PL. Cytochalasin B-induced structural changes in the anterior ocular segment of the cynomolgus monkey. *Invest Ophthalmol Vis Sci* 1978;17:718–734.
18. Ritch R, Mulberg A, Rosen C, Chubak G, Pokorny K, Yablonski ME. The effect of colchicine on aqueous humor dynamics. *Exp Eye Res* 1981;32:143–150.
19. Bhattacherjee P, Eakins KE. The intraocular pressure lowering effect of colchicine. *Exp Eye Res* 1978;27:649–653.
20. McClure WO, Paulson JC. The interaction of colchicine and some related alkaloids with rat brain tubulin. *Mol Pharmacol* 1977;13:560–575.
21. Rothstein A. Sulfhydryl- groups in membrane structure and function. In: Brenner F, Kleinzeller A, eds. *Current topics in Membrane Transport,* vol 1. New York: Academic Press, 1970;135–176.
22. Epstein DL, Hashimoto JM, Anderson PJ, Grant WM. Effect of iodoacetamide perfusion on outflow facility and metabolism of the trabecular meshwork. *Invest Ophthalmol Vis Sci* 1981;20:625–631.
23. Epstein DL, Patterson MM, Rivers SC, Anderson PJ. N-ethylmaleimide increases the facility of aqueous outflow of excised monkey and calf eyes. *Invest Ophthalmol Vis Sci* 1982;22:752.
24. Epstein DL, Freddo TF, Bassett-Chu S, Chung M, Karageuzian L. Influence of ethacrynic acid on outflow facility in the monkey and calf eye. *Invest Ophthalmol Vis Sci* 1987;28:2067–2075.
25. Schultz EM, Cragoe EJ, Bicking JB, Bolhofer WA, Sprague JM. Unsaturated ketone derivatives of aryloxyacetic acid a new class of diuretics. *J Med Pharm Chem* 1962;5:660–662.
26. Erickson-Lamy K, Schroeder A, Epstein DL. Ethacrynic acid induces reversible shape and cytoskeletal changes in cultured cells. *Invest Ophthalmol Vis Sci* 1992;33:2631–2640.
27. Xu S. Roychowdhury S, Gaskin F, Epstein DL. Ethacrynic acid inhibition of microtubule assembly in vitro. *Arch Biochem Biophysics* 1992;296:464–467.
28. Tripathi RC, Tripathi BJ. Functional anatomy of the human anterior chamber angle. In: Duane T, Jaeger E, eds. *Biomedical Foundations of Ophthalmology,* vol 1. Hagerstown, Maryland: Harper and Row, 1982;1–88.

29. Epstein DL, Rohen JW. Morphology of the trabecular meshwork and inner-wall endothelium after cationized ferritin perfusion in the monkey eye. *Invest Ophthalmol Vis Sci* 1991;32:160–171.
30. Allingham RR, de Kater AW, Ethier CR, Anderson PJ, Hertzmark E, Epstein DL. The relationship between pore density and outflow facility in human eyes. *Invest Ophthalmol Vis Sci* 1992;33:1661–1669.
31. Alvarado JA, Murphy CG. Outflow obstruction in pigmentary and primary open angle glaucoma. *Arch Ophthalmol* 1991;110:1769–1778.
32. Franse-Carman L, Alvarado JA, Murphy CG, Neufeld AH. Dose response, hydraulic conductivity (HC), and toxicity studies with ethacrynic acid (ECA) in cultured human trabecular (TM) cells. *Invest Ophthalmol Vis Sci* 1994;35:1847.
33. Tingey DP, Ozment RR, Schroeder A, Epstein DL. The effect of intracameral ethacrynic acid on the intraocular pressure of living monkeys. *Am J Ophthalmol* 1992;113:706–711.
34. Liang L-L, Epstein DL, de Kater AW, Shahsafaei A, Erickson-Lamy KA. Ethacrynic acid increases facility of outflow in the human eye in vitro. *Arch Ophthalmol* 1992;110:106–109.
35. Tingey DP, Schroeder A, Epstein MPM, Epstein DL. Effects of topical ethacrynic acid adducts on intraocular pressure in rabbits and monkeys. *Arch Ophthalmol* 1992;110:699–702.
36. Melamed S, Kotas-Neumann R, Barak A, Epstein DL. The effect of intracamerally injected ethacrynic acid on intraocular pressure in patients with glaucoma. *Am J Ophthalmol* 1992;113:508–512.
37. Wise JB, Witter SL. Argon laser therapy for open-angle glaucoma: a pilot study. *Arch Ophthalmol* 1976;94:61–64.
38. Acott TS, Samples JR, Bradley JMB, Bacon DR, Bylsma SS, Van Buskirk EM. Trabecular repopulation by anterior trabecular meshwork cells after laser trabeculoplasty. *Am J Ophthalmol* 1989;107:1–6.
39. Neufeld AH. Oral presentation at the American Academy of Ophthalmology, November 1, 1995.
40. Epstein DL, Roberts BC, Skinner LL. Non-sulfhydryl reactive phenoxyacetic acids increase outflow facility and disrupt the trabecular and endothelial cell cytoskeleton. *Invest Ophthalmol Vis Sci* 1996;37(suppl):S894.

Textbook of Ocular Pharmacology,
edited by T.J. Zimmerman, et al.
Lippincott–Raven Publishers, Philadelphia © 1997.

CHAPTER 31

Physiologic Aspects of Glaucoma and Its Current and Future Management

Laszlo Z. Bito

The chapters in this section discuss specific aspects of currently used glaucoma drugs as well as some potential new ones. This chapter provides physiologic perspectives on the nature of glaucoma and considers the established and theoretical advantages and disadvantages of current and possible future approaches to glaucoma management. Instead of reiterating traditional concepts that have already been reviewed effectively by others (1–4), the emphasis is on the more recently explored aspects of ocular physiology, as well as some of the resulting and new hypotheses concerning the causes and management of glaucomatous optic neuropathy (GON).

The pathophysiology of GON is generally assumed to be related to one or more of the following factors: mechanical damage of otherwise normal ganglion cell axons or their supporting cells caused directly by intraocular pressure (IOP) or by the distortion of the lamina cribrosa; an inherent or acquired insufficiency of the neural elements; neuronal damage secondary to chronic or periodic compromise, either diffuse or focal, of blood flow to the optic nerve head (ONH) caused by vascular abnormalities or by maintained or intermittent IOP increases. Pharmacologic protection against glaucomatous damage, therefore, may be achievable through direct protection of neuronal elements, strengthening of the lamina cribrosa, and protection against compromise of blood flow through the use of vasoactive agents or reduction of IOP.

Weakening of the lamina cribrosa, rather than being the cause of the neuropathy, is likely to occur secondarily to vascular insufficiencies or to the loss of axons, which are integral parts of this structure. In addition, pharmacologic strengthening of the lamina cribrosa does not appear to be a realistic goal for the foreseeable future.

L. Z. Bito: Department of Ophthalmology-Research, Columbia College of Physicians and Surgeons, New York, New York 10032.

PHARMACOLOGIC NEUROPROTECTION IN THE MANAGEMENT OF PRIMARY OPEN-ANGLE GLAUCOMA

The use of a membrane stabilizer, diphenylhydantoin (5), was explored more than two decades ago. Although no useful drug of this type has emerged, several other neuroprotective approaches have recently been considered for the management of primary open-angle glaucoma (POAG) (6,7), including calcium channel blockers, heat-shock proteins, growth factors, and inhibitors of the release or actions of excitatory neurotransmitters. To date, however, no neuroprotective agent has been described that affects only and specifically the ONH or its ganglion cell axons. It is most unlikely, therefore, that safe dosages or methods of administration can be found that will allow such agents to protect these axons without causing side effects that may impair other neuronal functions.

Even the most profound side effects, such as loss of consciousness or motor control, may be acceptable when these drugs are used for a few hours or a few days to reduce the risk of permanent damage caused by acute events, such as asphyxia caused by heart attacks or strokes (6,8,9). It cannot be expected, however, that drugs with such side effects, or even with much more moderate ones, could be used chronically for years or decades for the prevention of neuronal damage in POAG that presumably affects directly only the ONH, which represents in tissue volume <0.0001% of the central nervous system (CNS).

Induction of the intracellular release of heat-shock proteins has also been suggested as an alternate approach to glaucoma management (7), but their protective effect lasts only a few hours (10); in the case of POAG, damage to the ONH may occur gradually over years or decades. Even if this damage proves to be incremental, it cannot be predicted exactly when such protection may be required, whereas the synthesis of heat-shock proteins had to be induced 10 to 18 hours before light damage to provide effective neuroprotection in the retina.

Whereas delivery of drugs specifically to the ONH could circumvent some generalized side effects, it is unlikely that such targeted delivery systems will be sufficiently refined in the near future to allow their long-term use. On the other hand, it is possible that we will learn to use or to enhance the apparent neuroprotective effects of naturally occurring local hormones (see also the section on ocular hypotensive local hormones) (11,12).

Despite these problems, neuroprotection of ganglion cell axons eventually may become a primary treatment in some acute forms of glaucoma and may become a useful adjunct to ocular hypotensive therapy in POAG. The foregoing clearly indicates that application of this approach to the long-term management of POAG faces many hurdles. Thus, expectations, such as the statement that "soon after the turn of the century," glaucoma medications aimed at the reduction of IOP may be replaced by direct neuroprotective treatments (7) seem overly optimistic. In fact, such unsubstantiated statements may be counterproductive because they have the potential of shifting limited research funding away from the development of better, physiologically more acceptable ocular hypotensive agents. This concern is particularly important now, when a large investment over the past three decades into the understanding of aqueous humor dynamics and its pharmacology can be expected to yield a new generation of ocular hypotensive agents without local or systemic side effects negating their beneficial effect with respect to glaucoma.

Pharmacologic means of suppressing programmed cell death (*apoptosis*) has also been mentioned as a possible alternative to IOP control in the medical management of glaucoma (6,13). Advocacy of such an approach can be based only on the assumption that induction of programmed cell death is the cause, rather than the ultimate consequence, of GON. It is, however, difficult to comprehend why a mechanism would have evolved to destroy ganglion cells just because IOP is elevated. From a physiologic point of view, it is more reasonable to assume that programmed cell death occurs in glaucoma because a particular ganglion cell can no longer maintain its normal function. As in fetal development, superfluous neurons, which cannot form functional connection, self-destruct by apoptosis (14,15).

Apoptosis, a recently popularized process of cellular self-destruction, does indeed seem to be involved in ganglion cell death in glaucoma (13,16); however, this does not imply that the use of agents that antagonize this cellular response will prevent the development of GON irrespective of the extent of IOP elevation or vascular insufficiency. Such an approach to POAG management may be like taking away implements of self-destruction from a person suffering from suicidal depression: The person deprived of all means of self-destruction is likely to live, but without any benefit to society, unless the depression itself is treated.

The foregoing considerations suggest that even means of neuroprotection that may prove to be highly effective in preventing or reducing permanent damage after acute brain injuries or vascular events, such as stroke or heart attack, may not be readily applicable to chronic management of POAG. Our ultimate goal must be, therefore, to identify the causes or the "causative risk factors" (17) of this neuropathy and to eliminate or at least minimize them.

ROLE OF INTRAOCULAR PRESSURE

The use of ocular hypotensive agents will almost definitely remain a part of glaucoma management, because without effective IOP control, maintained ocular hypertension or periodic IOP elevations may eventually exceed, in most patients, the tolerance of the neuronal elements of the ONH or even the pressure tolerance of other ocular tissues. This event is particularly likely to occur in light of increasing life expectancy. Indeed, if IOP is left uncontrolled, its effect on the ONH may eventually exceed even the most optimistic expectations regarding therapeutic increases in the tolerance of its neuronal elements.

Clearly, unless we assume that neuroprotection can render these axons impervious to, and thus completely independent of, their chemical environment, we must accept the basic physiologic assumption that focal or generalized interference with ONH blood flow will eventually jeopardize the survival of its neuronal elements. The importance of a well-maintained vascular supply is particularly relevant to the ONH in view of this tissue's high metabolic demand (18).

The foregoing should not be interpreted, however, as advocacy of current approaches to IOP management. Instead, glaucoma management must, in years to come, shift away from the pragmatic approach of reducing IOP by any means to a more rational approach that considers the means of IOP reduction as well as its extent (19,20). We also must consider the mechanisms by which different IOP abnormalities contribute to the pathophysiology of GON and may respond to different ocular hypotensive agents. Thus, we have to examine the types of IOP abnormalities that may cause, or may contribute to, the alterations in functions that can lead to GON and the physiologic parameters that can be sufficiently affected by such IOP abnormalities to cause permanent neuronal damage.

Over the years, dozens of ocular or systemic parameters ranging from abnormal steroid metabolism to connective tissue disorders, have been associated with GON. Vascular mechanisms seem to be consistent with, and may actually account for, most of these putative risk factors, associations, or vulnerabilities. These include the decline in capillary density (21); the pattern of ONH vascularization (3); episodes of nocturnal arterial hypotension (3);

vasospastic syndrome (22); abnormal blood rheology (23–25); abnormal platelet aggregation (26); the reperfusion-induced formation of free radicals (6); and temporary focal hemostasis followed by microscopic areas of no-reflow leading to capillary obstruction and loss (19,27).

The fact that baseline IOP, even in the normal IOP range (28), as well as periodic IOP elevations (19,29–31) is a well-established risk factor with respect to POAG, underscores the role of blood flow parameters in POAG. Clearly, no other physiologic parameters can be expected to be affected by pressures within the very narrow range known to occur in most cases of POAG, especially true in so-called normal-tension glaucoma (NTG), in which the maintained IOP represents <3% of the atmospheric pressure to which we are continuously exposed. In trying to identify the cause of the neuropathy, we must focus on physiologic parameters that can be affected by IOP maintained in the 15 to 25 mm Hg IOP range, which is most commonly associated with POAG, or by transient IOP elevations up to 30 to 60 mm Hg, which may occur in any form of open-angle glaucoma but are too short (i.e., a fraction of a minute in duration) to be clinically detectable (19).

Hydrostatic pressure in this range, or even hundredfold greater pressures, have not been found to have deleterious effects on cells or cellular functions (19,31,32). In contrast, blood flow is driven and affected by pressures in the normal and glaucomatous IOP range.

Autoregulation normally may minimize the impact of ocular hypertension on ONH and retinal blood flow (18,33,34); however, it has recently been considered (31) that even very small increases in IOP can have large effects on some parameters of venous drainage. Furthermore, exaggerated or pharmacologically induced arterial vasodilation or enhanced autoregulation (as a predisposing factor in POAG) may be a predisposing factor for glaucomatous damage (31). These vascular factors and their vulnerability to IOP are considered in this chapter in some detail, but first we must examine current concepts and misconceptions regarding the type of IOP abnormalities that can contribute to vascular insufficiencies and glaucomatous damage.

The role of "office IOP" in the pathophysiology of glaucomatous damage needs to be examined. Clearly, the measurement of IOP in a comfortably seated patient by a reassuring, highly skilled ophthalmologist gives a highly reproducible numerical value. With regard to the progression of glaucomatous damage, however, this may be the least relevant pressure in the patient's eye during the varied activities and stresses of a typical day (19).

Therefore, IOP, as currently measured, should not be referred to as *the* IOP of the patient, but rather as the patient's *office* IOP or *baseline* IOP. Whereas it is clear that even a moderately elevated baseline IOP is a risk factor with respect to POAG (28), this finding may simply reflect a patient's vulnerability to transient IOP elevations (19,29,30).

The types of IOP elevations that may contribute to glaucomatous damage were recently examined (19) and classified according to their time course:

1. *Maintained ocular hypertension,* in which IOP is sufficiently high around the clock to increase the probability of ONH damage, especially when systemic blood pressure declines.
2. *Episodic ocular hypertension* (EPOCH), lasting for a fraction of an hour or a few hours, possibly associated with an activity, a physiologic or psychologic state, a behavior pattern, or an exaggerated circadian hypertensive phase.
3. *IOP spiking,* or sharp IOP increases lasting for a fraction of a minute to a couple of minutes, reaching peak values of 30 to 90 mm Hg, and even more likely to be behavior related than EPOCHs.

Spikes in IOP that last for a fraction of a minute could occur with some regularity in patients who never show any signs of IOP elevation in the office (19). Because of the immediate effect of IOP on the transmural pressure of intraocular blood vessels, such brief IOP elevations may cause focal microcirculatory collapse. According to a recently proposed hypothesis (19), some fraction of such extremely small areas of even momentary microvascular collapse may lead to capillary obstruction through the well-established no-reflow phenomenon (27), possibly combined with reperfusion-associated oxidative damage (6,19).

Examination of the physiologic mechanisms most vulnerable to EPOCH or maintained pressure, within the normal IOP range, also suggested that IOP-driven oscillations in the pressure within the central retinal vein (CRV) (34) can increase the chances of such focal microvascular obstruction (31).

The sequence of events that can lead to no-reflow and subsequent permanent capillary dropout following IOP spike-induced focal microcirculatory hemostasis or collapse may include increased blood viscosity, accumulation of autacoids within the capillary lumen, cellular (red blood cell, leukocytic, or endothelial) interactions, platelet aggregation, and blood clotting (19,31). Thus, even brief IOP spikes such as those associated with any form of pressure on the globe (e.g., those which occur in response to squeezing of the lids, extreme lateral gaze, or uncoordinated extraocular muscle contraction) may contribute significantly to or be the primary cause of the glaucomatous damage in some forms of so-called NTG (19,31).

Age must be considered a risk factor for the accumulation of microvascular occlusions or defects. In a youthful eye, microscopic areas of capillary obstruction or dropout may be revascularized before repeated insults would affect a large enough area to cause perceptible neuronal damage. Thus, detectable field loss can be expected to occur as a consequence of IOP spikes or exaggerated CRV pulsatility due to the waterfall effect (31) (see below) only when the frequency of focal microcirculatory collapse or the extent of capillary obstruction and dropout overwhelms the regenerative capacity of the microvascular system.

According to this model of focal vascular insufficiency, low perfusion pressure is a risk factor because it can exaggerate the no-reflow phenomenon (19). Therefore, IOP spikes superimposed on maintained or episodic ocular hypertension (19,31) are expected to result in great vulnerability to GON, especially when combined with periods of (nocturnal) arterial hypotension.

An association between the occurrence of IOP peaks and the progression of glaucomatous damage has already been demonstrated (29,30). Unfortunately, the home tonometer used was not suitable to achieve effective definition of the time course of the so-called IOP peaks. We can assume, however, that most of these represented EPOCHs rather than IOP spikes such as those caused by momentary compression of the globe by, for example, lid squeezing (35) or events occurring during sleep (19). Such IOP spikes cannot be detected even with the type of home tonometry used in that study (30) because the use of this tonometer requires the interruption of sleep or the patient's activities that can cause IOP spikes.

The contribution of maintained IOP to the pathophysiology of glaucoma is harder to understand in physiologic terms because the maintained pressure in most glaucomatous eyes, as measured by routine tonometry during office hours, is in the 15 to 25 mm Hg range, which obviously is not damaging to ocular tissues, unlike the IOP "peaks" (30), especially the IOP spikes, which can reach values of 60 to 90 mm Hg (19).

A maintained elevation of IOP from 15 mm Hg to 25 mm Hg theoretically could reduce perfusion pressure by only 10% to 20%, an amount likely to be well within the typical biological safety margin. Moreover, such an increase in IOP is expected to have no significant effect on perfusion pressure because of the well-demonstrated autoregulatory mechanisms that maintain blood flow in the retina and ONH, despite elevated IOP in this range (18,33). Nevertheless, the maintained IOP, even within the normal range, as measured in the office by routine tonometric techniques, is clearly a risk factor with respect to the development and progression of glaucomatous damage (28).

Only continuous IOP monitoring[1] can determine whether maintained IOP in the 14 to 20 mm Hg range of NTG is a risk factor by itself or whether IOP in this range is only an indication of the vulnerability to EPOCH or IOP spiking. As we shall see, however, baseline IOP in this range may have a dramatic effect on venous outflow (31). Furthermore, the level of baseline IOP should be a determinant of the amount of permanent damage caused by IOP spikes (19) because the extent of permanent damage following focal microcirculatory collapse depends on the magnitude of the postasphyxic perfusion pressure (27,36) and also because the time course of the IOP spike is too short to induce an autoregulatory response (19).

These considerations clearly suggest that IOP can well be the underlying cause of the pathophysiologic process in both normal tension and hypertensive POAG. For these reasons, the proposed vascular mechanism that can contribute to and may even account for the pathophysiologic processes leading to GON, even in NTG (19,31), will be discussed in some detail. First, however, we must examine whether there is a physiologic basis for dividing POAG into two separate entities based on IOP.

"Normal-tension glaucoma" is an inappropriate term inasmuch as it suggests that the development of glaucomatous damage is *known* to occur in patients whose IOP never exceeds the so-called normal range. *Normal baseline tension* or *normal office tension* glaucoma would be more appropriate terms to apply to patients whose IOP is never observed to exceed the perceived upper limit of the normal range as measured clinically in the office under resting conditions during daytime hours. This pressure is, however, unlikely to be representative of the patient's daily IOP history (19).

Until continuous IOP monitoring devices become available, we cannot be sure that true NTG exists; if it does, we cannot begin to estimate its prevalence (19). Even the phrase *normal baseline tension glaucoma* should not be used to include patients with recorded IOPs of up to 22 mm Hg, as has been reported in some recent publications (26), much less patients in whom such high IOPs are maintained despite glaucoma medication (42).

Even if true NTG does exist and, in the unlikely event that we are dealing with two distinctly different pathophysiologic mechanisms in normotensive and hypertensive glaucoma, it is most unlikely that the separation between these two mechanisms can be drawn at an IOP value of 22 mm Hg. On the contrary, there must be a gray zone in which either presumed mechanism may contribute to glaucomatous damage. Thus, it may be prudent for studies on the mechanisms and treatment of normotensive glaucoma to include only patients with IOPs up to the normal mean IOP + 1SD, or $\leq$19 mm Hg,[2] and in studies aimed at elucidating the mechanism or treatment of hypertensive glaucoma, only patients with IOP values greater than the normal mean IOP + 2SD, or $\geq$22 mm Hg should be included.

It is possible that the use of continuous IOP monitoring devices eventually will reveal some cases of progressive glaucomatous neuropathy in eyes that never exhibit maintained IOPs exceeding 16 to 18 mm Hg and do not experience sufficient episodic or spiking IOP abnormalities to account for the

[1]Several IOP monitoring devices have been described over the years (37–41); however, the extent of effort invested in developing a clinically acceptable design has not reflected the importance of such a device for the understanding of the true role of IOP, especially transient IOP abnormalities, in the glaucomatous process, and for the evaluation of the true, around-the-clock ocular hypotensive efficacy of glaucoma drugs (19).

[2]By rounding off to 16 $\pm$ 3 mm Hg, the value of 15.9 $\pm$ 2.89 mm Hg given for the mean $\pm$1 SD IOP of a large normal population (43).

neuropathy. Even in these cases, however, we should not assume that IOP is not a "causative risk factor" (17) because there are parameters of ocular blood flow that can be drastically affected by pressures within the normal IOP range (31).

THE EXIT OF THE CENTRAL RETINAL VEIN (CRV) FROM THE GLOBE AS A POINT OF GREAT VULNERABILITY TO IOP-DEPENDENT VASCULAR DAMAGE

The effects of IOP on the venous drainage of the ONH have generally been overlooked, as advocates of the vascular theory of glaucomatous damage have focused their attention on the arterial aspects of the vascular bed. As pointed out recently (31), the venous drainage of the ONH is not even mentioned in some otherwise thorough reviews (3,4). Even perfusion pressure is generally given as the difference between arterial pressure and IOP (3) rather than the actual perfusion pressure, which is the difference between the arterial and venous pressures within any vascular system (34).

Bill, in his excellent review of the ocular circulation (34), pointed out that an intravascular waterfall effect is created at the point where the pressure in a vein undergoes a precipitous drop as it leaves the high-pressure area of the globe and enters the low-pressure area of the orbit. This pressure difference accelerates the flow, making the vein partially collapse, which in turn increases the resistance to flow at the affected site until pressure builds again to exceed the IOP, giving rise to an oscillating or pulsatile and highly turbulent venous outflow (34).

Problems associated with the venous drainage of the globe could be regarded simply as the opposite side of the problem encountered with respect to the arterial blood supply entering the globe from a low-pressure to a high-pressure environment; however, arterial pressure typically is severalfold greater than IOP. Thus, even a 5 or 10 mm Hg increase in IOP has little effect on the ability of arterial blood to enter the globe, especially given the fact that the autoregulation of arterial tone may compensate for any pressure effect (33,34). In contrast, pressure in the venous side of the ONH circulation is approximately equal to IOP. Thus, an extremely small change in IOP can have a great effect on the magnitude of the waterfall effect (31).

The impact of IOP on venous drainage from the globe can be illustrated by the following example. Let us assume that in a supine subject pressure in the orbital portion of the CRV is 10 mm Hg, whereas in its prelaminal intraocular portion it is equal to the IOP, which is 14 mm Hg. Thus, there is a waterfall effect of 4 mm Hg. If, in the same eye at a later time, or in the other eye of the same subject at the same time, the IOP is 18 mm Hg, which is still within the domain of so-called NTG, then the magnitude of the waterfall effect is doubled, to 8 mm Hg.

The pathophysiologic significance of the waterfall effect can be appreciated if we bear in mind that turbulence in venous blood flow, which is proportional to the pressure drop at the site of the waterfall, has been considered the cause of endothelial damage leading to CRV occlusion (44). Venous occlusion, in turn, has been linked to glaucoma (45). One would expect, however, that more moderate or more localized compromises in venous drainage will occur well before frank CRV occlusion becomes clinically apparent.

Restriction to Venous Outflow from the Globe

In considering the problem posed by venous drainage from the high-pressure environment within the globe into the low-pressure environment of the orbit, Bill in 1984 (34) apparently assumed that the veins have the same cross-sectional area and shape in their intraocular, intrascleral, and orbital segments in all persons. A recent review of the relevant literature (31) led to the conclusion that this is not the case with respect to the CRV. The cross-sectional area and shape of this vein at its passage through the lamina cribrosa have been reported to show great individual-to-individual variation (44). This passage is relatively unrestricted in some eyes, whereas in other eyes the CRV is compressed by the central retinal artery into a narrow crescent shape at the point of their side-by-side passage through a connective tissue channel across the lamina cribrosa (44).

Considering the effects of this variability in CRV dimensions at the lamina cribrosa and, hence, in resistance to flow, it was concluded (31) that, depending on the extent of CRV restriction at the lamina cribrosa, individual eyes can be expected to have different vulnerabilities to IOP abnormalities and, consequently, different vulnerabilities to different pathologic effects (45). We can consider three categories of restrictions of the lamina cribrosa within the range of described CRV configurations (44): a highly restricted passage, a moderately restricted passage, and an essentially unrestricted passage for venous drainage.

The moderately restricted passage can be regarded as a CRV configuration that confers the least vulnerability to IOP, even well above its normal range. Such moderate restriction or "throttling" (46) can be sufficient to minimize pulsation without increasing the resistance to venous drainage to the point at which it reduces perfusion pressure below the value compatible with normal function. Eyes with this optimal morphologic arrangement may be unaffected by IOPs, even in the 20 to 30 mm Hg range, which may help to explain the fact that some eyes with elevated IOPs never develop GON (28,43).

An overly restricted lamina cribrosa passage can maintain pressure within the prelaminal CRV significantly above the IOP (31,46,47), which has two potentially pathologic consequences: First, the high intraocular venous pressure lowers the perfusion pressure below that calculated by the usual formula of arterial pressure minus IOP (3), which can lead to insufficient perfusion, especially in regions of lowest arterial pressure, such as a watershed zone that typically includes the ONH (3). In addition, the high intraocular venous pressure greatly increases the magnitude of the waterfall effect, causing a great acceleration of blood flow through the narrowest part of the CRV. This acceleration, in turn, causes turbulent flow past this restriction, causing endothelial damage, and ultimately may cause venous occlusion (44).

The CRV can be compressed and compromised further by the autoregulatory or pharmacologic relaxation of arterial tone: Dilation of the central retinal artery will compress the low-pressure CRV within the connective tissue channel they share (31). It can be predicted, therefore, that in some eyes pharmacologic arterial vasodilatation will actually reduce, rather than increase, perfusion pressure (31).

On the other hand, a completely unrestricted passage of the venous outflow through the lamina cribrosa leads to an extremely unstable situation in which the unthrottled acceleration of blood flow toward the low-pressure orbital region of the vein causes intermittent partial collapse, or oscillations, in the prelaminal portion of the CRV (34). The result is wear and tear on its wall and adjacent connective tissue elements (31).

The magnitude of these oscillations or pulsations is proportional to the difference between IOP and the pressure in the postlaminal segment of the CRV; however, the CRV itself is most unlikely to collapse completely, even if the IOP is elevated well above normal levels in an eye with unthrottled venous drainage. As the diameter of this vein begins to decrease in response to a momentarily negative transmural pressure, the pressure within it increases and, at one point, equalizes with the IOP (34). A few adjacent small-diameter venules occasionally may collapse completely, especially when the venous pulsations are compounded by the microvascular effects of transient IOP spikes (31).

The Predictable Prognostic Value of CRV Configuration and Restriction at its Passage Through the Lamina Cribrosa

These considerations suggest that the extent of laminal restriction or throttling of CRV blood flow may be important in determining the vulnerability of a particular eye to the pathophysiologic consequences of maintained ocular hypertension and transient IOP abnormalities (31). This hypothesis can be tested by using one of the rapidly improving imaging techniques (48). Such a study could elucidate the association between vulnerability to GON and the extent of restriction to flow at the site where the CRV passes through the lamina cribrosa.

Imaging techniques revealing the shape and cross-sectional area of the CRV at its passage through the lamina cribrosa, therefore, may turn out to be, in years to come, an important diagnostic means of determining the vulnerability of a particular patient to various types of IOP abnormalities. An appreciation of these differences in the vulnerability of the venous drainage to IOP also may lead to the development of a rational approach to the selection of appropriate means of IOP management for individual patients.

Even the most effective pharmacologic neuroprotection, therefore, is unlikely to prevent this type of axonal damage unless it can render the axons completely insensitive to their chemical environment. As long as the protected axons still require some metabolic exchanges, the accumulation of underperfused or ischemic foci or the gradual enlargement of such foci, due to repeated pressure transients and accumulating microvascular defects, eventually will jeopardize axonal survival.

Hemorrhagic Events and the Effects of Vasoactive Drugs

For patients whose glaucomatous neuropathies can be linked to cardiovascular insufficiency or deficiency in autoregulation, the use of drugs to overcome these deficiencies seems a logical approach (6,49). The maintenance of high intraocular arteriolar pressure by vasodilator agents can result in excessive microvascular transmural pressures, however. Under this condition, transmural pressure may exceed the tensile strength of some vascular walls when IOP declines. Transmural pressure and the consequent risk of microvascular hemorrhages can be further increased if the venous pressure is increased because of the compression of the CRV by the pharmacologic dilatation of the central retinal artery.

The vulnerability to hemorrhagic incidents also may be increased by drugs that enhance deficient autoregulation without causing permanent arterial vasodilatation. This occurs because ineffective autoregulation, or its complete inhibition in some ONH tissues, actually may be due to its physiologic suppression by endogenous vasoconstrictory autacoids, which are known to be released in the brain, for example, following a hemorrhagic incident (50,51), Thus, a lack of autoregulation may not be the sign of a deficiency but rather may reflect a physiologic response to limit the extent of bleeding or to prevent further hemorrhagic incidents after hemorrhaging has already occurred in a tissue.

These considerations are particularly important because hemorrhagic incidents in the ONH precede the progression of glaucomatous damage in some eyes and actually may be a cause of the neuropathy (45,52–54). Thus, drugs that prevent vasoconstriction may prove beneficial in some (nonhemorrhagic) forms of glaucoma but be detrimental in others.

It should be noted that some authorities have questioned the role of hemorrhagic events in the progression of this neuropathy. Maumenee (55) pointed out, for example, that splinter hemorrhages are located "in the retinal nerve fiber layer of the optic disc, and not in the area of the lamina cribrosa where axonal damage occurs in glaucoma." This may well be the case, but it is not known exactly where the axonal damage is initiated in any given eye, even if it is primarily expressed morphologically at the lamina cribrosa.

Moreover, the shape and size of a hemorrhage are obviously affected by the compactness and organization of the tissue around it, and the likelihood of a hemorrhage being noted also depends on its location and size, especially considering that, depending on its size and location, a small hemorrhage may be absorbed within days or weeks. Thus, the chances are small that highly restricted hemorrhages deep in the densely packed laminar region of the ONH will be detected during quarterly or semiannual examinations compared with the chances of detecting a larger hemorrhage in the less densely packed superficial layers of the disk.

IOP spikes can be expected to play an important role in, and may be the primary cause of, microhemorrhagic events. Hemorrhage is most likely to occur *after* IOP spikes of longer than typical duration or a sequence of brief IOP spikes because such events can lead to an autoregulatory increase in arteriolar pressure. Although capillary transmural pressure is minimized *during* an IOP spike by the elevated pressure within the globe, the precipitous postspike drop in IOP, too rapid to be paralleled by the reversal of autoregulatory increase in arteriolar pressure, possibly may cause high enough transmural pressure to rupture some microvessels.

This, together with a drop in IOP below its prespike baseline level, due to loss of choroidal blood volume during the IOP spikes, may increase transmural pressure to the point that it exceeds the tensile strength of some small blood vessels. The occurrence of such microhemorrhages is likely to be increased in the vicinity of previous episodes of no-reflow-induced capillary or venular thrombosis or dropout, which increases pressure in the adjacent capillaries.

OTHER PHYSIOLOGIC PARAMETERS THAT MAY CONTRIBUTE TO GLAUCOMATOUS DAMAGE

The relative contribution of diurnal[3] versus nocturnal IOP elevations to glaucomatous damage has not been adequately explored despite the fact that it has been known for many decades that IOP shows considerable circadian variation (56). The existence of such variation has been confirmed repeatedly, although the high and low IOP values have been reported at different times (29,57–59), possibly reflecting, in part, differences in sleep patterns (60).

The management of nocturnal IOP and IOP elevations or IOP spikes are of particular concern (19) because they may be associated with periods of greatest vulnerability to vascular compromises during nocturnal episodes of systemic hypotension (3). Furthermore, there is no reason to assume that either the diurnally measured parameters of aqueous humor dynamics or the effects of drugs on those parameters are directly applicable to the greatly different physiologic states that exist during sleep.

The fact that aqueous humor flow is reduced during sleep (63) clearly implies that other parameters of aqueous humor dynamics also are affected during sleep to reflect or compensate for reduced secretion. Indeed, we must assume that several coordinated changes in aqueous humor dynamics have evolved to facilitate daily maintenance and repair functions within the anterior segment, including the conventional outflow route (19).

Periodic reflux of blood into the collecting ducts and Schlemm's canal must be required to bring platelets into these vessels for the maintenance and repair of their endothelial lining (64,65). It is likely that a temporary increase in episcleral venous pressure (66) is required for this periodic reflux of blood to occur (19), which is achieved by the opening of some of the arteriovenous anastomoses that are known to exist in the episcleral and intrascleral plexuses (67,68). Such events may be reflected in the conjunctival hyperemia observed in many people on waking. During periods of increased episcleral venous pressure resulting from postural or vasodynamic effects, the reflux of blood into Schlemm's canal can be further facilitated by the shunting of aqueous humor outflow toward the uveoscleral outflow routes (19).

Alternatively, the periodic delivery of platelets to these unique parts of the vascular system, which are filled with aqueous humor most of the time, may be achieved by opening up only occasionally expressed anastomoses (69) between the canal of Schlemm, which should be regarded as part of the vascular system (64,65,67,68), and the adjacent arterial circle of the chamber angle. Such periodic arterialization of the canal of Schlemm implies drastic periodic changes in aqueous humor dynamics.

Interestingly, the stable analogue of the platelet-associated eicosanoid, thromboxane A_2, has a profound contractile effect on isolated strips of bovine trabecular meshwork (70). Furthermore, in the perfused bovine anterior segment, this analogue, U-46619, decreased outflow facility (71). This finding suggests that platelets that reflux into Schlemm's canal can release a local hormone to reduce, possibly block, outflow in a segment of the conventional outflow route to facilitate repair processes. This hypothesis is worthy of study because of its implications with respect to the maintenance of normal conventional outflow facility.

[3]Some glaucomatologists use the word *diurnal* to refer to daytime observations only (61), whereas others report under *diurnal* IOP values obtained over 24 hours (62). In this chapter, *diurnal* and *nocturnal* are used to describe events or observations pertaining to day and to night, respectively, and *circadian* to describe events or observations over an approximately 24-hour period. For the sake of uniformity, it is urged that this usage, which conforms to the first definitions of these terms in *Stedman's Medical Dictionary*, be generally adopted or that other terminology that clearly distinguishes between daytime and nighttime events, be adopted.

The vulnerability of tissues of the anterior segment to altered aqueous humor flow must also be considered in understanding the shortcomings of current means of IOP management and appreciating some basic requirements for the development of a rational physiologic approach to the management of IOP.

Based on the recent advocacy of as yet unproven neuroprotective approaches (6,7), it might be argued that glaucoma management optimally should begin in the future with direct pharmacologic protection of ONH functions and that IOP control should be employed only when general damage becomes apparent. This argument, however, overlooks the fact that the outflow channels are also located within the globe and are also vulnerable to IOP elevations (72–76). Furthermore, the trabecular meshwork is an avascular tissue that depends on the flow of aqueous humor for its metabolic exchanges. Consequently, one of the most imminent challenges to ocular pharmacology is the development of means of IOP control that will ensure the maintenance or restoration of the nutritional supply and functional normalcy of outflow channels.

Surgical techniques for IOP reduction clearly have improved during recent decades; however, the tools available to ophthalmic surgeons still look, from a cellular perspective, like meat cleavers and battering rams. Presumably, laser technology also alters only the general proximity of the apparently afflicted area, although improved laser delivery has helped to limit the tissue destruction to specific structures, thus reducing collateral damage. Such techniques can be sight saving when pharmacology fails and unquestionably will improve with time.

However, as long as glaucoma surgery depends on altering rather than restoring physiology, it will be necessary to use pharmacologic or even toxicologic antifibrotic agents (see Chapter 28) even if, because of their low therapeutic index, they provide a narrow safety margin (77). From a physiologic perspective, we can only admire the determination of surgeons to use the Trojan Horse of antimetabolites (77) to overcome the self-restorative capacity of the ocular tissues and the resilience of the biological system in resisting such chemical warfare.

Suppression of wound healing and the tissue damage caused by the antifibrotic agent is not the only physiologic concern regarding glaucoma surgery, however. An even more fundamental concern is the creation of a single pathway of flow of least resistance, particularly when combined with a peripheral iridectomy. Such procedures must shunt aqueous humor flow away from most anterior segment tissues, including most of the trabecular meshwork, which normally depend on it for their metabolic exchanges (76).

Compromise of the metabolic exchanges of the avascular tissues of the anterior segment is also a primary physiologic concern when using drugs that reduce aqueous humor production. Carbonic anhydrase inhibitors (CAIs), in particular, are expected to alter the chemical composition of aqueous humor (78), besides reducing the rate of aqueous flow below its already lowered circadian value at night.

This circadian variation is apparently the result of stimulation of aqueous humor production by circulating catecholamines or other mediators during waking hours (63, 79). This finding suggests that a mechanism has evolved to increase aqueous humor flow during the day and may be particularly important in diurnal species, which may require a more rapid turnover of aqueous humor during the day to minimize photooxidation-induced accumulation of potentially toxic substances in the anterior chamber (93).

Although the specifics of the effects of reduced aqueous flow on intraocular tissues will require study, it seems more physiologic to reduce daytime aqueous humor flow to its unstimulated, nighttime value, as achieved by timolol and other beta-adrenergic blocking agents than to reduce this flow rate below its nighttime low value by CAIs. Thus, the combined use of a beta-blocker and a CAI, having an additive effect on the reduction of aqueous humor flow, is important with respect to the potential compromise of the metabolic exchanges of the avascular anterior chamber tissues, including the trabecular meshwork (76,80).

From a physiologic point of view, reduction of the resistance to outflow is clearly preferable to the reduction of aqueous humor production as a means of achieving the required IOP reduction. We must not assume, however, that all drugs that reduce this resistance are equally effective in providing around-the-clock protection against all forms of IOP abnormalities that can contribute to glaucomatous damage (19).

PHYSIOLOGIC PERSPECTIVES ON CURRENTLY USED GLAUCOMA DRUGS AND ON THE DEVELOPMENT OF A RATIONAL APPROACH TO THE MEDICAL MANAGEMENT OF GLAUCOMA

Until now, IOP management has focused on the use of drugs that reduce "office IOP" by mimicking or blocking the effects of neurotransmitters, which is not surprising because neurotransmitters and some of their functions already had been discovered in the nineteenth century and drugs that mimic or inhibit their effects have dominated pharmacology during the first half of the twentieth century. It is time to explore the ocular hypotensive utility of new classes of biologic mediators that were discovered in the first half of the twentieth century and whose diverse pharmacologic properties still are being explored.

The manipulation of aqueous humor dynamics can be achieved by three distinctly different types of drugs: receptor-mediated agonists (pilocarpine, epinephrine) or antagonists (timolol and other beta blockers); directly acting agents, such as enzyme inhibitors (acetazolamide and other CAIs); and directly acting enzyme inhibitors that cause the accumulation of a substance that reduces IOP by a receptor-mediated mechanism (DFP, phospholine iodide) (see Chapter 20). These three drug types can be expected to have different specificity and side-effect profiles as well as different pharmacokinetic and pharmacodynamic properties (19,20).

Directly acting drugs, such as enzyme inhibitors, are likely to produce severe side effects given the fact that a unique enzyme responsible for ocular hypertension or glaucomatous damage has not been identified. Indeed, extensive side effects have greatly limited the use of systemic CAIs.

Drugs that have a direct effect on the cytoarchitecture or on cell-to-cell adhesion, such as ethacrynic acid and Na_2 EDTA (64), presumably reduce IOP by creating a pharmacologic trabeculocanulotomy. Such drugs are likely to lack specificity toward cells of the outflow channels. Thus, their long-term topical use is likely to be limited by local side effects.

The topical CAIs are expected to be free of the most common systemic side effects of oral CAIs because a smaller daily dose is used even in the course of bilateral treatment two or three times a day (80). It should be noted, however, that the often-raised question of how much of the topically applied drug is systemically absorbed is unwarranted from a physiologic perspective. We must assume that all the applied amount is systemically absorbed because it has nowhere else to go except when some of it runs down the patient's cheek or ends up on the fingers during punctal compression and is wiped or washed off. Herein may lie at least a partial answer to the otherwise unexplained claim that punctal occlusion reduces by 60% the amount of timolol absorbed systemically after its topical application (82).

Thus, the possibility of some systemic side effect occurring during long-term use of topical CAIs must be considered. Of the side effects reportedly associated with systemic CAIs, aplastic anemia is of particular concern because the incidence of this rare (83) but potentially lethal affliction is not directly related to the dose of the sulphonamide used (84).

Local side effects are more likely to occur with the topical application of CAIs because this route of delivery circumvents the blood-aqueous barrier. Thus, topical CAIs will cause much greater local inhibition of carbonic anhydrase activity, especially at the ocular surface, including the trabecular meshwork, than systemic CAIs.

The hydration of otherwise normal corneas is not expected to be adversely affected, however, even if endothelial carbonic anhydrase activity is completely blocked, because only about 30% of the fluid transport capacity of the corneal endothelium is bicarbonate dependent (85). We would expect that in a completely healthy cornea, this transport capacity has at least a 30% safety margin. It is not surprising, therefore, that a clinical study with topical CAIs on selected patients has not revealed a "clinically significant" increase in corneal thickness (81). However, these considerations suggest that corneas that are compromised by low endothelial cell counts, old age, or pathologies might not have sufficient reserve in their fluid transport capacity and must be carefully monitored when chronically exposed to topical CAIs.

These considerations also suggest that even if the observed statistically significant increase in corneal thickness after topical CAI treatment is judged to be "not clinically significant" (80), reports on such studies should include the range of corneal thickness or the number of corneas that exhibited "clinically significant" increases in thickness or decreases in endothelial cell count to allow evaluation of the impact of topical CAI treatment on eyes that may have greater than average vulnerability to inhibition of endothelial fluid transport.

However, from a physiological perspective, the greatest concern is not the side effects of these drugs but the mechanism of their IOP-lowering effect, which is presumably the same as that of oral CAIs (i.e., the nonphysiologic reduction of aqueous humor production) already considered above and elsewhere (76,80).

Receptor-mediated drugs have the great theoretical advantage that they can diffuse from the ocular surface to the sites of IOP control without affecting cells in the intervening tissues that do not express the particular receptor. Furthermore, receptor-mediated agonists should be preferred because they have the potential to restore normal function by stimulating or enhancing physiologic processes.

In contrast, receptor-mediated antagonists, such as timolol and other beta-blockers, which reduce IOP by blocking physiologic processes, can be expected to hinder normal function. With regard to the development of a rational physiologic approach to IOP management, we also must distinguish different subclasses of receptors that can exhibit very different properties, depending on their functions and the nature of their biologic agonists.

Three basic classes of substances are produced in the body, called *autacoids*; they mediate or modulate physiologic processes through their interaction with specific receptors: neurotransmitters, hormones, and local hormones. It has already been suggested that among the three corresponding classes of potential receptor-mediated drugs, those that mimic local hormones can be expected to offer the greatest advantage for glaucoma management. The underlying physiologic and pharmacokinetic principles have already been discussed in detail (19,20,86) and are reviewed here only briefly.

Neurotransmitters can exert unrelated or even antagonistic effects within the same organ system or even the same tissue. Their physiologically required selectivity is achieved by selective innervation. For example, through selective innervation, both the extension and the flexion of the arm are mediated by acetylcholine. Similarly, pilocarpine has been shown to have antagonistic effects on IOP control, increasing conventional outflow facility while hindering uveoscleral outflow (74,87,88).

In addition, neurotransmitters have evolved to have effects lasting only a fraction of a second to a few minutes. Consequently, their receptors typically become subsensitive or undergo "downregulation" during the course of prolonged exposure, as occurs, for example, during the course of daily application of cholinomimetic miotics or cholinesterase inhibitors to the eye (86,89). The question then arises of whether the efforts to develop slow-release technologies (see Chapter 10), such as the pilocarpine Ocusert for the continuous delivery of such drugs, are based on sound physiologic principles or on unexamined pharmacokinetic assumptions (20,86).

Hormones have evolved to maintain their effects continuously over days, months, or even years. Therefore, their receptors typically do not show downregulation, even after long-term exposure to their agonists. Furthermore, in contrast to neurotransmitters, *hormones* have evolved to be carried by the circulation to all parts of the body, simultaneously affecting many organ systems. Therefore, they are expected to have consonant, even if not the same, effects on all parts of the body. Because of their effective distribution through the circulation, however, they reach all parts of the body, and their topical application to the eye is likely to cause systemic side effects (19,86).

Local hormones, on the other hand, are autacoids that have evolved to affect cells or tissues in the vicinity of their site of release but are prevented from affecting other parts of the body by their rapid systemic metabolism or renal excretion. Given these physiologic principles, local hormones that have a limited range of action and consonant effects within their diffusional domain offer the best approach to the development of a new generation of topically applied ocular hypotensive agents (20,86).

Ocular hypotensive local hormones that enhance outflow offer special theoretical advantages for glaucoma management because we can expect them, or their appropriate analogues, to have effects within the globe that are consonant with and ancillary to the physiologic processes or requirements associated with IOP control. For example, some ocular hypotensive local hormones and their exogenous analogues can be expected not only to have beneficial effects on outflow structures but to offer protection against the adverse effect of increased IOP on other intraocular tissues, which can be regarded as physiologic effects consonant with their ocular hypotensive effects.

Protection of the ONH against IOP-induced damage also can be expected to be one such consonant effect. Conversely, we can expect that metabolic or mechanical stressing of the ONH may lead to the release of local hormones aimed at restoring normal IOP. Regarding the delivery of such local hormones from the ONH to the ciliary body to influence various aspects of aqueous humor dynamics, it should be noted that a transport mechanism has been described that provides for the essentially quantitative delivery of one class of local hormones, the prostaglandins, into the ciliary body from the posterior chamber and the vitreous body (90,91).

Although the local hormone approach offers the possibility of simultaneously mobilizing several consonant mechanisms for protection of the neuronal elements of the papillary area, the delivery to the ONH of a topically applied local hormone or its analogue appears to present a currently insurmountable pharmacokinetic challenge, as already discussed, with respect to the delivery of other neuroprotective agents to this site.

The spectrum of consonant effects of a topically applied exogenous local hormone or its analogue may, however, include the local release of the same or other endogenous local hormones from intraocular tissues. These local hormones in turn may reach the posterior pole of the eye. Alternatively, the consonant effects of such local hormones may be extended even more rapidly and over even greater distances through axon reflexes.

Indeed, the heavy sensory innervation of the anterior border layer of the iris (92), a site that is normally well protected from touch or mechanical irritation, is likely to reflect the physiologic and pathophysiologic significance of such axon reflex mechanisms that can cause the release of neuropeptides and other mediators required for the maintenance of normal homeostasis and physiologic protective responses.

These mechanisms may include the control of melanogenesis or other melanocytic functions within the iris in response to corneal irritation, for example (93). In turn, the intimate association of sensory and autonomic nerves with the melanocytes of the anterior border layer of the iris (92,94) may reflect communication between cells of the anterior uvea and other ocular structures through such axon reflexes and the consequent release of autacoids from neuronal components at remote intraocular sites.

Our knowledge of the spectrum of functional autacoids, in particular the spectrum of local hormones involved in the coordination of normal functions and in the biological responses to stress and injury, is still rudimentary. New local hormones are discovered yearly and, based on past experience, it may take decades to gain a reasonable comprehension of their biological effects. For example, prostaglandins were discovered in the 1930s, but their ubiquitous local hormone nature was not realized until the 1960s, whereas their protective effects, including ocular hypotensive effects, were not generally appreciated until the 1980s (95–97). This class of local hormones only recently yielded clinically useful ocular hypotensive agents (98) (see Chapter 29). Their other protective effects in the eye with regard to maintenance of the normal corneal endothelial morphology, facilitation of wound healing, and their neuroprotective effects only began to be appreciated recently (11,93,95,99), 60 years after their discovery.

Attaining a full appreciation of the advantages of the local hormone approach in the field of general pharmacology may be an even slower process because the selective delivery of such drugs to most target tissues presents a much greater problem than does their selective delivery to intraocular tissues. Therefore, we can expect that ocular pharmacology will take the lead in taking full advantage of this therapeutic approach, not only for the management of POAG but also for the management of other ocular disorders, including conditions such as rubeosis, pigment dispersion, and formation of synechiae that may lead to secondary glaucomas.

A Physiologic Perspective on the Combined Use of Ocular Hypotensive Agents

Gaining a better insight into the physiologic and pathophysiologic processes through which IOP abnormalities ultimately can lead to GON can be expected to allow the development of new, more effective, and more selective ocular hypotensive agents. The tendency has been to prescribe more and more ocular hypotensive agents as the glaucomatous process progresses, ultimately achieving so-called maximal medication of some patients only when nothing else is available on the pharmacist's shelves. Such an addition of ocular hypotensive agents might have started out as a reasonable approach when the number and the potency of glaucoma drugs were very limited. However, considering the delicate balance of the dozens of endogenous mediators required for the coordination of physiologic functions, as well as the complex and sometimes antagonistic effects and potentially synergistic adverse side effects of drugs, *multiple drug therapy* can be a pharmacologic nightmare.

On the other hand, the selection of one optimal drug for a given patient's glaucoma is a particularly difficult task because this neuropathy does not offer the rapid feedback that would let us know whether the alteration in aqueous humor dynamics achieved with therapy A is more beneficial for a given patient than therapy B, especially when the two therapies have comparable ocular hypotensive efficacy. In contrast, the failure of an antibiotic to achieve effective control of infection within a few days would, for example, lead to its replacement with another antibiotic with a different bactericidal spectrum but almost never to the addition of a second antibiotic. Moreover, with respect to antibiotics, the physician's job is made even easier by the in vitro techniques available to select the best treatment for a particular infection.

Perhaps the next generation of ophthalmologists will have diagnostic tools that will allow them to perform consecutive evaluations of the beneficial effects of several ocular hypotensive agents on the neuropathy within the course of a few months or even to select the best agent based on in vitro tests on the patients' platelets, leukocytes, or fibroblasts. Until then, many new glaucoma drugs will become available. As that happens, it will become increasingly counterproductive, from both pharmacodynamic and pharmacokinetic perspectives, to apply more and more drugs on top of each other to achieve only a little more IOP reduction.

Thus, from physiologic and pharmacologic perspectives, the most important trend in glaucoma management in the foreseeable future should be a move away from prescribing multiple ocular hypotensive agents toward substituting one drug for another. Combining drugs for glaucoma management should be done only when there is a theoretical or demonstrated mechanism by which their beneficial effect can be expected to have greater additivity than their adverse effects.

Only through a better understanding of the particular IOP abnormality that may predominate in a particular patient, and through the selective use of the appropriate ocular hypotensive agent, can we expect to achieve ocular hypotensive therapy that effectively prevents the development or slows the progression of visual loss. Only after such a rational approach to IOP management has been instituted will it be meaningful to evaluate the impact of pharmacologic IOP control on the glaucomatous process or to compare it with that achieved by surgical IOP reduction.

REFERENCES

1. Ritch R, Shields MB, Krupin T, eds. *The Glaucomas.* St. Louis: CV Mosby, 1989.
2. Shields MB. *Textbook of Glaucoma.* Baltimore: Williams & Wilkins, 1992.
3. Hayreh SS. Progress in the understanding of the vascular etiology of glaucoma. *Curr Opin Ophthalmol* 1994;5:26–35.
4. Fechtner RD, Weinreb RN: Mechanisms of optic nerve damage in primary open angle glaucoma. *Surv Ophthalmol* 1994;39:23–42.
5. Becker B, Stamper RL, Asseff C, Podos SM. Effect of diphenylhydantoin on glaucomatous field loss: a preliminary report. *Trans Am Acad Ophthal Otol* 1972;76:412–422.
6. Schumer RA, Podos SM. The nerve of glaucoma! *Arch Ophthalmol* 1994;112:37–44.
7. Neufeld AH. Protection of the optic nerve in glaucoma. In: Drance SM, van Buskirk EM, Neufeld AH, eds. *Pharmacology of Glaucoma.* Baltimore: Williams & Wilkins, 1992;292–321.
8. Levey DI, Lipton SA. Comparison of delayed administration of competitive and uncompetitive antagonists in preventing NMDA receptor-mediated neuronal death. *Neurology* 1990;40:852–855.
9. George CP, Goldberg MP, Choi DW. Dextromethorphan reduced neocortical ischemic neuronal damage in vivo. *Brain Res* 1988;440: 375–379.
10. Barbe MF, Tytell M, Gower DJ, Welch WJ. Hyperthermia protects against light damage in the rat retina. *Science* 1988;241:1817–1820.
11. Cazevieille C, Muller A, Meyner F, Dutrait N, Bonne C. Protection by prostaglandins from glutamate toxicity in cortical neurons. *Neurochem Int* 1994;24:395–398.
12. Cazevieille C, Muller A, Bonne C. Prostacyclin (PGI_2) protects rat cortical neurons in culture against hypoxia/reoxygenation and glutamate-induced injury. *Neurosci Lett* 1993;160:106–108.
13. Quigley HA, Nickells RW, Zack DJ, Kerrigan LA, Thibault DJ, Pease ME. Ganglion cell death in experimental monkey glaucoma and axotomy occurs by apoptosis. *Invest Ophthalmol Vis Sci* 1994;35(suppl): 2083.

14. Ilschner SU, Waring P. Fragmentation of DNA in the retina of chicken embryos coincides with retinal ganglion cell death. *Biochem Biophys Res Comm* 1992;183:1056–1061.
15. Oppenheim RW, Prevette D, Tytell M, Homma S. Naturally occurring and induced neuronal death in the chick embryo in vivo requires protein and RNA synthesis: evidence for the role of cell death genes. *Dev Biol* 1990;138:104–113.
16. Garcia-Valenzuela E, Shareef S, Walsh J, Sharma SC. Programmed cell death of retinal ganglion cells during experimental glaucoma. *Exp Eye Res* 1995;61:33–44.
17. Drance SM. Glaucoma—Changing concepts. *Eye* 1992;6:337–345.
18. Bill A. Vascular physiology of the optic nerve. In: Varma R, Spaeth GL, Parker K, eds. *The Optic Nerve in Glaucoma.* Philadelphia: JB Lippincott, 1993;37–50.
19. Bito LZ. Glaucoma: a physiologic perspective with Darwinian overtones. *J Glaucoma* 1992;1:193–205.
20. Bito LZ. A physiologic approach to the development of new drugs for glaucoma. *Ophthalmol Clin North Am* 1989;2:175–186.
21. Francois J, Neetens A. Vascularity of the eye and the optic nerve in glaucoma. *Arch Ophthalmol* 1964;71:219–225.
22. Gasser P, Flammer J. Short- and long-term effect of nifedipine on the visual field in patients with presumed vasospasm. *J Int Med Res* 1990;18:334–339.
23. Weinreb RN. Blood rheology and glaucoma. *J Glaucoma* 1993; 2:153–154.
24. Klaver JHJ, Greve EL, Goslinga H, Geijssen HC, Heuvelmans JHA. Blood and plasma viscosity measurements in patients with glaucoma. *Br J Ophthalmol* 1985;69:765–770.
25. Mary A, Serre I, Brun J-F, Arnaud B, Bonne C. Erythrocyte deformability measurements in patients with glaucoma. *J Glaucoma* 1993; 1:155–157.
26. Hoyng PFJ, de Jong N, Oosting H, Stilma J. Platelet aggregation, disc haemorrhage and progressive loss of visual fields in glaucoma. *Int Ophthalmol* 1992;16:65–73.
27. Ames A, Wright RL, Kowada M, Thurston JM, Majno G. Cerebral ischemia. II. The no-reflow phenomenon. *Am J Pathol* 1968;52: 437–447.
28. Sommer A. Intraocular pressure and glaucoma. *Am J Ophthalmol* 1989;107:186–188.
29. Zeimer RC. Circadian variations in intraocular pressure. In: Ritch R, Shields MB, Krupin T, eds. *The Glaucomas.* St. Louis: CV Mosby, 1989;319–335.
30. Zeimer RC, Wilensky JT, Gieser DK, Viana MAG. Association between intraocular pressure peaks and progression of visual field loss. *Ophthalmology* 1991;98:64–69.
31. Bito LZ. The impact of intraocular pressure on venous outflow from the globe: A hypothesis regarding IOP-dependent vascular damage in normal-tension and hypertensive glaucoma. *J Glaucoma* 1996;5: 127–134.
32. Goldinger JM, Kang BS, Choo YE, Paganelli CV, Hong SK. Effect of hydrostatic pressure on ion transport and metabolism in human erythrocytes. *J Appl Physiol* 1980;49:224–231.
33. Weinstein JM, Duckrow RB, Beard D, Brennan RW. Regional optic nerve blood flow and its autoregulation. *Invest Ophthalmol Vis Sci* 1983;24:1559–1565.
34. Bill A. Circulation in the eye. In: Renkin EM, Michel CC, eds. *The Handbook of Physiology: Cardiovascular System IV.* Bethesda: American Physiological Society, 1984;1001–1029.
35. Coleman DJ, Trokel S. Direct-recorded intraocular pressure variations in a human subject. *Arch Ophthalmol* 1969;82:637–640.
36. Pomfy M, Huska J. The state of the microcirculatory bed after total ischaemia of the brain: an experimental ultrastructural study. *Funct Dev Morp* 1992;2:253–259.
37. Maurice DM. A recording tonometer. *Br J Ophthalmol* 1958;42: 321–335.
38. Collins CC. Miniature passive pressure transensor for implanting in the eye. *IEEE Trans Biomed Eng* 1967;2:74–83.
39. Cooper RL, Beale DG, Constable IJ, Grose GC. Continual monitoring of intraocular pressure: effect of central venous pressure, respiration, and eye movements on continual recordings of intraocular pressure in the rabbit, dog, and man. *Br J Ophthalmol* 1979;63:799–804.
40. Flower RW, Maumanee AE, Michelson EA. Long-term continuous monitoring of intraocular pressure in conscious primates. *Ophthalmic Res* 1982;14:98–106.
41. Svedbergh B, Backlund Y, Hok B, Rosengren L. The IOP-IOL: a probe into the eye. *Acta Ophthalmol Scand* 1992;70:266–268.
42. Netland PA, Chaturvedi N, Dreyer EB. Calcium channel blockers in the management of low-tension and open-angle glaucoma. *Am J Ophthalmol* 1993;115:608–613.
43. Hart WM Jr. The epidemiology of primary open-angle glaucoma and ocular hypertension. In: Ritch R, Shields MB, Krupin T, eds. *The Glaucomas.* St. Louis: CV Mosby, 1989;789–795.
44. Green RW, Chan CC, Hutchins GM, Terry JM. Central retinal vein occlusion: A prospective histopathologic study of 29 eyes in 28 cases. *Trans Am Ophthalmol Soc* 1981;79:371–422.
45. Krakau CET. Disk hemorrhages and retinal vein occlusions in glaucoma. *Surv Ophthalmol* 1994;38(suppl):S18–S22.
46. Taylor AW, Sehu W, Williamson TH, Lee WR. Morphometric assessment of the central retinal artery and vein in the optic nerve head. *Can J Ophthalmol* 1993;28:320–324.
47. Attariwala R, Giebs CP, Glucksberg MR. The influence of elevated intraocular pressure on vascular pressures in the cat retina. *Invest Ophthalmol Vis Sci* 1994;35:1019–1025.
48. Schuman JS, Noecker RJ. Imaging of the optic nerve head and nerve fiber in glaucoma. *Ophthalmol Clin North Am* 1995;8:259–279.
49. Flammer J, Gasser P, Prunte C, Yao K. The probable involvement of factors other than intraocular pressure in the pathogenesis of glaucoma. In: Drance SM, van Buskirk EM, Neufeld AH, eds. *Pharmacology of Glaucoma.* Baltimore: Williams and Wilkins, 1992;273–283.
50. Kessell NF, Sasaki T, Colohan ART, et al. Cerebral vasospasm following aneurysmal subarachnoid hemorrhage. *Stroke* 1985;16:562–572.
51. Nakagami T, Kessell NF, Sasaki T, et al. Effect of subarachnoid hemorrhage on endothelium-dependent vasodilation. *J Neurosurg* 1987; 66:915–923.
52. Drance SM. Disc hemorrhages in the glaucomas. *Surv Ophthalmol* 1989;33:331–337.
53. Hitchings RA, Spaeth GL. Chronic retinal vein occlusion in glaucoma. *Br J Ophthalmol* 1976;60:694–699.
54. Luntz MH, Shenker HI. Retinal vascular accidents in glaucoma and ocular hypertension. *Surv Ophthalmol* 1980;25:163–167.
55. Maumenee AE. Causes of optic nerve damage in glaucoma. *Ophthalmology* 1983;90:741–752.
56. Ericson LA. Twenty-four hourly variations of the aqueous flow. *Acta Ophthalmol* (suppl 50). Copenhagen: Ejnar Munksgaard, 1958.
57. Henkind P, Leitman M, Weitzman E. The diurnal curve in man: new observations. *Invest Ophthalmol* 1973;12:705–707.
58. Frampton P, Da Rin D, Brown B. Diurnal variation of intraocular pressure and the overriding effects of sleep. *Am J Optom Physiol Opt* 1987;64:54–61.
59. Brown B, Burton P, Mann S, Parisi A. Fluctuations of intraocular pressure with sleep. II. Time course of IOP decrease after waking from sleep. *Ophthalmol Physiol Opt* 1988;8:249–252.
60. Buguet A, Py P, Romanet JP. 24-Hour (Nyctohemeral) and sleep-related variations of intraocular pressure in healthy white individuals. *Am J Ophthalmol* 1994;117:342–347.
61. David R, Zangwill L, Badarna M, Yassur Y. Epidemiology of retinal vein occlusion and its association with glaucoma and increased intraocular pressure. *Ophthalmologica* 1988;197:69–74.
62. Yamagami J, Araie M, Aihara M, Yamamoto S. Diurnal variation in intraocular pressure of normal-tension glaucoma eyes. *Ophthalmology* 1993;100:643–650.
63. Reiss GR, Lee DA, Topper J, Brubaker RF. Aqueous humor flow during sleep. *Invest Ophthalmol Vis Sci* 1984;25:776–778.
64. Hamanaka T, Bill A. Morphological and functional effects of Na_2EDTA on the outflow routes for aqueous humor in monkeys. *Exp Eye Res* 1987;44:171–190.
65. Hamanaka T, Bill A, Ichinohasama R, Ishida R. Aspects of the development of Schlemm's canal. *Exp Eye Res* 1992;55:479–488.
66. Weinreb RN, Jeng S, Goldstick BJ. Glaucoma secondary to elevated episcleral venous pressure. In: Ritch R, Shields MB, Krupin T, eds. *The Glaucomas.* St. Louis: CV Mosby, 1989;1127–1140.
67. Dvorak-Theobald G. Schlemm's canal: its anastomoses and anatomic relations. *Trans Am Ophthalmol Soc* 1934;32:574–595.
68. Dvorak TG. The limbal area: with particular reference to the trabecular meshwork in health and disease. *Am J Ophthalmol* 1960;50:543–557.
69. Phelps CD. Arterial anastomosis with Schlemm's Canal: A rare cause of secondary open-angle glaucoma. *Trans Am Ophthalmol Soc* 1985; 83:304–315.

70. Krauss AH-P, Wiederholt M, Sturm A, Woodward DF. Prostaglandin effects on contractility of bovine ciliary muscle and trabecular meshwork. *Invest Ophthalmol Vis Sci* 1994;35(suppl):1996.
71. Woodward DF, Regan JW, Lake S, Ocklind A. The molecular biology and ocular distribution of prostanoid receptors. *Surv Ophthalmol* 1997;41 (Suppl):515–522.
72. Johnstone MA, Grant WM. Pressure-dependent changes in structures of the aqueous outflow system of human and monkey eyes. *Am J Ophthalmol* 1973;75:365–383.
73. Brubaker RF. The effect of intraocular pressure on conventional outflow resistance in the enucleated human eye. *Invest Ophthalmol Vis Sci* 1975;14:286–292.
74. Bill A. Uveoscleral drainage of aqueous humor: Physiology and pharmacology. *Prog Clin Biol Res* 1989;312:417–427.
75. Lutjen-Drecoll E, Kaufman PL. Morphological changes in primate aqueous humor formation and drainage tissues after long-term treatment with antiglaucomatous drugs. *J Glaucoma* 1993;2:316–328.
76. Becker B. Does hyposecretion of aqueous humor damage the trabecular meshwork? *J Glaucoma* 1995;4:303–305.
77. Weinreb RN. Riding the Trojan Horse of glaucoma surgery. *J Glaucoma* 1995;4:2–4.
78. Davson H, ed. *The Eye,* vol 1. London: Academic Press, 1969;164–171.
79. Brubaker RF. Flow of aqueous humor in humans. *Invest Ophthalmol Vis Sci* 1991;32:3145–3166.
80. van Buskirk EM. Admonitions of the oracle. *J Glaucoma* 1995;4: 149–150.
81. Serle JB, Podos SM. Topical carbonic anhydrase inhibitors in the treatment of glaucoma. *Ophthalmol Clin North Am* 1995;8:315–325.
82. Zimmerman TJ, Kooner KS, Kandarakis AS, Ziegler LP. Improving the therapeutic index of topically applied ocular drugs. *Arch Ophthalmol* 1984;102:551–553.
83. Zimran A, Beutler E. Can the risk of acetazolamide-induced aplastic anemia be decreased by periodic monitoring of blood cell counts: *Am J Ophthalmol* 1987;104:654–658.
84. Hurvitz LM, Kaufman PL, Robin AL, Weinreb RN, Crawford K, Shaw B. New developments in the drug treatment of glaucoma. *Drugs* 1991;41:514–532.
85. Fischbarg J, Lim JJ. Fluid and electrolyte transports across corneal endothelium. *Curr Top Eye Res* 1984;4:201–223.
86. Bito LZ. A physiological approach to glaucoma management: the use of local hormones and the pharmacokinetics of prostaglandin esters. *Prog Clin Biol Res* 1989;312:329–348.
87. Bill A, Phillips CI. Uveoscleral drainage of aqueous humor in human eyes. *Exp Eye Res* 1971;12:275–281.
88. Kaufman PL, Crawford K. How $PGF_{2\alpha}$ lowers intraocular pressure. *Prog Clin Biol Res* 1989;312:387–416.
89. Bito LZ, Dawson MJ, Petrinovic L. Cholinergic sensitivity: normal variability as a function of stimulus background. *Science* 1971;172: 583–585.
90. Bito LZ, Salvador EV. Intraocular fluid dynamics. III. The site and mechanism of prostaglandin transfer across the blood intraocular fluid barriers. *Exp Eye Res* 1972;14:233–241.
91. Bito LZ, Wallenstein MC. Transport of prostaglandins across the blood-brain and blood-aqueous barriers and the physio-logical significance of these absorptive transport processes. *Exp Eye Res* 1977;25 (suppl):229–243.
92. Yamamoto R, McGlinn A, Stone RA. Brain natriuretic peptide-immunoreactive nerves in the porcine eye. *Neurosci Lett* 1991;122: 151–153.
93. Bito LZ. Prostaglandins: a new approach to glaucoma management—with a new, intriguing side effect. *Surv Ophthalmol* 1997;41 (Suppl): S1–S14.
94. Ringvold A. An electron microscopic study of the iris stroma in monkey and rabbit with particular reference to intercellular contacts and sympathetic innervation of anterior layer cell. *Exp Eye Res* 1975;20:349–365.
95. Cohen MM, ed. *Biological Protection with Prostaglandins.* Toronto: CRC Press Inc., 1985.
96. Stjernschantz J, Bito LZ. The ocular effects of eicosanoids and other autacoids: historic background and the need for a broader perspective. *Prog Clin Biol Res* 1989;312:1–14.
97. Bito LZ, Stjernschantz J, eds. *The Ocular Effects of Prostaglandins and Other Eicosanoids.* New York: Alan R. Liss, 1989.
98. Lichter PR. Another blockbuster glaucoma drug? *Ophthalmology* 1993;100:1281–1282.
99. Jumblatt MM, Paterson CA. Prostaglandin E_2 effects on corneal endothelial cyclic adenosine monophosphate synthesis and cell shape are mediated by a receptor of the EP_2 subtype. *Invest Ophthalmol Vis Sci* 1991;32:360–365.

SECTION III

Retina

Section Editors: David V. Weinberg and Lee M. Jampol

OVERVIEW

The chapters in this section describe diverse pharmacologic approaches to clinical problems. In some cases, these represent fresh approaches to old problems, and in other cases they represent responses to new clinical problems.

Diabetic retinopathy and macular degeneration are two of the most common and frustrating conditions faced by clinicians. Laser treatment has improved the outcomes for patients with these problems, but collectively they still account for most new cases of blindness in the United States. Improved understanding of the pathophysiology of these diseases offers the possibility of pharmacologic intervention. Neovascularization in the posterior segment is common to several blinding vitreoretinal diseases, including diabetic retinopathy and macular degeneration. In the past few years, we have seen an explosive growth in our understanding of the origin and natural course of neovascularization. These developments offer hope for therapies that are more physiologic and less destructive than laser therapy.

A few years ago, a chapter on antiviral drugs for retinal diseases probably would not have earned a place in this textbook. The emergence of AIDS and cytomegalovirus retinitis has forced a major research effort to seek drugs to treat this devastating infection (see Chapter 33, Antivirals in the Treatment of Retinal Disease). This effort has resulted in a growing armamentarium of therapies for cytomegalovirus retinitis.

The chapters on the pharmacology of proliferative vitreoretinopathy and the use of drugs affecting the coagulation cascade represent the efforts of a few clinicians and scientists in ophthalmology who have applied existing pharmacologic technology to novel clinical applications. The information in these chapters raises the possibility of expanding the scope of vitreoretinal surgery and supplementing the skills of vitreoretinal surgeons.

The two remaining chapters describe therapy for cystoid macular edema and endophthalmitis. Slow, steady progress over many years has improved our ability to treat these common, and frequently iatrogenic, diseases in many but not all cases. On behalf of all the authors in this section, we hope that we have provided information, insight, and inspiration to our readers.

Textbook of Ocular Pharmacology,
edited by T.J. Zimmerman, et al.
Lippincott–Raven Publishers, Philadelphia © 1997.

CHAPTER 32

Antibiotics and Antifungals

Travis A. Meredith

Antimicrobial therapy for infections of the retina and vitreous cavity presents special problems because of the unique anatomy and physiology of the eye. Infections of the vitreous cavity are most commonly caused by bacteria and occasionally by fungi. They usually result from the introduction of microorganisms into the eye during ocular surgery or penetrating injuries of the globe. Infectious retinitis may be caused by parasites, such as *Toxoplasmosis gondii* or *Toxocara canis;* by viruses, such as cytomegalovirus or herpes zoster; or by fungi. These organisms usually are spread hematogenously to the retina. Bacterial retinitis most often accompanies endophthalmitis but rarely is detected as a manifestation of bacteremia.

Therapy for retinitis and endophthalmitis almost always must be instituted without a culture-proven identity of the organism, and positive identification often is not possible for organisms causing retinitis. Treatment of endophthalmitis may be difficult because blood–ocular barriers limit penetration of antimicrobials into the vitreous cavity after intravenous or oral administration. Direct injection into the vitreous cavity is thus used for severe infections within the vitreous, whereas treatment of retinitis typically relies on oral or intravenous antimicrobials. The blood–retinal barrier is apparently sufficiently disrupted to allow successful therapy of toxoplasmosis and fungal infections that are localized to the retina. When these organisms spread from the retina into the vitreous cavity, however, intravitreal drug delivery may be necessary.

The goal of antimicrobial therapy for endophthalmitis is to provide intravitreal concentrations of appropriate antimicrobials for a sufficient time to eradicate microorganisms, while avoiding concentrations of drug that can produce iatrogenic tissue damage. Although this statement appears straightforward, pursuing this goal leads to many complex problems.

T. A. Meredith: Department of Ophthalmology, St. Louis University School of Medicine, St. Louis, Missouri 63110.

Intravitreal injection of antimicrobials is now regarded as the mainstay of therapy of endophthalmitis. Early in the modern antibiotic era, sulfa compounds and penicillin were injected into the vitreous cavity (1,2), but 35 years elapsed until full acceptance of this route of administration (3).

Because endophthalmitis usually progresses quickly, rapid eradication of organisms is important. Bacterial infections in particular often progress quickly, destroying the eye if left untreated. Antimicrobials must therefore almost always be initiated before identification of the infecting organism. The spectrum of bacteria that may cause acute endophthalmitis includes both gram-positive and gram-negative organisms; so injection of two antimicrobials at the same time is usually necessary to cover the most likely pathogens.

A single injection of antimicrobials is sufficient to kill invading bacteria in some, but not all, cases. In both laboratory studies (4–7) and clinical series (8,9), there may be persistence of certain microorganisms after a single intravitreal injection of an appropriate antimicrobial. This lack of effectiveness is seen against slowly replicating organisms (*Propionibacterium acnes* and fungi) (10) and in infections created by organisms considered more virulent, such as *Streptococcus* species (11) and gram-negative pathogens (12).

The duration of potentially effective concentrations of antimicrobials within the vitreous cavity depends on a number of factors, including original dose, route of egress from the eye, surgical status of the eye, and the presence or absence of inflammation. Little is known about dose-response relationships and the necessary duration of antimicrobials within the vitreous cavity for the various agents used in endophthalmitis therapy.

Because a single intravitreal injection is insufficient to eradicate all invading pathogens, many authorities advocate intravenous therapy for treatment of endophthalmitis. Penetration of antimicrobials into the eye after intravenous or oral administration is blocked by several blood–ocular barriers, although inflammation may decrease the effectiveness of these barriers for some agents. Subconjunctival injections are commonly administered, although penetration into the vitreous cavity is limited (13); some authors advise repeated intravitreal injections (8,14).

Prophylaxis of intraocular infection is usually directed against bacterial pathogens. The incidence of postoperative endophthalmitis is approximately 0.08% (15), depending on the operative procedure; so the aggressiveness of prophylactic measures must be measured against this risk. In traumatic cases, however, the incidence of infection may vary from 1% to 30%, depending on the circumstance of injury (16,17), and prophylaxis may be a more important issue. After elective surgery or traumatic repair, subconjunctival antimicrobials often are given despite restricted penetration into the vitreous cavity. The ability to achieve bactericidal levels in the anterior chamber, which is the site of implantation of most organisms in anterior segment surgery, may justify their use despite the paucity of studies demonstrating clinical efficacy. Intravenous administration is used more commonly for prophylaxis after penetrating trauma than after elective surgery, but its efficacy has not been demonstrated for this approach either. Undoubtedly, poor antimicrobial penetration into the vitreous cavity limits their prophylactic effectiveness. Adding antimicrobials into the infusion fluid has been advocated as a prophylactic measure in anterior and posterior segment surgery (18), but it is unclear whether the risk-to-benefit ratio or cost-effectiveness analyses support this strategy.

Most available literature on endophthalmitis treatment comes from retrospective clinical series, and few laboratory studies are available to guide appropriate therapy. Because there is a much broader scientific base for the treatment of meningitis, and meningitis and endophthalmitis share a significant number of characteristics, the relationship between the two entities deserves some consideration when contemplating therapeutic issues.

Meningitis and endophthalmitis are analogous in a number of their features. In both instances, infection takes place in a closed space, carrying significant implications for treatment and outcome. Bacterial replication and inflammation may cause tissue destruction quickly in both cases, leading to significant functional loss despite successful eradication of the invading organism (19–21). In both conditions, it is necessary to choose antibiotics and start therapy empirically before identification of the organism to attempt to control the infection as quickly as possible (20).

Penetration of antimicrobials into the cerebrospinal fluid (CSF) and into the vitreous cavity after intravenous administration is limited by the blood–brain barrier (19,21–23) and blood–ocular barriers (24–26), respectively. Certain antimicrobials are ineffective because of inadequate penetration. Furthermore, bacterial killing in the CSF may require higher concentrations of antimicrobials (19,27,28), a requirement not yet studied in the vitreous cavity. Higher concentrations may be necessary, in part because of the immune privilege of the CSF, a characteristic also found in the eye (19). A relative immune privilege was demonstrated for the anterior chamber, known as *anterior chamber autoimmune deviation,* and has been suggested for the posterior segment as well (29,30). Immune privilege with regard to infections within the vitreous cavity as yet has not been well defined.

PHARMACOKINETIC CONSIDERATIONS

Therapeutic Concentration Range

The therapeutic concentration range or therapeutic window is the range of drug concentration associated with effective therapy without undue toxicity (31). For most drugs, the therapeutic concentration range in plasma is narrow and the upper and lower limits differ by a factor of only 2 or 3. The upper limit of the concentration may be a result of diminishing effectiveness of the drug at higher concentrations or may be established by toxicity. Toxicity, in turn, may be an extension of the pharmacologic properties of the drug or may be disassociated totally from its therapeutic effect. The narrower the range within which the chances of successful therapy are high, the more difficult the maintenance of values within this range. The issue of toxicity as the limiting factor in the upper range of drug concentrations is particularly meaningful with regard to intravitreal injections, as high initial concentrations are achieved and, in most other tissues, toxicity is often related to peak dose. On the other hand, the blood–ocular barriers create difficulties when attempting to reach potentially effective concentrations in the vitreous cavity after intravenous or oral antimicrobial administration.

Blood–ocular Barriers

Penetration of drug into the eye from plasma is restricted by several barriers. The permeability restriction between blood and aqueous, which excludes certain substances either actively or passively, is termed the *blood–aqueous barrier* (25,32). The blood–aqueous barrier is thought to be similar to the blood–brain barrier because of the apparent active inward and outward transport of some substances in addition to the exclusionary properties. In the posterior pole, there are two major barriers to penetration: the retinal capillary endothelial cells (also called the inner blood–retinal barrier) and the tight junctions of the retinal pigment epithelium (RPE, sometimes termed the outer blood–retinal barrier) (24,25). The epithelium of the ciliary body where it faces the vitreous also may serve a barrier function (32).

The blood–brain barrier has been studied extensively, but less information is available on the blood–retinal barriers, although they are thought to have similar properties because of similar anatomic features (19,24,25). In the retinal capillaries, the tight junctions between endothelial cells create the blood–retinal barrier. Most other capillaries in the body, except in the central nervous system and prostate, are fenestrated and have pores large enough to admit substances of molecular weight up to 1,000 daltons. Retinal capillaries have tight junctions and are nonfenestrated, creating an obstruction to movement of substances from plasma into the retina and vitreous. The outer blood–retinal barrier is produced by the tight junctions between the RPE cells. There is a high rate of blood flow to the choriocapillaris, and its surface area is estimated to be about 2½ times the surface of the choroid (25). These capillaries are extremely permeable, but substances leaking out encounter the barrier of the junctional complexes between RPE cells and the pigment epithelium cells of the pars plana.

When drugs must pass through epithelial cells, they must cross cell membranes that create selective barriers to penetration. Most cellular membranes have a central layer that is predominantly lipoidal in nature, bound on each side by protein layers (19,31). Drug penetrations throughout the body are results of passive diffusion across barriers of this kind. The rate of penetration equals the permeability times the surface area times the concentration gradient (25). Higher lipid solubility allows antimicrobials to pass more easily through lipid membranes of capillary epithelium. Lipid-soluble drugs include minocycline, doxycycline, chloramphenicol, trimethoprim, and metronidazole. Drugs that are less lipid soluble include those more commonly given locally and systemically for endophthalmitis (i.e., the beta-lactams and the aminoglycosides) (19,24).

The pH of the system also influences the barrier effect in that ionized molecules are more polar than nonionized molecules and therefore are less soluble in the lipid membrane (21,31). Molecules that are more ionized are therefore less able to travel across the blood–retinal barrier (31). There is an increased accumulation of drug on the side of the membrane whose pH favors greater ionization. The pH partition hypothesis states that only nonionized, nonpolar drugs penetrate membranes and that the concentration of nonionized species is equal on both sides of the membrane (31). This affects the penetration of cephalosporins, for example, which are more ionized than many drugs at physiologic pH (33).

Molecular weight affects the penetration of drugs across barriers. The larger the molecule and the higher the molecular weight, the less readily the molecule can cross the blood–retinal barrier. The ability to pass through membranes is related to the square root of the molecular weight, and most drugs fall in a narrow range of molecular weight between 100 and 400 daltons. In general, this effect is less important in determining the crossing of barriers (19, 21,25).

Protein binding also can restrict passage of molecules out of a vascular compartment, as it is generally held that only unbound antimicrobials can pass through membranes (19,21,25). Many antimicrobial agents are bound extensively to serum proteins, particularly albumin. Most protein binding is reversible and rapid, reaching an equilibrium quickly. In the case of cephalosporins, there is variable protein binding of the third-generation cephalosporins, and the degree of protein binding correlates inversely to the percentage of penetration into CSF (34).

Active transport mechanisms achieve net movement of drug against a concentration gradient and, as mentioned, are involved in transporting some microbials both out of and into the CSF and aqueous humor; transport may thus be bidirectional. There is evidence of active transport of ceftriaxone, an important cephalosporin, into the CSF, but transport into the eye was not demonstrated in a similar fashion.

Inflammation may play a major role in the breakdown of the blood–brain barrier by disrupting tight junctions and increasing transendothelial vesicles, increasing pinocytosis, and enhancing the formation of microvilli by endothelial cell luminal membranes (19). Many drugs penetrate into the CSF more easily when the meninges are inflamed, and inflammation also increases the penetration of antimicrobials into the eye. Cefazolin, for example, does not penetrate into the phakic noninflamed eye even after repeated doses, but levels gradually increase to an average of 10.9 mcg/ml in the inflamed eye after seven intravenous doses administered every 8 hours (35). This effect on permeability may be important early in the course of infection, but as inflammation decreases during the course of the disease, permeability and thus antibiotic penetration also may decrease (24).

Other factors also affect antimicrobial penetration into the vitreous cavity. By removing the lens and vitreous, the inner eye is converted to a single chamber. In this configuration, drug can enter the vitreous cavity through both the aqueous and posterior structures. After removal of the vitreous and lens, the concentration of cefazolin was higher in the vitreous cavity after intravenous administration than in eyes without the vitreous removed, presumably as a result of removal of a physical barrier to diffusion added to a contribution from aqueous humor (phakic = 0 mcg, aphakic-vitrectomized = 3.9 μg/ml) (35). Coupled with inflammation, this effect was more striking, and in the inflamed eye with the vitreous removed, a significantly higher concentration is achieved in the vitreous cavity than in eyes with intact vitreous (phakic inflamed 10.6 μg/ml versus aphakic/vitrectomized 24.9 μg/ml) (35).

When repeated intravenous doses are given, intravitreal drug concentrations may increase progressively with time because the barrier to diffusion increases the time needed to reach a point of equilibrium (31). This effect is potentially important because in most studies of drug penetration, a single bolus dose of antimicrobial is given intravenously, followed by subsequent sampling 1 to 2 hours later. Studies on gentamicin and cefazolin demonstrated progressively higher concentrations over time with repeated intravenous drug administration (35,36).

The penetration of an antibiotic into the eye or the CSF usually is expressed in terms of the percentage of the drug at a given time compared with the amount of concentration of the drug in serum

$$(\text{CSF} \div \text{plasma} \times 100).(23)$$

Problems exist in this determination, however, because drug concentrations may change slowly in the vitreous and other body cavities but change rapidly in the plasma. The precise time of sampling of drugs is therefore significant in establishing a percentage. The area under the curve may be a better denominator than a single determination when calculating this parameter.

Aminoglycosides (37,38), beta-lactam agents (38), and vancomycin (39–42) are probably the antimicrobials most commonly administered intravenously for endophthalmitis. Penetration studies in animals and humans are summarized in Table 32-1. A number of studies of aminoglycosides indicate little if any vitreous-cavity penetration under various conditions. Studies of vitreous sampling in humans after single intravenous doses do not demonstrate therapeutic levels of gentamycin in the vitreous cavity (43). Barza studied phakic-infected rabbit eyes and was able to demonstrate concentrations of 2.6 μg/ml after continuous intravenous infusion of gentamycin for 6 hours, reaching slightly higher levels and a penetration ratio of 42% after 18 hours (36). Yoshisumi studied a model of traumatized eyes in the rabbit and could not demonstrate a therapeutic level of gentamycin in the vitreous cavity after intravenous injection (44). In our laboratories, intermittent intravenous doses of amikacin produced maximum concentrations of approximately 5.5 μg/ml in aphakic/vitrectomized inflamed rabbit eyes after more than 48 hours; these levels are less than the minimum inhibitory concentration (MIC) for staphylococci and pseudomonades. Similar studies of gentamicin produced maximum concentrations in inflamed aphakic-vitrectomized eyes of 1.8 μg/ml after 69 hours; this value is below the MIC for Pseudomonas spp. (45).

Cephalosporins have moderate penetration into eyes altered by surgery, inflammation, or disease. Cefazolin penetrates into aphakic and aphakic-vitrectomized rabbit eyes; penetration is enhanced by inflammation (35). Third-generation cephalosporins have the property of increased CSF penetration, and ceftazidime demonstrates superior penetration into the vitreous cavity after intravenous administration, especially in aphakic-vitrectomized eyes. Concentrations of 35.4 μg/ml were found 2 hours after in-

TABLE 32-1. *Intraocular penetration of antibiotics after systemic administration (μ/ml)*

			Phakic			Aphakic			Aphakic/vitrectomized			
Drug	Model	Dose	1–3	24–25 h	49 h	1–3 h	24 h	49 h	1–3 h	25 h	49 h	Reference
Cefazolin	Rabbit, control	50 μ/kg q8h ×48h	0	0	0				4.2	3.7	2.1	35
	Rabbit, inflamed	50 μ/kg q8h ×48h	3.0	6.3	10.6				6.7	19.0	24.9	35
	Human, vitrectomy	2 g i.v.	0.84–1.6									44
Ceftriaxone	Human, vitrectomy	1–2 g i.m.	5.9	11.5								44
Ceftazidime	Rabbit, control	50 mg/kg ×1	0.5–0	0	0	0	0	0	8.5	2.0	8.3	47,61
	Rabbit, inflamed	50 mg/kg ×1	3.1–0	11.3	4.6	0	1.4	5.1	35.4	9.4	10.7	47,61
Amikacin	Rabbit, control	15 mg/kg				0.9						114
	Rabbit, inflamed	15 mg/kg				Variable						114
Gentamicin	Human, vitrectomy	1.6 mg/kg i.m.	<0.2									43
	Rabbit, trauma	2.29 mg	0.25									115
	Rabbit, infected	4.6 mg/kg i.m. q3h×5		2.8								36
Ciprofloxacin	Human, vitrectomy	750 mg po		0.04–0.49								50
Imipenem	Human, vitrectomy	1 g i.v.	2.53									49
Vancomycin	Rabbit, control	15 mg/kg	0.67	0	0	2.2	4.5	5.6	3.5	6.8	8.7	46
	Rabbit, inflamed	15 mg/ml	0	0	1.3	1.2	5.1	6.0	5.4	9.2	10.3	46

i.v., intravenously; i.m., intramuscularly; q3h, every 3 hours.

travenous administration in these eyes, although no penetration was detected in phakic and aphakic eyes even after 48 hours of intermittent dosing (46,47).

Studies have been done of human samples obtained by vitrectomy at various intervals after a single intravenous bolus dose of cefazolin, methicillin, cephalothin, oxacillin, and nafcillin (48). Only cefazolin produced vitreous concentrations consistently above the MIC for *Staphylococcus epidermidis,* but it did not reach potentially effective levels for *Staphylococcus aureus.* Similar studies demonstrated inadequate penetration of moxalactam to achieve levels above the MIC for *S. aureus* or *S. epidermidis;* cefamandole did not reach therapeutic concentrations for gram-negative pathogens consistently (49). Imipenem tested under similar circumstances exceeded the MIC for *S. aureus* and *S. epidermidis* for some but not all patients, but did not reach the MIC levels for methicillin-resistant *S. aureus* or for many important gram-negative pathogens causing endophthalmitis (50).

Vancomycin is not generally thought to penetrate the CSF well, but it had surprising penetration into aphakic and aphakic-vitrectomized eyes in rabbit studies. Concentrations considered inhibitory for gram-positive organisms were achieved in these eyes after 24 hours of intermittent intravenous administration. No vancomycin could be detected in phakic eyes under the same experimental conditions (46).

In studies of human vitreous samples after oral administration of ciprofloxacin in patients undergoing vitrectomy for various indications, the average vitreous concentrations did not consistently exceed the MIC for *S. aureus, Streptococcus pyogenes* or *Pseudomonas aeruginosa* (51,52). Most eyes on which human studies have been performed did not have infections, but many had conditions, such as trauma and proliferative diabetic retinopathy, that might be expected to break down the blood–ocular barriers. Similar low values are found in animal studies, although inflammation increases the degree of penetration.

Clearance of Antimicrobials from the Vitreous Cavity

The intravitreal concentration of antibiotic at a given time after intravitreal injection is governed by several factors (31). The initial concentration is a result of the dose and the extent of distribution. Afterward, the concentration of the drug at a given time is determined by the volume of distribution, the dose of initial injection, and the rate of elimination. The elimination phase of the drug may be characterized by two parameters: (a) the apparent volume of distribution and (b) the elimination half-life.

The volume of distribution is a direct measure of the extent of distribution of the drug but rarely corresponds to a real volume. The volume of distribution may be many times higher than the actual physical volume or may be lower, depending on a number of factors. The *half-life* ($T_{1/2}$) is defined as the time required for the drug concentration to fall by half. Elimination of a drug from the body, a tissue, or a compartment is usually a first-order process; by definition, the rate of the elimination is proportional, therefore, to the amount of drug present. When plotted on semilog paper, the elimination of drug is usually a linear function. *K,* the elimination constant, is a definition of the fractional rate of drug removal. *K* is a first-order rate constant with a dimension of time (−1). *K* may be defined as the rate of elimination divided by the amount of drug in the body. The half-life then may be expressed as $T_{1/2} = 0.693/K$.

Clearance is the parameter which relates to the concentration to the rate of drug elimination. The rate of elimination equals clearance multiplied by concentration. The units of clearance are given in volume per unit of time, and the half-life may be expressed as

$$T_{1/2} = 0.693 \times \text{volume of distribution} \div \text{clearance}.$$

Both the half-life and elimination-rate constant reflect, rather than control, the volume of distribution and the clearance of the drug.

Implicit in the concept of the half-life as a first-order process is that less drug is eliminated with each succeeding half-life. On a practical level, all drug (97%) can be regarded as being eliminated within five half-lives. In systemic administration, the interval chosen for dosing is approximately every 4 half-lives, as concentrations usually fall below effective levels before the fifth half-life is reached. After intravenous injection of antimicrobials, the rate of distribution of the drug between blood and tissue is limited by either perfusion or permeability, depending on the organ being analyzed. The choroid has the highest blood flow rate in the body (53,54), but there are significant barriers to the movement of drugs into the retina and vitreous. The entry of drug into the vitreous cavity, therefore, is predominantly a permeability-limited function. If the concentration of the drug in blood is maintained long enough, any drug should reach a distribution equilibrium in which the concentration in tissue and plasma are equal; however, equality is not always observed for reasons such as active transport out of the tissue (a factor with beta-lactam antibiotics in the eye) (13,24,35) and pH gradients across cell membranes. When there is a decreased rate of entry into the tissue (e.g., because of the blood–brain barrier), the time to reach a distribution equilibrium is increased; the point of this equilibrium, however, is independent. The approach to the plateau concentration within a cavity such as the eye is determined only by the tissue distribution half-life and may be expressed by the following formula:

$$\text{half-life} = 0.693 \div k_t = 0.693\, k_p \div Q/v_t,$$

where k_t = fractional rate of exit with units of reciprocal time, k_p = equilibrium distribution ratio, Q = blood flow, and v_t = volume of tissue.

Within the eye, the concentration of drug at any given time is a combination of the amount given by intravitreal injection plus the inflow of drug through aqueous or posterior structures, reduced by the outflow through the trabecular meshwork, across retinal structures by passive diffusion, and across retinal structures by active transport.

Once antibiotics are injected into the eye, they diffuse through the vitreous cavity without significant barriers and are eliminated from the eye by either an anterior route or a posterior route (24,25,55). Drugs exiting from the anterior route are removed by the flow of the aqueous humor or by diffusion across the iris surface. Drug must move through the vitreous cavity, around the lens when it is present, into the anterior chamber, and exit through the trabecular meshwork into the canal of Schlemm (Fig. 32-1). Aminoglycosides, streptomycin, vancomycin, and sulfacetamide are thought to be eliminated anteriorly (24,25). The posterior route, or retinal route, is the alternative pathway for drug elimination from the vitreous cavity (Fig. 32-2). The first- and second-generation cephalosporins, clindamycin, and dexamethasone are believed to be eliminated posteriorly (24). Posteriorly, there is a barrier between the vitreous humor and the retina that is believed to be shared between the retinal capillaries and the pigment epithelium (24,25,32,55). This barrier is normally impermeable to materials of high molecular weight, but there is active transport of numerous substances out of the vitreous by the retinal structures. Both anterior and posterior routes of egress may come into play for some substances; ceftriaxone has been suggested as one example.

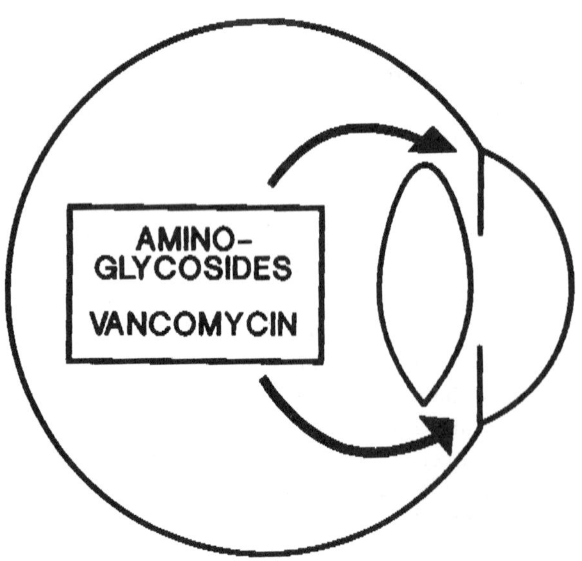

FIG. 32-1. Anterior route of clearance by which some antimicrobials, including aminoglycosides and vancomycin, leave the eye through the anterior chamber after intravitreal injection.

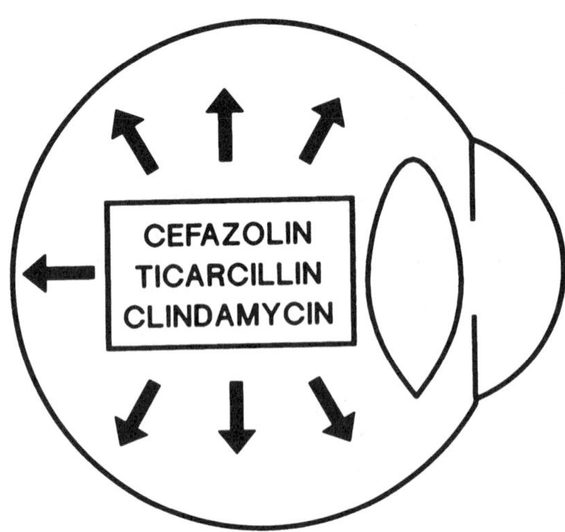

FIG. 32-2. Posterior route of elimination of drugs after intravitreal injection. Clindamycin and first- and second-generation cephalosporins leave the eye by this route.

According to Maurice, antibiotics diffuse through the vitreous rapidly after intravitreal injection, although this may take several hours (25,55). Lack of resistance to diffusion of drugs within the vitreous cavity is due to low-average concentration (0.01%) of collagen in the vitreous gel, and fluid flow is thought to be less important than movement by molecular action. Maurice states that if elimination is entirely through the anterior chamber, the amount of drug lost from the vitreous body in one hour equals

$$(k_v) \times (c_v) \times (v_v) = f \cdot c_a,$$

where k_v is the fraction lost every hour, c_v is the average concentration of the vitreous body, v_v is the volume in the vitreous body, f is the volume of the aqueous flow in 1 hour, and c_a is the concentration of drug in the aqueous. The rate of loss in this situation is thought to be controlled almost entirely by the rate of diffusion within the vitreous body, which is determined predominantly by geometric factors. Maurice calculated that injecting 100 times the therapeutic concentration of a drug into the central vitreous cavity allows it to reach the therapeutic concentration at the retinal surface within about 3 hours.

On the other hand, recent studies of drug elimination from rabbit eyes demonstrated that removal of the vitreous significantly shortens the half-life of several types of antimicrobials, suggesting the importance of the vitreous for retaining an antibiotic after it has been injected. In studies of amikacin, the half-life was reduced from 14.3 hours after injection of 400 mcg into the aphakic eye to 7.9 hours after removal of the lens and vitreous (56). Martin demonstrated a reduction in half-life from 8.3 hours to 6.0 hours when comparing clearance of intravitreal cefazolin from phakic versus aphakic-vitrectomized eyes (Table 32-2)

TABLE 32-2. *Antibiotic clearance after intravitreal injection (mg/ml)*

			Phakic			Aphakic			Aphakic/vitrectomized			
Drug	Model	Dose	24 h	48 h	T½ h	24 h	48 h	T½ h	24 h	48 h	T½ h	Reference
Carbenicillin	Monkey, normal	1 mg	50[a]	11[a]	10[b]							59
Cefazolin	Monkey, normal	1 mg	350[a]	30[a]	7[c]							59
	Rabbit, infected	2.25 mg	8.7	3.15								110
	Rabbit, control	2.25 mg	147	8.97	6.5	183.3	17.7	8.3	25.7	3.7	6	60
	Rabbit, inflamed	2.25 mg	340	57.4	10.4	242.5	31.9	9.0	33.4	5.7	6.7	60
Cefriaxone	Rabbit, normal	2 mg	200	45								77
	Monkey, normal	2 mg	434	59								111
Vancomycin	Rabbit	2 mg	>100	>100					90[d]	16[d]		109
Ceftazidime	Rabbit, control	2 mg	399	139	13.8	185.6	48.5	11.8	60.7	0	4.7	61
	Rabbit, inflamed	2 mg	532	56.5	10.1	135.7	19.1	8.7	8.1	1.6	5	61
Amikacin	Rabbit, normal	250 μg	19	7								112
	Rabbit, control	400 μg	100.9	55.6	25.5	25.3	15.3	14.3	15.5	3.0	7.9	56
	Rabbit, inflamed	400 μg	97.6	31.4	15.5	7.6	1.5	7.4	7.2	1.4	7.7	56
Gentamicin	Human, infected	100 μg					4.6					58
	Monkey, normal	100 μg	10.5	6.5	34							59
	Cat, normal	400 μg	50									113
	Cat, infected	400 μg	11									113
	Rabbit, control	71 μg/ml[a]	75	40	32	25	7	12				58
	Rabbit, infected	40–65 μg/ml[a]	35	18	19	20	6	14				58

Modified from ref 117.
[a]Estimated from graphic representation.
[b]With probenecid T½ = 20 hours.
[c]With probenecid T½ = 30 hours.
[d]Without intact capsule.

(35). Doft et al. noted that the half-life of intravitreal amphotericin was reduced from 4.7 days in aphakic eyes to 1.4 days in eyes with both lens and vitreous removed (57).

Maurice suggested that as drug leaves the vitreous by the anterior route, the lens creates a bottleneck, slowing removal from the eye. For this reason, half-lives of anteriorly excreted drugs are longer than those of posteriorly excreted drugs. Subsequent experiments have shown that removal of the lens in rabbits decreases the half-life of intravitreal amikacin from 25.5 hours to 14.3 hours (56) and of intravitreal gentamicin from 32 hours to 12 hours (58) (Table 32-2). Vancomycin has a shorter half-life in aphakic than in phakic eyes; the half-life is intermediate between these two values when the lens is removed but the posterior capsule left intact (39).

Inflammation also decreases the half-life of anteriorly excreted drugs, although the mechanism that accounts for this decrease is not clear. In phakic rabbit eyes, the half-life of amikacin is decreased from 25.5 hours to 15.5 hours by inducing inflammation (56), and the half-life of gentamicin is decreased from 32 to 19 hours (58). The same effect was noted in aphakic rabbit eyes for amikacin; the half-life was reduced from 14.3 hours to 7.4 hours by induction of inflammation (56). No prolongation of half-life was noted for gentamicin in aphakic rabbit eyes by inducing infection (58). Inflammation may increase posterior permeability, and these drugs then may be eliminated by both anterior and posterior routes, accounting for the observed increase in rate of elimination.

Substances removed posteriorly are thought to exit through the retinal vasculature or RPE. For these drugs, Maurice (25,55) suggests that the diffusional path through the vitreous is shortened, and the anterior bottleneck provided by the lens is now replaced by a wide surface area available for absorption. Because active transport may be involved in the excretion of some substances posteriorly, and there is a wide surface area for absorption, posteriorly excreted drugs usually have a significantly shorter half-life than anteriorly excreted ones (24). The system may demonstrate the properties of saturation kinetics; competitive inhibition and metabolic inhibition have been demonstrated in the case of beta-lactam antibiotics. It has been suggested that there is some correspondence between the extent of renal tubular excretion of drugs in humans and the vitreous half-life in rabbits (13,25). Probenicid administration, for example, prolongs the half-life of intravitreal carbenicillin from 5 hours to 13 hours in the rabbit and from 10 hours to 20 hours in the monkey (59). The half-life of cefazolin is prolonged from 7 hours to 30 hours in the monkey by probenecid (59).

Inflammation also increases the half-life of cefazolin injected intravitreally, probably by interfering with active transport. In phakic rabbit eyes, the half-life was increased from 6.5 hours to 10.4 hours by inflammation (60). As the posterior route is blocked by metabolic or competitive inhibition, the anterior route of removal may become more important or even become the major route of elimination from the eye. The half-life for cefazolin in the monkey, for example, in the presence of probenecid is 30 hours (59), a value essentially the same as the half-life of gentamicin (58). Inflammation may have more complex effects, however, because the permeability of the posterior structures may be increased, offsetting the effect of disabling active transport. In the case of cefazolin, aphakic and aphakic/vitrectomized eyes have similar half-lives when comparing control to inflammation (60). The effect of vitreous removal appears to predominate over inflammation for cefazolin, ceftazidime, and amikacin in aphakic and aphakic/vitrectomized eyes. The half-life values are 6 to 8 hours for both inflamed and control eyes for these antibiotics (56,60,61).

No information is available on the elimination times of antimicrobials after direct injection in the human eye. Some data are derived from studies in monkeys, but most information is available from studies done in the rabbit eye (Table 32-2). Typically, in these studies, the animal eyes are injected with the dose used in the human eye; however, the volume of the vitreous cavity has considerable intraspecies differences (Table 32-3). Because the volume of the human eye is approximately 4 cc and that of the rabbit is 1.4 cc, the initial concentration of the drug is approximately 2.8 times higher in the rabbit than would be expected in the human. Maurice postulated that because the vitreous cavity volume is significantly greater in the human than in the rabbit, the times of diffusion to the retinal surface are expected to be greater. He estimates that the half-life of a drug in a human may be 1.7 times that in the rabbit vitreous cavity (25,55). Recommended initial dosage of antimicrobials for intravitreal injection range from 100 μg for gentamicin to 2.25 μg/ml for cefazolin. Assuming an average vitreous volume of 4 cc, initial concentrations therefore vary from 25 μg/ml for gentamicin to 562 μg/ml for cefazolin.

TABLE 32-3. *Interspecies differences in vitreous volume and aqueous flow*

Species	Vitreous volume (ml)	Aqueous flow (μl/min)
Rabbit	1.4–1.7	3.6
Cat	2.4	13.0
Dog	3.2	
Monkey	3.0–4.0	3.0
Man	3.9–5.0	2.5–3.0

Modified from Barza, ref 26.

As a theoretical example, 100 mcg of a drug injected into the rabbit vitreous with a volume of 1.4 cc creates an initial concentration of 71 mcg/ml. If the half-life of drug is 20 hours, the concentration of drug in the eye after 100 hours (five half-lives) is approximately 2.1 μg. The same amount of drug injected into the human eye with a volume of 4 cc yields an initial concentration of 25 μg/ml. If the half-life is 1.7 times longer for the human than the rabbit, it will be 34 hours. After 100 hours (three half-lives), the concentration will be approximately 3.1 μg/ml. Therefore, data obtained from the rabbit approximate the values to be expected in the human for the time for drug to fall to low concentrations, although other factors, such as differences in protein binding, between the rabbit and human may cause further discrepancies.

SPECTRUM OF ACTIVITY

In treatment of retinitis, toxoplasmosis is probably the organism encountered most frequently in the patient who is not immune compromised. In other cases, systemic manifestations and laboratory testing may guide the choice of antimicrobial. In empiric endophthalmitis therapy, particularly for acute postoperative or posttraumatic infection, the spectrum of activity required is dictated by the clinical circumstances. A broad range of gram-positive and gram-negative organisms has been identified in producing endophthalmitis. The particular distribution depends on the clinical setting. Staphylococcal organisms are predominant in essentially all series of endophthalmitis (62–65). In postoperative cases, coagulase-negative staphylococci account for at least 50% of cases and *S. aureus* for about one third of the cases. Bacillus organisms are leading causes of endophthalmitis in traumatic cases (17,66,67). Among gram-negative organisms, *Pseudomonas* is the most frequent cause of endophthalmitis, and *P. aeruginosa* accounted for 23% of a recent series of gram-negative cases, with other Pseudomonas species represented somewhat less frequently. *Hemophilus influenzae* was present in 19% of the cases. *Proteus* species, *Serratia marcescens, Morganella morganii, Citrobacter diversus, Escherichia coli, Klebsiella pneumoniae, Enterobacter cloacae,* and *Moraxella non-liquefaciens* were also identified in this series (12). Among the fungi, *Candida* is the most common organism encountered, with *Aspergillus* also isolated in certain cases, especially among intravenous drug abusers (10).

TYPE OF ANTIMICROBIAL EFFECT

The eye, like the CSF, is an immune-privileged site (29,30). The host responses to infection in the eye may be somewhat different, therefore, from responses to infections elsewhere. In the brain, the blood–brain barrier excludes many macromolecules, including immunoglobulins and complement from the CSF, creating a localized host-defense deficiency. For this reason, in the treatment of meningitis the choice of a bactericidal drug is strongly recommended, and such a recommendation seems appropriate by analogy in the treatment of endophthalmitis (19,21,22).

TOXICITY OF INTRAVITREAL ANTIBIOTICS

Tissue toxicity defines the upper end of the therapeutic range (31). Because intravitreal injections often result in intraocular concentrations much higher than routinely achieved elsewhere in the body by intravenous dosing, toxicity considerations are particularly important in the eye.

Concentrations of gentamicin within the CSF after single intrathecal injection are reported to be between 27 and 81 μg/ml. Estimated intravitreal concentrations are 100 mcg/ml when 400 μg of gentamicin is injected into the vitreous cavity or 25 μg/ml when 100 μg is injected. In one prospective study of neonatal gram-negative bacillary meningitis, infants treated with intrathecal injection and systemic medications had a higher mortality than those treated with systemic medication alone. Possible explanations for the higher mortality with intrathecal therapy are either iatrogenic damage or gentamicin toxicity resulting from higher concentrations after intrathecal injection (22).

Within the eye, criteria for toxicity in the posterior segment have not been completely defined. Histopathologic criteria are most frequently employed and involve demonstration of changes in the retina or RPE some time after injection of intravitreal antimicrobials. The rabbit was chosen for most toxicity studies, usually for reasons of expense and convenience. It has been demonstrated, however, that the rabbit may be an inadequate model because its retina is merangiotic, with less vasculature compared with the holangiotic retina of higher-level primates. In testing for toxicity of aminoglycosides, this difference in structure led to a failure to recognize the vascular obliterative complications, which now are thought to be not only the most common sign of toxicity but also the most damaging complication after intraocular aminoglycoside administration (38,68).

The electroretinogram (ERG) may also be used as a criterion for toxicity, but its efficacy is complicated by the fact that surgical invasion of the eye can lower the ERG response. Therefore, it is important to include careful concurrent controls in which placebo is injected (69).

Toxicity may be attributable to the antimicrobial itself, to the vehicle, or to the preservatives associated with it. Marmor also suggested that changes in pH or osmolality may create iatrogenic tissue damage to the retina (70). This risk probably is minimized by the low volumes of drug injected, typically only 0.1 ml.

Peyman et al. hypothesized that injection of antibiotic into the eye in which the vitreous has been removed may increase the risk of toxicity (71), possibly because the antibiotic settles on the retinal surface, causing a high dose at the retinal surface rather than mixing completely within the vitreous cavity. Comparison of the rates of toxicity in vitrectomized versus nonvitrectomized eyes was made in studies of aminoglycosides (72), and no difference in toxicity was demonstrated using histopathologic criteria.

Aminoglycosides are the antibiotics that have been studied most carefully for their toxic potential after intraocular injection. Gentamicin has been most completely characterized. Zachary and Forster (73) noted dose-related damage to the outer retina, with marked disruption of the outer nuclear layer and prominent loss of outer segment with doses exceeding 0.2-mg injections in the rabbit. Ophthalmoscopically, RPE mottling and clumping and scattered areas of depigmentation were noted. The ERG became extinguished with 0.4- to 0.5-mg doses. D'Amico studied electron microscopy specimens from the rabbit after gentamycin intravitreal injections and noted lamellar lysosomal inclusions similar to drug-induced lipid-storage problems. These changes were similar to findings in the kidney and were thought to suggest that RPE is the primary site of toxicity for gentamicin (37).

Initially, no vascular abnormalities were noted on animal testing until Conway and Campochiaro identified a syndrome of infarction of macular vessels in humans resulting from intraocular injection of gentamicin (68). A subsequent survey of retinal specialists identified a number of similar cases secondary to both gentamicin and amikacin administration (38). To characterize this complication in the primate more fully, Conway et al. injected 1,000 mcg of gentamicin in *Cebus navrigatus* monkeys (74). Three days later, the clinical picture of macular infarction, with cotton-wool spots and intraretinal hemorrhages, was noted. Electron microscopy revealed striking damage to the inner retinal layers, mainly the nerve fiber, ganglion cell, inner plexiform, and nuclear layers. There were less severe changes in the outer layers. Despite the picture of macular infarction clinically, no apparent vascular changes were seen. The authors suggested that neurotoxic changes can lead to shutdown of regional blood flow, perhaps through granulocytic plugging.

D'Amico et al. studied five aminoglycosides by examining the clinical picture, histopathology, and electron microscopy after intravitreal injection (75). They noted that the first abnormalities produced were lysosomal overloading of the RPE with lamellar lipid material. At doses of amikacin 1,500 μg and gentamicin 400 μg, toxic reactions in the outer retina were noted that consisted of macrophages in the subretinal space with storage lysosomes, disorganization of the photoreceptor outer segments with preservation of the inner segments, and focal necrosis of the RPE. There were areas of focal disappearance of photoreceptors and RPE, with reactive gliosis as a late finding. Doubling these dosages led to full-thickness retinal necrosis marked ophthalmoscopically by gray-white areas in the RPE corresponding to destruction of the photoreceptor-RPE complex. In this model, the relative toxicities established were gentamicin > netilmicin = tobramycin > amikacin = kanamycin.

Repeated doses of intraocular antibiotics may increase the risk of complications. In other systems in the body, the antibiotic toxicity is often related to the peak dose. With multiple intraocular injections, high peak doses are repeated. Oum et al. injected 1 mg of vancomycin along with amikacin 400 μg or gentamicin 100 μg, demonstrating no toxicity after one injection (76). After two injections of each antibiotic spaced 48 hours apart, 5 of 6 of the gentamycin eyes and 3 of the 6 amikacin-injected eyes demonstrated abnormalities of the RPE, disorganization of the outer segments of the photoreceptors, and a mild loss of RPE photoreceptor interdigitation. A third injection given 48 hours later caused multiple white dots to appear from the posterior pole to the equator at the level of the RPE in 4 of 9 eyes with gentamicin and vancomycin and in 2 of 9 eyes with amikacin and vancomycin, findings not demonstrated in control eyes. The RPE disturbance was followed by disorganization of the photoreceptor outer segments, with focal disorganization of the RPE with hyperpigmentation and hypopigmentation.

Shockley et al. studied ceftriaxone and found no ERG or histopathologic changes after 5-mg injections (77). After injection of 7.5 mg or 20 mg, the ERG B-wave was diminished but recovered subsequently. There were no abnormal findings on ophthalmoscopic examination or histopathology. After injection of 50 mg in the vitreous cavity of the rabbit, lens opacification and corneal clouding were noted transiently. There was retinal edema, and the B-wave was flat at 24 hours and had not fully recovered after 2 weeks. There was generalized retinal edema on histopathologic examination, with disruption of the retinal layers. Schenk et al. studied carbenicillin disodium and found that 10, 15, or 20 mg produced cataracts, which cleared within 4 to 5 weeks (78). Campochiaro injected ceftazidime in various concentrations in squirrel monkey eyes and found no evidence of toxicity after injection of 2.25 mg. In eyes injected with 10 mg, full-thickness macular holes developed. The outer retina demonstrated photoreceptor detachment from the RPE and damage to photoreceptors, with many clear cystic spaces in the outer plexiform layer of the parafoveal areal. Electron microscopic studies showed significant damage to photoreceptors.

Systemic toxicities are a significant consideration in the choice of oral and intravenous antibiotics for the treatment and prophylaxis of intraocular infection and should be balanced against the poor penetration ratios for many drugs now used in endophthalmitis therapy. Because of the poor penetration of drug into the eye, higher concentrations may be given, thereby increasing the risk of systemic toxicity.

DOSE-RESPONSE RELATIONSHIPS IN THE VITREOUS CAVITY

Intravitreal injection of antibiotics creates a high concentration of drug within the vitreous cavity initially, with persistence for a variable time. The concentration and duration of exposure of the antimicrobial necessary for successful effect are unknown. The minimal inhibitory *concentration,* or MIC, is the lowest concentration of an antimicrobial agent that prevents visible growth of bacteria after an 18- or 24-hour period of incubation in vitro. In antimicrobial therapy, it is believed that the drug level should, at a minimum, reach a concentration that at least exceeds the MIC of the target organism. The MIC values for common organisms causing endophthalmitis are given in Table 32-4 for reference. The *minimal bactericidal concentration* (MBC) is the lowest concentration of antimicrobial that totally suppresses growth on antibiotic-free media or results in a 99.9% or greater decline in colony count after overnight (18- or 21-hour) incubation. The MIC may be the same as the MBC, but the MBC may be several multiples of the MIC, in which case the organism is said to be *resistant.* Research indicates that the MBC is the more critical level in the therapy of meningitis, but the MBC determinations for given organisms are less readily available than the MIC levels.

In the treatment of bacterial meningitis, there is a positive correlation between the bactericidal rate and the concentration of the antibiotic in the CSF in studies of beta-lactam treatment of pneumococcal meningitis. Bacterial killing in the CSF is dose dependent but is incompletely understood (27,28,79–82). As a general rule, in the CSF, concentrations in the range slightly above the MBC are bacteriostatic or minimally bactericidal; however, large

TABLE 32-4. *In vitro susceptibility of various bacteria causing endophthalmitis to selected antibiotics*

	Cefazolin	Ceftriaxone	Ceftazidime	Ciprofloxacin	Gentamicin	Amikacin	Imipenem
Gram-Positive[a]							
Staphylococcus epidermidis	0.8	16.0	32.0	0.25			0.2
Staphylococcus aureus	1.0	4.0	16.0	1.0	0.8	3.1	0.1
Streptococcus pyogenes	0.1	0.03	0.25	1.0			0.1
Streptococcus pneumoniae			1.0	1.0		0.01	
Enterococcus				2.0	6.2	50	0.8
Bacillus	>100	>64	>64	1.0			
Gram-Negative[b]							
Pseudomonas aeruginosa	>100	>32	4	0.5	3.1	12.5	12.5
Klebsiella pneumoniae	6.0	0.1	0.5	0.125	1.6	6.2	0.4
Serratia	>100	4.0	1.0	1.0	1.6	6.2	6.3
Proteus			0.12	0.06	3.1	12.5	0.6
Enterobacter		0.1	1.0	0.125	1.6	6.2	0.4
Escherichia coli	5.0	0.1	0.5	0.03	6.2	12.5	
Haemophilus influenza	10.0		0.1				0.1

Adapted from Schenk, et al., ref 78; Bennett, ref 96; Andriole, ref 101; and Neu, ref 116.
[a]Minimum inhibitory concentration (μg/ml) for 90% of strains (MIC_{90}).
[b]Minimum inhibitory concentration (μg/ml) for 100% of strains (MIC_{100}) except ciprofloxacin (MIC_{90}).

bolus doses of antibiotic are effective in meningitis treatment because the most important variable in cure rate of meningitis in some studies was the peak CSF antibiotic concentration. As CSF concentrations are increased tenfold to 100-fold that of the MBC, the bactericidal rate increases until it plateaus at a maximal killing rate of approximately a log (10) colony-forming units (CFU)/m/hour. Beyond this time, a postantibiotic effect has been noted, probably mediated by low residual levels of drug that are even lower than the MIC. It is thus recommended that CSF concentrations in meningitis should reach levels at least ten times the MBC for effective killing. For effective killing in the vitreous cavity, these may also be desirable target levels.

Davey et al. studied the rate of bacterial killing in models of experimental gram-negative endophthalmitis (6). Although CSF antimicrobial concentrations reach a maximal effective concentration, this effect was not noted in treatment of gram-negative endophthalmitis, even when concentrations were 100 times the MBC. Appropriate antimicrobials given after the infection was established for 48 hours failed to eradicate the infection. Exact causes for this lack of effective killing in the model of gram-negative endophthalmitis were not clear.

Factors in the activity of antimicrobials in vivo that may make their effects different from in vitro measurements include (a) a decrease in pH due to the infective process, which may cause aminoglycosides to lose activity; (b) slow growth rates of bacteria, which reduce the effectiveness of beta-lactam activity; (c) reduction of bacterial doubling times by fever (i.e., pneumococci in meningitis). Davey et al. also hypothesized that consumption of nutrients might be a limiting factor, but they were unable to demonstrate this as a significant factor in their model of gram-negative endophthalmitis (6).

Although in the past some authors suggested that a single injection of intravitreal antibiotic in the laboratory and clinical setting may be sufficient to eradicate bacterial infections (83–87), it is clear that this is not universally true. *P. acnes* infections, presumably the cause of slow growth rates of the organism, are notoriously resistant to single injections of antibiotic even when coupled with vitrectomy (10). In a laboratory study of experimental *S. aureus* endophthalmitis, Aguilar demonstrated residual bacteria were growing in 25% of the eyes after 48 hours when treatment was given with either vancomycin or cefazolin (4). Gram-negative organisms and streptococcal organisms (11) have been shown to be resistant to single-dose therapy, as have even staphylococcal organisms on occasion (9). Fungal organisms are also extremely difficult to eradicate with a single dosage of intraocular medication.

PHARMACOKINETICS OF SUBCONJUNCTIVAL INJECTIONS

Because the RPE is a barrier to diffusion, antimicrobials enter the vitreous cavity poorly after subconjunctival injection (24). There is evidence for higher levels of antimicrobials in the aqueous after subconjunctival injection, but insufficient levels are produced in the vitreous cavity to enhance significantly the antimicrobial effects of most antibiotics (88–93). In studies of subconjunctival injections of third-generation cephalosporins, the corneal levels achieved were fourfold higher than aqueous concentrations. Concentrations in the choroid were fivefold to 15-fold higher than for the retina; retinal concentrations were about tenfold higher than vitreous cavity. Thus, there is a significant concentration gradient from choroid to retina and from retina to vitreous. When the eyes were inflamed in this study, the barriers appeared to be preserved. This report suggested that subconjunctival injections cannot replace intravitreal injections in the treatment of endophthalmitis (13).

SELECTED ANTIMICROBIALS

Individual antimicrobials commonly used to treat endophthalmitis and retinitis are summarized below. A discussion of general principles of pharmacokinetics, as well as more specific discussions of pharmacokinetics and toxicities of these antimicrobials, is found in previous sections of this chapter.

AMINOGLYCOSIDES

History and Source

The aminoglycoside antibiotics are products of the actinomycetes fungi or semisynthetic analogues of these products. During the 1980s and early 1990s, the aminoglycosides were the most frequently used antimicrobials for the treatment and prophylaxis of endophthalmitis. Many surgeons administered an aminoglycoside subconjunctivally at the completion of elective surgery. Amikacin and gentamicin were frequently administered intravenously for prophylaxis after penetrating trauma and for treatment of intraocular infection. Intraocular injections of either gentamicin or amikacin often were administered for therapy of endophthalmitis, and amikacin was the drug chosen for intraocular and intravenous administration in the Endophthalmitis Vitrectomy Study (94).

Official Name and Chemistry

The aminoglycoside family of antibiotics is defined by the presence of an aminocyclitol ring linked by glycosidic bonds to two or more aminosugars. The six-member aminocyclitol ring is 2-deoxystreptamine in neomycin, gentamicin, tobramycin, amikacin, netilmicin, and kanamycin. Gentamicins and netilmicin have been isolated from *Micromonospora* species, whereas neomycin, kanamycin, neomycin, and tobramycin have each been isolated from a different species of *Streptomyces.* Amikacin is the 1-N-hydroxyaminobutyric acid derivative of kanamycin A.373

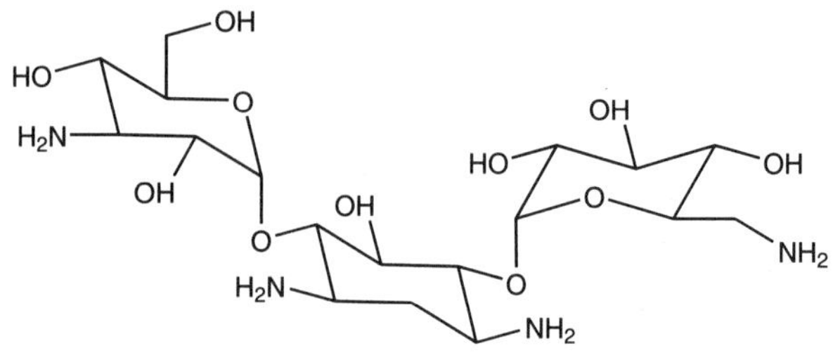

KANAMYCIN A

Gentamicin contains the sulfate salts of three components, gentamicin C_1, C_2, and C_{1A}. All three components have similar antimicrobial activity.

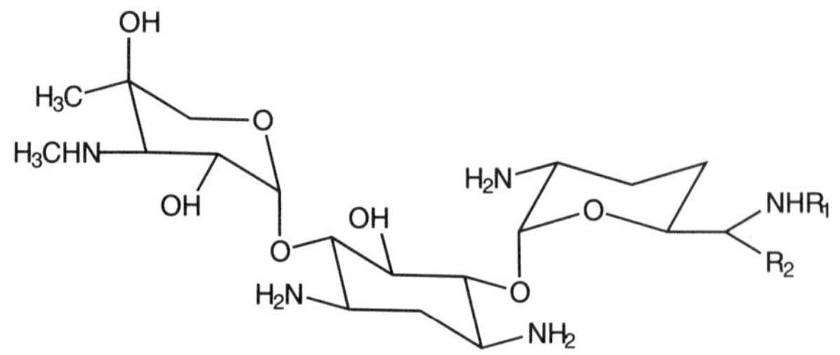

GENTAMICIN

Tobramycin sulfate has the chemical formula $(C_{18}H_{37}N_5O_9)_2 \cdot 5H_2SO_4$. The molecular weight is 1,425.39.

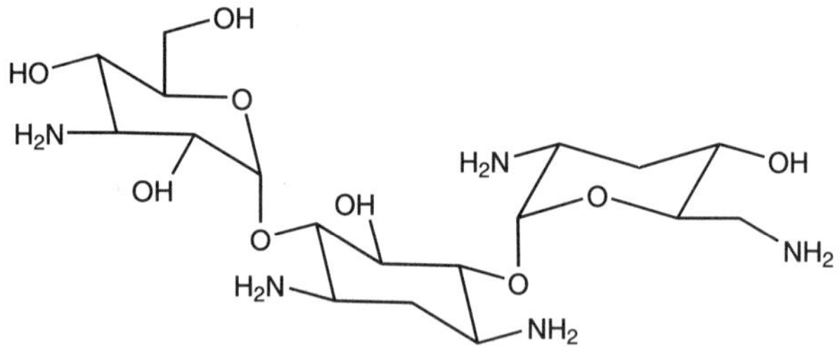

TOBRAMYCIN

Amikacin sulfate has the chemical formula $C_{22}H_{43}N_5O_{13} \cdot 2H_2SO_4$. The molecular weight is 781.75.

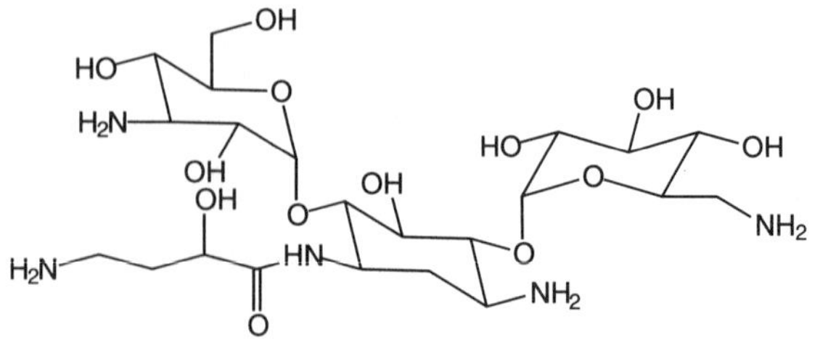

AMIKACIN

Pharmacology

The aminoglycosides are used because they are active against aerobic gram-negative bacilli, especially *Pseudomonas,* coupled with relatively low cost. Although not generally employed systemically against staphylococci, their ability to be bactericidal against gram-positive pathogens in higher concentration, especially staphylococcal species, is advantageous in ophthalmic practice.

The exact mechanism of action is unknown. Aminoglycosides inhibit protein syntheses, but this action may be insufficient to explain their effect. They also interact with ribosomal binding sites, demonstrating energy-dependent transport into cells. The MBC is generally near the MIC for aminoglycosides. Aminoglycosides demonstrate concentration-dependent killing, so higher doses usually give progressively greater degrees of bactericidal action. They additionally have a postantibiotic effect against *Pseudomonas* spp. and possibly *E. coli* and *K. pneumonia,* wherein there is not an immediate rebound of bacterial growth once the antibiotic concentration falls below the MIC for the given organism. Aminoglycosides may exhibit synergy with other antibiotics against some organisms. Vancomycin and gentamicin, for example, are synergistic against enterococci.

Pharmaceutics

Gentamicin (Garamicin, Shering) is available as 2 mg/ml solution for intramuscular, intrathecal, or intravenous use and as 10 mg/ml and 40 mg/ml solutions for intramuscular or intravenous use. Tobramycin (Nebcin, Lilly) is available as 10 mg/ml and 40 mg/ml solutions for intramuscular and intravenous use. Amikacin (Amikin, Bristol) is available as 50 mg/ml and 250 mg/ml solutions for intramuscular or intravenous use. These concentrated aminoglycoside solutions must be diluted before intravenous administration.

Pharmacokinetics, Concentration-effect Relationship, and Metabolism

Absorption after oral administration is poor. The usual route is intravenous, although absorption after intramuscular administration is good. Intrathecal injection also has been used. Aminoglycosides cross membranes without transport systems poorly.

Penetration of aminoglycosides into the vitreous cavity after intravenous administration is marginal and may not reach concentrations above the MIC for *Pseudomonas* or staphylococci. Barza et al. administered gentamicin continuously for 12 hours and achieved vitreous concentrations of 2.8 μg/ml in infected rabbit eyes (36). In a model using a traumatized rabbit eye, concentrations of only 0.25 μg/ml were attained after 1 to 3 hours (44). Aphakic-vitrectomized inflamed eyes have greater permeability to antimicrobials than eyes that have not been surgically altered. In studying this circumstance in the rabbit, gentamicin was given every 8 hours for 72 hours and amikacin was administered every 12 hours for 72 hours. The maximum concentration achieved for gentamicin was 1.8 mcg/ml, which is below the MIC for both *Pseudomonas* spp. and staphylococcal organisms. A higher concentration of amikacin was established but also remained below the MIC for staphylococci and *Pseudomonas* because amikacin is somewhat less potent on a weight basis (45).

The clearance of gentamicin after intravitreal injection was studied in several animal models and in humans. In the monkey, the half-life in the normal eye was 34 hours (59) and in the rabbit 32 hours (58), consistent with an anterior route of elimination. Rendering the eye aphakic had a dramatic effect on half-life, reducing it to 12 hours in control animals and 14 hours in infected animals. Cobo and Forster suggest that reinjection of the antimicrobial be considered after 48 hours because by then the concentrations had fallen to levels that might not produce a bactericidal effect in humans (58).

Amikacin is also eliminated anteriorly and demonstrates a long half-life after injection into the phakic eye of the rabbit. The control half-life of 25.5 hours is reduced to 15.5 hours when the eye is inflamed by injection of heat-killed *S. epidermidis* (56). Removing the lens reduced the half-life by 40% to 50%. Removing lens and vitreous reduced the half-life to slightly less than 8 hours in both the inflamed and control eyes.

Therapeutic Use

Recommended doses for intravitreal injection of amikacin are 0.2 to 0.4 mg and for gentamicin 0.1 mg. Vascular occlusive toxicity has been reported in these dosage ranges on occasion. For intravenous dosing, a variety of regimens have been used. A loading dose of 1.5 to 2.0 mg/kg for gentamicin and 7.5 to 8.0 mg/kg for amikacin is usually employed. Maintenance dosing is individualized, taking into consideration the dosing intervals, the patient's size, the size of individual doses, and renal status. Dosages must be reduced in patients who have decreased renal function. Typical dosage regimens administer gentamicin 1.5–2.0 mg/kg every 8 hours and amikacin 7.5 to 8 mg/kg every 12 hours. Plasma aminoglycoside levels are determined and dosing adjusted. Target plasma levels 30 to 60 minutes after intravenous infusion or intramuscular injection are 5–10 μg/ml for gentamicin and 20–40 μg/ml for amikacin.

Side Effects and Toxicity

The toxicities of intravitreal aminoglycoside administration have been studied extensively and were already reviewed. The three principal systemic toxic effects of aminoglycosides are nephrotoxicity, ototoxicity, and neuromuscular paralysis (95). Ototoxicity is relatively uncommon but is frequently irreversible and may occur even after the drug has been discontinued. The incidence of ototoxicity with hearing loss on audiometric testing has been reported to be 0.5% to 5% of patients given the aminoglycosides. Auditory toxicity tends to be cumulative and increases after repeated aminoglycoside courses even during carefully monitored therapy. Nephrotoxicity occurs as a result of proximal tubular cell damage. The onset of glomerular dysfunction usually occurs several days after the beginning of therapy and increases in severity over several days. Gentamicin is thought to be more nephrotoxic than tobramycin or amikacin. Renal function must be monitored carefully because renal damage is reversible and severe nephrotoxicity rarely occurs if the aminoglycoside dosage is adjusted. Neuromuscular paralysis has been noted when systemic administration is rapid; it may be treated with calcium infusion.

Drug Interactions

Aminoglycosides may interact with beta-lactam antibiotics in vitro and, to a lesser extent, in vivo, causing inactivation of both compounds; the aminoglycosides are more affected by this reaction. This interaction is probably more significant if the antimicrobials are mixed together than as an in vivo phenomenon. Concomitant administration of vancomycin or other nephrotoxic drugs may potentiate nephrotoxic effects. Concurrent use of diuretic agents also may potentiate the nephrotoxicity of the aminoglycosides.

AMPHOTERICIN B

History and Source

Amphotericin B is a polyene antibiotic derived from *Streptomyces nodosus.*

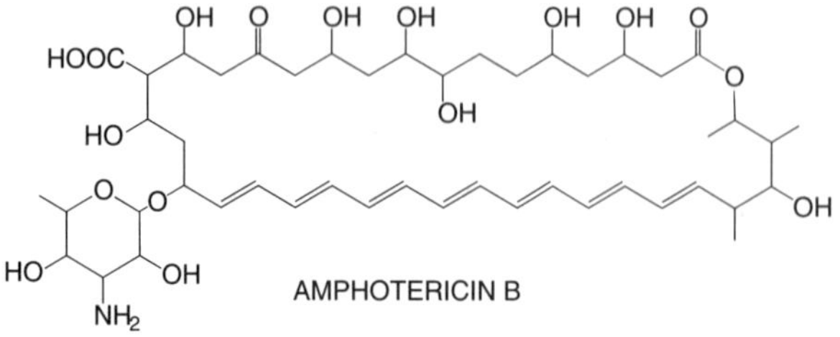

AMPHOTERICIN B

Pharmacology

Amphotericin B exerts its effects through combination with ergosterol, fungisterol, or other sterols in the fungal cytoplasmic membrane, thereby altering membrane permeability. Systemically, it is used for blastomycosis, candidiasis, histoplasmosis, cryptococcosis, aspergillosis, mucormycosis, and coccidioidomycosis. Combination therapy with flucytosine, rifampin, or tetracycline sometimes improves the therapeutic response (96). Because of the systemic complications of amphotericin and its uncertain intraocular penetration, therapy with only intraocular injections with or without vitrectomy is often chosen for endophthalmitis. Good clinical results are reported as a result of this strategy (10). Isolated retinitis in association with systemic fungemia is usually managed with intravenous therapy, often with successful eradication of the infection.

Pharmaceutics

Amphotericin B (Fungizone IV, Bristol-Myers Squibb) is available in vials containing 50 mg of lyophilized drug, which must be reconstituted before use. The vial must be refrigerated and protected from light. Reconstituted solutions should be used promptly and protected from light.

Pharmacokinetics, Concentration-effect Relationship, and Metabolism

After intravenous administration, amphotericin leaves the circulation rapidly and is stored in the liver, from which it is slowly released. Penetration into inflamed and normal meninges is poor. Penetration into both aqueous humor and vitreous is poor, achieving concentration of only two-thirds the plasma trough level of 0.2 to 0.5 μg/ml (97). Retention in phakic eyes is excellent after intravitreal injection, and the half-life is 4.7 days. Vitrectomy and lensectomy markedly reduce the half-life to 1.4 days (57).

Therapeutic Use

Amphotericin B remains the antimicrobial of choice for the vast majority of fungal infections. For treatment of fungal endophthalmitis, the usual intraocular dose is amphotericin B 0.005 mg; miconazole 0.025 mg has also been recommended. Systemic administration is not always necessary, but consultation with a specialist familiar with amphotericin B is advisable. A small test dose is often given initially, followed by administration of a larger dose in conjunction with corticosteroid.

Side Effects and Toxicity

Systemic complications of intravenous amphotericin are significant. According to one authority, azotemia is considered normal, and the creatinine rises to 2.0 to 3.0 mg/dl. The hematocrit may drop 20% to 30%, and hypokalemia necessitating supplementation is common. Weight loss of 15 pounds during a course of therapy is frequently encountered (96).

OTHER ANTIFUNGALS

Flucytosine and the imidazoles are other agents used for antifungal therapy, but there are limited data on their efficacy against intraocular infection. Flucytosine is thought to be inferior in activity to amphotericin for most infections, but its toxicity is less, and it may be administered orally with good absorption from the gastrointestinal tract. Flucytosine is usually used in combination with amphotericin B.

The imidazoles are synthetic organic compounds whose imidazole ring confers their antifungal activity. Ketaconazole has variable absorption after oral dosing and poor meningeal penetration. It is active against coccidiomycosis, candidiasis, blastomycosis, and histoplasmosis but not against aspergillosis. Fluconazole has good oral absorption and a half-life of 25 hours with 70% CSF penetration. There is no broad experience with its use, but cryptococcal meningitis has been reported to respond clinically (96).

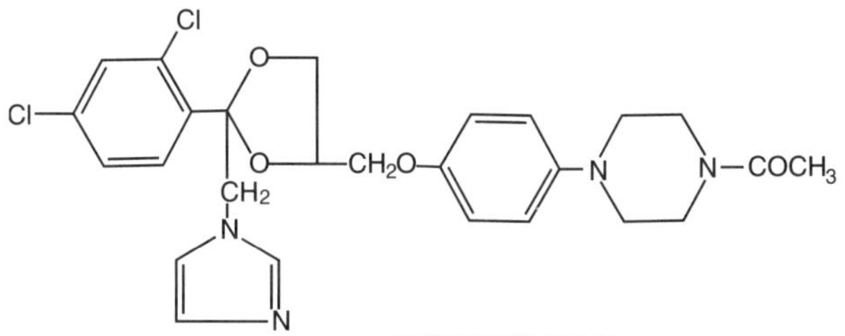

KETOCONAZOLE

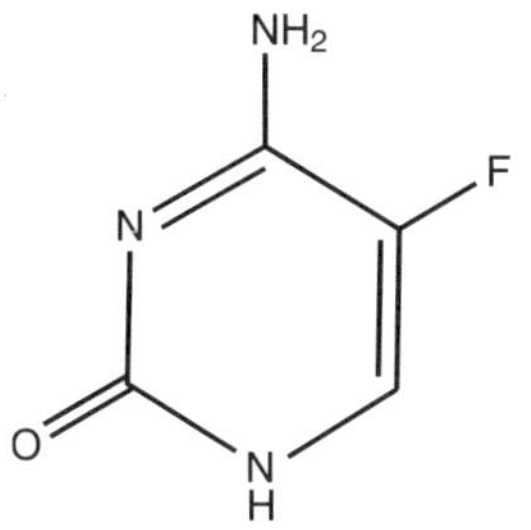

5-FLUOROCYTOSINE

CEPHALOSPORINS

History and Source

Active fermentation products of *Cephalosporium acremonium* were discovered in the 1940s to have antibacterial effects. Subsequently, one of these products, cephalosporin C, was hydrolyzed to 7-aminocephalosporanic acid, and modification of this compound with different side chains has given rise to the large family of cephalosporin antibiotics.

Official Drug Name and Chemistry

The cephalosporins are beta-lactam antibiotics and resemble penicillin, except the 5-member thiazolidine ring characteristic of penicillin is replaced by a 6-member dihydrothiazine ring.

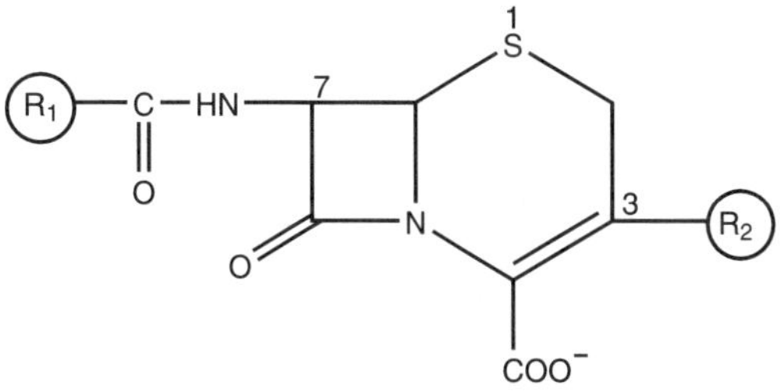

In general, modifications at position 7 of the 7-aminocephalosporanic acid nucleus are associated with alterations in antibacterial activity. Substitutions at position 3 of the dihydrothiazine ring are associated with changes in pharmacokinetics and metabolic parameters of the drugs (98).

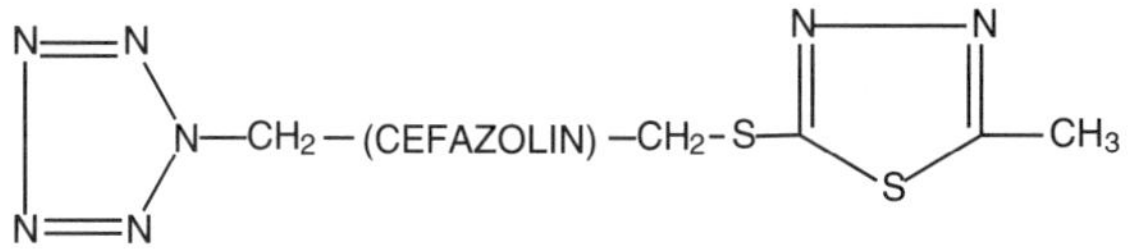

The chemical formula of cefazolin sodium is $C_{14}H_{13}N_8NaO_4S_3$. The molecular weight is 476.5.

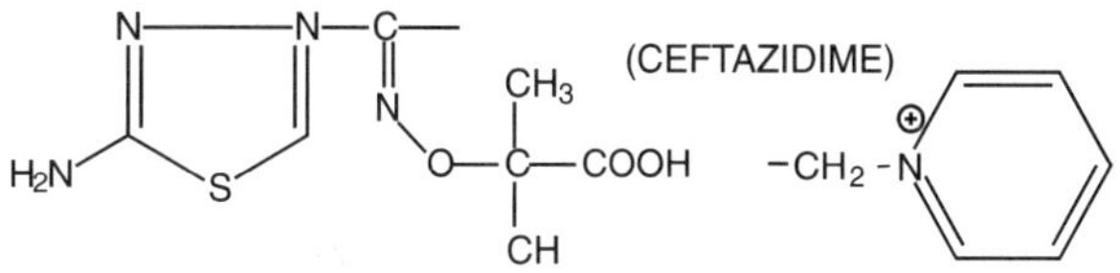

The chemical formula of ceftazidime is $C_{22}H_{32}N_6O_{12}S_2$. The molecular weight is 636.6.

Pharmacology

The mechanism of action of cephalosporins is complex and incompletely understood. They are known to bind to and inactivate specific targets on the inner aspect of bacterial cell membranes. The sites of binding are called penicillin-binding proteins (PBPs) and are enzymes important for biosynthesis of the peptidoglycan component of the bacterial cell wall. Different beta-lactams have different binding affinities for various PBPs, and their activity is related to the specific PBPs that are bound. Cephalosporins are bactericidal (98).

The activity of cephalosporins depends on their ability to penetrate the cell wall, to resist inactivation by bacterial enzymes (beta-lactamases), and to bind and inactivate PBPs. Resistance to their action can develop at any of these steps. Cephalosporins demonstrate time-dependent killing. After the MIC is reached, large increases in concentration will not necessarily increase the bactericidal effect, but the duration of exposure will remain an important factor in their ability to eradicate bacteria.

The cephalosporins are divided into three "generations" based on their antimicrobial activity. The first-generation agents are active against gram-positive cocci, including *S. aureus* and streptococci, but not including methicillin-resistant staphylococci and penicillin-resistant *S. pneumoniae.* They have moderate activity against aerobic gram-negative bacilli. From this group, cefazolin has been used against endophthalmitis but is less frequently employed because a significant percentage of staphylococci causing endophthalmitis are resistant to it (41). Second-generation agents are more potent than first-generation agents against *E. coli, Klebsiella,* and indole-negative *Proteus.* Certain members have extended activity against *Hemophilus influenzae, Neisseria, Serratia,* and many gram-negative bacilli. They have no significant activity against *Pseudomonas* species. The third-generation agents have the broadest spectrum and most potent activity against gram-negative organisms. They are divided into two groups based on their Pseudomonas activity. Their activity against gram-positive organisms is diminished compared with first- and second-generation agents.

Of third-generation agents, ceftazidime is the most widely employed in treatment of endophthalmitis. Ceftazidime is safe in doses up to 2.25 mg after injection into the monkey vitreous cavity. The spectrum of coverage against gram-negative organisms is equivalent to that of the aminoglycosides (12,99), and a small clinical series has been reported with good results and no recognized toxic side effects (100).

Pharmaceutics

Cefazolin sodium (Ancef, Smithkline Beecham) is available as a lyophilized form in 500 mg, 1-, 5-, and 10-g vials and as a frozen solution. Ceftazidime (Fortaz, Glaxo) is available as a powder in vials of 500 mg, 1, 2, and 6 g. It is available as a frozen solution in 1- and 2-g containers.

Pharmacokinetics, Concentration-effect Relationships, and Metabolism

Peak serum concentrations after intravenous administration are similar for most of these agents for a given dose and route of administration; a 2-g dose produces approximately 100 μg/ml serum concentrations. Penetration into the CSF varies but is best for cefuroxime among the second-generation agents. Third-generation agents have been designed for improved CSF penetration; moxalactam, ceftoxime, ceftriaxone, and ceftazidime all penetrate well (98). Most cephalosporins are excreted primarily by the kidneys. Cefoperazone and ceftriaxone are eliminated via the liver.

After systemic administration, several cephalosporins have been demonstrated to have reasonable degrees of penetration into the vitreous cavity when the eye is altered by surgery, disease, or inflammation. Ceftriaxone was given intramuscularly in humans with various conditions requiring vitrectomy and the concentration sampled at the time of subsequent surgery. Average concentrations of 5.9 mcg/ml 1 to 3 hours after intramuscular injection were demonstrated, and concentrations of 11.5 μg/ml were documented 24 hours after injection (48). Cefazolin was administered in the rabbit and the concentration studied in normal and surgically altered eyes, both with and without inflammation. No penetration was demonstrated into phakic eyes without inflammation, but concentrations reached 10.6 μg/ml in inflamed eyes after intravenous administration every 8 hours for 48 hours (35). In aphakic/vitrectomized control eyes, concentrations between 2.1 and 4.2 mcg/ml could be achieved after the same administration schedule. In eyes with inflammation, concentrations continued to rise over 48 hours, reaching 24.9 μg/ml 49 hours after the first injection.

In similar experiments in rabbits, ceftazidime had a more rapid penetration, achieving higher ratios to serum values. Peak concentrations ranged from 21.2 to 35.4 mcg/ml in inflamed aphakic/vitrectomized eyes 2 hours after administration and from 8.5 to 12 μg/ml in control eyes. Essentially no drug entered either phakic or aphakic control eyes. Inflammation in these eyes produced concentrations of approximately 5 μg/ml after 48 hours of intermittent intravenous administration (47,61).

Clearance of first-generation cephalosporins after intravitreal injection is consistent with a posterior route of clearance, whereas recent studies of new agents suggest an anterior route or combined posterior and anterior route (13). In phakic eyes, studies of cefazolin in the monkey and rabbit demonstrate a half-life of 6.5 to 7 hours (35,59). Inflammation increases the half-life of cefazolin, probably by interfering with active transport across posterior structures. Removal of the lens and vitreous produced half-lives similar to the phakic model (35). Studies of third-generation agents demonstrated increasing half-life values in infected rabbit eyes compared with controls (ceftizoxime 5.7 versus 9.4 hours; ceftriaxone 9.1 versus 13.1 hours) (13). In control eyes, ceftazidime had a half-life of 13.8 (61) to 20 hours (13). Removing the lens and vitreous dramatically lowers the half-life to approximately 5 hours, consistent with an anterior route of elimination (61).

After subconjunctival administration of ceftazidime, ceftizoxime, and ceftriaxone in normal rabbit eyes, vitreous concentrations ranged from 3.0 to 7.3 μg/ml. Vitreous concentrations were doubled in infected eyes for ceftazidime and ceftizoxime and increased nine times for ceftriaxone, but the half-life was inexplicably short (13).

Therapeutic Use

Ceftazidime (Fortaz, Tazicef, Tazidime) is recommended by many authorities for gram-negative coverage by intravitreal injection in acute postoperative, endogenous, traumatic, and bleb-related endophthalmitis. Doses of 2 mg in the monkey have been safe; for dilution simplicity, a human dose of 2.25 mg is often administered. Systemic dosage for adults is generally 1 g administered intravenously every 8 to 12 hours, but 2 g every 8 hours is recommended for serious systemic infections and may be advisable for endophthalmitis therapy. Cefazolin (Ancef, Kefzol) is given in adult doses of 0.5 to 1.5 g every 6 to 8 hours intravenously, but it is given less frequently for gram-positive coverage because of the possibility of the emergence of resistant staphylococci. The usual intravitreal dose is 2.25 mg.

Side Effects and Toxicity

Cephalosporins are considered relatively safe. They are known to have a low level of toxic side effects, but there is cross-reactivity with penicillin allergy. The recommendation of most authorities is to avoid cephalosporins if the patient has had an immunoglobulin E (IgE)-mediated reaction, such as hives, or has had anaphylaxis. The true risk of allergy is estimated at only 1% to 2% of individual patients (33). Most hypersensitivity reactions produce a maculopapular rash. Anaphylaxis, bronchospasm, and urticaria are rarer. Nephrotoxicity or bleeding abnormalities may be noted occasionally (33).

CIPROFLOXACIN

Official Drug Name and Chemistry

Ciprofloxacin (Cipro) is member of the 4-quinolone group of agents. Structural features common to these drugs include a carboxyl group at the 3 position and a piperazine ring at the 7 position of the quinolone nucleus. Ciprofloxacin is similar in structure to nalidixic acid. Its chemical formula is $C_{17}H_{18}FN_3O_3$, and its molecular weight is 331.4.

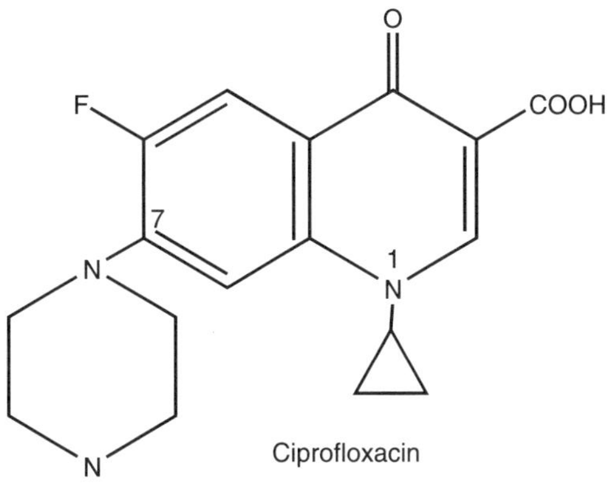

O
F
COOH
7
N
1
N
N

Ciprofloxacin

Pharmacology

The mechanism of action is inhibition of DNA synthesis in susceptible bacterial cells while sparing mammalian cells. The quinolones are thought to inhibit DNA gyrases, which are required to supercoil strands of intracellular bacterial DNA. Initially, ciprofloxacin was believed to be active against most strains of gram-negative and gram-positive bacteria that are ocular pathogens, including *Klebsiella, E. coli, Proteus mirabilis, Pseudomonas, Serratia, H. influenzae, Neisseria, S. aureus* (including methicillin-resistant strains), *S. epidermidis,* and streptococci (101). Unfortunately, with increased use, resistant strains are emerging.

Pharmaceutics

Ciprofloxacin (Cipro I.V., Miles) for intravenous infusion is available as a 1% solution (must be diluted before use) in 200-mg (20 ml) and 400-mg (40 ml) containers and as a .2% solution in 200-mg (100 ml) and 400-mg (200 ml) containers. Ciprofloxacin hydrochloride (Cipro, Miles) is available in 250-, 500-, and 750-mg tablets.

Pharmacokinetics, Concentration-effect Relationship, and Metabolism

Ciprofloxacin has good absorption from the gastrointestinal tract, with peak plasma levels reached in 1 to 1.5 hours, and it has excellent tissue distribution. After an oral dosage of 750 mg, vitrectomy specimens obtained from humans 24 hours later demonstrated a concentration of 0.04 to 0.49 μg/ml (51,52). At these concentrations, only 60% of organisms causing endophthalmitis tested in one laboratory would be inhibited. All 6 gram-negative bacteria would have been inhibited, but the gram-positive susceptibility was variable. The authors concluded that systemic ciprofloxacin alone is insufficient for empiric therapy of endophthalmitis (102). Ciprofloxacin may also be administered intravenously. The oral dose is 500 to 750 mg every 12 hours. Intravenously, 200 to 300 mg may be given slowly over 30 minutes every 12 hours.

After intraocular injection in rabbits, the clearance of ciprofloxacin was extremely rapid. The values determined for the half-life after intravitreal injection were 2.2 hours in phakic eyes and 1 hour in aphakic vitrectomized eyes (103).

Side Effects and Toxicity

Retinal toxicity has been documented at doses of 250 mcg/ml and corneal toxicity at 100 μg/ml after injection into the aphakic vitrectomized rabbit eye (104). The combination of short half-life and toxicity at relatively low concentrations restricts usefulness of intraocular injection of ciprofloxacin.

Ciprofloxacin is relatively safe systemically. Gastrointestinal side effects are the most common problem. Central nervous system symptoms such as headache, dizziness, and hallucinations also have been reported. Skin reaction may occur in up to 2.4% of patients. Ciprofloxacin is not recommended in pediatric patients (101).

CLINDAMYCIN

History and Source

Clindamycin (Cleocin) is a modification of lincomycin and was originally derived from *Streptomyces lincolnesis.* Modification to clindamycin increased the antibacterial potency and absorption.

Official Name

Clindamycin is methyl 7-chloro-6,7,8-trideoxy-6-(1 methyl-*trans*-4propyl-L-2pyrrolidinecarboxamido)-1thio-L-*threo-α*-D-*galacto*-oc-topyranoside. It is prepared as the hydrochloride salt for oral use and the phosphate salt for parenteral use.

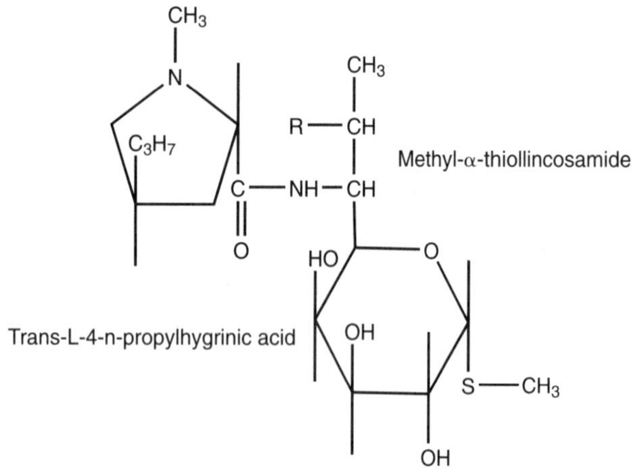

CH_3 N C_3H_7 C=O NH R—CH CH_3 CH HO O OH S—CH_3 OH

Trans-L-4-n-propylhygrinic acid

Methyl-α-thiollincosamide

Pharmacology

Clindamycin interferes with protein synthesis in microorganisms. The spectrum of action of clindamycin includes toxoplasmosis of the eye and brain and *Bacillus* species. It is also active against anaerobic bacteria, staphylococci, pneumococci, *S. pyogenes,* streptococci of the viridans group, and *Bacteroides fragilis.*

Pharmaceutics

Clindamycin hydrochloride (Cleocin HCl, Upjohn) is available for oral use in 75-, 150-, and 300-mg capsules. Clindamycin phosphate (Cleocin Phosphate, Upjohn) is available for parenteral use as a 150 mg/ml solution in 2-, 4-, and 5-ml vials or in 50-ml containers with 300, 600, or 900 mg of clindamycin.

Pharmacokinetics, Concentration-effect Relationship, and Metabolism

Clindamycin may be given intravenously, intravitreally, subconjunctivally, or orally. After oral administration, clindamycin has 90% absorption in the gastrointestinal tract, and a half-life of 2.4 hours. In usual concentrations, it is bacteriostatic. Clindamycin has little cerebrospinal penetration. There are no data on penetration into the vitreous cavity, but clinical responses to oral treatment of toxoplasmic retinitis have been observed.

Therapeutic Use

Dosages of clindamycin in adults depend on the severity of infection and condition of the patient. Oral doses are generally 150 to 300 mg every 8 hours, and parenteral doses of 900 mg given every 8 hours or 600 mg every 6 hours to a maximum daily dose of 8 g are employed. Intramuscular doses of 600 mg every 6 hours may also be administered, creating peak serum values within 3 hours. The normal half-life is 2.4 hours, and most of the absorbed drug is thought to be metabolized by the liver. After parenteral administration, there is a significant reduction of the population of sensitive bacteria in the colon that may last up to 14 days. The half-life and peak serum levels are increased in patients with severe renal failure, and modification of the dose should be considered in the presence of renal failure, particularly if liver disease is present, as prolongation of clindamycin activity in the serum is noted in patients with liver disease. Dosages of 1 mg for intraocular injection have been recommended. Intraocular efficacy may be limited because the drug is generally bacteriostatic.

Side Effects and Toxicity

Adverse reactions to clindamycin limit its use in general infectious disease. Diarrhea occurs in up to 20% of patients and is more common with oral administration. Pseudomembranous colitis may occur and is caused by a toxin secreted by *Clostridia difficile,* which overgrows in 0.01 to 10% of patients taking clindamycin; the syndrome may continue after the clindamycin is stopped. The resulting diarrhea and colitis may be not only protracted but fatal. Oral vancomycin is the treatment of choice. Additional side effects include allergic rashes and fever and rare cases of erythema multiforme and anaphylaxis. Occasionally, cases of minor reversible elevation of transaminase level and isolated cases of reversible neutropenia, thrombocytopenia, and agranulocytosis have been reported (105).

SULFONAMIDES

History and Source

Sulfonamides used clinically are derived from sulfanilamide, which is similar in structure to para-aminobenzoic acid (PABA), a factor required by bacteria for folic acid synthesis.

Official Name and Chemistry

Sulfadiazine is 2-sulfanilamidopyrimidine.

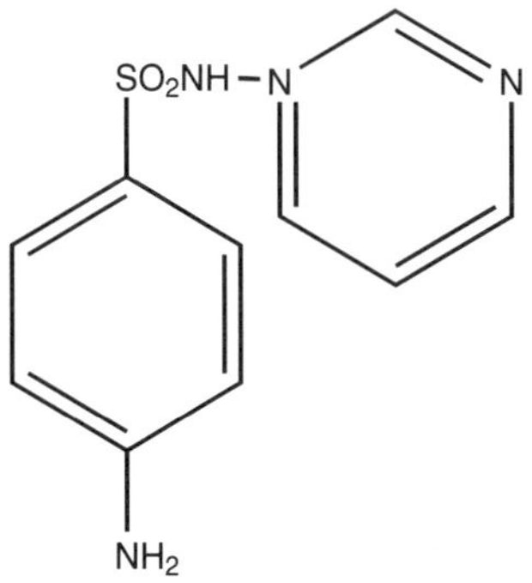

Sulfadiazine

Pharmacology

The sulfonamide commonly used for retinal infections is sulfadiazine USP (2-sulfanilamidopyridine, Sulfadyne), usually chosen for its activity against toxoplasmosic retinitis. Sulfonamides are also effective against *Nocardia asteroides.* Sulfadiazine is one of the short-acting sulfonamides and is highly active, attaining high blood and CSF levels, due to low protein binding. Sulfonamides are bacteriostatic and inhibit bacterial growth through interference with microbial folic acid synthesis. They competitively inhibit incorporation of PABA into tetrahydropteroic acid. Sulfonamides have in vitro inhibitory activity against a broad spectrum of gram-positive and gram-negative organisms, although resistance among many classes of organisms is increasingly being encountered.

Sulfonamides are usually administered orally, but sulfadiazine is also available for intravenous administration, although rarely used in this form. Short- and medium-acting sulfonamides are absorbed rapidly from the stomach and intestine and generally are well distributed throughout the body, including penetration into the CSF, depending on the degree of protein binding of the individual agent. Glucuronidation and acetylation occur in the liver. Metabolized and free drug appears in the urine, probably through glomerular filtration. Dosages must be reduced in renal failure.

Pharmaceutics

Sulfadiazine (Goldline) is available in 500-mg tablets.

Therapeutic Use

Sulfadiazine is usually prescribed for ocular toxoplasmosis. A loading dose of 2 to 4 g is followed by doses of 0.5 to 1 g every 6 hours. Drinking multiple glasses of water daily while taking the medication is encouraged to prevent deposition of renal crystals.

Side Effects and Toxicity

Sulfonamides may cause a variety of adverse reactions, including acute hemolytic anemia, aplastic anemia, leukopenia, thrombocytopenia, and agranulocytosis. Significant hypersensitivity reactions may also occur. In addition, they may cause fever, headache, depression, jaundice, nausea, vomiting, diarrhea, and rash, among other side effects.

TRIMETHOPRIM/SULFAMETHOXAZOLE

Official Name and Chemistry

Trimethoprim is 2,4-diamino-5-(3′,4′,5′-trimethoxybenzyl) pyrimidine. The molecular weight is 290.3.

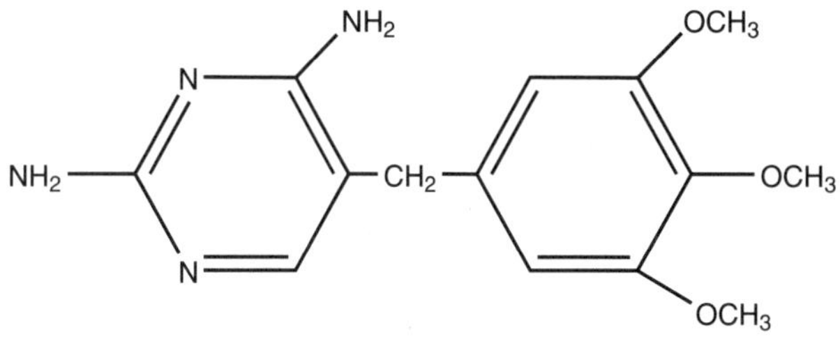

Trimethoprim

Sulfamethoxazole is N^1-(5-methyl-3-isoxazolyl)sulfanilamide. The molecular weight is 253.28.

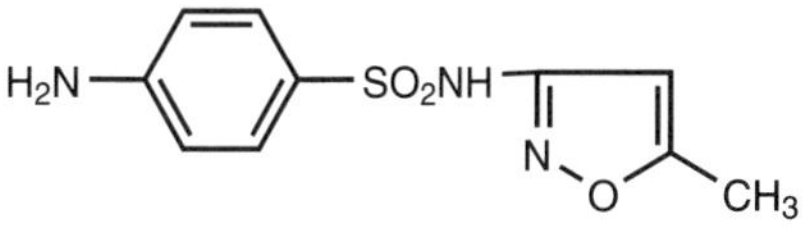

Pharmacology

Trimethoprim's activity is the result of inhibition of bacterial dihydrofolate reductase, the enzymatic step following the step in folic acid synthesis blocked by sulfonamides. It is 50,000 to 100,000 times more active against the bacterial enzyme than against its human counterpart. By interfering with the conversion of dihydrofolate to tetrahydrofolate, the precursor of folinic acid and ultimately purine and DNA synthesis, trimethoprim produces a high degree of synergistic activity against many organisms when used with sulfonamides (106).

Pharmaceutics

Trimethoprim is available in fixed combinations with sulfamethoxazole in a 1 : 5 ratio (by weight). Bactrim I.V. Infusion (Roche) is available as a solution of trimethoprim

(16 mg/ml) and sulfamethoxazole (80 mg/ml) in 5-ml ampules, and 5-, 10-, and 30-ml vials.

Bactrim (Roche) is available as tablets containing 80 mg trimethoprim and 400 mg of sulfamethoxazole. Bactrim DS tablets contain 160 mg of trimethoprim and 800 mg of sulfamethoxazole. Bactrim is also available as a suspension and pediatric suspension.

Pharmacokinetics, Concentration-effect Relationship, and Metabolism

Trimethoprim is excreted through the kidney.

Side Effects and Toxicity

Complications are similar to the sulfonamides.

Therapeutic Use

The adult oral dosage is trimethoprim 80 mg and sulfamethoxazole 400 mg (Bactrim, Septra). Pediatric suspension and intravenous combinations are also available. This combination has been reported effective in treating endophthalmitis caused by *Listeria monocytogenes* (107). It has also been recommended for treatment of intraocular *Nocardia.*

VANCOMYCIN

History and Source

Vancomycin is a bactericidal agent derived from *Streptomyces orientalis.*

Official Name and Chemistry

The chemical formula for vancomycin is $C_{66}H_{75}Cl_2 H_9O_{24}\cdot HCl$. The molecular weight is 1,486.

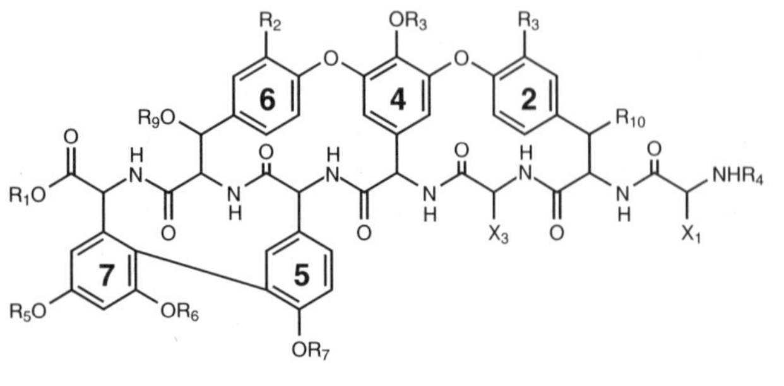

Pharmacology

Vancomycin inhibits synthesis and assembly of the second stage of bacterial cell wall peptidoglycan polymers by complexing with D-alanyl-D-alanine precursors. Additionally, it impairs RNA synthesis and injures protoplasts by damaging the permeability of their cytoplasmic membranes.

Vancomycin has a narrow spectrum of activity and is useful only against gram-positive organisms. Its action is against only replicating organisms with no lag period, and concentrations of 1 to 5 μg/ml are almost invariably inhibitory. Vancomycin is the drug of choice against methicillin-resistant staphylococci; with resistant staphylococci becoming more common, it assumes ever increasing importance (108). Vancomycin is active against almost all gram-positive organisms causing endophthalmitis, including *Bacillus* species, *P. acnes,* and streptococci (41). *Enterococcus* is relatively resistant.

Pharmaceutics

Vancomycin hydrochloride (Vancocin HCL, Lilly) is available in lyophilized form in 500-mg and 1-g vials and as a frozen solution in 500-mg containers.

Pharmacokinetics, Concentration-effect Relationship, and Metabolism

Vancomycin is poorly absorbed after oral administration and is usually given intravenously. No preparation is available for intramuscular injection because pain at the injection site is so significant. Vancomycin is eliminated from the body almost exclusively by glomerular filtration, and the dosage in patients with renal impairment must be reduced.

After intravenous administration, no vancomycin is absorbed in the phakic uninflamed eye. When the lens is removed and vancomycin is given intravenously every 12 hours, concentrations of 4.5 μg/ml may be achieved after 24 hours of administration, increasing to 5.6 μg/ml after 48 hours. Vitreous removal further enhances penetration. After 24 hours, the concentration is 6.8 μg/ml and after 49 hours it is 8.7 μg/ml in aphakic/vitrectomized eyes. Inflammation slightly enhances penetration in aphakic eyes; the effect is more significant in aphakic-vitrectomized eyes (46).

Clearance of vancomycin from the vitreous cavity after intravitreal injection is compatible with an anterior route of elimination. The half-life in the phakic eye is 25.5 hours, lengthened to 31.5 hours by ocular inflammation. A significant lowering of half-life occurs on lens removal to 9.8 hours in the control eye and 6.5 hours in the inflamed eye. Vitrectomy further shortens the half-life to 5.2 hours in the noninflamed eye (109).

Therapeutic Use

Vancomycin should be diluted in 100 to 250 ml of dextrose 5% or NaCl 0.9% and infused slowly over 30 to 60 minutes. More rapid administration may cause histamine release and produce the "red man syndrome" characterized by flushing, anaphylactoid reactions, and even cardiac arrest (108). Intravenous administration in patients with normal renal function usually begins with a loading dose of 15 mg/kg, followed by 1 g every 12 hours or 500 mg every 6 hours. The dosage must be reduced in patients with renal failure. Vancomycin is incompatible with many drugs in intravenous solutions and is best given by itself. Mixing with high concentrations of heparin may inactivate vancomycin. The usual intravitreal dose in the treatment of endophthalmitis is 1 mg.

Side Effects and Toxicity

In addition to the "red man syndrome," systemic complications include fever, chills, and phlebitis at the injection site. Vancomycin, like the aminoglycosides, may cause neurotoxicity, leading to auditory nerve damage and hearing loss (108). Hearing loss occasionally improves when the drug is discontinued but more often deteriorates and is permanent. Nephrotoxicity is now uncommon, but serum levels should be monitored carefully when other nephrotoxic drugs, such as the aminoglycosides, are given. Intravitreal doses of 2 mg in rabbits (producing intraocular concentrations of approximately 1,400 μg/ml) have been reported to be free of toxic effects on the retina (39).

ACKNOWLEDGMENT

Supported by NIH grant RO1 EY 05974-04A1 from the National Institutes of Health and in part from a department grant from Research to Prevent Blindness. Portions of this chapter were published previously as a thesis to fulfill the requirements for membership in the American Ophthalmological Society.

REFERENCES

1. Duguid JP, Ginsberg M, Fraser IS, Macaskill J, Michaelson I, Robson JM. Experimental observations on the intravitreous use of penicillin and other drugs. *Br J Ophthalmol* 1947;31:193.
2. Leopold IH, Scheie HG. Studies with microcrystalline sulfathiazole. *Arch Ophthalmol* 1943;29:811.
3. Baum J, Peyman GA, Barza M. Intravitreal administration of antibiotic in the treatment of bacterial endophthalmitis. III. Consensus. *Surv Ophthalmol* 1982;26:204.
4. Aguilar HE, Meredith TA, Drews CD, Sawant A, Gardner S, Wilson LA. Treatment of experimental *S. aureus* endophthalmitis with vancomycin, cefazolin and corticosteroids. *Invest Ophthalmol Vis Sci* 1990;31(suppl):308.
5. Forster RK. Experimental postoperative endophthalmitis. *Trans Am Ophthalmol Soc* 1992;90:505.
6. Davey PG, Barza M, Stuart M. Dose response of experimental Pseudomonas endophthalmitis to ciprofloxacin, gentamicin, and imipenem: evidence of resistance to "late" treatment of infections. *J Infect Dis* 1987;155:518.
7. Stern GA. Factors affecting the efficacy of antibiotics in the treatment of experimental postoperative endophthalmitis. *Trans Am Ophthalmol Soc* 1993;93:775.
8. Shaarawy A, Grand MG, Meredith TA, Ibanez H. Persistent infection after intravitreal antibimicrobial therapy. (In Press).
9. Stern GA, Engel HM, Driebe WT. Recurrent postoperative endophthalmitis. *Cornea* 1990;9:102.
10. Fox GM, Jooneph BC, Flynn HW. Delayed-onset pseudophakic endophthalmitis. *Am J Ophthalmol* 1991;111:163.
11. Mao LK, Flynn HW Jr, Miller D, Pflugfelder SC. Endophthalmitis caused by streptococcal species. *Arch Ophthalmol* 1992;119:798.
12. Irvine WD, Flynn HW Jr, Miller D, Pflugfelder SC. Endophthalmitis caused by gram-negative organisms. *Arch Ophthalmol* 1992;110:1450.
13. Barza M, Lynch E, Baum JL. Pharmacokinetics of newer cephalosporins after subconjunctival and intravitreal injection in rabbits. *Arch Ophthalmol* 1993;111:121.
14. Pavan PR, Oteiza EE, Hughes BA, Avni A. Exogenous endophthalmitis initially treated without systemic antibiotics. *Ophthalmology* 1994;101:1289.
15. Kattan HM, Flynn HW, Pflugfelder SC, Robertson C, Forster RK. Nosocomial endophthalmitis survey: current incidence of infection following intraocular surgery. *Ophthalmology* 1991;98:227.
16. Brinton GS, Topping TM, Hyndiuk RA, Aaberg TM, Reeser FH, Abrams GW. Posttraumatic endophthalmitis. *Arch Ophthalmol* 1984;102:547.
17. Boldt HC, Pulico JS, Blodi CS, Folk JC, Weingeist TA. Rural endophthalmitis. *Ophthalmology* 1989;96:1722.
18. Borhani H, Peyman GA, Wafapoor H. Use of vancomycin in vitrectomy infusion solution and evaluation of retinal toxicity. *Int Ophthalmol* 1993;17:85.
19. Scheld WM. Drug delivery to the central nervous system: general principles and relevance to therapy for infections of the central nervous system. *Reviews of Infectious Diseases* 1989;11:1669.
20. Quagliarello V, Scheld WM. Bacterial meningitis: pathogenesis, pathophysiology, and progress. *N Engl J Med* 1992;327:864.
21. Tauber MG, Sande MA. General principles of therapy of pyogenic meningitis. *Infect Dis Clin North Am* 1990;4:661.
22. Thea D, Barza M. Use of antibacterial agents in infections of the central nervous system. *Infect Dis Clin North Am* 1989;3:553.
23. Rich DS, Peter G, Jeffrey LP. Cerebrospinal fluid concentration of antibiotics. *Hosp Pharm* 1981;16:382.
24. Barza M. Antibacterial agents in the treatment of ocular infections. *Infect Clin North Am* 1989;3:533.
25. Maurice DM, Mishima S. Ocular pharmacokinetics. In: Sears ML, ed. *Pharmacology of the Eye.* New York: Springer-Verlag, 1984;19.
26. Barza M. Animal models in the evaluation of chemotherapy of ocular infections. In: Zak O, Sande MA, eds. *Experimental Models in Antimicrobial Chemotherapy,* 1st ed, vol 1. London: Harcourt Brace Jovanovich, 1986;187.
27. Scheld WM, Sande MA. Bactericidal versus bacteriostatic antibiotic therapy of experimental pneumococcal meningitis in rabbits. *J Clin Invest* 1983;71:411.
28. Tauber MG, Doroshow CA, Hackbarth CJ, et al. Antibacterial activity of beta-lactam antibiotics in experimental pneumococcal meningitis. *J Infect Dis* 1984;149:568.
29. Streilein JW. Anterior chamber associated immune deviation: the privilege of immunity in the eye. *Surv Ophthalmol* 1990;35:67.
30. Streilein JW, Wilbanks GA, Cousins SW. Immunoregulatory mechanisms of the eye. *J Neuroimmunol* 1992;39:185.
31. Rowland M, Tozer TN. *Clinical Pharmacokinetics: Concepts and Applications.* Philadelphia: Lea and Febiger, 1989.
32. Novak GD, Leopold IH. The blood-aqueous and blood–brain barriers to permeability. *Am J Ophthalmol* 1988;105:412.
33. Donowitz GR. Third generation cephalosporins. *Infect Dis Clin North Am* 1989;3:595.
34. Norrby SF. Role of cephalosporins in the treatment of bacterial meningitis in adults: overview with special emphasis on ceftazidime. *Am J Med* 1985;79(suppl 2A):56.
35. Martin DF, Ficker LA, Aguilar HA, Gardner SK, Wilson LA, Meredith TA. Vitreous cefazolin levels after intravenous injection: effects of inflammation, repeated antibiotic doses, and surgery. *Arch Ophthalmol* 1990;108:411.
36. Barza M, Kane A, Baum J. Comparison of the effects of continuous and intermittent systemic administration on the penetration of gentamicin into infected rabbit eyes. *J Infect Dis* 1983;147:144.
37. Talamo JH, D'Amico J, Kenyon KR. Intravitreal amikacin in the treatment of bacterial endophthalmitis. *Arch Ophthalmol* 1986;104:1483.
38. Campochiaro PA, Conway BP. Aminoglycoside toxicity: a survey of retinal specialists. *Arch Ophthalmol* 1991;109:946.

39. Pflugfelder SC, Hernandez E, Fleisler SJ, Alvarez J, Pflugfelder M, Forster RK. Intravitreal vancomycin. *Arch Ophthalmol* 1987;105: 831.
40. Davis JL, Koidou-Tsiligianni A, Pflugfelder SC, et al. Coagulase-negative Staphylococcal endophthalmitis: increase in antimicrobial resistance. *Ophthalmology* 1988;95:1404.
41. Flynn HW, Pulido JS, Pflugfelder SC. Endophthalmitis therapy: changing antibiotic sensitivity patterns and current therapeutic recommendations. *Arch Ophthalmol* 1991;109:175.
42. Smith MA, Sorenson JA, Lowy FD. Treatment of experimental methicillin-resistent staphylococcus epidermidis endophthalmitis with intravitreal vancomycin. *Ophthalmology* 1986;93:1328.
43. Rubinstein E, Goldfarb J, Keren G, Blumenthal M, Treister G. The penetration of gentamicin into the vitreous humor in man. *Invest Ophthalmol Vis Sci* 1983;24:637.
44. Yoshizumi MO, Leinwand MJ, Kim J. Topical and intravenous gentamicin in traumatically lacerated eyes. *Graefes Arch Clin Exp Ophthalmol* 1992;230:175.
45. El-Massry A, Meredith TA, Aguilar HE, Shaarawy A. Aminoglycoside concentrations in the vitreous cavity after intravenous administration. *Am J Opthalmol* 1996;122:684.
46. Meredith TA, Aguilar HE, Shaarawy A, Kincaid M, Dick J, Niesman MR. Vancomycin levels in the vitreous cavity after intravenous administration. *Am J Ophthalmol*; (In press).
47. Aguilar HE, Meredith TA, Shaarawy A, Kincaid M, Dick J. Vitreous cavity penetration of ceftazidime after intravenous administration. *Retina*; In press.
48. Axelrod JL, Klein RM, Bergen RL, Sheikh MZ. Human vitreous levels of selected antistaphylococcal antibiotics. *Am J Ophthalmol* 1985;100:570.
49. Axelrod JL, Klein RM, Bergen RL, Sheikh MZ. Human vitreous levels of cefamanadole and moxalactam. *Am J Ophthalmol* 1986; 101:684.
50. Axelrod JL, Newton JC, Klein RM, Bergen RL, Sheikh MZ. Penetration of imipenem into human aqueous and vitreous humor. *Am J Ophthalmol* 1987;104:649.
51. Keren G, Alhalel A, Bartov E. The intravitreal penetration of orally administered ciprofloxacin in humans. *Invest Ophthalmol Vis Sci* 1991;32:2388.
52. El Baba FZ, Trousdale MD, Gauderman WJ, Wagner DB, Liggett PE. Intravitreal penetration of oral ciprofloxacin in humans. *Ophthalmology* 1992;99:483.
53. Bill A. Blood circulation and fluid dynamics in the eye. *Physiol Rev* 1975;55:383.
54. Alm A, Bill A. Ocular and optic nerve flow at normal and increased intraocular pressures in monkeys (*Macaca irus*): a study with radioactively labelled microspheres including flow determinations in brain and some other tissues. *Exp Eye Res* 1973;15:15.
55. Maurice DM. Injection of drugs into the vitreous body. In: Leopold IJ, Burns RP, eds. *Symposium on Ocular Therapy,* vol 9. New York: John Wiley, 1976;59.
56. Mandell BA, Meredith TA, Aguilar E, El-Massry A, Sawant A, Grardner S. Amikacin levels after intravitreal injection. *Am J Ophthalmol* 1993;115:770–774.
57. Doft BH, Weiskopf J, Nillson-Ehle I, Wingard L. Amphotericin clearance in vitrectomized versus non-vitrectomized eyes. *Ophthalmology* 1985;92:1601.
58. Cobo LM, Forster RK. The clearance of intravitreal gentamicin. *Am J Ophthalmol* 1981;92:59.
59. Barza M, Kane A, Baum J. Pharmacokinetics of intravitreal carbenicillin, cefazolin, and gentamicin in rhesus monkeys. *Invest Ophthalmol Vis Sci* 1983;24:1602.
60. Ficker LA, Meredith TA, Gardner SK, Wilson LA. Cefazolin levels after intravitreal injection: effects of inflammation and surgery. *Invest Ophthalmol Vis Sci* 1990;31:502.
61. Meredith TA. Antimicrobial pharmacokinetics in endophthalmitis treatment; studies of ceftazidime. *Trans Am Ophthalmol Soc* 1993; 90:655.
62. Driebe WT Jr, Mandelbaum S, Forster RK, Schwartz LK, Culbertson WW. Pseudophakic endophthalmitis: diagnosis and management. *Ophthalmology* 1986;93:442.
63. Diamond JG. Intraocular management of endophthalmitis: a systematic approach. *Arch Ophthalmol* 1981;99:96.
64. Bohigian GM, Olk RJ. Factors associated with a poor visual result in endophthalmitis. *Am J Ophthalmol* 1986;101:332.
65. Olson JC, Flynn WH Jr, Forster RK, Culbertson WW. Results in the treatment of postoperative endophthalmitis. *Ophthalmology* 1983; 90:692.
66. O'Day DM, Smith RS, Gregg CR, et al. The problem of Bacillus species infection with special emphasis on the virulence of *Bacillus cereus. Ophthalmology* 1981;88:833.
67. Davey RT, Tauber WB. Posttraumatic endophthalmitis: the emerging role of *Bacillus cereus* infection. *Rev Infect Dis* 1987;9:110.
68. Conway BP, Campochiaro PA. Macular infarction after endophthalmitis treated with vitrectomy and intravitreal gentamicin. *Arch Ophthalmol* 1986;104:367.
69. Meredith TA, Lindsey DT, Edelhauser HF, Goldman AI. Electroretinographic studies following vitrectomy and intraocular silicone oil injection. *Br J Ophthalmol* 1985;69:254.
70. Marmor MF. Retinal detachment from hyperosmotic intravitreal injection. *Invest Ophthalmol Vis Sci* 1979;18:1237.
71. Peyman GA, Vastine DW, Raichand M. Postoperative endophthalmitis: experimental aspects and their clinical application. *Ophthalmology* 1978;85:374.
72. Talamo JH, D'Amico DJ, Hanninen LA. The influence of aphakia and vitrectomy on experimental retinal toxicity of aminoglucoside antibiotics. *Am J Ophthalmol* 1985;100:840.
73. Zachary IG, Forster RK. Experimental intravitreal gentamicin. *Am J Ophthalmol* 1976;82:604.
74. Conway BP, Tabatabay CA, Campochiaro PA, D'Amico DJ, Hanninen LA, Kenyon KR. Gentamicin toxicity in the primate retina. *Arch Ophthalmol* 1989;107:107.
75. D'Amico DJ, Caspers-Velu L, Libert J, et al. Comparative toxicity of intravitreal aminoglycoside antibiotics. *Am J Ophthalmol* 1985; 100:264.
76. Oum BS, D'Amico DJ, Wong KW. Intravitreal antibiotic therapy with vancomycin and aminoglycoside: an experimental study of combination and repetitive injections. *Arch Ophthalmol* 1989;107:1055.
77. Shockley RK, Jay WM, Friberg TR. Intravitreal ceftriaxone in a rabbit model: dose and time dependent toxic effects and pharmacokinetic analysis. *Arch Ophthalmol* 1984;102:1236.
78. Schenk AG, Peyman GA, Paque JT. The intravitreal use of carbenicillin (GEOPEN) for treatment of Pseudomonas endophthalmitis. *Acta Ophthalmol* 1974;52:707.
79. Spivey JM. The postantibiotic effect. *Clin Pharmacol* 1992;11:865.
80. Vogelman B, Craig WA. Kinetics of antimicrobial activity. *J Pediatr* 1986;108:835.
81. Zhanel GG, Hoban DJ, Harding GKM. The postantibiotic effect: a review of in vitro and in vivo data. *DICP, Ann Pharmacother* 1991;25:153–163.
82. Gerber AU, Craig WA, Brugger H-P, Feller C, Vastola AP, Brandel J. Impact of dosing intervals on activity of gentamicin and ticarcillin against *Pseudomonas aeruginosa* in granulocytopenic mice. *J Infect Dis* 1983;147:910.
83. Pavan PR, Brinser JH. Exogenous bacterial endophthalmitis treated without systemic antibiotics. *Am J Ophthalmol* 1987;104:121.
84. Peyman GA, Nelson P, Bennett TO. Intravitreal injection of kanamycin in experimental induced endophthalmitis. *Can J Ophthalmol* 1974;9:322.
85. Peyman GA, Vastine D, Crouch E, Herbst R. Clinical trials with intravitreal injection of antibiotics in treatment of endophthalmitis. *Trans Am Acad Ophthalmol Otolaryngol* 1974;78:862.
86. Pague JT, Peyman GA. Intravitreal clindamycin phosphate in the treatment of vitreous infection. *Ophthalmic Surg* 1974;5:34.
87. Peyman GA. Antibiotic administration in the treatment of bacterial endophthalmitis. II. Intravitreal injections. *Surv Ophthalmol* 1977;21:332.
88. Jay WM, Shockley RK, Aziz AM, Aziz MZ, Rissing JP. Ocular pharmacokinetics of ceftriaxone following subconjunctival injection in rabbits. *Arch Ophthalmol* 1984;102:430.
89. Barza M, Kane A, Baum J. Ocular penetration of subconjunctival oxacillin, methicillin, and cefazolin in rabbits with staphylococcal endophthalmitis. *J Infect Dis* 1982;145:899.
90. Barza M, Kane A, Baum J. Intraocular penetration of gentamicin after subconjunctival retrobulbar injection. *Am J Ophthalmol* 1978; 85:541.
91. Barza M, Kane A, Baum JL. Intraocular levels of cefamandole compared with cefazolin after subconjunctival injection in rabbits. *Invest Ophthalmol Vis Sci* 1979;18:250.

92. Barza M, Kane A, Baum J. Oxacillin for bacterial endophthalmitis: subconjunctival, intravenous, both, or neither? *Invest Ophthalmol Vis Sci* 1980;19:1348.
93. Rubinstein E, Triester G, Avin I. The intravitreal penetration of cefotaxime in man following systemic and subconjunctival administration. *Ophthalmology* 1987;94:30.
94. Doft BH. The endophthalmitis vitrectomy study. *Arch Ophthalmol* 1991;198:487.
95. Lietman PS. Aminoglycosides and spectinomycin: aminocyclitols. In: Mandell GL, Douglas RG, Bennett JE, eds. *Principles and Practice of Infectious Disease,* 3rd ed. New York: Churchill Livingstone, 1990;269.
96. Bennett JE. Antifungal agents. In: Mandell GL, Douglas RG, Bennett JE, eds. *Principles and Practice of Infectious Diseases,* 3rd ed. New York: Churchill Livingstone, 1990;361.
97. Fisher JF. Penetration of amphotericin B into the human eye. *J Infect Dis* 1983;147:164.
98. Donowitz GR, Mandell GL. Cephalosporins. In: Mandell GL, Douglas RG, Bennett JE, eds. *Principles and Practice of Infectious Diseases,* 3rd ed. New York: Churchill Livingstone, 1990;246.
99. Donahue S, Kowalski R, Eller A, DeVaro J, Jewart B. Empiric treatment of endophthalmitis. *Arch Ophthalmol* 1994;112:45.
100. Aaberg TJ, Flynn HJ, Murray T. Intraocular ceftazidime as an alternative to the aminoglycosides in the treatment of endophthalmitis. *Arch Ophthalmol* 1994;112:18.
101. Andriole VT. Quinolones. In: Mandell GL, Douglas RG, Bennett JE, eds. *Principles and Practice of Infectious Diseases,* 3rd ed. New York: Churchill Livingstone, 1990;337.
102. Kowalski RP, Karenchak LM, Eller AW. The role of ciprofloxacin in endophthalmitis therapy. *Am J Ophthalmol* 1993;116:695.
103. Pearson PA. Clearance and distribution of ciprofloxacin following intravitreal injection. *Retina* 1993;13:326.
104. Stevens SX, Fouraker BD, Jensen HG. Intraocular safety of ciprofloxacin. *Arch Ophthalmol* 1991;109:1737.
105. Steigbigel NH. Erythromycin, lincomycin and clindamycin. In: Mandell GL, Douglas RG, Bennett JE, eds. *Principles and Practice of Infectious Disease,* 3rd ed. New York: Churchill Livingstone, 1990;308.
106. Zinner SH, Mayer KH. Sulfonamides and trimethoprim. In: Mandell GL, Douglas RG, Bennett JE, eds. *Principles and Practice of Infectious Diseases,* 3rd ed. New York: Churchill Livingstone, 1990;325.
107. Maloney JM, Nolte GS, Meredith TA. Listeria monocytogenes endophthalmitis. *Emory Journal of Medicine* 1990;4:201.
108. Fekety R. Vancomycin and teicoplanin. In: Mandell GL, Douglas RG Jr, Bennett JE, eds. *Principles and Practice of Infectious Diseases.* New York: Churchill Livingstone, 1990;317.
109. Aguilar HE, Meredith TA, El-Massry A, et al. Vancomycin levels after intravitreal injection. *Retina* 1995;15:428.
110. Fisher JP, Civiletto SE, Forster RK. Toxicity, efficacy and clearance of intravitreally injected cefazolin. *Arch Ophthalmol* 1982;110:650.
111. Jay WM, Azia MZ, Rissing JP. Pharmacokinetic analysis of intravitreal ceftriaxone in monkeys. *Arch Ophthalmol* 1985;103:121.
112. Nelson P, Peyman GA, Bennett TO. BB-K8. A new aminoglycoside for intravitreal injection in bacterial endophthalmitis. *Am J Ophthalmol* 1974;78–82.
113. Ben-Num J, Joyce DA, Cooper RL. Pharmacokinetics of intravitreal injection: assessment of a gentamicin model by ocular dialysis. *Invest Ophthalmol Vis Sci* 1989;30:1055.
114. Kasbeer RT, Peyman GA, May DR. Penetration of amikacin into the aphakic eye. *Graefes Arch Clin Exp Ophthalmol* 1975;196:85.
115. Yannis RA, Rissing JP, Buxton TB. Multistrain comparison of three antimicrobial prophylaxis regimens in experimental postoperative *Pseudomonas endophthalmitis. Am J Ophthalmol* 1985;100:404.
116. Neu HC. Other beta lactam antibiotics. In: Mandell GL, Douglas RG Jr, Bennett JE, eds. *Principles and Practice of Infectious Diseases,* 3rd ed. New York: Churchill Livingstone, 1989;257–263.
117. Gardner S. Treatment of bacterial endophthalmitis: III. *Ocular Therapeutics and Management* 1991;2:141–149.

Textbook of Ocular Pharmacology,
edited by T.J. Zimmerman, et al.
Lippincott–Raven Publishers, Philadelphia © 1997.

CHAPTER 33

Antivirals in the Treatment of Retinal Diseases

Ramana S. Moorthy and David V. Weinberg

Known viral diseases of the posterior segment of the eye are generally caused by members of the herpesvirus family and represent only a small portion of the spectrum of human diseases caused by viruses. Although the antiviral drug acyclovir was adopted for the treatment of acute retinal necrosis, until recently retinal infection has not been a major target for antiviral drug research.

The importance of viral disease of the retina has been elevated by the growing prevalence of the acquired immune deficiency syndrome (AIDS) and the devastating infections that accompany it. A previously obscure retinal infection, cytomegalovirus (CMV) retinitis, has emerged as one of the most common opportunistic infections in patients with AIDS. A great deal of recent activity in research and development of antiviral drugs have been a response to this dreaded infection.

At present, treatment of most viral retinal diseases must be initiated without the benefit of cultures or other laboratory confirmation. Fortunately, most of these infections are sufficiently distinctive in setting and appearance that appropriate therapy can be selected empirically.

Current therapy is limited by several factors. The number of available antiviral agents is limited. Among the available drugs, therapeutic choices are limited by the significant toxicities of these agents. Viral resistance is a growing problem. All currently available agents are virustatic. The limitations of current therapy have been less significant for patients with healthy immune systems because the spectrum of disease is narrower and also because therapy seems to be necessary only until host defenses can control the infection. Among patients with AIDS, relapsing disease despite life-long therapy seems to be the rule.

R. S. Moorthy and D. V. Weinberg: Department of Ophthalmology, Northwestern University Medical School, Chicago, Illinois 60611.

ACYCLOVIR

History and Source

In the late 1960s to mid 1970s, compounds effective against viral infections of the external eye and skin, particularly those caused by herpes simplex virus (HSV) and herpes zoster virus, were introduced for topical use and included compounds such as methisazone, idoxuridine, vidarabine, and trifluorothymidine. These medications had significant systemic toxicities that prohibited their oral or intravenous use. In 1978, however, Schaeffer and colleagues (1) introduced the drug acyclovir based on earlier research showing that the intact cyclic carbohydrate moiety on nucleosides was not necessary to mimic nucleoside binding to enzymes necessary for DNA synthesis. They synthesized a range of nucleoside analogs that had an acyclic side chain attached to the heterocyclic base of a biglycosidic linkage, replacing the usual cyclic carbohydrate moiety (1–3). This group of compounds possessed good antiviral activity and low host toxicity. Acyclovir, the first of these compounds, was subsequently introduced for systemic use in 1982 after Phase III clinical trials. Soon after its introduction, acyclovir was found to be useful in the treatment of several viral retinal infections, including herpes zoster ophthalmicus, acute retinal necrosis syndrome, HSV retinitis, and possibly progressive outer retinal necrosis.

Official Drug Name and Chemistry

The full name of acyclovir is 9-(2-hydroxyethoxymethyl)guanine. It may also be called acycloguanosine. The molecular formula is $C_8H_{12}N_5O_3$ (4). Its molecular weight is 225.21 and that of its intravenous formulation, acyclovir sodium, is 247.

Acyclovir

Pharmacology

The selectivity of acyclovir for herpesviruses rather than host cells was evaluated by extensive work done by Biron and Elion (5). Using acyclovir synthesized with radioactive carbon 14 in the 8 position of guanine or tritium in the acyclic side chain, Vero cells that were either infected or uninfected with HSV then were incubated with this acyclovir for 6 hours at 0.5 m*M* concentrations. The cells were isolated, and high-pressure liquid chromatography (HPLC) was used to separate the components of the cellular extracts. Extracts from uninfected cells showed only one peak, corresponding to the acyclovir; however, those from cells infected with HSV-1 revealed three additional radioactive peaks. This result was the same for both the carbon 8-substituted as well as the tritium-substituted acyclovir. These three radioactive compounds were identified as monophosphate, diphosphate, and triphosphate derivatives of acyclovir proven by enzymatic conversion back to free acyclovir.

The enzyme responsible for the conversion of the acyclovir was identified by Fyfe and co-workers (6) in 1978 to be herpesvirus-specific thymidine kinase (HSV-TK). This enzyme converts thymidine deoxycytidine and other deoxyuridines to monophosphates and recognizes acyclovir as a substrate. Thus, HSV-TK, the target for acyclovir, was largely responsible for the high selectivity of acyclovir for infected cells and for the virus; HSV-TK has a higher affinity for guanine as a purine substrate than thymidine. Once the HSV-TK converts the acyclovir to a monophosphate derivative, the guanine monophosphate (GMP) kinase converts it to a diphosphate entity. Cellular kinases then convert it to a triphosphate entity. It is the acyclovir triphosphate that is then the active antiviral agent (Figure 33-1). It behaves as a deoxynucleoside triphosphate and competes with deoxyguanosine triphosphates (dGTP) for viral DNA polymerase. Thus, as the DNA chain begins to elongate, DNA polymerase incorporates a molecule of acyclovir triphosphate at a position opposite cytosine on the template. When this happens, the replication process is terminated because the acyclic side chain does not have the 3′-hydroxyl group that is necessary to form the phosphodiester bond between the two nucleosides (2). Thus, in this manner, acyclovir is a very active and selective agent against herpes simplex as well as varicella zoster virus (VZV); both have specific thymi-

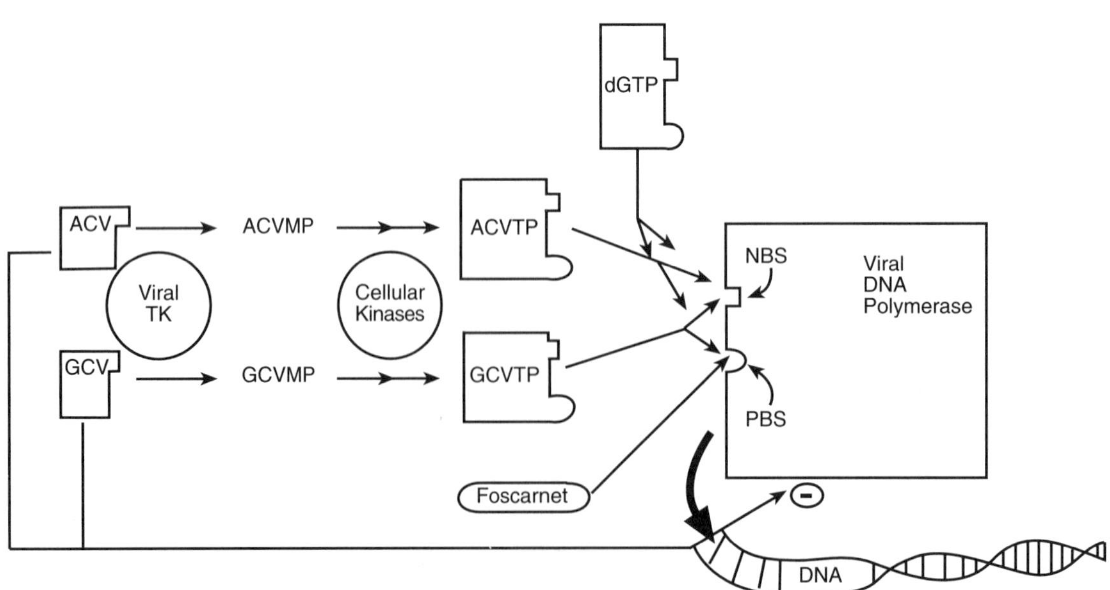

FIG. 33-1. Mechanism of action of acyclovir (ACV), ganciclovir (GCV), and foscarnet. MP, monophosphate; TP, triphosphate; NBS, nucleoside-binding site; PBS, phosphate-binding site.

dine kinases that use acyclovir as a substrate. Once viral DNA replication is halted, the production of more virus particles is also arrested. Acyclovir also inactivates the viral DNA polymerase but not the cellular polymerases. The reasons for acyclovir being active and selectively toxic to cells infected by HSV and VZV are the activation by an HSV- or VZV-specific thymidine kinase, the greater sensitivity of viral DNA polymerase than of cellular polymerases to acyclovir triphosphate, the inactivation of viral DNA polymerase by acyclovir triphosphate but not the cellular polymerases, and the chain termination of viral DNA by incorporation of acyclovir monophosphate (7). Neither the Epstein-Barr virus (EBV) nor the human CMV is as sensitive to acyclovir as the HSV and VZV virus. The EBV has a viral polymerase that can be inhibited by very low levels of acyclovir triphosphate, but there is no selective activation of acyclovir in infected cells. In the human CMV, acyclovir activation is quite poor; but, again, the viral polymerases are more sensitive to acyclovir triphosphate than the cellular polymerases (8,9).

Clinical Pharmacology

As in in vitro studies, acyclovir has the same mechanism of action among human tissues and cells infected with HSV or VZV. The concentration of acyclovir necessary for 50% inhibition (ID_{50}) of HSV-1 is 0.1 μM and for HSV-2, 1.6 μM (10). The VZV strains have an ID_{50} of 3.5 μM (2,10). Reproduction of EBV in superinfected Raji cells is suppressed 50% by an acyclovir concentration of 1.5 μg/ml (9). Human CMV is inhibited by an ID_{50} quite similar to that of human cells. Clinical trials have failed to establish any clear benefit of acyclovir in the treatment of patients with CMV infections (11,12).

There are three mechanisms of resistance of HSV to acyclovir. The most common is alteration or deletion of the gene for thymidine kinase, which makes it impossible for HSV to induce production of this enzyme. These strains of viruses have reduced infectivity and less virulence than the wild-type viruses (13). Another mechanism that has been shown in laboratory evaluation, but not in vitro, is the alteration of DNA polymerase chain gene that makes the herpes simplex DNA polymerase resistant to acyclovir. These mutants are as virulent as the wild-type virus. The final mechanism of resistance, demonstrated in the laboratory but not clinically, is the altered substrate specificity of viral-induced thymidine kinase, which results from a mutation in the structural gene for viral thymidine kinase. These genes then induce only a partial amount of the normal thymidine kinase, making the enzyme a less efficient phosphorylator of acyclovir. There may be some reduction in neurovirulence of these types of viruses (14). Herpes simplex virus-2 strains that are resistant to acyclovir are rare but increasing in frequency among patients with AIDS (15). Early investigations suggest that foscarnet may be a reasonable alternative antiviral agent in cases of acyclovir resistance (15).

Pharmaceutics

Acyclovir is available in both oral and parenteral forms. Oral forms include a 200-mg capsule, an 800-mg tablet, and a suspension of oral acyclovir 200 mg/500 ml of diluent. The parenteral forms of intravenous acyclovir are available in 500-mg vials that may be diluted with 10 ml of sterile water for injection. The recommended final concentration for intravenous injection is 50 mg/ml of acyclovir (product information, Zovirax, 1992). The intravenous solution has a pH of 10.5 to 11.6 (16). Because of the high pH of the solution, intravenous solution should not be stored in syringes, as to do so may cause interaction with the rubber plunger tips. Both the oral acyclovir tablets and the vials should be protected from light. Refrigeration of tablets is recommended; however, refrigeration of intravenous acyclovir may result in formation of a precipitate that dissolves at room temperature; this does not affect chemical stability (product information, Zovirax, 1992). Acyclovir vials, once reconstituted, are stable for 12 hours. The high pH of the solution can etch the glass vial over more prolonged storage periods. Acyclovir in large-volume intravenous solutions can be stable for up to 24 hours at room temperature. A reconstituted or diluted sample of the drug should be stored in a closed system to prevent the atmospheric CO_2 from lowering the pH and decreasing the solubility of the drug. There are no antimicrobial preservatives in the acyclovir vial; hence, if the normal clarity of the intravenous solution in a vial is lost, it should be discarded (product information, Zovirax, 1992).

Pharmacokinetics, Concentration-effect Relationship, and Metabolism

Much work on the onset and duration of action of acyclovir on cutaneous herpetic lesions has been done; however, in the case of retinal diseases, the most convincing work has been the observations made by Blumenkranz and associates in acute retinal necrosis syndrome (17). In these cases, acyclovir was given at 1500 mg/m^2/day in three divided doses, given over 7 to 21 days (average, 10 days). Regression of the lesions could be seen as early as 4 days but was complete at 1 month. Thus, the onset of action seems to be about 4 to 5 days, which is quite similar to the onset of action of medication in the treatment of cutaneous lesions (17,18).

The therapeutic responses to acyclovir when used systemically have correlated with plasma concentrations of 66.6 μM/ml at 15 minutes after infusion, and 35.3 μM/ml 1 hour after infusion (19). As an extension of this study, Pepose and Biron determined that the median effective dose (ED_{50}) of VZV recovered from the vitreous of a patient with acute retinal necrosis was 5.3 μM (20). This vitreous level, and the plasma levels that were suggested earlier, can be achieved by intravenous medication. Pediatric patients aged more than 1 year achieve plasma levels similar to those of adults when administered similar doses based on body surface area (21). The bioavailability of acyclovir is excellent when administered intravenously, but oral bioavailability is poor. Acyclovir is slowly and poorly absorbed from the gastrointestinal tract. Peak concentrations in plasma are achieved 1.5 to 2 hours after the oral dose is given. With multiple-dose administration, steady-state plasma levels are reached within 1 to 2 days. Estimated bioavailability in humans is between 15% and 30% for oral acyclovir, and it appears to decrease with increasing dose (22–25). Bioavailability data on oral acyclovir used in the eye are limited; however, aqueous humor levels of 3.26 μM, above the ED_{50} for HSV-1, have been achieved after five doses of 400 mg of oral acyclovir (26). The volume of distribution of acyclovir is 45 to 50 L/1.73m^2 of body surface area (27).

In patients with renal insufficiency, the dose of acyclovir may be the same as in patients with normal renal function, but the dosing interval should be adjusted. If creatinine clearance is > 50 ml/min/1.73 m^2, the dosing interval should be 8 hours; if it is 25 to 50, the interval should be 12 hours; and, if 10 to 25, the interval should be 24 hours (product information, Zovirax, 1992). In cases of end-stage renal disease with creatinine clearances < 10 ml/min/1.73 m^2, Laskin et al. recommend a loading dose of 37% of the standard dose (250–500 mg/m^2) and a maintenance dose of 14% of the standard every 8 hours or the standard dose every 48 hours given intravenously (28).

Metabolism

Up to 91% of plasma acyclovir is excreted unchanged in the urine (29). About 9% to 14% of the dose of acyclovir is metabolized to 9-carboxymethoxymethylguanine (29). About 0.2 to 1% of acyclovir is metabolized to 8-hydroxy-9-(2-hydroxyethylmethyl)guanine (30). It is also excreted in breast milk, but the American Academy of Pediatrics found this level to be compatible with breast-feeding and not a contraindication for use of acyclovir in breast-feeding mothers as long as the infant has normal renal function (31).

Therapeutic Use

Both oral and intravenous forms of acyclovir have been used in the treatment of HSV retinitis in otherwise healthy and immunosuppressed patients, occasionally retinitis caused by varicella zoster virus in patients with AIDS, and the acute retinal necrosis syndrome.

Herpes simplex virus retinitis that occurs in otherwise healthy persons has been treated successfully with intravenous acyclovir (32); HSV retinitis also can occur in immunosuppressed patients in whom it is difficult to distinguish CMV from VZV retinitis. If the infection is not sight threatening, high-dose intravenous acyclovir may be attempted (33,34). If there is no response to therapy and the lesions are sight-threatening, foscarnet or ganciclovir should be used (35).

Progressive outer retinal necrosis is a syndrome seen in immunocompromised patients and is due to VZV. This syndrome is marked by often bilateral, outer retinitis beginning in the periphery as confluent punctate lesions or macular lesions in eyes with minimal inflammation. The disease is rapidly progressive and poorly responsive to intravenous acyclovir. Little is known about the relative efficacy of other antivirals in this disease. Foscarnet or a combination of foscarnet and ganciclovir may be the preferred antiviral regimen in this disorder (36–38).

In a review of the treatment of acute retinal necrosis syndrome, Duker and Blumenkranz (35) recommended 1500 mg/m^2/day of intravenous acyclovir in three divided doses for 7 to 10 days, which is equivalent to 10 to 15 mg/kg given every 8 hours. Oral acyclovir at a dosage of 400 to 600 mg five times daily should be continued for 6 to 14 weeks after intravenous treatment because this is the period of greatest risk for bilateral involvement. Prednisone should not be started until after acyclovir therapy has been initiated (38). Prophylactic vitrectomy and intravitreal infusion of 10 to 40 μg of acyclovir have had variable success in the treatment of acute retinal necrosis. This therapy is not routinely recommended (17,34,38,39). Acyclovir has not been approved for use during pregnancy, but anecdotal reports describe its successful use in the treatment of acute retinal necrosis in the third trimester of pregnancy (40).

Side Effects and Toxicity

Acyclovir may cause transient renal impairment (41). The renal dysfunction is a result of crystalline nephropathy in which the drug exceeds its maximum solubility and free drug is precipitated in the kidney. This problem usually occurs with rapid bolus intravenous injection; however, concurrent uses of nephrotoxic drugs, preexisting renal disease, and dehydration can predispose to the development of renal impairment, which is usually reversible (42). Oral acyclovir also caused renal failure in one case (43). Renal function should be monitored closely in patients who are receiving intravenous acyclovir. Adequate hydration should be maintained to ensure high urine output. If renal insufficiency develops, the drug can be discontinued temporarily and restarted at lower doses after the renal function has normalized.

Diarrhea has been reported to occur in 8.8% of patients on oral acyclovir (product information, Zovirax, 1992).

Nausea and vomiting are the most frequent side effects of short-term acyclovir therapy. Diarrhea is more frequent after 6 months of systemic acyclovir use (44).

About 1% of patients receiving acyclovir manifest lethargy, tremors, confusion, hallucination, agitation, seizures, or coma (44). High doses of acyclovir or concomitant use of neurotoxic drugs may produce agitation, tremor, disorientation, hallucinations, delusions, myoclonus, slurred speech, and hyperacusis. These central nervous system complications are more common with intravenous than with oral acyclovir. Extravasation of intravenous infusion of acyclovir may result in phlebitis and inflammation at the site of injection. Tissue necrosis has been reported to occur in neonates (45). Arthralgia may occur in 3.6% of patients (product information, Zovirax, 1992).

Teratogenicity

The Acyclovir in Pregnancy Registry has provided useful information on the fetal and maternal safety of this drug; however, despite 239 monitored, first-trimester exposures to acyclovir, the sample size was not large enough to determine reliably the safety of acyclovir use during pregnancy (46). Similarly, second- and third-trimester exposures have been documented, but no conclusions could be drawn from the small sample size (46). The trends in this registry suggest, however, that during pregnancy acyclovir should be reserved for severe, life-threatening, or disseminated herpes virus infections.

High-risk Groups

Neonates in particular may be at risk for extravasation of intravenously administered acyclovir to the skin, resulting in necrosis. It is recommended that infusion be carried out using a peripherally inserted central venous catheter (45). Neonates should be given intravenous infusions of 10 mg/kg every 8 hours for 5 to 10 days, depending on the severity of infection, with each infusion carried out over a 1-hour period. Fourteen-day treatment is recommended for HSV encephalitis. To avoid nephrotoxicity following intravenous acyclovir therapy, it is recommended that the patient have a daily urine output of 1 ml for every 1.3 mg of acyclovir administered (47), and this is true for both neonates and children. Acyclovir has been detected in breast milk, but the American Association of Pediatrics has not considered this finding to be a contraindication for continuing acyclovir if the renal function of the neonate is normal. Meyer and colleagues reported that acyclovir is excreted in breast milk but that only about 1 mg of drug is absorbed daily by the neonate from maternal doses of 200 mg five times daily (48). Among elderly, no specific recommendations for treatment have been made, except adequate hydration and slow infusion to avoid the complications of renal insufficiency. Immunocompromised patients appear to tolerate the medication well. There are no specific contraindications for the use of acyclovir in immunocompromised patients.

Drug Interactions

Cyclosporine

Concomitant administration of cyclosporine and acyclovir can increase nephrotoxicity (49); however, when cyclosporine levels were monitored closely, nephrotoxicity was not increased. Renal function and cyclosprine blood levels must be monitored closely when acyclovir is administered concomitantly with cyclosporine.

Meperidine

Concomitant administration of intramuscular meperidine and high-dose acyclovir may result in neurologic deterioration, as evidenced in a case study by Johnson and co-workers (50). Careful monitoring is suggested in patients receiving concomitant therapy of these two drugs.

Probenecid

Probenecid has been reported to increase the plasma concentration of acyclovir by reducing renal clearance by 32%. It also may increase the acyclovir half-life by 18%. If concurrent therapy is necessary, the acyclovir dose interval should be extended (51).

Varicella Vaccine

Acyclovir has been reported to reduce live, attenuated varicella vaccine effectiveness, especially with the Oka varicella virus strain used in experimental vaccines. The virus apparently is sensitive to acyclovir; thus, the effectiveness of the vaccine is reduced (52).

Zidovudine

Acyclovir may potentiate lethargy and fatigue in patients concomitantly treated with zidovudine; despite this side effect, acyclovir does not seem to alter the disposition of zidovudine (53). In fact, a Phase I study of concomitant zidovudine and acyclovir therapy in 20 patients over a 24-week period revealed no drug interaction (54).

Major Clinical Trials

Randomized, controlled, prospective clinical trials evaluating the efficacy of acyclovir in retinal disorders have not been performed. In particular, acute retinal necrosis, progressive outer retinal necrosis, and herpes simplex retinitis are relatively rare entities, which makes it quite difficult to perform high-quality, randomized, controlled clinical trials; however, the extensive review of patients with acute retinal necrosis by Duker and Blumenkranz, cited earlier, provides the best evidence of the efficacy of parenteral and oral acyclovir in the treatment of patients with acute retinal necrosis syndrome (35).

Acyclovir treatment also may protect the other eye from involvement in acute retinal necrosis. Palay and colleagues (55) reviewed the course of 54 patients with unilateral acute retinal necrosis at their initial examination. Thirty one of these patients were treated for 7 to 10 days with 1,500 mg/m²/day of intravenous acyclovir followed by 2 to 4 weeks of 800 mg five times daily of oral acyclovir; 23 were not treated with the drug. Of the 31 patients treated with acyclovir, 27 (87.1%) had fellow eyes that remained disease free throughout the median follow-up of 1 year. Of the 23 patients not treated with acyclovir, 30.4% had fellow eyes that remained disease free over a median follow-up of 11 months. Survival analysis indicated that the fellow eyes of the group of patients treated with acyclovir were more likely to remain disease free than the fellow eyes of the group not treated with acyclovir. The difference between the two groups was highly statistically significant, particularly at 14 weeks after diagnosis. After 2 years, the percentage of disease-free eyes was 75% in the group treated with acyclovir compared with 35% in the group not treated with acyclovir. The authors concluded that acyclovir treatment reduces the risk of involvement of the fellow eye in patients with acute retinal necrosis syndrome (55). They recommended treatment of acute retinal necrosis with 7 to 10 days of 1,500 mg/m²/day of intravenous acyclovir followed by oral acyclovir (800 mg five times daily) for up to 14 weeks after intravenous therapy (55).

GANCICLOVIR

History and Source

The antiherpetic activity of the acyclic nucleoside 9-[1,3-dihydroxy-2-propoxymethyl]guanine was first described in early 1983 by Smee and colleagues (56). These investigators reported that in 50% plaque-reduction assays in Vero cells, both ganciclovir and acyclovir inhibited HSV-1 and HSV-2 thymidine kinase positive strains at relatively low concentrations; however, ganciclovir was markedly more active than acyclovir against human CMV. Human CMV 50% inhibitory doses were 7 μM for ganciclovir compared with 95 μM for acyclovir. In addition, the mortality of mice with herpes simplex 2 encephalitis and vaginitis was reduced by 50% with daily doses of 7–10 mg/kg of ganciclovir, equally effective as daily doses of 500 mg/kg of acyclovir. Subsequently, Mar and colleagues (57) in early 1983 reported similar results on human CMV replication using very low concentrations of ganciclovir with ID_{50} of 1 to 5 μM. At these concentrations, the drug seemed to inhibit the synthesis of 6 viral-specific polypeptides with molecular weights between 27,000 and 200,000 daltons up to 96 hours after infection of cell lines by human CMV. In addition, removal of this inhibitor allowed viral DNA synthesis to resume, and infected cells reappeared. This finding indicated that ganciclovir inhibition is virostatic and reversible.

In 1984 Mar and colleagues (58) reported that in human fibroblast cell lines infected with human CMV, ganciclovir and the monohydroxy version of this medication both preferentially bound with greater affinity to viral DNA polymerase, making the viral DNA polymerase much more sensitive to inhibition by nucleoside triphosphates than the cellular counterpart. The competitive inhibition of deoxyguanosine triphosphate incorporation into DNA by ganciclovir triphosphate results in inhibition of viral replication (58). Independently, in 1984 Tyms and colleagues (59) of Burroughs-Wellcome reported that an analog of acyclovir, BWB759U, synonymous with ganciclovir, inhibited human CMV replication in fibroblast cell lines. These three separate groups of investigators independently discovered the anti-CMV activity of ganciclovir, the new acyclovir analog. The discovery of this drug represented a natural evolution of the discovery of other acyclic nucleoside analogs used to treat viral infections.

Official Drug Name and Chemistry

The official drug name of ganciclovir is 9-[1,3-dihydroxy-2-propoxymethyl]guanine, also called ganciclovir. Other synonyms of this medication include Biolf-62, BWB 759U, BW759, 2-NDG, or 2 Nor-deoxyguanosine (56–61). This medication is an acyclic nucleoside analog of deoxyguanosine. Compared with acyclovir, the only structural difference in that ganciclovir has a terminal hydroxymethyl group. The chemical formula for ganciclovir is $C_8N_4O_4H_{15}$. The molecular weight of ganciclovir is 255.23 and that of its sodium salt is 278.2.

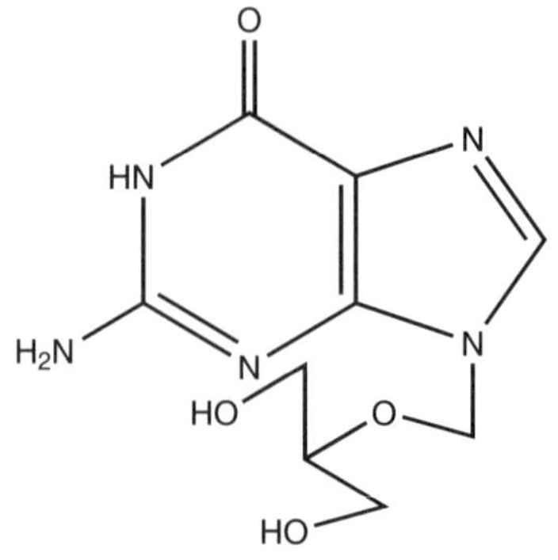

O
HN
N
H2N
N
N
HO
O
HO

Ganciclovir

Pharmacology

In CMV-infected cells, ganciclovir becomes phosphorylated to ganciclovir triphosphate by cellular kinases. This medication is selectively phosphorylated with tenfold greater affinity among virus-infected cells than in normal cells. The triphosphate form of ganciclovir then is incorporated into viral DNA, thus competitively inhibiting deoxyguanosine triphosphate binding to DNA polymerase (see Figure 33-1), resulting in inhibition of DNA synthesis and termination of DNA elongation in viral replication (57,60,61). Compared with acyclovir, ganciclovir is 10 to 25 times more active against CMV and equally as active as acyclovir against HSV-1 and -2, VZV, and EBV.

In humans, ganciclovir appears to work exactly the same as it does in vitro, preferentially affecting CMV-infected cells more than uninfected cells. Myeloid cells, because of their rapid mitotic rates, however, are uniquely sensitive to ganciclovir, which explains the risk of pancytopenia, the most important toxic side effect of ganciclovir (62).

Pharmaceutics

Ganciclovir sodium is available in lyophilized form in 500-mg vials. It should be reconstituted with 10 ml of sterile water to form a final concentration of 50 mg/ml of parenteral solution, which may be added to either normal saline or to dextrose 5% and water solution and stored at approximately 4°C (63). The manufacturer of ganciclovir recommends that the medication, once reconstituted, be used within 12 hours to avoid the possibility of contamination. These solutions of ganciclovir should not be reconstituted with solutions containing parabens, as precipitation can occur (product information, Cytovene, 1993). Following reconstitution, the pH of the solution is approximately 11.0 (product information, Cytovene, 1993) (63). Manufacturer recommendations suggest that ganciclovir be disposed of in the same manner as other cytotoxic drugs (product information, Cytovene, 1993).

Oral ganciclovir is also available. Jacobson and colleagues (64) administered 10 mg/kg/dose of oral ganciclovir four or five times daily and found that therapeutic levels could be achieved in plasma (64). Phase III clinical trials of oral ganciclovir in the prevention of CMV retinitis are in progress.

Preparation of ganciclovir solution for intravitreal injection has been outlined by Henry and colleagues (65). Ganciclovir is initially reconstituted with 2.5 mm of sterile normal saline in 500-mg vials, yielding a concentration of 200 mg/ml; 0.1 ml of this solution is then further diluted with 9.9 ml of sterile normal saline, yielding a final concentration of 2 mg/ml. Before injection, the solution is filtered through a 0.22 μm filter. In this manner, an intravitreal dose of approximately 200 μg in 0.1 ml of solution may be obtained (65). Intravitreal ganciclovir has been useful in the treatment of CMV retinitis and has been used in doses of 200 μg or 400 μg in 0.1-ml solutions at varying intervals. Injections may be given once, twice, or three times weekly; however, in general, it is agreed that 200 μg/0.1 ml or 400 μg/0.1 ml injections be given approximately twice weekly for 2 to 3 weeks or until the retinitis regresses, followed by once-weekly maintenance of the same dosage of injection (66,67). Intravitreal doses of up to 2 mg were reported to be safe and effective in a small clinical series (68).

Sanborn et al. (69) developed a device containing a 6-mg pellet of ganciclovir covered with a coating of polyvinyl alcohol that could be implanted into the vitreous cavity through the pars plana. This device was designed to release ganciclovir over 4 to 5 months. In a series of eight patients, CMV retinitis resolved in all eyes with the ganciclovir implant (69). In a recent randomized, controlled clinical trial evaluating the safety and efficacy of a 1 μg/hour ganciclovir implant, Martin and colleagues (70) randomized 26 patients (30 eyes) with previously untreated peripheral CMV retinitis to immediate treatment with the ganciclovir implant or deferred treatment. The median time to progression of retinitis was 15 days in the deferred treatment group compared with 226 days in the immediate treatment group ($p < 0.00001$) (70). They reported postoperative complications of late retinal detachments or tears in eight patients. Visceral CMV disease developed in 31% of patients. The estimated risk of development of CMV retinitis in the fellow eye was 50% at 6 months. In addition, the median survival time for these patients was 295 days (70). The authors concluded that the ganciclovir implant is effective in the treatment of CMV retinitis but that fellow eyes are likely to develop CMV retinitis and visceral CMV infections may develop in some patients (70). This clinical trial was the first to establish clearly the safety and efficacy of the ganciclovir implant in the treatment of CMV retinitis. This device provides another alternative route by which ganciclovir may be delivered and may be particularly useful for patients who cannot tolerate systemic antiviral therapy or for patients receiving concomitant zidovudine, which may increase myelosuppression. Additionally, the ganciclovir implant, Vitrasert (Chiron), was approved by the U.S. Food and Drug Administration (FDA) for clinical use in March 1996.

Pharmacokinetics: Concentration-effect, Relationship, and Metabolism

The human pharmacokinetics of ganciclovir have been well studied. In an evaluation of 21 patients with life- or sight-threatening CMV infections (71), several aspects of clinical pharmacokinetics were outlined. Using HPLC and radioimmunoassay methods for quantifying ganciclovir levels, patients receiving intravenous infusions of 5 mg/kg of ganciclovir over 1 hour twice daily for a 2-week period had a bioexponential decay of ganciclovir from plasma with an initial distribution half-life of approximately 0.76 hours and a termination half-life of about 3.6 hours. In patients with renal insufficiency receiving the same dosage, the termination half-life was markedly increased to 11.5 hours. In addition, they found that hemodialysis efficiently reduced the levels of ganciclovir in plasma by 53% (71). In another study by Fletcher and colleagues (72), six patients receiving 2.5 or 5 mg/kg of ganciclovir every 8 or 12 hours were examined. They obtained similar results, with a mean distribution half-life of 2.3 hours and a termination half-life of 2.53 hours. In addition, the mean volume of distribution at steady state was 32.8 L/1.73 m^2 of body surface area. In patients receiving 2.5 mg/kg doses, peak concentrations were well above the ID_{50} of human CMV (72). In addition, 24% to 67% of the drug penetrated the cerebrospinal fluid (CSF) (71,72). Both studies found that the clearance of ganciclovir was substantially higher than the estimated creatinine clearance (71,72). This observation confirms that the drug is eliminated from the kidney by both tubular secretion and glomeralar filtration.

The pharmacokinetics of oral ganciclovir also was studied. Jacobson et al. (64) studied four patients with AIDS and CMV retinitis who received 10 to 20 mg/kg of oral ganciclovir every 6 hours. They tolerated these doses quite well. With a 20 mg/kg dose given every 6 hours, mean steady-state peak and trough levels were 2.96 and 1.05 μM, respectively. Calculated absorption was about 3% based on the amount of urinary excretion. Because the levels of ganciclovir achieved in the plasma approximated those required for inhibition of CMV in vitro, a trial of oral maintenance therapy was suggested (64). Again, results of in vitro studies showed that for most strains of human CMV, the concentration of ganciclovir required to reduce plaque formation by 50% (ED_{50}) is 1.0 to 6.4 μM (73,74). Thus, when administered intravenously and, to some extent, orally, plasma levels of ganciclovir approach or surpass the ED_{50} for human CMV.

Although therapeutic drug monitoring may be performed using the methods outlined above, this is not done routinely in clinical practice. Because patients with normal renal function tend to tolerate ganciclovir well and have normal clearance of the medication, renal function and hematologic parameters are the most important parameters that are routinely monitored in patients receiving ganciclovir therapy.

The therapeutic effects of ganciclovir have been studied extensively in humans as well. Laskin and colleagues (75) studied 97 patients with AIDS and serious CMV infections. These patients received 3 to 15 mg/kg/day of ganciclovir. Viremia cleared during drug therapy in up to 88% of patients. Viral shedding for urine and throat became apparent during the treatment in 78% and 68% of patients, respectively. Among patients with CMV retinitis, 87% had improvement or stabilization of their disease; however, when the drug was discontinued, progression or recurrence of the disease always occurred. This study found that long-term suppressive therapy with intravenous 5 mg/kg of ganciclovir given daily five to seven times per week prevented the recurrence of CMV retinitis disease at a highly statistically significant level. Thus, ganciclovir seems to halt progression of disease, but it does not eradicate CMV in immunosuppressed patients, necessitating long-term maintenance therapy.

The distribution of ganciclovir was studied in humans as well. As outlined earlier, Fletcher and colleagues (72) noted a variable but definite penetrance of the drug into the CSF. Serum distribution of this drug also was studied and was already described herein. Patients receiving intravenous therapy for ganciclovir have had evaluation of levels of the drug in the subretinal fluid as well. In one patient, ganciclovir concentration in subretinal fluid was 7.16 μM when simultaneous plasma concentration was 8.16 μM. In addition, 8 hours after beginning a 5 mg/kg infusion of ganciclovir, the drug level reached 2.58 μM in the subretinal fluid with simultaneous plasma levels of 1.28 μM (76). This study suggested that penetration of ganciclovir into the eye from the blood and effective drug levels within the eye can be achieved.

The metabolism of ganciclovir has also been studied in humans. Clinical trials have indicated that 81% to 100% of the dose is eliminated unchanged in the urine (75). Intravenous ganciclovir is not hepatically metabolized. It is not known whether ganciclovir is excreted in human breast milk; however, because of the potential adverse reactions from ganciclovir in nursing infants, it has been recommended that mothers receiving intravenous ganciclovir discontinue nursing. Breast-feeding should not be resumed until 72 hours after the last dose of ganciclovir (product information, Cytovene, 1993).

Therapeutic Use

Of the retinal diseases, ganciclovir has been used almost exclusively for the treatment of CMV retinitis in immunocompromised patients. More recently, ganciclovir has been used to treat patients with progressive outer retinal necrosis. This zoster-mediated retinitis occurs primarily in immunocompromised persons, is often resistant to acyclovir therapy, and requires the use of ganciclovir; however, no treatment has been shown to be very effective for this infection.

The most extensive experience with therapeutic use of ganciclovir has been in the treatment of CMV retinitis. For the treatment of CMV retinitis as well as colitis and esophagitis, the recommended dose of ganciclovir for induction is 5 mg/kg given intravenously over 1 hour every 12 hours for 14 to 21 days (77). There may be variation in dosing from 2.5 to 5 mg/kg/dose given over 1 hour every 8 to 12 hours. This dose may be given from 10 days to 35 days, depending on the clinical response of the patient. Because of the high rate of recurrence of CMV retinitis among AIDS patients with CMV retinitis, if therapy is discontinued (75), long-term intravenous ganciclovir maintenance therapy with 5 mg/kg/dose over 1 hour once daily 7 days a week or, alternatively, 6 mg/kg/dose given over 1 hour once daily for 5 days of the week is recommended (77). Various maintenance regimens of ganciclovir for the suppression of CMV infections have been attempted, including the use of doses from 2.1 mg/kg/day to 6 mg/kg/day given intravenously daily, three times weekly, or five times weekly (75,78,79).

An alternative to intravenous therapy has been the use of intravitreal ganciclovir, but this alternative is reserved for patients who have developed severe neutropenic side effects from ganciclovir, who cannot tolerate the medication because of the idiosyncratic side effects, or who require concurrent retroviral therapy. The details of intravitreous ganciclovir preparation already have been discussed. There is disagreement in terms of the number of times intravitreal ganciclovir needs to be given during induction and how often it needs to be given for maintenance therapy. As discussed, the usual dose is 200 to 400 μg in 0.1 ml, which may be injected using a 27- or 30-gauge needle through the pars plana and into the midvitreous cavity. Twice-weekly or three-times-weekly injections of intravitreal ganciclovir are recommended for induction therapy. Injections given once weekly serve as maintenance therapy once the retinitis has become quiescent or has responded to the initial induction treatment.

Although oral ganciclovir has been approved by the FDA for use as maintenance therapy for stable CMV retinitis in patients with AIDS, results of clinical trials comparing oral and intravenous maintenance ganciclovir therapy have been inconsistent (80,81). Drew and colleagues (80) studied 123 patients with stable CMV retinitis after 3 weeks of intravenous ganciclovir therapy. They randomized 60 patients to intravenous maintenance (5 mg/kg/day) and 63 patients to oral maintenance (3,000 mg daily) ganciclovir therapy in an open-label study. After 20 weeks of follow-up with fundus photography every other week, masked assessment of photographs revealed no statistical difference in mean time to progression of retinitis between the two groups (62 days for the intravenous group and 57 days for the oral group). When mean time to progression was evaluated by ophthalmologists who knew the treatment assignments, however, mean time to progression was significantly shorter for the oral group (68 days for the oral group compared with 96 days for the intravenous group) (80). Similar results were obtained by the Oral Ganciclovir European and Australian Cooperative Study Group in a 20-week, randomized, multicenter, open-label study of 159 patients with stable CMV retinitis (81) in which 112 patients were randomized to oral ganciclovir maintenance therapy (500 mg six times daily while awake) and 47 patients to intravenous ganciclovir (5 mg/kg/day). Fundoscopy showed that CMV retinitis progressed in a mean period of 86 days for the oral ganciclovir group compared with 109 days for the intravenous ganciclovir group, a statistically significant difference (81). It appears that although effective serum ED_{50} levels may be attained with oral ganciclovir, it may not be quite as effective as intravenous ganciclovir for maintenance therapy in stable CMV retinitis.

Dose adjustments of intravenous and oral ganciclovir should be made for patients who have renal impairment. Chachoua et al. (78) administered intravenous ganciclovir in patients with renal dysfunction using the following guidelines. If the creatinine clearance is 25 to 50 ml/minute/1.73 m^2 of body surface area, 3 mg/kg of ganciclovir may be given every 12 hours for induction. If the creatinine clearance is 10 to 25, 3 mg/kg of ganciclovir may be given intravenously once daily. If the creatinine clearance is 0 to 10, 1.5 mg/kg of intravenous ganciclovir may be given once daily (78). Because 50% of the drug may be eliminated during hemodialysis, the drug should be given after hemodialysis (71).

Pediatric use of intraveous ganciclovir has been limited mainly to its use in patients with CMV retinitis. Because of the possibility of long-term carcinogenicity and reproductive toxicity, the use of ganciclovir in children necessitates caution and careful evaluation. With normal renal function, typical induction doses of 5 mg/kg given twice daily may be used in children. Maintenance therapy may be given 5 days per week at 6 mg/kg/day or 7 days per week at 5 mg/kg/day as in adults. Various doses from 7.5 mg/kg/day to 19 mg/kg/day divided into three times daily doses have been given to pediatric patients with serious CMV infections following bone marrow transplantation (82,83).

Side Effects and Toxicity

Ganciclovir is contraindicated in patients who are hypersensitive to the product or its inactive ingredients. It is also contraindicated in patients who are hypersensitive to acyclovir.

Adverse reactions from ganciclovir are mainly hematologic. The most prominent and severe side effect is myelosuppression. Up to 25% of patients receiving ganciclovir will develop some degree of myelosuppression (84). Among 219 patients treated with intravenous ganciclovir in two different clinical trials, the incidence of leukopenia varied from 19.5% to 32%. Neutropenia occurred in 14.6% to 60% of patients (60,75,78,79,85,86). In addition to myelosuppression, in vitro studies showed that ganciclovir also may inhibit lymphocyte proliferation (87). When neutropenia or leukopenia does occur, some investigators recommend reduction of induction doses of ganciclovir from 5 to 3 mg/kg/dose given every 12 hours when the neutrophil count falls to < 50% of baseline or < 1,000 cells/m^3 (78). The concomitant use of granulocyte colony stimulating factor or granulocyte–monocyte colony stimulating factor has profoundly influenced the management of patients who become neutropenic on ganciclovir. These two medications may preferentially stimulate bone marrow production of myeloid progenitor cells, thereby allowing aggressive dosing of parenteral ganciclovir to control CMV infections.

Intravenous ganciclovir therapy can result in elevated liver enzymes in up to 23% of patients (60). Significant elevations of aspartate aminotransferase (AST), alanine aminotransferase (ALT), gamma-glutamyltransferase (GGT), and alkaline phosphatase have been observed among these patients. Skin rash occurs in fewer than 5% of patients (product information, Cytovene, 1989) (78). Fewer than 5% of patients may develop gastrointestinal side effects (i.e., nausea and anorexia) with intravenous ganciclovir therapy (60,75), and fewer than 5% of patients may develop central nervous system toxicity, including headaches, disorientation, and mental status changes (60,75).

Other minor side effects have included arrhythmias, hypertension, and hypotension in fewer than 1% of patients; endocrine and metabolic disturbances in fewer than 1% of patients; and respiratory distress in fewer than 1% of patients. Rare case reports of myalgias have also been noted. Animal studies suggest that the drug may inhibit spermatogenesis (product information, Cytovene, 1993), and carcinogenic effects of the medication are being studied currently. Ganciclovir is a potential carcinogen in humans (product information, Cytovene, 1989).

High-risk Groups

Ganciclovir is relatively contraindicated in pregnancy. Animal studies of ganciclovir in rabbits demonstrated fetal growth retardation, embryonal lethality, teratogenicity, and maternal toxicity (product information, Cytovene, 1989). Ganciclovir is classified by the FDA as pregnancy category C (product information, Cytovene, 1993).

Adequate hydration is necessary to avoid nephrotoxicity when administering intravenous ganciclovir to patients. Thus, high-risk patients may include elderly patients who may be dehydrated or patients who have had significant diarrhea and dehydration. Administration of drug with patients with severe dehydration may result in high levels of the drug in the plasma. Ganciclovir should not be administered to patients who are profoundly neutropenic, with absolute neutrophil counts < 500 cells/mm^3, or platelet counts < 25,000/mm^3 (product information, Cytovene, 1989). Because of the possible carcinogenicity and reproductive toxicity, ganciclovir should be used with great caution in children.

Drug Interactions

In general, drugs that inhibit replication of rapidly dividing cell populations, such as bone marrow, spermatogonia, dermal layers of the skin, and gastrointestinal mucosa, may have additive toxicity when administered concomitantly with ganciclovir. These drugs should be given concomitantly only if the potential benefits outweigh risks. These drugs include amphotericin B, cotrimoxazole, dapsone, doxorubicin, flucytosine, pentamidine, vinblastine, and vincristine.

Ganciclovir may increase the nephrotoxicity of cyclosporin when it is concomitantly administered with this drug (49). Imipenim or cilastatin used in combination with ganciclovir may produce generalized seizures (88). The seizures may be of rapid onset and may be severe.

The concomitant use of ganciclovir and zidovudine has resulted in hematologic toxicity in up to 80% of patients (89). Foscarnet may be the preferred antiviral when zidovudine is required.

Major Clinical Trials

The efficacy of ganciclovir in the treatment of CMV disease has been explored by several clinical trials, in particular, for the treatment of CMV retinitis. The most important of these trials are summarized herein. (Table 33-1.)

In 1986 the Collaborative Ganciclovir Treatment Study Group, in conjunction with the Syntex Corporation, re-

TABLE 33-1. *Summary of prospective clinical trials of ganciclovir for the treatment of CMV retinitis*

Author (ref)	No. of patients	Response (%)	Relapse if therapy stopped (%)	Time to relapse (days)
Collaborative DHPG (60)	13	85	79	14–42
Jabs (90)	18	78	71	14–90
Holland (91)	41	55	45	NA
Laskin (75)	67	87	100, no maintenance	<30
			73, 2.5mg/kg/d maintenance	
			0, 5mg/kg/d maintenance	
Buhles (94)	108	84	50, no maintenance	47
			15, 5mg/kg/d maintenance	105
Henderly (92)	18	100	30	138
SOCA (95)	127	NA	NA	56

CMV, cytomegalovirus; NA, data not available.

leased its first prospective study of 26 patients with severe immunodeficiency, 22 of whom had AIDS (60). Of these 22 patients, 13 had CMV retinitis. These patients were treated with 5 mg/kg of body weight of ganciclovir infused intravenously over 1 hour at 8- to 12-hour intervals for a median period of 14 days. Nearly 85% of patients with CMV retinitis had a favorable response with clinical improvement of the CMV retinitis; however, virologic relapses occurred in 79% of patients when ganciclovir was discontinued. Neutropenia was the most frequent adverse reaction.

In 1986 a 15-month prospective study of 109 patients with AIDS or AIDS-related condition (ARC) was conducted. Cytomegalovirus retinitis developed in 18 of these patients (90), and they were all treated with ganciclovir. Five other patients with CMV retinitis who were not part of this prospective study were also treated with ganciclovir. All 23 patients treated with ganciclovir showed clinical regression of retinitis. Breakthrough retinitis occurred in seven patients while they were on maintenance therapy with ganciclovir. During treatment, the most common complication was neutropenia, which developed in 13% of the patients. Recurrences occurred at an average of 4.6 months, ranging from 2 to 7 months after initiation of treatment (90).

Jabs and colleagues (91) performed an open-labeled, compassionate-care, protocol-based prospective trial of intravenous ganciclovir for CMV retinitis in 18 patients, 17 of whom had AIDS. All patients received induction doses of 5 mg/kg every 12 hours for 2 to 3 weeks and maintenance doses of 5 to 6 mg/kg daily, 5 of every 7 days. They found that 14 of 18 patients had a complete (11 of 18) or partial (3 of 18) response of retinitis with this regimen. Furthermore, maintenance therapy was required: 5 of 7 patients, after interruptions in their treatment, developed recurrent retinitis. Reversible neutropenia was the major side effect of the treatment (91).

A controlled retrospective study of ganciclovir for CMV retinitis was undertaken by Holland and colleagues (92). Using fundus photography and a masked system for assessing progression, 24 ganciclovir-treated patients and 17 untreated patients with CMV retinitis were evaluated. A masked assessment of the disease revealed progression in 10 patients (43%) treated with ganciclovir over a period of 22 days compared with 16 untreated patients (94%) who had progression of disease during a median of 25 days. Despite its retrospective basis, this particular study at least suggests that ganciclovir is beneficial in the treatment of patients with AIDS and CMV retinitis (92).

In another randomized, prospective trial of ganciclovir maintenance therapy for CMV retinitis, Jacobson et al. (93) evaluated 11 patients with CMV retinitis and AIDS. They found that in these 11 patients who had received a 10-day course of induction therapy and then were randomized to receive either immediate daily ganciclovir maintenance or deferred maintenance therapy of 5 mg/kg given at hourly infusion 5 days per week, the median time to retinitis progression was 42 days for the immediate maintenance group compared with 16 days for the deferred maintenance group. This difference was statistically significant. After crossing over to maintenance therapy, the patients in the deferred group had a median time of retinitis progression of 58 days compared with 16 days while on maintenance therapy. This difference approached clinical significance as well. Only 9% of cultures obtained while patients received maintenance therapy were positive for CMV versus 40% of cultures obtained from patients off maintenance therapy. The difference also was highly significant statistically. These authors concluded that although maintenance therapy of ganciclovir delays progression of CMV retinitis and suppresses the virus, it does not eradicate CMV shedding or halt the progression of CMV retinitis.

Buhles and colleagues (94) reported their experience of 314 immunocompromised patients treated with ganciclovir sponsored by the Syntex Corporation in 1988. This was an extension of the earlier study from the Syntex group in 1986 (60). Of the 314 immunocompromised patients with CMV infections, 108 had CMV retinitis, 84% of whom had a favorable clinical response to ganciclovir therapy. This therapy consisted of 5 mg/kg of ganciclovir given twice daily or 2.5 mg/kg given three times daily for 10 to 14 days. Maintenance therapy consisted of 5 mg/kg daily 2 to 3 days per week (low-dose maintenance: 10–15 mg/kg weekly) or high-dose maintenance 5 to 6 mg/kg given 5 to 7 days per week (high-dose maintenance: 25 to 35 mg/kg given weekly). From the original group of 108 patients with CMV retinitis, 61 were eligible for evaluation of maintenance therapy. In this group, the median time to relapse of retinitis was 47 days in patients not receiving maintenance treatment compared with 105 days in patients treated with the higher dose maintenance period. This difference was highly statistically significant. In addition, adverse effects of the treatment in this study included neutropenia in 42% and thrombocytopenia in 19%, central nervous system side effects in 18%, and less common reactions (e.g., nausea, fever, rash, diarrhea, vomiting, infusion-site reaction, and anemia) in fewer than 10% of patients (94).

The foscarnet-ganciclovir CMV retinitis trial performed by the Studies of Ocular Complications of AIDS (SOCA) (95) research group was designed to evaluate the relative efficacy of foscarnet and ganciclovir for the treatment of CMV retinitis in patients with AIDS. It was also designed to compare the relative benefits of immediate treatment versus deferral of treatment for patients with disease not involving the posterior pole. Ganciclovir induction doses were 5 mg/kg given every 12 hours for 2 weeks. Maintenance therapy was started after completion of induction therapy and was at a dosage of 5 mg/kg/day. The doses were adjusted for renal function. Foscarnet induction consisted of 60 mg/kg given every 8 hours for 2 weeks. Maintenance therapy was begun after completion of induction therapy. Initial full-dose maintenance therapy was 90 mg/kg/day along with hydration of 1 L of normal saline solution. This multicenter randomized, open-label clinical trial was suspended in 1992 per recommendations of the policy and data-monitoring board of the study. At that time, about 234 patients were enrolled, 127 randomly assigned to ganciclovir and 107 to foscarnet. At the time of study closure, 65 patients assigned to ganciclovir had died compared with 36 of those assigned to foscarnet. This difference in mortality was highly significant statistically (relative risk, 1.79). The median survival was 8.5 months in the ganciclovir group and 12.6 in the foscarnet group. Although patients assigned to ganciclovir received less antiretroviral therapy on average than those assigned to foscarnet, the excess mortality could not be explained entirely on the differences in exposure to antiviral drugs. In the foscarnet group, the only subgroup of patients identified as having excessive mortality were those whose renal function was compromised at entry. There was no difference between the two treatment groups in the rate of progression of retinitis. The median time to disease progression was 56 days in the ganciclovir group and 59 days in the foscarnet group. This difference was not statistically significant. There were no significant differences in visual outcome and visual field scores between the two groups (95). This clinical trial established the position of ganciclovir in the scheme of CMV retinitis therapy in patients with AIDS.

FOSCARNET

History and Source

Foscarnet was originally developed as a topical preparation for the treatment of herpes simplex infection. It has a very broad spectrum of activity against many viral DNA kinases and is the second most active agent known against the reverse transcriptase of the human immunodeficiency virus (HIV). In the early 1980s, research by Eriksson and colleagues (96) revealed that of all 16 pyrophosphate analogs tested, foscarnet was the most effective analog against the CMV DNA polymerase. Subsequently, Oberg (97) described the antiviral effects of phosphornoformate (foscarnet) and the efficacy of foscarnet against a number of viral polymerases, including RNA polymerase of the influenza virus, a reverse transcriptasis of the mammalian retroviruses, and the DNA polymerase of animal and human herpes viruses (97). After this drug was shown to be effective against CMV and retrovirus infections, it was widely used in the treatment of human CMV infections in patients who were immunosuppressed following bone marrow transplantation and renal transplantation. It became an alternative agent to ganciclovir in the treatment of CMV infections in AIDS patients.

Official Drug Name and Chemistry

The full name of foscarnet is trisodium phosphonoformate. It is also known as phosphonoformate, phosphonoformic acid, PFA, and foscarnet sodium. It has a molecular weight of 191.95. Its chemical structure is CPO_5Na_3 (97).

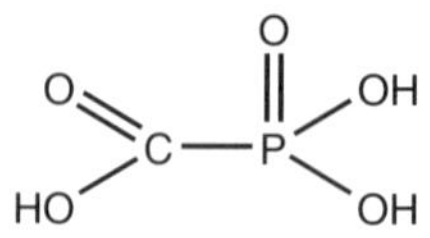

Foscarnet

Pharmacology

Foscarnet appears to inhibit reversibly and noncompetitively the activity of CMV DNA polymerase (see Fig. 33-1). It does not require phosphorylation to be efficacious against this polymerase. As already stated, of 16 pyrophosphate analogs studied by Eriksson and colleagues, foscarnet was the most effective, especially against the CMV DNA polymerase (96). In this study, a concentration of foscarnet of 0.3 μM caused a 50% inhibition of DNA polymerase activity in CMV strain AD169. In another study, 18 clinical CMV isolates were used to infect human embryonic fibroblasts. With the use of the enzyme-linked immunosorbent assay (ELISA) system for detection of production of CMV antigens, the mean ID_{50} for 16 sensitive clinical isolates to foscarnet was 323 μM. Two isolates were found to be resistant (98). Intravenous infusions of foscarnet can achieve plasma levels that surpass the ID_{50} of most strains of human CMV. Foscarnet is a virustatic agent (99).

Clinical Pharmacology

In humans, plasma concentrations during and after intravenous infusion of foscarnet are best described by a three-compartment model. In a study of six patients infected with HIV-1 virus who were treated with intravenous foscarnet, the mean half-life of this drug using this triphasic model was 0.45, 3.3, and 18 hours (100). The highest plasma concentrations were consistently found after 72 hours of continuous intravenous infusion of 16,000 mg/day. Concentrations in plasma reached levels of 75 to 265 μM. When intermittent 2-hour intravenous infusions of 60 mg/kg of foscarnet were administered three times daily for 2 weeks, peak and trough levels reached 557 and 155 μM, respectively (101). These levels were certainly in the range required to achieve 50% inhibition of viral DNA polymerase activity in vitro. In fact, most strains of human CMV are inhibited by foscarnet concentrations of 100 to 300 μM. Replication of HIV is inhibited almost completely at a concentration of 132 μM (102). In another pharmacokinetic study by Taburet and colleagues (103), 11 patients with AIDS were administered 2-hour infusions of 90 mg/kg of foscarnet twice daily for 2 weeks. The mean steady-state concentrations of foscarnet at 7 days and 14 days were 207 and 218 μM, respectively. Again, these plasma concentrations approximate the levels of foscarnet necessary for in vitro inhibition of most strains of human CMV.

Pharmaceutics

The parenteral form of foscarnet is available in an undiluted solution of 24 mg/ml, which has a shelf life of about 2 years (104). Because the solution will crystallize when refrigerated, it should be stored at room temperature, and should be protected against excessive heat and freezing (product information, Foscavir, 1992). The administration technique for intravenous foscarnet is to give it in a 24 mg/ml solution through a central venous catheter. It may be diluted to 12 mg/ml for administration through a peripheral vein. Diluents can include dextrose 5% in water or normal saline. The rate of administration should be controlled by using an infusion pump (product information, Foscavir, 1992) (104,105). When administering intravenous foscarnet, it is extremely important to hydrate the patient with approximately 2.5 L of normal saline daily, which may be begun the night before infusion and continued throughout the course of infusion. This step drastically reduces the incidence and nephrotoxicity from continuous infusion of foscarnet (106).

Intravitreal foscarnet also may be administered for CMV retinitis. The intravenous 24 mg/ml solution of foscarnet may be passed through a 0.22-μm filter, and 0.05 ml of the solution containing approximately 1,200 μg of foscarnet trisodium may be delivered into the midvitreous cavity (107). Little information on clinical experience with intravitreal foscarnet has been reported.

Foscarnet has poor oral bioavailability. The plasma concentrations achieved after oral dosing do not appear to be adequate for inhibiting HIV replication or treating CMV infections in AIDS patients (100,108). Peak plasma levels < 50 μM after a 4,000-mg oral dose have been reported (100,108). Thus, foscarnet is used mainly intravenously and occasionally intravitreally for the treatment of CMV retinitis.

Pharmacokinetics, Concentration-effect, and Relationship with Metabolism

Clinical studies detailing the onset and duration of action in humans treated with intravenous foscarnet suggest that peak plasma levels of foscarnet are achieved by day 3 or beyond. In one study, 60 mg/kg of foscarnet infused every 8 hours achieved mean plasma levels of 509 μM on day 3 immediately after infusion. With this regimen, steady-state peak plasma levels on day 14 reached 485 μM (102). In 11 patients with AIDS who received 90 mg/kg of foscarnet twice daily for 2 weeks, steady-state peak plasma concentrations reached 605 μM (103). Trough levels at steady state were approximately 52 μM. Mean steady-state concentrations of foscarnet on day 14 were approximately 218 μM (103). Although continuous intravenous infusion is not often used, in the early studies it could achieve levels of 100 to 500 μM at an infusion rate of 0.14 to 0.19 mg/kg/min (109). Estimated steady-state concentrations in this study ranged from 115 to 458 μM. These plasma concentrations appear to be therapeutic. As noted, most CMV strains are inhibited by foscarnet concentrations of 100 to 300 μM (102).

With induction therapy, significant improvement in CMV infection, particularly retinitis, occurs within 3 to 7 days after initiation of the drug (110,111). It should be noted that the duration of this effect rests on the continuation of maintenance doses of this medication. After discontinuation of intravenous induction of foscarnet, CMV retinitis appears to recur rapidly, within 3 to 4 weeks in most patients (110,111).

There may be several distribution sites for foscarnet. The average volume of distribution at steady state is 0.3 to 0.6 L/kg (103). When intermittent intravenous infusion is used, the volume of distribution appears to be 0.74 L/kg (102). During continuous intravenous infusion of foscarnet, however, the mean volume of distribution at steady state is 0.52 L/kg using the two-compartment model or 1.29 L/kg using the three-compartment model (100). There may be two separate distribution sites for foscarnet: bone and CSF. Foscarnet has been reported to be retained in bone in animals (97). Pharmacokinetic studies by Sjovall and colleagues (100,109) have shown that 3% to 28% of the cumulative intravenous dose was not recovered in the urine. These investigators suggest that this unrecovered portion may indeed be deposited in bone. Cerebrospinal fluid is variably penetrated by foscarnet; CSF concentrations of foscarnet range from 13% to 103% of plasma levels. In other clinical studies, during continuous intravenous infusion of foscarnet, CSF levels varied from 13% to 68% (mean, 43%) of plasma concentrations (109). All these patients have had elevated CSF proteins, suggesting some breakdown of the blood–brain barrier. This disease-related breakdown in the blood–brain barrier results in a variable penetrance of the drug into the CSF (product information, Foscavir, 1991).

Foscarnet does not undergo any significant metabolic transformation in humans (100,108,109). It is eliminated unchanged by the kidney and undergoes both glomerular filtration and tubular secretion, as clearance of foscarnet seems to exceed creatinine clearance. Recent evidence has been found that the clearance of foscarnet in some instances is less than the creatinine clearance, indicating that some tubular reabsorption of this drug may take place (product information, Foscavir, 1991) (100,102,103). In one clinical study by Sjovall (100), renal clearance accounted for most of the plasma clearance; however it was apparent that nonrenal clearance was about 40 ml/minute/ 1.73 m^2 of the body surface area. The investigators believed this finding may represent sequestration of foscarnet in bone. The mean plasma half-life of foscarnet is 3 to 6 hours in patients with normal renal function (100,102,103) and it may be prolonged in patients with decreased creatinine clearance (100,102,103). The extracorporeal clearance rate of foscarnet in hemodialysis is 80 ml/minute during the first hemodialysis session in a patient with foscarnet-induced renal failure (112). In another patient, the plasma half-life of foscarnet during dialysis was 3 hours, and between dialysis sessions the half-life was 86.6 hours (113).

Drug levels are not obtained routinely for intravenously administered foscarnet. Weekly or biweekly evaluation of electrolytes and renal function, along with complete blood counts, is recommended for patients who receive intravenous foscarnet therapy.

Intravitreal foscarnet pharmacokinetics were studied in one patient by Diaz-Llopiz and colleagues (107). After administering intravitreal injections of 1200 μg of foscarnet, the plasma and vitreous foscarnet levels were measured by HPLC. These authors found no evidence of systemic absorption of foscarnet after intravitreal injection. Elimination half-life from the vitreous after one injection was 54 hours. Levels of foscarnet in the vitreous cavity remained above the ID_{50} for CMV for approximately 56 hours and above the ID_{50} of HIV for approximately 241 hours after injection. The authors suggest an induction regimen of two injections weekly for 3 weeks followed by a maintenance regimen of one injection per week (107).

Therapeutic Use

Foscarnet is used primarily for the control of CMV retinitis in patients with AIDS and other causes of immune suppression. Patients with CMV retinitis require induction doses of 60 mg/kg of foscarnet infused intravenously over 1 hour in 8-hour intervals for 2 to 3 weeks. If there is relapse of retinitis during maintenance therapy, induction doses may be reinstituted (product information, Foscavir, 1992). Intermittent infusions of 60 mg/kg every 8 hours or 100 mg/kg every 12 hours have been associated with a lower incidence of nephrotoxicity than continuous intravenous infusions (105,110,111,114,115). A maintenance regimen of 90 mg/kg to 120 mg/kg given once daily is the most effective maintenance regimen of foscarnet for the treatment of CMV retinitis (115). When patients do not receive maintenance therapy, relapses can occur 2 to 4 weeks after induction (114). Despite maintenance therapy, relapse rates for CMV retinitis are still high. Higher foscarnet doses of approximately 200 mg/kg/day or greater have been suggested to suppress CMV activity in the retina; however, these doses have been associated with a higher incidence of nephrotoxicity (115). The induction and maintenance doses of foscarnet should be adjusted according to creatinine clearance in patients with renal insufficiency (product information, Foscavir, 1992) (102). Dosage may be estimated during dialysis. MacGregor and colleagues (113) administered 60 mg/kg of foscarnet after each dialysis session to treat a patient with CMV infection and renal failure, which allowed peak plasma levels of the medication to reach a range of 500 to 800 μM. The drug, however, did accumulate and required a decrease in the dosage over a 90-day period (113).

Side Effects and Toxicity

Contraindications to foscarnet are hypersensitivity to foscarnet and a creatinine clearance that drops below 0.4 ml/min/kg during therapy (product information, Foscavir, 1992). Foscarnet should be used cautiously in the presence of renal insufficiency, which requires dose reductions, concomitant administration of other potentially nephrotoxic medications, and concomitant use of intravenous pentamidine therapy, which may result in severe hypocalcemia. In addition, patients should be adequately hydrated during therapy to reduce the possibility of nephrotoxicity.

The most common adverse reactions to foscarnet are nephrotoxicity and various electrolyte abnormalities. Nephrotoxicity, which results in increased plasma creatinine and acute renal failure, is the most commonly observed side effect. Most patients develop some degree of renal insufficiency while on foscarnet (product information, Foscavir, 1991) (106,111,115,116). Nephrotoxicity may be reduced by adequate hydration. The extent of renal damage appears to be directly proportional to the cumulative dose of foscarnet, a function of both the plasma concentration as well as the duration of exposure (product information, Foscavir, 1991) (106). In one series of patients treated with continuous infusions of foscarnet, increases in plasma creatinine at least 25% above baseline were reported in 66% of patients, and some patients developed acute renal failure. Renal biopsy in one patient demonstrated evidence of extensive tubular necrosis (106). Some investigators suggest that nephrotoxicity may be less frequent and less severe with intermittent intravenous infusions of foscarnet compared with continuous intravenous infusions (114).

Foscarnet may cause several electrolyte disturbances: hyperphosphatemia, hypocalcemia, hypokalemia, and hypomagnesemia. Hyperphosphatemia is the most frequent foscarnet-induced abnormality of phosphate metabolism (114). In their series, Jacobson and colleagues reported that 9 of 10 patients developed hyperphosphatemia when given intermittent infusions of induction therapy with foscarnet for CMV retinitis. Mean baseline levels of phosphate increased from 3.6 mg/dl to 4.4 mg/dl during week 2 of treatment. Increases in parathyroid hormone subsequently occurred, which ultimately normalized calcium and phosphorus levels. It has been surmised that hyperphosphatemia, although generally asymptomatic, is probably related to the deposition of foscarnet in bone with the release of phosphorus from bone stores or to foscarnet-induced inhibition of phosphate and sodium transport in the renal epithelium (100,114). Hypocalcemia and hypercalcemia also have been reported during foscarnet administration (100,114). These changes may represent foscarnet incorporation into bone (100,111). Profound hypocalcemia can occur in patients receiving concomitant foscarnet and pentamidine. Hypokalemia has been reported with foscarnet therapy within 2 weeks of initiation of therapy. Oral potassium supplementation may not be effective in correcting this electrolyte disorder (117). Hypomagnesemia has also been reported in association with foscarnet therapy (117).

Several cases of penile ulcerations related to foscarnet administration have been reported in patients with AIDS (118–121). This condition may occur between 1 and 4 weeks after the initiation of foscarnet treatment. Resolution of ulceration occurs after withdrawal of foscarnet and recurrence upon rechallenge with the medication. This problem appears to be a fixed drug eruption caused by high concentrations of the unaltered drug in urine.

Hematologic abnormalities also may be seen with foscarnet. Reversible decreases in hemoglobin have been observed in up to half of patients treated with foscarnet (110, 111,115,116). Granulocytopenia, leukopenia, and thrombocytopenia are quite rare with foscarnet compared with ganciclovir. Occasional reports of congestive heart failure have been noted in association with intravenous foscarnet administration (122). Central nervous system side effects may include tremor and intermittent muscle twitching among patients receiving foscarnet (110,114). Nausea, vomiting, and diarrhea have also been associated with intravenous foscarnet administration. Nausea and vomiting occur more frequently with plasma foscarnet concentrations exceeding 350 μM (109).

Teratogenicity and effects of foscarnet in pregnancy are unknown, but the drug has been classified as FDA pregnancy category C by the manufacturer (product information, Foscavir, 1991).

High-risk Groups

Patients with renal insufficiency are at high risk when administered intravenous foscarnet. Little experience with the use of foscarnet in neonates, children, pregnant women, and nursing mothers has been reported.

Drug Interactions

Other nephrotoxic drugs, such as aminoglycoside antibiotics, amphotericin B, neomycin, netilmicin, and streptomycin, should not be used concomitantly with foscarnet because the combination potentially increases the incidence of nephrotoxicity. The following medicines should not be used concomitantly with foscarnet because they may lower plasma levels of ionized calcium: clodronate, edetate disodium, etidronate, pamidronate, and pentamidine, the last of which is known to cause severe drops in plasma calcium when used with foscarnet. The drop in calcium levels may be delayed. Four patients receiving systemic pentamidine and foscarnet were reported to have developed severe hypocalcemia, but calcium levels returned to normal in three of these four patients when one of the drugs was discontinued. The fourth patient died of severe hypocalcemia. Additive hypocalcemia is not observed when foscarnet is used with aerosolized pentamidine (product information, Foscavir, 1991) (123).

Zidovudine has been used safely in combination with foscarnet and generally is well tolerated; however, a higher incidence of anemia has been observed in patients being treated concomitantly with zidovudine and foscarnet. There is no increased incidence of myelosuppression (product information, Foscavir, 1991).

Major Clinical Trials

Several clinical trials have assessed the efficacy of foscarnet in the treatment of CMV retinitis (see Table 33-2). Walmsley and colleagues (110) reported the outcomes of a series of 14 patients from four centers with CMV retinitis who were treated with initial bolus intravenous infusion of 20 mg/kg of foscarnet over 30 minutes, followed by continuous intravenous infusion of 0.16 mg/kg/minute. This continuous infusion was dose adjusted for creatinine elevations. These investigators found partial or complete response of the CMV retinitis to foscarnet in 100% of the patients. Complete resolution of the retinitis occurred in 36% of patients and partial resolution in 64%; however, because none of these patients received maintenance foscarnet therapy, 91% relapsed within 4 weeks of discontinuation of induction treatment.

Jacobson and colleagues (114) prospectively treated 10 patients with CMV retinitis using induction doses of 60 mg/kg given every 8 hours for 14 days. The CMV retinitis stabilized or improved in 90% of the patients. Eight patients who presented into the study with positive blood or urine CMV cultures all had negative cultures at the end of induction. Seven of the 10 patients received maintenance therapy of 60 mg/kg of foscarnet 5 days per week. Six patients relapsed at 2 to 32 weeks after beginning maintenance therapy.

In a larger series of patients, LeHoang and colleagues (111) enrolled and prospectively treated 31 patients with CMV retinitis with foscarnet. Induction therapy consisted of 20 mg/kg bolus infusion of foscarnet over 30 minutes followed by continuous infusion of 0.16 mg/kg/minute over 3 weeks to achieve plasma levels of 100 to 150 μg/ml. All patients were monitored to the end of induction ther-

TABLE 33-2. *Summary of prospective clinical trials of foscarnet for the treatment of CMV retinitis*

Author (ref)	No. of patients	Response (%)	Relapse rate (%)	Time to relapse (days)
SOCA (95)	107	NA	NA	59
Walmsley (110)	13	100	77	6–60
LeHoang (111)	31	94	100 - no maintenance	<21
			50, 1/3 induction dose	<35
Jacobson (114)	10	90	86 - 60 mg/kg/d maintenance	14–214
Palestine (124)	24			
	13 Treated	100	92 at 1 yr	93
	11 Untreated	0		22
Jacobson (125)	32	100	NA	60 mg/kg/d 35
				90 mg/kg/d 56
				120 mg/kg/d 171

CMV, cytomegalovirus; SOCA, Studies of Ocular Complications of AIDS.

apy. Three patients died of AIDS-related diseases within 11 days after completion of 3 weeks of induction. After 3 weeks of induction therapy, retinitis improved in 29 of 31 patients, or 94%. More than 61% of patients had complete resolution, and more than 32% of patients had partial resolution. Slightly more than 6% of patients failed to respond to treatment. Maintenance therapy was later given to six patients after completion of induction treatment because, as the study progressed, it was noted that the patients who had stopped treatment after induction therapy had reactivation of retinitis. These 6 patients received daily 2-hour intravenous infusions of foscarnet containing a third of the induction dose which was given 5 days per week. All patients without maintenance therapy relapsed within 3 weeks after completion of induction. The rate of relapse on maintenance therapy was 50% within the first 5 weeks. These investigators suggested a controlled clinical trial of foscarnet and ganciclovir to determine their relative effectiveness in the treatment of CMV retinitis.

Another prospective randomized controlled trial of foscarnet for the treatment of CMV retinitis among patients with AIDS was conducted by Palestine and co-workers (124). Twenty-four patients with previously untreated CMV retinitis who were at low risk for loss of visual acuity were enrolled in the study. These patients were randomly assigned to a control group that received no antiviral therapy or to an immediate treatment group that received 60 mg/kg of intravenous foscarnet three times daily for 3 weeks of induction followed by maintenance therapy of 90 mg/kg once daily. This study also evaluated patients for the presence of cytomegalovirus in blood and urine, plasma levels of P24 antigen of HIV-1, and total CD4 lymphocyte counts over the course of the study. This group of investigators concluded that the mean time of progression of retinitis was 3.2 weeks in the control group compared with 13.3 weeks in the treatment group. There was a highly statistically significant difference between the two groups. In addition, 9 of the 13 treatment patients who had positive blood cultures for CMV had cleared their blood of CMV by the end of induction. This was also significant, as only one of the six patients in the control group had cleared his blood of CMV infection. The untreated group had no reduction in P24 levels, whereas the treated group demonstrated a more than 50% reduction. The authors concluded that the administration of foscarnet decreases the rate of progression of CMV retinitis in patients with AIDS. It should be noted that this study enrolled only patients with non-sight-threatening peripheral CMV retinitis lesions.

To evaluate the efficacy of maintenance intravenous foscarnet therapy, Jacobson and colleagues (125) enrolled 32 AIDS patients with previously untreated CMV retinitis. All these patients completed a course of induction of foscarnet of 60 mg/kg every 8 hours for 14 days and had stabilization of retinitis; then they were randomly assigned to receive foscarnet maintenance at either 90 or 120 mg/kg/day administered over 2 hours intravenously. This group of investigators found a median survival of 157 and 336 days for the 90 and 120 mg/kg/day groups, respectively. An independent masked analysis of retinal photographs taken over the course of the follow-up of these patients revealed that the median time of progression of retinitis was 31 days compared with 95 days for the 90 and 120 mg/kg/day groups, respectively. They concluded that daily intravenous foscarnet at a dose of 120 mg/kg/day resulted in significantly longer patient survival times and significantly increased the time to retinitis progression compared with standard 90 mg/kg/day maintenance. They also concluded that the size of the population of patients studied did not allow them to detect differences in toxicity between the two groups that might be clinically important (125). Again, the most frequent toxicities noted in all of these studies included nephrotoxicity, which was often transient, and electrolyte abnormalities, specifically hypocalcemia and hypomagnesemia.

The SOCA Research Group (95) performed a clinical trial to determine the efficacy of foscarnet versus ganciclovir in the treatment of CMV retinitis. The results of this study were detailed in the earlier section on ganciclovir. This study showed that patients with AIDS and CMV retinitis had a survival advantage if treated with foscarnet rather than ganciclovir; however, in terms of disease progression, both treatment groups had similar rates of progression of retinitis, suggesting that both drugs had similar efficacy in controlling CMV retinitis. Median time to disease progression was 56 days for ganciclovir and 59 days for foscarnet, a difference that is not statistically significant. Visual acuity and visual field scores and outcomes were also similar in both groups (95).

Foscarnet is an inhibitor of reverse transcriptase in a number of retroviruses. Specifically, it has a dose-related inhibitory effect on human T-cell lymphotropic virus type-3 (HTLV-3 or HIV) replication in the H9 cell line in vitro (126). In addition, Sandstrom and co-workers found that reverse transcriptase activity in HIV particles was inhibited completely by 5.0 μM levels of phosphornoformate in vitro. Two independent reports of in vivo efficacy of foscarnet against HIV have subsequently followed. Jacobson and colleagues (127) reported the effect of the use of zidovudine combined with foscarnet in the treatment of patients infected with HIV. Six symptomatic HIV-infected patients who had persistently quantifiable plasma HIV P24 antigen, despite having up to 27 weeks of full-dose oral zidovudine therapy (up to 1,200 mg/day), were enrolled. These patients were subsequently given 30 mg/kg of intravenous foscarnet every 8 hours with oral zidovudine for 14 days, followed by zidovudine alone for 6 months. They found plasma P24 antigen concentration decreased by a mean of 53% in all six patients over this period of combined therapy, a highly statistically significant reduction. After discontinuation of combination therapy, however, P24 antigen levels again increased to the baseline value in four patients after 14 weeks (127). In another series of 11 HIV-infected patients with CMV retinitis being treated with foscarnet, P24 antigen levels appeared to have decreased by 58% after a 14-day course of induction therapy with foscarnet therapy alone. None of these patients received zidovudine during this period, again suggesting in vivo efficacy of foscarnet on reducing retroviral reverse transcriptase activity (101). These studies all confirm the findings of the SOCA trial, suggesting that the antiretroviral activity of foscarnet in itself may play a role in prolonging the life expectancy of patients with CMV retinitis and AIDS (95).

Combination Foscarnet and Ganciclovir Therapy for Cytomegalovirus Retinitis

Ganciclovir resistance among patients with CMV retinitis has been well documented. Resistant clinical isolates of CMV are most commonly ganciclovir resistant. Stanat and colleagues (128) discovered nine ganciclovir-resistant clinical isolates of CMV in which ganciclovir phosphorylation could not be induced in virus-infected cells. Virally encoded DNA polymerase did not appear to play a role in ganciclovir resistance; however, the inability of cells infected with resistant isolates to phosphorylate ganciclovir appeared to be the major role for ganciclovir resistance (128). Foscarnet-resistant human CMV strains have been more difficult to detect (129). Sullivan and Coen (129) suggested that clinically important foscarnet-resistant infections could emerge based on the results of their in vitro studies (125). Clinically, evidence of ganciclovir-resistant CMV infection has been found in patients with AIDS as well. In a study of 72 patients with AIDS and serious CMV disease (130) treated with ganciclovir, 7.6% were excreting CMV resistant to ganciclovir (130). When ganciclovir resistance is documented, foscarnet is the drug of choice for treatment of resistant CMV retinitis (130,131).

In addition to ganciclovir resistance, there have been reports of patients who have had CMV retinitis that has been resistant to ganciclovir and foscarnet individually, necessitating the use of combination therapy. Indeed, combination ganciclovir and foscarnet therapy has synergistic effects in vitro against CMV as well as against HSV-2 replication (132,133). Clinically, several reports have described patients with CMV isolates resistant to both ganciclovir and foscarnet separately who responded to combination therapy (134–137). One report concluded that combination ganciclovir and foscarnet therapy appeared to be as effective as standard therapy for cytomegaloviral diseases. The rate of anemia, however, was significantly greater with combination therapy than with single-agent regimen. The rates of thrombocytopenia and neutropenia, although higher in the combination therapy group, were not statistically significantly different (137).

There are preliminary reports on the efficacy of the use of both of these agents in clinically resistant disease among patients with CMV retinitis appeared promising. In one report (138) of nine patients (14 eyes) with clinically resistant CMV retinitis who had progression of retinitis despite extended intravenous induction of single-drug therapy or alternating therapy with induction doses of ganciclovir or foscarnet, complete healing of retinitis on combination ganciclovir and foscarnet occurred in 12 of 14 eyes and partial healing in the other two eyes. A second small series (139) enrolled seven patients who had CMV retinitis and AIDS, all of whom demonstrated multiple progressions of retinitis on ganciclovir or foscarnet therapy alone. In all patients, the progression-free interval was longer while on combination therapy compared with monotherapy (139). There were no toxic side effects attributed to the drugs that required cessation of therapy in either study (138,139).

The SOCA Research Group performed a multicenter, randomized clinical trial for patients with persistent or relapsed CMV retinitis (140) in which 279 patients were randomly assigned to receive foscarnet 90 mg/kg twice a day for 2 weeks followed by 120 mg/kg/day maintenance, intravenous ganciclovir 5 mg/kg twice daily for 2 weeks followed by 10 mg/kg/day maintenance, or combination therapy consisting of continuation of existing maintenance therapy plus induction doses of the other drug for 2 weeks followed by maintenance intravenous therapy with both drugs (foscarnet 90 mg/kg/day plus ganciclovir 5 mg/kg/day).

The median times to retinitis progression as determined by a masked Fundus Photograph Reading Center were 1.3 months, 2.0 months, and 4.3 months for the foscarnet, ganciclovir, and combination groups, respectively ($p < 0.001$). Combination therapy showed a distinct advantage over monotherapy for the control of relapsing CMV retinitis; however, combination therapy was also associated with the greatest negative impact on quality-of-life measures (140).

INVESTIGATIONAL DRUGS

The drugs in this group are of limited usefulness to ophthalmologists today. Most are currently being evaluated in Phase II or Phase III clinical trials for nonophthalmic viral infections but may be useful in the future for the treatment or prevention of viral retinitis.

HPMPC (Cidofivir)

HPMPC, or (S)-1-(3-hydroxy-2-phosphonylmethoxypropyl)cytosine, is a newer cytosine analog that has both in vitro and in vivo efficacy against herpes viridae (141–143). The pharmacokinetics of intravenous HPMPC in patients with HIV infection has been studied (144). Dose proportional serum levels of HPMPC can be obtained over the dose range of 1.0 to 10.0 mg/kg of body weight. The serum half-life of HPMPC is 2.6 hours. Approximately 90% of the drug is recovered unchanged in urine. Active tubular secretion of the drug plays a significant role in its clearance. The approximate volume of distribution of HPMPC is 500 ml/kg, which suggests that the drug is distributed in total body water. Oral probenecid appears to block tubular secretion of HPMPC at higher doses (> 3.0 mg/kg dose) (144). Phase III trials of intravenous HPMPC in the treatment of CMV retinitis are ongoing.

More research has been published on intravitreal than intravenous HPMPC for the treatment of CMV retinitis. Intravitreal HPMPC is not morphologically or electrophysiologically retinotoxic in doses up to 1000 μg (145). The intravitreal half-life of 100 μg of HPMPC is 24.4 hours (145). Phase I and II clinical trials have been completed for intravitreal HPMPC in the treatment of CMV retinitis in patients with AIDS (146,147). Kirsch and colleagues (146) conducted an unmasked consecutive-case series of intravitreal HPMPC injections in patients with AIDS and active CMV retinitis in at least one eye despite intravenous ganciclovir or foscarnet therapy. In the preliminary safety study, all eyes received one injection of 20 μg of intravitreal HPMPC while concurrently receiving maintenance intravenous ganciclovir. Mean time to retinitis progression was 78 days. In the dose-escalating study, intravitreal cidofivir was the sole treatment for retinitis. In this study, the mean time to retinitis progression in eyes treated with 20 μg of HPMPC was 64 days. Hypotony occurred in one of three eyes that received a 40 μg injection and in the two eyes that received a 100 μg injection. The authors concluded that HPMPC may be a safe and effective local treatment for CMV retinitis that provides a long duration of antiviral effect (146). In addition to hypotony, these investigators also reported iritis in 20% of eyes receiving intravitreal HPMPC (147).

A novel liposomal, intravitreal delivery mechanism for HPMPC also has been investigated for the treatment of experimental viral retinitis in rabbits (148). A 1,000 μg liposome-encapsulated, intravitreal dose of HPMPC may provide antiviral activity for 8 months (148). This technique has potential for future local therapy for CMV retinitis.

Valacyclovir

Valacyclovir is the L-valyl ester of acyclovir. It is a prodrug of acyclovir with greater oral bioavailability that enables acyclovir to reach higher concentrations in plasma; this is accomplished without increased toxicity. Phase I pharmacokinetic studies of valacyclovir have been completed. This medication may have a role in the prevention of CMV retinitis, as high concentrations of acyclovir have been found to inhibit the replication of the CMV in vitro (149).

In healthy human volunteers, single oral doses of 100 to 1,000 mg of valacyclovir resulted in dose-dependent increases of acyclovir in plasma. Plasma levels of acyclovir achieved 5–6 μg/ml after a 1,000-mg dose; the plasma valacyclovir levels peaked at < 0.3 μg/ml. The prodrug was undetected in the plasma 3 hours after administration of the oral medication. Multiple doses of valacyclovir of 250 to 2,000 mg given four times daily for 10 days have resulted in dose-proportional increases in plasma acyclovir. No serious adverse or unexpected events or laboratory abnormalities were reported after use of the medication; however, common side effects included nausea, vomiting, diarrhea, and abdominal pain. Jacobson (149) concluded that valacyclovir is well absorbed and rapidly converted to acyclovir, with 3 to 4 times higher levels of acyclovir detected in the plasma compared with oral acyclovir of the same dosage; this was possible even in patients with advanced HIV disease. No evidence of nephrotoxicity or neurotoxicity was found with this medication (149). This drug may be useful in the treatment of acute retinal necrosis.

882C

This new drug was developed by Burroughs-Wellcome researchers and has been used in healthy human volunteers as a specific inhibitor of VZV. A recent clinical study by

Crooks and colleagues showed that 882C was effective and well tolerated in the treatment of herpes zoster among immunocompetent patients. The study suggested that potentially effective plasma concentrations of 882C can be maintained well above the in vitro ID_{50} of the VZV using a once- or twice-daily oral regimen of this agent (Crooks et al., International Congress of Chemotherapy 298: June, 1993).

The 882C compound was discovered by examining the antiviral activity of a large number of 5-substituted pyrimidines against human CMV and VZV; 882C was selected from about 80 analogs. It is one of the most potent drugs against VZV and had the least toxic side effects. This compound, however, did not have significant activity against HSV or human CMV. It is clear that both valacyclovir as well as 882C may be useful in VZV infections; however, clinical trials are pending (150,151).

Immunoglobulins

Immunoglobulins infused intravenously may be of value as prophylactic agents against certain CMV infections, particularly CMV pneumonia. These immunoglobulins, however, have no value or little efficacy in the treatment of CMV retinitis. These immunoglobulins may be combined with ganciclovir in the treatment of CMV pneumonia; however, their efficacy is not additive in the treatment of CMV retinitis (152).

Interferons

Interferons are immunomodulatory proteins that have nonspecific antiviral activity in cells by inducing RNA and protein synthesis. The three major classes of interferons (interferon-alpha, which is leukocyte interferon; interferon-beta, derived from fibroblasts; and interferon-gamma, which is immune interferon) have all been synthesized genetically using recombinant DNA techniques and also have been identified in nature (153). These compounds may be given intramuscularly or subcutaneously. They almost always cause systemic flulike illness. They have been used successfully in the treatment of hepatitis B and hepatitis C virus infections and other AIDS-related viral infections (40,154).

There is currently no FDA-labeled ophthalmic indication for interferons. Systemic interferon-alpha is not effective in preventing or in treating CMV retinitis in patients with AIDS (155). In addition, beta-interferon administered along with the ganciclovir at reduced maintenance doses did not seem to prevent retinitis recurrence despite in vitro synergistic activities of ganciclovir and beta-interferon (156). Interferons continue to be experimental adjuncts to the treatment of various viral infections, specifically CMV retinitis. They are of limited usefulness to ophthalmologists and internists.

REFERENCES

1. Schaffer HJ, Beaucham L, de Miranda P, Elion GB, Bauer DJ, Collins P. 9-(2-Hydroxyethoxymethyl)guanine activity against viruses of the herpes group. *Nature* 1978;272:583–585.
2. Elion GB. Acyclovir: discovery, mechanism of action, and selectivity. *J Med Virol* 1993;1(suppl):2–6.
3. Whitley RJ. Antiviral therapy: the time has come. *J Med Virol* 1993;1(suppl):1.
4. Dorsky DI, Crumpacker CS. Drugs five years later: acyclovir. *Ann Intern Med* 1987;107:859–874.
5. Biron KK, Elion GB. In vitro susceptibility of varicella-zoster virus to acyclovir. *Antimicrob Agents Chemother* 1980;18:443–447.
6. Fyfe JA, Keller PM, Furman PA, Miller RL, Elion GB. Thymidine kinase from herpes simplex virus phosphorylates the new antiviral compound 9-(2-hydroxyethoxymethyl)guanine. *J Biol Chem* 1978; 253:8721–8727.
7. Whitley RJ, Gnann JW Jr. Acyclovir: a decade later. *N Engl J Med* 1992;327:782–789.
8. Colby BM, Furman PA, Shaw JE, Elion GB, Pagano JS. Phosphorylation of acyclovir [9-(2-hydroxyethoxymethyl)guanine]in Epstein-Barr virus-infected lymphoblastoid cell lines. *J Virol* 1981;38: 606–611.
9. Datta AK, Colby BM, Shaw JE, Pagano JS. Acyclovir inhibition of Epstein-Barr virus replication. *Proc Natl Acad Sci USA* 1980;77: 5173–5176.
10. Crumpacker CS, Schnipper LE, Zaia JA, Levin MJ. Growth inhibition by acycloguanosine of herpesviruses isolated from human infections. *Antimicrob Agents Chemother* 1979;15:642–645.
11. Balfour HH, Bean B, Mitchell CD, Sachs GW, Boen JR, Edelman CK. Acyclovir in immunocompromised patients with cytomegalovirus disease. *Am J Med* 1982;73:241–248.
12. Wade JC, Hintz M, McGuffin RW, et al. Treatment of cytomegalovirus pneumonia with high-dose acyclovir. *Am J Med* 1982;73:249–256.
13. Field HJ, Wildy P. The pathogenicity of thymidine kinase deficient mutants of herpes simplex virus in mice. *J Hyg* (Lond) 1978;81: 267–277.
14. Balfour HH. Resistance of herpes simplex to acyclovir. *Ann Intern Med* 1983;98:404–406.
15. Erlich KS, Mills J, Chatis P, et al. Acyclovir-resistant herpes simplex virus infections in patients with the acquired immunodeficiency syndrome. *N Engl J Med* 1989;320:293–296.
16. Forman JK, Lachs JR, Souney PF. Visual compatibility of acyclovir sodium with commonly used intravenous drugs during simulated Y-site injection. *Am J Hosp Pharm* 1987;44:1408–1409.
17. Blumenkranz MS, Culbertson WW, Clarkson JG, Dix R. Treatment of the acute retinal necrosis syndrome with intravenous acyclovir. *Ophthalmology* 1986;93:296–300.
18. Meyers JD, Wade JC, Mitchell CD, et al. Multicenter collaborative trial of intravenous acyclovir for treatment of mucocutaneous herpes simplex virus infection in the immunocompromised host. *Am J Med* 1982;73:229–235.
19. Cupps TR, Straus SE, Waldmann TA. Successful treatment with acyclovir of an immunodeficient patient infected simultaneously with multiple herpes viruses. *Am J Med* 1981;70:882–886.
20. Pepose JS, Biron K. Antiviral sensitivities of the acute retinal necrosis syndrome virus. *Curr Eye Res* 1987;6:201–205.
21. Blum MR, Liao SHT, DeMiranda P. Overview of acyclovir pharmacokinetic disposition in adults and children. *Am J Med* 1982; 73:186–192.
22. Laskin OL. Clinical pharmacokinetics of acyclovir. *Clin Pharmacokinet* 1983;8:187–201.
23. McKendrick MW, McGill JI, White JE, Wood MJ. Oral acyclovir in acute herpes zoster. *Br Med J* 1986;293:1529–1532.
24. McKendrick MW, McGill JI, Bell AM, Hickmott E, Burke C. Oral acyclovir in herpes zoster [Letter]. *Lancet* 1984;2:925.
25. McKendrick MW, Care C, Burke C, Hickmott E, McKendrick GDW. Oral acyclovir in herpes zoster. *J Antimicrob Chemother* 1984;14:661–665.
26. Hung SO, Patterson A, Rees PJ. Pharmacokinetics of oral acyclovir (Zovirax) in the eye. *Br J Ophthalmol* 1984;68:192–195.

27. de Miranda P, Whitley RJ, Blum MR. Acyclovir kinetics after intravenous infusion. *Clin Pharmacol Ther* 1979;26:718–728.
28. Laskin OL, Longsterth JA, Whelton A, et al. Effect of renal failure on the pharmacokinetics of acyclovir. *Am J Med* 1982;73:197–201.
29. de Miranda P, Good SS, Connor JD, et al. Metabolic fate of radioactive acyclovir in humans. *Am J Med* 1982;73:215–220.
30. King DH. History, pharmacokinetics, and pharmacology of acyclovir. *J Am Acad Dermatol* 1988;18:176–179.
31. Anonymous. Committee on Drugs, American Academy of Pediatrics: transfer of drugs and other chemicals into human milk. *Pediatrics* 1989;84:924–936.
32. Grutzmacher RD, Henderson D, McDonald PJ, Coster DF. Herpes simplex chorioretinitis in a healthy adult. *Am J Ophthalmol* 1983;96:788–796.
33. Uninsky E, Jampol LM, Kaufman S, Nuraqi S. Disseminated herpes simplex infection with retinitis in a renal allograft recipient. *Ophthalmology* 1983;90:175–178.
34. Peyman GA, Goldberg MF, Uninsky E, et al. Vitrectomy and intravitreal antiviral drug therapy in acute retinal necrosis syndrome: report of two cases. *Arch Ophthalmol* 1984;102:1618–1621.
35. Duker JS, Blumenkranz MS. Diagnosis and management of acute retinal necrosis (ARN) syndrome. *Surv Ophthalmol* 1991;35:327–343.
36. Engstrom RE Jr, Holland GN, Margolis TP, et al. The progressive outer retinal necrosis syndrome: a variant of necrotizing herpetic retinopathy in patients with AIDS. *Ophthalmology* 1994;101:1488–1502.
37. Hellinger WC, Bolling JP, Smith TF, Campbell RJ. Varicella-zoster virus retinitis in a patient with AIDS-related complex: case report and brief review of the acute retinal necrosis syndrome. *Clin Infect Dis* 1993;16:208–212.
38. Duker JS, Shakin EP. Rapidly progressive outer retinal necrosis in the acquired immunodeficiency syndrome. *Am J Ophthalmol* 1991; 111:255–256.
39. Carney MD, Peyman GA, Goldberg MF, Packo K, Pulido J, Nicholson D. Acute retinal necrosis. *Retina* 1986;6:85–94.
40. Teich SA, Cheung TW, Friedman AH. Systemic antiviral drugs used in ophthalmology. *Surv Ophthalmol* 1992;37:19–53.
41. Keeney RE, Kirk LE, Brigden D. Acyclovir tolerance in humans. *Am J Med* 1982;73:176–181.
42. Peterslund NA, Esmann V, Ipsen J, et al. Oral and intravenous acyclovir are equally effective in herpes zoster. *J Antimicrob Chemother* 1984;14:185–189.
43. Eck P, Silver SM, Claark EC. Acute renal failure and coma after a high dose of oral acyclovir [Letter]. *N Engl J Med* 1991;325:1178.
44. Arndt KA. Adverse reactions to acyclovir: topical, oral, and intravenous. *J Am Acad Dermatol* 1988;18:188–190.
45. Robbins MS, Stromquist C, Tan LH. Acyclovir pH- possible cause of extravasation tissue injury [Letter]. *Ann Pharmacother* 1993;27: 238.
46. Andrews EB, Yankaskas BC, Cordero JF, et al. Acyclovir in pregnancy registry: six years' experience. *Obstet Gynecol* 1992;79:7–13.
47. Balfour HH, McMonigal KA, Bean B. Acyclovir therapy of varicella-zoster virus infections in immunocompromised patients. *J Antimicrob Chemother* 1983a;12(suppl B):169–179.
48. Meyer LJ, de Miranda P, Sheth N, et al. Acyclovir in human breast milk. *Am J Obstet Gynecol* 1988;158:586–588.
49. Lake KD. Management of drug interactions with cyclosporine. *Pharmacotherapy* 1991;11:110s–118s.
50. Johnson R, Douglas J, Corey L, et al. Adverse effects with acyclovir and meperidine [Letter]. *Ann Intern Med* 1985;103:962–963.
51. Laskin OL, de Miranda P, King DH, et al. Effects of probenicid on the pharmacokinetics and elimination of acyclovir in humans. *Antimicrob Agents Chemother* 1982;21:804–807.
52. Grabenstein JD. Drug interactions involving immunologic agents. Part 1. Vaccine-vaccine, vaccine-immunoglobulin, and vaccine-drug interactions. *DICP* 1990;24:67–81.
53. Bach MC. Possible drug interaction during therapy with azidothymidine and acyclovir for AIDS [Letter]. *N Engl J Med* 1987; 316:547.
54. Hollander H, Lifson AR, Maha M, et al. Phase I study of low-dose zidovudine and acyclovir in asymptomatic human immunodeficiency virus seropositive individuals. *Am J Med* 1989;87:628–632.
55. Palay DA, Sternberg P Jr, David J, et al. Decrease in the risk of bilateral acute retinal necrosis by acyclovir therapy. *Am J Ophthalmol* 1991;112:250–255.
56. Smee DF, Martin JC, Verheyden JPH, Matthews TR. Anti-herpesvirus activity of the acyclic nucleoside 9-(1,3-dihydroxy-2-propoxymethyl)guanine. *Antimicrob Agents Chemother* 1983;23: 676–682.
57. Mar E-C, Cheng Y-C, Huang E-S. Effect of 9-(1,3-dihydroxy-2-propoxymethyl)guanine on human cytomegalovirus replication in vitro. *Antimicrob Agents Chemother* 1983;24:518–521.
58. Mar E-C, Patel PC, Cheng Y-C, Fox JJ, Watanabe KA, Huang E-S. Effects of certain nucleoside analogues on human cytomegalovirus replication in vitro. *J Gen Virol* 1984;65:47–53.
59. Tyms AS, Davis JM, Jeffries DJ, Meyers JD. BWB759u, an analogue of acyclovir, inhibits human cytomegalovirus in vitro. *Lancet* 1984;2:924–925.
60. Collaborative Ganciclovir Treatment Study Group: Treatment of serious cytomegalovirus infections with 9-(1,3-dihydroxy-2-propoxymethyl)guanine in patients with AIDS and other immunodeficiencies. *N Engl J Med* 1986;314:801–805.
61. Balfour HH Jr. Management of cytomegalovirus disease with antiviral drugs. *Rev Infect Dis* 1990;12(suppl 7):s849–s859.
62. Matthews T, Boehme R. Antiviral activity and mechanism of action of ganciclovir. *Rev Infect Dis* 1988;10(suppl 3):s490–s494.
63. Visor GC, Lin L-H, Jackson SE, et al. Stability of ganciclovir sodium (ganciclovir sodium) in 5% dextrose or 0.9% sodium chloride injections. *Am J Hosp Pharm* 1986;43:2810–2812.
64. Jacobson MA, de Miranda P, Cederberg DM, et al. Human pharmacokinetics and tolerance of oral ganciclovir. *Antimicrob Agents Chemother* 1987;31:1251–1254.
65. Henry K, Cantrill H, Kish MA. Intravitreous ganciclovir for patients receiving zidovudine. *JAMA* 1987;257:3066.
66. Cantrill HL, Henry K, Melroe H, Knobloch WH, Ramsay RC, Balfour HH Jr. Treatment of cytomegalovirus retinitis with intravitreal ganciclovir: long term results. *Ophthalmology* 1989;96:367–374.
67. Cochereau-Massin I, Lehoang P, Lautier-Frau M, et al. Efficacy and tolerance of intravitreal ganciclovir in cytomegalovirus retinitis in acquired immune deficiency syndrome. *Ophthalmology* 1991;98: 1348–1355.
68. Young SH, Morlet N, Heery S, Hollows FC, Coroneo MT. High dose intravitreal ganciclovir in the treatment of cytomegalovirus retinitis. *Med J Aust* 1992;157:370–373.
69. Sanborn GE, Anand R, Torti RE, et al. Sustained-release ganciclovir therapy for treatment of cytomegalovirus retinitis: Use of an intravitreal device. *Arch Ophthalmol* 1992;110:188–195.
70. Martin DF, Parks DJ, Mellow SD, et al. Treatment of cytomegalovirus retinitis with an intraocular sustained-release ganciclovir implant: a randomized controlled clinical trial. *Arch Ophthalmol* 1994;112:1531–1539.
71. Sommadossi J-P, Bevan R, Ling T, et al. Clinical pharmacokinetics of ganciclovir in patients with normal and impaired renal function. *Rev Infect Dis* 1988;10(suppl 3):s507–s514.
72. Fletcher C, Sawchuk R, Chinnock B, de Miranda P, Balfour HH. Human pharmacokinetics of the antiviral drug ganciclovir. *Clin Pharmacol Ther* 1986;40:281–286.
73. Field AK, Davies ME, DeWitt C, et al. 9-([2-hydroxy-1-(hydroxymethyl)ethoxy]methyl)guanine: a selective inhibitor of herpes group virus replication. *Proc Natl Acad Sci USA* 1983;80:4139–4143.
74. Tocci MJ, Livelli TJ, Perry HC, Crumpacker CS, Field AK. Effects of the nucleoside analog 2′-nor-2′-deoxyguanosine on human cytomegalovirus replication. *Antimicrob Agents Chemother* 1984;25:247–252.
75. Laskin OL, Cederberg DM, Mills J, Eron LJ, Mildvan D, Spector SA, and the ganciclovir Study Group. Ganciclovir for the treatment and suppression of serious infections caused by cytomegalovirus. *Am J Med* 1987;83:201–207.
76. Jabs DA, Wingard JR, de Bustros S, de Miranda P, Saral R, Santos GW. BWB759U for cytomegalovirus retinitis: intraocular drug penetration. *Arch Ophthalmol* 1986;104:1436–1437.
77. Drugs for AIDS and associated infections. *Med Lett Drugs Ther* 1991;33:95–102.
78. Chachoua A, Dieterich D, Krasinski K, et al. 9-(1,3-dihydroxy-2-propoxymethyl)guanine (ganciclovir) in the treatment of cy-

tomegalovirus gastrointestinal disease with the acquired immunodeficiency syndrome. *Ann Intern Med* 1987;107:133–137.
79. Erice A, Jordan C, Chace BA, et al. Ganciclovir treatment of cytomegalovirus disease in transplant recipients and other immunocompromised hosts. *JAMA* 1987;257:3082–3087.
80. Drew WL, Ives D, Lalezari JP, et al. Oral ganciclovir as maintenance treatment for cytomegalovirus retinitis in patients with AIDS. Syntex Cooperative Oral Ganciclovir Study Group. *N Engl J Med* 1995;333:615–620.
81. Intravenous versus oral ganciclovir: European/Australian comparative study of efficacy and safety in the prevention of cytomegalovirus retinitis recurrence in patients with AIDS: the Oral Ganciclovir European and Australian Cooperative Study Group. *AIDS* 1995;9:471–477.
82. Rosecan LR, Laskin OL, Kalman CM, et al. Antiviral therapy with ganciclovir for cytomegalovirus retinitis and bilateral exudative retinal detachments in an immunocompromised child. *Ophthalmology* 1986;93:1401–1407.
83. Shepp DH, Dandliker PS, de Miranda P, et al. Activity of 9-[2-hydroxy-1-(hydroxymethyl)ethoxymethyl]guanine in the treatment of cytomegalovirus pneumonia. *Ann Intern Med* 1985;103: 368–373.
84. Drucker JL, King DH. Management of viral infections in AIDS patients. *Infection* 1987;15:S32–S33.
85. Reed EC, Dandliker PS, Meyers JD. Treatment of cytomegalovirus pneumonia with 9-(2-hydroxy-1-(hydroxymethyl)ethoxymethyl) guanine and high-dose corticosteroids. *Ann Intern Med* 1986;105: 214–215.
86. Masur H, Lane HC, Palestine A, et al. Effect of 9-(1,3-dihydroxy-2-propoxymethyl)guanine on serious cytomegalovirus disease in eight immunosuppressed homosexual men. *Ann Intern Med* 1986;104: 41–44.
87. Bowden RA, Digel J, Reed EC, et al. Immunosuppressive effects of ganciclovir on in vitro lymphocyte responses. *J Infect Dis* 1987;156: 899–903.
88. Faulds D, Heel RC. Ganciclovir: a review of its antiviral activity, pharmacokinetic properties and therapeutic efficacy in cytomegalovirus infections. *Drugs* 1990;39:597–638.
89. Hochster H, Dieterich D, Bozzette S, et al. Toxicity of combined ganciclovir and zidovudine for cytomegalovirus disease associated with AIDS: an AIDS Clinical Trials Group Study. *Ann Intern Med* 1990;113:111–117.
90. Henderley DE, Freeman WR, Causey DM, Rao NA. Cytomegalovirus retinitis and response to therapy with ganciclovir. *Ophthalmology* 1987;94:425–434.
91. Jabs DA, Newman C, de Bustros S, Polk BF. Treatment of cytomegalovirus retinitis with ganciclovir. *Ophthalmology* 1987;94: 824–830.
92. Holland GN, Buhles WC, Mastre B, Kaplan HJ, the UCLA CMV Retinopathy Study Group. A controlled retrospective study of ganciclovir treatment for cytomegalovirus retinopathy. *Arch Ophthalmol* 1989;107:1759–1766.
93. Jacobson MA, O'Donnell JJ, Brodie HR, Wofsy C, Mills J. Randomized prospective trial of ganciclovir maintenance therapy for cytomegalovirus retinitis. *J Med Virol* 1988;25:339–349.
94. Buhles WC Jr, Mastre BJ, Tinker AJ, Strand V, Koretz SH, Syntex Collaborative Ganciclovir Treatment Study Group. Ganciclovir treatment of life- or sight-threatening cytomegalovirus infection: experience in 314 immunocompromised patients. *Rev Infect Dis* 1988;10(suppl 3):s495–s504.
95. Studies of Ocular Complications of AIDS (SOCA) Research Group in collaboration with the AIDS Clinical Trials Group (ACTG). Mortality in patients with the acquired immunodeficiency syndrome treated with either foscarnet or ganciclovir for cytomegalovirus retinitis. *N Engl J Med* 1992;326:213–220.
96. Eriksson B, Oberg B, Wahren B. Pyrophosphate analogues as inhibitors of DNA polymerases of cytomegalovirus, herpes simplex virus and cellular origin. *Biochem Biophys Acta* 1982;696:115–123.
97. Oberg B. Antiviral effects of phosphonoformate (PFA, foscarnet sodium). *Pharmacol Ther* 1983;19:387–415.
98. Wahren B, Wahren P, Harmenberg J, Sundqvist V-A. Computer-based virus sensitivity assay and neutralization method: applications for herpesviruses. *J Virol Methods* 1983;6:271–282.
99. Wahren B, Oberg B. Reversible inhibition of cytomegalovirus replication by phosphonoformate. *Intervirology* 1980;14:7–15.
100. Sjovall J, Karlsson A. Ogenstad S, Sandstron E, Saarimaki M. Pharmacokinetics and absorption of foscarnet after intravenous and oral administration to patients with human immunodeficiency virus. *Clin Pharmacol Ther* 1988;44:65–73.
101. Jacobson MA, Crowe S, Levy J, et al. Effect of foscarnet therapy on infection with human immunodeficiency virus in patients with AIDS. *J Infect Dis* 1988;158:862–865.
102. Aweeka F, Gambertoglio J, Mills J, et al. Pharmacokinetics of intermittently administered intravenous foscarnet in the treatment of acquired immunodeficiency syndrome patients with cytomegalovirus retinitis. *Antimicrob Agents Chemother* 1989;33:742–745.
103. Taburet AM, Katlma C, Blanshard C, et al. Pharmacokinetics of foscarnet after twice-daily administrations for treatment of cytomegalovirus disease in AIDS patients. *Antimicrob Agents Chemother* 1992;36:1821–1824.
104. Minor JR, Baltz JK. Foscarnet sodium. *DICP* 1991;25:41–47.
105. Chrisp P, Clissold SP. Foscarnet: a review of its antiviral activity, pharmacokinetic properties and therapeutic use in immunocompromised patients with cytomegalovirus retinitis. *Drugs* 1991;41:104–129.
106. Deray G, Martinez F, Katalma C, et al. Foscarnet nephrotoxicity: mechanism, incidence, and prevention. *Am J Nephrol* 1989;9:316–321.
107. Diaz-Llopis M, Chipont E, Sanchez S, España E, Navea A, Menezo JL. Intravitreal foscarnet for cytomegalovirus retinitis in a patient with acquired immunodeficiency syndrome. *Am J Ophthalmol* 1992;114:742–747.
108. DeTorres O. Focus on foscarnet: a pyrophosphate analog for use in CMV retinitis and other viral infections. *Hosp Formul* 1991;26: 929–947.
109. Sjovall J, Bergdahl S, Movin G, et al. Pharmacokinetics of foscarnet and distribution to cerebrospinal fluid after intravenous infusion in patients with human immunodeficiency virus infection. *Antimicrob Agents Chemother* 1989;33:1023–1031.
110. Walmsley SL, Chew E, Read SE, et al. Treatment of cytomegalovirus retinitis with trisodium phosphonoformate hexahydrate (foscarnet). *J Infect Dis* 1988;157:569–572.
111. Lehoang P, Girard B, Robinet M, et al. Foscarnet in the treatment of cytomegalovirus retinitis in acquired immune deficiency syndrome. *Ophthalmology* 1989;96:865–874.
112. Deray G, Caroub P, Lehoang P, et al. Foscarnet-induced acute renal failure and effectiveness of hemodialysis [Letter]. *Lancet* 1987; 2:216.
113. MacGregor RR, Graziani AL, Weiss R, et al. Successful foscarnet therapy for cytomegalovirus retinitis in an AIDS patient undergoing hemodialysis: rationale for empiric dosing and plasma level monitoring. *J Infect Dis* 1991;164:785–787.
114. Jacobson MA, O'Donnell JJ, Mills J. Foscarnet treatment of cytomegalovirus retinitis in patients with the acquired immunodeficiency syndrome. *Antimicrob Agents Chemother* 1989;33:736–741.
115. Fanning MM, Read SE, Benson M, et al. Foscarnet therapy of cytomegalovirus retinitis in AIDS. *J Acquir Immune Defic Syndr Hum Retrovirol* 1990;3:472–479.
116. Farthing CF, Dalgleish AG, Clark A, et al. Phosphonoformate (foscarnet): a pilot study in AIDS and AIDS related complex. *AIDS* 1987;1:21–25.
117. Gearhart MO, Sorg TB. Foscarnet-induced severe hypomagnesemia and other electrolyte disorders. *Ann Pharmacother* 1993;27:285–289.
118. Connoly GM, Gazzard BG, Hawkins DA. Fixed drug eruption due to foscarnet. *Genitourin Med* 1990;66:97–98.
119. Fegueux S, Salmon D, Picard C, et al. Penile ulcerations with foscarnet [Letter]. *Lancet* 1990;335:547.
120. Van Der Pijl JW, Frissen PHJ, Reiss P, et al. Foscarnet and penile ulceration [Letter]. *Lancet* 1990;1:286.
121. Jacobson MA. Review of the toxicities of foscarnet. *J Acquir Immune Defic Syndr Hum Retrovirol* 1992;5:S11–S17.
122. Brown DL, Sather S, Cheitlin MD. Reversible cardiac dysfunction associated with foscarnet therapy for cytomegalovirus esophagitis in an AIDS patient. *Am Heart J* 1993;125:1439–1441.
123. Youle MS, Clarbour J, Gazzard B, Chanas A. Severe hypocalcemia in AIDS patients treated with foscarnet and pentamidine. *Lancet* 1988;1:1455–1456.

124. Palestine AG, Polis MA, De Smet MD, et al. A randomized, controlled trial of foscarnet in the treatment of cytomegalovirus retinitis in patients with AIDS. *Ann Intern Med* 1991;115:665–673.
125. Jacobson MA, Causey D, Polsky B, et al. Dose-ranging study of daily maintenance intravenous foscarnet therapy for cytomegalovirus retinitis in AIDS. *J Infect Dis* 1993;168:444–448.
126. Sandstrom AG, Byington RE, Kaplan JC, Hirsch MS. Inhibition of human T-cell lymphotropic virus type III in vitro by phosphonoformate. *Lancet* 1985;1:1480–1482.
127. Jacobson MA, van der Horst C, Causey DM, Dehlinger M, Hafner R, Mills J. In vivo additive antiretroviral effect of combined zidovudine and foscarnet therapy for human immunodeficiency virus infection (ACTG Protocol 053). *J Infect Dis* 1991;163:1219–1222.
128. Stanat SC, Reardon JE, Erice A, Jordan MC, Drew WL, Biron KK. Ganciclovir-resistant cytomegalovirus clinical isolates: mode of resistance to ganciclovir. *Antimicrob Agents Chemother* 1991;35:2191–2197.
129. Sullivan V, Coen DM. Isolation of foscarnet-resistant human cytomegalovirus patterns of resistance and sensitivity to other antiviral drugs. *J Infect Dis* 1991;164:781–784.
130. Drew WL, Miner RC, Bush DF, et al. Prevalence of resistance in patients receiving ganciclovir for serious cytomegalovirus infection. *J Infect Dis* 1991;163:716–719.
131. Jacobson MA, Drew WL, Feinberg J, et al. Foscarnet therapy for ganciclovir-resistant cytomegalovirus retinitis in patients with AIDS. *J Infect Dis* 1991;163:1348–1351.
132. Manischewitz JF, Quinnan GV, Lane HC, Wittek AE. Synergistic effect of ganciclovir and foscarnet of cytomegalovirus replication in vitro. *Antimicrob Agents Chemother* 1990;34:373–375.
133. Freitas VR, Fraser-Smith EB, Matthews TR. Increased efficacy of ganciclovir in combination with foscarnet against cytomegalovirus and herpes simplex virus type 2 in vitro and in vivo. *Antiviral Res* 1989;12:205–212.
134. Knox K, Drobyski W, Carrigan D. Cytomegalovirus isolate resistant to ganciclovir and foscarnet from a marrow transplant recipient. *Lancet* 1991;337:1292.
135. Nelson MR, Barter G, Hawkins D, Gazzard BG. Simultaneous treatment of cytomegalovirus retinitis with ganciclovir and foscarnet. *Lancet* 1991;338:250.
136. Butler KM, De Smet MD, Husson RN, et al. Treatment of aggressive cytomegalovirus retinitis with ganciclovir in combination with foscarnet in a child infected with human immunodeficiency virus. *J Pediatr* 1992;120:483–486.
137. Dieterich DT, Poles MA, Lew EA, et al. Concurrent use of ganciclovir and foscarnet to treat cytomegalovirus infection in AIDS patients. *J Infect Dis* 1993;167:1184–1188.
138. Kuppermann BD, Flores-Aguilar M, Quiceno JI, Rickman LS, Freeman WR. Combination ganciclovir and foscarnet in the treatment of clinically resistant cytomegalovirus retinitis in patients with acquired immunodeficiency syndrome. *Arch Ophthalmol* 1993;111:1359–1366.
139. Weinberg DV, Murphy R, Naughton K. Combined daily therapy with intravenous ganciclovir and foscarnet for patients with recurrent cytomegalovirus retinitis. *Am J Ophthalmol* 1994;117:776–782.
140. Studies of Ocular Complications of AIDS Research Group in Collaboration with the AIDS Clinical Trials Group. Combination foscarnet and ganciclovir therapy vs monotherapy for the treatment of relapsed cytomegalovirus retinitis in patients with AIDS: the cytomegalovirus retreatment trial. *Arch Ophthalmol* 1996;114:23–33.
141. Chatterjee S, Burns P, Whitley RJ, Kern ER. Effect of (S)-1-[(3-hydroxy-2-phosphonyl methoxy)propyl]cytosine on the replication and morphogenesis of herpes simplex virus type I. *Antiviral Res* 1992;19:181–192.
142. Moore MR, Hamzeh FM, Lee FE, Lietman PS. Activity of (S)-1-(3-hydroxy-2-phosphonylmethoxypropyl)cytosine against human cytomegalovirus when administered as single-bolus dose and continuous infusion in invitro cell culture perfusion system. *Antimicrob Agents Chemother* 1994;38:2404–2408.
143. Bravo FJ, Stanberry LR, Kier AB, Vogt PE, Kern ER. Evaluation of HPMPC therapy for primary and recurrent genital herpes in mice and guinea pigs. *Antiviral Res* 1993;21:59–72.
144. Cundy KC, Petty BG, Flaherty J, et al. Clinical pharmacokinetics of cidofovir in human immunodeficiency virus-infected patients. *Antimicrob Agents Chemother* 1995;39:1247–1252.
145. Dolnak DR, Munguia D, Wiley CA, et al. Lack of retinal toxicity of the anti-cytomegalovirus drug (S)-1-(3-hydroxy-2-phosphonylmethoxypropyl)cytosine. *Invest Ophthalmol Vis Sci* 1992;33:1557–1563.
146. Kirsch LS, Arevalo JF, De Clercq E, et al. Phase I/II study of intravitreal cidofovir for the treatment of cytomegalovirus retinitis in patients with the acquired immunodeficiency syndrome. *Am J Ophthalmol* 1995;119:466–476.
147. Kirsch LS, Arevalo JF, Chavez de la Paz E, et al. Intravitreal cidofovir (HPMPC) treatment of cytomegalovirus retinitis in patients with acquired immune deficiency syndrome. *Ophthalmology* 1995;102:533–542.
148. Besen G, Flores-Aguilar M, Assil KK, et al. Long-term therapy for herpes retinitis in an animal model with high-concentrated liposome-encapsulated HPMPC. *Arch Ophthalmol* 1995;113:661–668.
149. Jacobson MA. Valaciclovir (BW256U87): the L-valyl ester of acyclovir. *J Med Virol* 1993;1(suppl):150–153.
150. Purifoy DJM, Beauchamp LM, de Miranda P, et al. Review of research leading to new anti-herpesvirus agents in clinical development: valaciclovir hydrochloride (256U, the L-valyl ester of acyclovir) and 882C, a specific agent for varicella zoster virus. *J Med Virol* 1993;1(suppl):139–145.
151. Wood MJ, McKendrick MW, Bannister B, et al. Preliminary pharmacokinetics and safety of 882C87 in patients with herpes zoster. *J Med Virol* 1993;1(suppl):154–157.
152. Jacobson MA, O'Donnell JJ, Rousell R, et al. Failure of adjunctive cytomegalovirus intravenous immune globulin to improve efficacy of ganciclovir in patients with acquired immunodeficiency syndrome and cytomegalovirus retinitis: a phase I study. *Antimicrob Agents Chemother* 1990;34:176–178.
153. Committee on Interferon Nomenclature. Interferon nomenclature. *Nature* 1980;286:110.
154. Davis GL, Hoofnagle JH. Interferon in viral hepatitis: role in pathogenesis and treatment. *Hepatology* 1986;6:1038–1041.
155. Chou S, Dylewski JS, Gaynon MW, et al. Alpha interferon administration in cytomegalovirus retinitis. *Antimicrob Agents Chemother* 1984;25:25–28.
156. El Baba FZ, Causey DM, Baruch D, et al. Combination of ganciclovir and beta-interferon for prevention of relapse of AIDS-associated cytomegalovirus retinitis: preliminary report [Abstract]. *Ophthalmology* 1989;96(suppl):112.

Textbook of Ocular Pharmacology,
edited by T.J. Zimmerman, et al.
Lippincott–Raven Publishers, Philadelphia © 1997.

CHAPTER 34

Pharmacologic Therapy for Cystoid Macular Edema

Lee M. Jampol

The retina is separated from the plasma by a barrier with restricted permeabilities. This barrier is anatomically located at the tight junctions between retinal vascular endothelial cells (the inner blood–retinal barrier) and the tight junctions between adjacent retinal pigment epithelial cells (the outer blood–retinal barrier). Normal functioning of the retina requires this barrier.

The extracellular space of the retina is normally minimal; the retina remains in a state of deturgescence because of the active transport of electrolytes and larger molecules by the pigment epithelium from the retina to the choroid. Thickening of the retina in the macular area can occur either from disruption of the blood–retinal barrier or decreased transport of fluid from the retina to the choroid. With thickening of the macula area, cystic spaces are seen opthalmoscopically, so-called cystoid macular edema (CME). A wide variety of conditions can be associated with the development of macular edema (1), many of which are listed in Table 34-1. Treatment of CME requires either stimulating transport out of the retina or diminishing the leakage of fluid into the retina and is important in restoring normal retinal function.

THERAPY FOR CYSTOID MACULAR EDEMA

The conditions noted in Table 34-1 have in common increased thickness of the retina with cystic spaces; however, the pathogenic mechanisms of these conditions vary. In circumstances where the leakage is due to abnormal retinal vascular leakage, such as diabetes mellitus and branch retinal vein occlusion, focal or grid-type of photocoagulation is often of benefit. Some of the effect of this treatment may be due to a closure of the abnormal leaking vessels, but most clinicians believe the photocoagulation also affects the pigment epithelium, somehow improving its transport function and thereby contributing to a clearing of the retinal edema. Photocoagulation also has been used in some patients with central retinal vein occlusion, retinitis pigmentosa, radiation retinopathy, Von Hippel's disease, Coats' disease, macroaneurysm, and parafoveal telangiectasia. Disruption of the outer blood–retinal barrier by underlying choroidal diseases, such as choroidal tumors (e.g., hemangioma or melanoma) can cause CME. Therapy for the underlying tumor can improve the macular edema. In patients with choroidal neovascularization (secondary to age-related macular degeneration and other diseases) and CME, closure of the abnormal choroidal vessels by photocoagulation is of benefit.

In other circumstances, treatment of underlying systemic or ocular conditions can improve cystoid macular edema. Examples include hypertension (treatment-lowering blood pressure), epinephrine maculopathy (treatment is discontinuation of the medication), and epiretinal membranes (treatment is surgical removal of abnormal tissue).

In many patients, the increased permeability of the blood–retinal barrier is secondary to inflammation. Examples include pseudophakic or aphakic cystoid macular edema, uveitis, and CME following retinal detachment of vitreous surgery. In these circumstances, the mainstay of therapy has been antiinflammatory therapies, including corticosteroids and nonsteroidal antiinflammatory drugs (NSAIDs). In addition, carbonic anhydrase inhibitors have been reported to be of benefit for patients with retinitis pigmentosa, Irvine-Gass syndrome, and perhaps in other circumstances. In this chapter, we review the use of NSAIDs, corticosteroids, other antiinflammatory drugs, oxygen, and carbonic anhydrase inhibitors in the therapy for CME.

L. M. Jampol: Department of Ophthalmology, Northwestern University Medical School, Chicago, Illinois 60611.

TABLE 34-1. *Macular edema*

Cause of macular edema	Site of disruption of barrier	Treatment
Diabetes mellitus	I, ?O	Focal, grid photocoagulation
Branch retinal vein occlusion	I	Grid photocoagulation
Central retinal vein occlusion	I	None proven, ?photocoagulation, ?corticosteroids
Aphakic, pseudophakic CME	I	Corticosteroids, nonsteroidal drugs, CAI
Hypertension	I	Control of blood pressure
Retinitis pigmentosa	I, O	?Grid photocoagulation, CAI
Uveitis	I, O?	Antiinflammatory drugs, CAI
Radiation retinopathy	I	?Photocoagulation
Von Hippel's disease, Coats' disease, macroaneurysm	I	Photocoagulation, cryopexy
Parafoveal telangiectasia	I, O?	None proven, ?photocoagulation
Retinal detachment, vitrectomy surgery	I	?Antiinflammatory drugs, ?CAI
Epinephrine	I	Discontinue medication
Autosomal dominant CME	I, O?	CAI
Age-related macular degeneration	O	Photocoagulation
Choroidal tumors	O	Treatment of tumor
Epiretinal membranes	I	Surgery, ?CAI

From Jampol and Po, ref 1, with permission.
CME, cystoid macular edema; I, inner blood–retinal barrier; O, outer blood–retinal barrier; CAI, carbonic anhydrase inhibitor.

Nonsteroidal Antiinflammatory Drugs

The NSAIDs comprise a variety of compounds that inhibit the synthesis of prostaglandins, primarily through the inhibition of the cyclooxygenase pathway (Figure 34-1). (Other noncorticosteroid antiinflammatory agents will be reviewed subsequently.) A number of NSAIDs have been introduced for clinical use. Some of these compounds are listed in Table 34-2. Prostaglandins are 20-carbon metabolites of arachidonic acid that are biosynthesized by the ocular tissues and are involved in human ocular inflammation. Prostaglandins can be released in response to ocular

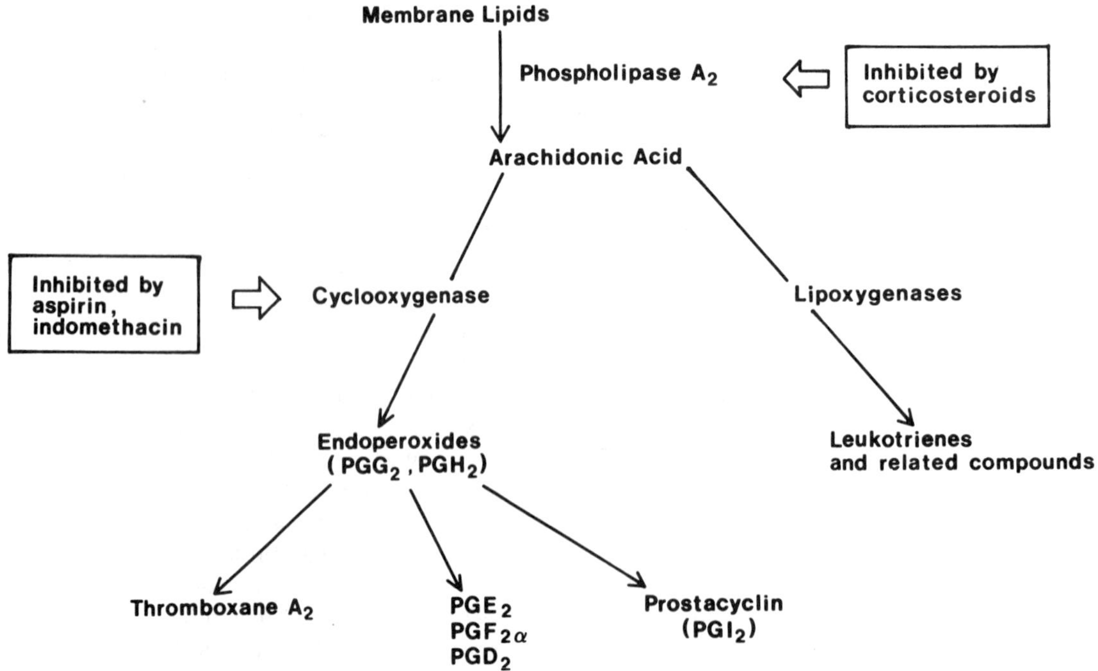

Fig. 34-1. Pathways of synthesis of prostaglandins (PG) and related compounds. From *Ophthalmology* 1982;89:894, with permission of the American Academy of Ophthalmology.

TABLE 34-2. *Nonsteroidal agents*

Phenylalkanoic acids
Ibuprofen (Motrin, Rufen, Advil, Nuprin, others)
Naproxen (Naprosyn)
Naproxen sodium (Anaprox)
Oxaprozin (Daypro)
Fenoprofen (Nalfon)
Ketoprofen (Orudis)
Flurbiprofen (Ocufen)
Suprofen (Profenal)
Ketorolac tromethamine (Acular, Toradol)
Salicylates
Aspirin
Diflunisal (Dolobid)
Salsalate
Acetic acids
Indomethacin (Indocin)
Diclofenac sodium (Voltaren)
Tolmetin (Tolectin)
Sulindac (Clinoril)
Fenamic acids
Mefenamic acid (Ponstel)
Meclofenamic acid (Meclomen)
Enolic acids
phenylbutazone (Butazolodin, Azolid)
piroxicam (Feldene)

trauma, ocular surgery, or other forms of ocular inflammation, including uveitis. Prostaglandins may contribute to disruption of the blood–aqueous barrier, miosis, and the development of CME. Largely because of their inhibition of the synthesis of prostaglandins, NSAIDs are effective in treating human ocular inflammation. Some of these compounds (e.g., diclofenac sodium) may also have an inhibitory effect on the lipoxygenase pathway (see Figure 34-1). This pathway, another major pathway of arachidonic acid metabolism, is being studied in hopes of developing inhibitors that may also be antiinflammatory. NSAIDs can be used systemically or topically.

Systemic NSAIDs

Before topical NSAIDs were available as therapy for CME, attempts were made to use systemic medications, including indomethacin. Systemic NSAIDs have significant toxicity with chronic use. Upper gastrointestinal bleeding, ulceration, and perforation can occur, sometimes without warning. Dyspepsia, nausea, vomiting, and constipation have been reported. Systemic NSAIDs also decrease the synthesis of renal prostaglandins, which can result in a decrease in renal blood flow with fluid retention and renal failure. These agents can also cause an allergic interstitial nephritis and nephrotic syndrome, which are reversible on discontinuation.

Rarely, NSAIDs can precipitate asthma or an anaphylactoid reaction in patients who are sensitive to aspirin. The effects of most NSAIDs on bleeding are less than those of aspirin, but platelet function can be affected, resulting in increased bleeding with ocular surgery or trauma. Other potential adverse effects include hepatotoxicity, central nervous systemic effects, hematologic toxicity, and skin reactions.

Topical NSAIDs

Because of the excellent penetration of newly developed topical NSAIDs, it is likely that systemic therapy will now be rarely used. New topical formulations, including flurbiprofen sodium, suprofen, ketorolac tromethamine, and diclofenac sodium, have been used to treat scleritis, uveitis, and postcataract inflammation (2). They can produce measurable levels of drug in the aqueous humor following topical administration with low or undetectable plasma levels. They may prevent miosis during intraocular surgery, treat external allergies causing itching, and be effective for the prophylaxis or treatment of cystoid macular edema, especially following cataract surgery. Flach reviewed the uses of these compounds for eye disease, including CME therapy (2). The U.S. Food and Drug Administration (FDA) approved the use of several topical NSAIDs in ophthalmology. So far, these approvals have been limited to specific indications. Flurbiprofen sodium and suprofen have been approved only for the prophylaxis of surgical miosis; ketorolac tromethamine, for the relief of itching due to occasional allergic conjunctivitis and recently for the treatment of postcataract surgery inflammation; and diclofenac sodium, for the treatment of postcataract inflammation and recently for photophobia after refractive surgery. Studies with several NSAIDs to date, however, have shown considerable benefit for the prophylaxis and therapy for CME (2).

The earliest studies of postcataract CME concentrated on the use of topical indomethacin and occasionally other compounds. Well-controlled, randomized prophylactic studies demonstrated that topical indomethacin was effective in diminishing the rate of angiographic CME after cataract surgery. This work was reported by several major groups, including Miyaki in Japan (3), Yannuzzi and coworkers in New York (4), and Kraff et al. in Chicago (5). A stable, comfortable, and safe topical formulation of indomethacin was never widely available. In addition, any extended benefit (> 6 months) of this therapy for postcataract cystoid macular edema was never demonstrated. Long-term studies did not demonstrate either an improvement in visual acuity in treated eyes or a sustained (> 6 months) decrease in the angiographic CME. As a result, to date, the FDA has not approved the use of topical NSAIDs for the prophylaxis (or treatment) of CME.

Chronic, visually significant CME probably occurs in only about 1% to 2% of patients who undergo cataract surgery (6,7), representing, however, more than 10,000 patients annually in the United States. Angiographic CME may be present in ≥20% of patients who undergo planned extracapsular cataract extraction or phakoemulsification (6–8). It is therefore much easier to prove the benefit of these agents by using angiographic CME as an endpoint than by using visual acuity, especially visual acuity at 6 months or later. Usually, it cannot be predicted preoperatively which patients will develop CME; consequently, prophylaxis of large numbers of patients with topical agents is in general not being done. Even if CME does develop, it will usually resolve, and the long-term visual outcome is usually excellent.

Perhaps a better strategy than universal prophylaxis is the use of NSAIDs for the treatment of CME once it develops (9–11). Two prospective, masked, placebo-controlled randomized studies performed by Flach and co-workers demonstrated improvement in visual acuity of eyes with visually significant, long-standing, CME postcataract surgery that was treated with topical ketorolac tromethamine (9,10); however, these studies did not attempt to demonstrate benefit beyond 120 days after initiation of treatment. Topical ketorolac tromethamine is thus effective for the treatment of CME as judged by the benefit up to 120 days. No similar randomized trials with comparison to either NSAIDs or placebo have been performed with corticosteroids.

Ketorolac Tromethamine 0.5% (Acular)

Ketorolac tromethamine has significant analgesic, anti-inflammatory, and antipyretic activities. One of its current primary uses is as an analgesic agent following surgery. Parenteral or oral ketorolac tromethamine is administered as Toradol. Topical ketorolac tromethamine (Acular) has been used as an analgesic after refractive surgery with excimer laser. The mechanism of action of ketorolac tromethamine is thought to be due at least in part to its ability to inhibit prostaglandin synthesis. So far, topical ketorolac tromethamine has been approved by the FDA for the treatment of ocular itching caused by seasonal allergies and for the treatment of postcataract surgery inflammation. Studies have suggested that it also has benefit for both the prophylaxis and the treatment of postcataract cystoid macular edema (2,9,10). It also stabilizes the blood–aqueous barrier after cataract surgery (12,13). Ketorolac tromethamine is supplied as a sterilized isotonic (0.5%) aqueous solution with a pH of 7.4. Its osmolality is 290 mOsmol/kg. Studies have shown that in rabbits topical ketorolac tromethamine can prevent increased ocular pressure induced by topically applied arachidonic acid. Limited studies suggest that it does not enhance the spread of ocular infections by fungi or bacteria, but additional work is needed in this area. Adverse effects from the topical use of ketorolac tromethamine have been stinging and burning on instillation. Side effects include occasional superficial punctate keratitis. The usual recommended dosage for ketorolac tromethamine ophthalmic solution for the treatment of itching is one drop four times a day. In studies of CME, a similar dosage was used. Measurable levels of ketorolac tromethamine appear in most eyes in the aqueous humor following topical administration. Low levels are also detectable in the plasma in some patients.

Diclofenac Sodium 0.1% Ophthalmic Solution (Voltaren)

Diclofenac sodium is an NSAID that is available as a topical ophthalmic solution. Its pH is about 7.2 and its osmolality about 300 mOsmol/kg. The solution has a mild odor of castor oil.

The main action of diclofenac sodium, a phenylacetic acid, is probably inhibition of prostaglandin synthesis, which it does in a somewhat different manner from most NSAIDs. It reduces the intracellular level of free arachidonic acid by stimulating its incorporation into triglycerides, thereby reducing the formation of products of both the cyclooxygenase and lipoxygenase pathways. The significance for ocular inflammation is as yet uncertain. To date, studies have not indicated an effect on intraocular pressure following cataract surgery. Its effect on wound healing remains to be elucidated. To date, most published studies on diclofenac sodium have concentrated on its effect on postcataract inflammation (2,14). Diclofenac sodium was more effective than topical prednisolone in protecting or reestablishing the blood–aqueous barrier after cataract surgery, as measured by fluorophotometry (14). The dosage in most studies has been one drop four times a day for 2 or more weeks following cataract surgery.

Patients who wear soft contact lenses and use diclofenac sodium may complain of an ocular irritation, redness, and burning. Tearing, burning, and stinging have been reported in 15% of patients treated with topical diclofenac sodium. In postcataract studies, keratitis developed in 28% of patients. Its effect on intraocular pressure after surgery is uncertain. Systemic absorption is limited. Plasma levels following topical administration are <10 ng/ml over a 4-hour period. However, exacerbation of asthma from topical diclofenac sodium has been reported.

Other NSAIDs

Flurbiprofen sodium 0.03% (available as Ocufen) and suprofen 1% (Profenal) are cyclooxygenase inhibitors that have been approved by the FDA for the prevention of surgical miosis. Studies have demonstrated that the instillation of these medications before cataract surgery results in a larger pupil both during and after the procedure.

Studies have also been performed using flurbiprofen sodium for the prophylaxis of postcataract cystoid macular edema and visual loss from CME, although the results have not been published in peer-reviewed journals as yet. A beneficial effect was found.

Side Effects and Penetration

The availability of a variety of topical NSAIDs, many of which have been used to treat CME, requires a careful examination of their possible adverse effects. To date, however, there is little literature on most of these topics.

1. Do topical NSAIDs significantly affect wound healing? There is presently very little objective data on this issue.
2. Do topical NSAIDs reactivate or worsen herpes simplex or fungal keratitis? Again, definitive studies are awaited.
3. Does clinical use of NSAIDs affect intraocular pressure? To date, clinical studies indicate no evidence of a pressure-raising effect similar to that seen with corticosteroids; but, again, trials have been limited.
4. Do topical NSAIDs affect platelet function in the eye and result in an increased risk of bleeding? It is unclear whether ocular surgical or trauma patients might have an increased risk of bleeding following the use of topical NSAIDs.

The use of topical NSAID therapy for CME after cataract surgery is being investigated, but the exact target site of the therapy is unclear. It may be that the prostaglandins are synthesized primarily by the uvea (the iris-ciliary body), although a role for retinal synthesis has not been ruled out. Penetration to the iris-ciliary body area with topical therapy has been demonstrated, and a therapeutic effect on preserving or reestablishing a blood-aqueous barrier has been demonstrated. Whether topical NSAIDs can penetrate to the vitreous and retina to establish posterior therapeutic levels in phakic, aphakic, or pseudophakic eyes remains uncertain.

Corticosteroids

Cystoid macular edema often accompanies intraocular inflammation. In patients with pars planitis, sarcoidosis, multifocal choroiditis, HLA-B-27-positive uveitis, idiopathic retinal vasculitis, Behçet's disease and many other situations, CME may be a major cause of visual loss. Corticosteroids have potent antiinflammatory activity, and CME often improves or resolves with the use of topical, periocular, or systemic corticosteroids (see Chapter 59). Besides the obvious antiinflammatory effect of corticosteroids, they also raise the intraocular pressure in many eyes. This pressure-raising effect has been hypothesized to play a role in the beneficial effect on postcataract surgery CME (Irvine-Gass syndrome) (15). It is also logical that the combined use of corticosteroids and NSAIDs should be more potent than either class of medication alone. As shown in Figure 34-1, they should act synergistically to inhibit the synthesis of inflammatory mediators from arachidonic acid. It is interesting that, despite many randomized clinical trials of NSAIDs for CME following cataract surgery and vitreoretinal surgery, no randomized trials have compared NSAIDs and corticosteroids or placebo and corticosteroids, partially because of the accepted potent antiinflammatory effect of corticosteroids and a hesitancy not to treat eyes with CME with these drugs.

Other Antiinflammatory Drugs

In situations where corticosteroids cannot control idiopathic intraocular inflammation or are not tolerated, more potent systemic antiinflammatory drugs may be used. These drugs include cytoxan, chlorambucil, 6-mercaptopurine, methotrexate, and others. The CME in these situations often responds to control of the inflammation. These drugs may have severe toxicity (See Chapter 59) and should be used only when necessary. In the early 1980s, Nussenblatt and co-workers demonstrated that cyclosporine is an alternative drug for treatment of CME secondary to severe intraocular inflammation (16). Cyclosporine was developed to control organ rejection in organ transplant recipients. Nussenblatt reported on 16 patients unresponsive to or intolerant of corticosteroids, 15 of whom (many had intermediate uveitis) responded, and visually significant CME often improved (16). Cyclosporine does, however, have significant potential toxicity. It can cause renal impairment and hypertension. An ophthalmologist using this drug should work with a specialist physician who is familiar with its use. In a recent randomized trial, Nussenblatt compared cyclosporine to corticosteroids in 56 patients with sight-threatening noninfectious uveitis (17), many of whom had CME. The patients were treated either with 3 months of 10 to 15 mg/kg/day of oral cyclosporine or 64 mg per day of oral prednisolone. The same number of patients in each group had improved vision (13 of 28). In the cyclosporine group, seven of 15 patients showed improvement in CME versus 10 of 16 treated with prednisolone. The study concluded that systemic corticosteroids should be the first line of drugs for severe ocular inflammation (and CME) but that cyclosporine is effective if the patient does not respond or has significant corticosteroid toxicity.

Oxygen Therapy

Because of its ability to constrict retinal vessels, oxygen administration has been suggested as a possible therapy for CME secondary to a variety of conditions. Studies have investigated the effects of hyperbaric oxygen on CME following cataract surgery (18). Reports (mostly in non–peer-reviewed journals) have described a beneficial effect of oxygen on postcataract cystoid macular edema, implying at least a temporary, and perhaps a permanent, effect on the edema. To date, however, well-controlled clinical trials have not appeared in peer-reviewed journals. Oxygen can be administered to the eye through the cornea using goggles (100% oxygen) (19,20), systemically by inhalation of increased concentrations of oxygen, or using a hyperbaric chamber. The hyperbaric chamber can also augment transcorneal delivery of oxygen.

Studies of oxygen therapy for CME secondary to a branch-vein occlusion have demonstrated some benefit (21), but it is not clear whether this effect is sustained. Hyperbaric oxygen also is reported to have a therapeutic effect on CME following cataract surgery (18). Mieler (personal communication, 1993) noted a temporary benefit for CME from severe ischemic radiation retinopathy in one patient.

Carbonic Anhydrase Inhibitors and CME

In 1989 a beneficial effect of systemic administration of acetazolamide (Diamox) on CME from a wide variety of causes was reported (22). This publication suggested that the benefit was present for patients with CME secondary to disruption of the outer blood–retinal barrier (e.g., retinitis pigmentosa and uveitis) but not for patients with disruption of the inner blood–retinal barrier (e.g., diabetes mellitus). An effect of carbonic anhydrase inhibitors on CME has been confirmed by well-controlled randomized, masked clinical trials of patients with retinitis pigmentosa (23). Acetazolamide and methazolamide may produce both improvement in vision and a decrease in leakage on the fluorescein angiogram (23–25). Interestingly, the dose of acetazolamide or methazolamide required appears to be less than that usually administered for glaucoma. A therapeutic effect has been reported with a dosage as low as 25 mg of methazolamide twice a day (25). There is some suggestion that with prolonged therapy the therapeutic benefit may disappear, at least with methazolamide (25).

Acetazolamide also was reported to affect CME in a single patient with epiretinal membrane and CME (26), in a patient with serpiginous choroiditis and CME (27), and in patients with uveitis (28). In our clinical experience, a beneficial effect in some patients with macular edema from juvenile diabetes mellitus has been noted, although it is not effective in patients with extensive leakage.

The mechanism of action of acetazolamide and other carbonic anhydrase inhibitors for CME is not clear. In some animal models, acetazolamide is known to produce vasoconstriction. Another explanation is an effect on transport by the retinal pigment epithelium. Some experimental evidence suggests that acetazolamide may be effective in reversing the direction of aberrant transport across the pigment epithelium in patients with ocular inflammation.

It has been suggested that acetazolamide may play a crucial role in eyes where there is only a slight imbalance between inflow of fluid and the ability of the pigment epithelium to transport fluid out (26). By increasing somewhat the transport by the pigment epithelium, it may be possible to dehydrate retinas that otherwise would be decompensated. If this is the case, then the use of carbonic anhydrase inhibitors should be of potential benefit for diseases associated with breakdown of either the inner or outer blood–retinal barrier.

REFERENCES

1. Jampol LM, Po SM. Macular edema. In: Ryan SJ, ed. *Retina,* 2nd ed. St. Louis: CV Mosby, 1994;999–1008.
2. Flach AJ. Cyclo-oxygenase inhibitors in ophthalmology. *Surv Ophthalmol* 1992;36:259–284.
3. Miyake K, Sakamura S, Miura H. Long term follow-up study on prevention of aphakic cystoid macular edema by topical indomethacin. *Br J Ophthalmol* 1980;64:324–328.
4. Yannuzzi LA, Landau AN, Turts AI. Incidence of aphakic cystoid macular edema with the use of topical indomethacin. *Ophthalmology* 1981;88:947–954.
5. Kraff MC, Sanders DR, Jampol LM, et al. Prophylaxis of pseudophakic cystoid macular edema with topical indomethacin. *Ophthalmology* 1982;89:885–890.
6. Jampol LM. Cystoid macular edema following cataract surgery. *Arch Ophthalmol* 1988;106:894–895.
7. Jampol LM. Pharmacologic therapy of aphakic and pseudophakic cystoid macular edema: 1985, update. *Ophthalmology* 1985;92:807–810.
8. Jampol LM. Pharmacologic therapy of aphakic and pseudophakic cystoid macular edema: 1985 update. *Ophthalmology* 1985;92:807–810.
9. Flach AJ, Dolan BJ, Irvine AR. Effectiveness of ketorolac tromethamine 0.5% ophthalmic solution for chronic aphakic and pseudophakic cystoid macular edema. *Am J Ophthalmol* 1987;103: 479–486.
10. Flach AJ, Jampol LM, Weinberg D, et al. Improvement in visual acuity in chronic aphakic and pseudophakic cystoid macular edema after treatment with topical 0.5% ketorolac tromethamine. *Am J Ophthalmol* 1991;112:514–519.
11. Jampol LM, Jain S, Pudzisc B, Weinreb RN. Non-steroidal antiinflammatory drugs and cataract surgery. *Arch Ophthalmol* 1994; 112:891–893.
12. Flach AJ, Graham J, Kruger LP, et al. Quantitative assessment of postsurgical breakdown of the blood-aqueous barrier following administration of 0.5% ketorolac tromethamine solution. *Arch Ophthalmol* 1988;106:344–347.
13. Flach AJ, Kraff MC, Sanders DR, Tannenbaum L. The quantitative effect of 0.5% ketorolac tromethamine solution and 0.1% dexamethasone sodium phosphate solution on postsurgical blood-aqueous barrier. *Arch Ophthalmol* 1988;106:480–483.
14. Kraff MC, Sanders DR, McGuigan L, et al. Inhibition of blood-aqueous barrier with diclofenac: a fluorophotometric study. *Arch Ophthalmol* 1990;108:380–383.
15. Melberg NS, Olk RJ. Corticosteroid-induced ocular hypertension in the treatment of aphakic or pseudophakic cystoid macular edema. *Ophthalmology* 1993;100:164–167.
16. Nussenblatt RB, Palestine AG, Char CC. Cyclosporine: a therapy in the treatment of intraocular disease resistant to systemic corticosteroids and cytotoxic agents. *Am J Ophthalmol* 1983;96:275–282.
17. Nussenblatt RB, Palestine AG, Chen CC, et al. Randomized, double-masked study of cyclosporine compared to prednisolone in the treatment of endogeneous uveitis. *Am J Ophthalmol* 1991;112:138–146.
18. Pfoff DS, Thom SR. Preliminary report on the effect of hyperbaric oxygen on cystoid macular edema. *J Cataract Refract Surg* 1987; 13:136–140.
19. Benner JD, Xiaoping M. Locally administered hyperoxic therapy for aphakic cystoid macular edema. *Am J Ophthalmol* 1992;113:104–105.
20. Jampol LM, Orlin C, Cohn SB, et al. Hyperbaric oxygen treatment for chronic cystoid macular edema after branch retinal vein occlusion. *Am J Ophthalmol* 1983;104:301–302.
21. Ogura Y, Takahashi M, Ueno S, Honda Y. Hyperbaric oxygen treatment for chronic cystoid macular edema after branch retinal vein occlusion. *Am J Ophthalmol* 1983;104:301–302.

22. Cox SN, Hay E, Bird AC. Treatment of chronic macular edema with acetazolamide. *Arch Ophthalmol* 1988;97:1190–1995.
23. Fishman GA, Gilbert LD, Fiscella RG, et al. Acetazolamide for treatment of chronic macular edema in retinitis pigmentosa. *Arch Ophthalmol* 1989;107:1445–1452.
24. Chen JC, Fitzke FW, Bird AC. Long-term effect of acetazolamide on a patient with retinitis pigmentosa. *Invest Ophthalmol Vis Sci* 1991; 31:1914–1918.
25. Fishman GA, Glenn AM, Gilbert LD. Rebound of macular edema with continued use of methazolamide in patients with retinitis pigmentosa. *Arch Ophthalmol* 1993;111:1640–1646.
26. Marmor MF. Hypothesis concerning carbonic anhydrase treatment of cystoid macular edema: example with epiretinal membrane. *Arch Ophthalmol* 1990;108:1524–1525.
27. Steinmetz RL, Fitzke FW, Bird AC. Treatment of cystoid macular edema with acetazolamide in a patient with serpiginous choroidopathy. *Retina* 1991;11:412–415.
28. Farber MD, Lam S, Tessler HH, et al. Reduction of macular edema by acetazolamide in patients with chronic iridocyclitis: A randomized prospective crossover study. *Br J Opthalmol* 1994;78:4–7.

Textbook of Ocular Pharmacology,
edited by T.J. Zimmerman, et al.
Lippincott–Raven Publishers, Philadelphia © 1997.

CHAPTER 35

Proliferative Vitreoretinopathy: Biology and Pharmacology

Glenn J. Jaffe and P. Andrew Pearson

Proliferative vitreoretinopathy (PVR), a disorder characterized by an intraocular wound-healing response, is a potential cause of blindness. It is the leading cause of failure of retinal detachment surgery and occurs in about 5% to 7% of otherwise uncomplicated scleral buckling procedures (1). It also may occur in a particularly aggressive manner in some cases of penetrating ocular injury in which a tear has been created in the neurosensory retina. In the United States and other developed countries, retinal detachments are usually repaired soon after the onset of symptoms, and it is relatively uncommon to detect advanced PVR at the initial presentation of a primary rhegmatogenous retinal detachment. In these cases, PVR typically develops approximately 6 weeks after the surgical procedure. In underdeveloped countries, however, in which primary rhegmatogenous retinal detachments may be neglected for long periods before the patient obtains ophthalmic care, it is much more common to detect advanced proliferative vitreoretinopathy in eyes that have not yet undergone surgical repair.

CELL BIOLOGY OF PROLIFERATIVE VITREORETINOPATHY

An understanding of the cell biology of proliferative vitreoretinopathy is crucial to the development of strategies to prevent or treat this disease. Proliferative vitreoretinopathy is most easily thought of as an intraocular wound-healing response. After the initial insult (retinal detachment, penetrating trauma, or surgical manipulation), there is breakdown of the blood–retinal barrier (2). Disruption of this barrier allows an influx of serum components into the vitreous cavity (3,4). Additionally, fluid in the vitreous cavity has access to the subretinal space through open breaks, where it may contact retinal pigment epithelial cells and cells in the outer retina. Early in the course of the disease, cells migrate and proliferate onto the surface and undersurface of detached retina (5). Several cell types have been implicated in the disease process on the basis of histopathologic and immunohistochemical analysis of preretinal and subretinal membranes from patients with PVR (6–10). Retinal pigment epithelial cells are a key cell type identified in these membranes. Glial cells, cells resembling fibroblasts, monocytes, and T lymphocytes also have been observed. Proliferative vitreoretinopathy differs somewhat from wound healing in other parts of the body; neovascularization, normally found in granulation tissue, is not a prominent component of PVR membranes, and, unlike other forms of wound healing, an early neutrophil influx is not a prominent feature. An extracellular matrix is produced by cells within the membranes. A variety of matrix molecules have been identified, including collagen (6), fibronectin (11), laminin (6), thrombospondin (12), vitronectin (13), and tenascin (14). Together, these components form the fibrocellular tissue constituting epiretinal and subretinal membranes. Cell-mediated contraction of these membranes may lead to traction retinal detachment or may produce or reopen retinal tears, producing a detachment with combined traction and rhegmatogenous components. Ultimately, this detachment may lead to loss of vision.

There is increasing evidence that cytokines are involved in the pathogenesis of proliferative vitreoretinopathy. Typically, cytokines are small peptides with multiple biological effects. They are potent and, as such, are often biologically active at low concentrations. They may exert their effect locally by autocrine or paracrine control mechanisms or may travel via the bloodstream to reach their effector site(s). Cytokines comprise a wide variety of peptides, in-

G. J. Jaffe and P. A. Pearson: Department of Ophthalmology, Duke University, Durham, North Carolina 27710.

cluding proteins typically thought of as growth factors, such as acidic and basic fibroblast growth factor (aFGF, bFGF), epidermal growth factor (EGF), platelet-derived growth factor (PDGF), and insulin-like growth factor (IGF); they also include interleukins, tumor necrosis factor α (TNF-α), colony stimulating factors, transforming growth factor β (TGF-β) and others. There are several lines of evidence implicating cytokines in PVR. Many cytokines are secreted by key cell types involved in the disease process. For example, the retinal pigment epithelial cell produces TGF-β (15), macrophage colony stimulating factor (M-CSF) (16), interleukin-1 (IL-1) (17), IL-6 (18,19), IL-8 (20), acidic and basic FGF (21), monocyte chemotactic and activating factor/monocyte chemoattractant protein (MCAF/MCP) (22), and melanoma growth stimulating activity/gro (MGSA/gro) (23). Increased levels of IL-6, IL-1, TNF-α, TGF-β, M-CSF, and MCAF/MCP are found in the vitreous cavity of patients with PVR (24–27). Acidic and basic FGF, PDGF, EGF, and IL-1 are found in epiretinal membranes and cells from the eyes of patients with PVR (28–34). Proliferative vitreoretinopathy can be induced in animal models by injection of specific cytokines. For example, coinjection of TGF-β and fibronectin can induce PVR in a rabbit model (24). Cytokines can influence virtually all aspects of the wound-healing response in PVR, including the migration and proliferation of cells and the production and breakdown of collagen and other extracellular matrix components. Recently, cytokines have been shown to influence cell-mediated contraction of collagenous matrices (35).

MODELS OF PROLIFERATIVE VITREORETINOPATHY

Several models have been developed to evaluate the efficacy of potentially useful drugs in the management of PVR. Both in vitro assays and animal models have been described. Each model has potential advantages and disadvantages, and ideally the agent should be tested using several different models before initiating clinical trials.

In Vitro Models

In vitro assays are useful for several reasons. It is possible to assess specific aspects of the wound-healing response, for example, proliferation or migration of cells in isolation. In vitro models are generally less expensive than animal models and provide useful baseline data regarding the toxicity and efficacy of the drug. This information then can be used to plan in vivo experiments more efficiently to minimize the number of animals used and to maximize the information obtained. In vitro assays are extremely useful in the initial evaluation of a therapeutic agent; however, they have several important limitations. Because a specific response is usually evaluated in isolation from other responses, and because the cells are not present in a milieu identical to that of PVR, results obtained using in vitro assays may not be a true reflection of the efficacy of a drug in vivo.

Cell proliferation assays are used to study the antiproliferative activity of a drug. Different cell types can be used for these assays. Generally, cells involved in the pathogenesis of PVR are chosen. Typically, these experiments have been performed using cultured retinal-pigment epithelial cells or cultured fibroblasts. Cell proliferation is usually assayed in one of two ways. Drug is added to cells grown on a two-dimensional support or in a three-dimensional matrix in wells of replicate plates for varying durations and at varying concentrations. To measure cell proliferation directly, cells are counted at varying times after the drug is added. Usually, these assays are conducted over a period of several days (36,37). Cell proliferation also can be measured indirectly using tritiated thymidine incorporation assays. Tritiated thymidine is incorporated in the cell during the S phase of the cell cycle. During this phase, DNA is synthesized, and the degree of tritiated thymidine incorporation is a measure of cell proliferation. Tritiated thymidine incorporation is generally measured over a period of 6 to 24 hours (38,39). Other in vitro assays assess the effect of the drug on protein synthesis. For example, uptake of tritiated leucine can be used as a measure of protein synthesis. Cell migration, another important component of the wound-healing response, can be measured using in vitro assay systems. To determine the effect of a drug on cell migration, a chemotactic stimulus is applied and the directed migration of cells is measured in the presence and absence of varying concentration of drug (40). Gel contraction assays are used to mimic cell-mediated contraction of fibrocellular scars occurring on the surface and undersurface of the retina in PVR. For these assays, cells are seeded in a three-dimensional matrix. Cells such as retinal pigment epithelial cells, retinal glial cells, or fibroblasts will contract the collagenous matrix (35,41,42). The ability of cells to contract the matrix can be determined in the presence and absence of drug.

In Vivo Models

Several animal models have been used to evaluate the efficacy, toxicity, and pharmacokinetics of drugs that are potentially useful in the treatment of PVR. The ideal animal model would closely resemble human PVR. Additionally, the drug effect should be similar in the animal model and human disease. Furthermore, it should be possible to produce PVR reproducibly in a high percentage of untreated eyes so that differences between treated and untreated eyes can be identified readily. Currently, there is no animal model that completely fulfills these criteria; therefore, available models represent a compromise between what is optimal and what is practical.

Rabbit models of PVR have been used most commonly as a means of evaluating the effect of various drugs. There are several advantages to using rabbits: The eye is large, and it is therefore relatively easy to perform surgical procedures on it. Rabbits are easy to handle and are much less expensive than primates; however, rabbit eyes differ anatomically from human eyes in several important respects. The blood vessels are confined to the region of the medullary ray, and the retina is not vascularized in other regions. There is no true macula in the rabbit, and the rabbit vitreous is more firmly adherent to the retina in regions other than the optic nerve than is human vitreous. Furthermore, there is some evidence that rabbit eyes may be more susceptible to drug toxicity than human eyes (41). This last point may not actually be a disadvantage, as a drug that produced no toxicity in the rabbit eye might be even less likely to do so in humans. The mechanism of drug clearance may differ in the rabbit eye compared with the human eye. Therefore, pharmacokinetic studies performed in the rabbit will only be an approximation to pharmacokinetics in the human. Most rabbit models of PVR are actually models of angiogenesis and epiretinal membrane formation. In particular, neovascularization is frequently observed in association with epiretinal membrane formation along the medullary ray. Because proliferative vitreoretinopathy in humans usually does not include a significant neovascular component, this feature is an important difference between rabbit models of PVR and human PVR.

With these caveats in mind, several models of PVR have been developed in the rabbit. An eye with intact vitreous or an eye that has undergone a vitrectomy can be used to create the animal model. The intact vitreous model simulates PVR that occurs after a rhegmatogenous retinal detachment (43,44); however, the vitrectomized model more closely simulates human PVR that occurs following vitrectomy surgery (45). The distinction between the two models is important when interpreting the results of drug studies performed in rabbit eyes. In general, it has been more difficult to inhibit pharmacologically PVR in the vitrectomized model (46). The most commonly used rabbit models of PVR involve injection of cells into the vitreous cavity. Proliferative vitreoretinopathy can be created with any of several different types of cells, including human and bovine retinal pigment epithelial cells (47), macrophages (48), rabbit (43,45,46,49), and rabbit corneal fibroblasts (50). Recently, a model of PVR was created by injecting monocytes in conjunction with the creation of a transscleral incision (51). Proliferative vitreoretinopathy can also be created by injecting cytokines into the vitreous cavity. For example, it can be created in the rabbit by coinjection of TGF or PDGF with fibronectin (24,52). Basic FGF has also been used to create PVR in a rabbit model (53). Injection of platelet-rich plasma in conjunction with cryopexy and vitrectomy leads to epiretinal membrane formation in the rabbit (54). Similarly, when gas injection is combined with the creation of a large retinal hole, PVR results (55). Finally, Zymosan has been injected to create a rabbit model of proliferative vitreoretinopathy (56).

Studies of drug toxicity complement studies of the efficacy of the drug in models of PVR. Typically, these studies have been conducted in normal rabbit eyes because it is difficult to distinguish between the effects of the disease process from possible toxic effects if toxicity were to be assessed in an eye in which proliferative vitreoretinopathy had been produced. This point must be kept in mind when interpreting the results of toxicity studies; it is possible that a given drug may be more toxic to the eye when administered in the presence of a retinal detachment or retinal hole and associated proliferating cells compared with an intact eye.

Generally, several parameters are used to evaluate retinal toxicity. Clinically, toxicity may be manifested by anterior segment or posterior segment inflammation, retinal edema, retinal necrosis, or retinal detachment. Electroretinography is a useful adjunct to the clinical evaluation of toxicity. When interpreting electroretinographic studies in the rabbit, significant variability among rabbit eyes should be accounted for. Because of this variability, it is common practice to compare the drug-treated eye to the sham-treated fellow eye. Because of eye-to-eye variability, subtle electroretinographic evidence of retinal toxicity may be impossible to identify. Finally, histopathologic analysis also is frequently used in combination with clinical evaluation and electroretinography to assess drug toxicity. Often, these studies may be confounded by artifacts of histologic specimen preparation, rendering it difficult to identify true toxicity.

SURGICAL TREATMENT OF PROLIFERATIVE VITREORETINOPATHY

Currently, PVR is managed with vitreoretinal surgery. Surgery is undertaken to remove preretinal and occasionally subretinal membranes to release traction on the retina to allow retinal reattachment. Using current techniques, this type of surgery is generally successful in the repair of primary PVR, and recent reports suggest that up to 90% of patients in this group will have a favorable outcome (57). For patients who have suffered ocular injuries and have subsequently developed PVR, however, or in eyes in which regrowth of fibrocellular membranes has occurred after initial surgery to repair retinal detachment complicated by PVR, the success rate is much worse (57–59). It is likely that we are approaching the limits of what we can accomplish mechanically with vitreoretinal surgical intervention. Further advances will require adjunctive forms of therapy specifically designed to address the underlying disease pathogenesis. With these concepts in mind, we now turn to a discussion of the pharmacologic management of proliferative vitreoretinopathy.

SPECIFIC DRUGS USED IN THE TREATMENT OF PROLIFERATIVE VITREORETINOPATHY

For most of the drugs to be discussed, efficacy, toxicity, and pharmacokinetics have been evaluated using in vitro and in vivo animal models. To date, only a handful of drugs have been tested in humans. An ideal agent would inhibit the pathologic processes contributing to the wound-healing response in PVR but would not affect normal cell functions. An optimal agent would have favorable pharmacokinetics; that is, it would remain in the eye and exert its effect over a time course sufficient to inhibit the disease process and would not be cleared from the eye before exerting this effect. As a corollary, a drug that is cleared from the eye before it has a chance to exert its effect may require multiple dosages to maintain adequate levels. Ideally, it should be possible to deliver the drug in a safe manner and one that does not incur significant systemic side effects. In addition to the choice of specific drug, several different drug-delivery methods have been developed in an attempt to achieve these goals.

Minoxidil

Mechanism of Action

Minoxidil is a drug used to treat refractory hypertension. A piperidinopyrimidine derivative, minoxidil has gained recent notoriety for its ability to stimulate hair growth. Recently, it was shown that minoxidil inhibits the proliferation of cultured dermal fibroblasts (60). The exact mechanism by which the antiproliferative effect occurs is not known; however, there are data to support the notion that it is mediated by the conversion of minoxidil to minoxidil sulfate by an enzyme termed *minoxidil sulfotransferase* (61). For example, minoxidil sulfate is significantly more potent than the parent compound. Furthermore, minoxidil derivatives that are not converted to the sulfated form are ineffective antimitogenic agents.

Minoxidil also inhibits the production of lysyl hydroxylase, a posttranslational modifying enzyme involved in the cross-linking of collagen (60). Collagen fibers devoid of hydroxy lysine-derived cross-links are unstable and thus cannot provide adequate tensile strength to tissue. Inhibition of lysyl hydroxylase occurs, at least in part, on a transcriptional level; minoxidil inhibits expression of lysyl hydroxylase mRNA (62). Although minoxidil inhibits cell proliferation and collagen cross-linking, potentially beneficial effects in the treatment of PVR, as will be discussed, it also has unwanted side effects, including hirsutism and hypotension.

In addition to the inhibitory effect of minoxidil on dermal fibroblasts described above, the antiproliferative effect of minoxidil also has been studied on human retinal pigment epithelial (RPE) cells and human Tenon's fibroblasts. Minoxidil exerted a dose- and time-dependent inhibition of proliferation, assayed by cell counting and tritiated thymidine incorporation in RPE cells and by cell counting in human Tenon's fibroblasts (63). The antiproliferative effect persisted even after minoxidil was removed from the culture medium.

Minoxidil was an effective antiproliferative agent for actively proliferating cells, but it did not inhibit proliferation of density-arrested confluent cells in culture. The differential effect of minoxidil on proliferating versus nondividing cells would be advantageous in the treatment of PVR. It has been proposed that this differential effect is the result of higher concentrations of minoxidil sulfotransferase in actively proliferating cells compared with their nondividing counterparts (64).

Minoxidil effectively inhibited lysyl hydroxylase activity in human RPE (63). In PVR, the tensile strength of epiretinal membranes contributes to tractional forces sufficient to detach the retina. It has been hypothesized that inhibition of lysyl hydroxylase, in turn, would decrease the tensile strength of epiretinal membranes by destablilizing collagen cross-links. This effect would be beneficial in the treatment of PVR because epiretinal membranes with low tensile strength would exert less traction on the retina, thereby decreasing the tendency for retinal detachment.

Minoxidil is a less potent antiproliferative agent than some of the other drugs discussed in this chapter. The half maximal effect (ED_{50}) is 1.5 mM and 2.5 mM on RPE cells and human Tenon's fibroblasts, respectively. In contrast, several other agents described in this chapter are effective in the nanomolar or micromolar range. Recently, the antiproliferative effect of two minoxidil derivatives, 5-hydroxy minoxidil and 3-hydroxy minoxidil, was evaluated (65). These derivatives were significantly more potent than the parent compound and have the potential for fewer side effects. Neither of the derivatives causes systemic hypotension, a potentially harmful side effect. Like minoxidil, each of these agents exerted a selective inhibitory effect on proliferating cells and not on density-arrested cells. Together with the decreased side effects, the selectivity of these agents could further widen the therapeutic index. Although minoxidil and its derivatives are promising antiproliferative agents, to date, results of animal studies and human trials have not yet been reported.

Immunotoxins

Immunotoxins contain monoclonal antibodies directed against a specific antigenic determinant on the target cell. The monoclonal antibody can be linked to a toxin, drug, or radioactive molecule to achieve selective inhibition of the cell population of interest. One immunotoxin, directed against human transferrin receptors, has been tested as an antiproliferative agent on human RPE cells. This immunotoxin is composed of a monoclonal antibody that specifically recognizes human transferrin receptors (but not transferrin receptors from other species) conjugated to a ribosomal inhibitor, ricin A chain. Ricin is a plant toxin composed of A and B chains. The ricin A chain does not exert its toxic effect until it is internalized by the cell, a process facilitated by the B chain. In the absence of its natural carrier B chain, ricin A chain does not have facilitated access to the cell interior. By coupling recombinant ricin A chain to an antitransferrin receptor monoclonal antibody, recombinant ricin A chain gains access to the cell cytoplasm by way of the transferrin receptor. The transferrin receptor, the primary target of this drug, is present on several cells implicated in PVR. Transferrin receptors have been identified on epiretinal membranes removed from patients with PVR, on cells obtained from the vitreous and subretinal fluid from patients with PVR, and on RPE cells (66). Initially, it was demonstrated that the antitransferrin receptor immunotoxin inhibited actively proliferating corneal endothelial cells, but it did not inhibit nonproliferating cells (67). This selective activity, together with the presence of the transferrin receptor on the target cells involved in the disease process, led to the rationale for testing this agent using in vitro and in vivo models of PVR.

Antitransferrin receptor immunotoxin exerts a dose and time-dependent inhibition of human retinal pigment epithelial cells (36,38). This effect can be achieved with only a short treatment with immunotoxin, as significant cell killing occurs after only 5 minutes of drug exposure. Cell death begins within the first 2 days after exposure to the agent, and a sustained antiproliferative effect persists at least 1 week after the drug is removed from the medium. Relative to other agents, antitransferrin receptor immunotoxin is extremely potent. The half-maximal effect is observed at approximately 0.06 ng/ml (2.5×10^{-12} mol/L). Despite the efficacy on actively proliferating cells, the drug does not kill nondividing cells (36).

Immunotoxins have been less potent cytoxic agents in vivo than in vitro. The slow onset of action is one factor limiting their efficacy. Lysomotropic agents like monensin have been used to potentiate the effect of immunotoxins. Monensin is a carboxylic ionophore that augments the cytotoxicity of immunotoxins against proliferating cultured cells and increases the effectiveness of immunotoxins in localized malignancy (69). Accordingly, monensin was tested for its ability to potentiate the effect of antitransferrin receptor immunotoxin in proliferating human RPE cells. Monensin enhanced the potency of the immunotoxin approximately fourfold and shortened the time to onset of cell kill from 48 hours to 24 hours (70).

The antitransferrin receptor immunotoxin specifically inhibits the proliferation of human RPE cells but not RPE cells from other species. Ideally, it would be possible to test the efficacy of an antiproliferative agent in vitro and in an animal model of disease before using the agent in humans. In the most commonly used animal model of PVR, a host-cell proliferative response is induced (71). In animal models of PVR, therefore, the effectiveness of an antiproliferative drug is dependent on its ability to inhibit host cell proliferation. Appropriate in vivo investigation of the antitransferrin receptor immunotoxin is limited by the specificity of the monoclonal antibody component for human tissue. Thus, it will not be possible to obtain detailed information about the safety and efficacy of this agent using an animal model of PVR. To address this problem, a transferrin–toxin conjugate was developed. This agent is composed of rabbit transferrin linked to recombinant ricin A chain. The agent exerts its effect by binding to transferrin receptors in a manner similar to that of the antitransferrin receptor immunotoxin; however, transferrin binds much less specifically to transferrin receptors from different species. Therefore, it would be possible to test the efficacy of this drug both in vitro using human cells and in vivo using animal models of PVR. Recently, it was shown that the transferrin receptor immunotoxin, like the antitransferrin receptor immunotoxin, exerts a dose- and time-dependent antiproliferative effect on proliferating human RPE cells but not nondividing cells (72). The drug had a similar effect on rabbit dermal fibroblasts; like the antitransferrin receptor immunotoxin, the effect was potentiated by monensin.

The toxicity of the antitransferrin receptor immunotoxin and the transferrin-toxin conjugate have been evaluated in the rabbit. When the immunotoxin and transferrin-toxin conjugate were injected into the anterior chamber of rabbits, there were no clinical signs of toxicity after 30 days of follow-up (Frank Murchison and associates, unpublished results, 1990).

In pharmacokinetic studies, the clearance of immunotoxin from the vitreous cavity was biphasic (73). There was a rapid disappearance of immunotoxin during the first 24 hours and a slow clearance thereafter. After a 1000-ng injection, 85 ng/ml was measured in the vitreous cavity. The vitreous fluid from eyes treated with immunotoxin recovered at 10 minutes, 24 hours, and 96 hours killed 98%, 97% and 48% of RPE cells in culture, respectively, compared with controls. Thus, the immunotoxin is cleared slowly from a gas-vitrectomized phakic eye, and the immunotoxin recovered from the vitreous cavity fluid is biologically active. Low levels of immunotoxin were present in the serum following intravitreal injection. The results of the pharmacokinetic studies indicate that following a single intravitreal injection, actively proliferating cells would be exposed to drug for several days. Coupled with the in vitro data that demonstrates a sustained effect from the drug, the results suggest that a single injection of immunotoxin should effectively inhibit cell proliferation for at least 1 or 2 weeks. Although it will not be possible to test the efficacy of the antitransferrin receptor immunotoxin using a rabbit model of PVR as described, it should be possible to do so using the transferrin-toxin conjugate. Results of these types of experiments have not yet been published.

Retinoic Acid

Retinoids, a group of compounds related to vitamin A, have an inhibitory effect on cellular proliferation (74) and have been implicated in cellular differentiation (75,76). It has been proposed that these effects are mediated through an interaction with intracellular nuclear retinoid-binding proteins and resultant modulation of gene expression (77). Retinoic acid (RA), a derivative of vitamin A, inhibits migration (78) of RPE cells and inhibits their proliferation in a density-dependent manner (79). Cells grown in the presence of 1 μM of retinoic acid maintain a contact-inhibited monolayer and demonstrate characteristics associated with the morphologic appearance of mature RPE cells in vivo. In cell culture, human RPE cells are depleted of retinoids (80). It has been suggested that depletion of RA secondary to retinal detachment may result in the morphologic and proliferative changes in the RPE that ultimately lead to PVR (81). Retinoic acid also markedly reduces the production of TGF-β (82). In the eyes of patients with PVR (24) TGF-β is increased, and it has been hypothesized that decreased levels of TGF-β, mediated by RA, would be beneficial in the treatment of PVR (83).

The efficacy of RA in PVR has been evaluated in animal models. A single intravitreal injection of RA used in conjunction with silicone oil reduces the incidence of traction retinal detachment (83). This effect was seen with doses as low as 5 μg. To prolong the intravitreal half-life, RA has been incorporated into poly(DL-lactide-co-glycolide) microspheres (84). The in vitro release of RA following incorporation in microspheres was relatively linear, with no significant early washout of the drug. These release kinetics may be attributable to the relative lipophilicity of RA compared with other drugs that have been evaluated in this type of system. Use of microsphere encapsulated RA reduced the incidence of PVR in a rabbit model by 64%.

The effect of orally administered RA in humans was investigated in a limited retrospective trial involving 21 patients (85). This study evaluated the redetachment rate (defined as detachment requiring surgical intervention) in patients operated on for PVR. Eleven of the 21 patients received RA (Accutane 40 mg orally twice a day for 4 weeks) and 10 patients served as controls. The redetachment rate was 60% in the control group and 9% in the group receiving RA. There was no difference in the incidence of macular pucker in the two groups. A randomized clinical trial is currently under way.

Colchicine

Colchicine is a phenanthrene derivative that is commonly used in the treatment of gout. Colchicine causes depolymerization of microtubules, which results in the inhibition of cellular migration, proliferation, and contraction. In vitro, colchicine inhibits RPE, astrocyte and fibroblast migration, and proliferation at doses as low as 10^{-7} M (86). In a similar study using cultured dermal fibroblasts (87), colchicine inhibited cellular migration, proliferation, and contraction at low levels (5×10^{-8}, 5×10^{-7}, 6×10^{-8} M, respectively). Contraction of collagen gels by human RPE cells has been used as a model for the inhibitory effect of colchicine. Doses of 10^{-7} M and 10^{-6} M colchicine caused near complete inhibition of gel contraction, whereas doses of 10^{-8} M had a significant, but less pronounced, effect (42). Toxicity of intravitreal colchicine has been evaluated by several investigators (88,89). Retinal atrophy occurs in monkeys after a single injection of 1 μg (90).

Intravitreally administered colchicine at doses of 1,000 nmol and 10 nmol (339 μg and 3.9 μg respectively) did not influence the development of PVR in a rabbit fibroblast model (43). The effect of oral colchicine was investigated using a rabbit model in which PVR was induced by the intravitreal injection of PDGF and fibronectin. The incidence of retinal detachment was reduced from 74% in controls to 29.6% in animals treated with about 1 mg/kg of colchicine (91). In a recent report, colchicine could not be detected in the vitreous following oral administration in rabbits (92).

Oral colchicine was evaluated in a prospective human trial involving 22 patients (93). Colchicine (1.2 mg/kg/day) or placebo was administered following various procedures for complications of proliferative diabetic retinopathy, sickle cell retinopathy, venous occlusive disease, globe rupture (one cohort), and rhegmatogenous retinal detachment (one cohort). Although the authors found no statistically significant difference between the colchicine and control groups, only two of the cohorts had disease processes classic for the development of PVR (globe rupture and retinal detachment). Because of poor patient selection and the small number of patients evaluated, no valid conclusions regarding the effectiveness of colchicine in human PVR can be drawn from this study.

Taxol

Taxol is a plant isolate that has demonstrated antitumor activity. In vitro, taxol inhibits both the contraction and proliferation of rabbit chorioretinal fibroblasts at concentrations of 2×10^{-8} M and 3×10^{-9} M, respectively (94). Additional studies have supported these findings and also demonstrated an inhibitory effect of taxol on cell migration (87). The mechanism of this inhibitory effect has not been well characterized. In contrast to colchicine, taxol appears to promote microtubule assembly and, in so doing, displaces intermediate and microfilaments (95). This disruption of the contractile apparatus is presumably the basis for the drug's effect on contraction, migration, and proliferation.

The effect of taxol was studied in a rabbit model of PVR (94). Doses of 0.5 μg (3×10^{-7} M) and 35 μg (2.3×10^{-5} M) equally inhibited the development of PVR following fibroblast injection. A dose of 0.05 μg (3×10^{-8} M) did not inhibit the development of retinal detachment in this model. Evidence of optic nerve toxicity occurred in 25% of those eyes receiving 35 μg of taxol. Detailed ocular clearance and ocular toxicity studies have not been performed to date.

Corticosteroids

Corticosteroids may be effective in the treatment of PVR based on either direct inhibition of mitosis (96,97) or suppression of inflammation (98), with a resultant decrease in fibrous proliferation. Inhibition of fibroblasts in vitro has been reported with dexamethasone concentrations as low as 0.01 μg/ml (97). Blumenkranz et al., in contrast, reported a bimodal effect of corticosteroids, including dexamethasone, on both dermal and conjunctival fibroblasts in culture. Dexamethasone in concentrations ranging from 1 to 30 mg/L (1–30 μg/ml) stimulated fibroblast proliferation. At concentrations >100 mg/L (100 μg/ml), proliferation of both dermal and conjunctival fibroblasts was inhibited (99). Sustained dexamethasone levels of 1 μg/ml inhibit phospholipase activity in perfused organs (100). Phospholipase is essential for the biosynthesis of prostaglandins, and the generation of prostaglandins is closely linked with inflammation.

Several investigators have demonstrated that corticosteroids effectively inhibit PVR in animal models. Dexamethasone alcohol reduced the incidence of retinal detachment from 57% to 24% in a rabbit model (101). In a similar model, triamcinolone acetonide decreased the rate of retinal detachment from 84% to 24% (102). Both these compounds have the advantage of being relatively lipophilic and, therefore, may be administered as a suspension. The crystalline drug then acts as a depot, providing relatively long-term intraocular levels of steroid that can be given at doses of 1 mg without apparent retinal toxicity (103). Chandler et al. demonstrated a better effect if the steroids are given before the injection of fibroblasts (98) and that doses >2 mg do not provide any additional therapeutic benefit (46). Using irradiated fibroblast injections, Chandler at al. (104) also showed that the injection of triamcinolone acetonide does not affect the contraction of preretinal membranes.

Although animal studies have demonstrated corticosteroids to be both safe and effective in the treatment of PVR, few controlled studies have been performed in humans. In the single trial performed to date (105), 141 patients were randomized to either oral prednisone (100 mg for 5 days, 50 mg for 10 days, and then 50 mg every other day for 40 days) or placebo. Six-month follow-up was done to detect any evidence of PVR. The results of this trial suggested an inhibitory effect of oral corticosteroids on postoperative retinal fibrosis, especially for subtle signs in the posterior pole. There was no difference between the two groups regarding the incidence of advanced retinal fibrosis or in the occurrence of peripheral retinal fibrosis. The authors concluded that higher tissue concentrations and a larger number of patients need to be evaluated before a definitive statement can be made regarding the efficacy of corticosteroids in the development of PVR.

Daunomycin

Daunorubicin hydrochloride (daunomycin hydrochloride) is an anthracycline antibiotic that inhibits cellular proliferation by a variety of mechanisms, including DNA binding, free radical formation, membrane binding, and metal ion chelation (106). Daunorubicin's multiple sites of action result in an antiproliferative effect that is not cell-cycle specific. Daunorubicin inhibits the proliferation and migration of cultured dermal fibroblasts at relatively low doses (4×10^{-8} M and 5×10^{-9} M, respectively) (87). In other in vitro studies, exposure of fibroblasts to 10^{-6} M daunorubicin for 1 hour or 500 nM for 5 hours significantly inhibited cellular proliferation (107). Exposure of cultured porcine RPE cells to 7.5 μg/ml daunorubicin for 5 to 10 minutes completely inhibited cellular proliferation (108).

Following an intravitreal injection of 10 nmol, the half-life of daunorubicin is about 2 hours (107). Daunorubicin appears to have toxic effects on the retina at relatively low doses. In the rabbit, a 9-nmol intravitreal injection is non-toxic. A single 15-nmol intravitreal injection, although demonstrating no clinically apparent toxicity, causes photoreceptor damage (109). In an intact vitreous model of PVR in rabbits, a single injection of 10 nmol of daunorubicin reduced the incidence of retinal detachment from 81% in controls to 8% in the treatment group (43). In this study, the administration of drug was simultaneous to the injection of fibroblasts. In a gas-compression model of PVR in the rabbit (110), an injection of 15 nmol of daunorubicin at the time of fibroblast injection reduced the incidence of retinal detachment from 100% in controls to 10% in experimental eyes. In an effort to determine the effectiveness of daunorubicin after the development of PVR, this study also evaluated the effect of drug administration 3 days after the injection of fibroblasts. The timing of the drug injection was based on studies that indicated that the host proliferative response was maximal 3 days subsequent to the injection of the fibroblasts (71). Two injections of 10 nmol and 5 nmol, given 4 hours apart, 3 days after the fibroblast injection, reduced the incidence of retinal detachment from 100% to 20%. Interestingly, a single dose of 15 nmol given on day 3 did not significantly reduce the incidence of retinal detachment (110).

There has been some experience in humans with administration of daunorubicin for the treatment of PVR. In one trial, after vitrectomy in patients with PVR or in patients believed to be at high risk for the development of posttraumatic PVR, a solution containing 7.5 μg/ml of daunorubicin was infused for 10 minutes and then removed. Anatomic success was obtained in 14 of 15 patients, and no toxic effects were attributed to the use of the drug (111). Daunorubicin, administered in a similar fashion, also has been employed in patients undergoing surgery for the repair of retinal detachment secondary to PVR (112). In the 68 eyes included in this study, 73% had no evidence of retinal detachment at 18 months. The authors believe this represented an improvement over the results they achieved in similar patients without the use of daunorubicin. They noted no toxicity directly attributable to the use of daunomycin.

Some authors (113) question the use of daunorubicin because of high mutagenic and carcinogenic potential (114–116). Aclacinomycin A is a dimethylated oligosaccharide anthracycline that is similar to daunorubicin in structure, but it does not appear to have carcinogenic effects (117–119). Aclacinomycin A has been evaluated in several trials for the treatment of malignancies, but it has received limited attention for the treatment of ocular disease (113). In a rabbit model of PVR, aclacinomycin A inhibited the development of retinal detachment at relatively low doses (113). There was a 62% reduction in the development of PVR after a single dose of 30 nmol administered 2 days after fibroblast injection. In addition, 60 nmol of aclacinomycin A, given as a divided dose 3 days after fibroblast injection, reduced the incidence of PVR by 73%. There appeared to be transient toxicity based on electronretinographic recordings 3 days after the 60-nmol injection. The authors suggest that aclacinomycin A may be a reasonable alternative to daunorubicin for the treatment of human PVR but that further evaluation is necessary.

5-Fluorouracil

5-Fluorouracil is a synthetic pyrimidine analog that has been investigated extensively for use in the treatment of PVR. It is formed by the substitution of a fluorine atom for a hydrogen atom at position 5 of the uracil ring. Then 5-fluorouracil can be enzymatically converted into a deoxyribose (5-fluorodeoxyuridine monophosphate), a molecule that inhibits thymidylate synthetase, an enzyme necessary for DNA synthesis. It also may be converted into a ribose (5-fluorouridine or 5-fluorouridine triphosphate), with subsequent incorporation into messenger and ribosomal RNA, resulting in coding errors.

In cell culture, 5-fluorouracil inhibits the growth of both rabbit dermal and conjunctival fibroblasts with a median effective dose (ID_{50}) of 0.2 to 0.3 μg/ml (99). An antiproliferative effect also was shown on human dermal fibroblasts and human RPE at concentrations of 0.35 μg/ml and 0.39 μg/ml, respectively (120). 5-Fluorouracil appears to have little effect on cell contraction as evaluated in a gel contraction model using human fibroblasts (41).

The toxicity of 5-fluorouracil, if given systemically, led to the investigation of other forms of administration. Subconjunctival injection of 6.25 mg in 0.5 ml resulted in peak vitreous levels of 10.5 μg/ml (121). Following a 1-mg intravitreal injection in the normal rabbit eye, a peak level of 664 μg/ml was achieved with a half-life of 7.7 hours (122). In aphakic/vitrectomized eyes, a similar peak vitreous level was obtained; however, the half-life was considerably shorter (122). 5-Fluorouracil appears to be relatively nontoxic when administered into the eye. Intravitreal injections of 1 mg are nontoxic as assessed by histopathology, electroretinography, and protein synthesis assays (123, 124). In contrast, injections of 2.5 mg (124) and 5 mg (99) resulted in toxicity. In a monkey model, injections of 0.75 mg into the vitreous were not toxic (125). Because of the relatively short half-life following intravitreal administration, repeat injections may be necessary to maintain therapeutic intraocular levels. In the vitrectomized eye, injections of 0.5 mg of 5-fluorouracil every 24 hours for 7 days is well tolerated in the rabbit, whereas doses of 1.25 mg per day for 7 days produce toxicity (126).

5-Fluorouracil has been tested in animal models of PVR. In a rabbit intact vitreous model using 250,000 fibroblasts, a single injection of 1 mg decreased the incidence of retinal detachment from 74% in controls to 32% in treated eyes (123). These authors also noted an enhanced effect with the addition of either intravitreal indomethacin or subconjunctival 5-fluorouracil. Daily injections of 0.5 mg of 5-fluorouracil in vitrectomized eyes reduced both the frequency and the height of traction retinal detachments induced by the injection of 200,000 cultured RPE cells (127). The effectiveness of a biodegradable device providing sustained release of 5-fluorouracil into the vitreous cavity also has been assessed (128). The device contained 1 mg of drug, which was released over several weeks and resulted in sustained intravitreal concentrations between 1 and 13 μg/ml for 2 weeks. Following gas compression vitrectomy, a retinal break was created and then treated with cryopexy. Retinal detachment occurred in 89% of controls versus 11% of animals implanted with the drug-delivery device.

Treatment of PVR in humans using 5-fluorouracil has been limited. Blumenkranz and associates used 5-fluorouracil in a group of 22 patients with advanced forms of PVR (129). Following surgical repair of the retinal detachment, 5-fluorouracil was administered either as repeated subconjunctival injections of 10 mg or as one or more intravitreal injections of 1 mg. Four of the 22 patients underwent both intravitreal and subconjunctival injections. Six months after surgery, 60% of the patients remained attached. The authors believed this represented an improved success compared with other studies of the reattachment rate following surgery for advanced PVR and that it was comparable to the reattachment rate achieved in studies using silicone oil tamponade.

Active metabolites of 5-fluorouracil as potential treatments for PVR have also been evaluated. 5-Fluorouradine, which interferes with RNA production (130), is approximately 100 times more potent than 5-fluorouracil as an antiproliferative agent (41). In addition, 5-fluorouridine has a significant anticontractile effect on fibroblasts in tissue culture (41,131). After intravitreal injection, 5-fluorouridine has a half-life of approximately 4 hours (132). Although 5-fluorouridine is significantly more potent, it also causes toxicity at much lower doses. Studies assessing toxicity based on ERG and histopathology found intravitreal injections of 0.1 mg to be well tolerated (120); however, other reports described the inhibition of protein synthesis in the retina for at least 8 days after a 0.1-mg intravitreal injection (124). Intravitreal injection of 0.1 mg of 5-fluorouridine in an animal model of PVR resulted in a significant reduction in traction retinal detachments compared with either control eyes or eyes treated with 1 mg of 5-fluorouracil (44). In an attempt to minimize toxicity while prolonging the intravitreal half-life, 5-fluorouridine 5′-monophosphate (a metabolite of 5-fluorouridine) has been incorporated into liposomes (133). Using this delivery method, drug half-life was extended to 124 hours; in a rabbit cell-injection model, 0.1 mg of 5-fluorouridine 5′-monophosphate in liposomes reduced the incidence of tractional retinal detachment by 92%.

Doxorubicin Adriamycin

Doxorubicin (Adriamycin), an anthracycline antineoplastic agent, is a potent inhibitor of cell proliferation. It is significantly more potent than 5-fluorouracil (134) and reduced the incidence of tractional retinal detachment in an experimental model of PVR (135). Even at intravitreal doses as low as 5.8 μg, however, it appears to be toxic (135). To avoid this toxicity, the use of microsphere delivery of Adriamycin has been studied (136). A 40% reduction in the incidence of traction retinal detachment was reported following the injection of 10 μg of Adriamycin in microspheres. When delivered in this fashion, there was no evidence of toxicity based on ERG or histopathology. To date, human studies have not been reported.

FUTURE DIRECTIONS

Although many drugs appear to be effective in animal models of PVR, as discussed above, relatively little testing has been done in humans. This paucity of human data may be the result of an inability to identify patients at risk for PVR, concerns about potential drug toxicity (ocular or systemic), or complications associated with repeated intravitreal administration. Because surgical therapy of PVR is fairly effective, to demonstrate the additional benefit of an adjunctive pharmalogic agent in a nonselected patient population, it would be necessary to randomize large numbers of patients. A more rational approach would be to develop better methods to identify prospectively those patients at risk of a poor surgical outcome when pharmalogical therapy is not used. With such a group of patients, it would be easier to demonstrate a drug treatment effect with a smaller sample size. Some progress in this area has been reported. Yang and associates have shown in an experimental model of PVR that the proliferative state of cells obtained from the vitreous cavity and the proliferation-inducing capacity of the vitreous itself may be useful parameters for evaluating eyes at risk of PVR (131,132). Recently, in preliminary studies, this approach was applied to patients undergoing vitrectomy for retinal detachment to identify those patients with favorable and unfavorable outcomes (133).

Sustained delivery techniques have the potential for providing intraocular drug levels for extended periods, avoiding systemic toxicity and maintaining levels of drug within the eye that are above therapeutic but well below toxic levels. As discussed, liposomes (133), microspheres, and bioerodible implants (128) have been evaluated. Recently, a delivery system that uses dexamethasone as the "delivery device" for 5-fluorouracil was reported (137). This delivery system is composed entirely of covalently linked dexamethasone and 5-fluorouracil. The compound formed is relatively insoluble and can be administered either as a solid or a suspension. As the solid dissolves and the codrug enters solution, the covalent bond is cleaved, resulting in the delivery of dexamethasone and 5-fluorouracil. By delivering a combination of drugs, each targeting different aspects of the wound-healing response, the codrug may prove more efficacious than treatment with 5-fluorouracil or dexamethasone alone. Furthermore, this type of system has the potential for extended delivery without the risk of complications of the delivery device itself. With further refinements in drug-delivery techniques, by determining the most efficacious and safe drug or combination of drugs, and by identifying patients at risk, it will be possible to inhibit or prevent the development of PVR.

ACKNOWLEDGMENT

This work was supported by EYO 9106, Adler Foundation, Heed Foundation, Research to Prevent Blindness.

REFERENCES

1. Bonnet M. Clinical findings associated with the development of postoperative PVR in primary rhegmatogenous retinal detachment. In: Heimann K, Wiedemann P, eds. *Proliferative Vitreoretinopathy.* Heidelberg: Kaden Verlag, 1989;18.
2. Ando N, Sen HA, Berkowitz BA, Wilson CA, de Juan E, Jr. Localization and quantitation of blood-retinal barrier breakdown in experimental proliferative vitreoretinopathy. *Arch Ophthalmol* 1994;112:117.

3. Clausen R, Weller M, Wiedemann P, Heimann K, Hilgers RD, Zilles K. An immunochemical quantitative analysis of the protein pattern in physiologic and pathologic vitreous. *Graefes Arch Clin Exp Ophthalmol* 1991;229:186.
4. Grisanti S, Wiedemann P, Heimann K. Proliferative vitreoretinopathy. On the significance of protein transfer through the blood-retina barrier. *Ophthalmologe* 1993;90:468.
5. Glaser BM, Lemor M. Pathobiology of proliferative vitreoretinopathy. In: Ryan SJ R, ed. *Retina.* St. Louis: Mosby, 1988;369.
6. Jerdan JA, Pepose JS, Michels RG, Hayashi H, deBustros S, Sebag M, Glaser BM. Proliferative vitreoretinopathy membranes: an immunohistochemical study. *Ophthalmology* 1989;96:801.
7. Charteris DG, Hiscott P, Robey HL, Gregor ZJ, Lightman SL, Grierson I. Inflammatory cells in proliferative vitreoretinopathy subretinal membranes. *Ophthalmology* 1993;100:43.
8. Vinores SA, Campochiaro PA, Conway BP. Ultrastructural and electronimmunocytochemical characterization of cells in epiretinal membranes. *Invest Ophthalmol Vis Sci* 1990;31:1428.
9. Baudouin C, Fredj-Reygrobellet D, Gordon WC, Peyman G, Lapalus P, Gastaud P, Bazan NG. Immunohistologic study of epiretinal membranes in proliferative vitreoretinopathy. *Am J Ophthalmol* 1990;110:593.
10. Nicolai U, Eckardt C. The occurrence of macrophages in the retina and periretinal tissues in ocular diseases. *Ger J Ophthalmol* 1993;2:195.
11. Grisanti S, Heimann K, Wiedemann P. Origin of fibronectin in epiretinal membranes of proliferative vitreoretinopathy and proliferative diabetic retinopathy. *Br J Ophthalmol* 1993;77:238.
12. Weller M, Esser P, Bresgen M, Heimann K, Wiedemann P. Thrombospondin: a new attachment protein in preretinal traction membranes. *Eur J Ophthalmol* 1992;2:10.
13. Weller M, Wiedemann P, Bresgen M, Heimann K. Vitronectin and proliferative intraocular disorders. I. A colocalisation study of the serum spreading factor, vitronectin, and fibronectin in traction membranes from patients with proliferative vitreoretinopathy. *Int Ophthalmol* 1991;15:93.
14. Hagedorn M, Esser P, Wiedemann P, Heimann K. Tenascin and decorin in epiretinal membranes of proliferative vitreoretinopathy and proliferative diabetic retinopathy. *Ger J Ophthalmol* 1993;2:28.
15. Connor T, Roberts A, Sporn M, Davis J, Glaser B. RPE cells synthesize and release transforming growth factor-beta, a modulator of endothelial cell growth and wound healing. *Invest Ophthalmol Vis Sci* 1988;29(suppl):307.
16. Jaffe GJ, Peters WP, Roberts W, Kurtzberg J, Stuart A, Wang AM, Stoudemire JB. Modulation of macrophage colony stimulating factor in cultured human retinal pigment epithelial cells. *Exp Eye Res* 1992;54:595–603.
17. Jaffe GJ, Van Le L, Valea F, Haskill S, Roberts W, Arend WP, Stuart A, Peters WP. Expression of interleukin-1 alpha, interleukin-1 beta, and an interleukin-1 receptor antagonist in human retinal pigment epithelial cells. *Exp Eye Res* 1992;55:325.
18. Elner VM, Scales W, Elner SG, Danforth J, Kunkel SL, Strieter RM. Interleukin-6 (IL-6) gene expression and secretion by cytokine-stimulated human retinal pigment epithelial cells. *Exp Eye Res* 1992;54:361.
19. Planck SR, Dang TT, Graves D, Tara D, Ansel JC, Rosenbaum JT. Retinal pigment epithelial cells secrete interleukin-6 in response to interleukin-1. *Invest Ophthalmol Vis Sci* 1992;33:78.
20. Elner VM, Strieter RM, Elner SG, Baggliolini M, Lindley I, Kunkel SL. Neutrophil chemotactic factor (IL8) gene expression by cytokine treated human retinal pigment epithelial (RPE) cells. *Am J Pathol* 1990;136:745.
21. Schweigerer L, Malerstein B, Neufeld G, Gospodarowicz D. Basic fibroblast growth factor is synthesized in cultured retinal pigment epithelial cells. *Biochem Biophys Res Commun* 1987;143:934.
22. Elner SG, Strieter RM, Elner VM, Rollins BJ, Del Monte MA, Kunkel SL. Monocyte chemotactic protein gene expression by cytokine-treated human retinal pigment epithelial cells. *Lab Invest* 1991;64:819.
23. Jaffe GJ, Richmond A, Van Le L, Shattuck RL, Cheng Q-C, Wong F, Roberts W. Expression of three forms of melanoma growth stimulating activity (MGSA)/growth in human retinal pigment epithelial cells. *Invest Ophthalmol Vis Sci* 1993;x:xx.
24. Connor TB, Roberts AB, Sporn MB, Danielpour D, Dart LL, Michels RG, de Bustros S, Enger C, Kato H, Lansing M, Hayashi H, Glaser BM. Correlation of fibrosis and transforming growth factor-type 2 levels in the eye. *J Clin Invest* 1989;83:1661.
25. Limb GA, Little BC, Meager A, Ogilvie JA, Wolstencroft RA, Franks WA, Chignell AH, Dumonde DC. Cytokines in proliferative vitreoretinopathy. *Eye* 1991;5(Pt 6):686.
26. Little BC, Limb GA, Meager A, Ogilvie JAE, Wolstencroft RA, Franks WA, Chignell AH, Dumonde DC. Cytokines in proliferative vitreoretinopathy. *Invest Ophthalmol Vis Sci* 1991;32(suppl): 768.
27. Jaffe GJ, Elner S, Elner V. Levels of macrophage colony stimulating factor, macrophage chemotactic and activating protein, and interleukin 8 in human vitreous. *Invest Ophthalmol Vis Sci* 1993;34: 1211.
28. Fredj-Reygrobellet D, Baudouin C, Negre F, Caruelle JP, Gastaud P, Lapalus P. Acidic FGF and other growth factors in preretinal membranes from patients with diabetic retinopathy and proliferative vitreoretinopathy. *Ophthalmic Res* 1991;23:154.
29. Baudouin C, Fredj-Reygrobellet D, Brignole F, Negre F, Lapalus P, Gastaud P. Growth factors in vitreous and subretinal fluid cells from patients with proliferative vitreoretinopathy. *Ophthalmic Res* 1993; 25:52.
30. Earley O, Limb GA, Jones S, Kapur S, Chignell AH, Dumonde DC. Expression of cytokine mRNA by cells infiltrating retinal membranes in proliferative vitreoretinopathy. *Invest Ophthalmol Vis Sci* 1993;34:951.
31. Malecaze F, Mathis A, Arne JL, Raulais D, Courtois Y, Hicks D. Localization of acidic fibroblast growth factor in proliferative vitreoretinopathy membranes. *Curr Eye Res* 1991;10:719.
32. Planck SR, Andresevic J, Chen JC, Holmes DL, Rodden W, Westra I, Wu SC, Huang XN, Kay G, Wilson DJ, et al. Expression of growth factor mRNA in rabbit PVR model systems. *Curr Eye Res* 1992;11:1031.
33. Robbins SG, Wilson DJ, Hart CE, Robertson JE, Westra I, Rosenbaum JT. Immunologic detection of platelet-derived growth factor-like activity in epiretinal membranes. *Invest Ophthalmol Vis Sci* 1992;33(suppl):820.
34. Westra I, Robbins SG, Wilson DJ, Robertson JE, O'Rourke LM, Hart CE, Rosenbaum JT. Time course of basic fibroblast growth factor (bFGF), platelet derived growth factor (PDGF) and proliferating cell nuclear antigen (PCNA) staining in a rabbit proliferative vitreoretinopathy model. *Invest Ophthalmol Vis Sci* 1993;34:1024.
35. Hunt RC, Pakalnis VA, Choudhury P, Black EP. Cytokines and serum cause contraction of gels by cultured retinal pigment epithelial cells. *Invest Ophthalmol Vis Sci* 1994;35:955.
36. Jaffe GJ, Earnest K, Fulcher S, Lui GM, Houston LL. Antitransferrin receptor immunotoxin inhibits proliferating human retinal pigment epithelial cells. *Arch Ophthalmol* 1990;108:1163–1168.
37. van Bockxmeer FM, Martin CE, Constable IJ. Models for assessing scar tissue inhibitors *Retina* 1985;5:47.
38. Burke JM. Stimulation of DNA synthesis in human and bovine RPE by peptide growth factors: the response to TNF-α and EGF is dependent upon culture density. *Curr Eye Res* 1989;8:1279.
39. Leschey KH, Hackett SF, Singer JH, Campochiaro PA. Growth factor responsiveness of human retinal pigment epithelial cells. *Invest Ophthalmol Vis Sci* 1990;31:839.
40. Compochiaro P, Bryan III JA, Conway BP, Jaccoma EA. Intravitreal chemotactic and mitogenic activity: implication of blood-retinal barrier breakdown *Arch Ophthalmol* 1986;104:1685.
41. Hartzer MK, Blumenkranz MS, Hajek AS, Dailey WA, Cheng M, Margherio AR. Selection of therapeutic agents for intraocular proliferative disease 3: effects of fluoropyrimidines on cell-mediated contraction in human fibroblasts. *Exp Eye Res* 1989;48:321.
42. Raymond MC, Thompson JT. RPE-mediated collagen gel contraction. Inhibition by colchicine and stimulation by TGF-beta. *Invest Ophthalmol Vis Sci* 1990;31:1079.
43. Kirmani M, Santana M, Sorgente N, Wiedemann P, Ryan SJ. Antiproliferative drugs in the treatment of experimental proliferative vitreoretinopathy. *Retina* 1983;3:269.
44. Ward T, Hartzer M, Blumenkranz M, Lin LR. A comparison of 5-fluorouridine and 5-fluorouracil in an experimental model for the treatment of vitreoretinal scarring. *Curr Eye Res* 1993;12:397.

45. Hida T, Chandler DB, Sheta SM. Classification of the stages of proliferative vitreoretinopathy in a refined experimental model in the rabbit eye. *Graefes Arch Clin Exp Ophthalmol*1987;225:303.
46. Chandler DB, Rozakis G, Dejuan E, Machemer R. The effect of triamcinolone acetonide on a refined experimental model of proliferative vitreoretinopathy. *Am J Ophthalmol* 1985;99:686.
47. Moorhead LC, Sepahban S, Armeniades CD. Evaluation of drug treatments for proliferative vitreoretinopathy using vitreous microtensiometry. *Ann Ophthalmol* 1991;23:349.
48. Hui YN, Liang HC, Cai YS, Kirchhof B, Heimann K. Corticosteroids and daunomycin in the prevention of experimental proliferative vitreoretinopathy induced by macrophages. *Graefes Arch Clin Exp Ophthalmol* 1993;231:109.
49. Fastenberg DM, Diddie KR, Delmage JM, Dorey K. Intraocular injection of silicone oil for experimental proliferative vitreoretinopathy. *Am J Ophthalmol* 1983;95:663.
50. Joondeph BC, Peyman GA, Khoobehi B, Yue BY. Liposome-encapsulated 5-fluorouracil in the treatment of proliferative vitreoretinopathy. *Ophthalmic Surg* 1988;19:252.
51. Planck SR, Andresevic J, Chen JC, et al. Expression of growth factor mRNA in rabbit PVR model systems. *Curr Eye Res* 1992;11:1031.
52. Yeo JH, Sadeghi J, Campochiaro PA, Green WR, Glaser BM. Intravitreous fibronectin and platelet-derived growth factor: new model for traction retinal detachment. *Arch Ophthalmol* 1986;104:417.
53. Baudouin C, Fredj-Reygrobellet D, Ettaiche M, Barritault D, Gastaud P, Lapalus P. Induction of experimental proliferative vitreoretinopathy in the rabbit eye by intravitreal injections of fibroblast growth factor. *Lens Eye Toxicology Research* 1992;9:505.
54. Pinon RM, Pastor JC, Saornil MA, Goldaracena MB, Layana AG, Gayoso MJ, Guisasola J. Intravitreal and subretinal proliferation induced by platelet-rich plasma injection in rabbits. *Curr Eye Res* 1992;11:1047.
55. Iwasaki T. Experimental proliferative vitreoretinopathy in rabbits after intravitreous gas injection and creation of retinal hole: ophthalmic findings and localization of fibronectin. *Nippon Ganka Gakkai Zasshi* 1992;96:613.
56. Kain HL. Experimental studies of proliferative vitreoretinopathy. *Fortschr Ophthalmol* 1991;88:671.
57. Lewis H, Aaberg TM, Abrams GW. Causes of failure after initial vitreoretinal surgery for severe proliferative vitreoretinopathy. *Am J Ophthalmol* 1991;111:8.
58. Kampik A, Hoing C, Heidenkummer HP. Problems and timing in the removal of silicone oil. *Retina* 1992;12(3 suppl):S11.
59. Bonnet M, Fleury J. Management of retinal detachment after penetrating eye injury. *Graefes Arch Clin Exp Ophthalmol* 1991;229:539.
60. Murad S, Pinnell S. Suppression of fibroblast proliferation and lysyl hydroxylase activity by minoxidil. *J Biol Chem* 1987;262:11973.
61. Handa JT, Jaffe GJ, Johnson GA. The mechanism of antiproliferation by minoxidil on cultured human retinal pigment epithelial cells. *J Cell Biol* 1991;115:212.
62. Yeowell HN, Ha V, Walker LC, Murad S, Pinnell SR. Regulation of lysyl hydroxylase mRNA in human skin fibroblasts by minoxidil and hydralazine. *Invest Dermatol* 1992;99:864.
63. Handa JT, Murad S, Jaffe GJ. Minoxidil inhibits ocular cell proliferation and lysyl hydroxylase activity. *Invest Ophthalmol Vis Sci* 1993;34:567.
64. Johnson GA, Handa JT, Baker CA, Jaffe GJ. Minoxidil inhibits human RPE cells by a mechanism dependent on the conversion to minoxidil sulfate. *Invest Ophthalmol Vis Sci* 1993;34:1426.
65. Handa JT, Murad S, Jaffe GJ. Inhibition of cultured human RPE cell proliferation and lysyl hydroxylase activity by hydroxy derivatives of minoxidil. *Invest Ophthalmol Vis Sci* 1994;35:463.
66. Baudouin C, Brignole F, Gastaud P. Transferrin receptor expression by retinal pigment epithelial cells in proliferative vitreoretinopathy [Letter; Comment]. *Arch Ophthalmol* 1991;109:1195.
67. Fulcher S, Lui G, Houston LL, et al. Use of immunotoxin to inhibit proliferating human corneal endothelium. *Invest Ophthalmol Vis Sci* 1988;29:755.
68. Davis AA, Whidby DE, Privette T, Houston LL, Hunt RC. Selective inhibition of growing pigment epithelial cells by a receptor-directed immunotoxin. *Invest Ophthalmol Vis Sci* 1990;31:2514.
69. Marks A, Ettenson D, Bjorn MJ, Lei M, Baumal R. Inhibition of human tumor growth by intraperitoneal immunotoxins in nude mice. *Cancer Res* 1990;50:288.
70. Handa JT, Houston LL, Jaffe GJ. Monensin enhances the cytotoxic effect of antitransferrin receptor immunotoxin on cultured RPE cells. *Curr Eye Res* 1993;12:45.
71. Hatchell DL, McAdoo T, Sheta S, King RT, Bartolome JV. Quantification of cellular proliferation in experimental proliferative vitreoretinopathy. *Arch Ophthalmol* 1988;106:669.
72. Handa JT, Houston LL, Jaffe GJ. The antiproliferative effect of a transferrin-toxin on human retinal pigment epithelial cells and rabbit fibroblasts. *Invest Ophthalmol Vis Sci* 1993;34:3419.
73. Handa JT, Pearson PA, Stuart A, Jaffe GJ. Intravitreal clearance of antitransferrin receptor immunotoxin in the gas vitrectomized phakic eye. *Invest Ophthalmol Vis Sci* 1993;34:1425.
74. Lotan R, Nicolson GL. Inhibitory effects of retinoic acid or retinyl acetate on the growth of untransformed, transformed, and tumor cells in vitro. *J Natl Cancer Inst* 1977;59:1717.
75. Strickland S, Smith KK, Marotti KR. The induction of differentiation in teratocarcinoma stem cells by retinoic acid. *Cell* 1980;21:347.
76. Jones-Villeneuve EMV, Rudnicki MA, Harris JF, McBurney MW. Retinoic acid-induced neural differentiation of embryonal carcinoma cells. *Mol Cell Biol* 1983;3:2271.
77. Giguere V, Ong ES, Sequi P, Evans RM. Identification of a receptor for the morphogen retinoic acid. *Nature* 1987;330:624.
78. Verstraeten TC, Wilcox DC. Effect of vitamin A on migration of human RPE cells in vitro. *Invest Ophthalmol Vis Sci* 1987;28(suppl):208.
79. Doyle JW, Dowgiert RK, Buzney SM. Factors modulating the effect of retinoids on cultured retinal pigment epithelial cell proliferation. *Curr Eye Res* 1992;11:753.
80. Das SR, Gouras P. Retinoid metabolism in cultured human retinal pigment epithelium. *Biochem J* 1988;250:459.
81. Campochiaro PA, Hackett SF, Conway BP. Retinoic acid promotes density-dependent growth arrest in human retinal pigment epithelial cells. *Invest Ophthalmol Vis Sci* 1991;32:65.
82. Davis BH, Kramer RT, Davidson NO. Retinoic acid modulates rat Ito cell proliferation, collagen, and transforming growth factor β production. *J Clin Invest* 1990;86:2062.
83. Araiz JJ, Refojo MF, Arroyo MH, Leong FL, Albert DM, Tolentino FI. Antiproliferative effect of retinoic acid in intravitreous silicone oil in an animal model of proliferative vitreoretinopathy. *Invest Ophthalmol Vis Sci* 1993;34:522.
84. Giordano GG, Refojo MF, Arroyo MH. Sustained delivery of retinoic acid from microspheres of biodegradable polymer in PVR. *Invest Ophthalmol Vis Sci* 1993;34:2743.
85. Fekrat S, de Juan E, Campochiaro PA. The effect of oral 13-cis-retinoic acid on retinal attachment after surgical repair in eyes with proliferative vitreoretinopathy (PVR). *Invest Ophthalmol Vis Sci* 1994;35(suppl):1532.
86. Lemor M, de Bustros S, Glaser BM. Low-dose colchicine inhibits astrocyte, fibroblast, and retinal pigment epithelial cell migration and proliferation. *Arch Ophthalmol* 1986;104:1223.
87. Verdoorn C, Renardel de Lavalette VW, Delma-Weizhausz J, Orr GM, Sorgente N, Ryan SJ. Cellular migration, proliferation, and contraction: an in vitro approach to a clinical problem—proliferative vitreoretinopathy. *Arch Ophthalmol* 1986;104:1216.
88. Vaccarezza OL, Pasqualini E, Saavedra JE. Retinal alteration induced by intravitreous colchicine. *Virchows Arch Cell Pathol* 1973;12:159.
89. Karlsson JO, Hansson HA, Sjostrand J. Effect of colchicine on axonal transport and morphology of retinal ganglion cells. *Z Zellforsch Mikrosk Anat* 1971;115:265.
90. Davidson C, Green WR, Wong VG. Retinal atrophy induced by intravitreous colchicine. *Invest Ophthalmol Vis Sci* 1983;24:301.
91. Lemor M, Yeo JH, Glaser BM. Oral colchicine for the treatment of experimental traction retinal detachment. *Arch Ophthalmol* 1986;104:1226.
92. Huna R, Moisseiev J, Dany S, Ezra D. Intraocular penetration of colchicine after oral administration. *Invest Ophthalmol Vis Sci* 1994;35(suppl):2217.
93. Berman DH, Gombos GM. Proliferative vitreoretinopathy: does oral low-dose colchicine have an inhibitory effect? A controlled study in humans. *Ophthalmic Surg* 1989;20:268.

94. van Bockxmeer FM, Martin CE, Thompson DE, Constable IJ. Taxol for the treatment of proliferative vitreoretinopathy. *Invest Ophthalmol Vis Sci* 1985;26:1140.
95. Antin PB, Forr-Schaudies S, Friedman TM, Tapscott SJ, Holtzer H. Taxol induces hostmitotic myoblasts to assemble interdigitation microtubule-myosin arrays that exclude actin. *J Cell Biol* 1981;90:300.
96. Grossfield H, Ragan C. Action of hydrocortisone on cells in tissue culture. *Proc Soc Exp Biol Med* 1954;86:63.
97. Ruhmann A, Berliner D. Effect of steroids on growth of mouse fibroblasts in vitro. *Endocrinology* 1965;76:916.
98. Chandler DB, Hida T, Sheta S, Proia AD, Machemer R. Improvement in efficacy of corticosteroid therapy in an animal model of proliferative vitreoretinopathy by pretreatment. *Graefes Arch Clin Exp Ophthalmol* 1987;225:259.
99. Blumenkranz MS, Claflin A, Hajek AS. Selection of therapeutic agents for intraocular proliferative disease: cell culture evaluation. *Arch Ophthalmol* 1984;102:598.
100. Flower RJ, Blackwell GJ. Anti-inflammatory steroids induce biosynthesis of a phospholipase A2 inhibitor which prevents prostaglandin generation. *Nature* 1979;278:456.
101. Tano Y, Sugita G, Abrams GW, Machemer R. Inhibition of intraocular proliferations with intravitreal corticosteroids. *Am J Ophthalmol* 1980;89:131.
102. Tano Y, Chandler D, Machemer R. Treatment of intraocular proliferations with intravitreal injection of triamcinolone acetonide. *Am J Ophthalmol* 1980;90:810.
103. McCuen BW, Bressler M, Tano Y, Chandler D, Machemer R. The lack of toxicity of intravitrealy administered triamcinolone acetonide. *Am J Ophthalmol* 1981;91:785.
104. Chandler DB, Hida T, Rozakis G, Forbes VS, Machemer R. The lack of an effect of intraocular steroids on irradiated fibroblasts in experimental proliferative vitreoretinopathy. *Graefes Arch Clin Exp Ophthalmol* 1992;230:188.
105. Koemer F, Merz A, Gloor B, Wagner E. Postoperative retinal fibrosis—a controlled clinical study of systemic steroid therapy. *Graefes Arch Clin Exp Ophthalmol* 1982;219:268.
106. Myers C. In: Chabner B, ed. *Pharmacologic Principles of Cancer Treatment.* Philadelphia: WB Saunders, 1982;416.
107. Wiedemann P, Sorgente N, Bekhor C, Patterson R, Tran T, Ryan S. Daunomycin in the treatment of experimental proliferative vitreoretinopathy. *Invest Ophthalmol Vis Sci* 1985;26:719.
108. Weller M, Heinmann K, Wiedemann P. Cytotoxic effects of daunomycin on retinal pigment epithelium in vitro. *Graefes Arch Clin Exp Ophthalmol* 1987;225:235.
109. Santana M, Wiedemann P, Kirmani M, Minckler D, Patterson R, Sorgente N, Ryan S. Daunomycin in the treatment of experimental proliferative vitreoretinopathy: retinal toxicity of intravitreal daunomycin in the rabbit. *Graefes Arch Clin Exp Ophthalmol* 1984;221:210.
110. Khawly JA, Saloupis P, Hatchell DL, Machemer R. Daunorubicin treatment in a refined experimental model of proliferative vitreoretinopathy. *Graefes Arch Clin Exp Ophthalmol* 1991;229:464.
111. Wiedemann P, Lemmen K, Schmiedl R, Heinmann K. Intraocular daunorubicin for the treatment and prophylaxis of traumatic proliferative vitreoretinopathy. *Am J Ophthalmol* 1987;104:10.
112. Wiedemann P, Leinung C, Hilgers RD, Heinmann K. Daunomycin and silicone oil for the treatment of proliferative vitreoretinopathy. *Graefes Arch Clin Exp Ophthalmol* 1991;229:150.
113. Steinhorst UH, Chen EP, Hatchell DL, Samsa GP, Saloupis PT, Westendorf J, Machemer R. Aclacinomycin A in the treatment of experimental proliferative vitreoretinopathy: efficacy and toxicity in the rabbit eye. *Invest Ophthalmol Vis Sci* 1993;34:1753.
114. Bucciarelli E. Mammary tumor induction in male and female Sprague-Dawley rat by Adriamycin and daunomycin. *J Natl Cancer Inst* 1981;66:81.
115. Sternberg S, Philips F, Cronin AP. Renal tumors and other lesions in rats following a single intravenous injection of daunomycin. *Cancer Res* 1972;32:1029.
116. Marquardt H, Philips F, Sternburg S. Tumorigenicity in vivo and induction of malignant transformation and mutagenesis in cell cultures by adriamycin and daunomycin. *Cancer Res* 1976;36:2065.
117. Suzuki H, Kawashima K, Yamada K. Aclacinomycin A, a new antileukemic agent. *Lancet* 1979;2:870.
118. Umezawa KSM, Matsushima T, Sugimura T. Mutagenicity of aclacinomycin A and daunomycin derivatives. *Cancer Res* 1978;32:1782.
119. Westendorf J, Marquardt H, Ketkar MB, Mohr U, Marquardt H. Tumorigenicity in vivo and induction of mutagenesis and DNA repair in vitro by aclacinomycin A and marcellomycin: structure-activity relationship and predictive value of short-term tests. *Cancer Res* 1983;43:5248.
120. Blumenkranz MS, Hartzer MK, Hajek AS. Selection of therapeutic agents for intraocular proliferative disease. II. Differing antiproliferative activity of the fluoropyrimidines. *Arch Ophthalmol* 1987;105:396.
121. Rootman J, Tisdall J, Gudauskas G, Ostrey A. Intraocular penetration of subconjunctivally administered ^{14}C-fluorouracil in rabbits. *Arch Ophthalmol* 1979;97:2375.
122. Jarus G, Blumenkranz M, Hernandez E, Sossi N. Clearance of intravitreal fluorouracil: normal and aphakic vitrectomized eyes. *Ophthalmology* 1985;92:91.
123. Blumenkranz MS, Ophir A, Claflin AJ, Hajek A. Fluorouracil for the treatment of massive periretinal proliferation. *Am J Ophthalmol* 1982;94:458.
124. Leon JA, Britt JM, Hopp RH, Mills RP, Milam AH. Effects of fluorouracil and fluorouridine on protein synthesis in rabbit retina. *Invest Ophthalmol Vis Sci* 1990;31:1709.
125. Barrada A, Peyman G, Case J, et al. Evaluation of intravitreal 5-fluorouracil, vincristine, VP 16, doxorubicin, and thiotepa in primate eyes. *Ophthalmic Surg* 1984;15:767.
126. Stern WH, Guerin CJ, Erickson PA, Lewis GP, Anderson DH, Fisher SK. Ocular toxicity of fluorouracil after vitrectomy. *Am J Ophthalmol* 1983;96:43.
127. Stern WH, Lewis GP, Erickson PA, Guerin CJ, Anderson DH, Fisher SK, O'Donnell JJ. Fluorouracil therapy for proliferative vitreoretinopathy after vitrectomy. *Am J Ophthalmol* 1983;96:33.
128. Rubsamen PE, David PD, Hernandez E, O'Grady GE, Cousins SW. Prevention of experimental proliferative vitreoretinopathy with a biodegradable intravitreal implant for the sustained release of fluorouracil. *Arch Ophthalmol* 1994;112:407.
129. Blumenkranz M, Hernandez E, Ophir A, Norton EWD. 5-Fluorouracil: new applications in complicated retinal detachment for an established antimetabolite. *Ophthalmology* 1984;91:122.
130. Wilkinson DS, Pitot HC. Inhibition of ribosomal ribonucleic acid maturation in Novikoff hepatoma cells by 5-fluorouracil and 5-fluorouridine. *J Biol Chem* 1973;248:63.
131. Heath TD, Lopez NG, Lewis GP, Stern WH. Fluoropyrimidine treatment of ocular cicatricial disease. *Invest Ophthalmol Vis Sci* 1986;27:940.
132. Huang D, Blumenkranz M, Hernandez E, Hartzer M. Uptake and clearance of 5-fluorouridine following subconjunctival and intravitreal injection. *Retina* 1988;8:205.
133. Assil KK, Hartzer M, Weinreb RN, Nehorayan M, Ward T, Blumenkranz M. Liposome suppression of proliferative vitreoretinopathy. Rabbit model using antimetabolite encapsulated liposomes [see comments]. *Invest Ophthalmol Vis Sci* 1991;32:2891.
134. Peyman GA, Schulman J. Proliferative vitreoretinopathy and chemotherapeutic agents. *Surv Ophthalmol* 1985;29:434.
135. Sunalp M, Wiedemann P, Sorgente N, Ryan SJ. Effects of cytotoxic drugs on proliferative vitreoretinopathy in the rabbit cell injection model. *Curr Eye Res* 1984;3:619.
136. Moritera T, Ogura Y, Yoshimura N, Honda Y, Wada R, Hyon SH, Ikada Y. Biodegradable microspheres containing adriamycin in the treatment of proliferative vitreoretinopathy. *Invest Ophthalmol Vis Sci* 1992;33:3125.
137. Berger AS, Cheng CK, Pearson PA, Ashton P, Jaffe GJ. Intravitreal sustained release dexamethasone/5FU device in the treatment of experimental PVR. *Invest Ophthalmol Vis Sci* 1994;35(suppl):1923.

Textbook of Ocular Pharmacology,
edited by T.J. Zimmerman, et al.
Lippincott–Raven Publishers, Philadelphia © 1997.

CHAPTER 36

Drugs Affecting the Coagulation/Fibrinolysis Pathways

George A. Williams

HEMOSTATIC SYSTEM

An understanding of the pharmacology of hemostasis requires a review of the coagulation and fibrinolytic pathways. Although the major components of these pathways will be discussed independently, their complex interdependence in vivo must be recognized. The hemostatic system maintains blood in a fluid state under normal physiologic conditions; however, it is primed to react to vascular injury in an explosive manner. Hemostatic events involve (a) the vascular endothelium, (b) platelets, (c) coagulation, and (d) fibrinolysis. The interplay between these four portions of hemostasis may be pharmacologically manipulated in either the normal state or disease states.

Endothelium

The vascular endothelium is an integral component in hemostasis. In the normal state, the endothelium maintains blood fluidity by producing inhibitors of coagulation and platelet aggregation. The endothelium serves as a non-thrombogenic surface separating the blood components from reactive subendothelial structures and also modulates vascular tone and permeability. These functions are mediated by the production of a variety of substances. The endothelium inhibits coagulation by producing thrombomodulin and heparin sulfate, which interact with coagulation factors. Platelet aggregation is controlled by the release of prostaglandins such as prostacyclin and nitric oxides. Vascular tone is regulated by vasoconstrictive endothelins and vasodilatory prostacyclin. The endothelium also participates in the fibrinolytic system by producing plasminogen activators and plasminogen activator inhibitors. Endothelial dysfunction can therefore result in thrombotic or hemorrhagic conditions.

G. A. Williams: Department of Vitreoretinal Surgery, William Beaumont Hospital, Royal Oak, MI 48073, and Department of Biomedical Sciences, Eye Research Institute, Oakland University, Rochester, Michigan 48067.

Platelets

Platelets are a fundamental component throughout hemostasis. They contribute to the initial homostatic plug in vascular injury and provide membrane surfaces for amplification of coagulation and fibrin formation. Platelets also contribute to clot contraction. Platelet activation is categorized into four processes: (a) platelet adhesion, (b) platelet aggregation, (c) platelet secretion, and (d) procoagulant properties.

Platelets normally do not adhere to the endothelium. Exposure of subendothelial structures results in platelet binding to adhesive proteins, collagen, fibronectin, and von Willebrand factor (vWF). This adhesion is mediated by specific glycoprotein receptors in the platelet membrane. Once platelets adhere to the subendothelial extracellular matrix, they undergo conformational changes and spread out. This conformational change exposes additional membrane receptors which bind fibrinogen. The divalent structure of fibrinogen allows the formation of platelet-to-platelet aggregation. Additional molecules such as fibronectin and thrombospondin bind to platelet receptors, which stabilizes the otherwise friable platelet aggregates.

As platelet activation proceeds, several platelet agonists bind to specific membrane receptors. The most important agonists are thrombin, adenosine diphosphate (ADP), collagen, arachidonic acid, and epinephrine. These agonists contribute to aggregation and induce secretion. The agonist–receptor complexes interact with proteins in the platelet membrane controlling calcium ion flux and protein kinase activity, which are critical for activation of the platelet cytoskeletal contractile apparatus and the production of thromboxane A_2.

Platelets contain three types of granules: (a) dense bodies containing serotonin, ADP and calcium, (b) α granules containing Factor V, fibrinogen, vWF, fibronectin, platelet factor 4, platelet-derived growth factor, and β-thromboglobulin, and (c) lysosomes containing acid hydrolases. Activation of cytoskeletal contraction results in secretion of the granule contents. Some of the contents such as ADP bind to specific receptors that mediate additional platelet aggregation and shape change. Others such as thrombomodulin, a powerful thrombin inhibitor, act as feedback inhibitors of platelet activation.

The most important regulatory factor in platelet activation is cyclic 3′, 5′adenosine monophosphate (cyclic AMP), which is produced from adenosine triphosphate (ATP) by adenylate cyclase. Adenylate cyclase, and thereby cyclic AMP, is stimulated by the arachidonic acid products prostaglandin D_2 and prostacyclin (PGI_2), which are produced by endothelial cells. Platelet phosphodiesterases cleave cyclic AMP to AMP, thereby lowering intracellular cyclic AMP. Cyclic AMP removes calcium from the cytosol through protein kinase phosphorylation of a calcium pump. Thus, cyclic AMP inhibits platelet adhesion aggregation and secretion. The procoagulant properties of platelets are mediated by the expression of membrane receptors for specific clotting Factors, particularly Factors V, IX, and X.

Coagulation

Coagulation classically has been divided into the intrinsic and extrinsic pathways (Fig. 36-1). Although this construct is useful for laboratory testing, it is not an accurate description of in vivo events because of the interaction that occurs between the two pathways. This section reviews the intrinsic and extrinsic pathways separately while emphasizing their interdependence and interaction.

Extrinsic Pathway

The extrinsic pathway is the primary initiating pathway of in vivo coagulation. The major plasma component of the extrinsic pathway is Factor VII. The central precipitating event is the exposure of the blood to tissue factor, an intrinsic membrane protein, which functions as a cofactor with activated Factor VII (VIIa). The VIIa–tissue factor complex has two principal substrates, Factor IX and Factor X. Activated Factor X (Xa) is the beginning of the final common pathway. In conjunction with Factor V and membrane phospholipids derived from platelets, Xa converts prothrombin into thrombin.

Intrinsic Pathway

The intrinsic pathway provides a pathway independent of Factor VII for coagulation. The initiating protein in the intrinsic pathway is Factor XII, which is autoactivated by binding to negatively charged surfaces. Activated Factor XII (XIIa) in turn activates Factor XI (XIa), which may also be activated by high molecular weight kininogen–Factor XIII complex. Factor XIa converts Factor IX to IXa. Factor IXa converts Factor X to Xa in the presence of Factor VIII and platelet phospholipids. Formation of Xa begins the formation of thrombin through the common pathway.

Interaction between the intrinsic and extrinsic pathways occurs at several points in the clotting cascade, with both positive and negative feedback. For example, the Factor VIIa–tissue factor complex can activate Factor IX. Although the extrinsic pathway can bypass Factor IX and Factor VIII-mediated activation of Factor X, deficiency of either Factor IX or Factor VIII results in the clinical bleeding disorder hemophilia.

Common Pathway

Once Factor Xa is formed by either the extrinsic or intrinsic pathway, it converts prothrombin to thrombin. This conversion is accelerated in the presence of Factor V, phospholipid, and calcium, which constitute a "prothrombinase complex." Factor V is derived from platelet α-granules and serves as a membrane receptor for the binding of Factor Xa to the platelet phospholipid membrane. Conversion of prothrombin to thrombin occurs on the membrane surface. After prothrombin is cleaved into thrombin by Factor Xa, thrombin detaches from the membrane surface.

Thrombin is a relatively nonspecific protease with multiple substrates, including fibrinogen, Factors XIII, V, VIII, protein S, protein C, and platelet membrane glycoproteins. Through a complex interplay of positive and negative feedback effects, it influences fibrin formation.

The formation of fibrin is the second phase of hemostasis (platelet activation is the first phase). Fibrinogen is a large glycoprotein present in both plasma and platelets. Thrombin binds to fibrinogen, resulting in fibrin monomer and subsequent polymer formation. Progressive lengthening of the polymer chain occurs by sequential approximation of the fibrin monomers and cross-linking mediated by Factor XIIIa. Two fibrin polymer chains combine to form a protofibril. The two-stranded protofibrils interact to form fibrin sheets or strands.

The fibrin meshwork binds platelets together and interacts with other adhesive proteins such as fibronectin and thrombospondin. These proteins also link fibrin to the extracellular matrix, thereby stabilizing the clot.

Multiple mechanisms exist for the regulation of hemostasis, including the effects of hemodilution and vascular flow,

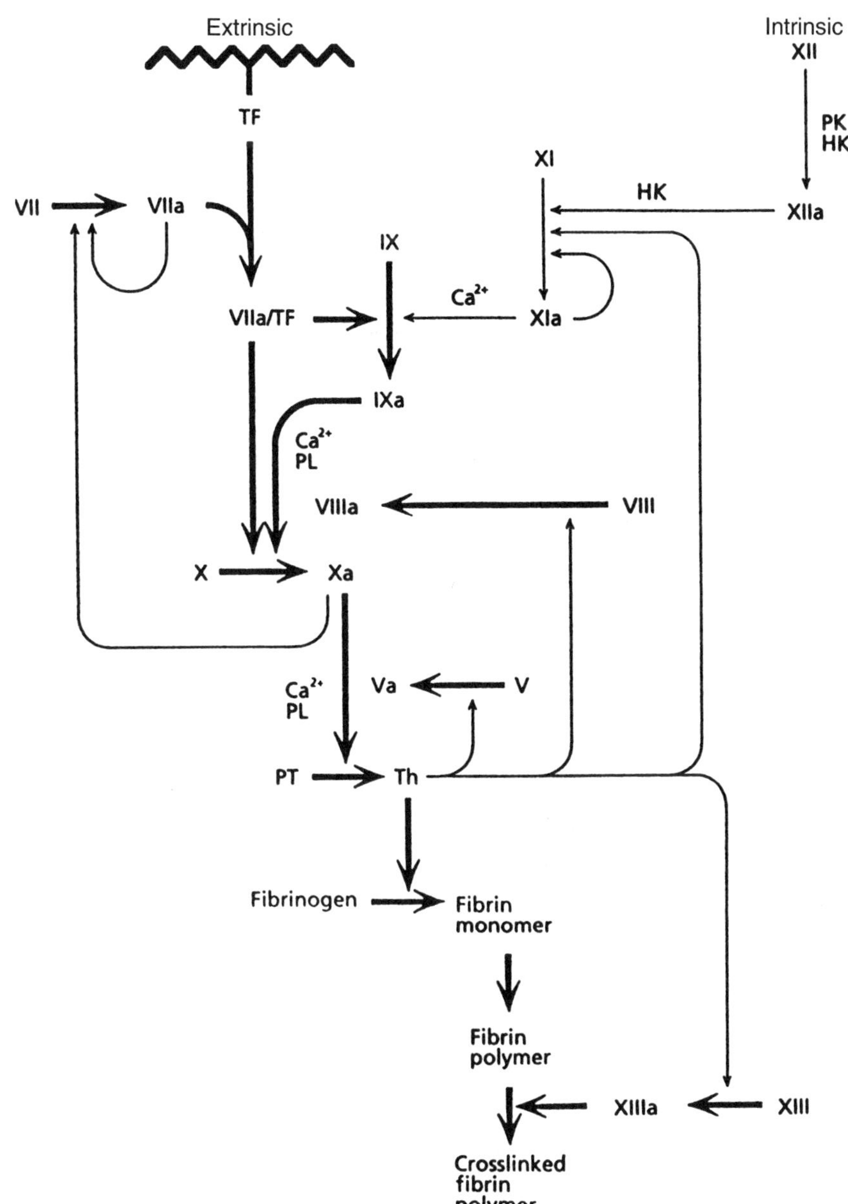

FIG. 36-1. The coagulation cascade. HK, high molecular weight kininogen; PK, prekallikrein; PL, phospholipid; PT, prothrombin; TF, tissue factor; Th, thrombin. (Adapted from Schafer AI. Coagulation cascade: an overview. In: Loscalzo J, Schafer AI, eds. *Thrombosis and hemorrhage.* Boston: Blackwell Scientific Publications, 1994;1–12.)

proteolytic feedback, inhibitory plasma proteins, and fibrinolysis. Vascular flow washes away inadequately secured platelets from the vascular wall. Hemodilution diminishes the concentration of procoagulant species that are not receptor bound and also delivers plasma inhibitors to the site of clot formation. The primary plasma inhibitor is antithrombin III (ATIII), which inhibits Factors IXa, Xa, and thrombin. This inhibition is potentiated by heparin. Other inhibitors include heparin co-Factor II, which inhibits thrombin but not Factors IXa or Xa, and α_1-protease inhibitor, which inhibits Factor XIa.

Thrombin-mediated proteolysis acts to inhibit fibrin formation in a negative-feedback manner. Initially, thrombin activates Factors V and VIII, but ultimately dampens this effect. Thrombin activates protein C through the endothelial protein thrombomodulin. Activated protein C in turn inhibits Factors Va and VIIIa, thereby slowing thrombin production.

Fibrinolysis

Fibrinolysis regulates fibrin formation and fibrin degradation. Like the coagulation pathways, fibrinolysis is a complex cascade of enzyme activations, feedback potentiation and inhibition, and balance between activators and inhibitors.

The inactive zymogen of fibrinolysis is plasminogen, which circulates in plasma. Plasminogen is converted to the active protease plasmin by plasminogen activators (PA). There are two primary endogenous PA, tissue plasminogen activator (t-PA), and urokinase-type plasminogen activator u-PA). t-PA is the primary operative PA in hemostasis. PA are regulated by PA inhibitors (PAI). Three primary PAIs have been described: PAI-1, PAI-2, and PAI-3. PAI-1 is the primary inhibitor of t-PA and circulates in plasma. Net plasmin production is the result of a balance between PA and PAI. During the initial period of hemostatic plug formation, endothelial cells and platelets release PAI, facilitating fibrin formation. As hemostasis proceeds, a poorly understood but precisely orchestrated sequence of stimuli results in endothelial cell production of PA, initiating the regulatory effects of fibrinolysis.

Once plasmin is produced, fibrin degradation begins. Again an intricate balance of the simultaneous forces of coagulation, platelet activation, inhibition of coagulation, profibrinolytic events, and cellular mechanisms mediates the gradual dissolution of the clot. The usual source of plasmin is plasminogen that is incorporated into the initial fibrin clot. Free circulating plasmin is rapidly inactivated by its inhibitor, α_2-antiplasmin, thereby limiting plasmin-mediated proteolysis to the site of the clot.

Plasmin has trypsin-like specificity with an affinity for the hydrolysis of lysl and arginyl bonds. The net result is the degradation of fibrinogen or fibrin into distinct fragments of the original molecule. Cross-linked fibrin is degraded more slowly.

The hemostatic system consists of endothelial cells, platelets, clotting factors, and fibrinolysis acting in concert to generate appropriate hemostasis. Dysfunction of any portion of this intricate process may result in disease. Pharmacologic intervention in this process is optimized by an understanding of the mechanisms of hemostasis.

PLASMINOGEN ACTIVATORS

PA are thrombolytic agents that result in the pharmacologic production of the serine protease plasmin, which in turn degrades fibrin. Ophthalmologists have long recognized the therapeutic potential of thrombolytic agents in thrombotic and hemorrhagic ocular disease such as hyphema and vitreous hemorrhage (1,2). Unfortunately, ocular toxicity due to impure preparations of thrombolytic drugs limited the utility of these agents. More recently, recombinant DNA technology and improved pharmacologic preparation have resulted in renewed interest in ocular thrombolytic therapy (3).

There are two endogenous PA: t-PA and u-PA. Streptokinase is an exogenous PA produced by hemolytic streptococci.

Tissue Plasminogen Activator

History and Source

t-PA is the primary physiologic PA in hemostasis, first identified as a product of melanoma cells in 1980 (4) and then purified in 1981 (5). Subsequent identification of the complementary DNA coding and recombinant DNA manufacturing techniques allowed pharmacologic production of t-PA. Currently, recombinant t-PA is produced by suspension-culture methods. The utility of recombinant t-PA in ophthalmology was first described in 1988 for the treatment of postoperative fibrin formation after posterior vitrectomy surgery (6).

Official Drug Name and Chemistry

The generic name of recombinant t-PA is alteplase. Currently, Activase (Genentech) is the only form of t-PA approved by the Food and Drug Administration (FDA). Activase has a variable molecular weight of 63,000 to 65,000 Da due to heterogenous glycosylation during production. The specific activity ranges from 550,000 to 667,000 IU/mg. Activase is produced primarily (60% to 80%) as a single-chain protein molecule with the remainder as a double-chain form (7).

The structure of t-PA is classified into five domains (Fig. 36-2). These domains are named according to conformational characteristics. The finger domain extends from amino acid residues 6 to 43 and is involved in the binding of t-PA to fibrin. The next domain is the epidermal growth factor domain extending from residues 44 to 92. This domain may mediate recognition of t-PA by receptors in the liver and thereby be involved in clearance of t-PA. There are two kringle domains, so named because of their conformational similarity to a Danish pastry. Kringle domains mediate binding to fibrin. The catalytic domain of t-PA consists of 239 amino acids with a 3-amino acid active site similar to other serine proteases.

Pharmacology

t-PA proteolytically converts the zymogen plasminogen to the protease plasmin by cleaving the Arg 561–Val 562 peptide bond in plasminogen, resulting in a two-chain plasmin molecule (8) (Fig. 36-3). Plasmin is the operative pharmacologic protease.

Clinical Pharmacology

In the absence of fibrin, t-PA is a relatively inefficient activator of plasminogen. However, in the presence of fibrin, the activation of plasminogen is increased more than 400-fold (7,8). This enhancement is the result of a conformational change in t-PA induced by fibrin binding to the finger and kringle domains. The conformational change facilitates the interaction between the catalytic domain and plasminogen. Secondarily, fibrin-induced conformational changes also occur in plasminogen. The net effect is enhanced production of plasmin.

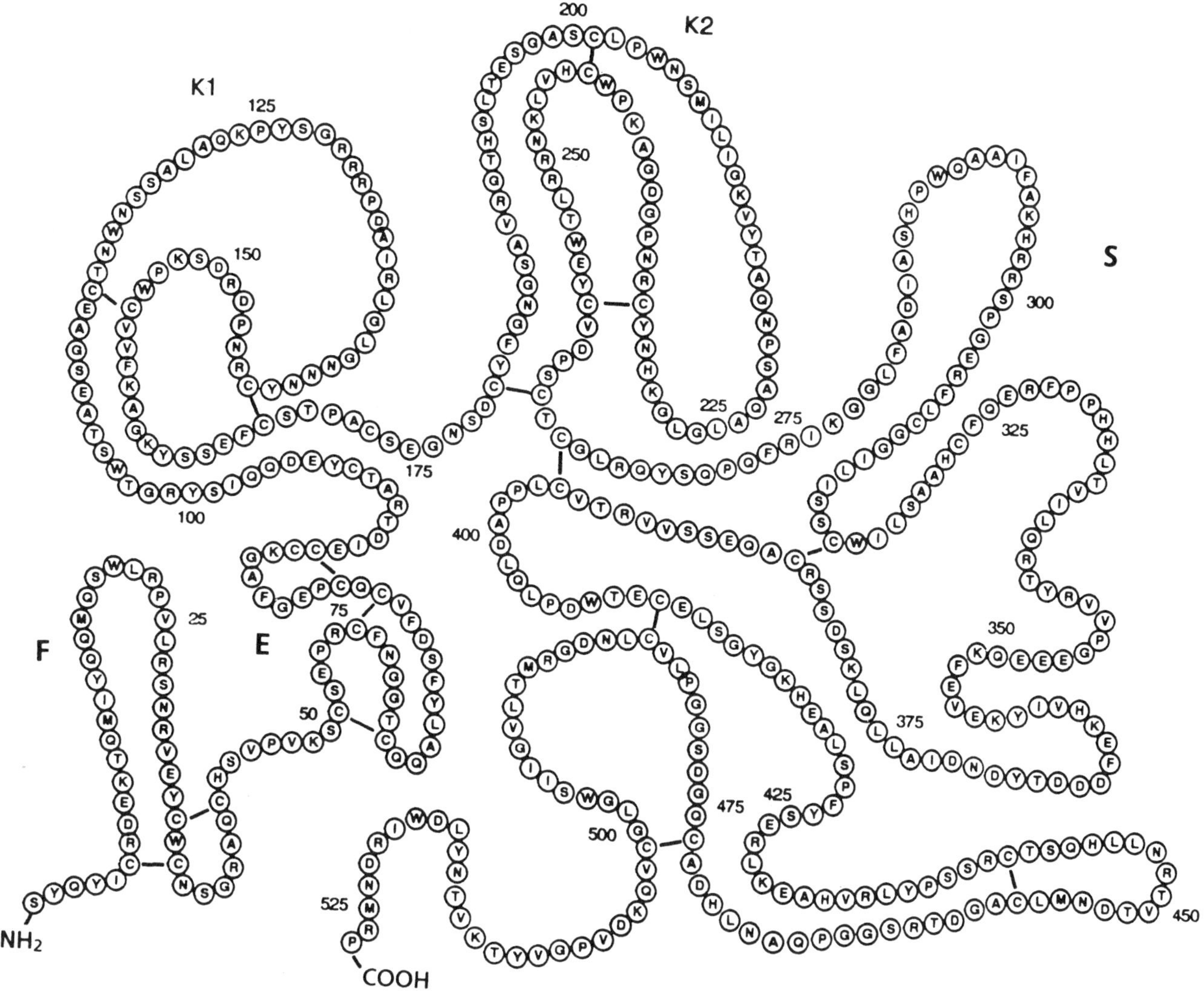

FIG. 36-2. Structure of tPA. F, finger domain; E, epidermal growth factor domain; K1 and K2, Kringle domains; S, serine protease domain. (Adapted from Pennica D, Holmes WE, Kohr WJ, et al. Cloning and expression of human tissue-type plasminogen activator cDNA in *E. Coli. Nature* 1983; 301:214–216.)

Pharmaceutics

Recombinant t-PA is available only as Activase in 20-mg or 50-mg vials. Activase is provided as a lyophilized powder and an accompanying diluent. When prepared according to the manufacturer's instructions, a concentration of 1 mg/ml is obtained. At room temperature, this concentration is stable for as long as 8 hours. When t-PA is prepared for ophthalmic use, further dilution is required. Currently recommended concentrations range from 100 μg/ml to 250 μl/ml. Dilution is performed with balanced saline solution or normal saline. Diluted Activase can be stored at a low temperature of −7°C to −70°C with maintenance of activity. At −70°C, Activase at a concentration of 250 μg/ml remained stable for 1 year (9). At −7°C, (the temperature of most commercial freezers) a concentration of 250 μg/ml is stable for as long as 4 months (10).

Pharmacokinetics, Concentration-effect and Metabolism

After intravenous administration, alteplase has an initial half-life (t½) in plasma ranging from 3.6 to 4.6 minutes. Its terminal t½ is 39 to 53 minutes (7). Because of this short t½, alteplase must be administered as a continuous intravenous infusion for 3 hours to maintain an intravascular fibrinolytic effect. The total volume of distribution is 27 to 40 L. Plasma clearance is primarily through hepatic uptake, but the endogenous inhibitor type 1 PAI may also have some effect. The plasma clearance is 520 to 1,000 ml/min.

The data on the ocular pharmacokinetics of t-PA are sparse and confined to the phakic rabbit model (11,12). With human fibroblast t-PA and a spectrophotometric solid-phase fibrin activity assay, the t½ of an intravitreal injection of 25 μg in 0.1 ml is related to the presence or ab-

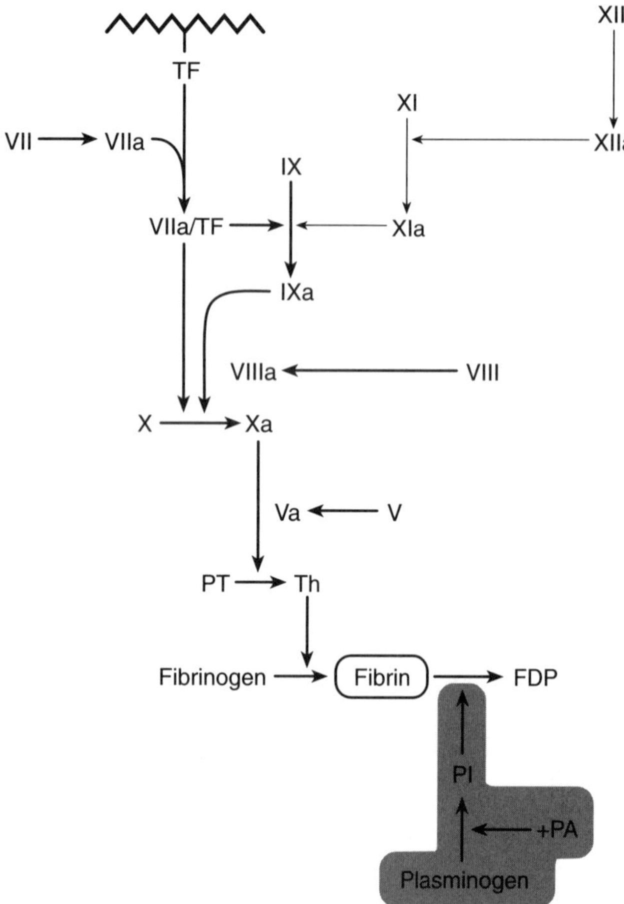

FIG. 36-3. Location of the action of tPA in the coagulation cascade. PT, prothrombin; Th, thrombin; FDP, fibrin(ogen) degradation products; PI, plasmin. (Adapted from Schafer AI. Coagulation cascade: an overview. In: Loscalzo J, Schafer AI, eds. *Thrombosis and hemorrhage.* Boston: Blackwell Scientific Publications, 1994;1–12.)

sence of fibrin. In the absence of vitreal fibrin, the t½ is 4.3 hours, whereas in the presence of fibrin the t½ is 9.8 hours. This prolongation of activity by fibrin is probably due to the fibrin-binding effect of t-PA, but may also be related to nonspecific effects of fibrin on aqueous clearance. The prolonged clearance of t-PA in the eye as compared with the clearance in plasma probably reflects the absence of hepatic circulation. A second explanation of the prolonged clearance may be the diminished level of PAI-1 in the eye (3). In rabbits, ocular clearance of t-PA occurred, at least in part, through the anterior chamber.

Therapeutic Use

Fibrin Formation

Intraocular fibrin formation after ocular surgery is a potentially serious complication that may lead to surgical failure. Fibrin formation most commonly occurs after vitrectomy for complicated retinal detachment, as in diabetes, proliferative vitreoretinopathy (PVR), retinopathy of prematurity, or trauma (3). Fibrin also forms subsequent to endophthalmitis and to glaucoma filtration surgery, penetrating keratoplasty and, rarely, cataract surgery (3,13,14).

Fibrin contributes to several pathophysiologic processes in the eye. Fibrin and fibrinogen-derived peptides modulate leukocyte influx into the eye, damage the corneal endothelium, and increase microvascular permeability. In vitro, fibrin stimulates retinal pigment epithelium (RPE) migration and may contribute to hypocellular gel contraction and recurrent detachment (3).

Intraocular t-PA is indicated for progressive fibrin formation that does not respond to aggressive antiinflammatory therapy with topical and periocular corticosteroids and topical nonsteroidal antiinflammatory agents. t-PA is not indicated for every case of fibrin formation because most cases will resolve with antiinflammatory therapy. In approximately 32% of posterior vitrectomies, some fibrin formation will develop (3). However, in the largest series reported to date, only 6% of 350 consecutive vitrectomies required t-PA therapy (15). Indications for t-PA include (a) massive fibrin response on the first postoperative day, (b) progressive worsening of fibrin formation in 48 to 72 hours despite antiinflammatory therapy, (c) pupillary membrane with pupillary block (16), (d) fibrin-induced traction retinal detachment, (e) glaucoma filtration fistula or tube closure by fibrin, and (f) severe nonclearing fibrin formation after cataract extraction. t-PA will clear fibrin formation in most eyes but not in eyes with long-standing fibrin formation. Fibrin membranes that have been present for 20 days or more are usually resistant to fibrinolysis (17), probably due to (a) progressive cross-linking of fibrin, (b) elimination of plasminogen from the fibrin, and (c) cellular infiltration of the fibrin. In most cases, t-PA will lyse ocular fibrin 1 to 3 hours and sometimes in a few minutes.

Intraocular t-PA is administered as an injection through the limbus or pars plana. A concentration of 100 to 250 μg/ml is used, with a total initial dose of 3 to 5 μg injected (18). If fibrin fails to clear after 24 hours, a second dose of 10 μg can be administered (3,19,20).

Although t-PA usually lyses ocular fibrin, it does not affect the underlying pathogenesis of fibrin formation. Therefore, once the fibrinolytic effect of t-PA has resolved, fibrin formation may recur if the underlying conditions that initially precipitated fibrin formation persist. Recurrent fibrin formation most commonly occurs 5 to 10 days after t-PA injection, but occasionally occurs 2 to 4 weeks later. Risk factors for recurrent fibrin formation include extensive anterior neovascularization such as rubeosis iridis and/or anterior hyaloidal fibrovascular proliferation. Endophthalmitis and anterior PVR also predispose to recurrent fibrin formation. Although recurrent fibrin can usually by lysed with repeat t-PA injection, the final visual outcome is often poor (3).

Subretinal Hemorrhage

In conjunction with vitrectomy techniques, t-PA can be injected into the subretinal space to facilitate removal of subretinal hemorrhage. Although this technique is most commonly used for large subretinal hemorrhages in age-related macular degeneration, it can be used for subretinal hemorrhage of any etiology. The details of the surgical approach are beyond the scope of this text and have been previously described (21). A standard three-port vitrectomy is performed with removal of any adherent posterior vitreous cortex. t-PA is then slowly injected into the clot through a transretinal approach with a small-gauge cannula (30 to 36 gauge). A total volume of 0.1 to 0.2 ml is injected, delivering a total initial dose of 10 to 20 μg. The t-PA remains in the subretinal space for 30 to 45 minutes, after which time the hemorrhage is aspirated or irrigated from the subretinal space. The retina is then reattached with a fluid–gas exchange.

Many questions remain concerning subretinal thrombolytic therapy. The optimal dose and concentration of t-PA are not known, nor are the optimum method of delivery and the required duration of exposure of the t-PA to the clot. Experimental animal work suggests that continuous or repeated irrigation of t-PA may more effectively lyse larger clots (22). To date, subretinal thrombolytic therapy has developed from empirical clinical observation and animal studies in rabbits and cats suggesting that t-PA reduces photoreceptor damage after subretinal hemorrhage. Although the initial results are promising, further clinical and laboratory investigations are warranted before the utility of this technique can be established.

Hyphema

Experimental animal studies have suggested the possibility of using t-PA to speed the clearance of hyphema (18,23). These studies suggest that t-PA does accelerate the clearance of experimental hyphema with use of either a blood injection model or laser trauma model. In the trauma model, the rate of rebleeding is increased if t-PA is administered sooner than 72 hours after the injury. To date, there have been no clinical reports of ocular t-PA for hyphema.

Retinal Vascular Occlusions

Intravenous t-PA has been suggested for the management of central retinal vein occlusion (24) and experimental branch retinal artery occlusion (25). To date, only small pilot studies have been reported.

Side Effects and Toxicity

The most serious potential complication of fibrinolytic therapy is hemorrhage. When t-PA is used intravenously for myocardial infarction, as many as 30% of patients have a significant bleeding episode (7). The incidence of bleeding with ocular therapy appears to be lower. In the 43 eyes reported by the group of investigators at the Medical College of Wisconsin, hemorrhage occurred in two eyes (3). In both eyes, rubeosis was present. The hemorrhages were hyphemas which spontaneously cleared.

Dabbs et al. described severe hemorrhagic complications after injection of 25 μg t-PA in 7 diabetic eyes (26). Although t-PA lysed the fibrin in each case, fibrin recurred and six of seven eyes developed no light perception. Risk factors for bleeding with ocular t-PA probably include rubeosis and anterior hyaloidal fibrovascular proliferation.

After t-PA injection, a turbid fluid phase often develops in the eye, resulting from the formation of fibrin degradation products and the mobilization of erythrocytes that were enmeshed in the fibrin. Sometimes these cells will layer out as a hyphema or disperse into the vitreous cavity. It is important to realize that this does not represent new bleeding. Fibrin degradation products can also exacerbate ocular inflammation. Therefore, a fluid–gas exchange may be indicated 24 to 48 hours after t-PA therapy.

The ocular toxicity of t-PA has not been studied in humans. Based on results of preliminary rabbit studies, an initial dose of 25 μg was used. Although this dose appeared to be clinically nontoxic, subsequent toxicity studies suggested that in an aphakic, vitrectomized, gas-filled rabbit eye, 25 μg is at the threshold for retinal toxicity (27). Because minimizing the dose of t-PA should decrease possible toxicity, lower doses have been studied. The dose–response curves of the rabbit model (11) indicate that doses as low as 3 μg are effective (20).

The toxicity of subretinal t-PA has also been studied only in animals. Such research suggests that subretinal t-PA is nontoxic to the retina at doses of 50 μg or less and concentrations of 500 μg/ml or less. A concentration of 1,000 μg/ml is toxic (21,22). At a dose of 25 μg, intraocular t-PA shows no evidence of corneal endothelial toxicity as measured by a corneal endothelial perfusion technique (28).

High-risk Groups

No high-risk groups have been described.

Drug Interactions

No drug interactions resulting from ocular t-PA have been described.

Major Clinical Trials

The efficacy of ocular t-PA has not been examined in any randomized, controlled clinical trials.

EPSILON-AMINOCAPROIC ACID (EACA)

History and Source

EACA was first reported in 1976 in the management of hyphema to prevent rebleeding (29). It is a synthetic lysine analogue.

Official Drug Name and Chemistry

EACA (Amicar) is a 6-amino hexanoic acid. The chemical formula is $C_6H_{13}NO_2$, and the molecular weight is 131.17.

Pharmacology

EACA inhibits fibrinolysis by binding to the lysine binding sites of plasminogen, resulting in a conformational change which inhibits the binding of plasminogen and plasmin to fibrin and fibrinogen (Fig. 36-4). The net effect is to inhibit fibrinolysis (30).

Clinical Pharmacology

Plasminogen is normally converted to plasmin by PA, which causes a proteolytic cleavage at the serine-histidine active site. Conversion of Glu-plasminogen to Lys-plasminogen by plasmin promotes the binding of plasminogen to a fibrin or fibrinogen substrate by binding between lysine sites on plasminogen and lysine residues of the substrate. Disruption of this binding inhibits proteolysis. EACA has a three-dimensional structure similar to that of lysine, which results in steric inhibition of the binding of lysine residues on fibrin or fibrinogen with the lysine binding sites of plasmin or plasminogen. The net effect is to inhibit fibrinolysis by plasmin (30).

Pharmaceutics

EACA is available as both intravenous and oral preparations. The intravenous preparation contains 250 mg/ml. The oral preparations are a syrup containing 250 mg/ml and a 500-mg tablet.

Pharmacokinetics, Concentration–Effect Relationship and Metabolism

EACA is rapidly absorbed from the gastrointestinal (GI) tract, with an absorption rate of 5.2 g/hr. The volume of distribution is estimated to be 23.1 ± 6.6 L after oral administration and 30.0 ± 8.2 L after intravenous administration. Peak plasma levels occur 2 hours after oral administration with chronic administration. EACA distributes throughout the intravascular and extravascular compartments (31). At the dose of 50 mg/kg orally every 4 hours, the mean peak plasma concentration (±SD) is 8.38 ± 2.37 mg/100 mL, the trough concentration is 6.16 ± 2.03 mg/100 mL, and the mean concentration is 7.27 ± 1.94 mg/100 mL. At a dose of 100 mg/kg orally every 4 hours with a maximum dose of 5 g, the mean peak concentration (±SD) is 15.1 ± 4.399 mg/100 mL (32). The trough concentration is 10/5 ± 3.41 mg/100 mL, and the mean concentration is 12/8 ± 3.7 mg/100 mL. Plasma levels of 1.3 mg/100 mL are adequate to inhibit in vivo fibrinolysis, but a level of 13 mg/100 mL is considered optimal (30). Experimental work in rabbits demonstrates a dose-dependent relationship between plasma levels and aqueous humor levels of EACA (33). After a 50-mg/kg intravenous dose, the mean peak aqueous level is 14 mg/100 mL and the mean trough aqueous level is 2 mg/100 mL.

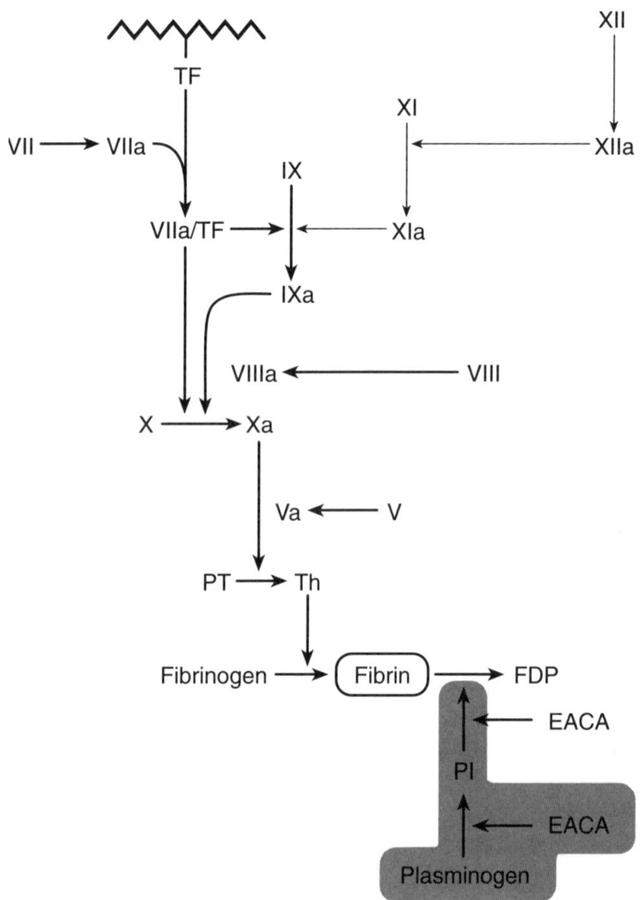

FIG. 36-4. Location of the action of EACA in the fibrinolytic portion of the coagulation cascade. PT, prothrombin; Th, thrombin; FDP, fibrin(ogen) degradation products; PI, plasmin. (Adapted from Schafer AI. Coagulation cascade: an overview. In: Loscalzo J, Schafer AI, eds. *Thrombosis and hemorrhage.* Boston: Blackwell Scientific Publications, 1994;1–12.)

EACA is rapidly excreted by the kidneys, with a t½ of approximately 2 hours. Approximately 80% of an intravenous dose is cleared in 3 hours or less, but because of its high volume of distribution, urinary excretion can be detected for as long as 12 to 36 hours after an intravenous dose. Most EACA is excreted unchanged; the remainder is excreted as the metabolite adipic acid. The renal clearance is 116 mL/min (31).

Therapeutic Use

Hyphema

EACA is used in the management of traumatic hyphema to decrease the incidence of secondary hemorrhage. The therapeutic rationale is that plasminogen activation to plasmin causes fibrinolysis at the traumatized bleeding site, which poses the risk of secondary hemorrhage. Inhibition of plasmin retards fibrinolysis, allowing more time for restoration of vascular integrity. The recommended dose of EACA is 50 to 100 mg/kg orally every 4 hours to a maximum of 5 g per dose or 30 g/day (32,34,35). In patients unable to tolerate oral administration, intravenous therapy may be administered as 50 to 100 mg/kg in 250 mL isotonic diluent in 1 hour. Thereafter, 1 g EACA is administered each hour by continuous infusion in 50 mL isotonic diluent. Rapid injection of undiluted EACA should be avoided.

EACA is contraindicated in the presence of the disseminated intravascular coagulation (DIC). The possibility of DIC should be considered in patients who have sustained significant trauma, particularly head trauma.

Prevention of Postoperative Vitreous Hemorrhage

Vitreous hemorrhage after vitrectomy surgery is a common postoperative problem, particularly after surgery for proliferative diabetic retinopathy. Potential sources of hemorrhage include recently dissected fibrovascular proliferation, anterior hyaloidal fibrovascular proliferation, and fibrovascular ingrowth at the sclerotomies. Antifibrinolytic therapy with EACA has been suggested to avoid premature clot lysis at potential bleeding sites and thus possibly decrease the chance of postoperative bleeding (36). EACA is administered with a 5 gram intravenous loading dose one hour before surgery. Postoperatively, EACA is administered intravenously until oral medication can be tolerated. Thereafter, oral EACA is administered at 100 mg/kg every 4 hours to a maximum of 30 g/day. Oral EACA treatment is continued for 4 days. In cases of renal failure, the dose of EACA must be adjusted.

Side Effects of Toxicity

The most common side effects of oral EACA are nausea or vomiting in approximately 25% of patients. Dizziness and systemic hypotension occur in approximately 20% of patients. The incidence of dizziness and hypotension is less at a 50-mg/kg oral dose, with no apparent decrease in efficacy. Less frequent side effects include diarrhea, rash, syncope, and myalgia. The mechanism of the nausea, vomiting, and diarrhea is probably gastrointestinal irritation since these side effects rarely occur with intravenous therapy (29,32,34,35).

Overdosage

There are no reports of the signs, symptoms, and complications of acute overdosage of EACA. Animal work suggests that the LD_{50} of EACA is high. In rats and mice, the oral LD_{50} is 12.0 to 16.0 g/kg. Although no treatment protocols for overdosage of EACA are reported, EACA is cleared by hemodialysis.

High-risk Groups

EACA should be avoided in pregnancy. Whether EACA is excreted in human milk is not known. EACA should be administered with caution to patients with renal disease and, if administered, the dose should be adjusted according to the degree of renal impairment.

Drug Interactions

No drug interactions occur with EACA.

Major Clinical Trials

Hyphema

The efficacy of EACA in lowering the incidence of secondary hemorrhage has been demonstrated in four clinical trials (29,32,34,35). However, EACA therapy has not gained universal acceptance primarily because of the high incidence of side effects, the cost, and the apparent population-dependent variability in rate of secondary hemorrhage.

Postoperative Hemorrhage

The efficacy of EACA on postvitrectomy hemorrhage has been examined in only one randomized trial. EACA significantly reduced vitreous hemorrhage during the first 4 postoperative days. However, there was no difference in the severity of postoperative hemorrhage between EACA-treated eyes and control eyes at either 2 weeks or 6 weeks after surgery (36).

THROMBIN

History and Source

Thrombin was first introduced into ophthalmology in 1951 for the control of anterior chamber bleeding (37). It was reintroduced in 1986 for the control of bleeding during diabetic vitrectomy (38). Thrombin is a naturally occurring procoagulant protease that converts fibrinogen to fibrin. Pharmacologic thrombin is a bovine-derived product produced by the conversion of prothrombin by tissue thromboplastin in the presence of calcium chloride.

Official Drug Name and Chemistry

Bovine thrombin is a large protease consisting of a two-chain enzyme composed of an A chain of 49 amino acid residues and a B chain of 259 amino acid residues. The A chain is subsequently cleaved to create the stable form of thrombin consisting of an A chain of 37 residues (39). Thrombin is available under the brand names Thombinar, Thrombostat, and Thrombogen.

Pharmacology

In vivo, thrombin is formed by the conversion of prothrombin by the prothrombinase complex, which consists of Factor Xa, Factor V, platelet membrane phospholipids, and calcium. Thrombin possesses a wide range of biologic activity beyond the conversion of fibrinogen to fibrin. Thrombin also activates platelets, activates various coagulation procofactors, stimulates fibrinolysis, regulates vascular tone, and participates in wound repair as a growth factor (GF).

Clinical Pharmacology

Thrombin is approved for human use only as a topical agent. Its strong procoagulant activity requires that it never be injected into the intravascular space. Because of the "closed space" nature of intraocular surgery, thrombin can be administered into the eye by ocular-infusion solutions without causing systemic complications.

Pharmaceutics

Thrombin is supplied as a lyophilized powder with calcium chloride, sodium chloride, and glycine. It is supplied with isotonic saline as a diluent. Thrombin is supplied in 5,000-U, 10,000-U, and 20,000-U vials. A unit is defined as the amount required to clot 1 ml standardized fibrinogen solution in 15 seconds. Approximately 2 U are required to clot 1 ml oxalated human plasma in 15 seconds.

Pharmacokinetics

The pharmacokinetics of intraocular thrombin have been studied only in a rabbit vitrectomy model (40). In this model, thrombin, at a concentration 100 U/ml in balanced salt solution (BSS), reduced the bleeding time from transected retinal vessels from a control average of 180 seconds (SD 23.7 seconds) to 27.6 seconds (SD 7.2 seconds).

Therapeutic Use

Thrombin has been reported to be effective in reducing intraoperative hemorrhage in eyes undergoing vitrectomy for proliferative diabetic retinopathy (38), trauma (41), and stage V retinopathy of prematurity (42). In these studies, a concentration of 100 U/ml in a BSS infusion was used. In the study of diabetic retinopathy, bleeding time after transection of fibrovascular tissue was measured. Although substantial case-to-case variability could be expected, the eyes treated with thrombin showed a significant decrease in bleeding time as compared with that in randomized, mashed placebo controls; 12.3 $\pm$ 14 versus 111.5 $\pm$ 17 seconds (mean $\pm$ SD). A more recent report suggests that lower concentrations of thrombin between 5 and 10 U/ml may also be effective in preventing or controlling intraoperative hemorrhage (43).

Side Effects and Toxicity

The only reported side effect of intraocular thrombin is excessive postoperative inflammation with hypopyon in 20% of patients (38); this occurred only in phakic eyes. The inflammation can be minimized by irrigating the thrombin solution from the eye at completion of surgery. The inflammation usually clears with hourly topical corticosteroids administration. Lower concentrations of thrombin (5 to 10 U/ml) may alleviate this inflammation (43). The etiology of the inflammation is unknown, but is speculated to be an immune response to the bovine product.

The toxicologic data on intraocular thrombin is limited. In the rabbit model, there is no evidence of histologic retinal toxicity or corneal endothelial toxicity (40,44). Electroretinographic studies show no effect on b-wave amplitudes at 3 days and 4 weeks after surgery. However, intensity–response function analysis revealed residual sensitivity reductions in thrombin-treated eyes (40).

High-risk Groups

Intraocular thrombin has been used in neonates and adults.

Drug Interactions

Absolute care must be taken to ensure that the thrombin solution is not inadvertently administered intravenously. Fatal systemic thrombosis could result.

Major Clinical Trials

No major clinical trials of thrombin have been conducted.

HEPARIN

History and Source

The reported use of heparin in ophthalmology is limited. Heparin supplementation of vitrectomy infusion solution to decrease postoperative fibrin formation has been described in diabetes (45) and retinopathy or prematurity (46). Experimental work suggests additional potential therapeutic applications of heparin in vitreoretinal surgery (47). Heparin is a naturally occurring glycosaminoglycan. Pharmacologic heparin is derived from bovine lung tissue or porcine intestinal mucosa.

Official Drug Name and Chemistry

Heparin is a mixture of sulfated glycosaminoglycans derived from a large proteoglycan (48). The proteoglycan consists of a core protein, termed serglycin, with carbohydrate linkage regions connecting to multiple polysaccharide chains. During synthesis, the polysaccharide chains are isolated and purified. Commercial heparin consists of a heterogenous mixture of polysaccharides. Isoelectric focusing identifies 21 single polysaccharide chains with molecular weights that vary from 3,000 to 35,000, with a mean of about 12,000. The polysaccharide chains consist of alternating residues of uronic acid and glucosamine. These monosaccharides have many possible arrangements. The uronic acid groups may exist as iduronic acid-2-sulfate, glucuronic acid-2-sulfate, nonsulfated glucuronic acid, or nonsulfated iduronic acid. The glucosamine residues may be *N*-sulfated, or *N*-acetylated or may have free amino groups. The actual structure of the polysaccharides varies according to the source of the commercial heparin preparation. Therefore, a great variety of possible glucosamine-uronic acid sequences exists in a heparin molecule.

Pharmacology

Heparin exerts its anticoagulant effect by binding to antithrombin, thereby potentiating this protease inhibitor, which inactivates the hemostatic enzymes thrombin and Factor Xa (49) (Fig. 36-5). Although heparin is a complex carbohydrate, only a small fraction of the commercial polysaccharide is responsible for the anticoagulant activity (Fig. 36-6). An oligosaccharide of approximately 16 residues accelerates the thrombin–antithrombin and Factor Xa–antithrombin interactions. This oligosaccharide binds to antithrombin, leading to a conformational change in antithrombin that accelerates the neutralization of thrombin and Factor Xa 2,000- to 10,000-fold (48).

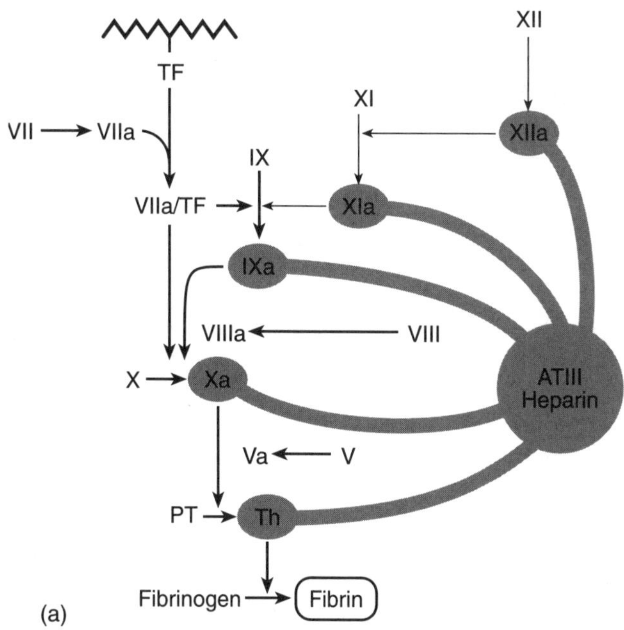

FIG. 36-5. Location of action of heparin and antithrombin III in the coagulation cascade. PT, prothrombin; Th, thrombin, AT-III, antithrombin III. (Adapted from Schafer AI. Coagulation cascade: an overview. In: Loscalzo J, Schafer AI, eds. *Thrombosis and hemorrhage.* Boston: Blackwell Scientific Publications, 1994;1–12.)

Heparin possesses a wide variety of biologic activities that are independent of its anticoagulant properties, including interactions with GF, inhibition of RPE proliferation, and inhibition of cell-mediated collagen-gel contraction (50). Heparin binds to platelets and causes platelet aggregation. This effect is due to a domain of the heparin molecule different from the domain responsible for the anticoagulant effect (48).

Clinical Pharmacology

The clinical pharmacology of ocular heparin therapy in humans is limited. Only a few reports exist of heparin supplementation to ocular irrigation solutions (45,46,51). The rationale of ocular heparin therapy is to inhibit the coagulation cascade and thus inhibit postoperative fibrin formation.

Pharmaceutics

Heparin is supplied as a sterile solution of heparin sodium. It is available in vials of 1,000 U, 5,000 U, and 10,000 U.

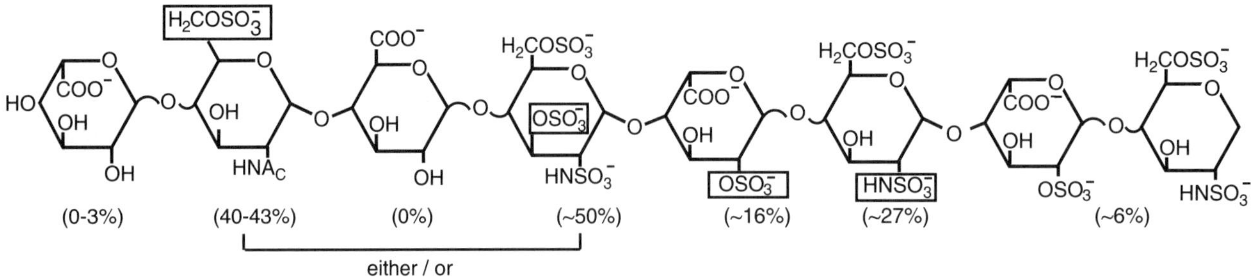

(0-3%) (40-43%) (0%) (~50%) (~16%) (~27%) (~6%)

either / or

FIG 36-6. Structure of anticoagulantly active heparin. The relative importance of the various residues in binding to AT-III is provided. (Adapted from Rosenberg RD. Prothrombinase generation. In: Loscalzo J, Schafer AI, eds. *Thrombosis and hemorrhage.* Boston: Blackwell Scientific Publications, 1994;25.)

Pharmacokinetics Concentration–Effect Relationship, and Metabolism

Human data on the pharmacokinetics of ocular heparin therapy is sparse. Reported doses are 1 U/ml, 5 U/ml, 10 U/ml, and 20 U/ml in BSS infusion. Only the concentrations of 5 U/ml and 10 U/ml have been compared for efficacy in preventing postoperative fibrin (45). The 10 U/ml dose demonstrated decreased fibrin formation as compared with controls. The 5-U/ml dose was not effective. In the same study, an intravenous dose of 10,0000 U at completion of surgery had no beneficial effect in preventing postoperative fibrin formation (45).

Animal work demonstrates a dose-dependent effect in the rabbit model. A concentration of 4 U/ml was more effective than 2 U/ml in preventing fibrin formation. A concentration of 0.5 U/ml had no effect on fibrin formation (52). There are no human or animal data on the metabolism or clearance of heparin in the eye.

Therapeutic Use

Ocular heparin therapy has been designed to limit fibrin formation and, more recently, to reduce reproliferation in PVR. In retinopathy of prematurity, a dose of 20 U/ml is reported to be effective in limiting intraoperative fibrin formation during open sky vitrectomy without bleeding complications (46). In a small series, a dose of 10 U/ml in the vitrectomy infusion solution eliminated fibrin formation after vitrectomy. This dose was associated with increased intraoperative bleeding (45).

In a recent study of patients undergoing vitrectomy for PVR, a combination of heparin, 1 U/ml and dexamethasone 4 μg/ml in the infusion solution reduced the rate of reproliferation, reoperation, and hypotony (51).

Side Effects and Toxicity

The major reported side effect of ocular heparin therapy is increased intraoperative and postoperative hemorrhage. This complication may not be due to the anticoagulant effect of heparin but rather to heparin-induced platelet dysfunction. Low molecular weight heparin fragments can dissociate the anticoagulant (antifibrin) effect from the hemorrhagic side effects (48). Experimental work suggests that low molecular weight heparin fragments may be useful in ocular disease (50).

High-risk Groups

No high-risk groups have been reported.

Drug Interactions

Platelet inhibitors such as aspirin, dypyridamole, and nonsteroidal antiinflammatory agents should be used with caution in patients receiving heparin systemically. Whether such drugs pose an increased risk of hemorrhage when used with ocular heparin therapy is unknown.

Major Clinical Trials

No multicenter, randomized trials have been reported.

REFERENCES

1. Friedman MW. Streptokinase in ophthalmology. *Am J Ophthalmol* 1952;35:1184–1187.
2. O'Rourke JF. An evaluation of intraocular streptokinase. *Am J Ophthalmol* 1955;39:119–136.
3. Williams GA. Pathogenesis and management of postvitrectomy fibrin formation. In: Lewis H, Ryan S, eds. *Medical and Surgical Retina. Advances, controversies and management.* St. Louis: CV Mosby, 1994;182–189.
4. Wilson EL, Becker MLB, Hoal EG, Dowdle EB. Molecular species of plasminogen activators secreted by normal and neoplastic human cells *Cancer Res* 1980;40:933–938.
5. Rijken DC, Collen D. Purification and characterization of the plasminogen activator secreted by human melanoma cells in culture *J Biol Chem* 1981;256:7035–7041.
6. Williams GA, Lambrou FH, Jaffe GA, et al. Treatment of postvitrectomy fibrin formation with intraocular tissue plasminogen activator. *Arch Ophthalmol* 1988;106:1055–1058.
7. Loscalzo J, Braunwald E. Tissue plasminogen activator. *N Engl J Med* 1988;319:925–931.

8. Hoylaerts M, Rijken DC, Lijnen HR, Collen D. Kinetics of the activation of plasminogen by human tissue plasminogen activator; role of fibrin. *J Biol Chem* 1982;257:2912–2919.
9. Jaffe GJ, Green GDJ, Abrams GW. Stability of recombinant tissue plasminogen activator. *Am J Ophthalmol* 1989;108:90–91.
10. Ko PC, Wagner DG, Cupples HP. Stability of recombinant tissue plasminogen activator. *Invest Ophthalmol Vis Sci* 1994;35(suppl):2217.
11. Snyder RW, Lambrou FH, Williams GA. Intraocular fibrinolysis with recombinant human tissue plasminogen activator: experimental treatment in a rabbit model. *Arch Ophthalmol* 1987;105:1277–1280.
12. Jaffe GJ, Green GDJ, McKay BS, Hartz A, Williams GA. Intravitreal clearance of tissue plasminogen activator in the rabbit. *Arch Ophthalmol* 1988;106:969–972.
13. Ortiz JR, Walker SD, McManos PE, Martinez LA, Brown RH, Jaffe GJ. Filtering bleb thrombolysis with tissue plasminogen activator. *Am J Ophthalmol* 1988;106:624–625.
14. Moon J, Chung S, Myong Y, et al. Treatment of postcataract fibrinous membranes with tissue plasminogen activator. *Ophthalmology* 1992; 99:1256–1259.
15. Jaffe GJ, Abrams GW, Williams GA, Han DP. Tissue plasminogen activator for postvitrectomy fibrin formation. *Ophthalmology* 1990;97: 184–189.
16. Jaffe GJ, Lewis H, Han DP, Williams GA, Abrams GW. Treatment of postvitrectomy fibrin pupillary block with tissue plasminogen activator. *Am J Ophthalmol* 1989;108:170–175.
17. Folk JC, Hershey JM, Rivers MB. Lack of effectiveness of tissue plasminogen activator 20 or more days after vitrectomy. *Arch Ophthalmol* 1991;109:614.
18. Lambrou FH, Snyder RW, Williams GA. Use of tissue plasminogen activator in experimental hyphema. *Arch Ophthalmol* 1987;105:995–997.
19. Williams DF, Bennett SR, Abrams GW, et al. Low dose tissue plasminogen activator for treatment of postvitrectomy fibrin formation. *Am J Ophthalmol* 1990;109:606–607.
20. Boldt HC, Abrams GW, Murray TG, Han DP, Mieler WF. The lowest effective dose of tissue plasminogen activator for fibrinolysis of postvitrectomy fibrin. *Retina* 1992;12:575–579.
21. Lewis H. Management of submacular hemorrhage. In: Lewis H, Ryan S, eds. *Medical and surgical retina. Advances, controversies and management.* St. Louis: CV Mosby, 1994;54–62.
22. Johnson MW, Olsen KR, Hernandez E. Tissue plasminogen activator thrombolysis during surgical evacuation of experimental subretinal hemorrhage. *Ophthalmology* 1992;99:515–521.
23. Williams DF, Han DP, Abrams GW. Rebleeding in experimental traumatic hyphema treated with intraocular tissue plasminogen activator. *Arch Ophthalmol* 1990;108:264–266.
24. Elman MJ, Quinlan P, Fine SL, et al. Thrombolytic therapy for central retinal vein occlusion. *Invest Ophthalmol Vis Sci* 1988;29(suppl):68.
25. Vine AK, Maguire PT, Martony C, Kincaid MC. Recombinant tissue plasminogen activator to lyse experimentally induced retinal arterial thrombi. *Am J Ophthalmol* 1988;105:266–270.
26. Dabbs CK, Aaberg TM, Aquilar HE, et al. Complication of tissue plasminogen activator therapy after vitrectomy for diabetes. *Am J Ophthalmol* 1990;110:354–360.
27. Irvine WD, Johnson MW, Hernandez E, Olsen KR. Retinal toxicity of human plasminogen activator in vitrectomized rabbit eyes. *Arch Ophthalmol* 1991;109:718–722.
28. McDermott ML, Edelhauser HF, Hyndiuk RA, Koenig SB. Tissue plasminogen activator and the corneal endothelium. *Am J Ophthalmol* 1989;108:91–92.
29. Crouch ER Jr, Frenkel M. Aminocaproic acid in the treatment of traumatic hyphema. *Am J Ophthalmol* 1976;81:355–360.
30. Griffin JD, Ellman L. Epsilon-aminocaproic acid (EACA). *Semin Thromb Hemost* 1978;5:27–40.
31. McNicol GP, Fletcher AP, Alkjaersig N, Sherry S. The absorption, distribution, and excretion of epsilon-aminocaproic acid following oral or intravenous administration to man. *J Lab Clin Med* 1962; 59:15–24.
32. Palmer DJ, Goldberg MF, Frenkel M, Fiscella R, Anderson RJ. A comparison of two dose regimens of epsilon-aminocaproic acid in the prevention and management of secondary traumatic hyphemas. *Ophthalmology* 1986;93:102–108.
33. Loewy DM, Williams PB, Crouch ER, Cooke WJ. Systemic aminocaproic acid reduces fibrinolysis in aqueous humor. *Arch Ophthalmol* 1987;105:272–276.
34. McGetrick JJ, Jampol LM, Goldberg MF, Frenkel M, Fiscella RG. Aminocaproic acid decreases secondary hemorrhage after traumatic hyphema. *Arch Ophthalmol* 1983;101:1031–1033.
35. Kutner B, Fourman S, Brein K, et al. Aminocaproic acid reduces the risk of secondary hemorrhage in patients with traumatic hyphema. *Arch Ophthalmol* 1987;105:206–208.
36. deBustros S, Glaser BM, Michels RG, Aver C. Effect of epsilon-aminocaproic acid on postvitrectomy hemorrhage. *Arch Ophthalmol* 1985;103:219–221.
37. Hughes WL. Use of thrombin in the anterior chamber to control hemorrhage. Sixteenth Concilium Ophthalmologicum, 1950. Britannia, 1951;1299–1306.
38. Thompson JT, Glaser BM, Michels RG, deBustros S. The use of intravitreal thrombin to control hemorrhage during vitrectomy. *Ophthalmology* 1986;93:279–282.
39. Downing MR, Butkowski RJ, Clark MM, Mann KG. Human prothrombin activator. *J Biol Chem* 1975;250:8897–8902.
40. deBustros S, Glaser BM, Johnson MA. Thrombin infusion for the control of intraocular bleeding during vitreous surgery. *Arch Ophthalmol* 1985;103:837–839.
41. deBustros S. Intraoperative control of hemorrhage in penetrating ocular injuries. *Retina* 1990;10:555–558.
42. Blacharski PA, Charles ST. Thrombin infusion to control bleeding during vitrectomy for stage V retinopathy of prematurity. *Arch Ophthalmol* 1987;105:203–205.
43. Eaton AM, Gehrs K, Handa JT, Machemer R. Low dose thrombin effectively controls intraocular hemorrhage. *Invest Ophthalmol Vis Sci* 1993;34(suppl4):948.
44. Mannis MJ, Sweet E, Landers MB, Lewis RA. Uses of thrombin in ocular surgery. Effect on the corneal endothelium. *Arch Ophthalmol* 1988;106:251–253.
45. Johnson RN, Blankenship G. A prospective randomized clinical trial of heparin therapy for postoperative intraocular fibrin. *Ophthalmology* 1988;95:312–317.
46. MacDonald SG, Buzney SM, Hirose T, Schepens CL. Inhibition of intraocular fibrin. *Invest Ophthalmol Vis Sci* 1985;26(suppl):24.
47. Blumenkranz MS, Hartzer MK, Iverson D. An overview of potential applications of heparin in vitreoretinal surgery. *Retina* 1992;12: 571–574.
48. Fareed J. Heparin, its fractions, fragments and derivatives. Some newer perspectives. *Semin Thromb Hemost* 1985;11:1–8.
49. Esmon CT. The regulation of natural anticoagulant pathways. *Science* 1987;235:1348–1352.
50. Blumenkranz MS, Hartzer MK. Pharmacologic treatment of proliferative vitreoretinopathy; interrelationship with the coagulation cascade. In: Lewis H, Ryan S, eds. *Medical and surgical retina. Advances, controversies and management.* St. Louis: CV Mosby, 1994; 172–181.
51. Williams RG, Chang S, Comaratta MR, Simone G. Does heparin and dexamethasone in the vitrectomy infusate reduce reproliferation in proliferative vitreoretinopathy? *Ophthalmology* 1992;99(suppl):111.
52. Johnson RN, Balyeat E, Stern WH. Heparin prophylaxis for intraocular fibrin. *Ophthalmology* 1987;94:597–601.

Textbook of Ocular Pharmacology,
edited by T.J. Zimmerman, et al.
Lippincott–Raven Publishers, Philadelphia © 1997.

CHAPTER 37

Ocular Pharmacology of Diabetic Retinopathy

Lawrence I. Rand

Diabetic retinopathy is an ocular manifestation of a systemic disease, diabetes mellitus. No ocular pharmacologic agent has been proven effective in the treatment of this condition. Retinal photocoagulation with laser energy is effective in reducing moderate visual loss from macular edema and severe visual loss from proliferative retinopathy (1–3). It may also be effective in eyes with severe non-proliferative retinopathy. In 1993, The Diabetes Control and Complications Trial (DCCT) proved that a treatment strategy whose goal was to keep a patient's blood sugar as near-normal for as long as possible effective in preventing or slowing development of retinopathy in patients without it, and preventing or delaying progression in those already having it (4–6).

Insulin, the pharmacologic agent used in the DCCT, has been used routinely to treat insulin-dependent diabetes mellitus (IDDM) since its discovery in 1922. It is a 51-amino acid polypeptide secreted by the B cells in the Islets of Langerhans of the pancreas. The details of the pharmacology (7) and mechanisms of action (8) of insulin are well known. Since the 1920s, animal insulins have been used, primarily bovine and porcine. In the last decade, synthesized human insulin has been available commercially. Without insulin, persons with IDDM die. With insulin they live, but almost all later develop one or more of the microvascular complications of diabetes: retinopathy, nephropathy, or neuropathy (9), which are the most common conditions leading to laser treatment, dialysis or kidney transplantation, and amputation. Because these entities were uncommon before insulin was discovered, some investigators have suggested that exogenous insulin administration may contribute to the development of diabetic complications (10). This is unlikely, given the results of the DCCT. However, neither is insulin alone responsible for the reduction in complications observed in that study, since both groups of patients received insulin and the total dose of insulin was less than 10% higher in intensively treated patients (11). The balance between the patient's metabolic state; dietary intake; activity level; and dose, timing, and type of insulin apparently influences metabolic control and secondarily, over time, influences the development and progression of retinopathy and other complications. Because the entirety of the intensive therapy regimen appears to be the only quasipharmacologic agent that influences development and progression of retinopathy, this is described in detail, along with metabolic and retinopathy outcomes of such therapy as documented in the DCCT.

L. I. Rand: 164 Bigelow Rd., West Newton, Massachusetts 02165.

INTENSIVE TREATMENT REGIMEN

Intensive treatment was a comprehensive, flexible program that allowed variation within prescribed guidelines to achieve glycemic goals as near the nondiabetic range as possible while minimizing severe hypoglycemia. Goals for blood glucose levels, measured with home glucose monitoring with meters at least four and as many as seven times daily were fasting and preprandial 70 mg/dl to 120 mg/dl, postprandial less than 180 mg/dl (90–120 minutes after a meal), and 3:00 a.m. more than 65 mg/dl (measured weekly). The goal for HgbA1c measured monthly was less than 6.05% (within 2 SD of nondiabetic mean). Patients and their physicians could select a multiple (three or more) daily injection (MDI) regimen or continuous subcutaneous insulin infusion (CSII, pump). Both types of regimens constituted an attempt to simulate a natural pattern of insulin release and involved establishing a low or basal level of insulin release using regular insulin in an infusion pump or intermediate (NPH or Lente) or long-acting (Ultralente) subcutaneous insulin, to facilitate ongoing metabolic tasks. Approximately 50% of daily insulin is given as basal. The regimen was supplemented by boluses of short-acting regular insulin 15 to 45 minutes before meals (approximately 20% breakfast, 10% lunch, 20% dinner), administered with the pump or by separate injections (frequently with a pen injector), mimicking the pancreatic release of insulin brought on by ingestion of food, and allowing nutrients to be incorporated into the body in a more physiologic manner. Insulin dosage and timing was adjusted using the results of the home glucose monitoring. More patients used the MDI than the pump regimen (58% to 70% as compared with 29% to 42% depending on the year). The most common MDI regimen included premeal regular insulin and one or more injections of NPH or Lente insulin (60%) (12). Most of the other MDI regimens were UltraLente-based, with regular insulin taken before meals. About 25% of patients switched between MDI and pump during the study; some did so several times. After initiation of intensive therapy in the hospital for 2 to 4 days, patients were monitored weekly until they were well versed in the implementation of the treatment regimen. Thereafter, they were monitored monthly with telephone contact at least weekly to review glycemic control and principles of intensive management and adjust the components of the regimen including diet, insulin dose and timing, exercise, and glucose monitoring to achieve the desired glycemic goals. Various commercially available meters were used in the trial to monitor glycemia.

Monitoring alone, without appropriate adjustment of insulin, does not result in substantial improvement in glycemic control. Ninety percent of intensively treated patients (86% to 92%) reported monitoring blood glucose at least three times a day during the study. Management of diet was another major tool used to achieve near-normoglycemia. Strict adherence to an isocaloric American Dietary Association (ADA) diet can make insulin adjustment easier. However, intensive therapy in a well-educated patient, particularly one with access to expert consultation from diabetes nurse clinicians and physicians, can allow considerable flexibility in the amount and types of food permitted and in the timing of its consumption while still maintaining excellent diabetes control. Intensive therapy included extensive nutritional counseling and as many visits with the dietitian as appeared to be helpful. Meeting glycemic goals took precedence over dietary goals. If weight gain became a problem, as it frequently did, every attempt was made to address the weight gain without compromising glycemic goals. Most patients realized that if their diabetes control was poor they could eat more without gaining weight or could lose weight without eating less. It took considerable time and effort to deal with these issues and the effort was not always successful.

Intensively treated patients received no specific exercise prescription, but it was encouraged. Although exercise can be a very important tool in managing diabetes and is certainly an important factor in maintaining overall health, it proved to be a frequent source of anxiety in many intensively managed patients because of the risk and common occurrence of hypoglycemia. If exercise was incorporated into an intensive regimen, it had to be performed regularly and at a fairly constant time to allow proper adjustment of diet and insulin. Monitoring before and after exercise was helpful initially, and a rapidly absorbed source of glucose had to be available in case a hypoglycemic episode occurred.

METABOLIC AND ADVERSE EFFECTS OF INTENSIVE TREATMENT

Intensive therapy was effective in improving glycemic control, reducing HgbA1c about 20% (9.0 at baseline to an average of 7.2 as compared to 9.1 for conventional patients). Median blood glucose profiles were reduced from 225 mg/dl to 155 mg/dl. Although 44% of intensively treated patients reached the target HgbA1c goal of less than 6.05 at least once, only 5% maintained that level throughout the study. Severe hypoglycemia occurred three times as often in these patients as in patients receiving conventional treatment and was the most important adverse effect (AE) of intensive treatment. Seventy-three percent (459) of intensively treated patients had 2,896 events (62/100 patient-years) as compared with 41% of conventional patients (255) with 892 events (19/100 patient-years). Neurobehavioral testing demonstrated no decrease in function that might be attributable to this excess hypoglycemia. Patients on intensive regimens were more likely to gain weight. Twice as many intensively treated patients were overweight (20% heavier than ideal body weight) by the end of the study (34% vs. 17%). Catheter infections from CSII therapy ranged from 7 to 11/100 patient-years.

Comparisons between various intensive treatment regimens were not randomized and, therefore, were less scientifically rigorous. Patients using pumps had lower HgbA1c at annual visits (−0.27%) than did patients on MDI. In addition, patients who used only pumps during the study had HgbA1c levels 0.2 to 0.4% lower than patients who used only MDI, who in turn had HgbA1c levels 0.1 to 0.2% lower than patients who used both regimens during the study. There were no differences in severe hypoglycemia; however, more episodes of coma or seizure occurred in patients using a pump. Diabetic ketoacidosis was also more common in patients using a pump. There was no difference in degree of excess weight between MDI and CSII patients.

RETINOPATHY OUTCOMES

Intensive therapy reduced the development of microaneurysms by only 27% in patients who had none at baseline, as demonstrated by grading of fundus photographs. However, after an average of 6.5 years of follow-up, intensively treated patients were 76% less likely to develop more severe forms of retinopathy, measured as a three-step change in the retinopathy scale. If no retinopathy is evident on fluorescein angiogram at baseline or if the patient has had diabetes for less than 2.5 years, the risk reduction approaches 90%, i.e., almost complete elimination of significant retinopathy. These results suggest that almost all cases of vision-threatening retinopathy might be eliminated if intensive therapy can be implemented soon after onset of diabetes. Certainly, this is a goal to which we should all aspire. For patients who already manifested some retinopathy, intensive treatment reduced any significant progression by 65% and progression to severe nonproliferative retinopathy or proliferative retinopathy by 47 to 64% in the average follow-up of 6.5 years. Need for laser treatment was reduced almost 60%. For reasons which remain unclear, the effect of treatment on macular edema was not as great. Nevertheless, all subgroups of retinopathy studied benefited from intensive treatment.

Initiation of intensive treatment can be associated with an early worsening of retinopathy, as noted in DCCT patients, particularly patients already manifesting retinopathy. It may have accounted in part for the delay in onset of the beneficial effect of intensive treatment for 2 to 3 years. In addition, retinopathy, like a moving train, has a momentum of its own and continues to progress even if the engine of progression, i.e., glycemic control, is changed. Once the beneficial effect of treatment was apparent, it appeared to increase with time, primarily because the condition of intensively treated patients did not become worse and actually frequently improved with time, whereas retinopathy in conventionally treated patients continued to progress.

SUMMARY AND FUTURE DIRECTIONS

The only pharmacologic agent with a proven beneficial effect on diabetic retinopathy is insulin, when used as part of an intensive treatment regimen. Use of such regimens reduces development and progression and increases regression of diabetic retinopathy. Other pharmacologic agents may soon play a role in treating or preventing diabetic retinopathy. Of greatest potential are drugs aimed at preventing the basic metabolic defects of diabetes itself, in some ways mimicking the effects of intensive diabetes control. One such class of drugs consists of aldose reductase inhibitors, which inhibit the conversion of glucose to sorbitol, a pathway that is activated in conditions of hyperglycemia and may be a mechanism of diabetes cellular damage. In the one major published clinical trial of aldose reductase inhibitors, they had no beneficial effect on retinopathy (12). Other clinical trials using more potent compounds are in progress. A clinical trial of an inhibitor of protein kinase C (PKC) is also in progress and is of great interest. Increased PKC is stimulated by hyperglycemia, and inhibition of isoform B in a rat model of diabetes ameliorates many pathologic effects on the vasculature of the glomeruli and retina (13). Vascular endothelial growth factor (VEGF) is another possible mediator of diabetic retinopathy and a condition in which pharmacologic intervention could prove of great value (see Chapter 38, Medical Therapy for Macular Degeneration.)

REFERENCES

1. DRS Research group, Diabetic Retinopathy Study Report No. 1. Preliminary report on effects of photocoagulation therapy. *Am J Ophthalmol* 1976;81:1–14.
2. DRS Research Group. Diabetic Retinopathy Study Report No. 3. Four risk factors for severe visual loss in diabetic retinopathy. *Arch Ophthalmol* 1979;97:658.
3. ETDRS Research Group. Photocoagulation for diabetic macular edema. Early Treatment Diabetic Retinopathy Study report number 1. *Arch Ophthalmol* 1985;103:1986–1996.
4. DCCT Research Group. The effect of intensive treatment of diabetes on the development and progression of long-term complications in insulin dependent diabetes. *N Engl J Med* 1993;329:977–986.
5. DCCT Research Group. The effect of intensive diabetes treatment on the progression of diabetic retinopathy in insulin dependent diabetes mellitus: the Diabetes Control and Complications Trial. *Arch Ophthalmol* 1995;113:36–51.
6. DCCT Research Group. Progression of retinopathy with intensive versus conventional treatment in the Diabetes Control and Complications Trial. *Ophthalmology* 1995;102:647–661.
7. Shoelson SE, Halban PE. Insulin biosynthesis and chemistry. In: Kahn CR, Weir GC, eds. *Joslin's Diabetes Mellitus.* Philadelphia: Lea & Febiger, 1994;29–55.
8. White MF, Kahn CR. Molecular aspects of insulin action. In: Kahn CR, Weir GC, eds. *Joslin's Diabetes Mellitus.* Philadelphia: Lea & Febiger, 1994;139–176.
9. Krolewski AS, Warram JH, Rand LI, Kahn CR. Epidemiologic approach to the etiology of type 1 diabetes mellitus and its complications. *N Engl J Med* 1987;317:1390–1398.
10. Shabo AL, Maxwell DS. Insulin-induced immunogenic retinopathy resembling the retinitis proliferans of diabetes. *Trans Am Acad Ophthalmol Otolaryngol* 1975;81:497–507.
11. DCCT Research Group. Implementation of treatment protocols in the Diabetes Control and Complications Trial. *Diabetes Care* 1995;18: 361–376.
12. The Sorbinil Retinopathy Trial Research Group. A randomized trial of Sorbinil, an aldose reductase inhibitor in diabetic retinopathy. *Arch Ophthalmol* 1990;198:1234–1244.
13. Ishii, H, Jirouseh MR, Koya D, King GL. Amelioration of vascular disfunction in diabetic rats by an oral PKC B inhibitor. *Science* 1996;272:728–731.

Textbook of Ocular Pharmacology,
edited by T.J. Zimmerman, et al.
Lippincott–Raven Publishers, Philadelphia © 1997.

CHAPTER 38

Medical Therapy for Macular Degeneration

Johanna M. Seddon and Joan W. Miller

Age-related macular degeneration (AMD) is the leading cause of irreversible blindness in the United States (1). Approximately 25% of people aged 65 years and older have some manifestation of this disease, including large or confluent drusen, retinal pigmentary changes, geographic atrophy, and exudative disease (2). Because the elderly constitute an increasing proportion of the population, it is estimated that the burden of this disease will increase and that more than 6 million persons will have AMD by the year 2030. This disease, therefore, has important implications for individual patients as well as for the general public.

At present, the causes of AMD are unknown; therefore, we cannot prevent it. Because we do not fully understand factors leading to its progression, its early stages cannot be arrested. The only proven method of treatment, laser photocoagulation, is effective for only a small fraction of patients, and vision is often impaired despite treatment (3). For these reasons, antioxidant vitamins and minerals represent particularly attractive possibilities for prevention and treatment of AMD. The evidence concerning supplements, however, although promising, is preliminary, and has led prematurely to their widespread use as an ocular therapy. On the other hand, dietary intake of antioxidants and other nutrients from foods may be beneficial. The potentially toxic drug, interferon, was also publicized as a treatment for the exudative or neovascular form of AMD before the drug's effect was rigorously tested. In this chapter, we summarize the status of the evidence regarding medical treatments for AMD, particularly nutritional factors, interferon, and other antiangiogenic drugs.

NUTRITIONAL FACTORS

The evidence regarding nutrition and AMD includes basic research (4–10), a few descriptive and observational epidemiologic studies (11–14), and one small randomized trial (15), which in aggregate support the need for further research, including prospective cohort studies and large-scale trials, to provide reliable data on this issue. Basic research concerning oxidative metabolism has provided plausible mechanisms for the benefits of certain nutrients that counteract the oxidative process. Light and even normal metabolic processes within cells can generate free radicals in the formation of highly reactive species of oxygen. These oxygen species can react with and damage innocent bystander molecules such as DNA, proteins, lipids, and carbohydrates. The retina is prone to oxidative damage because of the high level of polyunsaturated fatty acids in the photoreceptor outer-segment membranes (16). Despite the body's attempts, oxidative damage is constantly occurring. Vitamins and minerals that have the capacity to act as antioxidants may therefore be beneficial, including vitamins E, C, carotenoids, selenium, zinc, and enzymes that are involved in the oxidative process.

Several animal studies have been conducted that support the need for studies in humans (4–10). Animals fed diets supplemented with antioxidant-containing foods had less retinal degeneration, and animals fed diets deficient in antioxidants were more likely to develop retinal degeneration when exposed to bright light (4–8). Other studies involving clinical/pathologic assessment of eyes or cell cultures suggest that some antioxidants in ocular tissues decrease with age and that adding certain nutrients stimulates their activity (9,10). Such basic studies are useful for setting priorities in human research, but the doses of supplementation, level of deficiency, or the intense light exposure used in these experiments may be out of the range of the lifetime exposure of humans.

Only a few epidemiologic studies dealing with this subject have been published (11–14). Epidemiologic studies are either descriptive (case reports, correlational studies, cross-sectional surveys) (11,12) or analytic (observational studies, either case-control (13,14) or cohort, and experimental studies or randomized trials) (15). Descriptive stud-

J. M. Seddon and J. W. Miller: Department of Ophthalmology, Epidemiology Unit and Retina Service, Massachusetts Eye and Ear Infirmary, Harvard Medical School, Boston, Massachusetts 02114.

ies are primarily useful for the formulation of hypotheses, whereas analytic studies are useful for hypothesis testing.

Data from the Baltimore Longitudinal Study of Aging were used to assess the association between plasma antioxidants and AMD, which was primarily of the dry type (11). Plasma data were available for 55% to 68% of the population. Macular status was assessed once in participants at varying intervals from the time of the blood analyses, ranging from macular assessment concurrent with blood analyses (19% of subjects included in the analyses) to macular assessment 2 (69%) to 4 years (12%) later. In this descriptive, cross-sectional study, supplement use, in general, was not beneficial. Plasma vitamin E level was inversely associated with nonsevere AMD. There were similar, but nonsignificant, associations for plasma levels of vitamin C and β-carotene. The very few cases of severe AMD (n = 11) precluded any firm conclusions about this subgroup.

In another cross-sectional study using the National Health and Examination Survey, which was performed at several sites throughout the United States (12), persons diagnosed as having macular degeneration, combining atrophic and exudative types, were compared with subjects who were not diagnosed as having this disease. The study evaluated dietary intake of fruits and vegetables rich in vitamins A and C. Low intake of foods rich in vitamin A was significantly associated with a higher risk of AMD. Carotenoids, which are also found in these same foods, were not specifically addressed in that study.

In a multicenter eye disease case-control study (EDCCS), conducted from 1986 through 1990, 421 patients with recently diagnosed exudative macular degeneration were compared with 615 controls without macular degeneration with regard to plasma levels of nutrients (13). Nutrient values were divided into quintiles; the highest quintile was compared with the middle three quintiles and the lowest quintile (the referent). Persons with the highest plasma levels of carotene were shown to have a reduced risk of exudative macular degeneration. This effect was present after other factors such as age, sex, clinical center, education, hypertension, and smoking were controlled for in the analyses. Carotenoids were also divided into their fractions, and all but one (lycopene) were associated with a reduced risk of exudative macular degeneration in comparisons of the highest and the lowest blood levels. Vitamins C and E were evaluated similarly. A reduced risk of exudative AMD was shown for persons with high levels of these nutrients, but the effect was smaller and not statistically significant. There was no association between selenium intake and exudative AMD. Finally, evaluation of zinc levels did not show a protective effect for subjects with the highest blood level of zinc. Indeed, there was a nonsignificant trend for higher risk of AMD with increasing levels of serum zinc, which persisted even when persons who recently had begun to take zinc supplements were excluded from the analyses.

Dietary indicators of antioxidant status were also evaluated in the EDCCS population (14), including nutrient intake, supplement use, and consumption of specific foods. The relative risk for AMD was estimated according to dietary indicators of antioxidant status, controlling for smoking and other known and potential risk factors. A higher dietary intake of carotenoids was independently associated with a lower risk for AMD. Those who consumed the highest amounts of carotenoids in their foods had the lowest estimated relative risk as compared with those who consumed the least. There was a statistically significant dose–response effect; i.e., the greater the intake, the lower the risk. Among all carotenoids evaluated, lutein and zeaxanthin in combination were associated with the lowest risk. Specific foods rich in carotenoids were also analyzed. The dark green leafy vegetables, spinach and collard greens, were most strongly associated with a reduced risk for AMD, and the results indicated a significantly greater effect for more frequent intake of these specific vegetables. Supplementation with Vitamin A, E, or C pills did not have a significant beneficial effect. A small, nonsignificant association with Vitamin C from foods was noted. Overall, the strongest association with AMD thus far is that of dietary intake of carotenoids.

Results of these epidemiologic studies have led to important inferences and are compatible with a possible benefit of antioxidants or other nutritional factors on risk of AMD. Although known confounding factors, such as smoking and hypertension, were adjusted for in some analyses (13,14), other unknown confounders may have existed that were not measured and were therefore not controlled for in these studies. In addition, in cross-sectional studies (11,12), it is not possible to determine whether the exposure being evaluated is a cause or consequence of the disease. Prospective observational data are also needed. Furthermore, reliable data on whether antioxidant vitamins affect risk of AMD will emerge from large-scale randomized trials in which investigators allocate subjects at random to either the group receiving supplements or a placebo group. If these trials are sufficiently large, the randomization process will evenly distribute both known and unknown variables among treatment and placebo groups and will also distinguish reliably between the null hypothesis and the most plausible alternatives.

One small randomized trial has been reported that studied the effect of zinc on macular degeneration as defined by "ophthalmoscopically visible drusen with varying degrees of pigmentary change" (15). Eighty patients were treated with zinc, and 71 patients were in the placebo group. Patients in the placebo group had a greater decrease in visual acuity than persons in the zinc group. Significantly more eyes in the zinc-treated group remained in stable condition or showed less accumulation of visible drusen as compared with eyes in the placebo group. However, the degree to which the study group is representative of other populations is not clear, since the placebo group had a higher rate of visual loss than that reported in other natural history studies of AMD. Visual acuity was the important outcome in this trial (15), but it was not measured according to a standardized protocol. As stated in the article, "Because of the pilot nature of the study and the possible toxic effects and complications of oral zinc administration, widespread use of zinc in macular degeneration is not now warranted." These data reinforce the need for a randomized trial of sufficiently large sample size and sufficient duration to test the risks and benefits of zinc.

For most hypotheses, randomized trials are neither necessary nor desirable, particularly when the effect of a drug or agent is very great (17). However, when effects are small to moderate, i.e., 20% to 30%, evidence regarding a potential intervention is derived most reliably from randomized trials. Patients with optic neuritis had been treated with oral prednisone until a randomized trial demonstrated the therapy to be ineffective and, indeed, to increase the risk of recurrent optic neuritis (18). Similarly, the most plausible effect of antioxidant vitamins and minerals on AMD may be a slight to moderate effect. A benefit of even this magnitude, however, would have great clinical relevance and public health impact for such a common and serious disease.

The Age Related Eye Disease Study is a large, multicenter randomized trial that has enrolled more than 5,000 patients at 11 centers across the country to study the important question regarding supplements (Age Related Eye Disease Study, Manual of Procedures, National Eye Institute, Bethesda, MD). Study pills include vitamins E, C, β-carotene, and zinc. Patients at lower risk of developing visual loss due to AMD are randomized into two groups: high-dose antioxidants or placebo. Patients at higher risk of developing visual loss due to AMD are randomized into four groups in a factorial design: antioxidant vitamins, zinc, antioxidant vitamins and zinc, or placebo. Other ongoing large-scale randomized trials also provide an opportunity to evaluate eye disease.

The data from published studies regarding nutrients and AMD are important and promising but at present are insufficient to support a clinical recommendation regarding supplement use. There are several caveats to consider before treating eye disease with vitamin and mineral supplements. In the United States, most people prefer prescription of a preventive agent far more than proscription of harmful lifestyles. It would be unfortunate if the elderly took supplements while continuing to smoke or while not complying with therapy for hypertension, both of which factors, smoking and hypertension, appear to be associated with advanced AMD and are certainly determinants of overall mortality. In addition to the lack of definitive evidence regarding the effectiveness of vitamin pills, it is unclear what dose should be taken or how long the vitamins should be taken to demonstrate any effect. Antioxidant-rich foods appear protective (14), but the benefit may result not from their antioxidant properties but from some other component that these foods have in common. Supplements in that particular circumstance would not be helpful. People who take pills or supplements may rely on them to such an extent that they do not eat a "balanced diet" containing foods that are currently recommended by the National Cancer Institute and the National Academy of Sciences. Based on accumulating evidence, it seems prudent to recommend increasing the frequency and diversity of our intake of vegetables and to include the dark-green leafy variety.

The possible toxic effects of supplements need to be considered; e.g., zinc can cause copper-deficiency anemia and may lower levels of high density lipoprotein (19,20). High doses of vitamin E can lead to fatigue, muscle weaknesses, blurred vision, and decreased thyroid function. In people who do not have sufficient vitamin K, high doses of vitamin E may slow the time it takes for blood to clot (21). People who have had kidney stones or hemochromatosis should not take large doses of vitamin C (22,23).

Cost is also an issue. Patients who might not even be able to afford a proper diet may spend hundreds of dollars a year on vitamin and mineral supplements. What we do not yet know with certainty is whether beneficial effects on eye disease are attributable to this already widespread practice. No one would disagree that nutritional deficiency should be corrected, and some elderly patients may indeed need supplements to meet their recommended daily allowance of nutrients.

AMD is a significant clinical and public health problem. As already discussed, results of animal and other laboratory studies, cross-sectional studies, and case-control studies, as well as those of one small randomized clinical trial, together raise the possibility that nutritional factors are potentially related to the development or prevention of macular degeneration.

Additional basic research is needed to define further the mechanisms of oxidation and its effect on the eye and the degree to which oxidative effects occur in vivo. Better markers of oxidative stress may be helpful to identify people at higher risk who may benefit from antioxidants. Additional observational studies, particularly prospective studies, are important to assess the strength and consistency of the recent findings regarding diet and supplement use. Finally, randomized clinical trials will provide the most conclusive data about the nutrients which are evaluated as interventions in the trials. Results of all these efforts combined will form a totality of evidence on which rational clinical decision making can be based. At present, the hypothesis regarding antioxidant or other dietary therapy for AMD is promising, but not proven. Based on available evidence, it seems prudent to limit our recommendations to improving our dietary habits by increasing our vegetable intake, rather than consuming supplements, at least until we have further information.

ANTIANGIOGENIC AGENTS

Current treatment of exudative macular degeneration relies on thermal laser closure of the neovascular tissue. This treatment might damage the neural retina which one would wish to preserve. Clinicopathologic correlation suggests that laser-treated choroidal neovascularization (CNV), which appears to be quiescent clinically, may harbor neovascular tissue (24). This may be an important factor in the etiology of recurrences, which occur with a frequency of approximately 50% in 2 years (25). Finally, laser treatment of subfoveal CNV may be associated with vision loss. These factors motivate investigations directed at finding a more selective therapy. One such approach would be to develop a pharmacologic agent that would act directly on the neovascular tissue. Antiangiogenic agents might provide such a selective therapy.

Angiogenic modulators have been isolated from several systems. Typically, these modulators are first investigated in vitro, using endothelial cell cultures. The drug can also be screened in a simple in vivo model, the chick chorioallantoic membrane (chick CAM) bioassay, to assess its effect on developing blood vessels (26,27). The next step is to investigate the effect in a simple animal model of neovascularization, such as the rabbit corneal micropocket (28). However, the limitation of the various rabbit corneal models is that the neovascularization is either inflammatory (endotoxin), or relies on the implantation of large quantities of a particular growth factor (GF), and does not model a clinical disease. Other models that may more closely resemble human disease are the monkey model of iris neovascularization and the pig model of retinal neovascularization. Both these models simulate human diseases characterized by ischemic retina and may be useful in investigation of the control of pathologic neovascularization and in testing potentially useful pharmacologic agents (29–31). Results from even these models, however, may not be directly applicable to CNV in AMD. Preliminary studies in the monkey model of iris neovascularization have investigated the effect of angiostatic steroids, systemic interferon-α (IFN-α), and AGM-1470 (30,32). Many potential antiangiogenic agents have been described, and only a partial list with some applicability to ocular disease is discussed herein.

Angiostatic Steroids

Angiostatic steroids are a class of steroids shown to inhibit angiogenesis independent of any glucocorticoid activity. Their antiangiogenic property is enhanced in the presence of heparin and heparin analogues (27,33,34). Angiostatic steroids complexed with heparin analogues have been demonstrated to inhibit experimental corneal neovascularization and lead to the regression of newly formed vessels. Recently, a clinical trial of β-cyclodextrin (BCD) complexed with hydrocortisone-21-P was initiated for patients with corneal neovascularization not responding to steroid therapy. Application of these agents to choroidal neovascularization (CNV) in age-related macular degeneration would probably require some form of local delivery.

Platelet Factor 4

Platelet factor 4 (PF4) is an α-granule protein which is released from platelets during aggregation. PF4 inhibits the proliferation and migration of endothelial cells in vitro and inhibits angiogenesis in the chick CAM (35). PF4 has been investigated in the rat model of retinopathy of prematurity, in which it led to an increase in the area of avascular retina in rats exposed to high levels of O_2 (36). It may have a role in therapy for ocular neovascularization.

Prolactin Fragment 16k

The 16K fragment of prolactin, which is formed in tissues by cleavage of prolactin, has been demonstrated to inhibit basal and basic fibroblast growth factor (bFGF)-stimulated proliferation of endothelial cells (37). The prolactin fragment is another potential antiangiogenic agent.

Cartilage-derived Inhibitor (CDI)

CDI is a polypeptide isolated from cartilage that inhibits the proliferation and migration of endothelial cells in vitro and inhibits angiogenesis in the chick CAM model (38). The protein is also an inhibitor of mammalian collagenase, suggesting that it may exert an effect on the degradation of extracellular matrix which occurs early in angiogenesis. The polypeptide is currently being cloned and will soon be available in sufficient quantities to allow testing of the inhibitor in animal models.

Corneal Angiogenesis Inhibitor (CAI)

A cornea angiogenesis inhibitor (CAI) that inhibits endothelial cell proliferation and migration in vitro and has been shown to inhibit angiogenesis in the chick CAM has been demonstrated in normal cornea. The molecule has been only partially purified and remains to be identified (39).

Interferon

IFN-α is a polypeptide secreted by all eukaryotic cells (40). Among their many cellular effects, the interferons inhibit the proliferation and migration of endothelial cells in vitro (41). IFN-α has also been shown to inhibit neovascularization of murine or human tumors implanted in mouse cornea or skin (42) and has been used clinically with excellent results to treat life-threatening hemangiomas (43). IFN-α has also been shown to inhibit the proliferation of human Tenon's fibroblasts and may have application in the control of ocular fibrosis (44,45). IFN-α has also been described in case reports to be effective therapy for Behcet's disease with severe ocular involvement (46).

IFN-α was investigated in a monkey model of iris neovascularization modified from that of Virdi and Hayreh (47). When the drug was administered systemically to animals with neovascularization, it led to regression of iris neovascularization (32). Iris neovascularization was monitored angiographically, and treatment with IFN-α was instituted only after iris neovascularization was evident angiographically. Animals in the treatment group received systemic IFN-α by subcutaneous injection, with dosages based on those used in the trials for treatment of clinical hemangiomas in children (43). The first animal treated received 3 million U/m^2 for 1 week, and the neovascularization worsened. The dose was then increased to 5 million U/m^2 nightly, and the vessels regressed. Subsequently treated animals received 6 million U/m^2 nightly. Eight of eight eyes in the treatment group demonstrated regression of iris neovascularization with IFN-α treatment, whereas three of three of the control eyes demonstrated progression of iris neovascularization or developed neovascular glaucoma necessitating sacrifice of the animal. Histologic examination of the control eyes demonstrated a fibrovascular membrane over the anterior surface of the iris, with multiple, branching vessels. Light microscopy of the treated irises showed remnants of a membrane on the anterior surface, composed of fibrous tissue with rare, patent vessels.

An earlier report on the effectiveness of systemic IFN-α for choroidal neovascularization sparked great interest in patients and ophthalmologists with regard to the use of interferon in macular degeneration (48). Several groups of investigators published case reports and small series with mixed results (49–54).

As ophthalmologists began to use interferon for exudative AMD, concern arose regarding the side effects in the elderly population. IFN-α can have side effects involving many organ systems, including a flu-like syndrome with fever and myalgias; neutropenia; thrombocytopenia; liver dysfunction; cardiovascular and central nervous system events, such as chest pain, arrhythmia, dizziness, and numbness; nausea and diarrhea; autoimmune disorders such as thyroiditis or polyarthropathy; alopecia; dry skin and mouth; anorexia and weight loss; and depression (55). The severity of side effects appears to be somewhat dose-related, and side effects appear to be more severe in an older patient population. Early pilot studies suggested that older patients may not tolerate moderate doses (higher than 6 million IU every other day) because of leukopenia, extreme fatigue, and depression (56). In the series of Thomas et al., side effects were common, and two patients reported suicidal ideation (52). Other groups of investigators administering lower doses reported minor side effects (53,54). Gillies et al. (50) reported common minor side effects and several more serious side effects, including a cardiac arrest and death, a perforated ulcer, and an acute bowel obstruction. These more serious side effects occurred in patients treated with 3 million IU of IFN-α daily. The accumulated experience regarding IFN-α in the elderly has led to the recommendation that the drug be investigated in clinical trials with close supervision of the patients and with the involvement of an oncologist or internist familiar with IFN-α. Ocular side effects have also been described, primarily cotton wool spots and small intraretinal hemorrhages, although a more pronounced retinal vasculopathy has been observed rarely (57).

There are several problems with all reports to date regarding interferon therapy in patients with AMD, generally recognized by the researchers themselves. All of the series involved very few patients, including those which randomized patients, making any analysis of the effect of therapy impossible at the onset. Any attempt to draw conclusions from these studies is speculative at best. A definitive answer requires a large randomized clinical trial with adequate followup. Such a trial was undertaken in 45 centers in the United States, Europe, and other countries. Four hundred and eighty one patients were enrolled in a prospective, randomized, placebo-controlled, FDA-approved Phase III trial to assess the effect of IFN-α on subfoveal CNV. (The Phase III trial demonstrated that IFN-α-2a provides no benefit as a treatment for CNV secondary to age-related macular degeneration, and may be associated with a poorer visual outcome. The experience with interferon demonstrates the necessity of a well-designed, large, randomized prospective study to investigate therapies in AMO.) The treatment doses were 1.5, 3.0, and 6.0 million IU of IFN-α, administered subcutaneously 3 times a week for 52 weeks. Clinical experience with IFN-α in other diseases suggested that treatment effects may require weeks to months, and therapy probably must be continued longer than the several-week course described in most of the small series.

Thrombospondin

Thrombospondin is an adhesive glycoprotein produced by many cell types, including endothelial cells and macrophages, and is the most abundant protein in the platelet α-granule (59). Thrombospondin suppresses endothelial cell migration and tube formation in vitro. In vivo, it has been shown to inhibit neovascularization in a rat cornea model (59); other investigators have demonstrated it to be angiogenic in vivo (60). Its role in ocular neovascularization remains to be elucidated.

AGM-1470

AGM-1470 is another antiangiogenic drug with potential application to ophthalmic disease. AGM-1470 is a synthetic derivative of fumagillin, an antibiotic produced by a species of Aspergillus which was found serendipitously to inhibit endothelial cells in vitro (61). However, further investigation in a mouse tumor model demonstrated that fumagillin itself was too toxic. Subsequently, a fumagillin analogue, termed AGM-1470 or TNP-470, was developed that retains the antiangiogenic properties of fumagillin without its side effects (61). AGM-1470 inhibits proliferation of endothelial cells in vitro and also inhibits fibroblast proliferation and several tumor cell lines with varying degrees of sensitivity. Preliminary data suggest that AGM-1470 may act by suppressing expression of certain cdks and cyclins (62) and that it may prevent entry of endothelial cells into the G1 phase of the cell cycle, ensuring their quiescence (63).

AGM-1470 has been demonstrated to reduce the growth and neovascularization in four mouse tumor lines by 55% to 77% when administered subcutaneously every other day at a dose of 30 mg/kg (64). The drug was effective in both male and female mice and in mice immunosuppressed by irradiation. Similar results were obtained using intravenous administration in mouse and rat models with other tumor types (65). No significant toxic effects were noted. AGM-1470 has been shown to be effective in experimental models of rheumatoid arthritis, another angiogenic disease (66,67). AGM-1470 is currently undergoing phase I trials in patients with Kaposi's sarcoma and AIDS. AGM-1470 has also been shown to inhibit rabbit corneal neovascularization at doses of 5 mg/kg administered daily (68).

Preliminary results in the monkey iris model of neovascularization indicate that it may be effective in accelerating regression of iris neovascularization (30). Preliminary data from studies in which a dose of 6 mg/kg administered intravenously was used indicate that the number of days to regression tended to be shorter in the AGM-1470-treated group than in the control group. Some mild systemic toxicity was noted, with the treated animals losing 10% to 20% of their weight during 5 weeks of treatment.

Thalidomide

Thalidomide is a potent teratogen. This fact was missed in preclinical trials based on rodent models in the 1950s, with devastating results. D'Amato et al. (69) postulated that the teratogenic effect was secondary to inhibition of angiogenesis and began investigations of thalidomide and thalidomide analogues in the chick CAM assay and the rabbit corneal micropocket model. Thalidomide itself had no effect on the chick CAM, which was not surprising since it has been postulated that thalidomide must be metabolized by the liver to produce an active compound. Thalidomide analogues did have some weak antiangiogenic activity, although mild scarring frequently resulted. Thalidomide was then tested in the rabbit cornea model induced by bFGF and sucralfate pellets. When a teratogenic dose of thalidomide (200 mg/kg) was used, inhibition of the vascularized cornea ranged from 30% to 51%. This effect was also observed in immunosuppressed animals (which received whole body irradiation), suggesting that the effect is not immune mediated. Based on these preclinical data, a trial of thalidomide for AMD has been proposed.

Angiostatin

An angiogenesis inhibitor, which is produced by the primary tumor and inhibits neovascularization at distant sites, was recently identified in a Lewis mouse lung tumor model (70). Serum and urine from tumor-bearing mice specifically inhibit endothelial cell proliferation. The inhibitor was purified and sequenced and was demonstrated to have greater than 98% identity with an internal fragment of plasminogen. The plasminogen fragment, termed angiostatin, also inhibits endothelial cell proliferation, but not Lewis lung tumor cell growth.

Angiogenesis in the Lewis lung tumor is mediated mainly by vascular endothelial GF (VEGF), which undergoes rapid clearance from the circulation. In contrast, the inhibitory activity of angiostatin is present in the circulation for as long as 5 days (half-maximal activity is 2.5 days). The researchers (70) postulate that the primary tumor drives angiogenesis in its own vascular bed with an excess of VEGF and other angiogenic factors over angiostatin, while circulating angiostatin acts to inhibit neovascularization in the vascular bed of metastases. Preliminary data from their study suggest that systemic administration of angiostatin may inhibit the growth of primary tumors as well. This potent inhibitor warrants further investigation in nonneoplastic models of angiogenesis.

GF Blockers

Angiogenic factors and GF have been implicated in ocular neovascular processes such as diabetic retinopathy and AMD; these are discussed more fully in another chapter. As the pathogenesis of neovascularization in clinical disease is better elucidated, it may be possible to inhibit specifically a particular GF and interrupt the disease process. Antibodies to VEGF were shown to inhibit tumor growth in mice (71) and to prevent iris neovascularization in a monkey model (72). For such an approach to be clinically viable, one would have to be sure that blockage of the angiogenic factor did not lead to other undesired effects and that the blocking therapy (monoclonal antibodies, antisense DNA) was not toxic.

Pharmacological modulation of angiogenesis is a potential new approach to the complications of neovascularization in diseases such as AMD. To date there is no systematic approach to selecting the drugs that may be most appropriate to investigate in a clinical trial. One would hope that after evaluation in vitro, and in simple in vivo systems, drugs would be tested and compared in a model that best simulates the disease to be treated. Drug toxicity must be evaluated, particularly when treatment of an older patient population is considered, such as patients with AMD. Local drug delivery may be a viable alternative to avoid systemic toxicity. It is hoped that continued investigations will yield a pharmacologic agent for CNV in AMD.

REFERENCES

1. National Advisory Eye Council. *Report of the Retinal and Choroidal Diseases Panel. Vision research—a national plan: 1983–1987.* Bethesda, MD: U.S. Department of Health and Human Services; 1984;NIH publication no 83–2471.
2. Klein R, Klein B, Linton KLP. Prevalence of age-related maculopathy. The Beaver Dam study. *Ophthalmology* 1992;99:933–943.
3. Macular Photocoagulation Study Group. Argon laser photocoagulation for neovascular maculopathy. Five-year results from randomized clinical trials. *Arch Ophthalmol* 1991;109:1109–1114.
4. Katz ML, Parker KR, Handelman GJ, et al. Effects of antioxidant nutrient deficiency on the retina and retinal pigment epithelium of albino rats: a light and electron microscopic study. *Exp Eye Res* 1982; 34:339–369.
5. Hayes KC. Retinal degeneration in monkeys induced by deficiencies of vitamin E or A. *Invest Ophthalmol* 1974;13:499–510.
6. Organisciak DT, Wang HM, Li Z, et al. The protective effect of ascorbate in retinal light damage of rats. *Invest Ophthalmol Vis Sci* 1985;26:1580–1588.
7. Tso MOM, Woodford BJ, Lam KW. Distribution of ascorbate in normal primate retina and after photic injury: a biochemical, morphological correlated study. *Curr Eye Res* 1984;3:181–191.
8. Ham WT, Mueller HA, Ruffolo JJ, et al. Basic mechanisms underlying the production of photochemical lesions in the mammalian retina. *Curr Eye Res* 1984;3:165–174.
9. Liles MR, Newsome DA, Oliver PD. Antioxidant enzymes in the aging human retinal pigment epithelium. *Arch Ophthalmol* 1991;109: 1285–1288.
10. Oliver PD, Tate DJ Jr, Newsome DA. Metallothionein in human retinal pigment epithelial cells: expression, induction and zinc uptake. *Curr Eye Res* 1992;11:183–188.
11. West S, Vitale S, Hallfrisch J, et al. Antioxidants and supplements: protective for age-related macular degeneration? *Arch Ophthalmol* (in press).
12. Goldberg J, Flowerdew G, Smith E, et al. Factors associated with age-related macular degeneration: an analysis of data from the First National Health and Nutrition Examination Survey. *Am J Epidemiol* 1988;128:700–710.
13. The Eye Disease Case-Control Study Group. Biochemical antioxidant status and neovascular age-related macular degeneration. *Arch Ophthalmol* 1993;111:104–109.
14. Seddon JM, Ajani UA, Sperduto R, et al. Dietary carotenoids, vitamins A, C, and E, and advanced age-related macular degeneration. *JAMA* 1994;272:1413–1420.
15. Newsome DA, Swartz M, Leone NC, et al. Oral zinc in macular degeneration. *Arch Ophthalmol* 1988;106:192–198.
16. Young RW. Solar radiation and age-related macular degeneration. *Surv Ophthalmol* 1988;32:252–269.
17. Hennekens CH, Buring JE. *Epidemiology in medicine* Boston: Little, Brown, 1987.
18. Beck RW, Cleary PA, Anderson MM, et al. A randomized, controlled trial of corticosteroids in the treatment of acute optic neuritis. *N Engl J Med* 1992;326:581–588.
19. Broun ER, Greist A, Tricot G, Hoffman R. Excessive zinc ingestion. A reversible cause of sideroblastic anemia and bone marrow depression. *JAMA* 1990;264:1441–1443.
20. Hooper PL, Visconti L, Garry PJ, Johnson GE. Zinc lowers high-density lipoprotein-cholesterol levels. *JAMA* 1980;244:1960–1961.
21. Roberts HJ. Commentary: Perspective on vitamin E as therapy. *JAMA* 1981;246:1129–1331.
22. Herbert V. Risk of oxalate stone from large doses of vitamin C. *N Engl J Med* 1978;298:856.
23. Herbert V. The vitamin craze. *Arch Intern Med* 1980;140:173.
24. Green WR. Clinicopathologic studies of treated choroidal neovascular membranes: a review and report of two cases. *Retina* 1991;11: 328–356.
25. Macular Photocoagulation Study Group. Recurrent choroidal neovascularization after argon laser photocoagulation for neovascular maculopathy. *Arch Ophthalmol* 1986;104:503–512.
26. Folkman J, Klagsbrun M. Angiogenic factors. *Science* 1987;235:442–447.
27. Folkman J, Ingber DE. Angiostatic steroids: method of discovery and mechanism of action. *Ann Surg* 1987;206:374–383.
28. Li WW, Grayson G, Folkman J, D'Amore PA. Sustained-release endotoxin, a model for inducing corneal neovascularization. *Invest Ophthal Vis Sci* 1991;32:2906–2911.
29. Miller JW, Adamis AP, Shima D, et al. Vascular endothelial growth factor/vascular permeability factor is temporally and spatially correlated with ocular angiogenesis in a primate model. *Am J Pathol* 1994;145:574–584.
30. Miller JW, O'Reilly MS, Moulton RS, Folkman J. Treatment of experimental intraocular neovascularization using AGM-1470. *Invest Ophthalmol Vis Sci* 1993;34(suppl):1441.
31. Pournaras CJ, Tsacopoulos M, Strommer K, Gilodi N, Leuenberger PM. Experimental retinal branch vein occlusion in miniature pigs induces local tissue hypoxia and vasoproliferative microangiopathy. *Ophthalmology* 1990;97:1321–1328.
32. Miller JW, Stinson WG, Folkman J. Regression of experimental iris neovascularization with systemic alpha-interferon. *Ophthalmology* 1993;100:9–14.
33. Crum R, Szabo S, Folkman J. A new class of steroids inhibits angiogenesis in the presence of heparin or a heparin fragment. *Science* 1985;230:1375–1378.
34. Li WW, Casey R, Gonzalez EM, Folkman J. Angiostatic steroids potentiated by sulfated cyclodextrins ihibit corneal neovascularization. *Invest Ophthal Vis Sci* 1991;32:2898–2905.
35. Maione TE, Gray GS, Petro J, et al. Inhibition of angiogenesis by recombinant human platelet-4 and related peptides. *Science* 1990;247: 77–79.
36. Reynaud S, Knisely TL, Curtis A, Maione TE, Dorey CK. Inhibition of retinal vascular growth by systemic administration of recombinant human platelet factor 4 (rPF4) in the rat model of ROP. *Invest Ophthal Vis Sci* 1993;34:838.
37. Ferrara N, Clapp D, Weiner R. The 16K fragment of prolactin specifically inhibits basal or fibroblast growth factor stimulated growth of capillary endothelial cells. *Endocrinology* 1991;129:896–900.
38. Moses MA, Sudhalter J, Langer R. Identification of an inhibitor of neovascularization from cartilage. *Science* 1990;248:1408–1410.
39. Mun EC, Doctrow SR, Carter R, Ingber DE, Folkman J. An angiogenesis inhibitor from the cornea. *Invest Ophthal Vis Sci* 1989;30: 151.
40. Pober JS, Cotran RS. Cytokines and endothelial cell biology. *Physiol Rev* 1990;70:427–451.
41. Brouty-Boye D, Zetter BR. Inhibition of cell motility by interferon. *Science* 1980;208:516–518.
42. Sidky YA, Borden EC. Inhibition of angiogenesis by interferons: effects on tumor- and lymphoctye-induced vascular responses. *Cancer Res* 1987;47:5155–5161.
43. Ezekowitz RAB, Mulliken JB, Folkman J. Interferon alpha-2a therapy for life threatening hemangiomas of infancy. *N Engl J Med* 1992;326:1456–1463.
44. Gillies M, Su T, Sarossy M, Hollows F. Interferon-alpha 2b inhibits proliferation of human Tenon's capsule fibroblasts. *Graefes Arch Clin Exp Ophthalmol* 1993;231:118–121.
45. Wong J, Wang N, Miller JW, Schuman JS. Modulation of human fibroblast activity by selected angiogenesis inhibitors. *Exp Eye Res* 1994;58:439–451.

46. Feron EJ, Rothova A, van Hagen PM, Baarsma GS, Suttorp-Schulten MSA. Interferon-alpha 2b for refractory ocular Behcet's disease. *Lancet* 1994;343:1428.
47. Virdi PS, Hayreh SS. Ocular neovascularization with retinal vascular occlusion. I. Association with experimental retinal vein occlusion. *Arch Ophthalmol* 1982;100:331–341.
48. Fung WE. Interferon alpha 2a for treatment of age-related macular degeneration. *Am J Ophthalmol* 1991;112:349–350.
49. Poliner LS, Tornambe PE, Michelson PE, Heitzmann JG. Interferon alpha-2a for subfoveal neovascularization in age-related macular degeneration. *Ophthalmology* 1993;100:1417–1424.
50. Gillies MC, Sarks JP, Beaumont PE, et al. Treatment of choroidal neovascularisation in age-related macular degeneration with interferon alfa-2a and alfa-2b. *Br J Ophthalmol* 1993;77:759–764.
51. Lewis ML, Davis J, Chuang E. Interferon alfa-2a in the treatment of exudative age-related macular degeneration. *Graefes Arch Clin Exp Ophthalmol* 1993;231:615–618.
52. Thomas MA, Ibanez HE. Interferon alfa-2a in the treatment of subfoveal choroidal neovascularization. *Am J Ophthalmol* 1993;115:563–568.
53. Kirkpatrick JNP, Dick AD, Forrester JV. Clinical experience with interferon alfa-2a for exudative age-related macular degeneration. *Br J Ophthalmol* 1993;77:766–770.
54. Engler CB, Sander B, Koefoed P, Larsen M, Vinding T, Lund-Andersen H. Interferon alpha-2a treatment of patients with subfoveal neovascular macular degeneration. *Acta Ophthalmol* 1993;71:27–31.
55. Renault PF, Hoofnagle JH. Side effects of alpha-interferon. *Semin Liver Dis* 1989;9:273–277.
56. Lane AM, DeRosa JT, Egan KM, et al. Safety and tolerance of interferon-alfa-2a therapy for choroidal neovascularization. *Invest Ophthal Vis Sci* 1993;34:1159.
57. Guyer DR, Tiedeman J, Yanuzzi LA, et al. Interferon-associated retinopathy. *Arch Ophthalmol* 1993;111:350–356.
58. Pharmacological Therapy for Macular Degeneration Study Group. Interferon Alfa-2a is ineffective for patients with choroidal neovascularization secondary to age-related macular degeneration: results of a prospective randomized placebo-controlled clinical trial. *Arch Ophthalmol* 1997; in press.
59. Good DJ, Polverini PJ, Rastinejad F, et al. A tumor supressor-dependent inhibitor of angiogenesis is immunologically and functionally indistinguishable from a fragment of thrombospondin. *Proc Natl Acad Sci USA* 1990;87:6624–6628.
60. BenEzra D, Griffin BW, Maftzir G, Aharonov O. Thrombospondin and in vivo angiogenesis induced by basic fribroblast growth factor or lipopolysaccharide. *Invest Ophthal Vis Sci* 1993;34:3601–3608.
61. Ingber D, Gujita T, Kishimoto S, et al. Synthetic analogues of fumagillin that inhibit angiogenesis and suppress tumour growth. *Nature* 1990;348:555–557.
62. Abe J, Zhou W, Takuwa N, et al. A fumagillin derivative angiogenesis inhibitor, AGM-1470, inhibits activation of cyclin-dependent kinases and phosphorylation of retinoblastoma gene product but not protein tyrosyl phosphorylation or protooncogene expression in vascular endothelial cells. *Cancer Res* 1994;54:3407–3412.
63. Antoine N, Greimers R, De Roanne C, et al. AGM-1470, a potent angiogenesis inhibitor, prevents the entry of normal but not transformed endothelial cells into the G1 phase of the cell cycle. *Cancer Res* 1994;54:2073–2076.
64. Brem H, Folkman J. Analysis of experimental antiangiogenic therapy. *J Pediatr Surg* 1993;28:445–451.
65. Yamaoka M, Yamamoto T, Masaki T, Ikeyama S, Sudo K, Fujita T. Inhibition of tumor growth and metastasis of rodent tumors by the angiogenesis inhibitor *O*-(chloroacetyl-carbamoyl)fumagillol (TNP-470; AGM-1470). *Cancer Res* 1993;53:4262–4267.
66. Peacock DJ, Banquerigo ML, Brahn E. Angiogenesis inhibition suppresses collagen arthritis. *J Exp Med* 1992;175:1135–1138.
67. Oliver SJ, Banquerigo ML, Brahn E. Suppression of collagen-induced arthritis using an angiogenesis inhibitor, AGM-1470, and a microtubule stablilizer, Taxol. *Cell Immunol* 1994;157:291–299.
68. Gonzalez EM, Adamis AP, Folkman J. Systemic administration of an angiogenesis inhibitor (AGM-1470), inhibits bFGF-induced corneal neovascularization. *Invest Ophthalmol Vis Sci* 1992;33:777.
69. D'Amato RJ, Loughnan MS, Flynn E, Folkman J. Thalidomide is an inhibitor of angiogenesis. *Proc Natl Acad Sci USA* 1994;91:4082–4085.
70. O'Reilly MS, Holmgren L, Shing Y, et al. Angiostatin: a novel angiogenesis inhibitor that mediates the suppression of metastases by a Lewis lung carcinoma. *Cell* 1994;79:1–20.
71. Kim KJ, Li B, Winer J, et al. Inhibition of vascular endothelial growth factor-induced angiogenesis suppresses tumour growth in vivo. *Nature* 1993;362:841–844.
72. Adamis AP, Shima DT, Tolentino MJ, Gragoudas ES, Ferrara N, Folkman J, D'Amore PA, Miller JW. Inhibition of VEGF prevents ocular neovascularization in a primate. *Arch Ophthalmol* 1996;114: 66–71.

Textbook of Ocular Pharmacology,
edited by T.J. Zimmerman, et al.
Lippincott–Raven Publishers, Philadelphia © 1997.

CHAPTER 39

Angiogenesis and Growth Factors

Joan W. Miller and Patricia A. D'Amore

OVERVIEW OF ANGIOGENESIS

Many ophthalmic diseases are characterized by neovascularization, or the growth of new blood vessels that is abnormal either in timing or location. Depending on their location, the new vessels may bleed, leading to the formation of fibrous tissue and the destruction of the neural retina, as occurs in diabetes and age-related macular degeneration (AMD). Alternatively, they may grow over and impede normal structures, as in neovascular glaucoma or interstitial keratitis. New vessel growth or angiogenesis is a complex process, with multiple steps occurring in a patterned fashion (1). Endothelial cells are normally in a quiescent growth state, but in a pathologic process they can begin to proliferate rapidly (2). Activated endothelial cells secrete proteolytic enzymes which dissolve basement membrane around the parent vessel. Endothelial cells migrate from the parent vessel and align themselves to form a new capillary sprout, while proliferating and migrating to elongate the sprout. By curving and elongating, the sprouts form tubes with lumens and then anastomose to form a loop. Finally, a mesenchymal cell is recruited, it becomes a pericyte, and new basement membrane is deposited.

Control of the angiogenic process appears to be maintained by a balance of local modulators, or angiogenic stimulators and inhibitors. Many stimulators have been identified and include polypeptide factors such as vascular endothelial growth factor (VEGF), basic fibroblast growth factor (bFGF), transforming growth factor-α (TGF-α), interleukin-8 (IL-8), platelet-derived growth factor (PDGF), and insulin growth factor (IGF-I and IGF-II). Potential growth inhibitors include transforming growth factor-β (TGF-β), thrombospondin, and corneal angiogenesis inhibitor (CAI) (3). These growth-modulating molecules can act in multiple ways, as diffusible soluble factors or bound to the extracellular matrix. The modulators are likely to be regulated at several different levels; e.g., the synthesis of VEGF appears to be regulated by oxygen levels in the local environment (4,5), as well as by factors such as estrogen and epidermal growth factor (EGF). bFGF may be controlled primarily by its release from cells through injury and death and by sequestration and release from heparan sulfate either in the matrix or on the cell surface. TGF-β may be controlled primarily by its activation rather than synthesis. Given the redundancy of the system, with multiple stimulatory and inhibitory factors, and the multiple sites of regulation possible, it is likely that the initiating events may vary in different disease processes and in different capillary beds.

ETIOLOGY OF ANGIOGENESIS IN OPHTHALMIC DISEASES

Hypoxia

Clinically, iris and retinal neovascularization in diabetic retinopathy, retinal vein occlusion, and radiation retinopathy are associated with areas of retinal capillary closure and ischemic retina. This has led to the hypothesis that a factor diffusing from ischemic retina is responsible for neovascularization (6,7). Hypoxia appears to be the component of ischemia that stimulates angiogenesis. The retina has been demonstrated to be hypoxic in an experimental model of retinal neovascularization in miniature pigs after laser occlusion of a branch retinal vein (8,9). Using O_2-sensitive microelectrodes, Pournaras et al. showed that the intervascular zones of the normal retina had a pO_2 of 27.3 ± 2.9 mm Hg, which decreased to 13.7 ± 1.1 mm Hg after retinal vein occlusion. The pO_2 nadir was at 50% of

J. W. Miller: Massachusetts Eye and Ear Infirmary, Department of Ophthalmology, Harvard Medical School, Boston, Massachusetts 02114.

P. A. D'Amore: Department of Surgery and Pathology, Children's Hospital Medical Center, Department of Surgery, Harvard Medical School, Boston, Massachusetts 02115.

the retinal depth, corresponding to the interface of the inner nuclear layer and the outer plexiform layer.

Clinically, panretinal photocoagulation leads to regression of retinal and optic nerve neovascularization in diabetic retinopathy (10) and to regression of iris neovascularization in diabetic retinopathy or retinal vein occlusion (11,12). Explanations for this effect include reversal of hypoxia, destruction of cells producing angiogenic factors, and stimulation of cells capable of producing angiogenic inhibitors. Data in the miniature pig model suggest that hypoxia may be involved, since scatter laser photocoagulation in the region of the previous vein occlusion led to reversal of hypoxia of the inner retina; Pournaras et al. (13) observed that photocoagulation did not prevent neovascularization in the model and postulated that photocoagulation had affected only a portion of the hypoxic retina.

Injury

Hypoxia or ischemia may not be the mechanism that underlies other forms of neovascularization, such as choroidal neovascularization (CNV), which may be a response to injury. Hypoxia is not as obviously relevant to CNV since the choroid has a very high blood flow per tissue weight. Furthermore, in diseases in which the choriocapillaris is destroyed, CNV does not occur. In radiation retinopathy, there is vascular occlusion of retinal and choroidal capillaries (14). Yet, whereas neovascularization of the retina, disc, and iris occurs commonly, true CNV has not been described (15). A single case of subretinal neovascularization has been described, in which new vessels originating from telangiectatic retinal vessels were located between the neurosensory retina and the retinal pigment epithelium (RPE) of a patient treated with external beam radiation (16). Some alterations of the choriocapillaris have been observed in age-related macular degeneration (AMD), with thickening of the intercapillary septae and loss of the choriocapillaris endothelium (17). However, it is not clear that these changes would result in hypoxia of the outer retina.

Laser injury to the outer retina and choroid can lead to the development of CNV (18,19). Macrophages have been observed in these lesions and also in histologic studies of eyes with AMD, suggesting that inflammatory cells (which secrete angiogenic factors) may be involved in stimulating CNV (20,21). Inflammatory cells might be recruited in response to local tissue injury.

A model of AMD proposed by Friedman et al. (22) that is consistent with many of the clinical observations centers on the loss of scleral elasticity that occurs in cases of AMD (22) (E. Friedman, personal communication). The loss of elasticity may be attributable to deposition of lipids in the sclera and Bruch's membrane and may be similar to the loss of vascular compliance observed in arteriosclerosis; sphingomyelins and cholesterol esters are believed to be involved in both processes. Doppler studies have demonstrated that the pulsatility of the arteries perfusing the eye is greater in AMD cases than in age-matched controls (23). The greater pulsatility may be evidence of an increase in the resistance of the choroidal circulation. This increased resistance could result in decreased perfusion and RPE dysfunction. RPE dysfunction could lead to accumulation of degradation products of photoreceptor outer segments, including phospholipids. The accumulated deposits may themselves be angiogenic, may lead to the release of angiogenic substances, or may attract inflammatory cells, which would in turn release angiogenic substances.

Clinically, CNV is associated with large, soft drusen and with focal hyperpigmentation (24). Nongeographic atrophy, or RPE stippling, is associated with CNV, whereas geographic atrophy does not imply an increased risk for new vessel formation. Histopathologically, large, soft drusen represent either amorphous material located between a detached, thickened inner aspect of Bruch's membrane and the remainder of Bruch's, or diffuse thickening of the inner aspect of Bruch's membrane from accumulation of abnormal basement membrane with associated hypopigmentation of the overlying RPE (17). Histologically, choroidal capillary ingrowth occurs adjacent to these areas (17,25), which supports the hypothesis that the accumulated amorphous substance and basement membrane, or a process associated with its accumulation, leads to the production or release of angiogenic substances.

Although the pathogenesis of ocular neovascularization is not completely understood, the importance of modulators of angiogenesis, both stimulators and inhibitors, is generally accepted. A complete description of all the known angiogenic factors is beyond the scope of this article, but an overview of several factors is provided, followed by a discussion of three key factors, bFGF, VEGF, and IGF, and their relation to ocular neovascularization. Finally, a possible model of the interplay between stimulators and inhibitors is presented.

ANGIOGENIC FACTORS

FGF

Acidic FGF (aFGF) and bFGF are the prototypic members of the FGF family. The original mitogenic activity was partially purified from brain and pituitary extracts (26). bFGF was named because of its demonstrated mitogenic effect on fibroblasts and its high (basic) isoelectric point (9.6), which distinguished it from aFGF (pI 5.6). Purification to homogeneity from tumor extracts was accomplished by taking advantage of the high heparin affinity of these two factors (27,28). Basic and acidic FGF share a 53% absolute sequence homology (27).

Among the members of the FGF family are several oncogenes that encode for proteins with a 40% to 50% homology to bFGF and aFGF, including int-2, an oncogene activated by a mouse mammary tumor virus (29); hst/k-fgf, isolated from human stomach cancers (30); FGF-5, isolated from a human bladder tumor (31); and FGF-6, isolated from a mouse cosmid library by screening with the hst gene (32). There are three additional members of the FGF family; these share sequence homology and heparin affinity with the other family members but are distinguished by their target cell specificity. Whereas the FGF described are mitogens for vascular endothelial cells, these other factors are specific for epithelial cells (keratinocyte growth factor, KGF) (33), mouse mammary carcinoma cells (androgen-induced growth factor, AIGF) (34), and glial cells (glia-activating factor, FGF-9) (35).

Basic FGF

Because bFGF is the best characterized of the FGFs and has been most strongly implicated in the angiogenic process, the remainder of this section is confined to a discussion of bFGF.

Purification, Biochemistry and Distribution

The bFGF that was first purified had a molecular weight of 18 kD (36). Higher molecular weight forms of bFGF (22, 23, and 25 kD) are generated by alternative translation initiation involving the unusual CUG start codons lying further upstream from the usual AUG start codons. The relative amounts of the various forms of bFGF differ substantially in various cell lines, suggesting that the alternative translation initiation process may be regulated (37).

bFGF has been isolated from many mesoderm- and neuroectoderm-derived normal tissues and tumors (for review, see 38–41), as well as a variety of normal and tumor cells in culture (38). Biosynthetic studies in many cell types demonstrate that bFGF remains cell associated rather than secreted, an observation consistent with the lack of signal sequence. One of the features distinguishing the FGF from other GF is their high affinity for heparin and heparan sulfate. bFGF binds tightly to heparin-sepharose and is eluted with approximately 1.5 M NaCl, whereas other growth factor, such as PDGF (which has a pI similar to that of bFGF) is eluted with 0.5 M NaCl (41). The affinity for heparin is specific, since bFGF does not bind other glycosaminoglycans such as chondroitin sulfate and dermatan sulfate (42). Heparin protects bFGF from inactivation by acid and heat (43) and from degradation by proteases such as trypsin and chymotrypsin (44). Furthermore, several observations indicate that a significant portion of the cell-associated bFGF proteins is associated with the extracellular matrix (45), from which it can be released by treatment with high salt, heparin, heparitinase, or heparinase. Collectively, these observations have led to the concept of matrix-associated bFGF as a "stored growth factor" (41).

Biologic Activity

Mitogenesis, Chemotaxis and Survival. bFGF is mitogenic and chemotactic in vitro for many cell types of mesodermal and neuroectodermal lineages in vitro (for review, see 39,40) at concentrations as low as 1 pg/ml, with half-maximal effect occurring at 22 to 53 pg/ml, and with saturation occurring at 140 to 280 pg/ml (40). Although the actions of bFGF in vivo have not been systematically studied, several reports suggest that bFGF stimulates local cell proliferation in injured/lesioned articular cartilage (46), severed sciatic nerve (38), and denuded artery (47). bFGF has also been shown to modulate the differentiation of several cell types (for review, see 39); skeletal muscle and neural cells the best characterized. bFGF has also been shown to promote both survival and differentiation of a variety of cells derived from neural crest (39). Administration of bFGF delays the senescence of many cultured cells and extends their lifespan for many generations (40). In addition, bFGF has been shown to induce retinal regeneration in vivo and to enhance photoreceptor survival in inherited retinal dystrophy (48,49). Although the mechanism through which bFGF promotes cell survival is not known, studies in which BALB/c 3T3 (murine fibroblast cells) was used have demonstrated that protection by bFGF is not associated with cell-cycle traverse into S phase (50). In addition, protein synthesis is required for bFGF to exert its survival function.

Development. Several lines of experimental evidence suggest that bFGF or molecules closely related to bFGF play an important role in vertebrate development. Administration of bFGF to stage 8 *Xenopus* oocytes mimics the effects of ventrovegetal signal and mesoderm formation (51,52). Similarly, *Xenopus* oocytes contain a store of FGF polypeptides derived from maternal RNA sufficient to induce mesoderm. Definitive demonstration of bFGF's role in development derives from studies in which explants from embryos expressing dominant negative FGF receptors fail to induce mesoderm in response to FGF.

Angiogenesis. One of the biologic activities of bFGF that has been intensively investigated is its involvement in angiogenesis. bFGF has been shown to stimulate endothelial cell proliferation and migration, two likely functions of an angiogenic factor. bFGF also induces the production by endothelial cells of collagenase and plasminogen activator (PA), proteases capable of degrading basement membrane (53), and induces capillary endothelial cells to migrate into three-dimensional collagen matrices to form capillary-like tubes (54). bFGF at levels as low as 10 ng to 100 ng is angiogenic in vivo in the chick chorioallantoic membrane (CAM) and cornea bioassays (55–57). The potency of bFGF in the in vivo angiogenic assay suggests that it could also play an important role in normal physiologic angiogenesis. Moreover, bFGF has been isolated from corpus luteum, adrenal gland, kidney, and retina, all tissues with strong angiogenic properties (40). bFGF has also been proposed to play a role in tumor-mediated angiogenesis. The link between bFGF activity and vascularization of tumors has not been firmly established in all tumor systems (41). Possibly not all of the tumors depend solely on bFGF for angiogenic activity or growth. However, in certain cases in which bFGF was the sole mediator of angiogenesis, neutralizing antibodies against bFGF were demonstrated to block solid tumor growth by suppressing bFGF-induced angiogenesis (58).

Receptors

Chemical cross-linking was used to detect receptors ranging in molecular weight from 110 kD to 150 kD for bFGF in various cell types (38). These receptors bind bFGF with K_d values ranging from 11 pM to 270 pM, and the number of these receptors present on the cell surface vary from 0.2 to 1 $\times 10^5$ per cell (41). A 130-kD bFGF receptor was purified from chicken embryos by affinity chromatography on immobilized bFGF, and the corresponding cDNA was cloned with an oligonucleotide coding for a tryptic peptide fragment (59). This cDNA was homologous to a human cDNA (457*flg*/FGFR1), which is related to the *fms* gene (60). A second bFGF receptor (*bek*/FGFR2) cDNA was isolated by screening a mouse liver expression cDNA library with antiphosphotyrosine antibodies (61). Subsequently, full-length cDNA clones were isolated for both *flg* and *bek,* and their complete amino acid sequence was deduced (62). Screening of a chicken embryo fibroblast expression cDNA library with antiphosphotyrosine antibodies resulted in the isolation of a third FGF receptor, *cek 2* (63). In addition, FGFR3, the probable human homologue of *cek* 2, was cloned from K-562 erythroleukemia cells (64). In the case of *flg* and *bek* genes, multiple forms of the FGF receptor are generated by alternative splicing (65–68). The in vivo expression of these differentially spliced products is regulated in a tissue-specific fashion (68). Alternative splicing of the FGF receptor gene products appears to generate receptor proteins with different ligand-binding specificities (68).

The FGF receptor appears to require the cooperation of low-affinity receptors (for review, see 69). These receptors bind to bFGF with K_d values of about 2 nM, and the number of low-affinity receptor sites ranges from 0.5 to 2 $\times 10^6$ per cell (70). The ability of heparin and heparin-degrading enzymes to disrupt this low-affinity binding suggests that these may be heparan sulfate proteoglycans (71). In vitro binding assays have demonstrated that these low affinity heparin-like molecules are required for binding of bFGF to high affinity receptor sites (72) and that heparin is also required for cell-free binding of bFGF to a soluble FGF receptor (73) Further experimental evidence suggests that the nature of the glycosaminoglycan side chains of the heparan sulfate proteoglycans apparently determines the FGF binding specificity (74). However, a recent study has raised questions concerning the absolute requirement of heparin for high affinity interactions of bFGF with its receptor; Roghani et al. (75) reported that although heparin increases the affinity between bFGF and FGFR-1 two- to fourfold, it is not required for the binding of bFGF to its receptor. The discrepancy between these data may be attributed to different labeling methods used to prepare bFGF for binding analysis.

Release of bFGF

In light of the diverse biologic roles of bFGF, it is very perplexing that bFGF does not possess a consensus signal peptide for secretion (76). The lack of a signal sequence suggests that bFGF is not secreted by conventional means. Consistent with this is the finding that bFGF is not detected in the conditioned media of cultured cells (45) (P-T. Ku and P.A. D'Amore, unpublished observations). However, examination of bFGF localization in corneal endothelial cells (45) and capillary endothelial cells (77) has shown bFGF to be associated with or within the extracellular matrix. How the factor gains access to the matrix is unclear. In addition, bFGF is not glycosylated despite possessing a potential glycosylation site (38).

Collectively, these observations as well as others (reviewed in 78) have led investigators to believe that no FGF is released from cells under normal circumstances. However, increasing evidence shows that this belief is not entirely accurate. Schweigerer et al. (77) reported measurable amounts of bFGF in the conditioned media of adrenal cortical capillary endothelial cells. Consistent with this observation, bFGF was shown to be released from astrocytoma cell lines and bovine corneal endothelial cells in a density dependent manner (79). Using a transgenic mouse model of dermal fibrosarcomas, Kandel et al. observed that bFGF remains cell associated in dermal fibroblast cells derived from an avascular stage of fibromatosis, whereas it is apparently exported into the conditioned media by dermal fibroblast cells derived from highly vascular fibrosarcomas (80). Moreover, neutralizing antibodies against bFGF suppress the baseline growth of growing capillary endothelial cells 20% to 35% (81). Neutralizing antibodies against bFGF also block endothelial cell migration and DNA synthesis after a wound is sustained (82). In an elegant series of studies, extracellular matrix prepared from cells expressing bFGF has been shown to be capable of stimulating endothelial cell proliferation and PC12 cells differentiation. This stimulatory activity associated with the extracellular matrix is abolished by neutralizing antibodies against bFGF (83). The release of bFGF was demonstrated further in single, isolated NIH 3T3 cells transfected with bFGF cDNA. In these cells, migration is modulated by neutralization bFGF (84). The release of bFGF from these cells appears to occur through a pathway that is independent of the endoplasmic reticulum–Golgi complex (85). This observation, although of interest, might simply reflect an artifact of tissue culture. Several alternative pathways for bFGF release have been postulated, including selective exocytosis (86), the involvement of ATP-binding cassette (ABC)-transport proteins (for review, see 87), and cell death or injury (88) (for detailed discussion, see 78).

Of these alternative pathways, the most evidence is available for the last. The work of McNeil et al. suggests that sublethal injury of cells might provide a physiologically relevant route for the release of bFGF (for review, see 88,89). In sublethal injury cells incur transient disruption of the plasma membrane, from which they survive and recover. Sublethal injury appears to be a common occurrence among tissues normally subjected to mechanical stress in vivo (89). Both in vitro and in vivo studies support the notion of bFGF release through sublethal injury. Using cultured aortic endothelial cells as a model system, we demonstrated that mechanical wounding of cells by scraping leads to efficient release of bFGF from injured cells (88,90). Sublethal injury to the endothelium of the aorta has been demonstrated (91). With albumin used as a marker, approximately 6.5% of the endothelial cells of the undisturbed, normal rat aorta were shown to be wounded, with most of the wounded cells in clusters around vessel bifurcations, regions subjected to greater hemodynamic forces such as shear stress and turbulent flow, and as streaks aligned with the long axis of the vessel. Nearly 80% of the mitotic figures identified in the endothelium of the aorta corresponded to cells that had been identified as wounded, a finding consistent with observations of higher labeling index of endothelial cells at vessel bifurcations as compared with unbranched regions (92). Cell proliferation is mediated at least in part by polypeptide growth factor, and it has been proposed that bFGF might couple the mechanical stimulus with cell growth (89).

Evidence to date indicates that bFGF may act as a "wound hormone," both in the routine maintenance of tissue integrity and during repair after injury (90). In support of this concept, bFGF expression has been shown to be increased at the site of injury in several experimental models. After mechanical lesion to the cerebral cortex, bFGF immunoreactivity markedly increased (93). Similarly, isoproterenol-induced cardiomyocyte injury leads to an increase in both bFGF mRNA and protein within 24 hours (94). Finally, optic nerve crush in mice has been shown to result in a dramatic increase in bFGF immunostaining in the photoreceptor layer of the retina (95). The retinal ischemia that occurs in several types of ocular pathology may change the local environment sufficiently to cause frank tissue damage that would lead to release of bFGF.

VEGF

VEGF, also known as vascular permeability factor and vasculotropin, was first identified and purified on the basis of its ability to induce increased microvascular permeability (96). Subsequently VEGF was shown to stimulate vascular endothelial cell proliferation in vitro and vascular permeability and angiogenesis in vivo (97–100). A wide variety of cells has been demonstrated to produce VEGF in vitro, including RPE (101,102), vascular smooth muscle cells (103), and AIDS-associated Kaposi's sarcoma cells (104). VEGF has been shown to induce expression of plasminogen activator (PA) and plasminogen activator inhibitor (PAI-1) in microvascular endothelial cells (105). In these cells, urokinase-type PA (u-PA) and tissue-type PA (t-PA) were increased by VEGF in a dose-dependent manner. PA are believed to be involved in degradation of extracellular matrix during angiogenesis. Recombinant VEGF produces neovascularization in the corneal micropocket (106), stimulates angiogenesis in the chick CAM bioassay (107), and may lead to disc neovascularization in the rabbit after intravitreal injection (108). A single intraarterial bolus of VEGF stimulated angiogenesis and collateralization in a rabbit ischemic hindlimb model, suggesting that VEGF might have a role in collateral formation in vivo (109). VEGF and basic FGF may act synergistically to promote angiogenesis, as suggested by their synergistic effect on endothelial cells in culture (110,111).

VEGF comprises a group of four related heparin-binding polypeptides of 121, 165, 189, and 206 amino acids derived by alternative splicing (103). They exist as dimeric glycoproteins composed of disulfide-linked subunits and possess 21% and 24% homology with the A and B chains of PDGF respectively (112). The four forms differ in their affinity for heparin and in their solubility (113,114). The smaller forms (121 and 165 amino acids) have a lower affinity for heparin, with the 121 form failing to bind to heparin-sepharose and the 165 form eluting at 0 to 0.9 M NaCl. The larger forms (189 and 206 amino acids) bind heparin avidly, with only 20% to 30% of the 189 form eluting at 0.9 M NaCl, and the remainder eluting at 2.0 M NaCl. $VEGF_{165}$ appeared to be the predominantly expressed form when human cDNA libraries were screened, although multiple types were usually detected (114). Unlike aFGF and bFGF, all VEGF forms are efficiently secreted, endothelial-specific mitogens (100,106). However, the different forms of VEGF display different behaviors as secreted factors. $VEGF_{121}$ is entirely soluble, almost all $VEGF_{189}$ is bound to extracellular matrix or cell surface sites, and $VEGF_{165}$ is intermediate, with 50% to 70% bound (114).

Three high-affinity tyrosine kinase VEGF receptors have been identified: KDR, *flt-1,* and *flt-4* (115–118). The three receptors are structurally similar. All are tyrosine kinases, with seven immunoglobin-like domains in their extracellular region, and all are strongly related by sequence similarities. They are also related by sequence similarity to other members of the class III receptors, including the receptors for PDGF (116).

Increasing evidence shows that VEGF and its receptors serve an important role in various angiogenesis-dependent processes. High-affinity VEGF binding and mRNA expression during development suggest that VEGF and *flk-1* (the mouse KDR homologue) are major regulators of blood vessel development (119,120). High levels of VEGF mRNA have been demonstrated in the rat corpus luteum as compared with the mural granulosa cells at a time corresponding to maximal angiogenesis, suggesting a physiologic role for VEGF in ovulation (113). VEGF may have a role in maintaining normal vasculature, where binding sites have been demonstrated on adult rat heart valves and aorta, suggesting a reparative function in areas of high turbulence (113,121). High levels of VEGF mRNA have been demonstrated in various tumors, including human adenocarcinoma and glioblastoma, a highly vascularized tumor, in which VEGF mRNA expression was particularly high in tissue adjacent to necrotic centers, presumed to be hypoxic (5,122,123). In tumor models, systemically administered anti-VEGF monoclonal antibodies inhibited tumor angiogenesis and tumor growth (124). In a glioblastoma model, researchers demonstrated inhibition of tumor angiogenesis and growth by infecting endothelial cells in the tumor model with a retrovirus encoding a dominant-negative mutant of the Flk-1 VEGF receptor (125). The mutant Flk-1 receptor lacked the amino acids of the intracellular kinase domain, making it signal-incompetent.

Carmellet et al. (126) and Ferrara et al. (127) recently reported that formation of blood vessels was abnormal in heterozygous VEGF-deficient embryos and severely impaired in homozygous VEGF-deficient embryos, resulting in death of homozygotes and heterozygotes at midgestation. VEGF deficiency led to impairment of many aspects of vascular development, including differentiation of blood islands, vascular sprouting, lumen formation, the formation of large vessels, and the interconnection and organization of vascular networks. Heterozygotes were also noted to have vascular elements present in mesenchyme but not in neuroepithelium, with accompanying apoptosis and disorganization of neuroepithelial cells (127).

VEGF appears to play an important role in development, in physiologic maintenance of vessels, in physiologic ovulation, and in pathologic tumor growth. Its characteristics, including being a secreted mitogen, specific for endothelial cells, and its regulation by hypoxia, make it a prime candidate for an ocular angiogenesis factor and have led to recent investigations in ocular models and patients with ocular neovascularization.

TGF-α

TGF-α is one of a group of proteins related to EGF. These are membrane-bound glycoproteins that are cleaved, yielding soluble growth factors. They are implicated in cell growth and differentiation through specific protein–protein interactions. Pro–TGF-α is a 160-amino acid polypeptide with a hydrophobic transmembrane sequence of 23 amino acids. The proteolytic process which cleaves pro–TGF-α is inefficient in most cells, and pro–TGF-α accumulates on cell surfaces. Membrane bound pro–TGF-α binds EGF receptors with high affinity, with a subsequent rapid increase in cytosolic calcium levels, and may function as a mediator of cell–cell adhesion and interaction (128). This biologic activity of pro–TGF-α is in contrast to classical polypeptide prohormones that have very low biologic activity until they are cleaved to generate the active hormone. Cleavage of pro–TGF-α apparently switches between two active forms.

The soluble form of TGF-α is a 50-amino acid cleavage product of pro–TGF-α and was first detected in culture media from various oncogenically transformed cells (129,130). TGF-α was initially identified owing to its ability to induce fibroblast proliferation, an effect which was later shown to depend on TGF-β. TGF-α expression is most prevalent in tumor-derived cell lines and in cells transformed by cellular oncogenes, retroviruses, and tumor promoters (128–130). TGF-α cDNA transfected into fibroblasts and epithelial cells transforms the cell lines, suggesting that TGF-α may play a role in the generation or progression of neoplasia. TGF-α mRNA is also expressed during mouse and rat embryogenesis, including the optic vesicle. TGF-α binds to endothelial cells and stimulates DNA synthesis, as measured by radioactive thymidine uptake. Assessed in the hamster cheek pouch model, TGF-α stimulated angiogenesis without inflammation and was more effective than EGF (131).

IL-8

IL-8 belongs to a new class of chemotactic cytokines, known as chemokines, which are capable of attracting and activating leukocytes and act as mediators of inflammation and angiogenesis (132,133). IL-8 mRNA expression, and release of biologically active cytokine, have been reported for endothelial cells; fibroblasts; keratinocytes; synovial cells; chondrocytes; epithelial cells from various tissues, including RPE; tumor cells; and neutrophils (132,134, 135). IL-8 is chemotactic for neutrophils, lymphocytes and endothelial cells (136–138) and is also an endothelial cell mitogen (133). IL-8 may also be involved in modulating neutrophil emigration from the vasculature (139, 140). IL-8 bound to endothelial cells may upregulate neutrophil adhesion to endothelium by inducing the translocation of integrins (140). Conversely, soluble IL-8 can downregulate neutrophil/endothelial adhesion by binding to circulating neutrophils and leading to shedding of L-selectin, which inhibits neutrophil adhesion to the endothelium (140,141).

IL-8 induces angiogenesis in the rabbit corneal micropocket without signs of nonspecific inflammation and has been implicated, together with tumor necrosis factor-α (TNF-α), as the major factor responsible for the monocyte/macrophage-associated angiogenic response in inflammatory joint disease (133). When IL-8 is injected intradermally, it induces local accumulation of neutrophils and plasma exudation (132). IL-8 is resistant to inactivation by plasma peptidases, is only very slowly degraded by proteases (136), and appears to interact with tissue matrix glycosaminoglycans, confining it to the site of injection.

PDGF

PDGF was originally isolated from platelets as a mitogen for arterial smooth muscle cells (142). More recently, PDGF was shown to be produced by many different cell types and appears to have a broad range of functions (143). PDGF refers to a family of 30-kD dimers of structurally related A and B polypeptide chains linked by disulfide bonds (143,144). All three possible dimeric forms of PDGF have been isolated in whole blood serum: Human PDGF is believed to be an AB heterodimer, and PDGF-BB appears to be the predominant isoform from all other species. Certain tumors may secrete different isoforms, such as the AA homodimer purified from a glioma cell line.

Two PDGF receptors, α and β, have been identified (145). Cells of fibroblast origin express both α- and β-receptors, as do vascular smooth muscle cells and placental trophoblasts (143,144). Only α-receptors exist on oligodendrocyte progenitor cells, mesothelial cells, and liver capillary endothelial cells, whereas β-receptors exist only on brain capillary endothelial cells, neurons, and meningeal and Schwann cells (143). The α-receptor binds all three isoforms (PDGF-AA, BB, AB) with similarly high affinities, but the β-receptor binds only PDGF-BB with high affinity. The two receptor types are structurally and functionally related. They have five immunoglobin-like domains in their extracellular ligand-binding region, with a transmembrane segment and an intracellular tyrosine kinase. Apparently each subunit of the dimeric PDGF molecule binds one receptor molecule on the cell surface, with the ligand forming a bridge between the two receptors (143,144). The kinase is subsequently activated, possibly through a process of "autophosphorylation" between the two receptors. The ligand–receptor complex is then internalized, transferred to the lysosomes, and degraded.

Receptors are activated in three different manners: endocrine, paracrine, and autocrine (144). Circulating cells, such as platelets or monocytes, may release PDGF near an injured blood vessel where PDGF can interact in an endocrine manner with receptors on vascular smooth muscle cells. Endothelial cells lining blood vessels may release PDGF to act on nearby smooth muscle cells in a paracrine manner. Certain tumor cells release PDGF-like compounds and bear PDGF receptors, with PDGF thereby acting in an autocrine manner. PDGF may have an important role in neurobiologic processes, since it has been shown to be produced in the nervous system by neurons (PDGF-B), type 1 astrocytes (PDGF-A), and Schwann cells (PDGF-B), and may have a trophic effect on brain tissue in vivo (143).

IGF

IGF-1 and IGF-II are growth-promoting peptides with multiple biologic effects (146). IGF-1 was initially identified as a circulating factor that appeared to mediate the effects of growth hormone on cartilage development in rats (147). The IGF-I and IGF-II precursors contain A and B domains that are homologous to the A and B chains of insulin, but unlike that of insulin, the C domain of IGF-I and IGF-II precursors is not removed during processing. The mature IGF peptides are single-chain polypeptides. IGF-I and IGF-II mRNA is expressed in multiple tissues, but IGF-II appears to predominate during fetal development, and IGF-I is expressed primarily postnatally. The IGF peptides interact primarily with the IGF-I receptor, a transmembrane tyrosine kinase with structural similarity to the insulin receptor.

IGF action is also influenced by IGF-binding proteins (IGFBPs), which have been detected in the circulation and in extracellular fluids and affect IGF half-life (t½) and receptor interactions (146). In the eye, IGF and related peptides have been shown to have a variety of functions in the sensory retina and may also be expressed by RPE.

TGF-β

TGF-β is a dimeric protein of 25,000 kD, with multiple cellular targets and activities. Three isoforms exist in mammalian species, TGF-β 1, 2, and 3, occurring principally as homodimers, although heterodimeric forms exist in low abundance (148). The most abundant isoform is TGF-β1 in mammalian species. TGF-β1 and TGF-β2 have many similar characteristics, but when tested for their ability to inhibit DNA synthesis in bovine aortic endothelial cells, TGF-β2 was only 1% to 2% as potent as TGF-β1 (149).

TGF-β appears to play a major role in wound repair, inducing angiogenesis, fibrosis, and collagen formation (150). Because TGF-β is secreted by almost all cultured cells in an inactive or latent form, its action as a growth modulator appears to be regulated at the level of its activation. Latent TGF-β is activated by extremes of pH, treatment with chaotropic agents, plasmin, and cathepsin D. In vivo, acidic environments proteases such as plasminogen activator and type IV collagenase may activate TGF-β

(151). In wound repair, TGF-β released from degranulating platelets may be activated by a combination of these factors. The activated TGF-β recruits inflammatory cells, leading to formation of new blood vessels and synthesis of collagen. In this setting, TGF-β is secondarily angiogenic through the action of inflammatory cells.

In vitro, however, TGF-β is one of the most potent inhibitors of endothelial cell proliferation, which suggests a role for TGF-β in maintaining the normally quiescent state of the vasculature, a role which is supported by results of coculture experiments. When endothelial cells and cells of the vessel wall (smooth muscle cells or pericytes) are grown in an in vitro coculture system, pericytes inhibit endothelial cell proliferation in a contact-dependent manner. The mechanism of this inhibition is the production of an activated form of TGF-β (151). In pathologic states, such as diabetic retinopathy, pericyte loss precedes the development of new vessels. From the coculture experiments one may postulate that the loss of pericytes leads to loss of active TGF-β, releasing endothelial cells to respond to angiogenic factors, with subsequent proliferation and formation of new blood vessels.

In experimental systems, TGF-β has been demonstrated to promote wound healing, including experimentally induced retinal tears in rabbits (152,153). These results have been used as a rationale to treat full-thickness macular holes in patients (154). TGF-β may also lead to excessive scarring in some instances and, in an experimental model of incisional wounding in rats, neutralizing antibodies to TGF-β applied early in the healing process, reduced dermal scarring without affecting tensile strength (155). The antibody-treated wounds exhibited fewer macrophages, fewer blood vessels, and lower collagen and fibronectin contents. Unregulated production or activation of TGF-β, with resulting excessive production of connective tissue, may be involved in processes such as proliferative vitreoretinopathy (PVR), and pulmonary fibrosis. Vitreous aspirates from eyes with intraocular fibrosis and PVR had a threefold greater amount of TGF-β (mostly TGF-β2) than eyes with uncomplicated retinal detachments without fibrosis (156).

TGF-β may have a protective role in tissues affected by ischemia or infarction. TGF-β may also mediate the effects of the retinoic/vitamin D/steroid family of nuclear receptors. TGF-β has important immunomodulatory effects, suppressing the proliferation and differentiation of most cells of B and T cell lineages in vitro and antagonizing the effects of inflammatory cytokines (148).

ANGIOGENIC FACTORS: ROLE IN OCULAR NEOVASCULARIZATION

FGF

For several reasons, the role of FGF in ocular angiogenesis has been more difficult to study than that of VEGF (discussed herein). First, FGF does not possess a signal sequence. As a result, demonstration of aFGF (157,158) and bFGF (159) in the retina does not necessarily mean that the factors are exerting any action at that moment. In contrast, because VEGF is a secreted protein, identification of VEGF in a tissue is more likely to indicate that it is playing an active role. Similarly, there does not appear to be a strong correlation between bFGF mRNA and protein levels (160). Therefore, although bFGF mRNA and protein levels were reported to be increased in some circumstances, as in studies of the retinas of newborn mice exposed to hyperoxia (161), the RPE of retinas subjected to krypton laser treatment (162) and the retinas of animals in which the optic has been crush-injured (95), it is difficult to extrapolate findings of these descriptive studies to a physiologic role for bFGF in the eye. Similarly, investigators have examined various ocular fluids from persons with proliferative diabetic retinopathy for the presence of bFGF. The results of these studies are inconsistent, most likely due to a variety of effects, including the lability of bFGF and the variability in the sensitivity of the bFGF assays.

VEGF

VEGF has several characteristics that make it a prime candidate for an ocular angiogenesis factor, particularly in ischemic diseases: it appears to be regulated by hypoxia, it is a secreted mitogen, and it acts directly on endothelial cells. Preliminary data also showed VEGF expression in the retina (163). Recent observations in experimental models and in clinical studies substantiate its role in ocular neovascular disease.

VEGF levels correlate both spatially and temporally with the iris neovascularization in a monkey model of neovascularization (164). In this model, the branch retinal veins are occluded by dye yellow laser, producing an ischemic retinopathy angiographically similar to clinical central retinal vein occlusion (164). Iris neovascularization develops in the first week after laser treatment, increasing in the first 3 weeks and then typically regressing after 3 weeks unless neovascular glaucoma intervenes. The severity of iris neovascularization can be graded by use of standardized photographs and angiograms, analyzing the vessel density and degree of fluorescein leakage.

In a pilot experiment, four eyes were monitored for 35 days after laser vein occlusion. Fluorescein angiography was performed and aqueous samples were obtained every 6 days to measure the development of iris neovascularization and the aqueous VEGF levels. VEGF levels were assayed with a sensitive time-resolved immunofluorometric assay (165,166). Although there was substantial variability from monkey to monkey, both measures varied over time and there appeared to be a temporal association between changing aqueous VEGF level and changing iris neovascularization. Aqueous VEGF was undetectable before laser vein occlusion, increased to more than 30 pM as iris neovascularization developed, and then decreased as the new vessels regressed.

A second set of experiments was performed with a control, in which one eye underwent laser vein occlusion and the second eye received "sham" laser in which laser spots were placed adjacent to the retinal vessels. Serial iris angiograms were graded, and serial aqueous VEGF measurements were made for 12 to 14 days. Because each animal contributed both an ischemic and a nonischemic sham measure of VEGF and iris grade at each timepoint, the measures were summarized as paired differences (i.e., ischemic vs. nonischemic value for each animal at each time point). The corrected VEGF level (ischemic minus nonischemic) increased significantly with time ($p \leq 0.001$). Similarly, the corrected iris grade increased significantly during the period measured ($p \leq 0.01$). Finally, there was a statistically significant relationship ($p \leq 0.001$) between increasing VEGF level and increasing neovascularization.

The evidence for ischemic retina as the source of the increased aqueous VEGF is both indirect and direct. Serum VEGF was undetectable in the monkeys in the experiment, making it unlikely that VEGF was derived from blood. Vitreous levels of VEGF were equal to or higher than aqueous levels in eyes with neovascularization, consistent with VEGF being released from a posterior location in the eye. More direct evidence that the ischemic retina is the source of VEGF was provided by Northern analysis and in situ hybridization (ISH). Northern analysis of total RNA isolated from ischemic retina demonstrated two transcripts, a distinct and high-abundance band at 3.6 kilobases (kb), and a faint, low-abundance band at approximately 3.9 kb. The monkey retina VEGF was subsequently demonstrated by polymerase chain reaction (PCR) analysis to be the 121 and 165 forms of VEGF (167). In the nonischemic retina, VEGF mRNA was barely detectable. ISH showed VEGF mRNA to be localized to the inner nuclear layer and ganglion cell layer of the ischemic retina (164, 167). Increased VEGF expression was observed as early as day 1 after laser vein occlusion, and peak expression was observed at 14 days, corresponding to the peak severity of iris neovascularization. By 28 days, VEGF expression was still increased, but to a lesser degree. Minimal labeling was noted in the nonischemic retinas.

Correlation of VEGF with retinal neovascularization was seen in mice (168) and rats (169). In the neonatal mouse model, a high oxygen environment after birth leads to extensive capillary nonperfusion in the peripheral retina, with subsequent neovascularization of the posterior pole when the animals are again exposed to room air (168). VEGF mRNA levels were increased threefold in the retinas of animals after they were reexposed to room air but before the development of neovascularization. ISH demonstrated VEGF mRNA in the inner nuclear layer and ganglion cell layer of the retinas.

To determine if VEGF is sufficient to produce neovascularization in normal eyes, physiologic doses of human recombinant VEGF were injected into the vitreous of normal monkey eyes (170). Bioactive VEGF was injected into the vitreous of five monkey eyes, with doses ranging from 0.25 μg to 2.5 μg/injection. Equal amounts of inactivated human recombinant VEGF (rhVEGF) (two eyes) or vehicle (one eye) were injected into contralateral control eyes. Eyes were assessed by slit-lamp biomicroscopy, iris color photography and fluorescein angiography, histopathology, and immunostaining with antibodies against proliferating cell nuclear antigen (PCNA). All five bioactive VEGF-injected eyes developed iris neovascularization, but none of the three control eyes exhibited vascular changes. A dose response to VEGF was observed in one animal receiving 2.5 μg VEGF in the right eye and 0.25 μg in the left eye. Repeated VEGF injections produced severe iris neovascularization and neovascular glaucoma. Iris vessel endothelial cells were PCNA positive in the bioactive VEGF-injected eyes only.

In further investigations, we studied the effect of VEGF-blocking antibodies on ischemia-induced neovascularization (171). Eighteen eyes of nine animals underwent laser vein occlusion, followed by randomization to VEGF-blocking monoclonal antibody or to a control antibody. Antibody injections were administered intravitreally by sterile technique every other day for 14 days, and serial iris fluorescein angiograms were graded in a masked fashion. Control eyes developed typical iris neovascularization, whereas all eyes receiving VEGF-blocking monoclonal antibodies demonstrated inhibition of neovascularization. Northern blot of retinal RNA from eyes receiving either antibody demonstrated increased expression of VEGF mRNA, indicating that antibody injection did not interfere with the upregulation of VEGF mRNA in ischemia. Therefore, inhibition of VEGF in the monkey model of iris neovascularization prevents intraocular neovascularization and suggests that therapies directed at blocking the production or action of VEGF could be effective in eye diseases characterized by ischemia.

Studies of VEGF-blocking agents have also been conducted in the neonatal mouse model, with use of soluble VEGF receptors or chimeric proteins consisting of the exoplasmic domain of high-affinity VEGF receptors linked to the heavy chain of IgG by molecular biologic techniques (172). Single intravitreal injection of human Flt-IgG and murine Flk-1–IgG chimeric proteins reduced histologically evident retinal neovascularization in 25 of 25 (100%) and 21 of 22 (95%) animals studied ($p < 0.001$) (173). One eye of each animal received the VEGF-blocking protein; the other eye acted as a control and received an intravitreal injection of a control chimeric protein.

The role of VEGF in ischemic diseases has been evaluated in clinical studies. In one study, vitreous VEGF levels were measured in undiluted vitreous obtained at vitrectomy from eight patients with proliferative diabetic retinopathy and from 12 patients undergoing vitrectomy for other indications without proliferative retinopathy (174). VEGF levels were significantly increased in the eyes of patients with proliferative diabetic retinopathy ($p = 0.006$). The median vitreous concentration in the eyes with proliferative diabetic retinopathy was 29.1 pM, as compared with 6.1 pM in the controls. In a second study, both aqueous and vitreous fluids in 164 patients, including diabetics with and without proliferative disease, patients with other proliferative disorders, and nondiabetic controls, were evaluated (175). VEGF levels were significantly increased in either aqueous, vitreous, or subretinal fluid from patients with active proliferative diabetic retinopathy, iris neovascularization, ischemic central retinal vein occlusion, and chronic retinal detachment. Six patients with intraocular VEGF levels measured before and after panretinal photocoagulation had a 75% decrease in VEGF levels and a clinical decrease in the extent of neovascularization.

In another study, the presence of angiogenic growth factors expressed in neovascular membranes obtained from diabetic patients was evaluated. Only VEGF was consistently detected (176). Pe'er et al. demonstrated high VEGF mRNA levels in the retinas of enucleated eyes from patients with neovascularization secondary to diabetes central vein occlusion retinal detachment and intraocular tumors (177).

VEGF appears to have an important role in ocular angiogenesis, particularly in conditions in which retinal ischemia is part of the pathogenesis. The degree to which VEGF is involved in CNV and in corneal neovascularization remains to be determined, as does its possible role in maintenance of the normal vasculature. Treatment strategies directed at blocking the production or action of VEGF may have clinical application.

IGF

The role of growth hormone and its associated factors was first suggested by the clinical observation of regressing proliferative diabetic retinopathy after infarction of the pituitary during pregnancy (Sheehan's syndrome) (178). This observation led to experimental and clinical observations that hypophysectomy reduced the severity of diabetes and led to remission of diabetic retinopathy (179,180). The complications of hypophysectomy were frequent and often severe and, with the advent of laser photocoagulation, such therapy was largely abandoned. However, an association of growth hormone abnormalities and diabetic retinopathy had been demonstrated (181,182). Subsequently, growth hormone was demonstrated to mediate many of its effects through production of IGF-I and IGF-II and investigations were directed toward these factors.

In vitro studies support a role for IGF-I in retinal neovascularization. IGF-I receptors are present on retinal microvascular cells and demonstrate a fivefold increase in DNA synthesis in response to IGF-I (183). IGF-I stimulates migration and proliferation of bovine aortic endothelial cells, retinal capillary endothelial cells (184), and RPE cells in vitro (185). IGF-I stimulated a significant increase of t-PA production in vitro in human retinal endothelial cells from patients with diabetes, but not from control subjects (186). IGF-I was also shown to stimulate secretion of PA in RPE cells in vitro and also to cause a shape change to a more fibroblast-like morphology (185). Grant et al. speculate that in PDR and proliferative vitreoretinopathy IGF-I may act on RPE cells to form fibrovascular membranes.

IGF-I has been demonstrated to be angiogenic in vivo. When rhIGF-I was incorporated into Elvax pellets and implanted in rabbit cornea, neovascularization developed, with 100% of corneas responding when 10 μg IGF-I was used (187). Intravitreal injection rhIGF-I in a single dose of 600 μg (10^5 times the levels measured in clinical neovascularization), led to vascular tortuosity, hemorrhage, and hyperemia surrounding the optic disc in 100% of eyes by 7 days after injection. Leakage of fluorescein on angiography suggested the presence of neovascularization, and electron microscopy demonstrated retinal capillary basement-membrane thickening and reduplication. Slow-release devices containing 500 ng IGF-I were also placed on the surface of the retina, with no gross vascular abnormality evident during the 21-day course of the experiment. Histologically microvascular changes were evident along the medullary ray (187). These results support the hypothesis that IGF-I is angiogenic in vivo and may play a role in ocular neovascularization.

Grant et al. measured IGF levels in undiluted vitreous and serum from patients with proliferative diabetic retinopathy (188). In 23 patients with proliferative diabetic retinopathy, the mean vitreous concentration of IGF was 6.3 ± 0.93, as compared with 2.7 ± 0.96 ng/ml in vitreous from controls. IGF-II levels were not significantly different between diabetic patients and controls. In diabetic patients, the vitreous concentrations of both IGF-I and IGF-II correlated significantly with serum concentrations, but this did not hold true for controls. A large proportion of the IGF-II in the vitreous was shown to be bound to a 40- to 50-K protein, with a smaller amount of IGF-I bound. The significance of protein binding of IGF-I was unclear. Finally, a large population-based study of 928 diabetic patients demonstrated that increased levels of serum IGF-I correlated with an increased frequency of proliferative diabetic retinopathy (189).

ANTIANGIOGENIC AGENTS

Because growth factors appear to have a major role in ocular diseases characterized by neovascularization, there is growing interest in treatment strategies directed at their inhibition. A more complete discussion of antiangiogenic agents is provided in Chapter 38 Medical Therapy for Macular Degeneration. These antiangiogenic strategies could involve stimulating naturally occurring inhibitors, developing growth factor-blocking agents, or using agents proven to be antiangiogenic in other systems. An example of an inhibitor normally present in the eye is CAI, a molecule that has been partially purified and demonstrated to inhibit angiogenesis in the chick CAM (3). One might devise a treatment that stimulates production of such an endogenous inhibitor. TGF-β has also been demonstrated in ocular tissue and in vitro is an inhibitor of endothelial cell proliferation, but its effects in vivo appear to be more complicated (150,156). It may also be possible to use growth factor-blocking agents such as VEGF-blocking antibodies, which have been shown to inhibit experimental tumor growth (124), and experimental iris neovascularization (171).

Other naturally occurring agents that may have anti-angiogenic effect include IFN-α, angiostatin, thrombospondin, platelet factor 4, the 16K prolactin fragment, and cartilage-derived inhibitor. Finally, pharmacologic agents that have been identified as antiangiogenic include the angiostatic steroids AGM-1470 and thalidomide. The pharmacologic modulation of angiogenesis is a potentially new approach to the complications of ocular neovascularization. Antiangiogenic agents must be carefully screened in appropriate animal models and carefully evaluated for potential toxicity, particularly when the targeted patient

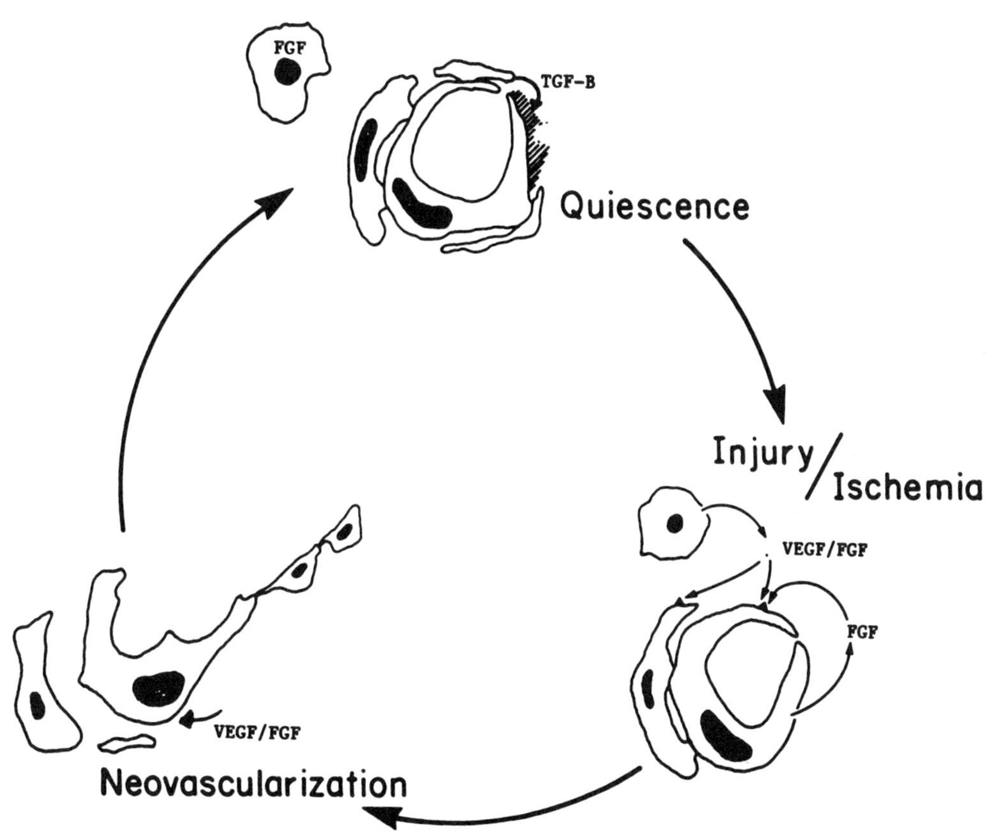

FIG. 39-1. Schematic of possible mechanisms involved in microvascular growth control. **Top middle:** The microvasculature consists of two cell types: the endothelial cell which junctions with itself or another endothelial cell to form the vessel lumen and the ablumenal pericyte or mural cell. The cells of the microvasculature are normally quiescent with respect to growth. The single cell shown outside the microvessel in this schematic is intended to represent the parenchymal cell of the tissue in question. For the purposes of this discussion, this cell may represent a retinal ganglion cell or a Mueller cell. **Bottom right:** Although the cells of the microvasculature seldom divide, in some conditions, such as proliferative diabetic retinopathy, vessel proliferation does occur. These conditions are usually characterized by the presence of ischemia (and therefore hypoxia) and/or tissue injury. We propose that hypoxia and/or injury lead to local increases in the levels of growth factors, including VEGF and FGF. In diabetic retinopathy, the loss of pericytes, which presumably exert an inhibitory influence on capillary growth, makes the microvascular network more vulnerable to local growth stimulators. **Bottom left:** Locally high concentrations of growth stimulators act either directly on the vascular endothelium to induce neovascularization (including proliferation, migration, and protease production) or recruit accessory cells such as macrophages, which release additional stimulatory factors that amplify the angiogenic process. (From *Invest Ophthalmol Vis Sci* 1994;35: 3975, Lippincott-Raven Publishers, Hagerstown, MD, with permission)

population is elderly, such as patients with AMD, or has other medical complications, such as diabetes mellitus.

SUMMARY

In trying to assimilate the list of angiogenic stimulators and inhibitors and the accumulated observations of their patterns of expression, secretion, and regulation in vitro and in vivo, one may feel overwhelmed. Scientists are forced to approach a complex process, such as proliferative diabetic retinopathy, and separate it into approachable problems. This usually requires the question first to an in vitro system, in which one can test simpler, defined relations between the cells and their milieu. Inherent in cell culture work is the understanding that the very act of growing cells in culture creates an artificial environment which may lead to erroneous conclusions. Nevertheless, to build a framework of understanding, certain hypotheses can be developed and tested in vitro. The next logical step is to test these hypotheses in an in vivo system, each animal model having strengths and weaknesses which must be considered when one interprets results. Animal models do permit an assessment of the system constituted by the tissue of interest and by the animal as a whole. Finally, one considers applying the approach to clinical diseases, which are often more chronic than any animal model and are affected by a broader range of genetic and environmental factors.

One can suggest a partial model of ocular angiogenesis for diseases associated with ischemia, such as proliferative diabetic retinopathy. The state of the endothelial cell in any tissue is probably determined by a balance of inhibitors and stimulators, presented locally, and from a distance (Fig. 1). Certain growth factors such as bFGF are produced constitutively and are stored in the extracellular matrix and on the cell surface. Others are produced by neighboring cells only in response to injury or hypoxia, such as VEGF. Finally, in pathologic states, some GF, such as IGF, may be circulating at increased levels in the serum.

The retinal capillary endothelial cell may be kept in its normally quiescent state through the cell–cell interaction with the pericyte, which secretes TGF-β, a potent inhibitor of endothelial cell proliferation, when the pericyte contacts endothelial cells. Other matrix components such as thrombospondin may also exert an antiproliferative effect on the endothelial cell (190). Pericytes are lost in diabetes during the course of the disease. Loss of pericytes may place the endothelial cell in a more responsive state by removing the inhibitory effect of TGF-β. As capillary closure occurs in the diabetic retina, possibly as the result of capillary occlusions by monocytes (191), the inner retina may become hypoxic, leading to the production of VEGF. Soluble VEGF may then act on the "receptive" capillary endothelial cell, stimulating proliferation. Serum IGF-I, circulating at increased levels in persons with diabetes, may act on the endothelial cell to increase levels of t-PA, producing plasmin and permitting dissolution of basement membrane. Disturbances in the local environment secondary to ischemia may lead to release of bFGF from the extracellular matrix. VEGF and bFGF may act synergistically to affect PA activity and lead to dissolution of the basement membrane. bFGF is also a potent endothelial cell mitogen and may act synergistically with VEGF to stimulate further endothelial cell proliferation.

Such a model is still incomplete, but by combining in vitro and reproducible animal models, and with the availability of well-characterized factors and strategies to neutralize them, one should be able to design experiments to further our understanding of these complex processes. The roles that these angiogenic modulators play in clinical disease, and the potential development of therapeutic strategies based on their effects, make them an important area of investigation for those concerned with ophthalmic disease.

REFERENCES

1. Ausprunk DH, Folkman J. Migration and proliferation of endothelial cells in preformed and newly formed blood vessels during tumor angiogenesis. *Microvasc Res* 1977;14:53–65.
2. Denekamp J. Vascular endothelium as the vulnerable element in tumours. *Acta Radiol Oncol* 1984;23:217–225.
3. Mun EC, Doctrow SR, Carter R, Ingber DE, Folkman J. An angiogenesis inhibitor from the cornea. *Invest Ophthal Vis Sci* 1989;30: 151.
4. Shima DT, Adamis AP, Yeo K-T, Yeo T-K, Berse B, Brown L. Hypoxic regulation of vascular permeability factor (vascular endothelial growth factor) mRNA and protein secretion by human retinal pigment epithelial cells. *Invest Ophthal Vis Sci* 1993;34(suppl):990.
5. Shweiki D, Itin A, Soffer D, Keshet E. Vascular endothelial growth factor induced by hypoxia may mediate hypoxia-initiated angiogenesis. *Nature* 1992;359:843–845.
6. Ashton N. Retinal vascularization in health and disease. *Am J Ophthalmol* 1957;44:7–24.
7. Michaelson IC. The mode of development of the vascular system of the retina, with some observations on its significance for certain retinal disease. *Trans Ophthalmol Soc UK* 1948;68:137–180.
8. Pournaras CJ, Tsacopoulos M, Riva CE, Roth A. Diffusion of O2 in normal and ischemic retinas of anesthetized miniature pigs in normoxia and hyperoxia. *Graefes Arch Clin Exp Ophthalmol* 1990;228: 138–142.
9. Pournaras CJ, Tsacopoulos M, Strommer K, Gilodi N, Leuenberger PM. Experimental retinal branch vein occlusion in miniature pigs induces local tissue hypoxia and vasoproliferative microangiopathy. *Ophthalmology* 1990;97:1321–1328.
10. The Diabetic Retinopathy Study Research Group. Photocoagulation treatment of proliferative diabetic retinopathy: the second report of Diabetic Retinopathy Study findings. *Ophthalmology* 1978;85:82–105.
11. Little HL, Rosenthal AR, Dellaporta A, Jacobson DR. The effect of pan-retinal photocoagulation of rubeosis iridis. *Am J Ophthalmol* 1976;81:804–809.
12. Wand M, Dueker DK, Aiello LM, Grant WM. Effects of panretinal photocoagulation on rubeosis iridis, angle neovascularization, and neovascular glaucoma. *Am J Ophthalmol* 1978;86:332–339.
13. Pournaras CJ, Tsacopoulos M, Strommer K, Gilodi N, Leuenberger PM. Scatter photocoagulation restores tissue hypoxia in experimental vasoproliferative microangiopathy in miniature pigs. *Ophthalmology* 1990;97:1329–1333.
14. Irvine AR, Wood IS. Radiation retinopathy as an experimental model for ischemic proliferative retinopathy and rubeosis iridis. *Am J Ophthalmol* 1987;103:790–797.
15. Brown GC, Shields JA, Sanborn G, Augsburger JJ, Savino PJ, Schatz NJ. Radiation retinopathy. *Ophthalmology* 1982;89:1494–1501.

16. Boozalis GT, Schachat AP, Green WR. Subretinal neovascularization from the retina in radiation retinopathy. *Retina* 1987;7:156–161.
17. Green WR, McDonnell PJ, Yeo JH. Pathologic features of senile macular degeneration. *Ophthalmology* 1985;92:615–627.
18. Ohkuma H, Ryan SJ. Experimental subretinal neovascularization in the monkey. *Arch Ophthalmol* 1983;101:1102–1110.
19. Wallow I, Johns K, Barry P, Chandra S, Bindley C. Chorioretinal and choriovitreal neovascularization after photocoagulation for proliferative diabetic retinopathy. *Ophthalmology* 1985;92:523–532.
20. Green WR, Enger C. Age-related macular degeneration histopathologic studies. The 1992 Lorenz E. Zimmerman lecture. *Ophthalmology* 1993;100:1519–1535.
21. Penfold PL, Provis JM, Bilson FA. Age-related macular degeneration: ultrastructural studies of the relationship of leucocytes to angiogenesis. *Graefes Arch Clin Exp Ophthalmol* 1987;225:70–76.
22. Friedman E, Ivry M, Ebert E, Glynn R, Gragoudas E, Seddon J. Increased scleral rigidity and age-related macular degeneration. *Ophthalmology* 1989;96:104–108.
23. Krupsky S, Friedman E, Lane AM, Oak SS, Gragoudas ES. Ocular blood flow in age related macular degeneration. *Invest Ophthal Vis Sci* 1994;35:1817.
24. Bressler SB, Maguire MG, Bressler NM, Fine SL, Macular Photocoagulation Study Group. Relationship of drusen and abnormalities of the retinal pigment epithelium to the prognosis of neovascular macular degeneration. *Arch Ophthalmol* 1990;108:1442–1447.
25. Sarks SH, Van Driel D, Maxwell L, Killingsworth M. Softening of drusen and subretinal neovascularization. *Trans Ophthalmol Soc UK* 1980;100:414–422.
26. Gospodarowicz D. Purification of fibroblast growth factor from bovine pituitary. *J Biol Chem* 1975;250:2515–2520.
27. Esch F, Baird A, Ling N, et al. Primary structure of bovine pituitary basic fibroblast growth factor (FGF) and comparison with the amino-terminal sequence of bovine brain acidic FGF. *Proc Natl Acad Sci USA* 1985;82:6507–6511.
28. Shing Y, Folkman J, Sullivan R, Butterfield C, Murray J, Klagsbrun M. Heparin affinity: purification of a tumor-derived capillary endothelial cell growth factor. *Science* 1984;223:1296–1298.
29. Moore R, Casey G, Brookes S, Dixon M, Peters G, Dickson C. Sequence, topography and protein coding potential of mouse int-2: a putative oncogene activated by mouse mammary tumor virus. *EMBO J* 1986;5:919–924.
30. Sakamoto H, Mori M, Taira M, et al. Transforming gene from human stomach cancers and a noncancerous portion of stomach mucosa. *Proc Natl Acad Sci USA* 1986;83:3997–4001.
31. Zhan X, Bates B, Hu XG, Goldfarb M. The human FGF-5 oncogene encodes a novel protein related to fibroblast growth factors. *Mol Cell Biol* 1988;8:3487–3495.
32. Marics I, Adelaide J, Raybaud F, et al. Characterization of the HST-related FGF.6 gene, a new member of the fibroblast growth factor gene family. *Oncogene* 1989;4:335–340.
33. Finch PW, Rubin JS, Miki T, Ron D, Aaronson SA. Human KGF is FGF-related with properties of a paracrine effector of epithelial cell growth. *Science* 1989;245:752–755.
34. Tanaka A, Miyamoto K, Minamino N, et al. Cloning and characterization of an androgen-induced growth factor essential for the androgen-dependent growth of mouse mammary carcinoma cells. *Proc Natl Acad Sci USA* 1992;89:8928–8932.
35. Miyamoto M, Naruo K-I, Seko C, Matsumoto S, Kondo T, Kurokawa T. Molecular cloning of a novel cytokine cDNA encoding the ninth member of the fibroblast growth factor family which has a unique secretion property. *Mol Cell Biol* 1993;13:4251–4259.
36. Ueno N, Baird A, Esch F, Ling N, Guillemin R. Isolation of an amino terminal extended form of basic fibroblast growth factor. *Biochem Biophys Res Commun* 1986;138:580–588.
37. Prats A-C, Vagner S, Prats H, Amalric F. *cis*-Acting elements involved in the alternative translation initiation process of human basic fibroblast growth factor mRNA. *Mol Cell Biol* 1992;12:4796–4805.
38. Baird A, Böhlen P. Fibroblast growth factors. In: Roberts AB, Sporn MB, eds. *Handbook of experimental pharmacology: peptide growth factors and their receptors.* Berlin: Springer-Verlag, 1990;369–418.
39. Burgess WH, Maciag T. The heparin-binding (fibroblast) growth factor family of proteins. *Annu Rev Biochem* 1989;58:575–606.
40. Gospodarowicz D. Fibroblast growth factors. In: Pimental E, Perucho M, eds. *Critical reviews in oncogenesis.* Boca Raton, FL: CRC Press, 1989;1–26.
41. Klagsbrun M. The fibroblast growth factor family: structural and biological properties. *Prog Growth Factor Res* 1989;1:207–235.
42. Sullivan R. Klagsbrun M. Purification of cartilage-derived growth factor by heparin affinity chromatography. *J Biol Chem* 1985; 260:2399–2403.
43. Gospodarowicz D, Cheng J. Heparin protects basic and acidic FGF from inactivation. *J Cell Physiol* 1986;128:475–484.
44. Sommer A, Rifkin DB. Interaction of heparin with human basic fibroblast growth factor: protection of the angiogenic protein from proteolytic degradation by a glycosaminoglycan. *J Cell Physiol* 1989;138:215–220.
45. Vlodavsky I, Folkman J, Sullivan R, et al. Endothelial cell-derived basic fibroblast growth factor: synthesis and deposition into subendothelial extracellular matrix. *Proc Natl Acad Sci USA* 1987;84: 2292–2296.
46. Davidson JM, Klagsbrun M, Hill KE, et al. Accelerated wound repair, cell proliferation, and collagen accumulation are produced by a cartilage-derived growth factor. *J Cell Biochem* 1985;100:1219–1227.
47. Lindner V, Majack R, Reidy M. Basic FGF stimulates endothelial regrowth and proliferation in denuded arteries. Effect of bFGF on endothelial recovery following injury. *J Clin Invest* 1990;85: 2004–2008.
48. Faktorovich EG, Steinberg RH, Yasumura D, Matthes MT, LaVail MM. Photoreceptor degeneration in inherited retinal dystrophy delayed by basic fibroblast growth factor. *Nature* 1990;347:83–86.
49. Hollenberg MJ, Park CM. Basic fibroblast growth factor induces retinal regeneration *in vivo*. *Dev Biol* 1989;134:201–205.
50. Tamm I, Kikuchi T, Zychlinsky A. Acidic and basic fibroblast growth factors are survival factors with distinctive activity in quiescent BALB/c3T3 murine fibroblasts. *Proc Natl Acad Sci USA* 1991;88:3372–3376.
51. Kimelman D, Kirschner M. Synergistic induction of mesoderm and FGF and TGF-β and the identification of an mRNA coding for FGF in the early *Xenopus* embryo. *Cell* 1987;51:869–877.
52. Slack JM, Darlington BG, Heath JK, Godsave SF. Mesoderm induction in early *Xenopus* embryos by heparin-binding growth factors. *Nature* 1987;326:197–200.
53. Mignatti P, Tsuboi R, Robbins E, Rifkin DB. *In vitro* angiogenesis of the human amniotic membrane: requirement for basic fibroblast growth factor-induced proteinases. *J Cell Biol* 1989;108:671–682.
54. Montesano R, Vassali JD, Baird A, Guillemin R, Orci L. Basic fibroblast growth factor induces angiogenesis *in vitro*. *Proc Natl Acad Sci USA* 1986;83:7297–7301.
55. Esch F, Ueno N, Baird A, et al. Primary structure of bovine brain acidic fibroblast growth factor. *Biochem Biophys Res Commun* 1986;133:554–562.
56. Lobb RR, Alderman EM, Fett JW. Induction of angiogenesis by bovine brain derived class I heparin-binding growth factor. *Biochemistry* 1985;24:4969–4973.
57. Shing Y, Folkman J, Haudenschild C, Lund D, Crum R, Klagsbrun M. Angiogenesis is stimulated by a tumor-derived endothelial cell growth factor. *J Cell Biochem* 1985;29:275–287.
58. Hori A, Sasada R, Matsutani E, et al. Suppression of solid tumor growth by immuno-neutralizing monoclonal antibody against human basic fibroblast growth factor. *Cancer Res* 1991;31:6180–6184.
59. Lee PL, Johnson DE, Cousens LS, Fried VA, Williams LT. Purification and complementary DNA cloning of a receptor for basic fibroblast growth factor. *Science* 1989;245:57–60.
60. Ruta M, Burgess W, Givol D, et al. Receptor for acidic fibroblast growth factor is related to the tyrosine kinase encoded by the fms-like gene (FLG). *Proc Natl Acad Sci USA* 1989;86:8722–8726.
61. Kornbluth S, Paulson KE, Hanafusa H. Novel tyrosine kinase identified by phosphotyrosine antibody screening of cDNA libraries. *Mol Cell Biol* 1988;8:5541–5544.
62. Dionne CA, Crumley G, Bellot F, et al. Cloning and expression of two distinct high-affinity receptors cross-reacting with acidic and basic fibroblast growth factors. *EMBO J* 1990;9:2685–2692.
63. Pasquale EB. A distinctive family of embryonic protein-tyrosine kinase receptors. *Proc Natl Acad Sci USA* 1990;87:5812–5816.

64. Keegan K, Johnson DE, Williams LT, Hayman MJ. Isolation of an additional member of the fibroblast growth factor receptor family, FGF R3. *Proc Natl Acad Sci USA* 1991;88:1095–1099.
65. Eisemann A, Ahn JA, Graziani G, Tronick SR, Ron D. Alternative splicing generates at least five different isoforms of the human basic-FGF receptor. *Oncogene* 1991;6:1195–1202.
66. Johnson DE, Lee PL, Lu J, Williams LT. Diverse forms of a receptor for acidic and basic fibroblast growth factors. *Mol Cell Biol* 1990;10:4728–4736.
67. Johnson DE, Lu J, Chen H, Werner S, Williams LT. The human fibroblast growth factor receptor genes: a common structural arrangement underlies the mechanisms for generating receptor forms that differ in their third immunoglobulin domain. *Mol Cell Biol* 1991;11:4627–4634.
68. Werner S, Duan D-SR, DeVries C, Peters KG, Johnson DE, Williams LT. Differential splicing in the extracellular region of fibroblast growth factor receptor 1 generates receptor variants with different ligand-binding specificities. *Mol Cell Biol* 1992;12:82–88.
69. Klagsbrun M, Baird A. A dual receptor system is required for basic fibroblast growth factor activity. *Cell* 1991;67:229–231.
70. Moscatelli D, Quarto N. Transformation of NIH 3T3 cells with basic fibroblast growth factor or the hst/K-fgf oncogene causes downregulation of the fibroblast growth factor receptor: reversal of morphological transformation and restoration of receptor number by suramin. *J Cell Biol* 1989;109:2519–2527.
71. Moscatelli D. High and low affinity binding sites for basic fibroblast growth factor on cultured cells: absence of a role for low affinity binding in the stimulation of plasminogen activator production by bovine capillary endothelial cells. *J Cell Physiol* 1987;131:123–130.
72. Yayon A, Klagsbrun M, Esko JD, Leder P, Ornitz DM. Cell surface, heparin-like molecules are required for binding of basic fibroblast growth factor to its high affinity receptor. *Cell* 1991;64:841–848.
73. Ornitz DM, Yayon A, Flanagan JG, Svahn CM, Levi E, Leder P. Heparin is required for cell-free binding of basic fibroblast growth factor to a soluble receptor and for mitogenesis in whole cells. *Mol Cell Biol* 1992;12:240–247.
74. Nurcombe V, Ford MD, Wildschut JA, Bartlett PF. Developmental regulation of neural response to FGF-1 and FGF-2 by heparan sulfate proteoglycan. *Science* 1993;260:103–106.
75. Roghani M, Mansukhani A, Dell'Era P, et al. Heparin increases the affinity of basic fibroblast growth factor for its receptor but is not required for binding. *J Biol Chem* 1994;269:3976–3984.
76. Abraham JA, Mergia A, Whang JL, et al. Nucleotide sequence of a bovine clone encoding the angiogenic protein, basic fibroblast growth factor. *Science* 1986;233:545–548.
77. Schweigerer L, Neufeld G, Friedman J, Abraham JA, Fiddes JC, Gospodarowicz D. Capillary endothelial cells express basic fibroblast growth factor, a mitogen that promotes their own growth. *Nature* 1987;325:257–259.
78. D'Amore PA. Modes of FGF release in vivo and in vitro. *Cancer Metastasis Rev* 1990;9:227–238.
79. Sato Y, Murphy PR, Sato R, Friesen HG. Fibroblast growth factor release by bovine endothelial cells and human astrocytoma cells in culture is density dependent. *Mol Endocrinol* 1989;3:744–748.
80. Kandel J, Bossy-Wetzel E, Radvany F, Klagsbrun M, Folkman J, Hanahan D. Neovascularization is associated with a switch to the export of bFGF in the multistep development of fibrosarcoma. *Cell* 1991;66:1095–1104.
81. D'Amore PA, Antonelli A, Smith SR, Herman IM. Basic fibroblast growth factor (bFGF) is an autocrine regulator of microvascular endothelial cell proliferation. *Invest Ophthal Vis Sci* 1990 (abstract); 31:199.
82. Sato Y, Rifkin DB. Autocrine activities of basic fibroblast growth factor: regulation of endothelial cell movement, plasminogen activator synthesis, and DNA synthesis. *J Cell Biol* 1988;107:1199–1205.
83. Rogelj S, Klagsbrun M, Atzmon R, et al. Basic fibroblast growth factor is an extracellular matrix component required for supporting the proliferation of vascular endothelial cells and the differentiation of PC12 cells. *J Cell Biol* 1989;109:823–831.
84. Mignatti P, Morimoto T, Rifkin DB. Basic fibroblast growth factor released by single, isolated cells stimulates their migration in an autocrine manner. *Proc Natl Acad Sci USA* 1991;88:11007–11011.
85. Mignatti P, Morimoto T, Rifkin DB. Basic fibroblast growth factor, a protein devoid of secretory signal sequence, is released by cells via a pathway independent of the endoplasmic reticulum-Golgi complex. *J Cell Physiol* 1992;151:81–93.
86. Cooper DNW, Barondes SH. Evidence for export of a muscle lectin from cytosol to extracellular matrix and for a novel secretion mechanism. *J Cell Biol* 1990;110:1681–1691.
87. Kuchler K. Unusual routes of protein secretion: the easy way out. *Trends Cell Biol* 1993;3:421–426.
88. McNeil PL, Muthukrishnan L, Warder E, D'Amore PA. Growth factors are released by mechanically wounded endothelial cells. *J Cell Biol* 1989;109:811–822.
89. McNeil PL. Cellular and molecular adaptations to injurious mechanical stress. *Trends Cell Biol* 1993;3:302–307.
90. Muthukrihnan L, Warder E, McNeil PL. Basic fibroblast growth factor is efficiently released from a cytosolic storage site through plasma membrane disruptions of endothelial cells. *J Cell Physiol* 1991;148:1–16.
91. Yu QC, McNeil PL. Transient disruptions of aortic endothelial cell plasma membranes. *Am J Pathol* 1992;141:1349–1360.
92. Wright HP. Endothelial mitosis around aortic branches in normal guinea pigs. *Nature* 1968;220:78–79.
93. Finklestein SP, Apostolides PJ, Caday CG, Prosser J, Philips MF, Klagsbrun M. Increased basic fibroblast growth factor (bFGF) immunoreactivity at the site of focal brain wounds. *Brain Res* 1988; 460:253–259.
94. Padua RR, Kardami E. Increased basic fibroblast growth factor (bFGF) accumulation and distinct patterns of localization in isoproterenol-induced cardiomyocyte injury. *Growth Factors* 1993;8:291–306.
95. Kostyk SK, D'Amore PA, Herman IM, Wagner JA. Optic nerve injury alters basic fibroblast growth factor localization in the retina and optic tract. *J Neurosci* 1994;14:1441–1449.
96. Senger DR, Galli SJ, Dvorak AM, Perruzzi CA, Harvey VS, Dvorak JF. Tumor cells secrete a vascular permeability factor that promotes accumulation of ascites fluid. *Science* 1983;219:983–985.
97. Clauss M, Gerlach M, Gerlach H, et al. Vascular permeability factor: a tumor-derived polypeptide that induces endothelial cell and monocyte procoagulant activity, and promotes monocyte migration. *J Exp Med* 1990;172:1535–1545.
98. Ferrara N, Henzel WJ. Pituitary follicular cells secrete a novel heparin-binding growth factor specific for vascular endothelial cells. *Biochem Biophys Res Commun* 1989;161:851–858.
99. Keck PJ, Hauser SD, Krivi G, et al. Vascular permeability factor, an endothelial cell mitogen related to PDGF. *Science* 1989;246:1309–1312.
100. Leung DW, Cachianes G, Kuang W-J, Goeddel DV, Ferrara N. Vascular endothelial growth factor is a secreted angiogenic mitogen. *Science* 1989;246:1306–1309.
101. Adamis AP, Shima DT, Yeo K-T, et al. Synthesis and secretion of vascular permeability factor/vascular endothelial growth factor by human retinal pigment epithelial cells. *Biochem Biophys Res Commun* 1993;193:631–638.
102. Yang Q, Zwijsen A, Slegers H, Vanden Berghe D. Purification and characterization of VEGF/VPF secreted by human retinal pigment epithelial cells. *Endothelium* 1994;2:73–85.
103. Tischer E, Mitchell R, Hartman T, et al. The human gene for vascular endothelial growth factor. Multiple protein forms are encoded through alternative exon splicing. *J Biol Chem* 1991;266:11947–11954.
104. Weindel K, Marme D, Weich HA. AIDS-associated Kaposi's sarcoma cells in culture express vascular endothelial growth factor. *Biochem Biophys Res Commun* 1992;183:1167–1174.
105. Pepper MS, Ferrara N, Orci L, Montesano R. Vascular endothelial growth factor (VEGF) induces plasminofen activators and plasminogen activator inhibitor-1 in microvascular endothelial cells. *Biochem Biophys Res Commun* 1991;181:902–906.
106. Connolly DT, Heuvelman DM, Nelson R, et al. Tumor vascular permeability factor stimulates endothelial cell growth and angiogenesis. *J Clin Invest* 1989;84:1470–1478.
107. Plouet J, Schilling J, Gospodarowicz D. Isolation and characterization of a newly identified endothelial cell mitogen produced by AtT-20 cells. *EMBO J* 1989;8:3801–3806.

108. Netzer E, Miller H, Neufeld G, Miller B. The in vivo effect of VEGF on the vasculature of the rabbit. *Invest Ophthal Vis Sci* 1994;35: 1587.
109. Takeshita S, Zheng LP, Brogi E, et al. Therapeutic angiogenesis. A single intraarterial bolus of vascular endothelial growth factor augments revascularization in a rabbit hind limb model. *J Clin Invest* 1994;93:662–670.
110. Goto F, Goto K, Weindel K, Folkman J. Synergistic effect of vascular endothelial growth factor and basic fibroblast growth factor on the proliferation and cord formation of bovine capillary endothelial cells within collagen gels. *Lab Invest* 1993;69:508–517.
111. Pepper MS, Ferrara N, Orci L, Montesano R. Potent synergism between vascular endothelial growth factor and basic fibroblast growth factor in the induction of angiogenesis in vitro. *Biochem Biophys Res Commun* 1992;189:824–831.
112. Tischer E, Gospodarowicz D, Mitchell R, et al. Vascular endothelial growth factor: a new member of the platelet-derived growth factor gene family. *Biochem Biophys Res Commun* 1989;165:1198–1206.
113. Ferrara N, Houck KA, Jakeman LB, Winer J, Leung DW. The vascular endothelial growth factor family of polypeptides. *J Cell Biochem* 1991;47:211–218.
114. Houck KA, Leung DW, Rowland AM, Winer J, Ferrara N. Dual regulation of vascular endothelial growth factor. *J Biol Chem* 1992;267:26031–26037.
115. De Vries C, Escobedo JA, Ueno H, Houck K, Ferrara N, Williams LT. The *fms*-like tyrosine kinase, a receptor for vascular endothelial growth factor. *Science* 1992;255:989–991.
116. Galland F, Karamysheva A, Pebusque M-J, et al. The FLT4 gene encodes a transmembrane tyrosine kinase related to the vascular endothelial growth factor receptor. *Oncogene* 1993;8:1233–1240.
117. Terman BI, Carrion ME, Kovacs E, Rasmussen BA, Eddy RL, Shows TB. Identification of a new endothelial cell growth factor receptor tyrosine kinase. *Oncogene* 1991;6:1677–1683.
118. Terman BI, Dougher-Vermazen M, Carrion ME, et al. Identification of the KDR tyrosine kinase as a receptor for vascular endothelial cell growth factor. *Biochem Biophys Res Commun* 1992;187:1579–1586.
119. Breier G, Albrecht U, Sterrer S, Risau W. Expression of vascular endothelial growth factor during embryonic angiogenesis and endothelial cell differentiation. *Development* 1992;114:521–532.
120. Millauer B, Wizigmann-Voos S, Schnurch H, et al. High affinity VEGF binding and developmental expression suggest Flk-1 as a major regulator of vasculogenesis and angiogenesis. *Cell* 1993;72: 835–846.
121. Jakeman LB, Winer J, Bennett GL, Altar A, Ferrrara N. Binding sites for vascular endothelial growth factor are localized on endothelial cells in adult rat tissues. *J Clin Invest* 1992;89:244–253.
122. Brown LF, Berse B, Jackman RW, et al. Expression of vascular permeability factor (vascular endothelial growth factor) and its receptors in adenocarcinomas of the gastrointestinal tract. *Cancer Res* 1993;53:4727–4735.
123. Plate KH, Breier G, Weich HA, Risau W. Vascular endothelial growth factor is a potential tumour angiogenesis factor in human gliomas in vivo. *Nature* 1992;359:845–848.
124. Kim KJ, Li B, Winer J, et al. Inhibition of vascular endothelial growth factor-induced angiogenesis suppresses tumour growth in vivo. *Nature* 1993;362:841–844.
125. Millauer B, Shawver LK, Plate KH, Risau W, Ullrich A. Glioblastoma growth inhibited in vivo by a dominant-negative Flk-1 mutant. *Nature* 1994;367:576–579.
126. Carmellet P, Ferreira V, Breier G, et al. Abnormal blood vessel development and lethality in embryos lacking a single VEGF allele. *Nature* 1996;380:435–439.
127. Ferrara N, Carver-Moore K, Chen H, et al. Heterozygous embryonic lethality induced by targeted inactivation of the VEGF gene. *Nature* 1996;380:439–442.
128. Massague J. Transforming growth factor-a: a model for membrane-anchored growth factors. *J Biol Chem* 1990;265:21393–21396.
129. De Larco JE, Todaro GJ. Growth factors from murine sarcoma virus-transformed cells. *Proc Natl Acad Sci USA* 1978;75:4001–4005.
130. Todaro GJ, Fryling C, De Larco JE. Transforming growth factors produced by certain human tumor cells: polypeptides that interact with epidermal growth factor receptors. *Proc Natl Acad Sci USA* 1980;77:5258–5262.
131. Schreiber AB, Winkler ME, Derynck R. Transforming growth factor-a: a more potent angiogenic mediator than epidermal growth factor. *Science* 1986;232:1250–1253.
132. Baggiolini M. Novel aspects of inflammation: interleukin-8 and related chemotactic cytokines. *Clin Invest* 1993;71:812–814.
133. Koch AE, Polverini PJ, Kunkel SL, et al. Interleukin-8 as a macrophage-derived mediator of angiogenesis. *Science* 1992;258:1798–1801.
134. Cubitt CL, Tang Q, Monteiro CA, Lausch RN, Oakes JE. IL-8 gene expression in cultures of human corneal epithelial cells and keratocytes. *Invest Ophthalmol Vis Sci* 1993;34:3199–3206.
135. Elner VM, Strieter RM, Elner SG, Baggiolini M, Lindley I, Kunkel SL. Neutophil chemotatic factor (IL-8) gene expression by cytokine-treated retinal pigment epithelial cells. *Am J Pathol* 1990; 136:745–750.
136. Baggiolini M, Walz A, Kunkel SL. Neutophil-activating peptide-1/interleukin 8, a novel cytokine that activates neutrophils. *J Clin Invest* 1989;84:1045–1049.
137. Larsen CG, Anderson AO, Appella E, Oppenheim JJ, Matsushima K. The neutrophil-activating protein (NAP-1) is also chemotactic for T lymphocytes. *Science* 1989;243:1464–1466.
138. Matsushima K, Morishita K, Yoshimura T, et al. Molecular cloning of a human monocyte-derived neutrophil chemotactic factor (MDNCF) and the induction of MDNCF mRNA by interleukin 1 and tumor necrosis factor. *J Exp Med* 1988;167:1883–1893.
139. Huber AR, Kunkel SL, Todd RF III, Weiss SJ. Regulation of transendothelial neutrophil migration by endogenous interleukin-8. *Science* 1991;254:99–102.
140. Rot A. Endothelial cell binding of NAP-1/IL-8: role in neutrophil emigration. *Immunol Today* 1992;13:291–294.
141. Gimbrone MA Jr, Obin MS, Brock AD, et al. Endothelial interleukin-8: a novel inhibitor of leukocyte-endothelial interactions. *Science* 1989;246:1601–1603.
142. Ross R, Glomset J, Kariya B, Harker L. A platelet-dependent serum factor that stimulates the proliferation of arterial smooth muscle cells in vitro. *Proc Natl Acad Sci USA* 1974;71:1207–1210.
143. Westermark B, Heldin C-H. Platelet-derived growth factor. Structure, function and implications in normal and malignant cell growth. *Acta Oncol* 1993;32:101–105.
144. Benito M, Lorenzo M. Platelet derived growth factor/tyrosine kinase receptor mediated proliferation. *Growth Regul* 1993;3:172–179.
145. Matsui T, Heidaran M, Miki T, et al. Isolation of a novel receptor cDNA establishes the existence of two PDGF receptor genes. *Science* 1989;243:800–804.
146. LeRoith D, Roberts CT Jr. Insulin-like growth factors. *Ann NY Acad Sci* 1993;692:1–9.
147. Salmon WD Jr, Daughaday WH. A hormonally controlled serum factor which stimulates sulfate incorporation by cartilage in vitro. *J Lab Clin Med* 1957;49:825–836.
148. Roberts AB, Sporn MB. Physiological actions and clinical applications of transforming growth factor-B (TGF-B). *Growth Factors* 1993;8:1–9.
149. Jennings JC, Mohan S, Linkhart TA, Widstrom R, Baylink DJ. Comparison of the biological actions of TGF beta-1 and TGF beta-2: differential activity in endothelial cells. *J Cell Physiol* 1988;137:167–172.
150. Roberts AB, Sporn MB, Assoian RK, et al. Transforming growth factor type B: rapid induction of fibrosis and angiogenesis in vivo and stimulation of collagen formation in vitro. *Proc Natl Acad Sci USA* 1986;83:4167–4171.
151. Antonelli-Orlidge A, Saunders KB, Smith SR, D'Amore PA. An activated form of transforming growth factor B is produced by cocultures of endothelial cells and pericytes. *Proc Natl Acad Sci USA* 1989;86:4544–4548.
152. Smiddy WE, Glaser BM, Green R, et al. Transforming growth factor beta. A biologic chorioretinal glue. *Arch Ophthalmol* 1989; 107:577–580.
153. Sporn MB, Roberts AB, Shull JH, Smith JM, Ward JM. Polypeptide transforming growth factors isolated from bovine sources and used for wound healing in vivo. *Science* 1983;219:1329–1331.

154. Glaser BM, Michels RG, Kuppermann BD, Sjaarda RN, Pena RA. Transforming growth factor-B2 for the treatment of full-thickness macular holes. A prospective randomized study. *Ophthalmology* 1992;99:1162–1173.
155. Shah M, Foreman DM, Ferguson MWJ. Control of scarring in adult wounds by neutralising antibody to transforming frowth factor B. *Lancet* 1992;339:213–214.
156. Connor TB, Roberts AB, Sporn MB, et al. Correlation of fibrosis and transforming growth factor-B type 2 levels in the eye. *J Clin Invest* 1989;83:1661–1666.
157. Caruelle D, Groux MB, Gaudric A, et al. Immunological study of acidic fibroblast growth factor (aFGF) distribution in the eye. *J Cell Biochem* 1989;39:117–128.
158. D'Amore PA, Klagsbrun M. Endothelial mitogens derived from retina and hypothalamus: biological and biochemical similarities. *J Cell Biol* 1984;99:1545–1549.
159. Gao H, Hollyfield JG. Basic fibroblast growth factor (bFGF) immunolocalization in the rodent outer retina demonstrated with an anti-rodent bFGF antibody. *Brain Res* 1992;585:355–360.
160. Ku P-T, D'Amore PA. Regulation of bFGF in endothelial cells following injury-induced bFGF release. *J Cell Biochem* 1995;58:328–343.
161. Nyberg F, Hahnenberger R, Jakobson AM, Terenius L. Enhancement of FGF-like polypeptides in the retinae of newborn mice exposed to hyperoxia. *FEBS Lett* 1990;267:75–77.
162. Zhang NL, Samadani EE, Frank RN. Mitogenesis and retinal pigment epithelial cell antigen expression in the rat after krypton laser photocoagulation. *Invest Ophthalmol Vis Sci* 1993;34:2412–2424.
163. McGookin E, Stopa E, Kuo-LeBlanc A, et al. Vascular endothelial growth factor (VEGF) has a different distribution than basic fibroblast growth factor (bFGF) in the adult human retina. *Invest Ophthal Vis Sci* 1992;33:651.
164. Miller JW, Adamis AP, Shima D, et al. Vascular endothelial growth factor/vascular permeability factor is temporally and spatially correlated with ocular angiogenesis in a primate model. *Am J Pathol* 1994;145:574–584.
165. Yeo K-T, Sioussat TM, Faix JD, Senger DR, Yeo T-K. Development of time-resolved immunofluorometric assay of vascular permeability factor. *Clin Chem* 1992;38:71–75.
166. Yeo K-T, Wang HH, Nagy JA, et al. Vascular permeability factor (vascular endothelial growth factor) in guinea pig and human tumor and inflammatory effusions. *Cancer Res* 1993;53:2912–2918.
167. Shima D, Gougos A, Miller J, et al. Cloning and mRNA expression of VEGF in ischemic retinas of *Macaca fascularis. Invest Ophthal Vis Sci* 1996;37:1334–1340.
168. Pierce EA, Avery R, Foley E, Aiello L, Smith LEH. Vascular endothelial growth factor/vascular permeability factor expression in a mouse model of retinal neovascularization. *Proc Natl Acad Sci USA* 1995;92:905–909.
169. Dorey CK, Aouididi S, Reynaud X, Dvorak HF, Brown LB. Correlation of vascular permeability factor/vascular endothelial growth factor with extraretinal neovascularization in the rat. *Arch Ophthalmol* 1996;114:1210–1217.
170. Adamis A. Vascular endothelial growth factor is sufficient to produce iris neovascularization and neovascular glaucoma in a nonhuman primate. *Arch Ophthalmol* 1996;(suppl):S402.
171. Adamis A, Shima D, Tolentino M, et al. Inhibition of VEGF prevent ocular neovascularization in a non-human primate. *Arch Ophthalmol* 1996;114:66–71.
172. Park J, Chen H, Winer J, Houck K, Ferrara N. Placenta growth factor. Potentiation of vascular endothelial growth factor bioactivity in vitro and in vivo, and high affinity binding to Flt-1 but not to flk-1/KDR. *J Biol Chem* 1994;269:25646–25654.
173. Aiello L, Pierce E, Foley E, et al. Inhibition of vascular endothelial growth factor suppresses retinal neovascularization in vivo. *Proc Natl Acad Sci USA* 1995;92:10457–10461.
174. Adamis AP, Miller JW, Bernal MT, D'Amico DJ, Folkman J, Yeo,T-K. Elevated vascular permeability factor/vascular endothelial growth factor levels in the vitreous of eyes with proliferative diabetic retinopathy. *Am J Ophthalmol* 1994;118:445–450.
175. Aiello L, Avery R, Arrigg P, et al. Vascular endothelial growth factor in ocular fluid of patients with diabetic retinopathy and other retinal disorders. *N Engl J Med* 1994;331:1480–1487.
176. Malecaze F, Clamens S, Simorre-Pinatel V, et al. Detection of vascular endothelial growth factor messenger RNA and vascular endothelial growth factor-like activity in proliferative diabetic retinopathy. *Arch Ophthalmol* 1994;112:1476–1482.
177. Pe'er J, Shweiki D, Itin A, Hemo I, Gnessin H, E K. Hypoxia-induced expression of vascular endothelial growth factor by retinal cells is a common factor in neovascularization ocular diseases. *Lab Invest* 1995;72:638–645.
178. Poulsen JE. The Houssay phenomenon in man. Recovery from retinopathy in a case of diabetes with Simmonds' disease. *Diabetes* 1953;2:7–12.
179. Luft R, Olivecrona H, Ikkos D, Kornerup T, Ljunggren H. Hypophysectomy in man: further experiences in severe diabetes mellitus. *Br Med J* 1955;2.
180. Sharp P, Fallon T, Brazier O, Sandler L, Joplin G, Kohner E. Long-term follow-up of patients who underwent Yttrium-90 pituitary implantation for treatment of proliferative diabetic retinopathy. *Diabetologia* 1987;30:199–207.
181. Merimee T. A follow-up study of vascular disease in growth-hormone-deficient dwarfs with diabetes. *N Engl J Med* 1978;298:1217–1222.
182. Poulsen J. Diabetes and anterior pituitary insufficiency. Final course and postmortem study of a diabetic patient with Sheehan's syndrome. *Diabetes* 1966;15:73–77.
183. Schultz GS, Grant MB. Neovascular growth factors. *Eye* 1991;5: 170–180.
184. Grant M, Jerdan J, Merimee TJ. Insulin-like growth factor-I modulates endothelial cell chemotaxis. *J Clin Endocrinol Metab* 1987; 65:370–371.
185. Grant MB, Guay C, Marsh R. Insulin-like growth factor I stimulates proliferation, migration and plasminogen activator release by human retinal pigment epithelial cells. *Curr Eye Res* 1990;9:323–335.
186. Grant MB, Guay C. Plasminogen activator production by human retinal endothelial cells of nondiabetic and diabetic origin. *Invest Ophthalmol Vis Sci* 1991;32:53–64.
187. Grant MB, Mames RN, Fitgerald C, et al. Insulin-like growth factor I as an angiogenic agent. In vivo and in vitro studies. *Ann NY Acad Sci* 1993;692:230–242.
188. Grant M, Russell B, Fitgerald C, Merimee TJ. Insulin-like growth factors in vitreous. Studies in control and diabetic subjects with neovascularization. *Diabetes* 1986;35:416–420.
189. Dills DG, Moss SE, Klein R, Klein BEK. Association of elevated IGF-1 levels with increased retinopathy in late-onset diabetes. *Diabetes* 1991;40:1725–1730.
190. Dameron KM, Volpert OV, Tainsky MA, Bouck N. Control of angiogenesis in fibroblasts by p53 regulation of thrombospondin-1. *Science* 1994;265:1582–1585.
191. Schroder A, Palinski W, Schmid-Schonbein G. Activated monocytes and granulocytes, capillary nonperfusion, and neovascularization in diabetic retinopathy. *Am J Pathol* 1991;139:81–100.

SECTION IV

Cornea and External Diseases

Section Editors: George R. John and Herbert E. Kaufman

OVERVIEW

Ocular therapeutics has a long and colorful history, one which parallels the changing beliefs in pathophysiology of diseases. Many of the early reports linked therapy to religious beliefs about the eye and/or substances used in the eye. As described in Duke-Elder's *System of Ophthalmology,* the Assyrians, Egyptians, and Hindus, at different times, used pastes and powders consisting of plant and animal parts which were applied to the eye. The Romans used a "collyrium" consisting of several different agents incorporated in a gum, forming a cake-like substance which was broken down and dissolved for use in the eye. The rituals and sorcery associated with early therapeutics gave way to experimentation in the fifteenth to seventeenth centuries. Concepts of humoral imbalances were replaced by a more active participation of the physician in the patient's care and, as a result, increased surgical intervention. Progress in surgery has also altered ocular therapeutics, separating and defining what can be managed medically from what can be surgically corrected. An increased understanding of disease processes was the key to development of ocular therapies. There is an inverse correlation between the understanding of a disease process and the variety of treatments available for that condition. By the eighteenth century, drugs aimed at specific disease processes, such as silver nitrate, belladonna, and physostigmine, were used routinely. Current concepts of topical drug delivery took root in the nineteenth century, with drops and ointments playing the major role in ocular therapy.

The treatment of corneal and anterior segment diseases relies almost exclusively on topical therapy, with the cornea being the primary penetration site and the main limiting barrier. This membrane, which is anatomically divided into five layers, has been simplified for pharmacokinetic purposes into a three-layered sandwich consisting of the hydrophilic stroma between the lipid-rich epithelium and the endothelium. Ideal topical agents are weak bases capable of transforming between ionized and nonionized forms, which then either passively diffuse or are actively transported across this barrier.

Therapy of cornea and anterior segment diseases is unique in several respects. First, its accessibility, as with other mucous membranes, allows delivery of drugs to various tissues in the eye without requiring a large quantity of drug. This factor has essentially eliminated the need for oral administration of agents, with their associated side effects and higher costs. Only about 1% to 2% of each topically delivered drug actually penetrates into the anterior chamber and intraocular tissues. Second, because of the visibility of the compartments, more rapid assessment of therapeutic efficacy and toxicity is possible. Adjustments in dosing can thus be made without prolonging unnecessary therapy. Third, the avascularity of the cornea allows penetration of drugs without their encountering vascular compartments. Conjunctival and episcleral vessels and the choroid are major restrictions to scleral penetration.

Of major physiologic importance in drug access and the overall health of the cornea is the tear film, including its secretion, turnover, production, and excretion. Associated with topical therapy is the lack of consistency in therapeutic levels delivered to the anterior segment due to variables such as the blink rate, the volume of the tear compartment, induced reflex tearing, and rate of elimination. Inadequacy of quantity and quality of tear film can result in breakdown of the corneal epithelium, with defects in this hydrophobic epithelium altering the penetration of certain agents.

Despite the many advantages of topical therapy, therapeutic options for the anterior segment rely heavily on two drug categories: antiinfective and antiinflammatory. Steroids and antibiotic agents are used for a wide variety of disease processes. In most conditions, such as conjunctivitis and uveitis, the therapy is not specifically aimed at the underlying etiologic process. Recently, interest in tailoring therapy to selective biochemical processes has grown and has led to the use of drugs such as antimitotics, growth factors, metalloproteinase inhibitors, and mast cell stabilizers.

The chapters in this section on the pharmacology of the cornea and anterior segment deal with all current clinically used, Food and Drug Administration (FDA)-approved pharmacologic agents in the treatment of diseases of the cornea, conjunctiva, and lids. A few select agents that are widely clinically used or are undergoing clinical trials but do not have FDA approval as of this writing are also discussed. Although topical agents are the mainstay of anterior segment therapy, the systemic preparations that may have anterior segment therapeutic applications will also be addressed. Therapy for uveitis, including all steroid preparations, is discussed in the Uveitis section and intravenous antibiotic preparations used for treatment of endophthalmitis are discussed in the Retina section. The section on diagnostic drugs is presented separately and includes all agents except vital tissue dyes, which are included in this section.

In addition to all of these topics, we discuss the pharmacology of all agents used during cataract surgery, such as irrigating solutions and viscoelastics. All material in the chapters on the pharmacology of the cornea and anterior segment is intended to serve as a reference on specific drugs—their history, pharmacology, indications, and toxicity—and not as a review of pathologic disease processes.

The future of anterior segment therapy may include gains in therapeutic efficacy with prodrugs, soft drugs, and improved drug delivery. Prodrugs and soft drugs allow less drug to be delivered and, as a result, fewer side effects. As variables in drug delivery such as systemic vascular absorption and drug excretion are better controlled, consistency and predictability may be achieved in anterior segment therapy. Methods of delivery such as iontophoresis are discussed widely in the literature but fail to achieve the combined ease and efficacy of topical therapy. Improvements in preservatives, drug preparations, and drug-delivery vehicles can also be anticipated. The future of topical drug delivery may include the use of agents to treat systemic conditions. We know that β-blockers can cause systemic side effects through their absorption by mucous membranes. If significant absorption can be achieved, systemic therapy for conditions outside the anterior segment may be considered.

Textbook of Ocular Pharmacology,
edited by T.J. Zimmerman, et al.
Lippincott–Raven Publishers, Philadelphia © 1997.

CHAPTER 40

Penicillins and Cephalosporins

Adam H. Kaufman and Jules Baum

While working with staphylococcus variants, a number of culture-plates were set aside on the laboratory bench and examined from time to time. In examinations, these plates were necessarily exposed to the air and they became contaminated with various micro-organisms. It was noticed that around a large colony of a contaminating mold the staphylococcus colonies became transparent and were obviously undergoing lysis.

Alexander Fleming, F.R.C.S., 1929

In 1929, Sir Alexander Fleming introduced the world to the antibiotic action of penicillin with these words in his historic paper (1). Fleming documented penicillin's efficacy against Staphylococcus, hemolytic Streptococcus, Pneumococcus, Gonococcus, and *Bacillus diphtheriae,* and demonstrated its ineffectiveness against *Escherichia coli* and *B. influenzae.* Remarkably, to this day, penicillin remains a highly used mode of treatment for the same susceptible bacterial species, and along with its close and distant synthetic relatives, penicillin continues to be an important therapeutic agent in multiple ophthalmic infectious diseases. The penicillins and the more recently developed cephalosporins may be formulated for topical use from parenteral products. They have never been available as a commercially prepared eye drop or ointment because of their relative instability. In this chapter, we describe the ocular pharmacology of the major penicillins and cephalosporins and provide therapeutic guidelines for common uses in cornea and external disease.

A. H. Kaufman: Department of Ophthalmology, University of Cincinnati College of Medicine, Cincinnati, Ohio 45219.

J. Baum: Department of Ophthalmology, Tufts University School of Medicine, Boston, MA, and Boston Eye Associates, Chestnut Hill, Massachusetts.

PENICILLIN G

History and Source

Penicillin was introduced into clinical medicine by Florey, et al. in 1941 (2). It was initially produced as an extract from cultured *Penicillium notatum,* which contained a mixture of penicillins (designated F, G, X, and K); it also contained impurities. Penicillin G (benzyl-penicillin) was the most satisfactory of the four for clinical use, and although it is now produced in a purified form, its dosage is still frequently described in units rather than milligrams.

As shown in Fig. 1, the essential structure of a penicillin consists of a thiazolidine ring that is connected to a β-lactam ring. Penicillin G has a benzyl group for a side chain; it is an unstable acid and is produced for clinical use in the more stable salt forms. Sodium penicillin G and potassium penicillin G are often termed "crystalline penicillin G," although all forms of penicillin currently made are pure and crystalline. Sodium penicillin G and potassium penicillin G are both highly soluble in water. Potassium penicillin G is preferred to sodium penicillin G. Procaine penicillin G and benzathine penicillin G are less soluble salts that are used for intramuscular injections as long-acting depot forms. Benzathine penicillin G is more slowly absorbed from an intramuscular injection and its serum level is more

Names and Chemistry

Penicillin G potassium tablets	(multiple manufacturers)	Oral
Penicillin G potassium powder	(Pfizerpen: Roerig)	IV, topical, subconjunctival
	(generic: Apothecon)	IV, topical, subconjunctival
	(generic: Lilly)	IV, topical, subconjunctival
Penicillin G sodium powder	(generic: Apothecon)	IV
Penicillin G potassium (frozen)	(generic: Galaxy)	IV
	(generic: Baxter)	IV
Penicillin G procaine	(Pfizerpen-AS: Roerig)	IM
	(Wycillin: Wyeth)	IM
	(Wycillin: Elkins-Sinn)	IM
Penicillin G benzathine	(Bicillin-LA: Wyeth)	IM
	(Bicillin-LA: Elkins-Sinn)	IM
Penicillin G benzathine/procaine	(Bicillin-C-R: Wyeth)	IM
	(Bicillin-C-R: Elkins-Sinn)	IM

prolonged than that of procaine penicillin G. Probenicid (Benemid), which may be administered orally in combination with intramuscular procaine penicillin G, inhibits tubular excretion of penicillin and thus increases serum level of procaine penicillin G. Probenicid also acts directly on the retina and ciliary pump to sustain intraocular penicillin concentration.

Pharmacology

Penicillin inhibits the biosynthesis of mucopeptides in the bacterial cell wall and has a bactericidal effect while organisms are dividing. The exact mechanisms of action remain incompletely elucidated since multiple cell membrane components bind to penicillin, although an integral penicillin G-sensitive transpeptidase may be essential for cell wall stability (3). Cell death subsequent to exposure to penicillin may require endogenous peptidoglycan hydrolases (autolysins), and lack of these enzymes may lead to antibiotic tolerance (4).

Clinical Pharmacology and Spectrum of Activity

Penicillin G remains effective against many gram-positive organisms, although resistance to *Staphylococcus aureus* and *S. epidermidis* is common (5). Penicillin G remains useful for the treatment of *S. pyogenes* (group A β-hemolytic streptococcus), Groups C, G, and F β-hemolytic streptococcus, *S. viridans* (α-hemolytic streptococcus), anaerobic gram-positive cocci (Peptococcus, Peptostreptococcus, and anaerobic streptococci), gram-positive bacilli (*Corynebacterium diphtheriae, Bacillus anthracis,* some Listeria strains, Clostridium species, Actinomyces, and Propionibacterium), and gram-negative cocci (*Neisseria meningitidis* and *N. gonorrhoeae*). Penicillin G is usually the agent of choice in spirochetal infections such as syphilis (*Treponema pallidum*), Lyme disease (*Borrelia burgdorferi*), pinta (*T. carateum*), and yaws (*T. pertenue*) (5). Sensitivity testing is usually indicated. Other entities such as erysipeloid (*Erysipelothrix rhusiopathie*), Fuscobacterium infections (e.g., *Leptotrichia buccalis*) and rat-bite fever (*Streptobacillus moniliformis* or *Spirillum minus*) may also be treated with penicillin G.

Pharmaceutics

1. Topical: 100,000–333,000 Units/ml
   a. Pediatric (for neonatal gonococcal conjunctivitis) 10,000 to 20,000 U
2. Subconjunctival: 0.5–1.0 million U
3. Intravitreal: 2,000 U and Probenecid 0.5 g orally four times daily (p.o. q.i.d.), possible retinal toxicity (discussed in Pharmacokinetics section)
4. Oral: 400,000 U q.i.d. Rarely used. Poorly absorbed from stomach. See section on Penicillin V.
5. IV: Two to 6 million Units every 4 hours (and Probenecid 0.5 g p.o. q.i.d.)
   a. Pediatric (for neonatal gonococcal conjunctivitis) 50,000 U/kg/day in two to three doses
6. IM: Variation per preparation

Pharmacokinetics

Topical application of penicillin G leads to high concentrations on the corneal surface but yields only low aqueous levels (6). Topical application of penicillin G may be curative in treating keratitis caused by sensitive organisms, but its use in intraocular infections is only adjunctive. Subconjunctival injection of penicillin G may result in therapeutic levels in the cornea and aqueous but in subtherapeutic levels in the vitreous (7–9). It is difficult to achieve high levels in the vitreous after topical, periocular, or intravenous administration (7–11). Intravitreal injection of penicillin is possible, but a half-life ($t_{\frac{1}{2}}$) of about 3 hours results in a rapidly diminishing concentration (12). Retinal toxicity may occur at low concentrations such as 5,000 U and there

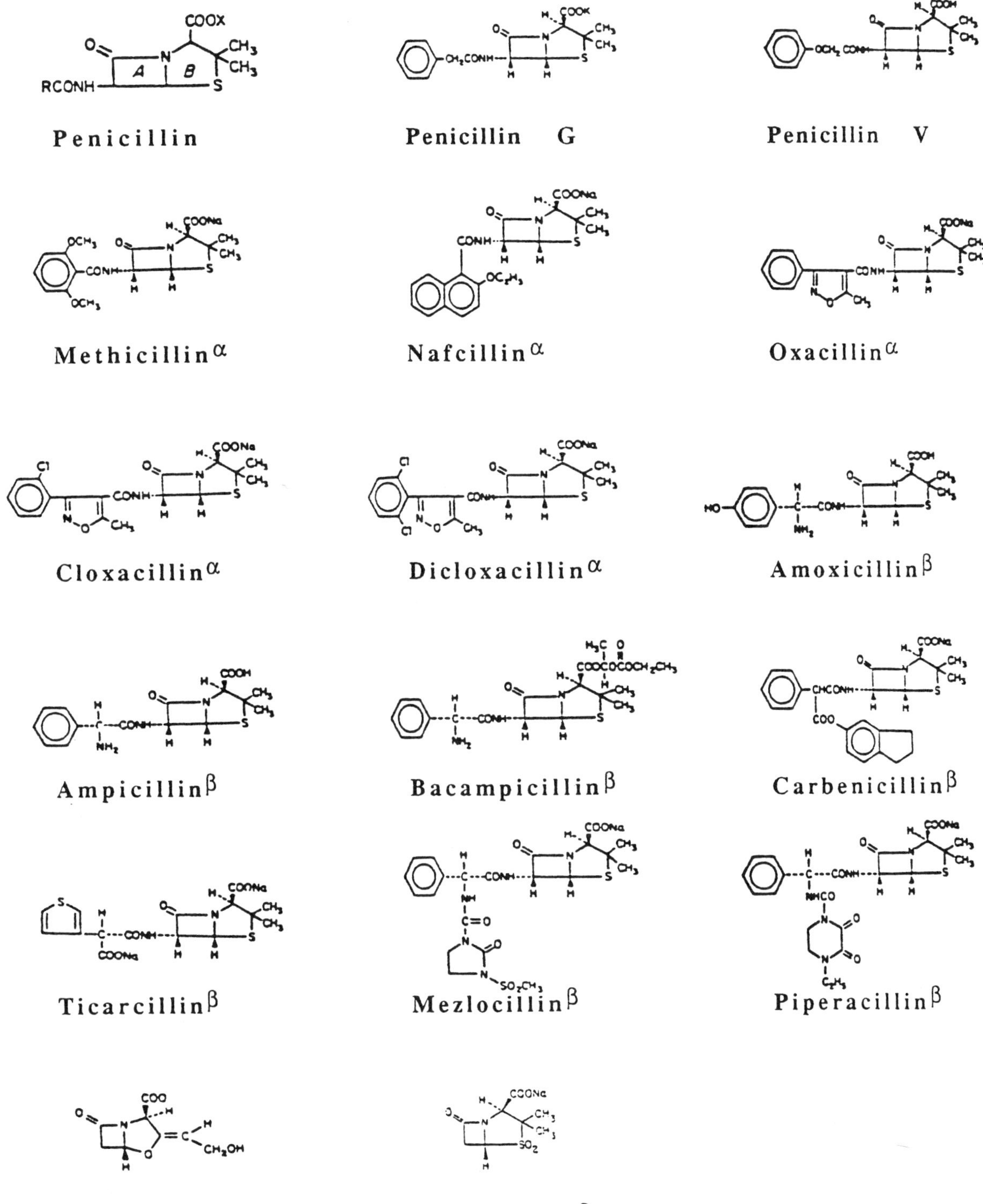

FIG. 40-1. A: β-lactam ring. **B:** Thiazolidine ring. *α:* Penicillinase-resistant penicillin. *β:* Extended-spectrum penicillin. *χ:* β-lactamase inhibitor, combined with amoxicillin and ticarcillin. *δ:* β-lactamase inhibitor, combined with ampicillin.

is currently no standard accepted dose for intravitreal penicillin. Penicillins are rarely administered intravitreally; antibiotic combinations such as vancomycin plus amikacin or ceftazidime are preferred. The Retina section further discusses usage of intravitreal penicillins.

Intravenous penicillin G penetrates well into subcutaneous tissue, joints, and well-vascularized tissue. Intraocular penetration is limited by the blood–ocular barriers, but inflammation may increase bioavailability of penicillins. Although penicillin G may be administered orally, it is unstable at low pH and only a third of the dose is absorbed under favorable conditions (13).

Plasma penicillin G is predominantly eliminated by the kidney, with most excreted by tubular secretion and only about 10% excreted through glomerular filtration. Six hours after an injection of penicillin G, more than 70% of the drug has been excreted into the urine (5). Probenecid is used to block renal tubular secretion and can result in significant increase in plasma penicillin levels. Probenicid also has a direct effect on the retina and ciliary body and aids in the retention of penicillin in the eye by blocking the pump that excretes intraocular antibiotic agent (11,14,15). A small percentage of penicillin is eliminated into the bile; the balance is emanated by the liver.

Ophthalmic Therapeutic Uses (Examples)

Bacterial Keratitis

Primary treatment is topical, although adjunctive treatment with subconjunctival injection is possible. Although treatment is usually initiated empirically with cefazolin, plus gentamicin or tobramycin, therapy may be changed to penicillin G after the pathogen and its sensitivity pattern are identified and a deteriorating clinical course is apparent (16).

Gonococcal Conjunctivitis

Although penicillin has been used in the past, the Center for Disease Control (CDC) currently recommends ceftriaxone for the treatment of adult or neonatal gonococcal conjunctivitis (see Cephalosporin section) (17). If gonococcal keratitis ensues, topical fortified penicillin (or ceftazidime) drops may be used; if no corneal ulceration exists, irrigation with saline drops is recommended.

Canaliculitis

If actinomyces infection is documented from material regurgitated from the punctum, penicillin G may be irrigated through the lacrimal outflow system several times weekly for several weeks. Infection may be recalcitrant and difficult to treat if there is obstruction to outflow. Adjunctive oral penicillin may be considered (discussed in section on penicillin V).

Lyme Disease

Ophthalmologists may encounter cases of Lyme disease with ocular inflammation such as conjunctivitis, keratitis, uveitis, or sixth nerve palsy. Although therapeutic regimens abound, two suggested treatment regimens for stage II or III lyme disease with significant ocular manifestations are IV ceftriaxone 2 g daily for 21 days or IV penicillin G 3 to 4 million Units every 4 hours. When corneal involvement exists, typically a nummular keratitis, the addition of topical steroid therapy alone may be curative.

Syphilitic Eye Disease

Because syphilitic eye disease (e.g., uveitis, neuroretinitis, optic neuritis) is often associated with neurosyphilis, patients with such conditions should be treated according to neurosyphilis guidelines (17). In all patients with syphilitic eye disease, cerebrospinal fluid (CSF) should be evaluated (17). The CDC continues to recommend penicillin G for treatment of neurosyphilis (17). No clinical data to date assure the efficacy of treatment other than with penicillin G. Three to 4 million U penicillin G is administered IV every 4 hours for 10 to 14 days. An alternative regimen is procaine penicillin G IM 2.4 million U daily plus probenicid 500 mg p.o. q.i.d. for 10 to 14 days. If the patient is allergic to penicillin, desensitization may be performed.

Side Effects and Toxicity

Hypersensitivity reactions are common with penicillin treatment; however, anaphylactic reactions are quite rare. Two to 4% of persons have dermatologic reactions such as urticaria or a maculopapular rash (18,19). Fever, chills, and eosinophilia may occur. Serum sickness may occur in as many as 2% of patients treated with penicillin G (18,19). Symptoms of serum sickness include fever, malaise, urticaria, joint pains, and lymphadenopathy. Rarely, Stevens-Johnson syndrome may occur. Contact dermatitis may occur from topical penicillin, possibly with local reaction around an injection site. Inadvertent IV injection of procaine penicillin G may result in severe reactions and even death. Jarisch-Herxheimer reaction is an acute febrile reaction that may occur in the first 24 hours of penicillin treatment in a patient with early syphilis. Nephropathy and hemolytic anemia occur in a few patients. Four to 10% of patients with hypersensitivity reactions to penicillin will also have hypersensitivity reactions to cephalosporins (19).

Type I hypersensitivity testing may be performed if alternative antibiotic therapy is not indicated (as in tertiary

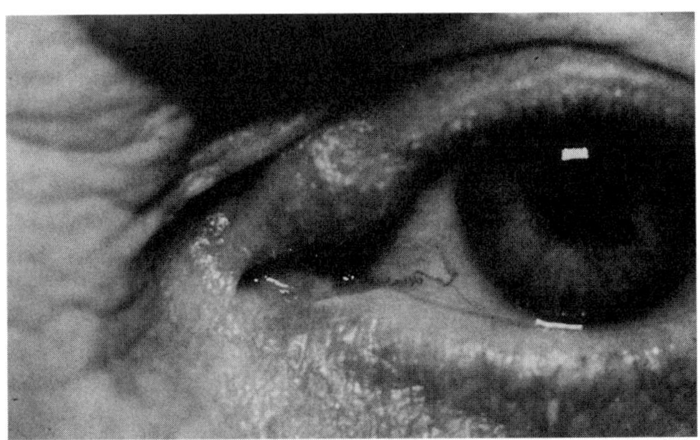
A

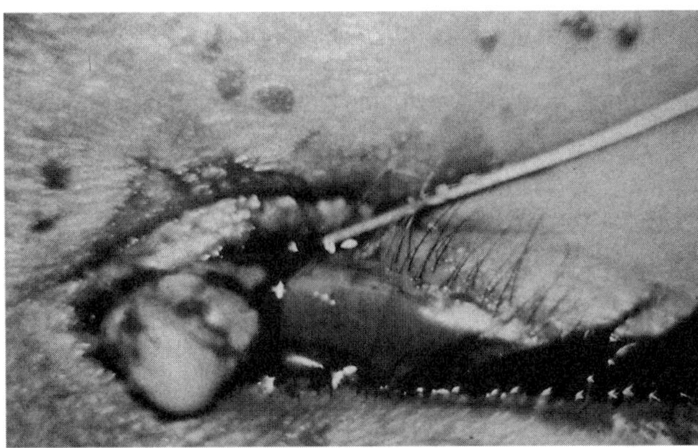
B

FIG. 40-2. Chronic actinomyces canaliculitis. (Photographs courtesy of Robert Kersten, M.D.)

syphilis) and penicillin allergy is suspected. Only 10% of patients who report a history of severe allergy to penicillin are still allergic when tested (17). Penicillin degradation products known as the "major" and "minor" antigenic determinants are used first in epicutaneous tests (scratch test) and then as intradermal tests to assess hypersensitivity. The major antigenic determinant is the penicilloyl derivative, formed by breaking of the β-lactam ring; the penicilloyl derivative is conjugated with polymerized lysine for safety reasons and is commercially available as penicilloyl-polylysine (PPL) 6×10^{-5} (Pre-Pen, Schwarz Pharmaceutical) (18). The minor antigenic determinants (MDM) consist of penicilloic acid, penilloic acid, and penicillin G. Unfortunately, a commercial preparation of MDM is currently unavailable. Penicillin G 6,000 U/ml alone may be substituted for an MDM preparation to help identify patients requiring desensitization (17). Some patients with skin testing negative to PPL and penicillin G are found to be allergic when treated with penicillin G (3% to 10%); if therapy is initiated in such patients, it should begin with oral test doses in a monitored setting to allow for possible anaphylactic reaction (17).

High-risk Groups

Animal studies have not shown evidence of teratogenic effects, and extensive use of penicillin G has not yielded reports of teratogenic effects in humans (18,19). However, because no controlled studies have been made in humans, use in pregnancy should be limited to cases in which there is clear need. Long-term studies on carcinogenesis, mutagenesis, or impairment of fertility caused by penicillin are lacking (18,19).

Drug Interactions

Because penicillin works most effectively on dividing bacteria, coadministration of a bacteriostatic agent may diminish the bactericidal effects of penicillin. Although aminoglycosides and penicillins may act synergistically, preparing these agents in the same bottle may lead to their inactivation. Aspirin and nonsteroidal antiinflammatory agents are highly protein bound and may compete with penicillins for available binding sites; prolonged serum $t_{\frac{1}{2}}$ may result. Probenicid prolongs blood levels by blocking renal tubule secretion of penicillin G (see Pharmacokinetics section).

PENICILLIN V

History and Source

Penicillin V is phenoxymethylpenicillin and was introduced in the early 1950s. It is a natural penicillin produced biosynthetically by the addition of phenoxyacetic acid to the fermentation medium.

Names and Chemistry

Penicillin V potassium (multiple manufacturers) is an *oral* preparation (tablets/solution). The structure of penicillin V is shown in Fig. 1.

Pharmacology and Spectrum of Activity

The range of antimicrobial activity of penicillin V is similar to that of penicillin G. Penicillin G is about four times more active against meningococci, gonococci, and *Hemophilus influenzae* (5).

Pharmaceutics

Recommended pharmaceutics is administration of penicillin V 250–500 mg p.o. q.i.d.; Pediatric pharmaceutics consists of 15–62.5 mg/kg/day administered in three to six divided doses.

Pharmacokinetics

Penicillin V is more stable in gastric acid and is thus the form preferred for oral therapy. Penicillin V is well absorbed, with good blood levels achieved 1 hour after ingestion of an oral dose. After its absorption from the intestine, the pharmacokinetics of penicillin V is similar to that of penicillin G.

Ophthalmic Therapeutic Uses (Examples)

Preseptal Cellulitis

Mild to moderate cellulitis and impetigo considered due to streptococcus species may be treated with penicillin V. Broader coverage can be achieved with an extended-spectrum penicillin with a β-lactamase inhibitor or with a second-generation cephalosporin.

Infected Cutaneous Laceration

An infected laceration with sensitive organisms identified may be treated with penicillin V. An oral first-generation cephalosporin such as cephalexin may be preferred as an initial treatment choice due to its superior coverage against staphylococcal species.

Chronic Actinomyces Canaliculitis

Use of adjunctive oral penicillin V may be considered in combination with intracanalicular penicillin G for chronic actinomyces canaliculitis.

Side Effects and Toxicity

Hypersensitivities, adverse effects (AE), and toxicity of penicillin V are similar to those of penicillin G.

High-risk Groups

As with penicillin G, there have been no controlled studies in humans with regard to use of penicillin V in pregnancy. Its use should be limited to cases in which it is clearly needed. Similarly, there have been no long-term studies of carcinogenesis, mutagenesis, or the impairment of fertility due to penicillin V (18,19).

Drug Interactions

Drug interactions occurring with penicillin V are the same as those occurring with penicillin G. Concomitant use of penicillin V and oral contraceptives may reduce efficacy of the contraceptive and increase the incidence of breakthrough bleeding.

PENICILLINASE-RESISTANT PENICILLINS

History and Source

Penicillinase-resistant penicillins are a group of semisynthetic agents that are resistant to hydrolysis by staphylococcal penicillinase (β-lactamase) and are often the first choice of drugs used to treat staphylococcal disease. They were developed in the early 1960s and, with the exception of methicillin (which is highly nephrotoxic), are still widely used (20–22). In general, these agents are less effective than penicillin G against nonstaphyloccal strains such as streptococcal and Neisseria species. In the last several years, the incidence of *S. aureus* and *S. epidermidis* resistance to this group of agents has increased (i.e., "methicillin" resistance: MRSA or MRSE) in nonsocomial infections. The first line of treatment for MRSA and MRSE infections is usually vancomycin.

Names and Chemistries

Methicillin	(Staphcillin, Apothecon)	IV
Nafcillin	(Multiple manufacturers)	IV (and oral)
Oxacillin	(Multiple manufacturers)	IV, oral
Cloxacillin	(Multiple manufacturers)	Oral
Dicloxacillin	(Multiple manufacturers)	Oral

The structures for the pencillinase-resistant penicillins are shown in Fig. 1. These semisynthetic penicillin derivatives are produced by acylation of 6-aminopenicillanic acid. Bulky side chains on the penicillin nucleus cause steric hindrance that helps prevent attachment of staphylococcal penicillinases to the β-lactam ring. Oxacillin, cloxacillin, and dicloxacillin are isoxazolyl penicillins that have heterocyclic side chains and greater stability in gastric acid. Oxacillin, cloxacillin, and dicloxacillin differ only in the number of chlorine atoms (0, 1, and 2, respectively). In general, addition of chlorine atoms increases in vitro antibacterial activity, gastrointestinal (GI) absorption, protein binding, and serum $t_{\frac{1}{2}}$. All penicillinase-resistant penicillins are available as sodium salts.

Pharmacology

The mechanism of action of penicillinase-resistant penicillins is similar to that of other penicillins.

Clinical Pharmacology and Spectrum of Activity

In general, the penicillinase-resistant penicillins are active against gram-positive cocci such as *S. aureus, S. epidermidis,*

S. pyogenes, S. pneumoniae, and *S. viridans.* These penicillins are active against some gram-positive aerobic and anaerobic bacilli but are inactive against gram-negative aerobic and anaerobic bacilli. These agents also are inactive against mycobacteria, spirochetes, mycoplasma, and rickettsia.

Pharmaceutics

1. Topical	Methicillin (50 mg/ml)
	Oxacillin (66 mg/ml)
2. Subconjunctival	Methicillin (75–100 mg)
	Oxacillin (75–100 mg)
3. Intravitreal	Methicillin (2 mg) + probenicid 0.5 g p.o. q.i.d.)
	Oxacillin (500 μg)
4. Oral	Oxacillin (500–1,000 mg q4–6h)
	Cloxacillin (250–500 mg q6h)
	Dicloxacillin (125–250 mg q6h)
5. IV	Methicillin (1,000 mg q6h)
	Nafcillin (500–1,000 mg q4h)
	Oxacillin (500 mg q6h)

Pharmacokinetics

Topical application of methicillin or oxacillin will lead to high concentrations on the corneal surface but only low aqueous levels (23,24). As with other penicillins, topical application of penicillinase-resistant penicillins may effectively treat sensitive organisms causing keratitis. However, their topical use is limited in intraocular infection due to the poor penetration of the drug into the aqueous humor. Multiple studies have documented effective inhibitory concentrations in the aqueous after subconjunctival administration of methicillin or oxacillin (24–27). Although vitreal penetration is generally poor after subconjunctival administration, inflamed eyes may achieve more significant vitreous levels of methicillin and oxacillin (28,29). Intravitreal injection of methicillin or oxacillin is possible but, as with penicillin G, their short $t_{\frac{1}{2}}$ and spectrum of activity limit their intravitreal use (30,31). Probenicid may be used to enhance the $t_{\frac{1}{2}}$ (32). Use of intravitreal antibiotic agents is discussed further in the Retina section.

Similar to other penicillins, orally administered penicillinase-resistant penicillins are absorbed in the duodenum and upper jejunum; extent of absorption depends on gastric acid stability and presence of food. Because methicillin is very susceptible to acid inactivation and nafcillin is poorly absorbed from the GI tract, neither drug is generally administered orally. After oral administration of oxacillin, cloxacillin, and dicloxacillin, 30% to 75% of the dose is absorbed, and a peak serum concentration is reached between 30 minutes and 2 hours (19). As do other penicillins, systemically administered penicillinase-resistant penicillins penetrate well into vascularized tissue but penetrate poorly into CSF and into the eye. Penetration into aqueous after intravenous or intramuscular administration has been extensively studied for this group of agents and has consistently shown to be poor (24–28,33,34). Methicillin, oxacillin, cloxacillin, and dicloxacillin are predominantly eliminated by the kidney and their serum $t_{\frac{1}{2}}$ is prolonged by probenicid. Nafcillin, on the other hand, is largely metabolized in the liver and is mainly eliminated by bile and the enterohepatic circulation.

Ocular Therapeutic Uses (Examples)

Bacterial Keratitis

Treatment of bacterial keratitis is usually initiated topically with cefazolin, plus gentamicin or tobramicin; therapy may be changed to methicillin or oxacillin after the pathogen and its sensitivity pattern are identified and a deteriorating clinical course becomes apparent.

Preseptal Cellulitis

Mild to moderate cellulitis and impetigo that is believed to be due to sensitive staphylococcal or streptococcal species may be treated with the penicillinase-resistant penicillins. Broader coverage can be obtained with an extended-spectrum penicillin combined with a β-lactamase inhibitor or a second-generation cephalosporin. Although discussion of the treatment of orbital cellulitis is beyond the scope of this chapter, initial treatment may include nafcillin plus chloramphenicol (if anaerobic or *H. influenza* infection is suspected).

Side Effects and Toxicity

In general, the penicillinase-resistant penicillins share the side effects, toxicity, and hypersensitivity potential of other penicillins. Acute interstitial nephritis occurs with a significant incidence with methicillin treatment and this toxicity has led to a decrease in its systemic use. An increased incidence of hepatotoxicity has been reported to occur with intravenously administered oxacillin.

High-risk Groups

The high-risk groups for the penicillinase-resistant penicillins are the same as those for penicillin G.

Drug Interactions

Drug interactions with the penicillinase-resistant penicillins are the same as those that occur with penicillin G.

EXTENDED-SPECTRUM PENICILLINS

History and Source

Agents in the group of extended-spectrum penicillins are penicillinase-sensitive penicillins, all of which have a broad gram-positive activity plus various activity against gram-negative organisms. Ampicillin was developed in the early 1960s and amoxicillin, with a similar spectrum but better GI absorption, was developed in the early 1970s (35,36). Bacampicillin is a prodrug that is rapidly hydrolyzed to ampicillin by esterases in the intestinal wall and in serum. Carbenicillin, ticarcillin, mezlocillin, and piperacillin have a broader gram-negative spectrum of activity that includes Pseudomonas species; they were developed in the late 1960s and 1970s (37–40).

Names and Chemistries

Amoxicillin	(Multiple manufacturers)	Oral
Ampicillin	(Multiple manufacturers)	Oral, IV
Bacampicillin	(Spectrobid, Roerig)	Oral
Carbenicillin	(Geocillin, Roerig)	Oral
Mezlocillin	(Mezlin, Miles)	IV
Ticarcillin	(Ticar, SmithKline Beecham)	IV
Piperacillin	(Pipracil, Lederle)	IV

Structures for these agents are shown in Figure 1. Aminopenicillins (amoxicillin, ampicillin, and bacampicillin) have a free amino group at the α-position on the benzene ring that results in increased gram-negative activity that includes some species of Hemophilus. The α-carboxypenicillins (carbenicillin and ticarcillin) have a carboxylic acid group at the α-position, which results in activity against some strains of Pseudomonas and Proteus. Acylaminopenicillins (mezlocillin and piperacillin) have a basic group at the α-position, which results in activity against enterobacteriaceae and strong activity against Pseudomonas species.

Pharmacology

The mechanism of action of extended-spectrum penicillins is similar to that of other penicillins. The extended spectrum is due to better penetration of the outer membranes of gram-negative bacteria and greater resistance to β-lactamases produced by gram-negative bacteria.

Pharmacology and Spectrum of Activity

Extended-spectrum penicillins are not effective against penicillinase-producing staphylococcal species. These agents have a broad gram-positive spectrum of activity that includes nonpenicillinase-producing staphylococcal species; groups A, B, C, and G streptococci; *S. pneumoniae,* viridans streptococci, and some strains of enterococci. Amoxicillin, ampicillin, and bacampicillin activity against aerobic gram-negative bacteria include neisseria (non-β-lactamase-producing strains), hemophilus (non-β-lactamase-producing strains), *E. coli, Proteus mirabilis,* salmonella, and shigella. Carbenicillin, ticarcillin, mezlocillin, and piperacillin have a further extended gram-negative spectrum that includes *Pseudomonas aeruginosa* (especially piperacillin), *P. vulgaris,* enterobacter species, *Serratia marcescens, Morganella morganii,* and *Klebsiella pneumoniae* (piperacillin).

Pharmaceutics

1. Topical	Ampicillin (50 mg/ml) Ticarcillin (6–20 mg/ml) Piperacillin (6–20 mg/ml)
2. Subconjunctival	Ampicillin (100 mg/ml) Ticarcillin (100 mg/ml) Piperacillin (100 mg/ml)
3. Intravitreal	Ampicillin (5,000 μg) Carbenicillin (1,000–2,000 μg)
4. Oral	Amoxicillin (250–500 mg q.i.d.) Ampicillin (250–500 mg q.i.d.) Bacampicillin (400–800 mg twice daily, b.i.d.) Carbenicillin (382–764 mg q.i.d.)
5. IV	Ampicillin (1–3 g q.i.d.) Ticarcillin (3 g every q4h, 4 g q6h) Mezlocillin (1–4 g q6h) Piperacillin (2–4 g q6h)

Pharmacokinetics

As with other penicillins, topical application of ampicillin, ticarcillin, or piperacillin will lead to high concentrations on the corneal surface but will not result in significant aqueous levels. Topical application of extended-spectrum penicillins may effectively treat sensitive organisms causing keratitis. However, the efficacy of topical extended-spectrum penicillins is limited in intraocular infection due to the poor penetration into aqueous. Effective inhibitory concentrations in the aqueous after subconjunctival administration of ampicillin or carbenicillin (with epinephrine) have been demonstrated (24,26,41–43). As with other penicillins, vitreal penetration after subconjunctival administration of extended-spectrum penicillins is likely to be poor. Intravitreal injection of carbenicillin has been well studied, and with concomitant use of probenicid, a $t_{\frac{1}{2}}$ of 20 hours may be attained (15,44). Unfortunately, an intravenous form of carbenicillin is not currently available; therefore, compounded forms for intraocular or topical use are not possible. Ampicillin may be used for intravitreal injection, but its spectrum of activity is inferior to that of carbenicillin. Probenicid may be used to enhance the $t_{\frac{1}{2}}$ of intravitreal ampicillin. For further discussion of intravitreal antibiotics use, see the Retina section.

Similar to other penicillins, amoxicillin, ampicillin, bacampicillin, and carbenicillin, orally administered, are absorbed in the duodenum and upper jejunum; extent of absorption depends on gastric acid stability and presence of food. As do other penicillins, systemically administered extended-spectrum penicillins penetrate well into vascularized tissue but poorly into CSF and into the eye. Penetration into aqueous after intravenous and intramuscular administration in animals has been extensively studied for ampicillin (24,26,41,42,45). Unlike most penicillins, ampicillin produced acceptable levels in the aqueous after intravenous and intramuscular administration in the studies. Animal studies by Kurose and Leopold (41) suggest that oral dosing of ampicillin leads to low aqueous levels. Faigenbaum et al. (46) demonstrated in a rabbit study that oral amoxicillin (which is better absorbed than ampicillin) may attain slightly higher aqueous levels. Intravenous ampicillin and oral amoxicillin may achieve inhibitory aqueous concentrations due to the low proportion (15% to 25% and 17% to 20%, respectively) that is protein bound; therefore, a resultant higher proportion of free ampicillin or free amoxicillin can cross the blood–aqueous barrier. Piperacillin also has a low proportion that is protein bound (16% to 22%). Adequate inhibitory levels of piperacillin were attained in the aqueous and tears after a single 4-g intramuscular injection (47). The extended-spectrum penicillins are predominantly eliminated by the kidney, and their serum $t_{\frac{1}{2}}$ is prolonged by probenicid. Probenicid's action on the ciliary body and retina also sustains intraocular concentrations of the extended spectrum penicillins.

Ocular Therapeutic Uses (Example)

Bacterial Keratitis

As already described, treatment for bacterial keratitis is usually initiated topically with cefazolin, plus gentamicin or tobramycin. If Pseudomonas is highly suspected initially, treatment may begin with tobramycin combined with either piperacillin or ticarcillin.

Side Effects and Toxicity

In general, the extended-spectrum penicillins share the side effects, toxicity, and hypersensitivity potential of other penicillins. In addition to the urticarial hypersensitivity observed with treatment with other penicillins, ampicillin and amoxicillin often cause a generalized erythematous, maculopapular rash.

High-risk Groups

The groups at high risk in treatment with extended-spectrum penicillins are the same as those at high risk with penicillin G treatment.

Drug Interactions

Drug interactions with extended-spectrum penicillins are the same as those that occur with penicillin G. Concomitant use of ampicillin and oral contraceptives may reduce efficacy of the contraceptive and increase the incidence of breakthrough bleeding.

β-LACTAMASE INHIBITORS WITH EXTENDED-SPECTRUM PENICILLINS

History and Source

Clavulonic acid is a potent, naturally occurring β-lactamase inhibitor that was isolated from *Streptomyces clavuligerus* (48). Clavulonic acid contains a β-lactam ring but has only low antibacterial activity. Sulbactam, a semisynthetic β-lactamase inhibitor that is similar to clavulonic acid, also has a low antibacterial activity (49). Clavulonic acid is commercially available in combination with amoxicillin and ticarcillin, and sulbactam is available in combination with ampicillin.

Names and Chemistries

Amoxicillin/ clavulonic acid	(Augmentin, Smith Kline Beecham)	Oral
Ampicillin/sulbactam	(Unasyn, Roerig)	IV
Ticarcillin/ clavulonic acid	(Timentin, Smith Kline Beecham)	IV

The structures of clavulonic acid and sulbactam are shown in Fig. 1.

Pharmacology

Clavulonic acid and sulbactam act as competitive inhibitors of β-lactamases. Concurrent administration of clavulonic acid and sulbactam does not alter the mechanism of amoxicillin, ampicillin, or ticarcillin.

Clinical Pharmacology and Spectrum of Activity

The further expanded spectrum with the combination of clavulonic acid and sulbactam include β-lactamase producing strains of *S. Aureus, S. epidermidus, H. influenzae, N. gonorrheae, E. coli, K. pneumoniae,* and proteus species.

Pharmaceutics

The pharmaceutics of β-lactamases is as follows: 250–500 mg amoxicillin/125 mg clavulonic acid p.o. every 8 hours, 1–2 g ampicillin/0.5 to 1 g sulbactam IV every 6 hours, and 3 g Ticarcillin/100 mg clavulonic acid IV every 4 to 6 hours.

Pharmacokinetics

Clavulonic acid is stable in gastric secretions and is relatively well absorbed after oral administration. Although a significant percentage of clavulonic acid is eliminated by the kidney, it is excreted largely by glomerular filtration rather than by tubular secretion (50). In addition, a significant percentage of clavulonic acid is metabolized in the body before it is excreted. Therefore, probenicid does not affect the serum $t_{\frac{1}{2}}$ of clavulonic acid. Sulbactam is poorly absorbed from the GI tract and is available only for intravenous administration in combination with ampicillin. Sulbactam is primarily eliminated by the kidney in its active form through tubular secretion, and its serum level is prolonged and enhanced by probenicid.

Ocular Therapeutic Uses (Examples)

Cellulitis

Mild to moderate cellulitis and impetigo that is believed to be due to sensitive staphylococcal, streptococcal, or hemophilus species may be treated with the combination of clavulonic acid and sulbactam. The combination of good anaerobic coverage plus activity against Hemophilus species makes these agents an excellent first-line choice for cellulitis. Good coverage can also be achieved with a second-generation cephalosporin.

Eyelid Bite Prophylaxis

Although a wide spectrum of potential pathogens prevent selection of a universally effective bite prophylaxis, extended-spectrum penicillins with a β-lactamase inhibitor are an excellent first-line choice.

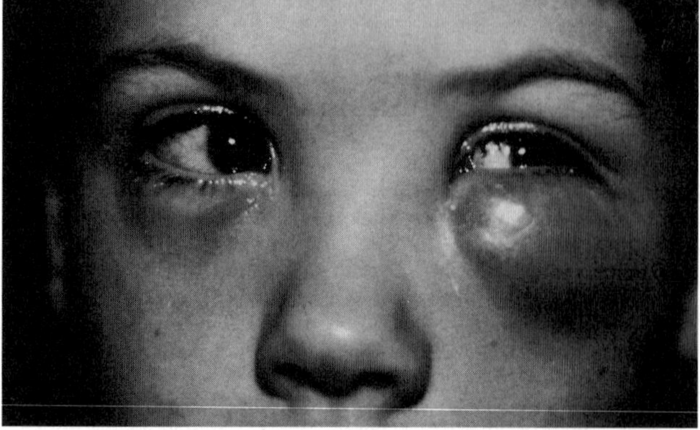

FIG. 40-3. Preseptal cellulitis. (Photograph courtesy of Robert Kersten, M.D.)

Intraorbital Foreign Body Prophylaxis

A small, "clean," well-tolerated intraorbital foreign body (e.g., stone, glass, plastic, steel, or aluminum) may be left in place, and the patient may be treated with amoxicillin/clavulonic acid. When surgical intervention is required (e.g., wood, vegetable matter, copper >85%, large size, sharp-edged, signs of infection), systemic antibiotics are combined with hospitalization and ampicillin/sulbactam or treatment with ticarcillin/clavulonic acid may be considered. Antibiotics may be adjusted with the culture results when possible.

Side Effects and Toxicity

Clavulonic acid and sulbactam do not appear to add additional side effects. However, GI symptoms such as nausea, vomiting, and diarrhea may occur more frequently with amoxicillin/clavulonic acid than with amoxicillin alone (52).

High-risk Groups

The groups at high risk for β-lactamases are the same as those at high risk with penicillin G.

Drug Interactions

Drug interactions with β-lactamases are the same as those that occur with penicillin G.

CEPHALOSPORINS

History and Source

The cephalosporins derive their name from a fungus known as *Cephalosporium acremonium* (the original source of the cephalosporins). *C. acremonium* was isolated by Brotzu in 1948 from a sewer outlet off the Sardinian coast (53). Crude broth-culture extracts of the fungus were shown to have antibiotic activity, and from the extracts three distinct compounds were isolated (cephalosporins P, N, and C) (54). Cephalosporin N is a penicillin, cephalosporin P is an antibiotic steroid, and cephalosporin C is a weak antibiotic that differs from the penicillins by having an additional carbon atom in the A ring (Fig. 2). Substitution of synthetic side chains to the nucleus of cephalosporin C (7-aminocephalosporanic acid) has yielded the family of cephalosporin antibiotics. The cephalosporins were first introduced for clinical use in the early 1960s; currently, multiple compounds with a range of antibiotic activity are available.

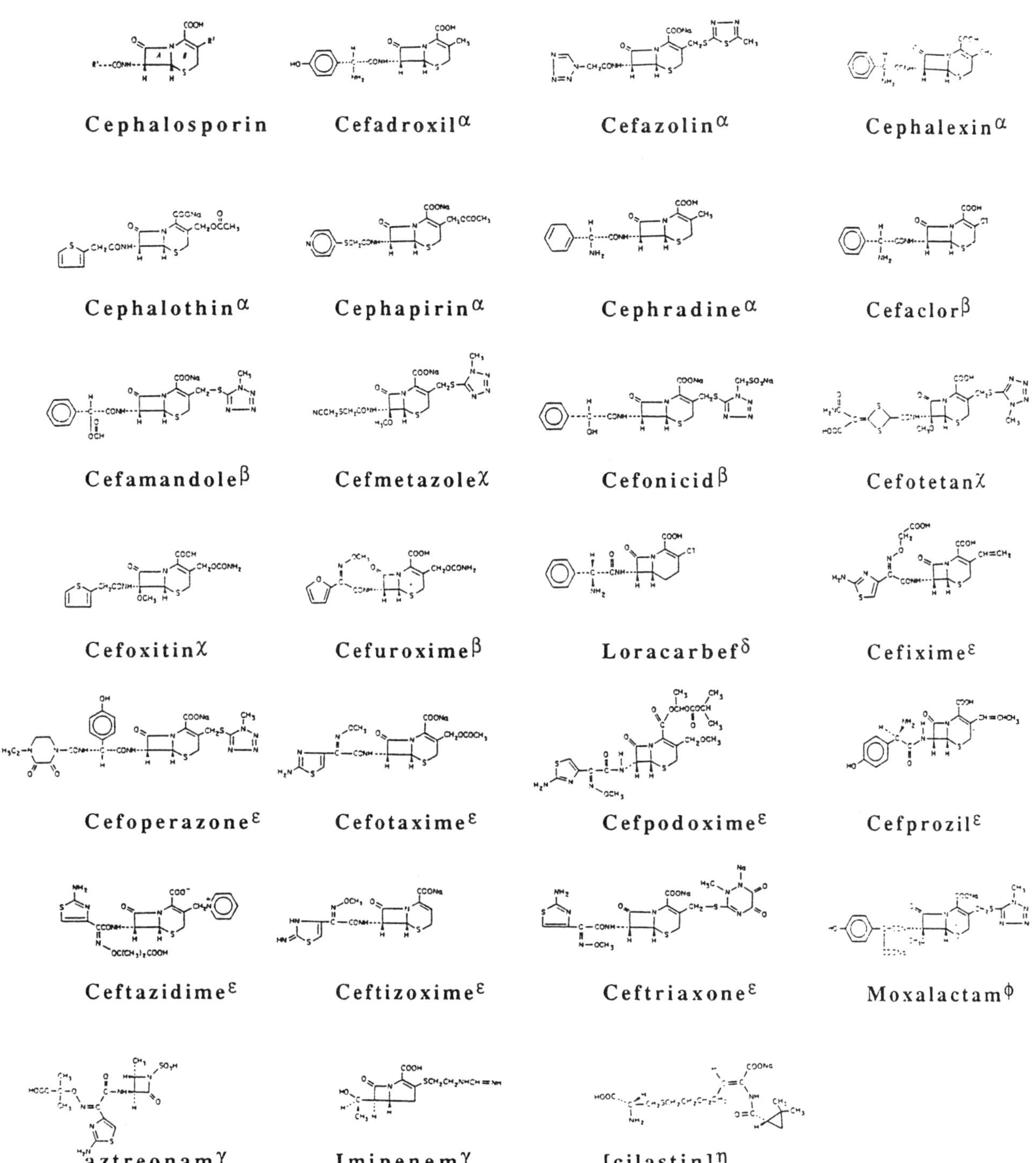

FIG. 40-4. **A:** β-lactam ring. **B:** Dihydrothiazine ring. *α:* First-generation cephalosporin. *β:* Second-generation cephalosporin. *χ:* Cephamycin; may be classified with second-generation cephalosporins. *δ:* Carbacephem; may be classified with second-generation cephalosporins. *ε:* Third-generation cephalosporin. *Φ:* 1-oxa-β-lactam; may be classified with third-generation cephalosporins. *γ:* Miscellaneous β-lactam antibiotic agents. *η:* Inhibitor of dehydropeptidase I, combined with imipenem.

Names and Chemistries

In general, modifications of the side chain at position 7 of the β-lactam ring result in modifications of antibiotic activity, and modifications at position 3 of the dihydrothiazine ring result in alterations of the pharmacokinetic properties (55). The cephamycins (cefmetazole, cefotetan, and cefoxitin) are categorized with the second-generation cephalosporins but have a methoxy group at position 7 of the β-lactam ring. Loracarbef is a carbacephem that may be classified with the second-generation cephalosporins but has a methylene group substituted for the sulfur atom at the 1-position in the dihydrothiazine ring. Moxalactam is no longer generally available; it is a 1-oxa-β-lactam that has been categorized with the third-generation cephalosporins, but it has an oxygen atom substituted for the sulfur atom at the 1-position in the dihydrothiazine ring.

The cephalosporins are classified into three "generations" on the basis of their spectrum of activity. This grouping does not necessarily reflect their chronology of development, and significant differences may exist between two agents in the same category. The general antibiotic activity of each generation is discussed in the Clinical Pharmacology and Spectrum of Activity section. The names and mode of administration of the currently available cephalosporins are listed below (18). The chemical structures are shown in Fig. 2.

First-generation cephalosporins		
Cefadroxil	(Duricef, Princeton)	Oral
Cefazolin	(Ancef, SmithKline)	IV
	(Kefzol, Lilly)	IV
Cephalexin	(Keflex/Keftab, Dista)	Oral
Cephalothin	(Keflin, Lilly)	IV
Cephapirin	(Cefadyl, Apothecon)	IV
Cephradine	(Velosef, Apothecon)	Oral
Second-generation cephalosporins		
Cefaclor	(Ceclor, Lilly)	Oral
Cefamandole	(Mandol, Lilly)	IV
Cefmetazole	(Zefazone, Upjohn)	IV
Cefonicid	(Monocid, SmithKline)	IV, IM
Cefotetan	(Cefotan, Stuart)	IV, IM
Cefoxitin	(Mefoxin, Merck)	IV, IM
Cefuroxime	(Ceftin, Allen and Hanburys)	Oral
	(Kefurox, Lilly)	IV, IM
	(Zinacef, Glaxo)	IV, IM
Loracarbef	(Lorabid, Lilly)	Oral
Third-generation cephalosporins		
Cefixime	(Suprax, Lederle)	Oral
Cefoperazone	(Cefobid, Roerig)	IV, IM
Cefotaxime	(Claforan, Hoechst-Roussel)	IV, IM
Cefpodoxime	(Vantin, Upjohn)	Oral
Cefprozil	(Cefzil, Bristol)	Oral
Ceftazidime	(Multiple manufacturers)	IV, IM
Ceftizoxime	(Cefizox, Fujisawa)	IV, IM
Ceftriaxone	(Rocephin, Roche)	IV, IM
Moxalactam	(Not available in the United States)	

Pharmacology

The mechanism of action of the cephalosporins, like the penicillins, results from the inhibition of mucopeptide synthesis in the bacterial cell wall. Varying affinities of the individual cephalosporins and penicillins for enzymes in the bacterial cytoplasmic membrane (e.g., transpeptidases) may explain differences in their speFctrum of activity.

Clinical Pharmacology and Spectrum of Activity

Overall, the cephalosporins are active against many gram-positive aerobic bacteria, some gram-negative aerobic bacteria, and some anaerobic bacteria. There is a wide range of activity among the cephalosporins, and traditionally they are divided into three groups or generations. Like the penicillins, none of the cephalosporins are effective against methicillin-resistant staphylococcal species. Although most of the penicillins are effective against *Enterococcus faecalis* (i.e., nafcillin and ticarcillin are at times resistant), none of the cephalosporins are effective. Similarly, penicillins are generally effective against *Lysteria monocytogenes,* but none of the cephalosporins are effective.

The first-generation cephalosporins have excellent activity against gram-positive cocci, including penicillinase-producing *S. aureus,* penicillinase-producing *S. epidermidis,* group A b-hemolytic streptococci (*S. pyogenes*), and Group B streptococci (*S. agalactiae*) and *S. pneumoniae.* The first-generation drugs are ineffective against *Bacteroides fragilis* and have only weak activity against gram-negative organisms.

The second-generation cephalosporins have excellent activity similar to that of the first-generation cephalosporins against gram-positive cocci. Unlike the first-generation cephalosporins, the second-generation cephalosporins are active against most strains of *H. influenzae.* The second-generation cephalosporins have greater gram-negative activity than the first-generation cephalosporins and may be effective against some strains of Acinetobacter, Citrobacter, Enterobacter, *E. coli,* Klebsiella, Neisseria, Proteus, Providencia, and Serratia. Cefotetan, cefoxitin, and cefamandole have some activity against *B. fragilis.*

The third-generation cephalosporins usually have less activity against staphylococcal species than do the first- or second-generation cephalosporins. They have significant activity against gram-negative bacteria and are usually active against Citrobacter, Enterobacter, *E. coli,* Klebsiella, Neisseria, Proteus, Morganella, Providencia, and Serratia. The intravenous agents are active against pseudomonas species, but the oral agents are generally ineffective against Pseudomonas. Most of the third-generation cephalosporins have some activity against *B. fragilis.*

Pharmaceutics

1. Topical	Cefazolin (133 mg/ml)
	Ceftazidime (50 mg/ml)
2. Subconjunctival	Cefazolin (100 mg/ml)
	Ceftazidime (200 mg/ml)
3. Intravitreal	Cefazolin (2.25 mg) + probenicid 0.5 g p.o. q.i.d.)

	Ceftazidime (2.2 mg)
	Ceftriaxone (3 mg)
4. Oral	Cefadroxil 1stG (500–1,000 mg b.i.d.)
	Cephalexin 1stG (250–500 mg q.i.d.)
	Cephradine 1stG (250–500 mg q.i.d.)
	Cefaclor 2ndG (250–500 mg t.i.d.)
	Cefuroxime 2ndG (250–500 mg b.i.d.)
	Loracarbef 2ndG (200–400 mg b.i.d.)
	Cefixime 3rdG (400 mg qd)
	Cefpodoxime (200 mg b.i.d.)
	Cefprozil 3rdG (250–500 mg b.i.d.)
5. IV/IM	Cefazolin 1stG (500–1,000 mg q6 h)
	Cephalothin 1stG (500–1,000 mg q4–6 h)
	Cephapirin 1stG (500–1,000 mg q4–6 h)
	Cefamandole 2ndG (500–1,000 mg q4–6 h)
	Cefmetazole 2ndG (2 g q8 h IV only)
	Cefonicid 2ndG (1 g q24 h)
	Cefotetan 2ndG (1–2 g q12 h)
	Cefoxitan 2ndG (1–2 g 6–8 h)
	Cefuroxime 2ndG (250–500 mg q12 h)
	Cefoperazone 3rdG (1–2 g q12 h)
	Cefotaxime 3rdG (1–2 g q6–8 h)
	Ceftazidime 3rdG (1–2 g q12 h)
	Ceftizoxime 3rdG (1–2 g q8–12 h)
	Ceftriaxone 3rdG (1–2 g q24 h)

In certain instances, the dosing regimens of the cephalosporins may be adjusted for severity of infection, alternate frequencies of administration, and renal insufficiency. Pediatric dosing schedules are usually available. The *Physicians Desk Reference* or equivalent drug evaluation source should be reviewed before one selects a dosing regimen (18).

Pharmacokinetics

As with the penicillins, topical application of cephalosporins will yield high concentrations on the ocular surface and in the cornea (56). Therefore, topical application of cephalosporins may be curative in treating keratitis caused by sensitive organisms. Certain cephalosporins may penetrate better than the penicillins. Topical application of cefazolin may generate therapeutic levels in the aqueous (56). In this study, rabbits with *S. aureus* keratitis were treated hourly with topical cefazolin (33 mg/ml). Aqueous concentrations of 17.7 μg/ml and 6.5 μg were generated by 9 hours and 17 hours, respectively (56). As a rule, vitreous concentrations of most antibiotics do not reach therapeutic levels after eyedrop delivery.

Multiple studies have demonstrated that subconjunctival injection of cephalosporins provide therapeutic levels in the aqueous humor, but levels in the vitreous are likely to be subtherapeutic (29,56–70). Cefazolin and ceftazidime are the cephalosporins most commonly used for subconjunctival injection, and both have been studied in rabbits and in humans undergoing cataract surgery (29,56, 60–63,67–69). In general, these agents achieve effective minimum inhibitory concentrations (MIC) for their respective sensitivity patterns in the aqueous but not in the vitreous humor. Ceftriaxone has also been shown to achieve adequate levels in the aqueous in rabbit studies (65,69). One group of investigators has demonstrated therapeutic vitreous concentrations that are further increased by aphakia after subconjunctival injection of ceftazidime or ceftriaxone in rabbits (65,68). However, other investigators have shown subtherapeutic vitreous concentrations after subconjunctival injection of these agents in rabbits (67,69). Barza et al. (69) showed that inflammation combined with repeated subconjunctival injection achieved higher vitreous concentrations of ceftazidime and ceftriaxone in rabbits (69). Previous studies have shown lower concentrations of cephalosporins in the vitreous of inflamed eyes (29,62,64), suggesting that the increased vitreous concentration in the study of Barza et al. (69) likely resulted from the repeated injections rather than from the inflammation.

Intravitreal injection of several cephalosporins has been investigated in rabbits and non-human primates (15,69, 71–76). Safe therapeutic doses have been established based on animal studies for cefazolin, ceftriaxone, and ceftazidime (72,74–76). Oral probenecid can significantly prolong the vitreal $t_{1/2}$ of cefazolin by acting on the cilioretinal pump (15). The $t_{1/2}$ of cefazolin after intravitreal injection in rabbits with noninflamed eyes is 7 hours; when oral probenecid is administered concomitantly, the $t_{1/2}$ is 30 hours (15). Ceftriaxone and ceftazidime are third-generation cephalosporins that are less efficiently secreted by the renal tubule (77) and possibly by the retina and ciliary body (69). After intravitreal injection in rabbits, the $t_{1/2}$ of ceftrixone is 9.1 hours in normal eyes and 13.1 hours in inflamed eyes (69). After intravitreal injection in rabbits, the $t_{1/2}$ of ceftazidime is 20 hours in normal eyes and 21.5 hours in infected eyes (69).

Oral cephalosporins are well absorbed from the GI tract and penetrate subcutaneous tissue well (18,19). They will likely penetrate eyelid and periocular tissues at concentrations adequate to treat minor infections caused by sensitive organisms effectively. The cephalosporins, like the penicillins, generally have poor intraocular penetration when administered orally. Cephalexin, an oral first-generation cephalosporin, has been shown to produce low levels in the aqueous (0.7–2 μg/ml) in rabbits and in humans undergoing cataract surgery (78,79). However, these low aqueous levels are below the median MIC for most organisms sensitive to cephalexin (5). Cefaclor, an oral second-generation cephalosporin, has also been shown to produce low levels in the aqueous (0.72 μg/ml) in humans undergoing cataract surgery (80). As with cephalexin, the aqueous cefaclor levels obtained are below the median MIC against most ocular pathogens (81).

Intravenous administration of the cephalosporins provides adequate tissue concentration to treat more serious infections of the eyelid and periocular tissues caused by sensitive organisms (18,19). Like the penicillins, the cephalosporins have relatively poor intraocular penetration into noninflamed normal rabbit and human eyes when administered intravenously (58,67,81–88). However, inflammation and repeated intravenous dosing may allow adequate intraocular penetration of cephalosporins. In a rabbit model, Martin et al. (88) showed that standardized sterile inflammation induced by heat killed *S. epidermidis,* and combined with intravenous dosing of cefazolin every 8 hours resulted in therapeutic levels in the vitreous by 48 hours (10.6 mg/L) (88). They also demonstrated in the same model that in inflamed aphakic and vitrectomized eyes even higher vitreal levels of cefazolin can be achieved by 48 hours (24.9 mg/L) (88).

After intravenous administration or absorption of oral forms from the GI tract, the cephalosporins are widely distributed to tissues and extracellular spaces. First- and second-generation cephalosporins penetrate poorly into the cerebrospinal fluid (CSF). However, the third-generation cephalosporins generally penetrate well into the CSF after intravenous or intramuscular injection. Ceftazidime has a low level of protein binding (5% to 24%) and penetrates well into the CSF after intravenous administration (19). Cephalosporins cross the placenta and are distributed in low concentrations in milk. Like the penicillins, most cephalosporins are rapidly excreted through the kidney by both glomerular filtration and tubular secretion. However, ceftazidime and ceftriaxone are primarily excreted by glomerular filtration and will be less affected by probenicid.

Ocular Therapeutic Uses (Examples)

Bacterial Keratitis

One current regimen for the initial therapy of bacterial keratitis consists of the empiric administration of fortified eyedrops of cefazolin, plus gentamicin or tobramycin (16). Therapy may be changed after the pathogen and its sensitivity pattern are identified. Ceftazidime has recently been considered as an alternate initial choice for topical therapy of bacterial keratitis (89). Ceftazidime may be used alone or in combination with an aminoglycoside or vancomycin, depending on the initial suspected pathogen. In a rabbit corneal ulcer study, ceftazidime was as effective as tobramycin against *P. aeruginosa,* and was as effective as cefazolin against *S. aureus* and *S. pneumoniae* (90). Ceftazidime's lower epithelial toxicity makes it an attractive substitute for aminoglycosides.

Gonococcal Conjunctivitis

The current treatment of choice for uncomplicated gonococcal conjunctivitis in the adult is a single injection of ceftriaxone 1 g IM (17). If gonococcal keratitis ensues, topical fortified penicillin has traditionally been added. However, topical ceftazidime may be a superior initial choice since it is usually effective against penicillinase-producing *N. gonococcus* (19). If there is no corneal involvement, topical irrigation with saline drops is adequate. For neonatal gonococcal ophthalmia, a single injection of ceftrixone (25–50 mg/kg, not to exceed 125 mg IM) may be used (17).

Lyme Disease

Because Lyme disease is usually in its late stages when corneal manifestations present, therapy is usually intensive. Intravenous ceftriaxone 2 g daily for 21 days or IV penicillin G 3–4 million Units every 4 hours are each considered effective treatments, but *B. burgdorferi* is more sensitive to ceftriaxone. Adjunctive topical steroid therapy may be required if nummular keratitis is present.

Preseptal Cellulitis

Cellulitis and impetigo may be treated with a second-generation cephalosporin. An extended-spectrum penicillin with a β-lactamase inhibitor may have superior anaerobic coverage and may be the preferable initial empiric agent.

Eyelid Laceration

A "clean" eyelid laceration may not require systemic antibiotic therapy and may be treated locally with antibiotic ointment (example: erythromycin or bacitracin/polymyxin B). Oral antibiotic coverage is indicated when wound contamination is suspected. Cephalexin 250 mg q.i.d. (children: 50 mg/kg/day in four doses) is a good choice due to its excellent coverage of Staphylococcus and Streptococcus species. Antibiotic coverage may be adjusted after culture results are obtained.

Prophylactic Postoperative Subconjunctival Antibiotics

A reduction in the incidence of postoperative endophthalmitis after prophylactic subconjunctival antibiotic injection has not been proven and remains controversial (91).

However, well-documented instances of substantial aqueous concentrations of drug have led many surgeons to administer subconjunctival antibiotic injection routinely after ocular surgery. Subconjunctival cefazolin (50–100 mg) is often used as a single agent or it may be combined with subconjunctival gentamicin for broad coverage. Reports of retinal toxicity with 400 μg intravitreal gentamicin or 20 to 80 mg subconjunctival gentamicin have led to a decrease in the subconjunctival and intraocular use of gentamicin (92–94). Some surgeons believe that the development of sutureless wound closure has shifted the risk/benefit ratio away from routine postoperative subconjunctival injections immediately after cataract surgery due to the theoretically increased possibility of antibiotic entering the eye through the sutureless wound. Low-concentration vancomycin and gentamicin in the irrigating solution for cataract surgery have been advocated by some surgeons as an alternative to subconjunctival injection (95). Routine usage of vancomycin may result in the emergence of vancomycin-resistant bacteria, however, and gentamicin may cause retina toxicity. For all intraocular surgeries with secure wounds, the use of prophylactic subconjunctival antibiotics remains a viable option.

Treatment of Significant Ruptured Globe Injuries

Preoperative. Because 2% to 7% of ruptured globe injuries result in bacterial endophthalmitis (96,97), antibiotic prophylaxis is indicated. Owing to potential toxicity, topical antibiotics are contraindicated for an open eye before surgical repair is undertaken. The eye should be protected with a shield, and primary repair of the corneal or scleral laceration should be performed soon after the injury. Systemic antibiotics may be initiated in the emergency room. Pooled data show the causative organisms in traumatic endophthalmitis to be *S. epidermidis* 24%, Bacillus species 22%, Streptococcus species 13%, gram-negative species 11%, mixed flora 10%, *S. aureus* 8%, fungi 8%, and anaerobes 3% (98,99). Intravenous antibiotics are recommended, since inflammation and repeated dosing may allow therapeutic intraocular levels. Although various intravenous antibiotic regimens have been recommended, broad antibacterial coverage can be obtained with ceftazidime (1 g IV every 12 hours) and vancomycin (1 g IV every 12 hours) (100). Alternatively, cefazolin (1 g IV every 6 hours) is often selected as a single intravenous agent. Although cefazolin provides inadequate coverage of Bacillus species, intraocular penetration in inflamed eyes has been best documented with cefazolin (see Pharmacokinetics section). Indiscriminate usage of vancomycin should be discouraged to prevent development of resistant bacterial strains. Fungi are not routinely covered prophylactically.

Intraoperative. In surgical repair of corneoscleral lacerations that do not involve lensectomy or vitrectomy, intraocular antibiotics are generally not used. However, some authorities advocate routine injection of an antibiotic agent or agents in the anterior chamber if the lens is not involved and into the vitreous if the lens or vitreous is violated (101). No prospective clinical study has determined the benefit of prophylactic intraocular antibiotics in this setting. If intraocular bacterial contamination is suspected, the surgeon should administer intraocular antibiotic agents. If surgical repair of the ruptured globe has been delayed and clinical signs of traumatic endophthalmitis are already present, injection of intravitreal antibiotic agents at the conclusion of surgery is mandatory. Cultures should be obtained when possible. Intraocular injections of vancomycin 1.0 mg and ceftazidime 2.25 mg or amikacin 400 μg provide appropriate coverage for likely bacterial pathogens. In secure wounds, subconjunctival injections of vancomycin 25 mg and ceftazidime 100 mg can be performed at the conclusion of surgery. Alternatively, subconjunctival injections of cefazolin 100 mg and gentamicin 20 to 40 mg may be considered; however, cefazolin provides inadequate coverage for Bacillus species and gentamicin increases the risk of retinal toxicity.

Postoperative. Hourly fortified antibiotics (i.e., vancomycin 25 mg/ml (or cefazolin 133 mg/ml) plus ceftazidime 50 mg/ml (or tobramycin 14 mg/ml) are administered topically for adjunctive therapy. Intravenous antibiotics are continued for 2 to 4 days. Antibiotic agents are adjusted if culture results are positive or if the clinical condition worsens.

Side Effects and Toxicity

Approximately 5% of patients have a hypersensitivity reaction to the cephalosporins; 3% of patients have positive direct and indirect Coombs' test results. Various rare hematologic effects of cephalosporins have been reported. Prolonged prothrombin time (PT), prolonged activated partial thromboplastin time (PTT) and/or hypothrombinemia have been rarely reported with cefixime, cefoperazone, cefotaxime, cefotetan, cefoxitin, ceftizoxime, ceftriaxone, cephalothin, and moxalactam. Nephrotoxicity has been reported with cephalothin, cephalexin, and cefazolin. Orally administered cephalosporins may result in nausea, vomiting, and diarrhea. Rarely, *Clostridium difficile* pseudomembranous colitis may occur.

High-risk Groups

Animal studies have not shown evidence of teratogenic effects, and extensive use of cephalosporins has not yielded reports of teratogenic effects in humans (18,19). However, cephalosporins should be used with caution in pregnant women and in lactating women since the use of

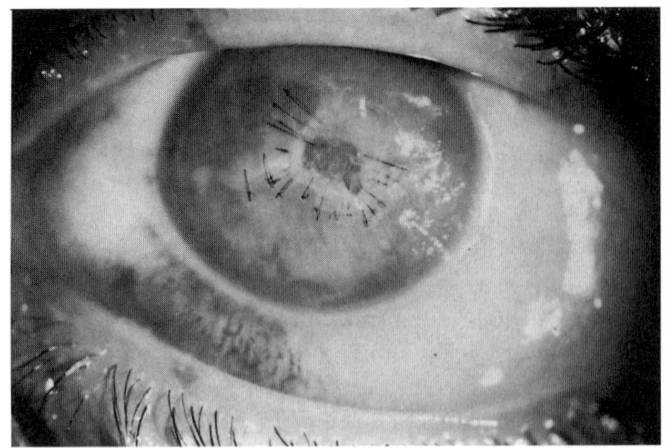

FIG. 40-5. Repair of severe corneal laceration.

cephalosporins in these groups has not been evaluated in controlled studies. Adverse testicular effects have been documented in prepubertal rats that received β-lactam antibiotics containing a tetrazolethiomethyl side chain (e.g., cefamandole, cefoperazone, cefotetan, and moxalactam).

Drug Interactions

Ingestion of alcohol after administration of agents containing a tetrazolethiomethyl side chain (e.g., cefamandole, cefoperazone, cefotetan, and moxalactam) can result in a disulfiram-like reaction. Probenicid prolongs the serum concentration of most cephalosporins.

Miscellaneous β-Lactam Antibiotics

Imipenem/cilastatin (primaxin, MSD) and aztreonam (Azactam, Squibb) are new β-lactam antibiotics that may have a role in treating pathogens resistant to traditional therapy.

SUMMARY

The enormous number of available β-lactam antibiotics, the paucity of prospective clinical studies (Tables 1 and 2), the wide range of potential pathogens, the various patterns of microbial resistance, the continual evolution of treatment patterns, and the possibility of patient antibiotic-agent

Table 40-1. *Ocular penetration of selected penicillins and cephalosporins: rabbit studies*

Penicillins	Concentration	Reference	Cephalosporins	Concentration	Reference
Cornea					
SC Penicillin G	3,277	(9)	TOCefazolin	75	(56[a])
IV Penicillin G	8.7	(9)	SC Cefazolin	624	(62[a])
SC Methicillin	542–874	(29[a])			
P.O. Amoxicillin	20.4–23.6	(46[b])			
Aqueous					
SC Penicillin G	682	(9)	TO Cefazolin	17.7	(56[a])
IV Penicillin G	3.1	(9)	SC Cefazolin	8,2–128	(56[a],60,61,62[a],63)
TO Methicillin	1.4–3.5	(24)	IV Cefazolin	4–70	(60,88[a])
SC Methicillin	12–166	(24–27,29[a])	OA Cephalexin	2.35	(78)
IV Methicillin	0.6–5.2	(24,25,26)	SC Cephalothin	2(58)	
TO Ampicillin	0.9–12.8	(24,41)	IV Cephalothin	54	(58)
SC Ampicillin	12–1,000	(24,26,41–43)	SC Ceftazidime	40.2	(68)
P.O. Ampicillin	0–0.6	(41)	IV Ceftazidime	8.4	(67)
IV Ampicillin	0–35	(24,26,41)	SC Ceftriazone	159.2	(65)
P.O. Amoxicillin	0.8–1.5	(46[b])	SC Cefuroxime	30	(70)
Vitreous					
SC Penicillin G	17	(9)	SC Cefazolin	0,24–18	(60,61,62[a])
IV Penicillin G	0.5	(9)	IV Cefazolin	10.6	(88[a])
TO Methicillin	<1.4	(24)	SC Ceftazidime	7.3–14.7	(68,69[a,c]
SC Methicillin	<1.4	(24,29[a])	SC Ceftizoxime	6.3–12.3	(69[a,c])
IV Methicillin	<1.4	(24)	SC Ceftriaxone	3–27.3	(65,69[a,c])
TO Ampicillin	<0.02	(24)	SC Cefuroxime	2	(70)
IV Ampicillin	<0.02–0.15	(24)			

TO, topical; SC, subconjunctival; P.O., oral; IV, intravenous.
Corneal concentrations are in micrograms per gram; aqueous and vitreous concentrations are in micrograms per milliliter.
All summarized data were from rabbit studies.
Only data from phakic eyes are tabulated.
Concentrations are the peak level obtained.
Some studies were performed on inflamed eyes.
[a]Study rabbits include inflamed eyes.
[b]Concentrations from doses of 50 mg/kg and 100 mg/kg were tabulated.
[c]Study rabbits received multiple subconjunctival injections.

Table 40-2. *Ocular penetration of penicillins and cephalosporins: human studies*

Site	Route of administration, agent	Reference
Tears	IV Piperacillin	5.6 (47)
Aqueous	IV Piperacillin	2.8 (47)
	SQ Cefazolin	80 (63)
	P.O. Cephalexin	0.7–2 (79)
	SQ Cephalothin	20 (59)
	IV Cephalothin	0.55 (81)
	P.O. Cefaclor	0.72 (80)
	IV Cefoxitin	3 (85)
	IV Ceftazidime	11 (67)
	IV Cefuroxime	1.7 (83)

Abbreviations as in Table 1.

intolerance prevents the development of a universal treatment guideline for their use. Nevertheless, a basic guideline for the use of penicillins and cephalosporins is helpful for designing initial empirical therapy. The regimens described below are recommendations for initial therapy that will require modifications based on history, clinical situation, and culture results. Indiscriminate usage of vancomycin should be discouraged to prevent development of resistant bacterial strains. Dosage and other issues are described in the appropriate chapter section.

Bacterial keratitis: (1) Topical cefazolin/tobramycin or (2) topical ceftazidime/vancomycin
Gonococcal conjunctivitis: Systemic ceftriaxone + saline irrigation
With keratitis: Add topical ceftazidime or penicillin
Chronic actinomyces canaliculitis: Intracanalicular penicillin G + penicillin V
Mild to moderate preseptal cellulitis: Oral amoxicillin/clavulonic acid
Eyelid laceration: Oral cephalexin
Eyelid bite prophylaxis: Oral amoxicillin/clavulonic acid
Prophylaxis for a "clean," well-tolerated intraorbital foreign body: Oral amoxicillin/clavulonic acid
Prophylactic postoperative subconjunctival antibiotics: Cefazolin and/or gentamicin
Treatment for significant ruptured globe injuries; (i.e., vitreal involvement with or without foreign body). Note—Indiscriminate usage of vancomycin is discouraged
Topical (after repair): Vancomycin plus ceftazidime or cefazolin plus tobramycin
Subconjunctival aftersuture closure: Vancomycin plus ceftazidime or cefazolin plus gentamicin
Intravitreal: Vancomycin plus ceftazidime or amikacin
Intravenous: Vancomycin plus ceftazidime (in certain clinical settings); cefazolin is alternative
Lyme disease (late stages): Intravenous ceftriaxone or penicillin G
Syphilitic eye disease: Intravenous or intramuscular penicillin G

CONCLUSION

In the years since the discovery of penicillin G by Alexander Fleming in 1929, the ever-enlarging penicillin and cephalosporin families of antibiotics have become an integral part of the treatment of corneal and external ocular diseases and intraocular infections. New β-lactam antibiotics certainly will be developed in the future, and potential applications for their use in the treatment of ocular infection will be identified.

ACKNOWLEDGMENT

Dr. Kaufman is a recipient of a Career Development Award from Research to Prevent Blindness, New York, NY.

REFERENCES

1. Fleming A. On the antibacterial action of cultures of a penicillium, with special reference to their use in the isolation of *B. influenzae. Br J Exp Pathol* 1929;10:226–236.
2. Chain E, Florey HW, Gardner AD, et al. Penicillin as a chemotherapeutic agent. *Lancet* 1940;2:226–228.
3. Shockman GD, Daneo-Moore L, Cornett JB, et al. Does penicillin kill bacteria? *Rev Infect Dis* 1979;1:787.
4. Handwerger S, Tomasz A. Antibiotic tolerance among clinical isolates of bacteria. *Rev Infect Dis* 1985;7:368.
5. Kucers A, McK Bennet N. *The use of antibiotics.* Philadelphia: JB Lippincott, 1987.
6. Sorsby A, Unger J. Pure penicillin in ophthalmology. *Br J Ophthalmol* 1946;114:4480.
7. Sorsby A, Unger J. Distribution of penicillin in the eye after injections of 1,000,000 units by subconjunctival, retrobulbar, and intramuscular routes. *Br J Ophthalmol* 1948;32:864.
8. Paterson CA. Intraocular penetration of ^{14}C-labeled penicillin after sub-tenon's or subconjunctival injection. *Ann Ophthalmol* 1973; 171–174.
9. Bloome MA, Golden B, McKee AP. Antibiotic concentration in ocular tissues: penicillin G and streptomycin. *Arch Ophthalmol* 1970; 83:78–83.
10. Leopold IA. Intravitreal penetration of penicillin and penicillin therapy of infections of the vitreous. *Arch Ophthalmol* 1945;33:211–216.
11. Barza M, Baum J. Penetration of ocular compartments by penicillin: analysis of factors affecting concentration and half life. *Surv Ophthalmol* 1973;18:71.
12. Duguid JP, Ginsberg M, Fraser IC, et al. Experimental observations on the intravitreous use of penicillin and other drugs. *Br J Ophthalmol* 1947;31:193–211.
13. Mandell GL, Sande MA. Penicillins, cephalosporins, and other beta-lactam antibiotics. In: Gilman AG, Rall TW, Nies AS, Taylor P, eds. *Goodman and Gilman's the pharmacological basis of therapeutics,* Chapter 46. New York: Pergamon Press.
14. Barza M, Baum J, Birkley B, Weinstein L. Intraocular penetration of carbenicillin in the rabbit. *Am J Ophthalmol* 1973;75:307.
15. Barza M, Kane A, Baum J. Pharmacokinetics of intravitreal carbenicillin, cefazolin, and gentamicin in rhesus monkeys. *Invest Ophthalmol Vis Sci* 1983;12:1602–1606.
16. Baum J. Antibiotic use in ophthalmology. In: Tasman W, Jaeger EA, eds. *Duane's clinical ophthalmology,* vol. 4. Philadelphia: JB Lippincott, Chapter 26.
17. Centers for Disease Control and Prevention: *MMWR* 1993;42(suppl RR-14).
18. *Physicians' Desk Reference* NJ: Medical Economics, 1995.
19. McEvoy GK, ed. *American Hospital Formulary Service Drug Information.* Bethesda, MD: American Society of Hospital Pharmacists, 1994.

20. Knudsen ET, Rolinson GN. Absorption and excretion of a new antibiotic (BRL 1241). *Br Med J* 1960;2:690.
21. Knudsen ET, Brown DM, Rolinson GN. A new orally effective penicillinase-stable penicillin-BRL 1621. *Lancet* 1962;2:632.
22. Klein JO, Finland M, Wilcox C. Nafcillin. Antibacterial action in vitro and absorption and excretion in normal young men. *Am J Med Sci* 1963;246:10.
23. Tanaka M. Studies on the ophthalmic use of penicillin derivatives: V. Stability of methyl-phenyl-isoxozolyl penicillin solution and its ocular penetration. *Acta Soc Ophthalmol Jpn* 1963;67:1756.
24. Faris BM, Uwaydah MM. Intraocular penetration of semisynthetic penicillins: methicillin, cloxacillin, ampicillin, and carbenicillin studies in experimental animals with a review of the literature. *Arch Ophthalmol* 1974;92:501–505.
25. Green WR, Leopold IH. Intraocular penetration of methicillin. *Am J Ophthalmol* 1965;60:800–804.
26. Records RE, Ellis PP. The intraocular penetration of ampicillin, methicillin, and oxacillin. *Am J Ophthalmol* 1967;64:135–143.
27. Deur HA, Mass ER. The penetration of several new penicillins into the tissues of the eye. *Ophthalmologica* 1962;144:316–322.
28. Barza M, Kane A, Baum J. Oxacillin for bacterial endophthalmitis: subconjunctival, intravenous, both, or neither? *Invest Ophthalmol Vis Sci* 1980;19:1348–1354.
29. Barza M, Kane A, Baum J. Ocular penetration of subconjunctival oxacillin, methicillin, and cefazolin in rabbits with staphylococcal endophthalmitis. *J Infect Dis* 1982;145:899–903.
30. Daily MJ, Peyman GA, Fishman G. Intravitreal injection of methicillin for treatment of endophthalmitis. *Am J Ophthalmol* 1973;76:343–350.
31. Kasbeer RT, Peyman GA. Intravitreal oxacillin in experimental staphylococcal endophthalmitis. *Albrecht Graefes Arch Klin Exp Ophthalmol* 1975;196:279–287.
32. Grant S. Probenecid and intraocular methicillin. *Ann Ophthalmol* 1981;13:209–211.
33. Uwaydah MM, Faris BM, Samara IN, et al. Cloxacillin penetration. *Am J Ophthalmol* 1976;82:114–116.
34. Records RE. Human intraocular penetration of sodium oxacillin. *Arch Ophthalmol* 1967;77:693–695.
35. Rolinson GN, Stevens S. Microbiological studies on a new broad-spectrum penicillin. 'Penbritin'. *Br Med J* 1961;2:191.
36. Sutherland R, Croydon EAP, Rolinson GN. Amoxicillin: a new semisynthetic penicillin. *Br Med J* 1972;3:13.
37. Knudsen ET, Rolinson GN, Sutherland R. Carbenicillin: a new semisynthetic penicillin active against *Pseudomonas pyocyanea. Br Med J* 1967;3:75.
38. Sutherland R, Burnet J, Rolinson GN. α-Carboxy-3-thienyl-methylpenicillin (BRL 2288), a new semisynthetic penicillin: in vitro evaluation. *Antimicrob Agents Chemother* 1970;390.
39. Bodey GP, Pan T. Mezlocillin: in vitro studies of a new broad-spectrum penicillin. *Antimicrob Agents Chemother* 1977;11:74.
40. Fu KP, Neu HC. Piperacillin, a new penicillin active against many bacteria resistant to other penicillins. *Antimicrob Agents Chemother* 1978;13:358.
41. Kurose Y, Leopold IH. Intraocular penetration of ampicillin: I. Animal experiment. *Arch Ophthalmol* 1965;73:361–365.
42. Goldman JN, Klein JO. Penetration of ampicillin and penicillin G into the aqueous humor. *Ann Ophthalmol* 1971;2:35–42.
43. McPherson SD Jr, Presley GD, et al. Aqueous humor assays of subconjunctival antibiotics. *Am J Ophthalmol* 1968;66:430–435.
44. Barza M, Kane A, Baum J. The effects of infection and probenicid on the transport of carbenicillin from the rabbit vitreous humor. *Invest Ophthalmol Vis Sci* 1982;22:720–726.
45. Goldman E, McLain JH, Smith JL. Penicillins and aqueous humor. *Am J Ophthalmol* 1968;65:717–721.
46. Faigenbaum AJ, Boyle GL, Prywes AS, et al. Intraocular penetration of amoxicillin. *Am J Ophthalmol* 1976;82:598–603.
47. Woo, FL, Johnson AP, Caldwell DR, et al. Piperacillin levels in human tears and aqueous humor. *Am J Ophthalmol* 1984;98:17.
48. Reading C, Cole M. Clavulonic acid: a beta-lactamase-inhibiting beta-lactam from *Streptomyces clavuligerus. Antimicrob Agents Chemother* 1977;11:852.
49. English AR, Retsema JA, Girard AE, et al. CP-45,899, a beta-lactamase inhibitor that extends the antibacterial spectrum of beta-lactams: initial bacteriological characterization. *Antimicrob Agents Chemother* 1978;14:414.
50. Staniforth DH, Jackson D, Clarke HL, Horton R. Amoxycillin/clavulonic acid: the effect of probenecid. *J Antimicrob Chemother* 1983;12:273.
51. Nilsson-Ehle I, Fellner H, Hedström SA, et al. Pharmacokinetics of clavulonic acid given in combination with amoxycillin in volunteers. *J Antimicrob Chemother* 1985;16:491.
52. Iravani A, Richard GA. Treatment of urinary tract infections with a combination of amoxicillin and clavulonic acid. *Antimicrob Agents Chemother* 1982;22:672.
53. Brotzu G. Richerche su di un nuovo antibiotico. *Lav Ist Iq Cagliari,* 1948, quoted by Abraham EP in The cephalosporins. *Pharmacol Rev* 1962;14:473–500.
54. Abraham EP. The cephalosporins. *Pharmacol Rev* 1962;14:473–500.
55. Huber FM, Chauvette RR, Jackson BG. Preparative methods for 7-aminocephalosporanic acid and 6-aminopenicillanic acid. In: Flynn EH, ed. *Cephalosporins and penicillins.* New York: Academic Press, 1972;27.
56. Baum J, Barza. Topical vs subconjunctival treatment of bacterial corneal ulcers. *Ophthalmology* 1983;90:162–168.
57. Mizukawa T, Azuma I, Kawaguchi S. Intraocular penetration of cephalothin and cephaloridine. *J Antibiot* 1965;18:525.
58. Records RE. Intraocular penetration of cephalothin: I. Animal studies. *Am J Ophthalmol* 1968;66:436–440.
59. Boyle Gl, Abel R, Lazachek GW, Leopold IH. Intraocular penetration of sodium cephalothin in man after subconjunctival injection. *Am J Ophthalmol* 1972;74:868–874.
60. Abel R, Boyle GL, Furman M, Leopold IH. Intraocular penetration of cefazolin sodium in rabbits. *Am J Ophthalmol* 1974;78:779–787.
61. Abel R, Boyle GL. Dissecting ocular tissue for intraocular drug studies. *Invest Ophthalmol* 1976;15:216–219.
62. Barza M, Kane A, Baum JL. Intraocular levels of cefamandole compared with cefazolin after subconjunctival injection in rabbits. *Invest Ophthalmol Vis Sci* 1979;18:250–255.
63. Saunders JH, McPherson SD. Ocular penetration of cefazolin in humans and rabbits after subconjunctival injection. *Am J Ophthalmol* 1980;89:564–566.
64. Kane A, Barza M, Baum J. Penetration of ocular tissues and fluids by moxalactam in rabbits with staphylococcal endophthalmitis. *Antimicrob Agents Chemother* 1981;20:595–599.
65. Jay WM, Shockley RK, Aziz AM, Aziz MZ, Rissing JP. Ocular pharmacokinetics of ceftriaxone following subconjunctival injection in rabbits. *Arch Ophthalmol* 1984;102:430–432.
66. Rubinstein E, Avni I, Tuizer M, et al. Cefsulodin levels in the human aqueous humor. *Arch Ophthalmol* 1985;103:426.
67. Walstad RA, Blika S. Penetration of ceftazidime into the normal rabbit and human eye. *Scand J Infect Dis* 1985;44(suppl):63–67.
68. Shockley RK, Fishman P, Aziz M, Yannis RZ, Jay WM. Subconjunctival administration of ceftazidime in pigmented rabbit eyes. *Arch Ophthalmol* 1986;104:266–268.
69. Barza M, Lynch E, Baum JL. Pharmacokinetics of newer cephalosporins after subconjunctival and intravitreal injection in rabbits. *Arch Ophthalmol* 1993;111:121–125.
70. Koul S, Philipson A, Philipson BT, Kock E, Nylen P. Intraocular levels of cefuroxime in uninflamed rabbit eyes. *Acta Ophthalmol* 1990;68:455–465.
71. Rutgard JJ, Berkowitz RA, Peyman GA. Intravitreal cephalothin in experimental staphylococcal endophthalmitis. *Ann Ophthalmol* 1978;293–298.
72. Fisher JP, Civiletto SE, Forster RK. Toxicity, efficacy and clearance of intravitreal injected cefazolin. *Arch Ophthalmol* 1982;100:650.
73. Leeds NH, Peyman GA, House B. Moxalactam (Moxam) in the treatment of experimental staphylococcal endophthalmitis. *Ophthalmic Surg* 1982;13:653–656.
74. Shockley RK, Jay WM, Friberg TR, Aziz AM, et al. Intravitreal ceftriaxone in a rabbit model. *Arch Ophthalmol* 1984;102:1236–1238.
75. Jay WM, Aziz MZ, Rissing JP, Shockley RK. Pharmacokinetic analysis of intravitreal ceftriaxone in monkeys. *Arch Ophthalmol* 1985;103:121–123.
76. Campochiaro AC, Green WR. Toxicity of intravitreous ceftazidime in primate retina. *Arch Ophthalmol* 1992;110:1625–1629.
77. Harding SM. Pharmacokinetics of the third-generation cephalosporins. *Am J Med* 1985;79(suppl):21–24.
78. Gager WE, Elsas FJ, Smith JL. Ocular penetration of cephalexin in the rabbit. *Br J Ophthalmol* 1969;53:403–406.

79. Boyle GL, Hein HF, Leopold IH. Intraocular penetration of cephalexin in man. *Am J Ophthalmol* 1970;69:868.
80. Axelrod JL, Kochman RS. Cefaclor levels in human aqueous humor. *Arch Ophthalmol* 1980;98:740–742.
81. Records RE. Intraocular penetration of cephalothin: II. Human studies. *Am J Ophthalmol* 1968;66:441–443.
82. Abel R, Boyle GL, Furman M, Leopold IH. Intraocular penetration of cefazolin sodium in rabbits. *Am J Ophthalmol* 1974;78:779–787.
83. Richards AB, Bron AJ, Rice NSC, Fells P, Marshall NJ, Jones BR. Intraocular penetration of cephaloridine. *Br J Ophthalmol* 1972;56:531–566.
84. Richards AB, Bron AJ, McLendon B, Kennedy MRK, Walker SR. The intraocular penetration of cefuroxime after parental administration. *Br J Ophthalmol* 1979;63:687–689.
85. Axelrod JL, Kochman RS. Cefoxitin levels in human aqueous humor. *Am J Ophthalmol* 1980;90:388–393.
86. Axelrod JL, Kochman RS. Moxalactam concentration in human aqueous humor after intravenous administration. *Arch Ophthalmol* 1982;100:1334–1336.
87. Quentin CD, Ansorg R. Penetration of cefotaxime into the aqueous humour of the human eye after intravenous application. *Graefes Arch Clin Exp Ophthalmol* 1983;220:245–247.
88. Martin DF, Ficker LA, Aguilar HA, et al. Vitreous Cefazolin levels after intravenous injection. *Arch Ophthalmol* 1990;108:411–414.
89. Jones DB. New horizons in antibacterial antibiotics. *Int Ophthalmol Clin* 1993;33:179–186.
90. Mills RA, Osato MS, Pyron M, Jones DB. Efficacy of topical ceftazidime in experimental bacterial keratitis. *Invest Ophthalmol Vis Sci* 1992;33:935.
91. McMillan JJ, Mead MD. Prophylactic subconjunctival antibiotics after cataract extraction—evaluation of their desirability and efficacy. *Int Ophthalmol Clin* 1994;34:43–49.
92. McDonald HR, Schatz H, Allen AW, et al. Retinal toxicity secondary to intraocular gentamicin injection. *Ophthalmology* 1986; 93:871–877.
93. Conway BP, Campochiaro PA. Macular infarction after endophthalmitis treated with vitrectomy and intravitreal gentamicin. *Arch Ophthalmol* 1986;104:367–371.
94. Campochiaro PA, Conway BP. Aminoglycoside toxicity—a survey of retinal specialists. *Arch Ophthalmol* 1991;109:946–949.
95. Gills JP. Filters and antibiotics in irrigating solution for cataract surgery. *J Cataract Refract Surg* 1991;17:385.
96. Brinton GS, Topping TM, Hyndiuk RA, et al. Posttraumatic endophthalmitis. *Arch Ophthalmol* 1984;102:547–550.
97. Forster RK. Endophthalmitis. In: Duane TD, ed. *Clinical Ophthalmology,* vol. 4, chap. 24, Philadelphia: JB Lippincott, 1987.
98. Parrish CM, O'Day DM. Traumatic endophthalmitis. *Int Ophthalmol Clin* 1987;27:112–119.
99. Levin MR, D'Amico DJ. Traumatic endophthalmitis. In: Shingleton BJ, Hersh PS, Kenyon KR, eds. *Eye Trauma,* chap. 23. St. Louis: CV Mosby, 1991.
100. Navon SE. Management of the ruptured globe. *Int Ophthalmol Clin* 1995;35:71–91.
101. Peyman GA, CArroll CP, Raichand M. Prevention and management of traumatic endophthalmitis. *Ophthalmology* 1980;87:320–324

Textbook of Ocular Pharmacology,
edited by T.J. Zimmerman, et al.
Lippincott–Raven Publishers, Philadelphia © 1997.

CHAPTER 41

Antiparasitic Agents

Lisa D. Kelly

SULFONAMIDES

History and Source

In 1932, Klarer and Mietzsch tested prontosil, an azo red dye, and found it ineffective against bacteria in vitro. In 1935, however, Domagk found that prontosil, when tested in vivo, had antibacterial activity, especially against hemolytic streptococci. This discovery ushered in the age of therapeutic antibiotic use. For his work, Domagk received the Nobel prize in 1938.

In vivo, prontosil is converted to its active metabolite, sulfanilamide. Since prontosil's initial introduction, more than 150 different sulfonamides have been marketed. The modified compounds have characteristics of increased potency, broader antibacterial spectrum, or enhanced solubility.

Sulfonamides were the first category of chemotherapeutic agents effective in the treatment of human infection. After the discovery of numerous other categories of antibiotics, the clinical use of sulfonamides decreased. Recently, in the last 10 to 15 years, recognition of their synergistic relationship with trimethoprim has resulted in increased interest in usage of the sulfonamides. Sulfonamides are an alternative treatment for urinary tract infection, bacillary dysentery, and meningococcal infection. However, due to the frequency of resistant strains, the role of sulfonamides is limited.

Official Drug Name and Chemistry

The term sulfonamide is a generic category name for sulfanilamide (aminobenzene sulfonamide).

All sulfonamides have the same parent nucleus. Substitution of the *R* radical in the amido group ($-SO_2$ NHR) or of the amino group (NH_2) results in alteration in the antibacterial spectrum, and in the chemical and physical properties of the sulfonamides. The amino group is critical for antibacterial activity, but the amido group is not. Sulfonamides typically are white, odorless crystalline powders that exhibit maximal solubility at alkaline pH. Because sulfonamide agents vary in solubility properties, therapy with a combination of sulfonamides such as trisulfapyrimidine allows a threefold greater concentration in urine than is achieved with single-agent therapy. The sodium salts of sulfonamides are readily soluble in water and are the form used for intravenous administration and in topical ophthalmic preparations.

Pharmacology

Although sulfonamides have a broad spectrum of antimicrobial activity against both gram-negative and gram-positive organisms, recent increases in rates of resistant strains has compromised clinical usefulness. Sulfonamides are bacteriostatic agents. The mechanism of action is as a structural analogue of paraminobenzoic acid (PABA). As a competitive antagonist of PABA in microorganisms, sulfonamides inhibit synthesis of folic acid. The most sensitive organisms are those incapable of using preformed folate. The bacteriostatic effect of sulfonamides is antagonized by administration of PABA.

Sulfonamides have a synergistic effect with trimethoprim against bacteria. The optimal antibacterial ratio of sulfonamide to trimethoprim for most bacteria is 20 : 1. Sulfonamides have a synergistic relationship with pyrimethamine against protozoa.

Pharmaceutics

Systemic Use

Sulfisoxazole (generic, Gantrisin, SK-Soxazole)
  Tablet 500 mg
  Syrup 500 mg/5 ml
  Oral use emulsion 1 g/5 ml
Sulfamethoxazole (generic, Gantanol)
  Tablet 500 mg

L. D. Kelly: University of Kansas, Leawood, Kansas 66209.

$H_2N-C_6H_4-SO_2NH_2$ (4 … 1)

Sulfanilamide

Sulfadiazine

Sulfamethoxazole

Sulfisoxazole

Sulfacetamide

Para-aminobenzoic Acid

500 mg/5 ml
Sulfadiazine (generic, Microsulfon)
  Tablet 500 mg
Sulfacytine (Renoquid)
  Tablet 250 mg
Trisulfapyrimidine (generic)
  Tablet 500 mg
Trimethoprim-Sulfamethoxazole (generic, Bactrim, Septra)
  Tablet 80 mg trimethoprim, 400 mg sulfamethoxazole
  Tablet 160 mg trimethoprim, 800 mg sulfamethazole
  40 mg trimethoprim, 200 mg sulfamethazole 5ml oral suspension
  80 mg trimethoprim, 400 mg sulfamethoxazole/5 ml for infusion

Topical Ophthalmic

Sulfisoxazole-Gantrisin (Roche)
  Sulfacetamide sodium
    Bleph-10 (Allergan) 10% suspension and ointment
    Sulamyd (Schering) 10%, 30% solution and 10% ointment
    Sulf-10 (IOLAB) 10% solution
    Sulfacetamide sodium 10%, 15%, and 30% solution
    Bausch and Lomb 10% ointment
    Ocu-Sul (Ocumed) 10%, 15%, and 30% solution and 10% ointment
  Sulfacetamide and steroid combination
    AK-cide (Akorn) solution and ointment: 0.5% prednisolone, 10% sulfacetamide
    Metimyd (Schering) suspension and ointment: 0.5% prednisolone and 10% sulfacetamide
    Sulpred (Bausch and Lomb) suspension: 0.2% prednisolone and 10% sulfacetamide
    Vasocidine (IOLAB) solution and ointment: 0.5% prednisolone and 10% sulfacetamide
    Ocu-lone-C (Ocumed) solution and ointment: 0.5% prednisolone and 10% sulfacetamide
    Cetapred (Alcon) ointment and suspension: 0.25% prednisone and 10% sulfacetamide
    FML-S (Allergan) suspension: 0.1 fluorometholone and 10% sulfacetamide

Pharmacokinetics

Topical

Sulfacetamide is the most commonly available topical ophthalmic sulfonamide and is the N'-acetyl-substituted derivative. The sodium salt is highly soluble as compared with other sulfonamides. At 30% solution, it has a pH of 7.4 and has good tissue penetration.

Systemic

When sulfonamides are administered orally, they are rapidly absorbed from the gastrointestinal (GI) tract. The drug distributes throughout tissues, including the CNS, cerebrospinal fluid (CSF), the placenta and fetus.

Absorbed sulfonamides are 20% to 90% protein bound. Once absorbed, the drug may be acetylated and/or metabolized. Techniques for measuring serum sulfonamide may measure free (active) or acetylated (inactive) drug. The therapeutic range is 8 mg to 12 mg of free drug.

Peak serum drug levels occur 2 to 3 hours after oral dosing. Soluble drug is excreted by glomerular filtration; insoluble drug is excreted in feces. Long-acting sulfonamides such as sulfadoxine are highly protein bound and have high levels of tubular reabsorption of the unacetylated form.

Therapeutic Use

Topical

Sulfacetamide sodium salts are used in the treatment of blepharitis, conjunctivitis, and corneal ulcers and may be used as a second-line agent in conjunction with systemic treatment for trachoma. Clinical usefulness may be limited by high rates of microorganism resistance.

Sulfacetamide solution is applied as 1 drop to the inferior cul-de-sac every 2 to 3 hours. Ointment is applied once to four times a day.

Systemic

Trachoma/Inclusion Conjunctivitis

Although the treatment of choice is a 3-week course of oral tetracycline or erythromycin, oral sulfonamides may be administered 30 mg/kg/day. Sulfonamides are ineffective against psittacosis.

Lymphogranuloma Venereum

Effective treatment for lymphogranuloma venereum is sulfisoxazole 1 gm four times a day for a 3-week course.

Toxoplasmosis

In adults, the treatment of choice for toxoplasmosis is combined therapy with oral pyrimethamine in a loading dose of 100 to 150 mg followed by 25 to 50 mg and sulfadiazine 4 to 6 mg/day in three divided doses for a 4- to 6-week course.

Side Effects

Topical

Local irritation, brow ache, blurred vision, transient burning and stinging, and sensitivity reactions, including rare cases of Stevens Johnson syndrome and exfoliative dermatitis, have been reported. GI upset and bone marrow depression have also been described.

Systemic

Hematologic disturbance, including agranulocytosis and aplastic anemia, are rare side effects of sulfonamide therapy. Patients with glucose 6-dehydrogenase deficiency are particularly at risk for hemolytic anemia. Hypersensitivity, photosensitivity, hepatotoxicity, and transient amblyopia and myopia are well-recognized adverse effects. Erythema nodusum and erythema multiforme have been reported in association with sulfonamide administration. Reversible bone-marrow suppression may occur in patients with AIDS.

Crystalluria may occur in patients with AIDS who are dehydrated. Hypersensitivity occurs in as many as 5% of patients. Nausea, vomiting, and fatigue occurs in 1% to 2% of patients.

High-risk Groups

The safety of use of sulfonamides in pregnant women and lactating mothers has not been established. Drug use should be reserved for clinical conditions in which the potential risk is clearly outweighed by the advantages of treatment.

Drug Interactions

Caution is advised when sulfonamides are administered in conjunction with the sulfonylurea hypoglycemic agents, hydantoin anticonvulsants, and oral anticoagulants. With each of these agents, sulfonamides potentiate drug effects by inhibiting drug metabolism. This may result in a need to alter dosing regimen.

Paraminobenzoic acid (PABA) is a potent antagonist of sulfonamides. PABA esters such as procaine may inhibit the antibacterial effect of these agents.

Trimethoprim is a potent synergist of sulfonamides. Use of these agents in combination results in blockage of sequential steps in microorganism synthesis of tetrahydrafolate.

Cross-allergenicity may occur with other sulfonamides, including carbonic anhydrase inhibitors, thiazides, and sulfonylurea hypoglycemic agents.

Clinical Trials

In a prospective multicenter trial, May et al. compared trimethoprim sulfamethoxazole (TMP-SMX) with aerosolized pentamidine prophylaxis for primary *Pneumocystis Carinii* pneumonia in AIDS patients. They concluded that both treatments were effective in decreasing incidence of pneumonia. Aerosolized pentamine was better tolerated, but TMP-SMX was less expensive and appeared to decrease risk of toxoplasmosis.

TRIMETHOPRIM

History and Source

TMP is a broad-spectrum antibiotic. Systematically, it is commonly used in combination with SMX because of the synergistic effect of the two agents. For topical ophthalmic use, TMP is combined with polymyxin B to achieve broader antibacterial spectrum.

Official Drug Name and Chemistry

TMP is a benzylpyrimidine 3, 4, 5-trimethaxybenzyl pyrimidine.

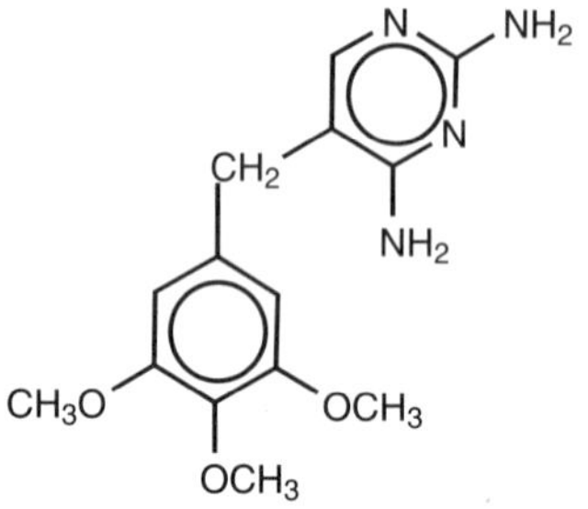

Trimethoprim

Pharmacology

The mechanism of action of TMP consists of disruption of folate synthesis. Specifically, the drug inhibits dihydrofolic acid reductase. This enzyme converts dihydrofolic to tetrahydrofolic acid, a step critical in purine synthesis. TMP inhibits bacterial dihydrofolic acid reductase 50,000 times more efficiently than mammalian enzyme.

The antibacterial spectrum of trimethoprim includes most gram-positive and gram-negative organisms, including *Staphylococcus aereus, S. epidermidis, Hemophilus influenzae, S. pneumococcus, S. viridans, Klebsiella pneumoniae* and *Escherichia coli;* with the notable resistance of *Pseudomonas aeruginosa, Bacteroides fragilis,* and neisseria species. Clinical usefulness as a single agent is limited by high rates of plasmid mediated resistance. TMP is synergistic in combination with sulfonamide because these agents interrupt sequential steps in folate synthesis. Sulfonamide inhibits incorporation of PABA in folic acid, and TMP inhibits conversion of dihydrofolate to tetrahydrofolate. The optimal drug ratio of SMX to TMP for synergy for most bacteria is 20 : 1.

Therapeutic Use

For urinary tract infection, oral TMP 100 mg twice daily for 10 days is effective, but resistance limits clinical usefulness. Oral TMP-SMX (160 to 800 mg) twice daily for a 10-day course achieves a high cure rate.

For GI tract infections, TMP-SMX (160 to 800 mg) is effective treatment for Shigella; for Salmonella, dosing is 1 tablet every 12 hours.

In pneumonia (e.g., severe pneumocystitis), intravenous TMP 20 kg/day and SMX 100 mg/kg in three divided doses is effective.

In moderate *Pneumocystis Carinii,* oral TMP-SMX (160 to 800 mg), one tablet every 12 hours, is effective. This dose may be used for *Pneumocystis* prophylaxis.

For ocular infection, TMP-polymyxin B offers excellent broad-spectrum antibacterial coverage in the treatment of conjunctivitis. Activity against *Hemophilus influenzae* is particularly useful in pediatric populations. Management of neonatal *H. influenzae* conjunctivitis should also include systemic antibiotic therapy.

Pharmaceutics

Systemic

TMP (Trimpex), 100- and 200-mg tablets, is used for systemic therapy.

Topical

TMP-polymyxin (Polytrim) ophthalmic solution is used for topical therapy.

Pharmacokinetics

TMP with SMX may be administered either orally (p.o.) or intravenously (IV). It is readily absorbed from the GI tract, and the peak serum concentration occurs at 2 hours with TMP and at 4 hours with TMP-SMX therapy. The half-life ($t_{\frac{1}{2}}$) is 10 hours for SMX and 11 hours for TMP. TMP is lipid soluble and penetrates tissue well, readily entering the cerebrospinal fluid (CSF). It is 40% protein bound in serum. TMP undergoes urinary excretion.

Clinical Pharmacology

TMP has minimal effect on mammalian cells since humans obtain preformed folate in a normal diet. When administered orally, TMP is absorbed from the gut and is 40% protein bound. The agent penetrates to the CSF and concentrates in prostatic and vaginal fluids.

Side Effects/Drug Interactions

Due to its antifolate effect, TMP may induce leukopenia, megaloblastic anemia, and thrombocytopenia. Folate-deficiency side effects may be avoided by administering folinic acid 6 to 8 mg/kg/day.

Most side effects are dermatologic. The combination of TMP-SMX results in a 5.9% rate of skin reaction (Arndt); occurrence of Stevens Johnson or Lyells syndrome is rare.

Other infrequent side effects include headache, nausea, fever, and renal damage. In particular, TMP-SMX treatment of *P. carinii*-infected AIDS patients has a high rate of adverse reaction. Wharton et al. reported a 90% rate of side effects. It may be possible to continue therapy at lower concentrations.

Clinical Trials

See section on clinical trials of TMP-SMX.

SURAMIN

History and Source

Suramin was introduced in the 1920s as a treatment for trypanosomiasis. Currently, it is the drug of choice in the treatment of *Trypanosoma brucei gambiense* and *T. brucei rhodesiense,* but it is ineffective against South American trypanosomiasis. Suramin is also an alternative treatment for *Onchocerca volvulus.* Suramin has recently been recognized as a protype of a new category of anticancer drug.

Official Name and Chemistry

Suramin is a polycyclic trypan dye derivative.

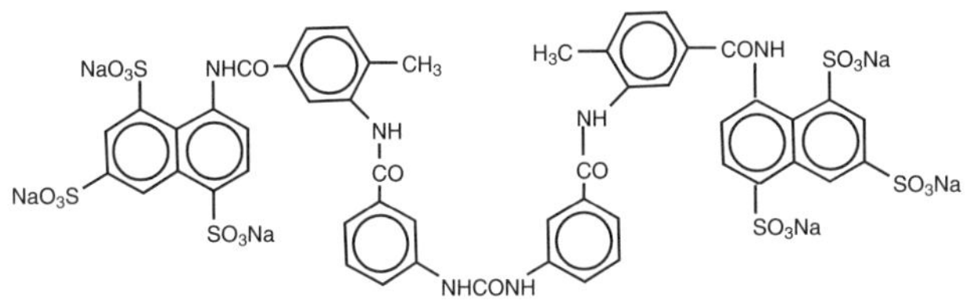

NaO3S NHCO CH3 H3C CONH SO3Na
NH CO NH CO
NaO3S SO3Na SO3Na SO3Na
NHCONH

Suramin Sodium

Pharmacology

The specific primary mode of action of suramin is not understood. A nonspecific inhibition of microorganism enzymes is the proposed mechanism of action, since suramin inhibits numerous tryponosomal enzymes. Suramin also appears to block parasite uptake of low density lipoprotein (LDL). Inhibition of glycerol phosphate oxides in trypanosoma has been correlated with activity in suramin derivatives.

Clinical Pharmacology

In plasma, 85% of suramin circulates binds to protein; approximately 15% of this is bound to LDL. Vansterkenburg et al. have suggested that LDL may serve as a carrier for microorganism uptake of the drug.

Pharmaceutics

Trade names for suramin are Germanin, Bayer 205, Moranyl, Belganyl, Forneau, Naphuride, and Antrypol, available as 0.5 g or 1 g powder to reconstitute as a 10% solution for immediate use. In the United States, suramin is available only from the Parasitic Disease Drug Service of the Centers for Disease Control (CDC).

Pharmacokinetics

Suramin is effective only when administered parenterally and is generally delivered by slow intravenous injection. Suramin has poor CNS penetration. Plasma $t_{\frac{1}{2}}$ is 48 hours, with final elimination at approximately 50 days. Renal excretion accounts for approximately 80% of elimination.

Therapeutic Use

Trypanosoma

For Trypanosoma, an intravenous test dose of 100 to 200 mg suramin should be administered, followed by treatment with 1 g IV on days 1, 3, 7, 14, and 21. The pediatric dose is 20 mg/kg given in the same schedule as that used in adults. In treatment of trypanosomiasis, adjunctive pentamidine 4 mg/kg/day for 10 days should be administered.

Onchocerca

For *Onchocerca,* after a 100 to 200 mg IV test dose, treatment is 1 g IV weekly for 5 weeks.

Side Effects

Suramin has a wide range of associated side effects that tend to be most severe in debilitated patients. Infrequent acute reactions (less than 1%) include nausea, vomiting, shock, and loss of consciousness. Common side effects include malaise, fever, rash, nausea, headache, and paresthesias. Palmar or plantar hyperesthesis may evolve to peripheral neuritis.

Twelve to 26% of patients with AIDS experience reversible leukopenia, agranulocytosis, thrombocytopenia, proteinuria, and increased creatinine, transamidases, and bilirubin levels. Patients with AIDS may also develop adrenal insufficiency and vortex keratopathy.

High-risk Groups

Suramin should be administered only when close observation is possible. Extreme caution should be used in patients with renal insufficiency; if casts appear in urinalysis, treatment should be discontinued.

Clinical Trials

Because of suramin's in vitro ability to inhibit retroviral reverse transcriptase, Cheson et al. recently conducted a multicenter trial in the treatment of AIDS; the drug was ineffective.

MEBENDAZOLE

History and Source

Mebendazole (benzimidazole) is a broad-spectrum anthelminthic and is an agent of choice in the treatment of *Trichinella spiralis* (trichinosis), *Enterobius vermicularis* (pinworm), *Trichuris trichiura* (whipworm), *Necator americanus* and *Ancylostoma deudenale* (hookworm), and *Ascaris lumbricoides* (roundworm).

Official Drug Name and Chemistry

Mebendazole is a benzimidazole structurally related to thiabendazole.

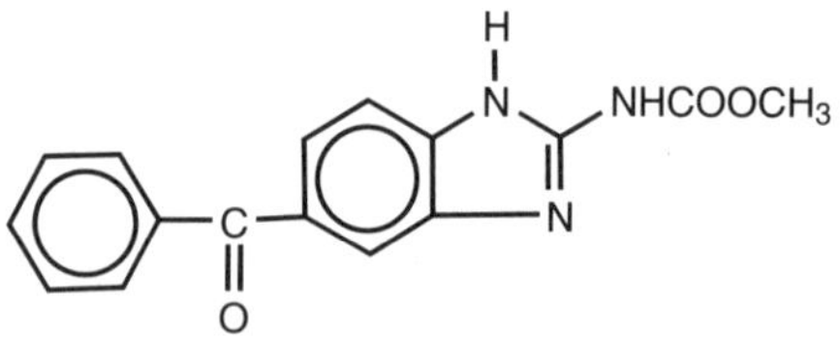

Mebendazole

Pharmacology

Mebendazole inhibits microtubule synthesis in nematodes. There is selective loss of cytoplasmic microtubules in parasite tegument and intestinal cells. Secretion of acetylcholinesterase and uptake of glucose are impaired, and glycogen is depleted.

Clinical Pharmacology

In human cells, mebendazole is almost inert. The agent has high affinity for parasite tubulin but does bind to host tubulin in vitro. The mechanism of selective activity is unknown. The efficacy of the drug depends on GI transit time.

Pharmaceutics

Trade names for mebendazole are Vermox, Mebutar, Neniasole, Pantelmin Sirben, Mebandecin, and Vermirax. In the United States, mebendazole is available as an oral 100-mg tablet; outside the United States, it is available as a 100-mg/5-ml oral suspension.

Pharmacokinetics

Mebendazole is poorly water soluble, and less than 10% of orally administered drug is absorbed by the GI tract. Peak plasma levels are achieved in 2 to 4 hours. The drug is readily metabolized and eliminated primarily by urinary excretion in 24 to 48 hours. A small amount of the drug is excreted in the bile, and drug absorption is enhanced if mebendazole is administered in conjunction with a high fat meal.

Therapeutic Use

For pinworm, treatment is 100 mg mebendazole; the dose is repeated at 2 and 4 weeks. Cure rates range from 90% to 100%.

For hookworm, roundworm, and whipworm, treatment is mebendazole 100 mg twice daily for 3 days. Treatment may be repeated at 2 to 3 weeks. Cure rates for roundworm and whipworm approach 100%. The cure rate for hookworm is lower, but treatment does result in significant decrease in nematode load.

Mebendazole is an alternative treatment for hydatid cyst. Surgery is the preferred treatment, but if a patient is not a candidate for surgery or if the cyst has ruptured, mebendazole should be administered 50 mg/kg in three divided doses daily for 3 months. Plasma levels of 100 ng/ml or greater at peak is required for nematode death.

Side Effects

Side effects of mebendazole are infrequent; however, abdominal pain, and mild diarrhea, nausea, and vomiting have been reported.

Treatment of hydatid disease with high-dose mebendazole occasionally induces reversible neutropenia, eosinophilia, fever, myalgia, rash, and pruritis. GI upset, liver dysfunction, glomerulonephritis, and agranulocytosis have also been reported.

High-risk Groups

Caution is advised in patients with hepatic dysfunction because mebendazole may be poorly detoxified. The drug should not be used during the first trimester of pregnancy and should be avoided later in pregnancy if alternative drugs are available. Mebendazole should be used with caution in the treatment of children aged less than 2 years because experience in such treatment is limited.

Clinical Trials

Bartoloni et al. compared a single dose of albendazole and mebendazole 400 mg in the treatment of pediatric nematode infection. Both agents had 100% cure rates for *Ascaris.* In treatment of trichuriasis, mebendazole produces a higher cure rate (60%) than does albendazole (33.3%).

Gocmen et al. reported that the recurrence rate for hydatid cyst in pediatric cases was less after mebendazole treatment than after surgery, but the difference was not statistically significant.

PRAZIQUANTEL

History and Source

Praziquantel is a derivative of the pyrazinoisoquinolines, a category of drugs determined in 1972 to have anthelminthic activity. It has broad-spectrum activity against cestodes and trematodes, but not against nematodes.

Official Name and Chemistry

Praziquantel is a synthetic isoquinoline-pyrazine derivative.

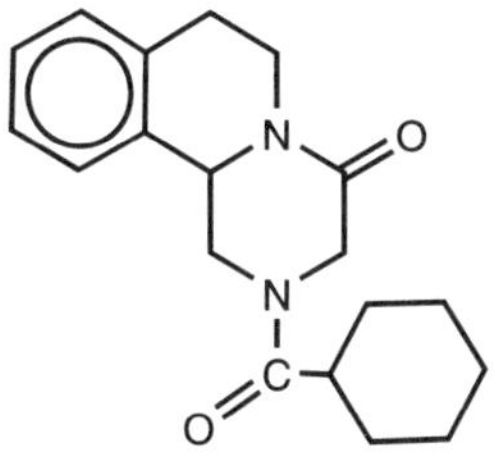

Praziquantel

Pharmacology

Praziquantel at low concentrations causes spastic paralysis in susceptible helminths. At higher concentrations, it causes vacuolization of parasite tegument. The molecular basis of effect is believed to be dependent on increased cell membrane permeability to calcium.

Clinical Pharmacology

The threshold serum concentration for activity is 0.3 μg/ml. It is effective against all species of schistosome, and against most other trematode and cestode infection as a single dose; in schistosomiasis, worms are immobilized and passively shifted to the liver.

Pharmaceutics

The trade name for praziquantel is Biltricide, which is available as an oral 600-mg tablet. Other strengths are available outside the United States.

Pharmacokinetics

Praziquantel is rapidly absorbed after oral administration. Peak plasma concentration of 0.2 to 2 μg/ml is achieved at 1 to 2 hours. CSF fluid concentration is 15% to 20% that of plasma concentration. Bioavailability of the agent is limited by rapid first-pass hepatic metabolism to hydroxylated and conjugated products.

The plasma $t_{\frac{1}{2}}$ of Praziquantel is 1.5 hours; that of its metabolites is 4 to 6 hours. Eighty percent of the dose of praziquantel is excreted in the urine as metabolites by day 4.

Therapeutic Use

Schistosomiasis

A single dose of 40 mg/kg or three doses of 20 mg/kg praziquantel 4 to 6 hours apart is effective treatment for *Salmonella mansoni* and *S. haematobium.* Two doses of 30 mg/kg several hours apart is treatment for *S. japonicum.* Resistance apparently does not occur; prophylactic benefit has not been established.

Neurocysticercosis

Neurocysticercosis requires hospitalization with observation by physicians with neurologic expertise. Treatment is 50 mg/kg/day praziquantel in three divided doses for a 14-day course. Response to treatment ranges from cure to no clinical improvement.

Side Effects

Transient, dose-related side effects of praziquantel include abdominal cramping, nausea, malaise, dizziness, drowsiness, and headache. Eosinophilia and skin rash have also occasionally been reported to occur several days after treatment. Minor electrocardiographic and transient liver function tests have been reported. Concurrent use of steroids decreases serum levels of praziquantel, but decreased efficacy has not been shown.

High-risk Groups

Numerous studies have been negative for carcinogenicity, mutagenicity, and teratogenicity. The drug is better tolerated by children than adults.

IVERMECTIN

History and Source

Ivermectin is the drug of choice in the treatment of onchocerciasis. It is a derivative of a soil actinomycete: *Streptomyces avermitilis.*

Official Drug Name and Chemistry

Ivermectin is a semisynthetic hydrogenated macrocyclic lactone.

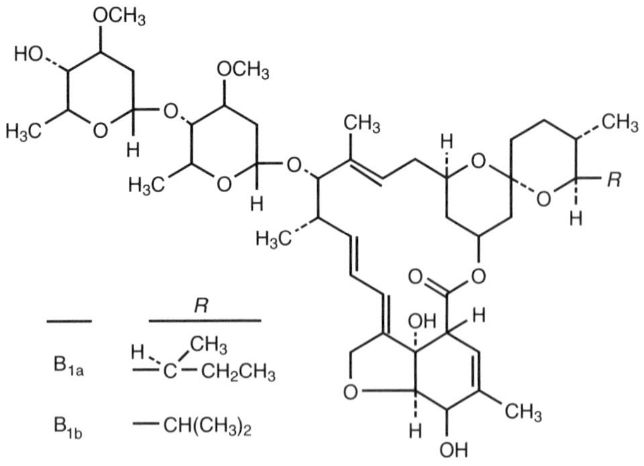

	R
B_{1a}	$-CH(CH_3)CH_2CH_3$
B_{1b}	$-CH(CH_3)_2$

Ivermectin

Pharmacology

Ivermectin acts by paralyzing nematodes by enhancing GABA-mediated signal transmission in peripheral nerves. Ivermectin is not active against adult worms in *O. volvulus.* Within 3 days of treatment, microfilaria counts decrease precipitously. In female worms, intrauterine microfilariae are also destroyed.

Clinical Pharmacology

In humans, γ-aminobutyric acid (GABA) signal transmission occurs only in the CNS. Because Ivermectin does not cross the blood–brain barrier (BBB), toxicity is minimal.

Pharmaceutics

Ivermectin is available as Mectizan in a 6 mg tablet but is not marketed in the United States. It is available from Merck Sharp and Dohme through physician compassionate use.

Pharmacokinetics

Ivermectin is administered orally and is readily absorbed by the GI tract. Peak serum concentration is achieved at 4 hours. Effective plasma concentration is 20 ng/ml. Plasma $t_{\frac{1}{2}}$ is 12 hours for the parent drug and 72 hours for drug metabolites. Ivermectin is excreted in feces; excretion is complete at approximately 12 days.

Therapeutic Use

Treatment with ivermectin consists of a single oral dose of 3 mg/15 to 25 kg body weight, 6 mg/26 to 44 kg body weight, 9 mg/45 to 64 kg body weight, and 15 mg/65 kg or greater body weight. Patients in endemic areas may require retreatment at a 6- to 24-month interval. Retreatment schedule depends on skin microfilarial load.

Side Effects and Toxicity

Ivermectin has far fewer side effects than diethylcarbamazine (DEC).

Ocular

Reported ocular side effects include conjunctivitis, punctate corneal opacities, uveitis, optic neuritis, and chorioretinitis. These conditions typically do not result in permanent visual loss.

Systemic

Systemic side effects typically are mild. Fewer than 15% of patients experience a mild Mazzotti allergic reaction. Approximately 1% have more severe reactions, including hypotension, tachycardia, joint and muscle pain, skin rash, lymphangitis, and lymphadenitis. Ivermectin may prolong prothrombin time (PT), but complications related to bleeding have not been reported.

High-risk Groups

Ivermectin should not be used in pregnant women or in children aged less than 5 years. Teratogenic effects have been observed in laboratory animals. The drug should not be used in patients with an impaired BBB (e.g., in meningitis).

Drug Interactions

Ivermectin should not be used in combination with agents that increase GABA activity, such as barbiturates, benzodiazapines, and valproate.

Clinical Trials

Zheng et al. conducted a randomized double-masked clinical study comparing single-dose ivermectin with full-course DEC in the treatment of microfilariasis. They concluded that ivermectin was a practical alternative to DEC.

In a randomized comparison of single-dose ivermectin (200 mg/kg) versus two-dose ivermectin (200 mg/kg) for 2 days versus thiabendazole (50 mg/kg) twice a day for 3 days in treatment of strongyloidiasis, Gann et al., observed that single-dose ivermectin had efficacy similar to that of thiabendazole, with fewer side effects.

DIETHYLCARBAMAZINE

History and Source

DEC was introduced 35 years ago as a treatment for onchocerciasis. It is the treatment of choice for *Wuchereria bancrofti* (filariasis), *Brugia Malayi* (filariasis), *Loa loa* (loisis), and tropical eosinophilia. It is an alternative treatment for *O. volvulus* (onchocerciasis).

Official Drug Name and Chemistry

The chemical structure of DEC, a synthetic piperazine derivative, is shown below.

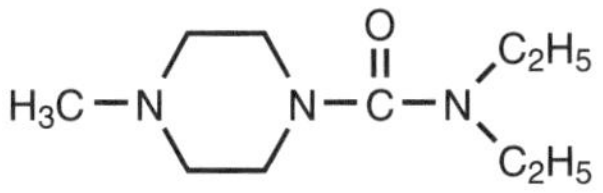

Diethylcarbamazine

Clinical Pharmacology

DEC immobilizes microfilariae and exposes the organism's surface antigens. This augments host immune-response efficacy in the destruction of microfilariae. The mechanism of action of DEC against adult worms is not known.

Pharmaceutics

DEC, available under the trade names Banocide, Notezine, and Hetrazan, is a citrate salt that contains 51% of the active base. It is formulated as a 50-mg tablet. No longer marketed in the United States, it is only available through physician compassionate use.

Pharmacokinetics

DEC is readily absorbed from the GI tract. An oral dose of 400 mg DEC citrate reaches a peak blood level of 1.6 μg/ml at 1 to 2 hours, which exceeds the minimal effective blood concentration of 0.1 to 1.0 μg/ml. The drug equilibrates with all tissues except fat. The plasma $t_{1/2}$ varies from 2 to 10 hours; shorter $t_{1/2}$ occurs in conjunction with acidic urine, whereas longer $t_{1/2}$ occurs with alkaline urine.

DEC is excreted in the urine within 30 hours. Even with multiple doses, the drug does not accumulate in patients with normal renal function.

Therapeutic Use

Filariasis and Loiasis

Infection is treated with 2 mg/kg three times a day for 3 weeks. Treatment is initiated with a test dose to assess the degree of allergic reaction to dying microfilariae. In treatment of *W. bancrofti,* a single dose of 2 mg/kg is given on day 1 followed by two doses of 2 mg/kg on day 2, followed by institution of full therapy of 2 mg/kg three times daily on day 3. In *L. loa* and *B. malayi,* therapy is initiated as a single dose of 1 mg/kg on day 1 and is increased to 2 mg/kg by day 6 of therapy.

Allergic reaction to microfilariae may be reduced by pretreatment with antihistamines. If severe allergic reaction occurs during treatment, a corticosteroid agent should be instituted and DEC should either be decreased or discontinued.

Multiple courses of treatment may be required for cure. Peripheral blood should be evaluated for microfilariae after treatment. The course of treatment may be repeated after 3 weeks.

O. volvulus

DEC is not the drug of choice for treatment of *O. volvulus* due to the high incidence of Mazzotti reaction and the inability of DEC to eradicate adult worms. Treatment consists of an initial dose of 0.5 mg/kg on day 1, 0.5 mg/kg twice daily on day 2, 1.0 mg/kg three times daily on day 3, and 2.0 mg/kg three times daily for treatment days 4 to 21.

Prophylaxis

DEC 50 mg monthly is effective prophylaxis against filariasis and 300 mg weekly is prophylaxis against loiasis.

Side Effects

Ocular

Numerous reported side effects of DEC include punctate corneal opacities due to dead intracorneal microfilariae and associated inflammation. Limbitis, uveitis, increased retinal vacular permeability, transient retinal pigment epithelialium (RPE) disturbance, white opacities under the internal limiting membrane, and papillitis have also been reported. Posterior segment findings occur in association with high levels of circulating immune complexes.

Systemic

The most notable systemic side effect of DEC is the Mazzotti reaction, a severe allergic reaction to dead microfilaria. Other side effects include skin rash, nausea, vomiting, and diarrhea. Almost all patients develop leukocytosis; eosinophilia and reversible proteinuria may also occur. Infrequent side effects reported are encephalopathy, headache, vertigo, dermatitis, and lymphadenopathy.

High-risk Groups

Caution should be used in treating patients with renal insufficiency or hypertension. Use of DEC in patients with untreated malaria should be avoided because it may provoke a relapse in asymptomatic malaria infected. Teratogenic effects have not been observed in laboratory animals.

Major Clinical Trials

See section on Clinical Trials of ivermectin.

THIABENDAZOLE

History and Source

Thiabendazole is the agent of choice in the treatment of strongyloidiasis and cutaneous larva migrans. It was discovered during screening hundreds of substituted benzimidazole compounds.

Official Name and Chemistry

Thiabendazole is a benzimidazole compound.

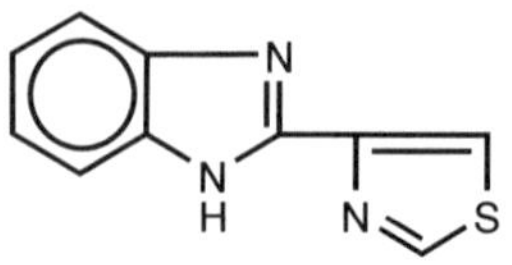

Thiabendazole

Pharmacology

The mechanism of action of thiabendazole is not known. The drug inhibits the mitochondrial filarial reductase system in helminths. In *Strongyloides,* thiabendazole inhibits microtubule assembly.

Clinical Pharmacology

Thiabendazole has low toxicity to mammalian cells. It is particularly effective against nematodes that infect the intestinal tract.

Pharmacokinetics

Thiabendazole is poorly water soluble and is rapidly absorbed on oral administration. Thiabendazole may also be absorbed though the skin. With oral administration, peak serum levels are achieved at 1 to 2 hours and final clearance occurs by 24 hours. The drug is metabolized to the 5-hydroxythiabendazole and is excreted in urine conjugated as the glucuronide or the sulfate.

Pharmaceutics

Thiabendazole (Mintezol) is available as a 500-mg chewable tablet and as a 500 mg/ml suspension. The drug should be ingested after meals.

Therapeutic Use

In the treatment of cutaneous larva migrans, the standard dose of thiabendazole is 25 mg/kg twice a day for two days. The course of treatment may be repeated in 2 days if active lesions are still present. The maximal daily dose is 3 g.

For trichinosis and strongyloidiasis, treatment is 25 mg/kg twice a day for a 5-day course. The cure rate is greater than 90% for strongyloidiasis. The efficacy in treatment of human trichinosis is unproven.

In visceral larva migrans, thiabendazole may be used in cases of severe infection, since milder cases tend to be self-limited. Treatment is 25 mg/kg thiabendazole twice daily until symptoms resolve. Prolonged courses of therapy may be limited by toxicity.

Side Effects

With standard thiabendazole treatment, 7% to 50% of patients experience adverse effects with onset typically at 3 to 4 hours and lasting 2 to 8 hours. The most common side effects are dizziness, anorexia, nausea, and vomiting. Less frequent side effects are somnolence, diarrhea, abdominal pain, headache, and pruritis. There are rare reports of bradycardia, hypotension, tinnitus, paresthesias, convulsions, hyperglycemia, visual disturbance, hematuria, crystalluria, leukopenia, and liver dysfunction. Hypersensitivity has been reported, including cases of fatal Steven Johnson syndrome.

High-risk Groups

Thiabendazole use should be avoided in pregnant women except in life-threatening infection and in children weighing less than 15 kg. The drug should be used with caution in patients with hepatic and renal insufficiency. Because of high rates of vomiting, an alternative agent should be sought for patients in whom emesis is medically contraindicated.

Hypocoagulation due to thiabendazole-acenocoumarol has been reported. Thiabendazole may also severely alter theophylline pharmacokinetics and decrease elimination.

Clinical Trials

See section on Clinical Trials of ivermectin.

PYRANTEL PAMOATE

History and Source

Originally introduced as a veterinary agent, pyrantel pamoate is a broad-spectrum anthelminthic agent. It is the treatment of choice for intestinal nematodes, *Ascaris,* and *Trichostrongylus orientalis.* It has moderate activity against hookworm species and is not effective against trichuriasis or strongyloidiasis.

Official Name and Chemistry

Pyrantel pamoate is a tetrahydropyrimidine derivative.

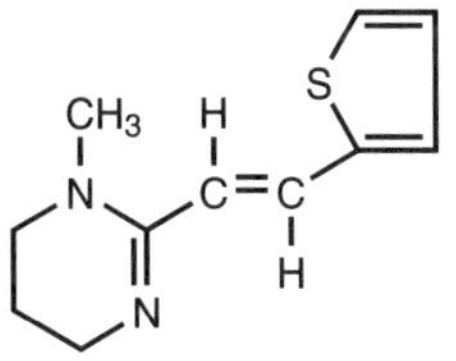

Pyrantel

Pharmacology

Pyrantel inhibits cholinesterases and exerts its effect by acting as a depolarizing neuromuscular blocking agent. This results in persistent nicotinic activation and spastic paralysis of the nematode. Pyrantel is not vermicidal or ovicidal.

Clinical Pharmacology

Pyrantel is effective against both mature and immature helminths in the intestinal tract but not against migratory stages in tissues. After drug-induced spastic paralysis occurs, worms are expelled through the host intestinal tract.

Pharmaceutics

Pyrantel pamoate (trade names: Antiminth and Combantrin) is available as a 50-mg/ml suspension. Outside the United States, it is available as a 125 mg chewable tablet.

Pharmacokinetics

Pyrantel pamoate is poorly absorbed from the GI tract. Peak plasma concentrations after oral administration is achieved at 1 to 3 hours. More than 50% of the administered dose is eliminated unmetabolized in feces. Approximately 15% of the drug is excreted in urine as parent compound and metabolites.

Therapeutic Use

Ascaris lumbricoides

For *A. lumbricoides,* pyrantel is administered as a single dose of 11 mg/kg (maximum dose 1 g) with or without food. Treatment is 85% to 100% effective; if eggs are still present 2 weeks after treatment, however, patients should receive a second course.

Hookworm

For hookworm, a single dose of pyrantel pamoate 11 mg/kg (maximum 1 g) results in a 90% cure rate for *Ancylostoma duodenale* and *T. orientalis.* In *north Americanus* infection, a 3-day course of treatment is required to achieve 90% cure rate. In patients with heavy hookworm infestation, eradication of infection may not be possible.

Side Effects

With oral administration of pyrantel pamoate, toxic effects are evident in 4% to 20% of patients. Parenteral administration in animals has resulted in complete neuromuscular blockage. Infrequent side effects observed include mild GI upset, headache, fever, and rash. No significant renal or hepatitic complications have been reported.

High-risk Groups

Myasthenia gravis may be aggravated by pyrantel pamoate therapy. Although teratogenic studies in animals have been negative, use of pyrantel pamoate in pregnant women and in children aged less than 2 years is not recommended. Combination therapy with pyrantel pamoate and piperazine is not recommended because of their antagonistic mechanisms of action.

LINDANE

History and Source

Benzene hexachloride is a mixture of eight isomers. Lindane is the γ-isomer of benzene hexachloride. It is used as a topical pediculocide and miticide, effective in the treatment of scabies; pediculosis pubic, capititis and corporis; and *Phthirus pubis.*

Official Name and Chemistry

Lindane is the γ-isomer of benzene hexachloride.

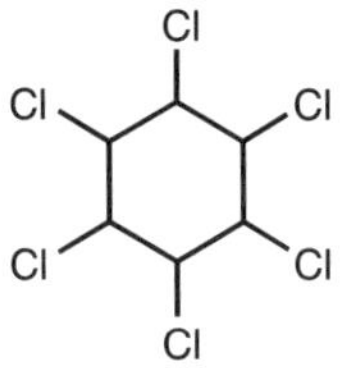

Pharmacology

Lindane is the most toxic isomer of benzene hexachloride. It acts by blocking GABA effects.

Clinical Pharmacology

Lindane is available under the trade names Kwell and Scabene. It is formulated as a 1% creme, as a lotion, and also as a shampoo for topical usage.

Therapeutic Use

Lindane is a miticide and pediculocide: A single layer of cream or lotion is applied to the skin from the neck down, with caution taken to avoid mucosal tissues. The cream is washed away after 8 to 12 hours. Relief from pruritis generally occurs in 24 hours. The cream or lotion may be applied a second time at 1 week if required.

Side Effects

Lindane is a cutaneous and mucous membrane irritant. Lindane poisoning results in tremor, ataxia, arrhythmia, and convulsions. It has been implicated in causing aplastic anemia, and hepatomas have been produced in exposed rodents.

High-risk Groups

Transplacental transport of lindane has been reported in rats. Extreme caution should be used in the treatment of pregnant women.

PENTAMIDINE

History and Source

Pentamidine is a member of the diamidine class of drugs. In 1938, the diamidines were discovered to have antiprotozoal activity. The most potent diamides are stilbamidine, propamidine, and pentamidine. Its relative stability makes pentamidine the most clinically useful of the group. It is the drug of choice in the treatment and prophylaxis of *Pneumocystis Carinii* infection.

Official Name and Chemistry

Pentamidine is 4,4′-diamidinophenoxypentane.

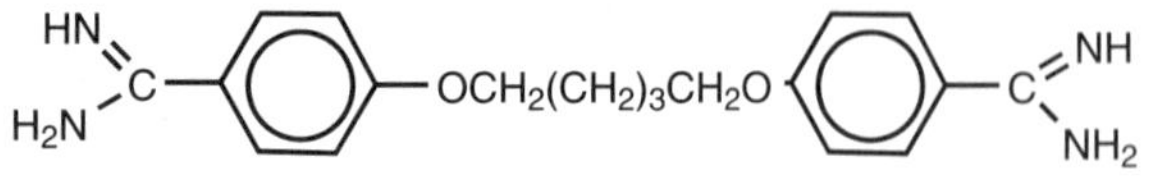

HN=C(H$_2$N)–C$_6$H$_4$–OCH$_2$(CH$_2$)$_3$CH$_2$O–C$_6$H$_4$–C(=NH)NH$_2$

Pentamidine

Pharmacology

Pentamidine is toxic to several protozoa, including *Trypanosoma rhodesiense* and *T. congolese.* It exerts a direct lethal effect on *P. carinii.* Pentamidine is also fungicidal. The mechanism by which the agent inhibits glucose metabolism in *P. carinii* is not known.

Pharmaceutics

Pentamidine isothionate is available as a 300-mg vial for injection (trade name: Pentam 300). It is also available as an aerosol (trade name: Nebupent) for inhalation.

Pharmacokinetics

After a single dose, pentamidine is eliminated with a plasma $t_{\frac{1}{2}}$ of approximately 6 hours. Pentamidine accumulates extensively in tissues, especially the liver, kidney, adrenals, and spleen. A higher concentration of drug can be delivered to the lungs by aerosol inhalation than by parenteral administration.

Therapeutic Use

For *P. Carinii,* treatment is pentamidine 4 mg/kg daily intramuscularly or intravenously for 14 days. The drug is administered as a slow infusion in 50 to 250 ml 5% dextrose in 60 minutes. Clinical improvement is apparent 4 to 6 days after initiation of therapy.

Pentamidine inhaled in aerosolized form is effective in prophylaxis against pulmonary infection when 300 mg in 5 to 10% nebulized solution is delivered in 30 to 45 minutes once a month. It is a second-line strategy for treatment of pneumocystic infection.

Side Effects

Acute side effects of pentamidine include tachycardia, shortness of breath, dizziness, headache, and vomiting. The mechanism of these effects may be associated hypotension or histamine release. Pancreatitis and hypoglycemia are well-established side effects and are potentially life-threatening. Reversible renal insufficiency and thrombocytopenia occur infrequently.

High-risk Groups

Sha et al. reported that 7 patients in a series of eight patients with *Pneumocystis* choroiditis had received aerosolized pentamidine. Pneumocystis choroiditis is a rare complication of advanced AIDS typically occurring in association with systemic dissemination. Patients frequently are receiving aerosolized pentamidine at the time of ocular diagnosis; therefore, aerosolized drug is not prophylaxis against ocular disease. Ocular disease may improve with systemic anti-*Pneumocystis* therapy.

Clinical Trials

In a multicenter clinical trial the PRIO study group evaluated the efficacy of dapsone-pyrimethamine (50 mg per week) and compared it with that of aerosolized pentamidine (300 mg per month) in primary prophylaxis of *P. carinii* pneumonia. The two patient groups had similar survival rates and similar incidence rates of pneumonia; however, aerosolized pentamidine therapy was better tolerated.

PYRIMETHAMINE

History and Source

Pyrimethamine is a folic acid analogue, effective in the treatment of *Toxoplasma gondii* and *Falciparum malaria.*

Official Name and Chemistry

Pyrimethamine, or 2,4-diaminopyrimidine, is structurally related to trimethoprim.

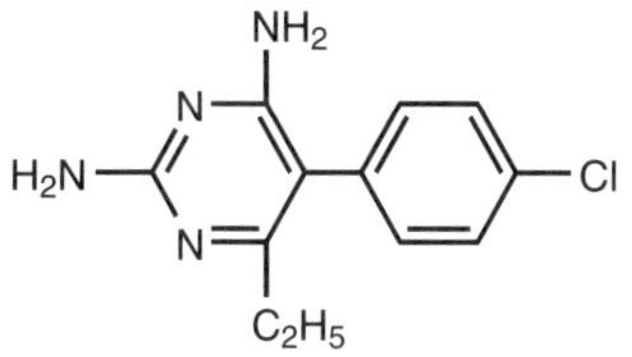

Pharmacology

Pyrimethamine penetrates a cell wall by diffusion and blocks the action of dihydrofolate reductase by substrate inhibition. Dihydrofolate reductase catalyzes reduction of dihydrofolate to tetrahydrofolate. This reaction is critical in purine and pyrimidine synthesis, and exposure to pyrimethamine results in genetically aberrant organisms. The onset of therapeutic action is slow and has no effect on nonreplicating organisms.

Clinical Pharmacology

Pyrimethamine binds with greater avidity to protozoan cells than to mammalian cells.

Pharmaceutics

Pyrimethamine is available under the trade name Daraprim as a 25-mg tablet and as an elixir.

Pharmacokinetics

Pyrimethamine is readily absorbed after oral administration. Elimination is slow, with a serum t1/2 of 4 days. Suppressive levels of the agent may be apparent as long as 2 weeks after treatment.

Therapeutic Use

Toxoplasmosis

For toxoplasmosis, optimal therapeutic effect is achieved when pyrimethamine is used in conjunction with sulfadiazine. Treatment is a loading dose of 100 to 150 mg, followed by 25 to 50 mg/day for 4 to 6 weeks. Folinic acid (leukovorin) should be administered orally or intramuscularly twice weekly throughout the course of treatment.

Prolonged use of pyrimethamine results in bone marrow suppression, leukopenia, thrombocytopenia, and megaloblastic anemia. Peripheral blood and platelet counts should be monitored once or twice weekly.

Malaria

For treatment of chloroquine-resistant *F. malaria,* a fixed pyrimethamine-sulfadoxine combination (trade name: Fansidar) is used in conjunction with quinine. Fansidar is not effective against *V. malaria,* and its efficacy against Movale and *Malariae malaria* has not been sufficiently investigated.

Treatment is chloroquine 650 mg three times a day for 3 to 7 days, with a one-time dose of 75 mg pyrimethamine/ 1,500 sulfadoxine (3 tablets Fansidar) or 25 mg pyrimethamine twice daily for 3 days and 500 mg sulfadoxine once daily for 5 days. Fansidar toxicity precludes use of a prophylactic agent.

Side Effects

Side effects are rare and include shock, nausea, vomiting, and rash. High dosages may result in megaloblastic anemia, which reverses with folinic acid administration. Toxicity may result in convulsions. The pyrimethamine/ sulfadoxine combination has been associated with Stevens-Johnson syndrome, toxic epidermal necrolysis, urticaria, and hepatitis.

High-risk Groups

Use of pyrimethamine in pregnant women should be avoided due to teratogenic risk.

Clinical Trials

Saba et al. prospectively evaluated treatment of acute toxoplasmosis in AIDS patients with a combination of azithromycin 500 mg and pyrimethamine 75 mg daily. The regimen was administered for a 14-day course. The investigators concluded that this combined therapy may be of value, but the optimum dosing of azithromycin is unclear. Jacobson et al. reported that pyrimethamine prophylaxis against toxoplasmic encephalitis is unnecessary in patients receiving trimethoprim-sulfamethoxazole. See Clinical Trials of pentamidine.

BIBLIOGRAPHY

Sulfonamides

1. Cockerill FR, Edson RS: Trimethoprim-sulfamethoxazole. *Mayo Clin Proc* 1987;62:92.
2. Drugs for parasitic infections. *Med Lett* 1990;32:23-32.
3. Drugs for parasitic infections. The Medical Letter on Drugs and Therapeutics. The Medical Letter, New Rochelle, New York 1988;30 (759): 15-22.
4. Gordin FM: Adverse reactions to trimethoprim sulfamethoxazole in patients with the acquired immunodeficiency syndrome. *Ann Intern Med* 1984;10:495.
5. May T, Beuscart C, Reynes J, Marchou B, LeClercq P, Borsa Lebas, F, Saba J, Micoud M, Mouton Y, Canton P: Trimethoprim sulfamethoxazole of pneumocystis pneumonia. LFPML Study Group. *J Acq Immune Def Syndromes* 1994; (5):457-62.
6. Rubin RH, Swartz MN: Trimethoprim-sulfamethoxazole. *N Engl J Med* 1980;303:426.
7. Webster L, Jr: Chemotherapy of parasitic diseases. In: Gilman AG, Goodman LL. Rall T, and Murad, eds. The Pharmacological Basis of Therapeutics. 7th ed. New York: MacMillan Publishers, 1990; pp 954-1012.

Trimethoprim

1. Gilman AG, Rall TW, Nies AS, Taylor P: *Goodman and Gilman: The Pharmacological Basis of Therapeutics.* New York: Pergamon Press 1990;1054-1057.
2. Jawetz E, Melnick JL, Adelberg EA, Brooks GF, Butel JS, Ornston LN: *Medical Microbiology.* East Norwalk, Connecticut: Appleton and Lange. 1989; pp. 170-1, 145-6.
3. Katzung BG: *Basic and Clinical Pharmacology.* East Norwalk, Connecticut: Appleton and Lange. 1992; pp. 664-5.
4. Pavan-Langston, DP, Dunkel EC: *Handbook of Ocular Drug Therapy and Ocular Side Effects of Systemic Drugs.* Boston: Little Brown 1991; pp. 73-6.
5. Trimethoprim-polymyxin B for Bacterial Conjunctivitis. Medical Letter on Drugs and Therapeutics. 1990;32(823):71-2.

Diethylcarbamazine

1. Awadzi K, Gilles HM: Diethylcarbamazine in the treatment of patients with onchocerciasis. *Brit J Pharmacol* 1992;34(4):281-8.
2. Fujimaki Y, et al: Deithylcarbamazine antifilarial drug, inhibits microtubule polymerization and disrupts preformed microtubules. *Biochem Pharmacol* 1990;39:851.
3. Hawking F: Diethylcarbamazine and new compounds for the treatment of filariasis. *Adv Pharmacol Chemother* 1979:16:129.
4. Mackenzie CD, Kron MA: Diethylcarbamazine: A review of its action in onchocerciasis, lymphatic filariasis and inflammation. *Trop Dis Bull* 1985:82.
5. Nutman TB, et al: Diethylcarbamazine Prophylaxis for human loiasis: Results of a double-blind study. *N Engl J Med* 1988;319-752.

Ivermectin

1. Bennett JL, Williams JS, Dave V: Pharmacology of Ivermectin. *Parasitology Today* 1988;4:226.
2. Dadzie KY, et al: Changes in Ocular Onchocerciasis four and twelve months after a community-based treatment with Ivermectin in a holoendemic onchocerciasis focus. *Tran R Soc Trop Med Hyg* 1990;84:103.
3. Gann PH, Neva FA, Gam AA: A randomized trial of single-and two-dose Ivermectin versus thiabendazole for treatment of strongyloidiasis. *J Inf Dis* 1994;169(5):1076-9.
4. Ottesen EA, et al: A controlled trial of Ivermectin and Diethylcarbamazine in lymphatic filariasis. *N Engl J Med* 1990;322:1113.
5. Zhen HJ, Piessenslof, Tao ZH, Cheng WF, Wang SH, et al: Efficacy of ivermectin for control of microfilaremia recurring after treatment with diethylcarbamazine. *I Clinical and Parasitologic Observations. Am J Trop Med Hygiene* 1991;45(2):168-74.

Praziquantel

1. El Masry NA, Bassily S, Farid Z: A comparison of the efficacy and side-effects of various regimens of praziquantel for the treatment of schistosomiases. *Trans Roy Soc Trop Med Hyg* 1988;82:719.
2. Groll E. Praziquantel. *Adv Pharmacol Chemother* 1984;20:219.
3. Vasquez ML, Jung H, Sotelo J: Plasma Levels of praziquantel decrease when dexamethasome is given simultaneously. *Neurology* 1987;37:1561.

Pyrantel Pamoate

1. Kale O: Controlled comparative study of the efficacy of pyrantel pamoate and a combined regimen of piperazine citrate in the treatment of intestinal nematodes. *Afr J Med Sci* 1981;10:63.
2. Sinniah B, Sinniah D: The anti-helmintic effects of pyrantel pamoate, oxantel-pyrantel pamoate, levamasole and mebendazote in the treatment of intestinal nematodes. *Ann Trop Med Parasitol* 1981;73:315.

Mebendazole

1. Gocmen A, Toppare MF, Kiper F: Treatment of hydatid disease in childhood with mebendazole. *European Respir J* 1963;6(2):253-7.
2. Kammerer WS, Schantz PM: Long term follow up of human hydatid disease (Echinococcus granulosus) treated with a high dose mebendazole regimen. *Am J Trop Med Hyg* 1984;33:132.
3. Mrzvak S, Schopp W, Bienzle U: Treatment of Strongyloidiasis with mebendazole. *Acta Tropica* 1983;40:93.
4. Van den Bossche, H, Rochette F, Horig C: Mebendazole and related anthelmintis. *Adv Pharmacol Chemother* 1982;19:67.

Suramin

1. Bartoloni A, Guglielmetti P, Cancrini G, Gamboa H, Roselli M, Nicoletti A, Paradisi F: Comparative efficacy of single 400mg dose of albendazole or mebendazole in the treatment of nematode infections in children. *Trop Geograph Med* 1993;45(3):114-6.
2. Cheson BD: Suramin therapy in AIDS and related disorders. Report of the U.S. Suramin Working Group. *JAMA* 1987;258:1347-51.
3. Vansterkenberg EL, Coppens I, Wilting J, Bos OH, Fischer MJ, Janssen LH, Opperdoes FR: The uptake of the trypanocidal drug suramin in combination with low-density lipoproteins by trypanosoma brucei and its possible mode of action. *Acta Tropica* 1993;54(3-4):237-50.

Thibendazole

1. Maquire AM, Zarbin MA, Connor TB, Justin J: Ocular penetration of thiabendazole. *Arch Ophthalmol* 1990;108(12):1675.

Pyrimenthamine

1. Saba J, Morlat P, Raffi F, Hazebroucg V, Joly V, Leport C, Vilde JL: Pyrimethamine plus azithromycin for treatment of acute toxoplasmosic encephalitis in patients with AIDS. *Eur J Clin Micro Inf Dis* 1993;12(11):853-6.
2. Jacobson MA, Besch CL, Child C, Hafner R, Matts JP, Muth K, Wentworth DN, Neaton JD, Abrams D, Rimland D: Primary prophylaxis with pyrimethamine for toxoplasmic encephalitis in patient with advanced human immuno deficiency virus disease: results of a randomized trial. *J Inf Disease* 1994;169(2):384-94.

Pentamidine

1. Dugel PU, Rao NA, Forster DJ, Chong LP, Frangieh GT, Sattler F: Pneumocystis carinii choroiditis after long-term aerosolized pentamidine therapy. *Am J Ophthalmol* 1990;110(2):113-7.
2. Girard PM, Landman R, Gaudebout C, Olivares R, Saimot AG, Jelazko P, Gaudebout C, Certain A, Boue F, Bouvet E: Dapsonepyrimethamine compared with aerosolized pentamidine as primary prophylaxis against pneumocystis carinii pneumonia and toxoplasmosis in HIV infection. The PRIO study group. *N Eng J Med* 1993;328(21):1514-20.
3. Sha BE, Benson CA, Deutsch T, Noskin GA, Murphy RL, Pottage JC, Finn WG, Roth SI, Kessler HA: Pneumocystis carinii choroiditis in patients with AIDS: Clinical features, response to therapy and outcome. *J Acq Immune Def* 1992;5(10):1051-8.

Textbook of Ocular Pharmacology,
edited by T.J. Zimmerman, et al.
Lippincott–Raven Publishers, Philadelphia © 1997.

CHAPTER 42

The Tetracyclines

Carol L. Karp and Eduardo C. Alfonso

THE TETRACYCLINES

History and Source

The tetracycline antibiotics were discovered as a result of soil screening for antibiotic-producing microorganisms. The first tetracycline to be introduced was chlortetracycline in 1948. A few years later, oxytetracycline became available, followed by tetracycline in 1952. Demethychlortetracycline, now termed demeclocycline, became available in 1959. Methacycline was developed in 1961, doxycycline in 1966, and minocycline in 1972 (1).

Currently six tetracycline analogues are in use in the United States. The basis of the tetracyclines derives from the Streptomyces species. Tetracycline, oxytetracycline, and demeclocycline are naturally derived compounds from the bacteria. Specifically, *Streptomyces aureofaciens* elaborates chlortetracycline and *S. rimosus* produces oxytetracycline. Demeclocycline is a product of a mutant strain of *S. aureofaciens*. Methacycline and doxycycline are derived semisynthetically from oxytetracycline, and minocycline is a chemical modification of tetracycline. Tetracycline can also be semisynthetically produced from chlortetracycline (2).

Official Drug Name and Chemistry

Chlortetracycline (Aureomycin)
Tetracycline: Achromycin V (Lederle), Achromycin V (Lederle), SK-Tetracycline (Smith Kline & French), Sumycin (Squibb), Cyclopar (Parke-Davis), Robitet (Robins), Tetracyn (Pfipharmecs), Panmycin (Upjohn)
Demeclocycline: Declomycin (Lederle)
Oxytetracycline: Terramycin (Pfipharmecs)
Methacycline: Rondomycin (Wallace)
Doxycycline: Vibramycin (Pfizer), Doryx (Parke-Davis), SK-Doxycycline Hyclate (Smith Kline & French)
Minocycline: Minocin (Lederle)

The basis of the tetracyclines is a four-ring naphthacenecarboxamide (Fig. 1). The differences in the various drugs are based on the modification of this basic structure (Table 1).

Pharmacology

Tetracyclines impede protein synthesis through attachment to the bacterial 30S ribosomal subunit, which blocks the attachment of aminoacyl transfer RNA to the acceptor site on the messenger RNA ribosome unit and prevents the addition of amino acids to a growing polypeptide chain. In gram negative bacteria, the tetracycline drug first enters by passive diffusion through the porin proteins in the outer cell membrane. The more lipophilic agents pass more easily through the lipid bilayer. The next barrier is the inner cytoplasmic membrane. The tetracyclines are transported with an active transport mechanism (3). The transport of the drug into gram-positive organisms also appears to involve an energy-dependent process. The binding of tetracyclines to the 30S ribosome is generally reversible, although a small percentage may remain irreversibly bound. Furthermore, in high doses, the drug may penetrate into mammalian cells; generally, however, mammalian cells lack the active transport mechanism to deliver the drug intracellularly. Differences in ribosomal sensitivity to tetracyclines may also play a role in the efficacy of the drug response.

Clinical Pharmacology

The tetracyclines are termed broad-spectrum antibiotics and are effective against a wide range of bacteria, includ-

C. L. Karp and E. C. Alfonso: Department of Ophthalmology, Bascom Palmer Eye Institute, University of Miami School of Medicine, Miami, Florida 33136.

ing gram-positive, gram-negative, aerobic, and anaerobic organisms. Furthermore, the tetracyclines are active against certain rickettsiae, mycoplasma, chlamydia, atypical mycobacteria, and some protozoa (3).

The tetracyclines are bacteriostatic in vitro. The sensitivity of the various tetracycline compounds is similar, although the newer compounds minocycline and doxycycline are more active and longer-acting than the other derivatives. Demeclocycline and methacycline are intermediate-acting and tetracycline and oxytetracycline are short-acting versions of the drug, requiring more frequent dosing.

In terms of gram-positive cocci, most strains of *Streptococcus pneumoniae* are susceptible to the tetracyclines, with minimum inhibitory concentration (MIC) 90 of 0.4 to 0.8 μg/ml. Other streptococci such as *S. pyogenes, S. agalactiae, S. viridans,* and some anaerobic streptococci are susceptible, but are generally not used because of the high incidence of resistance. Almost all strains of *S. faecalis* (group D, enterococcus) are resistant. *Staphylococcus aureus* is also generally resistant to the tetracyclines, with an MIC 90 of 25 μg/ml for tetracycline or doxycycline (1). The tetracyclines are active against several gram-positive bacilli such as *Bacillus anthracis, Clostridium tetani,* and *Listeria monocytogenes.*

Neisseria gonorrhoeae and *N. meningitis* are inhibited by the tetracyclines (MIC 90 is 1 to 2 μg/ml), but many resistant organisms have emerged in the United States, and the Center for Disease Control (CDC) no longer recommends tetracycline as the sole treatment for gonococcal infections (4,5).

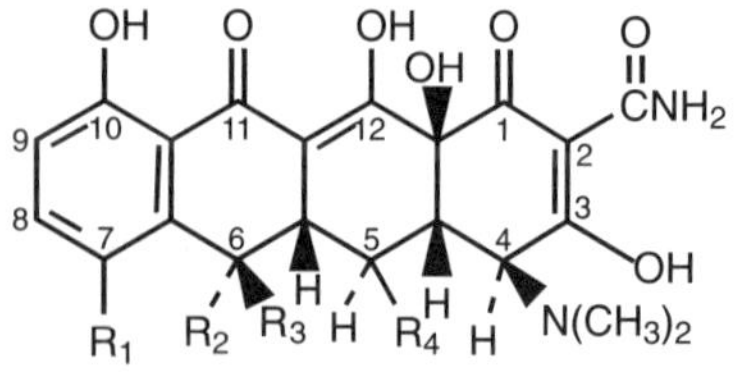

FIG. 42-1. Structural formula of the tetracyclines (see Table 1).

Table 42-1. *Modification of the basic structure of the tetracyclines*

Generic name	R_1	R_2	R_3	R_4
Short-acting				
Tetracycline	H	OH	CH_3	H
Oxytetracycline	H	OH	CH_3	OH
Intermediate-Acting				
Demeclocycline	Cl	OH	H	H
Methacycline	H	$=CH_3$		OH
Long-Acting				
Doxycycline	H	H	CH_3	OH
Minocycline	$N(CH_3)_2$	H	H	H

The tetracyclines are effective against certain gram-negative organisms, although resistances are increasing. *Haemophilus influenzae* may still be sensitive (6). Other susceptible organisms include *Pseudomonas pseudomallei, Campylobacter jejuni, Vibrio cholerae, Francisella tularensis, Pasteurella multocida, Leptotrichia buccalis, Bordetella pertussis, Yersinia pestis, Y. enterocolitica,* and Brucella. The tetracyclines are also effective against anaerobes such as Actinomyces and Fusobacterium. The activity against *Bacteroides fragilis* is unreliable (7).

The tetracyclines are highly effective against rickettsiae, which cause diseases such as Rocky Mountain spotted fever, murine typhus, rickettsial pox, and Q fever. They are also active against spirochetes including *Borrelia burgdorferi,* which causes Lyme disease, *Borrelia recurrentis, Treponema pallidum* (syphilis), and *T. pertenue.* They are the drug of choice for chlamydial disease (except in children and pregnant women). In high concentrations, the tetracyclines are active against *Entamoeba histolytica,* protozoans, and certain strains of *Plasmodium falciparum.* Minocycline is active against *Nocardia asteroides* (8). In addition to their antibiotic effects, tetracyclines also appear to possess anti-inflammatory and anticollagenase effects (9) and are used for acne, rosacea, blepharitis and gingivitis.

Resistance

Bacterial resistance has become a significant problem. Many staphylococci, streptococci, and Bacteroides are no longer susceptible to tetracycline. Similarly, many *Enterobacteriaceae, P. aeruginosa,* pneumococci, and *N. gonorrhoeae* are resistant.

The primary mechanism of resistance is probably due to alterations in the bacterial cell walls leading to decreased uptake of the tetracyclines by the energy-dependent transport process. In addition, some strains of *Escherichia coli* with ribosomal resistance have been isolated, and some bacteria may produce enzymes which degrade the antibiotic (10).

Pharmaceutics

The tetracyclines are available in oral, parental, and ophthalmic topical forms. Intrathecal, intramuscular, and topical skin use is not advised. The tetracyclines are available orally in tablet or capsular form. Some are also available in powders, syrups, and oral suspensions. The appropriate dose varies, depending on the existing pathology. Single doses vary from 50 to 500 mg depending on the preparation. The appropriate dose of tetracycline and oxytetracycline in adults and nonpregnant women is 1–2 g/day. Children aged more than 8 years should receive 25 to 50 mg/kg daily in two to four divided doses.

Ophthalmic preparations include chlortetracycline hydrochloride ophthalmic ointment, tetracycline hydrochloride ointment, and tetracycline hydrochloride ophthalmic suspension. The suspensions are usually in 1% concentrations.

Short-acting Tetracyclines

- Tetracycline
  - Generic: Suspension and syrup 125 mg/5 ml
  - Achromycin V (Lederle): Suspension 125 mg/5 ml
  - SK-Tetracycline (Smith Kline & French): Syrup 125 mg/5 ml, contains 1% alcohol
  - Sumycin (Squibb): Syrup 125 mg/5 ml, buffered with potassium metaphosphate
- Oral Tetracycline Hydrochloride
  - Generic (Mylan, Warner Chilcott): 250-mg and 500-mg capsules, 250-mg tablets
  - Achromycin V (Lederle), Cyclopar (Parke-Davis), Robitet (Robins), Tetracyn (Pfipharmecs): 250-mg and 500-mg capsules
  - Panmycin (Upjohn): 250-mg capsules
  - Sumycin (Squibb): 250-mg and 500-mg capsules and tablets
- Intravenous tetracycline
  - Achromycin IV (Lederle): 250 mg and 500 mg sterile powder with ascorbic acid 625 mg or 1.25 g to be diluted and injected at a rate not exceeding 2 mg/min.
- Intramuscular Tetracycline Hydrochloride
  - Achromycin IM (Lederle): 100 mg and 250 mg sterile powder with procaine hydrochloride 40 mg, magnesium chloride 46.84 mg, and ascorbic acid 250 or 275 mg
- Oral Oxytetracycline
  - Terramycin (Pfipharmecs): 250-mg film-coated tablets
- Oral Oxytetracycline Hydrochloride
  - Generic: 250-mg capsules
  - Terramycin (Pfipharmecs): 250-mg capsules
- Intravenous Oxytetracycline Hydrochloride
  - Terramycin IV (Pfipharmecs): 250 mg powder dissolved in 10 ml sterile water for injection, then diluted to 100 ml with sodium chloride or 5% dextrose.
- Intramuscular Oxytetracycline
  - Terramycin (Pfipharmecs): 50-mg/ml solution with 2% lidocaine in 2 ml and 10 ml or 125 mg/ml with 2% lidocaine in 2-mg containers

Intermediate-acting Tetracyclines

- Oral Demeclocycline Hydrochloride
  - Declomycin (Lederle): 150-mg capsules, 150-mg and 300-mg tablets.
- Oral Methacycline Hydrochloride
  - Rondomycin (Wallace): 150-mg and 300-mg capsules

Long-acting Tetracyclines

- Oral Doxycycline calcium
  - Vibramycin (Pfizer): 50 mg/5 ml
- Doxycycline Hyclate
  - Generic (Mylan, and Warner Chilcott): 50-mg and 100-mg tablets
  - Doryx (Parke-Davis): 100-mg capsules
  - SK-Doxycycline Hyclate (Smith Kline & French), Vibramycin (Pfizer): 50-mg and 100-mg capsules
- Doxycycline monohydrate
  - Vibramycin (Pfizer): 25 mg/5 ml or powder for oral suspension after reconstitution
- Intravenous Doxycycline Hyclate
  - Vibramycin IV (Pfizer): 100 mg or 200 mg powder with ascorbic acid 480 or 960 mg
- Oral Minocycline Hydrochloride
  - Minocin (Lederle): 50 mg and 100 mg base, oral suspension with 50 mg base/5 ml with 5% alcohol.
- Intravenous Minocycline Hydrochloride
  - Minocin IV (Lederle): 100 mg sterile powder.

Topical Products

- Topicycline (Roberts): Tetracycline hydrochloride 2.2 mg/ml, applied to affected skin area twice daily
- Achromycin 1% ophthalmic ointment (Lederle): 10 mg tetracycline hydrochloride per gram
- Achromycin 1% ophthalmic solution (Lederle): 10 mg tetracycline hydrochloride per milliliter
- Aureomycin 1% topical ophthalmic ointment 10 mg chlortetracycline HCl/gram lanolin-petrolatum base.

TERAK (Akorn) ophthalmic ointment: 5 mg oxytetracy tetracycline, 10,000 U of polymyxin B sulfate, white and liquid petrolatum per gram.

Ophthalmic preparations based on *Physicians Desk Reference for Ophthalmology* (PDR, 24th ed.). New Jersey: Medical Economics Data Production Company, 1996.

Oral Mixtures

- Urobiotic-250 (Roerig): Oxytetracycline hydrochloride 250 mg, sulfamethizole 250 mg, phenazopyridine hydrochloride 50 mg.
- Mysteclin-F (Squibb): Tetracycline hydrochloride 250 mg, amphotericin B 50 mg; syrup contains tetracycline hydrochloride 125 mg and amphotericin B 25 mg.

Pharmacokinetics, Concentration–effect Relationship, and Metabolism: Routes of Administration

The tetracyclines are usually administered orally, but as already described, may be administered in parental form. The longer-acting derivatives doxycycline and minocycline are generally better tolerated intravenously than are the shorter-acting derivatives tetracycline and oxytetracycline. The drug is rarely administered intramuscularly as it is very painful and poorly absorbed systemically through the muscles. Topical application is generally avoided except for ophthalmic use.

Absorption

Oral tetracyclines are primarily absorbed in the proximal small intestine. The short-acting tetracycline and oxytetracycline and intermediate-acting demeclocycline and methacycline are incompletely absorbed from the intestinal tract, and absorption is hindered by food. The longer-acting drugs are better absorbed and less affected by the presence of food. Barza and Scheife (11) have shown that the absorption of doxycycline and minocycline is almost 100% on an empty stomach, but that absorption of chlortetracycline is decreased to 30%. The tetracyclines form insoluble complexes with calcium, zinc, iron, aluminum, and other compounds. Coingestion of milk products, vitamins, antacids, bismuth subsalicylate (12), and minerals will result in decreased and unpredictable serum levels. Peak serum levels occur between 1 and 4 hours depending on the drug, and usually achieve 2 to 3 μg/ml. Duration depends on which formulation of tetracycline is used; the $t_{\frac{1}{2}}$ of tetracycline and oxytetracycline being 6 to 12 hours and that of demeclocycline, methacycline, doxycycline, and minocycline is 16 to 18 hours.

Ocular penetration of oxytetracycline and chlortetracycline is hindered by the corneal epithelium and therefore improved by the presence of a corneal defect (13). The more lipophilic derivatives of tetracycline, such as minocycline, appear to have better ocular penetration when administered systemically than do derivatives such as chlortetracycline.

Distribution

The tetracyclines are bound to plasma proteins in varying amounts. The volume of distribution of the tetracyclines is larger than that of the body water (5). All the tetracyclines are concentrated in the liver and excreted into the bile. The concentrations in the bile are 5 to 20 times that of serum. The bile is excreted into the intestine, where the drug may be partially reabsorbed. Impaired hepatic function or duct obstruction may lead to persistence of the drug in the blood.

The tetracyclines have an affinity for metabolically active tissue and therefore accumulate not only in the liver, but also in new bone and teeth, especially prenatally and in early life. The tetracyclines cross the placenta, and concentrations of tetracycline in the umbilical cord may reach 60% of the mother's serum level and 20% in the amniotic fluid.

The lipid solubility of the tetracyclines also varies depending on the preparation. The long-acting minocycline and doxycycline have excellent penetration into the tears, saliva, prostate, kidney, and endometrium. Oral minocycline penetrates well into the eye, and a study has shown aqueous levels of minocycline to be approximately half the plasma level (14). The more lipophilic structure of minocycline facilitates gastrointestinal (GI) absorption, and improves blood–brain and blood–eye penetration (15). Thus, the long-acting drugs are also helpful in eradicating pelvic inflammatory disease and can be used to sterilize the meningococcal carrier state.

Elimination

The tetracyclines have an enterohepatic circulation and are both recovered and excreted in the feces. The primary route of elimination, however, is through the kidneys. Impaired glomerular filtration significantly reduces the drug clearance. Minocycline has low renal clearance, and may be metabolized in the enterohepatic circulation. Its $t_{\frac{1}{2}}$ is not prolonged in patients with hepatic failure. Furthermore, the elimination of doxycycline is not affected by renal or hepatic failure. The drug is excreted in the feces, largely as a chelated product. Therefore, the drug has the significant advantage of not requiring modification in patients with kidney or liver failure.

Therapeutic Use

Prophylaxis of Ophthalmia Neonatorum

The Centers of Disease Control (CDC) and the Committee on Drugs, the Committee on Infectious Disease of the American Academy of Pediatrics, and the Committee on Fetus and Newborn include 1% tetracycline as an acceptable and effective prophylaxis of gonococcal ophthalmia neonatorum due to *N. gonorrhoeae* or *Chlamydia trachomatis* (16,17).

Treatment for Chlamydial Infections

The tetracyclines are effective in several diseases caused by Chlamydia, including conjunctivitis, urethritis, cervicitis, and pneumonitis. Trachoma is treated with oral doxycycline 2.5 to 4 mg/kg daily for 40 days (18). Acute trachoma may be treated with topical tetracycline for 2 to 4 weeks with the ointment vehicle (15). Adult inclusion conjunctivitis is treated with oral tetracycline 250 mg four times daily or doxycycline 100 mg twice daily for 3 weeks. Phlyctenular keratoconjunctivitis has been treated effectively with oral tetracyclines (19). Urethritis and endocervicitis caused by *C. trachomatis* also responds to tetracycline (20). The patient's sexual partner also should be treated.

Blepharitis, Acne, and Rosacea

The tetracyclines are helpful in cases of acne (21), blepharitis (22), and rosacea (23). This may be secondary to the effect on *Propionibacterium* in the skin follicles. The antiinflammatory effects of the tetracyclines may also play a role in its effectiveness. (See section on Gingivitis.) The doses recommended are generally tetracycline 250 mg orally four times daily for 6 weeks, then reduced to 250 mg twice daily for 6 more weeks (22).

Persistent Corneal Epithelial Defects/Gingivitis

The tetracyclines have anticollagenase (24) and antiinflammatory (25,26) properties in addition to their antibiotic properties and may be helpful in treating persistent epithelial defects. The basis of this effect is believed to be secondary to the tetracyclines' effect on anticollagenase and metalloproteinase activity after trauma to the corneal epithelium (27). Forms of gingivitis and periodontal disease may be treated similarly (24).

Other Uses

The tetracyclines are the drug of choice for cholera, brucellosis, melioidosis, leptospirosis, *M. pneumoniae,* and rickettsial infections. The tetracyclines may also provide effective therapy against tularemia, yaws, anthrax, traveler's diarrhea, Whipple's disease, pinworms, and molluscum contagiosum (15). Other uses of the tetracyclines include treatment for sexually transmitted diseases, including gonorrhea, syphilis, trichomonads, and lymphogranuloma venereum.

Tetracycline and minocycline may be effective for toxoplasmosis, with the suggested doses of minocycline 100 mg once or twice daily or tetracycline 250 mg four times daily (28,29) for 4 to 6 weeks. Lyme disease is also effectively treated with tetracycline 250 to 500 mg orally four times daily for 10 to 30 days depending on the response (15). (See Retina section for further information.)

Demeclocycline may also be helpful in cases of syndrome of inappropriate antidiuretic hormone (SIADH) (30).

Side Effects and Toxicity

Gastrointestinal

The tetracyclines produce gastrointestinal irritation in some patients. The side effects include abdominal discomfort, nausea, vomiting, epigastric burning, and flatulence. These effects are usually dose related and may occur in 10% of patients receiving 2 g or more tetracycline daily (2). The drugs may produce esophagitis or even pancreatitis (32,33).

The gastric irritation may be diminished by taking food with the drug but, as described, this may limit the absorption of the tetracycline compounds, especially in the presence of milk or calcium-containing products. The chemical/irritative diarrhea must be distinguished from pseudomembranous diarrhea, which would require immediate treatment with vancomycin.

Hepatic Toxicity

The tetracyclines may cause liver toxicity in patients receiving large doses of oral or intravenous tetracycline, usually 2 g or more of daily consumption. The damage can be detected by liver function studies. Histologic studies show a fatty metamorphosis with other cytoplasmic changes (34,35). Patients with preexisting hepatic or renal damage are especially susceptible to the fatty changes occurring with the tetracyclines. Pregnant women, who appear to be especially susceptible to tetracycline-induced damage, also constitute a high-risk group.

Renal Toxicity

All the tetracyclines can increase blood urea nitrogen (BUN) levels and produce a negative nitrogen balance. This is generally of no significance in patients with normal renal function, but the tetracyclines may exacerbate renal dysfunction in patients with renal failure. Tetracyclines other than doxycycline should probably be avoided in the setting of renal failure (2). Although the doxycycline analogue is believed to be safer in these settings because of its gastrointestinal excretion, the drug may indeed have renal side effects and should be used with care (36).

Nephrogenic diabetes insipidus has been documented in patients receiving demeclocycline. The syndrome is reversible with discontinuation of the antibiotic. This effect has been used therapeutically to treat chronic SIADH.

Outdated and degradation products of the tetracyclines have produced a Fanconi-like syndrome of emesis, polyuria, polydipsia, proteinuria, acidosis, glycosuria, and aminoaciduria due to toxicity of the proximal renal tubules. Outdated tetracyclines have also been known to produce a systemic lupus-like picture (2).

Toxicity to Bones and Teeth

Tetracyclines can chelate with calcium to form a tetracycline-calcium orthophosphate complex. Bone growth is depressed in the fetus and in young children receiving this treatment but can be reversed with discontinuation of the medication.

The tetracyclines can cause discoloration of developing deciduous and permanent teeth. The period of greatest risk to the teeth is from midpregnancy to 6 months postpartum for the deciduous anterior teeth, and from 4 to 6 months of age to 5 years of age for the permanent anterior teeth, the periods when the crowns are being formed. This damage can occur to age 8; therefore, use of these drugs should be avoided in this age group. Doxycycline and oxytetracycline may produce less tooth discoloration than other tetracycline formulations.

Nervous System Toxicity

The tetracyclines may cause pseudotumor cerebri in young infants and sometimes adults, even in appropriate doses (38). The spinal fluid composition is normal, but the pressure is increased. The pressure usually becomes normal on discontinuation of the drug (39). The tetracyclines have also been implicated in the unmasking or worsening of myasthenia gravis (40).

Vertigo is a common side effect in patients treated with minocycline. This tetracycline analogue is very lipid soluble and appears to concentrate in lipid cells of the vestibular system. The symptoms of lightheadedness, dizziness, nausea, and tinnitus usually begin 2 to 3 days after the initiation of the drug and is reversible with discontinuation. Patients taking minocycline should be advised of this possible side effect, and avoid operating machinery or driving.

Conjunctival deposits similar to those observed in epinephrine-treated glaucoma patients can be observed in patients treated with oral tetracycline. The pigment concentrations give a yellow fluorescence characteristic of tetracycline (41). Furthermore, myopia and altered color vision may be rare side effects (42).

Photosensitivity

Reactions subsequent to sun exposure can occur with treatment with any of the tetracycline analogues, but is especially common with democycline. Exaggerated sunburn and erythema are common. Bullae can also occur occasionally.

Hypersensitivity

Hypersensitivity reactions to the tetracyclines can occur and usually involve the skin. Manifestations include urticaria, exfoliative dermatitis, idiopathic nonthrombocytopenic purpura, angioedema, and asthma. Anaphylaxis has been reported rarely.

Hematologic

Tetracyclines can depress plasma prothrombin activity. Patients receiving anticoagulants may need to lower their doses. Other hematologic changes include possible eosinophilia, leukocytosis, atypical lymphocytes, and thrombocytopenia purpura.

Other Side Effects

Tetracyclines can produce thrombophlebitis when administered intravenously. Tetracyclines may cause discoloration of the thyroid gland (43). Pigmentation of the skin (44,45) nails, and mucous membranes has been reported (46).

High-risk Groups

The tetracyclines should be used with caution in children, pregnant women, and patients with renal failure or liver disease.

Drug Interactions

Magnesium, iron, zinc, aluminum, and calcium are divalent or trivalent cations and can chelate tetracyclines. Tetracyclines therefore should not be administered with milk products, antacids, cathartics, or vitamins containing these ions to avoid chelation and decreased absorption (47,48). Doxycycline and bismuth subsalicylate are often used to treat traveler's diarrhea, but to improve doxycycline's absorption should not be ingested together (49,50).

The half-life of doxycycline may be decreased by drugs that increase the hepatic metabolism, causing carbamazepine (Tegretol), phenytoin (Dilantin) (51), and other barbiturates (52).

Tetracyclines may interfere with the bactericidal action of penicillins. Tetracycline may lead to a change in the GI flora and therefore prevent inactivation of digoxin. Increased serum digoxin levels can occur (53). Breakthrough bleeding and pregnancy may occur in patients receiving oral contraceptives and antibiotics. Patients should be warned of this possibility and should seek additional contraceptive protection (54,55).

The tetracyclines increase BUN, and their combined administration with diuretic agents can also lead to an increase in BUN (56). A severe renal effect can occur with tetracyclines and methoxyflurane (penthrane), leading to renal failure and even death (57). Oxytetracycline has been reported to reduce insulin requirements and increase the hypoglycemic effect of tolbutamide. Diabetic patients receiving both tolbutamide and oxytetracycline should be monitored for signs of hypoglycemia (58). Tetracycline may cause lactic acidosis in patients receiving phenformin (59). Tetracyclines can potentiate warfarin; therefore, prothrombin time (PT) should be monitored in patients receiving both medications (60).

REFERENCES

1. Gilman AG, Rall TW, Nies AS, Taylor P, eds. *Goodman and Gilman's the Pharmacological Basis of Therapeutics,* 8th ed. New York: Pergamon Press, 1990.
2. Tetracyclines and chloramphenicol. In: *Drug Evaluations,* 6th ed. Chicago: American Medical Association, 1978;1409–1424.
3. Chopra I, Howe TGB. Bacterial resistance to the tetracyclines. *Microbiol Rev* 1978;42:707–724.
4. Knapp JS, Zenilman JM, Biddle JW, Perkins GH, DeWitt WE, Thomas ML, Johnson SR, Morse SA. Frequency and distribution in the United States of strains of *Neisseria gonorrhoeae* with plasmid-mediated, high-level resistance to tetracycline. *J Infect Dis* 1987; 155:819–822.
5. Jaffe HW, Biddle JW, Johnson SR, Wiesner PJ. Infections due to penicillinase-producing *Neisseria gonorrhoeae* in the United States: 1976–1980. *J Infect Dis* 1981;144:191–197.
6. Ringertz S, Dornbusch K. In vitro susceptibility to tetracycline and doxycycline in clinical isolates of *Haemophilus influenzae. Scand J Infect Dis* 1988 suppl; (53):7–11.
7. Park BH, Hendricks M, Malamy MH, Tally FP, Levy SB. Cryptic tetracycline resistance determinant (class F) from *Bacteroides fragilis* mediates resistance in *Escherichia coli* by actively reducing tetracycline accumulation. *Antimicrob Agents Chemother* 1987;31:1739–1743.
8. Dewsnup DH, Wright DN. In vitro susceptibility of *Nocardia asteroides* to 25 antimicrobial agents. *Antimicrob Agents Chemother* 1984; 25:165–167.
9. Rifkin BR, Vernillo AT, Golub LM. Blocking periodontal disease progression by inhibiting tissue-destructive enzymes: a potential therapeutic role for tetracyclines and their chemically-modified analogs. *J Periodont* 1993;64(suppl 8):819–827.
10. Speer BS, Shoemaker NB, Salyers AA. Bacterial resistance to tetracycline: mechanisms, transfer, and clinical significance. *Clin Microbiol Rev* 1992;5:387–399.
11. Barza M, Scheife RT. Antimicrobial spectrum, pharmacology, and therapeutic use of antibiotics. IV. Aminoglycosides. *J Maine Med Assoc* 1977;68:194–210.
12. Ericsson CD, Feldman S, Pickering LK, Cleary TG. Influence of subsalicylate bismuth on absorption of doxycycline. *JAMA* 1982;247: 2266–2267.
13. Douvas NG, Fetherstone RM, Bradey AE. Role of terramycin in ophthalmology. *Arch Ophthalmol* 1951;46:57.
14. Poirier RH, Ellison AC. Ocular penetration of orally administered minocycline. *Ann Ophthalmol* 1979;11:1859.
15. Mauger TF. Antimicrobials. In: Mauger TF, Craig EL, eds. *Havener's ocular pharmacology,* 6th ed. St. Louis: CV Mosby, 1994.
16. Periodic health examination, 1992 update: 4. Prophylaxis for gonococcal and chlamydial ophthalmia neonatorum. Canadian Task Force on the Periodic Health Examination. *Can Med Assoc J* 1992;147: 1449–1454.
17. American Academy of Pediatrics Committee. Prophylaxis and treatment of neonatal gonococcal infections. *Pediatrics* 1980;65:1047–1048.
18. Hoshiwara I, Ostler HB, Hanna L, Cignetti F, Coleman VR, Jawetz E. Doxycycline treatment of chronic trachoma. *JAMA* 1973;224:220–223.
19. Culbertson WW, Huang AJ, Mandelbaum SH, Pflugfelder SC, Boozalis GT, Miller D. Effective treatment of phlyctenular keratoconjunctivitis with oral tetracycline. *Ophthalmology* 1993;100:1358–1366.
20. Egerman RS. The tetracyclines. *Obstet Gynecol Clin North Am* 1992; 9:551–561.
21. Humbert P, Treffel P, Chapuis JF, Buchet S, Derancourt C, Agache P. The tetracyclines in dermatology. *J Am Acad Dermatol* 1991;25:691–697.
22. Dougherty JM, McCulley JP, Silvany RE, Meyer DR. The role of tetracycline in chronic blepharitis. Inhibition of lipase production in staphylococci. *Invest Ophthalmol Vis Sci* 1991;32:2970–2975.
23. Frucht-Pery J, Sagi E, Hemo I, Ever-Hadani P. Efficacy of doxycycline and tetracycline in ocular rosacea. *Am J Ophthalmol* 1993;116: 88–92.
24. Suomalainen K, Halinen S, Ingman T, Lindy O, Saari H, Konttinen YT, Golub LM. Tetracycline inhibition identifies the cellular sources of collagenase in gingival crevicular fluid in different forms of periodontal diseases. *Drugs Exp Clin Res* 1992;18:99–104.
25. Ingham E, Turnbull L, Kearney JN. The effects of minocycline and tetracycline on the mitotic response of human peripheral blood-lymphocytes. *J Antimicrob Chemother* 1991;27:607–617.
26. Gabler WL. Fluxes and accumulation of tetracyclines by human blood cells. *Res Commun Chem Pathol Pharmacol* 1991;72:39–51.
27. Perry HD, Kenyon KR, Lemberts DW, et al. Systemic tetracycline hydrochloride as adjunctive therapy in the treatment of persistent epithelial defects. *Ophthalmology* 1986;93:1320.
28. Engstrom RE Jr, Holland GN, Nussenblatt RB, Jabs DA. Current practices in the management of ocular toxoplasmosis. *Am J Ophthalmol* 1991;111:601–610.
29. Rollins DR, Tabbara KF, Ghosheh R, Nozik FA. Minocycline in experimental ocular toxoplasmosis in the rabbit. *Am J Ophthalmol* 1982;93:361–365.
30. Forrest JN Jr, Cox M, Hong C, Morrison G, Bia M, Singer I. Superiority of demeclocycline over lithium in the treatment of chronic syndrome of inappropriate secretion of antidiuretic hormone. *N Engl J Med* 1978;298:173–177.
31. Biller JA, Flores A, Buie T, Mazor S, Katz AJ. Tetracycline-induced esophagitis in adolescent patients. *J Pediatr* 1992;120:144–145.
32. Elmore MF, Rogge JD. Tetracycline induced pancreatitis. *Gastroenterology* 1981;81:1134–1136.
33. Nicolau DP, Mengedoht DE, Kline JJ. Tetracycline-induced pancreatitis. *Am J Gastroenterol* 1991;86:1669–1671.
34. Zimmerman HJ, Lewis JH. Hepatic toxicity of antimicrobial agents. In: Root RK, Sande MA, eds. *New dimensions in antimicrobial therapy.* New York: Churchill Livingstone, 1984;153–202. (Contemp Issues Infect Dis; vol. I.)
35. Timbrell JA. Drug hepatotoxicity. *Br J Clin Pharmacol* 1983;15: 3–14.
36. Orr LH Jr, Rudisill E Jr, Brodkin R, Hamilton RW. Exacerbation of renal failure associated with doxycycline. *Arch Intern Med* 1978; 138:793–794.
37. Cohlan SQ, Bevelander G, Tiamisic T. Growth inhibition of prematures receiving tetracycline: clinical and laboratory investigation. *Am J Dis Child* 1963;105:453–461.
38. Moskowitz Y, Leibowitz E, Ronen M, Aviel E. Pseudotumor cerebri induced by vitamin A combined with minocycline. *Ann Ophthalmol* 1993;25:306–308.
39. Walters BNJ, Gubbay SS. Tetracycline and benign intracranial hypertension: report of five cases. *Br Med J* 1981;282:19–20.
40. Kaeser HE. Drug-induced myasthenic syndromes. *Acta Neurol Scand* 1984;70:39.
41. *Ophthalmic drug facts.* St. Louis: Facts and Comparisons, 1993.
42. Fraunfelder FT. Drug-induced ocular side effects and drug interactions. Philadelphia: Lea & Febiger.
43. Purdue B. An incidental autopsy finding of black thyroid associated with minocycline therapy. *Med Sci Law* 1992;32:148–150.
44. Bridges AJ, Graziano FM, Calhoun W, Reizner GT. Hyperpigmentation, neutrophilic alveolitis, and erythema nodosum resulting from minocycline. *J Am Acad Dermatol* 1990;22:959–962.
45. Pepine M, Flowers FP, Ramos-Caro FA. Extensive cutaneous hyperpigmentation caused by minocycline. *J Am Acad Dermatol* 1993; 28:292–295.
46. Poliak SC, DiGiovanna JJ, Gross EG, Gantt G, Peck GL. Minocycline-associated tooth discoloration in young adults. *JAMA* 1985; 254:2930–2932.
47. Welling PG, Kock PA, Lau CC, Craig WA. Bioavailability of tetracycline and doxycycline in fasted and nonfasted subjects. *Antimicrob Agents Chemother* 1977;11:462–469.
48. Mattila MJ, Neuvonen PJ, Gothoni G, and Hackwon CR. Interference of iron preparations and milk with the absorption of tetracyclines. In: *European Society for the Study of Drug Toxicity: toxological problems of drug combinations.* Amsterdam: Exerpta Medica, 1972;129–133. (International Congress Series No. 254.)
49. Albert KS, Welch RD, DeSante KA, DiSanto AR. Decreased tetracycline bioavailability caused by a bismuth subsalicylate antidiarrheal mixture. *J Pharm Sci* 1979;68:586–588.
50. Ericsson CD, Feldman S, Pickering LK, Cleary TG. Influence of subsalicylate bismuth on absorption of doxycycline. *JAMA* 1982; 247:2266–2267.

51. Penttila O, Neuvonen PJ, Aho K, Lehtovaara R. Interaction between doxycycline and some antiepileptic drugs. *Br Med J* 1974;2:470–472.
52. Neuvonen PJ, Penttila O. Interaction between doxycycline and barbiturates. *Br Med J* 1974;1:535–536.
53. Lindenbaum J, Rund DG, Butler VP Jr, Tse-Eng D, Saha JR. Inactivation of digoxin by the gut flora: reversal by antibiotic therapy. *N Engl J Med* 1981;305:789–794.
54. Bacon JF, Shenfield GM. Pregnancy attributable to interaction between tetracycline and oral contraceptives. *Br Med J* 1980;280: 293.
55. Murphy AA, Zacur HA, Charache P, Burkman RT. The effect of tetracycline on levels of oral contraceptives. *Am J Obstet Gynecol* 1991; 164:28–33.
56. Tannenberg AM. Tetracycline and rises in urea nitrogen. *JAMA* 1972; 221:713–714.
57. Kuzucu EY. Methoxyflurane, tetracycline, and renal failure. *JAMA* 1970;211:1162–1164.
58. Miller JB. Hypoglycaemic effect of oxytetracycline. *Br Med J* 1966;2:1007.
59. Phillips PJ, Pain RW. Phenformin, tetracycline and lactic acidosis. *Ann Intern Med* 1977;86:111.
60. Westfall LK, Mintzer DL, Wiser TH. Potentiation of warfarin by tetracycline. *Am J Hosp Pharm* 1980;37:1620–1625.

Textbook of Ocular Pharmacology,
edited by T.J. Zimmerman, et al.
Lippincott–Raven Publishers, Philadelphia © 1997.

CHAPTER 43

Erythromycin, Clarithromycin, and Azithromycin

Robert E. Leonard II, Carol L. Karp, and Eduardo C. Alfonso

ERYTHROMYCIN, CLARITHROMYCIN, AND AZITHROMYCIN

History and Source

Erythromycin, along with the newer synthetic drugs azithromycin and clarithromycin, constitute the macrolide family of antibiotics. The compound erythromycin was discovered in 1952 by McGuire et al. (1) in the metabolic products of a strain of *Streptomyces erythreus,* originally obtained from a soil sample collected in the Philippine Archipelago.

Official Drug Name and Chemistry

Erythromycin (E-Mycin, ERYC), erythromycin estolate (Illosone), erythromycin ethylsuccinate (E.E.S., E-Mycin E), erythromycin gluceptate, erythromycin lactobionate, and erythromycin stearate (Erypar, Ethril) all have the same spectrum of antibacterial activity and uses. Erythromycin is one of the macrolide antibiotics, so termed because they contain a many-membered lactone ring to which are attached one or more deoxy sugars (2). Erythromycin contains a 14-membered lactone ring. Clarithromycin differs from erythromycin in chemical structure in that it contains a methylated hydroxyl group at position 6 in the ring structure. This confers stability in an acidic environment; thus, clarithromycin has greater bioavailability than erythromycin (3). Azithromycin differs from erythromycin in that it contains a nitrogen atom in the lactone ring structure. This so-called "azolide" configuration also confers stability under acidic conditions, enhances tissue penetration, and prolongs the half-life ($t_{\frac{1}{2}}$) of the drug (4). The structural formula of these three drugs are shown below (Fig 1).

Pharmacology

Erythromycin inhibits bacterial protein synthesis by reversibly binding to the 50S subunit of the bacterial ribosome (5). This prevents elongation of the bacterial peptide chain. Erythromycin does not bind to mammalian 80S ribosomes, which accounts for its selective toxicity. Competitive binding experiments demonstrate that the binding sites for the macrolides may overlap those of the lincosamides but are not identical to them. The binding of one of these antibiotics to the bacterial 50S ribosome may inhibit the reaction of the other; therefore, there are no clinical indications for the concurrent use of these antibiotics. Certain resistant microorganisms with mutational changes in components of this ribosomal subunit fail to bind to the drug. Erythromycin is believed not to inhibit peptide bond formation directly but rather to inhibit the translocation step wherein a newly synthesized peptidyl tRNA molecule moves from the acceptor site on the ribosome to the peptidyl (or donor) site (6).

Erythromycin may be bacteriostatic or bacteriocidal, depending on the concentration of drug, organism susceptibility, the growth rate, and the size of the innoculum. The antibacterial activity of erythromycin increases progressively over the pH range 5.5 to 8.5 for both gram-positive and gram-negative bacteria (7). This pH effect is also evident with both clarithromycin and azithromycin (8).

Clinical Pharmacology

Erythromycin is active in vitro against most gram-positive and some gram-negative bacteria, actinomycetes, my-

R. E. Leonard, C. L. Karp, and E. C. Alfonso: Department of Ophthalmology, Bascom Palmer Eye Institute, Miami, Florida 33136.

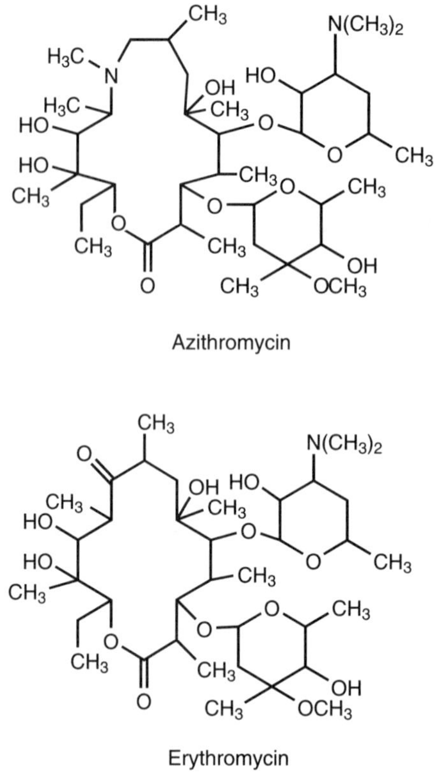

Azithromycin

Erythromycin

FIG. 43-1. Structural formulas of azithromycin and erythromycin.

coplasmas, spirochetes, chlamydiae, rickettsiae, and certain atypical mycobacteria. In general, clarithromycin and erythromycin appear to be more effective against gram-positive cocci than is azithromycin, whereas azithromycin appears to be more effective than the other two drugs against gram-negative organisms, particularly bacilli.

Among gram-positive cocci, *Streptococcus pyogenes* and *S. pneumoniae* are highly susceptible, although resistance does exist. Erythromycin also is active against most viridans and anaerobic streptococci. It is inhibitory against a number of strains of enterococcus. Most *Staphylococcus aureus* (80%) are susceptible; however, resistance in nosocomial *S. aureus* infections is reported to be as great as 12% (9). In addition, isolates of *S. aureus* that are resistant to methicillin are uniformly resistant to all the macrolide antibiotics (10). Coagulase-negative staphylococci are more susceptible to erythromycin and clarithromycin than to azithromycin, but are often resistant to all the macrolides (10).

Susceptible gram-positive bacilli include *Bacillus anthracis, Clostridium tetani, Corynebacterium diphtheriae,* and *Listeria monocytogenes.* Many strains of *C. perfringens,* anaerobic streptococci, and *Bacteroides fragilis* are only moderately susceptible to all three drugs. *Nocardia asteroides* has variable susceptibility to erythromycin alone, but may be quite sensitive to the combination of erythromycin and ampicillin.

Most strains of *N. gonorrhoeae* and *N. meningitidis,* gram-negative cocci, are susceptible to erythromycin, but azithromycin appears to be the most effective of the three drugs in treating such infections (11). *Moraxella catarrhalis* is also highly susceptible to all three drugs, but particularly to azithromycin (11).

Among gram-negative bacilli, most strains of *Bordatella pertussis, Campylobacter jejuni,* and *Haemophilus ducreyi* are susceptible, but *H. influenzae* is only moderately susceptible to erythromycin and clarithromycin. Azithromycin, however, has increased activity against *H. influenzae* (11). Most aerobic gram-negative bacilli, including Enterobacteriaceae, are resistant to erythromycin and clarithromycin, but azithromycin does have some appreciable activity against salmonellae, shegellae, and *Escherichia coli* (11).

The macrolides are active against *Mycoplasma pneumoniae, Ureaplasma urealyticum, Treponema pallidum, Legionella pneumophila,* and many strains of Rickettsia and Chlamydia. Against *Chlamydia trachomatis* and *U. urealyticum,* clarithromycin appears to be much more active than erythromycin and azithromycin (11). Some strains of nontuberculous mycobacteria are usually susceptible to the macrolide antibiotics in vitro, but others are resistant. In particular, clarithromycin appears to be particularly effective against the *Mycobacterium avium* complex (12) and *M. chelonae* (13). Both clarithromycin and azithromycin apparently have more activity than erythromycin against

M. fortuitum (13). Against *Borrelia burgdorferi,* recent studies indicate that azithromycin is more potent in vivo than either erythromycin or clarithromycin (14), although all three drugs have efficacy.

Pharmaceutics

All doses and strengths of erythromycin are expressed in terms of the base.

Erythromycin Compounds

Topical Ophthalmic Preparation

For external ocular infections involving the cornea and/or conjunctiva, apply ophthalmic preparation directly to the infected area one or more times daily depending on the severity of the infection.

Generic: Ointment, 5 mg/g (0.5%), in 3.5 and 3.75 g and UD 1 g

AK-Mycin (Akorn): Preservative-free ointment, 5 mg/g, 3.5 g

Illotycin (Dista): Ointment, 5 mg/ g, in 3.5 g and UD 1 g

Oral

For adults, dosage is 250 to 500 mg every 6 hours. Alternative schedules for the lower dosages are 333 mg every 8 hours (E-mycin and Ery-Tab only) or 500 mg every 12 hours.

Estolate: Adults, 250 to 500 mg every 6 hours. Alternative schedule for the lower dosage is 500 mg every 12 hours.

Ethylsuccinate: Adults, 400 to 800 mg every six hours. Alternative schedules for the lower dosages are 600 mg every 8 hours or 800 mg every 12 hours.

Stearate: Adults, 250 to 500 mg every 6 hours. Alternative schedule for the lower dosage is 500 mg every 12 hours. Preferably the drug is ingested on an empty stomach. See the manufacturers' recommendations for specific preparations.

All forms: For severe infections in adults, as much as 4 g may be prescribed daily in divided doses. For children, 30 to 50 mg/kg is prescribed daily in four divided doses; for severe infections, the dose may be doubled.

How Supplied:

Erythromycin

Generic: Powder; tablets (plain, enteric-coated) 250 and 500 mg

Erythromycin Base Filmtab (Abbott): Tablets (film-coated) 250 and 500 mg

E-Mycin (Upjohn): Tablets (enteric-coated) 250 and 333 mg

Erythromycin Estolate

Generic: Capsules, tablets 250 mg; suspension 125 and 250 mg/5 ml

Ilosone (Dista): Capsules 125 and 250 mg; drops 100 mg/ml; suspension 125 and 250 mg/5 ml; tablets (chewable) 125 and 250 mg; tablets 500 mg

Erythromycin Ethylsuccinate

Generic: Granules, powder for suspension 200 mg/5 ml after reconstitution; suspension 200 and 400 mg/5 ml; tablets 400 mg

E.E.S. (Abbott): Powder for oral suspension 100 mg/2.5 ml after reconstitution; granules for oral suspension 200 mg/5 ml after reconstitution; suspension 200 and 400 mg/5 ml; tablets (chewable) 200 mg, (film-coated) 400 mg

E-Mycin E (Upjohn), Wyamycin E (Wyeth): Suspension 200 and 400 mg/5 ml.

Pediamycin (Ross): Powder for oral suspension 100 mg/2.5 ml after reconstitution; granules for oral suspension 200 mg/5ml after reconstitution; suspension 200 and 400 mg/5 ml

Erythromycin Stearate

Generic: Tablets (film-coated) 250 and 500 mg, (enteric-coated) 250 mg

Erypar (Parke-Davis); Erythrocin Stearate Filmtab (Abbott); Ethril (Squibb); SK-Erythromycin (Smith Kline & French); Wyamycin S (Wyeth): Tablets (film-coated) 250 and 500 mg

Pfizer-E (Pfipharmecs): Tablets (film-coated) 250 mg

Intravenous

For severe infections, adults 1 to 4 g daily; children, 15 to 50 mg/kg daily (maximum 4 g daily). The larger doses are necessary for known or suspected *Legionella* infections. Continuous infusion is preferable, but administration in divided doses at intervals not longer than every 6 hours also is effective. Because of the irritating properties of erythromycin, intravenous push is not acceptable. An oral dosage form should be substituted as soon as possible.

How Supplied:

Erythromycin gluceptate

Ilotycin Gluceptate (Dista): Powder 250 and 500 mg and 1 g

Erythromycin lactobionate

Generic, Erythrocin Lactobionate-IV (Abbott): Powder (sterile, lyophilized) 500 mg and 1 g

Clarithromycin

Oral

For adults, the dosage is 250 mg to 500 mg every 12 hours. For children, the dosage is 15 mg/kg/day in divided doses every 12 hours.

How Supplied:

Biaxin Filmtab (Abbott): Tablets (film-coated) 250 mg and 500 mg

Biaxin Granules (Abbott): Clarithromycin granules for oral suspension, 125 mg/5 ml and 250 mg/ 5 ml after reconstitution

Azithromycin Dihydrate

Oral

For adults, 500 mg as a single dose on the first day, followed by 250 mg once daily on days 2 through 5. For the treatment of nongonococcal urethritis and cervicitis due to *Chlamydia tracomatis,* a single dose of 1 g (1,000 mg) may be given.

How Supplied:

Zithromax capsules (Pfizer). Capsules, 250 mg

Pharmacokinetics, Concentration-effect Relationship, and Metabolism

The only form of erythromycin known to be biologically active in vivo is the free base. Erythromycin base is incompletely but adequately absorbed from the upper part of the small intestine. Because it is inactivated by gastric juice, the drug is administered orally as protected tablets or capsules containing enteric-coated pellets that dissolve in the duodenum (15). Absorption of film-coated erythromycin base tends to be erratic, and administration under fasting conditions is required, as food in the stomach delays its ultimate absorption; however, other preparations provide excellent bioavailability in the fasting and nonfasting states (16). In general, the bioavailability of clarithromycin (55%) is more than twice that of erythromycin, and the bioavailability of azithromycin is 1.5 times (37%) that of erythromycin. Food slightly enhances the rate and extent of absorption of clarithromycin (11), whereas food decreases the rate and extent of absorption of azithromycin by approximately half (17). Peak serum concentrations (C_{max}) of all three drugs are attained 2 to 3 hours after an oral dose (11).

Various esters of erythromycin have been prepared in an attempt to improve stability and facilitate absorption. Erythromycin estolate is less susceptible than the parent compound to acid. It is better absorbed than other forms of the drug. A single, oral 250-mg dose of the estolate produces peak concentrations in plasma of approximately 1.5 μg/ml after 2 hours, and a 500 mg dose produces peak concentrations of 4 μg/ml (2). These peak values include both the ester and the free base, the latter constituting 20% to 35% of the total (2). Therefore, the actual concentration of the erythromycin base in plasma may be similar for the three preparations.

Erythromycin ethylsuccinate is another ester that is adequately absorbed after oral administration, particularly when the stomach is empty. Peak concentrations in plasma are 1.5 μg/ml (0.5 μg/ml base) 1 to 2 hours after administration of a 500-mg dose (2).

High concentrations of erythromycin can be achieved by intravenous administration. Values are approximately 10 μg/ml 1 hour after intravenous administration of 500 to 1,000 mg erythromycin lactobionate or gluceptate (2).

Only 2% to 5% of orally administered erythromycin is excreted in active form in the urine; 12% to 15% is excreted after intravenous infusion. The antibiotic is concentrated in the liver and excreted in active form in the bile, which may contain as much as 250 μg/ml when plasma concentrations are very high (2). Some of the drug may be inactivated by demethylation in the liver. The plasma $t_{\frac{1}{2}}$ of erythromycin is approximately 1.6 hours, whereas the plasma $t_{\frac{1}{2}}$ of clarithromycin is 4 to 7 hours (11). Azithromycin has a plasma $t_{\frac{1}{2}}$ of 48 to 72 hours after multiple doses, which allows once-daily administration (11).

The $t_{\frac{1}{2}}$ of azithromycin is considerably longer than that of clarithromycin because clarithromycin undergoes much more extensive hepatic metabolism than azithromycin and because azithromycin is accumulated in tissues, where it undergoes slow release into the plasma (11). Azithromycin is excreted either as the parent substance or as metabolites in the bile; these metabolites are antibacterially inactive (17). The remainder is excreted mainly as the parent substance unchanged in the urine (17).

Elimination of clarithromycin occurs mainly through a combination of hepatic metabolism (78%) and renal excretion. Only one of the metabolites, the 14-hydroxy moiety, has antibacterial activity (11). This metabolite is eliminated more slowly than the parent drug (11). Approximately 30% of the metabolite is excreted unchanged in the urine (11). These drugs are not removed significantly by either peritoneal dialysis or hemodialysis, and the dosing interval must be extended severalfold for clarithromycin in patients with renal impairment (11). No data are available regarding the effects of renal impairment on the pharmacokinetics of azithromycin.

Macrolide antibiotics diffuse readily into intercellular fluids, and antibacterial activity can be achieved at essentially all sites except the brain and the cerebrospinal fluid (CSF). The extent of binding of erythromycin to plasma proteins varies among the different forms of the drug, but probably exceeds 70% in all cases. Clarithromycin undergoes binding to plasma proteins in a fashion similar to erythromycin. Unlike other antibiotic agents, which are bound almost exclusively to albumin, the macrolides are bound to α_1-glycoproteins. Azithromycin appears to undergo the least protein binding of the three drugs (11). Erythromycin traverses the placental barrier, and the concentrations of the drug in fetal plasma are about 5% to 20% of those in the maternal circulation. Both clarithromycin and azithromycin are assumed to traverse the placental barrier similarly; however, the degree to which this occurs is uncertain (11). Macrolide antibiotics have been found detected in the breast milk of lactating animals, and although human studies are lacking for clarithromycin and azithromycin, these drugs should be presumed to be present in human breast milk (11).

Macrolide antibiotics cause several changes in the cytochrome P450 system. Both erythromycin and clarithromycin induce P450 isozymes that are more active in the metabolism of macrolide antibiotics than other P450 enzymes. Thus, both antibiotics induce their own metabolism. These metabolites then form complexes with the cytochrome P450 enzyme. These enzyme–metabolite complexes have a decreased ability to metabolize other drugs (18). Large interindividual differences affect the ability of erythromyin to inhibit P450 activity.

Ocular Pharmacology

In rabbit models, erythromycin penetrates ocular tissues poorly when administered intravenously. Topical solutions are well tolerated and nonirritating to ocular tissues, and they yield therapeutic drug levels. Subconjunctival injections of erythromycin can cause severe chemosis and corneal haze at higher doses, but yield high therapeutic levels at lower doses. Anterior chamber injections in rabbits of erythromycin 2.5 mg or more are destructive, resulting in prolonged keratitis and iritis (19). Intravitreal injections of 500 μg erythromycin are well tolerated, but are not associated with favorable outcome in the treatment of bacterial endophthalmitis in rabbit models (19).

Very little information exists on the ocular pharmacology of clarithromycin and azithromycin. A recent study in rabbits with topical administration of clarithromycin at concentrations of 10, 20, and 40 mg/ml suggests that tissue drug concentrations attained therapeutic levels (20). Further study is needed for topical use in humans.

Therapeutic Use

Ocular Indications

Erythromycin ointment (5 mg base/g [0.5%]) is indicated for the treatment of superficial ocular infections involving the conjunctiva and/or cornea caused by organisms susceptible to erythromycin. Erythromycin is also indicated for prophylaxis of ophthalmia neonatorum due to *N. gonorrhoeae* or *C. trachomatis.*

External Ocular Infections Involving the Cornea and/or Conjunctiva

For external ocular infections, apply directly to the infected area one or more times daily depending on the severity of the infection.

Prophylaxis of Neonatal Gonococcal or Chlamydial Conjunctivitis

For neonatal gonococcal or chlamydial infections, instill a thin line of ointment approximately 0.5 to 1 cm long into each conjunctival sac. Do not flush the ointment from the eye after application. Use a new tube for each infant. Administer to infants born by cesarian section and those delivered vaginally.

Adult Inclusion Conjunctivitis

Erythromycin is the drug of choice in children and pregnant women with inclusion conjunctivitis. Treatment of chlamydial conjunctivitis in infants consists of oral erythromycin suspension (ethylsuccinate or stearate) 50 mg/kg/day in four divided doses for 10 to 14 days. This treatment provides better and faster resolution of the conjuctivitis and also treats any concurrent nasopharyngeal infection, which will prevent the development of pneumonia (21). Additional topical therapy is not needed. The efficacy of this regimen is reportedly 80% to 90%; therefore, as many as 20% of infants may require another course of therapy (21). Erythromycin at the same dose for 2 to 3 weeks is the treatment of choice for chlamydial pneumonia in infants. Children aged more than 8 years may be treated with tetracycline. Pregnant women may be treated with 500 mg erythromycin base or stearate every 6 hours daily for 7 days and erythromycin ethylsuccinate 800 mg orally every 6 hours for 7 days (22). This regimen can cure the mother and also prevent neonatal infection (22).

Trachoma

Trachoma, a leading cause of blindness worldwide, is sometimes treated with oral erythromycin as an adjunct to topical tetracycline in severe cases (23). The treatment of choice is 1% topical tetracycline ointment applied twice daily for 6 weeks.

Supplementation with oral erythromycin stearate 250 mg every 6 hours for 2 weeks is often used in severe cases. Recently, a study evaluating the role of one-time administration of oral azithromycin (20 mg/kg) showed that cure rates of as much as 78% at 6 months can be attained with a single oral dose of this drug alone (23). Comparable cure rates of 72% were obtained with the standard regimen of tetracycline ointment, with careful compliance (23).

Nonocular Indications

Mycoplasma Pneumoniae Infections

Erythromycin (given orally in doses of 500 mg every 6 hours or, if not tolerated orally, intravenously) reduces the duration of fever caused by *M. pneumoniae.* In addition, the rate of clearing as noted in the chest roentgenogram is accelerated. Both azithromycin and clarithromycin have similar efficacy (11).

Legionnaires' Disease

Erythromycin is currently recommended for the treatment of pneumonia caused by *Legionella pneumophilia, L. micdadei,* or other Legionella species. The antibiotic may be given orally (0.5 to 1 g four times daily) or intravenously (1 to 4 g daily) for 3 weeks. Some researchers recommend the concurrent administration of rifampin for severe disease, but there are no controlled trials to support this practice. Clarithromycin in the treatment of *L. pneumophilia* infections was described in a Pakistani report, with success comparable to that achieved with erythromycin, but other studies are not available (24).

Chlamydia Infections

Chlamydia infections can be treated effectively with erythromycin, which is specifically recommended as an alternative to tetracycline in patients with uncomplicated urethral, endocervical, rectal, or epididymal infections (500 mg orally every 6 hours for at least 7 days). During pregnancy, erythromycin is the drug of choice for chlamydial urogenital infections; it is also preferred for chlamydial pneumonia of infancy (50 mg/kg daily in four divided doses for 14 days), when tetracyclines are contraindicated because of their effects on tissues that are calcifying (21). *Chlamydia pneumoniae,* a newly described agent that causes pneumonia, appears to respond to treatment with erythromycin (500 mg orally every 6 hours for 14 days) (25). Azithromycin, given in short-course regimens, is highly effective for the treatment of genital chlamydial infections. Stamm (26) compared a single 1-g dose of azithromycin with a standard regimen of doxycycline for 7 days for the treatment of uncomplicated genital chlamydial infections in 184 patients. The clinical cure rates were 77% with azithromycin and 63% with doxycycline.

Diphtheria

Erythromycin is very effective in eradicating the acute or chronic diphtheria bacillus carrier state. Erythromycin estolate (250 mg four times daily for 7 days) was effective in 90% of adults. However, neither erythromycin nor any other antibiotic agent alters the course of an acute infection with the diphtheria bacillus or the risk of complications.

Pertussis

If administered early in the course of pertussis (whooping cough), erythromycin may shorten the duration of illness. The drug has little influence on the disease once the paroxysmal stage is reached, although it may eliminate the microorganisms from the nasopharynx (27). Erythromycin can also prevent whooping cough in susceptible individuals who are exposed to the disease.

GI Infections

The treatment of gastroenteritis caused by *C. jejuni* with erythromycin (250 to 500 mg orally four times daily for 7 days) has been shown to hasten the eradication of the microorganism from the stools, and early treatment of children reduces the duration of symptoms.

Recently, use of clarithromycin has been advocated for eradication of *Helicobacter pylori,* in combination with ranitidine and metronidazole (28). Fifteen consecutive inpatients with *H. pylori*-positive peptic ulcer disease were treated with a 1-week course of 300 mg ranitidine twice daily combined with 500 mg clarithromycin three times daily and metronidazole 500 mg three times daily. In all patients, *H. pylori* was eradicated 4 weeks after discontinuation of study medication (28).

Azithromycin has also been advocated in the treatment of *H. pylori* infection. A new report of triple therapy with azithromycin, omeprazole, and amoxicillin has been published (29). In this randomized controlled trial, 91.6% of *H. pylori* infections were eradicated with the triple-therapy regimen as compared with 59.1% of those treated with conventional two-drug therapy consisting of omeprazole and amoxicillin (29).

Tetanus

Erythromycin (500 mg orally every 6 hours for 10 days) may be given to eradicate *C. tetani* in patients with tetanus who are allergic to penicillin. The mainstays of therapy are debridement, physiologic support, tetanus antitoxin, and drug control of convulsions.

Syphilis

Erythromycin in doses of 2 to 4 g/day for 10 to 15 days has been used successfully in the treatment of early syphilis in patients who are allergic to penicillin. Azithromycin appears to have efficacy similar to that of erythromycin in the treatment of *Treponema pallidum* (11).

Gonorrhea

Both erythromycin estolate and the base have been used in therapy of gonococcal urethritis. However, the relapse rate is nearly 25% after oral administration of 9 g in a 4-day period; this is unacceptably high for routine use. Erythromycin may be useful for disseminated gonococcal disease in pregnant patients who are allergic to β-lactam antibiotics. Patients treated with 500 mg erthromycin estolate or stearate orally every 6 hours for 5 days show rapid clinical and bacteriologic responses. Ceftriaxone is now the drug of choice for the treatment of all forms of gonorrhea. Azithromycin appears to be the most active of the macrolides against *N. gonorrheae* (11). Recent studies have shown a single 1-g dose of azithromycin to be an extremely effective method of treatment for gonorrhea, with a 95% clinical and bacteriologic cure rate (30). There is little correlation between β-lactamase production and susceptibility of *N. gonorrheae* to macrolides (11).

Upper Respiratory Tract Infections

All three drugs appear to be as effective as penicillin V for streptococcal pharyngitis in adults, but the incidence of GI side effects was markedly higher for the macrolides than for penicillin V (11).

Azithromycin has been compared with amoxicillin for the treatment of maxillary sinusitis. The incidence of combined clinical cure or improvement and of bacteriologic cure was 100% in the two groups (11).

Eisenberg and Barza (11) reported that in the treatment of acute exacerbations of chronic bronchitis, clarithromycin, erythromycin, and azithromycin appeared to have efficacy similar to that of ampicillin and cefaclor (11).

Community-acquired Pneumonia

All three drugs have similar efficacy in the treatment of community-acquired pneumonia, including the treatment of atypical pneumonia (11). Notably, azithromycin has the same cure rates as erythromycin in the treatment of atypical pneumonia, but only a 5-day treatment course is required, as compared with a required 10-day regimen with erythromycin (11).

Skin and Soft-tissue Infections

Clarithromycin was compared with erythromycin and cefadroxil in the treatment of skin and skin-structure infections, including impetigo, folliculitis, cellulitis, abscess, and wound infection (11). High rates of clinical cure and improvement were noted with all three drugs (11). The most common infecting species was *S. aureus.*

Azithromycin in a five-day course was compared with cephalexin in a 10-day course for the treatment of infections of the skin and skin structures (31). The major pathogens were *S. aureus, S. pyogenes,* and *S. agalactieae.* As in the clarithromycin trials, the incidences of cure and improvement and of bacteriologic eradication were high with both agents.

Side Effects and Toxicity

Serious adverse reactions are only rarely caused by the macrolide antibiotics. Side effects reported with macrolide antibiotics are characterized below.

Ocular

Erythromycin topical solutions are generally well tolerated and nonirritating to ocular tissues. Erythromycin has been reported to cause Stevens-Johnson syndrome and mydriasis when administered topically (32). Intercameral injection has been associated with severe intraocular inflammation, corneal edema, and lens damage (19). Subconjuctival or subtenons injection of erythromycin can cause severe chemosis and corneal haze, but yields higher therapeutic levels (19). Ocular side effects associated with systemic erythromycin include color vision abnormalities, allergic reactions, hyperemia, angioneurotic edema, urticaria, Stevens-Johnson syndrome, exfoliative dermatitis, and Lyell's syndrome (31). Myasthenic neuromuscular effects resulting in paralysis of extraocular muscles and ptosis have also been reported with systemic administration of erythromycin (31).

Clarithromycin has been implicated in the rifabutin-associated uveitis observed in patients with AIDS (33). Other ocular side effects have not been reported.

Gastrointestinal

The most common adverse reaction to erythromycin is GI disturbance. GI disturbance is less common in clarithromycin and azithromycin treatment. Studies have shown that the binding of clarithromycin to the putative motilin receptor is less than that of erythromycin, which may account for its decreased incidence of GI side effects (11). Oral administration of erythromycin, especially in large doses, is frequently accompanied by epigastric distress, which may be quite severe; intravenous administration may occasionally cause similar symptoms (34). Abdominal cramps, nausea, vomiting, and diarrhea are all dose-related and occur more commonly in children and young adults.

Hypersensitivity

Allergies to erythromycin range in severity from urticaria, fever, eosinophilia, and skin rash to anaphylaxis.

Hepatic

Erythromycin estolate can cause cholestatic hepatitis when administered systemically, but jaundice and abnormal liver function is unusual with the other forms of erythromycin (35). The illness has onset after about 10 to 20 days of treatment and is characterized initially by nausea, vomiting, and abdominal cramps. The pain often mimics that of acute cholecystitis, and unnecessary surgery has been performed. These symptoms are followed shortly thereafter by jaundice, which may be accompanied by fever, leukocytosis, eosinophilia, and increased activities of transaminases in plasma. All manifestations usually disappear within a few days after discontinuation of drug therapy and rarely are prolonged. The syndrome may represent a hypersensitivity reaction to the estolate ester (35).

Ototoxicity

Dose-related ototoxicity has been reported in some patients. This effect appears to be reversible and is usually associated with intravenous overdosage of gluceptate or lactobionate in these patients (36).

Other Side Effects

Erythromycin has been reported to cause false-positive increases in serum glutamate oxaloacetic transaminase (SGOT) concentrations measured by colorimetric methods (37). This finding must be distinguished from the aforementioned drug-induced hepatotoxicity (38). Erythromycin may also cause false elevations in urinary catecholamines and 17-hydroxycorticosteroid levels. Abnormalities of laboratory tests possibly related to clarithromycin are rare and include decreased white blood cell (WBC) counts in fewer than 1% of adult patients and increased liver function tests (11). These abnormalities disappear after discontinuation of the drug.

Headache and dizziness occurred in 1.3% and rash in 0.6% of all patients after administration of azithromycin. The only abnormalites in laboratory tests occurring in more than 1% of patients treated with azithromycin were an increase in alanine aminotransferase or aspartate aminotransferase levels and mild increases or decreases in leukocyte counts (39). All these effects were transient.

Drug Interactions

Erythromycin administration may cause cardiac arrhythmias in patients treated with terfenadine, as erythromycin appears to inhibit the metabolism of terfenadine to its carboxylic acid metabolite and may also inhibit the further metabolism of the metabolite (40). Therefore, patients receiving terfenadine should avoid concomitant use of erythromycin. Erythromycin and clarithromycin undergo extensive oxidation by the cytochrome P450 system in the liver. Therefore, both these drugs interfere with the metabolism of theophylline and can increase serum theophylline concentrations and produce toxicity (41). Because erythromycin can increase the effects of any drug metabolized by the cytochrome P450 system, including digoxin, carbamazepine, oral anticoagulants, ergotamine, triazolam, cyclosporine, hexobarbital, and phenytoin, there should be concern that the same kind of interaction could occur with clarithromycin. In contrast, azithromycin does not appear to form complexes with the cytochrome P450 system and has not been shown to interfere with the pharmacologic behavior of drugs metabolized by this system. Furthermore, according to a recent report (42), azithromycin apparently does not interact with terfenadine.

Erythromycin, along with other antibiotics that reduce bowel flora, may increase drug concentrations in certain patients. This effect has been demonstrated with the β-blocker nadolol (43) and digoxin compounds. Erythromycin has also been shown to increase serum concentrations of the calcium-channel blocker felodipine (44), although the mechanism through which this occurs is unknown.

Erythromycin, which is a bacteriostatic antibiotic under usual circumstances, may interfere with the bactericidal effect of penicillin compounds when administered concomitantly (45). This effect has not been sufficiently documented in clinical studies, however, and because the spectrum of activity is not enhanced by concurrent use of these two drugs, little clinical indication exists for concomitant administration.

High-risk Groups

High-risk groups include persons with a known hypersensitivity to any of the macrolide antibiotics or a history of an adverse reaction to the drugs. Administration of clarithromycin to pregnant animals produced fetal growth retardation in monkeys, cleft palate in mice, and cardiovascular abnormalities in rats (11). Because of these findings, clarithromycin is listed in pregnancy category C. Neither azithromycin nor erythromycin produce abnormalities in pregnant animals (11).

Major Clinical Trials

Major clinical trials are discussed herein.

REFERENCES

1. McGuire JM, Bunch RL, Anderson RC, et al. Ilotycin, a new antibiotic. *Antibiotic Chemother* 1952;2:281–283.
2. Gilman AG, Goodman LS, Rall TW, Murad F, eds. *Goodman and Gilman's the Pharmacological Basis of Therapeutics,* 8th ed. New York: Pergamon Press, 1990.
3. Neu HC. The development of the macrolides: clarithromycin in perspective. *J Antimicrob Chemother* 1991;27(Suppl A):1–9.
4. Peters DH, Friedel HA, McTavish D. Azithromycin: a review of its antimicrobial activity, pharmacokinetic properties and clinical efficacy. *Drugs* 1992;44:750–799.

5. Brisson-Noel A, Trieu-Cuot P, Courvalin P. Mechanism of action of spiramycin and other macrolides. *J Antimicrob Chemother* 1988;22 (Suppl B):13–23.
6. Gale EF, Cundliffe EC, Reynolds PE, Richmond MH, Waring MJ. *The molecular basis of antibiotic action,* 2nd ed. London: Wiley Interscience, 1981.
7. Sabath LD, Lorian V, Gerstein D, Lorder PB, Finland M. Enhancing effect on alkalinization of the medium on the activity of erythromycin against gram-negative bacteria. *Appl Microbiol* 1968;16:1288–1292.
8. Barry AL, Jones RN, Thornsberry C. *In vitro* activities of azithromycin (CP 62,993), clarithromycin (A-56268; TE-031), erythromycin, roxithromycin, and clindamycin. *Antimicrob Agents Chemother* 1988;32:752–754.
9. Washington JA II, Wilson WR. Erythromycin: a microbial and clinical perspective after 30 years of clinical use. *Mayo Clin Proc* 1985;60:271–278.
10. Hardy D, Hensey D, Beyer J, Voitko C, McDonald E, Fernandes P. Comparative in vitro activities of new 14-, 15-, and 16-membered macrolides. *Antimicrob Agents Chemother* 1988;32:1710–1719.
11. Eisenberg E, Barza M. Azithromycin and clarithromycin. *Curr Clin Top Infect Dis* 1994;14:52–79.
12. Naik S, Ruck R. *In vitro* activities of several new macrolide antibiotics against *Mycobacterium avium* complex. *Antimicrob Agents Chemother* 1989;33:1614–1616.
13. Brown BA, Wallace RJ Jr., Onyi GO, De Rosas V, Wallace R III. Activities of four macrolides, including clarithromycin, against *Mycobacterium fortuitum, Mycobacterium chelonae,* and *M. chelonae*-like organisms. *Antimicrob Agents Chemother* 1992;36:180–184.
14. Preac-Mursic V, Wilske B, Schierz G, Sub E, Grob B. Comparative antimicrobial activity of the new macrolides against *Borrelia burgdorferi. Clin Microbiol Infect Dis* 1989;8:651–653.
15. Nicholas P. Erythromycin: clinical review I. Clinical pharmacology. *NY State J of Med* 1977;77:2088–2094.
16. Fraser DG. Selection of an oral erythromycin product. *Am J Hosp Pharm* 1980;37:1199–1205.
17. Drew R, Gallis H. Azithromycin-spectrum of activity, pharmokinetics, and clinical applications. *Pharmacotherapy* 1992;12:161–173.
18. Ludden TM. Pharmacokinetic interactions of the macrolide antibiotics. *Clin Pharmacokinet* 1985;10:63–79.
19. Mauger TF, Craig EL, eds. *Havener's ocular pharmacology,* 6th ed. St. Louis: CV Mosby, 1994.
20. Gross RH, Holland GN, Elias SJ, Tuz R. Corneal pharmacokinetics of topical clarithromycin. *Invest Ophthal Vis Sci* 1995;36:965–968.
21. Hammerschlag MR. *Chlamydia trachomatis* in children. *Ped Ann* 1994;23:349–353.
22. Numazaki K, Wainberg MA, McDonald J. *Chlamydia trachomatis* infections in infants. *Can Med Assoc J* 1989;140:615–622.
23. Bailey RL, Arullendran P, Whittle HC, Mabey DC. Randomised controlled trial of single dose azithromycin in treatment of trachoma. *Lancet* 1993;342:453–456.
24. Hamedani P, Ali J, Hafeez S, et al. The safety and efficacy of clarithromycin in patients with *Legionella* pneumonia. *Chest* 1991; 100:1503–1506.
25. Grayston JT, Wang SP, Kuo CC, Campbell LA. Current knowledge on *Chlamydia pneumoniae,* strain TWAR, an important cause of pneumonia and other acute respiratory diseases. *Eur J Clin Microbiol Infect Dis* 1989;8:191–202.
26. Stamm WE. Azithromycin in the treatment of uncomplicated genital chlamydial infections. *Am J Med* 1991;91(suppl 3A):19–22.
27. Bass JW, Klenk EL, Kotheimer JB, et al. Antimicrobial treatment of pertussis. *J Ped* 1969;75:768–781.
28. Amdek RJ, Opferkuch W, Wegener M. Modified short-term triple therapy—ranitidine, clarithromycin, and metronidazole—for cure of *Helicobacter pylori* infection. *Am J Gastroenterol* 1995;90:168–169.
29. Bertoni G, Sassatelli R, Nigrisoli E, et al. Triple therapy with azithromycin, omeprazole, and amoxicillin is highly effective in the eradication of *Helicobacter pylori:* a controlled trial versus omeprazole plus amoxicillin. *Am J Gastroenterol* 1996;91:258–263.
30. Steingrimsson O, Olafsson JH, Thorarinsson H, Ryan RW, Johnson RB, Tilton RC. Single dose azithromycin treatment of gonorrhea and infections caused by *C. trachomatis* and *U. urealyticum* in men. *Sex Trans Dis* 1994;21:43–46.
31. Kiani R. Double blind, double-dummy comparison of azithromycin and cephalexin in the treatment of skin and skin structure infections. *Eur J Clin Microbiol Infect Dis* 1991;10:880–884.
32. Fraunfelder FT, Meyer SM, eds. *Drug-induced ocular side effects and drug interactions,* 3rd ed. Philadelphia: Lea & Febiger, 1989.
33. Tseng AL, Walmsley SL. Rifabutin-associated uveitis. *Ann Pharmacother* 1995;29:1149–1155.
34. Seifert CF, Swaney RJ, Bellanger-McCleery RA. Intravenous erythromycin lactobionate-induced severe nausea and vomiting. *Drug Intell Clin Pharm* 1989;23:40–44.
35. Tolman KG, Sannella JJ, Freston JW. Chemical structure of erythromycin and hepatotoxicity. *Ann Intern Med* 1974;81:58–60.
36. Karmody CS, Weinstein L. Reversible sensorineural hearing loss with intravenous erythromycin lactobionate. *Ann Otorhinolaryngol* 1977;86(1 Pt 1):9–11.
37. Sabath LD, Gerstein DA, Finland M. Serum glutamic oxalacetic transaminase. False elevations during administration of erythromycin. *N Eng J Med* 1968;279:1137–1139.
38. Ginsburg CM, Eichenwald HF. Erythromycin: a review of its uses in pediatric practice. *J Ped* 1976;89:872–884.
39. Hopkins S. Clinical toleration and safety of azithromycin. *Am J Med* 1991;91(suppl 3A):75–82.
40. Honig PK, Woosley RL, Zamani K, Conner DP, Cantilena LR Jr. Changes in the pharmacokinetics and electrocardiographic pharmacodynamics of terfenadine with concomitant administration of erythromycin. *Clin Pharmacol Ther* 1992;52:231–238.
41. Zarowitz BJ, Szefler SJ, Lasezkay GM. Effect of erythromycin base on the theophylline kinetics. *Clin Pharmacol Ther* 1981;29:601–605.
42. Harris S, Hilligoss DM, Colangelo PM, Eller M, Okerholm R. Azithromycin and terfenadine: lack of drug interaction. *Clin Pharmacol Ther* 1995;58:310–315.
43. DuSouich P. Enhancement of nadolol elimination by activated charcoal and antibiotics. *Clin Pharmacol Ther* 1983;33:585.
44. Liedholm H, Nordin G. Erythromycin-felodipine interaction. *Drug Intell Clin Pharm* 1991;25:1007–1008.
45. Garrod LP. Causes of failure in antibiotic treatment. *Br Med J* 1972;4:441–456.

Textbook of Ocular Pharmacology,
edited by T.J. Zimmerman, et al.
Lippincott–Raven Publishers, Philadelphia © 1997.

CHAPTER 44

Chloramphenicol

Carol L. Karp, Joseph R. Gussler, and Eduardo C. Alfonso

CHLORAMPHENICOL

History and Source

Chloramphenicol is a broad-spectrum bacteriostatic antibiotic originally derived from *Streptomyces venezuelae.* Chloramphenicol was initially used to treat an outbreak of typhus in Bolivia. Since then, chloramphenicol has been shown to be effective against many gram-positive and gram-negative bacteria, certain mycoplasma, rickettsiae, and Chlamydia (1). In the eye, chloramphenicol was first used to treat intraocular infections and was administered systemically.

Official Drug Name and Chemistry

The chemical names for chloramphenicol are (a) acetamide,2, 2-dichloro-*N*-[2-hydroxy-1-(hydroxymethyl)-2-(4-nitrophenyl) ethyl], and (b) D-threo-(-)-2,2-dichloro-*N*-[beta-hydroxy-alpha-(hydroxymethyl)-*p*-nitrophenethyl] acetamide. Chloramphenicol structure and molecular formula are shown below.

Chloramphenicol

Pharmacology

Chloramphenicol inhibits protein synthesis by reversibly binding to the 50S ribosomal subunit of bacteria and, to a lesser degree, to mammalian cells. Chloramphenicol appears to prevent the binding of the amino acid containing tRNA to the acceptor site on the 50S ribosome. Due to the reversible binding, chloramphenicol is bacteriostatic.

C. L. Karp, J. R. Gussler, and E. C. Alfonso: Department of Ophthalmology, Bascom Palmer Eye Institute, University of Miami School of Medicine, Miami, Florida 33136.

Clinical Pharmacology

Chloramphenicol inhibits protein synthesis in bacteria and, to a lesser degree, in eucaryotic cells. Chloramphenicol may inhibit mitochondrial protein synthesis since mitochondrial ribosomes closely resemble bacterial ribosomes. The drug is active against a broad spectrum of organisms, including gram-positive, gram-negative, aerobic, and anaerobic bacteria. Chloramphenicol is also effective against mycoplasma, chlamydiae, and rickettsia. It is also effective against gram-positive bacilli, including *Bacillus* species, *Listeria monocytogenes, Corynebacterium diptheriae,* and *Clostridium* species.

More specifically, chloramphenicol is usually active against *Streptococcus pneumoniae, S. pyogens, S. agalactiae,* and most strains of *Staphylococcus aureus.* Although usually bacteriostatic, chloramphenicol may be bactericidal to *Haemophilus influenzae.* It is also used to treat infections caused by *Neisseria meningitidis, N. gonorrhoeae, Bordetella pertusis, Pseudomonas pseudomallei, P. mallei, P. cepacia,* and several *Bacteroides* species. *Salmonella typhi* in the United States is usually susceptible, but some strains from Mexico may be resistant. Furthermore, almost all strains of *P. aeruginosa* are resistant.

Pharmaceutics

Chloramphenicol is available in oral, intravenous, and topical forms.

Oral

Generic: Capsules 250 and 500 mg
Chloromycetin (Parke-Davis): Capsules 250 mg
Mychel (Rachelle): Capsules 250 mg

Chloramphenicol palmitate (Parke-Davis): Suspension equivalent to 150 mg/5 ml.

Injection/Intravenous

Chloromycetin sodium succinate (Parke-Davis): 1 g; equivalent to 100 mg/ml chloramphenicol when reconstituted.

Mychel S (Rachelle): 1 gm; equivalent to 100 mg/ml chloramphenicol when reconstituted.

Ocular

Higher corneal penetration is obtained with the ointment form (2). The solution should be refrigerated until dispensed.

AK-Chlor (Akorn) 0.5% solution: Chloramphenicol 5 mg/ml

AK-Chlor Ointment (Akorn) 1.0%: Chloramphenicol 10 mg/g

Chloromycetin Hydrocortisone Ophthalmic (Parke-Davis): Chloramphenicol 2.5 mg/ml and hydrocortisone acetate 5 mg/ml

Chloromycetin Ophthalmic Ointment 1% (Parke-Davis): Chloramphenicol 10 mg/g

Chloromycetin Ophthalmic Solution 0.5% (Parke-Davis): Chloramphenicol 5 mg/ml.

Chloroptic 1% S.O.P. (Allergan): Chloramphenicol 10 mg/g

Chloroptic Sterile Ophthalmic Solution 0.5% (Allergan): Chloramphenicol 5 mg/ml

Ophthocort Ointment (Parke-Davis): Chloramphenicol 10 mg, polymixin B 10,000 U, and hydrocortisone 5 mg/g

Resistance

Resistance of certain gram-positive and gram-negative bacteria to chloramphenicol is of concern. Gram-negative bacilli appear to be resistant secondary to a plasmid-mediated acetyltransferase that inactivates the drug. Resistant strains of *H. influenzae* may also be resistant to tetracycline and ampicillin (3). *Escherichia coli* and *P. aeruginosa* may be resistant owing to decreased permeability of the drug into the organism (4–6). Resistance of certain staphlylococci has also been increasing and may be due to a chloramphenicol acetyltransferase (7).

Pharmacokinetics, Concentration-effect Relationship and Metabolism

Three preparations of chloramphenicol are available for systemic use: chloramphenicol base in capsules for oral use and the prodrug forms of chloramphenicol palmitate and chloramphenicol succinate. Ocular preparations are available in both solution and ointment form.

Absorption

Systemically, oral chloramphenicol base is rapidly absorbed by the gastrointestinal (GI) system. The prodrug, chloramphenicol palmitate must be hydrolyzed by pancreatic esterases in the small intestine. Bioavailability of chloramphenicol ester is approximately 80%. Once the drug is in the active form, peak plasma concentrations usually are obtained 2 to 3 hours after dosing (8). The usual dosage for adults is 3 to 5 g/day in divided doses every 4 hours.

The bioavailability of the chloramphenicol palmitate is decreased and unpredictable in patients with GI disease and in neonates, probably owing to incomplete hydrolysis of the prodrug. The parenteral, water-soluble form of chloramphenicol, chloramphenicol succinate, probably is hydrolyzed by the esterases of the liver, kidneys, and lungs. Decreased activity of the esterases in neonates may result in prolonged time to peak concentration (9).

Distribution

Chloramphenicol is distributed to all body fluids, including cerebrospinal fluid (CSF), due to its lipophilic character. The drug is present in bile, is secreted in milk and crosses the placenta. Chloramphenicol is 50% protein bound.

Ocular penetration of chloramphenicol occurs after systemic, subconjunctival, and topical application. After systemic administration, chloramphenicol penetrates the eye better than oxytetracycline, chlortetracycline, or penicillin (10). One hour after intravenous delivery of 50 mg/kg chloramphenicol in rabbits, levels of 12 μg/ml and 6 μg/ml were obtained in serum and aqueous, respectively (11). No drug was detectable in vitreous. Aqueous levels of 5 to 10 μg/ml were obtained in rabbits 1 to 4 hours after subconjunctival injection of 10 mg/kg chloramphenicol (12). In patients undergoing routine cataract surgery, aqueous levels of 3 to 6 μg/ml were obtained 2 hours after topical application of 0.5% chloramphenicol drops every 5 minutes for six doses (13). Enhanced penetration obtained with the ointment vehicle has also been demonstrated. Patients with cataracts received 1% chloramphenicol ointment every 30 minutes for 4 doses, which resulted in aqueous levels of 60 μg/ml (14).

Elimination

Chloramphenicol is metabolized mostly by the liver, with conversion to the inactive glucuronide. Chloramphenicol, the inactive glucuronide, and prodrug chloramphenicol succinate are cleared through the kidneys. In a 24-hour period, 75% to 90% of the orally administered drug is eliminated (1). Patients with renal insufficiency may experience increased levels of chloramphenicol succinate and chloramphenicol. Furthermore, patients with cirrhosis will have increased levels due to decreased metabolic inactivation.

Therapeutic Use

Due to its potential to cause aplastic anemia, chloramphenicol should only be considered when specifically indicated or when other potentially less toxic antibiotics are not available.

Ocular Infections

Topical chloramphenicol is effective against *H. influenzae; S. aureus; Streptococcus,* including *S. pneumonia; E. coli; Klebsiella; Enterobacter; Neisseria;* and *Moraxella* species. Chloramphenicol is particularly effective against *H. influenzae* and may be used after filtering surgery to prevent *H. influenzae* conjunctivitis and endophthalmitis. The usual dose of chloramphenicol solution is 1% drop to the affected eye two to six times a day or 1% ointment every 3 hours or less. The drug may be tapered as the clinical situation warrants. Chloramphenicol is generally ineffective against Pseudomonas and Serratia species.

Chloramphenicol has been reported to be effective in trachoma. The dose is 1 g orally daily for 9 days (15). Chloramphenicol and other antibiotic agents most likely treat the secondary bacterial infections that are common in trachoma. Disappearance of the conjunctival follicles in trachoma usually requires more time than that required to clear the cornea, and persistence of the conjunctival reaction does not mandate continued antibiotic treatment, as this will usually resolve.

Bacterial Meningitis

Chloramphenicol is highly effective in *H. influenzae* meningitis. Although usually a bacteriostatic drug, it is bactericidal to *H. influenzae* and some other meningeal pathogens (16). Chloramphenicol is also an effective treatment for *N. meningitidis* and *S. pneumoniae.* Some of the new cephalosporins will likely replace chloramphenicol because of their lesser toxicity.

Anaerobic Infections

Chloramphenicol is quite effective against many anaerobic bacteria, including *Bacteroides.* It may be used in conjunction with or instead of metronidazole or clindamycin for brain, abdominal, or pelvic abscesses. The treatment should include surgical drainage when feasible.

Other Systemic Uses

Chloramphenicol is an important agent in the treatment of typhoid fever and other salmonella infections. Unfortunately, organisms resistant to chloramphenicol are responsible for some epidemics (e.g., in Mexico). Chloramphenicol may be used for rickettsial disease and brucellosis when tetracycline cannot be used.

Side Effects and Toxicity

Hematologic

Chloramphenicol has its most serious side effect on the bone marrow. The first type of bone marrow effect is a predictable, dose-related, and reversible anemia with occasional leukopenia and thrombocytopenia and is usually evident as reticulocytopenia 5 to 7 days after initiation of chloramphenicol therapy. It occurs in patients receiving large doses (4 g/day or more) or having plasma levels greater than 25 μg/ml. The mechanism is believed to be secondary to inhibition of host mitochondrial protein synthesis (4). Blood count monitoring is essential for patients treated with systemic chloramphenicol. Chloramphenicol may also precipitate hemolytic anemia in patients with glucose-6-phosphate-dehydrogenase deficiency (G6PD).

The second type of bone marrow effects caused by chloramphenicol treatment is aplastic anemia, a serious form of anemia. The anemia is characterized by peripheral pancytopenia and aplastic bone marrow and is usually irreversible. This reaction is believed to be idiosyncratic, but may be dose related (17). The estimated risk of aplastic anemia from chloramphenicol is 1 in 13,000 to 1 in 50,000. The mechanism may be related to the bacterially mediated modifications of the nitro radical of chloramphenicol, which may cause bone marrow toxicity (18). Although more common after prolonged systemic use of chloramphenicol, aplastic anemia and death have been reported after a short course of topical chloramphenicol drops and ointment (19,20).

Ocular

Optic atrophy occurs in children with cystic fibrosis receiving more than 100 g chloramphenicol (21). The optic atrophy does appear to be dose related but does not negate the beneficial effect of chloramphenicol in such patients. Histologic examination of children treated with chloramphenicol has shown demyelination, especially of the papillomacular bundle. Optic neuritis has also been reported in such children (22).

Systemic administration can also lead to problems with color vision, allergic conjunctivitis, mydriasis, retinal edema, or retinal hemorrhages secondary to drug-induced anemia (23). Usually well tolerated on the ocular surface, topically applied chloramphenicol may induce a local hypersensitivity reaction associated with burning and stinging or, possibly, with depigmentation.

Neurologic

Prolonged chloramphenicol therapy may result in peripheral neuritis or delirium. Optic neuritis may occur and is described in the ocular section.

Gray Syndrome

The gray syndrome is a potentially fatal disorder associated with serum levels of chloramphenicol greater than 75 to 100 μg/ml. The syndrome usually presents 4 days after treatment is initiated and is heralded by vomiting, refusal to suck, abdominal distention, cyanosis, lethargy, gray stools, ashen color, and tachypnea. It may lead to metabolic acidosis and vasomotor collapse. Death may occur in 40% of patients. The syndrome is more common in neonates and premature infants. The mechanism is believed to be secondary to inhibition of host mitochondrial electron transport in the liver, myocardium, and skeletal muscle. The effect may be accentuated in neonates due to a decreased renal excretion of unconjugated chloramphenicol and inadequate hepatic deactivation of the drug. Children aged 2 weeks or younger should not receive more than 25 mg/kg (1).

Gastrointestinal

Vomiting, nausea, stomatitis, diarrhea may occur.

Hypersensitivity

Rarely, vesicular or macular rashes, fever, or angioedema may occur.

High-risk Groups

Neonates and children who receive large amounts of systemic chloramphenicol may develop gray syndrome, bone marrow suppression, optic neuritis, and optic atrophy. Chloramphenicol passes the placental barrier and is present in breast milk and should be avoided in lactating women or pregnant women near term.

Drug Interactions

Chloramphenicol irreversibily inhibits hepatic microsomal enzymes of the cytochrome P450 complex and may prolong the half-life of drugs that are metabolized by this system. These drugs include phenytoin (24), chlorpropamide (25), tolbutamide, and dicumarol. Conversely, other drugs may alter the elimination of chloramphenicol. Both rifampin and phenobarbital (26) shorten the half-life of chloramphenicol.

Chloramphenicol may inhibit the response to iron and B12 therapy in patients with anemia (27). Chloramphenicol acts at the same site as macrolide antibiotics such as erythromycin and therefore competitively inhibits their action.

Major Clinical Trials

To our knowledge, there are no clinical trials of chloramphenicol at present.

REFERENCES

1. Gilman AG, Rall TW, Nies AS, Taylor P, eds. *Goodman and Gilman's: the Pharmacological Basis of Therapeutics,* 8th ed. New York: Pergamon Press, 1990.
2. Leopold IH, Nichols AC, Vogel AW. Penetration of chloramphenicol U.S.P. (chloromycetin) into the eye. *Arc Ophthalmol* 1950;44:22–36.
3. Doern GV, Jorgensen JH, Thornsberry C, Preston DA, Tubert T, Redding JS, Maher LA. National collaborative study of the prevalence of antimicrobial resistance among clinical isolates of *Haemophilus influenzae. Antimicrob Agents Chemother* 1988;32:180–185.
4. Tetracyclines and chloramphenicol. In: *Drug evaluations,* 6th ed. Chicago: American Medical Association, 1978;1409–1422.
5. Baughman GA, Fahnestock SR. Chloramphenicol resistance mutation in *Escherichia coli* which maps in the major ribosomal protein gene cluster. *J Bacteriol* 1979;137:1315–1323.
6. Sompolinsky D, Samra Z. Mechanism of high-level resistance to chloramphenicol in different *Escherichia coli* variants. *J Gen Microbiol* 1968;50:55–66.
7. Sands LC, Shaw WV. Mechanism of chloramphenicol resistance in staphylococci: characterization and hybridization of variants of chloramphenicol acetyltransferase. *Antimicrob Agents Chemother* 1973;3: 299–305.
8. Ambrose PJ. Clinical pharmacokinetics of chloramphenicol and chloramphenicol succinate. *Clin Pharmacokinet* 1984;9:222–238.
9. Kauffman RE, Thirumoorthi MC, Buckley JA, Aravind MK, Dajani AS. Relative bioavailability of intravenous chloramphenicol succinate and oral chloramphenicol palmitate in infants and children. *J Pediatr* 1981;99:963–967.
10. Leopold IH. Clinical trial with chloramphenicol in ocular infections. *Arch Ophthalmol* 1951;45:44.
11. Furgiuele FP, Sery TW, Leopold IH. Newer antibiotics: their intraocular penetration. *Am J Ophthalmol* 1960;50:614–622.
12. Broughton W, Goldman JN. The intraocular penetration of chloramphenicol succinate in rabbits. *Ann Ophthalmol* 1973;5:71–74.
13. Beasley H, Boltralik JJ, Baldwin HA. Chloramphenicol in aqueous humor after topical application. *Arch Ophthalmol* 1975;93:184–185.
14. Havener WH. *Ocular pharmacology,* 6th ed. St. Louis: CV Mosby, 1994;275.
15. Thygeson P. Criteria of cure in trachoma, with special reference to provocative tests. *Rev Int Trachome* 1953;30:450–464.
16. Rahal JJ Jr, Simberkoff MS. Bactericidal and bacteriostatic action of chloramphenicol against meningeal pathogens. *Antimicrob Agents Chemother* 1979;16:13–18.
17. Daum RS, Cohen DL, Smith AL. Fatal aplastic anemia following apparent "dose-related" chloramphenicol toxicity. *J Pediatr* 1979;94: 403–406.
18. Jimenez JJ, Arimura GK, Abou-Khalil WH, Isildar M, Yunis AA. Chloramphenicol-induced bone marrow injury: possible role of bacterial metabolites of chloramphenicol. *Blood* 1987;70:1180–1185.
19. Abrams SM, Degnan TJ, Vinciguerra V. Marrow aplasia following topical application of chloramphenicol eye ointment. *Arch Intern Med* 1980;140:576–577.
20. Fraunfelder FT, Bagby GC Jr, Kelly DJ. Fatal aplastic anemia following topical administration of ophthalmic chloramphenicol. *Am J Ophthalmol* 1982;93:356–360.

21. Harley RD, Huang NN, Macri CH, Green WR. Optic neuritis and optic atrophy following chloramphenicol in cystic fibrosis patients. *Trans Am Acad Ophthalmol Otolaryngol* 1970;74:1011–1031.
22. Cocke JG Jr. Chloramphenicol optic neuritis; apparent protective effects of very high daily doses of pyridoxine and cyanocobalamin. *Am J Dis Child* 1967;114:424–426.
23. Fraundelder FT, Meyer SM. *Drug-induced ocular side effects and drug interactions,* 3rd ed. Philadelphia: Lea & Febiger, 1989.
24. Koup JF, Gibaldi M, McNamara P, Hilligoss DM, Colburn WA, Bruck E. Interaction of chloramphenicol with phenytoin and phenobarbital. Case report. *Clin Pharmacol Ther* 1978;24:571.
25. Petitpierre B, Fabre J. Chlorpropramide and chloramphenicol. *Lancet* 1970;1:789.
26. Bloxham RA, Durbin GM, Johnson T, Winterborn MH. Chloramphenicol and phenobarbitone. A drug interaction. *Arch Dis Child* 1979;54:76–77.
27. Saidi P, Wallerstein RO, Aggeler PM. Effect of chloramphenicol on erythropoiesis. *J Lab Clin Med* 1961;57:247–256.

Textbook of Ocular Pharmacology,
edited by T.J. Zimmerman, et al.
Lippincott–Raven Publishers, Philadelphia © 1997.

CHAPTER 45

Aminoglycosides in Ophthalmology

Steven M. Patalano and Robert A. Hyndiuk

AMINOGLYCOSIDES

History and Source

Aminoglycosides are widely used in ophthalmology to control both superficial and deep infections of the eye and ocular adnexa (1,2). They are potent bactericidal agents that are particularly useful against aerobic gram negative bacteria. They are commonly administered topically at commercially available concentrations or as fortified preparations subconjunctivally, intravenously, and intravitreally. The current available list of clinically important aminoglycosides includes gentamicin, tobramycin, amikacin, netilmicin, kanamycin, streptomycin, and neomycin. Tobramycin and gentamicin are by far those most commonly used in ophthalmology (3). Table 1 shows the currently available single-agent aminoglycosides for ophthalmic use and common trade names. Combination mixtures are also available (Table 2).

The first aminoglycoside, streptomycin, was isolated from *Streptomyces griseus* in 1943 in the laboratory of Selman A. Waksman at Rutgers University. A different species of Streptomyces was later shown to produce neomycin. Gentamicin and netilmicin were subsequently isolated from *Micromonospora purpurea.* That these two agents were isolated from Micromonospora instead of Streptomyces is reflected in their unique spelling (-micin instead of -mycin). In 1971, researchers isolated tobramycin from *S. tenebrarius* (4). More recently, semisynthetic aminoglycoside preparations have become available, including amikacin and netilmicin. Unfortunately, the emergence of streptomycin-resistant gram-negative bacilli and gram-positive cocci has significantly limited streptomycin's clinical usefulness.

Pharmacology

As a class, the aminoglycosides share many important characteristics. They are all polycations with poor oral absorption. They are rapidly absorbed after intramuscular and subcutaneous injection, with peak plasma concentration similar to those achieved with intravenous administration. Their polar nature results in poor CNS and ocular penetration, with CNS levels probably less than 10% of plasma concentrations. They are almost entirely excreted by glomerular filtration, and appropriate dosing adjustments are necessary in patients with renal impairment. Most important, they are rapidly bactericidal and are known to interfere with bacterial protein synthesis at the ribosomal level.

Side Effects

Reversible and irreversible vestibular, cochlear, and renal toxicity are the principal adverse effects of aminoglycosides. As many as 2% of patients receiving prolonged systemic aminoglycosides develop ototoxicity (5). High concentrations and long half-lives ($t\frac{1}{2}$) of aminoglycosides in the endolymph and perilymph of the inner ear probably contribute to this toxicity (6,7). A significant number of these cases are irreversible. High-pitched tinnitus and high-frequency hearing loss are the earliest signs of ototoxicity. Vestibular dysfunction may present as dizziness, vertigo, ataxia, or even nystagmus. Streptomycin and gentamicin have predominantly vestibular side effects. As many as 20% of patients receiving prolonged systemic streptomycin for endocarditis develop detectable, irreversible vestibular damage (8). Streptomycin has even been linked to hearing loss in children born to women who received the drug during pregnancy (9). Amikacin, ke-

S. M. Patalano: Department of Ophthalmology, Harvard Medical School, Boston, Massachusetts 02115.

R. A. Hyndiuk: Cornea and External Disease Service, Department of Ophthalmology, Medical College of Wisconsin, Milwaukee, Wisconsin 53226.

Table 45-1. *Aminoglycosides for ophthalmic use*[a]

Individual agents	Trade name	gtt concentration	ung concentration
Tobramycin	Tobrex, AKTOB	3 mg/ml	3 mg/g
Gentamicin	Genoptic SOS (allergan)	3 mg/ml	3 mg/g
	Gentacidin (IOLAB)		
	Gentak (Akorn)		
	Ocu-mycin (Ocumed)		
	Gentavision (Coopervision)		

Data from ref. 27, with permission.

namycin, and neomycin are believed to affect auditory function more commonly. Tobramycin probably adversely affects both the vestibular and cochlear systems equally.

Toxicity

Nephrotoxicity, which results from high concentration of aminoglycosides in proximal renal tubules, may present as mild proteinuria to severe azotemia. As many as 26% of patients receiving prolonged treatment with systemic aminoglycosides develop evidence of mild renal impairment (10). Risk of nephrotoxicity is increased with concurrent use of cephalosporins or other nephrotoxic agents. Gentamicin is more likely to cause toxicity than tobramycin (11). Patients receiving parental aminoglycosides should be closely monitored for changes in serum creatinine levels. Any increase in serum creatinine level should be promptly addressed by appropriate dosing adjustments or discontinuation of the drug.

Aminoglycoside antibiotic agents are also associated with neuromuscular blockade. This is a potentially life-threatening side effect and may include respiratory depression and cardiovascular arrest (12). Patients may present

Table 45-2. *Combination aminoglycoside preparations*[a]

Trade name	Individual agents
Pred-GSOP (Allergan)	Prednisolone acetate
Pred-G Liquifilm (Allergan)	Gentamicin sulfate
Tobradex suspension/ointment (Alcon)	Dexamethasone, tobramycin
AK-Spore solution (Akorn)	Neomycin sulfate
Ocutricin solution (Bausch & Lomb)	Polymyxin B sulfate
Neosporin solution (Burroughs-Wellcome)	Gramacidin
Ocu-Spor-G (Ocumed)	
Ocutricin ointment (Bausch & Lomb)	Neomycin sulfate
AK-Spore ointment (Akorn)	Polymyxin B sulfate
Ocu-Spor B (Ocumed)	Bacitracin
Neosporin ointment (Burroughs-Wellcome)	
Cortisporin ointment (Burroughs-Wellcome)	Polymyxin B sulfate
Neotricin HC ointment (Bausch & Lomb)	Bacitracin zinc
	Neomycin sulfate, hydrocortisone
Dexasporin (Bausch & Lomb)	Neomycin sulfate
Ocu-Trol (Ocumed)	Polymyxin B sulfate
Neopolydex (Medical Opthalmics)	Dexamethasone
Maxitrol (Alcon)	
Ak-Trol (Akorn)	
Dexacidin (iOLab)	
NeoDexair (Bausch & Lomb)	Neomycin sulfate
NeoDecadron (Merck & Co.)	Dexamethasone sodium
Neodexasone (Medical Ophthalmics)	
Ak-Neo-Dex (Akorn)	Phosphate
Ocutricin HC suspension (Bausch & Lomb)	Neomycin sulfate
Cortimycin (Medical Ophthalmics)	Polymyxin B sulfate, hydrocortisone
Poly-Pred	Prednisolone acetate, neomycin sulfate, polymyxin B sulfate

[a]Data from refs. 27 and 28, with permission.

with generalized muscular weakness, ptosis, or even extraocular muscle paralysis. Although usually associated with intraperitoneal and intrapleural administration, this effect has also been reported after intravenous, intramuscular, and even oral administration (13). The neuromuscular blocking action of aminoglycosides is more pronounced in patients with myasthenia gravis and hypokalemia. Extreme caution should by used in prescribing systemic aminoglycoside therapy in these groups of patients.

Topical

Despite the above adverse side effects, aminoglycosides have little allergenic potential. True anaphylaxis and rash are uncommon, but localized side effects after topical administration are common. Frequent dosing of fortified aminoglycoside preparations used to treat bacterial keratitis can result in severe corneal epithelial toxicity, including near-total epithelial defect. Occurrence of pseudomembranous conjunctivitis is common with fortified topical gentamicin and occasionally results from treatment with topical fortified tobramycin. Aminoglycosides, especially neomycin, are a frequent cause of allergic conjunctivitis and severe contact dermatitis of the lids.

Chemistry

The structure common to the aminoglycosides is two or more amino sugars joined in glycoside linkages to a hexose (aminocyclitol) nucleus. In the case of streptomycin, this nucleus is streptidine. In all other available aminoglycosides the hexose nucleus is 2-deoxystreptamine. The individual aminoglycoside families are determined by the specific amino sugars attached to the aminocyclitol ring. Most of the aminoglycosides are naturally occurring isolates derived from strains of bacteria. Newer semisynthetic aminoglycosides, including amikacin and netilmicin, are also available.

Pharmacokinetics

Aminoglycosides are bactericidal agents and are rapidly lethal to sensitive organisms. This effect is achieved in part by inhibition of bacterial protein synthesis through interference with translation of mRNA at the ribosomal level. The aminoglycosides enter aqueous channels in the outer membrane of susceptible gram-negative bacteria. Passage through the inner cytoplasmic membrane occurs by a process dependent on electron transport. This process is rate-limiting and can be inhibited under conditions of low pH, hyperosmolarity, presence of divalent cations (e.g., Ca^{++}), and anaerobiasis (14). Poor penetration into bacteria under anaerobic and low pH conditions results in limited usefulness of aminoglycosides in treatment of abscesses.

Once within the cytoplasm, the aminoglycoside binds to the 30s ribosomal subunit. The 30s subunit itself consists of 21 proteins and a single 16s subunit. The nature of the binding is aminoglycoside specific. For example, streptomycin is believed to bind to at least three of the 30s ribosomal proteins and possibly to the 16s molecule of RNA. Any alteration in the protein sequence in the 30s ribosomal proteins can significantly affect binding and subsequently the activity of the agent. Other aminoglycosides bind to the 30s at specific protein sites and may also bind to the 50s ribosomal subunit. This aminoglycoside–ribosomal binding results in interference with initiation of protein synthesis (15). Misreading of mRNA also occurs, resulting in the incorrect amino acid being incorporated into the growing polypeptide chain and chain termination (16). This effect is usually irreversible and results in bacterial cell death. The subunits of bacterial and mammalian ribosomes are sufficiently different from one another to allow selective inhibition of bacterial protein without significantly affecting host protein synthesis.

This effect on bacterial protein synthesis may not fully explain the rapidly lethal effect of aminoglycosides on susceptible bacteria. Most antibiotics that interfere with bacterial protein synthesis actually are merely bacteriostatic. Aminoglycosides have also been shown to cause a progressive disruption of the cell envelope, which may contribute to their lethal effect. Leakage of small ions has been shown to occur early, followed later by leakage of larger molecules. Leakage of proteins eventually occurs soon before cell death.

With the widespread use of aminoglycosides, microbial resistance is becoming more common. This resistance can be a result of several different factors. Most simply, the aminoglycosides may fail to penetrate the cytoplasm of the organism. Penetration of the bacterial cytoplasmic membrane is an oxygen-dependent, active process. Strictly anaerobic bacteria and facultative bacteria under anaerobic conditions are therefore highly resistant. Bacteria can produce enzymes that inactivate or destroy aminoglycosides. These enzymes are usually plasmid mediated and are termed aminoglycoside-modifying enzymes. These agents are analogous to β-lactamase (penicillinase), which hydrolyzes the β-lactam ring of some penicillins and cephalosporins. Genetic information for these inactivating enzymes is located on the bacterial chromosome itself or, more commonly, on pieces of extrachromosomal DNA termed plasmids. Many organisms contain a special plasmid segment, termed a resistance transfer factor, that allows the bacterium to mate with another organism through conjugation and pass the plasmid coding for the aminoglycoside-inactivating enzyme. Gram-negative bacteria that possess these inactivating enzymes can effectively prevent aminoglycosides from reaching their target ribosomes by maintaining a concentration of the enzymes in the periplasmic space between the cell membrane and the peptidoglycan cell walls. Any aminoglycoside trying to penetrate the bacterial cytoplasm will be inactivated before reaching the bacterial ribosomes. Many of these plasmid-mediated deactivating enzymes are not antibiotic specific and may confer resistance on multiple aminoglycosides. Many modifying enzymes have already been identified. Enzyme-mediated resistance to kenomycin is so widespread that the antibiotic has little clinical usefulness. Amikacin, a semisynthetic derivative of kenamycin, was developed to resist the effects of these enzymes. For this reason, many gram-negative bacilli that are resistant to tobramycin and gentamicin remain sensitive to amikacin.

Bacteria can also gain resistance to aminoglycosides through a random mutation in a protein that constitutes part of the aminoglycoside–ribosomal receptor site. Major changes in these critical proteins would likely be lethal to the bacteria. However, mutations that result in only a slight configurational change in the receptor site could prevent effective binding of the drugs and confer marked resistance to their action. Any mutation in the receptor site would be a random occurrence and probably is not a common mechanism for acquiring resistance. Because of the specific nature of aminoglycoside–ribosome binding, resistance would be expected to be specific for a single aminoglycoside only. As a result, this form of resistance is probably much less important clinically than is plasmid-mediated resistance.

Therapeutic Use

As a class, aminoglycosides share a similar spectrum of activity. They are clinically useful primarily against aerobic gram-negative organisms and pseudomonas. They have little activity against anaerobic organisms or facultative organisms under anaerobic conditions. They also have limited usefulness against gram-positive bacteria. Nevertheless, gentamicin and tobramycin are active in vitro against most strains of *Staphylococcus aureus* and *S. epidermidis.* Resistance, mediated by aminoglycoside-modifying enzymes, is increasingly making aminoglycosides unreliable for treatment of infections caused by these organisms (17). Most gram-negative organisms that possess plasmid-mediated aminoglycoside-modifying enzymes will be resistant to both tobramycin and gentamicin. However, 50% of *P. aeruginosa* species resistant to gentamicin remain sensitive to tobramycin (18). For this reason, tobramycin should be used instead of gentamycin for suspected cases of bacterial keratitis due to pseudomonas. Amikacin, a semisynthetic aminoglycoside, through resistance to aminoglycoside-inactivating enzymes, remains effective against most gentamicin- and tobramycin-resistant organisms. Streptomycin has no significant clinical use in ophthalmology. It is used only for the treatment of certain unusual infections, usually in combination with other agents. It is also infrequently used for tuberculosis.

Neomycin may have some special clinical usefulness in cases of *Acanthamoeba* keratitis. Prolonged and intensive triple antiamoebic therapy consisting of topical neomycin-polymyxin B-gramacidin, propamidine, and miconazole has shown promise in treating patients with documented *Acanthamoeba* keratitis (19,20).

Because of their broad spectrum of activity and bacteriocidal nature, aminoglycosides have proven useful for treatment of both superficial and deep infections of the eye and ocular adnexa. For less serious infections, such as bacterial conjunctivitis, commercially available concentrations of gentamicin and tobramycin will usually suffice. Bacterial corneal ulcers require significantly higher concentrations of topical drops than are commercially available. Highly concentrated, fortified preparations must be prepared, usually from concentrated intravenous preparations, soon before use, due to a limited shelf life.

Preparation of Fortified Aminoglycoside Drops for Topical Use

Tobramycin: Add 2.0 ml of 40 mg/ml solution of tobramycin to 3.0 cc sterile water or saline for a final concentration of 16 mg/ml; keep refrigerated; shelf life is 3 months (21).

Gentamicin: Dilute 2.0 ml of 40 mg/ml in 3.0 cc sterile water or saline for a final concentration of 16 mg/ml; keep refrigerated; shelf life is 3 months (21).

Neomycin: Reconstitute 500 mg powder neomycin in 15.0 ml sterile H_2O or saline for a final concentration of 33 mg/ml; keep refrigerated; shelf life is 3 days.

Table 2 shows preparations of fortified aminoglycosides. Although dosing of commercially available aminoglycoside preparation four times daily may suffice for conjunctivitis, fortified tobramycin or gentamicin is usually administered every 30 to 60 minutes. When the responsible bacterial agent is unknown, these concentrated preparations of aminoglycosides are usually alternated with a fortified preparation of cephalosporin (such as cephamandole 50 mg/ml). Because of the wide variety of possible ocular pathogens, the aminoglycoside is administered primarily to cover potential gram-negative pathogens, which is particularly important if Pseudomonas is suspected. The fortified cephalosporin is used to provide broad gram-positive coverage. This “shot gun” antimicrobial treatment will cover most bacterial ocular pathogens. If the offending bacteria can be isolated by culture, the topical regimen can be tailored according to sensitivity results.

The frequent dosing of fortified drops, in particular the aminoglycoside, can cause significant epithelial toxicity, conjunctival injection, pseudomembrane, eyelid-skin erythema, and even cicatricial changes in the eyelids. Because of the need for prolonged antimicrobial therapy of serious bacterial ulcers, these side effects can be problematic. Patients may even need oculoplastic procedures to correct entropion or ectropion that results.

Although the combination of a fortified aminoglycoside and fortified cephalosporin has traditionally been used for serious corneal ulcers, newer, less toxic agents have recently become available. Fluoroquinolones, an important new class of antibiotic agents in ophthalmology, include ciprofloxacin, norfloxacin, and ofloxacin. The activity of the fluoroquinolones varies slightly from agent to agent, but in general they have excellent activity against gram-negative organisms, including *P. aeruginosa* and penicillin-resistant *Neisseria gonorrhea,* and good activity against most gram-positive organisms (22–24). Many ophthalmologists now prefer ciprofloxacin 0.3% ophthalmic solution to fortified antibiotic agents as the drug of choice for initial treatment of bacterial keratitis. Ciprofloxacin is extremely well tolerated even at frequent doses. For more information on the usefulness of fluoroquinolones in ophthalmology, see Chapter 46, *this volume.*

Aminoglycosides are also administered intravitreally in the treatment of endophthalmitis (25). Most treatment regimens pair vancomycin hydrochloride and aminoglycoside such as amikacin sulfate. Caution must be used, however, because intravitreal injections of amikacin, tobramycin, and gentamicin have been associated with retinal toxicity, including macular infarction (26). Evidence suggests that intravitreal amikacin may be slightly safer than either tobramycin or gentamicin.

ACKNOWLEDGMENT: This work was supported in part by an unrestricted grant from Research to Prevent Blindness, Inc., New York, NY, and by Core Grant No. EYO1931 from the National Institutes of Health, Bethesda, MD.

REFERENCES

1. Glasser DB, Baum J. Antibacterial agents. In: Tabbara KF, Hyndiuk RA, eds. *Infections of the Eye,* 2nd ed. Boston: Little, Brown, 1994.
2. Glasser DB, Hyndiuk RA. Antibacterial agents. In: Tabbara KF, Hyndiuk RA, eds. *Infections of the eye.* Boston: Little, Brown, 1986;211–238.
3. Wilhelmus KR, Gibert ML, Osato MS. Tobramycin in ophthalmology. *Surv Ophthalmol* 1987;32:111–122.
4. Sande MA, Mandell GL. The aminoglycosides. In: *Gilman and Goodman's The pharmacological basis of therapeutics,* 8th ed. New York: Macmillan, 1994;1098–1116.
5. Phillips I. Good antimicrobial prescribing aminoglycosides. *Lancet* 1982;2:311.
6. Davies BD, Brummett RE, Bendrick TW, Hines DL. Dissociation of maximum concentration of kenamycin in plasma and perilymph from ototoxic effect. *J Antimicrob Chemother* 1984;14:291–302.
7. Huy PTB, Meutemans A, Wassef M, Manuel C, Sterkers O, Amiel C. Gentamicin persistence in rat endolymph and perilymph after a two-day constant infusion. *Antimicrob Agents Chemother* 1983;23:344–346.
8. Wilson WR, Wilkowske CJ, Wright AJ, Sande MA, Geraci JE. Treatment of streptomycin susceptible and streptomycin resistant enterococcal endocarditis. *Ann Intern Med* 1984;100:816–823.
9. Warkang J. Antituberculous drugs. *Teratology* 1979;20:133–138.
10. Smith CR, Lipshy JJ, Laskin OL, et al. Double-blind comparison of the nephrotoxicity and auditory toxicity of gentamicin and tobramycin. *N Engl J Med* 1980;302:1106–1109.
11. Waltz K, Margo CE. Intraocular gentamicin toxicity [Letter]. *Arch Ophthalmol* 1991;109:911.
12. Pittinger C, Adamson R. Antibiotic blockade of neuromuscular function. *Annu Rev Pharmacol* 1972;12:169–184.
13. Holtzman JL. Gentamicin neuromuscular blockage. *Ann Intern Med* 1976;84.
14. Mates SM, Patel L, Kaback HR, Miller MH. Membrane potential in anaerobically growing *Staphylococcus aureus* and its relationship to gentamicin uptake. *Antimicrob Agents Chemother* 1983;23:526–530.
15. Luzzatto L, Apirion D, Schlessinger D. Polyribosome depletion and blockage of ribosome cycle by streptomycin in *Escherichia coli. J Mol Biol* 1969;42:315–335.
16. Tai PC, Wallace BJ, Davis BD. Streptomycin causes misreading of natural messenger by interactions with ribosomes after initiation. *Proc Natl Acad Sci USA* 1978;75:275–279.
17. Kucers A, Bennett NMcK. Gentamicin. In: Kucers A, Bennett NMcK, eds. *The use of antibiotics,* 4th ed. Philadelphia: JB Lippincott, 1987; 619–674.
18. Symposium. Tobramycin. *J Infect Dis* 1976;134:S1–S234.
19. Berger ST, Mondino BJ, Hoft RH, et al. Successful medical management of *Acanthamoeba* keratitis. *Am J Ophthalmol* 1990;110:395–403.
20. John T, Lin J. *Acanthamoeba* keratitis successfully treated with prolonged propamidine isethionate and neomycin-polymyxin-gramicidin. *Ann Ophthalmol* 1990;22:20–23.
21. McBride HA, Martinez DR, Trang JM, Lander RD, Helmms HA. Stability of gentamicin sulfate and tobramycin sulfate in extemporaneously prepared ophthalmic solutions at 8 degrees C. *Am J Hosp Pharm* 1991;48:507–509.
22. Ogawa GSH, Hyndiuk RA. The fluoroquinolones: new antibiotics in ophthalmology. *Int Ophthalmol Clin* 1993;33:59–68.
23. Gwon A. Ofloxacin vs tobramycin for the treatment of external ocular infection. *Arch Ophthalmol* 1992;110:1234–1237.
24. Miller IM, Vogel R, Cook JJ, Wittrerch J. Topically administered norfloxacin compared with topically administered gentamicin for the treatment of external ocular bacterial infections. *Am J Ophthalmol* 1992;113:638–644.
25. Donahue SP, et al. Empiric treatment of endophthalmitis. *Arch Ophthalmol* 1994;112:45–47.
26. Campochiaro PA, Lim JI. Aminoglycoside toxicity in the treatment of endophthalmitis. *Arch Ophthalmol* 1994;112:48–53.
27. *Physicians Desk Reference for Ophthalmology*, 24th ed. Montvale, NJ: Medical Economics Data, 1996.
28. Baum J. Appendix 1, preparation of antibiotics for topical use. In: Lamberts D, Potter D, eds. *Clinical ophthalmic pharmacology.* Boston: Little, Brown, 1987;519–531.

Textbook of Ocular Pharmacology,
edited by T.J. Zimmerman, et al.
Lippincott–Raven Publishers, Philadelphia © 1997.

CHAPTER 46

Fluoroquinolones

Gregory S. H. Ogawa and Robert A. Hyndiuk

FLUOROQUINOLONES

History and Source

The fluoroquinolones are a new family of antibacterial agents based on the original 4-quinolone, nalidixic acid, a drug first marketed in 1962 for treatment of urinary tract infections. The fluoroquinolones were initially developed from nalidixic acid in the 1980s by adding a fluorine to the 6 position of the molecule. The newer fluoroquinolones have a much wider spectrum of antibacterial activity than nalidixic acid and also have a lower rate of development of resistant organisms.

Drug Names and Chemistry

Ciprofloxacin HCl [Cipro, oral form; Cipro I.V., intravenous (IV) form; Ciloxan, ophthalmic solution] is the monohydrochloride monohydrate salt of 1-cyclopropyl-6-fluoro-1,4-dihydro-4-oxo-7-(1-piperazinyl)-3-quinoline-carboxylic acid. The empirical formula is $C_{17}H_{18}FN_3O_3 \cdot HCl \cdot H_2O$. The structural formula of ciprofloxacin HCl is shown below.

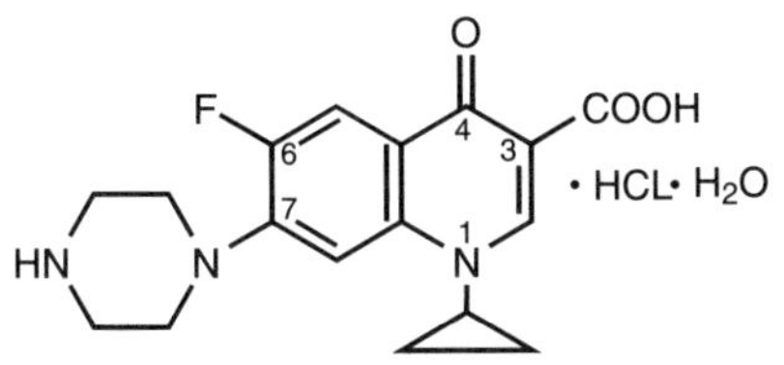

F
O
COOH
6
4
3
• HCL• H2O
7
1
HN
N
N

Norfloxacin (Noroxin tablets, for oral form; Chibroxin, for ophthalmic solution) is 1-ethyl-6-fluoro-1,4-dihydro-4-oxo-7-(1-piperazinyl)-3-quinoline-carboxylic acid. The empirical formula is $C_{16}H_{18}FN_3O_3$. The structural formula of norfloxacin is shown below.

O
F
COOH
H—N
N
N
C2H5

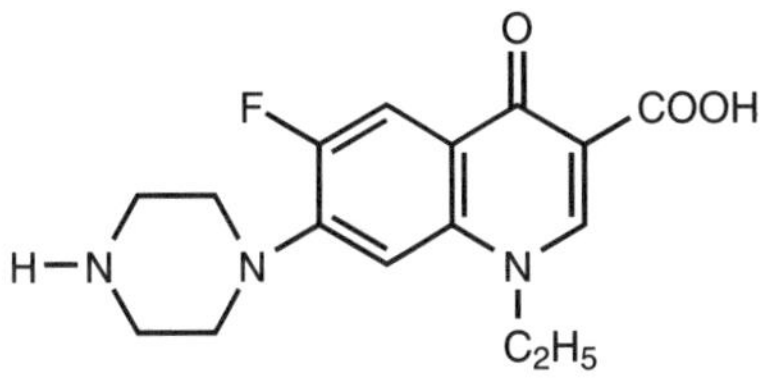

Ofloxacin (Floxin tablets, oral form; Floxin I.V., IV form; Ocuflox, ophthalmic solution) is the racemate: (±)-9-fluoro-2,3-dihydro-3-methyl-10-(4-methyl-1-piperazinyl)-7-oxo-7H-pyrido[1,2,3-de-]1,4 benzoxazine-6-carboxylic acid. The empirical formula is $C_{18}H_{20}FN_3O_4$. The structural formula of ofloxacin is shown below.

O
F
COOH
H3C—N
N
N
O
CH3

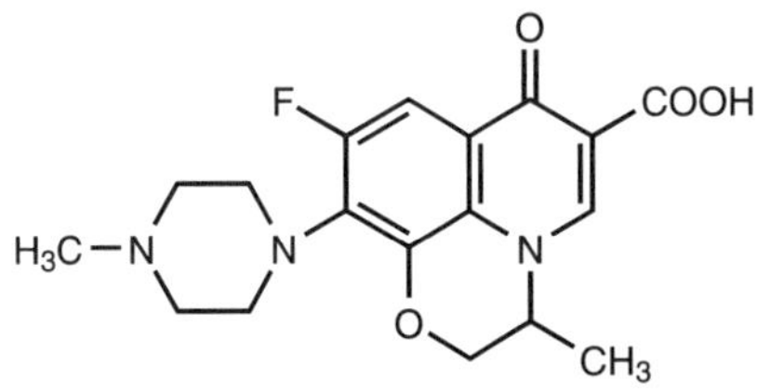

Enoxacin (Penetrex, oral form) is 1-ethyl-6-fluoro-1,4-dihydro-4-oxo-7-(piperazinyl)-1,8-naph-thyridine-3-carboxylic acid sesquihydrate. The empirical formula is $C_{15}H_{17}N_4O_3F \cdot 1\frac{1}{2}\ H_2O$. The structural formula of enoxacin is shown below.

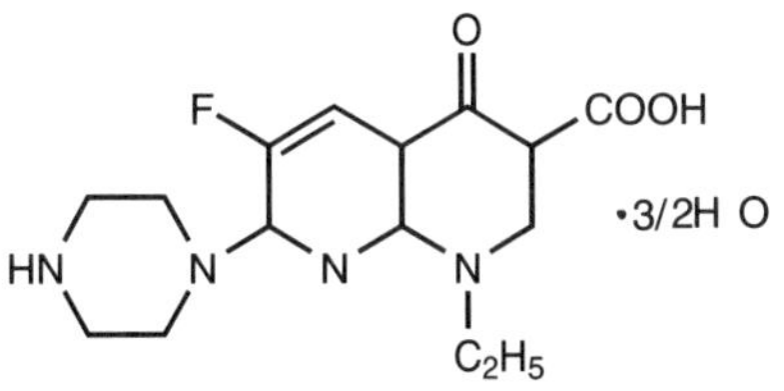

O
F
COOH
•3/2H O
HN
N
N
N
C2H5

Lomefloxacin HCl (Maxaquin, oral form) is the monohydrochloride salt of the racemate: (±)-1-ethyl-6,8,-difluoro-1,4-dihydro-7-(3-methyl-1-piperazinyl)-4-oxo-3-quin-

G. S. H. Ogawa: The Division of Ophthalmology, The University of New Mexico, Albuquerque, New Mexico 87131–5341.
R. A. Hyndiuk: The Department of Ophthalmology, Medical College of Wisconsin, Milwaukee, Wisconsin 53226.

oline-carboxylic acid. The empirical formula is $C_{17}H_{19}F_2N_3O_3.HCl$. The structural formula of lomefloxacin is shown below.

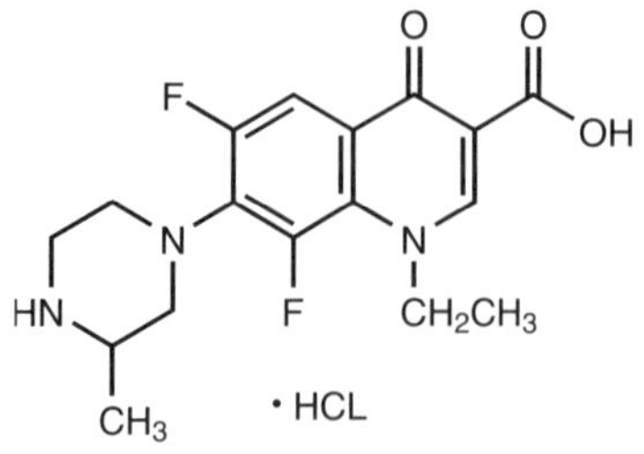

Pharmacology

The fluoroquinolones are bactericidal agents that inhibit DNA gyrase (bacterial topoisomerase II). Bacterial gyrase is a four-subunit enzyme that plays an important role in supercoiling of DNA for storage and in bacterial DNA replication, transcription, repair, and recombination. The effect of the fluoroquinolones is selective for bacteria since the agents do not inhibit the human topoisomerase II, which is composed of only two subunits and has a fundamentally different function (1). Bacteria not initially killed by the fluoroquinolones experience a postantibiotic effect of 2 to 6 hours, during which time the organism does not grow (2).

The fluoroquinolones probably have two basic mechanisms through which they enter the gram-negative bacterial cell. The first is a porin-mediated mechanism in which outer membrane proteins aid in the transport of the drug into the cell. The second is a self-promoted transport through which hydrophobic fluoroquinolones enter the cell by lipopolysaccharide transport after chelation of membrane-associated magnesium (3). The fluoroquinolones enter gram-positive organisms only by a hydrophobic route, so that the greater the hydrophobicity of the fluoroquinolone, the greater the bacterial accumulation. [Ofloxacin is more hydrophobic than ciprofloxacin (3).]

The current fluoroquinolones have a carboxylic acid substitution at position 3 and a ketocarboxyl group at position 4, which together help the drug bind to bacterial DNA gyrase (below). A fluorine at position 6 increases the DNA gyrase inhibitory activity of the drug. A piperazine group at position 7 increases a drug's activity against Pseudomonas, and a methylpiperazine group (as in ofloxacin) at position 7 increases a drug's activity against *Enterobacteriaceae* and also increases oral absorption and serum half-life ($t\frac{1}{2}$). A variety of side chain substitutions exist at position 1 (2,4).

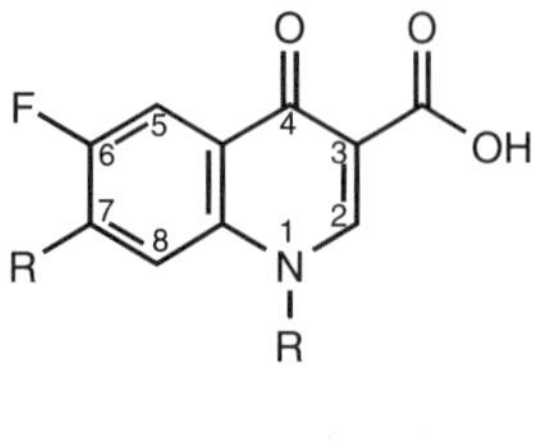

PHARMACEUTICS

The following is a list of the newer fluoroquinolones available in the United States, showing their forms, brand names, manufacturers, Food and Drug Administration (FDA) approval dates, and how they are supplied.

Fluoroquinolones

Ciprofloxacin
- Ciprofloxacin HCl 0.3% sterile ophthalmic solution, Ciloxan
  - Alcon Laboratories (Fort Wayne, TX); FDA approval 1990 2.5-ml and 5-ml bottles
- Ciprofloxacin HCl tablets, Cipro
  - Miles Pharmaceutical (West Haven, CT); FDA approval 1987 250 mg, 500 mg, 750 mg
- Ciprofloxacin HCl IV solutions, Cipro I.V.
  - Miles Pharmaceutical; FDA approval 1991
    - Vials: 20 ml with 200 mg in 1% solution; 40 ml with 400 mg in 1% solution; 120 ml with 1,200 mg in 1% solution
    - Flexible container: 100 ml with 200 mg in 0.2% solution in 5% dextrose; 200 ml with 400 mg in 0.2% solution in 5% dextrose

Ciprofloxacin in a 0.3% topical ophthalmic ointment form is currently an investigational drug but may be approved by the FDA in the future (5).

Norfloxacin
- Norfloxacin 0.3% sterile ophthalmic solution, Chibroxin
  - Merck & Co. (West Point, PA); FDA approval 1991 5-ml bottle
- Norfloxacin tablets, Noroxin tablets
  - Merck & Co.; FDA approval 1986 400 mg

Ofloxacin
- Ofloxacin 0.3% sterile ophthalmic solution, Ocuflox
  - Allergan (Irvine, CA); FDA approval 1993 5 ml
- Ofloxacin tablets, Floxin tablets
  - McNeil Pharmaceutical (Fort Washington, PA); FDA approval 1990 200 mg, 300 mg, 400 mg
- Ofloxacin IV solutions, Floxin I.V.
  - McNeil Pharmaceutical; FDA approval 1990
    - Vials: 10 ml with 400 mg 40-mg/ml solution; 20 ml with 400 mg 20-mg/ml solution
    - Bottles: 100 ml with 400 mg 4-mg/ml solution in 5% dextrose

Flexible container: 50 ml with 200 mg 4-mg/ml solution in 5% dextrose; 100 ml with 400 mg 4-mg/ml solution in 5% dextrose

Enoxacin

Enoxacin tablets, Penetrex

Rhone-Poulenc Rorer Pharmaceuticals (Collegeville, PA); FDA approval 1991

200 mg, 400 mg

Lomefloxacin

Lomefloxacin HCl tablets, Maxaquin

Searle (Chicago IL); FDA approval 1992

400 mg

Other fluoroquinolones available abroad or still under development include fleroxacin, levofloxacin, pefloxacin, clinafloxacin, Bay y3118, and sparfloxacin. The latter three of these fluoroquinolones have particularly enhanced activity against gram-positive organisms.

Pharmacokinetics

Systemic Pharmacokinetics

Orally administered fluoroquinolones achieve 50% to 95% absorption with peak serum levels at 1 to 3 hours, with a wide tissue distribution. Systemic doses of most fluoroquinolones are metabolized hepatically and excreted renally, whereas ofloxacin is principally excreted renally. For systemic elimination, $t_{\frac{1}{2}}$ ranges from 3 to 11 hours, allowing once-daily to twice-daily systemic dosing. Oral ofloxacin has a longer $t_{\frac{1}{2}}$ than ciprofloxacin, and oral doses achieve higher serum levels (6,7).

Ocular Penetration: Topical

All the topically available fluoroquinolones have much better penetration into the cornea and anterior chamber when the epithelium is compromised or disrupted; therefore, they more readily achieve adequate tissue and anterior chamber drug levels in treatment of active ocular infections or other ocular conditions in which epithelium is impaired.

Hourly drops of 0.3% solution topical ciprofloxacin produce corneal stromal levels of 5.28 ± 3.4 μg/g through intact human corneal epithelium. These drug levels may not exceed the minimum inhibitory concentration at 90% (MIC_{90}) for some gram-positive organisms, but the augmented tissue levels possible with compromised epithelium are likely to cover most corneal pathogens (8). Human aqueous-humor levels of ciprofloxacin 30 minutes after two doses of hourly 0.3% drops with intact epithelium range from 0.02 to 0.153 μg/ml (9). These levels are lower than those needed to offer adequate broad-spectrum coverage reliably, but they may have been higher if a more aggressive dosing protocol was used. Topical ciprofloxacin drops achieve anterior chamber levels two to three times greater if the epithelium is compromised than if it is intact, as demonstrated experimentally by O'Brien et al. (10) in uninflamed rabbit eyes with ciprofloxacin levels of 13 μg/ml 30 minutes after the last dose with epithelial debridement versus 5 μg/ml with intact corneal epithelium. Ciprofloxacin is less lipophilic than ofloxacin (3), which may make it less effective in penetrating intact epithelium. The elimination $t_{\frac{1}{2}}$ for ciprofloxacin from the aqueous humor appears to be 1 to 2 hours (10).

Peak aqueous humor levels of norfloxacin after topical dosing in eyes with intact epithelium range from <0.04 μg/ml to approximately 0.6 μg/ml, which may be above the MIC_{90} for some gram-negative organisms but below that of many gram-positive organisms (9,11,12).

Topical 0.3% ofloxacin applied hourly to intact epithelium for two doses produces a wide range of aqueous humor levels from 0.078 to 0.626 μg/ml 30 minutes after the last dose (9). These levels are higher than those achieved with ciprofloxacin using the same protocol, but they still are not reliable for adequate broad-spectrum coverage of organisms in the anterior chamber.

When the epithelium is not intact in an experimental rabbit model, the tear film level, corneal tissue level, and anterior chamber level of the three topical fluoroquinolones become comparable and are significantly increased as compared with those obtained in intact epithelium (10); therefore, in treatment of ulcerative bacterial keratitis, the important factor becomes potency of the fluoroquinolone rather than penetration data based on intact epithelium models.

Hatano et al. (13) demonstrated good penetration of topical lomefloxacin into the eye and applied the drug experimentally in the treatment of *Pseudomonas aeruginosa* endophthalmitis (13).

Ocular Penetration: Subconjunctival Administration

Subconjunctival doses of ciprofloxacin in rabbits result in rapid anterior chamber levels of the drug (14). Subconjunctival ciprofloxacin achieves good aqueous humor levels (approximately 1.0 μg/ml), but its clinical safety and efficacy have not yet been defined (15).

Ocular Penetration: Iontophoresis

Iontophoresis is a process through which ions are driven into cells by direct current. Cationic drugs are driven into cells by an anode, whereas anionic drugs are delivered by a cathode. Most of the ocular studies of this type delivery system have been performed in either humans or animals. Ocular iontophoresis of antibiotics may be performed through the cornea or sclera. Transcorneal iontophoresis produces high drug levels in the anterior chamber and cornea, but cannot penetrate the lens into the vitreous. Transscleral iontophoresis avoids the lens and can deliver therapeutic doses of antibiotic agent to the vitreous (16).

Initial research with transcorneal iontophoresis and ciprofloxacin in a rabbit experimental model demonstrated excellent drug levels in the anterior chamber. Transcorneal ciprofloxacin anodal iontophoresis produces anterior chamber drug levels more than twice as high as those achieved with topically administered drops (16).

Ocular Penetration: Systemic Administration

After systemic doses of ciprofloxacin, intraocular penetration in uninflamed eyes occurs with levels of at least 0.25 μg/ml, which is greater than the MIC_{90} for almost all gram-negative organisms but does not cover all gram-positive organisms (15,17–19). (See the Endophthalmitis section.)

Resistance

Bacterial resistance to fluoroquinolones can occur through one or both of the following mechanisms: (a) bacterial DNA gyrase modifications to decrease or eliminate inhibition by fluoroquinolones, and (b) cell membrane modifications to decrease the amount of fluoroquinolone that can enter the bacteria (3,4). The former mechanism is the one responsible for high-level resistance when it occurs in gram-negative or gram-positive organisms (3,20). Gram-negative organisms can alter their outer membrane proteins to decrease penetration by the hydrophilic fluoroquinolones that rely on transport by porins to enter the bacteria. Gram-negative and gram-positive organisms may alter other factors such as lipopolysaccharides to decrease the activity of the hydrophobic transport mechanism for fluoroquinolones into the cell (3). Chromosome mutations are required to produce resistance to the fluoroquinolones; therefore, the rate of resistance to newer fluoroquinolones generally is low. Resistance mechanisms with drug destruction and/or drug modification have not yet been identified, and plasmid-mediated resistance has not been reported.

The development of resistance to fluoroquinolones varies with the bacteria and the particular quinolone agent. As with other antibiotics, drug-resistant mutants are selected more commonly in tissues with low or borderline drug levels than in tissues with high drug levels. For the fluoroquinolones, this is particularly true of *P. aeruginosa* and methicillin-resistant *Staphylococcus aureus* (MRSA). Therefore, resistant mutants are much more likely to be selected in some infections treated systemically than in external ocular infections aggressively treated topically since very high peak ocular surface drug levels are achieved with topical treatment. A few strains of ciprofloxacin-resistant *P. aeruginosa* and *S. aureus* (including MRSA) have emerged from the use of oral ciprofloxacin, but no data are yet available regarding the development of resistant organisms from the use of topical ophthalmic ciprofloxacin (21–23). In experimental *S. aureus* keratitis, no evidence of development of resistance was detected after 5 hours of treatment with topical ciprofloxacin solution, since surviving organisms had the same MIC as nonchallenged organisms (24,25).

Clinical Pharmacology and Therapeutic Uses

Antibacterial Activity

The antimicrobial activity of fluoroquinolones varies from agent to agent but, as a class, they have excellent activity against gram-negative organisms, including *P. aeruginosa* and penicillin-resistant *N. gonorrhoeae,* with good to excellent activity against most gram-positive organisms and variable activity against anaerobes (4,26) (Table 1). Although some of the fluoroquinolones are relatively less active against *Streptococcus* organisms (Table 1), ciprofloxacin and ofloxacin have sufficient activity to be used as initial monotherapy for bacterial keratitis against these organisms. We have successfully used ciprofloxacin topically as monotherapy for *α-streptococcus* infectious crystalline keratopathy, effecting a cure medically. This is normally a very difficult infection to treat and usually requires keratoplasty for eradication of the organism (Fig. 1) (Hyndiuk RA, Tabbara KF. Infectious Crystalline Keratopathy, Third International Symposium on Ocular Inflammation; Ocular Infection and Antibiotics Symposium, Fukuoka, Japan, October 23, 1994) Fluoroquinolone activity against *S. pneumoniae* is not affected by the organism's penicillin-susceptibility status (27).

The fluoroquinolones have increasing bactericidal activity as the drug concentration increases to an optimum (the optimum bactericidal concentration [OBC]), after which increasing the drug concentration produces paradoxically less bactericidal activity. The OBC for newer fluoroquinolones is generally 10 to 20 times higher than the MIC of the drug against *S. aureus* and *S. epidermidis* (20). How significant this phenomenon is in treating clinical infections is unclear.

Ciprofloxacin is the most potent of the fluoroquinolones (1). It has extended broad-spectrum activity, with excellent in vitro activity against *P. aeruginosa, Chlamydia trachomatis, Haemophilus influenzae, N. gonorrhoeae, S. aureus, S. epidermidis,* and *Enterobacteriaceae. S. pneumoniae* is also inhibited, but at antibiotic concentrations higher than those needed for inhibition of *Enterobacteriaceae* (2,28). In vitro and experimental evidence suggest that ciprofloxacin is quite effective against most aminoglycoside resistant strains of *P. aeruginosa* (29).

Table 46-1. *In vitro activity of fluoroquinolones and gentamicin for common ocular pathogens*[a]

Bacteria	MIC$_{90}$ (μg/ml)								
	Ciprofloxacin	Enoxacin	Fleroxacin	Lomefloxacin	Norfloxacin	Ofloxacin	Pefloxacin	Sparfloxacin	Gentamicin
Bacillus cereus	0.25	—	—	—	—	—	—	—	2
Chlamydia trachomatis	0.5–2	8	3.1	0.25	8	1	—	—	—
Escherichia coli	0.08	0.25	0.25	0.25	<0.25	≤0.25	<0.25	0.06	≤1
Haemophilus influenzae	0.03	<0.12	8	8	<0.12	4	0.06	<0.02	1–4
Klebsiella pneumoniae	0.24	0.25	0.50	0.50	0.50	0.25	2	—	2–16
Moraxella lacunata	≤0.25	—	—	—	0.50	—	0.50	—	≤1
Neisseria gonorrhoeae	0.004	<0.12	0.12	0.12	<0.12	<0.12	0.125	<0.02	4
N. meningitidis	<0.06	<0.12	0.12	0.12	<0.12	<0.12	0.03–1.0	—	—
Proteus mirabilis	0.18	0.8	0.50	0.25	≤0.25–0.5	≤0.25	1	0.50	2
Pseudomonas aeruginosa	0.50	2	0.50	0.50	2	4	2	2	4–32
Serratia marcescens	0.12	0.25–2	0.50	0.25–4	≤0.25	4	<0.25	—	≤1–8
Staphylococcus aureus	0.61	2	2	4	1	0.5–1	<0.25	0.25	≤1
S. epidermidis	0.49	8	2	2	4	1–2	0.50	0.25	16
Streptococcus pneumoniae	1.97	16	16	16	4–16	1–2	4	1	8–32

MIC$_{90}$, minimum inhibitory concentration at 90%.

Data from Neu (2), Wolfson and Hooper (4,26), Baba et al. (18), King and Phillips (28), Cokingtin and Hyndiuk (37), and Wiederman and Atkinson (49).

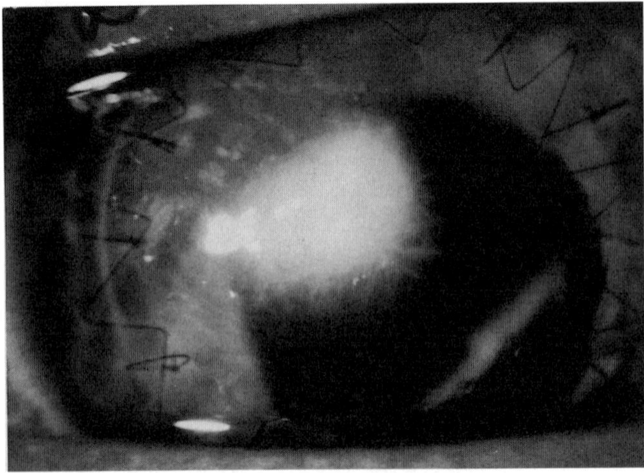

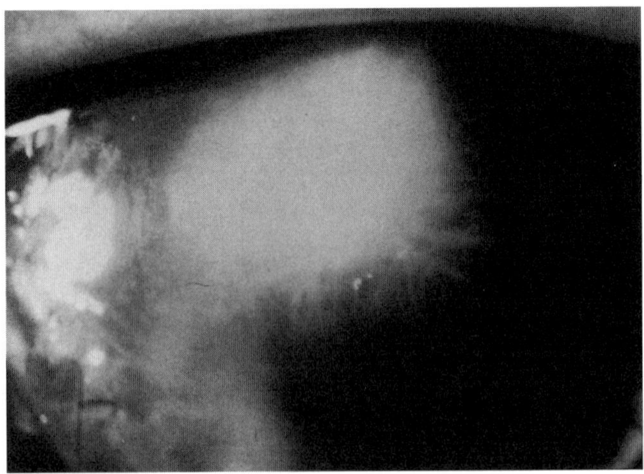

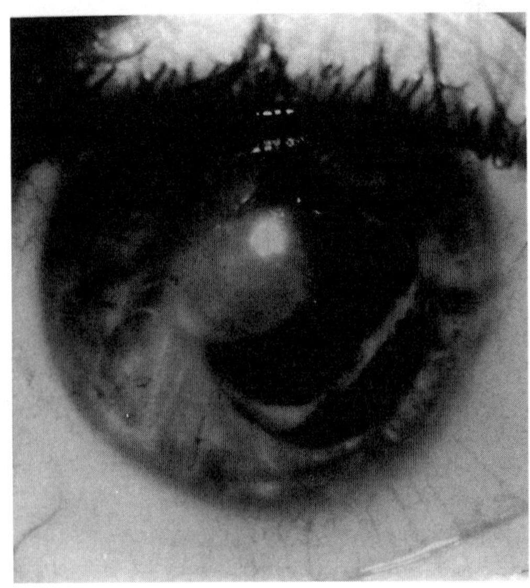

A B C

FIG. 46-1. *α-Streptococcus* crystalline keratopathy in a corneal transplant. **A.** Low magnification. **B.** High magnification. **C.** Medical cure of the infectious keratopathy with a residual scar. The infection was treated aggressively with ciprofloxacin 0.3% topical ophthalmic solution monotherapy for 7 weeks.

Norfloxacin is the least potent of the fluoroquinolones available topically in the United States. Its greatest activity is against gram-negative organisms, although it is significantly less active than ciprofloxacin against *P. aeruginosa.* Norfloxacin is relatively less active against anaerobic organisms and gram-positive organisms, especially *Streptococcus* and *Staphylococcus* (26,28–30).

Ofloxacin has a wide spectrum of activity (31); however, it is not as potent as ciprofloxacin against gram-negative organisms such as *P. aeruginosa, H. influenzae,* and *Serratia.* Ofloxacin has better activity than ciprofloxacin (32) against MRSA and has activity comparable to that of ciprofloxacin against other gram-positive organisms, except against *S. viridans,* against which ciprofloxacin is more active.

Enoxacin has an antimicrobial profile similar to norfloxacin.

Levofloxacin is the *S*-(-) optical isomer of ofloxacin and was scheduled for release in Japan in 1995 (33). Levofloxacin is more active than enoxacin, norfloxacin or ciprofloxacin against coagulase-negative *Staphylococcus* and is 8 to 128 times more active than the *R*-(-) optical isomer (33,34). Some other investigational fluoroquinolones have increased activity against gram-positive organisms such as *S. pneumoniae* and offer the hope of even broader-spectrum drugs that may be more effective in ocular infections (27).

Bacterial Keratitis

Ciprofloxacin 0.3% ophthalmic solution has become the antibiotic of choice of many ophthalmologists for initial monotherapy of mild, moderate, or the most severe ulcerative bacterial keratitis (35). It is effective against almost all important corneal pathogens, is very well tolerated even with aggressive dosing regimens, is effective at its commercial, nonfortified strength, and has been approved by the FDA for the treatment of bacterial keratitis (36,37). Topical ciprofloxacin has demonstrated excellent experimental and clinical efficacy in treatment of bacterial corneal ulcers (10,24,35,36). Ciprofloxacin is a very good choice for the treatment of bacterial keratitis because of its high potency, broad spectrum, excellent activity against *P. aeruginosa,* and good activity against Streptococcus species.

Ofloxacin 0.3% ophthalmic solution is now beginning to be used in the treatment of bacterial keratitis. This agent has a very broad spectrum of activity, with excellent potency against most ocular pathogens, although it is not as effective as ciprofloxacin against gram-negative organisms. The Bacterial Keratitis Study Research Group showed ofloxacin to be as effective as a combination of fortified tobramycin and cefazolin for bacterial corneal ulcers in their multicenter study (38). At the time of this writing, ofloxacin is not approved by the FDA for the treatment of bacterial keratitis.

Norfloxacin showed good results in the treatment of bacterial keratitis in one small study (39), but because it is significantly less potent than either ciprofloxacin or ofloxacin and its gram-positive spectrum is variable, we do not consider it a good choice for monotherapy in the treatment of bacterial keratitis.

When treating bacterial corneal ulcers with ciprofloxacin or ofloxacin, we load the cornea with one drop of antibiotic agent every 5 minutes for six doses to achieve peak corneal drug levels quickly. We then administer one drop every 15 minutes for 6 hours before changing to one drop every 30 minutes (or every hour for mild ulcers) for the rest of day 1 of treatment. If the infection is stable or improving on day 2 or 3, we switch to hourly dosing. We taper the frequency of drops during the rest of the treatment course, basing frequency on the clinical response. We do not discontinue the antibiotic agent until all signs of active infection have cleared and the epithelial defect has healed.

A useful way to maximize corneal drug-level peaks and minimize the drug level troughs when dosing frequency is being tapered is to group the doses in a technique we call "bunching," which is a method of loading the cornea with high drug levels on an intermittent basis. We often use one drop every 5 minutes for five doses as one "bunch." In the therapeutic course of an ulcer that is responding well to treatment, bunching can be used to allow a patient to awaken for medication administration just once during the night or to sleep through the night. The patient loads the cornea with drug, using one bunch before going to sleep, another bunch halfway through the night if needed, and an additional bunch on awakening. The patient can continue hourly dosing or some other frequent dosing regimen during the day combined with the night time bunches. When factors limit the times of the day when medications can be administered (such as when a patient is dependent on someone else to administer drops), bunching can be used for all doses administered. Bunching works best with drugs like ciprofloxacin that have a low toxicity level, since the peak drug levels achieved with this technique can maximize a drug's toxic effects.

Topical ocular use of fluoroquinolones is not known to have promoted the development of new resistant bacteria, but pretreatment-resistant bacteria do exist and have been reported to cause bacterial keratitis occasionally (40). Ophthalmologists should culture cases of bacterial ulcerative keratitis before initiating any antibiotic treatment (35,41). The sensitivity results can then be used in selecting another antibiotic agent if the infection does not respond clinically to treatment and the organism is discovered to be resistant to the first antibiotic agent used.

Ciprofloxacin 0.3% ophthalmic ointment showed very good efficacy in treatment of corneal ulcers in clinical trials in Milwaukee (Ogawa GSH, Cokingtin CD, Hyndiuk RA, Koenig SB. Early clinical data on ciprofloxacin ointment in the treatment of bacterial keratitis. Presented at the Annual Eye Institute Meeting, Medical College of Wisconsin, Milwaukee, WI, June 13, 1992) and elsewhere (5), even though other nonfortified, topical ophthalmic antibiotic ointments have been demonstrated to be ineffective in bacterial corneal ulcers (42). Topical ciprofloxacin ophthalmic ointment may have true advantages in certain patients with ocular surface disease for treatment and for prophylaxis since it is extremely well tolerated by the corneal and conjunctival epithelium even when used aggressively.

Nontuberculous Mycobacterium Keratitis

Topical ciprofloxacin drops have experimentally demonstrated good efficacy against *M. fortuitum* stromal keratitis and variable activity against *M. chelonae* keratitis (43).

Bacterial Conjunctivitis

Bacterial conjunctivitis is generally a self-limited infection, but more rapid resolution usually is achieved with use of topical antibiotics. Bacterial agents commonly causing conjunctivitis include *H. influenzae, S. pneumoniae, S. aureus,* and *S. epidermidis* (35). Two other important causes of conjunctivitis that do not cause self-limited infection are *N. gonorrhoeae* and *C. trachomatis* (44). The fluoroquinolones vary from agent to agent in their MIC_{90} value against the common causes of conjunctivitis (Table 1). Clinically, however, large randomized studies have demonstrated the efficacy and safety of topical ciprofloxacin 0.3%, ofloxacin 0.3%, and norfloxacin 0.3% in the treatment of bacterial conjunctivitis (45–48). For the self-limited types of bacterial conjunctivitis, these topical fluoroquinolones are used every 2 hours for 1 to 2 days while the patient is awake, and then every 4 hours for the next 5 to 6 days while the patient is awake, with frequency of administration tailored to the clinical response.

N. gonorrhoeae is exquisitely sensitive to the fluoroquinolones (49). Early studies demonstrated excellent results with ciprofloxacin, norfloxacin, pefloxacin, and fleroxacin in the treatment of urogenital gonococcus infection

(50–52). A preliminary small study of norfloxacin in a single oral dose for treatment of gonococcal conjunctivitis and keratoconjunctivitis also demonstrated efficacy (53). Regardless of the systemic antibiotic used to treat gonococcal keratoconjunctivitis, we believe that concomitant, aggressive topical treatment with a fluoroquinolone will probably be beneficial in more rapidly halting the ocular destruction caused by the infection. Speed of resolution is important in gonococcal keratoconjunctivitis since this infection can rapidly cause corneal perforation. Rare reports of *N. gonorrhoeae* with less sensitivity to the fluoroquinolones (MIC 2.0 for ciprofloxacin and ofloxacin) have recently emerged (54). These less sensitive strains may cause difficulties in systemic fluoroquinolone treatment of gonococcal disease in the future, but topical fluoroquinolones achieve sufficiently high surface drug levels to ensure that they would still be useful against these strains as an adjunct in the treatment of gonococcal conjunctivitis.

The fluoroquinolones vary from agent to agent in their MIC_{90} for *C. trachomatis,* but ofloxacin is very active against this organism. Ofloxacin 300 mg orally twice daily for 7 days is recommended as an alternative to doxycycline for *C. trachomatis* conjunctivitis, urethritis, cervicitis, or proctitis (55).

Endophthalmitis

Fluoroquinolones may eventually play a significant role in the treatment of and prophylaxis against bacterial endophthalmitis. Oral doses of ciprofloxacin achieve intravitreal levels of 0.4 μg/ml in uninflamed eyes after a single dose of 750 mg ciprofloxacin (18), and levels of about 0.6 μg/ml are achieved in aqueous humor (15,19). These levels are greater than the MIC_{90} for many intraocular pathogens, but not all (Table 1). Intraocular drug levels after oral administration may be higher in eyes inflamed owing to trauma or infection. Combined oral and topical ciprofloxacin have been used by some ophthalmologists to prevent infectious endophthalmitis after penetrating ocular trauma. This method of prophylaxis may be particularly appealing for trauma cases at risk for the devastating endophthalmitis from *Bacillus cereus,* since the MIC_{90} of *B. cereus* (approximately 0.25 μg/ml) is well below achievable intravitreal levels. Pefloxacin achieves a peak aqueous level of 1.5 μg/ml after a 400-mg intravenous dose (56), and ofloxacin reaches aqueous levels of approximately 1.0 μg/ml after a 400-mg oral dose (57,58). Because of the rarity of postoperative endophthalmitis and the variability in trauma-induced endophthalmitis, no clinical studies have been conducted to demonstrate the effectiveness of the fluoroquinolones for this purpose. Intravitreal ciprofloxacin has been shown to be safe in rabbit eyes at a dose of 100 μg or greater (59). In the future, intravitreal ciprofloxacin could become a helpful agent in the treatment of endophthalmitis if human safety is demonstrated.

If a systemic fluoroquinolone is used for endophthalmitis prophylaxis or treatment, the maximal oral or intravenous doses indicated in the Nonophthalmic Uses section should be used, with duration of use determined by the clinical situation or response.

Perioperative Infection Prophylaxis

The role of perioperative antibiotics in the prophylaxis against endophthalmitis is very controversial. Because of the low incidence of postoperative endophthalmitis, the disease entity is very difficult to evaluate in quality studies. Preparing the ocular surface with 5% povidone-iodine solution (60) does help decrease the incidence of postoperative endophthalmitis, and using adhesive plastic drapes to cover the lid margins and lashes may also be of benefit. Currently, the medicolegal indication is probably a stronger reason to use perioperative topical antibiotics than is the theoretical benefit to the patient.

If one uses a perioperative antibiotic, the fluoroquinolones have several characteristics that make them attractive. These agents have good efficacy against gram-positive organisms, which are the most common cause of postoperative endophthalmitis and wound infections, as well as excellent activity against gram-negative organisms, which less commonly infect the eye postoperatively. Topically, the fluoroquinolones have minimal epithelial toxicity and, with aggressive dosing, effective corneal and sometimes anterior-chamber drug levels may be achieved. Because none of the fluoroquinolones penetrate intact epithelium very well, drug levels in routine prophylaxis of preoperative cases can be variable. Of the three available topical agents, ofloxacin may achieve the best penetration of intact epithelium (9,61). Ciprofloxacin is another good choice for perioperative prophylaxis because of its potency against most important pathogens, with excellent gram-negative coverage, and because it probably has the lowest epithelial toxicity of the three agents. The potential for formation of a ciprofloxacin precipitate should be borne in mind when one aggressively doses a postoperative patient with a persisting epithelial defect. In perioperative use, both ciprofloxacin and ofloxacin have demonstrated efficacy in significantly decreasing external ocular flora (62,63). Of the three topically available fluoroquinolones, norfloxacin is probably the least desirable for perioperative prophylaxis since it has less potency against gram-positive organisms than the other two agents and does not penetrate the epithelium as well as ofloxacin.

Surgeons who use perioperative antibiotics can use a topical fluoroquinolone as a single agent for perioperative ocular infection prophylaxis in place of another topical antibiotic agent. For example, one drop of the agent can be administered every 5 to 15 minutes for five doses, beginning 1 to 1½ hours preoperatively. The same agent can be continued postoperatively four times daily for 5 to 7 days.

Nonophthalmic Uses

The systemic fluoroquinolones have FDA indications that vary from agent to agent, but include urinary tract infections, lower respiratory tract infections, skin and skin structure infections, bone and joint infections, infectious diarrhea, uncomplicated gonorrhea, *C. trachomatis* urethritis, and cervicitis. The original 4-quinolone, nalidixic acid, has no ophthalmic uses but continues to have approval for uncomplicated lower urinary tract infections.

The systemic dose range for each agent is as follows:

Ciprofloxacin 250 to 750 mg orally twice daily or 200 to 400 mg IV twice daily
Norfloxacin 400 mg p.o. twice daily
Ofloxacin 200 to 400 mg p.o. or IV two twice daily
Enoxacin 200 to 400 mg p.o. twice daily
Lomefloxacin 400 mg p.o. twice daily

The dosage of each of these antibiotic agents must be decreased for patients with renal impairment with creatinine clearance rates less than 30 ml/min to less than 50 ml/min.

Side Effects and Toxicity

The fluoroquinolones are generally well tolerated topically or systemically and have a low incidence of severe adverse effects (64). Adverse effects from systemic use include gastrointestinal (GI) symptoms such as nausea/vomiting, abdominal pain, dyspepsia, flatulence, and diarrhea (3% to 8%); CNS symptoms including headache, drowsiness, agitation, insomnia, and dizziness (rarely depression, psychosis, hallucinations, and convulsive seizures) (5%); and allergic reactions such as skin rashes (1%), skin photosensitivity, pseudomembranous colitis, interstitial nephritis, vasculitis, myalgia, arthralgia, arthritis, tendinitis and, very rarely, possibly Achilles tendon rupture (4,65,66). A case of reversible toxic optic neuropathy was also reported in a patient treated with 1.5 g/day of ciprofloxacin for 4 months for osteomyelitis (67). One should be cautious in administering these drugs in patients with epilepsy or cerebral arteriosclerosis. Infrequent, minor laboratory abnormalities may occur but are reversible with discontinuation of the drug. The abnormalities include increases in liver enzymes (ALT and AST), eosinophilia, leukopenia, blood urea nitrogen (BUN) level increases, and serum creatinine level increases (66). The intravenous forms of the fluoroquinolones must be administered as a 60-minute slow infusion to avoid hypotension with ofloxacin and local skin reaction with ciprofloxacin.

The currently available topical ocular fluoroquinolones are all well tolerated, but ciprofloxacin is probably the gentlest on the ocular epithelium. In experimental (noncommercial) formulations of the topical fluoroquinolones, the epithelial toxicity of ciprofloxacin was shown to be very low; that of ofloxacin and norfloxacin was similar to the epithelial toxicity of a combination of an aminoglycoside and a cephalosporin (68). One study of topical ofloxacin showed it to be well tolerated, with a very low rate of systemic side effects (47).

The most common untoward event with topical ciprofloxacin treatment for bacterial corneal ulcers is the formation of a white ciprofloxacin precipitate, usually in the region of the epithelial defect, in about 16% of patients (36) (Fig. 2). This precipitate has the advantage of providing a depot of the drug at the site of infection and occasionally slowing the healing of the epithelial defect for improved corneal drug penetration. The ciprofloxacin precipitate has

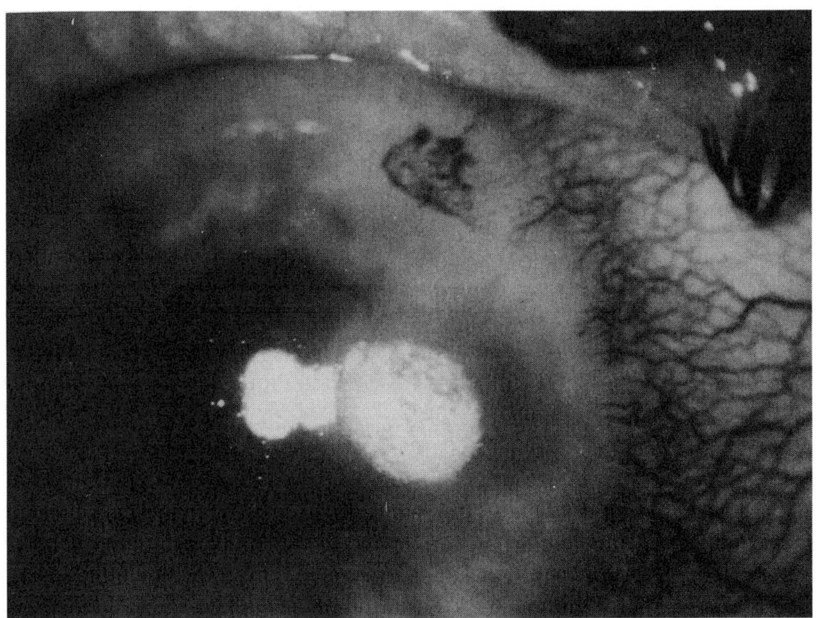

FIG. 46-2. Ciprofloxacin precipitate in the epithelial defect of patient with a *Pseudomonas aeruginosa* corneal ulcer. Photograph was taken on day 8 of treatment with topical ciprofloxacin.

the disadvantage of sometimes decreasing visualization of the corneal infiltrate immediately deep to the precipitate, but this generally does not interfere with management of the infection (Hyndiuk RA, Tabbara KF, Ophthalmic fluoroquinolones, Third International Symposium on Ocular Inflammation; Ocular Infection and Antibiotics Symposium, Fukuoka, Japan, October 23, 1994). The precipitate appears to form more frequently in patients requiring the more aggressive dosing of antibiotic agent and spontaneously resolves with continued treatment. Kanellopoulos et al. published a single report of an adherent, nonclearing, white corneal plaque that formed after topical ciprofloxacin treatment of a penetrating keratoplasty suture abscess in a patient with dry eyes and chronic postoperative hemorrhage and inflammation (69). The report does not make clear whether this plaque was actually crystallized ciprofloxacin or some other substance. Clinicians should be alerted to this type of plaque formation in diseased dry eyes; however, the occurrence of a nonclearing plaque in association with topical ciprofloxacin use must be extremely rare, given the widespread use of this drug and the dearth of similar reports.

The investigational ophthalmic ointment form of ciprofloxacin appears to be as well tolerated topically as the solution. The most common side effect is the formation of a superficial white ciprofloxacin precipitate in 13% of patients, which almost always spontaneously resolves without treatment (5) (Fig. 2). High-performance liquid chromatography has proven this precipitate to be actual ciprofloxacin material. In a multicenter trial of ciprofloxacin ointment, none of 32 patients with ciprofloxacin precipitate had any residual ocular sequelae (5). Other reported adverse events include ocular burning (2%), blurred vision (1.2%), punctate epitheliopathy (0.4%), and tearing (0.4%).

High-risk Groups

The topical and systemic fluoroquinolone preparations are in FDA Pregnancy Category C and should be used during pregnancy only if the potential benefit to the mother justifies the potential risk to the fetus. Systemic fluoroquinolones should be avoided in children and lactating women due to the potential risk of damage to immature cartilage, which may produce arthropathy. Arthropathy is not considered a risk with the ophthalmic topical forms of the fluoroquinolones in children, however. The ophthalmic topical fluoroquinolones should be used with caution in lactating women since it is not known whether the topically applied drug is excreted in breast milk.

Drug Interaction

Drug interaction studies have not been performed with the topical ophthalmic form of ciprofloxacin, norfloxacin, or ofloxacin. Systemic administration of fluoroquinolones may decrease metabolism of theophylline, leading to increased theophylline levels; interfere with the metabolism of caffeine; enhance the effect of warfarin oral anticoagulant; and increase serum creatinine levels with concomitant use of cyclosporine. Probenecid slows renal tubular secretion of the fluoroquinolones and causes an increase in fluoroquinolone serum levels. Use of nitrofurantoin with norfloxacin may antagonize the antibacterial effect of norfloxacin in the urinary tract. Disturbances of blood sugar may result from use of a fluoroquinolone with an antidiabetic agent (either insulin or an oral agent). Because sucralfate, antacids, and metal ions in multivitamins may chelate the fluoroquinolones, these agents should not be ingested with the fluoroquinolones or for 8 hours before fluoroquinolone administration and at least 2 hours after fluoroquinolone administration. Systemic administration of nonsteroidal antiinflammatory agents and some fluoroquinolones may lead to excessive CNS stimulation and cause seizure activity.

Clinical Trials

Topical ciprofloxacin solution 0.3% has had excellent therapeutic effect in multicenter clinical trials in both bacterial keratitis (91.9% success rate) and bacterial conjunctivitis (94% rate of reduction or eradication of bacteria) (36,45).

When used as a single agent, topical 0.3% ciprofloxacin ointment demonstrated clinical success in 135 (93%) of 145 patients culture-positive with bacterial keratitis. The agent was very well tolerated, with no significant adverse effects (5).

In a double-masked, multicenter study (38), topical ofloxacin solution 0.3% proved as efficacious in the treatment of bacterial keratitis as a combination of 1.5% tobramycin and 10.0% cefazolin solutions; the healing rate was 89% with ofloxacin and 86% with the combined fortified antibiotic agents in the 140 patients who were culture positive. There was a lower incidence of ocular toxicity in the ofloxacin group (38).

Clinically, large randomized studies have demonstrated the efficacy and safety of topical ciprofloxacin 0.3%, ofloxacin 0.3%, and norfloxacin 0.3% in the treatment of bacterial conjunctivitis (45–48).

ACKNOWLEDGMENT

This work was supported in part by Core Grant No. EY01931 from the National Eye Institute and by an unrestricted grant from Research to Prevent Blindness, Inc., New York, NY.

REFERENCES

1. Smith JT. The mode of action of 4-quinolones and possible mechanisms of resistance. *J Antimicrob Chemother* 1986;18(suppl D): 21–29.

2. Neu HC. Microbiologic aspects of fluoroquinolones. *Am J Ophthalmol* 1991;112:15S–24S.
3. Denis A, Moreau NJ. Mechanisms of quinolone resistance in clinical isolates: accumulation of sparfloxacin and of fluoroquinolones of various hydrophobicity, and analysis of membrane composition. *J Antimicrob Chemother* 1993;32:379–392.
4. Wolfson JS, Hooper DC. The fluoroquinolones: clinical and laboratory considerations. *Clin Microbiol Newslett* 1992;14:1–7.
5. Wilhelmus KR, Hyndiuk RA, Caldwell DR, Abshire RL, Folkens AT, Godio LB. 0.3% Ciprofloxacin ophthalmic ointment in the treatment of bacterial keratitis. *Arch Ophthalmol* 1993;111:1210–1218.
6. Belliveau P. Ofloxacin vs. ciprofloxacin: a comparison. *Conn Med* 1992;56:261–263.
7. Monk JP, Campoli-Richards DM. Ofloxacin. A review of its antibacterial activity, pharmacokinetic properties and therapeutic use. *Drugs* 1987;33:346–391.
8. McDermott ML, Tran TD, Cowden JW, Bugge CJL. Corneal stromal penetration of topical ciprofloxacin in humans. *Ophthalmology* 1993; 100:197–200.
9. Donnenfeld ED, Schrier A, Perry HD, Aulicino T, Gombert ME, Snyder R. Penetration of topically applied ciprofloxacin, norfloxacin, and ofloxacin into the aqueous humor. *Ophthalmology* 1994;101:902–905.
10. O'Brien TP, Sawusch MR, Dick JD, Gottsch JD. Topical ciprofloxacin treatment of Pseudomonas keratitis in rabbits. *Arch Ophthalmol* 1988;106:1444–1446.
11. Bergogne-Berezin E. Pefloxacin. *Int J Antimicrob Agents* 1991;1:29–46.
12. Huber-Spitzy VN, Czejka M, Georgiew L, et al. Penetration of norfloxacin into the aqueous humor of the human eye. *Invest Ophthalmol Vis Sci* 1992;33:1723–1726.
13. Hatano H, Inoue K, Shia S, Liping W. Application of topical lomefloxacin against experimental Pseudomonas endophthalmitis in rabbits. *Acta Ophthalmol* 1993;71:666–670.
14. Behrens-Baumann W, Martell J. Ciprofloxacin concentration in the rabbit aqueous humor and vitreous following intravenous and subconjunctival administration. *Infection* 1988;16:54–57.
15. Wilhelmus KR. Ciprofloxacin for ophthalmic infections. *Ocular Ther Manage* 1990;1:10–14.
16. Hill JM, O'Callaghan RJ, Hobden JA. Ocular iontophoresis. In: Mitra AK, ed. *Ophthalmic drug delivery systems.* New York: Marcel Dekker, 1993;331–354.
17. Kowalski RP, Karenchak LM, Eller AW. The role of ciprofloxacin in endophthalmitis therapy. *Am J Ophthalmol* 1993;116:695–699.
18. Baba FZ, Trousdale MD, Gauderman WJ, et al. Intravitreal penetration of oral ciprofloxacin in humans. *Ophthalmology* 1992;99:483–486.
19. Sweeney G, Fern AI, Lindsay G, Doig MW. Penetration of ciprofloxacin into the aqueous humor of the uninflamed human eye after oral administration. *J Antimicrob Chemother* 1990;26:99–105.
20. Piddock LJV. New quinolones and gram-positive bacteria. *Antimicrob Agents Chemother* 1994;38:163–169.
21. Kaatz GW, Seo SM. Mechanism of ciprofloxacin resistance in *Pseudomonas aeruginosa. J Infect Dis* 1988;158:537–541.
22. Trucksis M, Hooper DC, Wolfson JS. Emerging resistance to fluoroquinolones in staphylococci: an alert [Editorial]. *Ann Int Med* 1991; 114:424–426.
23. Abramowicz M. Ophthalmic ciprofloxacin. *Med Lett Drugs Ther* 1991;33:52–53.
24. Callegan MC, Hobden JA, Hill JM, et al. Topical antibiotic therapy for the treatment of experimental *Staphylococcus aureus* keratitis. *Invest Ophthalmol Vis Sci* 1992;33:3017–3023.
25. Callegan MC, Hill JM, Insler MS, Hobden JA, O'Callaghan RJ. Methicillin-resistant *Staphylococcus aureus* keratitus in the rabbit: therapy with ciprofloxacin, vancomycin and cefazolin. *Curr Eye Res* 1992;11:1111–1119.
26. Wolfson JS, Hooper DC. The fluoroquinolones: structures, mechanisms of action and resistance, and spectra of activity in vitro. *Antimicrob Agents Chemother* 1985;28:581–586.
27. Spangler SK, Jacobs MR, Appelbaum PC. Comparative activity of the new fluoroquinolone bay y3118 against 177 penicillin susceptible and resistant pneumococci. *Eur J Clin Microbiol Infect Dis* 1993;12: 965–967.
28. King A, Phillips I. The comparative in vitro activity of eight newer quinolones and nalidixic acid. *J Antimicrob Chemother* 1986; 18(suppl D):1–20.
29. Reidy JJ, Hobden JA, Hill JM, et al. The efficacy of topical ciprofloxacin and norfloxacin in the treatment of experimental Pseudomonas keratitis. *Cornea* 1991;10:25–28.
30. Heessen FW, Muytjens HL. In vitro activities of ciprofloxacin, norfloxacin, pipemidic acid, cinoxacin, and nalidixic acid against *Chlamydia trachomatis. Antimicrob Agents Chemother* 1984;25:123–124.
31. Jones RN, Reller LB, Rosati LA, et al. Ofloxacin, a new broad-spectrum fluoroquinolone. Results from a multicenter, national comparative activity surveillance study. The Ofloxacin Surveillance Group. *Diagn Microbiol Infect Dis* 1992;15:425–434.
32. Peterson LR, Cooper I, Willard KE, et al. Activity of twenty-one antimicrobial agents including *l*-ofloxacin against quinolone-sensitive and -resistant, and methicillin-sensitive and -resistant *Staphylococcus aureus. Chemotherapy* 1994;40:21–25.
33. Hayakawa I, Furuhama K, Takayama S, Osada Y. Levofloxacin, a new quinolone antibacterial agent. *Arzneimittel Forschung Drug Res* 1992;42:363–364.
34. Foleno B, Fu KP. In vitro activity of *l*-ofloxacin against norfloxacin-resistant coagulase-negative staphylococci. *Diagn Microbiol Infect Dis* 1992;15:557–559.
35. Ogawa GSH, Hyndiuk RA. Bacterial keratitis and conjunctivitis: clinical disease. In: Smolin G, Thoft R, eds. *The Cornea.* Boston: Little, Brown, 1994;125–167.
36. Leibowitz HM. Clinical evaluation of ciprofloxacin 0.3% ophthalmic solution for treatment of bacterial keratitis. *Am J Ophthalmol* 1991; 112:34S–47S.
37. Cokingtin CD, Hyndiuk RA. Insights from experimental data on ciprofloxacin in the treatment of bacterial keratitis and ocular infections. *Am J Ophthalmol* 1991;112:25S–28S.
38. O'Brien TP, Maguire MG, Fink NE, Alfonso E, McDonnell P, Bacterial Keratitis Study Research Group . Efficacy of ofloxacin vs cefazolin and tobramycin in the therapy for bacterial keratitis. *Arch Ophthalmol* 1995;113:1257–1265.
39. Vajpayee RB, Gupta SK, Angra SK, Munjal A. Topical norfloxacin therapy in Pseudomonas corneal ulcerations. *Cornea* 1991;10:268–271.
40. Snyder ME, Katz HR. Ciprofloxacin-resistant bacterial keratitis. *Am J Ophthalmol* 1992;114:336–338.
41. Hyndiuk RA, Skorich D, Burd E. Bacterial keratitis. In: Tabbara K, Hyndiuk RA, eds. *Infections of the Eye.* Boston: Little, Brown, 1986; 303–330.
42. Hyndiuk RA, Skorich DN, Davis SD, et al. Fortified antibiotic ointment in bacterial keratitis. *Am J Ophthalmol* 1988;105:239–243.
43. Lin R, Holland GN, Helm CJ, Elias SJ, Berlin OGW, Bruckner DA. Comparative efficacy of topical ciprofloxacin for treating *Mycobacterium fortuitum* and *Mycobacterium chelonae. Am J Ophthalmol* 1994;117:657–662.
44. Syed NA, Hyndiuk RA. Infectious conjunctivitis. *Infect Dis Clin North Am* 1992;6:789–805.
45. Leibowitz HM. Antibacterial effectiveness of ciprofloxacin 0.3% ophthalmic solution in the treatment of bacterial conjunctivitis. *Am J Ophthalmol* 1991;112:29S–33S.
46. Miller IM, Wittreich JM, Cook T, Vogel R. The safety and efficacy of topical norfloxacin compared with chloramphenicol for the treatment of external ocular bacterial infections. *Eye* 1992;6:111–114.
47. Gwon A, for the Ofloxacin Study Group II. Ofloxacin vs. tobramycin for the treatment of external ocular infection. *Arch Ophthalmol* 1992;110:1234–1237.
48. Miller IM, Vogel R, Cook TJ, et al. Topically administered norfloxacin compared with topically administered gentamicin for the treatment of external ocular bacterial infections. *Am J Ophthalmol* 1992;113:638–644.
49. Wiedermann B, Atkinson BA. Susceptibility to antibiotics: species incidence and trends. In: Lorian V, ed. *Antibiotics in Laboratory Medicine.* 3rd ed. Baltimore: Williams & Wilkins, 1991;962–1208.
50. Lassus A, Abagh Filho L, Santos MF, Belli L. Comparison of fleroxacin and penicillin G plus probenecid in the treatment of acute uncomplicated gonococcal infections. *Genitourin Med* 1992;68:317–320.
51. Cheong LL, Chan RK, Nadarajah M. Perfloxacin and ciprofloxacin in the treatment of uncomplicated gonococcal urethritis in males. *Genitourin Med* 1992;68:260–262.
52. Balachandran T, Roberts AP, Evans BA, Azadian BS. Single-dose therapy of anogenital and pharyngeal gonorrhoea with cipfofloxacin. *Int J STD AIDS* 1992;3:49–51.

53. Kestelyn P, Bogaerts J, Stevens AM, et al. Treatment of adult gonococcal keratoconjunctivitis with oral norfloxacin. *Am J Ophthalmol* 1989;108:516–523.
54. Ohye R, Higa H, Vogt R, et al. Decreased susceptibility of *Neisseria gonorrhoeae* to fluoroquinolones—Ohio and Hawaii, 1992–1994. *MMWR* 1994;43:325–327.
55. Abramowicz M. Drugs for sexually transmitted diseases. *Med Lett Drugs Ther* 1994;36:1–6.
56. Salvanet A, Fisch A, Lafaix C, et al. Pefloxacin concentrations in human aqueous humor and lens. *J Antimicrob Chemother* 1986;18:199–201.
57. Fisch A, Lafaix C, Salvanet A, et al. Ofloxacin in human aqueous humor and lens. *J Antimicrob Chemother* 1987;20:453–454.
58. Mournier M, Ploy MC, Chauvin M, et al. Study of intraocular diffusion of ofloxacin in humans and rabbits. *Pathol Biol* 1992;40:529–533.
59. Stevens SX, Fouraker BD, Jensen HG. Intraocular safety of ciprofloxacin. *Arch Ophthalmol* 1991;109:1737–1743.
60. Speaker MG, Menikoff JA. Prophylaxis of endophthalmitis with topical povidone-iodine. *Ophthalmology* 1991;98:1769–1775.
61. Diamond JP, White L, Leeming JP, Hoh HB, Easty DL. Topical 0.3% ciprofloxacin, norfloxacin, and ofloxacin in treatment of bacterial keratitis: a new method for comparative evaluation of ocular drug penetration. *Br J Ophthalmol* 1995;79:606–609.
62. Leeming JP, Diamond JP, Trigg R, White L, Hoh HB, Easty DL. Ocular penetration of topical ciprofloxacin and norfloxacin drops and their effect upon eyelid flora. *Br J Ophthalmol* 1994;78:546–548.
63. Kirsch LS, Jackson WB, Goldstein DA, Discepola MJ. Perioperative ofloxacin vs. tobramycin: efficacy in external ocular adnexal sterilization and anterior chamber penetration. *Can J Ophthalmol* 1995;30:11–20.
64. Ball AP. Overview of clinical experience with ciprofloxacin. *Eur J Clin Microbiol* 1986;5:214–219.
65. Ribard P, Audisio F, Kahn M-F, et al. Seven Achilles tendinitis including 3 complicated by rupture during fluoroquinolone therapy. *J Rheumatol* 1992;19:1479–1481.
66. Miscellaneous Antibacterial Drugs. In: Bennett DR, ed. *Drug Evaluations annual 1991,* 7th ed. Milwaukee: American Medical Association, 1991;1353–1387.
67. Vrabec TR, Sergott RC, Jaeger EA, Savino PJ, Bosley TM. Reversible visual loss in a patient receiving high-dose ciprofloxacin hydrochloride (Cipro). *Ophthalmology* 1990;97:707–710.
68. Cutarelli PE, Lass JH, Lazarus HM, et al. Topical fluoroquinolones: antimicrobial activity and in vitro corneal epithelial toxicity. *Curr Eye Res* 1991;10:557–563.
69. Kanellopoulos AJ, Miller F, Wittpenn JR. Deposition of topical ciprofloxacin to prevent re-epithelialization of corneal defect. *Am J Ophthalmol* 1994;117:258–259

Textbook of Ocular Pharmacology,
edited by T.J. Zimmerman, et al.
Lippincott–Raven Publishers, Philadelphia © 1997.

CHAPTER 47

Peptide Antibiotics: Vancomycin, Bacitracin, and Polymyxin B

Gerard D'Aversa and George A. Stern

VANCOMYCIN

History and Source

Vancomycin is a tricyclic glycopeptide derived from *Amycolatopsis orientalis.* Purification of this drug and its chemical and antibicrobial properties were first described by McCormick et al. in 1956 (1). The ophthalmic uses of vancomycin include treating methicillin-resistant *Staphylococcus epidermidis* and *S. aureus* (MRSE, MRSA) keratitis, conjunctivitis, and blepharoconjunctivitis. Initial reports of successful treatment of these conditions with topical and subconjunctival administration of vancomycin have led to the widespread use of this drug in ophthalmology (2–5). In addition, vancomycin has become the drug of choice for intravitreal treatment of endophthalmitis caused by gram-positive bacteria.

Official Drug Name and Chemistry

Vancomycin hydrochloride (Vancocin HCl, U.S.P., Lilly) has a chemical formula of $C_{66}H_{75}C_{12}H_9O_{24}$ HCl. Its molecular weight is 1,486 (6).

Pharmacology

Vancomycin is a bactericidal antibiotic that inhibits cell wall biosynthesis and alters the permeability of the cell membrane. Unlike penicillin, which inhibits the cross-linking of glycopeptides which constitute the bacterial cell wall, vancomycin specifically inhibits utilization of lipid intermediates in the process of cell wall formation (7). Vancomycin also inhibits RNA synthesis. There is no cross-resistance between vancomycin and other antibiotic agents.

Clinical Pharmacology

Vancomycin is active against gram-positive bacteria, including methicillin-resistant coagulase-negative staphylococci, *S. aureus, S. pyogenes, S. pneumoniae,* other α-hemolytic streptococci, enterococci, *Clostridium difficile,* corynebacteria, and *Propionibacterium* sp. In vitro activity also exists against *Listeria monocytogenes, Lactobacillus* sp, *Clostridium* sp, and *Bacillus* sp. Vancomycin is not active against gram-negative bacilli, mycobacteria, or fungi.

Pharmaceutics

Vancocin HCl (Lilly): Intravenous
- 500-mg vial, 10-ml size
- 1-g vial, 20-ml size
- 10-g vial, 100-ml size

Vancocin HCl (Abbott): Intravenous
- 500-mg vial, 15-ml size*
- 1-g vial, 15-ml size*
- *Note: Vials must be stored at room temperatures of 15°to 30°C

Vancocin HCl (Lilly): Oral solution
- 10 g
- 1 g
- *Note: Must be stored at room temperature of 15° to 30°C

G. D'Aversa and G. A. Stern: Department of Ophthalmology, University of Florida College of Medicine, Box 100284 JHMHC, Gainesville, Florida 32610-0284.

This work was supported in part by an unrestricted departmental grant from Research to Prevent Blindness, Inc.

Vancocin HCl (Lilly): Pulvules
125 mg, blue and brown
250 mg, blue and lavender
*Note: Must be stored at room temperature of 15° to 30°C

Pharmacokinetics, Concentration-effect Relationship, and Metabolism

Vancomycin is poorly absorbed from the gastrointestinal (GI) tract. Because intramuscular administration is extremely painful, parenteral use is limited to intravenous (IV) administration. Ocular uses include topical, subconjunctival, and intravitreal administration.

In patients with normal renal function, multiple dosing of vancomycin 500 mg IV produces mean plasma concentrations of approximately 19 μg/ml 2 hours after infusion and approximately 10 μg/ml 6 hours after infusion. Doses of 1 g produce plasma concentrations of 23 μg/ml at 1 hour and of 8 μg/ml at 11 hours after infusion (6).

The half-life ($t_{\frac{1}{2}}$) of vancomycin in the circulation is 4 to 6 hours in patients with normal renal function. Approximately 80% of each dose is excreted in the urine. Renal dysfunction slows the excretion of vancomycin and may lead to the accumulation of dangerously high blood levels. Total systemic and renal clearance of vancomycin may also be reduced in the elderly. Serum concentrations of vancomycin should be monitored to detect potentially toxic levels. Renal function tests must also be monitored to adjust dosing, as well as to identify vancomycin-related nephrotoxicity.

Vancomycin is 55% bound by serum protein. After intravenous administration, inhibitory levels of vancomycin are present in pleural, pericardial, ascitic, and synovial fluids, in urine and in aqueous humor. Vancomycin does not readily cross the blood–brain barrier (BBB) into the cerebrospinal fluid (CSF), except in the presence of inflammation (8).

Studies in rabbits have demonstrated good penetration into the aqueous humor, in both normal and inflamed eyes, when vancomycin is administered as a 5% topical solution, 25 mg subconjunctival injection, or intravenous dosage of 20 mg per pound (9). Pflugfelder et al. (10) also demonstrated in rabbits that intravitreal vancomycin is cleared most slowly in phakic eyes, most rapidly in aphakic/vitrectomized eyes without an intact lens capsule, and at an intermediate rate in aphakic/vitrectomized eyes with an intact lens capsule.

Therapeutic Use

Vancomycin is used in the treatment of infections caused by vancomycin-sensitive bacteria that are resistant to other antimicrobial agents, including methicillin-resistant strains of staphylococci, and in treatment of patients with hypersensitivity to penicillins and cephalosporins.

Intravenous administration of vancomycin is used in the treatment of systemic infections caused by gram-positive organisms, including endocarditis caused by streptococci or corynebacteria, or in combination with an aminoglycoside in treating other types of endocarditis such as those caused by enterococci. Intravenous vancomycin may also be used to treat orbital infections in patients allergic to penicillin and as an adjunct in the treatment of endophthalmitis. In adults, the usual daily intravenous dose of vancomycin is 2 g, divided as 500 mg every 6 hours or 1 g every 12 hours. In severe infections, the dose may be increased to 1 g every 8 hours. Intravenous infusions should be administered in at least 60 minutes to avoid inducing hypotension.

In elderly patients, premature infants, and patients with impaired renal function, the dosage must be adjusted. Vancomycin serum concentrations should be monitored to optimize treatment and limit toxicity. Vancomycin peak and trough levels and renal function tests must be evaluated periodically. In patients with impaired renal function, the intravenous dose should be approximately 15 times the glomerular filtration rate (11). The dosage in children is usually 10 mg/kg administered every 6 hours.

The intravenous solution is prepared by adding 10 ml sterile water to a 1-g vial. This reconstitutes a solution of 50 mg/ml, which has been used as a 5% topical solution. The reconstituted solution, which has a pH of 2.5 to 4.5, may be stored in a refrigerator for 14 days without significant loss of potency.

Vancomycin may also be administered orally (p.o.) for the treatment of staphylococcal enterocolitis or pseudomembranous colitis caused by *C. difficile*. The usual oral dose is 500 mg to 1 g every 6 hours for 7 to 10 days. In children, the recommended daily dose is 40 mg/kg in three to four divided doses for 7 to 10 days.

Vancomycin is used topically, subconjunctivally, and intravitreally for the treatment of ocular infections caused by gram-positive organisms not susceptible to other antibiotics. It is commonly used for the treatment of infectious and posttraumatic endophthalmitis (intravitreal, subconjunctival) and keratitis (topical, subconjunctival), as well as for other ocular/orbital infections that require aggressive coverage of gram-positive bacteria.

Solutions of vancomycin for topical ophthalmic use are stable for 2 weeks. Concentrations ranging from 5 to 50 mg/ml can be prepared by mixing the powder with sterile water, sodium chloride 0.9%, or phosphate-buffered saline (PBS). At higher concentrations, the solution is more toxic to the ocular surface and is symptomatically less well tolerated (2). In our experience, patients rarely tolerate a 5% solution for any length of time, whereas a 1% to 2% solution is tolerated well and is effective. In treatment of corneal ulcers caused by methicillin-resistant staphylococci, topical vancomycin 1% to 2% should be the first line of treatment. This solution should be used every 30 minutes initially and tapered as clinical improvement occurs.

Subconjunctival injections should be administered at a concentration of vancomycin 25 mg/0.5 ml. These injections may be used as an adjunct in the treatment of severe keratitis or endophthalmitis. Because subconjunctival injections of vancomycin are painful, they should be limited to injections once or twice daily for no more than 5 to 7 days.

Vancomycin has been demonstrated to be effective in the treatment of experimental endophthalmitis caused by gram-positive bacteria in rabbits (10,12,13). It has more uniform coverage against staphylococci (especially methicillin-resistant strains), streptococci (including enterococci), and *Bacillus* sp than cefazolin or aminoglycosides (12,14,15). Pflugfelder et al. (10) reported that intravitreal dosages of 2 mg or less were not toxic to the retina, and a 1-mg intravitreal dosage of vancomycin has become the standard for treatment of endophthalmitis caused by gram-positive organisms. Intravitreal vancomycin should be considered in the treatment of perforating ocular trauma, especially in the presence of an intraocular foreign body, in which *Bacillus* sp predominates as the most common organism (16–18). Intravenous, subconjunctival, and topical administrations of vancomycin do not result in detectable vitreous levels.

Side Effects and Toxicity

Intravenous Administration

After rapid infusion, an anaphylactoid reaction, characterized by hypotension, wheezing, urticaria, or pruritis, may occur. Rapid infusion may also cause flushing of the upper body ("red neck" syndrome) or pain and muscle spasm of the chest and back. These reactions usually resolve in 30 to 60 minutes but may last for hours. To prevent these reactions, intravenous vancomycin should be administered slowly in 30 to 60 minutes.

Nephrotoxicity

Renal failure and interstitial nephritis have been associated with administration of large doses of vancomycin. Patients who developed these complications usually had preexisting renal dysfunction or were treated concurrently with an aminoglycoside. Azotemia usually resolves when the drug is discontinued. Periodic renal function tests should be performed when patients are treated with parenteral vancomycin, and the drug should be discontinued if renal function begins to deteriorate.

Ototoxicity

Sensorineural hearing loss has been associated with the parenteral use of vancomycin. In most cases, high serum levels were detected. Hearing loss has occurred in patients with preexisting renal dysfunction or preexisting hearing defects and in patients treated concomitantly with other ototoxic drugs. The hearing loss may continue to progress even after vancomycin treatment is discontinued.

Ocular

Topical application of vancomycin is often painful, related to its low pH (2.5 to 4.5) and its concentration (higher concentrations cause more ocular discomfort). Toxicity may be manifest as superficial punctate keratopathy, conjunctival injection, chemosis, or papillary conjunctivitis. Topical administration has also been shown to retard epithelial wound healing in rabbits (18).

Hematopoietic

Reversible neutropenia, thrombocytopenia, and agranulocytosis have been associated with use of vancomycin, generally with cumulative doses greater than 25 g.

Miscellaneous

Phlebitis and pain can occur at the intravenous infusion site. Other side effects include Stevens-Johnson syndrome, nausea, chills, fever, eosinophilia, skin rashes, and vasculitis.

Overdosage

In the presence of an overdose, initial supportive care is essential, including maintenance of an adequate glomerular filtration rate. Hemofiltration and hemoperfusion with polysulfone resin may increase the clearance of vancomycin (19).

High-risk Groups

Renal Insufficiency

Patients with renal dysfunction should not be treated with nephrotoxic agents such as vancomycin unless such treatment is absolutely medically indicated. When treating such patients, one must adjust the dose according to the patient's creatinine clearance (11). It is imperative to monitor serum vancomycin levels and renal function tests.

Hearing Dysfunction

Patients with hearing dysfunction should have baseline and serial auditory function tests performed before and during vancomycin treatment.

Pregnancy

Animal reproductive studies have not been conducted with vancomycin. In a controlled study, potential ototoxicity or nephrotoxicity was assessed in infants after vancomycin was administered to pregnant women. The study did not demonstrate any sensorineural hearing loss or renal damage associated with vancomycin use (8). It is recommended that vancomycin not be given to pregnant women unless treatment is absolutely indicated.

Nursing

Vancomycin is excreted in human milk. If vancomycin is administered to a nursing mother, cessation of nursing is recommended.

Pediatrics

In neonates and infants, serum vancomycin concentrations should be monitored. Concomitant administration of vancomycin with anesthetic agents has been associated with erythema and histamine-like flushing in children.

Elderly

Decreased creatinine clearance rates associated with aging may lead to elevated concentrations of vancomycin. Dosing should be adjusted according to the creatinine clearance rate.

Drug Interactions

Systemic

Concomitant administration of vancomycin with anesthetic agents may cause erythematous, histamine-like flushing and anaphylactoid reactions in children. Concurrent or sequential use of potentially ototoxic or nephrotoxic agents may lead to sensorineural or renal toxicity, respectively.

Ocular

Intravitreal dexamethasone, when injected concomitantly with vancomycin, has been shown to reduce the level of intravitreal vancomycin in a rabbit model of endophthalmitis (20). Vancomycin may precipitate when combined with ceftazidime (21).

Major Clinical Trials

Smith et al. (12) studied the toxicity, clearance, and efficacy of intravitreal vancomycin in the treatment of experimental MRSE endophthalmitis in rabbits. There was no retinal toxicity, and therapeutic levels of vancomycin were present for 6 days after intravitreal injection. The treated rabbit eyes showed a marked beneficial effect as compared with the untreated eyes. Smith et al. (12) recommend that vancomycin be considered the drug of choice in treatment of MRSE endophthalmitis.

Pflugfelder et al. (10) identified gram-positive isolates from exogenous bacterial endophthalmitis resistant to cefazolin and gentamicin, but sensitive to vancomycin. They evaluated the retinal toxicity and clearance of intravitreal vancomycin in pigmented rabbits and reported that doses of 2 mg or less were nontoxic in both phakic and aphakic-vitrectomized eyes. They also reported that vancomycin and gentamicin were synergistic against the gram-positive isolates. They recommended that a combination of intravitreal vancomycin and an aminoglycoside be used as the initial therapy for exogenous endophthalmitis.

Goodman and Gottsch (4) and Eiferman et al. (5) reported corneal ulcers caused by staphylococci that were resistant to methicillin and did not respond to treatment with fortified gentamicin and cefazolin. Their five cases all responded to treatment with topical vancomycin. These reports stressed the increased frequency of methicillin-resistant staphylococci and the need to use an alternative agent such as vancomycin to eradicate the infection.

BACITRACIN

History and Source

Bacitracin is a polypeptide antibiotic produced by *Bacillus subtilis* and *B. licheniformis.* It was introduced into use in ophthalmology in the 1940s when Bellows and Farmer reported the successful treatment of acute conjunctivitis and blepharoconjunctivitis with bacitracin (22).

Official Drug Name and Chemistry

The bacitracins are a group of antibiotics containing a thiazolidine ring structure. The antibiotic consists of three separate compounds, bacitracin A, B, and C. Bacitracin A ($C_{66}H_{103}N_{17}O_{16}S$) is the major constituent of the antibiotic.

Pharmacology

Bacitracin is a bactericidal antibiotic agent whose exact mechanism of action is unknown. Bacitracin causes an accumulation of cell-wall precursor nucleotides and suppresses the multiplication of lysozyme-induced protoplasts. The drug may also act as a chelating agent.

Clinical Pharmacology

Bacitracin is bactericidal against most gram-positive organisms, as well as spirochetes, *N. gonorrheae, Entamoeba histolytica, Actinomyces,* and *Fusobacterium.* Whereas most staphylococci are not susceptible to penicillin, most remain susceptible to bacitracin. Gram-positive organisms are generally inhibited by concentrations of 0.1 to 0.5 U/ml. Bacitracin is ineffective against gram-negative organisms. It is not inactivated by blood, pus, necrotic tissue, large inocula, or bacterial enzymes such as penicillinase.

Pharmaceutics

Ophthalmic Preparations

1. Bacitracin Ophthalmic Ointment (bacitracin zinc) U.S.P (E. Fougera) AK-Tracin (bacitracin zinc) (Akorn)
   Tube: 1/8 oz; 500 U/g
2. Corticosporin Ophthalmic Ointment (polymyxin B sulfate, bacitracin zinc, neomycin sulfate, hydrocortisone acetate) (Burroughs Wellcome)

Tube: 1/8 oz

3. Neosporin Ophthalmic Ointment (polymyxin B sulfate, bacitracin zinc, neomycin sulfate) (Burroughs Wellcome)
   Tube: 1/8 oz
4. Polysporin Ophthalmic Ointment (polymyxin B sulfate, bacitracin zinc) (Burroughs Wellcome)
   Tube: 1/8 oz.

Nonophthalmic Preparations

5. Aquaphor Antibiotic Formula (polymyxin B sulfate, bacitracin zinc) (Biersdorf)
   Tube: 5 oz
6. Corticosporin Ointment (polymyxin B sulfate, bacitracin zinc, neomycin sulfate, hydrocortisone acetate) (Burroughs Wellcome)
   Tube: 7.5 g
7. Neosporin Ointment (polymyxin B sulfate, bacitracin zinc, neomycin sulfate) (Burroughs Wellcome)
   Tubes: 1/2 oz and 1 oz
8. AK-Tracin (Bacitracin) (Upjohn)*
   Vial containing 50,000 U
   *Note: Once prepared, solutions must be refrigerated
9. Bacitracin tablets
   Soluble tablet: 2,500 U

Bacitracin is stable at room temperature for more than 1 year when incorporated with petrolatum in ointment form.

Pharmacokinetics, Concentration-effect Relationship, and Metabolism

Bacitracin is not absorbed from the GI tract in appreciable amounts. After intramuscular injection, absorption is rapid and complete and the drug is widely distributed in the body. Maximal blood levels are reached 1 to 2 hours after intramuscular injection. Bactericidal plasma concentrations may be present for as long as 4 to 6 hours after a single intramuscular injection.

Bacitracin is slowly excreted by glomerular filtration. Twenty-four hours after a single intramuscular injection, only 10% to 40% of the bacitracin dose can be detected in the urine. If ingested orally, all of the drug is excreted in the feces.

Topically applied bacitracin has poor penetration through the cornea. Corneal penetration may be enhanced in the presence of an epithelial defect (22).

Therapeutic Use

Bacitracin may be administered topically, orally, or intramuscularly. It is not administered intravenously. Because the drug produces systemic toxicity, its use is limited to topical application.

Bacitracin is available as a single drug in an opthalmic ointment or as part of a multidrug ophthalmic antibiotic preparation. All these preparations contain 500 U bacitracin per gram of ointment. Ocular use of topical bacitracin may include treatment of hordeola, chalazia, blepharitis, eyelid burns, corneal abrasions, bacterial conjunctivitis, infectious corneal ulcers, or other external ocular infections caused by susceptible gram-positive bacteria. The drug is usually administered one to four times daily, but may be used as often as hourly to treat more severe infections such as bacterial keratitis or hyperacute suppurative conjunctivitis.

Bacitracin ointments are also used for a number of dermatologic conditions, including furunculosis, pyoderma, carbuncle, impetigo, superficial and deep abscesses, infected eczema, dermal ulcers, and infected traumatic and surgical wounds. The ointments may be applied several times daily to the affected areas.

There is little role for parenteral use of bacitracin. It should be reserved for treating infections caused by organisms susceptible to bacitracin and resistant to other antibiotic agents. When used parenterally, the total daily intramuscular dose must not exceed 100,000 U. The solution for intramuscular injection is prepared by adding sterile isotonic saline to the vials to produce concentrations ranging from 100 to 10,000 U/ml (23). Solutions are stable at pH levels of 5 to 7. If refrigerated, the solutions remain stable for as long as 3 weeks. Lack of refrigeration leads to loss of activity. Renal function tests should be performed frequently during systemic use of bacitracin because of its nephrotoxicity. Any sign of renal insufficiency should lead to discontinuation of the drug.

Bacitracin has been used in oral form to treat intestinal infections such as enterocolitis caused by *Entamoeba histolytica.* A soluble tablet that is not destroyed by the gastric juices is available (2,500 U).

Side Effects and Toxicity

Ocular

Concentrations of bacitracin ranging from 500 to 1,000 U/g are nonirritating to the eye and other surfaces and do not produce any systemic side effects.

Renal

Bacitracin in doses greater than 200 to 400 U/kg may lead to renal damage. Repeated doses of the drug may lead to decreased glomerular filtration and tubular function, proteinuria, and hematuria. If drug levels rapidly accumulate in the blood due to renal dysfunction, uremia may ensue. Death due to progressive renal failure and acute tubular necrosis has been reported.

Gastrointestinal

Epigastric distress, nausea, vomiting, diarrhea, rectal itching, and burning are associated with oral use.

Miscellaneous

Hypersensitivity reactions, generally occurring as skin eruptions, can occur with oral or parenteral use. Topical application has also been associated with acute anaphylactic reaction (24). Local pain, induration, heat, and petechiae can develop at an injection site.

High-risk Groups

Renal Insufficiency

Bacitracin should not be administered parenterally to patients with renal insufficiency because of its nephrotoxicity.

Hypersensitivity

Patients with known hypersensitivity should avoid use of topical and parenteral bacitracin.

Pregnancy

Information regarding the use of bacitracin in pregnancy and in nursing mothers is not available.

Elderly

Parenteral dosing must be modified in patients with decreased creatinine clearance associated with aging.

Other

Combination preparations containing a corticosteroid should not be used in patients who have a steroid contraindication.

Major Clinical Trials

Meleny et al. (25) described the history, properties and uses of bacitracin in 1945. Bellows and Farmer reported 42 cases of conjunctivitis and blepharoconjunctivitis which were treated with bacitracin with favorable results. They also reported a *Pseudomonas* corneal ulcer in which the organism was sensitive to bacitracin and which responded well to treatment. This introduced the use of bacitracin into ophthalmic practice (22).

POLYMYXIN

History and Source

Polymyxin B is one of a group of polypeptide antibiotics derived from *Bacillus polymyxa* (*B. aerosporous*). The polymyxins were discovered as antimicrobial agents in 1947 (27–29). Polymyxin came into opthalmic use in the 1950s after Wiggins (30) demonstrated the effectiveness of polymyxin B in treating experimental *Pseudomonas* corneal ulcers in rabbits. Early reports of clinical success in treating *Pseudomonas* corneal ulcers in human patients were described by Moorman and Harber (31) and McNeel et al. (32).

Official Drug Name and Chemistry

Polymyxin B sulfate (Aerosporin, Burroughs Wellcome) is the most common polymyxin in clinical usage. The polymyxins are simple, basic polypeptides with molecular weights of about 1,000 that act as cationic detergents. They readily form water-soluble salts with mineral acids. Of the polymyxins, polymyxin B is the antibiotic that is used clinically because it is less nephrotoxic.

Pharmacology

Polymyxin B is a bactericidal antibiotic. It adheres to the lipoprotein membrane of bacteria and causes permeability changes in the membrane, allowing cell contents to escape. Sensitivity to polymyxin B is determined by the phospholipid fraction of the bacterial cell wall. There is complete cross-resistance between colistin derivatives and polymyxin B.

Clinical Pharmacology

Polymyxin B is bactericidal agent against most gram-negative bacilli except *Proteus, Providencia, Serratia,* and *Brucella.* Sensitive organisms are inhibited by concentrations of polymyxin B ranging from 0.05 to 2.0 μg/ml. All gram-positive bacteria, fungi, and gram-negative cocci, including *N. gonorrhea* and *N. meningitidis,* are resistant.

Polymyxin B is used to treat infections of the urinary tract, CNS, and blood caused by susceptible strains of *Pseudomonas.* Ocular use includes topical application and subconjunctival injection for the treatment of ocular infections caused by *Pseudomonas.*

Pharmaceutics

Ophthalmic Preparations

1. Polytrim Ophthalmic Solution (Allergan): Trimethoprim sulfate and polymyxin B sulfate
   Dropper bottle: 10 ml
2. Polysporin Ophthalmic Ointment (Burroughs Wellcome); AK-Poly-Bac (Akorn); Ocumycin (Bausch & Lomb): Polymyxin B sulfate and bacitracin zinc
   Tube: 1/8 oz
3. Neosporin Ophthalmic Ointment (Burroughs Wellcome); AK-Spore (Akorn); Neocidin (Major); Neotal (Hauck); OcuSpor-B (Ocumed); Ocutricin (Bausch & Lomb): Neomycin sulfate, polymyxin B sulfate, and bacitracin zinc
   Tube: 1/8 oz
4. Neosporin Ophthalmic Solution (Burroughs Wellcome): Neomycin sulfate, polymyxin B sulfate, and gramicidin
   Dropper bottle: 10 ml
5. Cortisporin Ophthalmic Ointment (Burroughs Wellcome); Coracin Ophthalmic Ointment (Hauck): Neomycin sulfate, polymyxin B sulfate, bacitracin zinc, and hydrocortisone
   Tube: 1/8 oz
6. Terramycin Ophthalmic Ointment (Roerig): Oxytetracycline HCl and polymyxin B sulfate
   Tube: 1/8 oz

Nonophthalmic Preparations

7. Aerosporin (Burroughs Wellcome, Roerig): Polymyxin B sulfate sterile powder
   U Vial: 500,000
8. Aquaphor Antibiotic Formula (Beiersdorf): Polymyxin B sulfate and bacitracin zinc
   Tube: 5 oz
9. Cortisporin Cream (Burroughs Wellcome): Polymyxin B sulfate, neomycin sulfate, hydrocortisone acetate
   Tube: 7.5 g
10. Cortisporin Otic Solution or Suspension (Burroughs Wellcome): Neomycin sulfate, polymyxin B sulfate, hydrocortisone
    Dropper bottle: 7.5 or 10 ml
11. Neosporin Ointment (Burroughs Wellcome): Neomycin sulfate, polymyxin B sulfate, and bacitracin zinc
    Tubes: 1/2 oz and 1 oz
12. Neosporin GU Irrigant (Burroughs Wellcome): Neomycin sulfate and polymyxin B sulfate
    Ampules 1 ml
    Multidose vial: 20 ml
13. Lazersporin-C (Pedinol): Neomycin sulfate, polymyxin B sulfate, and hydrocortisone
    Dropper bottle: 10 ml

Pharmacokinetics, Concentration-effect Relationship, and Metabolism

Polymyxin B is not significantly absorbed from the GI tract. It is also poorly absorbed from the conjunctiva and the surface of large burns. It has poor corneal penetration in the presence of an intact epithelium but has good stromal penetration through an epithelial defect, whether administered topically or subconjuctivally.

The drug loses 50% of its activity in the presence of serum. Active blood levels are therefore low. Repeated injections of the drug may lead to an accumulation in the circulation. Peak blood concentrations occur about 2 hours after injection. Higher blood levels occur in infants, children, and patients with renal insufficiency.

Polymyxin B is excreted slowly by the kidneys. Elimination of the drug may continue for 1 to 3 days after the drug has been discontinued. Therefore, careful monitoring of the patients' renal status is necessary in all patients receiving this drug parenterally. Tissue diffusion is poor with polymyxin B, and the drug does not readily pass the blood–brain barrier (BBB) or the blood–aqueous barrier.

Therapeutic Use

Topical or subconjunctival administration of compounds containing polymyxin B may be useful in the treatment of external ocular infections caused by susceptible gram-negative organisms, especially *Pseudomonas.* Topical solutions consist of 500,000 U of polymyxin B dissolved in 20 to 50 ml sterile distilled water or physiologic saline, yielding a concentration of 10,000 to 25,000 U/ml. Ophthalmic ointments contain 10,000 U/g polymyxin B in combination with other antibiotic and/or steroid agents. Depending on the severity of the infection, these topical preparations may be applied every half hour to hourly and then tapered as clinical improvement is noted. Subconjunctival injections of 10,000 U/day or less may also be used in treating more severe external ocular infections. To prevent systemic side effects, ophthalmic doses greater than 25,000 U/kg/day should be avoided.

Polymyxin B is effective in treating urinary tract infections caused by *Pseudomonas* and other gram-negative bacilli. This drug should be reserved for treating disease caused by susceptible organisms and infections involving the kidneys (pyelonephritis). Doses of 20,000 to 25,000 U/kg/day administered intramuscularly in three to four divided doses often achieves clinical cure.

Polymyxin B may also be used in the treatment of systemic infections caused by susceptible gram-negative bacilli. Such infections may be treated by intramuscular or intravenous administration of the drug. Total daily intramuscular doses range from 25,00 to 30,000 U/kg/day in infants and to 40,000 U/kg/day or less in adults. The intramuscular solution is prepared by dissolving 500,000 U Polymyxin B in 2 ml sterile distilled water, saline, or 1% procaine HCl.

Intravenous solutions should be prepared by dissolving 500,000 U polymyxin B in 300 to 500 ml of 5% dextrose in water. Usual doses for adults and children are 15,000 to 25,000 U/kg/day in two divided doses daily. Infants may receive as much as 40,000 U/kg/day (33).

Meningeal infections caused by susceptible gram-negative bacilli that are not sensitive to other antibiotic agents may also be treated with polymyxin B. Treatment of meningitis requires intrathecal injections because polymyxin B penetrates the BBB poorly, even when the meninges are inflamed. Intrathecal solutions are prepared by dissolving 500,000 U polymyxin B in 10 ml sterile 0.9% sodium chloride solution. Dosing varies according to age. Starting doses for children aged 2 years or younger is 20,000 U/day; for older children and adults, the starting dose is 50,000 U/day (33). Patients receiving parenteral treatment require hospitalization so that they can be monitored for possible renal toxicity.

Side Effects and Toxicity

Nephrotoxicity

Polymyxin B may cause proteinuria, cylinduria, albuminuria, azotemia, acute tubular necrosis, and interstitial nephritis. It is recommended that a baseline renal function survey be performed before this drug is initiated and that periodic renal function tests be performed during the course of treatment. It is also recommended that other nephrotoxic agents be avoided during treatment with polymyxin B.

Neurotoxicity

Facial flushing, dizziness, ataxia, paresthesias, diplopia due to external ophthalmoplegia, ptosis, slurred speech, generalized areflexia, blurred vision, dysphagia, dyspnea, and apnea can occur in patients treated with polymyxin B. These neurotoxic reactions usually evolve in patients who have high serum levels of polymyxin B due to impaired renal function and/or nephrotoxicity. Respiratory paralysis may occur in association with concurrent use of anesthesia or muscle relaxants.

Ocular

Topical administration of polymyxin B may cause hypersensitivity reactions, and chronic use may lead to toxic conjunctivitis. Subconjunctival injections of 10 mg polymyxin B in rabbits caused severe chemosis, localized necrosis, and bloody discharge, whereas 0.5 mg injections are well tolerated (34).

Other

Fever and skin rashes occur infrequently with parenteral administration. GI side effects in patients treated systemically include nausea, vomiting, and diarrhea. Intramuscular injections can be painful, and phlebitis can occur at the site of intravenous infusion. Intrathecal administration may cause meningeal irritation, and patients may demonstrate an increase in cerebrospinal fluid (CSF) cells and protein.

High-risk Groups

Use of polymyxin B should be avoided in patients with renal insufficiency unless it is absolutely required. Reduced dosage and monitoring of serum drug levels are required in patients with renal insufficiency.

The safety of polymyxin B in pregnancy has not been established. In animal studies, polymyxin B impairs the motility of equine sperm, and its effects on human fertility are unknown. The carcinogenic potential of polymyxin B has not been established.

Drug Interactions

Increased nephrotoxicity is associated with the use of other nephrotoxic drugs. Apnea can occur with the concurrent use of curariform muscle relaxants and drugs such as ether, tubocurarine, succinylcholine, gallamine, decamethonium, and sodium citrate.

Clinical Trials

In 1952, Wiggins (30) demonstrated the effectiveness of polymyxin B against *P. aeruginosa* corneal ulcers in rabbit eyes. This first introduced the use of polymyxin B in the treatment of corneal ulcers. In 1955, Moorman and Harber (31) successfully treated two patients with *Pseudomonas* corneal ulcers. Both patients recovered visual acuities of 20/30 (31). Polytrim Ophthalmic Solution has proved effective in the treatment of bacterial conjunctivitis in both adult and pediatric populations (35,36).

REFERENCES

1. McCormick MH, Stark WM, Pittinger GE, Pittenger RC, McGuire JM. Vancomycin, a new antibiotic. I. Chemical and biologic properties. In: *Antibiotics annual, 1955–56.* New York: Medical Encyclopedia, Inc., 1956;606–611.
2. Fleischer AB, Hoover DL, Khan JA, Parisi JT, Burns RP. Topical vancomycin formulation for methicillin-resistant *Staphylococcus epidermidis* blepharoconjunctivitis. *Am J Ophthalmol* 1986;101:283–287.
3. Ross J, Abate MA. Topical vancomycin for the treatment of *Staphylococcus epidermidis* and methicillin-resistant *Staphylococcus aureus* conjunctivitis. *Ann Pharmacother* 1990;24:1050–1053.
4. Goodman DF, Gottsch JD. Methicillin-resistant *Staphylococcus epidermidis* keratitis treated with vancomycin. *Arch Ophthalmol* 1988; 106:1570–1571.
5. Eiferman FA, O'Neill KP, Morrison NA. Methicillin-resistant *Staphylococcus aureus* corneal ulcers. *Ann Ophthalmol* 1988;23:414–415.
6. *Physicians Desk Reference,* 47th ed. Montvale, NJ: Medical Economics Data, 1993;1341–1342.
7. Strominger JL, Tipper DJ. Bacterial cell wall synthesis and structure in relation to the mechanism of action of penicillins and other antibacterial agents *Am J Med* 1965;39:707–721.
8. *Physicians Desk Reference,* 47th ed. Montvale, NJ: Medical Economics Data, 1993;1342–1343.
9. Pryor JG, Apt L, Leopold IH. Intraocular penetration of vancomycin *Arch Ophthalmol* 1962;67:608–611.
10. Pflugfelder SC, Hernandez E, Fliesler SJ, Alvarez J, Pflugfelder ME, Forster RK. Intravitreal vancomycin. Retinal toxicity, clearance and interaction with gentamicin. *Arch Ophthalmol* 1987;105:831–837.
11. Moellering RC, Krogstad DJ, Greenblarr DJ. Vancomycin therapy in patients with impaired renal function. A nomogram for dosage. *Ann Intern Med* 1981;94:343.
12. Smith MA, Sorenson JA, Lowy FD, Shakin JL, Harrison W, Jadobiec FA. Treatment of experimental methicillin-resistant *Staphylococcus epidermidis* endophthalmitis with intravitreal vancomycin. *Ophthalmology* 1986;93:1328–1335.
13. Homer P, Peyman GA, Koziol J, Sanders D. Intravitreal injection of vancomycin in experimental staphylococcal endophthalmitis. *Acta Ophthalmol* 1975;53:311–320.
14. Lambert SR, Stern WH. Methicillin- and gentamicin-resistant *Staphylococcus epidermidis* endophthalmitis after intraocular surgery. *Am J Ophthalmol* 1985;99:725–726.
15. Davis JL, Koidov-Tsiligianni A, Pflugfelder SC, Miller D, Flynn HW, Forster RK. Coagulase-negative staphylococcal endophthalmitis. Increase in antimicrobial resistance. *Ophthalmology* 1988;95:1404–1410.
16. Hemady R, Zaltas M, Paton B, Foster CS, Baker AS. *Bacillus*-induced endophthalmitis: new series of 10 cases and review of the literature. *Br J Ophthalmol* 1990;74:26–29.
17. Affeldt JC, Flynn HW Jr, Forster RK, Mandelbaum S, Clarkson JG, Jarus GD. Microbial endophthalmitis resulting from ocular trauma *Ophthalmology* 1987;94:407–413.
18. Gigantelli JW, Torres-Gomez J, Osato MS. *In vitro* susceptibility of ocular *Bacillus cereus* isolates to clindamycin, gentamicin, and vancomycin alone or in combination. *Antimicrob Agents Chemother* 1991;35: 201–202.
19. Petroutos G, Guimarres R, Pouliquen Y. The effect of concentrated antibiotics on the rabbit's corneal epithelium. *Int Ophthalmol* 1984;7: 65–69.
20. Smith MA, Sorenson JS, Smith C, Miller M, Borenstein M. Effects of intravitreal dexamethasone on concentration of intravitreal vancomycin in experimental methicillin-resistant *Staphylococcus epidermidis* endophthalmitis. *Antimicrob Agents Chemother* 1991;35:1298–1302.
21. Trissel LA. Vancomycin HCl. In: *Handbook of injectable drugs,* 7th ed. Bethesda: American Society of Hospital Pharmacists, 1992;905–910.
22. Bellows JG, Farmer CJ. The use of bacitracin in ocular infections. Part II. Bacitracin therapy of experimental and clinical ocular infections. *Am J Ophthalmol* 1948;37:1211–1216.
23. *Physicians desk reference,* 47th ed. Montvale, NJ: Medical Economics Data, 1993;685,774–775, 813–814, 819.
24. Schecter JF, Wilkinson RD, Del-Carpio J. Anaphylaxis following the use of bacitracin ointment. Report of a case and review of the literature. *Arch Dermatol* 1984;120:909–911.
25. Meleny FL, Johnson BA, Balbina A. Bacitracin. *Am J Med* 1949; 7:794–806.
26. Goodman LS, Gillman LA. *The pharmacologic basis of therapeutics,* 4th ed. New York: MacMillan, 1970;1293–1294.
27. Ainsworth GC, Brown AM, Brownlee G. Aerosporin, an antibiotic produced by *Bacillus aerosporus. Nature* 1947;160:263.
28. Benedict RG, Langlykke AF. Antibiotic activity of *Bacillus polymyxa. J Bacteriol* 1947;54:24–25.
29. Stansly PG, Sheperd RG, White HJ. Polymyxin: a new chemotherapeutic agent. *Bull Johns Hopkins Hosp* 1947;81:43–54.
30. Wiggins RL. Experimental studies on the eye with polymyxin B. *Am J Ophthalmol* 1952;35:83–99.
31. Moorman LT, Harber F. Treatment of *Pseudomonas* corneal ulcers. *Arch Ophthalmol* 1955;53:345–346.
32. McNeel JW, Wood RM, Senterfit LB. Effect of polymyxin B sulfate on *Pseudomonas* corneal ulcers. *Arch Ophthalmol* 1961;66:646–648.
33. *Physicians desk reference,* 47th ed. Montvale, NJ: Medical Economics Data, 1993;592, 685, 774–777, 813–819, 1826, 2053.
34. Williams RK, Hench ME, Guerry D. Pyocyaneus ulcer. *Am J Ophthalmol* 1954;37:538–544.
35. Behrens-Baumann W, Quentin CD, Gibson JR, Calthrop JG, Harvey SG, Booth K. Trimethoprim-polymyxin B sulphate ophthalmic ointment in the treatment of bacterial conjunctivitis: a double-blind study vs. chloramphenicol ophthalmic ointment. *Curr Med Res Opin* 1988; 11:227–231.
36. Lohr JA, Austin RD, Grossman M, Hayden GF, Knowlton FM, Dudley SM. Comparison of three topical antimicrobials for acute bacterial conjunctivitis. *Pediatr Infect Dis J* 1988;7:626–629.
37. Goodman LS, Gillman LA. *The pharmacologic basis of therapeutics,* 4th ed. New York: MacMillan, 1970;1287–1290.
38. Havener W. *Ocular pharmacology,* 4th ed. St Louis: CV Mosby, 1978;159–160.

Textbook of Ocular Pharmacology,
edited by T.J. Zimmerman, et al.
Lippincott–Raven Publishers, Philadelphia © 1997.

CHAPTER 48

Rifampin

W. Craig Fowler, James E. Arena, and Mark J. Iacobucci

RIFAMPIN

History and Source

Rifampin is of interest in ophthalmology because of its wide range of activity against gram-positive bacteria, gram-negative bacteria, Mycobacteria, and mollicutes or organisms with no cell walls. Rifampin is derived from rifamycin B, a macrolytic compound first isolated from the fungus *Streptomyces mediterranei* at the Lepetit Research Laboratories in Milan, Italy, in 1960 (1,2). Rifampin was introduced for clinical systemic use in 1968 as a potent antituberculous agent (3). In 1969, Sana et al. (4) first reported the successful ophthalmologic use of topical 1% rifampin to treat gram-positive and gram-negative acute and subacute conjunctivitis. Although an animal study by Feldman et al. (5) indicated that topical application of 1% rifampin produced therapeutic concentrations in rabbit aqueous, topical rifampin is not commercially available in the United States at present.

Official Drug Name and Chemistry

The chemical name of rifampin is 3-(4-methyl-1-piperazinyl-1-iminomethyl)-rifamycin SV (6). Rifampin is also known as rifampicin (B.P.), rifadazine, rifampicinium, and rifamycin AMP. Rifampin is sold under the trade names Rifadin and Rimactane. Rifampin is soluble in water at acidic pH (7). The molecular formula of rifampin is $C_{43}H_{58}N_4$ (8,9); and the structural formula of rifampin (10) is shown below:

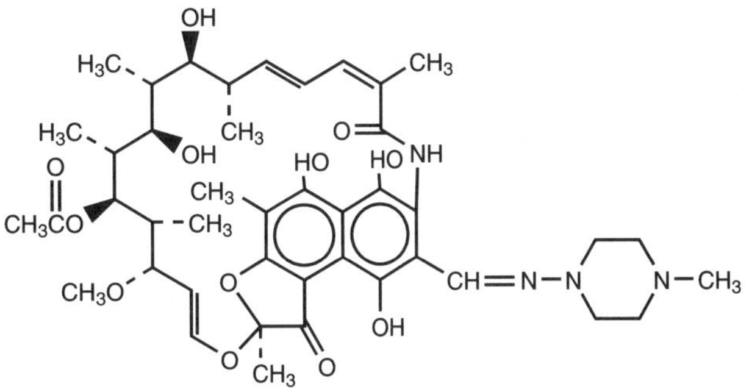

W. C. Fowler, J. E. Arena, and M. J. Iacobucci: Department of Ophthalmology, Duke University Eye Center, Box 3802, Durham, North Carolina 27710.

OH, H_3C, CH_3, H_3C, OH, CH_3, O, HO, HO, NH, CH_3CO, CH_3, $-CH_3$, CH_3O, O, $CH{=}N{-}N$, $N{-}CH_3$, OH, O, CH_3, O

Pharmacology (Main Action)

Rifampin forms a stable complex with bacterial DNA-dependent RNA polymerase and is bactericidal by preventing nucleic acid synthesis (11). Mammalian DNA synthesis is not affected by rifampin (12).

Clinical Pharmacology (Effect in Humans)

Rifampin is effective against *Mycobacterium tuberculosis, M. kansasii, M. marinum, M. avium-intracellulare, M. xenopi, M. ulcerans, M. scofulaceum,* and *M. leprae* (3). Drug resistance to rifampin among *M. tuberculosis* strains is less than 1% (13). Rifampin-resistant bacterial isolates have an altered DNA-dependent RNA polymerase that has less affinity for rifampin binding (14,15). Reportedly, rifampin has no in vitro activity against *M. fortuitum* and *M. chelonei,* but use of rifampin in combination with other agents for long-term therapy of *M. fortuitum* has been reported (16).

Pharmaceutics

Rifampin is available in 150-mg and 300-mg capsules (Rifadin, Rimactane) and in a powder for injection (600 mg, Rifadin). A combination fixed-dose capsule containing

300 mg rifampin and 150 mg isoniazid is also commercially available (Rifamate). The injection is reconstituted with 10 ml sterile water and is stable at room temperature for 24 hours. The calculated dose is diluted further in 500 ml dextrose 5% in water and infused in 3 hours. Solutions should be used within 4 hours of preparation because a precipitate may form after 4 hours. An oral (p.o.) suspension with a stability of 4 weeks may be prepared using the capsules and syrup (10).

Pharmacokinetics

Bioavailability

Oral rifampin is reported to have a bioavailability of 90% to 95% after a single oral dose of 600 mg. Peak serum levels of 7 to 9 μg are attained in 2 to 4 hours (9). Eighty percent of serum rifampin is protein bound, and decreased plasma protein levels in malnourished patients increases the bioavailability of rifampin. The biologic half-life ($t_{\frac{1}{2}}$) is about 3 hours and is dose dependent. The $t_{\frac{1}{2}}$ is increased to 5 hours with higher dosing (900 mg) and is reduced to 2 to 3 hours with repeated administration. Liver dysfunction can increase the $t_{\frac{1}{2}}$ to as long as 13 hours (17); $t_{\frac{1}{2}}$ is unaffected by peritoneal dialysis or hemodialysis. Intravenous (IV) administration of 600 mg rifampin infused in 30 minutes produces a mean peak plasma concentration of 17.4 μg/ml 30 minutes after infusion and one of 3.5 μg/ml at 8 hours. As does oral dosing, larger doses and repeated administration affect the $t_{\frac{1}{2}}$ of rifampin. The bioavailability of topical ophthalmic preparations is dependent on the vehicle used. Feldman et al. (5) reported that topical application of 1% rifampin in dimethyl sulfoxide (DMSO) provided bactericidal levels of rifampin in the aqueous humor of rabbits.

Absorption

Rifampin is almost completely absorbed from the gastrointestinal (GI) tract after oral administration; however, absorption may be decreased by taking rifampin with food. After a 600-mg oral dose in tuberculosis patients, food doubled the time required to attain peak serum levels and decreased the peak serum level by 25% (18). Rifampin should be ingested 1 hour before or 2 hours after a meal to ensure maximal absorption (10). Concurrent administration of aminosalicylic acid delays the absorption of rifampin and may prevent achievement of adequate plasma concentrations of rifampin (19).

Distribution

Rifampin is highly lipid soluble and is distributed in effective concentrations to the lungs, liver, bone, and cerebrospinal fluid (CSF) in the presence of inflamed meninges (20). Rifampin distributes readily into body fluids and produces an orange-red color of the urine, feces, saliva, sputum, sweat, and tears. The distribution of rifampin into tears may cause permanent discoloration of soft contact lenses (8,9).

Excretion

Rifampin is metabolized by the liver to its active metabolite and is primarily eliminated in the bile. As much as 30% of unmetabolized rifampin is cleared by the kidney. The remaining 60% to 80% of rifampin undergoes enterohepatic metabolism. Enterohepatic circulation deacetylates rifampin almost completely in 6 hours or less to its active primary metabolite, 25-deacetyl-rifampin, which is excreted into the bile, has reduced intestinal reabsorption, and is therefore cleared through the GI tract (21). Girling (22) reported that doses of 150 mg rifampin were excreted almost completely in the bile, whereas larger doses (300 mg or more) were cleared by hepatic as well as renal mechanisms.

Concentration-effect Relationship

The minimum inhibitory concentrations (MIC) for various pathogenic bacteria are shown in Table 1. Rifampin has bactericidal activity at concentrations of 3 to 12 μg/ml

Table 48-1. *Rifampin MIC for various organisms*[a]

Organism	MIC (μg/ml)
Staphylococcus aureus	0.002–0.005
S. albus	0.002
Streptococcus faecalis	0.01–0.5
S. hemolyticus	0.02
Diplococcus pneumoniae	0.01
Sarina lutea	0.01
Bacillus subtilus	0.02
Clostridium perfringens	0.002
Haemophilus influenzae	0.02
Neiserria catarrhalis	0.001
N. gonorrhoeae	0.02
Pseudomonas aeruginosa	10.0
Escherichia coli	1.0–10.0
Aeobacter aerogens	5.0
Klebsiella pneumoniae	5.0–10.0
Proteus vulgaris	5.0
Proteus morganii	10.0
Salmonella typhi	5.0
Shigella sonnei	10.0
Legionella pneumophila	0.03
Mycobacterium tuberculosis	0.5
M. fortuitum	1.0

MIC, minimum inhibitory concentration.
[a]From Arioli et al. (25).

against gram-positive cocci such as *Staphylococcus aureus,* including methicillin-resistant strains (23). Rifampin is also effective against *Neisseria gonorrhoeae, N. menigitidis, Haemophilus influenzae, Legionella pneumophila, Escherichia coli, Pseudomonas, Proteus,* and *Klebsiella.* Rifampin has subclinical activity against *Vaccinia* virus, with minimum bactericidal concentrations (MBC) of 100 μg/ml (24).

Therapeutic Use

Rifampin is most commonly used in combination with other agents to treat *M. tuberculosis* infections. Rifampin increases the in vitro activity of streptomycin and isoniazid (26). Rifampin also may be used for prophylaxis of meningococcal disease and meningitis secondary to *H. influenzae* in household contacts (3). In addition, rifampin has broad-spectrum activity and is effective in treating ocular leprosy, ocular staphylococcus infections, *Moraxella* conjunctivitis, chlamydial trachoma, and idiopathic chronic uveitis.

Ocular Tuberculosis

Most cases of ocular tuberculosis occur in patients aged less than 20 years; females are affected twice as often as males. Infection may involve the lid, conjunctiva, cornea, or uveal tract. Lupus vulgaris may spread to involve the eyelids and is characterized by small, soft, jelly-like nodules (27). Granulomatous conjunctivitis and *M. fortuitum* keratitis have been reported after injury or surgery and occur more commonly in compromised hosts. Conjunctival phylctenulosis may also occur and is sometimes sensitive to topical corticosteroids. Tuberculous uveitis should be suspected in the setting of chronic uveitis or granulomatous uveitis of unknown etiology. Diagnosis is made by acid-fast smear culture in Lowenstein-Jensen or Middlebrook media and a positive purified protein derivative (PPD) test. A chest roentgenogram and sputum culture may be obtained to exclude possible concurrent active pulmonary tuberculosis. Treatment consists of rifampin 600 mg/day p.o. in combination with isoniazid (5 mg/kg/day) for 9 months. If isoniazid-resistant organisms are suspected, a third drug such as ethambutol (15 mg/kg) should be added while susceptibility tests are performed (28). Lazar et al. (16) reported that one of three patients with *M. fortuitum* keratitis responded to the use of 1% topical rifampin in addition to rifampin 600 mg/day p.o. Lin et al. (29) reported effective treatment of 10 of 13 cases of atypical mycobacterial keratitis with systemic rifampin 600 mg/day p.o. Currently, however, we prefer to use topical amikacin 20 mg/ml as first-line drug for treatment of corneal involvement.

Ocular Leprosy

Hansen's disease is a chronic granulomatous disease of the eyelids caused by *M. leprae.* There are two types of Hansen's disease which are designated tuberculoid and lepromatous. The tuberculoid type is manifest by loss of eyebrows and eye lashes and is associated with skin tuberculoid lesions. The lepromatous type presents with thickening of the supraciliary ridge and nodular thickening of the tarsal area, with locally anesthetized, hypopigmented areas. Blepharochalasis and ptosis from bacterial infiltration of the skin may also be evident; some researchers believe that iris pearls are pathognomonic (27). Diagnosis is made based on clinical signs and biopsy. Treatment consists of rifampin 300 mg p.o. twice daily (b.i.d.) in combination with dapsone (100 mg/day) or another antileprosy drug (27).

Infectious Conjunctivitis

Infectious conjunctivitis secondary to *N. gonorrhoeae* and *N. menigitidis* may also be treated with rifampin in combination with appropriate topical agents. Rifampin may be used for *N. menigitidis* prophylaxis in household contacts. Adult nonsymptomatic contacts of *N. menigitidis*-infected patients may receive rifampin 600 mg p.o. b.i.d. for 4 days as prophylaxis. The prophylaxis dose in children is 10 to 20 mg/kg/day for 4 days (30). Emergence of rifampin resistance in *N. menigitidis* strains is rapid, however, and rifampin should not be used to treat active meningococcal disease.

Ocular Staphylococcus Infections

Oral rifampin 300 mg p.o. b.i.d. may be used supplementally to treat staphylococcal endophthalmitis in combination with appropriate topical, subconjunctival, and or intravenous therapy. Vancomycin is still the preferred drug for methicillin-resistant *S. Aureus* (MRSA) infections. In combination with trimethoprim-sulfamethoxazole, rifampin can also be used to treat MRSA infections in patients who are allergic to β-lactam antibiotics. Mikuni et al. (31) reported that rifampin 600 mg p.o. daily was effective in treating hordeolum secondary to *S. auerus.*

Moraxella Conjunctivitis

Moraxella conjunctivitis is characterized by acute angular conjunctivitis with mucopurulent discharge and maceration of the skin at the canthi. *Moraxella* conjunctivitis may also present as chronic follicular conjunctivitis. *Moraxella*-associated conjunctivitis is more common in women secondary to use of contaminated eye makeup. Schwartz et al. (32) reported use of systemic rifampin to treat a culture-proven outbreak of *Moraxella* conjunctivitis at a Navajo boarding school. Treatment with rifampin 600 mg p.o. b.i.d. for 2 months led to eradication of *Moraxella* from the conjunctiva in 91% of symptomatic patients and eradication from the nares of all of the asymptomatic carriers.

Trachoma

Trachoma is caused by *Chlamydia* trachomatis and is characterized by tearing and serous discharge, with linear and stellate scarring of the tarsal conjunctiva. Conjunctival scrapings may disclose large macrophages (Leber cells) and intracytoplasmic inclusions (27). Topical and systemic tetracycline or erythromycin is current accepted therapy for trachoma; however, in a limited number of trials, topical rifampin was efficacious. Topical rifampin is commercially available in the United States, but can be compounded using Rifadin powder for injection (16). A clinical trial in schoolchildren with active hyperendemic trachoma in Tunisia demonstrated that 1% rifampin eye ointment twice daily for 10 weeks was substantially more beneficial than boric acid treatment and potentially as effective as 1% tetracycline ointment (33). In a clinical trial, treatment with 1% rifamycin ointment for 6 to 7 weeks in 63 patients with *Chlamydia* trachomatis yielded 90% clinical and microbiologic cure rate (34).

Mycotic Keratitis

In addition to amphotericin B, flucytosine, ketoconazole, and micononazole, combination therapy with rifampin may be of value in treating certain strains of *Candida* and *Aspergillis* (35). Results of investigations (36,37) have suggested that the combination of amphotericin B and rifampin is synergistic against 90% of *C. albicans.* Lou et al. (38) reported successful resolution of one case of *Candida* endophthalmitis after combination therapy with amphotericin B and rifampin.

Mollicutes

Mollicutes are pleomorphic organisms without cell walls that pass through bacteria-retaining filters and are sometimes confused with viruses. Extracellular mollicutes cause human lung disease characterized by lymphoid infiltrates, immunosuppression, and autoantibody production. Mollicutes have been implicated in causing chronic keratitis, scleritis, experimental uveitis in mice, and other related idiopathic ocular inflammatory conditions. In one study, rifampin treatment reduced the morbidity in a mice mollicute uveitis model (39). Rifampin is also a potentially useful therapeutic option in treating idiopathic chronic uveitis (40).

Viral Infections

Rifampin is not currently approved for use in treating viral infections. However, the *Vaccinia* virus contains a DNA-directed RNA polymerase. Heller et al. (24) reported that 100 μg/ml rifampin inhibited *Vaccinia* growth in vitro. Rifampin also inhibited replication of Herpessimplex and Adenovirus, but inhibition occurred at concentrations greater than those typically reached in the serum with oral rifampin therapy (41).

Contraindications

Rifampin is contraindicated in patients with a known hypersensitivity to rifamycin or those with significant preexisting liver disease. Rifadin injection contains sodium formaldehyde sulfoxylate, a sulfite that may cause a severe hypersensitivity reaction. Pregnancy is also a relative contraindication to the use of rifampin. Rifampin use in the first trimester of pregnancy has been associated with isolated cases of fetal malformation (10).

Side Effects

Rifampin is usually well tolerated; less than 4% of patients with tuberculosis report adverse reactions. The most common side effect is nausea and vomiting (1.5%), followed by fever (0.5%) and rash (0.4%) (7). Rifampin-induced hepatitis occurs in less than 1% of patients and is more common in patients receiving multiple potentially hepatotoxic drugs. Asymtomatic elevation of liver enzymes may occur in as many as 14% of patients, however (42). Therefore, baseline clinical chemistries must be obtained and liver function must be tested before rifampin therapy is initiated and every 2 weeks during rifampin therapy. High-dose intermittent therapy is associated with a flu-like hypersensitivity syndrome (43), which may progress to include interstitial nephritis, acute tubular necrosis, thrombocytopenia, hemolytic anemia, and shock (44). The following ocular side effects have been reported with systemic rifampin use: soft contact lens stain/discoloration, decreased vision, red/green color defects, increased lacrimation, retinal hemorrhages, blepharoconjunctivits, subconjunctival hemorrhage, and optic neuritis (rare) (30).

Acute Toxicity

Nonfatal overdoses with as much as 12 g rifampin and a fatality occurring after self-administration of 60 g rifampin have been reported (10). Rifampin overdose causes symptoms that are extensions of common side effects such as nausea, vomiting, and liver dysfunction. Treatment of rifampin overdose includes gastric lavage, followed by activated charcoal slurry and diuresis. Bile drainage and hemodialysis may be indicated if serious hepatic impairment lasts longer than 48 to 72 hours (6).

High-risk Groups

Chronic liver disease, alcoholism, and old age appear to increase the incidence of rifampin-induced hepatotoxicity (45). The safe use of rifampin during pregnancy has not been established. Rifampin is teratogenic in rodents at 15 to 25 times the oral dose. Rifampin is highly lipophilic and is excreted in breast milk at therapeutic concentrations. However, rifampin combined with isoniazid and or ethambutol has been used to treat tuberculosis in pregnant women. When administered in the last weeks of pregnancy, rifampin may cause postpartum hemorrhage.

Drug Interactions

Drug interactions with rifampin have been reported previously (10,46,47). Rifampin is primarily metabolized by the liver and subsequently induces hepatic microsomal enzymes and thus interacts with drugs that are primarily metabolized by the liver. Rifampin increases the rate of metabolism of the following drugs:

Warfarin
Chloramphenicol
Oral contraceptives
Corticosteroids
Cyclosporin
Estrogen
Methadone
Quinidine
Sulfones
Sulfonylureas
Verapmil
Ketoconazole

Rifampin therapy may result in decreased concentration and effect of the above drugs when coadministered. Because rifampin enhances the breakdown of various steroids (48), patients receiving oral contraceptives should be instructed to use nonhormonal methods of birth control while receiving rifampin.

Concurrent administration of rifampin has also been reported to diminish the effects of the following drugs:

Acetaminophen
Benzodiazepines
Barbituates
β-Blockers
Clofibrate
Disopramide
Hydantoins
Mexiletine
Theophylline
Tocanide

Rifampin should also be used with caution in steroid- or theophylline-dependent asthmatic patients because rifampin may decrease steroid and theophylline effects and precipitate an asthma attack. The use of rifampin and isoniazid in combination also increases the risk of hepatoxicity. Aminosalicylic acid decreases the absorption of rifampin, and aspirin should be ingested 8 to 12 hours after the rifampin daily dose if it is used concurrently.

Clinical Trials

No ophthalmologic clinical trials involving rifampin are currently in progress. Pertinent historical clinical trials with rifampin are described in the Therapeutic Use section.

Other Antituberculous Agents

Other antituberculous agents include INH, ethambutol, PAS, streptomycin, cycloserine, and capreomycin and have been used for systemic tuberculous therapy; a few selective agents have been used in treatment of uveitis or posterior segment therapy. The only agent used for topical therapy is INH. In 1954, Kratka (49) noted that 100 mg/cc INH delivered topically every hour resulted in an aqueous concentration of 5 μg/ml, whereas the ointment form (200 mg/g) resulted in aqueous levels of 30 μg/ml. Oral and intramuscular delivery of INH resulted in aqueous levels greater than 10 μg/ml. A keratitis model was also treated with INH topically and intramuscularly but was believed to be bacteriostatic and not bactericidal. Currently, none of these agents are recommended for anterior segment clinical use.

REFERENCES

1. Sensi P, Greco M, Ballootta R. Rifamycin I. Isolation and properties of rifamycin B and rifamycin complex. *Antibiot Ann* 1960;250:262.
2. Sensi P, Maggi N, Furesz S, Maffii G. Chemical modiciation and biological properties of rifamycins. *Antimicrob Agents Chemother* 1966; 699–714.
3. Balows A, Hausler W, Herrmann K, Isenberg H, Shadomy J, eds. *Manual of Clinical Microbiology,* 5th ed. Washington, D.C.: American Society for Microbiology, 1991.
4. Sanna G. Ricerche cliniche preliminari sull' impiego della rifampicina in ofthalmogia. *Arch Maragliano Pat Clin* 1969;25:345.
5. Feldman MF, Moses RA. Corneal penetration of rifampin. *Am J Ophthalmol* 1977;83:862–865.
6. Barnhart E. *Physician's Desk Reference,* 44th ed. Oradell, NJ: Medical Economics, 1990;1473.
7. Mandell GL, Sande MA. Antimicrobial agents. Drugs used in the chemotherapy of tuberculosis and leprosy. In: Gillman AG, Rall TW, Nies AS, Taylor P, eds. *The Pharmacological Basis of Therapeutics,* 8th ed. New York: Pergamon Press, 1990.
8. Reynolds EF, Prosad AB, eds. *The Extra Pharmacopoeia,* 28th ed. London: The Pharmaceutical Press, 1982.
9. Patti RF. *Drugdex Revision 08/93,* vol. 82. Micromedix, 1994.

10. Package Insert, Rifadin. Merrel Dow, 1990.
11. Konno K, Oizumi K, Oka S. Mode of action of rifampin on mycobacteria. *Am Rev Resp Dis* 1973;107:1006–1012.
12. Wehrli W, Knusel K, Schmid K, Staehelin M. Interaction of rifamycin with bacterial RNA polymerase. *Proc Natl Acad Sci USA* 1968;61: 667–663.
13. Collins CH, Yates MD. Low incidence of rifampin resistant tubercle bacilli. *Thorax* 1982;37:526–527.
14. Wehrli W. Rifampin: mechanisms of action and resistance. *Rev Infect Dis* 1983;5(suppl 3):S407–S411.
15. Yamada T, Nagata A, Ono Y, Suzuki Y, Yamanouchi. Alterations of ribosomes and RNA-polymerase in drug resistant clinical isolates of Mycobacterium tuberculosis. *Antimicrob Agents Chemother* 1985;27: 921–924.
16. Lazar M, Nemet P, Bracha R, Campus A. *Mycobacterium fortuitum* keratitis. *Am J Ophthalmol* 1974;78(3):530–532.
17. Acocela G, Bomolla P, Garimoldi M, et al. Kinetics of rifampicin and isoniazid administered alone and in combination to normal subjects and patients with liver disease. *Gut* 1972;13:47.
18. Siegler DI, Bryant M, Burley DM, et al. Effect of meals on rifampicin absorption. *Lancet* 1974;2:197–198.
19. Radner DB. Toxicologic and pharmacologic aspects of rifampin. *Chest* 1973;64:213–216.
20. De Rautlin de la Roy, et al. Rifampicin serum and cerebrospinal fluid concentrations in children. *Nouv Presse Med* 1973;2:2000.
21. Acocella G. Clinical pharmacokinetics of rifampicin. *Clin Pharmacokinet* 1978;3:108.
22. Girling DJ. Adverse effects to rifampin in antituberculous regimens. *J Antimicrob Chemother* 1977;3:115–132.
23. Thornsberry C, Hill B, Senson J, McDougal L. Rifampin: spectrum of antibacterial activity. *Rev Infect Dis* 1983;5(suppl 3):S412–S417.
24. Heller F, Aragaman M, Levy H, Goldblum N. Selective inhibition of vaccinia virus by the antibiotic rifampicin. *Nature* 1969;222:273.
25. Arioli V, Pallanza R, Furesz S, Carnitti G. Rifampicin: a new rifamycin. *Arzneimittelforschung* 1967;17:529.
26. Hobby GL, Lenert TF. Observations on the action of rifampin and ethambutol alone and in combination with other anti-tuberculous drugs. *Am Rev Respir Dis* 1972;105:292–295.
27. Ostler BH. *Diseases of the external eye and adnexa, a text and atlas.* Baltimore: Williams & Wilkins, 1993.
28. Ellis PP. *Ocular Therapeutics and Pharmacology,* 7th ed. St. Louis: CV Mosby, 1985.
29. Lin H, Chen C, Sheu M, Wang H, Chue P. Clinicoetiological observation of 13 cases of mycobacterial keratitis. *Kasohsiung J Med Sci* 1989;5:676–682.
30. Pavan-Langston D, Dunkel EC. *Handbook of Ocular Drug Therapy and Ocular Side Effects of Systemic Drugs.* Boston: Little, Brown, 1991; 66.
31. Mikuni M, Ohishi M, Suda S, Imal M, Takahashi T. Rifampicin in ophthalmology. *Acta Med Biol* 1970;18:201–210.
32. Schwartz B, Harrison L, Motter JS, Motter RN, Hightower AW, Broome CV. Investigation of an outbreak of *Moraxella* conjunctivitis at a Navajo boarding school. *Am J Ophthal* 1989;107:341–347.
33. Daghfous T, Messadi M, Vastine D, Schachter J. Topical tetrcycline and rifampicin therapy of endemic trachoma in Tunisia. *Am J Ophthalmol* 1975;79:803–811.
34. Dargougar S, Viswalingam M, Kinnison J. Treatment of TRIC infection of the eye with rifampicin or chloramphenicol. *Br J Ophthalmol* 1977;61:255–259.
35. Stern GA. In vitro antibiotic synergism against ocular fungal isolates. *Am J Ophthalmol* 1978;86:359–367.
36. Begs WHO, Sarosi GA, Andrew WS. Synergistic action of amphotericin B and rifampin against *Candida albicans. Am Rev Respir Dis* 1974;110:671–673.
37. Stern GA, Okumoto M, Smolin G. Combined amphotericin B and rifampin treatment of experimental *Candida albicans* keratitis. *Arch Ophthalmol* 1979;97:721–722.
38. Lou P, Kazdan J, Bannatyne RM, Cheung R. Successful treatment of *Candida* endophthalmitis with a synergistic combination of amphotericin B and rifampin. *Am J Ophthalmol* 1977;83:12–15.
39. Wirostko E, Johnson L. The inducation of mouse uveitis by human idiopathic uveitis aqueous humor and treatment by certain anti-tuberculous drugs. *Trans NY Acad Sci* 1974;36:693.
40. Wirostko E, Johnson L, Wirostko B. Crohn's disease—rifampin treatment of ocular and gut disease. *Hepatogastroenterology* 1978;34:90–93.
41. Subak-Sharpe JH, Tunbury MD, Williams JF. Rifampicin inhibits the growth of some mammalian viruses. *Nature* 1969;222:273.
42. Furesz S, Scotti R. Rifamycin IV laboratory and clinical experiences with rifamycin B. *Antibiot Ann* 1959–1960;285.
43. Flynn CT, Rainford DJ, Hoppe E. Acute renal failure and rifampin: danger of unsuspected intermittent dose. *Br Med J* 1974;2:82.
44. Groset J, Leventis S. Adverse effects of rifampin. *Rev Infect Dis* 1983; 5(suppl 3):S440–S446.
45. Gronhagen-Riska C, Hellstrom PE, Froseth B. Predisposing factors in hepatitis induced by isoniazid-rifampin treatment of tuberculosis. *Am Rev Respir Dis* 1978;118:461–466.
46. Sewester CS, Olive BR, Hebel SK, Domebek CE, Kastrup EK, eds. *Drug Facts and Comparisons,* 1994 edition. St. Louis: JB Lippincott, 1994.
47. McEvoy GK, Litvok K, eds. *AHFS Drug Information.* Washington, D.C.: American Society of Hospital Pharmacists, 1992.
48. Buffington GA, Dominguez JH, Piering WF, Herbert L, Kouggman HM, Lemann J. Interaction of rifampin and glucocorticoids. *JAMA* 1976;36:1958–1960.
49. Kratka. *Arch Ophthalmol* 1955;54:330.

Textbook of Ocular Pharmacology,
edited by T.J. Zimmerman, et al.
Lippincott–Raven Publishers, Philadelphia © 1997.

CHAPTER 49

Amebic Disease of the Eye

Hassan Alizadeh, Jerry Niederkorn, and James P. McCulley

AMOEBA

Acanthamoeba sp are extracellular protozoan organisms that have been isolated from a variety of environments. Free-living amoebae are present in hot tubs, fresh water, swimming pools, salt water, soil, and emergency eye wash stations in medical and industrial laboratories (1–4). The organisms can also be isolated from the nasopharyngeal passages of healthy individuals (5,6). The trophozoite (active stage) is 10 to 25 μm long and is characterized by a large single nucleus and by spindle-like pseudopodia termed "acanthapodia." In an unfavorable environment, trophozoites become encysted. The cysts are double walled, with the inner wall having a variety of polygonal shapes depending on the species of organism (Fig. 1). Previously, differences in cyst morphology were used to identify different species of *Acanthamoeba.* More recently, isoenzyme analysis has been used to classify different strains of *Acanthamoeba.* Restriction enzyme analysis of either mitochondrial DNA or cellular DNA often has not correlated with morphologic characteristics of different species (7). At present, the identification and classification of *Acanthamoeba* is based on morphology and on biologic and physiologic characteristics.

History of *Acanthamoeba* Keratitis

Acanthamoeba keratitis is a sight-threatening corneal disease caused by pathogenic free-living amoebae. The first case of *Acanthamoeba* keratitis was reported by Jones et al. (8). The patient was a 59-year-old cattleman from southern Texas with a history of ocular trauma (caused by straw) and exposure to contaminated water. However, approximately 10 additional cases of *Acanthamoeba* keratitis were reported between 1973 and 1981 (3). Since 1981, the number of *Acanthamoeba* keratitis cases has increased gradually, and more than 100 cases were reported during the late 1980s in the United States. The disease is closely associated with contact lens wear, which appears to be an important risk factor in infection. In a recent study, more than 80% of the cases of *Acanthamoeba* keratitis occurred in contact lens wearers (9). Considering the ubiquity of the parasite and the large population of contact lens wearers, it is somewhat surprising that fewer than 300 cases of *Acanthamoeba* keratitis have been reported since its initial description in 1973, although the true incidence of *Acanthamoeba* keratitis may be higher than that reported to the Centers for Disease Control (CDC).

Clinical Features of *Acanthamoeba* Keratitis

Acanthamoeba keratitis occurs in immunocompetent, healthy young individuals, many of whom are contact lens wearers. The disease occurs with equal frequency in males and females. Daily-wear soft contact lenses account for approximately 75% of the cases. Most patients who develop *Acanthamoeba* keratitis have at least three risk factors associated with the disease: corneal trauma, contaminated water or solutions, and contact lenses. Stehr-Green et al. (10), who studied 189 cases of *Acanthamoeba* keratitis, reported that many patients had at least one risk factor for *Acanthamoeba* keratitis.

Acanthamoeba keratitis can have many appearances, but the signs of disease at an early stage (1 to 2 weeks) include eyelid-reactive ptosis, conjunctival hyperemia, and lack of discharge. In addition to these signs, chemosis and nodules appear at later stages (1 to 3 months) of the disease. In more advanced stages of disease (3 to 6 months), not only do these signs remain unchanged but episcleritis and scleritis become more easily recognizable.

One of the specific and important symptoms of *Acanthamoeba* keratitis is the severity of the pain in the early stage of infection. This initial symptom nonetheless is atyp-

H. Alizadeh, J. Niederkorn, J. P. McCulley: Department of Ophthalmology, University of Texas Southwestern Medical Center at Dallas, Dallas, Texas 75235–9057.

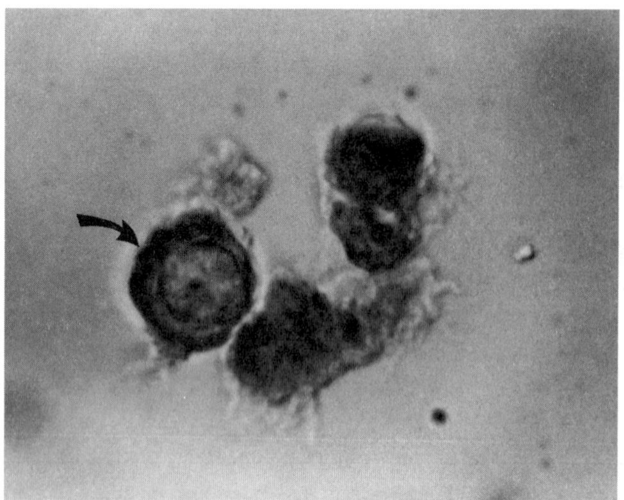

FIG. 49-1. Two-stage life cycle of *Acanthamoeba* trophozoite and cyst (arrow).

ical as compared with that of other categories of infectious keratitis (e.g., Herpes simplex keratitis). Corneal epithelium and sometimes stromal tissue are affected in the early stage of infection. Vesicular epithelium and pseudodendritic epithelial lesions are changes that occur superficially in the cornea. Moreover, the occurrence of patchy stromal infiltrates in the subepithelium and stroma indicates early-stage *Acanthamoeba* keratitis. Subsequently, the patchy stromal infiltrates extend and form crescents or ring infiltrates. The rings initially located in the central cornea become more circumscribed and dense at later stages of infection (Fig. 2). Furthermore, other later symptoms of *Acanthamoeba* keratitis are the occurrence of lacuna-like changes in the ring, satellite lesions, necrotizing inflammation, and stromal abscess formation. Mannis et al. (11) reported that severe anterior and posterior scleritis with a nodular component is involved in *Acanthamoeba* keratitis. Corneal neovascularization is rare, however. At present, radial neuritis or infiltrate along the corneal nerve by the organisms is pathognomonic for *Acanthamoeba* (12). Therefore, the severity of the pain in *Acanthamoeba* infection probably arises from parasite infiltration and neuritis. More recently, in vitro studies showed that *Acanthamoeba* trophozoites are chemotaxically more attracted to the tissues such as endothelium that arise from neural crest than to epithelium (13). The other features of *Acanthamoeba* keratitis include recurrent epithelial breakdown and overlying ring infiltrates which may cause abscesses. These manifestations are indistinguishable from the ring abscesses caused by Herpes simplex virus. Indeed, many previously misdiagnosed herpes ring abscesses probably were caused by *Acanthamoeba.* The development of a ring abscess and involvement of stroma vary and manifest differently. These features include formation of dense single or multiple anterior stromal infiltrates and nummular keratitis that appear at one or all levels of the stroma.

The stroma become more affected at late stages of the disease, characterized by a ring infiltrate or abscess consisting of dense single, multiple, or overlapping rings. The cause of the dense ring infiltrates in the corneas of patients with *Acanthamoeba* keratitis is not known. The ring infiltrates have been suggested to result from release of various proteolytic enzymes by infiltrating neutrophils that cause collagenolysis of the stroma. Other investigators have suggested that the ring infiltrates are due to the presence of the organisms and minimal inflammatory reaction at the site of infection. We have reported, however, that elaboration of collagenolytic enzymes by *Acanthamoeba* not only degrades collagen in vitro but also produces ring infiltrates in

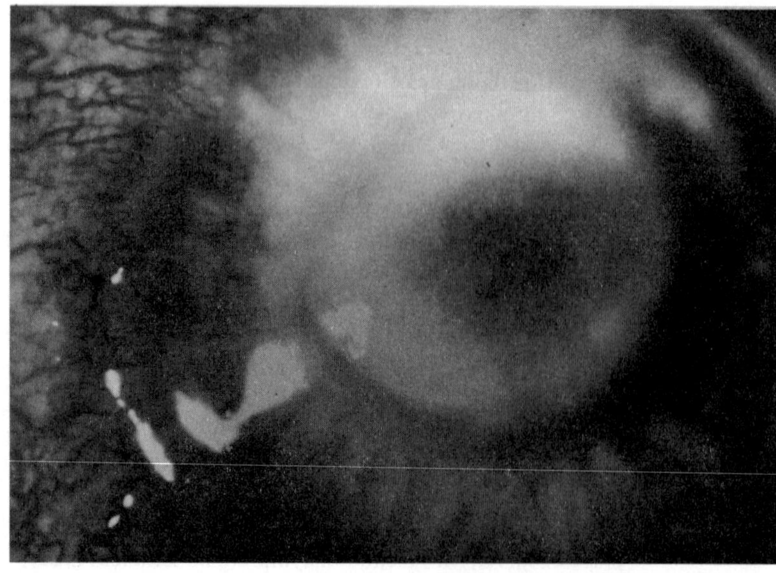

FIG. 49-2. Complete ring formation, indicating progressive stromal infiltrate (courtesy of Dr. ZM Husseini, Dallas, TX).

the corneas of rats that mimic *Acanthamoeba* keratitis in human patients (14).

Laboratory Diagnosis of *Acanthamoeba* Keratitis

It is very important to perform a laboratory test for *Acanthamoeba* as soon as possible, because therapy for the disease is quite extensive and very long treatment is required. Moreover, the extensive treatments must be continued for at least 1 year. Several diagnostic tests are available for culture and recognition of *Acanthamoeba.* Because the parasite is difficult to identify in a tissue section, the organism should be cultured in vitro. In the laboratory *Acanthamoeba* can be diagnosed with greatest accuracy through culture of the specimen on a confluent lawn of *Escherichia coli* or *Enterobacter* sp in nonnutrient agar (Fig. 3). In such culture plates, the *E. coli* serve as a food source for *Acanthamoeba* which will, in effect, eat the bacteria and leave a little path through the lawn of *E. coli.* Because the culture contains nonnutrient agar, the *E. coli* do not proliferate to fill the path (15). In this culture and under the microscope, trophozoites can be identified by the presence of the contractile vacuoles, which will disappear and reappear very quickly.

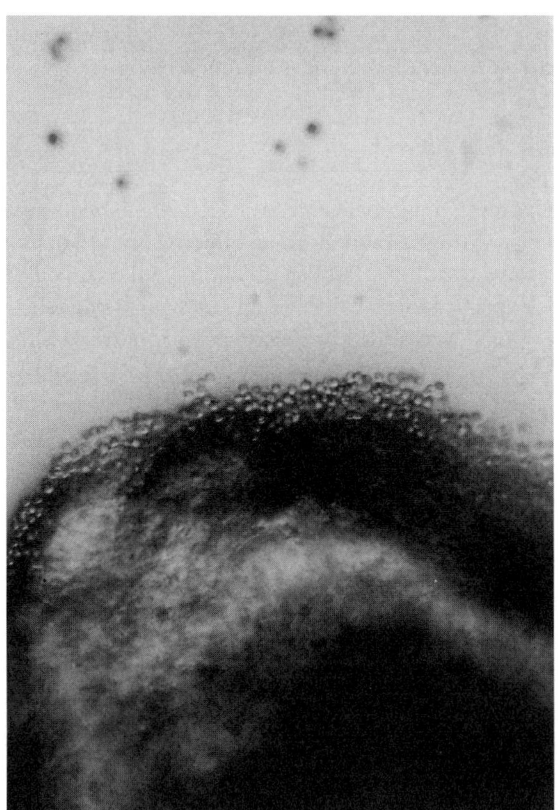

FIG. 49-3. Day-10 culture of *Acanthamoeba* cyst from patient corneal biopsy in nonnutrient agar (courtesy of R. Silvany, Dallas, TX).

Medical Treatment of *Acanthamoeba* Keratitis

Successful medical treatment is one of the goals in management of *Acanthamoeba* keratitis. In vitro sensitivity testing has identified agents that are inhibitory to the trophozoites; however, higher concentrations of these agents are required to kill the cysts (4). Medical control of *Acanthamoeba* keratitis was reported by several investigators (9), yet the preferred treatment of this disease has not been determined. However, *Acanthamoeba* keratitis has been successfully treated with the following drugs either alone or in combination.

PROPAMIDINE ISETHIONATE

History and Source

Propamidine isethionate (May and Baker, Dagenham, Essex, England) was used as early as 1900 to treat ocular infection. It has been used to treat blepharitis and superficial skin infection. In addition to their amoebicidal effect, the compounds show antibacterial and antifungal properties.

Propamidine isethionate belongs to the diamidine group and is available only in England as an over-the-counter antibiotic for treatment of external ocular infection. It is available either as a drop (Brolene solution) (Fig. 4) or as ointment (Brolene ointment).

Drug Name and Chemistry

Brolene is the trade name for the generic propamidine isethionate (plus other unknown ingredients), a 4,4′-diamidino-α ω-diphenoxypropane isethionate (Fig. 5). It is commercially available as 0.1% solution with preservatives such as methyl paraben (0.023% wt/vol) and propyl paraben (0.011% wt/vol). Dibromopropamidine isethion-

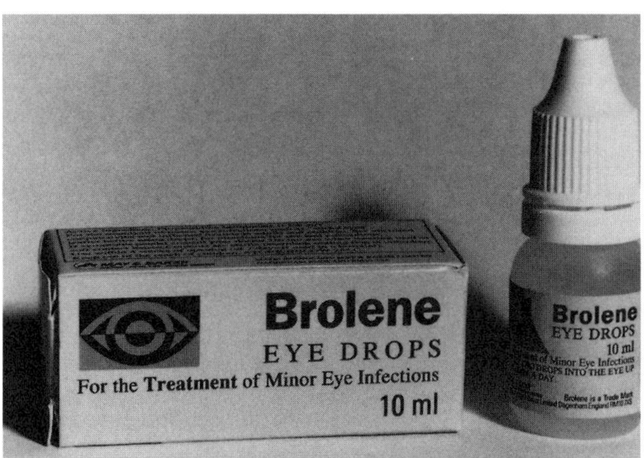

FIG. 49-4. Brolene drops.

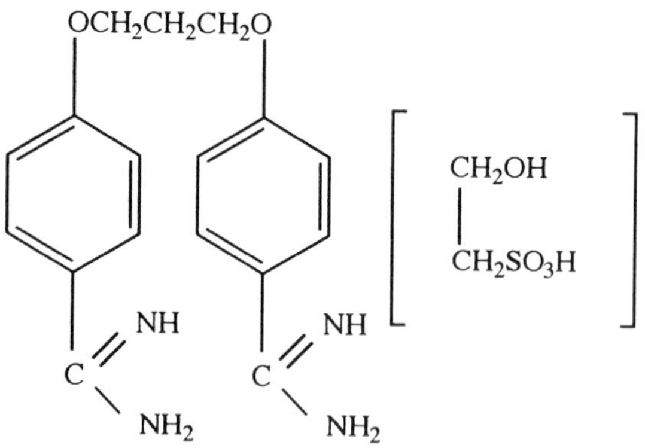

FIG. 49-5. Propamidine isethionate.

ate (Brolene ointment) is similar to the Brolene eye drops but is more water soluble; it is commercially available as 0.15% in water (Table 1).

Pharmacology

The mechanism of action of propamidine isethionate is not known; the drug is believed to inhibit or interfere with DNA, RNA, phospholipid, and protein synthesis. It is reported to be effective against pyrogenic cocci, *Staphylococcus aureus,* gram-negative organisms including *E. coli* and *Proteus vulgaris,* and some strains of *Pseudomonas.*

Table 49-1. *Description and history of Brolene*

Trade name:	Brolene
Generic name:	Propamidine isethionate plus other unknown ingredients
Concentration:	Ophthalmic solution 0.1%
Chemistry:	4,4′ Diamidinodiphenoxypropane, an aromatic diamidine
Preservatives:	Methylparaben 0.023% wt/vol, propylparaben 0.011% wt/vol
First used:	In early 1900s in England to treat ocular parasitic infection
First advocated:	In 1983 by Peter Wright in England to treat *Acanthamoeba* keratitis
First published and confirmed:	In 1987 by Mary Beth Moore and James P. McCulley in the United States
Properties:	Has antibacterial, antifungal and antiparasitic properties

Pharmaceutics

Topical Ophthalmic

Brolene eye drops
  Propamidine isethionate soluble 1 in 5 in water. One tenth percent solution.
Brolene ointment
  Dibromopropamidine soluble 1 in 2 in water. 0.15% solution.

Therapeutic Use

Brolene is administered as 1 drop every 30 minutes in 24 hours for 3 days. Early maintenance therapy is continued for 3 or 4 weeks, during which time the dosage is gradually decreased to one drop every 2, 3, or 4 hours while the patient is awake. The late maintenance therapy is continued for 1 year, during which time Brolene is administered four times daily (Table 2).

Side Effects and Drug Interaction

Brolene drops and ointment have been reported to have very serious adverse effects on the eye. Local irritation and superficial necrosis of granulation tissue were observed in some patients after topical application to the wounded cornea for more than 10 days. Moreover, drug toxicity to intensive usage of Brolene is common but reversible.

Clinical Trials

The limited number of cases of *Acanthamoeba* keratitis makes it difficult to organize an effective trial to determine definitive treatment. Published reports in the United States and England indicate that treatment with Brolene is very effective in controlling *Acanthamoeba* keratitis (15,16).

NEOSPORIN OPHTHALMIC SOLUTION

Neosporin ophthalmic solution (Burroughs Wellcome, Research Triangle Park, NC, U.S.A.) is an antimicrobial solution. Each milliliter contains 10,000 U polymyxin B, 1.75 mg neomycin sulfate, and 0.025 mg gramicidin. A combination of Brolene and Neosporin solution was used successfully to treat *Acanthamoeba* keratitis (15). The treatment regimen used for Neosporin solution was the same as that used for Brolene (Table 2). Neosporin has a wide range of antibacterial action against most bacterial pathogens of the eye. Neomycin is bactericidal for many gram-positive and gram-negative organisms. It inhibits protein synthesis by binding with ribosomal RNA. Neosporin ophthalmic solution also contains polymyxin B,

Table 49-2. *Treatment protocol for Brolene and Neosporin*[a]

Initial intensive therapy: 6 days	
First 3 days:	Brolene and Neosporin 1 drop every 30 minutes for 24 hours, with alternating drops at each administration
Second 3 days:	Brolene and Neosporin 1 drop every hour while the patient is awake and 1 drop every 2 hours during the night, with alternating drops at each administration
Early maintenance therapy:	4 weeks
Brolene and Neosporin:	Week 1, every 2 hours while awake; Week 2, every 3 hours while awake; Week 3, every 4 hours while awake; Week 4, every 4 hours while awake
Late maintenance therapy:	One year
Brolene and Neosporin:	Both drops 4 times a day: For early and late maintenance therapy, both Brolene and Neosporin drops are administered at each time interval, allowing a 5-minute interval between the administration of Brolene and that of Neosporin
Follow-up visits	
Days:	1, 2, 3, 5, 7, 14, 21 and 28 days
Months:	At 2, 3, 4, 6, 7, and 12 months
Post treatment:	Month 15
For patients who are allergic to neomycin, the same treatment regimen should be followed using Brolene only.	

[a]Brolene study by Dr. ZM Husseini, Dallas, Texas.

which is bactericidal for a variety of gram-positive organisms. It increases cell membrane permeability by interacting with the phospholipid components of the membrane. Gramicidin also is bactericidal for many gram-positive organisms. It increases the cell membrane permeability through the cation channels in cell membranes. The manifestations of allergy to neomycin are itching, reddening, and edema of the conjunctiva and eyelid. Patients should be examined periodically for such allergic reactions to neomycin treatment and should be advised to discontinue the product if these reactions are observed. (See the Aminoglycoside section for further details.)

Therapeutic Use

One drop of neosporin solution (10,000 Units polymyxin B, 1.75 mg neomycin sulfate, 0.025 mg gramicidin) is applied to the inferior cul-de-sac (Table 2).

PENTAMIDINE ISETHIONATE

Pentamidine isethionate (Pentam 300, Lyophomed, Rosemont, IL, U.S.A.) is an antiprotozoal agent that has activity against *Pneumocystis carinii.* Pentamidine is a white crystalline powder soluble in water and glycerin. The mode of action of pentamidine is not fully understood. In vitro studies with mammalian tissue and the protozoan *Crithidia oncopelti* indicate that the drug interferes with nuclear metabolism, producing inhibition of the synthesis of DNA, RNA, phospholipids, and proteins. Brolene and pentamidine belong to the diamidine group; however, pentamidine is more toxic than Brolene and can be used temporarily to treat *Acanthamoeba* keratitis until Brolene becomes available. (See the Diamidine section for further details.)

Therapeutic Use

Pentamidine powder can be mixed with an artificial tear to obtain a 0.05% to 0.1% solution and can be applied as a drop.

MICONAZOLE

Miconazole (Monistat I.V., Janssen Pharmaceutical, Piscataway, NJ, U.S.A.) is an antifungal agent. Each milliliter of the sterile solution contains 10 mg miconazole with 0.115 ml polyethylene glycol (PEG) 40 castor oil, 1.0 mg lactic acid USP, 0.5 mg methylparaben USP, and 0.05 mg propylparaben USP in water. Miconazole is an irritant to the eye, and some patients do not tolerate it well. It is unstable at room temperature and should be stored at 4°C or on ice; it should be replaced weekly. (See chapter on Imidazoles for further details.)

Therapeutic Use

Miconazole is supplied as a sterile solution for intravenous infusion; however, one drop of this solution can be applied topically to the cornea every 2 hours (4,15,17).

KETOCONAZOLE

Ketoconazole (Nizoral, Janssen Pharmaceutical) is a broad-spectrum synthetic antifungal agent that inhibits in vitro growth of many organisms by altering the permeability of the cell membrane and interrupting the synthesis of ergosterol. Although not difficult to tolerate, it has some side effects. Mean peak plasma levels of approximately 3.5 μg/ml are reached 1 to 2 hours after oral administration of a single 200-mg dose taken with food. Neither the half-life ($t_{\frac{1}{2}}$) of the drug nor level of the drug that reaches the cornea is known, however. Prompt recognition of liver injury is essential. Liver function should be tested before and every week during treatment with ketoconazole. (See chapter on Imidazoles for further details.)

Therapeutic Use

Ketoconazole is administered orally as a single dose of 200 to 600 mg/day (4,15).

CLOTRIMAZOLE

Clotrimazole (Lotrimin, Schering, Kenilworth, NJ, U.S.A.) is also a synthetic antifungal agent that causes breakdown of cellular nucleic acids. In vitro clotrimazole exhibits amoebolytic activity against *Acanthamoeba.* It is a nonsterile crystalline substance that is insoluble in water and very soluble in lipid. Clotrimazole is available as a 1% solution and cream (ointment) for dermatologic use; however, this lotion is not recommended for topical use in the eye. (See chapter on Imidazoles for further details.)

Therapeutic Use

Clotrimazole solution 1% can be mixed with artificial tears and applied topically (4,15).

POLYHEXAMETHYLENE BIGUANIDE (PHMB)

History and Source

Biguanidnes have been long recognized as potent antimicrobial agents (18); bisbiguanide salts are in use as disinfectants, preservatives, and antiseptics. The antimicrobial activity of polyhexamethylene biguanide is greater than that of bisbiguanide and monomeric biguanides.

PHMB (Arlagard E. ICI Specialty Chemicals, Kortenberg, Belgium) is an active ingredient of Vantocil IB and has a broad spectrum of activity against both gram-positive and gram-negative bacteria. It is also a disinfectant agent and, although it has not yet been reported in the treatment of infectious disease, it has been used as a contact lens disinfectant at a very low concentration and as an antimicrobial agent in various ophthalmic products. More recently, PHMB has been used topically to treat *Acanthamoeba* keratitis (19,20).

Drug Name and Chemistry

PHMB is a heterodispersed mixture containing polymers, as shown in Fig. 49-6. (The value of *n* varies from 2 to 35, with a mean of 5.5.)

Pharmacology

Little is known of the mechanism of action of PHMB, but the drug has been suggested to bind to the surface of the cells, then to cause alteration of membrane structure, and subsequently to lead to loss of cytoplasmic contents.

Therapeutic Use

Sterile 0.02% solution can be prepared from 20% stock solution by diluting PHMB 1 : 1,000 with 0.3% hypromellose (without preservative). The optimum treatment of *Acanthamoeba* keratitis with PHMB has not yet been established. Larkin et al. (19) and Elder et al. (20) reported that a 0.02% concentration of PHMB was sufficient to achieve medical cure of *Acanthamoeba* keratitis. Patients with *Acanthamoeba* keratitis were treated topically with PHMB. Initially, the drug was administered one to three times hourly (from 6 to 24 times daily) for 3 to 4 weeks. Subsequently, the frequency of application of PHMB was gradually reduced in 3 months. The patients were treated with PHMB three times daily for 3 to 88 weeks until they were medically cured. The patients had received treatment with corticosteroids or other anti-*Acanthamoeba* drugs be-

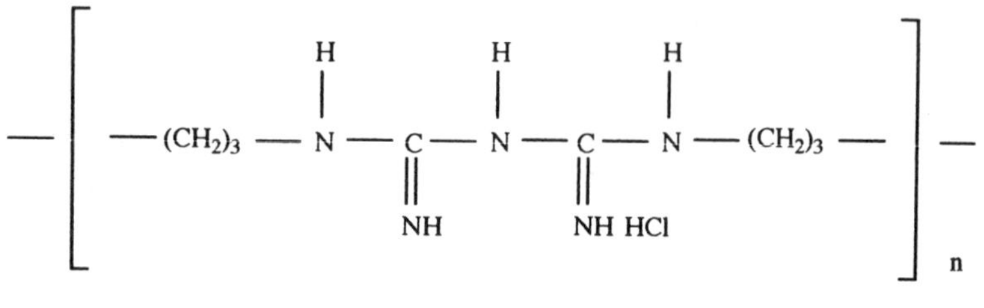

$$-\left[-(CH_2)_3-\overset{H}{\overset{|}{N}}-\underset{NH}{\underset{\|}{C}}-\overset{H}{\overset{|}{N}}-\underset{NH\,HCl}{\underset{\|}{C}}-\overset{H}{\overset{|}{N}}-(CH_2)_3-\right]_n-$$

FIG. 49-6. General formula of polyhexamethylene biguanides.

fore PHMB was administered. Because *Acanthamoeba* keratiis is a recently recognized disease, the treatment should be tailored for each patient depending on the previous treatment and the severity of the disease.

Side Effects and Drug Interactions

Topical administration of PHMB for treatment of *Acanthamoeba* keratitis has been reported only by Larkin et al. (19) and Elder et al. (20), who reported that the drug was not toxic to corneal epithelium even when used for a long time. Because PHMB is a new drug and has been used only in limited studies, more clinical trials are needed to verify the drug's toxicity and sensitivity.

Clinical Trials

In the studies of Larkin et al. (19) and Elder et al. (20), the patients with *Acanthamoeba* keratitis who failed to respond to other antiamoebic drugs were treated with topical PHMB (19,20). Eight of ten patients were medically cured. However, corneal cultures from two patients were still positive for *Acanthamoeba* after 28 and 41 weeks of treatment with PHMB. The investigators also concluded that the clinical results were correlated with the in vitro drug sensitivity assay against 23 *Acanthamoeba* isolates cultured from *Acanthamoeba*-infected patients (19,20).

SULINDAC

History and Source

Sulindac (Clinoril, Merck, Sharp and Dohme, West Point, PA, USA) is a nonsteroidal antiinflammatory drug (NSAID) that also has analgesic and antipyretic activities. It is chemically related to indomethacin, which inhibits prostaglandin synthesis systems (21).

Drug Name and Chemistry

Clinoril is the trade name for sulindac. The pharmacologic activity of the drug apparently resides in the sulfide metabolite (Fig. 49-7).

FIG. 49-7. Sulindac.

Pharmacology

Studies in an animal model of inflammation indicate that sulindac has antiinflammatory activity. However, its activity is less than half that of indomethacin. Because sulindac is a prodrug, most of its activity is related to its sulfide metabolite. The sulfide metabolite is more than 500 times as potent as sulindac as an inhibitor of cyclooxygenase. Sulindac 200 mg inhibited collagen-induced platelet aggregation and prolonged bleeding time in healthy subjects; however, the effect was less than that produced by the same dosage of aspirin. The incidence of gastrointestinal (GI) hemorrhage and toxicity also was less than that caused by indomethacin.

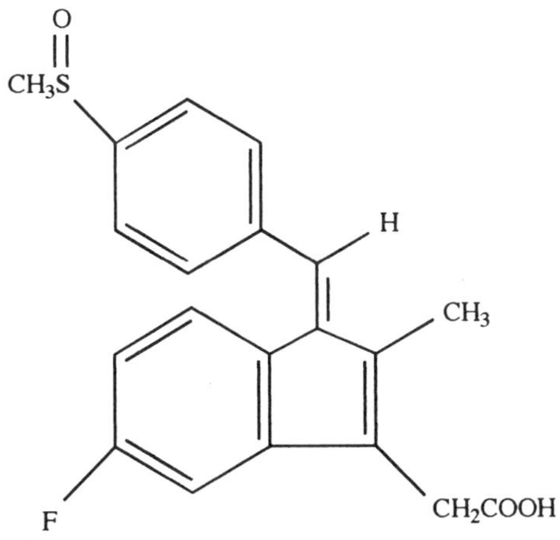

Therapeutic Use

Sulindac (Arthrocin, Artribid, Clinoril) is very effective in controlling pain in patients with acutely painful eyes (22). It is available as 150- to 200-mg tablets. Sulindac should be administered orally in 200-mg doses four times daily (21,22), although dosage can be optimized for each patient. The maximum dosage is 400 mg daily and should be ingested with food if GI complication has occurred.

Side Effects, Toxicity, and Drug Interactions

At the dosage generally used in treatment of rheumatic arthritis, sulindac has been well tolerated in either short- or long-term administration. GI side effects are common, occurring in approximately 20% of patients. GI side effects such as abdominal pain, nausea, and constipation are the most frequently reported effects; in general, however, sulindac has side effects less severe than those of aspirin and similar to those of ibuprofen. CNS side effects such as dizziness, drowsiness, headaches, and nervousness occur in 10% of patients. Skin rash and pruritus are common side effects. Increased hepatic enzymes in plasma is common. Significant drug interactions have not been observed with sulindac (21).

SURGICAL THERAPY

Epithelial debridement has been used for clinical management and treatment of *Acanthamoeba* keratitis, but this procedure may not be successful if the parasites have already penetrated into the corneal stroma. Surgical debridement has been suggested to improve the penetration of the drugs into the cornea, however, and to facilitate the removal of pathogens from the lesion (4). Epithelial debridement is effective in the early phase of *Acanthamoeba* keratitis if it is used in combination with antiamoebic drugs (4).

Rapid freezing of the cornea (cryotherapy) has been used either with or without penetrating keratoplasty (4). Cryotherapy has been used during performance of penetrating keratoplasty to destroy any remaining parasites before corneal transplantation. The rationale for these combinations of treatment was prevention of recurrence of *Acanthamoeba* in recipients of corneal grafts. In vitro experiments have shown, however, that trophozoites were killed when they were exposed to temperatures ranging from −50° to −130°C. By contrast, cysts survived when they were subjected to freezing temperatures. Cryotherapy treatment itself may cause extensive damage to the cornea, including opacification, thinning of corneal epithelium, increased inflammation, necrosis, and vascularization of the cornea. Therefore, cryotherapy is not a very successful treatment for *Acanthamoeba* keratitis.

Penetrating keratoplasty has been recommended for treatment of *Acanthamoeba* keratitis, but the proper timing of penetrating keratoplasty is controversial. If parasites are not completely eradicated before penetrating keratoplasty is performed, *Acanthamoeba* often recurs in the transplanted cornea (Fig. 8). Therefore, the resulting keratitis in the wounded cornea would be more severe and far more difficult to control, possibly resulting in loss of vision or even the globe itself. Penetrating keratoplasty should not be performed unless the eyes become perforated or until the infection has cleared completely.

PREVENTION

The most important factor in *Acanthamoeba* keratitis is prevention. The frequent association between the disease and homemade saline prepared from distilled water and salt tablets has led several companies to withdraw salt tablets from the market. No one should use distilled water and salt tablets to make saline solution. The next step in prevention is provision of effective education to the patient regarding the care of contact lenses. Commercially available heat sterilization units are very effective methods of sterilizing contact lenses; they kill both *Acanthamoeba* trophozoites and cysts. Patients should be advised not to contaminate the lenses after heat sterilization and before reinsertion of the lenses in the eyes.

Exposure to hydrogen peroxide in its active state for 2 hours is also a very effective means of destroying both *Acanthamoeba* trophozoites and cysts (23,24). However, hydrogen peroxide should be deactivated with deactivating agents if the lens is placed in hydrogen peroxide for more than 2 hours.

Preservatives found in cold-sterilization solutions are also effective in killing the organisms; however, 4 hours of exposure to such solutions is necessary to kill *Acanthamoeba* (23). Preservatives that are very effective in destroying the organisms are thimerosal with ethylene diaminetetraacetic acid (EDTA), benzalkonium chloride, chlorhexidine, and polyaminopropyl biguanide at a concentration of 0.0015% (19,23).

ACKNOWLEDGMENT

This work was supported in part by an unrestricted grant from Research to Prevent Blindness, Inc., New York, New York, and by National Institutes of Health Grant No. R01-EY03650.

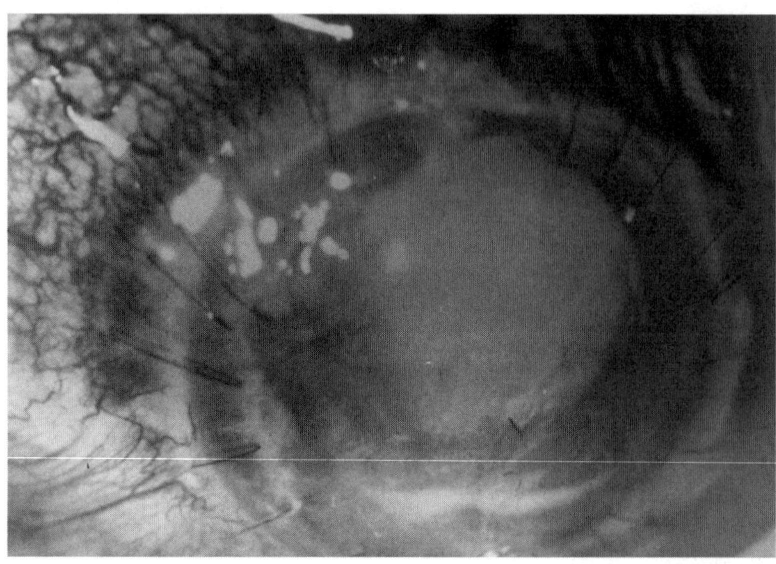

FIG. 49-8. Recurrence of *Acanthamoeba* keratitis in a human corneal graft (courtesy of Dr. ZM Husseini, Dallas, TX).

REFERENCES

1. John DT. Opportunistically pathogenic free-living amoeba.In: Kreier JP, Baker JR, eds. *Parasitic protozoa,* 2nd ed. California: Academic Press, Inc 1993;143–233.
2. Martinez AJ. Free-living amoeba: pathogenic aspect, a review. *Protozoal Abst* 1983;7:293–306.
3. Martinez AJ. *Free-Living Amoeba: Natural History, Prevention, Diagnosis, Pathology and Treatment of Disease.* Florida: CRC Press, 1985.
4. Auran JD, Starr MB, Jakobiec FA. *Acanthamoeba* keratitis. *Cornea* 1987;6:2–26.
5. Wang SS, Feldman HA. Isolation of *Hartmannella* species from human throats. *N Engl J Med* 1967;277:1147–1179.
6. Rivera F, Medina F, Ramirez P, Alcocer J, Vilaclara G, Robles E. Pathogenic and free-living protozoa cultured from the nasopharyngeal and oral regions of dental patients. *Environ Res* 1984;33:420–440.
7. Byers TJ, Bogler SA, Burianek LL. Analysis of mitochondrial DNA variation as an approach to systematic relationships in the genus *Acanthamoeba. J Protozool* 1983;30:198–203.
8. Jones DB, Visvesvara GS, Robinson NM. *Acanthamoeba polyphaga* keratitis and *Acanthamoeba* uveitis associated with fatal meningoencephalitis. *Trans Ophthalmol Soc UK* 1975;95:221–231.
9. Moore MB, McCulley JP, Newton C, et al. A growing problem in soft and hard contact lens wearers. *Ophthalmology* 1097;94:1654–1661.
10. Stehr-Green JK, Bailey TM, Visvesvara GS. The epidemiology of *Acanthamoeba* keratitis in the United States. *Am J Ophthalmol* 1989;107:331–336.
11. Mannis MJ, Tamaru R, Roth AM, Burns M, Thirkill C. *Acanthamoeba* sclerokeratitis: determining diagnostic criteria. *Arch Ophthalmol* 1986;104:1313–1317.
12. Moore MB, McCulley JP, Kaufman HE, Robin JB. Radial keratoneuritis as a presenting sign in *Acanthamoeba* keratitis. *Ophthalmology* 1986;93:1310–1315.
13. van Klink F, Alizadeh H, Stewart GL, et al. Characterization and pathogenic potential of a soil isolate and an ocular isolate of *Acanthamoeba castellanii* in relation to *Acanthamoeba* keratitis. *Curr Eye Res* 1992;11:1207–1220.
14. He YG, Niederkorn JY, McCulley JP, Stewart GL, Meyer DR, Silvany RE, Dougherty J. In vivo and in vitro collagenolytic activity of *Acanthamoeba castellanii. Invest Ophthalmol Vis Sci* 1990;31:2235–2240.
15. Moore MB. Management of *Acanthamoeba* keratitis. In Cavanagh HD, ed. *Cornea: transactions of the World Congress on the Cornea 111.* New York: Raven Press, 1988;517–521.
16. Wright P, Warhurst D, Jones BR. *Acanthamoeba* keratitis successfully treated medically. *Br J Ophthalmol* 1985;69:778–782.
17. Ishibashi Y, Matsumoto Y, Kabata T, et al. Oral itraconazole and topical miconazole with debridement for *Acanthamoeba* keratitis. *Am J Ophthalmol* 1990;109:121–126.
18. Rose FL, Swain G. Bisdiguanides having antimicrobial activity. *J Chem Soc* 1956;part IV:4422–4425.
19. Larkin DFP, Kilvington S, Dart JKG. Treatment of *Acanthamoeba* keratitis with polyhexamethylene biguanide. *Ophthalmology* 1992; 99:185–191.
20. Elder MJ, Kilvington S, Dart JKG. A clinicopathological study of in vitro sensitivity testing and *Acanthamoeba* keratitis. *Invest Ophthalmol Vis Sci* 1994;35:1059–1064.
21. Brogden RN, Heel RC, Speight TM, Avery GS. Sulindac: a reveiw of its pharmacological properties and therapeutic efficacy in rheumatic disease. *Drugs* 1978;16:97–114.
22. Koenig BS, Solomon JM, Hyndiuk RA, Sucher RA, Gradus MS. *Acanthamoeba* keratitis associated with gas-permeable contact lens wear. *Am J Ophthalmol* 1987;103:832.
23. Silvany RE, Dougherty JM, McCulley JP. The effect of contact lens preservatives on *Acanthamoeba. Ophthalmology* 1991;98:854–857.
24. Silvany RE, Dougherty JM, McCulley JP, Wood TS, Bowman WR, Moore MB. The effect of currently available contact lens disinfection systems on *Acanthamoeba castellanii* and *Acanthamoeba polyphaga. Ophthalmology* 1990;97:286–290.

Textbook of Ocular Pharmacology,
edited by T.J. Zimmerman, et al.
Lippincott–Raven Publishers, Philadelphia © 1997.

CHAPTER 50

Antivirals

James M. Hill, Richard J. O'Callaghan, and Bryan M. Gebhardt

More than 35 years ago, Kaufman first reported the use of idoxuridine for the treatment of herpes simplex virus (HSV) epithelial keratitis (1,2). Since then, 18 additional antivirals have been licensed in the United States (3); nine have been introduced in the last 5 years. Table 1 shows the six antivirals used to treat ocular viral infections. Two pairs of these compounds (acyclovir [ACV], and ganciclovir [DHPG], and idoxuridine [IDU], and trifluridine [TFT]) are actually derivatives of each other (Fig. 1). All these antivirals have therapeutic limitations and toxic side effects (4). We review the six commercially available ocular antivirals and present new drugs and novel approaches in therapy of viral infections of the eye.

In addition to these six approved drugs, newer compounds with higher bioavailability have received considerable interest. Penciclovir (PCV) and famciclovir (FCV) are acyclic nucleoside analogues that are currently being clinically evaluated for the treatment of ocular herpes infection (5,6). Valacyclovir (VACV) is a prodrug of ACV (7). These drugs are used to treat nonocular varicella zoster virus (VZV) infections but have the potential for chemotherapy of viral infections of the eye.

The route of administration of ocular antivirals is an important consideration. IDU, TFT, and vidarabine (Ara-A) are available for topical use. DHPG and foscarnet (PFA) can be administered intravenously and intravitreally; acyclovir (ACV) can be administered intravenously or orally. ACV has not been approved for topical ophthalmic use in the United States. FCV (an oral form of PCV) and VACV have improved oral bioavailability, a longer intracellular half-life ($t_{\frac{1}{2}}$), less cross-resistance than ACV, and potency equivalent to that of ACV. Six antivirals used to treat ocular infections are administered by a variety of routes. These antivirals are presented in the order in which they were approved by the Food and Drug Administration (FDA) for ophthalmic use.

J. M. Hill, R. J. O'Callaghan, and M. Gebhardt: Lions Eye Research Laboratories, LSU Eye Center; Department of Microbiology, Immunology, and Parasitology (R.J.O'C., B.M.G.); and Department of Pharmacology and Experimental Therapeutics (J.M.H.), Louisiana State University Medical Center, New Orleans, Louisiana 70112.

ANTIVIRAL AGENTS FOR OPHTHALMIC USE

Cornea (HSV)

Idoxuridine

IDU (5-iodo-2′-deoxyuridine, Herplex) is the first successful antiviral agent reported to be of value in treating HSV keratitis. It was originally synthesized by Prusoff as an antineoplastic agent in 1959 (8). Although IDU was not effective as an anticancer drug, it was shown to improve the healing of HSV keratitis in an animal model and in human HSV keratitis (9–12). Attempts by some investigators to treat HSV encephalitis with intravenous IDU were abandoned because of severe toxic reactions (13).

IDU is an analogue of thymidine and is metabolized by the same enzymatic pathways as the pyrimidine. IDU is activated after phosphorylation by cellular or virus-encoded thymidine kinase (14). Because HSV-infected cells contain both an active viral thymidine kinase and a cellular kinase, more IDU is phosphorylated to IDU-monophosphate in these cells than in uninfected cells. IDU-monophosphate is then rapidly converted to IDU-triphosphate by host cell kinases. IDU-triphosphate interacts with viral DNA polymerase, and the nucleotide analogue is incorporated into the viral DNA. The IDU-substituted virions were defective in their ability to synthesize viral-induced proteins, resulting in markedly reduced yields of progeny virions (12).

IDU also affects the metabolism of normal, uninfected cells. Toxic effects associated with the disruption of normal cellular DNA synthesis include pathologic changes in the cornea, conjunctiva, and eyelids. The cornea can show superficial punctate keratopathy, indolent ulceration, de-

Table 50-1. *Ophthalmic use of antivirals*

Ophthalmic disease	Generic name	Trade name	Route of administration	Principal mechanism of action
HSV epithelial keratitis	Idoxuridine (IDU)	Herplex	Topical	Abnormal base results in false mRNA and faulty viral proteins
HSV epithelial keratitis	Vidarabine (Ara-A)	Vira-A	Intravenous, topical	Abnormal sugar results in premature termination of viral DNA synthesis
HSV epithelial keratitis (drug of choice)	Trifluridine (TFT)	Viroptic	Topical	Similar to IDU
VZV ophthalmicus Pediatric HSV opithelial keratitis	Acyclovir	Zovirax	Oral Intravenous	Similar to Ara-A
CMV retinitis	Ganciclovir	Cytovene	Intravenous intravitreal	Similar to Ara-A
CMV retinitis	Foscarnet	Foscavir	Intravenous, intravitreal	Blocks pyrophosphate binding site of viral DNA poly merase

HSV, herpes simplex virus; VZV, varicella zoster virus; CMV, Cytomegalovirus.

layed epithelial healing, and superficial stromal opacification. Conjunctival changes include chemosis, hyperemia, punctate staining with fluorescein, and follicles in the lower tarsus. Lid symptoms include edema, plugging of the meibomian glands, and punctal occlusion.

IDU is relatively water-insoluble, and only a 0.1% solution is available. Furthermore, IDU does not readily penetrate the cornea. Viral resistance to IDU is common. The percentage of unsuccessful treatments is relatively high (24%) (15). TFT is more effective and is the drug of choice for HSV keratitis treatment in the United States. IDU is now seldom used in the United States; the drug is less frequently used in industrial countries, but is still in extensive use in developing countries. IDU is useful for therapy of primary and recurrent epithelial HSV keratitis in patients who cannot tolerate TFT or Ara-A.

Vidarabine

Vidarabine (9-β-D-arabinofuranosyladenine, Vira-A, adenine arabinoside, Ara-A) was the second drug approved for the treatment of acute and recurrent herpetic keratoconjunctivitis and keratitis (15–20). Ara-A was synthesized and studied in the early 1960s as an antitumor agent. Subsequently, Ara-A was shown to be active in vitro against HSV, VZV, Cytomegalovirus (CMV), vaccinia virus, and some RNA tumor viruses (21). In animal models, Ara-A was active against HSV and vaccinia virus (14,15,17,19).

Ara-A is a purine nucleoside analogue, which is phosphorylated by host cellular kinases to the active triphosphate form (Ara-ATP). Ara-ATP acts as a chain terminator for newly synthesized viral DNA after incorporation of its unusual sugar residue, arabinose. Unlike ACV and TFT, Ara-A does not require viral thymidine kinase for phosphorylation. Therefore, Ara-A is effective against thymidine kinase-deficient mutants of HSV that are resistant to ACV.

Topical Ara-A (3% Vira-A ointment) is indicated for the treatment of HSV epithelial keratitis in patients allergic to IDU or TFT. After an average of 7 to 9 days of treatment, corneal reepithelialization begins. In controlled trials, 3 weeks of treatment were required for complete reepithelialization. If there are no signs of improvement after 1 week or if complete reepithelialization has not occurred by 3 weeks of Ara-A application, other forms of therapy, such as TFT or IDU, should be considered.

Systemic Ara-A is beneficial in the treatment of HSV encephalitis, neonatal HSV infections, and VZV infections in immunosuppressed patients (22,23). However, ACV is more effective, less toxic, and has almost entirely replaced Ara-A for systemic therapies. In an extensive review, Teich et al. (4) reported that Ara-A toxicity includes gastrointestinal (GI) disturbances (e.g., anorexia, nausea, vomiting, and diarrhea, occurring in 10% to 15% of patients), CNS disturbances (i.e., dizziness, confusion, hallucinations, ataxia, myoclonus, and psychoses, occurring in 2% to 10% of patients), weakness, and weight loss. Such toxicities are not uncommon and have occurred in a relatively high proportion of treated patients (22,23).

Trifluorothymidine

Trifluorothymidine (F_3TdR, TFT, Viroptic, TFT, 5-trifluoromethyl-2′-deoxyuridine) is a fluorinated pyrimidine

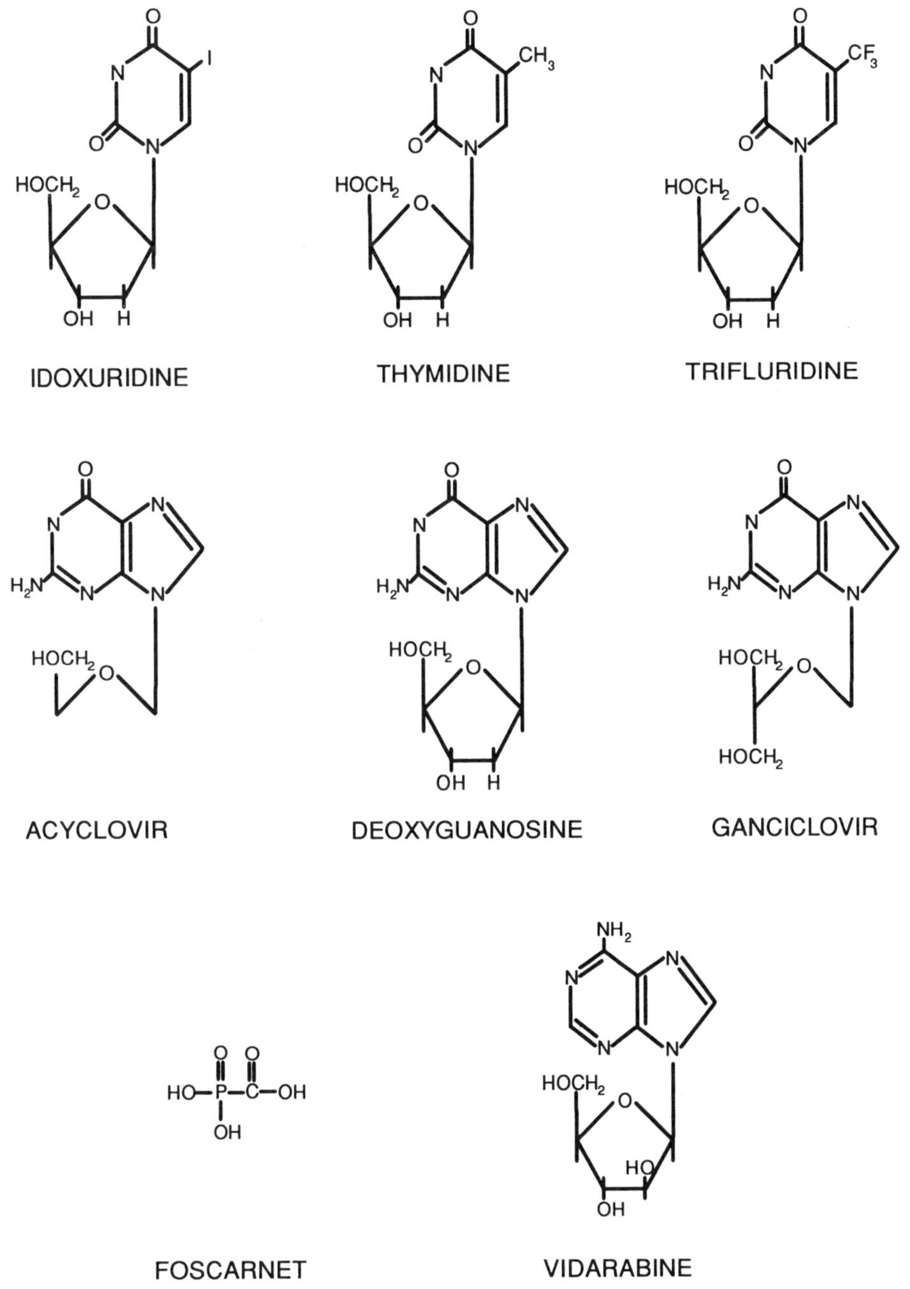

IDOXURIDINE THYMIDINE TRIFLURIDINE

ACYCLOVIR DEOXYGUANOSINE GANCICLOVIR

FOSCARNET VIDARABINE

FIG. 50-1. Structures of antiviral agents approved for ophthalmic use. Thymidine and deoxyguanosine, normal pyrimidine and purine nucleosides, are shown to allow comparisons.

nucleoside and the drug of choice for HSV keratitis. TFT was originally synthesized as an anticancer agent by Gottschling and Heidelberger in 1963 (24). The antiviral activity of TFT against HSV and its usefulness in the treatment of HSV keratitis were first reported by Kaufman and Heidelberger (25) in 1964. Although TFT appeared to be superior to other available antiviral agents, the cost of synthesizing the drug and the expense involved in obtaining clearance from the FDA delayed its licensing until 1978. Since then, TFT has become the drug of choice in the treatment of HSV keratitis (11,18,26).

Like IDU, TFT is a thymidine analogue and must be phosphorylated to the active triphosphate by either cellular or viral thymidine kinases. TFT monophosphate is a potent inhibitor of cellular thymidylate synthetase. Because of this enzyme inhibition, the formation of cellular deoxythymidine monophosphate (dTMP) is reduced. These cells produce little dTMP as they actively convert TFT to the phosphorylated form. Due to the activity of viral thymidine kinase, infected cells have a particularly high ratio of phosphorylated TFT to dTMP. TFT triphosphate is incorporated into viral DNA, with subsequent production of defective progeny virus. Viral DNA polymerase uses TFT triphosphate more efficiently as a substrate than does the host cell enzyme; therefore, the effect on viral DNA replication is much greater than the effect on cellular DNA replication.

Although TFT is much more abundant in virus-infected cells than in normal cells, the drug does have effects on the metabolism of normal cells. Adverse ocular reactions to TFT can occur with prolonged topical use. The drug can cause superficial punctate keratopathy. Additional side effects associated with TFT are mild transient burning or stinging on instillation, conjunctival hyperemia and edema, keratitis sicca, contact blepharodermatitis, delayed corneal wound healing, and increased intraocular pressure. Allergic responses to TFT are much less common than to IDU. These adverse reactions are generally reversible on discontinuation of the drug.

TFT, formulated as a topical preparation (Viroptic), is considerably more soluble than Ara-A or IDU. TFT is also lipid soluble; this biphasic solubility accounts for the relatively good corneal penetration of the drug. The effectiveness of TFT is evidenced by the healing of 97% of dendritic epithelial herpetic keratitis cases by TFT in 2 weeks as compared with only 80% of such cases treated with IDU (26). Furthermore, the development of drug-resistant HSV is extremely rare with TFT as compared with IDU, and some studies showed that TFT is less toxic than Ara-A in the corneal epithelium during wound healing.

ACV

ACV (9-[2-hydroxyethoxymethyl]guanine, Zovirax, acycloguanosine) is a selective inhibitor of herpesvirus replication, represents an important advance in antiviral therapy, and serves as the prototype for future antiviral drug development (27). ACV was first developed in 1971 (28). Later, Schaeffer et al. demonstrated the antiviral effects of ACV against HSV types 1 and 2, VZV, and Epstein-Barr virus (EBV) (29).

ACV is an acyclic nucleoside analogue of guanosine. The selective activity of ACV for cells infected with HSV is due to two herpes-specific enzymes: thymidine kinase and DNA polymerase. ACV is phosphorylated more efficiently to a monophosphate form by the herpes thymidine kinase than by cellular enzymes. Why a purine is phosphorylated by a pyrimidine (thymidine) kinase is not known. Cellular enzymes then convert ACV monophosphate to ACV diphosphate and ACV triphosphate. ACV triphosphate is present in HSV-infected cells at 40 to 100 times the concentration present in uninfected cells. ACV triphosphate has a greater affinity for viral DNA polymerase than for cellular DNA polymerase. ACV triphosphate is a selective substrate inhibitor of the Herpesvirus DNA polymerase. In addition, since ACV lacks the 3′-hydroxy group necessary for the continued elongation of newly synthesized DNA, incorporation into the viral DNA chain results in chain termination. CMV is relatively insensitive to ACV because the viral genome does not encode for viral thymidine kinase (30,31).

The selectivity of viral enzymes at both the phosphorylation and polymerization steps accounts in large degree for the great effectiveness of ACV. A series of reports of clinical trials showed that ACV was both a safe and an efficacious antiviral. ACV has excellent antiviral activity against HSV and VZV (32–35). The most dramatic results were observed in treatment of herpes infections in immunocompromised patients (36). Positive benefits were also observed in treatment of both ocular and genital infections in immunocompetent patients; symptoms were less severe and healing was more rapid (32,37). Oral ACV is effective in the treatment of HSV dendritic ulcers and should be considered in conditions in which delivery of eye drops is a problem. Oral ACV can also be a useful alternative for patients with topical ocular toxicity of TFT and/or IDU. Several groups of investigators have reported a beneficial effect of oral ACV combined with topical corticosteroids in the treatment of HSV stromal keratouveitis (38–41). ACV therapy, despite its effectiveness and low toxicity, does not reduce the recurrence rate once treatment is discontinued (42). ACV therapy is able to suppress clinical manifestations of disease without adding complications. Evaluated in a National Institutes of Health-supported, controlled clinical trial, ACV was not effective in treating stromal disease and iritis.

As compared with other antiviral agents, ACV is an extremely safe drug (4,5,43). Although in most respects ACV is an excellent drug, one drawback is its limited oral bioavailability. Efforts to improve the efficacy of ACV have led to the development of prodrugs with improved oral bioavailability. The major adverse effect is that on renal function, due to crystallization and deposition of the drug in the kidneys of patients whose hydration, renal function, or both are inadequate. Phlebitis and local injection site irritation have been observed. These lesions are not due to ACV's toxicity, but instead result from subcutaneous infiltration caused by the high pH of the infusing solution (pH 11). Nausea, vomiting, and abdominal pain can occur when ACV is administered orally, probably as a direct toxic effect on the GI tract. Because ACV can be incorporated into DNA, there has been some concern over possible mutagenicity; however, no significant evidence indicates that ACV is a carcinogen or a teratogen.

PCV/FCV (Famvir)

PCV {9-[4-hydroxy-3-(hydroxymethyl)butyl]guanine} is a potent and highly selective inhibitor of members of the herpesvirus family, including HSV, VZV, and EBV (44). Like other acyclic nucleoside analogues, PCV has poor oral bioavailability. To overcome this problem, a new oral form, FCV (the diacetyl 6-deoxy analogue of PCV) was developed (Fig. 2). FCV (Famvir) has been shown to be absorbed well and to be converted efficiently to PCV in mice, rats, and humans.

PCV is phosphorylated efficiently in HSV- or VZV-infected cells to form PCV-triphosphate; the interaction between penciclovir-triphosphate and the viral DNA polymerase results in inhibition of viral DNA synthesis. In cells infected with either HSV or VZV, PCV is phosphorylated to its triphosphate ester much more rapidly than ACV. After removal of PCV from the culture medium, PCV-triphosphate is trapped in the cells for a longer time than ACV (44). PCV and FCV show potent activity in a variety of cutaneous, genital, and systemic HSV infections in animals when administered either topically or systemically (subcutaneously, intravenously, or orally) (7). In addition, evidence suggests that virus replication in the CNS is reduced after treatment with either PCV or FCV. Moreover, a

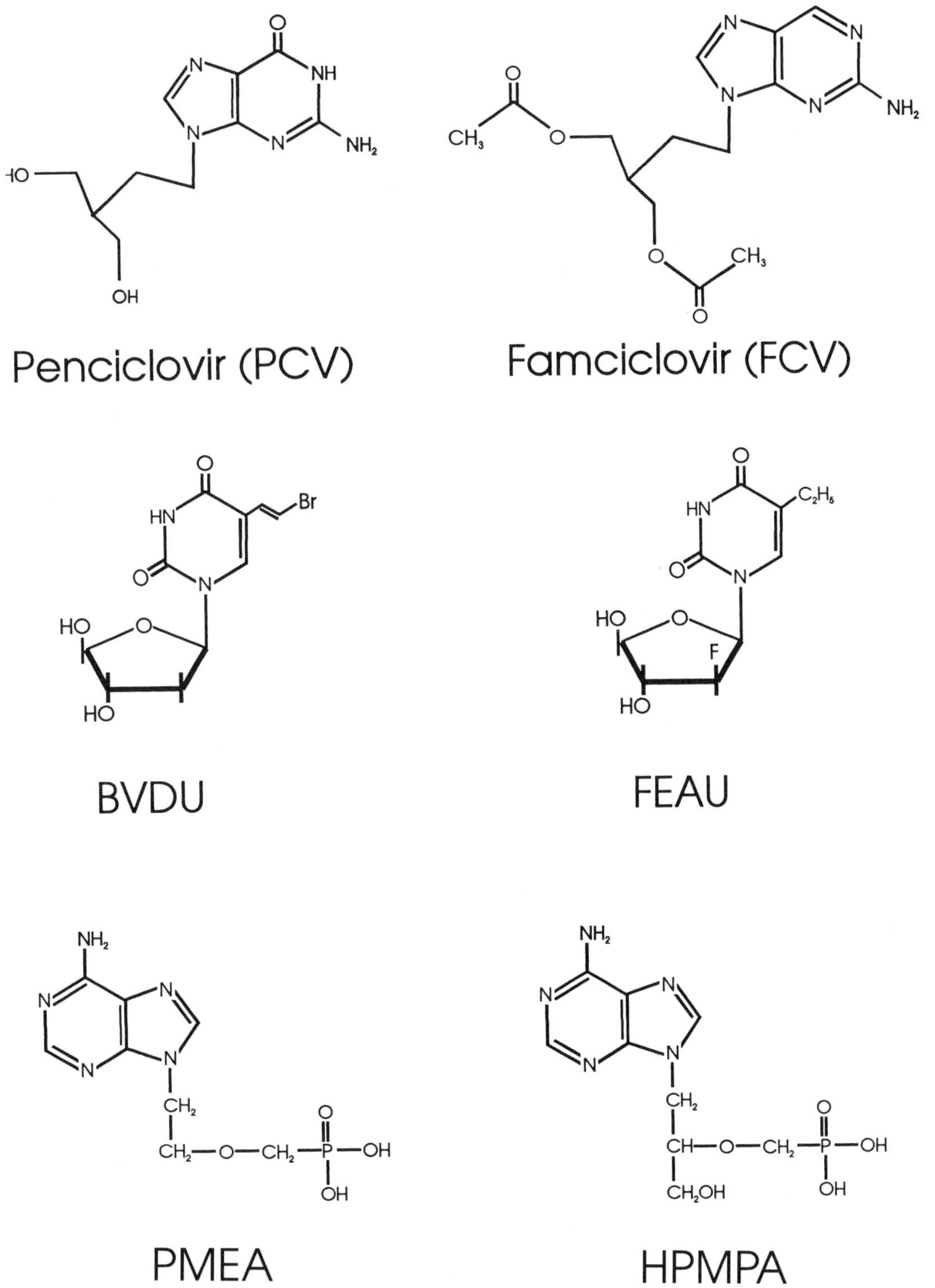

Penciclovir (PCV)

Famciclovir (FCV)

BVDU

FEAU

PMEA

HPMPA

FIG. 50-2. Structures of antivirals that have potential as ocular antivirals.

series of PFA- and ACV-resistant HSV isolates appear to be susceptible to PCV. In mice infected intraperitoneally with HSV-1, a lower dose of oral FCV relative to an oral dose of ACV was more effective, which is consistent with the stability of intracellular PCV-triphosphate in herpesvirus-infected cells and the prolonged antiviral activity of PCV in cell culture as compared with that of ACV.

The spectrum of activity of FCV is similar to that of ACV and has certain advantages over ACV, including improved oral bioavailability, a longer intracellular $t_{\frac{1}{2}}$, less cross-resistance, and potency equivalent to that of ACV.

FCV was well tolerated by healthy volunteers after oral administration (27). Adverse effects observed after administration of FCV include headache (19.4%) and diarrhea (5.6%). Diarrhea was reported in two dosing sessions (5.6%). There was no evidence of clinically significant interactions between FCV and a variety of other drugs, including allopurinol, cimetidine, theophylline, and digoxin.

FCV has been evaluated in clinical studies for the treatment of herpesvirus infections (45,46). The toxicity data on FCV indicated no incorporation of the drug into normal cellular DNA. Based on the mechanism of action and the pharmacology and toxicity data, FCV has the potential to be useful in the treatment of herpetic eye disease.

VACV (Valtrex)

L-Valine added to acycloguanosine produces VACV (Valtrex), which significantly increases the bioavailability of acycloguanosine. This oral prodrug of Zovirax can be used to treat nonocular VZV infections and recurrent HSV-2 genital infections. This newly formulated antiviral has the same mechanism of action as acycloguanosine (7). Valtrex may replace Zovirax as the oral form of ACV.

BVDU (Bromovinyldeoxyuridine, (E)-5-(2-Bromovinyl)-2′-Deoxyuridine)

In a randomized double-blind trial, 0.1% bromovinyldeoxyuridine (BVDU) was as efficacious as 1.0% TFT for therapy of herpetic dendritic keratitis with respect to lack of toxicity, the number of ulcers healed, and the mean healing time of the lesions (47). BVDU has not been tested in a clinical trial in the United States and is not licensed for use.

Retina (CMV)

DHPG

DHPG (9-[1-,3-dihydroxy-2-propoxy]methylguanine, Cytovene) was the first drug approved for treatment of CMV retinitis (48). DHPG is an acyclic purine nucleoside structurally related to ACV (Fig. 2), but differs by virtue of the presence of a methoxy group at the 3′carbon of the acyclic side chain. This minor chemical modification substantially enhances the antiviral activity, especially against herpesviruses, but unfortunately this change also increases the hematopoietic toxicity of DHPG. DHPG was the first available drug with significant activity against CMV, and in 1989 was approved for the treatment and maintenance therapy of CMV retinitis in immunocompromised patients. Human herpesviruses that are sensitive to DHPG include HSV types 1 and 2, VZV, CMV, and EBV. CMV is inhibited in vitro by DHPG concentrations of 5 to 10 μM (49,50).

Like that of ACV, the active form of DHPG that inhibits viral replication is a triphosphate. The initial phosphorylating reaction of DHPG to a monophosphate occurs through a cellular enzyme. The drug is then phosphorylated to a triphosphate by host ocular kinases. The triphosphate of DHPG competitively inhibits the binding of deoxyguanosine triphosphate to DNA polymerase, thereby inhibiting DNA synthesis and terminating DNA elongation.

DHPG is administered intravenously because of its poor absorption in the GI tract. This drug is excreted by the kidneys virtually unmetabolized. The elimination of DHPG correlates with creatinine clearance. When renal insufficiency exists, the $t_{\frac{1}{2}}$ and plasma concentrations of DHPG are increased; however, the drug is not nephrotoxic. Intravitreal use of DHPG can be considered for patients who are unwilling or unable to undergo intravenous therapy but who face progressive vision-threatening CMV retinitis. Studies investigating intravitreal liposomes for long-term release of DHPG are continuing (51). The treatment of CMV retinitis with DHPG incorporated into a sustained-release vehicle has also been reported (52). The disease generally recurs when DHPG is discontinued. Pollard (53) recently reported that DHPG combined with a monoclonal antibody showed promise. More studies are needed in this new combination antiviral therapy for CMV retinitis. This is especially important because of the emergence of drug-resistant CMV.

DHPG can be myelosuppressive. Other potential side effects include fever, phlebitis, nausea, and hepatocellular dysfunction.

PFA

PFA (Foscavir), the trisodium salt of phosphonoformic acid, has been approved by the FDA for treatment of CMV retinitis (54). PFA halts the progression of CMV retinitis in more than 80% of immunocompromised patients and appears to be as effective as DHPG. PFA is a pyrophosphate (Fig. 2) and differs structurally from ACV, DHPG, and Ara-A, all of which are nucleoside analogues. Therefore, PFA is effective against DHPG- or ACV-resistant CMV (55). Unlike DHPG, PFA does not cause severe myelosuppression. However, like DHPG, PFA must be administered intravenously and its rate of treatment failure is similar.

Because PFA is a pyrophosphate analogue, it does not require conversion to an active triphosphate by viral thymidine kinase. PFA inhibits viral DNA replication directly by blocking the pyrophosphate binding site of the viral DNA polymerase at a concentration that does not interfere with cellular DNA polymerase. Therefore, PFA is useful for treating ACV- and DHPG-resistant herpesviruses that are deficient in thymidine kinase (56).

PFA is not metabolized to any significant degree after intravenous administration and is eliminated by the kidneys (4). Oral administration yields poor absorption, and GI side effects are common. The most frequently reported adverse effect of PFA is nephrotoxicity (4). Other side effects include anemia, increase in hepatic enzymes, tremors and seizures, nausea, vomiting, diarrhea, abdominal pain, headaches, and local irritation at the infusion site.

In clinical trials, good results were obtained with PFA in the treatment of patients with AIDS who were infected with ACV-resistant HSV and VZV (55,56). With intravenous administration of PFA, approximately 90% of patients with CMV retinitis demonstrated clinical improvement (57). PFA is not myelosuppressive. Because relapses can occur in CMV retinitis patients within 1 month of discontinuation of therapy, a maintenance dosage should be used, but the optimal maintenance dosage has not yet been established. During treatment, adequate intravenous hydration is critical, and close monitoring and frequent dosage adjustments are important to avoid renal toxic effects.

NEW APPROACHES IN ANTIVIRAL THERAPY

To be useful as a chemotherapeutic agent, a drug must selectively inhibit a metabolic process of the invading pathogen without interfering with host cellular function. The multitude of available antibacterial agents can be attributed to the marked differences between bacterial and mammalian cell structure and physiology. Commercially available antiviral agents are few because viruses reproduce in mammalian cells and use host cell metabolic machinery in the process. The antiviral agents in use today (Table 1) primarily target viral DNA polymerase, an enzyme required for viral DNA synthesis. With the exception of PFA, all these drugs are nucleoside analogues. Early analogues, such as IDU and TFT, were too toxic to be used as systemic antiviral agents. More recently developed analogues, such as ACV and DHPG, are not quite as toxic and are administered intravenously. The search for even less toxic antiviral agents continues, with the development of new, more selective nucleoside analogues, as well as compounds that target key viral components other than DNA polymerase.

Other Ocular Antivirals

FEAU (1-2′-deoxy-2′-fluoro-β-D-arabinofuranosyl)-5-ethylurasil

A 1.0% solution of FEAU was as effective as 3.0% ACV in a rabbit model of HSV keratitis with respect to reducing the severity of symptoms, with no toxicity (58) (structure shown in Fig. 2). No clinical studies have been reported.

HPMPA and PMEA

(*S*)-9-(3-hydroxy-2-phosphonylmethoxypropyl) adenine (HPMPA) and 9-(2-phosphonylmethoxyethyl) adenine (PM EA) can be regarded as hybrid molecules combining 9-(2,3-dihydroxypropyl)adenine (DHPA) and phosphonoacetic acid (PAA). The antiviral properties of HPMPA and PMEA were first described in 1986 (59). PMEA was reported to be as active as HPMPA against HSV (including thymidine kinase negative HSV) but less active than HPMPA against other herpesviruses, such as VZV and CMV.

PAA and its derivative phosphonoformic acid (PFA) have long since been recognized as broad-spectrum antiviral agents active against herpesviruses, hepadonviruses, and retroviruses. This antiviral spectrum is preserved when the phosphonomethyl group of PAA is transferred to DHPA or the truncated form thereof 9-(2-hydroxyethyl)-adenine (HEA), resulting in formation of HPMPA and PMEA, respectively. Indeed HPMPA and PMEA (structures shown in Fig. 2) are much more potent in their antiviral action than is PAA or PFA. They offer substantial promise as broad-spectrum antiviral agents for treatment of various DNA virus and retrovirus infections.

HPMPA and PMEA are taken into cells and phosphorylated by cellular enzymes to diphosphorylphosphonates (i.e., HPMPApp, PMEApp). Therefore, for their intracellular phosphorylation, HPMPA and PMEA do not depend on the virus-encoded thymidine kinase, which explains why these compounds are equally effective against thymidine kinase-negative and thymidine kinase-positive HSV and VZV strains. HPMPApp and PMEApp are potent inhibitors of viral DNA polymerase (or retroviral reverse transcriptase). A PMEA-resistant HSV-1 strain has been isolated that is more susceptible than the wild-type virus to HPMPA. PMEA is strongly inhibitory to retroviruses, whereas HPMPA is not, and PMEA is a chain terminator, whereas HPMPA can also be incorporated into the interior of the DNA chain.

Both HPMPA and PMEA are effective in a large variety of experimental virus infections in animal models. These experimental infections are similar to the clinically important herpes-, pox-, and papovavirus infections in humans; therefore, the acyclic nucleoside phosphonate analogues could hold promise for treatment of such infections (60).

HPMPC (Cidofivir, Vistide)

The antiviral, HPMPC, (*S*)-1-(3-hydroxy-2-phosphonylmethoxypropyl)cytosine, is active against both adenovirus keratitis and herpes keratitis (61–64). Animal models of adenovirus infection developed by Gordon et al. (65) and Trousdale et al. (66) have greatly assisted in the study of new antiviral agents for chemotherapy of adenovirus keratitis. HPMPC is a broad-spectrum topical antiviral that has potential uses in inhibiting viral infections caused by DNA viruses. To date, no phase II clinical trials have been conducted. This area is one that needs attention because of the high incidence and highly contagious nature of adenovirus.

Inhibitors of Viral Thymidine Kinase

Under normal growth conditions, eukaryotic cells synthesize thymidine nucleotides required for DNA synthesis by a pathway in which thymidine monophosphate is synthesized from deoxyuridine monophosphate. Therefore, thymidine kinase is not required for normal cell growth, but the synthesis of a new species of thymidine kinase by HSV presumably is necessary to accommodate the increased demand for thymidine triphosphate to fuel viral DNA synthesis. The virus-encoded thymidine kinase is produced by virus-infected cells.

Inhibitors of thymidine kinase have a protective effect in animals. Kaufman et al. (10), using 5′ethynylthymidine, an inhibitor of viral thymidine kinase, were first to demonstrate that a thymidine kinase inhibitor can reduce ocular recurrences of HSV-1 in infected squirrel monkeys.

Inhibitors of Viral Ribonucleotide Reductase

One alternative antiviral drug target is the HSV-encoded ribonucleotide reductase. This enzyme catalyzes the reduction of ribonucleoside diphosphates to the corresponding deoxyribose counterparts. The HSV-encoded ribonucleotide reductase is not sensitive to feedback inhibition by dATP and dTTP; therefore, synthesis of deoxyribonucleoside triphosphates is unrestricted in virus-infected cells. This requirement for large amounts of deoxyribonucleotides strongly suggests that HSV ribonucleotide reductase could be essential for virus reproduction (67). Indeed, several reports have suggested that viral ribonucleotide reductase is required for virus replication in tissue culture. Selective inhibition of HSV ribonucleotide reductase is correlated with inhibition of HSV replication (67,68). Other investigators (67–69), using viruses with mutations in the genes for either the large or small subunit of ribonucleotide reductase, reported that HSV ribonucleotide reductase appears to be required for reactivation from latency and essential for pathogenicity in mice.

A potent peptidomimetic inhibitor of HSV ribonucleotide reductase has been shown to have significant antiviral activity in an in vivo ocular model of HSV keratitis (69). Synthetic peptides containing the amino acid sequences in the carboxy terminal of the ribonucleotide reductase have been shown to be critical for the inhibition of the viral enzyme. This new class of antiviral also strongly potentiated the antiviral activity of ACV. Therefore, the possibility of using the new peptidomimetic inhibitor in combination with another antiviral offers great promise.

Tumor Necrosis Factor (TNF)

Among the pleiotropic effects of TNF is a remarkable antiviral activity. Like the interferons (IFNs), TNF can exert its antiviral effects on cells directly, as well as indirectly, through the immune system. TNF has both a prophylactic value, protecting uninfected cells from viral infection, and a cytotoxic role, selectively killing virus-infected cells. Infection with either RNA or DNA viruses rapidly elicits the production of TNF. Several cell types are capable of producing TNF, including macrophages, mast cells, T lymphocytes, natural killer (NK) cells, polymorphonuclear leukocytes, and endothelial cells. The most striking antiviral action of TNF occurs in the presence of IFN-γ. In some circumstances, TNF and IFN-γ appear to have independent antiviral properties. However, dramatic antiviral activity is evident when both factors are used together (70). The antiviral activity of TNF is nonspecific; it is not limited to a few viruses or cell lines.

Experiments designed to test the antiviral activity of TNF in vivo have yielded contradictory results (71–73). Injection of TNF does not appear to protect mice already infected with virus. On the other hand, induction of TNF in mice, with use of vaccinia virus expression vectors, generates significant protection from viral infection. Therefore, TNF could be more useful prophylactically than as a therapeutic agent (74).

Antisense Oligonucleotides

Nucleoside analogues such as ACV and DHPG are selective enough in their inhibition of viral DNA polymerase to be useful as therapeutic agents. However, because of similarities between these analogues and conventional nucleosides, some degree of host cell toxicity is inevitable. Therefore, antisense oligonucleotides are being investigated as potential antiviral agents. These oligonucleotides, either DNA or RNA, are specific complementary sequences for viral genes such as HSV-1 IE (immediate early) and could disrupt viral transcription or translation (75–77). Antisense oligonucleotide research is progressing rapidly. The therapeutic applications of antisense oligonucleotides have been reviewed (19,78–80). Cantin et al. (78) discussed the efficacy of HSV-specific antisense oligonucleotides in suppressing HSV replication in cultured cells. Kulka et al. (77) reported the antiviral effects of antisense oligonucleotides directed against HSV-1 immediate early mRNAs in a mouse ear and footpad model of HSV infection.

In vivo models of viral infection have been shown to be susceptible to therapy with antisense oligonucleotides. These promising studies offer the possibility that this type of antiviral could be used alone or in combination with existing antivirals to treat serious viral infection (19,78, 81,82). Clinical trials of antisense molecules for ocular chemotherapy have not been reported.

Protease Inhibitors

Ritonavir, Invirase (saquinavir), and Indinavir (crixivan) are protease inhibitors recently used in clinical trials in combination with other antiviral agents such as Retrovir (AZT). These combinations have had considerable clinical success. The protease inhibitors act by blocking aspartic protease. This inhibition prevents the cleavage of a large precursor molecule to a small functional core viral protein. Although some success has been reported with protease inhibitors in treatment of patients with AIDS, numerous problems such as lack of potency, poor adsorption, and development of resistance have been reported (50,83,84). However, protease inhibitors in combination with two or more AIDS antivirals have shown efficacy. More controlled clinical studies are needed to verify efficacy, determine the best combinations, and assess the extent of drug resistance. Whether protease inhibitors can be used for any of the ocular viral diseases is unknown. However, combination antivirals are certainly a therapeutic strategy that could involve treatment of very severe and/or complicated cases of ocular infections.

COMBINATION THERAPY FOR HSV STROMAL DISEASE WITH TFT AND PREDNISOLONE

Although topically applied antivirals such as Ara-A and TFT are effective in controlling superficial epithelial HSV keratitis, these agents have limited therapeutic impact on stromal disease. Because the host immune system is an important contributor to the overall pathology of stromal keratitis, topical corticosteroids have been used to control the disease. Because corticosteroids can exacerbate epithelial disease, they have been used with topical antivirals. The possibility that steroid therapy could worsen clinical outcome has been noted.

To address the issue of the possible therapeutic benefits of combined corticosteroid and antiviral chemotherapy, the Herpetic Eye Disease Study (HEDS) Group has completed several clinical trials (41,85,86). In one trial, patients with HSV stromal keratitis were treated with either topical TFT and prednisolone phosphate of TFT plus a placebo. Patients treated with TFT and prednisolone had reduced symptoms and a shorter duration of stromal disease than did patients treated with TFT and a placebo. In another trial, two groups of patients with HSV stromal keratitis treated with topical prednisolone phosphate and TFT were also treated with oral ACV or a placebo. There was no significant difference in the therapeutic outcome of patients receiving oral ACV and that of patients receiving placebo. The coordinators of the HEDS Group concluded that a combination of topical TFT and prednisolone is beneficial in treating HSV stromal disease and that augmentation of this therapy with oral ACV is not useful (41).

NEW APPROACHES FOR DRUG DELIVERY OF OCULAR ANTIVIRALS

There are three traditional ways of delivering drugs to the eye: systemically, topically, and subconjunctivally. Systemic administration of drugs to treat ocular disease requires that high serum concentrations be achieved. For some drugs, excessive serum levels produce severe toxicity. Most of the topically applied drug is immediately diluted in the tear film and rapidly drained away from the ocular fornices to the nasal passage. To maintain adequate drug concentrations, frequent topical administration is often necessary. Subconjunctival injection is painful and has the potential for local toxicity.

New ocular drug delivery systems are aimed at circumventing these constraints so as to deliver a therapeutic dose of medication to diseased tissue while sparing healthy tissue and decreasing waste. Three new approaches (collagen shields, iontophoresis, and liposomes) are being refined and tested (87–89). Collagen shields are contact lens-like disks of porcine scleral collagen that dissolve in 12 to 72 hours on the surface of the eye. They are protective and promote wound healing (88) (similar to a bandage soft contact lens), while avoiding some of the disadvantages. Clinical studies show that patients with epithelial defects respond to use of the shield with improved epithelial healing, whereas patients with chronic epithelial erosions respond less well, probably because of damage to the stromal surface (88). When the shield is rehydrated in a solution containing an antiviral or other drug, it serves as a slow-release drug delivery system, dispersing the drug into the tear films as tears act on the shield and as the collagen matrix dissolves. Drugs can be incorporated into the collagen matrix during manufacture, as has been done with cyclosprine A, but no antiviral has been tested (43,89). Experimental studies have shown that drug delivery by collagen shield produces high concentrations of drug in the cornea and aqueous humor.

Iontophoresis, which drives the ionized drugs by the physical principle that ions are repelled by poles of the same charge and attracted by poles of the opposite charge, has been shown to greatly enhance penetration of antiviral drugs across the cutaneous and ocular surface barriers (90–92). The procedure minimizes systemic toxicity by targeting the drug to the area of viral infection. However, no chemotherapeutic ophthalmic applications have been developed for widespread use.

Liposomes, which encapsulate drugs in phospholipid bilayer vesicles, represent an approach to targeting relatively toxic drugs to specific areas, such as vascular blockages or tumors, while limiting systemic toxicity. The use of iontophoresis and liposomes in the eye for antiviral drug delivery is still in the developmental stages.

CONCLUSIONS

Antiviral research has entered an exciting and productive phase. With the advent of AIDS, the search for safe and effective antiviral agents has become critical. Ideally, an antiviral should specifically inhibit viral replication by irreversibly blocking some virus-mediated or virus-induced event without affecting host cell function. Unfortunately, no such agents yet exist. As research into the mechanisms of viral replication progresses, new targets for more selective chemotherapy are being discovered. Recent studies of the use of antiviral combinations (two or more drugs with different mechanisms) have offered great promise. Certainly, more efficient and rapidly acting antivirals will be developed in the future.

ACKNOWLEDGMENT

This work was supported in part by U.S. Public Health Service Grants No. EY06311 and EY09171 and by Core Grant No. EY02377 from the National Eye Institute, National Institutes of Health, Bethesda, MD.

REFERENCES

1. Kaufman HE. Clinical cure of herpes simplex keratitis by 5-iodo-2′-deoxyuridine. *Proc Soc Exp Biol Med* 1962;109:251–252.
2. Kaufman HE, Martola E-L, Dohlman CH. Use of 5-iodo-2′-deoxyuridine (IDU) in treatment of herpes simplex keratitis. *Arch Ophthalmol* 1962;68:235–239.
3. Bean B. Antiviral therapy: current concepts and practices. *Clin Microbiol Rev* 1992;5:146–182.
4. Teich SA, Cheung TW, Friedman AH. Systemic antiviral drugs used in ophthalmology. *Surv Ophthalmol* 1992;37:19–53.
5. Mader TH, Stulting RD. Viral keratitis. *Infect Dis Clin North Am* 1992;6:831–849.
6. Weiter JJ, Roh S. Viral infections of the choroid and retina. *Infect Dis Clin North Am* 1992;6:875–891.
7. Field HJ, Tewari D, Sutton D, Thackray AM. Comparison of efficacies of famciclovir and valciclovir against herpes simplex virus type 1 in a murine immunosuppression model. *Antimicrob Agent Chemother* 1995;39:1114–1119.
8. Prusoff WH. Synthesis and biological activities of iododeoxyuridine, an analog of thymidine. *Biochim Biophys Acta* 1959;32:295–296.
9. Kaufman HE, Rayfield MA. Viral conjunctivitis and keratitis. In: Kaufman HE, Barron BA, McDonald MB, Waltman SR, eds. *The Cornea.* New York: Churchill Livingstone, 1988;299–311.
10. Kaufman HE, Varnell ED, Cheng YC, Bobek M, Thompson HW, Dutschman GE. Suppression of ocular herpes recurrences by a thymidine kinase inhibitor in squirrel monkeys. *Antiviral Res* 1991;16: 227–232.
11. Kaufman HE. Management of herpetic keratitis. In: Bialasiewicz AA, Schaal KP, eds. *Infectious Disease of the Eye.* Buren, The Netherlands: Aeoulus Press Science Publishers, 1994;194–198.
12. Kaufman HE. Introduction: the first antiviral. In: Adams J, Merluzzi VJ, eds. *The Search for Antiviral Drugs.* Boston: Birkhauser, 1993; 1–21.
13. Boston Interhospital Viral Study Group. Failure of high-dose 5-iodo-2′-deoxyuridine in the therapy of herpes simplex virus encephalitis. Evidence of unacceptable toxicity. *N Engl J Med* 1975;292:559.
14. Prusoff WH, Chang PK. 5-Iodo-2′-deoxyuridine 5′-triphosphate, an allosteric inhibitor of deoxycytidylate deaminase. *J Biol Chem* 1968; 243:223.
15. Pavan-Langston D. Major ocular viral infections. In: Galasso GJ, Whitley RJ, Merigan TC, eds. *Antiviral Agents and Viral Diseases of Man,* 3rd ed. New York: Raven Press, 1990;183–233.
16. Brik D, Dunkel E, Pavan-Langston D. Herpetic keratitis: persistence of viral particles despite topical and systemic antiviral therapy. *Arch Ophthalmol* 1993;111:522–527.
17. de Jong MD, Boucher CAB, Calasso GJ, et al. Consensus symposium on combined antiviral therapy. *Antiviral Res* 1996;29:5–30.
18. Hill JM, Hobden JA, Liu WG, et al. Ocular antivirals. *Int Ophthalmol Clin* 1993;33:69–80.
19. Rossi JJ. Therapeutic antisense and ribozymes. *Br Med Bull* 1995;51: 217–225.
20. Whitley RJ, Gnann JW Jr. Antiviral therapy. In: Roizman B, Whitley RJ, Lopez C, eds. *The Human Herpesviruses.* New York: Raven Press, 1993;329–348.
21. Schabel FM Jr. The antiviral activity of 9-β-D-arabinofuranosyladenine(Ara-A). *Chemotherapy* 1968;13:321–338.
22. Whitley RJ, Soong SJ, Dolin R, Galasso GJ, Chien LT, Alford CA. Adenine arabinoside therapy of biopsy-proved herpes simplex encephalitis: National Institutes of Allergy and Infectious Diseases collaborative antiviral study. *N Engl J Med* 1977;297:289–294.
23. Whitley RJ, Soong SJ, Dolin R, Betts R, Linnemann C Jr, Alford CA Jr. Early vidarabine therapy to control the complications of herpes zoster in immunosuppressed patients. *N Engl Med* 1982;307:971–975.
24. Gottschling H, Heidelberger C. Fluorinated pyrimidines XIX. Some biological effects of 5-trifluoromethyl-2′-deoxyuridine on *Escherichia coli* and bacteriophage T4B. *J Mol Biol* 1963;7:541.
25. Kaufman HE, Heidelberger C. Therapeutic antiviral action of 5-trifluoromethyl-2′-deoxyuridine in herpes simplex keratitis. *Science* 1964;145:585.
26. Wellings PC, Awdry PN, Bors PH, et al. Clinical evaluation of trifluorothymidine in the treatment of herpes simplex corneal ulcers. *Am J Ophthalmol* 1972;73:932.
27. Daniels S, Schentag JJ. Drug interaction studies and safety of famciclovir in healthy volunteers: a review. *Antiviral Chem Chemother Suppl* 1993;4:57–64.
28. Schaeffer HJ, Gurwara S, Vince R, et al. Novel substrate of adenosine deaminase. *J Med Chem* 1971;4:367.
29. Schaeffer HJ, Beauchamp L, DeMiranda P, Elion GB, Baver DJ, Collins P. 9-(2-Hydroxyethoxymethyl)guanine activity against viruses of the herpes group. *Nature* 1978;272:583–585.
30. De Clercq E. Antivirals for the treatment of herpesvirus infections. *J Antimicrob Chemother* 1993;32:121–132.
31. De Clercq E. Antiviral agents: characteristic activity spectrum depending on the molecular target with which they interact. *Adv Virus Res* 1993;42:1–55.
32. Corey L. Herpes simplex virus infections during the decade since the licensure of acyclovir. *J Med Virol* 1993;1(suppl):7–12.
33. Darby G. The acyclovir legacy: its contribution to antiviral drug discovery. *J Med Virol* 1993;1(suppl):134–138.
34. Elion GB. Acyclovir: discovery, mechanism of action, and selectivity. *J Med Virol* 1993(suppl);1:2–6.
35. Karbassi M, Raizmand MB, Schuman JS. Herpes zoster ophthalmicus. *Surv Ophthalmol* 1992;36:395–410.

36. Meyers JD, Wade JC, Mitchell CD, et al. Multicenter collaborative trial of intravenous acyclovir for treatment of mucocutaneous herpes simplex virus infection in the immunocompromised host. *Am J Med* 1982;73:229–235.
37. Mertz GJ, Critchlow CW, Benedetti J, et al. Double blind placebo-controlled trial of oral acyclovir in first-episode genital herpes simplex virus infection. *JAMA* 1984;252:1147–1151.
38. Bialasiewicz AA, Jahn GJ. Systemische Acyclovir Therapie bei rezidivierender durch Herpes Simplex Virus bedingter Keratouveitis. *Klin Monatsbl Augenheilkd* 1984;185:539–542.
39. Colin J, Malet F, Chastel C. Acyclovir in herpetic anterior uveitis. *Ann Ophthalmol* 1991;23:28–30.
40. Porter SM, Patterson A, Kho P. A comparison of local and systemic acyclovir in the management of herpetic disciform keratitis. *Br J Ophthalmol* 1990;74:283–285.
41. Wilhelmus KR, Gee L, Hauck WW, et al., and the Herpetic Eye Disease Study Group: herpetic eye disease study. A controlled trial of topical corticosteroids for herpes simplex stromal keratitis. *Ophthalmology* 1994;101:1883–1896.
42. Schwab IR. Oral acyclovir in the management of herpes simplex ocular infections. *Ophthalmology* 1988;95:423–430.
43. Collum LMT, Benedict-Smith A, Hillary IB. Randomized double blind trial of acyclovir and idoxuridine in dendritic corneal ulceration. *Br J Ophthalmol* 1980;64:766–769.
44. Vere Hodge RA, Cheng YC. The mode of action of penciclovir. *Antiviral Chem Chemother* 1993;4(suppl):13–24.
45. Bacon TH, Schinazi RF. An overview of the further evaluation of penciclovir against HSV and varicella-zoster virus in cell culture highlighting contrasts with acyclovir. *Antiviral Chem Chemother* 1993;4:(suppl):25–36.
46. Sutton D, Kern ER. Activity of famciclovir and penciclovir in HSV-infected animals: a review. *Antiviral Chem Chemother* 1993;4(suppl): 37–46.
47. Power WJ, Benedict-Smith A, Hillery M, Brady K, Collum LMT. Randomized double-blind trial of bromovinyldeoxyuridine (BVDU) and trifluorothymidine (TFT) in dendritic corneal ulceration. *Br J Ophthalmol* 1991;75:649–651.
48. Matthews TR, Boehme R. Antiviral activity and mechanism of action of ganciclovir. *Rev Infect Dis* 1988;10:S490–S494.
49. Freitas VR, Smee DF, Chernow M, Boehme R, Matthews TR. Activity of 9-(1,3-dihydroxy-2-propoxymethyl)guanine compared with that of acyclovir against human, monkey, and rodent cytomegaloviruses. *Antimicrob Agents Chemother* 1985;28:240–245.
50. Markowitz M, Saag M, Powderly G, et al. A preliminary study of ritonavir, an inhibitor of HIV-1 protease, to treat HIV-1 infection. *N Engl J Med* 1995;333:1534–1539.
51. Peyman GA, Schulman JA, Khoobehi B, Alkan H, Tawakol ME, Mani H. Toxicity and clearance of a combination of liposome-encapsulated ganciclovir and trifluridine. *Retina* 1989;9:232–236.
52. Anand R, Font RL, Fish RH, Nightingale SD. Pathology of cytomegalovirus retinitis treated with sustained release intravitreal ganciclovir. *Ophthalmology* 1993;100:1032–1039.
53. Pollard RB. CMV retinitis: ganciclovir/monoclonal antibody. *Antiviral Res* 1996;29:73–76.
54. Brockmeyer NH, Hengge UR, Mertins L, Malessa R, Steinmetz R, Gooss M. Foscarnet treatment in various cytomegalovirus infections. *Int J Clin Pharmacol Ther Toxicol* 1993;31:204–207.
55. Safrin S, Crumpacker C, Chatis P, et al. A controlled trial comparing foscarnet with vidarabine for acyclovir-resistant mucocutaneous herpes simplex in the acquired immunodeficiency syndrome. The AIDS clinical trials group. *N Engl J Med* 1991;325: 551–555.
56. Flores-Aguilar M, Kuppermann BD, Quiceno JI, et al. Pathophysiology and treatment of clinically resistant cytomegalovirus retinitis. *Ophthalmology* 1993;100:1022–1031.
57. Walmsley SL, Chew E, Read SE, et al. Treatment of cytomegalovirus retinitis with trisodium phosphonoformate hexahydrate (foscarnet). *J Infect Dis* 1988;157:569–572.
58. Trousdale MD, Law JL, Yarber FA, Watanabe KA, Fox JJ. Evaluation of 1-(2′deoxy-2′-fluoro-β-D-arabinofuranosyl)-5-ethyluracil in a rabbit model of herpetic keratitis. *Antiviral Res* 1992;17:157–167.
59. De Clercq E, Holy A, Rosenberg I, Sakuma T, Balzarini J, Maudgal PC. A novel selective broad-spectrum anti-DNA virus agent. *Nature* 1986;323:464–467.
60. De Clercq E. Broad-spectrum anti-DNA virus and anti-retrovirus activity of phosphonylmethoxyalkylpurines and pyrimidines. *Biochem Pharmacol* 1991;42:963–972.
61. Gordon YJ, Romanowski EG, Araullo-Cruz T. HPMPC, a broad-spectrum topical antiviral agent, inhibits herpes simplex virus type 1 replication and promotes healing of dendritic keratitis in the New Zealand rabbit ocular model. *Cornea* 1994;13:516–520.
62. Gordon RJ, Romanowski E, Araullo-Cruz T, DeClercq E. Pretreatment with topical 0.1% (*s*)-1-(3-hydroxy-2-phosphonylmethoxypropyl)cytosine inhibits adenovirus type 5 replication in the New Zealand rabbit ocular model. *Cornea* 1992;11:529–533.
63. Gordon YJ, Romanowski E, Araullo-Cruz T, et al. Inhibitory effect of (*S*)-PMPC, (*S*)-HPMPA, and 2-nor-cyclicCMP on clinical ocular adenoviral isolates in serotype-dependent in vitro. *Antiviral Res* 1991;16: 11–16.
64. Maudgal PC, DeClercq E. (*S*)-1-(3-hydroxy-2-phosphonyl-methoxypropyl)cytosine in the therapy of thymidine kinase-positive and deficient herpes simplex virus experimental keratitis. *Invest Ophthalmol Vis Sci* 1991;32:1816–1820.
65. Gordon YJ, Romanowski E, Araullo-Cruz T. An ocular model of adenovirus type 5 infection in the NZ rabbit. *Invest Ophthalmol Vis Sci* 1992;33:574–580.
66. Tsai JC, Garlinghouse G, McDonnell PJ, Trousdale MD. An experimental animal model of adenovirus-induced ocular disease. *Arch Ophthalmol* 1992;110:1167–1170.
67. Liuzzi M, Scouten E, Ingemarson R. Inhibition of herpes simplex virus ribonucleotide reductase by synthetic nonpeptides: a potential therapy. In: Block TM, Jungkind D, Crowell RL, Denison M, Walsh LR, eds. *Innovations in Antiviral Development and the Detection of Virus Infection.* New York: Plenum Press, 1992;129–138.
68. Spector T, Averett DR, Nelson DJ, et al. Potentiation of antiherpetic activity of acyclovir by ribonucleotide reductase inhibition. *Proc Natl Acad Sci USA* 1985;82:4254–4257.
69. Liuzzi M, Deziel R, Moss N, et al. A potent peptidomimetic inhibitor of HSV ribonucleotide reductase with antiviral activity *in vivo. Nature* 1994;372:695–698.
70. Mestan J, Brockhaus M, Kirchner H, Jacobsen H. Antiviral activity of tumor necrosis factor. Synergism with interferons and induction of (2′-5′)A_n-synthetase. *J Gen Virol* 1988;69:3113–3120.
71. Aboulafia D, Miles SA, Saks SR, Mitsuyasu RT. Intravenous recombinant tumor necrosis factor in the treatment of AIDS-related Kaposi's sarcoma. *J AIDS Immune Defic* 1989;2:54–58.
72. Doherty PC, Allen JE, Clark IA. Tumor necrosis factor inhibits the development of viral meningitis or induces rapid death depending on the severity of inflammation at time of administration. *J Immunol* 1989;142:3576–3580.
73. Sambhi SK, Kohonen-Cornish MRJ, Ramshaw IA. Local production of tumor necrosis factor encoded by recombinant vaccinia virus is effective in controlling viral replication in vivo. *Proc Natl Acad Sci USA* 1991;88:4024–4029.
74. Wong GHW, Kamb A, Goeddel DV. Antiviral properties of TNF. In: Beutler B, ed. *The molecules and their emerging role in medicine.* New York: Raven Press, 1992;371–381.
75. Jacob A, Duval-Valentin G, Ingrand D, Thuong NT, Helene C. Inhibition of viral growth by an α-oligonucleotide directed to the splice junction of herpes simplex virus type-1 immediate-early pre-mRNA species 22 and 47. *Eur J Biochem* 1993;216:19–24.
76. Kean JM, Kipp SA, Miller PS, Kulka M, Aurelain L. Inhibition of herpes simplex virus replication by antisense oligo-2′-*O*-methyl-ribonucleoside methylphosphonates. *Biochemistry* 1995;34:14617–14620.
77. Kulka M, Wachsmand M, Miura S, et al. Antiviral effect of oligo(nucleoside methylphosphonates) complementary to the herpes simplex virus type 1 immediate early mRNAs 4 and 5. *Antiviral Res* 1993; 20:115–130.
78. Cantin EM, Podsakoff G, Willey DE, Openshaw H. Antiviral effects of herpes simplex virus specific anti-sense nucleic acids. In: Block TM, Jungkind D, Crowell RL, Denison M, Walsh LR, eds. *Innovations in Antiviral Development and the Detection of Virus Infection.* New York: Plenum Press, 1992;139–149.
79. Cohen JS. Oligonucleotides as therapeutic agents. *Pharmacol Ther* 1991;52:211–225.
80. Crooke ST. Therapeutic applications of oligonucleotides. *Annu Rev Pharmacol Toxicol* 1992;32:329–376.

81. Agrawal S, Temsamani J, Galbraith W, Tang J. Pharmacokinetics of antisense oligonucleotides. *Clin Pharmacokinet* 1995;28:7–16.
82. Jabs DA. Design of clinical trials for drug combinations: cytomegalovirus retinitis—foscarnet and ganciclovir. The CMV retinitis retreatment trial. *Antiviral Res* 1996;29:69–72.
83. Collier AC, Coombs RW, Schoenfeld DA, Bassett R, Baruch A, Corey L. Combination therapy with zidovudine, didanosine and saquinavir. *Antiviral Res* 1996;29:99–101.
84. Danner A, Carr A, Leonard M, et al. A short-term study of the safety, pharmacokinetics, and efficacy of ritonavir, an inhibitor of HIV-1 protease. *N Engl J Med* 1995;333:1528–1533.
85. Barron BA, Gee L, Hauck WW, et al., and the Herpetic Eye Disease Study Group: herpetic eye disease study. A controlled trial of oral acyclovir for herpes simplex stromal keratitis. *Ophthalmology* 1994; 101:1871–1882.
86. Dawson CR, Jones DB, Kaufman HE, Barron BA, Hauck WW, Wilhelmus KR. Design and organization of the herpetic eye disease study (HEDS). *Curr Eye Res* 1991;10:105–110.
87. Hill JM, O'Callaghan RJ, Hobden JA. Ocular iontophoresis. In: Mitra AK, ed. *Ophthalmic Drug Delivery Systems.* New York: Marcel Dekker, 1993;331–354.
88. Hill JM, O'Callaghan RJ, Hobden JA, Kaufman HA. Collagen shields for ocular drug delivery. In: Mitra AK, ed. *Ophthalmic Drug Delivery Systems.* New York: Marcel Dekker, 1993;261–273.
89. Reidy JJ, Gebhardt BM, Kaufman HE. The collagen shield, a new vehicle for delivery of cyclosporin A to the eye. *Cornea* 1990;9:196–199.
90. Hill JM, Kwon BS, Burch KD, et al. Acyclovir and vidarabine monophosphate: a comparison of iontophoresis and intravenous administration for the treatment of HSV-1 stromal keratitis in rabbits. *Am J Med* 1982;73:300–304.
91. Hill JM, Gangarosa LP, Park NH. Iontophoretic application of antiviral chemotherapeutic agents. Third Conference on Antiviral Substances. *NY Acad Sci* 1977;284:604–612.
92. Hill JM, Park NH, Gangarosa LP, et al. Iontophoresis of vidarabine monophosphate in rabbit eyes. *Invest Ophthalmol Vis Sci* 1978; 17:473–476.

Textbook of Ocular Pharmacology,
edited by T.J. Zimmerman, et al.
Lippincott–Raven Publishers, Philadelphia © 1997.

CHAPTER 51

Pharmacotherapy of Fungus Infections of the Eye

Terrence P. O'Brien and Peter Rhee

In many instances, the treatment of ocular fungal infections represents a therapeutic dilemma for ophthalmologists (1). Although ocular fungal infections are less common than bacterial infections in developed nations, the need to improve antifungal therapy is underscored by the potentially poor clinical outcomes in patients with severe ocular mycoses.

In the past few decades, an increased number of fungal infections of the eye have been reported, due in part to increased clinical awareness and improved laboratory techniques, but possibly more significantly reflecting the widespread use of antibiotics, immunosuppression, chemotherapy, and ocular prosthetic devices (2). Although the number of cases of ocular mycoses has increased, the number of antifungal agents available for therapy are few compared with the number of fungal pathogens capable of infecting the eye. Current treatment for systemic fungal infections is not always sufficiently effective for ocular mycoses. Part of the reason for the slow development in antifungal therapy as compared with that in antibacterial therapy is that fungal cells, unlike bacteria, are eukaryotic; therefore, any drug that is toxic to fungal cells might exert similar effects on mammalian cells. In addition, less financial incentive has been offered pharmaceutical companies to invest in the development of ocular antifungal agents.

Fungal infections can involve various regions of the eye and periocular tissues, including the lacrimal apparatus, conjunctiva, eyelids, and body orbit. The two most common sites for fungal infections of the eye are the cornea and retina or vitreous. Successful medical treatment of fungal keratitis and endophthalmitis does not depend solely on the spectrum of antifungal activity of the particular drug; it is also largely influenced by the pharmacokinetic properties of the agent (i.e., its ability to achieve therapeutic concentrations in the cornea and/or vitreous).

CLASSES OF ANTIFUNGAL AGENTS

Polyenes

The polyenes are the oldest group of antifungal agents. They work by bonding directly to ergosterol, a sterol unique to fungal cell membranes, thereby disrupting fungal cell membrane integrity (Fig. 1). The agents commonly used in this group for ocular mycoses are amphotericin-B and natamycin.

AMPHOTERICIN-B

History and Source

Amphotericin was discovered in 1956 by Gold et al., who were studying *Streptomyces nodosus,* an aerobic actinomycete. It was isolated by Vandeputte in the same year (3).

Drug Name and Chemistry

The chemical structure of amphotericin-B is shown below.

H_3C O 1 37 O OH OH OH OH OH OH O HO CH_3 COOH H_3C O OH NH_2 O OH CH_3

T. P. O'Brien and P. Rhee: Ocular Microbiology Laboratory, The Wilmer Eye Institute, Johns Hopkins University, School of Medicine, Baltimore, Maryland 21287-9121.

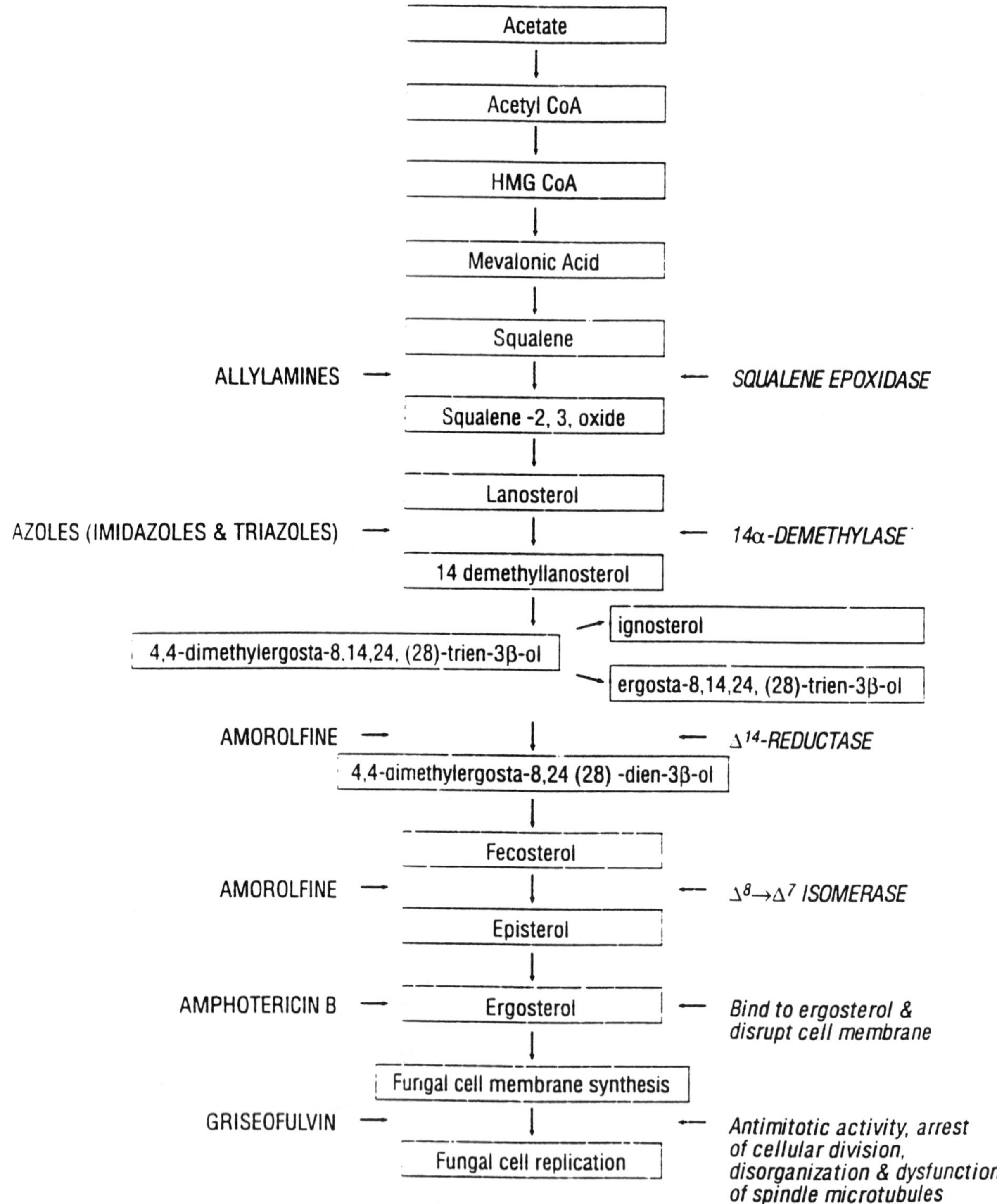

FIG. 51-1. Site of action of antifungal agents. (Reproduced with permission from Grupa AK, Sauder DN, Shear NH. *J Am Acad Dermatol* 1994;30:682.)

Pharmacology

Amphotericin-B works by binding ergosterol and forming ion channels which increase permeability of cell membranes (4). Amphotericin-B has been postulated to form pores in the ergosterol-containing membrane for forming a 1:1 ergosterol–amphotericin-B complex in the external leaflet of the membrane, with resultant removal of ergosterol from the lipid phase (5). Amphotericin-B may also cause direct oxidative damage to the cell membrane (6).

Recent studies suggest that amphotericin-B also accumulates in monocytes and macrophages and can confer on them a greatly increased killing capability without altering the respiratory burst or the number of cells involved in phagocytosis (7). Results obtained using human neutrophils are somewhat conflicting, but one study did show an increased degree of killing by neutrophils pretreated with very high concentrations of amphotericin-B (8).

Clinical Pharmacology

Due to the wide spectrum and efficacy of amphotericin, it is frequently considered the gold standard of antifungal agents with which others are compared. Topical amphotericin-B is generally effective against most cases of *Candida albicans* keratomycoses, against which it is superior in efficacy to solutions of 5% natamycin, 1% fluconazole, 1% miconazole, or 1% ketoconazole (9). The minimal inhibitory concentrations (MIC) for most of the yeasts and dimorphic or filamentous fungi that are pathogens in deep mycoses are generally in the range of 0.05 to 1 μg/ml (10). Amphotericin-B is either fungistatic or fungicidal, depending on the serum or tissue concentrations and the susceptibility of the pathogen, having maximal activity at pH ranging from 6.0 to 7.5 (11). It has been shown to have good activity against both yeast and mycelial phases of *C. albicans* (some *Candida* species are less susceptible), *Aspergillus sp, Cryptococcus neoformans, Histoplasma capsulatum, Coccidioides immitis, Paracoccidioides brasiliensis, Sporothrix schenkii,* and *Rhodotorula rubra,* but limited activity against *Fusarium* species and the agents of mucormycoses, and no significant activity against *Pseudallescheria boydii, Actinomyces,* and resistant strains of *C. albicans* or *C. lusitaniae* (11–13).

Antifungal resistance to the polyenes appears to be relatively rare. Even experimentally, resistance has been difficult to induce in *Candida* species (14). Polyene resistance among pathogenic fungi is probably not a significant clinical problem. Various mechanisms postulated for resistance, when it does occur, include an increased amount of ergosterol in the fungal cell membrane, mutation in the ergosterol biosynthetic pathway with accumulation of ergosterol precursors, the presence of enzymes that actually degrade polyenes, and endogenous fungal enzymes that modify the cell wall, such as the glucanases (14).

In treatment of fungal keratitis, tissue penetration of amphotericin-B is hindered by the effective barrier of corneal epithelium. Removal of the surface epithelium effectively increases aqueous humor and corneal stromal levels of the drug. However, this is probably not necessary, because solutions as dilute as 0.05% proved efficacious in a variety of keratomycoses (15). Animal experiments suggest that topical applications every 5 minutes for 1 hour can quickly achieve therapeutic levels for keratomycoses (16). For fungal keratitis confirmed by culture to be caused by yeast, the 0.15% topical solution is considered by some investigators to be the drug of choice (17). Animal experiments have suggested drug levels of amphotericin-B decrease rapidly after subconjunctival injection and also induce a severe inflammatory response (18). In humans, subconjunctival administration of amphotericin-B is extremely painful (17).

Although at least two cases of fungal endophthalmitis responding favorably to subconjunctival and intravitreal amphotericin without parenteral administration have been reported (19,20), most patients with fungal endophthalmitis require intravenous amphotericin-B, not only as an adjunct to local treatment, but also because of the high prevalence of concurrent systemic infection, especially in immunocompromised patients (20,21). Vitreous levels of the drug during systemic therapy alone are generally low, on the order of 0.04 to 0.17 μg/ml (22). Consequently, intravitreal injections of amphotericin-B are required for effective therapy of fungal endophthalmitis. An experimental study showed *C. albicans* endophthalmitis in a rabbit model to be cured with one intravitreal injection of 5 μg amphotericin-B administered for 4 days after inoculation of the organism (23). However, such deep-seated infections, including *Candida* endophthalmitis, are generally assumed to require high-dose and prolonged therapy with amphotericin-B (24).

Pharmaceutics

Amphotericin-B is available as a complex with sodium deoxycholate, a bile salt carrier that increases the relatively low aqueous solubility of amphotericin-B. The solution consists of 50 mg amphotericin B plus 41 mg sodium deoxycholate and $NaPO_4$ buffer in 10 ml sterile water. At concentrations of 1.4 g/L, this preparation is stable for at least 36 hours and for as long as 24 hours if exposed to light and room temperature (11). Commercial preparations are available in 50-mg vials of dry powder for intravenous use (Amphocin Adria) and Fungizone (Apothecon), as well as in 3% cream, lotion, or ointments (Fungizone).

Pharmacokinetics

When administered systemically, amphotericin-B is highly protein-bound, with 91% to 95% bound to β-lipoproteins (22). It rapidly leaves the blood compartment and exhibits a high degree of tissue binding (11). Due to this biphasic elimination process from the plasma (half-life [$t\frac{1}{2}$] 1 to 2 days), and then from the tissues ($t\frac{1}{2}$ 15 days), the practice of measuring serum levels of amphotericin-B can be misleading and is of little value (11,22). Amphotericin-B is excreted principally by the kidney. With intravenous administration, daily dosing is usually 0.5 to 0.6 mg/kg, with a maximum of 1.5 mg/kg, by slow infusion in 4 hours to avoid the increasing side effects caused by more rapid infusions (11). Oral administration results in poor (5%) absorption and is probably effective only for gastrointestinal (GI) infections.

Side Effects

Whether amphotericin-B is administered topically, subconjunctivally, or systemically, one of the major clinical problems is its toxicity. Topical 1% amphotericin-B solution was shown to retard healing of experimentally induced corneal epithelial defects and is also associated with increased corneal stromal haze, edema, and iritis; toxicities induced by the other antifungal agents—ketoconazole, fluconazole, and flucytosine—were far more modest or were nonexistent (25).

Subconjunctival administration of amphotericin-B is associated with severe pain, as well as reported conjunctival necrosis, yellow discoloration, and development of nodules (17,20,22). Some of these effects may be due to the solubilizing agent, deoxycholate, which has been shown to cause chemosis, burning, epithelial clouding, and punctate epithelial erosions (17). Another formulation of amphotericin, its methylester, has been associated with the development of leukoencephalopathy after systemic administration (26).

Because only low drug concentrations can be achieved by intravenous administration of amphotericin-B, intravitreal injections are usually considered for cases of fungal endophthalmitis. However, toxicity to the retina is a significant complication of intravitreal dosing. In an experimental toxicity study, doses as low as 1 μg amphotericin-B produced histopathologic signs of retinal necrosis in rabbit eyes; however, these results may differ from those in human eyes (27). Other investigators showed that 10 μg amphotericin-B or less is safe if injected into the midvitreous of rabbit eyes with the injecting needle oriented bevel up, whereas dosages greater than or equal to 25 μg produced signs of obvious retinal toxicity (28). Another report suggested that total intravitreal dosages of 5 to 50 μg in human eyes in the treatment of *Aspergillus, Candida,* and *Paecilomyces* endophthalmitis did not appear to cause retinal toxicity (29).

With systemic administration, a variety of deleterious side effects of amphotericin-B treatment have been reported. These include the general symptoms of fever, chills, nausea, and vomiting, as well as more specific conditions, such as thrombophlebitis and anemia, which may be manifest by a decrease of 18% to 35% in hemoglobin concentration (30). By far the most feared complication of amphotericin-B treatment, however, is nephrotoxicity, manifest by azotemia, decreased concentration ability, and renal tubular acidosis (31). Indeed, as many as 80% of patients receiving amphotericin-B therapy may experience a decrease in glomerular filtration rate (GFR) to about 40% of normal levels within 2 weeks of initiation of therapy, although this reduction usually stabilizes at about 20% to 60% of normal (31). Therefore, creatinine levels must be monitored in patients receiving amphotericin-B. Although some studies have suggested that these nephrotoxic effects may be long-lived, with the possibility of irreversible kidney damage being dose dependent (32), others have shown that duration of treatment does not necessarily correlate with renal impairment and that glomerular filtration can be rapidly restored with appropriate therapy (31). The renal toxicity of amphotericin-B may be related to its ability to potentiate the tubuloglomerular feedback, whereby increasing delivery of sodium to the distal tubule (possibly secondary to amphotericin-induced proximal tubular damage) causes afferent arteriolar vasoconstriction with decreased renal blood flow (33). Sodium depletion has been shown to enhance this mechanism, whereas sodium loading reduces it; correspondingly, sodium supplementation at approximately 150 mEq/day appears to lessen the degree of renal impairment in patients receiving amphotericin-B therapy (33,34).

Despite the ability of amphotericin-B to cross the placenta, no adverse effects have been reported in women who have received amphotericin-B during pregnancy (11).

Amphotericin-B has been assumed to react with cholesterol-containing membranes in essentially the same way it reacts with ergosterol containing membranes. At least one recent in vitro study suggests, however, that the two mechanisms may be fundamentally different, with leakage of cholesterol membranes dependent on achieving a critical concentration of amphotericin-B at about $5 \times 10^{-8} M$ at 23°C, whereas leakage in ergosterol membranes depends only on a specific amphotericin-B/lipid molar ratio, with no lower limit of amphotericin-B necessary (5). Bolard et al. (5) suggest that since in the former case amphotericin-B dimers or groups of dimers apparently are responsible for forming the membrane pore complex, whereas in the latter case the monomeric form is responsible. A possible method of decreasing toxicity to mammalian cells might include creating an amphotericin-B derivative with a low degree of self-association.

One of the newer methods reported as a means of decreasing amphotericin toxicity is enveloping the drug in lamellar lipids. A variety of formulations have been made with different types of lipid carriers encapsulating the amphotericin-B, including amphotericin-B lipid complex (ABLC), with the lipid carriers being dimyristoylphosphatidyl choline and dimyristoylphosphatidyl glycerol; ambizone (intralipid), with the carrier being distearoyophosphatidyl glycerol; and Amphocil (ABCD), with the carrier being cholesteryl sulfate (11). These intravenous formulations may have a greater therapeutic index than free amphotericin-B and theoretically could be given at similar or higher doses with sufficient therapeutic efficacy but with decreased toxicity (35–37). A study of ABLC given to rabbits at doses of 10 mg/kg demonstrated efficacy in treatment of *C. Albicans* pyelonephritis or endocarditis with no apparent toxicity (38). The efficacy of these special formulations of amphotericin-B in therapy of fungal endophthalmitis remains to be demonstrated. The reduced toxicity of these special formulations has been suggested to be due to decreased interaction of the liposomes with host membrane, concentration of the intercalated drug in the reticuloendothelial system (lung, liver, retinal epithelial cells), higher tissue/serum ratios, and/or inactivation of macrophages (10).

Because of the hypokalemia that often results from amphotericin-B-induced renal impairment, the actions of toxicities of neuromuscular blocking agents and cardiac glycosides, respectively, may be increased (11). Amphotericin-B may also increase renal toxicity of cyclosporine and aminoglycosides, and antineoplastic agents may actually increase the renal toxicity of amphotericin-B (22).

Drug Interaction

Although toxic drug reactions caused by amphotericin-B remain a concern to clinicians, several studies have suggested that synergistic antifungal interactions may exist between amphotericin-B and a variety of other drugs. Much research has been devoted to the possibility of synergy because theoretically it would allow lower dosages of amphotericin-B to be administered with the same or greater antifungal effect. Possibly the best characterized of these numerous interactions is that which exists between amphotericin-B and rifampin, an antibacterial agent which in itself is inactive against fungi. Amphotericin-B is postulated to alter the fungal cell membrane and allow rifampin to enter the cell, thereby altering RNA synthesis (39). A synergistic activity was shown between amphotericin-B and rifampin against *S. cerevisciae, C. albicans, H. capsulatum,* and *C. neoformans* (40–42). One in vitro study showed that more than half of 40 different *Candida* strains tested exhibited a fourfold or greater decrease in their MIC to amphotericin-B if rifampin was added at a concentration of 25 μg/ml (43). Another study of *C. albicans* keratitis in rabbits showed that the number of organisms isolated from corneas in rabbits treated with subconjunctival injections of rifampin, in addition to amphotericin-B treatment was significantly reduced in comparison to that in rabbits treated with amphotericin-B alone (44).

5-Fluorocytosine (5-FC) has also been suggested to have a sequential mode of action when combined with amphotericin-B, which actually inhibits 5-FC uptake into the fungal cell (45). When the two drugs were administered together in an in vitro system, 5-FC, its metabolites, or both were rapidly taken up only after a certain time, presumably when amphotericin-B had become nearly depleted but had also induced sufficient membrane damage to allow the uptake of 5-FC (45). Indeed, this time lag corresponded approximately to the $t_{\frac{1}{2}}$ of amphotericin in the system used (45). An in vitro study examining the effect of the amphotericin-B/5-FC combination on isolates of *Candida,* as well as *C. neoformans,* showed evidence of synergy in 9 of 32 *C. neoformans* strains and in 5 of 14 *Candida* sp (42).

The effects of combining amphotericin-B and another group of antifungals, the azoles, are somewhat equivocal. One study showed that combining amphotericin-and miconazole and ketoconazole resulted in antagonism or no effect, respectively, for short incubation times, but appeared to show synergistic effects with both drugs after longer incubation times, on the order of several days (46). In a single case study of anterior segment blastomycoses, the patient's condition was unresponsive to amphotericin-B treatment alone but completely resolved with a combination of amphotericin-B, miconazole, and ketoconazole (47). Obviously, more studies, especially in vivo experiments, are required to allow full assessment of the synergistic effect of amphotericin with other compounds. The effect of serum and its constituents on the overall effects of polyene antibiotics, for example, must be further elucidated, and a more standardized definition of synergy needs to be established.

PIMARICIN (NATAMYCIN)

History

The second member of the polyene antifungal group is natamycin which was isolated by Struyk et al. in 1958 from the fermentation process of *Streptomyces natalemsis* (48). It was the first antifungal specifically developed for topical ophthalmic use and is currently the only FDA-approved topical ophthalmic antifungal agent.

Drug Name and Chemistry

The chemical structure of natamycin is shown below:

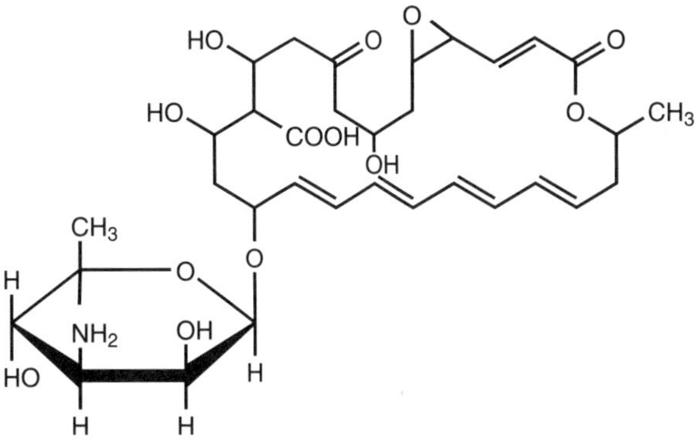

Pharmacology

The exact mechanism of action of natamycin, although not as extensively studied as that of amphotericin, most likely also involved binding of ergosterol to induce cell membrane damage.

Clinical Pharmacology

Natamycin has been recommended as the drug of choice against ocular infections with *Fusarium* sp (49,50). In one report, 18 of 18 patients with *F. solani* keratitis treated with topical 5% natamycin suspension showed improvement in vision, with 16 of 18 healing completely and 13 of 18 having visual acuities of 20/40 or better (50). In general, natamycin shows excellent activity against the filamentous fungi, including *Fusarium,* and against *Aspergillus, Acremonium (Cephalosporium),* and dematiacious fungi, such as *Curvularia* (49).

Pharmaceutics

The most common formulation of natamycin is a 5% suspension (Natacyn, Alcon), which can be stored at room temperature or refrigerated but which should not be frozen or exposed to light or high temperatures. The optimal dosing schedule for administration has not yet been established, but a loading dose in which one drop is applied every 30 minutes and gradually tapered to one drop every hour for 6 to 8 days appears to be sufficient (17).

Pharmacokinetics

Natamycin was initially believed to be poorly absorbed into cornea; recent radiolabeling studies, however, suggest that it actually penetrates well and instead has a low bioavailability, on the order of 2% (51). This study showed that the corneal concentration of natamycin was significantly increased by debridement of the corneal epithelium, with levels peaking at approximately 10 minutes after dosage. Thirteen topical applications every 5 minutes resulted in a drug concentration of approximately 2.5 mg/g cornea. Levels in nondebrided corneas with intact epithelium peaked earlier and were also far lower than those in corneas from which the epithelium had been removed.

Side Effects

Due to its low aqueous solubility, natamycin is not available for systemic administration. It has been shown to have a very low level of toxicity with topical administration, but has been reported to cause a punctate epithelial keratitis occasionally, without significantly affecting healing rate (17). Conjunctival necrosis precludes its administration by subconjunctival injection (49).

The Azoles

IMIDAZOLES

The imidazoles are a group of antifungal agents that were developed largely because of the need for a form of therapy that was effective and yet less toxic than amphotericin. Although amphotericin-B is still probably the preferable drug for serious deep-seated systemic infections, numerous members of the azole group have exhibited the potential to be as effective as or superior to treatment for ocular fungal infections (Table 1).

Pharmacology

The mechanism of action of azoles includes binding to a cytochrome P450 fungal enzyme involved in the 14-α demethylation of either lanosterol (in *C. glabrata, S. cerevisiae,* and mammalian cells), or 25-methylenedihydrolanosterol (in filamentous fungi, the yeast form of *H. capsulatum, C. neoformans,* and several *C. albicans* strains), which are steps in the formation of ergosterol (Fig. 1) (52). Binding to the cytochrome P450 is through the ferric heme iron to N3 of the imidazole or the N4 of the triazoles, as well as through a hydrophobic portion of the P450 apoprotein to N1 of the azole, with this latter bond determining relative affinity (53). As a result of the inhibition of the 14-α demethylation, ergosterol synthesis decreases and 14-methylated sterols accumulate, which appear to increase membrane permeability, inhibit growth, alter membrane enzymes, and induce cell death (52). Another notable change occurring after inhibition of ergosterol synthesis is the rapid accumulation of chitin over the entire cell wall, not just at the septa and growth tip; ergosterol is known to exert a regulatory function in cell proliferation (52,54). Precisely which mechanism is more important, the buildup of 14-methylated sterols or the decrease in ergosterol, has not yet been completely resolved.

The azoles have also been proposed to act by inhibiting cytochrome C oxidative and peroxidative enzymes, increasing concentrations of peroxidase (13). In addition, all azoles, except for fluconazole, apparently decrease immune cell function, especially lymphocyte function (55). Such a mechanism may affect the efficacy of the azoles in vivo as well as the degree of tissue damage that often results from inflammatory reactions. Although azoles have

Table 51-1. *Imidazole antifungal compounds*

Generic name/trade name(s)	Chemical structure	Formulations
Clotrimazole Canesten Mycelex Mycelex-G Lotrimin Gyne-Lotrimin	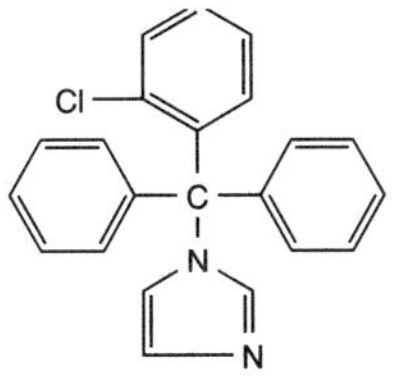	1% Cream and solution, 100-, 200-, and 500-mg vaginal tablets, 10-mg oral troches
Miconazole Monistat Monistat-Derm Monistat I.V.	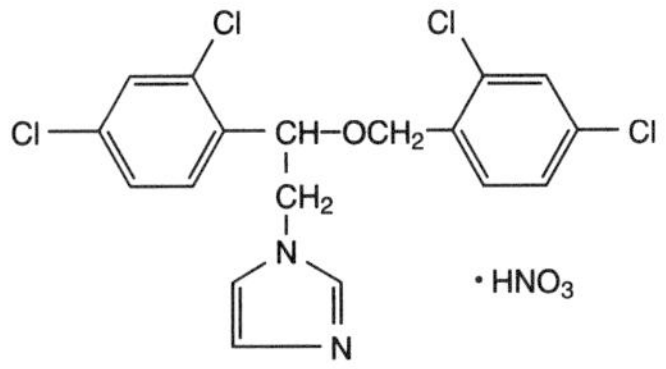	2% Cream and lotion 200-mg Vaginal suppositories 10-mg/ml Sterile solution for intravenous use
Econazole Spectazole Pevaryl	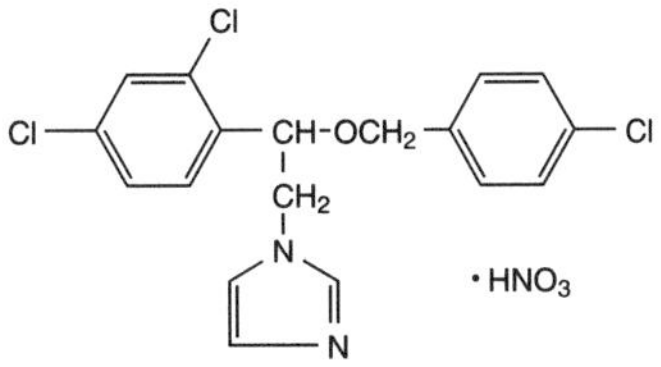	1% Topical and vaginal creams 1% solution, spray, and powder
Ketoconazole Nizoral Fungarol Fungarest Orifungal	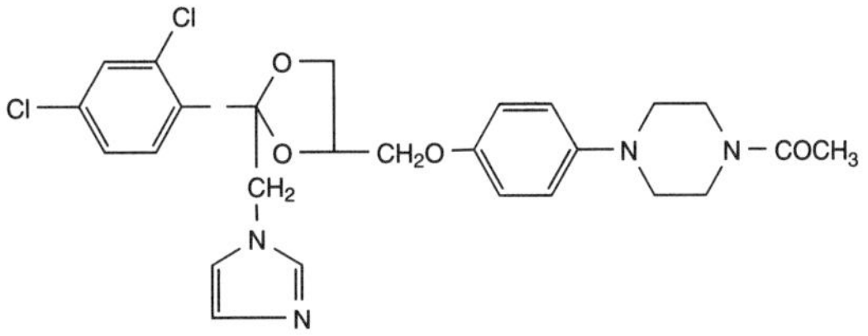	200-mg Tablets for oral use, 2% cream and solution
Bifonazole Mycospor Mycosporan	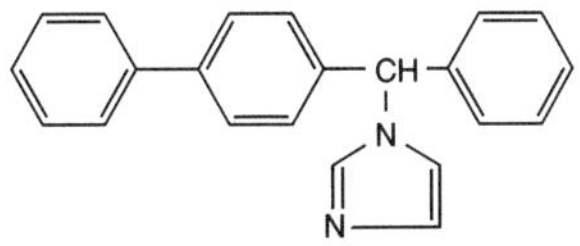	1% Cream and solution
Butoconazole Femstat	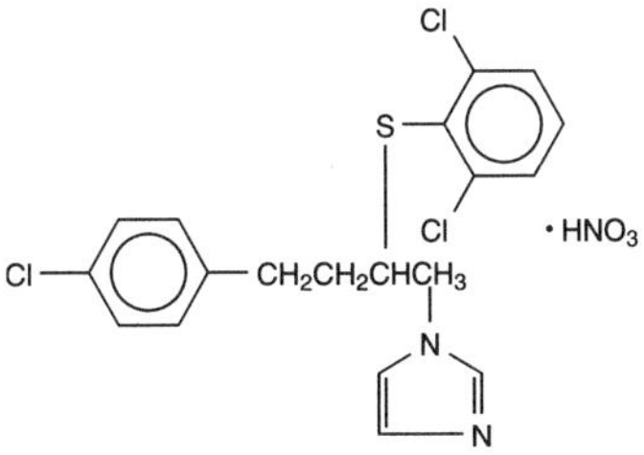	2% Vaginal cream, 100-mg vaginal ovules
Croconazole Pilzcin	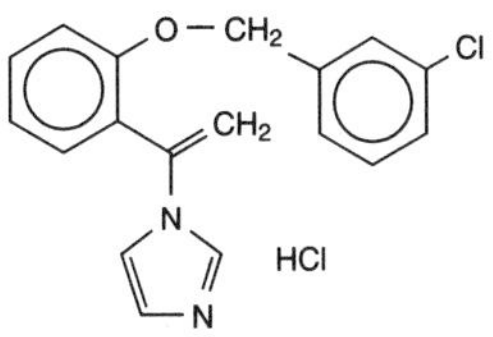	1% Cream and gel
Fenticonazole Lomexin	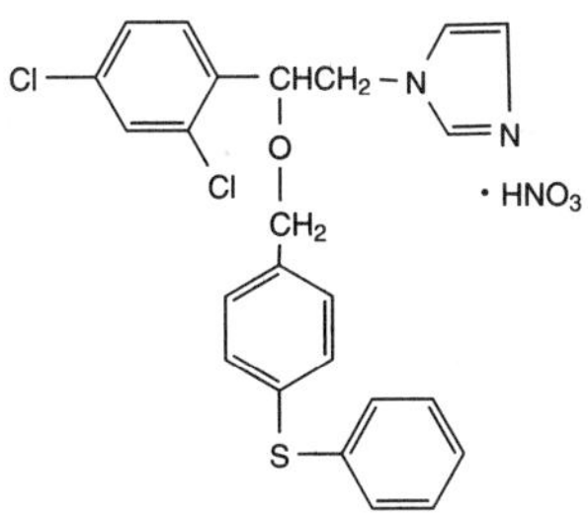	2% Topical and vaginal creams

Table 51-1. *Continued*

Generic name/trade name(s)	Chemical structure	Formulations
Isoconazole Travogen Gyne-Travogen	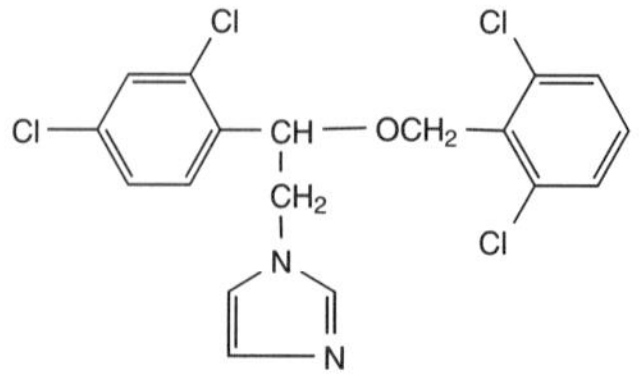	2% Topical and vaginal creams
Oxiconazole Oceral Myfungar Gyno-Myfungar Okinazole Derimine	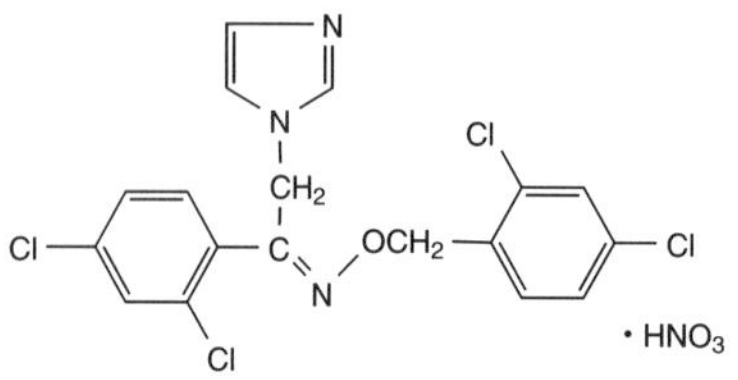 · HNO_3	1% Cream, spray, and powder
Sulconazole Exelderm Sulcosyn	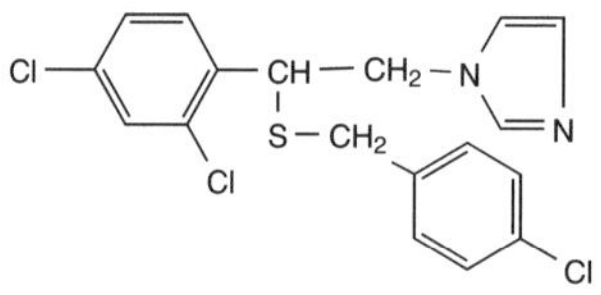	1% Cream
Troconazole Trosyd Gyne-Trosyd	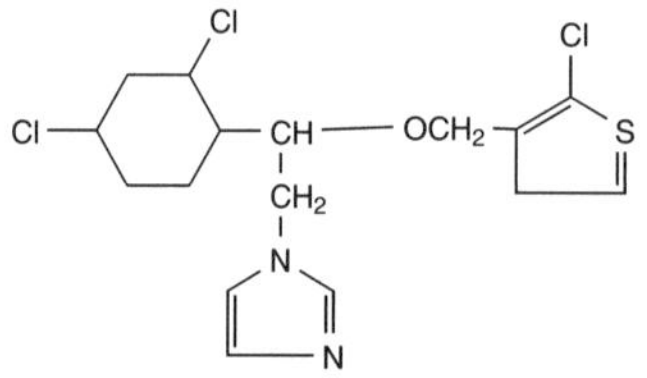	1% Cream, lotion, spray, and powder
Terconazole (triazole) Terazol Gyne-Terazol Fungistat	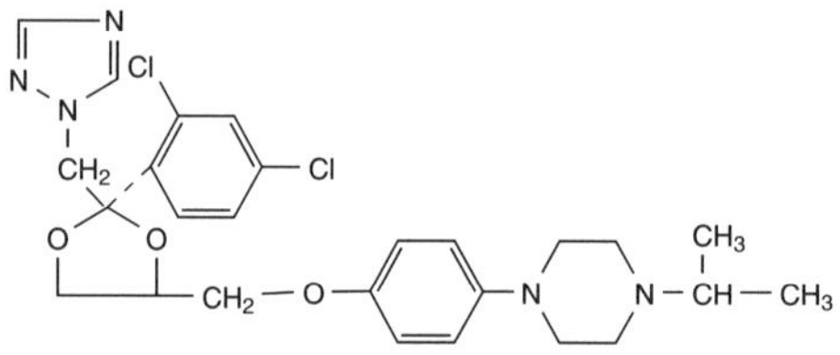	0.8% Vaginal cream, 40- and 80-mg vaginal ovules
Imidazoles Aliconazole (Knoll)	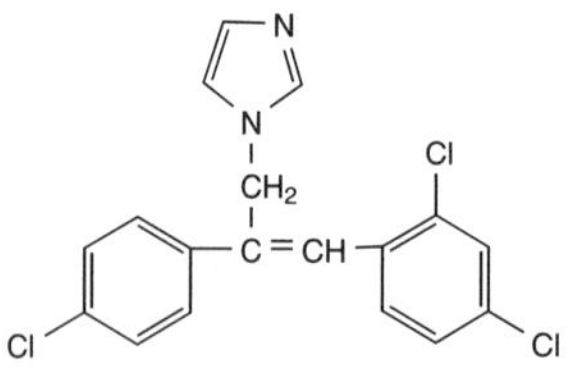	Topical
Omoconazole (Siegfried AG)	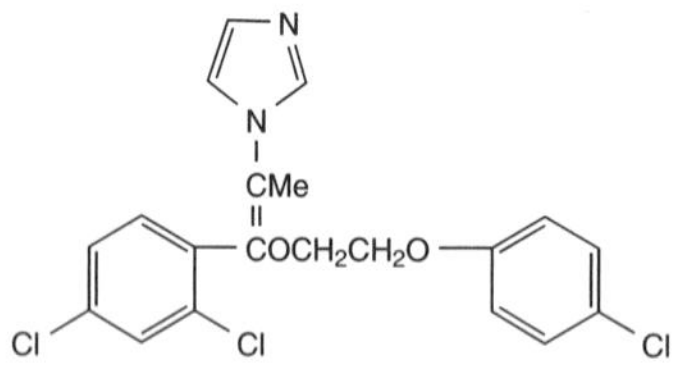	Topical

been suggested to exert a direct membrane-damaging affect, this mechanism probably exists only at high concentrations of the agents, greater than that which can be achieved in the eye. Therefore, for ocular fungal infections, azoles are probably best viewed as being fungistatic only (17).

Clinical Pharmacology

Testing a variety of azoles has shown them to be potent inhibitors of ergosterol biosynthesis in *C. albicans, C. glabrata, C. lusitaniae, P. ovale, T. mentagrophytes, P. brasiliensis, H. capsulatum,* and *A. fumigatus* (52). In vitro testing data of all azoles, however, should be viewed cautiously, because test conditions, such as type of media, solvent, temperature, and inoculation density can create discrepancies in apparent antifungal activity (56). Even in vivo experiments may provide misleading results if, for example, clearance mechanisms in an animal are significantly different from that in other animals or humans (57). The lack of correlation between in vitro and in vivo testing has been particularly problematic for the azoles; e.g., ketoconazole usually demonstrates MIC values higher than those of the first-generation azoles clotrimazole and miconazole, yet the antifungal activity of ketoconazole in vivo is not significantly lower than that of the other two azoles (58). The best example may be fluconazole, which shows activity against *C. albicans* far inferior to that of ketoconazole and miconazole in vitro but excellent activity in vivo. This may be explained by the low protein binding and longer $t_{\frac{1}{2}}$ of fluconazole in vivo, possibly resulting in fluconazole's greater bioavailability (58).

Resistance to most of the azoles is relatively rare, usually manifested only by severely debilitated patients receiving long-term treatment. In one study of patients with AIDS who had been treated with fluconazole, the frequency of resistance was approximately 5% (59). The mechanism of resistance is usually due to decreased susceptibility of the P450 demethylase enzyme or decreased permeability of the cells to the azole (60). Cross-resistance to azoles may be exhibited in resistant strains, which probably do not arise from mutation, but rather from selection from the susceptible population (60).

KETOCONAZOLE

History

Ketoconazole, introduced in 1979, was the first successful orally absorbable broad-spectrum antifungal azole. Although the initial enthusiasm following its development was later tempered by increasing reports of drug interactions and limited efficacy against infections, ketoconazole remains a mainstay of antifungal therapy, especially against mucosal candidosis, histoplasmosis, and blastomycosis.

Drug Name and Chemistry

The chemical structure of ketoconazole is shown below:

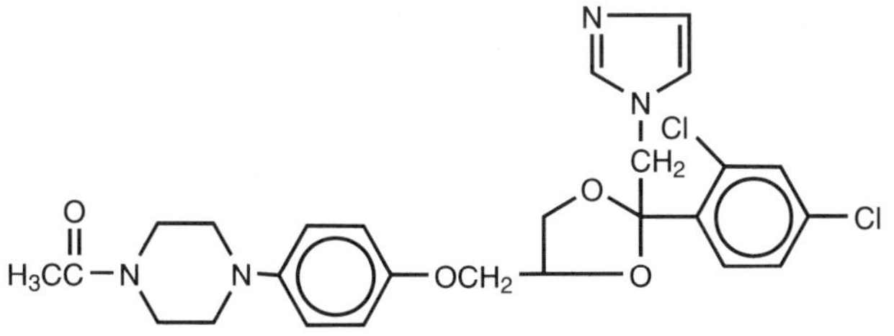

Pharmacology

In addition to inhibiting the P450-dependent demethylase, ketoconazole also may exert a direct inhibitory effect on the distal respiratory chain by inhibiting the cytochrome C-dependent NADH oxidase (61), an effect that may not be directly related to ergosterol biosynthesis, in either the plasma membrane or the mitochondrial membrane (62).

Clinical Pharmacology

Results of various studies examining the susceptibilities of specific fungal organisms to ketoconazole are somewhat conflicting. This may be due to use of different animal models and different drug preparations and concentrations and to the wide variation in susceptibility of organisms to ketoconazole (63). In general, ketoconazole is considered to have excellent activity against *C. albicans;* concentrations 10 to 100 times lower than the MIC have been shown to interfere with germ formation, the initial step in mycelial transformation and tissue invasion (10). Most pathogenic yeasts, dimorphic fungi (e.g., *C. immitis, B. dermititidis, H. capsulatum, P. brasiliensis*), and some filamentous fungi, such as *P. boydii,* and *F. solani,* are considered susceptible to ketoconazole (64). The susceptibility of *Aspergillus* appears to depend on the particular species of *Aspergillus* that is causing the infection. A study of experimentally established *A. flavus* keratomycoses in a rabbit model showed that topical dosing regimen of 1% ketoconazole in arachis (peanut) oil every hour for 10 hours for 16 days cleared all infections (65). In another study, however, treatment with oral or topical ketoconazole for *A. fumigatus* keratitis was unsuccessful (66). Such results agree with those obtained in MIC studies of the two different *Aspergillus* species (65). There is at least one case report, however, of an *A. fumigatus* infection successfully treated with topical ketoconazole 2% in an intensive dosing regimen (67). Ketoconazole has also been suggested to have prophylactic potential in inhibiting *A. flavus* keratitis to a significant degree (65). Therefore, Oji (65) suggested that ketoconazole could be administered as prophylaxis against fungal keratitis in areas or times of high risk.

Although no studies have detailed the efficacy of ketoconazole against ocular infections in immunocompromised hosts, systemic infections in such patients are largely resistant to ketoconazole treatment (68).

Pharmaceutics

Ketoconazole is commercially available as Nizural (Janssen) in 2% cream, 2% shampoo, and 200-mg tablets.

Pharmacokinetics

A 1% ketoconazole solution, administered subconjunctivally, topically, or orally to undebrided corneas having intact epithelium has been shown to achieve relatively high concentrations in the cornea, whereas levels in the vitreous were nondetectable (63). Debridement of the corneal epithelium resulted in greatly increased corneal drug levels, especially after topical administration, but with subconjunctival administration, corneal drug level was also significantly increased. Vitreous levels remained low.

Administered systemically, ketoconazole is highly bound to serum protein (90% to 95%), but it also has a high tissue distribution and a biphasic $t_{1/2}$: $t_{1/2}\alpha$ of approximately 2 hours and a $t_{1/2}\beta$ of approximately 9 hours (63). Ketoconazole is insoluble at neutral pH, but becomes highly soluble at pH values less than 2 to 3. As a result, it is well absorbed orally; a 200-mg oral dose yields a peak serum level in the range of 2 to 3 mg/L 2 to 3 hours after the dose (69). However, there is significant individual variability in absorption of ketoconazole and there is no clear relation between serum levels and clinical outcome (69). Because absorption is heavily dependent on gastric pH, any substances that decrease pH or inhibit gastric acid secretion, such as cimetidine or other antacids, will decrease absorption of orally administered ketoconazole (70).

Side Effects

Ketoconazole appears to have few toxic effects. Administered topically at 1%, 3%, and 5% solutions in arachis oil, it caused no toxicity in rabbit corneas except for some conjunctival hyperemia at 5% solution, which may have been due to the presence of undissolved drug (71). In rabbit studies in which the retinal toxicities of intravitreal ketoconazole dissolved in dimethyl sulfoxide (DMSO) were examined, injection of 540 μg was well tolerated, whereas 720 μg produced evidence of electroretinogram (ERG) abnormalities, and dosages of 2,240 μg resulted in loss of photoreceptor outer segments and degeneration of the retinal pigment epithelium (RPE) (72). Oral dosages of ketoconazole greater than 400 mg/day may cause nausea, vomiting, and transient increases in liver enzymes, with an incidence of clinical hepatitis of one in 10,000 to 50,000 patients overall, but in only 1 in 1,500 patients receiving long-term therapy (69, 73). Sexual impotence, hair loss, gynecomastia, and oligospermia are all most likely the result of decreased steroid synthesis (74). The concentration of ketoconazole is reduced by rifampin, but ketoconazole in itself can increase the concentration or effect of cyclosporine, coumarin, phenytoin, and sulfonylureas and decrease the concentration of theophyline (73).

CLOTRIMAZOLE

History

Clotrimazole, a chlorinated trityl imidazole, was developed in Germany by Bayer. It was the first imidazole derivative developed for human mycotic infection.

Drug Name and Chemistry

The chemical structure of clotrimazole is shown below:

Pharmacology

Clotrimazole has excellent activity against *Aspergillus* infections of the eye and is also active against *Candida, Paecilomyces, Dresch elera, Alternaria,* and *Fonsecae* sp, but not against *Fusarium* sp (1).

Although clotrimazole was the first azole meant for oral use, it became apparent that after only a week or so of treatment, liver microsomal enzymes were rapidly induced and serum concentration of clotrimazole decreased (75). As a result, clotrimazole is now mostly used as an antiamoebic agent. Because tissue drug levels after oral administration are initially high, however, at least one report has suggested a regimen combining a topical and oral clotrimazole dosing of 60 to 100 mg/kg/day, with discontinuance of the oral dosing after about 2 weeks, or as clinical response improves (1).

Side Effects

A case of punctate keratopathy and ocular irritation have been reported to result from long-term topical use of clotrimazole (17). Oral administration occasionally results in anorexia, nausea, vomiting, and mild hepatic toxicity (17). Clotrimazole is not recommended for treatment of women in the first trimester or pregnancy or for patients with severe adrenal or liver disease (1).

MICONAZOLE

History

Miconazole is another imidazole derivative first synthesized by Janssen Pharmaceutical of Belgium and introduced in 1969.

Drug Name and Chemistry

The chemical structure of miconazole is shown below:

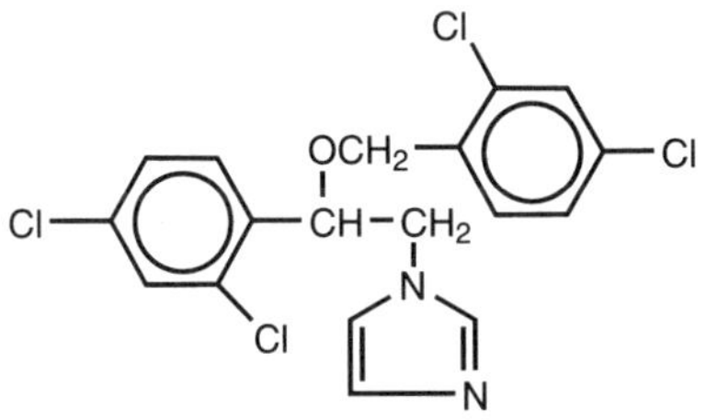

Pharmacology

Although miconazole inhibits C14-demethylation, like the other azoles, Fromtling (75) suggested that it also has a direct membrane-damaging effect.

Clinical Pharmacology

Miconazole has a relatively broad antifungal spectrum, showing clinical efficacy in patients with keratomycoses caused by *Fusarium, Asperigillus, Penicillium, Alternaria,* and *Rhodotorula* (1). Although many strains of *Pseudallescheria boydii* have been shown to be susceptible to miconazole, in the few case reports of endophthalmitis or keratitis due to this organism, miconazole treatment has not resulted in a clinically successful response (76,77).

In experiments in rabbit eyes, subconjunctivally and topically administered miconazole penetrated the cornea very well, resulting in high tissue concentrations that could be greatly increased by epithelial debridement; intravenous administration, on the other hand, resulted in no detectable drug concentrations in rabbit cornea or vitreous, whereas in the aqueous humor, drug concentrations were initially high but decreased rapidly in about 2 hours (78). Measured drug concentrations in humans after intravenous dosing also appeared to decrease rather rapidly (10). In two studies in which vitreous levels of miconazole were measured in the human eye after intravenous administration, concentrations of the drug in the vitreous were low; however, these concentrations were well below that required to be effective against *Candida* or *Aspergillus* endophthalmitis (78,79).

A 1% solution of miconazole nitrate appears successful in a variety of keratomycoses. There is some evidence that the nitrate derivative is superior to miconazole alone in treatment of *T. glabrata,* but the irritation caused by miconazole nitrate administration makes topical application difficult (1,80).

Pharmaceutics

Miconazole is available as a 2% cream (Geneva Pharm), and the nitrate derivative is available as a 2% cream (Clay-Park, Fougera, G&W, Major, H.L. Moore, NML Lab, Rugby, Taro) or Powder (A-A Spectrum, Coopley, H.L. Moore, Paddock).

Side Effects

Reported side effects after systemic administration of miconazole include phlebitis, pruritus, rash, fever, chills, nausea, vomiting, and diarrhea, as well as hyponatremia and hematologic or hepatic toxicities (10,13). Some of these effects may be due to the Cremophor El (poyoxyl 35 castor oil) vehicle, which has histamine-releasing properties and makes long-term intravenous use difficult (10). In a toxicity study, miconazole injected intravitreally in rabbit eyes produced damage to the lens and retina at dosages of 100 μg or more, with mild damage at 10 to 80 μg, whereas in monkey eyes no damage resulted from dosages of 80 μg or more (79). From these data, the researchers suggested that a dose of 40 μg be used in severe cases of fungal endophthalmitis.

ECONAZOLE

History

Econazole is another imidazole derivative that has been used extensively in Europe for many years for treatment of superficial mycotic infections. It is currently in use in the United States for treatment of skin infections.

Drug Name and Chemistry

The chemical structure of econazole is shown below:

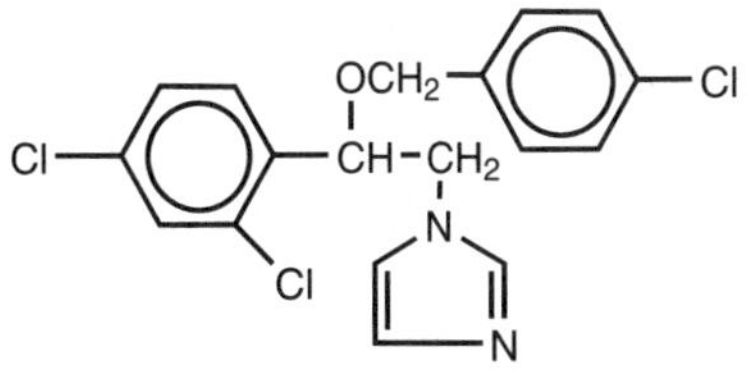

Pharmacology

The exact mechanism of the antifungal activity of econazole is not clearly defined; various suggested theories include mitochondrial damage, suppression of ATP production, or direct membrane damage (75).

Clinical Pharmacology

Of all the imidazoles, econazole is reported to have the broadest spectrum and is highly active against filamentous fungi such as *Aspergillus, Fusarium,* and *Penicillium* species (1,81).

Pharmaceutics

For skin fungal infections, econazole nitrate is available as a 1% cream (Spectazole, Ortho). The optimal preparation of econazole, like that of miconazole, is a 1% solution in arachis oil, which appears to be well tolerated in the eye.

Ketoconazole, econazole, and miconazole are the three imidazoles that have been used most extensively in the eye, although a variety of other imidazoles have exhibited varying degrees of efficacy in treating potential ocular fungal pathogens. Few or no pharmacologic data are available regarding the ophthalmic applications of these other azoles. Most of these agents were originally introduced for the treatment of dermatologic fungal infections. They are presented herein as a guide to antifungal agents that may play a significant role in the future treatment of ocular mycoses.

Other Agents

TIOCONAZOLE

History

Tioconazole (Table 1) is an imidazole that was synthesized by Pfizer Research Laboratories in the late 1970s. It is currently used for treatment of skin and nail infections.

Clinical Pharmacology

In vitro studies have shown tioconazole to be more active than miconazole against *Candida* species, *C. neoformans,* and *T. glabrata,* and to have activity comparable to that of miconazole against *Aspergillus* (75). Its in vitro killing activity is markedly decreased by even slightly acidic conditions, which may explain the discrepancies in MIC studies reported by some investigators (82).

Oxiconazole (Table 1), another imidazole, exhibits excellent activity against *A. fumigatus, C. neoformans, C. albicans,* and *T. mentagrophytes,* as well as *Rhizopus* species (75).

One study showed that 0.2% oxiconazole solution in DMSO and normal saline administered subconjunctivally achieved a complete cure in a rabbit model of *Aspergillus terreus* keratomycoses (83).

Omoconazole is a newer topical antifungal agent that was shown to have in vitro activity against yeasts comparable to that of clotrimazole, tioconazole, miconazole, econazole, and isoconazole and greater than that of ketoconazole (84). It was also shown to be the most active of the aforementioned antifungal agents against *C. neoformans* and *Pityrosporum* and against various strains of *A. fumigatus* (83).

Croconazole is an imidazole with an arylvinyl group at N1 rather than the alkyl group of other imidazoles (Table 1). It is used as topical treatment for dermatomycoses and candidiasis (75). In vitro studies showed activity against five *Aspergillus* species, two *Penicillium* species, *T. mentagrophytes, T. rubrum, Microsporum canis, M. gypseum,* and *E. floccosum* but lesser activity against yeasts such as *Candida* species and *C. neoformans* (75).

Sulconazole is an imidazole developed for the treatment of dermatomycoses, pityriasis versicolor, and cutaneous candidiasis (Table 1) (75). One in vitro study showed it to have moderate activity against *C. albicans* and *Aspergillus* species, with much greater activity against dermatophytes (85), although sulconazole also exerted fungicidal effects on *C. albicans* depending on the growth phase of the organism (86). The different methods used to measure antifungal activity, as well as the use of different strains of *C. albicans,* probably explain for the differing results of the two studies.

Isoconazole is an imidazole which has been shown in vitro to have activity against dermatophytes, yeasts, and fungi. One in vitro study showed isoconazole to be more active than econazole, miconazole, and ketoconazole against ten species of *Candida* (87). Damage to the cell membrane, with lowering of ATP concentration, appears to be its mechanism of action (75). Isoconazole is apparently effective only when administered topically (75).

Fenticonazole is an imidazole that has shown good activity against superficial mycoses and vaginal candidiasis (Table 1). In vitro, it is most active against dermatophytes, but in the presence of acid pH, it also appears to be active against *C. neoformans* and *C. albicans* (75). Electron microscopy studies have suggested that fenticonazole exerts a direct membrane-damaging effect on cytoplasmic organelles, such as the mitochondria, nuclear membrane, and endoplasmic reticulum (88).

Butoconazole (below) is an imidazole which was first developed for treatment of vaginal candidiasis. As compared with ketoconazole in vitro, it appears to have a similar level of activity against *Candida* but an inferior level of activity against *Aspergillus* (75).

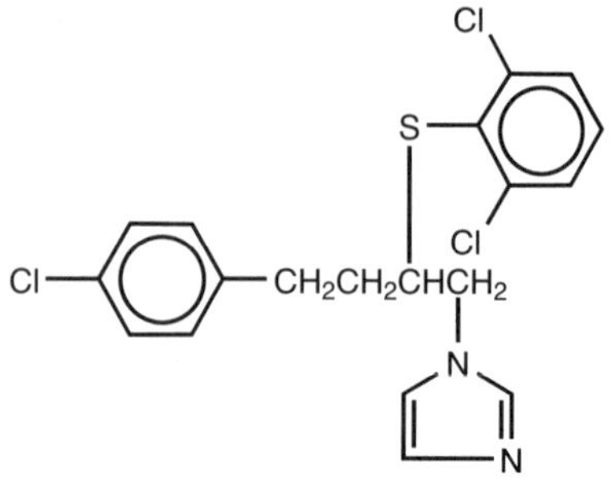

Bifonazole is an imidazole with a broad in vitro spectrum against pathogenic yeasts, dimorphic fungi, and some filamentous fungi (Table 1) (75). It appears to have weak in vitro activity against *Candida* and *Aspergillus* sp, however (85).

Triazoles

History

The second major group of azole antifungals consists of the triazole derivatives, which were developed approximately 10 years after the introduction of the imidazoles (Table 2). These drugs, the most important of which are terconazole, itraconazole, and fluconazole, were largely developed in response to increasingly evident shortcomings of ketoconazole, i.e., its limited spectrum and side effects (68).

Pharmacology

The mechanism of action of the triazoles is essentially the same as that of the imidazoles, but the replacement of the imidazole ring by the triazole ring offers several advantages, including increased affinity of the azole ring for the $P_{450}F_e$ atom, with improved selectivity and lowered toxicity, broader spectrum, increased stability, and lower rate of self-induced hepatic metabolism (75,89).

Table 51-2. *Triazoles*

Generic name (developer)	Chemical structure	Proposed route or routes of administration
Triazoles Fluconazole (Pfizer U.K.)	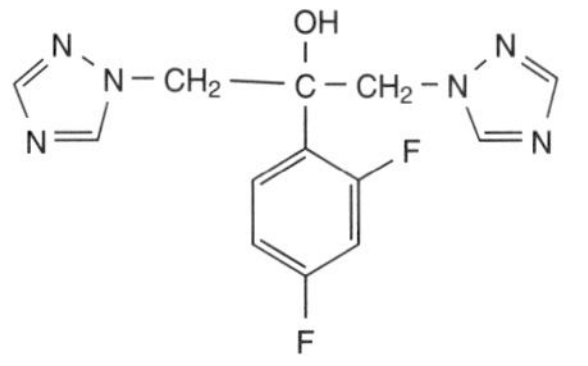	Oral, topical
Itraconazole (Janssen)	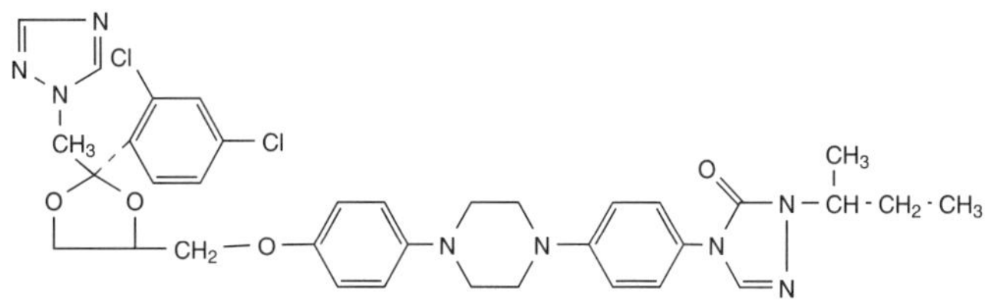	Oral, topical (?)
Vibunazole (Bayer AG)	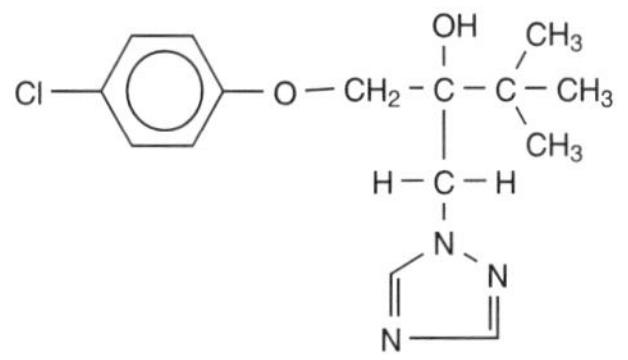	Oral, topical
Alteconazole (Knoll)	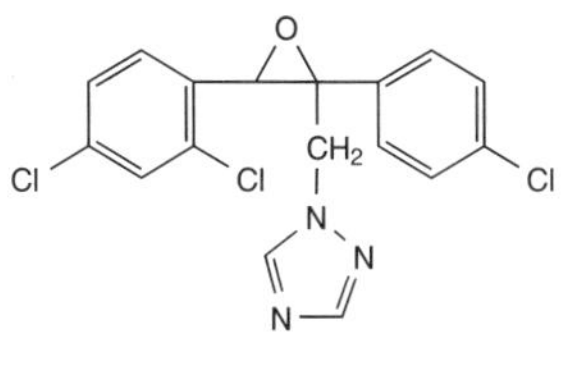	Oral, topical
ICI 195,739 (Imperial Chemical Industries)	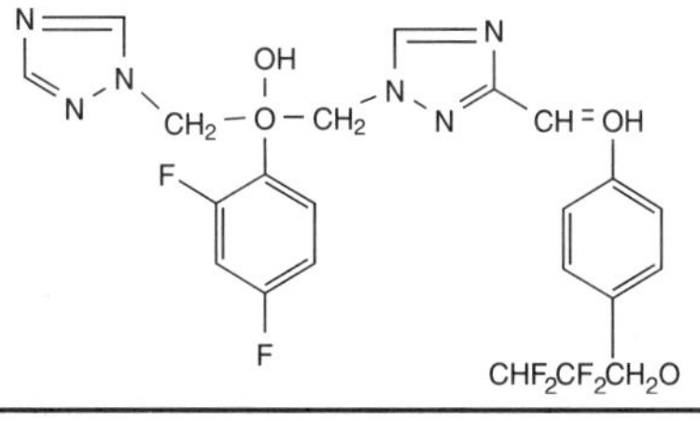	Oral, topical

TERCONAZOLE

The chemical structure of terconazole is shown below:

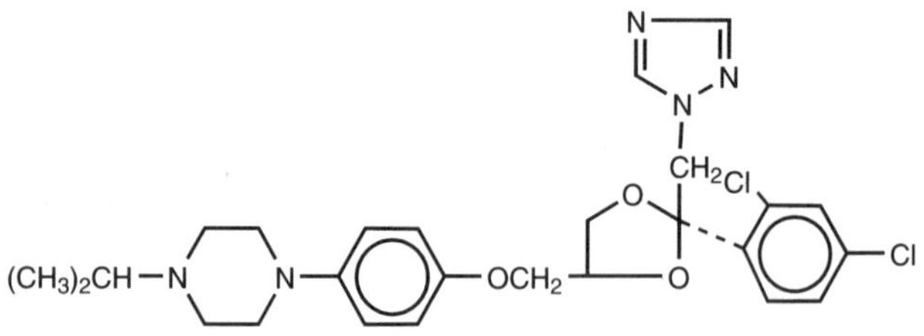

$$(CH_3)_2CH-N\langle\rangle N-C_6H_4-OCH_2-\text{(dioxolane, } CH_2\text{-triazole)}-C_6H_3Cl_2$$

Clinical Pharmacology

Terconazole is very effective in inhibiting the yeast to mycelium transformation in *C. albicans* (90). In vitro experiments with *C. albicans* showed terconazole 10 μM to cause a greater decrease in ergosterol content than did the other azoles, mainly clotrimazole, miconazole, and butoconazole (91). That same study showed chitin content to be increased most by terconazole (245%). A sterol, possibly ergosterol itself, has been proposed to play a role in regulation of chitin synthesis (92), which is normally localized to the site of fission in *C. albicans* yeast forms and to wall formation in the hyphal form (93). These effects, however, are observed at low concentrations; at high concentrations, terconazole probably works mainly by direct lysis.

Terconazole has also been reported to have excellent in vitro activity against dermatophytes and *C. neoformans* (75).

Pharmaceutics

Terconazole is available as a 0.4% cream [Terazol 7 (Ortho)] and a 0.8% cream for vaginal infection (Terazol 3, Ortho).

ITRACONAZOLE

The chemical structure of itraconazole is shown below:

$$\text{Triazole}-CH_2-\text{(dioxolane, H)}-CH_2O-C_6H_4-N\langle\rangle N-C_6H_4-\text{triazolone}-CHCH_2CH_3(CH_3)$$

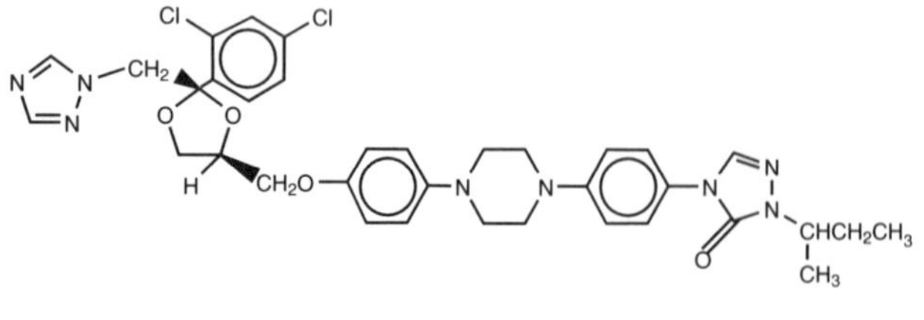

Pharmacology

The second major triazole in this group is itraconazole, which, in addition to decreasing ergosterol biosynthesis by inhibiting the cytochrome P450-dependent 14-α demethylase of lanosterol or 24-methylene-24,25-dihydrolanosterol, may also inhibit the NADPH-dependent keto-steroid reductase, which would increase the amount of 3-ketosteroids that could destabilize the lipid bilayer (54). In fungal cells, itraconazole induced morphologic changes, depending on the species and morphology of the organism (94). In *C. albicans,* itraconazole inhibited further elongation and branching of the germ tube, although spores continued to form. In *P. ovale* and *A. fumigatus,* the internal organelles were disrupted, with significant changes in the cell periphery, whereas in *P. brasiliensis* the effects of itraconazole were dependent on the phase of the organism, with the mycelium to yeast transformation most sensitive (94).

Clinical Pharmacology

Itraconazole has a broad spectrum, including *C. albicans, C. glabrata, C. lusitaniae, Paracoccidiodes, H. capsulatum, Paecilomyces,* and *Coccidioides,* and also exhibits excellent in vitro activity against *Aspergillus* species, unlike ketoconazole (10,68,94,95). Itraconazole, however, may not be as effective against *Fusarium* and some other filamentous fungi (76).

In a guinea pig model, oral intraconazole 1.25 mg/kg appeared superior to oral ketoconazole 10 mg/kg in treatment of *M. canis* skin infections (56). The study also showed that the activity of itraconazole was further enhanced when it was formulated in a polyethylene glycol (PEG) solution rather than an aqueous suspension. Systemic *C. albicans* infection also showed an excellent response to either oral or parenteral administration of itraconazole (56).

Pharmaceutics

Itraconazole is commonly available as 100-mg capsules (Sporanox, Janssen).

Pharmacokinetics

Itraconazole is highly concentrated in lipid-rich tissue, poorly soluble in aqueous solution, but well absorbed orally, especially when administered with a meal and formulated in PEG (96). A single 200-mg oral dose produces a peak serum level of about 0.3 μg/ml, far below that of ketoconazole or fluconazole (97). This low serum level can be substantially increased by multiple long-term dosing; the same 200-mg/day oral dose, when administered for 2 weeks, produced a 3.5 μg/ml serum level in the successful treatment of a patient with *A. flavus* scleritis (95). Although experiments with rabbits showed poor penetration of oral itraconazole at 80 mg/kg into the cornea, aqueous humor, and vitreous as compared with that of fluconazole and ketoconazole in a model of *Candida* endophthalmitis, itraconazole was at least as effective as the other two drugs when treatment was initiated 24 hours postinoculation (98).

The $t_{1/2}$ of itraconazole is approximately 15 hours and increases with both dose and duration of treatment, stabilizing at about 34 to 42 hours after 2 weeks of administration (73). Itraconazole has a very high affinity for tissues, which explains why it is just as effective as fluconazole, which produces a higher plasma concentration but a lower tissue distribution (97). It is extensively metabolized in the liver, and at least one of its metabolites, hydroxyitraconazole, has some antifungal activity (73).

Side Effects

Itraconazole has also shown a relatively low level of toxicity, with the most common side effect being GI upset, occurring in about 5% of patients treated with the drug (68). Dosages as high as 50 to 100 mg/day for 2 weeks had no effect on testosterone or cortisol levels in healthy male volunteers (96). In dog studies, dosages of 10 mg/kg were neither teratogenic nor embryotoxic; however, such effects were observed at dosages of 40 mg/kg or more (99). Unlike almost all other antifungal agents, itraconazole appeared to have no hepatic cytochrome P450 enzyme-inducing effects when tested in rodents, even at dosages as high as 160 mg/kg/day for 7 days (97). Indirect studies in human volunteers suggested similar findings for dosages as high as 200 mg/day for 35 days (97). However, other investigators have observed side effects such as hypertriglyceridemia, hypokalemia and, rarely, edema, decreased libido, and gynecomastia at dosages of about 400 mg/day; these effects may be endocrine related but do not appear to be dose dependent (68). Although itraconazole is transmitted in breast milk, the dose received by the baby is less than 1% of that received by the mother, suggesting that itraconazole is safe for nursing mothers (100).

FLUCONAZOLE

The chemical structure of fluconazole is shown below:

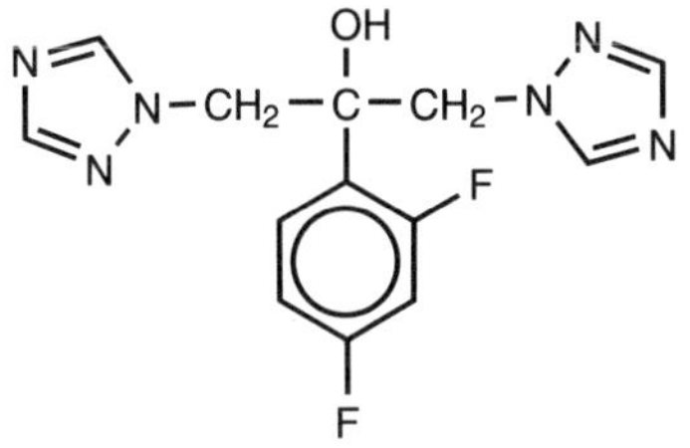

Clinical Pharmacology

Fluconazole is the third important member of the triazole antifungal group. In vitro determination of azole activity, and that of fluconazole in particular, has demonstrated poor correlation with in vivo results. Laboratory data have been compiled on the activity of fluconazole against a wide variety of fungi. Fluconazole is generally regarded as having good activity against *Candida* sp (101) and *C. neoformans,* but data on other types of fungi are so varied and/or discrepant with in vivo results that it is nearly impossible to establish a standard spectrum of activity for fluconazole. To complicate matters further, strong evidence shows that resistance subsequent to prolonged treatment with fluconazole in particular may make some fungal infections unresponsive to therapy (59,60, 102). In one study, the efficacy of fluconazole in treating endophthalmitis with disseminated candidiasis in rabbits decreased and was eventually lost between day 17 and day 24 of treatment, whereas amphotericin was able to maintain its therapeutic effect throughout the treatment (102). Filler et al. (102) suggested that this was due to the increasing prevalence of fungal pathogens resistant to fluconazole.

Pharmaceutics

Fluconazole is available commercially as 50-, 100-, and 200-mg tablets (Diflucan, Roerig) and as 2-mg/ml solutions in saline or dextrose (Diflucan IV, Roerig).

Pharmacokinetics

Fluconazole, because of its structural modifications, has pharmacokinetic properties that render it unique among the azoles. The substitution of a second triazole ring decreases protein binding and increases serum concentration, and the addition of a difluorophenyl group instead of the 2, 4-halo-substituted moiety increases water solubility (103). As a result of these modifications, fluconazole has a high body water distribution (V_d = 0.7 L/kg), a relatively long $t_{1/2}$ of at least 30 hours, and a bioavailability of approximately 90% after oral or intravenous dosing (104). Fluconazole is eliminated in the urine (80% renal excretion), and steady state concentrations are reached in 5 to 10 days. A 1-mg/kg oral dose in humans reaches a level of about 1.4 μg/ml in 4 hours, with absorption minimally affected by gastric pH (57,73). Oral fluconazole appears to penetrate well into the ocular fluids, reaching levels that are approximately 65% of serum levels in the presence of inflammation, but studies examining the response of endophthalmitis to fluconazole treatment are still limited (98). Fluconazole is available as a tablet and as a 2-mg/L aqueous solution for intravenous use, which should not exceed 200 mg/hour (13). It is also available as a 1% solution in sterile water for topical use. Dosages vary from 50 to 400 mg/day and should be decreased in the presence of renal failure to about 50% of the normal dose when creatinine clearance is measured at 21 to 50 ml/min and to about 25% of the normal dose when creatinine clearance is less than 21 ml/min (69).

Side Effects

Like itraconazole, fluconazole appears to be well tolerated by most patients. Indeed, it is generally recommended for patients who cannot tolerate amphotericin (69). The most common side effect is GI upset, reported by about 5% of all patients treated with fluconazole; other side effects include headaches, rash, diarrhea, vomiting, flatulence, and hepatotoxicity in a small percentage of patients (68). Overall, side effects are reported by about 16% of patients receiving between 50 and 400 mg fluconazole daily for 7 days or more (68). Extremely rare cases of anaphylaxis, Stevens-Johnson syndrome, and thrombocytopenia have been reported (105–107).

Fluconazole is generally considered intermediate between ketoconazole and itraconazole in its ability to interact with drug-metabolizing enzymes (13). At oral doses of 300 mg/day or more, fluconazole greatly increased cyclosporine's trough concentration : daily dose ratio in a dose-dependent manner in a renal transplant patient (108). Obviously, such an interaction is especially significant since transplant patients receiving intensive immunosuppressive therapy frequently require antifungal treatment. Fluconazole also appears to decrease the metabolism of warfarin at a dosage of 200 mg/day and phenytoin at a dosage of 400 mg/day (109,110). Other reported drug interactions include a significant increase in serum concentration of tolbutamide and glyburide in the presence of fluconazole, although not all patients became hypoglycemic (111). Rifampin has been reported to increase the metabolism of fluconazole (112).

Other Triazoles

Triazoles other than itraconazole and fluconazole include vibunazole, saperconazole, and ICI 195, 739 (Table 2). Vibunazole is a triazole that can be used both orally and topically. In vitro, it has shown activity against most pathogenic fungi, including *Fusarium,* but has shown less activity against *Aspergillus, Zygomycetes,* and *S. schenkii* (75). Contrasting with these data are reports that vibunazole may have activity in a murine model of experimental aspergillosis (113). Other models suggest vibunazole is not as effective as ketoconazole in treating disseminated *Coccidiomycoses, Paracoccidiodomycoses,* or *Blastomycoses* in mice, but was as effective as or more effective than ketoconazole in *A. fumigatus, C. albicans,* and *C. neoformans* systemic infections (75).

Vibunazole has been shown to be absorbed almost completely when administered orally. A 400-mg dose in humans is subject to first-order absorption and exhibits a peak serum concentration between 2 and 5 μg/ml with a $t_{\frac{1}{2}}$ of about 2.5 hours in the β-phase and of 12 to 15 hours in the γ-phase (114). Its serum levels do not appear to be affected by gastric pH, unlike those of ketoconazole (115).

In a study of dogs, vibunazole doses of 80 mg/kg or more produced no toxic effects; in men, plasma testosterone levels do not appear to be affected by the vibunazole and enzyme induction apparently does not occur, as shown by serial measurements of peak plasma concentrations of vibunazole in human volunteers (114).

Saperconazole is a triazole with a broad spectrum of activity against many yeasts, including most species of *Candida, Rhodotorula,* dermatophytes, and especially against the various *Aspergillus* species, but lacking activity, at least in vitro, against *Fusarium, Scopulariopsis,* and the zygomycetes (116).

Saperconazole is highly lipophilic and appears to penetrate the cornea well. A single drop of 0.25% saperconazole produced a peak level of 2.32 μg/g cornea with intact epithelium; in debrided corneas, the peak level was 13 μg/g. Subconjunctival administration of saperconazole resulted in higher concentrations for both normal and debrided corneas, whereas oral administration resulted in low concentrations in all ocular tissues (117). The bioavailability of the drug after topical administration in the cornea was estimated at approximately 44%.

ICI 195, 739 is a new triazole with fungicidal activity against experimental *B. dermatitidis* and greater potency than ketoconazole, fluconazole, and itraconazole in experimental murine candidiasis in mice (75). It also appears to have in vivo activity against *C. neoformans* and *A. fumigatus,* as well as *Trichophyton* species (75).

Although it most likely works by the same mechanism as the other azoles, ICI 195, 739 appears to penetrate host cells of *Candida* better than either ketoconazole or fluconazole and may also have a better safety profile (75).

In vitro studies showed that the concentrations of ICI 195, 739 causing 50% inhibition (IC_{50}) of the main enzymes involved in mammalian steroid metabolism (cholesterol side chain cleavage enzyme, steroid 17- and 11-hydroxylases, and placental aromatase) were greater than the respective IC_{50} values for ketoconazole, implying a greater specificity of ICI 195, 739 for the fungal α-demethylase (118).

D0870 is the enantiomer of ICI 195, 739. This drug has been demonstrated to prolong survival in cases of experimental murine blastomycoses and also shows good in vitro activity against *C. albicans* and *C. neoformans,* with about 90% of tested strains having MIC values of .03 μg/ml although, as the authors of this study noted, data were strongly influenced by testing conditions such as inoculum density, type of medium and buffer, and incubation time (119,120).

Antimetabolites

FLUCYTOSINE

History

Flucytosine is a fluorinated cytosine analogue first synthesized as a potential antineoplastic agent. Its chemical structure is shown below:

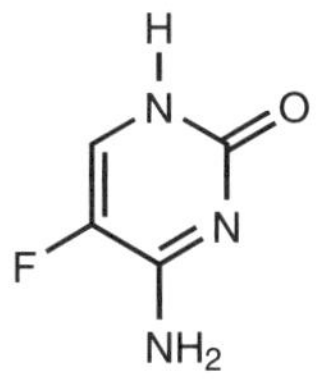

Pharmacology

Flucytosine is taken up into fungal cells by cytosine permease, deaminated by cytosine deaminase to 5-fluorouracil (5-FU), and converted to 5-fluorodeoxyuridine monophosphate, which is a competitive inhibitor of thymidylate synthetase, involved in DNA synthesis (121). By replacing uracil in the nucleotide pool, 5-FU also directly disrupts protein synthesis (69).

One of the major problems with the use of flucytosine has been the development of resistance among many strains of fungi. Resistance may be due to a decrease in the cytosine permease activity, a decrease in the enzymes involved in flucytosine metabolism, and/or constituents competing with flucytosine and its metabolites (69). As a result, flucytosine is usually not administered as a single agent, but instead is administered in combination with another antifungal agent, most commonly amphotericin-B. This combination has also been suggested to have synergistic effects.

Clinical Pharmacology

Flucytosine shows markedly selective activity against pathogenic yeasts (e.g., *Candida, C. neoformans*), and only moderate activity against *Aspergillus* and the agents of chromoblastomycoses (e.g., *Phialophora*) (10). Most strains of yeasts have MIC values that have been tested at less than or equal to 1 μg/ml (10). Resistance of common fungal pathogens has often been measured as unacceptably high. One study showed that the frequency of resistance among varied strains to a concentration of 64 μg/ml flucytosine was on the order of 10^{-7} for *C. albicans,* 10^{-6} for *C. neoformans,* and 10^{-4} for *A. fumigatus* (122). The same study showed no evidence of deficient cytosine permease in the resistant strains. Little or no cross-resistance of 5-flucytosine (5-FC) resistant strains has been observed with other antifungal agents (14).

Pharmaceutics

Flucytosine is available in 250- and 500-mg capsules (Ancobon, Roche).

Pharmacokinetics

5-FC has a low molecular weight and moderate aqueous solubility. It has a high bioavailability secondary to excellent GI absorption. Peak concentrations after an oral dose of 2 g are reached in 2 to 4 hours (10). The drug is excreted by the kidneys 90% unchanged; its $t_{1/2}$ is approximately 4 hours (10). Anterior chamber levels of 10 to 40 μg/ml have been measured after oral administration of 200 mg/kg/day (1). Despite flucytosine's moderate solubility in water and relatively high tolerance in the eye, its topical and subconjunctival administration has been reported to produce disappointingly low intraocular levels (1).

Side Effects

In general, toxicity of flucytosine is relatively low due to the fungal specificity of the deamination step required to convert 5-FC to 5-FU (123). However, cases of enterocolitis and bone marrow and hepatic toxicity may be secondary to 5-FU formation in the gut by endogenous *Escherichia coli* (10,17). Toxicity has been shown to correlate with plasma levels, which should be maintained between 20 and 100 μg/ml (124). Dosages of 150 mg/kg every 6 hours have been recommended, and yield a 50 to 80 mg/L serum concentration after 1 to 2 hours; the $t_{1/2}$ has been measured at 3 to 5 hours (69). Dosing should correspondingly be decreased in cases of renal failure.

Other Miscellaneous Antifungal Drugs

GRISEOFULVIN

The chemical structure of griseofulvin is shown below:

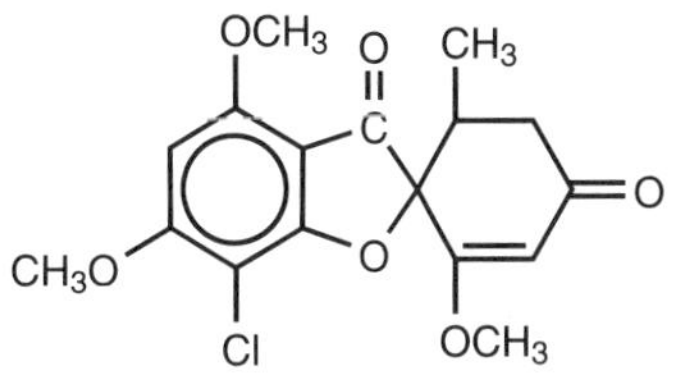

History

Griseofulvin was first discovered in 1939 by Oxford et al., who had received a strain of *Penicillium griseofulvum* from a colleague. Not until 20 years later, however, did the utility of griseofulvin become apparent, when Genteles

(125) showed it to be effective in treating ringworm in guinea pigs.

Pharmacology

Griseofulvin is believed to exert a fungistatic action by disrupting the mitotic spindle structure, thereby arresting the fungal cell in the M-phase (3).

Clinical Pharmacology

Griseofulvin remains the oral drug of choice for dermatophytoses, including tinea corporis, tinea pedis, tinea capitis, and tinea cruris (126). In addition, griseofulvin has been suggested to exert a therapeutic effect in cases of mycosis fungoids, eosinophilic fasciitis, lichen planus, progressive systemic sclerosis, and Raynaud's phenomenon (126).

Pharmaceutics

Griseofulvin is available in 125- and 250-mg capsules, in 250- or 500-mg tablets, and as an oral suspension (125 mg/5 ml). (Fulvicin-U/F, Grifulvin V, Grisactin). For enhanced absorption, griseofulvin also is available in an "ultra-microsized" particulate form with PEG added (Fulvicin P/G, Grisactin Ultra, Gris-PEG), but the microsize preparation may actually achieve higher concentrations over time than the ultra-microsize preparation (127).

Pharmacokinetics

After oral administration, Griseofulvin becomes highly concentrated in keratin precursor cells, especially in diseased skin (126), but is also present in high levels in liver, fat, and skeletal muscles (126). Its $t_{\frac{1}{2}}$ varies among individuals (9 to 24 hours), with most of the drug eliminated either in the urine or feces (126).

Side Effects

The most common side effects of griseofulvin are headaches, nausea, vomiting, abdominal cramps, and diarrhea. Ingesting the drug with meals usually relieves symptoms (126). A photosensitivity reaction has also been reported with griseofulvin (12).

SQUALENE EPOXIDASE INHIBITORS

Pharmacology

Another group of antifungal drugs consists of the squalene epoxidase inhibitors, which inhibit the transformation of squalene to 23 oxidosqualene, a step involved in ergosterol biosynthesis that is not dependent on cytochrome P450 (Fig. 1) Therefore, squalene epoxidase inhibitors are suggested to be less likely to cause the altered steroidal hormone levels caused by azole administration (128). The most extensively studied squalene epoxidase inhibitors are the allylamines, which include naftifine and terbinafine, and the thiocarbamates, which include tolnaftate and tolciclate. In addition, butenafine is a newer squalene epoxidase inhibitor that has shown a broad spectrum of activity. These inhibitors are considered highly fungicidal against dermatophytes, but are not clinically useful against *Candida* (129). Naftifine is a topical antimycotic with a wide range of activity against pathogenic fungi, including dermatophytes and yeasts. In addition to its direct antifungal effect, naftifine appears to have antiinflammatory properties. When added to human neutrophils, naftifine caused decreased chemotaxis and respiratory burst activity, perhaps by exerting the same effect on the neutrophil membrane as on the fungal cell membrane (130).

Terbinafine is characterized by the addition of a triple bond and branching of the adjacent alkyl side chain to form a tert-butylacetylene group, which increases potency (i.e., decreases K_i) and oral efficacy and broadens the spectrum (131). Terbinafine is fungicidal against dermatophytes (with MIC values far lower than those of naftifine, ketoconazole, or itraconazole), *Aspergillus* and *C. parapsilosis*, and also shows excellent activity against *H. capsulatum* and *C. neoformans* (128,131).

Unlike naftifine, both oral and topical terbinafine are well-absorbed. Terbinafine is metabolized in the liver, but does not appear to alter disposition of other hepatically metabolized drugs (131).

The squalene epoxidase inhibitors exhibit a high degree of selectivity. The ratio of the concentration of terbinafine needed to inhibit mammalian cholesterol synthesis to that required to inhibit ergosterol synthesis is about 4,000 to 1, whereas for ketoconazole it is only 160 to 1 (131). Animal studies have shown no embryotoxic or mutagenic effects of terbinafine (128).

Pharmaceutics

Naftifine is available as a 1% cream or gel (Naftin, Allergan, Herbert), and terbinafine is available as a 1% cream (below) (Lamisil, Sandoz Pharmaceutical).

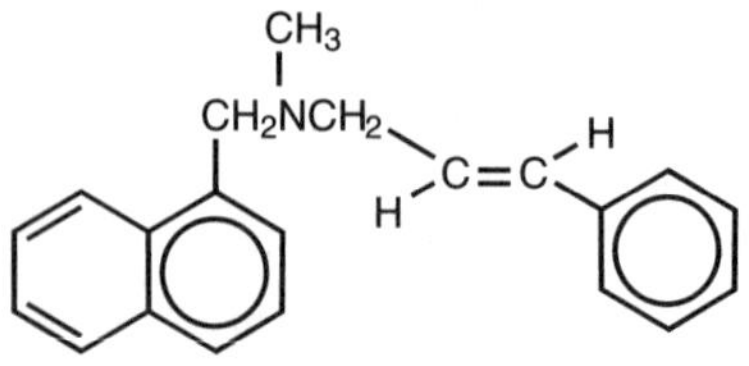

CH_3
CH_2NCH_2 H
H C=C

Tolnaftate (below) and tolciclate most likely have the same mechanism of activity as the allylamines, although in one in vitro study of *C. albicans,* the allylamines showed measurable growth inhibitory activity and the thiocarbamates did not (129). Georgopapadakou and Bertasso (129) also showed that the ability of tolnaftate and that of tolciclate to inhibit ergosterol synthesis varied greatly as did their abilities in comparison with those of allylamines.

S
NCO
H_3C
CH_3

Butenafine is a benzylamine squalene epoxidase inhibitor which, unlike both the allylamines and thiocarbamates, has shown good activity against *Candida* as well as *Cryptococcus* species and dimorphic fungi such as *S. schenkii.* At low concentrations (less than 0.1 μg/ml) butenafine markedly inhibits ergosterol biosynthesis, but only at higher concentrations (more than 12.5 μg/ml), when butenafine exerts a direct membrane-damaging effect, is a correlation apparent between anticandidal activity and drug levels (132). Therefore, this latter mechanism has been postulated to play the more important role in butenafine's anti-candidal activity, especially against species such as *C. glabrata,* which can survive with low ergosterol content (131).

MORPHOLINES

Morpholines are the last main group of antifungal agents. The two members of this group are fenpropimorph (currently marketed as an agrofungicide) and amorolfine, which has shown efficacy in vaginal candidiasis. These compounds act at two sites, the $\Delta^8\Delta^7$-isomerase and the Δ^{14}-reductase, to inhibit sterol synthesis, changing membrane fluidity and most likely altering chitin deposition as well (133). In vitro, they have shown good activity against the yeasts *C. albicans,* other *Candida* sp, and *C. neoformans,* as well as dimorphic fungi such as *H. capsulatum,* but lesser activity against *Fusarium, Aspergillus,* and *Zygomycetes* (133).

REFERENCES

1. Jones BR. Principles in the management of oculomycosis (Jackson Memorial Lecture). *Am J Ophthalmol* 1975;79:7119–7151.
2. O'Brien TP, Green WR. Fungus infections of the eye and periocular tissues. In: Garner A, Klintworth GK, eds. *Pathobiology of ocular disease: a dynamic approach,* part A, 2nd ed. New York: Marcel Dekker, 1994;299–333.
3. Goodman LS, Gilman AZ, Gilman AG, eds. *Goodman and Gilman's the pharmacological basis of therapeutics,* 8th ed. New York: MacMillan, 1990;1165–1181.
4. Braitberg J, Elberg S, Maddock J, Kobayashi G, Schlesinger D, Maddock G. Stimulatory, permeabilizing, and toxic effects of amphotericin B on L-cells. *Antimicrob Agents Chemother* 1984;26: 892–897.
5. Bolard J, Legrand P, Heitz F, Cybulska V. One-sided action of amphotericin B on cholesterol-containing membranes is determined by its self-association in the medium. *Biochemistry* 1991;30:5707–5715.
6. Braitberg J, Elberg S, Schwartz DR, Vertut-Croquin A, Schlesinger D, Kobayashi GS, Medoff G. Involvement of oxidative damage in erythrocyte lysis induced by amphotericin B. *Antimicrob Agents Chemother* 1985;27:172–176.
7. Martin E, Stuben A, Gorz A, Weller U, Bhakdi S. Novel aspect of amphotericin B action: accumulation in human monocytes potentiates killing of phagocytosed *Candida albicans. Antimicrob Agents Chemother* 1994;38:13–22.
8. Pallister CJ, Johnson EM, Warnock DW, Elliot PJ, Reeves DF. *In vitro* effects of liposome-encapsulated amphotericin-B (AmBisome) and amphotericin-B deoxycholate (Fungizone) on the phagocytic and candidacidal function of human polymorphonuclear leukocytes. *J Antimicrob Chemother* 1992;30:313–320.
9. O'Day DM, Robinson R, Head WS. Efficacy of antifungal agents in the cornea. *Invest Ophthalmol Vis Sci* 1983;24:1098–1102.
10. Drouhet E, Dupont B. Evolution of antifungal agents: past, present, and future. *Rev Infect Dis* 1987;9(suppl 1):4–14.
11. Khoo SH, Bond J, Denning DW. Administering amphotericin B: a practical approach. *J Antimicrob Chemother* 1994;32:203–213.
12. Patel A, Hemady R, Rodrigues M, Rajagopalan S, Elman M. Endogenous *Fusarium* endophthalmitis in a patient with acute lymphocytic leukemia. *Am J Ophthalmol* 1994;117:363–368.
13. Kowalski SF, Dixon D. Fluconazole: a new antifungal agent. *Clin Pharm* 1991;10:179–194.
14. Iwata TK. Drug resistance in human pathogenic fungi. *Eur J Epidemiol* 1992;8:407–421.
15. Wood TO, Tuberville AW, Monnett R. Keratomycosis and amphotericin-B. 1985;83:397–409.
16. O'Day DM, Head WS, Robinson RD, Clanton JA. Bioavailability and penetration of topical amphotericin-B in the anterior segment of the rabbit eye. *J Ocul Pharmacol* 1986;2:371–378.
17. Johns KJ, O'Day D. Pharmacologic management of keratomycoses. *Surv Ophthalmol* 1988;11:178–188.
18. O'Day DM, Smith R, Stevens JB, Williams TE, Robinson RD, Head WS. Toxicity and pharmacokinetics of subconjunctival amphotericin B. An experimental study. Department of Ophthalmology, Vanderbilt University School of Medicine, Nashville, Tennessee.
19. Brod RD, Flynn HW Jr, Clarkson JG, Pflugfelder SC, Culbertson WW, Miller D. Endogenous *Candida* endophthalmitis. Management without intravenous amphotericin B. *Ophthalmology* 1990;97:666–672.
20. Gross JG. Endogenous *Aspergillus*-induced endophthalmitis. *Redman* 1992;12:341–345.
21. McDonnell PJ, McDonnell JM, Brown RH, Green WR. Ocular involvement in patients with fungal infections. *Ophthalmology* 1985; 92:206–209.
22. Gallis HA, Drew R, Pickard W. Amphotericin B: 30 years of clinical experience. *Rev Infect Dis* 1990;12:308–329.
23. Axelrod AJ, Gholam P. Intravitreal amphotericin B treatment of experimental fungal endophthalmitis. *Am J Ophthalmol* 1973;76:584–588.
24. Sarosi GA. Amphotericin B. *Postgrad Med* 1990;88:151–166.
25. Foster C, Lass J, Moran-Wallace K, Giovanoni R. Ocular toxicity of topical antifungal agents. *Arch Ophthalmol* 1981;99:1081–1084.
26. Ellis W, Sobel R, Nielsen S. Leukoencephalopathy in patients treated with amphotericin B methylester. *J Infect Dis* 1982;146: 125–137.
27. Souri EN, Green WR. Intravitreal amphotericin B toxicity. *Am J Ophthalmol* 1974;78:77–81.
28. Axelrod AJ, Gholam P, Apple D. Toxicity of intravitreal injection of amphotericin B. *Am J Ophthalmol* 1973;76:578–583.
29. Ho PC, Tolentino FI, Baker AS. Successful treatment of exogenous *Aspergillus endophthalmitis:* a case report. *Br J Ophthalmol* 1984; 68:412–415.
30. Maddux MS, Barriere SL. A review of complications of amphotericin B therapy: recommendations for prevention and management. *Drug Intell Clin Pharm* 1980;177–181.
31. Butler WT, Bennett J, Alling D, et al. Nephrotoxicity of amphotericin B: early and late effects in 81 patients. *Ann Intern Med* 1964; 61:175–187.
32. Miller RP, Bates JH. Amphotericin-B toxicity. A follow-up report of 53 patients. *Ann Intern Med* 1969;71:1089–1095.

33. Branch RA. Prevention of amphotericin B-induced renal impairment. *Arch Intern Med* 1988;148:2389–2394.
34. Gardner ML, Godley PJ, Wasan SM. Sodium loading treatment for amphotericin-B-induced nephrotoxicity. *Drug Intell Clin Pharm* 1990;24:940–946.
35. Moreau P, Milpied N, Fayette N, Ramee JF, Harousseau JL. Reduced renal toxicity and improved clinical tolerance of amphotericin-B mixed with intralipid compared with conventional amphotericin-B in neutropenic patients. *J Antimicrob Chemother* 1992;30:535–541.
36. Ringden O, Meunier F, Tollemar J, Ricci P, et al. Efficacy of amphotericin-B encapsulated in liposomes (AmBisome) in the treatment of invasive fungal infections in immunocompromised patients. *J Antimicrob Chemother* 1991;28:73–82.
37. Gokhale PC, Barapatre RJ, Advani SH, Kshirsagar NA, Pandya SK. Successful treatment of disseminated candidiasis resistant to amphotericin-B by liposomal amphotericin-B: a case report. *J Cancer Res Clin Oncol* 1993;119:569–571.
38. Perfect J, Wright K. Amphotericin B lipid complex in the treatment of experimental cryptococcal meningitis and disseminated candidosis. *J Antimicrob Chemother* 1994;33:73–81.
39. Medoff G. Antifungal action of rifampin. *Rev Infect Dis* 1983;5 (suppl 3):S614–S619.
40. Medoff G, Kobayashi GS, Kwan CN, Schlessinger D, Venkov P. Potentiation of rifampicin and 5-fluorocytosine as antifungal antibiotics by amphotericin B. *Proc Natl Acad Sci USA* 1972;69:196–199.
41. Fujita NK, Edwards J. Combined *in vitro* effect of amphotericin B and rifampin on *Cryptococcus neoformans. Antimicrob Agents Chemother* 1981;19:196–198.
42. Shadomy S. *In vitro* and *in vivo* studies on synergistic antifungal activity. *Contrib Microbiol Immunol* 1977;4:147–157.
43. Edwards J, Morrison J, Henderson D, Montgomerie J. Combined effective amphotericin B and rifampin on *Candida* species. *Antimicrob Agents Chemother* 1980;17:484:487.
44. Stern GA, Okumoto M, Smolin G. Combined amphotericin B and rifampin treatment of experimental *Candida albicans* keratitis. *Arch Ophthalmol* 1979;97:721–722.
45. Beggs WH, Sarosi G. Further evidence for sequential action of amphotericin B and a 5-fluorocytosine against *Candida albicans. Chemotherapy* 1982;28:341–344.
46. Braitberg J, Kobayashi D, Medoff J, Kobayashi G. Antifungal action of amphotericin B in combination with other polyene or imidazole antibiotics. *J Infect Dis* 1982;146:138–146.
47. Mason J, Parker J. Subconjunctival miconazole and anterior segment blastomycosis. *Am J Ophthalmol* 1993;116:506–507.
48. Edwards G, LaTouche CJP. The treatment of bronchopulmonary mycoses with a new antibiotic—Pimaricin. *Lancet* 1964;1:1349–1353.
49. O'Day DM. Selection of appropriate antifungal therapy. *Cornea* 1987;6:235–245.
50. Jones DB, Forster R, Rebell G. *Fusarium solani* keratitis treated with natamycin (Pimaricin). *Arch Ophthalmol* 1972;88:147–154.
51. O'Day DM, Head WS, Robinson R, Clanton JA. Corneal penetration of topical amphotericin B and natamycin. *Curr Eye Res* 1986;15:877–882.
52. Vanden Bossche H, Marichal P. Mode of action of anti-*Candida* drugs: focus on terconazole and other ergosterol biosynthesis inhibitors. *Am J Obstet Gynecol* 1991;165:1193–1199.
53. Kelly SL, Rower J, Watson PF. Molecular genetic studies on the mode of action of azole antifungal agents. *Biochem Soc Trans* 1991;19:796–798.
54. Vanden Bossche H, Marichal P, le Jeune L, Coene MG, Garrens J, Cools W. Effects of itraconazole on cytochrome P-450-dependent sterol 14 α-demethylation and reduction of 3-ketosteroids in *Cryptococcus neoformans. Antimicrob Agents Chemother* 1993;37:2101–2105.
55. Yamaguchi H, Abe S, Tokuda Y. Immunomodulating activity of antifungal drugs *Ann NY Acad Sci* 1993;685:447–457.
56. Van Cutsem J, Van Gerven F, Janssen P. Activity of orally, topically and parenterally administered itraconazole in the treatment of superficial and deep mycoses: animal models. *Rev Infect Dis* 1987;9 (suppl 1):S15–S32.
57. Humphrey MJ, Jevons S, Tarbit MH. Pharmacokinetic evaluation of UK-49,858, a metabolically stable triazole antifungal drug in animals and humans. *Antimicrob Agents Chemother* 1985;28:648–653.
58. Odds FC, Cheesman SL, Abbott AB. Antifungal effects of fluconazole (UK 49858), a new triazole antifungal, *in vitro. J Antimicrob Chemother* 1986;18:473–478.
59. Sandver P, Bjorneklett A, Maeland A, Norwegians Yeast Study Group. Susceptibilities of Norwegian *Candida albicans* strains to fluconazole: emergence of resistance. *Antimicrob Agents Chemother* 1993;37:2443–2448.
60. Hitchcock TC, Pye GW, Troke PF, Johnson EM, Warnock DW. Fluconazole resistance in *Candida glabrata. Antimicrob Agents Chemother* 1993;37:1962–1965.
61. Shigematsu ML, Uno J, Arai T. Effect of ketoconazole on isolated mitochondria from *Candida albicans. Antimicrob Agents Chemother* 1982;21:919–924.
62. Uno J, Shigematsu M, Arai T. Primary site of action of ketoconazole on *Candida albicans. Antimicrob Agents Chemother* 1982;21:912–918.
63. Hemady RK, Chu W, Foster CS. Intraocular penetration of ketaconazole in rabbits. *Cornea* 1992;11:329–333.
64. Heel RC, Brogden RN, Carmine A, Morley P, Speight TM, Avery G. Ketoconazole: a review of its therapeutic efficacy in superficial and systemic fungal infections. *Drugs* 1982;23:1–36.
65. Oji EO. Ketoconazole: a new imidazole antifungal agent has both prophylactic potential and therapeutic efficacy in keratomycoses of rabbits. *Int Ophthalmol* 1982;5:163–167.
66. Komadina TG, Wilkes TD, Shock JP, Ulmer WC, Jackson J, Bradsher R. Treatment of *Aspergillus fumigatus* keratitis in rabbits with oral and topical ketoconazole. *Am J Ophthalmol* 1985;99:476–479.
67. Torres M, Mohamed J, Cavazos-Adams H, Martinez L. Topical ketoconazole for fungal keratitis. *Am J Ophthalmol* 1985;100:293–298.
68. Sugar A. Fluconazole and itraconazole: current status and prospects for antifungal therapy. *Curr Clin Top Infect Dis* 1993;74–98.
69. Lyman CA, Walsh TJ. Systemically administered antifungal agents. *Drugs* 1992;44:9–45.
70. Daneshmend T, Warnock DW, Ene MD, Johnson E, Potten MR, Richardson MD, Williams PJ. Influence of food on the pharmacokinetics of ketaconazole. *Antimicrob Agents Chemother* 1984;25:1–3.
71. Oji EO. Study of ketoconazole toxicity in rabbit cornea and conjunctiva. *Int Ophthalmol* 1982;5:169–174.
72. Yoshizumi M, Banihashemi A. Experimental intravitreal ketoconazole in DMSO. *Retina* 1988;8:210–215.
73. Bodey JT. Azole antifungal agents. *Clin Infect Dis* 1992;14(suppl 1):161–169.
74. Pont A, Graybill JR, Craven PC, Galgiani JN, Dismukes WE. High-dose ketoconazole therapy and adrenal and testicular function in humans. *Arch Intern Med* 1984;144:2150–2153.
75. Fromtling RA. Overview of medically important antifungal azole derivatives. *Clin Microbiol Rev* 1988;1:187–217.
76. Bloom PA, Laidlaw DA, Easty DL, Warnock DW. Treatment failure in a case of fungal keratitis caused by *Pseudallesheria boydii. Br J Ophthalmol* 1992;76:367–368.
77. Bouchard CS, Chacko B, Cupples H, Cavanagh HD, Mathers W. Surgical treatment for a case of postoperative *Pseudallesheria boydii* endophthalmitis. *Ophthalmic Surg* 1991;22:98–101.
78. Foster C, Stefanyszyn M. Intraocular penetration of miconazole in rabbits. *Arch Ophthalmol* 1979;97:1703–1706.
79. Tolentino F, Foster CS, Lahuv M, Lui AR. Toxicity of intravitreal miconazole. *Arch Ophthalmol* 1982;100:1504–1509.
80. Moody MR, Young VM, Morris MJ, Schimpff SC. *In vitro* activities of miconazole, miconazole nitrate, and ketaconazole alone and combined with rifampin against *Candida* species and *Torulopsis glabrata* recovered from cancer patients. *Antimicrob Agents Chemother* 1980;17:871–875.
81. Jones BR, Clayton YM, Oji EO. Recognition and chemotherapy of oculomycoses. *Postgrad Med J* 1979;55:625–628.
82. Beggs WH. Rapid fungicidal action of tioconazole and miconazole [Letter]. *Micropathology* 1987;97:187–188.
83. Singh SM, Sharma S, Chatterjee PK. Clinical and experimental mycotic keratitis caused by *Aspergillus terreus* and the effect of subconjunctival oxiconazole treatment in the rabbit model. *Mycopathologia* 1990;112:127–137.

84. Zirngibl L, Fischer J, Jahn U, Thiele K. Stucture-activity relationships of 2-(1H-imidazol-1-yl) vinyl ethers. *Ann NY Acad Sci* 1988;544:63–73.
85. Odds FC, Webster CE, Abbott AB. Antifungal relative inhibition factors: BAY1-9139, bifoconazole, butoconazole, isoconazole, itraconazole (R 51211), oxiconazole, R. 14-4767/002, sulconazole, terconazole, and vibunazole (BAY n-7133) compared *in vitro* with nine established antifungal agents. *J Antimicrob Chemother* 1984; 14:105–114.
86. Beggs WH. Influence of growth phase on the susceptibility of *Candida albicans* to butoconazole, oxiconazole, and sulconazole. *J Antimicrob Chemother* 1985;16:397–399.
87. Hernandez Molina JM, Llosa J, Martinez Brocal A, Ventosa A. *In vitro* activity of cloconazole, sulconazole, butoconazole, isoconazole, fenticonazole, and five other antifungal agents against clinical isolates of *Candida albicans* and *Candida* species. *Mycopathology* 1992;118:15–21.
88. Costa A, Veronese M, Ruggeri P, Valenti A. Ultrastructural findings of *Candida albicans* blastoconidia submitted to the action of fenticonazole. *Arzneimittelforschung* 1989;39:230–233.
89. Ernest JM. Topical antifungal agents. *Obstet Gynecol Clin North Am* 1992;19:587–607.
90. Tolman EL, Isaacson D, Rosenthall M, McGuire JL, Van Cutsem J, Borgers M, Vanden Bossche H. Anticandidal activities of terconazole, a broad spectrum antimycotic. *Antimicrob Agents Chemother* 1986;29:986–991.
91. Pfaller MA, Rile J, Koerner T. Effects of terconazole and other azole antifungal agents on the sterol and carbohydrate composition of *Candida albicans. Diag Microbiol Infect Dis* 1990;113:31–35.
92. Chiew Y, Sullivan P, Shepherd M. The effects of ergosterol and alcohols on germ tube formation and chitin synthase in *Candida albicans. Can J Biochem* 1982;60:15–20.
93. Braun P, Calderon R. Chitin synthesis in *Candida albicans:* comparison of yeast and hyphal forms. *J Bacteriol* 1978;133:1472.
94. Borgers M, Van de Ven M. Degenerative changes in fungi after intraconazole treatment. *Rev Infect Dis* 1987;9(suppl 1):33–43.
95. Carlson AN, Foulks J, Perfect J, Kim J. Fungal scleritis after cataract surgery. *Cornea* 1992;11:151–154.
96. Hay RJ. Antifungal therapy and the new azole compounds. *J Antimicrob Chemother* 1991;28(suppl A):35–46.
97. Heykants J, Peer A, Lavrijsen K, Meuldermans W, Woestenborghs R, Cauwenbergh C. Pharmacokinetics of oral antifungals and their clinical implication. *Br J Clin Pharmacol* 1990(suppl 71):50–57.
98. Savani D, Perfect J, Cobo LM, Durack D. Penetration of new azole compounds into the eye and efficacy in experimental *Candida* endophthalmitis. *Antimicrob Agents Chemother* 1987;31:6–10.
99. Van Cauteren H, Heykants J, DeCoster R, Cauwengergh G. Itraconazole: pharmacologic studies in animals and humans *Rev Infect Dis* 1987;9(suppl 1):S43–S46.
100. Heykants J. Discussion: topics of general interest. *Br J Clin Prac Sym Suppl* 1990;(suppl 71):57.
101. Brooks JH, O'Brien TP, Wilhelmus KR, et al. Comparative topical triazole therapy of experimental *Candida albicans* keratitis. *Invest Ophthalmol Vis Sci* 1990;31(suppl):2793.
102. Filler S, Crislip M, Mayer C, Edwards J. Comparison of fluconazole and amphotericin B for treatment of disseminated *Candidiasis* and endophthalmitis in rabbits. *Antimicrob Agents Chemother* 1991;35:288–292.
103. Richardson K, Cooper K, Marriott MS, Tarbit MH, Troke PF, Whittle PJ. Design and evaluation of a systemically active agent, fluconazole. *Ann NY Acad Sci* 1988;544:4–12.
104. Brammer KW, Farrow PR, Faulkner JK. Pharmacokinetics and tissue penetration of fluconazole in humans. *Rev Infect Dis* 1990; 12(suppl 3):S318–326.
105. Neuhaus G, Pavic N, Pletscher M. Anaphylactic reaction after oral fluconazole. *Br Med J* 1991;302:1341.
106. Gussenhoven MJE, Haak A, Peereboom-Wynia JDR, Van't Wout JW. Stevens-Johnson syndrome after fluconazole. *Lancet* 1991;338: 120.
107. Agarwal A, Sakhuja, Chugh KS. Fluconazole-induced thrombocytopenia. *Ann Intern Med* 1990;113:899.
108. Lopez-Gill, Arturo J. Fluconazole-cyclosporin interaction: a dose-dependent effect? *Ann Pharmacother* 1993;27:427–430.
109. Isulska B, Stanbridge T. Fluconazole in the treatment of candidal prosthetic valve endocarditis. *Br Med J* 1988;297:178.
110. Mitchel A, Holland J. Fluconazole and phenytoin: a predictable interaction. *Br Med J* 1989;298:1315.
111. Lazar JD, Wilner KD. Drug interactions with fluconazole. *Rev Infect Dis* 1990;12(suppl 3):S327–S333.
112. Apseloff G, Hilligoss D, Gardner MJ, et al. Induction of fluconazole metabolism by rifampin: *in vivo* study in humans. *J Clin Pharm* 1991;31:358–361.
113. Graybill JR, Kaster SR, Drutz DJ. A treatment of experimental murine aspergillosis with BAYn7133. *J Infect Dis* 1983;148:898–906.
114. Ritter W, Holmwood G, Ahr HJ, Detzer K, Kraatz U, Plempel M, Scherling D, Siefert HM. Vibunazole and its enantiomers. *Ann NY Acad Sci* 1987;544:74–85.
115. Gulpin C, Kelder O, Mattie H, van der Meer JWN, van't Wout J. Pharmacokinetics of vibunazole (BAYn7133) administered orally to healthy subjects. *J Antimicrob Chem* 1985;16:75–79.
116. Otcenasek M. Susceptibility of clinical isolates of fungi to superconazole. *Mycopathologia* 1992;118:179–183.
117. O'Day DM. Ocular pharmacokinetics of saperconazole in rabbits. *Arch Ophthalmol* 1992;110:550–554.
118. Barrett-Bee K, Lees J, Pinder P, Campbell J, Newboult L. Biochemical studies with a novel antifungal agent, ICI 195,739. *Ann NY Acad Sci* 1988;544:231–244.
119. Peng T, Galgiani J. *In vitro* studies of a new antifungal triazole, D0870, against *Candida albicans, Cryptococcus neoformans* and other pathogenic yeasts. *Antimicrob Agents Chemother* 1993;137: 2126–2131.
120. Clemons C, Hansen L, Stevens D. Activities of the triazole D 0870 *in vitro* and against murine blastomycosis. *Antimicrob Agents Chemother* 1993;37:1177–1179.
121. Diasio RB, Bennett JE, Myers CE. Mode of action of 5-fluorocytosine. *Biochem Pharmacol* 1978;27:703–707.
122. Polak A, Scholer HJ. Mode of action of 5-fluorocytosine and mechanisms of resistance. *Chemotherapy* 1975;21:113–130.
123. Polak A. 5-Fluorocytosine—current status with special references to mode of action and drug resistance. *Contrib Microbiol Immunol* 1977;4:158–167.
124. Stevens DA. Discussion: topics of general interest. *Br J Clin Pract* 1990;(suppl 71):57.
125. Genteles JC. Experimental ringworm in guinea pigs: oral treatment with griseofulvin. *Nature* 1958;182:476–477.
126. Araujo OE, Flowers FP, King MM. Griseofulvin: a new look at an old drug. *Drug Intell Clin Pharm* 1990;24:851–854.
127. Straughn AB, Meyer MC, Raghow G, Rotenberg K. Bioavailability of microsize and ultramicrosize griseofulvin products in man. *J Pharmacokinet Biopharm* 1980;8:347–362.
128. Stutz A. Synthesis and structure-activity correlations within allylamine antimycotics. *Ann NY Acad Sci* 1988;544:46–63.
129. Georgopapadakou NH, Bertasso A. Effects of squalene epoxidase inhibitors on *Candida albicans. Antimicrob Agents Chemother* 1992;1779–1781.
130. Solomon BA, Lee WL, Green SC, Suntharalingam K, Fikrig SM, Shakita AR. Modification of neutrophil functions by naftifine. *Br J Dermatol* 1993;128:393–398.
131. Birnbaum J. Pharmacology of the allylamines. *J Am Acad Dermatol* 1990;23:782–785.
132. Iwatani W, Tadashi A, Yamaguchi H. Two mechanisms of butenifine action in *Candida albicans. Antimicrob Agents Chemother* 1993;37: 785–788.
133. Polak A. Mode of action of morpholine derivatives. *Ann NY Acad Sci* 1988;544:221–229.
134. Pont A, Williams PL, Aghar S, Reitz RE, Bochra C, Smith ER, Stevens DA. Ketoconazole blocks testosterone synthesis. *Arch Intern Med* 1982;142:2137–2140.

Textbook of Ocular Pharmacology,
edited by T.J. Zimmerman, et al.
Lippincott–Raven Publishers, Philadelphia © 1997.

CHAPTER 52

Antiallergic Therapies

Mark B. Abelson, Paula J. McGarr, and Kevin P. Richard

Allergic diseases of the eye are among the most common clinical problems involving the external ocular adnexa. These conditions primarily involve the conjunctiva, the continuous mucous membrane lining the eyelids and covering the sclera. Ocular allergic disorders include seasonal and panseasonal allergic conjunctivitis, vernal keratoconjunctivitis (VKC), some cases of giant papillary conjunctivitis (GPC), atopic keratoconjunctivitis (AKC), and drug-induced allergy; patients with these conditions constitute a significant part of an ophthalmologist's practice (1). The atopic predisposition of many of these patients may prime them for ocular involvement. In some of the allergic diseases, such as VKC and AKC, corneal involvement is also part of the disease complex.

Immune hypersensitivity, the basis of allergic disease and other inflammatory disorders, has been divided into four major classes: types I, II, III, and IV (2). Type I hypersensitivity reactions include diseases in which antigen-specific immunoglobulin E (IgE) is responsible for the generation of the immune response through mast cell degranulation and the subsequent release of chemical mediators. Type II responses involve antibody-dependent cell killing by subtypes of T lymphocytes. Diseases associated with antigen–antibody complex deposition in body tissues are classified as type III hypersensitivity responses. Last, type IV reactions are characterized by activity of T lymphocytes and their cytokines, which results in a delayed response (3). As is the case systemically, ocular allergy is principally the result of a type I-mediated response, although type IV mechanisms have been implicated in some cases, such as VKC, drug-induced allergic reactions and GPC.

Type I hypersensitivity reactions, also termed anaphylactic, immediate, or IgE-mediated reactions, are responses to specific antigens such as pollen, animal dander, or dust mites. Whether airborne or carried to the eye by the hand or other vehicles, the offending antigen dissolves in the tear film and then traverses the conjunctiva to bind IgE antibodies attached to the $F_c\varepsilon$ receptors on the mast cell (Fig. 1). This antigen–antibody cross-linking triggers mast cell degranulation, the mechanism by which the chemical mediators of the allergic inflammatory response (4), including histamine, eosinophil chemotactic factors, neutrophil chemotactic factor, and platelet-activating factor (PAF) (5) are released. These cellular and biochemical changes result in conjunctival vasodilation, increased vasopermeability, leukocyte chemotaxis, and ocular surface destruction and subsequent repair (6). Clinically, they present as itching, tearing, hyperemia, chemosis, and eyelid swelling associated with allergic conjunctivitis (7).

Type IV hypersensitivity reactions, on the other hand, are delayed-type, or cell-mediated reactions. These reactions typically develop within hours or days of exposure to the offending antigen and differ from the three other types of hypersensitivity in that sensitized T lymphocytes, rather than antibodies, interact with antigen. The presence of antigen activates local T lymphocytes which secrete lymphokines, at least one of which, interferon-γ (IFN-γ) subsequently stimulates macrophages to release toxic compounds. The toxic compounds include interleukin-1 (IL-1), tissue necrosis factor-α (TNF-α), reactive oxygen intermediates, lysosomal enzymes, and collagenase (8). These compounds cause inflammation and tissue damage, resulting in the signs and symptoms of atopic keratoconjunctivitis, drug allergy, and some aspects of VKC and GPC (9).

Currently, the therapy for ocular allergic disease focuses on allergen elimination, modulation of the immune system, and pharmacologic inhibition of the chemical mediators involved in the immune response. Removal of the offending allergen or modification of the patient's environment are most effective, although rarely practical.

Basically, topical therapeutic agents belong to one of four classes: antihistamines (antihistamine/vasoconstrictor combinations), mast cell stabilizers, nonsteroidal antiinflammatory drugs (NSAIDs), and corticosteroids. Oral an-

M. B. Abelson, P. J. McGarr, and K. P. Richard: Ophthalmic Research Associates, North Andover, Massachusetts 01845.

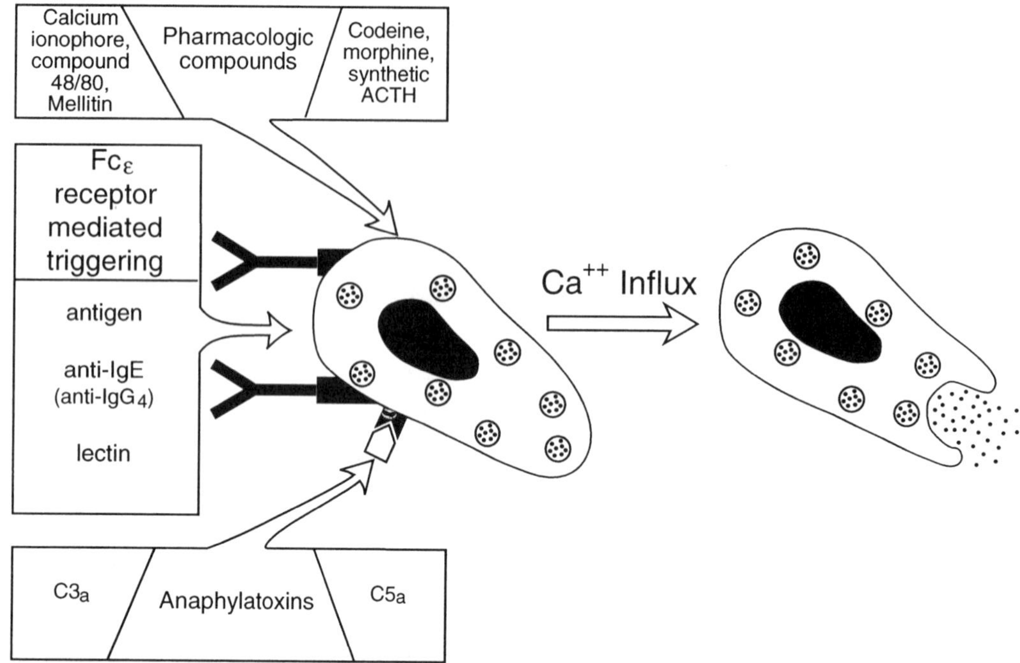

FIG. 52-1. Mast cell activation. Mast cells can be activated by (1) anaphlytoxins binding to the receptors on the mast cell surface, (2) a substance cross-linking F_c receptors on the mast cell surface, or (3) certain pharmacologic agents acting directly on the mast cell. Any of these mechanisms will activate the mast cell and result in an influx of calcium ions. This influx on calcium ions results in degranulation of the mast cell and release of preformed mediators.

tihistamines may be used, but these agents do not reliably relieve ocular symptoms and may exacerbate the problem by decreasing tear production. By removing the barrier that provides both protection and integrity to all ocular surfaces a normally functional tear system is affected. These effects may preclude their use. Topical corticosteroids are very effective at relieving itching, chemosis, and mucous discharge. However, long-term steroid use has been associated with serious side effects, which limits the use of these drugs to patients who are unresponsive to milder forms of therapy. Treatment with topical antihistamines usually provides symptomatic relief without systemic side effects. Mast cell stabilizers are purported to stabilize the mast cell plasma membrane, thereby preventing mast cell degranulation and mediator release. Finally, NSAIDs may also be used to treat ocular allergy (4).

This chapter briefly describes each ocular allergic disease and the drugs available as potential therapies.

ALLERGIC CONJUNCTIVITIS

Allergic conjunctivitis, also called hay fever conjunctivitis, is a recurrent condition, usually transient and self-limiting, that can be seasonal if due to pollens from trees, grasses, or weeds. The current body of research suggests that allergic conjunctivitis is essentially a pure type I hypersensitivity. Environmental allergens can vary depending on geographic and climactic variations. In New England, for example, tree pollens are dispersed in the early spring, grasses in May and June, and ragweed from mid-August to the first killing frost. If the antigen is abundant throughout the year (i.e., animal danders, dust or molds), allergic conjunctivitis may present as perennial and chronic or as single acute episodes separated by significant intervals.

Although the early phase of allergic conjunctivitis can be self-limiting, a reaction of this limited acute allergic response, considered "late phase," may present many hours later with cellular infiltration, inflammation, and further mast cell degranulation. This condition is rare in the eye, estimated to occur in only 2% of persons with ocular allergic disease. Clinically, late-phase disease has not yet been clearly recognized. In addition, the pathophysiology of the disease is uncertain, although some investigators believe that the mast cell mediator platelet activating factor (PAF) may play a role in setting the stage.

Clinical Presentation

Allergic conjunctivitis is the most common form of ocular allergic disease and accounts for 90% of all allergic disorders encountered by allergists (10). Ocular allergy is more common in males than in females and often presents by the time the patient is aged 20 years, but may first present at any age. Approximately 50% of affected persons have a positive family history of allergy (1).

Itching is the hallmark symptom of all ocular allergy. Clinical signs of hyperemia, chemosis, tearing, and lid swelling may not always be present. However, most patients have some conjunctival edema, dilation of the conjunctival vessels, or swelling of the lids. Reactions may be accompanied by a clear or white globular, mucous exudate. Excessive conjunctival chemosis can, in very rare instances, lead to corneal dellen which may result in pain, photophobia, and blurred vision (6).

Pathogenesis

The mast cell is the basic effector cell of allergic conjunctivitis. There are approximately 50 million mast cells in the ocular and adnexal tissues of the human eye (11). Each mast cell contains several hundred vesicles, within which are several types of chemical mediators of ocular allergy and inflammation. The surface of each mast cell contains approximately 500,000 IgE receptors, 10% of which are occupied in vivo by IgE antibody (12). When antigen binds to the IgE receptors, forming an antigen–antibody–mast cell complex, the F_c portion of the IgE molecule changes. This change initiates a chain of reactions in the mast cell plasma membrane, resulting in the degranulation of the mast cell and the consequent release of chemical mediators (3). These mediators attract eosinophils and neutrophils to the tissue. The eosinophils and neutrophils contain secondary mediators that can either restore homeostasis or, in more chronic allergic disease, cause tissue damage.

Homeostasis is achieved through various negative feedback mechanisms; for example, an activated mast cell will release several chemical mediators, one of which is histamine. Histamine will then bind to histamine receptors on the surface of the mast cell, resulting in an increase in the concentration of 3′,5′-cyclic adenosine monophosphate (cyclic AMP). This increased concentration of cyclic AMP "shuts off" the mast cell, thereby limiting the allergic response. Conversely, increasing the levels of 3′,5′-cyclic guanosine monophosphate (cyclic GMP) stimulates mediator release. There are several mechanisms by which cyclic AMP and cyclic GMP levels can be altered, and allergic symptoms clearly can be controlled by increasing cyclic AMP levels or by decreasing cyclic GMP levels (5). Indeed, a novel approach to the treatment of ocular allergic disease would be manipulation of these second messengers. Clinically, caffeine, acting in this manner by inhibiting phosphodiesterase (PDE), decreases conjunctival reactivity to topically applied allergens.

ATOPIC KERATOCONJUNCTIVITIS (AKC)

The etiology of AKC is unknown. This disease usually appears in late adolescence or early adulthood (13) and is rarely outgrown. AKC has a strong correlation to atopic dermatitis, and many patients with AKC are also concurrently treated by a dermatologist.

Clinical Presentation

AKC is a chronic condition characterized by intense itching; swollen, crusty, and excoriated lids; chemosis; and photophobia (14). The eyelids quite frequently develop edematous, eczematous lesions which become crusty and scaly, usually resulting in a loss of lashes. Conjunctival vessels are often dilated, and mucous discharge is common. Both papillae and follicles can occur in AKC (13). In more severe cases, corneal vascularization, corneal melting and scarring, anterior polar cataracts, and keratoconus may occur. Often, these signs and symptoms worsen in the winter months (4).

AKC patients are predisposed to secondary staphylococcal blepharitis, and *Staphylococcus aureus* can be cultured from the eyelids of many patients (15). In addition, depressed cell-mediated immunity makes these patients susceptible to viral and fungal diseases.

Pathogenesis

Serum IgE levels are elevated in patients with AKC, yet its distinct clinical and histopathologic presentation indicates that AKC is not strictly a type I hypersensitivity reaction. Indeed, it is characterized by cellular infiltration with lymphocytes in addition to mast cells, basophils, and eosinophils (6). Mechanisms of cellular immunity have been demonstrated to be diminished in AKC (16). Because the T cell regulates IgE production, alterations to the ratio between helper T and suppressor T cells have been postulated to be responsible for the inability to arrest IgE responses. The resultant overproduction of IgE antibody may result in continuous stimulation to release histamine and other mediators, with the subsequent clinical manifestations of atopic disease (17).

VERNAL KERATOCONJUNCTIVITIS (VKC)

The word vernal is derived from the Greek and means "occurring in the spring." VKC is a seasonally recurrent, bilateral inflammation of the conjunctiva. It is characterized by cobblestone papillae, usually on the superior tarsal conjunctiva, and by papillary hypertrophy of the limbal conjunctiva. The disease has precise epidemiologic characteristics, including a predilection for warm climates, a frequent family and personal history of atopic allergies, an incidence rate more than twice as high in males as in females, and an early onset; VKC rarely is present in patients aged less than 3 years or more than 25 years (18,19).

Although hereditary predisposition is an important epidemiologic characteristic of VKC, exogenous factors, such as climate, season, and allergen exposure determine the likelihood and severity of the disease. The Middle East, North Africa, Puerto Rico, and the Mediterranean regions of European countries, with arid climates and the high potential for wind and desert storms, have the highest incidence of VKC. These environmental conditions are often referred to as "nonspecific" factors that provoke exacerbations of the disease. In colder climates, this disease is usually at its worst in the spring and summer, presumably due to exposure to the airborne pollens of grasses, trees, and weeds.

Clinical Presentation

There are two clinical forms of VKC: palpebral and limbal. The two forms usually occur together, although one may predominate. Patients with the palpebral form usually present pink, raised conjunctival cobblestones over the superior tarsal plate; these may be discrete or clumped, crowding together as they develop. A distinct branching pattern of vessels is visible, growing through the center of the papillae. Due to pressure from the globe, the papillae often become flattened, resembling "a mosaic of flat-topped cobblestones" (19).

Thick, dirty, yellow or white cordlike mucus with highly elastic properties, described as the Maxwell Lyon sign, is highly characteristic of VKC. This lardaceous mucus contains dead epithelial cells, mononuclear and polymorphonuclear cells, and many eosinophils with their Charcot-Layden granules (20). By everting the upper lid with a cotton swab during ophthalmic examination, the ophthalmologist can often see a milky veil coating the cobblestones. The fine, stringy material can be removed from the conjunctiva by gently swabbing the surface with a cotton-tipped applicator.

The limbal form presents superficial translucent, gelatinous, globular deposits at the limbus that vary greatly in size and shape. These deposits can be a small circle, rarely larger than 3 mm, an arc with a predilection for the superior limbus, or a 360° limbal ring. Within this heaped-up tissue are Horner-Trantas dots, chalk-white infiltrates straddling the limbus that are virtually pathognomonic for VKC. Although classically reported to contain eosinophils, a large proportion of the cells in the dot are actually neutrophils.

In more severe cases, a diffuse epithelial keratitis is present. The shield ulcer, a well-defined, centrally located, white, fibrinous epithelial defect of the cornea, may be present, although it is a rarer manifestation.

Itching is the most common feature of VKC, in both limbal and palpebral forms. It is usually intense and persistent. Photophobia, indicating corneal involvement, and pain, described as a hot, tight, sensitive feeling of the eyes, are often debilitating in patients with VKC.

Pathogenesis

Although they differ in clinical appearance, both palpebral and limbal VKC undergo the same pathologic transformation (19). A prehypertrophic phase of hyperemia and a thin, milky-white pseudomembrane defines the first stage of development. After the initial stage, hypertrophic changes occur that are related to a stromal infiltration with papillae covered by an epithelial monolayer with mucoid degeneration in the crypts between papillae. Collagen deposition, hyaluronization, decreased vascularity, and an overall decrease in inflammatory cells replace the earlier cellular and vascular phase (18).

Mast cells play a central role in the pathogenesis of VKC. They are found in increased numbers in both the epithelium and the substantia propria of the conjunctiva. Approximately 80% of the mast cells are degranulated, exhibiting a greater presence of vacuoles, an expansion of the cytoplasm, and disappearance of the cytoplasmic extensions (21). That histamine levels are dramatically increased in patients with VKC—10-fold higher than those of normal subjects—suggests that this mediator plays a central role in the pathophysiology of the disease (22,23). A contributing factor to the increased histamine levels may be related to a dysfunction in the histamine-degrading enzymes, collectively termed histaminase. Histaminase inactivation in acute allergic conjunctivitis resulted in a 10-fold increase in recovery of histamine from tears (24). These levels are similar to those detected in patients with VKC (25). Blood samples of patients with VKC have exhibited reduced levels of histaminase, suggesting that histaminase dysfunction may play an important role in the elevation of histamine levels (26).

Eosinophils are also found in increased numbers in the epithelium and the substantia propria, which makes them readily available for recovery in scrapings. VKC is the only ocular surface disorder in which more than two eosinophils can be found per 25-power objective field (27). Eosinophil major basic protein (EMBP), the primary toxic mediator released by eosinophils, is believed to be the agent responsible for the resultant corneal damage in more severe cases of VKC (28). This theory is supported by the recovery of eosinophils and their granules from the mucoid plaque overlying the shield ulcer (29) and by elution of tear EMBP from the ulcer itself (28).

In addition to the presence of eosinophils and the increased number of mast cells, basophils and an increased total number of lymphocytes and plasma cells are evident in the conjunctival epithelium of patients with VKC. This cellular profile suggests that cutaneous basophil hypersensitivity mechanisms may be present (19).

GIANT PAPILLARY CONJUNCTIVITIS (GPC)

GPC is a disorder characterized by irritation, tearing, mucous discharge, blurred vision, itching (occasionally), and proliferation of subepithelial collagen, leading to the eruption of giant papillae on the superior palpebral conjunctiva. Contact lenses, surgical suture barbs, and ocular prostheses have been implicated as the causative factors or elements responsible for the signs and symptoms associated with GPC.

Our understanding of this condition is incomplete. Current theory suggests that GPC is essentially a type I hypersensitivity reaction, a type IV delayed hypersensitivity of the conjunctiva to antigens present on the surface of the contact lens, or both. This theory has been disputed, however, and alternative theories have suggested that induction of chronic trauma to the conjunctiva by the lens edge causes the condition. Disorders of the conjunctiva associated with the persistent presence of a foreign body on or in the eye are best explained by a combination of factors involving hyperactivity of local mast cells and lymphocytes, fibroblasts, and the consequent formation of conjunctival papillae (30).

GPC has no clear individual predilection. Patients with GPC who wear soft contact lenses have worn them for an average of 8 months whereas those who wear hard contact lenses have worn them for an average of 8 years before developing the clinical signs and symptoms that characterize the disorder (31). Occurrence of GPC is based on (a) personal predisposition, (b) presence of appropriate antagonist, (c) duration of exposure to the agent, (d) area exposed to the agent, and (e) geometry of exposure. Although GPC can result in scarring of the upper palpebral conjunctiva, no permanent visual loss has been reported to date.

Clinical Presentation

Contact lens-associated GPC has been observed in wearers of both rigid gas-permeable and soft lenses, although the incidence has been reported to be greater in wearers of soft contact lenses (30). GPC is a reversible ocular inflammatory disorder characterized by foreign-body sensation, blurred vision, excess mucus production, hyperemia, and the eruption of enlarged papillae.

Symptoms of GPC usually appear well before the signs, which can be easily overlooked, requiring a meticulous eye examination and a thorough patient history. Patients may experience increased accumulations of mucus in the nasal corner of the eye and discomfort of the lids after insertion or removal of the lenses. These signs and symptoms frequently go unreported because the patient considers them to be within normally expected sensations or because the symptoms just are not bothersome enough to prompt a visit (19). As the disease progresses, vision may become blurred due to coatings on the surface of the contact lens, mucus production becomes more severe, and lens movement may result from blinking. In more advanced cases of GPC, patients describe a foreign body sensation or pain associated with contact lens wear and mucus production sufficient to glue the eyes shut during sleep. This increased mucus production appears to be the result of increased secretory vesicles in the superficial non-goblet epithelial cells of the conjunctiva (32) and should be distinguished from the purulent discharge of bacterial conjunctivitis.

The most prominent sign of GPC is the presentation of enlarged papillae (0.3 mm or more in diameter) of the superior conjunctiva. The patient may present mild hyperemia of the upper tarsal conjunctiva, with strands of milky white discharge covering the areas of the giant papillae (30). Alterations in the conjunctival tissue become apparent, with thickening due to the infiltration of inflammatory cells.

Papillae differ from follicles clinically and histopathologically. Papillae are clear vascularized conjunctival elevations, often giving a velvety appearance to the affected surface. In contrast, follicles are white/yellow, translucent, avascular elevations of the conjunctiva. Histopathologic analysis of a papilla shows diffuse infiltration of acute and chronic inflammatory cells surrounding a central conjunctival vessel. Immature lymphocytes and macrophages with surrounding mature lymphocytes define the cellular profile of a follicle (7).

A personal history of atopy and the occurrence of GPC appear to be associated. Patients with GPC had a higher incidence of allergy to airborne allergens and to thimerosal. Begley et al. demonstrated that the number of patients diagnosed with GPC was not uniform throughout the year, but instead increased in the spring and spiked in the summer/early fall (33). Although immediate hypersensitivity alone cannot account for the etiology of GPC, atopy appears to play a predisposing role.

Pathogenesis

Analysis of contact lenses worn by GPC patients has revealed tear protein deposits (34). These lens surface deposits can be composed of lysozyme, IgA, lactoferrin, and IgG. These deposits may not act as the antigenic stimulus themselves, but help attach environmental allergens to the lens surface. The combination of trauma to the superior tarsal conjunctiva from the wear of contact lenses and the continuous exposure of the antigen to the compromised area may initiate the hypersensitivity response. Investigators have demonstrated that lenses first worn by GPC patients can induce an intense infiltration of neutrophils, lymphocytes, and plasma cells at the epithelial–stromal junction when placed on the eyes of cynomologus monkeys. Mast cells were observed in the epithelial layers. Tears from the two monkeys with GPC lenses showed increased levels of IgG, IgA, and IgE 35 to 75 days after lens placement. The study (34) suggests that some factor (or factors) in the lens coating from GPC patients was able to induce a tear immunoglobulin response and histopathologic changes in monkeys. These changes are similar to the histopathologic and immunologic findings in human patients with GPC (35).

Mechanical trauma is an important contributing factor in the pathogenesis of GPC. Abrasion of the upper palpebral conjunctiva by exposed suture ends and by epithelialized corneal foreign body has been reported (36–38). Removal or excision of the offending body resolved the papillary reaction. In both cases, the causative factor appeared to be physical trauma.

Inflammation induced by chronic irritation of the lids is the common component common to all patients with GPC. Indeed, patients with contact lenses of different edge design can develop unilateral GPC. The infrequency of itch, chemosis, or lid edema and the more frequent presence of irritation of the ocular surface, lens discomfort, and lid discomfort on removal of lenses present a distinct clinical picture. Histamine levels are not increased, and the cellular infiltration resembles chronic inflammation more than allergy. This does not mean that an allergic component may not play a role in some patients, but clearly allergy itself is insufficient and is probably never the major component.

Histologic analysis of tissue from patients with GPC and VKC showed differences in number but not in type of cellular mediators (21). Patients with VKC have a greater number of mast cells in the epithelium and substantia propria of the conjunctiva, which are more completely degranulated, than do patients with GPC. This difference may explain the higher tear histamine levels, the greater number of eosinophils, greater itching and inflammation, and more extensive corneal involvement in VKC.

Histologic analysis of conjunctiva from patients with GPC has shown that the clinically apparent increase in mucus production is not associated with an increase in goblet cell density of the upper tarsal conjunctiva, although proliferation of papillae can alter the conjunctival surface and increase the absolute number of goblet cells. Electron microscopy showed increased numbers of secretory vesicles in the superficial nongoblet epithelial cells, some of which appeared to discharge their contents into the conjunctival sac, supporting the premise that the superficial layers of nongoblet conjunctival epithelial cells can contribute to an increase in mucus production (32).

DRUG-INDUCED ALLERGIC CONJUNCTIVITIS

Drug-induced allergic conjunctivitis is usually a type IV (delayed type) hypersensitivity reaction. These reactions typically occur 36 to 48 hours after the offending drug is applied to the eye, but may occur after months or years of contact. Drug-induced allergic conjunctivitis is characterized by conjunctival hyperemia and corneal surface staining and, very rarely, by subepithelial peripheral infiltrates. This condition is frequently associated with contact dermatitis of the skin of the eyelids. The most commonly implicated drugs are neomycin, erythromycin, pilocarpine, and sulfa drugs (1,13).

The best therapy for drug-induced allergic conjunctivitis is identification and avoidance of the offending drug. This type of therapy is both practical and effective. If a patient absolutely requires use of the allergy-provoking drug, some practitioners have added an antiallergic agent or mild steroid into the medication regimen until the offending drug can be discontinued. However, for obvious reasons, this is the least desirable alternative.

THERAPIES

ANTIHISTAMINES

History and Source

The role of histamine in the acute allergic response has been well established. Histamine was first synthesized in 1907, and its biologic activity was discovered when it was detected as a uterine stimulant in extracts of ergot in 1910 (39). Later that year, histamine was observed to have bronchospastic and vasodilator activity in animals (40). Over the next 17 years, Dale et al. discovered that histamine applied locally produced redness, swelling, and edema and that large intravenous doses of histamine produced a symptom complex identical to that occurring in anaphylactic shock. These discoveries led to the deduction that histamine was the primary humoral mediator involved in acute allergic reactions (41).

In 1953, histamine was identified in the mast cells of human skin (42), but not until 1977 did Abelson et al. detect histamine in human tear film (23). In 1979, Abelson et al. demonstrated that topical instillation of histamine produced, in a dose-dependent fashion, the itching and redness associated with allergic conjunctivitis (43). Subsequently, identification of specific receptors on the ocular surface has made it possible to identify the pathologic effects of histamine selectively (Fig. 2). Stimulation of H_1 receptors, identified by Ash and Schild (44), with the highly selective H_1-receptor agonist 2-(2-aminoethyl) thiazoledihydrochloride elicits ocular itching (45). On the other hand, stimulation of H_2 receptors by dimethylaminopropylisothiourea, a highly selective H_2-receptor agonist, produces vasodilation of conjunctival vessels without itching (46).

Inactivation of histaminase and recovery of histamine from the tear film of patients with allergic conjunctivitis has been instructive. If sensitized patients are ocularly challenged with a pollen or dander, histamine levels increase by a factor of 60 from baseline in 3 minutes. By 8 minutes, histamine returns to three times baseline levels, which corresponds clinically with peak itching and onset of redness of the conjunctiva. The rapid peaked release of the preformed mediator histamine from the mast cell is rapidly hydrolyzed by histaminase to prevent an ongoing reaction or conver-

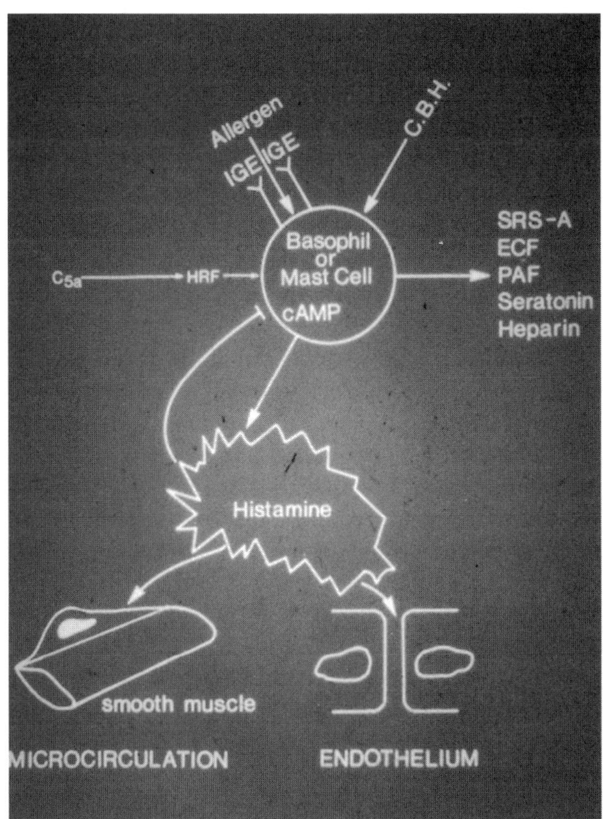

FIG. 52-2. The source and sites of activation of histamine. Mast cells and basophils, when activated by allergen, complement, or other secretagogues, release several mediators of inflammation, including histamine. The released histamine binds to receptors on smooth muscle and endothelial cells. Other mediators released by activated mast cells and basophils include slow-reacting substance of anaphylaxis (SRS-A, also termed leukotrienes C_4 and D_4), eosinophil chemotactic factor (ECF), platelet-activating factor (PAF), seratonin, and heparin.

sion to a more chronic disease with associated structural tissue changes. Such appears to be the case in VKC, in which tear histamine levels remain high and no significant histaminase activity has been detected in tears.

Official Drug Name and Chemistry

Histamine H_1-receptor antagonists compete pharmacologically with histamine at the H_1 site on the effector cell and have been classified by their chemical structures into seven groups: alkylamines, ethanolamines, ethylenediamines, phenothiazines, piperidines, piperazines, and a cyclohexylpiperidine. Structures of representatives from each of these seven groups are shown in Fig. 3. The H_1 receptor antagonists are composed of one or two aromatic (heterocyclic) rings connected by a nitrogen, carbon, or oxygen atom to the ethylamine group. The ethylamine group has a tertiary nitrogen atom attached. In contrast,

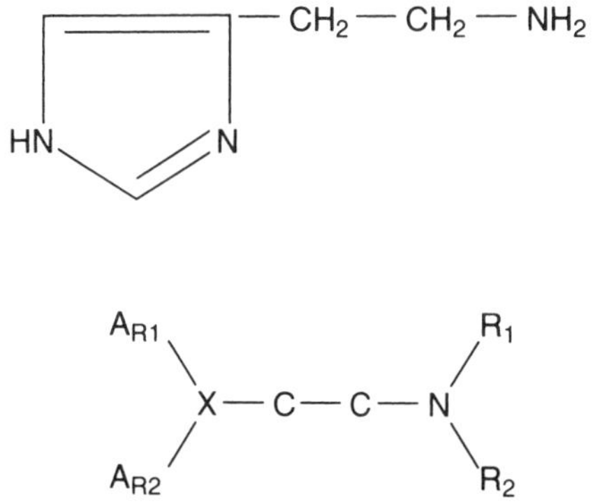

— CH_2 — CH_2 — NH_2
HN N

A_{R1} R_1
X — C — C — N
A_{R2} R_2

FIG. 52-3. A comparison of the chemical structure of histamine (**top**) and of H_1-receptor antagonists (**bottom**).

histamine consists of a single heterocyclic ring, imidazole, connected directly to the ethylamine group. The nitrogen atom in the ethylamine group of histamine is either primary or unsubstituted (3).

The multiple aromatic rings of the H_1 antihistamines make these compounds very lipophilic, which contributes to H_1 receptor binding (47). In addition, both histamine and the H_1 antihistamines have a positively charged amino group believed to be important in receptor recognition (48).

Histamine H_2 receptor antagonists are more similar in structure to histamine than are the H_1-receptor antagonists. H_2-Receptor antagonists have an imidazole ring and are polar, hydrophilic compounds. The imidazole or another heterocyclic side-chain ring is critical for H_2-receptor site recognition. These compounds are weak bases and are highly water soluble; therefore, they exist uncharged in aqueous solutions at physiologic conditions (pH 7.4) (47).

Topical ophthalmic preparations of H_1 antihistamines presently include an alkylamine (pheniramine maleate), two ethylenediamines (antazoline phosphate and pyrilamine maleate) (4), and a cyclohexylpiperidine (levocabastine hydrochloride) (49). Three of the classic H_1 antihistamines currently approved for use in ocular antiallergic preparations—pheniramine maleate, antazoline phosphate, and pyrilamine maleate—have been shown to inhibit ocular itching significantly but are available only in combination with α-adrenergic agents, which alleviate conjunctival redness. Of all approved topical ocular preparations for the treatment of ocular allergic disease, only levocabastine hydrochloride is effective in reducing both itching and redness in the absence of a vasoconstrictor. Currently, no H_2-receptor antagonists are approved for ocular use.

Pharmacology

The pharmacologic actions of both the H_1- and H_2-receptor antagonists are similar in that they block the effects of histamine by reversibly binding to the histamine receptor, thus preventing histamine–receptor interaction. Because the antagonists do not stimulate the H_1 and H_2 receptors responsible for dilating the small precapillary blood vessels and constricting the larger venules, the signs and symptoms of ocular allergy are prevented. However, neither H_1 nor H_2 blockers have an effect on the release of endogenous histamine (50).

Levocabastine hydrochloride, Livostin, is a long-acting, highly potent, and selective H_1-receptor antagonist (49). It is 15,000 times more potent than chlorpheneramine in the rat model of 48/80 induced mortality (51). In studies using radiolabeled markers, levocabastine specifically bound histamine H_1-receptor sites and dissociated from those sites very slowly; the dissociation of half-life ($t_{\frac{1}{2}}$) is 116 minutes (49). In contrast, levocabastine has a remarkably low affinity for dopamine, serotonin, α-adrenergic, β-adrenergic, and several other receptor sites. Furthermore, the small amounts of levocabastine that do bind to these sites dissociate rapidly and therefore display no pharmacodynamic effect.

Clinical Pharmacology

By competing with histamine for receptors on effector cells, both H_1 and H_2 antihistamines effectively prevent the immune response that results in manifestation of the clinical signs and symptoms of allergic disease.

Histamine affects the vascular system through both H_1 and H_2 receptors (52). Stimulation of the H_1 receptors causes systemic vasodilation and localized erythema and edema due to capillary dilation and increased permeability (53). In the eye, topically applied histamine induces ocular itching and vasodilation. H_1 antihistamines effectively reduce this histamine-induced itching (3), but the only antihistamine marketed that is also effective in relieving ocular redness is levocabastine hydrochloride. The mechanism by which this reduction in hyperemia is attained is probably related to the blocking of H_1 receptors to such an extent that minimal effects of H_1 receptors in mediating hyperemia are eliminated.

Pharmaceutics

Table 1 shows the currently available topical ocular antihistamines and their respective concentrations.

Topical H_1 antihistamines are the drugs most commonly used for treatment of ocular allergic conjunctivitis (3) and are also commonly used to quiet the manifestations associated with VKC and AKC. The usual recommended dose is 1 to 2 drops every 3 to 4 hours as needed, as many as four times daily, to relieve symptoms.

Although many oral antihistamines are available, they are not commonly used for treatment of ocular allergic disease and therefore are not included in this section.

Pharmacokinetics

Oral Antihistamines

The H_1 antihistamines are rapidly and completely absorbed after oral administration, and drug effects are observed within 30 minutes, with peak efficacy occurring between 1 and 2 hours after administration. Drug action usually lasts 4 to 6 hours, but some (i.e., the piperazines and the piperidines) have much longer lasting effects. These antihistamines are lipid soluble; therefore, they cross the blood–brain, blood–placental, and blood–ocular barriers. Oral H_1 antihistamines are widely distributed throughout the body, and most penetrate the CNS. In addition, they are all completely metabolized by the liver and all metabolites are excreted in the urine (9).

Although oral antihistamines are widely distributed throughout the body, resulting in a high incidence of systemic side effects, attaining adequate concentrations in ocular tissue is very difficult. For therapeutic doses to be de-

TABLE 52-1. *Topical antihistamines*

Trade name	Manufacturer	Composition	Concentration (%)
Livostin	Ciba	Levocabastine HCl	0.05
Vasocon-A	Ciba	Antazoline PO_4	0.5
		Naphazoline HCl	0.05
Naphcon-A	Alcon	Pheniramine maleate	0.3
		Naphazoline HCl	0.025
AK-Con-A	Akorn	Pheneramine maleate	0.3
		Naphazoline HCl	0.025
Opcon-A	Bausch & Lomb	Pheneramine maleate,	0.3
		Naphazoline HCl	0.025

Ciba, CibaVision ophthalmics
Alcon, Alcon Laboratories, Inc.
Bausch & Lomb, Bausch & Lomb Pharmaceuticals, Inc.

livered to the ocular tissue, high oral doses would be required. This problem, compounded by the problem of drying of the ocular surface, prevents common use of oral antihistamines in the treatment of ocular allergy.

Topical Antihistamines

With use of topically applied antihistamines, it is important to remember that the amount of drug administered to the ocular surface is not the amount that will be available to act at the targeted site. The final concentration of a compound is decreased by the following factors: (a) dilution by the tear film, (b) normal evaporation in the tear film, (c) systemic absorption by vessels in the conjunctiva, (d) nonproductive absorption by surrounding tissues, (e) normal drainage from the conjunctiva into the nasolacrimal duct, (f) breakdown by tear film enzymes, (g) overflow from the conjunctival sac and, finally, (h) binding with tear film proteins (54).

Levocabastine is incompletely absorbed after topical application. After repeated doses, topically applied levocabastine did not significantly inhibit the wheal and flare response to intradermal histamine, indicating that minimal systemic absorption occurs after topical administration. Steady-state plasma concentrations of 1.6 μg/L were achieved within 7 to 10 days after topical ocular application of 1 drop per eye three times daily. Peak plasma concentrations were observed in approximately 2 hours. The drug is rapidly distributed and has an elimination $t_{\frac{1}{2}}$ of 33 hours. Fifty-five percent of levocabastine is bound to protein, most of this being bound to albumin. Approximately 65% to 70% is excreted unchanged in the urine, 10% is excreted in the urine as the metabolite acylglucuronide, and the remaining 20% is excreted unchanged in the feces (49).

Therapeutic Use

Topical H_1 antihistamines are the drugs most commonly used for treatment of ocular allergic conjunctivitis (55). Topical H_1 antihistamines may also be used to treat the intense itching associated with AKC.

Like any other medication, topical H_1 antihistamines are contraindicated in any patient with a known allergy to any component of the medication. In addition, combination products containing antihistamines and vasoconstrictors are contraindicated in patients with poorly controlled hypertension, cardiovascular disease with arrhythmias, or poorly controlled diabetes mellitus, or in any patient concurrently treated with monoamine oxidase (MAO) inhibitors. Finally, no topical ocular medications are currently approved for use in patients wearing contact lenses.

Side Effects and Toxicity

Oral Antihistamines

Therapeutic doses of oral H_1 antihistamines are associated with several mild systemic side effects; occasionally, the response may necessitate discontinuation of the drug.

The most common adverse effect associated with oral H_1 antihistamines is sedation (9). Other CNS side effects include disturbed coordination, dizziness, fatigue, and difficulty in concentration. These effects result from a generalized depression of the CNS. In contrast, some patients may experience euphoria, nervousness, insomnia, or tremors.

Gastrointestinal (GI) adverse effects include loss of appetite, nausea, vomiting, epigastric distress, diarrhea, and constipation. These side effects occur less frequently than the CNS side effects and can sometimes be controlled by administering oral antihistamines with meals.

The anticholinergic properties of the oral H_1 antihistamines are responsible for dryness of the mucous membranes of the oropharynx and conjunctiva. The conjunctival involvement is responsible for the appearance of dry eye symptoms.

The atropine-like effects of the vasoconstrictor component in individual and combination products include mydriasis, which could precipitate an attack of acute angle-closure glaucoma in predisposed, untreated individuals. Ciliary muscle paresis, with an associated decrease in accommodation, may account for visual difficulties experienced by some patients.

Topical Antihistamines

On the other hand, topical ocular antihistamines are associated with an extraordinarily low incidence of systemic side effects. Indeed, blood levels are often not detectable after topical ocular application of antihistamines. Local irritation, including burning and/or stinging, may occur but usually resolves within a few seconds after instillation. Medicamentosa and punctate keratitis have been associated with the preservative benzalkonium chloride, a component of many topical antihistamines. Topical antihistamines are contraindicated in patients with narrow angle glaucoma. Furthermore, antihistamine/vasoconstrictor combination products should be used with caution in patients with poorly controlled hypertension, cardiovascular disease with arrhythmias, and poorly controlled diabetes mellitus (3).

Overdose

When used in the recommended therapeutic doses, the oral H_1 antihistamines are safe drugs. Systemically, massive doses result in CNS stimulation (i.e., convulsions) in children and in CNS depression (i.e., coma) followed by

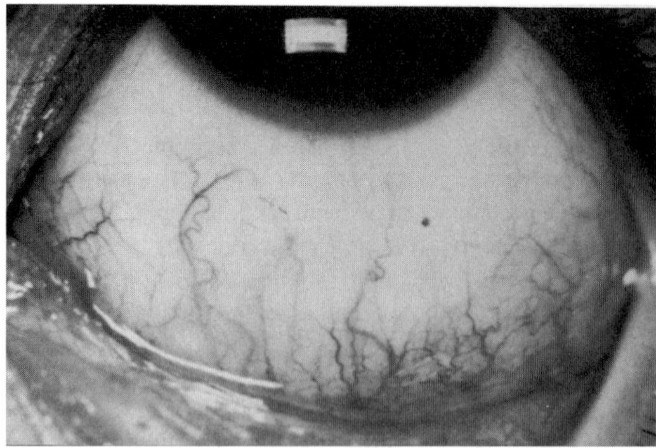
A

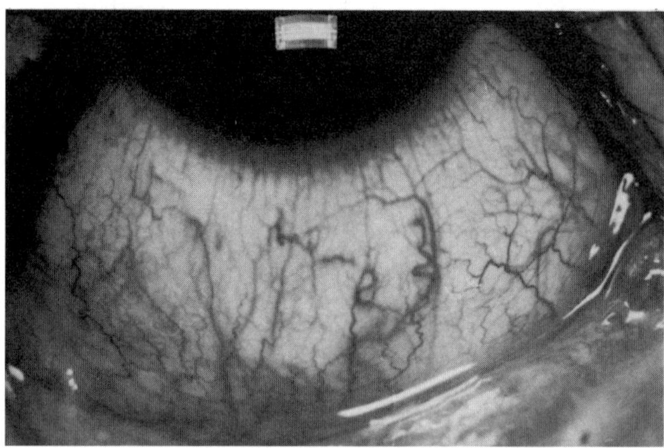
B

FIG. 52-4. A major clinical trial comparing the efficacy of levocabastine and that of cromolyn sodium Left (**A**) and right (**B**) eyes of one subject 10 minutes after ocular challenge with allergen. The left eye was pretreated with levocabastine, and the right eye was pretreated four times daily for 2 weeks with cromolyn sodium.

CNS stimulation in adults. In extremely severe systemic overdoses, coma, cardiorespiratory failure, and even death may occur. Treatment is supportive, and may include treatment with phenobarbital or diazepam during the convulsive phase (9). On the contrary, acute toxicity effects of topical antihistamines have not been observed.

High-risk Groups

The safety of H_1 antihistamines in infants, children, pregnant women, and nursing mothers has not been established. According to the *Physicians Desk Reference 1994* (48th edition), oral chlorcyclizine hydrochloride, a piperazine compound, has been shown to be teratogenic in animals. Long-term studies involving topical application have not been conducted.

Drug Interactions

There are no known drug interactions with respect to topical ocular antihistamines. MAO inhibitors have been suggested to have a potentially hazardous interaction with antihistamines. However, evidence fully supporting this claim is lacking.

Major Clinical Trials

The allergen (or antigen) challenge model, developed by Abelson et al. (56), has become the standard for demonstrating the efficacy of antiallergic compounds. It has been used successfully to show the efficacy of Livostin (levocabastine hydrochloride), Vasocon-A (naphazoline hydrochloride/antazoline phosphate), Naphcon-A, AK-Con-A, and Opcon-A (naphazoline hydrochloride/pheniramine maleate) in the treatment of seasonal allergic conjunctivitis (Fig. 4). In this model, the mechanism for allergic conjunctivitis is induced by directly exposing the conjunctiva to a topically applied dilution of antigen. This elicits the physiologic immune response, resulting in the classic picture of allergic conjunctivitis, including the cardinal signs and symptoms of allergy: itching, redness, chemosis, tearing and, to a lesser extent, lid swelling (56). With use of this model, the above drugs were shown to be clinically and statistically significantly better than placebo in inhibition of the signs and symptoms of allergic conjunctivitis (55,57–59).

Seasonal environmental studies have also been successfully used to demonstrate the efficacy of these compounds despite several variables. Environmental studies rely on conjunctival allergen contact, which varies diurnally and from day to day. This variable and intermittent stimulus and the resultant response do not provide a suitable baseline for evaluating the efficacy of potential antiallergic agents. In addition, the associated mechanical properties of placebo controls have been shown to elicit a "drug effect" in approximately 70% of treated subjects (56).

MAST CELL STABILIZERS

History and Source

The first mast cell-stabilizing compound was developed in the 1960s from khellin, a chromone (benzopyrone) derived from *Ammi visnaga,* an eastern Mediterranean plant (60), which was used by the ancient Egyptians as an antispasmotic agent (61). Successive modifications in structure yielded disodium cromoglycate (DSCG, cromolyn sodium or cromolyn) (3). The drug was first noted to have antiasthmatic properties when Altounyan used himself to demonstrate that cromolyn protected against a provoked asthmatic attack (62). In an attempt to discover cromolyn's mechanism of action as an antiasthmatic, Rall

(61) showed that cromolyn inhibits the release of histamine and other granule contents from sensitized mast cells (61). This led to the development of cromolyn as an ophthalmic preparation (Opticrom) for the treatment of ocular allergic disease.

Although Opticrom was widely used as a treatment for allergic conjunctivitis, AKC, and VKC, it was indicated only for treatment of VKC. Opticrom was never approved by the Food and Drug Administration (FDA) for use in treatment of seasonal allergic conjunctivitis, and there have been no placebo-controlled studies in which definitive criteria show cromolyn to be effective in treating this disease (4). Although Opticrom is no longer available in the United States, cromolyn sodium was recently released as Crolom by Bausch & Lomb. In addition, lodoxamide, a new mast cell-stabilizing agent which was shown to be 2,500 times more powerful than cromolyn sodium in inhibiting the signs and symptoms associated with allergic reactions (63), has been approved for the treatment of VKC.

Official Drug Name and Chemistry

Lodoxamide tromethamine (lodoxomide, Alomide) is a white, crystalline, water-soluble powder with a molecular weight of 553.91. The full chemical name is *N,N'*-(2-chloro-5-cyano-*m*-phenylene)dioxamic acid tromethamine salt. The empirical formula is $C_{19}H_{28}O_{12}N_5Cl$.

Cromolyn sodium (Crolom) is a clear, colorless solution with a molecular weight of 512.34. The full chemical name is disodium 5,5′-[(2-hydroxytrimethylene)dioxy]*bis*(4-oxo-4H-1-benzopyran-2-carboxylate). The empirical formula is $C_{23}H_{14}Na_2O_{11}$.

Pharmacology

Mast cell stabilizers inhibit the degranulation of mast cells, thereby preventing the release of histamine and other mediators of hypersensitivity reactions. Lodoxamide and cromolyn act only to prevent the degranulation of the mast cell and have no direct vasoconstrictor, antihistaminic, or antiinflammatory actions (Alomide package insert, Alcon Laboratories [Ft. Worth, TX]; Crolom package insert, Bausch & Lomb [Tampa, FL]).

Clinical Pharmacology

Both lodoxamide and cromolyn are mast cell stabilizers that inhibit type I hypersensitivity reactions. Although the specific mechanisms of action of these drugs are unknown, studies have shown that lodoxamide prevents the release of histamine, leukotrienes, and slow-reaction substances of anaphylaxis (SRS-A, or peptido-leukotrienes) and inhibits eosinophil chemotaxis. The *1993 PDR for Ophthalmology* reports that this is achieved through prevention of calcium influx into mast cells after antigen stimulation. Cromolyn acts by inhibiting the release of histamine and SRS-A through an as-yet-unknown pathway.

Pharmaceutics

Lodoxamide (Alomide) is available as a 0.1% topical ophthalmic solution. Cromolyn (Crolom) is available as a 4% topical ophthalmic solution.

Pharmacokinetics

Radiolabeled lodoxamide has been used to demonstrate that the elimination $t_{\frac{1}{2}}$ of this drug is approximately 8.5 hours. Urinary excretion is the major route of elimination. In addition, topical administration of 0.1% lodoxamide ophthalmic solution, one drop per eye four times daily for 10 days, did not result in any measurable plasma levels at a detection limit of 2.5 ng/ml (Alomide package insert, Alcon Laboratories).

Analysis of cromolyn excretion in normal volunteers shows that approximately 0.03% of this drug is absorbed after topical administration. Preclinical data show that after instillation of multiple doses of cromolyn into normal rabbit eyes, less than 0.07% is absorbed into the systemic circulation and less than 0.01% penetrates the aqueous humor. Clearance from the aqueous humor is complete within 24 hours after treatment is discontinued (Crolom package insert, Bausch & Lomb).

Therapeutic Use

Lodoxamide and cromolyn are indicated for the treatment of VKC (vernal conjunctivitis, or vernal keratitis). Lodoxamide is available as Alomide Ophthalmic Solution 0.1%, and the recommended dosage for adults and children aged more than 2 years is 1 to 2 drops per affected eye four times daily for as long as 3 months. Cromolyn is available as Crolom (Cromolyn Sodium Ophthalmic Solution USP, 4%); the recommended dosage is not to exceed 1 to 2 drops in each eye four to six times daily at regular intervals.

Like any medication, both lodoxamide and cromolyn are contraindicated in persons with a known allergy to any of the contents of these medications. Furthermore, due to the inclusion of the preservative benzalkonium chloride in these preparations, patients should be instructed not to wear contact lenses during their use (Alomide package insert, Alcon Laboratories and Crolom package insert, Bausch & Lomb).

Side Effects and Toxicity

Systemic absorption of lodoxamide appears to be negligible. Approximately 15% of patients participating in clinical trials of this drug experienced transient burning, stinging, and ocular discomfort after its instillation. Other adverse events occurring in 1% to 5% of patients included itching, hyperemia, blurred vision, tearing, dry eye symptoms, and foreign body sensation. Fewer than 1% of patients experienced corneal erosion, eye pain, ocular edema, chemosis, scaling of the lids/lashes, corneal abrasion, ocular warming sensation, ocular fatigue, blepharitis, keratopathy, allergy, stickiness, or epitheliopathy (Alomide package insert, Alcon Laboratories).

Systemic absorption of cromolyn also appears to be negligible. The most common adverse reaction to cromolyn is transient ocular burning or stinging on instillation. In addition, conjunctival hyperemia, tearing, itching, dryness around the eye, irritation, puffiness, and sties were reported as infrequent events (Crolom package insert, Bausch & Lomb).

Overdose

There have been no reported cases of overdose of topically applied lodoxamide or cromolyn. However, an overdose of an oral preparation of lodoxamide resulted in a sensation of temporary warmth, profuse sweating, diarrhea, light-headedness, and a feeling of stomach distention. No permanent adverse effects were observed. Treatment may include emesis in the case of overdose (Alomide package insert, Alcon Laboratories).

High-risk Groups

The safety and efficacy of lodoxamide has not been determined in pregnant women, nursing mothers, or children under the age of two years. Similarly, the safety and efficacy of cromolyn has not been established in pregnant women, nursing mothers, or in children aged less than 4 years.

Drug Interactions

There are no known drug interactions with respect to lodoxamide tromethamine or cromolyn sodium.

Major Clinical Trials

Major clinical trials comparing lodoxamide 0.1% with both placebo (64) and cromolyn sodium 4% (65) showed that lodoxamide is safe and efficacious in the treatment of VKC.

In particular, lodoxamide has demonstrated effectiveness in reversing the serious corneal complications associated with VKC (64). This is of particular importance because complications are typically resistant to treatment.

In addition, lodoxamide showed particularly powerful effects in preventing keratitis and shield ulcers in VKC. Although the mechanism of action of lodoxamide is unknown, it has been suggested to block the action of EMBP, thus preventing the release of eosinophils (64).

CORTICOSTEROIDS

History and Source

The physiologic importance of the adrenal glands began to be appreciated in 1855 when the clinical syndromes associated with their impaired function was described by Addison. Brown-Sequard published experiments on the effects of adrenalectomy in the following year, concluding that the adrenal glands are essential to life. By the 1930s, the adrenal cortex, rather than the medulla, was recognized to secrete physiologically important hormones, glucocorticoids, and mineralocorticoids (66).

By 1942, 28 steroids had been isolated from the adrenal cortex and their structures were established. Five of these compounds, cortisol, cortisone, corticosterone, 11-dehydro-corticosterone, and 11-desoxycorticosterone, exhibited biologic activity.

As early as 1929, Hench had recognized that arthritic patients experienced temporary remission when pregnant or jaundiced. Believing that the antirheumatic compound might be an adrenocortical hormone, Hench et al. tested cortisone in acute rheumatoid arthritis in 1949 (66a). The antiinflammatory response was dramatic. Soon, the therapeutic effects of adrenocorticotropic hormone (ACTH) were also demonstrated. By 1950, corticosteroids and ACTH were introduced into the clinical practice by Gordon and McLean (66b).

Official Drug Name and Chemistry

Cortisone, a 21-carbon four-ring structure, was the first steroid to be used in ocular therapy for its antiinflammatory effects (Fig. 5). Alterations made to the molecular structure at various sites result in modification of biologic potency, transcorneal penetration, protein binding, rate of metabolic transformation, rate of excretion, ability to traverse membranes, and intrinsic effectiveness of the molecule at its site of action (67). These alterations and modifications can be summarized as follows:

1. Prednisolone and prednisone have, in addition to the basic nucleus, a 1, 2 double bond in ring A. This modification increases their carbohydrate-regulating potency and prolongs their metabolism as compared with that of cortisol.
2. Methylation of carbon 6 in ring B leads to 6 α-methyl prenisolone. This compound has a slightly greater antiinflammatory effect than prednisolone.
3. Fluorination at a 9 α position in ring B, as in fluorocortisone (9 α-fluorocortisol) enhances its antiinflammatory property.
4. 11-Desoxycortisol has an oxygen function at the c-11 site of ring C, augmenting its antiinflammatory activity.
5. Methylation or hydroxylation at site 16 in ring D eliminates the sodium-retaining effects and has only a slight effect on the antiinflammatory potency.

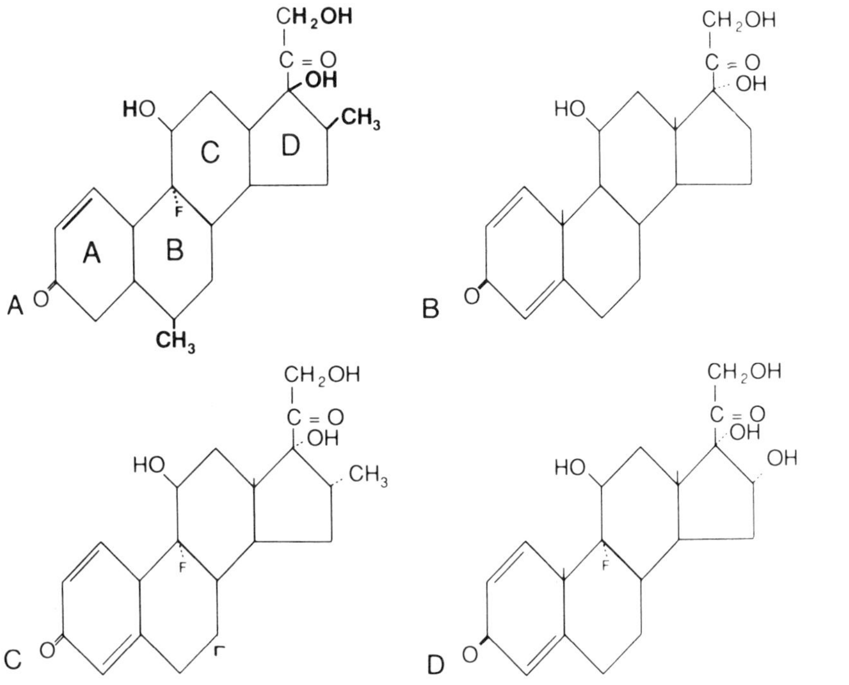

FIG. 52-5. Examples of different corticosteroids. **A:** The cortisol nucleus, showing sites at which the different chemical groups are added to form compounds with different potencies. **B:** Prednisolone. **C:** Dexamethasone. **D:** Triamcinolone.

6. In ring D, 17 α-hydroxylation is present in most of the antiinflammatory steroids.
7. Most of the active synthetic analogues and all natural corticosteroids have the hydroxyl group attached to carbon 21 in ring D (68).

Pharmacology

Corticosteroids act as both antiinflammatory and immunosuppressive agents, yet their precise mechanism of action is not well understood. They appear to work at the molecular and cellular levels. Corticosteroids freely penetrate the cell membrane and bind to a specific steroid-binding protein receptor in the cytoplasm, forming a steroid–receptor complex. This complex enters the nucleus, where it binds to chromatin, signaling the production of messenger RNA and coding for proteins that will determine the response of that cell to the hormone. The cytoplasmic steroid-binding receptor exhibits a high affinity for glucocorticoids. Glucocorticoid receptors have been identified in the iris, ciliary body, cornea, sclera, trabecular meshwork, and Schlemm's canal (68).

The molecular and cellular changes result in steroid-induced inhibition of all the cardinal signs of inflammation, such as pain, redness, swelling, and localized heat. This inhibition is accomplished through interference with leukocyte chemotaxis, arachidonic acid (AA) cascade, and normal function of immunocompetent cells. The antiinflammatory activity of corticosteroids is the result of a variety of mechanisms:

1. Constriction of blood vessels, which inhibit leakage of fluid, proteins, and inflammatory cells to the target site.
2. Stabilization of intracellular lysosomal membranes and inhibition of the expression of various damaging enzymes.
3. Stabilization of mast cells and basophils, which inhibits the degranulation process and subsequent release of histamine, bradykinin, PAF, proteases, and eosinophilic chemotactic factors.
4. Mobilization of polymorphonuclear leukocytes (PMN) from the bone marrow, which results in neutrophilic leukocytosis, corticosteroids simultaneously prevent adherence of PMN to the vascular endothelium, inhibiting infiltration from vessel to surrounding tissues.
5. Suppression of lymphocyte proliferation and lymphopenia; corticosteroids do not destroy T lymphocytes but rather affect their redistribution into circulation, concentrating them in the bone marrow.
6. Reduction of circulating eosinophils and monocytes.
7. Inhibition of macrophage recruitment and migration; steroids also interfere with macrophages' ability to process antigens.
8. Suppression of fibroplasia.
9. Depression of the bactericidal activity of monocytes and macrophages.
10. Inhibition of phospholipase A_2 by steroids, through a protein called macrocortin, resulting in inhibition of arachidonic acid degradation and subsequent synthesis of prostaglandins and leukotrienes by cyclooxygenase and lipoxygenase pathways (68).

Clinical Pharmacology

Corticosteroid preparations vary in their antiinflammatory potency. An attempt to compare the potency of these ophthalmic preparations should take into account the type of corticosteroid, formulation, concentration, and the model of inflammation used for comparison. An experimental model that mimics the clinical course of inflammation and allows determination of dose–response curves is desirable. However, in vivo models of ocular inflammation are difficult to design and standardize, and many animal models do not reflect the clinical action in humans.

Leibowitz and Kupferman attempted to determine the ocular antiinflammatory effectiveness of sodium phosphate, alcohol, and acetate derivatives of dexamethasone and prednisolone by measuring the decreased radioactivity of radiolabeled neutrophils in a rabbit keratitis model induced by injection of clove oil. Results demonstrated that, after a given period, corneal drug concentration with an intact corneal epithelium was highest with prednisolone acetate, followed by prednisolone sodium phosphate and dexamethasone alcohol suspension; dexamethasone sodium phosphate was not absorbed. Prednisolone sodium phosphate solution achieved highest concentration after topical application to a denuded epithelium, a circumstance that may more accurately represent the clinical circumstances in cases of keratitis. Under these conditions, the next highest concentration was achieved with the dexamethasone sodium phosphate solution, followed by prednisolone acetate, and last by the dexamethasone alcohol suspension (69,70).

The clove oil model used by Leibowitz and Kupferman was criticized because the oil causes greater absorption of lipophilic drugs than of lipophobic drugs. A pharmacokinetic model of absorption of lipophilic drugs, such as prednisolone acetate, and lipophobic drugs, such as prednisolone phosphate, was used to compare the drug elimination rate in the precornea and anterior chamber, the rate of drug dissolution, the rate of drug penetration in the cornea, and the rate of drug transport into the aqueous humor. In this model, the two forms of prednisolone had similar absorption capacity (71). Similar bioavailability was also determined in a rabbit eye model in vivo when prednisolone phosphate, acetate, and their metabolite prednisolone were directly quantitated in aqueous humor by reverse-phase high-performance liquid chromatography (HPLC) (72,73).

Evaluation of these steroid derivatives for antiinflammatory potency in a model of corneal inflammation showed that prednisolone acetate produced a significantly more potent antiinflammatory effect than the sodium phosphate solution in eyes with intact corneal epithelium. When the corneal epithelium was absent, no significant difference was noted among the three and dexamethasone alcohol. The dexamethasone sodium phosphate solution was clearly significantly inferior in eyes with the epithelium intact or absent (74,75).

Increasing the concentration of prednisolone acetate from 0.125% to 1.0% produces a significant increase in its corneal concentration and antiinflammatory effectiveness (74,76,77). However, antiinflammatory potency does not appear to be directly proportional to the concentration of drug obtained at the site of inflammation. Increasing the concentration of prednisolone acetate from 1.0% to 2% or 3% increases the corneal concentration but does not affect antiinflammatory potency (78). Similar results were obtained in comparisons of corneal bioavailability and antiinflammatory efficacy of three different dexamethasones. In one study, the acetate derivative achieved the lowest corneal concentration yet produced the greatest antiinflammatory effect (75).

The antiinflammatory potency of corticosteroids depend to a large degree on the frequency of instillation; e.g., hourly instillation of 1.0% prednisolone acetate produces much more effective suppression of corneal inflammation than does instillation every 4 hours (79). Maximum suppression is obtained if the drug is instilled every 5 minutes.

Two other topical corticosteroids available for ocular use are fluorometholone (FML) and medrysone (HMS). FML in 0.1% and 0.25% suspensions is far less efficacious than prednisolone in penetrating the cornea (80) but does have moderate antiinflammatory effects (81). FML acetate 0.1% has a therapeutic effect comparable to that of 1.0% prednisolone in alleviating corneal inflammation. FML is mildly hydrophobic, concentrating in the corneal epithelial layer, to the point of saturation, before passing through the hydrophilic layers of the stroma. This may explain why FML penetrates the cornea in comparatively low concentrations yet produces moderate but effective suppression of corneal inflammation (81). HMS, available in a 1.0% suspension, is used only for minor conjunctival inflammation due to its weak effect on the cornea.

As a result of their structural modifications, a new class of corticosteroids, termed the "soft steroids," may offer the therapeutic benefits of the existing steroid agents but with fewer side effects. Loteprednol etabonate, a steroid of this class, is a molecularly modified form of prednisolone. A labile ester functional group occupies the 17-β position and a stable carbonate group occupies the 17-α position. After topical application and corneal penetration, the soft steroid is rapidly hydrolized in the anterior chamber to the inactive 17-β carboxylic acid derivative (82). Animal studies have shown loteprednol to retain its antiinflammatory effects in the cornea (83), whereas a study in humans suggests that it may play a role in the treatment of GPC (84).

Rimexolone is a steroid with a unique molecular design which compares favorably with the strongest steroids available yet has a safer side-effect profile. Rimexolone 1.0% (Vexol) is currently approved for postsurgical inflammation and uveitis. A previous clinical trial demonstrated that rimexolone was clinically and statistically more effective than placebo in control of postcataract surgery inflammation and in reducing anterior chamber cells and flare at each follow-up visit. Furthermore, there were no treatment failures with rimexolone, and a significantly higher percentage of subjects had no anterior chamber inflammation (84a).

Corticosteroids are also available as an ointment. Although ointments increase contact time between the drug and the ocular surface, less drug is absorbed in the cornea and anterior chamber when dexamethasone phosphate ointment is used than when the solution form is used; the ointment may form a barrier that prevents rapid release of the drug into the tears (75). FML produced similar concentrations of drug in the aqueous humor whether suspended in water or ointment (85).

Pharmaceutics

Choice of corticosteroid therapy is largely determined by the physician's clinical experience and preference. Table 2 shows the common topical ocular preparations available.

In addition, various steroid antibiotic combinations are available. Table 3 shows selected topical ocular steroid antibiotic combination preparations currently available.

Pharmacokinetics

Corticosteroids are delivered into the eye topically, periocularly, orally, parenterally, or intravitreally. Topical preparations are available as solutions, suspensions, or ointments. Phosphate preparations are solutions because they are highly soluble in aqueous vehicles. Conversely, acetate and alcohol preparations are suspensions, which can penetrate the uninflamed cornea with intact epithelium. Corticosteroids can also be released by a drug depot placed on the ocular surface or by iontophoresis. One advantage of drug depots is the steady, sustained, and slow release of the corticosteroid over the ocular surface.

Factors influencing the penetration are relative water and lipid solubility, viscosity, concentration, pH, tonicity, condition of the corneal epithelium, size of particles in suspension, and addition of other compounds or vehicles, such as preservatives or methyl cellulose (86,87). Dexamethasone phosphate penetrates into the cornea and aqueous humor in 10 minutes or less. It reaches a peak in 30 to 60 minutes and remains inside the eye for several hours to 24 hours (88). The corneal tissue concentration of tritiated dexamethasone alcohol (Maxidex) reaches 14.79 μg/g cornea 7.5 minutes after instillation and then decreases to 1.86 μg/g cornea at 4 hours (89).

Prednisolone phosphate 1% (Inflamase) is a highly soluble compound with limited lipid solubility. Therefore, the compound was generally considered to have limited solubility through an intact cornea. Corneal concentrations, however, reach 10 μg/g and aqueous humor concentrations reach 0.5 μg/g 30 minutes after instillation. When the corneal epithelium is removed, the corneal concentration reaches 235 μg/g and levels in the aqueous humor reach 17 μg/g (71).

TABLE 52-2. *Common topical ocular preparations*

Name and preparation/trade name	Concentration (%)
Prednisolone acetate suspension	
Pred Mild	0.12
Econopred	0.125
AK-Tate	1.0
Econopred Plus	1.0
Pred Forte	1.0
Prednisolone sodium phosphate solution	
AK-Pred	0.125
Inflamase	0.125
AK-Pred	1.0
Inflamase Forte	1.0
Dexamethasone suspension	
Maxidex	0.1
Dexamethasone sodium phosphate solution	
AK-Dex	0.1
Decadron	0.1
Dexamethasone sodium phosphate ointment	
AK-Dex	0.05
Decadron	0.05
Maxidex	0.05
Fluorometholone suspension	
Fluor-Op	0.1
FML	0.1
FML Forte	0.25
Fluorometholone acetate suspension	
Flarex	0.1
Fluorometholone ointment	
FML S.O.P.	0.1
Medrysone suspension	
HMS	1.0
Rimexolone	
Vexol	1.0

Topically applied corticosteroid can drain through the upper and lower puncti into the nasolacrimal duct. Once exposed to the highly vascular nasal mucosa, it traverses into the circulatory system, where it binds to globulin and albumin. Eighty percent of circulating cortisol is bound to α-globulin as transcortin (corticosteroid-binding globulin), an inactive transport complex. A smaller portion is bound to albumin; it is this portion that can diffuse into the extravascular fluid and bathe tissue cells. Synthetic analogues of cortisol do not compete with cortisol for binding to transcortin. In addition, synthetic analogues are bound less tenaciously to albumin, enabling them to diffuse more completely into the extravascular tissue than cortisol (90).

All the biologically active corticosteroids and their synthetic derivatives have a double bond in the 4, 5 position and a ketone group at C 3. Reduction of the 4, 5 double bond occurs at both hepatic and extrahepatic sites, yielding an inactive component. The subsequent reduction of the 3-ketone substituent to a 3-hydroxyl, forming tetrahydrocortisol, has been demonstrated only in the liver. Most of the ring A-reduced metabolites are enzymatically coupled with

TABLE 52-3. *Topical ocular steroid antibiotic combination preparations (partial)*

Name and preparation	Trade name	Concentration
Sulfacetamide sodium, Prednisolone acetate suspension	Blephamide	10%, 0.2%
Sulfacetamide sodium, Prednisolone acetate solution	Vasocidin	10%, 0.25%
Sulfacetamide sodium, Prednisolone acetate ointment	Cetapred	10%, 0.25%
Sulfacetamide sodium, Fluorometholone suspension	FML-S	10%, 0.1%
Tobramycin, Dexamethasone suspension	Tobradex	0.3%, 0.1%
Neomycin sulfate, Dexamethasone sodium phosphate solution	Neodecadron	0.35%, 0.05%
Neomycin sulfate, Polymyxin B sulfate, Dexamethasone suspension	Dexasporin	3.5 mg/g, 10,000 U/g, 1 mg/g
Neomycin sulfate, polymyxin B sulfate, dexamethasone ointment	Dexacidin	3.5 mg/g, 10,000 U/g, 1 mg/g

sulfate or with glucuronic acid, through the 3-hydroxyl functional group, to form water-soluble sulfate esters or glucuronides, which are excreted as such. The conjugation reactions occur principally through the liver and to some degree in the kidney (67).

The metabolism of cortisol has been studied more extensively than that of all other corticosteroids, and the metabolism of its derivatives is generally assumed to be qualitatively similar. Cortisol has a plasma $t_{\frac{1}{2}}$ of approximately 1.5 hours. The metabolism of corticosteroids is greatly slowed by introduction of the 1, 2 double bond or a fluorine atom into the molecule, and the $t_{\frac{1}{2}}$ is correspondingly prolonged (67).

Therapeutic Use

Mild topical corticosteroids can be used for short-term management of ocular allergy when all other therapeutic modalities have been explored. Short trials of prednisolone 0.12% two to three times daily has resulted in few complications (19). However, safer alternatives to steroids should be used when possible.

The use of corticosteroids in the treatment of VKC can have dramatic results, yet the effects of chronic steroid therapy in this chronic disease must be delicately balanced. A pulse therapy of a topical steroid such as prednisolone phosphate 1.0% six to eight times daily for as long as 1 week, followed by rapid tapering to the lowest levels needed to allow the patient to function should be prescribed. Steroids should not be used to eliminate the last vestige of vasodilation or itching; neither should the clinician expect immediate resolution of the cobbles.

The relief afforded by steroids in GPC, even by the most aggressive of therapies, is not remarkable. A short course of topical steroids may quiet the associated inflammation before long-term management is undertaken, but since the wearing of contact lenses is elective and the disease resolves with the removal of the lenses, the use of steroids should be limited.

In severe cases of AKC, steroid therapy may be considered. Corticosteroid use can bring dramatic relief of symptoms, decreased corneal infiltrates, and vascularization. However, corticosteroids should be used in low doses for short times since long-term therapy can result in many unacceptable complications. Corticosteroid therapy should be avoided in cases of acute untreated purulent ocular infections, acute superficial herpes simplex, and other viral diseases of the cornea and conjunctiva, ocular tuberculosis, and fungal diseases of the eye.

Suspensions must be shaken. If particles are not evenly distributed, incorrect doses may be removed from the bottle. Patient compliance in shaking suspension eyedrops has been reported to be poor (91), and the risks of incorrect dosing and sudden discontinuation of steroid administration are well documented (92,93). The difficulty of predicting a steroid concentration in suspension drops suggests that the consistent dosing provided by solutions may be superior.

Side Effects and Toxicity

More than a decade after corticosteroids came into wide use for rheumatoid arthritis, Black et al. (94,95) reported a high incidence of cataracts in patients receiving long-term systemic therapy. Dosage and duration of steroid therapy correlated with the incidence of posterior subcapsular cataract (PSC) formation. Patients who received prednisone therapy for 1 to 4 years showed an 80% incidence when the dosage was more than 15 mg/day. If the dose was decreased to 10 mg/day, the chance of PSC formation decreased significantly to 11% incidence. These findings suggest that PSC formation is significantly related to the total cumulative steroid dose and the duration of steroid administration. Individual susceptibility to side effects of corticosteroids must be considered. Hispanics (96) and diabetic patients appear to be more susceptible to the complications of topical steroid administration. Discontinuation of corticosteroid therapy does not result in resolution of the opacity. The pathogenesis of corticosteroid-induced cataract formation has not been fully elucidated. Corticosteroids have been suggested to enter the lens and bind to its fibers. The steroid reacts nonenzymatically with the amino group of lysine in the lens crystallin, resulting in either exposure of protein sulfhydral groups or an increased susceptibility to oxidation. Disulfide cross-linking eventually occurs, generating complexes that refract light (steroid-induced cataracts).

Topical or systemic administration of steroids has been shown to produce increased intraocular pressure (IOP) (97–106). The increase in IOP and the reduction in outflow facility are generally reversible, but can lead to optic nerve damage and visual field changes similar to those observed in patients with chronic open-angle glaucoma. Factors contributing to pressure increases include genetic tendencies, age, diabetes, and corticosteroid used. Akingbehin (107) reported that 15 of 24 eyes treated with 0.1% dexamethasone showed an increase in IOP of more than 5 mm Hg, whereas only 2 of the 24 eyes treated with 0.1% FML showed such an increase. Mindel et al. (108) compared increases in IOP after application of 0.1% dexamethasone phosphate, 0.1% FML, and 1% HMS four times daily for 6 weeks. After the 6-week regimen, the mean IOP increases for dexamethasone, FML, and HMS were 63.1%, 33.8%, and 8.3%, respectively (108). The presence of glycosaminoglycans has been suggested to obstruct the trabecular meshwork, thereby causing resistance to aqueous outflow (109).

Corticosteroids substantially suppress the activation and migration of leukocytes, which is a major part of the cellular host defense against invading microorganisms and infection. Evidence shows that steroid administration increases susceptibility to viral, fungal, and bacterial infections (110). These secondary infections can take the form of bacterial conjunctivitis and keratitis, viral keratitis, or more serious vision-threatening infections such as fungal keratitis, fungal endophthalmitis, and toxoplasmic chorioretinitis. Management of these complications involves tapering, and eventually discontinuing, the corticosteroid while initiating therapy with appropriate antiinfective agents. Prophylactic coverage with appropriate antiviral or antibacterial agents can be considered.

Corticosteroid therapy can retard corneal epithelial and stromal healing, resulting in further corneal melting and perforation. Topical and systemic steroid administration has been shown to slow corneal regeneration time by as much as 30% after induced alkali corneal burns (111). The steroid's effect on the fibroblast results in delayed collagen synthesis, which can cause or exacerbate corneal melting (93,112).

Use of corticosteroids can result in acute anterior uveitis. Mydriasis, ptosis, and loss of accommodation have been reported after topical administration of steroids. Although some investigators suggest the cause to be related to the corticosteroid itself, studies comparing the effects of steroid, vehicle, and steroid/vehicle combination in monkey eyes suggest that a combination of agents in the vehicle mixture produces the observed effects by disturbing the selective semipermeability of the surface membrane, thereby altering the physiologic function of the muscle cell (113,114). In addition, transient ocular discomfort, refractive changes, blurring of vision, increased corneal thickness, and pseudotumor cerebri with papilledema and petechial conjunctival hemorrhages have been reported. It is recommended that patients who wear contact lenses avoid lens wear while using topical corticosteroids.

TABLE 52-4. *Systemic complications of corticosteroid therapy*[a]

Musculoskeletal
Myopathy
Osteoporosis, vertebral compression fractures
Aseptic necrosis of bone
Gastrointestinal
Peptic ulcer (often gastric)
Gastric hemorrhage
Intestinal perforation
Pancreatitis
Central nervous system
Psychiatric disorders
Pseudotumor cerebri
Ophthalmic
Glaucoma
Posterior subcapsular cataracts
Cardiovascular and renal
Hypertension
Sodium and water retention edema
Hypokalemic alkalosis
Metabolic
Precipitation of clinical manifestations, including ketoacidosis, diabetes mellitus
Hyperomolar nonketotic coma
Hyperlipidemia
Centripetal obesity
Endocrine
Growth failure
Secondary amenorrhea
Suppression of hypothalmic–pituitary–adrenal system
Inhibition of fibroplasia
Impaired wound healing
Subcutaneous tissue atrophy
Suppression of the immune response
Superimposition of a variety of bacterial, fungal, and viral infections in steroid-treated patients

Data from Melby JC. Systemic corticosteroid therapy: pharmacology and endocrinologic considerations. *Ann Intern Med* 1974;81:510, with permission.

Systemic absorption of steroids after topical treatment can be considerable. Six weeks of treatment with topical 0.1% dexamethasone sodium phosphate caused suppression of the adrenal cortex, reflected in a decrease in serum cortisol levels. Potential systemic complications of corticosteroid use are shown in Table 4.

High-risk Groups

No adequate, well-controlled studies have been performed to evaluate the possible effects of corticosteroids in neonates, children, pregnant women/nursing mothers, or the elderly. In rabbits, corticosteroids have been shown to be teratogenic and embryocidal. Topical application to the eyes of pregnant rabbits caused a significant dose-related increase in fetal abnormalities and in fetal loss. Pregnant women should use steroids only if the potential benefit significantly outweighs the potential risk to the fetus. Nursing mothers are advised not to nurse because corticosteroids do appear in breast milk. Potential effects to the infant are suppression of growth and interference with endogenous corticosteroid production. Studies in children have shown that long-term use of corticosteroids can retard skeletal maturation (115). Alternate-day therapy is recommended in children when possible, as such therapy appears to affect growth less.

Drug Interactions

Concurrent administration of other medications may interfere with metabolism and alter the pharmacologic effects of corticosteroids. Rifampin, used in the treatment of *Mycobacterium tuberculosis* infections, has been shown to interfere with the effects of steroids. Rifampin therapy induces a gradual proliferation of hepatic cell smooth endoplasmic reticulum, which is believed to be a locus of drug-metabolizing enzymes, making the usual therapeutic dose less effective (116). Phenobarbital, phenytoin, and ephedrine enhance the metabolic clearance of corticosteroids, thus reducing their antiinflammatory and immunosuppressive effects. Response to dicumarol and warfarin is inhibited when these drugs are taken concomitantly with steroids.

Major Clinical Trials

Prednisolone sodium phosphate 1% was evaluated for efficacy in alleviating the signs and symptoms of allergic conjunctivitis induced by allergen challenge. Instillation of drug four times daily for 2 full days before allergen challenge resulted in significant inhibition of hyperemia at all timed evaluations. Itching was significantly inhibited at 20 and 30 minutes, and chemosis was significantly inhibited at 10, 20, and 30 minutes after challenge. In addition to its acute effects, prednisolone significantly inhibited itching and hyperemia after a 4-hour rechallenge (117).

NSAIDs

History and Source

The therapeutic effects of willow bark was first noted in the mid-eighteenth century by Reverend Edmund Stone, who provided "an account of the success of the bark of willow in the cure of agues" (fever). In 1829, Leroux isolated the active ingredient in the willow bark, a bitter glycoside called salicin. Salicin, when hydrolized, yields glucose and salicylic alcohol, which can be converted to salicylic acid. By 1875, sodium salicylate was used therapeutically for the treatment of rheumatic fever and as an antipyretic. Based on the earlier work of Gerhardt, Hoffman, a chemist for Bayer, attempted to prepare acetylsalicylic acid. Demonstrating the antiinflammatory effects of this compound, Dreser introduced it into medicine at the end of the nineteenth century under the name of aspirin (118).

The chief therapeutic actions of aspirin were elucidated by the beginning of the nineteenth century. Synthetic analogues of the salicylates eventually replaced the more expensive natural derivatives. New compounds that shared some or all of the therapeutic actions of aspirin were discovered. Of these, only the derivatives of *para*-aminophenol are still in use today. Beginning with indomethacin, a host of new agents has been introduced into medicine in various countries in the past 20 years (118).

Official Drug Name and Chemistry

To some degree, all NSAIDs have antiinflammatory, antipyretic, and analgesic properties; however, there are some differences in their therapeutic properties. Acetaminophen, for example, is useful as an antipyretic and analgesic agent but does not have clinically significant antiinflammatory activity or any effect on platelets or bleeding time. Systemic NSAIDs at therapeutic doses can produce changes in the GI, respiratory, hepatic, endocrine, coagulation, and renal systems. This broad spectrum of pharmacologic properties is directly related to the diverse range of actions of the prostaglandins (PGs), whose production is inhibited by the NSAIDs. The NSAIDs can be divided into eight groups: salicylates, fenamates, and derivatives of indole, pyrazolone, propionic acid, *p*-aminophenol, phenylacetic acid, and oxicam (119).

Acular (ketorolac tromethamine), the only NSAID currently approved for the relief of itch due to seasonal allergic conjunctivitis, is a member of the pyrrolo-pyrolle group of NSAIDs. Its chemical name is (±)-5-benzoyl-2, 3-dihydro-1,H-pyrrolizine-1-carboxylic acid compound with 2-amino-2-(hydroxymethyl)-1,3-propanediol (1 : 1). Ketorolac is a white crystalline powder with a molecular weight of 376.41.

Pharmacology

AA, the primary precursor of PGs, leukotrienes (LTs), and related compounds, is bound to phospholipids in the plasma membrane and released by phospholipases. The currently marketed NSAIDs block PG biosynthesis by inhibiting the effects of cyclooxygenase, which is responsible for the conversion of AA to endoperoxides (PGG_2, PGH_2) in ocular and nonocular tissues (120). Correlation between the inhibitory activity of NSAIDs on cyclooxygenase and its antiinflammatory activity have been demonstrated (121). Experimental studies demonstrating that certain PGs are potent mediators of ocular inflammation have confirmed this view (122,123). Topical application of AA or certain PGs produces dilation of conjunctival vessels, with chemosis, changes in IOP, and miosis (124). Increased levels of PGs are present in aqueous humor after argon iridectomy (125), cataract surgery (126), and trauma (122). By inhibiting cyclooxygenase, NSAIDs have been shown to reduce the de novo synthesis of PGs (122,127,128) (Fig. 6). However, the NSAIDs do not generally inhibit the formation of eicosanoids such as the LTs, which also contribute to inflammation, as they are formed through the lipoxygenase arm of the AA pathway. Lipoxygenase blockers have yet to be developed for use in the eye.

When used as analgesic agents, the NSAIDs are usually effective only against pain of low to moderate intensity. Pain arising from integumental structures is well controlled, whereas pain originating from the hollow viscera is not relieved. Despite having a limited effect, NSAIDs do not change the perception of sensory modalities other than pain, as do the opioids.

As antipyretic agents, NSAIDs reduce the body temperature in febrile states. Fever, the result of a diseased state, enhances the formation of cytokines which induce the synthesis of PGE_2 in vascular organs in the preoptic hypothalmic area. The PG acts within the hypothalamus to produce the resultant increase in body temperature by processes that appear to be mediated by cyclic AMP. The NSAIDs suppress this response by inhibiting the synthesis of PGE_2 (118).

Clinical Pharmacology

The NSAIDs have been used in ophthalmic practice for the prevention of intraoperative miosis, postsurgical inflammation, and treatment of ocular inflammatory disorders. Surgical trauma that stimulates the production of PGs appears to play an integral role in the development of intraoperative miosis. Application of 0.03% flurbiprofen every 30 minutes, beginning 2 hours preoperatively, has been demonstrated to limit intraoperative miosis during anterior segment surgery in animal (129,130) and human eyes (131). The breakdown of the blood–aqueous barrier, assessed by fluorophotometry or slit-lamp biomicroscopy after cataract surgery, appears to be reduced by several topical NSAIDs, including ketorolac tromethamine, diclofenac sodium, and flurbiprofen (132–136). The only topical NSAID currently indicated for the treatment of inflammation after cataract surgery is diclofenac sodium 0.1% (137).

Treatment of inflammation associated with ocular infections may be useful but remains controversial. Two studies have demonstrated that topical NSAIDs do not worsen herpes simplex viral infections of the cornea (138,139), whereas one study suggests that the exacerbation of ocular herpes simplex viral infections caused by topical flurbiprofen is similar to that caused by topical dexamethasone (140). Preliminary trials have demonstrated that topical flurbiprofen 0.03% and suprofen 1.0% may play a role in the management of allergic conjunctivitis (141) and VKC (142), respectively. Oral aspirin has demonstrated efficacy as a primary therapy (143) as well as an adjunctive therapy

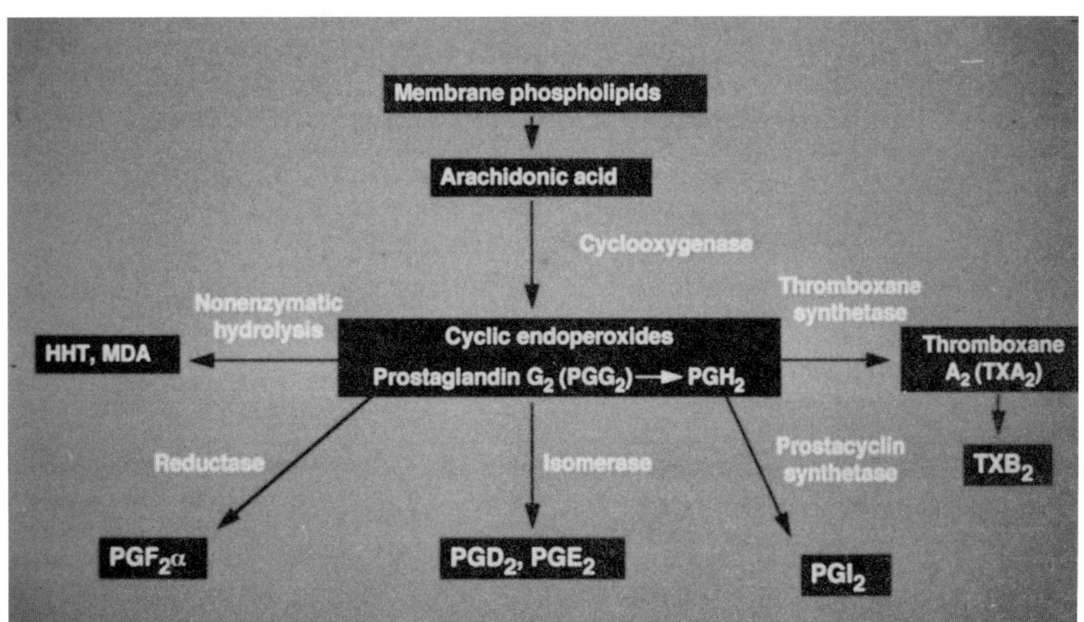

FIG. 52-6. Arachidonic acid (AA) metabolism: AA is converted (by cyclooxygenase) to the prostaglandins and thromboxanes. Nonsteroidal antiinflammatory drugs (NSAIDs) act by blocking the activity of cyclooxygenase, the enzyme responsible for the initiation of the AA cascade.

(144) with steroids in VKC. Although these NSAIDs show promise as therapies for the treatment of ocular allergies, ketorolac tromethamine is currently indicated for the relief of ocular itching associated with seasonal allergic conjunctivitis.

Pharmaceutics

A wide variety of NSAIDs is available for the treatment of ocular disease states. Choice of NSAID therapy is generally based on degree of therapeutic effect and the patient's tolerance to treatment. Table 5 shows the NSAIDs most commonly used in clinical practice today.

Pharmacokinetics

In general, orally ingested NSAIDs are rapidly and completely absorbed from the GI tract and distributed throughout most body tissues. The NSAIDs are extensively bound to plasma proteins, and peak concentrations may be detected in plasma 0.5 to 2 hours after administration. Unaltered NSAIDs and their metabolic products are usually eliminated in the urine. Therefore, patients with underlying liver or kidney dysfunction should be made aware of the risk of development of a wide range of toxic effects from therapeutic doses of systemic NSAIDs. As a result of their potential to cause systemic toxicity, oral NSAIDs appear on the whole to be significantly less safe than topical NSAIDs.

Therapeutic Uses

The NSAIDs currently available have shown promise in the management of allergic disorders of the eye. The only NSAID currently approved by the U.S. FDA for the relief of itch due to seasonal allergic conjunctivitis is ketorolac tromethamine 0.5%. When evaluated in the mouse writhing assay, ketorolac was 180 times more potent than aspirin (145). Topical application of ketorolac 0.5% four times daily for 1 week in patients with acute allergic conjunctivitis was significantly more effective than placebo at relieving itching and clinical signs of conjunctivitis, including hyperemia, edema, and mucous discharge (146,147). In addition to inhibiting the allergic inflammatory response effectively, ketorolac may be useful in the prophylaxis and treatment of cystoid macular edema (CME) after cataract surgery (147a).

The only topical NSAID currently indicated for treatment of postoperative inflammation is diclofenac sodium 0.1%. In a randomized, prospective, placebo-controlled clinical trial, eyes treated with diclofenac sodium showed significantly greater improvement from baseline in summed flare plus cell score than placebo-treated eyes at 2 to 5 days and 7 to 9 days after baseline measurement. In addition, diclofenac sodium-treated eyes had significantly less post-baseline conjunctival erythema and ciliary flush than placebo-treated eyes. By 5 to 7 days, significantly more diclofenac-treated subjects than placebo subjects had corrected visual acuities of 20/40 or better (147b).

Flurbiprofen 0.03% topical ophthalmic solution was superior to vehicle control at reducing conjunctival, ciliary, and episcleral hyperemia and ocular itching after topical antigen challenge (141). In addition, studies have suggested that flurbiprofen 0.03% may be useful therapy in treating and preventing CME after cataract surgery (147c and 147d).

Aspirin, piroxicam, and indomethacin have all showed promise as well. All three NSAIDs blocked lid closure and chemosis induced by topical challenge with 0.25% and 0.5% AA in humans and animals (124). New classes of NSAIDs, such as mixed cyclooxygenase and lipoxygenase antagonists (148–151) and lipoxygenase antagonists (152) are currently being investigated to determine their potential usefulness in ophthalmic practice.

Oral aspirin therapy has proven successful in the relief of conjunctival and episcleral hyperemia and resolution of keratitis and limbal infiltrates associated with VKC (144). Twenty-four of 27 patients with VKC who remained symptomatic after treatment with topical steroids and/or sodium cromoglycate showed a dramatic decrease in symptoms

TABLE 52-5. *Common NSAIDs*

Name and preparation	Trade name	Concentration (%)	Indication
Diclofenac solution	Voltaren	0.1	Postsurgical inflammation
Flurbiprofen solution	Ocufen	0.03	Inhibition of intraoperative miosis
Ketorolac solution	Acular	0.5	Relief of itch due to seasonal allergic conjunctivitis
Suprofen solution	Profenal	1	Inhibition of intraoperative miosis

NSAIDs, nonsteroidal antiinflammatory agents.

and signs after treatment with 1.5 g aspirin or less daily for 6 weeks (143). Oral aspirin appears to be useful as both primary and adjunctive therapy for recalcitrant cases of VKC. Because of required high doses, the side effects of aspirin should be given careful consideration.

As compared with vehicle, suprofen 1.0% provided symptomatic relief of the main symptoms of VKC (ocular itching, discomfort, and mucus strands) and suppressed the primary ocular signs (papillae and discharge). Indomethacin 1.0% caused highly significant reduction of itching, lacrimation, conjunctival injection, and papillae. Furthermore, three of four patients with corneal involvement obtained complete relief (153).

As compared with vehicle control, suprofen 1.0% also proved effective in management of contact lens-associated GPC (154). After 4 weeks of therapy four times daily, eyes treated with suprofen 1.0% showed more than twofold reduction in papillary and ocular discharge and mucus strand scores. With the development of better models in which to evaluate critically the efficacy of new NSAIDs and a better understanding of the pathogenesis of ocular allergic and inflammatory disorders, we can expect significant strides to be made in the development of more effective NSAIDs.

Cyclosporine, although not an NSAID in the classic sense, is a potent immunomodulator that has a selective inhibitory effect on helper T lymphocytes and on the expression of the HLA-DR determinant on the surface of cells involved in immunologically mediated inflammations. Studies have demonstrated that cyclosporine is effective in controlling the symptoms of both conjunctival tarsal and limbal forms of VKC; however, only minor changes in signs such as papillary hyperplasia were noticed (155,156). (A more comprehensive discussion of cyclosporine is provided in the chapter by Steven Foster, this volume).

Side Effects and Toxicity

Some patients have reported a stinging sensation after application of topical NSAIDs. The benefits of greater comfort cannot be overemphasized, since comfort is clearly an important factor in the patients' adherence to a therapeutic regimen. Although topical NSAIDs may cause increased bleeding time of ocular tissues in association with surgery, this increase has not been reported to be clinically relevant. Punctate keratitis has been associated with use of topical NSAIDs. Whether topical NSAIDs may be used safely in the presence of fungal, bacterial, or viral infections remains controversial and unclear. In addition, contact lens wear should be avoided during topical NSAIDs therapy.

Therapeutic use of oral NSAIDs can result in a variety of complications. The most common side effect is GI irritation, which can lead to nausea, vomiting, cramps, and gastric or intestinal ulceration, which in turn can result in significant blood loss and anemia (157,158). Because NSAIDs are potent inhibitors of PGs, which normally protect against erosion of the GI mucosa, oral administration of NSAIDs may inhibit certain key gastric PGs and contribute to local irritative effects; this has not been demonstrated to be an issue with use of topical NSAIDs. Furthermore, punctate keratitis has been associated with topical NSAID use.

The NSAIDs increase bleeding time by inhibiting platelet production of thromboxane A_2, a potent aggregating agent (159). A single dose of 0.65 g aspirin approximately doubles the mean bleeding time of normal persons for 4 to 7 days (118).

The NSAIDs can produce acute renal failure in patients with chronic renal disease, congestive heart failure, cirrhosis with ascites, volume depletion secondary to diuretic treatment, and hypotension secondary to hemorrhage. By stimulating vasodilation and maintaining renal perfusion, PGs protect the kidneys in disease states in which renal perfusion is compromised. The use of these aspirin-like drugs blocks this PG-mediated compensatory response (160); this is not considered an issue with topical NSAIDs therapy.

High-risk Groups

No adequate, well-controlled studies have been made in neonates, children, pregnant women/nursing mothers, and the elderly to evaluate the possible effects with NSAIDs. Reproductive studies performed in rabbits and rats at doses of 200 mg/kg/day and 80 mg/kg/day have resulted in an increased incidence of fetal resorption associated with maternal toxicity, increased stillbirths, and decreased postnatal survival. The NSAIDs should be used by pregnant women only if the potential benefit justifies the potential risk to the fetus. Use of the aspirin-like drugs should be discontinued during late pregnancy to avoid complications such as prolongation of labor, increased risk of postpartum hemorrhage, and intrauterine closure of the ductus arteriosus.

Orally administered NSAIDs have been detected in human breast milk after a single oral dose. Due to the potential for systemic absorption of topically applied NSAIDs, mothers should consider either discontinuation of nursing or of NSAID therapy since the safety of the aspirin-like drugs in human neonates has not been established.

At present, the safety of NSAIDs in neonates and children at this time is not certain. The association of Reye's syndrome in children with the administration of aspirin for treatment of febrile viral illnesses precludes its use in such circumstances. NSAIDs have been suggested to produce renal compromise in the elderly (161)—an important observation; however, such complications with NSAID use in ophthalmics have not been reported.

Drug Interactions

The NSAIDs bind firmly to plasma proteins, competing with certain other drugs for binding sites and often displacing them. Such competitive interactions can occur in patients treated with NSAIDs together with warfarin, a sulfonylurea hypoglycemic agent, or methotrexate. These types of interactions may also occur with some antibiotic agents. Either the dosage of such agents should be adjusted, or concurrent administration should be avoided (118).

Major Clinical Trials

The evaluation of ketorolac tromethamine in two separate seasonal environmental studies showed the 0.5% ophthalmic solution to be an effective and well-tolerated treatment in alleviating the signs and symptoms associated with seasonal allergic conjunctivitis. Ketorolac 0.5% ophthalmic solution was superior to placebo in reducing conjunctival inflammation, itching, swollen eyes, burning/stinging, discharge/tearing, foreign body sensation, and photophobia (146,147).

Diclofenac sodium 0.1% ophthalmic solution was compared with placebo in relieving ocular signs and symptoms in patients with acute seasonal allergic conjunctivitis. After 2 weeks of treatment (162), diclofenac was statistically and clinically superior to placebo in the physician's global evaluation and the primary composite score.

Flurbiprofen 0.03% topical ophthalmic solution was evaluated in the topical antigen challenge model. Flurbiprofen was significantly superior to vehicle control at reducing conjunctival, ciliary, and episcleral hyperemia and ocular itching (141).

REFERENCES

1. Butrus SI, Abelson MB, Allansmith MR. Ocular allergic disorders. In: Lockey R, Bukantz S, eds. *Principles of immunology and allergy.* Philadelphia: W.B. Saunders, 1987;165–176.
2. Gell PGH, Coombs RRA. In: Lachmann PJ and Peters DK, eds. *Clinical aspects of immunology,* 2nd ed. Oxford: Blackwell Scientific, 1968;575–596.
3. Berdy GJ, Abelson MB. Antihistamines and mast cell stabilizers in allergic ocular disease. In: Abelson M, Neufeld A, Topping T, eds. *Principles and practice of ophthalmology.* Philadelphia: W.B. Saunders, 1994;1028–1039.
4. Abelson MB, Schaefer K. Conjunctivitis of allergic origin: Immunologic mechanisms and current approaches to therapy. *Surv Ophthalmol* 1993;38(suppl):115–132.
5. Abelson MB, Smith LM. Mediators of ocular inflammation. In: Tasman W, ed. *Duane's foundation of clinical ophthalmology,* vol. 2. Philadelphia. J.B. Lippincott, 1991;1–10.
6. Allansmith MR, Abelson MB. Ocular allergies. In: Smolin G, Thoft R, eds. *The cornea: scientific foundations and clinical practice,* 2nd ed. Boston: Little, Brown, 1987;307.
7. Wallace W. Diseases of the conjunctiva. In: Bartlett J, Jaanus S, eds. *Clinical ocular pharmacology,* 2nd ed. Boston: Butterworths, 1989;515–566.
8. Atkinson JP, Eisen HN. Immunology. In: Eisen H, ed. *Microbiology,* 4th ed. Philadelphia: J.B. Lippincott, 1990;237–453.
9. Hegeman SL. Antihistamines. In: Bartlett J, ed. *Clinical ocular pharmacology,* 2nd ed. Boston: Butterworths, 1989;313–321.
10. Marrache F, Brunet D, Frandeboeuf J, et al. The role of ocular manifestations in childhood allergy syndromes. *Clin Rev Fr Allergol Immunol* 1978;18:151–155.
11. Allansmith MR. Immunology of the eye. In: Allansmith M, ed. *The eye and immunology.* St. Louis: C.V. Mosby, 1982;99–115.
12. Metzger H, Bach MK. The receptors for IgE in mast cells and basophils: studies on IgE binding and on the structure of the receptor. In: Bach M, ed. *Immediate hypersensitivity: modern concepts developments.* New York: Dekker, 1978;561.
13. Abelson MB, George MA, Garofalo C. Differential diagnosis of ocular allergic disorders. *Ann Allergy* 1993;70:95–113.
14. Allansmith MR. Diseases of the lids and the conjunctiva. In: *The eye and immunology.* St. Louis: C.V. Mosby, 1982;115.
15. Friedlaender MH, Masi RJ, Okumoto M, et al. Ocular microbial flora in immunodeficient patients. *Arch Ophthalmol* 1980;98:1211.
16. McGeady SJ, Buckley RH. Depression of cell-mediated immunity in atopic eczema. *J Allergy Clin Immunol* 1975;56:393.
17. Lobitz WC, Honeyman JF, Winkler NW. Suppressed cell-mediated immunity in two adults with atopic dermatitis. *Br J Dermatol* 1972;86:317.
18. Beigelman MN. *Vernal conjunctivitis.* Los Angeles: University of Southern California Press, 1950.
19. Allansmith MR. Vernal conjunctivitis. In: Duane TD, Jaeger EA, eds. *Clinical ophthalmology,* revised ed., vol. 1. Philadelphia: J.B. Lippincott, 1986.
20. Duke-Elder S. Allergic keratoconjunctivitis. In: Duke-Elder S, ed. *System of ophthalmology, diseases of the outer eye,* vol. 8., part 1. London: Henry Kimpton, 1965;475.
21. Henriquez AS, Kenyon KR, Allansmith MR. Mast cell ultrastructure: comparison in contact lens-associated giant papillary conjunctivitis and vernal conjunctivitis. *Arch Ophthalmol* 1981;99: 1266.
22. Abelson MB, Baird RS, Allansmith MR. Tear histamine levels in vernal conjunctivitis and ocular inflammations. *Ophthalmology* 1980;87:812.
23. Abelson MB, Soter NA, Simon MA, et al. Histamine in human tears. *Am J Ophthalmol* 1977;83:417.
24. Berdy GJ, Levene RB, Bateman ST. Identification of histaminase activity in human tears after conjunctival antigen challenge. *Invest Ophthalmol Vis Sci* 1990;31(suppl):65.
25. Abelson MB, Leonardi AA, Smith LM, Fregona IA, Secchi AG. *Histaminase activity in vernal keratoconjunctivitis.* Sarasota, Florida: The Association for Research in Vision and Ophthalmology, 1994;00–00.
26. Mukhopadhyay K, Pradhan SC, Mathur JS, et al. Studies on histamine and histaminase in spring catarrh (vernal conjunctivitis). *Int Arch Allergy Appl Immunol* 1981;64:464.
27. Abelson MB, Udell IJ, Weston JH. Conjunctival eosinophils in allergic ocular disease. *Arch Ophthalmol* 1983;101:631.
28. Udell IJ, Gleich GJ, Allansmith MR, et al. Eosinophil granule major basic protein and Charcot-Leydon crystal protein in human tears. *Am J Ophthalmol* 1981;92:824.
29. Golubovic S, Parunovic A. Vernal conjunctivitis—a cause of corneal mucoid plaques. *Fortschr Ophthalmol* 1986;83:272.
30. Abelson MB, Allansmith MR, Udell IJ, et al. Allergic and toxic disorders. In: *Principles and practice of ophthalmology: the Harvard system.* Philadelphia: W.B. Saunders, 1994;77–100.
31. Allansmith MR, Korb DR, Greiner JV, et al. Giant papillary conjunctivitis in contact lens wearers. *Am J Ophthalmol* 1977;86:697.
32. Greiner JV, Kenyon KR, Henriquez AS, et al. Mucus secretory vesicles in conjunctival epithelial cells of wearers of contact lenses. *Arch Ophthalmol* 1980;98:1843–1846.
33. Begley CG, Riggle A, Tuel JA. Association of giant papillary conjunctivitis with seasonal allergies. *Optom Vis Sci* 1990;67:192.
34. Gudmundsson OG, Woodward DF, Fowler SA, et al. Identification of proteins in contact lens surface deposits by immunofluorescence microscopy. *Arch Ophthalmol* 1985;103:196.
35. Ballow M, Donshik PC, Rapacz P, et al. Immune responses in monkeys to lenses from patients with contact lens-induced giant papillary conjunctivitis. *CLAO* 1989;15:64.
36. Jolson AS, Jolson SC. Suture barb giant papillary conjunctivitis. *Ophthalmic Surg* 1984;15:139.
37. Nirankari VS, Karesh JW, Richards RD. Complications of exposed monofilament sutures. *Am J Ophthalmol* 1983;95:515.
38. Greiner JV. Papillary conjunctivitis induced by an epithelialized corneal foreign body. *Ophthalmologica* 1988;196:82.
39. Windaus A, Vogt W. Synthese des imidazolylathylamins. *Berl Dtsch Chem Ges* 1907;3:3691.

40. Dale HH, Laidlaw PP. The physiologic action of beta-imidazolethylamine. *J Physiol (Lond))* 1910;41:318.
41. Dale HH, Laidlaw PP. Histamine shock. *J Physiol (Lond)* 1919;52: 355.
42. Riley JF, West GB. The presence of histamine in tissue mast cells. *J Physiol (Lond)* 1953;120:528.
43. Abelson MB, Allansmith MR. Histamine and the eye. In: Silverstein A, O'Connor G, eds. *Immunology and immunopathology of the eye.* New York: Masson, 1979;362–364.
44. Ash ASF, Schild HO. Receptors mediating some actions of histamine. *Br J Pharmacol Chemother* 1966;27:427.
45. Weston JH, Udell IJ, Abelson MB. H1 Receptors in the human ocular surface. *Invest Ophthalmol Vis Sci* 1981;20(suppl):32.
46. Abelson MB, Udell IJ. H2 Receptors in the human ocular surface. *Arch Ophthalmol* 1981;99:302.
47. Ganellin CR. Chemistry and structure-activity relationships of H2 receptor antagonists. In: Rocha, Silva M, eds. *Histamine II and anti-histaminics: chemistry, metabolism, and physiological and pharmacological actions. Handbook of experimental pharmacology,* vol. 18, part 2. New York: Springer-Verlag, 1978;251–294.
48. Ariens EJ, Simonis AM. Autonomic drugs and their receptors. *Arch Int Pharmacodyn* 1960;127:479.
49. Dechant KL, Goa KL. Levocabastine A review of its pharmacological properties and therapeutic potential as a topical antihistamine in allergic rhinitis and conjunctivitis. *Drugs* 1991;41:202–224.
50. Douglas WW. Histamine and 5-hydroxytryptamine (serotonin) and their antagonists. In: Gilman A, Goodman L, Gilman A, eds. *Goodman and Gilman's the pharmacological basis of therapeutics,* 6th ed. New York: MacMillan, 1980;609.
51. Abelson MB, Smith LM. Levocabastine: evaluation in the histamine and compound 48/80 models of ocular allergy in humans. *Ophthalmology* 1988;95:1494–1497.
52. Witiak DT, Lewis NJ. Absorption, distribution, metabolism, and elimination of antihistamines. In: Rocha, Silva M, eds. *Histamine II and anti-histaminics: chemistry, metabolism, and physiological and pharmacological actions. Handbook of experimental pharmacology,* vol. 18, part 2. New York: Springer-Verlag, 1978;513–560.
53. Harvey RP, Schocket AL. The effect of H1 and H2 blockade on cutaneous histamine response in man. *J Allergy Clin Immunol* 1980; 65:136.
54. Ueno N, Refojo MF, Abelson MB. Pharmacokinetics. In: Abelson M, Neufeld A, Topping T, eds. *Principles and practice of ophthalmology.* Philadelphia: W.B. Saunders, 1994;916–919.
55. Berdy GJ, Abelson MB, George MA, Smith LM, Giovanoni RL. Allergic conjunctivitis: a survey of new antihistamines. *J Ocul Pharmacol* 1991;7:313–324.
56. Abelson MB, Chambers WA, Smith LM. Conjunctival allergen challenge. A clinical approach to studying allergic conjunctivitis. *Arch Ophthalmol* 1990;108:84–88.
57. Abelson MB, Paradis A, George MA, Smith LM. The effects of Vasocon-A in the allergen challenge model of acute conjunctivitis. *Arch Ophthalmol* 1990;108:520–524.
58. Smith LM, Abelson MB, George MA, West L. A double-masked study on the effects of ophthalmic levocabastine vs placebo on the signs and symptoms of allergic conjunctivitis [Abstract]. *Invest Ophthal Vis Sci* 1992;33(suppl):1297.
59. Abelson MB, George MA, Schaefer K, et al. Evaluation of the new ophthalmic antihistamine 0.05% levocabastine in the clinical allergen challenge model of allergic conjunctivitis. J *Allerg Clin Immunol* 1994;94:458–64.
60. Cox JSG, Beach JE, Blair AMJN, et al. Disodium cromoglycate (Intal). *Adv Drug Res* 1970;5:115.
61. Rall TW. Drugs used in the treatment of asthma: the methylxanthines, cromolyn sodium, and other agents. In: Gilman A, Rall T, Nies A, Taylor P, eds. *Goodman and Gilman's the pharmacological basis of therapeutics,* 8th ed. New York: Pergamon Press, 1990; 619–637.
62. Altounyan REC. Inhibition of experimental asthma by a new compound, disodium cromoglycate, "INTAL." *Acta Allergol* 1967;22: 487.
63. Johnson HG, VanHout CA, Wright JB. Inhibition of allergic reactions by cromoglycate and by a new antiallergy drug U-42,585E. II. Activity in primates against aerosolized Ascrs suum antigen. *Int Arch Allergy Appl Immunol* 1978;56:481.
64. Santos CI, Huang AJ, Abelson MB, Foster CS, Friedlaender M, McCulley JP. Efficacy of lodoxamide 0.1% ophthalmic solution in resolving corneal epitheliopathy associated with vernal keratoconjunctivitis. *Am J Ophthalmol* 1994;117:488–497.
65. Caldwell DR, Verin P, Hartwich-Young R, Meyer SM, Drake MM. Efficacy and safety of lodoxamide 0.1% vs cromolyn sodium 4% in patients with vernal keratoconjunctivitis. *Am J Ophthalmol* 1992;113:632–637.
66. Jaanus SD. Anti-inflammatory drugs. In: Bartlett J, Jaanus S, eds. *Clinical ocular pharmacology,* 2nd ed. Boston: Butterworths, 1989; 163.
66a. Hench PS, Kendall EC, Slocumb CH, et al. The effect of a hormone of the adrenal cortex (17-hydroxy-11-dehydrocorticosterone, compound E) and of pituitary adrenocorticotropic hormone or rheumatoid arthritis. *Proc Staff Meet Mayo Clin* 1949;24:181.
66b. Gordon DM,. McLean JM. Effects of Pituitary adrenocorticotropic hormone (ACTH) therapy in ophthalmologic conditions. JAMA 1950;142:1271–1276.
67. Haynes RC. Adrenocorticotropic hormone; adrenocortical steroids and their synthetic analogs; inhibitors of the synthesis and actions of adrenocortical hormones. In: Gilman A, Rall T, Nies A, Taylor P, eds. *The pharmacological basis of therapeutics,* 8th ed. New York: Pergamon Press, 1990;1431.
68. Abelson MB, Butrus S. Corticosteroids in ophthalmic practice. In: *Principles and practice of ophthalmology: the Harvard system.* Philadelphia: W.B. Saunders, 1994;1013–1022.
69. Feldman D. The role of hormone receptors in the action of adrenal steroids. *Annu Rev Med* 1978;26:83.
70. O'Malley BW. Mechanisms of action of steroid hormones. *N Engl J Med* 1976;84:304.
71. Olejnick O, Weisbecker CA. Ocular bioavailability of topical prednisolone preparations. *Clin Ther* 1990;12:2.
72. Musson DG, Bidgood AM, Olejnick O. Assay methodology for prednisolone, prednisolone acetate and prednisolone sodium phosphate in rabbit aqueous humor and ocular physiological solutions. *J Chromatogr* 1991;565:89.
73. Musson DG, Bidgood AM, Olejnick O. An in vitro comparison of the permeability of prednisolone, prednisolone sodium phosphate, and prednisolone acetate across the NZW rabbit cornea. *J Ocul Pharmacol* 1992;8:139.
74. Kupferman A, Leibowitz HM. Antiinflammatory effectiveness of topically administered corticosteroid in the cornea without epithelium. *Invest Ophthalmol* 1975;14:352.
75. Leibowitz HM, Kupferman A. Bioavailability and therapeutic effectiveness of topically administered corticosteroids. *Trans Am Acad Ophthalmol* 1975;79:78.
76. Kupferman A, Leibowitz HM. Topically applied steroids in corneal disease IV. The role of drug concentration in stromal absorption of prednisolone acetate. *Arch Ophthalmol* 1974;88:377.
77. Leibowitz HM, Kupferman A. Antiinflammatory effectiveness of topically administered prednisolone. *Invest Ophthalmol Vis Sci* 1974;13:757.
78. Leibowitz HM, Kupferman A. Kinetics of topically administered prednisolone acetate optimal concentration for treatment of inflammatory keratitis. *Arch Ophthalmol* 1976;94:1387.
79. Leibowitz HM. Management of inflammation in the cornea and conjunctiva. *Ophthalmology* 1980;87:753.
80. Leibowitz HM, Kupferman A. Penetration of fluorometholone into the cornea and aqueous humor. *Arch Ophthalmol* 1975;93:-425.
81. Kupferman A, Leibowitz HM. Therapeutic effectiveness of fluorometholone in inflammatory keratitis. *Arch Ophthalmol* 1975;93: 1011.
82. Druzgala PD, Wu WM, Winwood D, et al. Ocular absorption and distribution of loteprednol etabonate: A "soft" steroid. *Current Eye Research* 1991;10(10):933–937.
83. Leibowitz HM, Ryan WJ, Kupferman A. Comparative anti-inflammatory efficacy of topical corticosteroids with low glaucoma-inducing potential. *Archives of Ophthalmol* 1992;110(1):118–120.
84. Labowitz RA, Ghormley NR, Insler MS, et al. Treatment of giant papillary conjunctivitis with loteprednol etabonate, a novel corticosteroid. *Invest Ophthalmol Vis Sci* 1991;32(suppl):734.
84a. Lehmann R, Assil K, Stewart R, et al. Comparison of rimexolone 1.0% ophthalmic suspension to placebo in control of post cataract surgery inflammation. IOVS 1995;36(suppl):3667 (abstr.)

85. Sieg J, Robinson J. Vehicle effects on ocular drug bioavailability. I. Evaluation of fluorometholone. *J Pharm Sci* 1975;64:931.
86. Gardner SK. Ocular drug penetration and pharmacokinetic principles. In: Lamberts D, Potter D, eds. *Clinical ophthalmic pharmacology.* Boston: Little, Brown, 1987;00–00.
87. Maurice DM. Factors influencing the penetration of topically applied drugs. In: Holly F, ed. *Clinical pharmacology of the anterior segment.* Boston: Little, Brown, 1980;00–00.
88. Jasami MK. Anti-inflammatory steroids: mode of action in rheumatoid arthritis and homograft rejection. In: Vane J, Ferriera S, eds. *Antiinflammatory drugs.* Berlin: Springer-Verlag, 1979;00–00.
89. Short C, Keates RH, Donovan EF, et al. Ocular penetration studies I. Topical administration of dexamethasone. *Arch Ophthalmol* 1966;75:689.
90. Melby JC. Systemic corticosteroid therapy: pharmacology and endocrinologic considerations. *Ann Intern Med* 1974;81:505.
91. Apt L, Henrick A, Silverman LM. Patient compliance with the use of topical ophthalmic corticosteroid suspensions. *Am J Ophthalmol* 1979;87:210.
92. Burch PG, Migeon CJ. Systemic absorption of topical steroids. *Arch Ophthalmol* 1968;79(2):174–176.
93. Aronson SB, Moore TE. Corticosteroid therapy in central stromal keratitis. *Am J Ophthalmol* 1969;67:873.
94. Black RL, Oglesby RB, Sallman L Von, et al. Posterior subcapsular cataracts induced by corticosteroids in patients with rheumatoid arthritis. *JAMA* 1960;174:166.
95. Spaeth GI, Sallman L Von. Corticosteroids and cataracts. *Int Ophthalmol Clin* 1966;6:915.
96. Loredo A, Rodriquez RS, Murillo L. Cataracts after short-term corticosteroid treatment. *N Engl J Med* 1972;286:160–163.
97. Francois J. Cortisone et tension oculaire. *Ann Ocul* 1954;187:805.
98. Stern JJ. Acute glaucoma during cortisone therapy. *Am J Ophthalmol* 1953;70:389.
99. Armaly M. Effect of corticosteroids on intraocular pressure and fluid dynamics: I. The effect of dexamethasone in the normal eye. *Arch Ophthalmol* 1963;70:482.
100. Armaly M. Effect of corticosteroids on intraocular pressure and fluid dynamics: II. The effect of dexamethasone in the glaucomatous eye. *Arch Ophthalmol* 1963;70:492.
101. Armaly M. Statistical attributes of the steroid hypertensive response in the clinically normal eye. *Invest Ophthalmol Vis Sci* 1965;4:187.
102. Armaly M. Heritable nature of dexamethasone-induced ocular hypertension. *Arch Ophthalmol* 1966;75:32.
103. Becker B, Mill SW. Corticosteroids and intraocular pressure. *Arch Ophthalmol* 1963;70:500.
104. Becker B, Hahn KA. Topical corticosteroids and heredity in primary open-angle glaucoma. *Am Ophthalmol* 1964;57:544.
105. Bernstein HN, Schwartz B. Effects of long term systemic steroids on ocular pressure and tonographic values. *Arch Ophthalmol* 1962; 68:742.
106. Covell LL. Glaucoma induced by systemic steroid therapy. *Am J Ophthalmol* 1954;45:108.
107. Akingbehin AO. Comparative study of the intraocular pressure effects of fluorometholone 0.1% versus dexamethasone 0.1%. *Br J Ophthalmol* 1983;67:661.
108. Mindel JS, Tovitian HO, Smith H, Walker EC. Comparative ocular pressure elevations by medrysone, fluorometholone, and dexamethasone phosphate. *Arch Ophthalmol* 1980;98:1577.
109. Godel V, Rogenbogen L, Stein R. On the mechanism of corticosteroid-induced ocular hypertension. *Ann Ophthalmol* 1978;10:191.
110. Leopold IH. The steroid shield in ophthalmology. *Trans Am Acad Ophthalmol Otolaryngol* 1967;71:273.
111. Leopold IH, Maylath F. Intraocular penetration of cortisone and its effectiveness against experimental corneal burns. *Am J Ophthalmol* 1952;35:1125.
112. Ashton N, Cook C. Effect of cortisone on healing of corneal wounds. *Br J Ophthalmol* 1951;35:708.
113. Kern R, Marci FJ. Steroid eye drops and their components. *Arch Ophthalmol* 1967;78:798.
114. Newsome DA, Wong VG, Cameron TP, Anderson RR. "Steroid-induced" mydriasis and ptosis. *Invest Ophthalmol* 1971;10:424.
115. Sturge RA, Beardwell C, Hartog M, et al. Cortisol and growth hormone secretion in relation to linear growth. *Br Med J* 1970;3:547.
116. Buffington GA, Dominguez JH, Piering WF, et al. Interaction of rifampin and glucocorticoids. *JAMA* 1976;236:1958.
117. George MA, Smith LM, Abelson MB. *Efficacy of 1.0% prednisolone sodium phosphate in alleviating the signs and symptoms of allergic conjunctivitis induced by allergen challenge.* Sarasota, FL: ARVO, 1991;00–00.
118. Insel PA. Analgesic-antipyretics and antiinflammatory agents: Drugs employed in the treatment of rheumatoid arthritis and gout. In: Gilman A, Rall T, Nies A, Taylor P, eds. *The pharmacologic basis of therapeutics,* 8th ed. New York: Pergamon Press, 1990; 638.
119. Rainsford KO. Anti-inflammatory and anti-rheumatic drugs. In: *Inflammation mechanisms and actions of traditional drugs,* vol. 1. Boca Raton: CRC Press, 1985.
120. Bhattacherjee P. The role of arachidonate metabolites in ocular inflammation. *Prog Clin Biol Res* 1989;312:211.
121. Vane JR, Botting R. Inflammation and mechanism of action of antiinflammatory drugs. *FASEB J* 1987;1:89.
122. Eakins KE. Prostaglandin and non-prostaglandin-mediated breakdown of the blood-aqueous barrier: in the ocular and cerebrospinal fluid. *Exp Eye Res* 1977;25:483.
123. Bhattacherjee P. Prostaglandin and inflammatory reactions in the eye. *Methods Find Exp Clin Pharmacol* 1980;2:17.
124. Abelson MB, Butrus SI, Kliman GH, et al. Topical arachidonic acid: a model for screening anti-inflammatory agents. *J Ocul Pharmacol* 1987;3:63.
125. Unger WG, Bass MS. Prostaglandin and nerve-mediated response of the rabbit eye to argon laser irradiation of the iris. *Ophthalmologica* 1977;175:153.
126. Miyake K, Sugiyama S, Norimatsu I, et al. Prevention of cystoid macular edema after lens extraction by topical indomethacin: (III) Radioimmunoassay measurement of prostaglandins in the aqueous during and after lens extraction procedures. *Graefes Arch Clin Exp Ophthalmol* 1978;209:83.
127. Conquet P, Plazonnet B, LeDouarec J. Arachidonic acid-induced elevation of intraocular pressure and anti-inflammatory agents. *Invest Ophthalmol* 1975;14:772.
128. Podos SM. Prostaglandin, nonsteroidal anti-inflammatory agents and eye disease. *Trans Am Ophthalmol Soc* 1976;74:637.
129. Anderson JA, Chen CC, Vita JB, et al. Disposition of topical flurbiprofen in normal and aphakic rabbit eyes. *Arch Ophthalmol* 1982;100:642.
130. Duffin RM, Camras CB, Gardner SK, et al. Inhibitors of surgically induced miosis. *Ophthalmology* 1982;89:966.
131. Keates RH, Jay WM. Clinical trial of flurbiprofen to maintain pupillary dilation during cataract surgery. *Ann Ophthalmol* 1984; 16:919.
132. Flach AJ, Kraff MC, Sanders DR, et al. The quantitative effect of 0.5% ketorolac tromethamine solution and 0.1% dexamethasone sodium phosphate solution on postsurgical blood aqueous barrier. *Arch Ophthalmol* 1988;106:480.
133. Araie M, Sawa M, Takase M. Topical flurbiprofen and diclofenac suppress blood-aqueous barrier breakdown in cataract surgery: a fluorophotometric study. *Jpn J Ophthalmol* 1983;27:535.
134. Kraff MC, Sanders DR, McGuigan L, et al. Inhibition of the blood-aqueous barrier breakdown with diclofenac. *Arch Ophthalmol* 1990;108:380.
135. Flach AJ, Graham J, Kruger LP, et al. Quantitative assessment of postsurgical breakdown of blood-aqueous barrier following administration of 0.5% ketorolac tromethamine solution: a double-masked, paired comparison with vehicle-placebo solution study. *Arch Ophthalmol* 1988;106:344.
136. Flach AJ, Lavelle CJ, Olander KW, et al. The effect of ketorolac tromethamine solution 0.5% in reducing postoperative inflammation after cataract extraction and intraocular lens implantation. *Ophthalmology* 1988;95:1279.
137. Vickers FF, McGuigan LJB, Ford C, et al. The effect of diclofenac sodium on the treatment of postoperative inflammation. *Invest Ophthalmol Vis Sci* 1991;32(ARVO suppl):793.
138. Fraser-Smith EB, Mathews TR. Effect of ketorolac on herpes simplex virus type on ocular infection in rabbits. *J Ocul Pharmacol* 1988;4:321.
139. Colin J, Bodin C, Malet F, et al. La kératite hépétique experimentale du lapin. *J Fr Ophthalmol* 1989;12:255.
140. Trousdale MD, Dunkel EC, Nesburn AB. Effect of flurbiprofen on herpes simplex keratitis in rabbits. *Invest Ophthalmol Vis Sci* 1980;19:267.

141. Bishop K, Abelson M, Cheetham J, et al. Evaluation of flurbiprofen in the treatment of antigen-induced allergic conjunctivitis. *Invest Ophthalmol Vis Sci* 1990;31(ARVO suppl):487.
142. Buckley DC, Caldwell DR, Reaves TA. Treatment of vernal conjunctivitis with suprofen, a topical non-steroidal antiinflammatory agent. *Invest Ophthalmol Vis Sci* 1986;27(ARVO suppl):29.
143. Meyer E, Kraus E, Zonis S. Efficacy of antiprostaglandin therapy in vernal conjunctivitis. *Br J Ophthalmol* 1987;71:497.
144. Abelson MB, Butrus SI, Weston JH. Aspirin therapy in vernal conjunctivitis. *Am J Ophthalmol* 1983;95:502.
145. Rooks WH, Maloney PJ, Shott LD, et al. The analgesic and antiinflammatory profile of ketorolac and its tromethamine salt. *Drugs Exp Clin Res* 1985;11:479.
146. Tinkelman D, Rupp G, Kaufman H, et al. Ketorolac tromethamine 0.5% ophthalmic solution in the treatment of seasonal allergic conjunctivitis: a placebo-controlled clinical trial. *Surv Ophthalmol* 1993;38(suppl):133.
147. Ballas Z, Blumenthal M, Tinkelman D, et al. Clinical evaluation of ketorolac tromethamine 0.5% ophthalmic solution for treatment of seasonal allergic conjunctivitis. *Surv Ophthalmol* 1993;38(suppl):141.
147a. Flach AJ, Jampol LM, Weinberg D, et al. Improvement in visual acuity in chronic aphakic and pseudophakic cystoid macular edema after treatment with topical 0.5% ketorolac tromethamine. *AJO* 1991;112(5):514–9.
147b. Kraff MC, Martin RG, Neumaan HC, et al. Efficacy of diclofenac sodium ophthalmic solution versus placebo in reducing inflammation following cataract and posterior chamber lens implantation. *J Cat Refr Surg* 1994;20(2):138–44.
147c. Ginsburg AP, Cheetham JK, Debrayse RZ, et al. Effects of flurbiprofen and indomethacin on acute cystoid macular edema after cataract surgery: functional vision and contrast sensitivity. *J Cat Refr Surg* 1995;21(1):82–92.
147d. Solomon LD. Efficacy of topical flurbiprofen and indomethacin in preventing pseudophakic cystoid macular edema. Flurbiprofen CME Study Group I. *J Cat Refr Surg* 1995;21(1):73–81.
148. Bhattacherjee P, Williams RN, Eakins KE. A comparison of the ocular anti-inflammatory activity of steroidal and nonsteroidal compounds in the rat. *Invest Ophthalmol Vis Sci* 1983;24:1143.
149. George MA, Greiner JV, Conway J, et al. The effects of a new nonsteroidal anti-inflammatory agent, 1% and 0.05% RMI 1068, in an animal model of anterior uveitis. *Invest Ophthalmol Vis Sci* 1989; 30(ARVO suppl):84.
150. Colin J, Bodin C, Malet F, et al. Experimental herpes simplex keratitis: evaluation of pro-infectious effects of topical nonsteroidal anti-inflammatory drugs. *J Fr Ophthalmol* 1989;12:255.
151. Conway J, Olejnik O. Therapeutic effect of the topical NSAID, RMI 1068, on experimental iritis in cats. *Invest Ophthalmol Vis Sci* 1990;31(ARVO suppl):61.
152. Chiou LY, Chiou GCY. Ocular anti-inflammatory action of a lipoxygenase inhibitor in the rabbit. *J Ocul Pharmacol* 1985;1: 383.
153. Gupta S, Khurana AK, Ahluwalia BK, Gupta NC. Topical indomethacin for vernal keratoconjunctivitis. *Acta Ophthalmol* 1991; 69:95.
154. Wood TS, Steward RH, Bowman RW. Suprofen treatment of contact lens associated GPC. *Ophthalmology* 1988;96:822.
155. Secchi AG, Tognon MS, Leonardi A. Topical use of cyclosporine in the treatment of vernal keratoconjunctivitis. *Am J Ophthalmol* 1990; 110:641.
156. BenEzra D, Peter J, Brodsky M, Cohen E. Cyclosporin eyedrops for the treatment of severe vernal keratoconjunctivitis. *Am J Ophthalmol* 1986;101:278.
157. Langman MJS. Peptic ulcer complications and the use of nonaspirin non-steroidal anti-inflammatory drugs. *Adverse Drug Reaction Bull* 1986;120:448.
158. Paulus HE. Arthritis Advisory Committee Meeting. Risks of agranulocytosis aplastic anemia, flank pain and adverse gastrointestinal effects with the use of nonsteroidal antiinflammatory drugs. *Arthritis Rheum* 1987;30:593.
159. Hamberg M, Svensson J, Samuelsson B. Thromboxane: a new group of biologically active compounds derived from prostaglandin endoperoxides. *Proc Natl Acad Sci USA* 1975;72:2994.
160. Clive DM, Stoff JS. Renal syndromes associated with nonsteroidal antiinflammatory drugs. *N Engl J Med* 1984;310:563.
161. Gurwitz JH, Avorn J, Ross-Degnan D, et al. Nonsteroidal antiinflammatory drug-associated azotemia in the very old. *JAMA* 1990;264:471
162. Laibovitz RA, Koester J,. Schaich L, et al. Safety and efficacy of diclofenac sodium 0.1% ophthalmic solution in acute seasonal allergic conjunctivitis. *J Occul Pharmacol Therap* 1995;11(3): 311–368.

Textbook of Ocular Pharmacology,
edited by T.J. Zimmerman, et al.
Lippincott–Raven Publishers, Philadelphia © 1997.

CHAPTER 53

Intraocular Irrigating Solutions

Henry F. Edelhauser, Roger Amass, and Richard Lambert

HISTORICAL OVERVIEW

By the 1950s, normal saline (Table 1) was the most commonly used intraocular irrigant for ophthalmic surgery. However, in vitro experiments published by Harper and Pomerat in 1958 (1) and Merrill et al. in 1960 (2) on rabbit and human intraocular tissues showed saline to be toxic. As an outgrowth of these studies, Merrill et al. (2) developed a balanced salt solution (BSS). BSS intraocular irrigating solution 15 ml (Table 1) in a plastic squeeze bottle to which a cannula could be attached became commercially available in 1962. This irrigating solution represented a significant advance and was widely accepted. At that time, BSS 15 ml was the only size needed because ophthalmic procedures (intracapsular cataract extraction, ICCE) required minimal amounts of irrigating fluid.

During the early 1970s, new, sophisticated intraocular surgical techniques were developed (i.e., vitrectomy, phacoemulsification, implantation of intraocular lenses, and anterior segment reconstruction). These surgical procedures, because of the need for prolonged irrigation, created a demand for an improved solution in a larger size bottle. The intraocular irrigating solutions surgeons originally used for these procedures were Plasma-Lyte 148, Ringer's solution, and lactated Ringer's solution, but these solutions resulted in corneal swelling, clouding, stria, and/or edema. Edelhauser et al. (3,4) established that both Plasma-Lyte 148 and lactated Ringer's normal saline solution damaged the corneal endothelium and that 15 ml BSS was a better tolerated irrigant. Table 1 shows the composition of these intraocular irrigating solutions.

Early research indicated that the ideal intraocular irrigating solution should contain concentrations of inorganic and organic constituents similar to those present in aqueous humor. Although BSS possessed the essential ions, it lacked other important constituents of intraocular fluids such as bicarbonate, glucose, and glutathione. It was also buffered with citrate and acetate substances, which are not the natural buffer salts of the intraocular fluid that bathes and nourishes the intraocular tissues. In 1972, Dikstein and Maurice (5) showed that the endothelia of isolated perfused rabbit cornea could maintain corneal thickness and cause temperature reversal if a Krebs-Henseleit bicarbonate Ringer's solution, with addition of adenosine and reduced glutathione, was used as the perfusate. (Stored corneas are generally maintained at 4°C. At these temperatures, the corneal endothelial pump is inoperative and the cornea is swollen. If the endothelial pump functions effectively when the cornea is returned to normal temperature, the cornea will de-swell [temperature reversal effect].) In 1973, similar studies by McCarey et al. (6) also confirmed that the composition of the perfusion media directly influenced functional and structural changes in the corneal endothelium. These studies further showed that a bicarbonate Ringer's solution fortified with glucose, adenosine, and glutathione prevented corneal swelling and effectively maintained the integrity of the endothelial monolayer.

The studies of Dikstein and Maurice (5) and McCarey et al. (6) led to development of a glutathione bicarbonate Ringer's (GBR) solution (Table 1). This solution contained the basic salts (NaCl, KCl, $CaCl_2$ $2H_2O$, and $MgCl_2$ $6H_2O$), as well as sodium bicarbonate, glucose, glutathione, and adenosine.

BSS was then the most tissue-compatible solution available; BSS 500 ml became available in 1976, and BSS Plus, enriched with bicarbonate, dextrose, and glutathione, was being clinically evaluated. BSS 500 ml became the standard for large-volume ophthalmic irrigation.

GBR, known as BSS Plus (500 ml), became commercially available in the United States in January, 1981. BSS Plus is similar to GBR except that it does not contain adenosine and oxidized glutathione is used instead of reduced glutathione. These changes in the BSS Plus formula

H. F. Edelhauser: Department of Ophthalmology, Emory University Eye Center, N.E., Atlanta, Georgia 30322.

R. Amass and R. Lambert: Alcon Laboratories, Inc., Fort Worth, Texas 76134-2099.

TABLE 53-1. *Composition of various intraocular irrigating solutions*[a]

Ingredient	Normal saline (0.9% NaCl)[b]	Lactated Ringer's[a] solution[b]	Hartmann's Lactated Ringer's	Plasma-Lyte 148[b]	BSS intraocular irrigating solution[b,c]	BSS PLUS intraocular irrigating solution[b,c]	GBR	S-MA$_2$[b]
Sodium chloride	154	102	111	86	110	122.2	111.6	112.9
Potassium chloride		4	5	5	10	5.08	4.8	4.8
Calcium chloride		3	2	–	3			
Magnesium chloride		—	—	1.5	1.5	0.98	0.78	—
Magnesium sulfate		—	—	—	—	—	—	1.2
Sodium lactate		28	29	—	—	—	—	—
Sodium acetate				27	29	—	—	4.4
Sodium gluconate				23	—	—	—	—
Sodium citrate					6	—	—	3.4
Sodium acid phosphate						—	0.86	—
Disodium phosphate						3.0	—	—
Sodium bicarbonate						25.0	29.2	25.0
Dextrose						5.11	5.01	8.3
Glutathione (reduced)						—	0.30	—
Glutathione (oxidized)						0.30	—	—
Adenosine						—	0.50	—
pH	4.5–7.2	6.0–7.2	6.4	7.4	7.4	7.4	7.4	7.3
Osmolality (mOsm)	290	277	258	299	305	305	274	290

BSS, balanced salt solution; GBR, glutathione bicarbonate Ringer's; pH adjusted by bubbling with mixture of 5% CO_2 and 95% air.
[a]All concentrations expressed in millimoles per liter of solution.
[b]Commercially available.
[c]ALCON Laboratories, Fort Worth, Texas.

TABLE 53-2. *Chemical composition of human aqueous humor, vitreous humor, BSS Plus intraocular irrigating solution, and BSS intraocular irrigating solution*[a]

Ingredient	Human aqueous humor	Human vitreous humor	BSS Plus intraocular irrigating solution	BSS intraocular irrigating solution
Sodium	162.9	144	160.0	155.7
Potassium	2.2–3.9	5.5	5.0	10.1
Calcium	1.8	1.6	1.0	3.3
Magnesium	1.1	1.3	1.0	1.5
Chloride	131.6	177.0	130.0	128.9
Bicarbonate	20.15	15.0	25.0	—
Phosphate	0.62	0.4	3.0	—
Lactate	2.5	7.8	—	—
Glucose	2.7–3.7	3.4	5.0	—
Ascorbate	1.06	2.0	—	—
Glutathione	0.0019	—	0.3	—
Citrate	—	—	—	5.8
Acetate	—	—	—	28.6
pH	7.38	—	7.4	7.6
Osmolality (mOsm)	304		305	298

[a]All concentrations expressed in millemoles per liter or milliequivalents per liter of solution.

were necessary to provide a stable solution with an acceptable shelf life. Table 1 compares the composition of BSS Plus with that of GBR; Table 2 compares the compositions of BSS and BSS Plus with that of human aqueous and vitreous humor.

PHARMACOLOGIC ACTION OF CHEMICAL CONSTITUENTS

The primary purpose of an intraocular irrigating solution is to maintain both the anatomic and physiologic integrity of intraocular tissues. Physiologic studies performed on the corneal endothelium (4), crystalline lens (7), trabecular meshwork (8), and retina (9) have confirmed that a solution with a chemical composition similar to that of aqueous and vitreous humor provides the best protection for intraocular tissues. An outline of the importance of the various ingredients necessary for ocular tissues to maintain their normal function follows.

Sodium, Potassium, and Magnesium

Sodium is the major extracellular ion of plasma and aqueous humor and is essential to maintenance of cellular tonicity. Sodium is also the major ion transported by cells for cell volume regulation and is essential for function of the metabolic pump (10) in the corneal endothelium. The sodium ion is involved in volume regulation of the lens and is essential for nerve transmission.

Potassium is the major intracellular ion of cells and is actively transported across the cell membrane to maintain the intracellular potential. The inward transport of K^+ is coupled with the outward transport of Na^+ by the enzyme Na^+/K^+ ATPase. Therefore, the potassium ion at a low concentration (3 to 6 m*M*) is essential for an intraocular irrigating solution.

Magnesium is an essential element for all cells. It is a co-factor for some ATPases and for many cellular biochemical reactions. Therefore, it should be included in an intraocular irrigating solution in a concentration similar to that present in aqueous humor.

Calcium

Calcium ion is essential to the corneal endothelium for maintenance of the barrier function and control of the apical junctional complexes (11). The ultrastructural integrity of the apical junctional complex is dependent on the availability of intracellular and extracellular Ca^{++} (12). An irrigating solution that lacks calcium will cause endothelial junctional breakdown and result in corneal edema (4, 11–13). Calcium is also an essential ion for the retina in regulating the visual cycle (14) and should be included as an ingredient in an irrigating solution for posterior segment use.

Bicarbonate

The natural extracellular buffer for human tissues is bicarbonate and plasma proteins. For tissues bathed by special body fluids in which protein is lacking [cerebrospinal fluid (CSF) and aqueous humor], bicarbonate is the major buffer. It is also a major constituent of aqueous humor and should be included as the most important buffer system of an intraocular irrigating solution. Much scientific evidence supports the use of HCO_3^- by the intraocular tissues.

Hodson (15,16) reported that corneal thickness could be maintained if the concentration of sodium bicarbonate in an endothelial perfusion medium was maintained at 24 m*M*. Later, Hodson and Miller (16) and Hull et al. (17) provided evidence that an active transport of HCO_3^- across the corneal endothelium contributes to the endothelial pump function. Wiederholt and Koch (18) and Hodson et al. (19) showed that the bicarbonate concentration of GBR was able to maintain the human corneal endothelial potential for extended periods of time.

Bicarbonate has similarly been shown to support retinal function. Winkler et al. (20) and Moorhead et al. (9) reported the beneficial effects on the electroretinogram (ERG) of an intravitreal bicarbonate buffered Ringer's solution used for irrigation during vitrectomy. Negi et al. (21,22) also concluded that bicarbonate and glucose are essential in maintaining retinal function during intraocular irrigation.

All these reports support the need for an intraocular irrigating solution to contain HCO_3^-. Solutions not containing bicarbonate do not adequately support the cellular metabolic processes vital to normal functioning of intraocular tissues.

Glucose

All cells metabolize glucose for the production of energy necessary for normal function (Fig. 1). The ocular tissues use glucose for production of ATP and maintenance of corneal and lens transparency and retinal function. Therefore, glucose is a necessary ingredient for an intraocular irrigating solution used in anterior and/or posterior segment surgery.

The corneal endothelium has a comparatively high rate of aerobic glycolysis, as suggested from the hexose monophosphate shunt studies of Geroski et al. (23). They concluded that 63% of all glucose oxidized to CO_2 occurs through aerobic glycolysis in the endothelium, as compared with 34% in the epithelium. In both cases, the remaining CO_2 is formed by the hexose monophosphate shunt. From their numerous mitochondria, endothelial

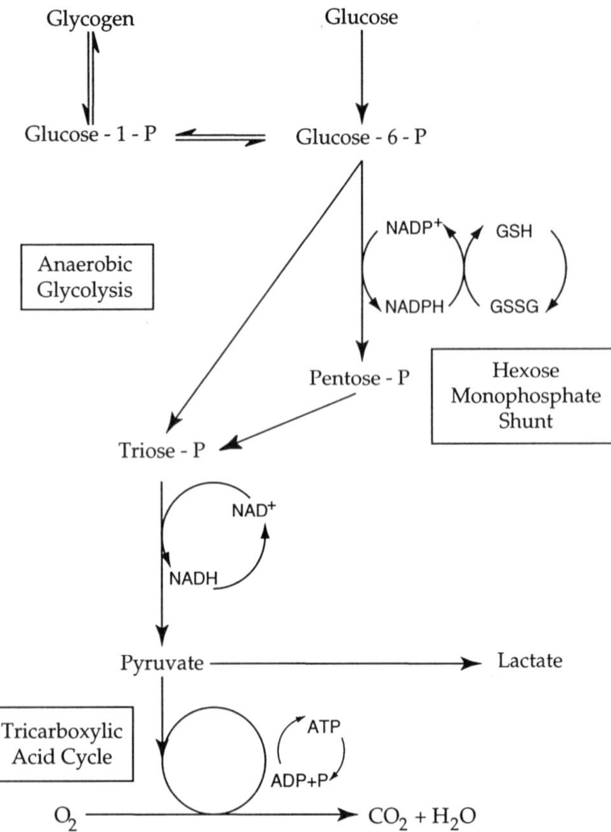

FIG. 53-1. Major metabolic pathways for glucose metabolism in ocular tissues.

cells can be inferred to have a high rate of aerobic glycolysis, higher than that of any other ocular cell type except retinal photoreceptors (24). The corneal endothelium receives both glucose and oxygen directly from the aqueous, which bathes the apical cellular membranes. Gaasterland et al. (25) reported an average value of 2.94 m*M* glucose in the aqueous of fasting Rhesus monkeys. Endothelial cells are especially vulnerable to interruptions in their source of nourishment for the control of corneal hydration and clarity. Therefore, these cells can be affected by the nature of an intraocular irrigating solution used in the course of anterior segment surgery (4).

Most of the energy requirements of the lens are met by anaerobic glycolysis (26), with aerobic glycolysis occurring only in the epithelial cells. Glucose serves as the main energy source of the lens, and its presence in tissue storage solutions has been demonstrated to assist in maintenance of lens clarity in rabbit lenses (7). The presence of glucose in the perfusion fluids was shown in several studies (9,22,27) to be essential for maintenance of normal metabolism and electrical activity (ERG amplitude) in isolated retinal tissue. Glucose is therefore an important constituent of any intraocular irrigating solution intended for use in anterior and posterior segment surgery and is especially needed to decrease the stress of these procedures.

Glutathione (GSH)

GSH, an important tripeptide (r-L-glutamyl-L-cysteinyl-glycine) with a reactive sulfhydryl group, is found in aqueous humor. The concentration of glutathione ranges from 1 to 10 μM in primates and dogs and from 10 to 30 μM in rabbits (28). Although the blood GSH concentration is high, GSH is mainly present in erythrocytes and the plasma at a concentration of 5 μM or less. Although aqueous GSH may be derived by diffusion from the blood or by an active transport system in the ciliary epithelium analogous to that of the lens, it probably also diffuses from the lens and cornea.

Dikstein and Maurice (5) first showed fluid transport in the isolated cornea to be influenced by the presence of GSH. Anderson et al. (29) reported that GSH (the reduced form), when added to a medium deficient in both glucose and adenosine, protected the endothelium from ATP depletion. However, later studies by Anderson et al. (30) showed that the addition of glucose alone was equal to GSH in maintaining ATP levels and that adenosine alone was superior.

In these studies, the presence of GSH was demonstrated to be more important than glucose or adenosine alone in inducing corneal de-swelling and improving corneal survival time. The effect on the endothelium could be maintained equally well by the addition of 240 μM GSH or 20 μM GSSG (the oxidized form of GSH).

Edelhauser et al. (31), however, reported that when intracellular endothelial cell GSH was completely oxidized with diamide, endothelial cells lost their barrier functions and the apical junctions became disrupted. Measurement of the endothelial cellular concentrations of GSH and GSSG after perfusion of corneas with media of varying glutathione content (32,33), showed endothelial fluid transport to be disrupted only when the total intracellular GSH level decreased below one third of the in vivo value. These studies also showed that corneal swelling was prevented and the intracellular level of GSH was maintained by addition of both GSH and GSSG to an irrigating solution. Similarly, Hodson and Wigham (34) and Hodson et al. (19) showed that the transendothelial potential across the human corneal endothelium is stabilized and maintained for as long as 6 hours in the presence of 0.5 m*M* reduced GSH, whereas a simple salt solution could not maintain this potential.

These data indicate that a critical level of GSH is required in the endothelial cells and that there is a need for a fraction of both the oxidized and reduced forms, suggesting that GSH functions as a redox buffer system to combat the effects of oxidizing free radicals (Fig. 2). A continuous supply of GSH in the aqueous humor or an irrigating solution could therefore effectively detoxify any injurious free radicals produced in the anterior segment or vitreous humor (10,35) during intraocular surgery, at which time the intraocular tissues are exposed to excessive light from the

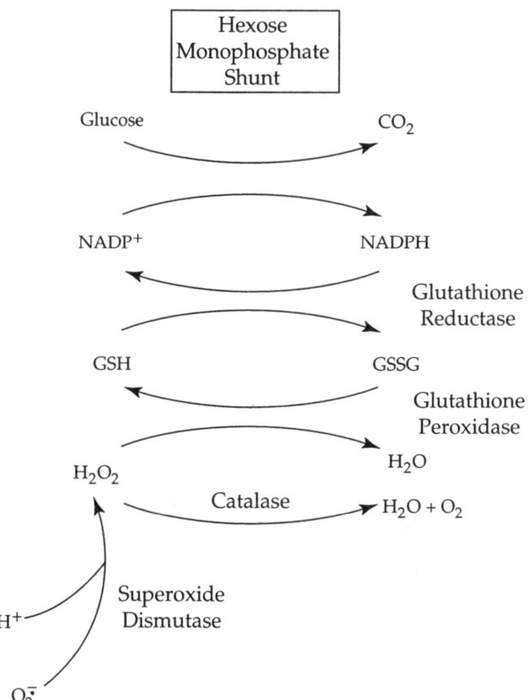

FIG. 53-2. Possible mechanisms for the removal of oxidizing free radicals(O_2^- and H_2O_2) in ocular tissues.

operating microscope, atmospheric oxygen, and either phacoemulsification (36,37) or vitrectomy capable of forming free radicals. Further in vitro studies by Nakamura et al. (38) compared the protective effects of GSSG and GSH on rabbit corneal endothelial barrier function, using permeability to carboxyfluorescein as a measure of barrier integrity. They noted that barrier function was better maintained by supplementation of the perfusion solution with 0.3 m*M* GSSG than with 0.6 m*M* GSH, suggesting that exogenous GSSG may be more readily taken up into corneal endothelial cells.

GSH is a natural constituent of the lens, serving to protect thiol groups involved in cation transport and other lens proteins from oxidative damage (39). Christiansen et al. (7) demonstrated that in the absence of GSH, isolated rabbit lenses could not be maintained in a clear state for prolonged periods, even when glucose and bicarbonate were present in the storage solution.

Araie (40) reported that the permeability index of the blood–aqueous barrier in rabbit eyes was more significantly reduced by perfusion with BSS Plus than by perfusion with a similar solution without GSSG. These results suggest that GSSG has a beneficial effect on the integrity of the blood–aqueous barrier. Such studies suggest that GSSG may be important in reducing postsurgical inflammation in the eye.

In studies using radiolabeled GSH ([^{35}S]-GSSG) contained in BSS Plus in pigmented rabbits, exogenous GSSG in an intraocular irrigating solution appeared to be beneficial in maintaining GSH homeostasis in both the retina and cornea (41). These studies showed that GSSG present in a intraocular irrigating solution is taken up by the retina, choroid, and corneal endothelium and readily converted to GSH.

The available evidence suggests that GSH is an important redox substrate in a variety of ocular tissues and is therefore an important component of a well-formulated intraocular irrigating solution. Although GSH is the form active in cells, it is unstable in an irrigating solution. GSSG in an irrigating solution will, however, be broken down into its individual amino acid components, which are transported by the enzyme γ-glutamyl transpeptidase into the cell to form GSH (42,43).

pH and Osmolality

The cornea can tolerate irrigation with physiologic solutions within an osmolality range of 200 to 400 mOsm (44) and within a pH range of 6.8 to 8.2 (45,46). An ideal irrigating solution should be isoosmotic with the intraocular tissues, (i.e., 305 mOsm) and should contain the essential ingredients to prevent corneal swelling and cellular destruction. Table 1 shows the pH variability of irrigating solutions. Both 0.9% NaCl and lactated Ringer's solution can fall below the pH tolerance of the intraocular tissues. The pH of the irrigating solutions can also be changed if antibiotic agents (47) or epinephrine (48) is added. Therefore, ophthalmic surgeons should be cautious with regard to additions to an irrigating solution used during intraocular surgery. This issue is addressed herein. The presence of both phosphate and bicarbonate buffer salts in an intraocular irrigating solution afford the solution a high buffer capacity, making it relatively resistant to pH changes caused by additives (47).

CONSIDERATIONS FOR ANTERIOR SEGMENT SURGERY

Comparison of Intraocular Irrigating Solutions

The effects of different intraocular irrigating solutions on the cornea are best compared by perfusing the endothelium of isolated rabbit, primate, or human corneal tissue. In this way, the effects of the irrigating solutions can be distinguished from those of surgical trauma and other variables.

Studies of this type have shown 0.9% NaCl to cause complete endothelial destruction within 1 hour of initiation of perfusion of the corneal endothelium (3). Figures 3 and 4 compare changes in corneal thickness of paired stumptailed monkey corneas after 1 hour of endothelial perfusion with 0.9% physiological saline and GBR (similar to BSS

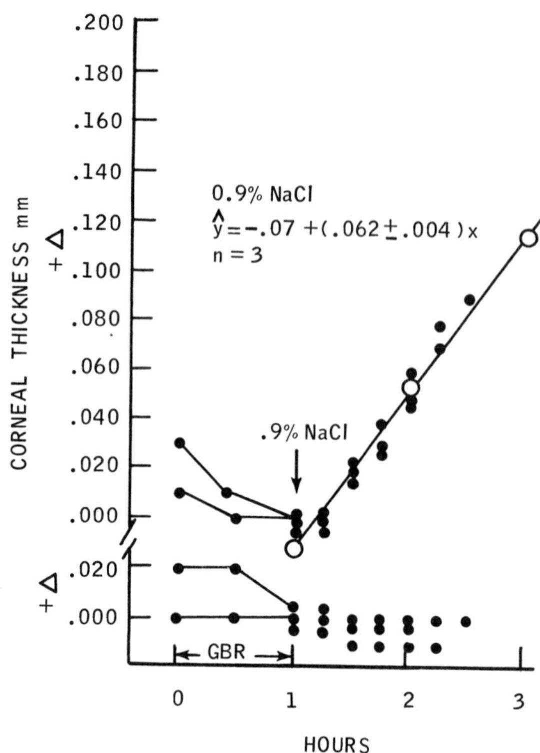

FIG. 53-3. Changes in corneal thickness of paired primate corneas perfused with 0.9% physiologic saline and GBR after initial 1-hour perfusion with glutathione bicarbonate Ringer's solution (GBR). Start of 0.9% saline perfusion (arrow). Regression line for swelling rate (62 μm/hr) with 0.9% saline (straight line). Corneas perfused with GBR did not swell. (From ref. 3, with permission.)

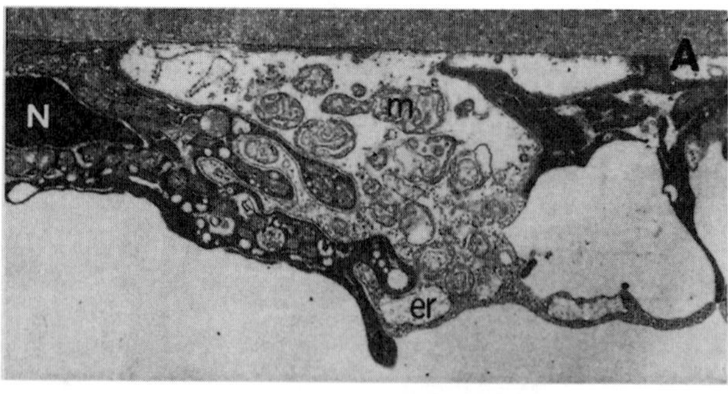

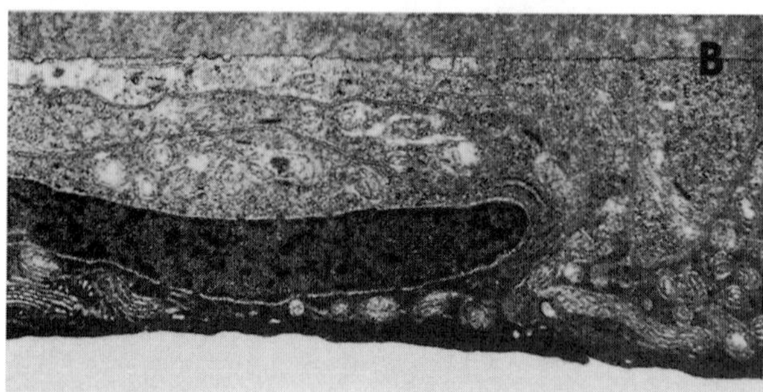

FIG. 53-4. A: Endothelium of primate cornea perfused with 0.9% physiologic saline for 1.5 hours. Some cells have dense cytoplasm, shrunken nuclei (N), and vesiculated cytoplasm. Other cells have swollen mitochondria (M) and endoplasmic reticulum (er) in clarified cytoplasm (×10,100). **B:** Endothelium of paired primate cornea perfused with glutathione bicarbonate Ringer's solution (GBR) for 1.5 hours (×10,100).(From ref. 3, with permission.)

Plus). GBR maintained corneal thickness, but 0.9% NaCl failed to maintain endothelial pump and barrier functions; and marked corneal swelling resulted.

Plasma-Lyte 148 (Table 1) was the first solution used for phacoemulsification because it had a stable pH of 7.4. However, it lacks the critical ion calcium. Perfusion of the endothelium with this solution causes the junctions between the endothelial cells to break down and marked corneal edema ensues (49) (Fig. 5).

Lactated Ringer's solution (Table 1) contains most of the essential ions to maintain the intraocular tissues; however, it contains 28 m*M* lactate, a much higher concentration than that present in intraocular fluids (Table 2). Lactated Ringer's is an intravenous solution, not an intraocular irrigating solution, and the high concentration of lactate was intended to supply the heart with a substrate that would serve as an energy source while it was under metabolic stress. Intraocular tissues do not use lactate as a major substrate for metabolism; therefore, the presence of 38 m*M* lactate is of questionable benefit to the intraocular tissues. Furthermore, lactated Ringer's has a variable pH (6.0 to 7.2). In vitro studies of isolated perfused human corneas showed that lactated Ringer's can cause various degrees of endothelial cell breakdown and corneal swelling during a 3-hour perfusion (Fig. 6).

In further studies (Figs. 7 and 8), Nuyts et al. showed that when isolated human corneas are perfused with Hartmann's solution, the cornea will not de-swell and the endothelial cells become edematous and vacuolated. These effects can be observed after as little as 15 minutes of perfusion, but can be reversed when the perfusate is changed to a more complete intraocular irrigating solution (50).

BSS has been demonstrated to be a better intraocular irrigating solution than the solutions described previously (3,6). In comparative clinical studies it maintained corneal clarity better than Hartmann's solution in extracapsular cataract surgery (51,52). However, BSS lacks the bicarbonate, glucose, and GSH present in aqueous humor. In a study designed to compare the effects of BSS and BSS Plus after anterior chamber infusion in cats, wide-field specular microscopy and computerized morphometric analysis of the individual endothelial cells were used (53). After short-term (15 and 30 minutes) and long-term (1 and 2 hours) irrigation, endothelial cell density remained unchanged, but corneal thickness increased significantly in the BSS group after 1 hour of irrigation. BSS Plus caused

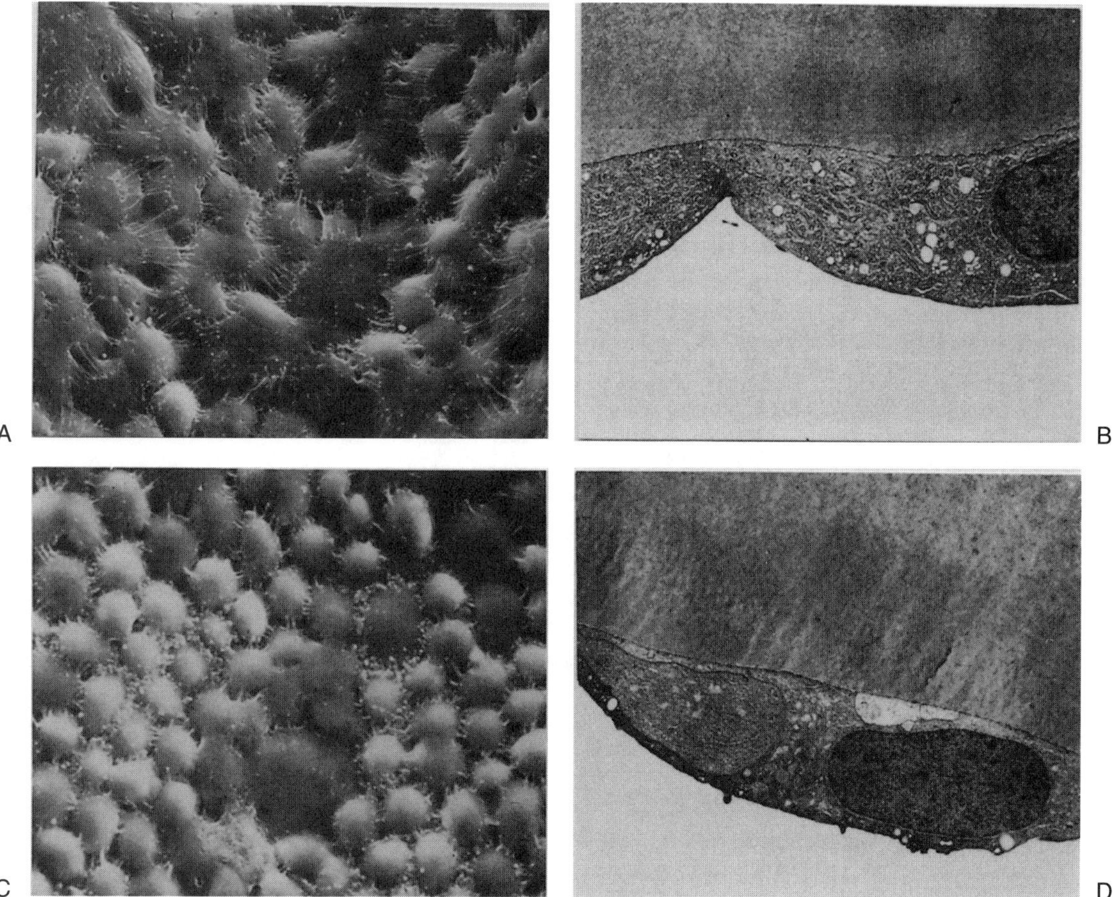

FIG. 53-5. A: Scanning electron microscopy (SEM) of human corneal endothelium (51 years old) perfused with Plasma-Lyte 148 for 1.5 hours. The endothelial cells are separating at their junctions, and the cells are becoming round. Original magnification ×1,000. **B:** Transmission electron microscopy (TEM) of the same cornea. The cells have rounded and are vacuolated, and the mitochondria are condensed. Original magnification ×4,400. **C:** SEM of a human corneal endothelium (97 years old) perfused with Plasma-Lyte 148 for 1.75 hours. The cells are separating at their junctions and becoming round. Original magnification ×1,000. **D:** Transmission electron microscopy (TEM) of the same cornea showing junctional breakdown, rounding of the nucleus, and some cytoplasmic vacuolization. Original magnification ×3,600. (From ref. 49, with permission.)

minimal changes in endothelial morphologic characteristics regardless of the irrigation time. By comparison, BSS caused a significant increase in the coefficient of variation of cell area (polymegathism) and a significant decrease in the percentage of hexagonal cells (pleomorphism). These changes were more prominent after the longer irrigation period (Figs. 9–11). The morphologic changes caused by BSS are indicative of a stressed endothelial monolayer, which may be more susceptible to additional surgical trauma.

Li et al. (54) evaluated the ability of BSS and BSS Plus to maintain the normal electrical potential difference across isolated rabbit corneal endothelium (transendothelial electrical potential difference, TEPD). The magnitude of the TEPD correlates with the rate of fluid transport by the corneal endothelium (55,56). Perfusion with BSS Plus maintained high TEPD values for as long as 8 hours, whereas perfusion with BSS caused a rapid decrease. These results are further evidence that an irrigating solution similar to aqueous humor is superior in maintaining normal corneal endothelial function.

Kline et al. (57) measured endothelial cell density pre- and postoperatively in 100 patients undergoing extracapsular cataract extraction (ECCE), 50 of whom were treated with BSS Plus and 50 with BSS. They reported a mean cell loss of 15.4% in BSS Plus-treated eyes compared with 22.7% in BSS-treated eyes, a statistically significant difference. They did not use viscoelastics in their study to protect the corneal endothelium.

S-MA_2 is an irrigating solution commercially available in Japan which contains glucose and is buffered by both acetate-citrate and bicarbonate (Table 1). In rabbits, Otori et

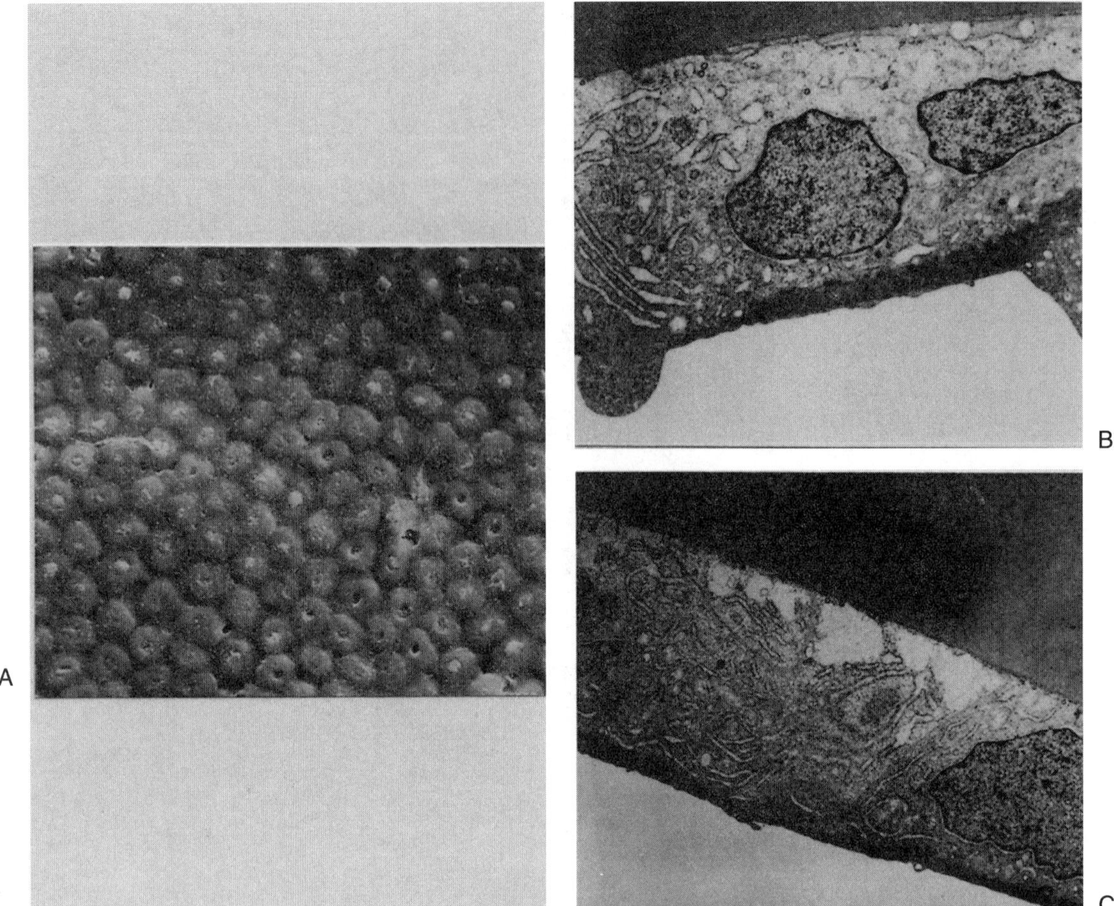

FIG. 53-6. A: Scanning electron microscoyp (SEM) of rabbit corneal endothelium perfused with lactated Ringer's solution for 3 hours. The endothelial cells are swollen, cytoplasmic blebbing has occurred, and areas of junctional breakdown and cell loss are apparent. Original magnification ×1,000. **B:** Transmission electron microscopy (TEM) of the same cornea perfused with lactated Ringer's for 3 hours shows cytoplasmic blebbing, dilation of the endoplasmic reticulum, and areas of clarified cytoplasm. Original magnification ×12,000. **C:** TEM of the same cornea showing the area of clarified cytoplasm adjacent to Descemet's membrane. Original magnification ×9,600. (From ref. 49, with permission.)

al. showed that this solution could protect the corneal endothelium and prevent corneal edema when perfused into the endothelium for extended time periods (58,59). Matsuda et al. also demonstrated the ability of this solution to prevent corneal complications after pars plana vitrectomy (60,61). Subsequently, Araie (60) showed that rabbit corneal endothelium perfused with S-MA_2 had an increased endothelial permeability (measured by uptake of carboxyfluorescein) as compared with a BSS Plus or GBR-perfused control.

Glasser et al. also compared the ability of BSS, S-MA2, and BSS Plus to protect the human corneal endothelium after in vitro perfusion (53). BSS maintained the cornea without swelling throughout a 2-hour perfusion period. By comparison, S-MA_2 caused the corneas to swell at 7 μm/hr; BSS Plus promoted temperature reversal, and the human corneas de-swelled at 13 μm/hr (Fig. 11). BSS maintained endothelial structure, but there was marked swelling of the endothelial cells. S-MA_2 caused a breakdown of the endothelial cell junctions, similar to that which occurs in a calcium-free medium (e.g., Plasma-Lyte 148) (47). These changes are shown in Figure 12.

In a further study, Glasser et al. compared the effects of S-MA_2 and BSS Plus in an in vitro cat model (46). The anterior chambers of both eyes of five adult cats were perfused for 70 minutes (BSS Plus in the right eye and S-MA_2 in the left eye), and the effects on morphologic characteristics of corneal endothelial cells were compared. The results of this study are summarized in Figure 13. S-MA_2 caused a significant decrease in the percentage of hexagonal endothelial cells and a marked increase in the coefficient of variation. Like BSS, S-MA_2 caused significant morphologic alterations of the endothelium.

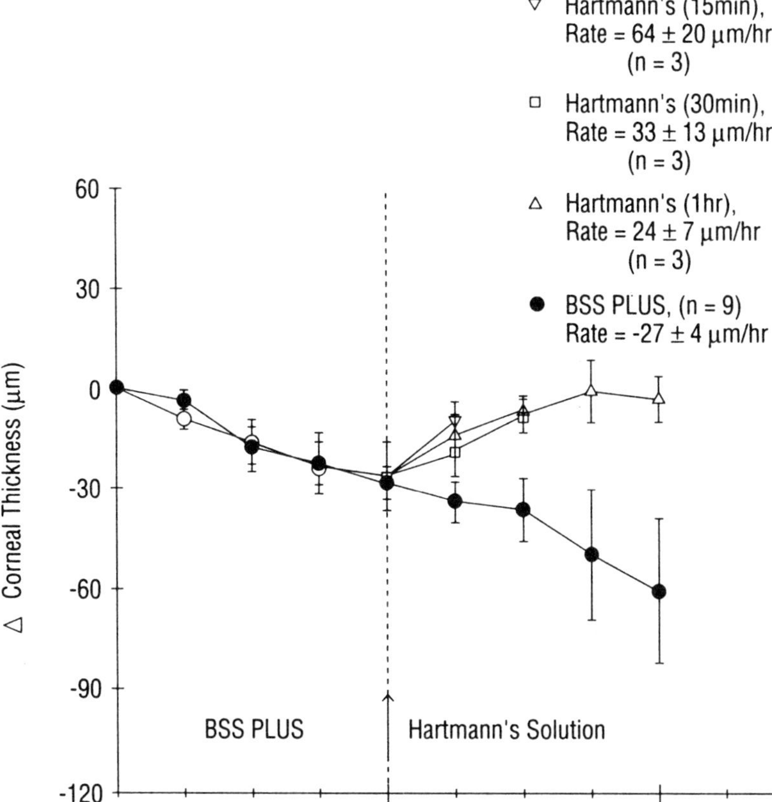

FIG. 53-7. Corneal thickness measurements after perfusion of human corneal endothelium with BSS Plus for 1 hour followed by Hartmann's solution. (From ref. 50, with permission.)

Matsuda et al. examined the effects of BSS Plus and S-MA_2 on the corneal endothelium of patients undergoing extracapsular cataract extraction (63). BSS Plus caused significantly less corneal swelling on the first postoperative day. S-MA_2 caused a significant loss of endothelial cells and a deviation from the normal hexagonal pattern whereas BSS Plus did not. S-MA_2 and BSS Plus both contain bicarbonate and glucose together with Na^+, K^+ and Ca^{++}. However, S-MA_2 has a lesser ability to maintain corneal thickness and endothelial barrier function than either BSS Plus or BSS. The main differences between S-MA_2 and BSS Plus are that S-MA_2 does not contain GSH and uses acetate-citrate as a major component of its buffering system. Araie (39) postulated that the acetate-citrate in S-MA_2 acts to chelate most of the Ca^{++}, giving it the characteristics and performance of a calcium-free solution. Figures 14 and 15 illustrate the effect of S-MA_2 and BSS Plus perfused to the corneal endothelium of a pair of isolated human corneas. The junctions between the endothelial cells have been disrupted by the S-MA_2. In vitro animal and clinical studies have clearly demonstrated that an irrigating solution that is similar in composition to aqueous humor will maintain corneal function and structure.

Irrigating Solutions in the Postoperative Eye

Of prime importance when one considers the effects of any irrigating solution on internal ocular tissues, is the length of time the solution remains in the eye after surgery before being replaced by aqueous humor. Although the duration of surgical irrigation is important, it nevertheless represents only a small fraction of the overall time the solution is in direct contact with the corneal endothelium and other intraocular structures.

Table 3 shows that 4 hours and 23 minutes are required for aqueous secretions to fill the fluid capacity of the normal nongeriatic eye [in which the crystalline lens has been replaced by a posterior chamber intraocular lens (IOL)]. Because surgery often reduces aqueous inflow and outflow by as much as 50%, a reforming solution frequently remains in the eye postoperatively for more than 8 hours before being replaced by aqueous humor (64).

Because of the amount of intraocular tissue contact time, the quality of solution used becomes critical. Based on the study of Glasser et al. (53), which showed that BSS Plus is more effective than BSS in protecting endothelial structural stability, and that of Mishima (65), who reported that time-

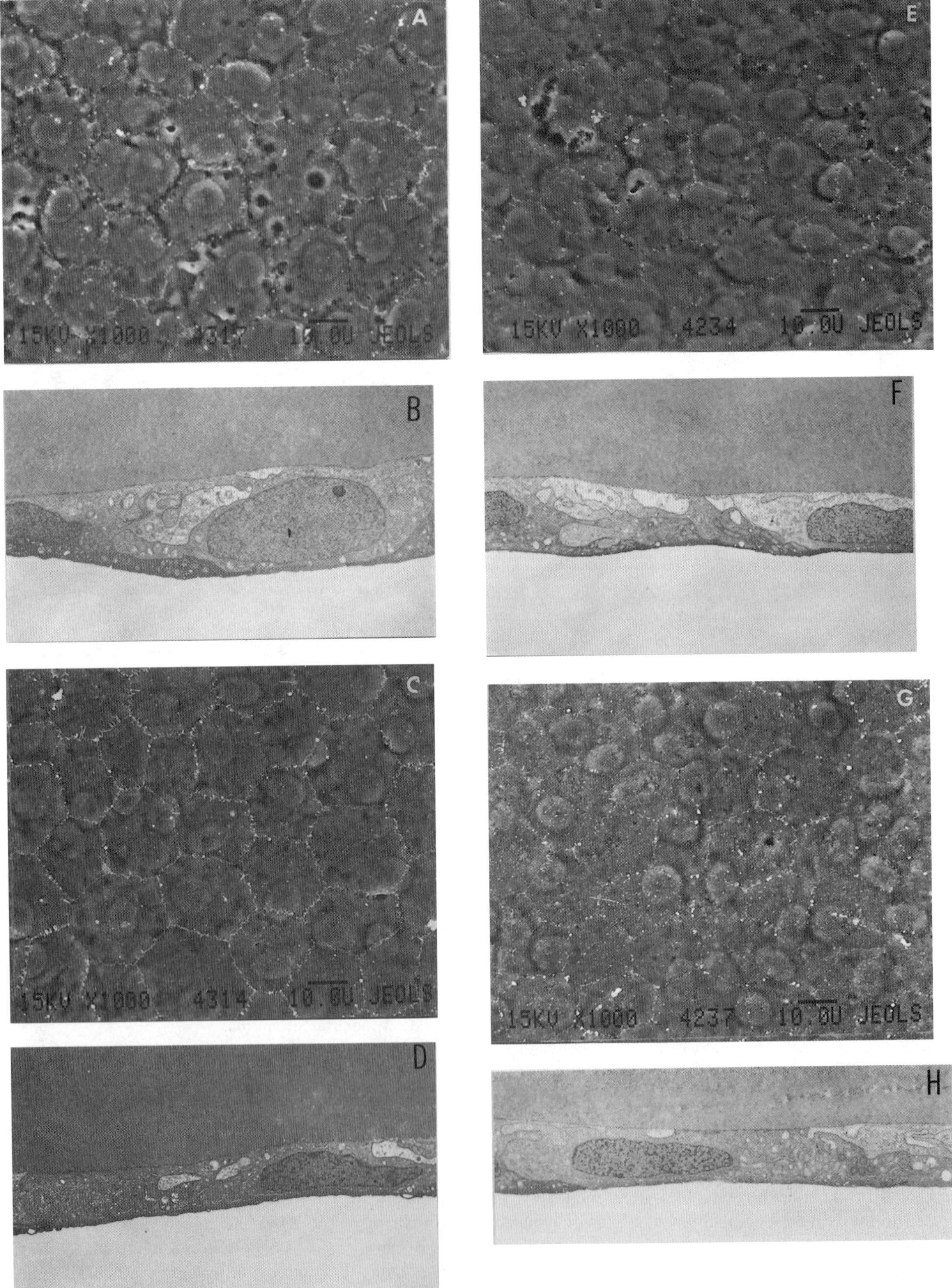
A
15KV X1000 4317 10.0U JEOLS
E
15KV X1000 4234 10.0U JEOLS
B
F
C
15KV X1000 4314 10.0U JEOLS
G
15KV X1000 4237 10.0U JEOLS
D
H

FIG. 53-8.

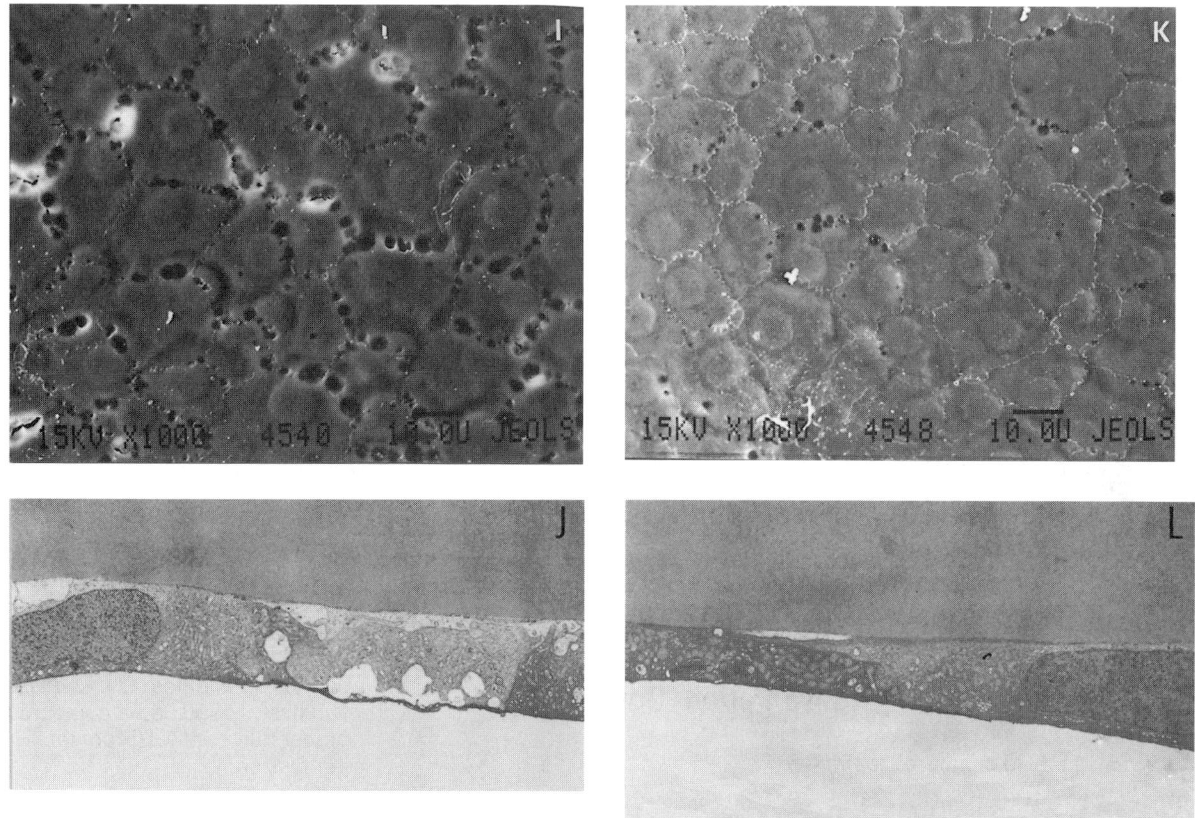

FIG. 53-8 ***Continued.*** **A:** Scanning electron microscopy (SEM) of human corneal endothelium after 15-minute perfusion with Hartmann's lactated Ringer's solution (HLR). Original magnification ×1,000. **B:** Transmission electron microscopy (TEM) of same human corneal endothelium after 15-minute perfusion with HLR shows endothelial cell swelling (×3,451). **C:** SEM of paired human corneal endothelium perfused with BSS Plus (original magnification ×1,000). **D:** TEM of same human cornea perfused with BSS Plus (×3,451). **E:** SEM of human cornea after 30-minute perfusion with HLR shows marked endothelial swelling (original magnification ×1,000). **F:** TEM of the same corneal endothelium shows a greater degree of endothelial edema (×2,261). **G:** SEM of paired human corneal endothelium perfused with BSS Plus (original magnification ×1,000). **H:** TEM of same human cornea perfused with BSS Plus (×3,451). **I:** SEM of human cornea perfused with HLR for 60 minutes shows endothelial cell swelling and junctional breakdown (original magnification ×1,000). **J:** TEM of same cornea perfused with HLR demonstrates progressive endothelial edema and vacuolization (×2,128). **K:** SEM of paired human corneal endothelium perfused for 60 minutes with BSS Plus (original magnification ×1,000). **L:** TEM of same cornea perfused with BSS Plus. The endothelial cell microstructure is maintained, and the cellular organelles are normal (×3,451). (From ref. 50, with permission.)

related postsurgical corneal decompensation is almost certain to occur, a complete intraocular irrigating solution is the solution of choice for all intraocular surgical irrigation.

CONSIDERATIONS FOR POSTERIOR SEGMENT SURGERY

Use of Irrigating Solutions in Pars Plana Vitrectomy

Pars plana vitrectomy was pioneered in the 1970s by surgeons such as Machemer, Parel, Beuttner, Aaberg, Peyman, and Dodich (66–68), with the development of combined infusion, suction, and cutting instruments. Instrumentation available for vitrectomy is now highly sophisticated; a typical system consists of a vitrectomy handpiece and console, an infusion line, and a light source. The infusion line is run from an irrigating solution bottle to an infusion cannula inserted in the eye at the pars plana and opening directly into the vitreous cavity.

The irrigating solution keeps the globe inflated and contributes to a normal pressure–volume relationship intraoperatively. When intraocular fluid or tissue is aspirated, the intraocular pressure decreases transiently and irrigating solution flows from the bottle into the vitreous cavity down a hydrostatic pressure gradient.

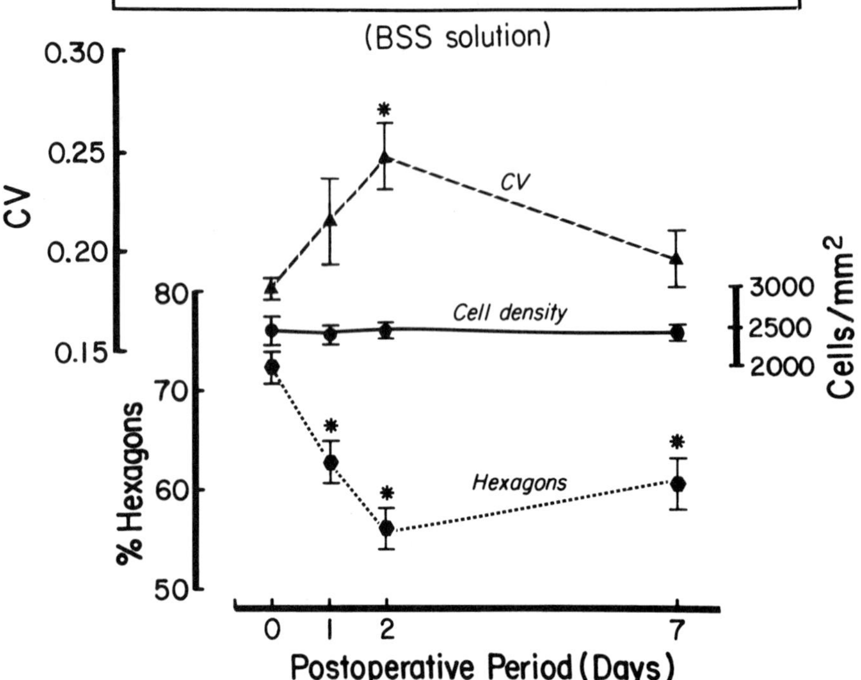

FIG. 53-9. Changes in morphologic characteristics of corneal endothelial cells in the cat after irrigation of anterior chamber with balanced salt solution (BSS) intraocular irrigating solution for 30 minutes. CV, coefficient of variation. *$p < 0.05$ as compared with preoperative value. (From ref. 53, with permission.)

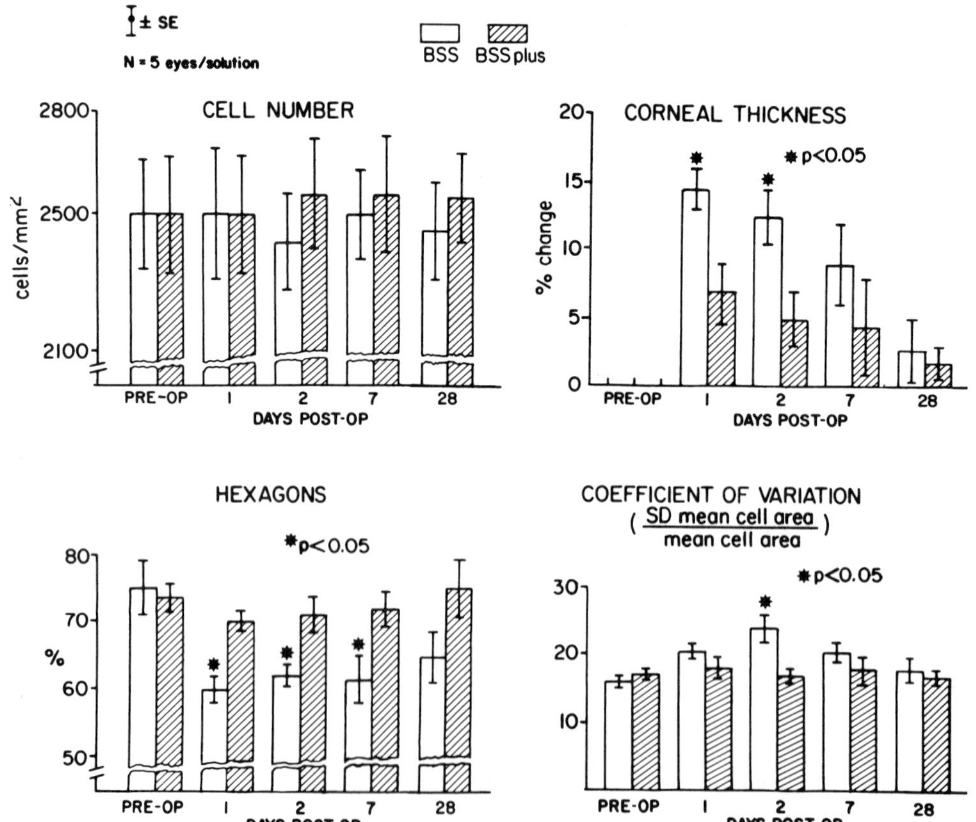

FIG. 53-10. Comparison of corneal endothelial cell changes in the cat after 60-minute irrigation of anterior chamber with balanced salt solution (BSS) (open bars) or BSS Plus (hatched bars). *$p < 0.05$. (From ref. 53, with permission.)

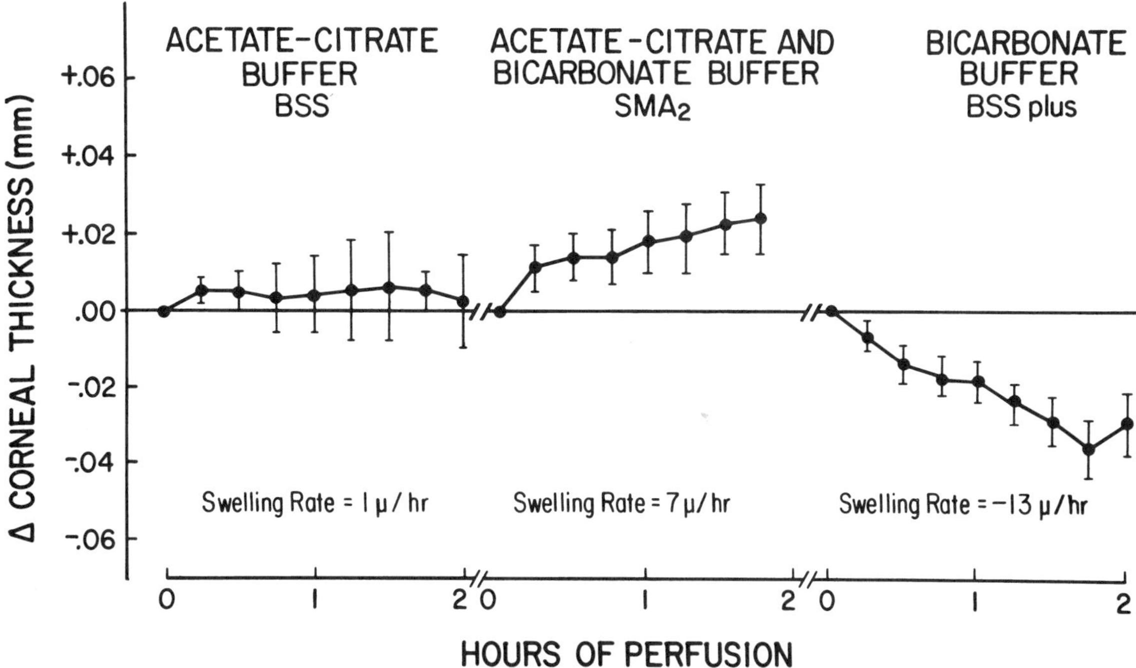

FIG. 53-11. Corneal swelling after in vitro corneal endothelial perfusion with balanced salt solution (BSS, n = 6), S-MA$_2$ (n = 8), and BSS Plus (n = 14). (From ref. 46, with permission.)

During vitrectomy, the irrigating solution will be in contact with the retina, lens (if present), cornea, and other ocular tissues such as the pars plana and ciliary body. For this reason, it is important that a tissue-compatible intraocular irrigating solution be used to ensure minimal physiological stress to the intraocular tissues during the procedure.

Effects on the Cornea

The potential for intraocular irrigating solutions to affect the cornea has already been discussed. In a prospective study, Benson et al. (69) observed that BSS-Plus caused significantly less ($p < 0.05$) corneal edema on the first day

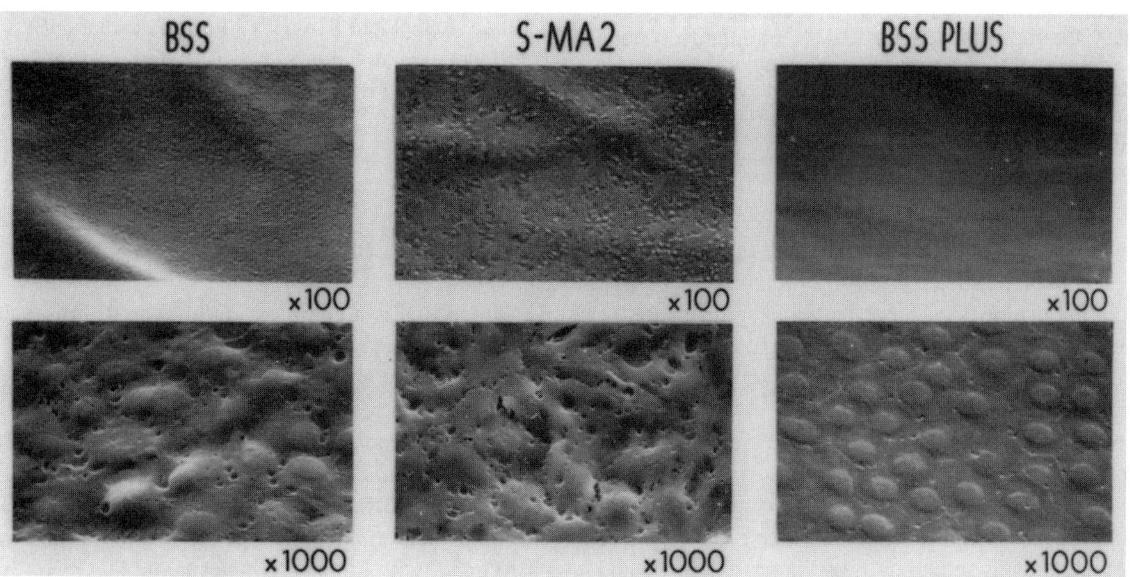

FIG. 53-12. Scanning electron microscopy of human corneas after 2 hours of endothelial perfusion with balanced salt solution (BSS) intraocular irrigating solution, S-MA$_2$, and BSS Plus. (From ref. 46, with permission.)

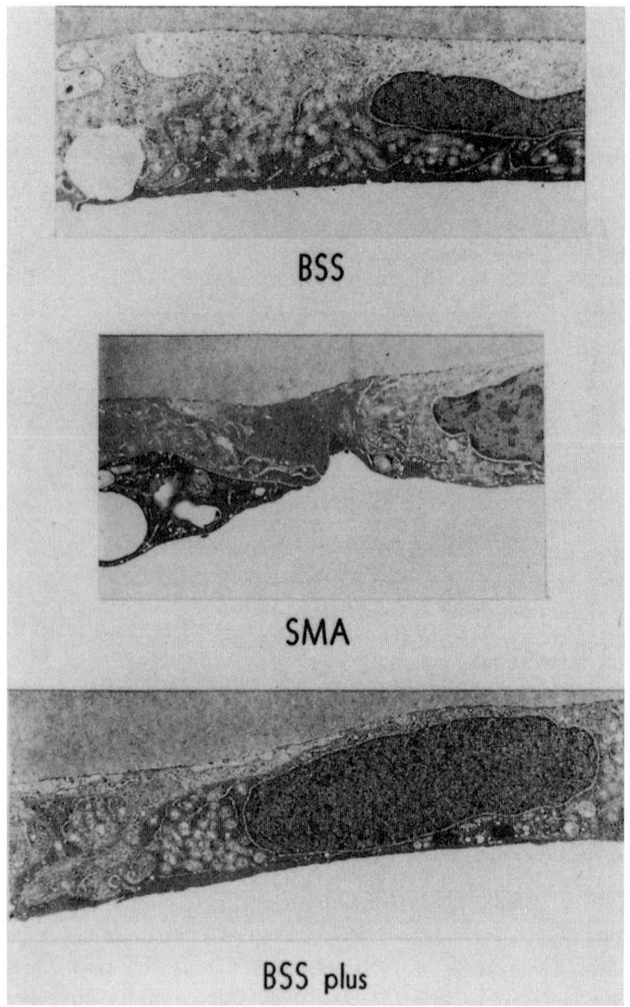

FIG. 53-13. Transmission electron micrographs of human corneal endothelium after perfusion with balanced salt solution (BSS), S-MA_2, and BSS Plus for 2 hours. Corneal endothelial cells perfused with BSS have clarified cytoplasm and dilated intercellular spaces; S-MA_2-perfused corneas show apical junctional breakdown and cytoplasmic vacuoles. Corneal endothelial cells perfused with BSS Plus show normal junctional complexes and normal intracellular organelles. (From ref. 46, with permission.)

after vitrectomy than lactated Ringer's solution. This finding is in accord with a later report by Matsuda et al. (61), who noted that use of BSS Plus resulted in significantly ($p < 0.05$) less endothelial cell loss after vitrectomy than did use of lactated Ringer's solution.

Effects on the Lens

The lens has a complex series of active and passive transport mechanisms to maintain its viability. Kinsey and Reddy (70) demonstrated that sodium is actively pumped from the lens by Na^+/K^+-ATPase in the epithelial layer and that water and chloride enter and leave the lens by simple diffusion through the posterior surface. Maintenance of lens volume is therefore an energy-requiring process.

The lens also actively pumps out calcium (71,72) and actively transports amino acids, necessary for lens growth and metabolism, into the lens (42,73). Sugars enter the lens by facilitated diffusion.

Being avascular, the lens receives all its nutrients from the aqueous humor. Glucose serves as the main source of energy for the lens. Most of the energy the lens requires is derived from anaerobic glycolysis, with approximately 78% of the available glucose being used by this pathway. About 14% of the available glucose passes through the hexose monophosphate shunt. This pathway produces pentoses needed for the synthesis of nucleic acids as well as for the production of NADPH, a necessary component of many biochemical reactions, including the production of reduced GSH from GSSG.

The cells of the lens are continually challenged by peroxides generated by light within the lens fibers and epithelial cells, as well as by H_20_2 in the aqueous humor (74,75). Studies of cultured lens epithelial cells have shown that enzymes in the GSH redox cycle are needed in the detoxification of H_20_2. A failure of this system may be involved in the formation of certain kinds of cataract, since much higher values of H_20_2 have sometimes been detected in the aqueous humor of cataractous patients (74). Therefore, an irrigating solution that maintains the intraocular tissues is needed for vitrectomy in phakic eyes if the clarity of the lens pre- and postoperatively is to be maintained.

Christiansen et al. (7) examined the effects of storing isolated Rhesus monkey lenses in different irrigating solutions at 37°C. GBR solution retained lens clarity for at least 48 hours. In contrast, only 10% of lenses incubated in lactated Ringer's solution remained clear at 4 hours and none were clear at 24 hours. Addition of glucose and bicarbonate to lactated Ringer's solution dramatically improved performance at 4 hours, but all lenses were opaque by 48 hours, indicating that this solution could not preserve lens function as well as GBR.

Effects on the Retina

The retina is a complex, multilayered tissue which, unlike the cornea and the lens, has its own blood supply. However, use of an improperly formulated irrigating solution during vitrectomy can have significant effects on retinal function and viability.

In vitro studies using rabbit and rat retinas (9,20) have shown that perfusion with irrigating solutions that do not contain bicarbonate and glucose results in changes to the ERG and, with longer term perfusion, can result in permanent retinal cell damage (22). Similar studies in rats have demonstrated a decrease in metabolic activity in retinal cells when glucose and bicarbonate are missing from the

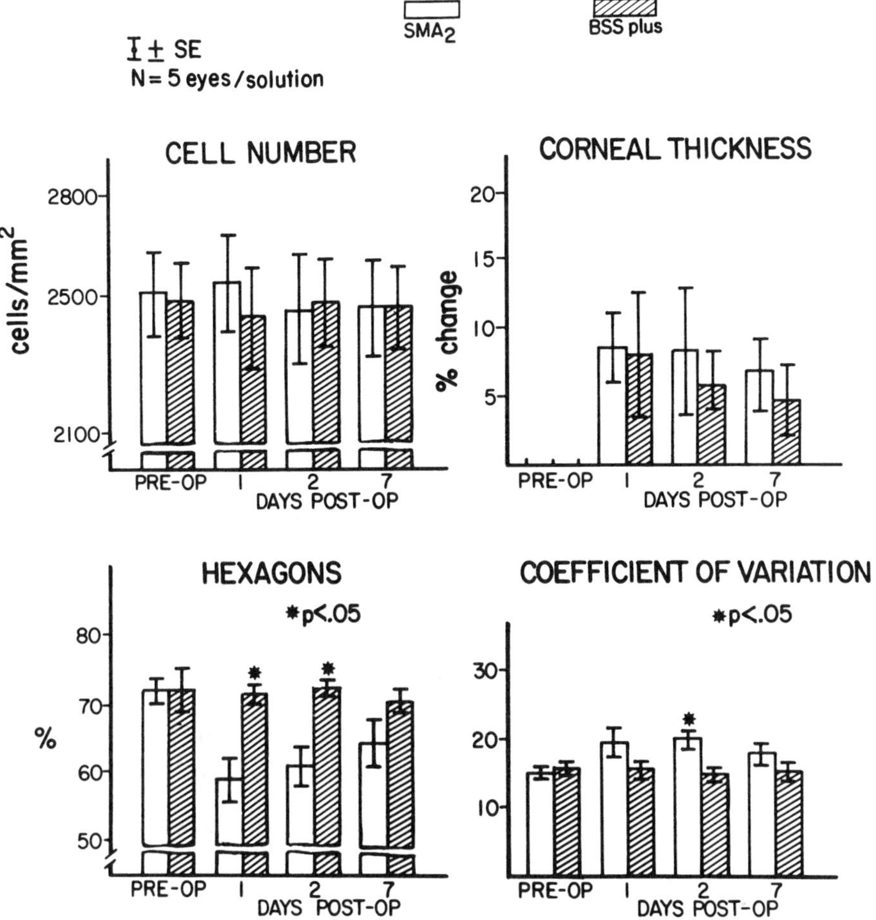

FIG. 53-14. Morphologic changes in corneal endothelial cell density, corneal swelling, percentage of hexagonal cells, and coefficient of variation, in cats after anterior chamber irrigation for 60 minutes with S-MA_2 (open bars) and balanced salt solution (BSS) Plus (hatched bars). $^*p < 0.05$. (From ref. 46, with permission.)

perfusate (27). Retinal edema, which is a complication of vitrectomy, has been shown in animal studies to be reduced when using BSS Plus compared to lactated Ringer's or saline (76).

SOLUTION ADDITIVES

The indiscriminate addition of adjunctive drugs to a bottle of intraocular irrigating solution may compromise the safety, as well as the chemical and physiological integrity, of the solution. Well-formulated intraocular irrigants are a delicately balanced mixture of ions and other essential constituents adjusted to a pH and osmolality compatible with ocular tissues.

Most additive drugs such as antibiotic agents, mydriatic agents, and epinephrine are not indicated for intraocular administration. They contain their specific vehicles, preservatives, solubilizers, and antioxidants. The introduction of these drugs into an irrigating solution may disrupt the chemical balance and alter the pH and osmolality: The resulting mixture from these additives can also have toxic effects on intraocular tissues. Additives to an intraocular irrigating solution are not FDA approved.

Epinephrine

Use of topical mydriatic agents to dilate the pupil before cataract surgery is a common practice that has been extended to adding epinephrine to irrigating solutions. Maintaining a dilated pupil aids visualization during lens nucleus and cortex removal and IOL insertion, thereby reducing the potential for ocular trauma and increasing the safety of the procedure.

After presurgical pupil dilation with tropicamide and phenylephrine, Freeman and Gettelfinger (77) reported the addition of epinephrine to BSS irrigating solution with additional dextrose and bicarbonate. The resulting epinephrine concentration of 0.57 ppm (0.000057%) maintained pupillary dilation in most cases during phacoemulsification or during irrigation/aspiration of lens remnants and manual expression of the nucleus.

In response to reports of corneal decompensation associated with epinephrine in irrigating solutions, Duffin et al. (78) studied the ocular response to intraocular epinephrine, injecting 0.1 ml epinephrine solution into the anterior chamber of 55 patients who had undergone lens extraction to redilate or maintain pupillary dilation of patients to

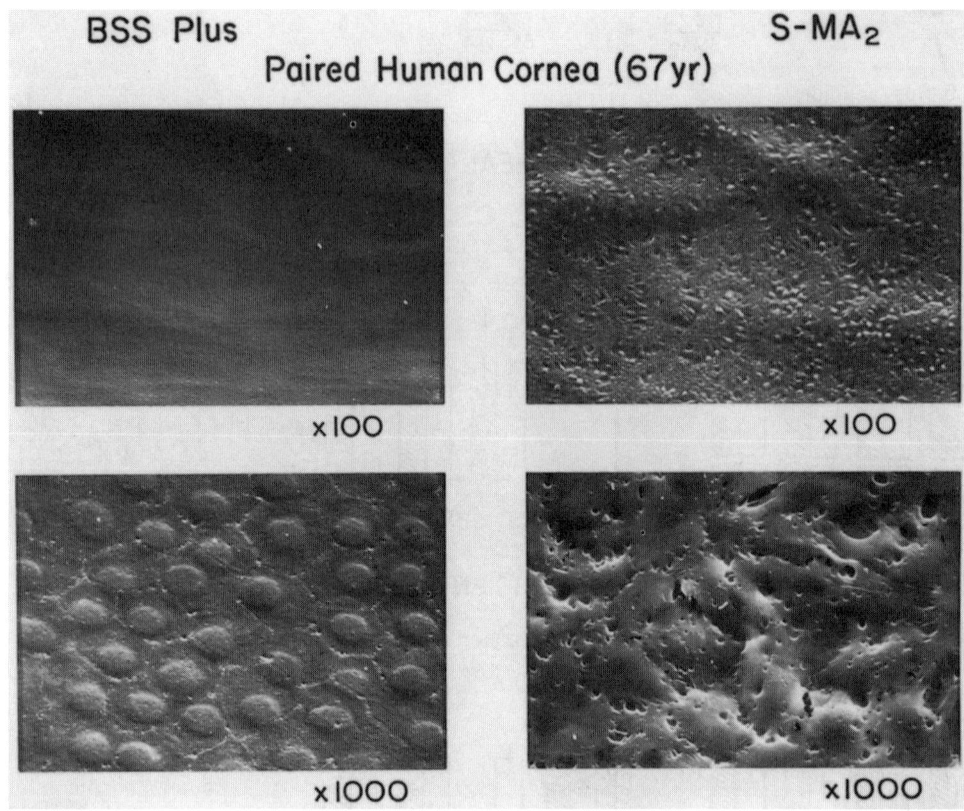

FIG. 53-15. Scanning electron microscopy of the corneal endothelium of paired human corneal endothelium cells after 1.5 hours of balanced salt solution (BSS) Plus and S-MA_2 endothelial perfusion in the in vitro specular microscope. The S-MA_2 endothelium has the characteristics of a calcium-free solution. (From ref. 46, with permission.)

whom topical drops of phenylephrine and cyclopentolate had been administered presurgically. The concentrations of epinephrine ranged from 62.5 ppm (0.00625%) to 10.4 ppm [0.001, (04%)]; however, 25% of the irides did not dilate further and 42% increased pupil area by less than 20% at 1 minute after injection. The pupils that responded poorly were generally those already dilated to 6.0 mm or more. Injection of another 0.1 ml of the high concentration of epinephrine (62.5 ppm) resulted in little, if any, additional mydriasis. There were no indications of adverse ocular effects from the epinephrine.

TABLE 53-3. *Irrigation solution in the postoperative eye: Aqueous replacement over time*

Fluid capacity (ml)	
Anterior chamber	0.250[a]
Posterior chamber	0.060
Space left by extracted crystalline lens	0.250
Subtotal fluid capacity	0.560
Posterior chamber IOL (average)	−0.035
Total fluid capacity	0.525
Aqueous flow rate	
Normal nongeriatric eye (average)	0.002 ml/min[a]
Aqueous replacement	
Minimum time $\frac{0.525 \text{ mL}}{0.002 \text{ mL/min}}$ = 262.5 min (4 hr, 23 min)	
Flow rate following surgery: Aqueous flow is nearly always reduced by surgery. A 50% reduction is not uncommon. Therefore, irrigation solution often remains in the eye postoperatively for as long as 8 hours 45 minutes.	

IOL, intraocular lens.

In a randomized, prospective, double-masked study, Elliott and Carter (79) measured pupil size pre- and postsurgically in patients who received 1 ppm epinephrine added to the irrigating solution during ECCE and IOL implantation. They reported significantly less pupillary constriction at the end of surgery in the epinephrine group as compared with the control group.

A concentration of 0.57 ppm epinephrine in the irrigating solution maintained mydriasis in patients during phacoemulsification and IOL implantation in a double-masked, placebo-controlled study (80). Pupil size was reduced 19% to 24% in patients not receiving epinephrine who were pretreated with Indocid or Ocufen.

In a controlled comparison, Corbelt and Richard (81) reported that patients receiving 1 ppm epinephrine in the irrigating solution had significantly larger mean pupil size during ECCE and after irrigation and aspiration of cortical remnants. The number of patients with pupil diameters less than 5.0 mm, which was associated with greater surgical difficulty, was significantly greater in the group not receiving epinephrine in the irrigating solution.

Other researchers have described adding less than 0.2 ml (0.4 ppm) (82) to 0.5 ml (1 ppm) (83) of a 1 : 1,000 solution of epinephrine to a 500-ml bottle of irrigating solution to be used as a constant infusion during cataract surgery. Use of 0.4 to 1 ppm epinephrine in the irrigating solution during cataract surgery did not significantly alter the subsequent response of the iris to the intracameral miotic acetylcholine (79,84).

Reports of corneal edema after use of epinephrine (1 : 1,000 and 1 : 10,000) during ocular surgery resulted in laboratory investigations which showed that the preservative (antioxidant) sodium bisulfite, low pH, and high buffer capacity was responsible (17,47). The corneal endothelium of the in vitro-perfused human cornea could tolerate the bisulfite antioxidant-preserved epinephrine if it was diluted to 1 : 5,000 (200 ppm) (85). Despite the problems that have been associated with preservatives in epinephrine, the structures of the anterior chamber, and particularly the corneal endothelium, appear to tolerate concentrations of epinephrine far in excess of those likely to be used in an irrigating solution. However, a sterile, preservative-free, sulfite-free epinephrine solution for injection (American Regent Laboratories, Shirley, NY) does provide a margin of safety for intraocular use (86).

Duffin et al. (78) also reported that injecting 0.1 ml epinephrine solution into the anterior chamber of 55 patients after lens extraction redilated the pupil and maintained pupillary dilation. They used concentrations ranging from 62.5 to 10.5 ppm, without adverse ocular responses or evidence of an increase in blood pressure (BP). Adams et al. (87), using a 1-ml solution containing 100 μg epinephrine (100 ppm) to flush the anterior chamber of patients, noted no adverse effects on the ocular structures or changes in plasma epinephrine concentration, heart rate (HR), or mean arterial BP.

Thirteen patients receiving an irrigating solution with 2 ppm epinephrine during cataract surgery did not experience an increase in plasma catecholamines or a statistical change in HR or BP (88). The maximal amount of ocular exposure to epinephrine was estimated at 1.3 μg/kg body weight (irrigation with 46 ml irrigating solution for a person weighing 70 kg). Neither HR nor systemic BP was altered in 62 patients who were exposed to 200 to 300 ml BSS with 1 ppm epinephrine during cataract surgery (89).

In a study of patients with hypertension diagnosed with senile cataracts who were undergoing ECCE with an irrigating solution containing either 1 or 2 ppm epinephrine, Yamaguchi et al. (90) reported no alteration in HR or BP. Neither were there any changes in HR, BP, or electrocardiograms in 12 patients who received 1 ppm epinephrine in the irrigating solution as compared with 200 control patients (81). Nevertheless, patients should be monitored for signs of systemic epinephrine toxicity such as headache, palpitations, tachycardia, or increased BP if they receive epinephrine in an intraocular irrigating solution.

Although several reports describe the addition of epinephrine to an irrigating solution, information on the concentration of epinephrine needed to ensure adequate mydriasis is minimal. Published information is inadequate to establish a minimum effective concentration of epinephrine in an irrigating solution. The limited information available indicates that the concentration of epinephrine should probably be greater than 0.6 ppm (0.00006% or a dilution of 1 : 1,166,666).

Glucose

Some surgeons have advocated the addition of supplemental glucose to BSS Plus to preserve lens clarity during vitrectomy in diabetic patients (91,92). Raising the glucose level from 100 to 400 mg/dl increases the solution's osmolality from 305 to 320 mOsm, which is consistent with the osmolality of the diabetic patient's aqueous humor (91,92). The addition of glucose has prevented the posterior subcapsular opacification that can occur during vitrectomy in diabetic patients. Other clinical experience presents a challenge to this assertion and shows that BSS Plus preserves lens clarity even in diabetic patients (92).

Antibiotics

Geroski et al., who investigated the effects of adding various antibiotics to BSS Plus (94), reported that addition of vancomycin and amikacin had no significant effect on the ability of the solution to maintain isolated rabbit corneal tissue for a 6-hour period whereas gentamicin was moderately toxic. In addition, bubbles formed when amikacin and gentamicin were added, and the presence of bubbles resulted in corneal swelling during perfusion.

Winkler and Trese (48) measured the pH of BSS, BSS Plus, and lactated Ringer's solution after the addition of commercial antibiotic preparations containing gentamicin, amikacin, methicillin, tobramycin, and vancomycin. Addition of the antibiotic agents caused a concentration-dependent decrease in pH of the irrigating solution in all cases. The decrease was least for BSS Plus and greatest for lactated Ringer's solution. They suggest that the shift in pH may contribute to retinal toxicity that occurs, for example, with intravitreal administration of gentamicin (95,96).

Although several in vitro studies and a large body of clinical experience suggests that a variety of pharmacologic agents can be added to intraocular irrigating solutions, the potential for ocular damage from the inappropriate use of additives remains. Formulation excipients such as preservatives, antioxidants, and pH adjusters may adversely affect the formulation of the irrigating solution or be directly toxic to ocular tissues.

Ophthalmic surgeons are advised that all intraocular irrigating solution products contain a label warning cautioning against the use of solution additives. The efficacy and safety of any additives have not been confirmed by well-controlled clinical studies; therefore, additions to intraocular irrigating solutions cannot be recommended by the various ophthalmic companies.

CONCLUSIONS

Intraocular irrigating solutions have a vital role in ocular surgery and can influence ultimate surgical outcome. The cornea and lens rely on aqueous humor for their nutritional requirement, even during brief surgical procedures. It may take longer than 8 hours for aqueous humor to fully replace an irrigating solution used to reconstitute the anterior chamber. Posterior segment surgery involving vitrectomy is a lengthy procedure and can expose the lens, retina, and corneal endothelium to high volumes of irrigant for a prolonged period. Therefore, it is important that the ideal intraocular irrigating solution be as close in composition to normal aqueous and vitreous humor as possible.

In vitro and clinical studies have demonstrated that ocular tissues are best maintained by an irrigating solution containing the five major aqueous humor ions (Na^+, K^+, Ca^{++}, Mg^{++}, Cl^-) and also containing glucose, GSH, and a bicarbonate buffer. GSSG apparently can be incorporated into the intraocular tissues and enhances the ability of the tissue to withstand the oxidative challenge of a surgical procedure. An intraocular irrigating solution should also have a pH and an osmolality similar to that of aqueous and vitreous humor. Caution must be used to avoid altering the pH, osmolality, or chemical composition of intraocular irrigating solutions when other drugs (epinephrine and antibiotics) are added to them.

ACKNOWLEDGMENT

This work was supported in part by NIH Grants No. P30 EY06360 (Departmental Core Grant) and R01 EY00933 and Research to Prevent Blindness, Inc. H.F.E. is a Research to Prevent Blindness Senior Scientific Investigator.

REFERENCES

1. Harper JY, Pomerat CM. In vitro observations on the behavior of conjunctival and corneal cells in relation to electrolytes. *Am J Ophthalmol* 1958;46:269–276.
2. Merrill DL, Fleming TC, Girard LJ. The effects of physiologic balanced salt solutions and normal saline on intraocular and extraocular tissues. *Am J Ophthalmol* 1960;49:895–898.
3. Edelhauser HF, Van Horn DL, Hyndiuk RA, Schultz RO. Intraocular irrigating solutions: their effects on the corneal endothelium. *Arch Ophthalmol* 1975;93:648–657.
4. Edelhauser HF, Van Horn DL, Schultz RO, Hyndiuk RA. Comparative toxicity of intraocular irrigating solutions on the corneal endothelium. *Am J Ophthalmol* 1976;81:473–481.
5. Dikstein S, Maurice DM. The metabolic basis to the fluid pump in the cornea. *J Physiol (Lond)* 1972;221:29–41.
6. McCarey BE, Edelhauser HF, Van Horn DL. Functional and structural changes in the corneal endothelium during in vitro perfusion. *Invest Ophthalmol* 1973;12:410–417.
7. Christiansen JM, Kollarits CR, Fukui H, Fishman ML. Intraocular irrigating solutions and lens clarity. *Am J Ophthalmol* 1976;82: 594–597.
8. Kahn MG, Giblin FJ, Epstein DL. Glutathione in calf trabecular meshwork and its relation to aqueous humor outflow facility. *Invest Ophthalmol Vis Sci* 1983;24:1382–1387.
9. Moorhead LC, Redburn DA, Merritt J, Garcia CA. The effects of intravitreal irrigation during vitrectomy on the electroretinogram. *Am J Ophthalmol* 1979;88:239–245.
10. Riley MV. Transport of ions and metabolites across the corneal endothelium. In: McDevitt DS, ed. *Cell biology of the eye.* New York: Academic Press, 1982;53–95.
11. Kaye GI, Mishima S, Cole JD, Kayen W. Studies on the cornea. VII. Effects of perfusion with a Ca^{++}-free medium on the corneal endothelium. *Invest Ophthalmol* 1968;7:53–66.
12. Stern ME, Edelhauser HF, Pederson HJ, Staatz WD. Effects of ionophores X537A and A23187 and calcium-free medium on corneal endothelial morphology. *Invest Ophthalmol Vis Sci* 1981;20:497–507.
13. Watsky MA, Edelhauser HF. Intraocular irrigating solutions: the importance of Ca^{++} and glass versus polypropylene bottles. *Int Ophthalmol Clin* 1993;33:109–125.
14. Lolley RN. Metabolism of retinal rod outer segment. In: Anderson RE, ed. *Biochemistry of the eye.* San Francisco: American Academy of Ophthalmology, 1983;178–188.
15. Hodson S. The regulation of corneal hydration by a salt pump requiring the presence of sodium and bicarbonate ions. *J Physiol (Lond)* 1974;236:271–302.
16. Hodson S, Miller F. The bicarbonate ion pump in the endothelium which regulates the hydration of rabbit cornea. *J Physiol (Lond)* 1976;263:563–577.
17. Hull DS, Chemotti MT, Edelhauser HF, Van Horn DL, Hyndiuk RA. Effect of epinephrine on the corneal endothelium. *Am J Ophthalmol* 1975;79:245–250.
18. Wiederholt M, Koch M. Effect of intraocular irrigating solutions on intracellular membrane potentials and swelling rate of isolated human and rabbit cornea. *Invest Ophthalmol Vis Sci* 1979;18:313–317.
19. Hodson S, Wigham C, Williams L, Mayes KR, Graham MV. Observations on the human cornea in vitro. *Exp Eye Res* 1981;32:353–360.
20. Winkler BS, Simson V, Benner J. Importance of bicarbonate in retinal function. *Invest Ophthalmol Vis Sci* 1977;16:766–768.
21. Negi A, Honda Y, Kawano S. Comparative studies on intraocular irrigating solutions. *Folia Ophthalmol Jpn* 1980;31:1452–1459.
22. Negi A, Honda Y, Kawano S. Effects of intraocular irrigating solutions on the electroretinographic B-wave. *Am J Ophthalmol* 1981;92: 28–37.
23. Geroski DH, Edelhauser HF, O'Brien WJ. Hexose-monophosphate shunt response to diamide in the component layers of the cornea. *Exp Eye Res* 1978;26:611–619.
24. Hogan MJ, Alvarado JA, Weddell JE. *Histology of the human eye.* Philadelphia: W.B. Saunders, 1971.
25. Gaasterland DE, Pederson JE, MacLellan HM. Rhesus monkey aqueous humor composition and a primate ocular perfusate. *Invest Ophthalmol Vis Sci* 1979;18:1139–1150.
26. Kinoshita JH. Pathways of glucose metabolism in the lens. *Invest Ophthalmol* 1965;4:619–628.
27. Winkler BS. Comparison of intraocular solutions on glycolysis and levels of ATP and glutathione in the retina. *J Cataract Refract Surg* 1988;14:633–637.
28. Riley MV, Meyer RF, Yates E. Glutathione in the aqueous humor of human and other species. *Invest Ophthalmol Vis Sci* 1980;19:94–96.
29. Anderson EI, Fischbarg J, Spector A. Fluid transport, ATP level and ATPase activities in isolated rabbit corneal endothelium. *Biochim Biophys Acta* 1973;307:557–562.
30. Anderson, EI, Fischbarg J, Spector A. Disulfide stimulation of fluid transport and effect on ATP level in rabbit corneal endothelium. *Exp Eye Res* 1974;19:1–10.
31. Edelhauser HF, Van Horn DL, Miller P, Pederson HJ. Effect of thiol-oxidation of glutathione with diamide on corneal endothelial function, junctional complexes and microfilaments. *J Cell Biol* 1976; 68:567–578.

32. Ng MC, Riley MV. Relation of intracellular levels and redox state of glutathione to endothelial function in the rabbit cornea. *Exp Eye Res* 1980;30:511–517.
33. Whikehart DR, Edelhauser HF. Glutathione in rabbit corneal endothelia: the effects of selected perfusion fluids. *Invest Ophthalmol Vis Sci* 1978;17:455–464.
34. Hodson SA, Wigham CG. Effect of glutathione on human corneal transendothelial potential difference. *J Physiol* 1980:301:34–35.
35. Riley MV. The chemistry of the aqueous humor. In: Anderson RE, ed. *Biochemistry of the eye.* San Francisco: American Academy of Ophthalmology, 1983;79–95.
36. Halst A, Rolfsen W, Sevensson B, Ollinger K, Lundgren B. Formation of free-radicals during phacoemulsification. *Curr Eye Res* 1993;12:359–365.
37. Shimmura S, Tsubata K, Oguchi Y, Fukumura D, Suematsu, Tsuchiya M. Oxiradical-dependent photoemission induced by a phacoemulsification probe. *Invest Ophthalmol Vis Sci* 1992;33:2904–2907.
38. Nakamura MT, Nakano T, Hikida M. Effects of oxidized glutathione and reduced glutathione on the barrier function of the corneal endothelium. *Cornea* 1994;13:493–495.
39. Jaffe NS, Horwitz J. Lens and cataract. In: Podos SM, Yanoff M, eds. *Textbook of ophthalmology.* New York: Gower Medical Publishing, 1992;4.1–4.13.
40. Araie M. Intraocular irrigating solutions and permeability of the blood aqueous barrier. *Arch Ophthalmol* 1990;108:882–885.
41. Mayer P, Mattern J, Parnell D, Hall K, Veltman J, Edelhauser HF. Distribution of [^{35}S-GSSG] into ocular tissues and its effect on ocular glutathione homeostasis. *Invest Ophthalmol Vis Sci* 1992;33(suppl): 1413.
42. Reddy VN, Unakar NJ. Localization of gamma-glutamyl transpeptidase in rabbit lens ciliary process and cornea. *Exp Eye Res* 1973;17: 405–408.
43. Reddy VN. Dynamics of transport systems in the eye. *Invest Ophthalmol Vis Sci* 1979;18:1000–1018.
44. Edelhauser HF, Hanneken AM, Pederson HJ, Van Horn DL. Osmotic tolerance of rabbit and human corneal endothelium. *Arch Ophthalmol* 1981;99:1281–1287.
45. Gonnering R, Edelhauser HF, Van Horn DL, Durant W. The pH tolerance of rabbit and human corneal endothelium. *Invest Ophthalmol Vis Sci* 1979;18:373–390.
46. Glasser DB, Matsuda M, Edelhauser HF. Comparison of corneal endothelial structural and functional integrity after irrigation with bicarbonate-buffered and acetate-citrate-buffered solutions. In: Cavanagh HD, ed. *The cornea: transactions of the World Congress on the Cornea III.* New York: Raven Press, 1988;101–106.
47. Edelhauser HF, Hyndiuk RA, Zeeb A, Schultz RO. Corneal edema and the intraocular use of epinephrine. *Am J Ophthalmol* 1982;93: 327–333.
48. Winkler BS, Trese MT. The pH of antibiotic vitreous infusion combinations: a potential cause of retinal toxicity. *Ophthalmic Surg* 1992; 23:622–624.
49. Edelhauser HF, MacRae SM. Irrigating and viscous solutions. In: Sears M, Tarkkanen A, eds. *Surgical pharmacology of the eye.* New York: Raven Press, 1985;363–388.
50. Nuyts RMMA, Edelhauser HF, Holley GP. Intraocular irrigating solutions: a comparison of Hartmann's lactated Ringer's solution, BSS and BSS Plus. *Graefes Arch Clin Exp Ophthalmol* 1995;233:655–661.
51. Claoue C, Rosen P, Stevens J, Steele A. A prospective randomized double-masked clinical comparison of Hartmann's solution and balanced salt solution in phacoemulsification. *Eur J Implant Refract Surg* 1994;6:54–56.
52. McDonnell PJ, Spalton DJ. Corneal clarity during extracapsular cataract surgery. *Implant Refract Surg* 1988;6:9–13.
53. Glasser DB, Matsuda M, Ellis JG, Edelhauser HF. Effects of intraocular irrigating solutions on the corneal endothelium after in vivo anterior chamber irrigation. *Am J Ophthalmol* 1985;99:321–328.
54. Li J, Akiyama R, Kuang K, Fischbarg J. Effects of BSS and BSS Plus irrigation solutions on rabbit corneal transendothelial electrical potential difference. *Cornea* 1993;12:199–203.
55. Barfort P, Maurice DM. Electrical potential and fluid transport across the corneal endothelium. *Exp Eye Res* 1974;19:11–19.
56. Fischbarg J, Lim JJ. Role of cations, anions and carbonic anhydrase in fluid transport across rabbit corneal endothelium. *J Physiol* 1974; 241:647–675.
57. Kline OR, Symes DJ, Lorenzetti OJ. Effect of BSS Plus on the corneal endothelium with intraocular lens implantation. *J Toxicol Cut Ocul Toxicol* 1983;2:243–247.
58. Otori T, Hohki T, Yamamoto Y, Mamamoto M, Ikeda M. Physiological studies on the intraocular irrigating solution for ophthalmic surgery: a preliminary report. *Acta Soc Ophthalmol Jpn* 1980;84:1272–1277.
59. Orori T, Hohki T, Nakao Y, et al. Studies on the intraocular irrigating solution for ophthalmic surgery: report 2: reappraisal of the role of bicarbonate concentration. *Acta Soc Ophthalmol Jpn* 1981;85:1237–1242.
60. Matsuda M, Tano Y, Inaba M, Sato M, Inone Y, Manabe R. Corneal complications after pars plana vitrectomy using S-MA_2 for an intraocular irrigating solution. *Folia Ophthalmol Jpn* 1983;34:1424–1428.
61. Matsuda M, Yano Y, Edelhauser HF. Comparison of intraocular irrigating solutions used for pars plana vitrectomy and prevention of endothelial cell loss. *Jpn J Ophthalmol* 1984;28:230–238.
62. Araie M. Barrier function of corneal endothelium and the intraocular irrigating solutions. *Arch Ophthalmol* 1986;104:435–438.
63. Matsuda M, Kinoshita S, Ohashi Y, et al. Comparison of the effects of intraocular irrigating solutions on the corneal endothelium in intraocular lens implantation. *Br J Ophthalmol* 1991;75:476–479.
64. McDermott ML, Edelhauser HF, Hock HM, Langston RHS. Ophthalmic irrigants: a current review and update. *Ophthalmic Surg* 1988;19:724–733.
65. Mishima S. Clinical investigations on the corneal endothelium. *Am J Ophthalmol* 1982;93:1–29.
66. Machemer R, Parel J-M, Beuttner H. A new concept for vitreous surgery. 1. Instrumentation. *Am J Ophthalmol* 1972;73:1–7.
67. Machemer R, Aaberg TM. *Vitrectomy.* New York, Grune & Stratton, 1979;1–245.
68. Peyman GA, Dodich NA. Experimental vitrectomy: instrumentation and surgical technique. *Arch Ophthalmol* 1971;86:548–551.
69. Benson WE, Diamond JG, Tasman W. Intraocular irrigating solutions for pars plana vitrectomy. *Arch Ophthalmol* 1981;99:1013–1015.
70. Kinsey VE, Reddy DVN. Studies on the crystalline lens. XI. The relative role of the epithelium and capsule in transport. *Invest Ophthalmol* 1965;4:104–116.
71. Borchman D, Paterson CA, Delamere NA. Ca^{++} ATPase activity in the human lens. *Curr Eye Res* 1989;8:1049–1054.
72. Hightower KR, Leverenz V, Reddy VN. Calcium transport in the lens. *Invest Ophthalmol Vis Sci* 1980;19:1059–1066.
73. Reddy VN. Transport of organic molecules in the lens. *Exp Eye Res* 1973;15:731–750.
74. Spector A, Garner WH. Hydrogen peroxide and human cataract. *Exp Eye Res* 1981;33:673–681.
75. Spector A. Oxidation and aspects of ocular pathology. *CLAO J* 1990; 16:8–10.
76. Saornil Alvarez MA, Pastor Jimeno JC. Role of the intraocular irrigating solutions in the pathogenesis of the postvitrectomy retinal edema. *Curr Eye Res* 1987;6:1369–1379.
77. Freeman JM, Gettelfinger TC. Maintaining pupillary dilation during lens implant surgery. *Am Intraocul Implant Soc J* 1981;7:172–173.
78. Duffin RM, Pettit TH, Straatsma BR. Maintenance of mydriasis with epinephrine during cataract surgery. *Ophthalmic Surg* 1983;14:41–45.
79. Elliott A, Carter C. Pupil size after extracapsular cataract extraction and posterior chamber lens implantation: a prospective randomized trial of epinephrine and acetylcholine. *Ophthalmic Surg* 1989;20: 591–594.
80. Gimbel HV. The effect of treatment with topical nonsteroidal antiinflammatory drugs with and without intraoperative epinephrine on the maintenance of mydriasis during cataract surgery. *Ophthalmology* 1989;96:585–588.
81. Corbett MC, Richards AB. Intraocular adrenaline maintains mydriasis during cataract surgery. *Br J Ophthalmol* 1994;78:95–98.
82. Abelson MB, Alfonso E. Pupillary update: mydriasis and miosis during surgery. *Excerpta Medica* 1986:10–12.
83. Steedle TO. Pupillary dilation. In: Abrahamson IA, ed. *Cataract surgery.* McGraw Hill, 1986;34–36.
84. Alfonso E, Abelson MB, Smith LM. Pharmacologic pupillary modulation in the perioperative period. *J Cataract Refract Surg* 1988;14: 78–80.

85. Schultz RO, Edelhauser HF, Van Horn DL, Hyndiuk RA. Hazards of intraocular irrigating solutions and epinephrine in cataract surgery. In: Emery JM, Paton D, eds. *Current concepts in cataract surgery.* Selected proceedings of the Fourth Biennial Cataract Surgical Congress. St. Louis: C.V. Mosby, 1976;269–276.
86. Slack JW, Edelhauser HF, Helenek MJ. A bisulfite-free intraocular epinephrine solution. *Am J Ophthalmol* 1990;110:77–82.
87. Adams HA, Nowak MR, Jung U, von Kavassey A, Hempelmann G. Absorption of adrenaline after local administration to the eye. *Fortschr Ophthalmol* 1991;88:852–856.
88. Fell D, Watson AP, Hindocha N. Plasma concentrations of catecholamines following intraocular irrigation with adrenaline. *Br J Anaesth* 1989;62:573–575.
89. Fiore PM, Cinotti AA. Systemic effects of intraocular epinephrine during cataract surgery. *Ann Ophthalmol* 1988;20:23–25.
90. Yamaguchi H, Matsumoto Y. Stability of blood pressure and heart rate during intraocular epinephrine irrigation. *Ann Ophthalmol* 1988;20:58–60.
91. Haimann MH, Abrams GW, Edelhauser HF, Hatchell DL. The effect of intraocular irrigating solutions on lens clarity in normal and diabetic rabbits. *Am J Ophthalmol* 1982;94:594–605.
92. Haimann MH, Abrams GW. Prevention of lens opacification during diabetic vitrectomy. *Ophthalmology* 1984;91:116–121.
93. Araki H, Kanai A, Nakajima A, Ninomiya H, Kobayashi Y, Tanaka M. BSS Plus does not cause lens opacification during vitrectomy in diabetic patients. XXVII International Congress of Ophthalmology, Toronto, June, 1994.
94. Geroski DH, Hadley A, Edelhauser HF. Antibiotics in intraocular irrigating solutions: effects on the corneal endothelium. *Invest Ophthalmol Vis Sci* 1994;35:1436.
95. Brown GC, Eagle RC, Shakin EP, Gruber M, Arbizio VV. Retinal toxicity of intravitreal gentamicin. *Arch Ophthalmol* 1990;108:1740–1744.
96. Conway BP, Tabatabay CA, Campochiaro PA, D'Amico DJ, Hanninen LA, Kenyon KR. Gentamicin toxicity in the primate retina. *Arch Ophthalmol* 1989;107:107–112.

Textbook of Ocular Pharmacology, edited by T.J. Zimmerman, et al.
Lippincott–Raven Publishers, Philadelphia © 1997.

CHAPTER 54

Surgical Viscoelastic Substances

Gavin J. Roberts and Robert A. Hyndiuk

SURGICAL VISCOELASTIC SUBSTANCES

The use of viscoelastic substances in ophthalmology began with the search for a vitreous substitute in the 1960s, as the importance of the role of the vitreous in retinal detachment began to be understood (1). Sodium hyaluronate used for this purpose was purified by Balazs et al. (2) and was successfully used in vitreoretinal surgery. Anterior segment surgeons began to explore the role of viscoelastics in protecting the corneal endothelium during cataract surgery. In 1983, Miller and Stegmann authored a definitive text on the use of sodium hyaluronate in opthalmic surgery (3). In the decade that followed, both the indications for use and the surgeon's choice of viscoelastic materials have expanded. A more recent extensive review was completed by Liesegang in 1990 (4).

In choosing the most appropriate viscoelastic for a particular application, surgeons must be aware of the differences in behavior of these unique substances. Different types of viscoelastic may be indicated for various types of surgeries and during various stages of cataract and anterior segment surgery. A basic understanding of the rheologic properties of the commonly available products is essential.

Rheologic Properties

Viscosity

Viscosity is defined as resistance to flow, and is measured in units termed "poises." A high viscous material placed between two parallel plates makes sliding one plate across the other more difficult. "Shear force" is that force required to move one plate across the other. A material of low viscosity between the plates requires less shear force to move one plate across the other. Comparison of the viscosities of the various viscoelastic substances is facilitated by use of a standardized unit of measurement (Table 1). Viscosity is dependent on the molecular weight and concentration of substances in solution.

Viscoelasticity

Elastic materials are those that tend to return to their original shape after deformation. This property is advantageous, for example, in anterior chamber maintenance, and allows protection of tissues such as corneal endothelium from ultrasonic energy or irrigating currents. Unlike for viscosity, no standardized units exist for comparison of viscoelasticity among different substances. Therefore, comparing the viscoelastic tendencies of these materials is more difficult than comparing their viscosity.

Pseudoplasticity

Pseudoplasticity refers to a change in viscosity with increasing shear rate. In the parallel plate model described above, the viscosity of an interposed pseudoplastic substance decreases as the plates are moved against each other more rapidly. This property is particularly important among opthalmic viscoelastic substances because it influences the ease with which the substance can be injected through a cannula or to leave the eye once injected. Materials that exhibit pseudoplastic behavior include sodium hyaluronate, methylcellulose, and polyacrylamide. Materials that do not exhibit such behavior include chondroitin sulfate and silicone oil.

Coatability

The ability of one material to coat another is dependent on the angle it makes on a flat surface (contact angle), sur-

G. J. Roberts and R. A. Hyndiuk: Department of Ophthalmology, Cornea and External Disease Service, Medical College of Wisconsin, Milwaukee, Wisconsin 53226.

TABLE 54-1. *Composition and properties of commercially available viscoelastics substances*

Parameter	Healon	Healon GV	Amvisc	Amvisc Plus	ProVisc	Viscoat	Occucoat
Source	Rooster combs	Rooster combs	Rooster combs	Rooster combs	Bacterial fermentation	Bacterial fermentation, shark fin cartilage	Wood pulp
Composition	1% NaHA	1.4% NaHA	1% NaHA	1.6% NaHA	1% NaHA	3.0% NaHA + 4.0% CDS	2%HPMC
Molecular weight (Daltons)	4.0 M	5.0M	1.0+ M	1.0+ M	1,9+ M	500 K, 25 K	NA
Pseudoplasticity index[a]	>1333	10,000	909	410	NA	210	NA

NaHA, sodium hyaluronate; HPMC, hydroxypropyl methylcellulose; CDS, chondroitin sulfate.
M, million; K, thousand.
[a]Viscosity at shear rate 0/viscosity at shear rate 1,000.

face tension, and molecular weight. Generally, sodium hyaluronate, which has a smaller contact angle, coats less well than solutions containing chondroitin sulfate or methylcellulose, which have larger contact angles and lower viscosities.

Cohesiveness

Materials that are highly cohesive tend to enter or leave the eye in a single, globular mass. If left in the eye, these substances may be more likely to clog the trabecular meshwork, causing increases in intraocular pressure (IOP). Cohesiveness is determined by both the molecular weight and the elastic properties of the substance. Defined standards of cohesiveness are not readily available, but sodium hyaluronate is the most cohesive of the popular viscoelastic substances.

SODIUM HYALURONATE

Drug Name, Chemistry, and Pharmaceutics

Sodium hyaluronate is a long-chain, naturally occurring mucopolysaccharide. It is present in high concentrations in the vitreous humor and in the trabecular meshwork (5), where it may have a role in the rate of aqueous humor outflow (6).

Preparations composed solely of sodium hyaluronate and commercially available are Healon, Healon GV, Amvisc, Amvisc Plus, and ProVisc. Healon (Pharmacia Pharmaceuticals) is 1% sodium hyaluronate derived from rooster combs, as is Amvisc (IOLAB). Healon and Amvisc differ principally in their viscosities (see Table 1): Amvisc is slightly less viscous (4). A higher viscosity Amvisc Plus is 1.6% sodium hyaluronate. Healon GV, composed of 1.4% sodium hyaluronate, was recently introduced. The production of Amvisc was halted temporarily in 1990 because of a legal dispute; its production has since resumed. Current efforts are being directed toward the manufacture of sodium hyaluronate through genetically engineered microbial fermentation which, theoretically, may enhance purification and lessen cost. ProVisc (Alcon) is a sodium hyaluronate recently introduced commercially that is produced by microbial fermentation.

An owl monkey model has been used to study the inflammatory potential of rooster comb-derived sodium hyaluronate preparations by injection into the vitreous cavity (7,8). These studies demonstrated that inflammation varies by batch and is not dependent on origin or concentration.

CHONDROITIN SULFATE

Drug Name, Chemistry, and Pharmaceutics

Chondroitin sulfate, like sodium hyaluronate, is a mucopolysaccharide found in nature. However, it is sulfated and carries a negative charge, in contrast to sodium hyaluronate. Because of its negative charge, it can better coat positively charged surfaces such as intraocular lenses and corneal endothelium (9,10).

Viscoat (Alcon Surgical) is a mixture of 4% chondroitin sulfate derived from shark fin cartilage and 3% sodium hyaluronate from microbial fermentation. Earlier production lots of Viscoat were shown to contain bacterial endotoxins; this has not been true in the last several years.

METHYLCELLULOSE

Drug Name, Chemistry, and Pharmaceutics

Hydroxypropyl methylcellulose (HPMC) is a wood pulp product consisting of long chains of glucose molecules with hydroxypropyl and methoxyl substitutions for hydroxyl groups, which lends increased hydrophyllicity (4). Methylcellulose has been used for surgical applications, in artificial tear preparations, and as a gonioscopic solution.

Some investigators have reservations about the use of methylcellulose in intraocular surgery because of its derivation from wood rather than animal products and because its ultimate fate in human tissues remains unknown (11,12). Vegetable particulate matter contaminants have been detected in hospital-prepared lots (11), and its use as a vitreous substitute produced marked inflammation in an animal model. Nonetheless, a large body of work collectively indicates that HPMC is a safe, useful viscoelastic agent (10–17).

Occucoat (Storz Pharmaceuticals) is a double-filtered preparation of 2% HPMC. Thus far, when used in intraocular surgery in humans, it has not been associated with problems unique to its derivation. One investigation showed that HPMC produced greater corneal thickness than sodium hyaluronate 1 day after phacoemulsification surgery (18), but no difference was observed after standard extracapsular surgery.

Clinically, HPMC, sodium hyaluronate, and chondroitin sulfate all appear to be tolerated well by the corneal endothelium if the contact time is not prolonged (10,19). If the contact time of a viscoelastic substance is prolonged, severe endothelial damage may occur in human eyes (20).

OTHER AGENTS

Orcolon (Optical Radiation Corporation) was a solution of 0.5% polyacrylamide withdrawn from the market after several reports of delayed, extremely high postoperative increases in intraocular pressure, some of which required filtration surgery (20).

Cellugell (Vision Biology) is a carbohydrate polymer undergoing clinical trials in England and South America (17).

Therapeutic Uses

Anterior Chamber Maintenance

The ability to maintain a physiologic depth of the anterior chamber during intraocular surgery increases the ease with which many procedures can be performed. All the viscoelastics mentioned provide a stable anterior chamber (16,17). Under conditions that compress the anterior chamber, such as posterior vitreous pressure, the elasticity of a compound may be the most important rheologic property determining whether or not depth will be maintained. Viscosity of the substance appears to be less important (21). Materials that lack pseudoplasticity are also more likely to maintain space. An animal model investigation showed that significantly more Viscoat than Healon was retained in eyes after phacoemulsification with and without traumatic lens implantation (22). Clinically, anterior segment surgeons rely on Viscoat when viscoelastic retention is important, as in phacoemulsification surgery and many complicated cataract or traumatic cataract cases.

Corneal Endothelial Protection

All currently available viscoelastics are effective in preventing mechanical damage from the pseudophakos to the corneal endothelium (15,20). Aside from protecting the endothelium from direct lens rubbing, viscoelastic substance must further protect against compressive forces directed perpendicular to the endothelium and against drag or shear forces generated parallel to it. A thicker endothelial coating transmits less compressive and shearing forces than does a thin layer of the same viscosity and pseudoplasticity.

Rheologic properties also became important in corneal endothelial protection. An "ideal" viscoelastic would have a high viscosity and elasticity to minimize compression but would also be pseudoplastic to minimize endothelial damage from shear forces (23).

Healon is a very viscous substance that allows greater transmission of shear force and coats the endothelium less well than Viscoat (23,24). An animal model of endothelial cell cultures demonstrated that Healon had greater cell toxicity than HPMC, Amvisc, or Viscoat (25). Aside from the rheologic properties of Healon, its lack of ability to bind calcium (unlike Viscoat) and thus supply calcium to endothelium may play a role in its increased endothelial toxicity.

Tissue Manipulation

Viscoelastics may be used during surgery to manipulate the capsular bag, iris, and Descemet's membrane and to hold wound edges in apposition. Rheologic properties enhancing the ability to move or manipulate tissue include high viscosity, elasticity, and pseudoplasticity. Therefore, when in a stationary position in the eye, more viscous materials such as Healon may be better able to maintain tissue position than can material of lesser viscosity.

Coating of Tissues and Implants

The coating ability of viscoelastic substances is an interplay of contact angle, surface tension, electrical charge, and other factors. Materials with a low contact angle and a low surface tension are better able to coat a surface than are materials with a high surface tension or contact angle.

Theoretically, materials with a charge opposite that of the surface to be coated would be better able to adhere to the surface. Because of its relatively high surface tension and contact angle, sodium hyaluronate (Healon) "beads" when applied to the pseudophakos and does not coat the lens or endothelium (20,24). HPMC coats well because of its low contact angle but is retained on the lens or endothelial surface less well because of its low viscosity (26). Viscoat provides more protection than Healon against controlled intraocular lens trauma and coats surfaces easily as compared with Healon (20,24). Viscoat, however, due to these properties, must be aspirated from the anterior chamber rather than simply being irrigated out. Viscoat has been considered to be more well suited to procedures in which coating and retention characteristics are highly desirable (20,24,27,28), such as phacoemulsification surgery. Retention properties are also important in surgical cases in which the surgeon must deal with management or prevention of problems such as vitreous presentation in possible or actual capsular or zonular rupture. In such cases, a more stable viscoelastic "patch" or "barrier" provided by Viscoat may be advantageous (when continued gentle phacoemulsification or low-infusion irrigation and aspiration may be appropriate and necessary).

Other Uses of Viscoelastic Substances

The use of viscoelastic substances is not confined to corneal or cataract surgery. The risks of a flat anterior chamber after filtration surgery may be lessened with viscoelastic use (29,30). To maintain anterior chamber depth, the viscoelastic material would have to be left in the eye at the conclusion of surgery. This should be done after the safest material possible is chosen to minimize the risks of intraocular pressure increase and corneal edema as described above.

The earliest use of viscoelastic substances in ophthalmic surgery was in retinal detachment surgery (1). High molecular weight sodium hyaluronate is still used by some posterior segment surgeons in the repair of retinal detachment (31), sometimes in conjunction with silicone oil (32). Silicon oil itself is not a viscoelastic material.

Additional uses for viscoelastic substances are many, including lubrication of fascia lata strips used in ptosis surgery and as lubricants in strabismus surgery. Dry eye conditions are often treated with substances such as methylcellulose to provide viscous lubrication to the ocular surface.

Side Effects of Viscoelastic Substances

Intraocular Pressure Increase

Apart from their cost, perhaps the biggest drawback to the use of viscoelastic substances is the risk of postoperative intraocular pressure elevation (20). Viscoelastic material that is not removed from the eye after surgery is not degraded to any significant degree when in the anterior chamber (4). The route of exit is principally through the trabecular meshwork into Schlemm's canal (33). Other routes of lesser importance have been shown to play a role in animal models, including iris and ciliary body resorption (34).

The mechanism involved in intraocular pressure elevation related to the use of Healon appears to be mechanical outflow obstruction that is relieved with the concomitant administration of hyaluronidase (33,35,36). The ability of viscoelastic materials to pass through rather than occlude the trabecular meshwork is a function of viscosity, chain length, molecular volume, molecular rigidity, and electrical charge (4,29). Any spike in intraocular pressure is more likely to occur in the early hours after surgery (maximal 4 to 7 hours) and often returns to baseline by 24 hours (10,15,20,30). This underscores the importance of early postoperative measurements of pressure in eyes in which even transient increases in pressure could have potentially damaging consequences, especially eyes with preexisting glaucomatous optic nerve damage. Patients with glaucoma or ocular hypertension often develop extremely high pressures after ocular surgery even if a "washout" is performed (20).

Animal studies have demonstrated that a replacement of the aqueous volume by less than one half its total by sodium hyaluronate resulted in no significant increase in IOP (5). Even after the IOP has returned to normal, the aqueous may be 3,500 times as viscous as normal, with 370 times the physiologic concentration of sodium hyaluronate (29).

Evidence regarding which viscoelastics provide the best margin of safety with regard to avoiding IOP spikes is conflicting. Some studies support a lower risk with HPMC (13), Viscoat (31), and Amvisc Plus (32), whereas others demonstrate no significant difference between Viscoat and Healon (37). One animal study demonstrated that an increase in IOP resulting from Viscoat, Healon, and 2% HPMC could be reduced by anterior chamber washout (15). At present, it is probably best to assume that all viscoelastic substances have the potential to increase IOP postoperatively and that careful removal may lessen the chance of a significant spike. The use of prophylactic acetazolamide may blunt but not eliminate any increase in IOP (38,39).

Corneal Edema

The residual effects of retained viscoelastic material in the anterior chamber should be considered in the differential diagnosis of postoperative corneal edema. Kim reported three cases of severe corneal edema due to thimerosal residues in reused viscoelastic cannulas (40). One of us (R.A.H.) reported five serial cases at a Wisconsin hospital of severe, persistent corneal edema requiring keratoplasty that was determined to be due to residues of viscoelastic and cleaning solutions in reused viscoelastic cannulas (20). No cases occurred after use of disposable cannulas was instituted.

Severe sectoral corneal edema associated with Healon retained in the anterior chamber and in contact with corneal endothelium has been observed (20). Lindstrom reported that human donor corneal endothelium exhibits significant cell death at 30 minutes and near-complete cell death at 2 hours if viscoelastic material remains in contact with corneal endothelium (R.L. Lindstrom, March 1990, personal communication).

To minimize the risk of viscoelastic-related corneal edema, surgeons should attempt thorough intraoperative washout. Some procedures are performed during which retention of the viscoelastic substance is planned to maintain stability of the anterior chamber (e.g., in certain keratoplasties with anterior chamber intraocular lens exchange and complicated anterior segment procedures). During these operations, the chance of corneal edema may be reduced by injecting a small amount of balanced salt solution at the viscoelastic–endothelium interface to reduce prolonged contact between the viscoelastic substance and the endothelium.

Drug Binding

To date, no evidence suggests that drugs in the intraocular milieu bind to viscous solutions to any significant degree. One study specifically found no evidence of drug binding (41).

Uses of Viscoelastic Cannulas

Reuse of cannulas in the delivery of viscoelastic solutions has been implicated as a cause of severe postoperative corneal edema (20,40). Nuyts et al. (42) reported retained detergent residue in irrigating cannulas that was responsible for marked corneal edema in 17 patients. All manufacturers now supply a disposable cannula with their viscoelastic solutions. In this regard, we recommend that cannulas *never* be reused with viscoelastic solutions.

Other Effects of Viscoelastic Substances

Several cases of acute calcific band keratopathy were reported several years ago (43–45) in association with intracameral Viscoat use. After the reduction of the phosphate-buffering content of Viscoat used in a rabbit model demonstrated no keratopathy as compared with stock commercially prepared Viscoat (44), the product was reformulated, and no subsequent cases of band keratopathy have been reported.

CONCLUSIONS

An increasing number of viscoelastics are available to ophthalmic surgeons. By understanding the unique pharmacology and rheology of each substance, physicians will be able to choose the most suitable product for a given application.

ACKNOWLEDGMENT

This work was supported in part by an unrestricted grant from Research to Prevent Blindness, Inc., New York, NY, and by Core Grant No. EY01931 from the National Institutes of Health, Bethesda, MD.

REFERENCES

1. Balazs EA. Physiology of the vitreous body. In: Schepens CL, ed. *Importance of the vitreous body in retina surgery with special emphasis on reoperations.* St. Louis: CV Mosby, 1960;29–48.
2. Balazs EA, Freeman MI, Klöti R, Meyer-Schwickerath G, Regnault F, Sweeny DB. Hyaluronic acid and the replacement of vitreous and aqueous humor. *Mod Probl Ophthalmol* 1972;10:3–21.
3. Miller D, Stegmann R, eds. *Healon: a guide to its use in ophthalmic surgery.* New York: Wiley Medical Publishers, 1983.
4. Liesegang TJ. Viscoelastic substances in ophthalmology. *Surv Ophthalmol* 1990;34:268–293.
5. Balazs EA. Sodium hyaluronate and viscosurgery. In: Miller D, Stegmann R, eds. *Healon: a guide to its use in ophthalmic surgery.* New York, Wiley Medical Publishers, 1983;00–00.
6. Barany EH. The action of different kinds of hyaluronidase on the resistance to flow through the angle of the anterior chamber. *Acta Ophthalmol* 1956;34:397.
7. Hultsch E. The scope of hyaluronic acid as an experimental intraocular implant. *Ophthalmology* 1980;87:706.
8. Balazs EA. Viscosurgery, features of a true viscosurgical tool and its role in ophthalmic surgery. In: Miller D, Stegmann R, eds. *Treatment of anterior segment ocular trauma.* Montreal: Medicopea, 1986;00–00.
9. Harrison SE, Soll DB, Shayegan M, Clinch T. Chondroitin sulfate; a new and effective agent for intraocular lens insertion. *Ophthalmology 1982;89:1254.*
10. MacRae SM, Edelhauser HF, Hyndiuk RA, Burd EM, Schultz RO. The effects of sodium hyaluronate, chondroitin sulfate and methylcellulose on the corneal endothelium and intraocular pressure. *Am J Ophthalmol* 1983;95:332–341.
11. Rosen ES, Gregory RPE, Barnett F. Is 2% methoxypropyl methylcellulose a safe solution for intraoperative clinical applications? *J Cataract Refract Surg* 1986;12:679.
12. Smith SG, Lindstrom RL, Miller RA, et al. Safety and efficacy of 2% methylcellulose in cat and monkey cataract implant surgery. *J Am Intraocul Implant Soc* 1984;10:160.
13. Arcu-Rosa D, Cohn JC, Aron JJ. Methylcellulose instead of Healon in extracapsular surgery with intraocular lens implantation. *Ophthalmology* 1983;90:1235.
14. Fecher PU, Fechner MU. Methylcellulose and lens implantation. *Br J Ophthalmol* 1983;67:259.
15. Glasser DB, Matsuda M, Edelhauser HF. A comparison of the efficacy and toxicity of and intraocular pressure response to viscous solutions in the anterior chamber. *Arch Ophthalmol* 1986;104:1819.
16. Kerr Muir MG, Sherrard ES, Andrews V, Steele AD. Air, methylcellulose, sodium hyaluronate and the corneal endothelium; endothelial protective agents. *Eye* 1987;1:480–486.
17. Liesegang TJ, Bourne WM, Ilstrup DM. The use of hydroxypropyl methylcellulose in extracapsular cataract extraction with intraocular lens implantation. *Am J Ophthalmol* 1986;102:723.
18. Pederson OO. Comparison of the protective effects of methylcellulose and sodium hyaluronate on corneal swelling following phacoemulsification of senile cataracts. *J Cataract Refract Surg* 1990;16: 594.
19. Graue EL, Polack FM, Balazs EA. The protective effects of methylcellulose and sodium hyaluronate on corneal swelling following phacoemulsification of senile cataracts. *Exp Eye Res* 1980;31:119.

20. Hyndiuk RA, Slack JW. Toxicology of surgical solutions and drugs. In: Albert D, Jakobiec F, eds. *Textbook of ophthalmology: the Harvard system.* Philadelphia: WB Saunders, 1994;00–00.
21. Miyauchi S, Iwata S. Evaluations on the usefulness of viscous agents in anterior segment surgery. I. The ability to maintain the deepness of the anterior chamber. *J Oculr Pharm* 1986;2:267–274.
22. Glasser DB, Osborn DC, Nordeen JF, Min YI. Endothelial protection and viscoelastic retention during phacoemulsification and intraocular lens implantation. *J Cataract Refract Surg* 1987;13:537.
23. Hammer ME, Burch TG. Viscous corneal protection by sodium hyaluronate, chondroitin sulfate, and methylcellulose. *Invest Ophthalmol Vis Sci* 1984;25:1329–1332.
24. Glasser DB, Katz HR, Boyd JE, Laugdon JD, Shobe SL, Peiffer RL. Protective effects of viscous solution in phacoemulsification and traumatic lens implantation. *Arch Ophthalmol* 1989;107:1047–1051.
25. Meyer DR, McCulley JP. Different prospects of risk management from *in vitro* toxicology and its relevance to the evolution of viscoelastic formulations. In: Rosen ES, ed. *Viscoelastic materials: basic science and clinical applications.* New York: Pergamon Press, 1989;00–00.
26. Hazariwala K, Mortimer CB, Slomovic AR, et al. Comparison of 2% hydroxypropyl methylcellulose and sodium hyaluronate in implant surgery. *Can J Ophthalmol* 1988;23:259.
27. Beesly RD, Olson RJ, Brady SE. The effects of prolonged phacoemulsification time on the corneal endothelium. *Ann Ophthalmol* 1986;18:216.
28. Glasser DB, Schultz RO, Hyndiuk RA. The role of viscoelastics, cannulas, and irrigating solution additives in post-cataract surgery corneal edema: a brief review. *Lens Eye Toxicity Res* 1992;9:351–359.
29. Denlinger JL, Balazs EA. The fate of exogenous viscoelastic hyaluron solutions in the primate eye. In: Rosen ES, ed. *Viscoelastic materials: basic science and clinical applications.* New York: Pergamon Press, 1989;00–00.
30. Denlinger JL, Schubert H, Balazs EA. Na hyaluronate of various molecular sizes injected into the anterior chamber of owl monkey: disappearance and effect on intraocular pressure. *Proc Int Soc Eye Res* 1980;1:88.
31. Embriano PJ. Postoperative pressure after phacoemulsification: sodium hyaluronate vs. sodium chondroitin sulfate-sodium hyaluronate. *Am J Ophthalmol* 1989;21:85.
32. Levy NS, Boone L. Effect of hyaluronic acid viscosity on IOP elevation after cataract surgery. *Glaucoma* 1989;11:82.
33. Berson FG, Patterson MM, Epstein DL. Obstruction of aqueous outflow by sodium hyaluronate in enucleated human eyes. *Am J Ophthalmol* 1983;95:668–672.
34. Miyauchi S, Iwata S. Biochemical studies on the use of sodium hyaluronate in the anterior eye segment. IV. The protective efficacy on the corneal endothelium. *Curr Eye Res* 1984;3:1063–1067.
35. Calder IG, Smith UH. Hyaluronidase and sodium hyaluronate in cataract surgery. *Br J Ophthalmol* 1986;70:418.
36. Hein SR, Keates RH, Weber RA. Elimination of sodium hyaluronate-induced decrease in outflow facility with hyaluronidase. *Ophthalmic Surg* 1986;17:731.
37. Barron BA, Busin M, Page C, Bergsma DR, Kaufman HE. Comparison of the effects of Viscoat and Healon on postoperative intraocular pressure. *Am J Ophthalmol* 1985;100:377.
38. Lewen R, Insler MS. The effect of prophylactic acetazolamide on the intraocular pressure rise associated with Healon-aided intraocular lens surgery. *Ann Ophthalmol* 1985;17:315–318.
39. Naeser K, Thim K, Hansen TE, Degn T, Madsen S, Skov J. Intraocular pressure in the first days after implantation of posterior chamber lenses with the use of sodium hyaluronate (Healon®). *Acta Ophthalmol (Copenh)* 1986;64:330–337.
40. Kim JH. Intraocular inflammation of denatured viscoelastic substance in cases of cataract extraction. *J Cataract Refract Surg* 1987; 13:537.
41. McDermott ML, Edelhauser HE. Drug binding of ophthalmic viscoelastic agents. *Arch Ophthalmol* 1989;107:261.
42. Nuyts RM, Edelhauser HF, Pels E, Breebart AC. Toxic effects of detergents on the corneal endothelium. *Arch Ophthalmol* 1990;108: 1158.
43. Binder PS, Deg JK, Kohl FS. Calcific band keratopathy after intraocular chondroitin sulfate. *Arch Ophthalmol* 1987;105:1243.
44. Nevyas AS, Raber IM, Eagle RC Jr, Wallace IB, Nevyas HJ. Acute band keratopathy following intraocular Viscoat. *Arch Ophthalmol* 1987;105:958.
45. Coffman MR, Mann PM. Corneal subepithelial deposits after use of sodium chondroitin. *Am J Ophthalmol* 1986;102:279.

Textbook of Ocular Pharmacology,
edited by T.J. Zimmerman, et al.
Lippincott–Raven Publishers, Philadelphia © 1997.

CHAPTER 55

Antiseptics and Disinfectants

Rajesh K. Rajpal and Stephen R. Glaser

Antiseptics are antimicrobial agents used on living tissues. Therefore, they must kill microorganisms or inhibit their reproduction and metabolic activities without destroying human tissue. The concentration of an antiseptic will always have a therapeutic window. This window may be very narrow. Antiseptics commonly used are ethyl and isopropyl alcohol, cationic surface-active agents (benzalkonium), biguanids (chlorhexidine), iodine compounds (iodine solution, iodine tincture, and povidone-iodine), and phenolic agents (hexachlorophene).

Disinfectants are used on inanimate objects to destroy microorganisms and to prevent infection. Some disinfectants may be used as antiseptics if diluted appropriately. Disinfectants most commonly used are the aldehydes (formaldehyde and glutaral), the hypochlorites, the phenolic compounds, and selected quaternary ammonium compounds.

Sterilization is the elimination of all viable microbes by a disinfectant. Frequently used compounds for chemical sterilization include ethylene oxide, glutaraldehyde, peroxyacetic acid, hydrogen peroxide, and sodium hypochlorite.

ALCOHOLS

History and Source

In 1834, Dumas and Peligot described the relationship between wood-spirit (methyl alcohol-CH_3OH) and spirit of wine (ethyl alcohol-C_2H_5OH). In 1894, Reinicke first described ethanol as an antiseptic. In 1903, Harrington and Walker showed that a 60% to 70% solution was most effective. In 1939, Price advocated using 65.5% alcohol as a surgical scrub. Today 70% ethyl alcohol is widely used as a skin preparation.

R. K. Rajpal, Cornea Consultants, George Washington University Medical Center, Washington, D.C. 20007.

S. R. Glaser: Center for Sight-7PHC, Georgetown University Medical Center, Washington, D.C. 20007.

General Information

Alcohols are antiseptics applied to reduce local microbial flora before use of needles or other sharp instruments and as a preoperative wash.

Pharmacology

The bactericidal effects of ethyl alcohol result from rapid coagulation of protein. The 70% aqueous solution is more effective than absolute alcohol in reducing the surface tension of bacterial cells. Isopropyl alcohol (used as a 60% to 70% solution) has slightly greater bactericidal activity than ethyl alcohol.

Uses and Indication

Ethyl alcohol is widely used for skin antisepsis. Both ethyl and isopropyl alcohol were more effective than chlorhexidine or povidone-iodine in producing antisepsis in the presence of blood (1).

Side Effects and Toxicity

Alcohols should not be used to disinfect wounds because they irritate tissues, resulting in painful burning and stinging. They may precipitate protein to form a coagulated mass from which secondary growth of bacteria can occur.

Preparations

Ethyl alcohol is available as alcohol, U.S.P. and diluted alcohol, U.S.P. Isopropyl alcohol is available as isopropyl alcohol, N.F. (nonprescription) and rubbing alcohol, N.F.

HYDROGEN PEROXIDE

History and Source

In 1818, Thenard discovered the chemical formula of hydrogen peroxide: H_2O_2. In 1858, B. W. Richardson first described hydrogen peroxide use as an antiseptic. The 3% solution first became popular in the 1920s.

General Information

Hydrogen peroxide is a weak antiseptic; however, it loosens masses of infected debris in wounds.

Pharmacology

Hydrogen peroxide in the presence of catalase (found in blood and most tissues) rapidly decomposes into oxygen and water. Its use is directed against anaerobes.

Uses/Indication

Hydrogen peroxide is used for antisepsis of minor wounds and mucous membranes (it is not for ophthalmic use). It is also a common disinfecting agent for use with contact lenses.

Side Effects and Toxicity

Hydrogen peroxide should never be instilled in closed body cavities or abscesses. Only preparations labeled for use with contact lens should be so instilled. Hydrogen peroxide should never be used directly in the eyes. Painful keratitis has been reported from failure of neutralizing contact lens disinfectant.

Preparations

Hydrogen peroxide is available in a 3% solution (nonprescription). Various brand names are labeled as "contact lens disinfectant."

CHLORHEXIDINE GLUCONATE

History and Source

Chlorhexidine was first synthesized in 1950 in England in the search for a proguanil antimalarial agent. It has gained usage in ophthalmic solutions.

General Information

Chlorhexidine is a chlorophenyl biguanide antiseptic with broad antimicrobial coverage, including that many gram positive and negative organisms such as *Pseudomonas aeruginosa* (2). Chlorhexidine has low potential for producing contact sensitivity and photosensitivity in long-term clinical use, and is not absorbed through intact skin.

Pharmacology

Chlorhexidine gluconate prevents bacterial spores from germinating. However, heat is required to kill the spores. Its antimicrobial efficacy is reduced by blood and other organic matter (3). Chlorhexidine has a slower onset of action than the alcohols, but has residual adherence.

Uses/Indication

Low concentrations of chlorhexidine are used as a preservative in ophthalmic formulations and contact lens solutions. Chlorhexidine gluconate 4% solutions are used as antiseptics for preoperative skin preparation and for handwashing.

Side Effects and Toxicity

Because chlorhexidine is cationic, formulations that contain anionic-based chemicals may neutralize its effect. *Serratia* organisms were detected in contact lens disinfectants with chlorhexidine (4). Corneal exposure to high concentrations of chlorhexidine for more than 5 minutes (as with preoperative skin preparations with 4% chlorhexidine) has resulted in serious keratopathy (5,6). Cases of anaphylaxis caused by the scrub have been reported. It is not recommended for periorbital and eyelid preoperative preparation; corneal neovascularization has been reported after accidental exposure.

Preparations

Chlorhexidine gluconate (Stuart, nonprescription) is available under the trade names of Hibiclens Skin Cleanser (4% with 4% isopropyl alcohol) and Hibistat Hand Rinse (0.5% chlorhexidine gluconate with 70% isopropyl alcohol).

CATIONIC SURFACTANTS (BENZALKONIUM CHLORIDE, BAC)

History and Source

Bipolar detergents have been used to sterilize opthalmic instruments, as preoperative scrubs, and as preservatives in ophthalmic solutions since the 1930s. BAC is a cationic hydrophilic detergent. Lauryl sulfate is an anionic hydrophilic detergent commonly used today as a hair shampoo.

General Information

Organic quaternary ammonium compounds are cationic surface-active agents. They have limited action against gram-positive and gram-negative organisms. BAC is the prototype of the organic quaternary ammonium compounds. It is a mixture of alkyldimethylbenzylammonium chlorides in which the alkyls range from C8H17 to C18H37.

Pharmacology

The method of action of the compounds is due to alteration of microbial membrane permeability. Any anionic agents including soap will inactivate these cationic surfactants.

Uses/Indications

Most artificial tear preparations, ocular decongestants, and ophthalmic irrigation solutions contain BAC as a preservative agent. BAC is a cationic wetting agent possessing detergent, kerolytic, and emulsifying action. It has a rapid onset and a relative long duration of action. It has limited coverage against gram-positive and gram-negative organisms and against some fungi and protozoa. BAC is ineffective against *Mycobacterium tuberculosis, Clostridium,* and other spore-forming bacteria and viruses.

BAC is used on minor wounds in a 1 : 750 dilution. Mucous membrane and diseased skin require at least a 1 : 5,000 dilution. In ophthalmic use (as an irrigant) the dilution should be 1 : 5,000 to 1 : 20,000. BAC is used in rigid gas permeable (RGP) and polymethylmethacrolate (PMMA) contact lens solutions, but should not be used with soft contact lenses (especially hydrophilic lenses).

Side Effects and Toxicity

Repeated topical application, in a dose-dependent fashion, may produce corneal cytotoxic effects (7) and punctate epithelial opacities and may retard corneal epithelial healing. Corneal edema and vascularization have been reported after application of 10% solution. Concentrated solutions may produce severe irritation, necrosis, and scarring. Muscle weakness has been reported after irrigating body cavities. Because solutions are prone to contamination by resistant bacteria and spores, they should be checked regularly.

Preparations

BAC is available in generic form (solution 1 : 750 or 17% concentrate) and under the trade names Benza (Century) 1 : 750 solution; Zephiran (Sanofi Winthrop) 1 : 750 solution, 17% concentrate, tincture, and tincture spray; and Ionax (Owen) foam aerosol and scrub paste.

IODINE COMPOUNDS

History and Source

During the Napoleonic wars, the French chemist Bernard Courtois isolated iodine from ashes of seaweed when he was trying to obtain nitrate for gunpowder (the British navy had blockaded nitrate shipments). The English chemists Davy and Faraday were consulted for identification of this new element and named the compound "iodine," from the Greek meaning "violet-colored." In the early 19th century, goiter was successfully treated with this new element. In 1821, Magendie popularized the use of iodine to treat almost any type of ailment. In 1839, John Davies, in his *Textbook of Surgery* first specifically advocated its use in the treatment of wounds. It was used to treat soldiers' wounds in the Civil War.

In 1863, Fano introduced iodine into the ophthalmic literature for irrigation of the lacrimal sac in dacryocystitis. Iodine gained popularity in ophthalmology for treatment of both infectious and noninfectious entities in the 1930s, including use for prophylaxis against cataracts.

General Information

Iodine is a nonmetallic element that forms salts with most other elements. Elemental iodine (I_2) is an omnipotent antimicrobial, effective against most bacteria, fungi, viruses, protozoa, and yeasts. Iodine tincture is a hydroalcoholic solution containing 2 g iodine and 2.4 g sodium iodide per 100 ml. Iodine solution contains approximately 2% iodine and 2.4% sodium iodide in water (2% available iodine and 0.03% free iodine).

Pharmacology

In aqueous solutions, iodine is present as seven different species, with elemental iodine, hypoiodic acid (HOI), and iodine cation ($H2OI^+$) showing the strongest antimicrobial activity. Soluble iodine is termed free iodine. Additional iodine can be made soluble only by conversion to triiodide ion with an iodide salt, such as sodium iodide and iodine tincture. This reaction is reversible when the concentration of elemental iodine falls below the saturation level.

Free and complexed elemental iodine (I_2) is organic idophors (i.e., povidone-iodine) together are termed "available iodine." However, only free iodine appears to have significant antimicrobial activity.

Free iodine is an avid collector of electrons to form iodide ion. Once iodine is converted to iodide ion, antimicrobial activity is lost. Iodine cannot penetrate tissue without undergoing rapid conversion to inactivate iodine ion.

Uses/Indications

Iodine solution is used to treat superficial lacerations. It is preferable to irrigate the wound with saline and apply iodine solution around the wound rather than apply it directly to the wound, because iodine is toxic to fibroblasts and epithelial cells and may retard healing. Iodine can be used to disinfect water. Three drops of tincture of iodine added to 1 quart water kills bacteria and amoebae in 15 minutes.

Side Effects and Toxicity

Iodine should not be used in patients with known hypersensitivity to iodine. Systemic absorption can occur, causing metabolic complications. It is not for opthalmic use, but external use only. Sodium thiosulfate is the most effective chemical antidote. Iodine should not be used under occlusive dressings.

Preparations

Iodine/sodium iodide is available as iodine solution, 2% iodine and 2.4% sodium iodide in water; strong iodine (trade name: Lugol's solution) is 5% iodine and 10% potassium iodide in water; iodine tincture is 2% iodine and 2.4% sodium iodide in 47% alcohol, water (2% available iodine and 0.03% free iodine); and strong iodine tincture is 7% iodine and 5% potassium iodide in 83% alcohol.

IODOPHORS

General Information

Iodophors are complexes of iodine and organic compounds that gradually release low concentrations of free iodine from a reservoir of available iodine. Medical use is limited to the nonsurfactant aqueous and alcohol-soluble polyvinylpyrrolidine–iodine complex (povidone-iodine).

Pharmacology

Povidone-iodine has no antimicrobial activity until free iodine is released in solution. The standard preparation is 10% aqueous povidone-iodine solution.

Uses/Indications

Povidone-iodine preparations are used as handwashes and skin preparations and are widely used for conjunctival antisepsis presurgically (8). Its use in preventing donor eye contamination has been suggested (9).

Side Effects and Toxicity

Iodophors should not be used in patients with known hypersensitivity to iodine. Systemic absorption can occur causing metabolic complications, including hypothyroidism. They are not for ophthalmic use, but for external use only. Sodium thiosulfate is the most effective chemical antidote. Unlike areas treated with iodine tincture, areas treated with iodophors may be bandaged.

Preparations

Povidone-iodine is available in generic 10% solutions and under the trade name Betadine, a 10%, 7.5% surgical scrub with nonoxynol-4-sulfate, lauramide DEA (Purdue Frederick).

PHENOLIC COMPOUNDS

History and Source

Lord Joseph Lister introduced phenol as an antiseptic in 1867. Phenol (carbolic acid-C_6H_5OH) was used in a 1% solution for nonspecific coagulation. In 1949, Von Oettingen used 5% solution to kill tubercle bacilli. Addition of alkyl groups (cresol-$C_6H_4HCH_3$) increases germicidal efficacy of phenol fourfold and was combined with a soap for form the popular disinfectant Lysol. Duke-Elder described phenol "cauterization" of corneal ulcers.

General Information

Dilute phenol is bacteriostatic; more concentrated solution are bactericidal and fungicidal. Phenol possesses local anesthetic and antipruritic activity in low concentrations.

Pharmacology

Hexachlorophene is a polychlorinated biphenol compound having action against most gram-positive bacteria, including staphylococci. It has little activity against most gram-negative bacteria or spores.

Uses/Indications

Hexachlorophene is used for handwashing and as a skin preparation. It may be used in combination with other soaps. Triclosan is a *bis*-phenol used as a skin cleanser. It is bacteriostatic and should not be used as a surgical scrub.

Side Effects and Toxicity

Hexachlorophene is not for opthalmic use and may cause extreme eye irritation. It also may have systemic side effects since it is absorbed through intact skin. Neurotoxicity and death have been reported with the use of hexachlorophene. Early treatment for hexachlorophene toxicity include gastrointestinal evacuation/emesis. Vegetable oil taken orally will delay absorption and this should be followed by a saline cathartic. Electrolyte balance must be maintained. Care should be taken to avoid prolonged contact time. Hexachlorophene should not be used in open wounds or on mucous membranes. Hexachlorophene should be stored in tight, light-resistant containers. The Food and Drug Administration (FDA) Category for pregnancy is C.

Preparations

Hexachlorophene is available under the trade name pHisoHex (Sanofi Winthrop), emulsion 3%; and Septisol (Calgon Vestal), foam 0.23% with alcohol 56%.

REFERENCES

1. Larson E. Effective hand degermination in the presence of blood. *J Emerg Med* 1992;10:7–11.
2. Sebben JE. Surgical antiseptics. *J Am Acad Dermatol* 1983;9:759–765.
3. Sheikh W. Comparative antimicrobial efficacy of Hibiclens and Betadine. *Curr Ther Res* 1986;40:1096–1102.
4. Gandhi PA. *Appl Environ Microbiol* 1993;59:183–188.
5. Phinney RB. Corneal edema related to accidental Hibiclens exposure. *Am J Ophthalmol* 106:210–215.
6. Hamed LM. Hibiclens keratitis. *Am J Ophthalmol* 1987;104:50–56.
7. Lemp MA, Zimmerman LE. Toxic endothelial degeneration in ocular surface disease treated with topical medications containing benzalkonium chloride. *Am J Ophthalmol* 1988;105:670.
8. Boes DA. *Ophthalmology* 1992;99:1569–1574.
9. Nash RW. *Arch Ophthalmol* 1991;109:869–873.
10. Zanoni D. *Clin Pediatr* 1992;295–298.
11. Mathys B. *Bull Soc Belg Ophthalmol* 1988;229:49–60.
12. Grass GM. *Invest Ophthalmol Vis Sci* 1985;26:110–113.
13. Leahey AB. *Ophthamology* 1993;100:173–180.

GENERAL TEXT REFERENCES

1. *AHFS drug information 1994,* Bethesda: American Society of Hospital Pharmacists, 1994.
2. *AMA drug evaluations,* American Medical Association, 1994.
3. Block S. *Disinfection, sterilization, and preservation,* 4th ed. Malvern, PA: Lea & Febiger, 1991.
4. *Drug facts and comparisons,* St Louis: Facts and Comparisons, 1994.
5. *Physicians' desk reference,* 48th ed. Montvale, NJ: Medical Economics Company, 1994.
6. Duke-Elder S. *System of ophthalmology,* St Louis: CV Mosby, 1962.

Textbook of Ocular Pharmacology,
edited by T.J. Zimmerman, et al.
Lippincott–Raven Publishers, Philadelphia © 1997.

CHAPTER 56

Mitomycin Treatment of Corneal Disease

Roswell R. Pfister

MITOMYCIN

History and Source

Mitomycin is a member of the group of antitumor antibiotic agents produced by *Streptomyces caespitasus.* Used extensively in chemotherapy for liver, gastrointestinal (GI) tract and bladder tumors, it found its way into ophthalmic use in 1969 when Kunitomo and Mori reported its efficiency in preventing the recurrence of pterygia after excision (1).

Official Drug Name and Chemistry

The chemical formula of mitomycin C (ametycine, MMC, Mutamycin), $C_{15}H_{18}N_4O_5$ is shown below

O
R3 CH2OCONH2
OR1
H3C N
N—R2
O

Pharmacology

Mitomycin C, like the other aziridine alkylating agents thiotepa and AZQ (diazoquone), are closely related to the nitrogen mustards. Alkalating agents exert their cytotoxic effects by cross-linking of DNA. At higher concentrations, RNA and protein synthesis is also suppressed.

Clinical Pharmacology

Reduction of the quinone and loss of the methoxy group within the cell converts mitomycin into a bifunctional or trifunctional alkylating agent (2). DNA is inhibited by cross-linking at the N_6 position of adenine and at the O_6 and N_2 positions of guanine (3). The cell cycle is most affected during the late G–1 and early S phases. A dose-response has not been determined for the use of mitomycin in external eye conditions.

R. R. Pfister: The Eye Research Laboratories, Brookwood Medical Center, Birmingham, Alabama 35209.

Pharmaceutics

There is considerable variation in and controversy over the selection of concentrations of mitomycin C and the duration of use. Because the solutions are not commercially available, the diluent and the presence or absence of preservatives varies depending on the pharmaceutical firm that formulates the drops. Mitomycin should be reconstituted in sterile water at neutral pH; the drug is inactivated in acidic solution (4). The drug should be stored under refrigeration to preserve its potency and, if it is mixed without a preservative, to maintain its sterility. Under these conditions, mitomycin is potent for a period of 2 weeks. The powder and solution are light-sensitive, requiring an amber container.

Singh et al. reported the 0.1% concentration to be more irritating than the 0.04% concentration, but the latter to be just as effective (5). Because of concerns about local mitomycin toxicity, Hayasaka et al. suggest decreasing the postoperative dose from 0.04% four times daily for 10 days to 0.02% twice daily for 5 days (6,7).

Pharmacokinetics, Concentration–Effect Relationship, and Metabolism

Because mitomycin is delivered to the eye in a completely solubalized form, often in the presence of a conjunctival and corneal epithelial defect, the drug is highly bioavailable to the target tissues. Little is known of its distribution in the tissues; however, its hydrophobic character favors its penetration into epithelially denuded cornea and conjunctiva while deterring its movement into or through intact epithelium. Most of the contents of any drop placed in the eye is lost by excretion through the drainage system.

Systemic administration results in rapid detoxification by the liver, but local metabolism is not known to make any contribution to drug elimination. The use of mitomycin eye drops, even at the highest dose used, does not result in any detectable levels of mitomycin in blood.

Therapeutic Use

Mitomycin has been shown to be a useful adjunct in ophthalmology in two distinct areas: glaucoma and corneal surgery. The section on glaucoma describes specifics of treatment in that condition.

In corneal disease mitomycin is used mainly in treatment of pterygium. Although a concentration of 0.04% and a 10- to 14-day duration of treatment were initially popular, lower concentrations are now preferred (i.e., 0.02% or even 0.005%) for shorter periods (i.e., 5 days). Although some reported series indicate no complications from higher dose therapy, clinicians in referral practices specializing in corneal diseases have noted serious complications (8).

Excision of the pannus associated with atopic keratoconjunctivitis was successful in two patients when the surgery was followed by mitomycin drops 0.4% four times daily for 10 days (9). Mitomycin was used as adjunctive therapy in correcting iatrogenic punctal stenosis in one patient (10). Combining mitomycin 0.04% in a pledget applied to the punctum for 5 minutes after opening by a one-snip procedure and followed by 1 week of mitomycin drops applied four times daily permanently reopened the punctum when surgery alone failed.

Topical treatment of conjunctival melanoma with mitomycin should be regarded as investigational (11). In the one case thus treated, 0.04% mitomycin drops and soaked sponges were used four times daily to debulk the majority of a lesion that had received laser treatments three times for recurrences in 5 years. Subsequent excision showed residual tumor only deep within a tarsal lesion hitherto not treated with anything other than mitomycin (11).

Another investigational use of mitomycin was reported in the treatment of corneal intraepithelial neoplasia (12). Treatment of three patients (two confirmed by biopsy) with 0.02% mitomycin four times daily for 2 weeks yielded biomicroscopically normal epithelium within 9 weeks. No recurrence was noted in the subsequent 4 to 12 months of follow-up. Surgical excision is the current standard of therapy.

Side Effects and Toxicity

The most serious side effect of mitomycin topical therapy after pterygium excision is the development of a persistent epithelial defect which progresses to scleral ulceration and potential loss of the eye (8). This finding is consistent with animal studies showing that mitomycin C was 125 times as potent as 5-fluorouracil (5-FU) in inhibiting corneal epithelial healing (13). Very serious complications were first reported in Japan years earlier, since mitomycin was first introduced there. The reports describe scleral ulceration (14–16), necrotizing scleritis (14,16,17), perforation (14,19,20), iridocyclitis (14,16,17), cataract (17), infection (14,16), glaucoma (16,17), scleral calcification (15,16), and loss of the eye (16). In the Western literature, less serious cases of symblephara (7) and calcification (21) have been reported.

Patients commonly report ocular pain and photophobia out of proportion to that produced by the operative procedure. This correlates to the higher concentrations of mitomycin used and endures not only for the period of treatment but for as long as 3 months. The strongest concentrations of mitomycin can result in conjunctival injection, delayed healing (3 to 4 weeks longer than that in controls), a moderate superficial keratitis, and anterior chamber reaction. When the bare sclera technique is used, the exposed sclera can develop a porcelin white appearance due to the absence of blood vessels.

Overdose

If topical ocular mitomycin is inadvertently used for a prolonged postoperative period, the opportunity for occurrence of any of the ocular complications previously mentioned is enhanced. Systemic levels of mitomycin have not been measured, and no untoward effects have been reported. Systemic administration is associated with the potential for bone marrow suppression, renal toxicity, and blurred vision (22). Instillation of 0.02% mitomycin every 8 hours for 3 weeks resulted in significant intraocular penetration, causing toxicity of the ciliary body, vitreous, and retina sufficient to produce hypotony, vitreitis, macular edema, and disk changes (23). Idiosyncratic reactions and hypersensitivity have also been reported.

High-risk Groups

Mitomycin therapy should be avoided in patients with conditions predisposing to ulceration or poor wound healing such as Sjogren syndrome, severe keratoconjunctivitis sicca, acne rosacea, atopic keratoconjunctivitis, or herpes keratitis (8). Although systemic absorption of mitomycin is miniscule, use of the drug in pregnant or nursing women is inadvisable.

Drug Interactions

When used in the topical form, mitomycin is not known to interact with any drug.

Major Clinical Trials

Singh et al. (5) reported a randomized clinical trial using 1.0 or 0.4 mg/ml mitomycin treatment or a control in primary or recurrent pterygia; 62 pterygia in 45 eyes of 38 patients were treated. Pterygia recurred in 88.9% of eyes in the control group (mean follow-up 6 weeks). A single pterygiun developed in one eye (5%) in the 1.0-mg/ml group (mean follow-up 23 weeks). There were no recurrences in the 0.04-mg/ml group.

In a follow-up study (23), Singh et al. (5) observed 48 patients for 7 to 21 months (mean 18 months) (24). Placebo-treated pterygia showed a 73% recurrence rate. One of 58 (1.7%) mitomycin-treated pterygia recurred.

Chayakul (24) detailed the outcome of primary pterygium excision in 72 eyes treated with two drops of 0.02% mitomycin three times daily for 2 weeks (25). The corneal recurrence rate was 1.4% in 6 months, and the conjunctival recurrence rate was 5.6% in 1 year. There were no serious complications.

Sixty-one patients with recurrent pterygia underwent operative excision and were subsequently divided into four treatment groups. The incidence of recurrence, with a follow-up of 4.1 to 5.7 years, was as follows: (a) excision alone in 11 patients, with recurrence in 5 eyes (45%); (b) excision and radiation in 9 patients, with recurrence in 3 eyes (33%); (c) excision and 0.02% mitomycin for 5 days in 22 patients, with recurrence in 2 eyes (9%); and (d) excision and 0.02% mitomycin in 19 patients, with recurrence in 1 eye (5%). Hayasaka et al. (7) concluded that topical 0.02% mitomycin used twice daily for 5 days was safe and effective in the treatment of recurrent pterygium.

In a series of 250 pterygia patients, 45 of whom had recurrent ptergia, Dash et al. (26) found that after excision recurrence rate was nil with 0.04% mitomycin treatment daily for 2 weeks, 2,000 rad beta rays, or buccal mucosal transplantation. The mitomycin-treated group also obtained the best cosmetic result. Simple excision or excision with carbolization yielded recurrence rates of 25% and 30.6%, respectively.

ACKNOWLEDGMENT

This work was supported by NEI Grant No. EY04716.

REFERENCES

1. Kunitomo N, Mori S. Studies on the pterygium: part 4, a treatment of the pterygium by mitomycin C installation. *Acta Soc Ophthalmol Jpn* 1969;67:601–607.
2. Goodman LS, Gilman AG, eds. *The pharmacological basis of therapeutics,* 8th ed. Elmsford, NY: Pergamon Press, 1990;1247–1248.
3. Dorr RT. New findings in the pharmacokinetic, metabolic, and drug-resistance aspects of mitomycin C. *Semin Oncol* 1988;15:32–41.
4. Fiscella RG, Proffitt DA, Weisbecker CA. Stability of mitomycin for ophthalmic use. *Am J Hosp Pharm* 1992;49:2440.
5. Singh G, Wilson MR, Foster CS. Mitomycin eye drops as treatment for pterygium. *Ophthalmology* 1988;95:813–821.
6. Hayasaka S, et al. Postoperative instillation of low-dose mitomycin C in the treatment of primary pterygium. *Am J Ophthalmol* 1988;106: 715–718.
7. Hayasaka S, et al. Postoperative instillation of mitomycin C in the treatment of recurrent pterygium. *Ophthalmic Surg* 1989;20:580–583.
8. Rubinfeld RS, et al. Serious complications of topical mitomycin-C after pterygium surgery. *Ophthalmology* 1992;99:1647–1654.
9. Akova YA, et al. Atypical ocular atopy. *Ophthalmology* 1993;100: 1367–1371.
10. Lam S, Tessler HH. Mitomycin as adjunct therapy in correcting iatrogenic punctal stenosis. *Ophthalmol Surg* 1993;24:123–124.
11. Finger PT, Milner MS, McCormick SA. Topical chemotherapy for conjunctival melanoma. *Br J Ophthalmol* 1993;77:751–753.
12. Frucht-Pery J, Rozenman Y. Mitomycin C therapy for corneal intraepithelial neoplasia. *Am J Ophthalmol* 1994;117:164–168.
13. Ando H, et al. Inhibition of corneal epithelial wound healing. *Ophthalmology* 1992;99:1809–1814.
14. Fukamachi LY, Hikita N. Ocular complications following pterygium operation and instillation of mitomycin C. *Folia Ophthalmol Jpn* 1981;32:197–201.
15. Yamanouchi U, et al. Scleromalacia presumably due to mitomycin C instillation after pterygium excision. *Jpn J Clin Ophthalmol* 1979;33: 139–144.
16. Yamanouchi U. A case of scleral calcification due to mitomycin C instillation after pterygium operation. *Folia Ophthalmol Jpn* 1978;29: 1221–1225.
17. Yamanouchi U, Mishima K. Eye lesions due to mitomycin C instillation after pterygium operation. *Folia Ophthalmol Jpn* 1967;18:854–861.
18. Fujitani A, et al. Corneoscleral ulceration and corneal perforation after pterygium excision and topical mitomycin therapy. *Ophthalmologica* 1993;207:162–164.
19. Dunn JP, et al. Development of scleral ulceration and calcification after pterygium excision and mitomycin therapy [Letter]. *Am J Ophthalmol* 1991;112:343–344.
20. Berkow R, ed. *Merck manual,* Merck, Sharp and Dohme Research Laboratories, 1987;1224.
21. Gupta S, Basti S. Corneoscleral, ciliary body and vitreoretinal toxicity after excessive instillation of mitomycin C. *Am J Ophthalmol* 1992;114:503–504.
22. Singh G, Wilson MR, Foster CS. Long-term follow-up study of mitomycin eye drops as adjunctive treatment of pterygia and its comparison with conjunctival autograft transplantation. *Cornea* 1990;9:331–334.
23. Chayakul V. Prevention of recurrent pterygium by mitomycin-C. *Fortschr Ophthalmol* 1987;84:422–424.
24. Dash R, Boparai S. Pterygium—evaluation of management. *Ind J Ophthalmol* 1986;34:7–10

Textbook of Ocular Pharmacology,
edited by T.J. Zimmerman, et al.
Lippincott–Raven Publishers, Philadelphia © 1997.

CHAPTER 57

Cyanoacrylate Tissue Adhesives

George R. John

History and Source

Cyanoacrylates were introduced as commercial plastic adhesives in the late 1950s (1) and were first used clinically in the 1960s (2,3). Various industrial polymers were used in early research involving tissue adhesives, but the Eastman 910 monomer (methyl 2-cyanoacrylate) is the most notable in the early literature (4). The growing interest in nonsuture repair of wounds spilled over from general and vascular surgery to ophthalmic surgery. Some of the earliest ocular uses involving this material were reported by Ellis and Levine in 1962 and included sutureless tarsorrhaphy, muscle surgery, and repair of corneal/scleral incisions (5).

The adhesive was composed of repeating monomers consisting of cyanoacetate and a hydrocarbon side chain. Through alteration of the hydrocarbon side chain, other synthetic monomers have been developed, and the higher alkyl chains have been shown to be less toxic to surrounding tissues. The most recent studies using cyanoacrylates have examined *n*-butyl 2-cyanoacrylate (Histacryl, Germany) and *N*-butyl cyanoacrylate (Nexacryl, TriPoint, Raleigh, NC) (6,7).

Official Drug Name and Chemistry

At present, the only cyanoacrylate agent under Food and Drug Administration (FDA) consideration is *N*-butyl cyanoacrylate (Nexacryl). Cyanoacrylates vary in the hydrocarbon side chain.

$$\begin{array}{c} \quad\quad CN \\ \quad\quad | \\ nCH_2 = C\text{-}COOR \end{array}$$

G. R. John: Department of Ophthalmology, University of Louisville, Louisville, Kentucky 40292.

Pharmacology

The cyanoacrylate monomer polymerizes anionically when combined with fluids containing water or weak bases, transforming from a clear liquid to a solid. In the process of polymerization, a bond is created with surrounding tissues (8). The cyanoacrylate polymer (in particular the higher alkyl side chain cyanoacrylates) is considered nonbiodegradablebecause it dissolves very slowly in water and tissue fluids. It has been shown to dissolve in acetone (9).

Cyanoacrylates are broken down into formaldehyde and alkyl cyanoacetate. The toxicity may be due to the monomer, breakdown products, or impurities or to the generation of free radicals. Most studies fail to show significant tissue penetration of the monomer, the polymer, or its products. Therefore, the toxicity is limited to surrounding tissues and effects are dose dependent (10).

Clinical Pharmacology/Therapeutic Uses

Cyanoacrylates are used to glue nonadherent surfaces or to provide a temporary protective surface. They are applied to a variety of corneal perforating and ulcerating disorders, either allowing healing to occur or allowing a more definitive procedure to be performed. Cyanoacrylates may be applied directly to the site; for larger defects, they may be applied with the use of a plastic drape (11). The polymer acts as a temporizing measure, stabilizing and supporting the tissue, allowing time for the normal wound-healing processes to repair a defect or for other definitive management. The adhesive then either falls off or is mechanically removed. Reported indications for cyanoacrylate adhesive use include immune corneal/scleral melts and corneal ulcerations, including infectious keratitis, herpetic stromal keratitis, neurotrophic ulcers, traumatic corneal/scleral perforations, and small lacerations (11). Treatment of scleral ulcers (12) and conjunctival buttonholes (13) has been successful in some cases. Other reported uses which are not prevalent include punctal occlusion (14), epikeratophakia (15), keratoplasty (16), strabismus surgery (4), choroidal perforations (17), retinal detachment repair (18,19), and treatment of alkali burns (20).

Pharmaceutics

The only experimental form of cyanoacrylates available in the United States is Nexacryl. It is shipped as a clear liquid in 0.4-cc sterile vials and will polymerize on contact with water or weak bases in less than 5 to 10 seconds. The rate of polymerization is dependent on the surface area exposed and the pH.

There is no evidence that cyanoacrylates are metabolized by the body. They may remain indefinitely (1 to 660 days) on the ocular surface (21) and can be removed mechanically or with acetone (9).

Side Effects

The polymerization of cyanoacrylates incorporates surrounding tissues and, in the process, causes localized tissue damage. There are several theories regarding mechanism of tissue injury, but one considered the most likely is the release of toxins such as formaldehyde, free radicals, impurities, and unreacted monomer. Minimal heat is released, particularly by the higher alkyl chain compounds (22,23). Inflammatory mediators are responsible for the resultant typical polymorphonuclear leukocyte infiltration and neovascularization. The inflammation subsides after the cyanoacrylate is removed, but a scar may result (11). Histopathologically, polymorphonuclear leukocyte infiltration and foreign body giant cell reaction have been observed (24).

The cyanoacrylate may not always be deposited at the intended site, and contact with conjunctiva may result in symblepharon (21). Either an irregular surface or the polymerized adhesive or the edges of the drape may cause mechanical irritation and even giant papillary conjunctivitis (25). This irritation often necessitates a bandage contact lens. Patients may also report burning, dryness, redness, or discharge.

Because the cyanoacrylate is nonbiodegradable, application to tissues other than the ocular surface causes the adhesive to remain indefinitely at its application site. In perforating injuries, iris incarceration and lens contact may cause damage to the tissues. Cataractogenesis is not common unless a larger dose of adhesive is used (8).

Application of the adhesive to an ocular surface defect, whether corneal or conjunctival, may result in the extension of the defect as the glue comes off (26). Anterior chamber reaction and cataractogenesis have been suggested to result from cyanoacrylate injection in the anterior chamber. Subconjunctival injection results in an inflammatory reaction (23). Cyanoacrylates on the ocular surface increase the risk of bacterial adhesion and secondary infection.

The cyanoacrylate monomer is considered sterile and does not support bacterial growth (7). Despite reports of the antibacterial effects of the adhesive, the irregularity of the polymer surface encourages bacterial colonization. Infectious keratitis has been reported to occur after glue application (6). The requirement of contact lenses is certainly a risk factor.

Other Tissue Adhesives

The study of alternative tissue adhesives has centered on human fibrinogen, often in combination with thrombin (27–31). Commercial preparations such as Tisseel and Beriplast-P have been described in the literature (32,33). Although the rapidity of adhesion and bond strength may be adequate, degradation of the bond and long-term stability have not been documented. In addition, the risk of transmitting infectious agents such as human immunodeficiency virus is significant with these pooled blood products (34). Neither has success been achieved in clinical trials with mussel adhesive protein (polypheolic protein combined with enzyme polymerizer), one of the few non-human biologically derived agents (35,36). Most studies of alternate forms of tissue adhesives have been performed in Europe and Japan.

REFERENCES

1. Coover HW Jr, Joyce FB, Shearer NH Jr, Wicker TH Jr. Chemistry and performance of cyanoacrylate adhesives. *SPE Tech Papers* 1959; 92.
2. Carton CA, Kessler LA, Seidenberg B, Hurwitt ES. A plastic adhesive method of small blood vessel surgery. *World Neurol* 1960;1:356.
3. Healy JE Jr, Brooks BJ, Gallager HS, et al. A technique for nonsuture repair of veins. *J Surg* 1961;1:267.
4. Bloomfield S, Barnert AH, Kanter PD. The use of Eastman 910 monomer as an adhesive in ocular surgery. I. Biologic effects on ocular tissue. *Am J Ophthalmol* 1963;55:742–748.
5. Ellis RA, Levine A. Experimental sutureless ocular surgery. *Am J Ophthalmol* 1963;55:733–741
6. Weiss JL, Williams JP, Lindstrom RL, et al. The use of tissue adhesives in corneal perforations. *Ophthalmology* 1983;90:610–615.
7. Eiferman RA, Snyder JW. Antibacterial effects of cyanoacrylate glue. *Arch Ophthalmol* 1983;101:958–960.
8. Refojo MF, Dohlman CH, Koliopoulos J. Adhesives in ophthalmology: a review. *Surv Ophthalmol* 1971;15:217–236.
9. Turss U, Turss R, Refojo MF. Removal of isobutyl cyanoacrylate adhesive from the cornea with acetone. *Am J Ophthalmol* 1970;70: 725–728.
10. Aronson SB, McMaster PRB, Moore TE Jr, Coon MA. Toxicity of cyanoacrylates. *Arch Ophthalmol* 1970;84:342–349.
11. Refojo MF, Dohlman CH, Ahmad B, et al. Evaluation of adhesives for corneal surgery. *Arch Ophthalmol* 1968;80:645–656.
12. Lin CP, Wu YH, Chen MT, Huang WL. Repair of a giant scleral ulcer with a scleral graft and a tissue glue [Letter]. *Am J Ophthalmol* 1991; 111:251.
13. Grady FJ, Forbes M. Tissue adhesive for repair of conjunctival buttonhole in glaucoma surgery. *Am J Ophthalmol* 1969;68:656–658.

14. Patten JT. Punctual occlusion with *N*-butyl cyanoacrylate tissue adhesive. *Ophthalmic Surg* 1976;7:24–26.
15. Rostron CK, Brittain GPH, Morton DB, Rees JE. Experimental epikeratophakia with biological adhesive. *Arch Ophthalmol* 1988;106: 1103–1106.
16. Cardarelli J, Basu PK. Lamellar corneal transplantation in rabbits using isobutyl cyanoacrylate. *Can J Ophthalmol* 1969;4:179–182.
17. Seelenfreund MH, Refojo MF, Schepus CL. Sealing choroidal perforations with cyanoacrylate adhesives. *Arch Ophthalmol* 1970;83:619–625.
18. Calabria GA, Pruett RC, Refojo MF, Stephens CL. Sutureless scleral buckling. An experimental technique. *Arch Ophthalmol* 1970;83: 613–618.
19. Sheta SM, Hida T, McCuen BW. Cyanoacrylate tissue adhesive in the management of recurrent retinal detachment caused by macular hole. *Am J Ophthalmol* 1990;109:28–32.
20. Kenyon KR, Berman M, Rose J, Gage J. Prevention of stromal ulceration in the alkali-burned rabbit cornea by glued-on contact lens. Evidence for the role of polymorphonuclear leukocytes in collagen degradation. *Invest Ophthalmol Vis Sci* 1979;18:570–587.
21. Leahey AB, Gottsch JD, Stark WJ. Clinical experience with *N*-butyl cyanoacrylate (Nexacryl) tissue adhesive. *Ophthalmology* 1993;100: 173.
22. Lehman RA, Hayes GJ, Leonard F. Toxicity of allyl 2-cyanoacrylates. *Arch Surg* 1966;93:441.
23. Gasset AR, Hood CT, Ellison ED, Kaufman HE. Ocular tolerance to cyanoacrylate monomers tissue adhesive analysis. *Invest Ophthalmol* 1970;9:3.
24. Ferry AP, Barnert AH. Granulomatous keratitis resulting from use of cyanoacrylate adhesive for closure of perforated corneal ulcer. *Am J Ophthalmol* 1971;72:538–541.
25. Carlson AN, Wilhelmus KR. Giant papillary conjunctivitis associated with cyanoacrylate glue. *Am J Ophthalmol* 1987;104:437–438.
26. Kajiwara K. Repair of a leaking bleb with fibrin glue. *Am J Ophthalmol* 1990;109:599–601.
27. Brown A, Nantz F. Corneal wound healing. II: variations in adhesive power of fibrin in vitro studies. *Tr Am Ophthalmol Soc* 1946; 44:85.
28. Town A, Naidoff D. Fibrin closure in eye surgery. *Am J Ophthalmol* 1950;33:879–882.
29. Katzin HM. Aqueous fibron fixation of corneal transplants in the rabbit. *Arch Ophthalmol* 1946;35:415–420.
30. Parry T, Lazzlo G. Thrombin technique in ophthalmologic surgery. *Br J Ophthalmol* 1946;30:176–178.
31. Tassman I. Experimental studies with physiological (autogenous plasma plus thrombin) for use in the eyes. *Am J Ophthalmol* 1950;33: 870–878.
32. Robin J, Picciano P, Salazar J, Benedict C. A preliminary evaluation of the use of mussel adhesive protein in epikeraplasty. *Arch Ophthalmol* 1988;106:973–977.
33. Robin JB, Lee CF, Riley JM. Preliminary evaluation of two experimental surgical adhesives in the rabbit cornea. *Refract Corneal Surg* 1989;5:302–306.
34. Hennis HL, Stewart WC, Jeter EK. Infectious disease risks of fibrin glue. 1992;23:640–00.
35. Henrick A, Gaster RN, Silverstone PJ. Organic tissue glue closure of cataract incisions. *J Cataract Refract Surg* 1991;13:551–553.
36. Henrick A, Kalpakian B, Gaster RN, Vanley C. Organic tissue glue closure of cataract incision in rabbit eyes. *J Cataract Refract Surg* 1991;17:551–555.

Textbook of Ocular Pharmacology,
edited by T.J. Zimmerman, et al.
Lippincott–Raven Publishers, Philadelphia © 1997.

CHAPTER 58

Future Developments in Corneal Therapy: Growth Factors

Gregory Schultz

OVERVIEW AND HISTORY OF GROWTH FACTORS

Growth factors (GF) are proteins that stimulate repeated cycles of mitosis by quiescent cells under conditions of complete nutritional support (1,2). This property distinguishes protein GF from essential nutritional factors such as vitamins, essential amino acids, and trace elements, which are required to support mitosis but are not capable of initiating mitosis in the absence of GF. Although protein GF were originally identified due to their ability to stimulate mitosis of cells, GF also can directly regulate many other physiologic functions of ocular cells, including migration and gene expression. Thus, GF have multiple effects on ocular cells.

There are five major families of protein GF that affect corneal cells (1,2). These are the epidermal GF (EGF) family, the fibroblast GF (FGF) family, the insulin-like GF (IGF) family, the platelet-derived GF (PDGF) family, and the transforming GF-β (TGF-β) family. Each family consists of several distinct proteins that are structurally related. Frequently the GF constituting a family have similar biologic effects on ocular cells, but the relative potencies may vary. EGF is the GF that has been investigated most extensively in the cornea.

All GF share some common properties (1,2). In general, GF are initially synthesized as precursor proteins that undergo proteolytic processing to generate the biologically active, secreted factor. In addition, GF do not typically function through the classic endocrine hormone pathway in which a protein is synthesized by a specialized cell type and secreted into the blood stream and acts on a distant target cell. Instead, GF typically are synthesized by a variety of cell types and act locally on the cell that synthesized the GF or on adjacent cells by autocrine or paracrine mechanisms. Finally, all GF act on cells by binding to specific, high-affinity receptor proteins located on the plasma membrane of target cells.

Each of the five general GF families has a different receptor protein or proteins that mediate their interaction with target cells. GF receptors typically are large transmembrane glycoproteins. The extracellular portion of a receptor selectively binds a specific GF which activates the kinase domain in the cytoplasmic region of the receptor. The receptor kinase phosphorylates tyrosine or serine/threonine residues on selected cellular proteins which activates the proteins. This initiates a cascade of events that eventually alters the migration, mitosis, and gene expression of the cell. Different GF receptors selectively phosphorylate different cellular proteins which regulate different signal transduction pathways in target cells. Working to balance the activation of proteins by phosphorylation are a group of enzymes known as phosphatases which inactivate proteins by removing phosphates from proteins. Therefore, GF generally stimulate cells by stimulating receptor kinases which activate cellular proteins by adding phosphate groups while phosphatases work to suppress these intracellular signals by removing phosphate groups from the proteins.

The ability of GF to directly regulate key cellular processes such as migration, mitosis, and synthesis of extracellular matrix proteins suggests that treatment with exogenous GF might enhance healing of corneal wounds (3,4). This has led to extensive in vitro experimentation and preclinical animal studies as well as initial clinical trials evaluating topical GF treatment of corneal epithelial defects.

G. Schultz: Departments of Ophthalmology and Obstetrics and Gynecology, J. H. Miller Health Center, Box 100294, University of Florida, Gainesville, Florida 32610.

EGF

History and Source

EGF was the first GF to be biochemically characterized. It was initially purified from extracts of mouse submaxillary gland in 1962 (5). Human EGF was purified 10 years later from human urine. EGF is synthesized by several ocular cells, including lacrimal gland cells, corneal epithelial cells, and endothelial cells (3,4). EGF is a normal constituent of tears and is present at an average concentration of approximately 6 ng/ml (3,4). Ocular surface disease is associated with a decreased concentration of EGF in tears (0.9 ng/ml) (3,4). Corneal epithelial cells express a high level of EGF receptors. Corneal stromal fibroblasts and endothelial cells also express EGF receptors, but at lower levels, as well as retinal pigmented epithelial cells, retinal neuronal cells, and lens cells. Therefore, many ocular cells are potential targets for EGF action.

The concentration of EGF and other GF in natural human sources is extremely low. However, mouse submandibular glands have a high concentration of EGF, and purified mouse EGF was used in several initial clinical trials. Recombinant DNA technologies, which typically utilize bacterial or yeast expression systems, can readily produce large amounts of human sequence EGF. Recombinant EGF should rapidly replace animal-derived EGF in routine clinical use.

Official Drug Name and Chemistry

Natural EGF is synthesized as a 1,217-amino acid, transmembrane glycoprotein precursor that is proteolytically processed to release a soluble 53-amino acid fragment (6,060 daltons) that is biologically active (5). EGF is a single-chain polypeptide folded into three loops by intrachain disulfide bonds that are essential for biologic activity (Fig. 1). Mouse EGF isolated from extracts of submandibular glands is available in Europe under the trade name Gentel (Inpharzam SA, Cadempino, Switzerland). Other major biotechnology companies that produce recombinant human EGF are Chiron Vision, Amgen and Creative Biomolecules. Mouse EGF and human EGF share approximately 70% amino acid sequence homology. Mouse and human EGF bind to human EGF receptors with almost equal affinity and produce indistinguishable biologic effects.

Pharmacology

EGF has several major actions on corneal cells. It stimulates migration and mitosis of all three types of corneal cells in vitro (epithelial cells, stromal fibroblasts, and endothelial cells) (6). In addition, EGF increases synthesis of extracellular matrix proteins such as fibronectin by corneal epithelial cells. The molecular mechanism by which EGF increases migration, mitosis, and gene expression in corneal cells is partially understood (5). EGF binds to the extracellular domain of its receptor, which activates kinase activity in the cytoplasmic domain. The EGF receptor kinase then autophosphorylates itself on tyrosine residues, which generates new binding sites for cellular proteins that bind and activate other kinase proteins. These activated proteins (such as the Ras kinase) then sequentially phosphorylate other protein kinases that eventually activate transcription factors (such as AP-1) which stimulate transcription of selected genes. Thus, EGF mediates its effects on cells by selectively phosphorylating cellular proteins which act in an amplifying cascade to phosphorylate other cellular proteins, eventually resulting in activation of selected genes.

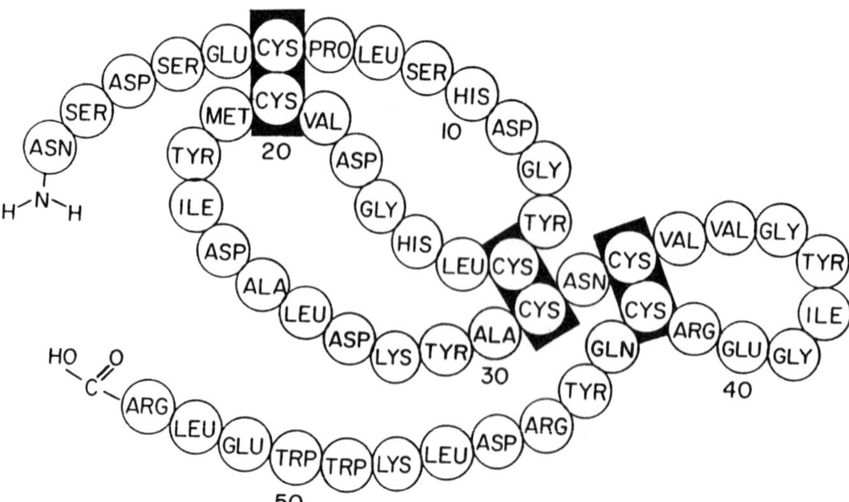

FIG. 58-1. Primary amino acid sequence of human epidermal growth factor.

Clinical Pharmacology

The ability of EGF to stimulate migration, mitosis, and synthesis of extracellular matrix proteins is the basis for its clinical use. In vitro experiments with primary cultures of human corneal epithelial cells with Boyden chambers showed that EGF stimulated a peak of migration at 20 ng/ml which decreased at higher concentrations (6). Dose-response trials of EGF in traumatic epithelial ulcers have not been performed. However, two properties of the EGF receptor system established from experiments with cells in culture and with animals indicate that the concentration and frequency of EGF dosing could have a major influence on the response of ocular cells. First, cells in culture become refractive to EGF after exposure to high concentrations of EGF due to downregulation of the EGF receptor. Second, cells must be continuously exposed to EGF for several hours to divide. Therefore, a continuous low level of EGF applied to the cornea should stimulate corneal cells better than would infrequent dosing with EGF eye drops containing high pharmacologic levels of EGF. These concepts are supported by results of preclinical studies in rabbits. A minimum of 4 hours of continuous perfusion was necessary to increase the rate of epithelial healing, and concentrations of EGF greater than 50 μg/ml reduced the rate of healing (7). Collagen shield lenses or soft contact lenses may provide a simple and inexpensive device to deliver lower levels of EGF for a more prolonged time.

Pharmaceutics

EGF typically is formulated as a solution for topical administration as an eye drop at concentrations varying between 10 μg/ml and 2 mg/ml. Gentel (mouse EGF 10 μg/ml) is formulated with 40 mg mannitol and 0.5 mg human serum albumin dissolved in 5 ml sterile 0.1 *M* phosphate-buffered saline (PBS), pH 7.2 (8). Human EGF is very stable in solution at −20°C in PBS or in 0.1 N acetic acid, with no degradation products detectable after 30 days by reverse-phase high-pressure liquid chromatography (HPLC) (9). Approximately 5% degradation was detected after 30 days of storage at 4°C in PBS. Human EGF is precipitated by several preservatives, such as benzalkonium chloride, commonly included in repetitive-dose eye drop formulations. This has led Chiron Vision to formulate EGF in unidose eye drop vials.

Pharmacokinetics, Concentration–Effect Relationship, and Metabolism

EGF is rapidly lost from the tear film of rabbits, with a half-life ($t_{\frac{1}{2}}$) of approximately 5 minutes (10). Whether physiologically significant amounts of EGF can penetrate an intact corneal epithelial layer into the cornea or anterior chamber is not known (11). The intact corneal epithelium is very resistant to penetration by hydrophilic ionized substances. Ocular pharmacokinetic studies of insulin (which is very similar in size and charge properties to EGF) instilled in rabbit eyes indicate that minuscule amounts of insulin penetrate the intact cornea (12). However, if the hydrophobic barrier of the epithelial layer were disrupted by trauma or disease, EGF would be expected to penetrate the hydrophilic environment of the stroma. The endothelium layer also would be expected to retard penetration of EGF into the anterior chamber due to similar high lipid content of the endothelial and epithelial layers (which is 100 times greater than that of the stroma).

Clearance and metabolic studies of EGF in humans have not been reported. However, studies in rats showed that EGF molecules are rapidly cleared from the systemic circulation by several tissues in a saturable process (13). The $t_{\frac{1}{2}}$ of EGF at low concentrations (0.05 nmol/kg) was 0.77 min and increased to slightly more than 2 min at high doses of EGF (20 nmol/kg). EGF is primarily cleared by the liver at both high and low doses of EGF, although other highly vascularized organs such as kidney and lung also contribute to clearance. EGF is not bound specifically by any serum protein, and the major route of metabolism of EGF appears to be destruction by intracellular proteases.

Therapeutic Use

EGF is used primarily to accelerate the rate of corneal epithelial regeneration in patients with epithelial ulcers (8,14,15). The most consistent results have been obtained in patients with traumatic epithelial ulcers and minimal stromal erosion. Treatment regimens typically consist of 2 drops EGF 10 μg/ml to be instilled into the lower conjunctival fornix four times daily (approximately every 3 hr) until healing is achieved. Treatment with topical antibiotics, either as solutions or ointment, are not contraindicated as long as dosing is staggered and preservatives that inactivate EGF are avoided. In one clinical study, researchers reported no beneficial effect of topical EGF treatment on the rate of epithelial regeneration after corneal transplantation (16).

Mouse EGF has been used to treat patients with severe corneal chemical burns (17). Results indicated that treatment with EGF 10 μg/ml five times daily in combination with conventional therapies, including corticosteroids, antibiotics, hyaluronic acid, and ascorbic acid, may enhance epithelial regeneration. Corneal ulcers resulting from thermal injuries and postherpetic infections may also respond to eye drops containing high concentrations of mouse EGF (2 mg/ml) administered every 4 hours, although the benefit of EGF treatment is reported to decrease with increased depth of stromal damage (15). At present, EGF is not approved for sale in the United States and remains an experimental drug.

Side Effects and Toxicity

No serious side effects of EGF eye drops have been reported in clinical trials. A transient burning sensation related to instillation of Gentel and lasting 1 to 2 minutes was experienced by 2% of patients in both the Gentel- and placebo-treated groups (8). Although mouse and human EGF share substantial sequence homology, rabbit antisera generated against mouse or human EGF are species specific, suggesting that mouse EGF might be antigenic in humans. However, ocular application of mouse EGF to rabbits did not produce antibody reaction or ocular inflammation (18).

High-risk Groups

No high-risk groups for EGF treatment have been identified. However, EGF effectiveness may be reduced in cases of corneal ulcers with substantial stromal involvement (15).

Drug Interactions

No potentially hazardous drug interactions have been identified for EGF treatment. However, EGF is inactivated by some preservatives present in eye drop formulations, and simultaneous dosing with solutions containing such preservatives should be avoided.

Major Clinical Trials

Two clinical trials evaluated the effect of topical EGF on the rate of epithelial regeneration of traumatic epithelial defects. In 1992, Pastor and Calonge (8) reported the results of a prospective, randomized, double-blind, placebo-controlled clinical trial conducted in five centers evaluating the safety, ocular tolerance, and efficacy of an ophthalmic solution of mouse EGF Gentel (Zambon Group, Inpharzam Laboratories, Cadempino, Switzerland) for traumatic epithelial defects. One hundred four patients completed the study: 47 received EGF eye drops 10 μg/ml in vehicle (formulated with 40 mg mannitol and 0.5 mg human serum albumin dissolved in 5 ml sterile 0.1 *M* PBS, pH 7.2), and 57 received vehicle. Patients received 1 drop five times daily. Gentamicin drops (1%, Colircust Gentamicina, Labporatoriios Cusi, Barcilona, Spain) were also prescribed five times daily, 10 min after the application of either EGF or placebo drops. Patients were examined daily by a masked observer using a slit lamp biomicroscope. Epithelial defects were detected by fluorescein staining, and the initial size was drawn on a 5 : 1 scale. Healing was considered complete when no staining was observed. At each visit, patients were evaluated for conjunctivitis, keratitis, stromal edema, corneal haze, and iritis and assigned a score of 0 to 3+ for ocular tolerance and adverse reactions.

The mean sizes of the epithelial defects at the baseline visit were 20.6 ± 11.7 mm^2 for the EGF-treated group and 20.2 ± 12.5 for the placebo-treated group ($p > 0.05$). Mean epithelial healing time was significantly decreased for the EGF-treated group (44.17 hr) as compared with the placebo-treated group (61.05 hours) ($p < 0.01$). The number of epithelial defects healed completely at 24, 48, and 72 hours after onset of treatment was significantly greater in the EGF-treated group. Local tolerance was adequate in both treatment groups.

In 1993, Scardovi et al. (14) reported the results of a prospective, randomized, double-blind, placebo-controlled clinical trial of mouse EGF treatment of traumatic corneal ulcers. Forty patients were equally assigned to two treatment arms to receive 2 drops mouse EGF at 10 μg/ml (Gentel) or vehicle four times daily at approximately every 3 hours until healing occurred or for 7 days. Patients also received approximately 1 cm standard antibiotic ointment administered four times daily to the lower conjunctiva fornix 1 hour after instillation of the study eye drops. Epithelial defects, detected by fluorescein staining and use of a slit lamp biomicroscope, covered at least 20% of the entire corneal surface. Patients were assigned a clinical score of 0 to 4 according to the adverse reactions experienced. On day 4 of treatment, all EGF-treated ulcers were healed and 85% of vehicle-treated ulcers were healed ($p < 0.05$, Gehean-Wilcoxon test). On day 6, all placebo-treated ulcers were healed. No adverse reactions were detected.

Kandarakis et al. (16) evaluated the efficacy of mouse EGF eye drops on epithelial healing after penetrating keratoplasty. All patients has 7.5-mm grafts placed in an 8-mm bed; during surgery, the epithelium was removed by vigorous scrubbing with a Paton scapula. At the end of the procedure, patients received methylprednisolone acetate, gentamycin, and cephalothin sodium in a sub-Tenon injection and the eye was pressure-patched. In the first study, 8 eyes were treated four times daily on the day of surgery and twice daily for the next 2 days with 1 drop mouse EGF 2-mg/ml solution containing chlorobutanol as a preservative. Eight patients received placebo eye drops. Eyes were stained with fluorescein and photographed twice daily for 2 days after surgery, and the area of epithelial defect was measured by planimetry. No difference in the percent of epithelial defect area was noted between the two treatment groups. In a second study, 9 eyes were treated with 1 drop mouse EGF 1 mg/ml with no preservative and 10 patients received placebo eight times daily beginning on preoperative day 1 and continuing until epithelial healing occurred. No difference in the percent of epithelial defect area was noted between the two treatment groups. Intraocular pressures were normal in all patients during the course of the study, and slit lamp biomicroscopy showed no evidence of toxicity.

ACKNOWLEDGMENT

This work was supported in part by funds from the National Institutes of Health, Grant No. EY05587.

REFERENCES

1. Bennett NT, Schultz GS. Growth factors and wound healing: biochemical properties of growth factors and their receptors. *Am J Surgery* 1993;165:728–737.
2. Bennett NT, Schultz GS. Growth factors and wound healing: part II. Role in normal and chronic wound healing. *Surgery* 1993;166:74–81.
3. Schultz G, Chegini N, Grant M, Khaw P, MacKay S. Effects of growth factors on corneal wound healing. *ACTA Ophthal* 1992;70: 60–66.
4. Schultz G, Khaw PT, Oxford K, Macauley S, van Setten G, Chigini N. Growth factors and ocular wound healing. *Eye* 1994;8:184–187.
5. Carpenter G, Cohen S. Epidermal growth factor. *J Biol Chem* 1990; 265:7709–7712.
6. Grant MB, Khaw PT, Schultz GS, Adams JL, Shimizu RW. Effects of epidermal growth factor, fibroblast growth factor, and transforming growth factor-β on corneal cell chemotaxis. *Invest Ophthalmol Vis Sci* 1992;33:3292–3301.
7. Sheradown H, Wedge C, Chou L, Apel R, Rootman DS, Cheng Y-L. Continuous epidermal growth factor delivery in corneal epithelial wound healing. *Invest Ophthalmol Vis Sci* 1993;34:3593–3600.
8. Pastor JC, Calonge M. Epidermal growth factor and corneal wound healing. *Cornea* 1992;11:311–314.
9. Araki F, Nakamura H, Nojima N, Tsukomo K, Sakamoto S. Stability of recombinant human epidermal growth factor in various solutions. *Chem Pharm Bull* 1989;37:404–406.
10. Schultz GS, Davis JB, Eiferman RA. Growth factors and corneal epithelium. *Cornea* 1988;7:96–101.
11. Chan KY, Lindquist TD, Edenfield MJ, Nicolson A, Banks AR. Pharmacokinetic study of recombinant human epidermal growth factor in the anterior eye. *Invest Ophthalmol Vis Sci* 1991;32:3209–3215.
12. Chiou GCY, Chuang CY, Chang MS. Systemic delivery of insulin through the eyes to lower the glucose concentration. *J Ocul Pharmacol* 1989;5:81–91.
13. Kim DC, Sugiyama Y, Satoh H, Fuwa T, Iga T, Hanano M. Kinetic analysis of vivo receptor-dependent binding of human epidermal growth factor by rat tissues. *J Pharm Sci* 1988;77:200–207.
14. Scardovi C, De Felice GP, Gazzaniga A. Epidermal growth factor in the topical treatment of traumatic corneal ulcers. *Ophthalmologica* 1993;206:119–124.
15. Daniele S, Frati L, Fiore C, Santoni G. The effect of the epidermal growth factor (EGF) on the corneal epithelium in humans. *Graefes Arch Clin Exp Ophthalmol* 1979;210:159–165.
16. Kandarakis AS, Page C, Kaufman HE. The effect of epidermal growth factor epithelial healing after penetrating keratoplasty in human eyes. *Am J Ophthalmol* 1984;98:411–415.
17. Reim M, Kehrer T, Lund M. Clinical application of epidermal growth factor in patients with most severe eye burns. *Ophthalmologica* 1988;197:179–184.
18. Meyers-Elliott RH, Elliott JH, Chitjian PA, Ho PC. Humoral and cell-mediated immune response to epidermal growth factor in the rabbit. *Invest Ophthalmol Vis Sci* 1981;20:86–99.

SECTION V

Uveitis

Section Editors: Albert Vitale and C. Stephen Foster

OVERVIEW

The problem of inflammation of the eye, including uveitis, was known to the ancients (Hippocrates, Galen, Aetius), but not until the 18th century did truly "modern" therapy for intraocular inflammation become well entrenched in the medical community. Scarpa, in his 1806 text (1), describes "a strong country-woman, 35 years old" who "was brought into this hospital towards the end of April 1796, on account of a violent, acute ophthalmia in both her eyes, with which she had been afflicted three days, with great tumefaction of the eyelids, redness of the conjunctiva, acute pain, fever, and watchfulness." Scarpa then described the presence of hypopyon and his treatment of same:

> I took away blood abundantly from the arm and foot, and also locally by means of leeches applied near both the angles of the eyes, and I also purged her. These remedies were attended with some advantage, inasmuch as they contributed to abate the inflammatory stage of the violent ophthalmia. Nevertheless an extravacation of yellowish glutinous lymph appeared in the anterior chamber of the aqueous humor, which filled out one-third of that cavity (1).

Adjunctive therapy, common to the times, was then used: "The uninterrupted application of small bags of gauze filled with emollient herbs boiled in milk, . . . and repeated mild purges with a grain of the antimonium tartarizatum dissolved in a pint of the decoction of the root of the triticum repens." The symptoms of the inflammation were entirely relieved, and "on the eleventh day the patient was able to bear a moderate degree of light." Additional therapies mentioned in Scarpa's text (1) include drops of vitriolic collyrium, with mucilage of quince-seed, bags of tepid mallows, a few grains of camphire, and blister production of the neck. Scarpa's text makes clear that these therapies were accepted as best medical practice for the time.

By 1830, as outlined in MacKenzie's text on diseases of the eye (2), dilation of the pupil with tincture of belladonna had been added to bloodletting, purging, and blistering therapy. Also added was the use of antimony and other nauseants, opiates for relief of pain, and mercury as an adjunctive antiphlogistic agent. Fever therapy, induced by intramuscular injection of milk or intravenous injection of triple typhoid H antigen, became fashionable in the first half of the 20th century. This "stimulatory" treatment, effective only if the patient's temperature were raised to about 40°C three or four times in succession, persisted into the early 1950s. Its effectiveness was undisputed, although its mechanism is unknown.

The next major advance in the care of patients with inflammatory disease was not made until 1952 with the discovery of the effectiveness of corticosteroid therapy. It is with this class of drugs that we begin our discussion of the pharmacology of treating intraocular inflammation. We then address the issue of cycloplegic therapy; then, in Chapters 61 and 62, we introduce the reader to the more modern advances in the care of patients with inflammatory disease: the use of nonsteroidal antiinflammatory drugs and of immunosuppressive agents.

Clearly, despite the advances made in the past 30 years with the discovery and development of these latter two additional classes of antiinflammatory agents, a significant proportion of patients with uveitis are still treated suboptimally by ophthalmologists unfamiliar with the effective and safe use of such drugs. It is regrettable that, still today, fully 10% of all blindness occurring in the United States alone results from inadequately treated uveitis.

It is our fervent hope that the following chapters will contribute to a "sea change" in the attitudes of ophthalmologists regarding tolerance or not of low-grade chronic inflammation which continues, eventually, to rob children and adults of precious vision. We believe strongly in a paradigm of zero tolerance for chronic intraocular inflammation and further believe that a stepwise algorithm to achieve that goal is highly effective in reducing ocular morbidity secondary to uveitis.

REFERENCES

1. Scarpa A. *Practical observations on the principle diseases of the eyes.* T. Cadell and W. Davies, London: Strand, 1806;292–321.
2. MacKenzie W. *A practical treatise on the diseases of the eye.* London: Longman, Rees, Orme, Brown & Green, 1830;422–457.

Textbook of Ocular Pharmacology,
edited by T.J. Zimmerman, et al.
Lippincott–Raven Publishers, Philadelphia © 1997.

CHAPTER 59

Pharmacology of Medical Therapy for Uveitis

Albert Vitale and C. Stephen Foster

CORTICOSTEROIDS

Introduction, History, and Source

The isolation of cortisone (compound E) in 1935 by Edward C. Kendall and the subsequent clinical demonstration of the dramatic beneficial effects of this compound and adrenocorticotropic hormone (ACTH) in the treatment of acute rheumatoid arthritis by Hench et al. (1) in 1948 marked a revolution in modern medical therapeutics. Today, the synthetic congeners of the naturally occurring corticosteroids produced by the adrenal cortex are as indispensable as antibiotics to medical practice.

In 1950, Gordon and McLean (2) extended the use of corticosteroids and ACTH to ophthalmic practice. Cortisone and hydroxycortisone were subsequently introduced for systemic and topical use by 1952 (3). The attendant success in the treatment of ocular inflammation catalyzed a search for better synthetic analogues of these steroids with more potent antiinflammatory effects, better ocular penetration, and bioavailability. A variety of formulations for topical, regional (subconjunctival and retrobulbar), and systemic use were developed in the next decade. By 1956, it had become evident that topical prednisolone minimized systemic side effects and was more efficacious in treatment of anterior segment inflammation, whereas systemic prednisone was preferable for posterior disease (4,5). As experience with these medications grew, an understanding of their potent antiinflammatory and immunosuppressive properties emerged, together with an appreciation of their capability of producing many potentially serious ocular and systemic complications. At present, corticosteroids remain the mainstay of management of ocular inflammatory and immune-mediated disease. A wide variety of synthetic preparations are currently available, the efficacy and toxicities of which depend on the formulation; the dose, frequency, and route of administration; and the therapeutic strategy used.

A. T. Vitale: Retina Specialists of Boston and The Massachusetts Eye and Ear Infirmary, Harvard Medical School, Boston, Massachusetts 02114.

C. S. Foster: Immunology and Uveitis Service, The Massachusetts Eye and Ear Infirmary, Harvard Medical School, Boston, Massachusetts 02114.

Official Drug Name and Chemistry

Corticosteroids (glucocorticoids and mineralocorticoids) may occur naturally in response to ACTH-induced conversion of cholesterol to pregnenolone in the adrenal cortex or as synthetic congeners of cortisol (hydroxycortisone). (Fig. 1) All corticosteroids are 21 carbon molecules consisting of a cyclopentoperhydrophenathrene nucleus, three hexane rings, and one pentane ring, designated A, B, C, and D. Modifications in this basic structure at various sites (Fig. 1) result in compounds with different biologic properties, (i.e., duration of action, relative antiinflammatory activity, sodium-retaining activity (Table 1), and transcorneal penetration). These alterations, in turn, determine their overall effectiveness in a particular clinical condition or route of administration and influence the occurrence of systemic or ocular side effects. Modifications in the structure–activity relationship include the following (6):

1. Most glucocorticoids are 17-α-hydroxy compounds, distinguishing them from androgenic steroids, which are 19 carbon, 17-α-keto molecules. Medrysone is an exception.
2. All naturally occurring steroids and most synthetic congeners have a hydroxyl group attached to carbon 21 (C-21), ring D.
3. In addition, all biologically active corticosteroids have a double bond at the C-4, 5 position and a ketone group at C-3, ring A. Cortisone, which is an inactive form, contains, in addition to the basic nucleus, a ketone group at C-11, ring C. It is converted to its active 11-hydroxyl form, cortisol (hydroxycortisone), through hepatic 11-B hydroxylation.
4. The addition of a 1, 2 double bond in ring A to the basic nucleus results in prednisolone and prednisone (with an

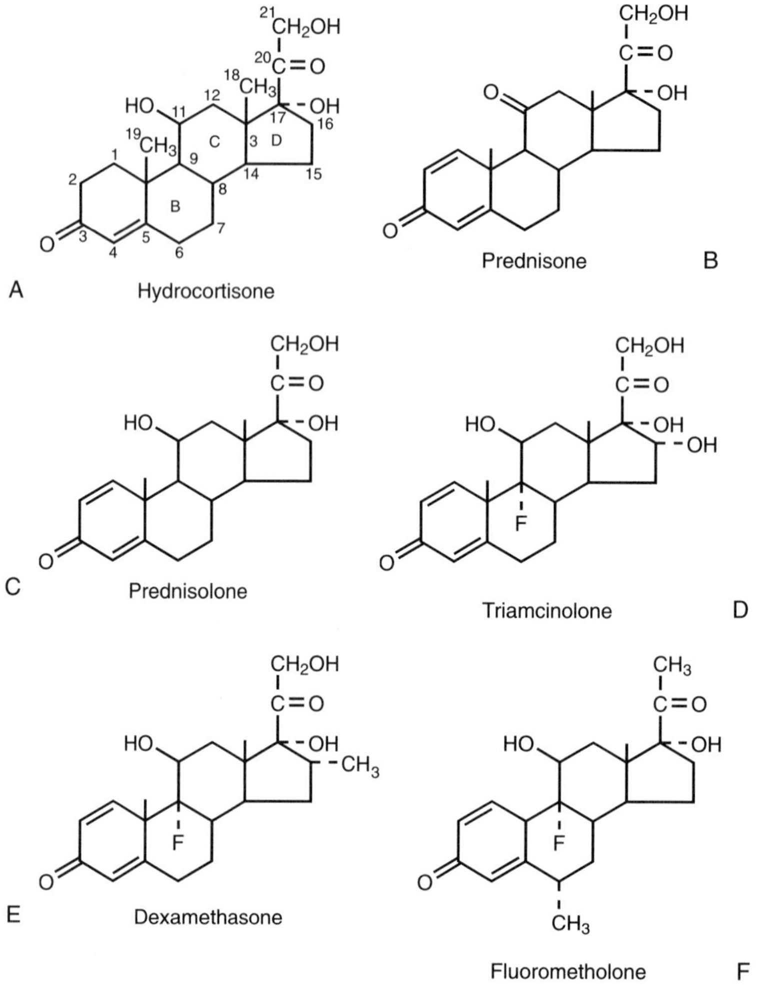

FIG. 59-1. (**A**) Structure of cortisol (hydroxycortisone). Synthetic congeners are derived from modifications in this basic structure; prednisone (**B**), prednisolone (**C**), triamcinolone (**D**), dexamethasone (**E**), and fluorometholone (**F**).

11-keto group). This modification results in a decreased rate of degradation (prolonged half-life, $t_{\frac{1}{2}}$) and enhanced carbohydrate regulating capacity.

5. Methylprednisolone is formed by the addition of a 6-methyl carbon group in ring B with slightly more antiinflammatory activity than prednisolone.
6. Although fluorination at the 9-α position in ring B leads to enhanced antiinflammatory potency, it produces excessive mineralocorticoid activity. Most fluorinated topical steroids have this basic structure, and the mineralocorticoid effect is diminished by masking the 16- or 17-hydroxy group with various esters (7).
7. 9-α Fluorohydrocortisone, together with the 1, 2 double bond in ring A, can be further modified by the addition of a 16-α-hydroxy, a 16-α-methyl, or a 16-β-methyl group to produce triamcinolone, dexamethasone, and betamethasone, respectively. Systemically, these glucocorticoids have enhanced antiinflammatory but minimal mineralocorticoid activity.

Pharmacology

The mechanism by which corticosteroids are believed to act ultimately entails control of the rate of protein synthesis at both a cellular and molecular level (6,8). After passively entering a target cell, the glucocorticoid molecule rapidly binds to a specific cytoplasmic steroid receptor protein (Fig. 2). The cytoplasmic steroid–receptor complex then becomes activated, undergoing a conformational change that allows it to cross the nuclear membrane and bind to DNA directly at sites known as glucocorticoid response elements (GRE). GRE binding controls the transcription of specific genes, which in turn either promote or inhibit the

TABLE 59-1. *Biological half-life, relative antiinflammatory activity, systemic equivalent, and sodium-retaining activity of systemic steroids*

Drug	Common trade name	Biologic half-life (hr)	Relative antiinflammatory activity	Systemic equivalent (mg)	Relative Na^+ retention
Short-Acting					
Hydrocortisone	Cortef (Upjohn, Kalamazoo, MI)	8–12	1.0	20	1.0
	Hydrocortone (MSD, West Point, PA)				
	Phosphate				
Cortisone	Cortone (MSD)	8–12	0.8	25	0.8
	Acetate				
Intermediate-acting					
Prednisone	Deltasone (Upjohn)	18–36	4.0	5	0.8
	Meticorten (Schering, Kenilworth, NJ)				
	Orasone (Solvay, Marietta, GA)				
Prednisolone	Delta-Cortef (Upjohn)	18–36	4.0	5	0.8
Methylprednisolone	Medrol (Upjohn)	18–36	5.0	4	0.0
Triamcinolone	Aristocort (Fujisawa, Deerfield, IL)	18–36	5.0	4	0.0
9-α-Fluorocortisol	Florinef (Apothecon, Princeton, NJ)	18–36	10	1.5	125
Long-acting					
Paramethasone	Haldrone (Lilly, Indianapolis, IN)	36–54	10	2	0.0
Dexamethasone	Decadron (MSD)	36–54	25	0.75	0.0
Betamethasone	Celestone (Schering)	36–54	25	0.75	0.0

production of specific mRNAs. As a consequence, the rate of translation and production of specific protein products encoded by their mRNAs is changed, thereby mediating the response of a particular cell to corticosteroids. Corticosteroid receptors have been identified in the iris, ciliary body, and adjacent corneoscleral tissue (9).

Clinical Pharmacology

Corticosteroids produce a multiplicity of important biochemical and physiologic effects on many tissues throughout the body. These effects mediate not only the antiinflammatory and immunosuppressive action of cor-

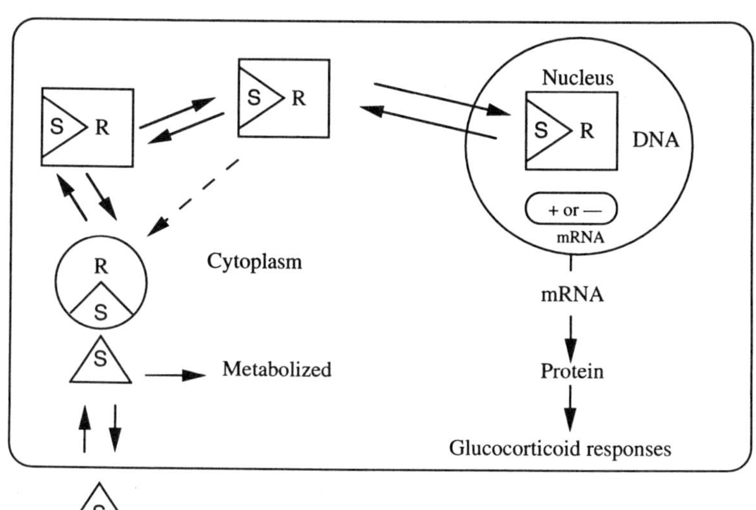

FIG. 59-2. After entry into the cell, a steroid or steroids bind to a cytoplasmic receptor (R) with subsequent translocation of steroid–receptor complex to the nucleus. Glucocorticoid response elements (GRE) binding to DNA promotes synthesis of specific MRNAs and thus specific target cell proteins. (Adapted from Polansky JR, Weinreb RN. Anti-inflammatory agents. In: Sears ML, ed. *Pharmacology of the eye.* New York: Springer-Verlag, 1984;515.)

ticosteroids, but also account for the potentially undesirable side effects in the course of systemic or topical therapy.

Hypothalamic–Pituitary–Adrenal (HPA) Axis

The exogenous administration of corticosteroids suppresses the release of both corticotropin-releasing factor (CRF) from the hypothalamus and ACTH from the anterior pituitary, resulting in a decrease in cortisol production by the adrenal cortex. This feedback inhibition is very sensitive, occurring within minutes after administration of systemic corticosteroid. It is progressive, in both a dose- and time-dependent manner, affects basal and stress-stimulated release, and is reversible (10). Administration of a large dose of corticosteroids may suppress the HPA axis for a few hours whereas more prolonged exposure is associated with profound suppression and an extended recovery time for normal HPA axis functioning.

Carbohydrate, Protein, and Lipid Metabolism

The principal biochemical actions of corticosteroids are stimulation and induction of protein synthesis and gluconeogenesis in the liver and inhibition of peripheral tissue protein synthesis (11). In addition, corticosteroids produce peripheral insulin resistance, inhibiting glucose uptake in most target tissues except brain, heart, and liver and in erythrocytes. Hepatic glycogen storage is enhanced, and lipid stores are stimulated to undergo lipolysis. The net effect is a corticosteroid-induced catabolic state with hyperglycemia, ketosis and hyperlipidemia which, in normal subjects, is blunted by a compensatory increase in insulin release (10). These physiologic effects of corticosteroids on intermediary metabolism may explain some of the more conspicuous manifestations of excessive and prolonged steroid therapy: fat redistribution characteristic of Cushing's syndrome, thinning of the skin, striae, osteoporosis, poor wound healing, and corticosteroid-induced myopathy.

Calcium Metabolism

Corticosteroids affect calcium metabolism in a complex manner, resulting in a net reduction in total body calcium stores and osteopenia. Corticosteroids inhibit intestinal absorption and promote renal excretion of calcium and inhibit osteoblast function. In addition, osteoblasts are stimulated by the compensatory increase in parathyroid hormone levels (10,12).

Central Nervous System

Transient mood disturbances ranging from euphoria to depression, anxiety, and frank psychosis are well-known complications of systemic glucocorticoid administration and vary considerably between patients. Although the mechanism or mechanisms underlying these changes are poorly understood, corticosteroids have been suggested to cross the blood–brain barrier (BBB) and act either directly on the brain or mediate these effects indirectly through changes in cerebral blood flow or through perturbations in local electrolyte concentrations (6).

Electrolyte and Fluid Balance

Synthetic corticosteroids with mineralocorticoid activity (Table 1) may significantly alter the patient's fluid and electrolyte balance. Aldosterone, the prototypical, naturally occurring mineralocorticoid hormone, stimulates active reabsorption of sodium in exchange for potassium at the proximal convoluted tubule in the kidney. Water follows sodium passively while potassium is excreted, which may produce hypokalemia when there is an excessive mineralocorticoid effect. The renin-angiotensin system (RAS) and plasma potassium levels are chiefly responsible for primary mineralocorticoid control (12).

Cardiovascular System

Systemic hypertension and increased cardiac output may occur after systemic administration of corticosteroids. Indeed, high-dose corticosteroids may restore circulatory function in various states of shock. Although these actions may be due in part to mineralocorticoid effects, myocardial tissue contains high-affinity glucocorticoid receptors and exhibits a positive ionotropic response to corticosteroids (10,11).

Gastrointestinal (GI) System

Corticosteroids inhibit DNA synthesis in the GI tract and enhance gastric secretions. This increases the risk of formation of duodenal ulcers and development of gastritis, particularly when higher doses are used (10).

Antiinflammatory and Immunosuppressive Effects

Corticosteroids have both antiinflammatory and immunosuppressive effects which are unspecific, i.e., they act to ameliorate the cardinal signs of inflammation (rubor, calor, dolor, and edema), irrespective of the inciting inflammatory stimulus or disease process. Corticosteroids mediate their antiinflammatory and immunosuppressive effects by many different mechanisms (6,11,13–16), as follows:

1. Induction of lymphocytopenia. In humans, corticosteroids are not cytotoxic to lymphocytes. Instead, the distribution of these cells, particularly the T-helper subset, is altered so that they are sequestered from the

intravascular circulation and concentrated in the bone marrow. Consequently, fewer immunoreactive cells are recruited to the site of inflammation. After administration of a single large dose of corticosteroid, blood lymphocytes are maximally reduced in 1 to 6 hr. Small to moderate doses preferentially affect T-lymphocytes, whereas high chronic dosing may affect B-lymphocytes and thus antibody production.

2. Neutrophilic leukocytosis. Corticosteroids simultaneously induce production of large numbers of neutrophils by the bone marrow while preventing the adherence of these cells to the vascular endothelium, impeding their migration from the intravascular space to the site of inflammation.
3. Reduction of circulating eosinophils and monocytes.
4. Inhibition of macrophage recruitment with consequent alterations in cell-mediated immune responses, (i.e., reduced skin-test reactivity).
5. Inhibition of macrophage migration and antigen-processing capability. Corticosteroids suppress the action of certain lymphokines, (i.e., macrophage migration inhibitory factor) and prevent vascular endothelial adhesion. In this way, the macrophage is denied access to sites where antigens are initially deposited.
6. Attenuation of bactericidal activity of macrophages and monocytes.
7. Stabilization of intracellular lysozomal membranes. With inhibition of neutrophil degranulation, the surrounding tissues are spared the potentially damaging effects of the liberated lysozomal enzymes.
8. Stabilization of mast cell and basophil membranes. Degranulation of these cells is inhibited, thereby preventing release of various inflammatory mediators such as histamine, bradykinin, platelet-activating factor (PAF), slow-reacting substance of anaphylaxis (SRS-A), and eosinophilic chemotactic factor (ECF).
9. Inhibition of prostaglandin synthesis. Corticosteroids, through a protein termed macrocortin, inhibit the enzyme phospholipase A_2 and thus conversion of phospholipid to arachidonic acid (AA). (See Fig. 2 in Chapter 61, Nonsteroidal Antiinflammatory Agents, *this volume.*) Consequently, the synthesis of both prostaglandins (though the cyclooxygenase pathway) and leukotrienes (through lipoxygenase pathway) is prevented.
10. Reduction of capillary permeability and suppression of vasodilation in the setting of acute inflammation. As a consequence, transudation of fluid, protein, and inflammatory cells into the target site is reduced.
11. Suppression of fibroplasia.

Pharmaceutics

Topical Corticosteroid Preparations

A variety of corticosteroid preparations is available for topical use in treatment of inflammatory ocular disease. These are listed in order of ascending antiinflammatory potency in Table 2 and are discussed briefly herein.

TABLE 59-2. *Ophthalmic topical corticosteroid preparations*

Drug/preparation	Common trade name	Formulation	
Dexamethasone			
Alcohol	Maxidex (Alcon)	0.1% 0.05%	suspension, ointment
Sodium phosphate	Decadron Phosphate (MSD)	0.1% 0.05%	solution, ointment
Prednisolone			
Acetate	Pred Forte (Allergan), Econopred Plus (Alcon), AK-Tate (Akorn)	1.0%	suspension
	Pred Mild (Allergan), Econopred (Alcon)	0.12%	suspension
Sodium phosphate	Inflamase Forte (Iolab), AK-Pred (Akorn)	1%	solution
	Metreton (Schering)	0.5%	solution
	Inflamase Mild (Iolab), AK-Pred (Akorn)	0.12%	solution
Phosphate	Hydeltrasol (MSD)	0.5% 0.25%	solution ointment
Fluoromethalone			
Alcohol	FML (Allergan)	0.1% 0.1%	suspension, ointment
Medroxyprogesterone			
Acetate	Provera	1%	suspension
Medrysone			
Alcohol	HMS (Allergan)	1.0%	suspension

Dexamethasone

Dexamethasone is formulated as a 0.1% alcohol suspension/0.1% sodium phosphate solution and as a 0.05% ointment. It is the most potent commercially available topical steroid, and thus poses a concomitant increased risk of untoward ocular side effects.

Prednisolone

Prednisolone is available as a 0.12% or 1% acetate suspension, as a 0.12%, 0.5%, or 1% sodium phosphate solution, and as a 0.25% phosphate ointment. Although acetate preparations, with their biphasic solubility, achieve better penetration into and through an intact cornea than do water-soluble phosphate vehicles, this difference is not clinically significant when intraocular inflammation exists, depending more on concentration and dosage frequency (17) (described in Pharmacokinetics section). Moreover, suspensions require thorough mixing to ensure maximal steroid concentrations with each delivery, introducing a potential compliance problem, which may make solutions preferable in clinical practice. The bioavailability and potency of prednisolone not only make it an efficacious antiinflammatory agent, but also increase the likelihood of dose-dependent ocular toxicity.

Fluorometholone (FML) and Medrysone (HMS)

FML (0.1% or 0.25%) and HMS (1.0%) are supplied as ophthalmic suspensions. Fluorometholone is also available as an 0.1% ointment. These are weak antiinflammatory agents and are the least likely to produce steroid-related ocular damage (cataract and glaucoma).

Medroxyprogesterone

Medroxyprogesterone is not available commercially for ophthalmic use, but may be prepared by the hospital pharmacy from a 1% solution used parenterally. This agent is particularly useful in certain peripheral ulcerative, inflammatory, external ocular diseases because it not only reduces inflammation, but also decreases the production of collagenase and interferes less with collagen synthesis than other steroids (18). Its relative potency is slightly less than 0.12% prednisolone.

Systemic and Regional Corticosteroid Preparations

Corticosteroids used in systemic and regional (subconjunctival, sub-Tenon, transseptal, and retrobulbar) therapy of ocular inflammatory disease are presented in order of increasing antiinflammatory potency in Tables 3 and 4, respectively and are discussed herein.

Hydrocortisone

Hydrocortisone is formulated in 5-, 10-, and 20-mg tablets or as a 10-mg/5-ml suspension for oral (p.o.) use. In addition, intramuscular (i.m.), intravenous (i.v.) and regional injectable preparations are available in concentrations ranging from 25, 50, 100, 250 to 1,000 mg/ml. Typical subconjunctival doses range from 50 to 125 mg, whereas systemic therapy may be initiated at 20 to 240 mg, depending on the severity of inflammation.

Prednisone

Prednisone is supplied in tablet form in doses of 1, 2.5, 5, 10, 20, 25, and 50 mg and as a 5-mg/ml oral solution. It is commonly used in therapy of severe ocular inflammatory diseases, with a typical initial dose of 1.0 to 1.5 mg/kg and subsequent taper, depending on the clinical response (described in Therapeutic Use section).

Prednisolone

Prednisolone is available in 5-mg tablets or as a 15-mg/ml syrup for oral use; however, it is used far more often as a topical agent. It has four times the inflammatory potency of hydrocortisone (Table 1), with common systemic dosages ranging from 5 mg every other morning to 50 mg daily in divided doses (19).

Methylprednisolone

Methylprednisolone is available in 2- to 32-mg tablets for oral use or as an acetate suspension (20 to 80 mg/ml) and as a sodium succinate (40- to 100-mg powder) solution for intramuscular or intravenous administration. Its relative inflammatory potency is four times that of hydrocortisone (Table 1). The sodium succinate formulation is used regionally, with typical doses ranging from 40 to 125 mg per injection. A methylprednisolone acetate depot is available for subconjunctival sub-Tenon, or retrobulbar administration in doses ranging from 40 to 80 mg/0.5 ml, providing prolonged local release of steroid. Finally, methylprednisolone sodium succinate is occasionally used in intravenous pulse therapy (1 g/day for 3 days) in cases of severe bilateral, sight-threatening uveitis (described in the Therapeutic Use section).

Triamcinolone

Triamcinolone tablets are available in strength of 1, 2, 4, and 8 mg and as a 4-mg/5 ml syrup for oral use. Triamcinolone has essentially no mineralocorticoid activity, yet has five times more antiinflammatory activity than hydrocortisone (Table 1). Triamcinolone acetonide and diacetate suspensions (10 to 40 mg/ml) are also available for intra-

TABLE 59-3. *Systemic corticosteroid preparations*

Drug	Common trade name	Oral	Formulation
Hydrocortisone	Cortef (Upjohn, Kalamazoo, MI)	5- to 20-mg tablet 10-mg/5-ml suspension	25- and 50-mg suspension i.m.
	Hydrocortone Phosphate (MSD, West Point, PA)		50-mg/ml solution i.m./i.v.
	Solu-Cortef (Upjohn)		100- to 1,000 mg powder i.m./i.v.
Prednisone	Deltasone (Upjohn)		
	Meticorten (Schering, Kenilworth, NJ)	1.0- to 50-mg tablet	
	Drasone (Solvay, Marietta, GA)		
	Liquid-Pred (Muro)	5-mg/ml solution	
Prednisolone	Delta-Cortef (Upjohn)	1- to 5-mg tablet	
	Prelone (Muro, Tewksbury, MA)	15-mg/ml syrup	
Acetate	Predalone (Forest, St. Louis, MO)		25- to 100-mg/ml suspension i.m.
Sodium phosphate	Hydeltrasol (MSD)		20-mg/ml Solution i.m./i.v.
Methylprednisolone	Medrol (Upjohn)	2- to 32-mg tablet	
Acetate	Depo-Medrol (Upjohn)		20- to 80-mg/ml suspension i.m.
Sodium succinate	Solu-Medrol (Upjohn)		40- to 1,000-mg powder i.m./i.v.
Triamcinolone diacetate	Kenacort (Apothecon, Princeton, NJ)	4-mg/5-ml syrup	
	Aristocort (Fujisawa, Deerfield, IL)	1- to 8-mg tablet	40-mg/ml suspension i.m.
Acetonide	Kenalog (Westwood-Squibb, Princeton, NJ)		10- and 40-mg/ml suspension i.m.
Dexamethasone sodium	Decadron (MSD)	0.25- to 6.0-mg tablet 0.5-mg/5-ml elixir 0.5-mg/5-ml solution	
Dexamethasone sodium phosphate	Decadron Phosphate (MSD)		4- to 24-mg/ml solution i.v.
Acetate	Decadron-LA (MSD)		8-mg/ml suspension i.m.
Betamethasone	Celestone (Schering)	0.6-mg tablet 0.6-mg/5-ml syrup	
Sodium phosphate	Celestone Phosphate (Schering)		3-mg/ml solution i.v.
Acetate and sodium phosphate	Celestone (Schering) Soluspan		3- and 6-mg/ml suspension i.m.

i.m., intramuscular; i.v., intravenous.

TABLE 59-4. *Regional corticosteroid preparations*

Drug	Common trade names	Formulation	Route and typical dose
Hydrocortisone	Hydrocortisone Sodium Succinate (MSD, West Point, PA)	100- to 1,000-mg powder	Subconjunctival/Tenon 50–125 mg
Methylprednisolone			
Sodium succinate	Solu-Medrol (Upjohn, Kalamazoo, MI)	40-mg/ml, 125-mg/2-ml, 2g/30-ml solution	Subconjunctival/Tenon 40–125 mg
Acetate	Depo-Medrol (Upjohn)	20- to 80-mg/ml depot) suspension	Transseptal, retrobulbar, 40–80 mg/0.5 ml
Triamcinolone			
Diacetate	Aristocort (Fugisawa, Deerfield, IL)	25- and 40-mg/ml suspension	Subconjunctival/Tenon 40 mg,
Acetonide	Kenalog (Westwood-Squibb, Princeton, NJ)	10 and 40 mg/ml	Transseptal 40 mg
Dexamathasone			
Acetate	Decadron-LA (MSD)	8- to 16-mg/ml suspension	Subconjunctival/Tenon 4–8 mg, Transseptal 4–8 mg
Sodium phosphate	Decadron Phosphate (MSD)	4-, 10-, 24-mg/ml solution	Retrobulbar, intravitreal 0.4 mg
Betamethasone acetate and sodium phosphate	Celestone Soluspan (Schering, Kenilworth, TX)	3-mg/ml suspension	Subconjunctival/Tenon, transeptal, 1 mg

Subconjunctival/Tenon, subconjunctival or sub-Tenon injection.

muscular injection and are frequently administered in 10-mg doses through the sub-Tenon, subconjunctival, and transseptal routes in the regional management of uveitis (Table 4).

Dexamethasone

Dexamethasone sodium tablets are formulated in strength of 0.25, 0,5 0.75, 1.5, 4, and 6 mg, as a 0.5-mg/ml elixir, and as a 0.5-mg/5 ml solution for oral use. Initial doses range from 0.75 mg to 9 mg p.o. daily, depending on the severity of inflammation (19). Dexamethasone acetate suspension (8 mg/ml) and sodium phosphate solution (4, 10, 24 mg/ml) are available for intramuscular and intravenous administration, respectively. The latter may also be injected regionally or intravitreally with initial doses of 40 mg and 0.4 mg, respectively (Table 4). Dexamethasone is 25 times more potent than hydrocortisone and has little sodium-retaining or potassium-wasting activity (Table 1).

Betamethasone

Betamethasone is the most potent synthetic steroid, with an antiinflammatory and mineralocorticoid profile similar to that of dexamethasone. It is formulated as 0.6-mg tablets and as a 0.6-mg/5 ml syrup for oral use. The sodium phosphate solution (3 mg/ml) and the acetate-sodium phosphate suspension (3 and 6 mg/ml) are available for intravenous and intramuscular administration, respectively. The latter may be given by the subconjunctival, sub-Tenon, or transseptal routes at a dose of 1 mg per injection (Table 4). Initial systemic doses range from 0.5 to 9 mg/day, depending on disease severity. As with all systemically administered steroids (orally or intravenously), GI prophylaxis should be instituted concomitantly (described in sections on Therapeutic Use, Side Effects, and Toxicity).

Pharmacokinetics, Concentration–Effect Relationship, and Metabolism

Systemic Corticosteroids

Orally administered corticosteroids (prednisone) are readily absorbed in the upper jejunum, have a bioavailability $\leq 90\%$, and reach peak plasma concentrations 30 min to 2 hr after ingestion. Parenteral (intramuscular) administration of corticosteroids in suspension have prolonged effects (8). Concomitant food ingestion delays, but does not reduce, the amount of drug absorbed. Corticosteroids are widely distributed throughout most body tissues. In the plasma, 80% to 90% of corticosteroids are protein bound; the remaining free fraction represents the biologically active form. Two steroid-binding proteins exist: a high-affinity, low-capacity, cortisol-binding globulin (CBG) and a low-affinity, high-capacity, binding protein, albumin. CBG levels are decreased by hypothyroidism, liver and kidney disease, and obesity, thereby increasing the free fraction. Conversely, the relative amount of free steroid is reduced by entities that increase CBG levels, (i.e., pregnancy, estrogen therapy, and hyperthyroidism) (6).

Corticosteroids compete with each other for binding sites on the CBG. Synthetic congeners or cortisol bind less avidly than the endogenous molecule, thereby increasing the available free fraction of steroid. Prednisolone reportedly binds with greater affinity than other synthetic compounds, resulting in the replacement of endogenous cortisol from the protein binding sites (12). Prolonged and/or high-dose corticosteroid therapy consequently produces a greater proportion of free steroid in the body.

All biologically active corticosteroids have a double bond in the C-4, 5 position and a ketone group at the C-3 position (Fig. 1). Cortisone and prednisone have no inherent glucocorticoid activity and depend on the reversible action of 11-β-hydroxy-dehydrogenase in the liver to convert them to the active analogues hydroxycortisone and prednisolone. Patients with hepatic disease may have impaired glucocorticoid interconversions and clearance. In such circumstances, administration of prednisolone rather than prednisone is more appropriate (6). Hepatic reduction of the C-4, 5 double bond and C-3 ketone group results in an inactive metabolite which is then conjugated with glucuronide to form a soluble product that is excreted by the kidney (6).

There is a poor correlation between the duration of biologic activity and the plasma $t_{\frac{1}{2}}$ of the various synthetic corticosteroids (8). Their biologic $t_{\frac{1}{2}}$ varies: short-acting hydrocortisone (8 to 12 hours), intermediate-acting triamcinolone (18 to 36 hours), and long-acting dexamethasone (36 to 54 hours) (Table 1). In contrast, the plasma $t_{\frac{1}{2}}$ ranges from 1 hour (cortisone and prednisone) to 5 hours (triamcinolone).

The intraocular penetration of systemically administered corticosteroids is limited by the blood–ocular barrier. Intramuscular administration of cortisone has been shown to penetrate the vitreous in appreciable quantities, though not quite reaching the aqueous concentrations after topical therapy (5). In contrast, topical applications yield the lowest vitreous concentrations. Peak concentrations of dexamethasone, triamcinolone, and methylprednisolone have been determined in the aqueous humor of rabbits 1 hour after intravenous administration of 25 mg steroid, with slightly higher levels of drug attained when it is applied topically (20).

Topical and Regional Corticosteroids

Several interdependent factors influence the overall efficacy of a particular topical steroid preparation in treatment of ocular inflammatory disease, including (a) its ability to penetrate into and through the cornea, sclera, or blood–ocular barriers; (b) the relative antiinflammatory potency and duration of action in the cornea, aqueous humor, or vitreous cavity; (c) the dose and frequency of administration; and (d) the side-effect profile (16,21).

Early ocular penetration studies demonstrated the presence of 0.97% prednisolone acetate in the aqueous humor of rabbits within 5 minutes of a single topical dose, a peak concentration by 30 minutes, and a nadir by 240 minutes (22). Similarly, radiolabeled 0.1% dexamethasone phosphate was shown to penetrate the intact cornea and aqueous of rabbits within 10 minutes and to remain in the eye for as long as 24 hours (23). In the same study, a surprising degree of systemic absorption was observed after topical application, as manifested by the presence of radioactivity in the urine, plasma, kidneys, and liver of the animals. With regard to ocular tissues, the highest concentrations of steroid 30 minutes after topical application have been detected in the cornea and conjunctiva, followed by the sclera, choroid, and aqueous, with very little drug detectable in the lens or vitreous (24,25).

Ocular tissues themselves may play an important role in local steroid metabolism and thus determine to some degree the efficacy of a particular topical preparation. Systemically administered cortisone is rendered biologically active (converted to hydroxycortisone) by hydroxylation at C-11 in the liver. The clinical antiinflammatory efficacy of topically applied cortisone and prednisone suggest inherent 11-hydroxylase activity in the cornea and, possibly, other ocular tissues (26). Phosphate derivatives may be converted into more active alcohol forms by corneal phosphatase activity (27). Steroid reaching the eye may depend in part on degradative enzyme systems such as "A" ring reductase in the iris, cornea, and ciliary body (28). Long-acting synthetic congeners such as dexamethasone are more resistant to such inactivation.

Variability in ocular penetration among topical steroids is due not only to differences in their formulation, but also in intrinsic properties of the cornea. Phosphate preparations, marketed as solutions, are highly water soluble and would be expected to penetrate lipophillic barriers (the corneal epithelium and endothelium) relatively poorly. In contradistinction, alcohol-based and, in particular, acetate suspensions exhibit biphasic solubility and thus theoretically are better able to penetrate all corneal layers to reach the anterior chamber. Similarly, the presence or absence of the corneal epithelium is expected to affect the intracorneal and intraocular bioavailability of various steroid preparations. The experimental data, however, are not as clear-cut as the theoretical expectations.

In one study, in which a rabbit model of clove oil-induced keratitis was used, the corneal drug concentration after topical administration, when epithelium was intact, was greatest for prednisolone acetate, followed by prednisolone sodium phosphate and dexamethasone alcohol, whereas in corneas denuded of epithelium the concentration of prednisolone phosphate was greatest, followed by prednisolone acetate and dexamethasone alcohol. For each condition, these trends were mirrored in the levels of specific drug detected in the aqueous (29–33). Results of another study supported the superior penetration of prednisolone sodium phosphate in rabbit corneas denuded of epithelium; however, equal corneal penetration by prednisolone acetate, sodium phosphate, and fluorometholone was demonstrated when epithelium was intact (34). More recent work, in which the potentially confounding effect of stromal clove oil was eliminated, has demonstrated better penetration of topically applied prednisolone phosphate through an intact rabbit corneal epithelium than might be expected, given its limited lipid solubility (35). Both in vivo and in vitro studies comparing the permeability of prednisolone phosphate and prednisolone acetate across intact corneal epithelium in rabbits have shown steady-state conditions for penetration and similar fluxes for both drugs with respect to prednisolone and similar bioavailability in the aqueous humor as measured directly by HPLC (36,37). With similar concentrations of drug in the anterior chamber, the differential penetration of phosphate solutions versus acetate suspensions themselves may not be the crucial determinant of therapeutic efficacy in the treatment of intraocular inflammation. Other factors, such as inherent antiinflammatory activity, glucocorticoid receptor-binding efficacy, metabolic interconversion, and intraocular clearance of a particular steroid preparation, as well as dosing frequency, may be more important in the therapy of uveitis.

The antiinflammatory activity of various corticosteroids varies considerably (Table 1). Potency is influenced by many factors, including glucocorticoid receptor-binding affinity, formulation, route of administration, and the experimental model used to evaluate the drug. These data on antiinflammatory potency were obtained from nonocular experimental models in which drug was systemically administered and thus cannot be directly extended to topical ocular human use (17). Therefore, Liebowitz and Kupferman (17) quantitatively evaluated the antiinflammatory effects of different topical steroid preparations in a rabbit model of clove oil-induced keratitis by measuring the decrease in radioactively labeled neutrophils in the cornea. Their work demonstrated that prednisolone acetate 1% was the most potent antiinflammatory agent for the suppression of inflammation in corneas with or without an intact epithelium (Table 5). The two commercially available forms of this drug were identical in their bioavailability in the cornea and in their antiinflammatory efficacy. Although it may be tempting to assume that increased bioavailability of a particular steroid preparation at the site of anterior segment inflammation will provide to proportionately enhanced antiinflammatory activity, Liebowitz and Kupferman showed that this is not the case with respect to intracorneal inflammation (38). For example, although the

TABLE 59-5. *Decrease in corneal inflammatory activity after topical therapy with various corticosteroid derivatives in rabbits*

	Corneal epithelium	
Preparation	Intact (%)	Absent (%)
Prednisolone acetate 1.0%	51	53
Dexamethasone alcohol 0.1%	40	42
Prednisolone phosphate 1.0%	28	47
Dexamethasone phosphate 0.1%	19	22
Dexamethasone phosphate 0.05% (ointment)	13	
Fluorometholone alcohol 0.1%	31	37

Adapted from Leibowitz HM, Kupferman A. *Int Ophthalmol Clin* 1980;20:117–134.

corneal concentrations of dexamethasone acetate and alcohol were significantly lower than that of the phosphate preparation, they demonstrated superior antiinflammatory activity irrespective of epithelial integrity (Table 6). These data suggest that different derivatives of the same corticosteroid base are not equivalent in their antiinflammatory properties in the therapy of keratitis. Indeed, when assayed for its ability to compete for glucocorticoid receptors, dexamethasone alcohol was shown to be 15 times more potent than dexamethasone phosphate (39), which may explain in part the apparent diminished topical antiinflammatory effect with phosphate preparations in a keratitis model (26). Extension of these findings to intraocular inflammation has yet to be confirmed experimentally. Ocular tissue phosphatases might convert the phosphate derivative to the more active alcohol form once the steroid has reached the anterior chamber, thus enhancing the antiinflammatory effect observed clinically.

More practical considerations may dictate the choice between derivatives of the same steroid base in clinical practice. Acetate suspensions must be adequately shaken to distribute insoluble drug particles so that the maximal concentration of steroid is delivered with each dose. Poor patient compliance has been demonstrated in persons who were instructed to shake their suspension eye drops before topical instillation (40). Therefore, there is a good rationale for preferring phosphate solutions that provide more consistent dosage of drug.

Increasing the concentration and dosage frequency of a particular steroid enhances both the bioavailability in the cornea and anterior chamber and its antiinflammatory efficacy. However, raising the concentration of a drug such as prednisolone acetate beyond 1% does not offer additional antiinflammatory benefit in the cornea but increases the potential for toxicity (41). Likewise, hourly administration of prednisolone acetate is five times more effective than instillation every 4 hours in suppressing corneal inflammation (Table 7) (42). Although it is clinically impractical, maximal inflammatory suppression was achieved with an every-5-minute regimen.

Two other less potent topical corticosteroids are commercially available for ocular use: FML and HMS. Although the corneal penetration of 0.1% FML is poor in comparison to that of 1% prednisolone acetate, no significant differences in antiinflammatory efficacy was observed between the two steroids in the treatment of corneal inflammation (43). The therapeutic efficacy of FML in the cornea, despite a reduced concentration, may be explained by its mildly hydrophobic properties, which allow achievement of saturation levels in the corneal epithelium before the drug is diffused through the more hydrophilic stroma (16). In addition, FML has a high affinity for the glucocorticoid receptor which, combined with its poor corneal penetration, may enhance its "local" corneal antiinflammatory effect while reducing the propensity for steroid-induced ocular complications (26). For the same reasons the poor corneal penetration of FML makes it less effective than other more potent steroids in treatment of intraocular inflammation.

HMS has weak antiinflammatory effects and poor corneal penetration and is the least likely of all topical ophthalmic steroid preparations to produce a steroid-induced increase in intraocular pressure (IOP). It has no place in treatment of intraocular inflammation.

The emergence of newly formulated "soft steroids" may provide enhanced antiinflammatory efficacy while minimizing the potential for untoward steroid-induced side effects. These agents are inert until activated locally in the eye and are rapidly degraded in the anterior chamber or bloodstream; thus, intraocular or systemic toxicity is limited (44). One such drug, loteprednol etabonate, a congener of prednisolone, has been shown to be useful in treatment of giant papillary conjunctivitis in humans (45).

TABLE 59-6. *Corneal bioavailability and antiinflammatory effectiveness of different dexamethasone preparations*

	Antiinflammatory effect (%)		Corneal bioavailability (mg/min/1g)	
Corticosteroid	Epithelium intact	Absent	Epithelium intact	Absent
Dexamethasone acetate 0.1%	55	60	111	118
Dexamethasone alcohol 0.1%	40	42	543	1,316
Dexamethasone sodium phosphate 0.1%	19	22	1,068	4,642

Adapted from Leibowitz HM, Kupferman A. *Int Ophthalmol Clin* 1980;20:117–134.

TABLE 59-7. *Ophthalmic indications for use of corticosteroids*

Eyelids
Contact dermatitis
Blepharitis
Discoid lupus
Chalazion
Chemical burns
Conjunctiva
Allergic disease (atopic, seasonal, vernal, GPC)
Viral (herpetic, EKC)
Mucocutaneous (graft vs. host, erythema multiforme, toxic epidermal necrolysis, ocular cicatricial pemphigoid
Chemical burns
Cornea
Keratitis
Herpes zoster
Disciform herpes simplex
Immune infiltrates
Interstitial
Superficial punctate
Peripheral ulcerative (Wegener's, polyarteritis nodosa, Mooren's)
Reiter's, Lyme disease, sarcoid
Acne rosaceae
Graft rejection
Chemical burns
Sclera
Scleritis
Orbit
Pseudotumor
Grave's orbitopathy
Uvea
Anterior uveitis
Intermediate uveitis (pars planitis)
Posterior uveitis
Sympathetic ophthalmia
Vogt-Koyanagi-Harada syndrome
Endophthalmitis
Retina
Cystoid macular edema
Vasculitis
Choroiditis
Retinitis
Acute retinal necrosis
Optic nerve
Optic neuritis
Temporal arteritis
Postoperative
Trauma
Extraocular muscles
Ocular myasthenia gravis

GPC, giant papillary conjunctivitis.

The drug vehicle has impact on the therapeutic efficacy of topically applied corticosteroids. Although ointments might be presumed to be superior to collyria because of the prolonged contact time between the drug and the ocular surface, dexamethasone phosphate ointment produces lower drug levels in the cornea and anterior chamber than does the solution. The petrolatum vehicle of the ointment is believed to retain drug and thus retard its release (46). Nevertheless, steroid ointments are a practical alternative to frequent dosing when use of the latter is impossible (during sleep).

Finally, high-viscosity gels (47) and depot preparations in the form of cotton pledgets (48) and collagen shields (49) have been used in an attempt to enhance the ocular bioavailability and antiinflammatory effects of topically applied corticosteroids. Depot preparations have the advantage of providing slow, steady release of drug over the ocular surface (16).

Regional therapy of ocular inflammatory disease may be instituted with periocular injection (subconjunctival, sub-Tenon, transseptal, or retrobulbar) of steroid, providing rapid delivery of high concentrations of drug to the target tissues. With the exception of hydrocortisone, the preparations shown in Table 3 are of moderate to high potency. Their formulation is likely to affect the rate of release and duration of action of drug administered as subconjunctival or sub-Tenon depots (26). Water-soluble preparations (methylprednisolone sodium succinate), which diffuse from the depot more rapidly, are short-acting, even when steroids with a prolonged biological $t_{\frac{1}{2}}$ (dexamethasone sodium phosphate) are used (50). Although less soluble formulations (methylprednisolone acetate and triamcinolone acetonide) have a longer duration of action, they pose an increased risk of development of steroid-induced ocular toxicity. The site of injection (subconjunctival vs. retrobulbar) and the distribution of drug into the surrounding tissues will also affect the duration of action and ocular bioavailability; e.g., in experiments in which radiolabeled methylprednisolone acetate (Depo-Medrol) was injected by the retrobulbar route, high levels of drug were produced in the sclera, choroid, retina, and vitreous for a week or more (51). Wine et al. (52) showed that higher intraocular concentrations and more rapid ocular penetration of hydrocortisone were achieved after subconjunctival administration than after injection into the anterior orbital fat.

Although the site of injection depends on the location of the inflammatory process (anterior vs. posterior segment) and the clinician's individual preference, the clear-cut superiority of a single method of regional injection has not been established. Even though hydroxycortisone may be detected in the anterior chamber almost immediately after subconjunctival injection, controlled experiments have demonstrated that topical instillation of steroids produces significantly greater reduction of neutrophils infiltrating the cornea than does subconjunctival injection (53). Concurrent administration of topical and subconjunctival steroid has an additive effect and thus would be expected to demonstrate enhanced therapeutic efficacy in cases of severe anterior segment inflammation. Sub-Tenon, transseptal, and retrobulbar injections were shown to deliver significant sustained levels of drug to the posterior uvea, retina, optic nerve, and vitreous, although these routes were not directly compared (54–57).

The mechanism of steroid delivery into intraocular tissues is unclear. McCartney et al. (58) propose that in rabbits transscleral diffusion is the major route of penetration after subconjunctival or sub-Tenon injection and emphasize the importance of placing the corticosteroid immediately adjacent to the site of intraocular inflammation. More recent work comparing subconjunctival and retrobulbar injection of dexamethasone in the rabbit eye showed that hematogenous absorption was primarily responsible for drug delivery to the choroid, aqueous, and vitreous for both routes, whereas a combination of hematogenous and transcleral mechanisms was operative in drug delivery to the retina. Retrobulbar injections provided sustained long-term steroid levels whereas hematogenous delivery of dexamethasone following subconjunctival injection peaked earlier in the choroid and presumably in other ocular tissues (59).

TABLE 59-8. *Nonocular complications of corticosteroid therapy*

Endocrines
Adrenal insufficiency
Cushing's syndrome
Growth failure
Menstrual disorders
Neuropsychiatric
Pseudotumor cerebri
Insomnia
Mood swings
Psychosis
Gastrointestinal
Peptic ulcer
Gastric hemorrhage
Intestinal perforation
Pancreatitis
Musculoskeletal
Osteoporosis
Vertebral compression fractures
Aseptic hip necrosis
Myopathy
Cardiovascular
Hypertension
Sodium and fluid retention
Metabolic
Secondary diabetes mellitus
Hyperosmotic, hyperglycemic, nonketotic coma
Centripetal obesity
Hyperlipidemia
Dermatologic
Acne
Striae
Hirsutism
Subcutaneous tissue atrophy
Immunologic
Impaired inflammatory response
Delayed tissue healing

Therapeutic Use

Steroids are the most widely used antiinflammatory and immunosuppressant drugs in ophthalmology in general and are the mainstay of therapy for patients with uveitis. Ophthalmic indications for use of corticosteroids are shown in Table 7; these indications may be grouped into three broad therapeutic categories: (a) postoperative inflammatory control, (b) abnormalities of immune regulation, and (c) entities with a combined immune and inflammatory mechanism (16).

Our philosophy concerning the longitudinal care of patients with uveitis has been one of complete intolerance of recurrent or persistent inflammation, coupled with implementation of a stepladder algorithm for control of inflammation in an effort to limit permanent structural damage to the ocular structures critical to good vision. Although this goal may be difficult to achieve in selected cases, it is almost always attainable through use of this stepladder approach to the aggressiveness of therapy. This algorithm consists of (a) steroids (topical, regional, and systemic), (b) nonsteroidal antiinflammatory drugs (NSAIDs), (c) peripheral retinal cryopexy in selected patients with pars planitis, (d) systemic immunosuppressive chemotherapy, and (e) pars plana vitrectomy with intraocular steroid injection.

The diagnosis of active inflammation should be based solely on the presence of inflammatory cells in the anterior chamber or vitreous. Aqueous flare should never guide therapy because it represents vascular incompetence from the iris and ciliary body and is usually chronic. Although anterior chamber inflammatory cells are relatively easy to detect, their presence in the vitreous may be extremely difficult to discern. Eyes with chronic or recurrent iridocyclitis or posterior uveitis usually have vitreous pathology that includes the presence of cells, fibrin, and cellular aggregates trapped in vitreous fibrils and fibers. These cannot be eliminated even with the most aggressive antiinflammatory therapy. The clear spaces, or lacunae, in the vitreous are typically devoid of cells in patients with inactive uveitis. Therefore, the diagnosis of active anterior vitreal inflammation is made by careful biomicroscopic examination of the lacunae for the presence of inflammatory cells and by an evaluation of the vitreous exudates, or "snowballs." (Sharp borders and no change with time are characteristic of old, inactive fixed clumps of material, whereas hazy edges of the exudates are more characteristic of acute inflammatory material.)

Topical steroids alone are usually effective in the management of anterior segment inflammation and have little activity against intermediate or posterior uveitis in the phakic eye. The anterior uveitides comprise a heterogenous group of diseases which include idiopathic anterior uveitis, traumatic and postoperative iritis, HLA-B27–associated diseases, lens-induced uveitis, juvenile rheumatoid arthritis, sclerouveitis, keratouveitis, Behçet's disease, and anterior chamber inflammatory "spillover" from primarily posterior segment disease. Although topical steroids are the first rung in the antiinflammatory stepladder for most of these entities, important exceptions include ocular inflammation associated with Behçet's disease, Wegener's granulomatosis, polyarteritis nodosa, relapsing polychondritis with renal involvement, sympathetic ophthalmia, Vogt-Koyanagi-Hadara (VKH) syndrome, and rheumatoid arthritis, in which systemic immunosuppression, alone or in combination with systemic steroids, is mandatory first-line treatment (50,60).

A sensible approach to the use of topical steroids in anterior uveitis is to treat the patient aggressively with a potent agent during the initial stage of inflammation, to reevaluate the patient at frequent intervals, and to taper the drug slowly, as dictated by the clinical response. In very severe cases of anterior uveitis, prednisolone acetate 1% or dexamethasone alcohol 0.1% may be required hourly around the clock, together with periocular and/or oral corticosteroids as adjunctive therapy. Although corticosteroid ointments may be used at night in lieu of 24-hour dosing, these preparations are less potent than steroid drops. In addition, if steroid suspensions (e.g., prednisolone acetate) are used, the patient must be instructed to shake the bottle sufficiently with each administration to ensure delivery of maximal concentration of steroid. We prefer to avert this potential compliance problem (particularly when frequent dosing is required) by using steroid solutions (e.g., prednisolone phosphate).

We and other investigators (15), believe that most treatment failures with topical steroids are due to poor patient compliance, inadequate dosing, or abrupt or rapid tapering schedules. The latter two factors may be due in part to the reluctance of some clinicians to expose their patients unduly to potential steroid-induced ocular complications such as cataract formation and glaucoma. Ironically, the effort to do no harm, with less frequent dosing or a switch to a "softer" agent allows low-grade inflammation to continue, the long-term consequence of which is permanent ocular structural damage, (i.e., cystic macula). Again, the goal of therapy is control of intraocular inflammation. Aggressive antiinflammatory therapy, together with use of antiglaucomatous agents in the short term and with cycloplegic agents to keep the pupil dilated, may limit irreversible damage that even the most elegant surgical procedure cannot repair.

One must be prudent in applying topical corticosteroids in cases of anterior uveitis in which the etiology is suspected to be infectious, since these agents may potentiate the underlying disease. Active herpetic dendritic keratitis and uveitis associated with suspected fungal keratitis are contraindications to use of topical corticosteroids. The reactivation of herpes keratitis is potentiated by use of topical agents, a problem of particular importance in patients undergoing penetrating keratoplasty. Topical steroids should be used judiciously in patients with anterior uveitis associated with disciform keratitis or bacterial corneal ulcers and always in conjunction with appropriate antibiotic or antiviral "cover."

Topical corticosteroids are not particularly effective in treatment of Fuchs' heterochromic iridocyclitis and should be used sparingly, if at all, in cases of episcleritis and scleritis (NSAIDs are first-line treatment for most cases of simple, diffuse, or nodular scleritis; immunosuppressive chemotherapy for scleritis that is necrotizing or associated with collagen vascular disease). Chronic flare associated with juvenile rheumatoid arthritis-associated iridocyclitis, as in any case of anterior uveitis, regardless of etiology, should never be an indication for treatment. Reflexive administration of topical steroids in the aforementioned instances merely increases the risk of steroid-induced ocular morbidity.

Because topical steroids penetrate the posterior segment poorly, they are ineffective in treatment of intermediate and posterior uveitis. Periocular corticosteroid injection (subconjunctival, anterior or posterior sub-Tenon, transseptal, and retrobulbar) is effective in such instances, particularly in unilateral cases, providing rapid delivery of high concentrations of drug to the site of inflammation. In cases of severe anterior uveitis, subconjunctival or anterior sub-Tenon injection of corticosteroid serves as a useful adjunct to topical therapy, maximizing the concentration of drug in the anterior segment. The purported superiority of posterior sub-Tenon versus transseptal versus retrobulbar administration for posterior segment inflammation has yet to be established; the choice of delivery is largely one of individual preference, with each route having its own particular advantage.

Retrobulbar injection, while providing high concentrations of drug to the posterior segment, poses the risk of inadvertent penetration of the globe, optic nerve, or both. Posterior sub-Tenon injection by the temporal approach as initially described by Schlaegel (61) and as detailed by Smith and Nozik (62) decreases the potential for ocular penetration and places the medication in contact with the sclera in the region of the macula. Indeed, proximity of repository steroid to the macular area has been shown to correlate with an improvement in macular function (63). We prefer the transseptal approach because it obviates the risk of ocular penetration, is better tolerated, and delivers high concentration of drug to the desired location. Steroid is thoroughly mixed with local anesthetic in a 3-ml syringe with a 30-gauge, $\frac{5}{8}$-inch needle. The patient is instructed to look superonasally, the globe is elevated above the inferior orbital rim with the nondominant index finger, and the needle is introduced between the globe and the lateral third of the orbital margin and advanced to the hub through the lower lid and orbital septum. A quick wiggle of the syringe assumes one, in the absence of any globe movement, of nonpenetrance of the globe. Steroid is then injected quickly to avoid precipitation, and mild pressure is held over the closed lid for approximately 2 minutes. To monitor any adverse reactions, the patient is observed for at least 1 hour if the injection is given in an outpatient setting, and a mild analgesic is administered as needed. As opposed to the posterior sub-Tenon method, in which a side-to-side circumferential motion of the needle is required to verify the proper location of the needle tip between Tenon's capsule and the sclera, no such movement is necessary with the transseptal approach, as the clinician is aware, tactilely, of the location of the needle tip beneath the globe. Although premedication with topical anesthesia such as proparacaine or tetracaine is sufficient for adults, periocular injection in children and infants usually requires general anesthesia.

Corticosteroids available for periocular injection are shown in Table 4; they range from short-acting preparations (methylprednisolone sodium succinate) to long-acting depots (methylprednisolone acetate or Depo-Medrol). Postinjection glaucoma syndrome is a potential hazard after sub-Tenon repository steroid injections which, in certain cases, may require surgical excision of the depot. In clinical practice, however, the occurrence of this complication after posterior sub-Tenon injection (rather than subconjunctival or anterior sub-Tenon injection) is distinctly uncommon, even in steroid responders (62). Nevertheless, we do not generally use depot preparations unless prior treatment with steroid drops and transseptal injections has not been associated with increase in IOP and shorter-action regional steroids have been only transiently effective. We prefer the aqueous suspension of triamcinolone acetonide (Kenalog) in a concentration of 40 mg/ml. This formulation has little tendency to cause scar formation, extraocular muscle fibrosis, or hypersensitivity to the vehicle (62).

After periocular injection with triamcinolone, a treatment effect is usually apparent in 2 to 3 days. Injections may be repeated every 2 to 4 weeks, as dictated by the clinical response. We administer a maximum of four injections in an 8 to 10-week period before declaring a treatment failure. Periocular injections are contraindicated in patients with uveitis associated with toxoplasmosis and in patients with necrotizing scleritis.

Systemic corticosteroids are used when, in the clinician's judgment, the inflammatory response is of such severe degree that it warrants this therapeutic approach, usually in cases of bilateral sight-threatening uveitis or in patients with severe unilateral disease who have failed or are intolerant of periocular injections. Although steroids in general remain the first-line agents for treatment of intraocular inflammatory disease, important exceptions exist which require immunosuppressive chemotherapy, alone or in combination with systemic steroids.

Our tolerance for the use of systemic steroids is extremely limited because of our experience (64), and the experience of other investigators with the highly undesirable effects of their prolonged use. Except in patients with steroid-dependent sarcoidosis, it is extremely unusual for us to continue administering systemic steroids for longer than 6 months. As we do when we initiate topical or periocular therapy, we inform the patient regarding the prognosis, duration, and potential side effects of systemic steroid administration for a given diagnosis.

The initial dosage and duration of treatment with systemic steroids depends on the nature and severity of the inflammatory disease and the clinical response. Gordon's (66) very early dictum, "use enough, soon enough, to accomplish the goal of complete suppression of inflammation, then taper and discontinue," is as sound today as it was in the early 1950s. Indeed, using too little, too late, and then gradually increasing the dose of steroids generally produces little benefit and potentiates adverse side effects.

Accordingly, we initiate therapy with 1.0 to 2.0 mg/kg of prednisone daily as a single morning dose, a regimen which is easily tolerated and produces less suppression of the HPA axis than do divided dose schedules. Other researchers advocate splitting the initial dose to enhance its therapeutic efficacy or dividing it in four (dosing every 6 hours) to facilitate a rapid taper if treatment is given for less than 2 weeks (62). Prednisone and triamcinolone are the preferred preparations because they offer maximal flexibility required for uveitis therapy by virtue of their antiinflammatory potency, their intermediate duration of action, and the lack of sodium-retaining activity in the latter.

This relatively high dose is maintained, barring untoward complications, for a short (7 to 14 days) time until a clinical response is noted. A slow and steady taper is then begun at a rate dictated by the clinical condition so that a recurrence of inflammation is not precipitated, until a dose of 20 mg/day prednisone is reached. Some patients require only a periodic short course of systemic steroids, but others require more protracted therapy. In the latter, if inflammatory quiescence has been achieved at the 20-mg/kg level, we frequently use an alternate-day dosage schedule, as described by Fauci (67). The daily maintenance dose of 20 mg/kg is doubled to 40 mg/kg every other day (q.o.d.), continued for at least 2 weeks, after which time it is further tapered to 30 mg q.o.d. for 2 more weeks. If there is no further recurrence of inflammation, the dose is reduced to 20 mg q.o.d. for 2 weeks, with continued tapering on an every-other-week basis to 15 mg q.o.d., 10 mg q.o.d., 7.5 mg q.o.d., and 5 mg q.o.d., after which time the drug is discontinued. Alternate-day therapy produces less severe and fewer steroid-induced side effects and does not disturb the HPA axis (19). Adrenal suppression is possible, however, and as with any long-term steroid regimen, the medication should never be abruptly discontinued owing to the risk of precipitating an Addisonian crisis.

When long-term therapy with systemic corticosteroids is anticipated, another useful approach entails addition of a second steroid-sparing agent. This strategy reduces the total amount of steroid required to maintain quiescence or to prevent inflammatory recurrence. We frequently use azathioprine or oral NSAIDs to this end; the latter have been shown to reduce ocular inflammation after cataract extraction and may help reduce cystoid macular edema (68). Systemic steroids combined with cyclosporine have also been shown to be effective in the treatment of noninfectious endogenous uveitis of various etiologies (69,70).

Finally, intravenous pulse steroid therapy is an alternative to daily therapy in patients with severe, bilateral, sight-threatening posterior uveitis. Patients receiving such treatment must undergo a thorough medical evaluation before pulse therapy is initiated because serious side effects such as perforation of a peptic ulcer, systemic hypertension, aseptic necrosis of the hip, and even sudden death have been reported (71). Pulse therapy may induce a rapid and prolonged therapeutic effect while avoiding some of the chronic side effects associated with daily therapy. A commonly used regimen consists of intravenous methylprednisolone 1 g/day for 3 days, repeated as frequently as once a month (72).

Patients treated with systemic steroids, particularly those receiving long-term therapy, in contrast to those receiving concomitant NSAIDs, are at risk of gastritis, GI mucosal ulceration, and bleeding. To prevent such side effects, patients should be instructed to take oral steroids with milk, food, antacids, or gastric mucosal coating material such as Carafate (sucralfate) and to take calcium supplements to reduce the drug's calcium-leeching effects. In treating patients with a past or current history of such symptoms we add an H_2 receptor blocker such as Zantac (ranitidine hydrochloride), and we add Cytotec (misoprostol) to the regimen of any patient with a documented history of peptic ulcer disease or any patient receiving concurrent NSAID therapy.

Systemic corticosteroids are absolutely contraindicated in patients with known or suspected systemic fungal infections and a known hypersensitivity to the components of the steroid formulation (73). As with topical or periocular therapy, systemic steroids should be avoided in patients in whom an infectious etiology for intraocular inflammation has not been adequately excluded or appropriately covered with antimicrobial therapy. Examples are ocular syphilis, toxoplasmosis, herpes, candidiasis, and tuberculosis, in which disease activity is reactivated or exacerbated by systemic steroids alone. In addition, use of systemic steroids before diagnostic vitrectomy in patients in whom intraocular lymphoma is suspected may confound cytologic interpretation and delay the diagnosis because steroids are cytotoxic to lymphoma cells (74). Other relative contraindications to systemic steroid therapy are severe cardiovascular (hypertension, congestive heart failure), psychiatric (depression, previous psychosis), GI (active peptic ulcer disease), metabolic (poorly controlled diabetes mellitus), musculoskeletal (osteoporosis) disease, and pregnancy (73).

Side Effects and Toxicity

Corticosteroid therapy produces both ocular and systemic side effects irrespective of the route of administration. Although after topical or periocular administration may result in significant systemic absorption, untoward systemic complications are far more likely after oral or parenteral therapy, and their frequency is both dose and duration dependent. These are shown in Table 8 and are discussed in the Clinical Pharmacology section.

In our experience in the care of 402 patients with ocular inflammatory disease treated with systemic corticosteroids alone or in combination with immunosuppressive agents, neuropsychiatric and endocrine side effects were the most common complications attributed to prednisone and were reversible. It is noteworthy that 17 of these patients developed pathologic fractures involving the hip and spine (64).

The most clinically significant ocular complication of corticosteroid therapy is development of cataract and secondary glaucoma. Other important side effects produced by all routes of corticosteroid administration include mydriasis, ptosis, susceptibility to infection, and impaired wound healing (Table 9).

Secondary open-angle glaucoma is most likely to occur after prolonged topical therapy with potent steroids. In one study, approximately 30% of normal volunteers treated for 6 weeks with topical betamethasone had an IOP of 20 mm Hg or more, and 4% had IOP greater than 31 mm Hg (75). IOP usually returns to baseline values within 2 weeks after drug discontinuation. A more pronounced steroid-induced IOP increase is noted in patients with open-angle glaucoma, diabetics, and high myopes (76). The increase in IOP may occur as early as 1 week or may be delayed for years after the initiation of therapy; therefore all patients

TABLE 59-9. *Ocular complications of topical, periocular, and systemic corticosteroid therapy*

Topical
Blurred vision
Allergy to vehicle
Punctate keratopathy
Paralysis of accommodation
Potentiation of collagenase
Altered corneal thickness
Anterior uveitis
Periocular
Globe penetration
Proptosis
Atrophy and fibrosis of extraocular muscles and periorbita
Central retinal artery occlusion
Hemorrhage
Optic nerve injury
Limbal dellen, cosmesis
Systemic
Myopia
Pseudotumor cerebri
Exophthalmia
Central serous chorioretinopathy
Common to all routes
Glaucoma
Cataract
Susceptibility to infection
Impaired wound healing
Mydriasis
Ptosis

treated with corticosteroid medications should be monitored periodically. The exact mechanism for this phenomenon is unclear; however, evidence shows that corticosteroids enhance the deposition of mucopolysaccharide in the trabecular meshwork (77). Although some topical preparations such as FML and HMS are less apt to produce an increase in IOP, their poor corneal penetration makes them less suitable for treatment of intraocular inflammation than are more potent steroids (described in the Pharmacokinetics section). Intractable glaucoma may result after repository steroid injections, requiring surgical excision of the depot (described in the Therapeutics section).

Posterior subcapsular cataracts (PSC) arise in a dose- and duration-dependent manner after long-term corticosteroid therapy, although individual susceptibility appears to vary. Children and patients with diabetes are more prone to develop this complication (78). In one study of patients treated with systemic prednisone for rheumatoid arthritis for 1 to 4 years, 11% treated with 10 to 15 mg/day developed cataracts, as did 78% of those receiving more than 16 mg/day (79). In another study, 50% of patients treated with topical steroids after undergoing keratoplasty for keratoconus developed PSC after receiving 765 drops of 0.1% dexamethasone in 10.5 months (80). Once established, the opacity is generally not reversible. However, regression of PSC has been reported in children after therapy is discontinued (78). The mechanism of corticosteroid-induced cataract formation is believed to involve the binding of glucocorticoids to lens fibers, leading to biochemical alterations with protein aggregation in the cells and a change in the refractive index (81).

Susceptibility to microbial infections is enhanced by corticosteroids, since these agents suppress the inflammatory response. Herpetic, bacterial (particularly pseudomonal), and fungal keratitis may be potentiated by corticosteroid therapy unless the appropriate antiviral or antibiotic is administered concomitantly. Likewise, posterior segment inflammatory conditions such as ocular syphilis, tuberculosis, and toxoplasmosis should always be treated with appropriate anti-infective agents before corticosteroid treatment is instituted.

Corneal epithelial and stromal healing is inhibited by all corticosteroids, with the possible exception of medroxyprogesterone. Manifestations may be as trivial as superficial punctate staining of the cornea to relentless corneal-scleral melting and perforation. Corticosteroids retard collagen synthesis by fibroblasts (82) and enhance collagenase activity (83). Cognizance of the effects of steroids on wound healing is particularly important in the presence of corneal-scleral ulceration or thinning or minor trauma and during the postoperative period.

Mild mydriasis and ptosis are more often common complications of topical steroids therapy (84). Increase in the pupillary diameter of 1 mm may be observed as early as 1 week after initiation of therapy, with return to normal diameter when steroid treatment is discontinued. Agents in the vehicle mixture rather than the steroids themselves have been suggested to mediate these effects (85).

After topical therapy, paradoxical anterior uveitis may be induced by the corticosteroid itself rather than the vehicle (86). The incidence is apparently greater in blacks than in whites (87), with patients presenting with signs and symptoms typical of acute iritis which abate once the steroid is discontinued. The development of corticosteroid-induced uveitis has been suggested to be related to an activation of latent spirochetes in the eye, although no direct proof substantiates this (18).

Other side effects of topical steroid therapy such as blurred vision and punctate keratopathy may relate to ocular irritation arising from mechanical effects of the steroid particles in suspension, allergy to the vehicle, or the underlying inflammatory condition. In addition, refractive changes, paralysis of accommodation, and altered corneal thickness have been reported (88). Central serous retinopathy has been reported in association with systemic steroid therapy (89), whereas pseudotumor cerebri, especially in children, may occur after abrupt discontinuation or reduction of therapy (90).

Periocular injection of steroids has side effects and complications unique to the mode of delivery in addition to those previously described for the drugs themselves. These are shown separately in Table 9 and include the following: (a) inadvertent penetration of the globe, (b) proptosis, (c) subdermal fat atrophy and fibrosis of the extraocular muscles and surrounding periorbital tissues, (d) central retinal artery obstruction from drug embolization, (e) subconjunctival or retrobulbar hemorrhage after anterior and posterior injections respectively, (f) optic nerve injury from retrobulbar injection, (g) limbal dellen after anterior injections, and (h) unsightly white steroid repository after anterior injections in the palpebral fissure (62).

High-risk Groups

Corticosteroids are contraindicated in patients with systemic fungal infections or known hypersensitivity to the drug formulation and should be used with great caution in patients with a history of excessive alcohol consumption, oral steroid use, peptic ulcer disease, various infectious diseases, diabetes mellitus, severe hypertension or congestive heart failure, psychiatric problems, and osteoporosis. Postmenopausal women and the elderly receiving prolonged therapy with corticosteroids are at particularly high risk of developing osteoporosis and attendant serious complications such as compression fractures of the vertebral column. Alternate-day regimens in normal adults and dosage reduction to as little as 10 mg/day in the elderly are still associated with insidious osteopenia (91,92). Routine screening of such patients with thoracolumbar spine roentgenograms and consideration of adjunctive therapy with vitamin D, calcium and/or estrogen is appropriate (8,91).

Use of corticosteroids in children suppresses normal growth, retarding both epiphyseal maturation and long bone growth, which is particularly problematic during puberty, when epiphyseal closure is accelerated under the influence of sex hormones and may result in permanent loss in height (8). Inhibition or arrest of growth cannot be overcome with exogenous growth hormone.

Newborns of mothers who have received systemic corticosteroids during pregnancy, although not at increased teratogenic risk, should be monitored for adrenal insufficiency during the neonatal period. Furthermore, systemic corticosteroids are excreted in breast milk, placing infants who are breast fed at risk of growth retardation and suppression of endogenous steroid production (73).

Drug Interactions

Concurrent administration of medications that increase microsomal enzymes, such as phenobarbital, phenytoin, carbamazepine, ephedrine, and rifampin, decrease the pharmacologic effects of corticosteroids by enhancing their metabolism (8). Cholestyramine and antacids decrease the GI absorption of corticosteroids (73). On the other hand, erythromycin may impair elimination of methylprednisolone, whereas cyclosporine reduces the clearance of prednisone in renal transplant patients. Likewise, the dose of corticosteroids should be reduced when isoniazid and ketoconazole, which reduce steroid metabolism, or oral contraceptives, which increase protein binding and impair elimination are administered concurrently (73). Corticosteroids increase the clearance of salicylates and reduce the activity of anticholinesterases and antiviral eye preparations (93). Finally, corticosteroids diminish the effectiveness of anticoagulant therapy by either increasing or decreasing clotting (6).

Major Clinical Trials

Although the efficacy of corticosteroid therapy in the control of intraocular inflammation is tacitly accepted by most clinicians, few well-controlled, randomized clinical trials have clearly demonstrated a treatment effect, much less an optimal dosing regimen. Postoperative inflammation is probably the most common indication for topical steroid use today; however, early randomized, controlled trials failed to demonstrate a significant reduction in intraocular inflammation after uncomplicated intracapsular cataract extraction in eyes treated with topical steroids once to three times daily versus placebo (94,95). Suggesting that a treatment benefit might be demonstrable with more frequent dosing, Corboy (90) conducted a randomized, double-blind, multicenter clinical trial, in which topical betamethasone phosphate 0.1% was used five times daily for 2 weeks after uncomplicated intracapsular cataract extraction. This regimen was more effective than placebo in the reduction of postoperative inflammation with no ocular complications of corticosteroid treatment.

The efficacy of topical corticosteroids in the treatment of acute unilateral nongranulomatous anterior uveitis was evaluated by Dunne and Travers (96), who conducted a controlled, double-blind trial comparing betamethasone phosphate 0.1%, clobetasone butyrate 0.1%, and placebo. Both steroids were equivalent in improving clinical symptoms during the initial stage of treatment; however, only betamethasone phosphate was significantly better than placebo in reducing signs of inflammation.

Godfrey et al. (97) retrospectively evaluated the effectiveness of corticosteroids in the treatment of 173 patients with pars planitis who received either no therapy, topical steroids only, systemic steroids, or periocular steroids. Although their findings were inconclusive, periocular administration of steroids appeared to be efficacious in treatment of cystoid macular edema associated with pars planitis, with a 70% improvement in vision (97).

The first controlled, double-masked clinical trial in the United States that provided therapeutic success data for systemic corticosteroids was conducted by Nussenblatt et al. (70): 56 patients were randomized to treatment with either cyclosporine-A or prednisolone for severe, noninfectious uveitis. Therapeutic efficacy was remarkably similar for both treatment groups; however, improvement in visual acuity in either group was less than 50%. A subgroup of patients who had failed monotherapy with either drug were subsequently treated with a combination of steroid and cyclosporine, and some exhibited improvement in visual acuity (70).

Most recently, a 28-day double-masked, randomized, active-controlled, parallel group, multicenter study was conducted to evaluate the efficacy of a new soft steroid, remexolone 1% ophthalmic suspension, as compared with 1% prednisolone acetate in 160 patients with uveitis for whom topical steroid was indicated (98). Rimexolone 1% suspension was equivalent to 1% prednisolone acetate in controlling anterior chamber inflammation and increased IOP (increased 10 mm Hg or more as compared with baseline) was reported approximately 50% less frequently in the rimexolone-treated patients. This promising agent is currently undergoing phase III clinical trials.

REFERENCES

1. Hench PS, Kendall EC, Slocomb CH, et al. Effects of cortisone acetate and pituitary ACTH on rheumatoid arthritis, rheumatic fever, and certain other conditions: study in clinical physiology. *Arch Intern Med* 1950;85:545–666.
2. Gordon DM, McLean JM. Effects of pituitary adrenocorticotropine hormone (ACTH) therapy in ophthalmologic conditions. *JAMA* 1950;142:1271–1276.
3. Thygeson P. Historical observations on herpetic keratitis. *Surv Ophthalmol* 1976;21:82–90.
4. Gordon DM. Prednisone and prednisolone in ocular disease. *Am J Ophthalmol* 1956;41:593–600.

5. Leopold IH, Maylath F. Intraocular penetration of cortisone and its effectiveness against experimental corneal burns. *Am J Ophthalmol* 1952;42:1125–1134.
6. Haynes RC. Adrenocorticotropic hormone; adrenocorticotropic steroids and their synthetic analogs; inhibitors of the synthesis and actions of adrenocortical hormones. In: Gilman AG, Rall TW, Nies AS, Taylor P, eds. *Goodman and Gilman's the pharmacological basis of therapeutics.* New York: Pergamon Press, 1990;1431–1462.
7. Gallant C, Kenny P. Oral glucocorticoids and their complications: a review. *J Am Acad Dermatol* 1986;14:161–177.
8. Feldman SR. The biology and clinical application of systemic glucocorticoids. In: Callen JP, ed. *Current problems in dermatology.* St. Louis: Mosby-Year Book, 1992;211–234.
9. Southren LA, Dominguez MO, Gordon GG, et al. Nuclear translocation of cytoplasmic glucocorticoid receptor in the iris-ciliary body and adjacent corneoscleral tissue of the rabbit following topical administration of various glucocorticoids. *Invest Ophthalmol Vis Sci* 1983;24:147–152.
10. Tyrell JB, Baxter JD. Disorders of the adrenal cortex. In: Wyngaarden JB, Smith LH, Bennett JC, eds. *Cecil textbook of medicine.* Philadelphia: WB Saunders, 1992;1271–1279.
11. Melby JC. Clinical pharmacology of systemic corticosteroids. *Annu Rev Pharmacol Toxicol* 1977;17:511–527.
12. Wolverton SE. Glucocorticosteroids. In: Wolverton SE, Wilkin JK, eds. *Systemic drugs for skin diseases.* Philadelphia: WB Saunders, 1991;86–124.
13. Friedlander MH. Corticosteroid therapy of ocular inflammation. *Int Ophthalmol Clin* 1983;23:175–182.
14. Mondino BJ, Alfuss DH, Farley MK. Steroids. In: Lamberts DW, Potter DE, eds. *Clinical ophthalmic pharmacology.* Boston: Little, Brown, 1987;157–162.
15. Nussenblatt RB, Palestine AF. *Uveitis, fundamental and clinical practice.* Chicago: Year Book Medical Publishers, 1989;107–117.
16. Abelson MB, Butrus S. Corticosteroids in ophthalmic practice. In: Albert DM, Jakobiec FA, eds. *Principles and practice of ophthalmology: basic sciences.* Philadelphia: WB Saunders, 1994;1013–1022.
17. Leibowitz HM, Kupferman A. Anti-inflammatory medications. *Int Ophthalmol Clin* 1980;20:117–134.
18. Friend J. Physiology of the cornea: metabolism and biochemistry. In: Smolon G, Thoft RA, eds. *The cornea, scientific foundations and clinical practice.* Boston: Little, Brown, 1987;16–38.
19. Pavan-Langston D, Dunkel EL. *Handbook of ocular drug therapy and ocular side effects of systemic drugs.* Boston: Little, Brown, 1991;182–217.
20. Kroman HS, Leopold IL. Studies upon methyl- and fluoro-substituted prednisolones in the aqueous humor of rabbit. *Am J Ophthalmol* 1961;52:77–81.
21. Leopold IH, Gaster BN. Ocular inflammation and anti-inflammatory drugs. In: Kaufman HE, Barron BA, McDonald MB, Waltman SR, eds. *The Cornea.* New York: Churchill Livingstone, 1988; 67–79.
22. Murdick PW, Keates RH, Donovan EF, Wyman M, Short C. Ocular penetration studies. II. Topical administration of prednisolone. *Arch Ophthalmol* 1966;76:602–603.
23. Rosenblum C, Denglor RE, Geoffory RF. Ocular absorption of dexamethasone sodium phosphate disodium by the rabbit. *Arch Ophthalmol* 1967;77:234–237.
24. Hamashige S, Potts A. The penetration of cortisone and hydrocortisone into the ocular structures. *Am J Ophthalmol* 1955;40:211–216.
25. James RG, Stiles JF. The penetration of cortisol into normal and pathologic rabbit eyes. *Am J Ophthalmol* 1963;56:84–90.
26. Polansky JR, Weinres RN. Anti-inflammatory agents, steroids as anti-inflammatory agents. In: Sears ML, ed. *Pharmacology of the eye.* Berlin: Springer-Verlag, 1984;460–538.
27. Sugar J, Burde RM, Sugar A, et al. Tetrahydrotriamcinolone and triamcinolone. I. Ocular penetration. *Invest Ophthalmol Vis Sci* 1972; 11:890–893.
28. Soutaren AL, Altman K, Vittek J, Bonvik V, Gordon GG. Steroid metabolism in ocular tissues of the rabbit. *Invest Ophthalmol Vis Sci* 1976;15:222–228.
29. Cox WV, Kupferman A, Leibowitz HM. Topically applied steroids in corneal disease. I. The role of inflammation in stromal absorption of dexamethasone. *Arch Ophthalmol* 1972;88:308–313.
30. Kupferman A, Pratt MV, Suckewer K, Leibowitz HM. Topically applied steroids in corneal disease. III. The role of drug derivative in stromal absorption of dexamethasone. *Arch Ophthalmol* 1974;91: 373–376.
31. Kupferman A, Leibowitz HM. Topically applied steroids in corneal disease. IV. The role of drug concentration in stromal absorption of prednisolone acetate. *Arch Ophthalmol* 1974;91:377–380.
32. Kupferman A, Leibowitz HM. Topically applied steroids in corneal disease. V. Dexamethasone alcohol. *Arch Ophthalmol* 1974;92:329–330.
33. Kupferman A, Leibowitz HM. Topically applied steroids in corneal disease. VI. Kinetics of prednisolone phosphate. *Arch Ophthalmol* 1974;92:331–334.
34. Hull DS, Hine JE, Edelhauser HF, Hyndiuk RA. Permeability of isolated rabbit cornea to corticosteroids. *Invest Ophthalmol Vis Sci* 1974;13:457–459.
35. Olejnick O, Weisbecker CA. Ocular bioavailability of topical prednisolone preparations. *Clin Ther* 1990;12:2–11.
36. Musson DG, Bidgood AM, Olejnick O. Assay methodology for prednisolone, prednisone acetate, and prednisolone sodium phosphate in rabbit aqueous humor and ocular physiologic solutions. *J Chromatogr* 1991;565:89–102.
37. Musson DG, Bidwood AM, Olejnick O. An in vitro comparison of the permeability of prednisolone, prednisolone sodium phosphate, and prednisolone acetate across the NZW rabbit cornea. *J Ocul Pharmacol* 1992;8:139–150.
38. Liebowitz HM, Stewart RH, Kupferman A. Evaluation of dexamethasone acetate as a topical ophthalmic formulation. *Am J Ophthalmol* 1978;86:418–423.
39. Ballard PL. Delivery and transport of glucocorticoids to target cells. In: Baxter JD, Rousseau GG, eds. *Glucocorticoid hormone action.* Berlin: Springer-Verlag, 1979;25.
40. Apt L, Henrick A, Silverman LM. Patient compliance with the use of topical ophthalmic corticosteroid suspensions. *Am J Ophthalmol* 1979;87:210–214.
41. Leibowitz HM, Kupferman A. Kinetics of topically applied prednisolone acetate optimal concentration for treatment of inflammatory keratitis. *Arch Ophthalmol* 1976;94:1387–1389.
42. Leibowitz HM. Management of inflammation in the cornea and conjunctiva. *Ophthalmology* 1980;87:753–758.
43. Kupferman A, Leibowitz HM. Therapeutic effectiveness of fluoromethalone in inflammatory keratitis. *Arch Ophthalmol* 1975;93: 1011–1014.
44. Liebowitz HM, Kupferman A, Ryan WJ, et al. Corneal anti-inflammatory steroidal "soft drug." *Invest Ophthalmol Vis Sci* 1991;32 (suppl):735.
45. Laibowitz RA, Ghormley NR, Insler MS, et al. Treatment of giant papillary conjunctivitis with loteprednol etabonate, a novel corticosteroid. *Invest Ophthalmol Vis Sci* 1991;32(suppl):734.
46. Cox WV, Kupferman A, Leibowitz HM. Topically applied steroids in corneal disease. II. The role of the drug vehicle in stromal absorption of dexamethasone. *Arch Ophthalmol* 1972;88:549–552.
47. Schoenwald RD, Boltralik JS. A bioavailability comparison in rabbits of two steroid formulations as high viscosity gels and reference aqueous preparations. *Invest Ophthalmol Vis Sci* 1979;18:61–66.
48. Katz IM, Blackman WM. A soluble sustained-release artificial ophthalmic delivery unit. *Am J Ophthalmol* 1977;83:728–734.
49. Hwang DG, Stern WH, Hwang PH, et al. Collagen shield enhancement of topical dexamethasone penetration. *Arch Ophthalmol* 1989;107:1375–1380.
50. Hemady R, Tauber J, Foster CS. Immunosuppressive drugs in immune and inflammatory disease. *Surv Ophthalmol* 1991;35:369–385.
51. Cloes RS, Krohn DL, Breslin H, Braunstein R. Depo-Medrol in the treatment of inflammatory diseases. *Am J Ophthalmol* 1962;54: 407–411.
52. Wine NA, Gornall AG, Bass RP. The ocular uptake of subconjunctivally injected C14 hydrocortisone. Part I. Time and major route of penetration in a normal eye. *Am J Ophthalmol* 1964;58:362–366.
53. Leibowitz HM, Kupferman A. Periocular injection of corticosteroids. *Arch Ophthalmol* 1977;95:311–314.
54. Hyndiuk RA, Reagan MG. Radioactive depot corticosteroid penetration into monkey ocular tissue. I. Retrobulbar and systemic administration. *Arch Ophthalmol* 1968;80:499–503.

55. Hyndiuk RA. Radioactive depot corticosteroid penetration into ocular tissue. II. Subconjunctival administration. *Arch Ophthalmol* 1969;82:259–263.
56. Levine ND, Aronson SB. Orbital infusion of steroids in the rabbit. *Arch Ophthalmol* 1970;83:599–607.
57. Jennings T, Rusin MM, Tessler HH, Cunha-Vaz JG. Posterior sub-Tenon's injections of corticosteroids in uveitis patients with cystoid macular edema. *Jpn J Ophthalmol* 1988;32:385–391.
58. McCartney HJ, Drysdale JO, Gornal AG, Basu PK. An autoradiographic study of the penetration of subconjunctivally injected mydrocortisone into the normal and inflamed rabbit eye. *Invest Ophthalmol Vis Sci* 1965;4:247–302.
59. Bodker FS, Ticho BA, Feist RM, Lam TT. Intraocular dexamethasone penetration via subconjunctival or retrobulbar injections in rabbits. *Ophthalmic Surg* 1993;24:453–457.
60. Biswas J, Rao NA. Management of intraocular inflammation. In: Ryan SJ, ed. *Retina,* vol. 2. St. Louis: CV Mosby, 1989;139–146.
61. Schlaegel TF Jr. *Essentials of uveitis.* Boston: Little, Brown, 1969;41–42.
62. Smith RE, Nozik RA. *Uveitis: a clinical approach to diagnosis and management.* Baltimore: Williams & Wilkins, 1989;51–76.
63. Freeman WR, Green RL, Smith RE. Echographic localization of corticosteroids after periocular injection. *Am J Ophthalmol* 1987; 103:281–288.
64. Tamesis RR, Rodriguez A, Akova YA, Mesmer E, Foster CS. Systemic drug toxicity trends in immunosuppressive therapy of immune and inflammatory ocular disease. *Ophthalmology* 1996;(103):769–775.
65. Dave VK, Vickers CHF. Azathioprine in the treatment of mucocutaneous pemphigoid. *Br J Ophthalmol* 1974;90:183–186.
66. Gordon DM. Diseases of the uveal tract. In: Gordon DM, ed. *Medical management of ocular disease.* New York: Harper and Row, 1964;245–271.
67. Fauci AS. Alternate-day corticosteroid therapy. *Am J Med* 1978;64: 729–731.
68. Flach AJ. Cyclo-oxygenase inhibitors in ophthalmology. *Surv Ophthalmol* 1992;36:259–284.
69. Towler HMA, Whiting PH, Forrester JV. Combination low dose cyclosporine A and steroid therapy in chronic intraocular inflammation. *Eye* 1990;4:514–520.
70. Nussenblatt RB, Palestine AG, Chan LC, et al. Randomized double masked study of cyclosporine compared to prednisolone in the treatment of endogenous uveitis. *Am J Ophthalmol* 1991;112:138–146.
71. Bocanegra TS, Castaneda MD, Espinoza LR, et al. Sudden death after methylprednisolone pulse therapy. *Ann Intern Med* 1981;95:122.
72. Rosenbaum JT. Immunosuppressive therapy of uveitis. *Ophthalmol Clin North Am* 1993;6:167–175.
73. *AMA drug evaluations.* Chicago: American Medical Association, 1994;1871–1913.
74. Whitcup SM, de Smet MD, Rubin BI, et al. Intraocular lymphoma, clinical and histopathologic diagnoses. *Ophthalmology* 1993;100: 1399–1406.
75. Becker B. Intraocular pressure response to topical corticosteroids. *Invest Ophthalmol Vis Sci* 1965;4:198–205.
76. Hoskins HD Jr. Kass M. *Becker-Schaffer's diagnosis and therapy of the glaucomas.* St. Louis: CV Mosby, 1989;115–116.
77. Francois J. The importance of the mucopolysaccharides in intraocular pressure regulation. *Invest Ophthalmol Vis Sci* 1975;14:173–176.
78. Urban RC Jr, Cotlier E. Corticosteroid-induced cataracts. *Surv Ophthalmol* 1986;31:102–110.
79. Black RL, Oglesby RB, von Sallmann L, et al. Posterior subcapsular cataracts induced by corticosteroids in patients with rheumatoid arthritis. *JAMA* 1960;174:166–171.
80. Donshik PL, Cavanaugh HD, Boruchoff DA, et al. Posterior subcapsular cataracts induced by topical steroids following keratoplasty for keratoconus. *Ann Ophthalmol* 1981;13:29–32.
81. Rubin B, Palestine AG. Complications of corticosteroids and immunosuppressive drugs. *Int Ophthalmol Clin* 1989;29:159–171.
82. Ashton N, Cook C. Effect of cortisone on healing of corneal wounds. *Br J Ophthalmol* 1951;35:708–717.
83. Leopold IH. The steroid shield in ophthalmology. *Trans Am Acad Ophthalmol Otolaryngol* 1967;71:273–289.
84. Armaly MF. Effects of corticosteroids on intraocular pressure and fluid dynamics. I. The effect of dexamethasone in the normal eye. *Arch Ophthalmol* 1963;70:482–491.
85. Newsome DA, Wong UG, Cameron TP, Anderson RL. "Steroid-induced" mydriasis and ptosis. *Invest Ophthalmol Vis Sci* 1971; 10:424–429.
86. Krupin T, LeBlanc RP, Becker B, et al. Uveitis in association with topically administered corticosteroid. *Am J Ophthalmol* 1970;70: 883–885.
87. Martins JC, Wilensky JT, Asseth CF, et al. Corticosteroid induced uveitis. *Am J Ophthalmol* 1974;77:433–437.
88. Jaanus SD. Anti-inflammatory drugs. In: Bartlett JD, Jaanus SD, eds. *Clinical ocular pharmacology.* Boston: Butterworths, 1989; 163–197.
89. Wakakura M, Ishikawa S. Central serous chorioretinopathy complicating corticosteroid treatment. *Br J Ophthalmol* 1984;68:329–331.
90. Corboy JM. Corticosteroid therapy for the reduction of postoperative inflammation after cataract extraction. *Am J Ophthalmol* 1976;82:923–927.
91. Thomas TPL. The complications of systemic corticosteroid therapy in the elderly. *Gerontology* 1984;30:60–65.
92. Gluck OS, Murphy WA, Hahn TJ, Hahn B. Bone loss in adults receiving alternate-day glucocorticoid therapy: a comparison with daily therapy. *Arthritis Rheum* 1981;24:892–898.
93. Fraunfelder FT. *Drug-induced ocular side effects and drug interactions,* ed 3. Philadelphia: Lea & Febiger, 1989;321–328.
94. Burde RM, Waltman SR. Topical corticosteroids after cataract surgery. *Ann Ophthalmol* 1972;4:290–293.
95. Mustakallio A, Kaufman HE, Johnston G, Wilson RS, Roberts MD, Harter JC. Corticosteroid efficacy in postoperative uveitis. *Ann Ophthalmol* 1973;6:719–730.
96. Dunne JA, Travers JP. Double-blind clinical trial of topical steroids in anterior uveitis. *Br J Ophthalmol* 1979;63:762–767.
97. Godfrey WA, Smith RE, Kimura SJ. Chronic cyclitis: corticosteroid therapy. *Trans Am Ophthalmol Soc* 1976;74:178–187.
98. Foster CS, Drake M, Turner FD, et al. Efficacy and safety of 1% rimexolone ophthalmic suspension vs. 1% prednisolone acetate (Pred Forte) for treatment of uveitis. *Am J Ophthalmol* 1996; 122(2):171–182.
99. Shin DH, Kass MA, Kolker AE, et al. Positive FTA-Abs tests in subjects with corticosteroid induced uveitis. *Am J Ophthalmol* 1976;82:259–260.
100. Walker AE, Adamkiewicz JJ. Pseudotumor cerebri associated with prolonged corticosteroid therapy. *JAMA* 1964;188:779–784.

Textbook of Ocular Pharmacology,
edited by T.J. Zimmerman, et al.
Lippincott–Raven Publishers, Philadelphia © 1997.

CHAPTER 60

Mydriatic and Cycloplegic Agents

Albert Vitale and C. Stephen Foster

MYDRIATIC AND CYCLOPLEGIC AGENTS

Introduction, History, and Source

Topical cycloplegics and/or mydriatics have a broad spectrum of clinical utility in diagnostic ophthalmology and serve as important adjunctive medications in the management of anterior chamber inflammation. Specifically, these agents, when used in concert with appropriate antiinflammatory therapy, are effective in prevention and treatment of debilitating ocular inflammatory sequelae (i.e., pain arising from ciliary spasm, anterior and posterior synechiae, iris bombé, pupillary block, and secondary angle closure).

The most commonly used drugs fall into two broad categories: those with antimuscarinic activity (cholinergic antagonists such as atropine, scopolamine, homatropine, cyclopentolate, and tropicamide) and the α_1-adrenergic agonists (i.e., phenylephrine). Because the mechanism of action is different for each of the two categories, in clinical practice these medications are frequently used in combination to achieve maximal therapeutic efficacy; however, for the sake of discussion, each group is considered separately herein.

The naturally occurring belladonna alkaloids, atropine (DL-hyoscyamine) and scopolamine (hyoscine), are derived from the Solanaceae plants: *Atropa belladonna* and *Hyoscyamus niger,* respectively (1). The pharmacologic, medicinal, and toxic properties of these drugs have been well known since antiquity to maidens, physicians, and villains alike. The name belladonna reflects the alleged use of atropine by Italian women to dilate their pupils, thereby imparting to them a flattering, "wide-eyed" appearance, whereas in the Middle Ages these drugs were the agents of choice of professional poisoners (2). Since the isolation of pure atropine by Mein in 1831 (1), the inhibitory effects of the belladonna alkaloids on the actions of acetylcholine (ACh) in the brain, heart, smooth muscle, and glands have been well characterized. In ophthalmology, these agents have been used since the middle of the 19th century to facilitate examination of the posterior segment and to paralyze accommodation so that a true estimate of the eye's total refractive power could be made (3). Since then, many semisynthetic congeners (homatropine) of the belladonna alkaloids and synthetic antimuscarinic compounds (cyclopentolate and tropicamide) have been prepared, primarily with the objective of providing adequate mydriasis and/or cycloplegia together with a faster onset, a relatively shorter duration of action, and a reduced side-effect profile as compared with their naturally occurring counterparts. Cyclopentolate was introduced into clinical practice in 1951 (4), and tropicamide became available for ocular use in 1959 (5). Phenylephrine, a synthetic sympathomimetic amine, was introduced in 1936 principally as a vasoconstrictor and mydriatic (6,7).

A. Vitale: Retina Specialists of Boston and The Massachusetts Eye and Ear Infirmary, Harvard Medical School, Boston, Massachusetts 02214.

C. S. Foster: Immunology and Uveitis Service, The Massachusetts Eye and Ear Infirmary, Harvard Medical School, Boston, Massachusetts 02214.

Official Drug Name and Chemistry

The full chemical, nonproprietary names of the most frequently used topical mydriatic cycloplegic agents are shown in Table 1 along with the common trade names, manufacturers, and available formulations. The corresponding structural formulas of these drugs are shown in Fig. 1.

The naturally occurring belladonna alkaloids atropine and scopolamine are organic esters formed by the combination of a tropic acid, an aromatic acid, and complex organic bases, either scopine or tropine (1). The intact ester of tropine and tropic acid and a free hydroxyl (OH) group in the acid portion of the ester are important for antimus-

TABLE 60-1. *Mydriatic-cycloplegic agents*

Generic name/trade name		Concentration (%)
Atropine SO_4		
Atropine Sulfate Ophthalmic	(Various)	Ointment (1)
Atropine Sulfate S.O.P.	(Allergan, Irvine, CA)	Ointment (0.5, 1)
Atropair	(Texas)	Solution (1)
Atropine-Care	(Akorn, Abita Springs, CA)	Solution (1)
Atropisol	(Iolab, Claremont, CA)	Solution (0.5, 1, 2)
Isopto Atropine	(Alcon, Fort Worth, TX)	Solution (0.5, 1, 3)
Ocuo Tropine	(Ocumed, Roseland, NJ)	Solution (1)
Scopolamine HBr		
Isopto Hyoscine	(Alcon)	Solution (0.25)
Homatropine HBr		
Homatropine Ophthalmic	(Various)	Solution (5)
AK-Homatropine	(Akorn)	Solution (5)
Isopto Homatropine	(Alcon)	Solution (2.5)
Cyclopentolate HCl		
Cyclogel	(Akorn)	Solution (0.5, 1, 2)
AK-Pentolate	(Akorn)	Solution (0.5, 1)
Ocu-Pentolate	(Ocumed)	Solution (1)
Pentolair	(Texas)	Solution (1)
Cyclopentolate HCl and phenylephrine HCl		Solution (1)
Cyclomydril	(Akorn)	Solution (0.2)
Tropicamide		
Mydriacil	(Alcon)	Solution (0.5, 1)
Mydriafair	(Texas)	Solution (0.5, 1)
Ocu-Tropic	(Ocumed)	Solution (0.5)
Tropicacyl	(Akorn)	Solution (0.5)
Phenylephrine HCl		
Ak-Dilate	(Akorn)	Solution (2.5, 10)
Dilatair	(Texas)	Solution (2.5)
Mydrifin	(Alcon)	Solution (2.5)
Neo-Synephrine	(Sanofi Winthrop, New York, NY)	Solution (2.5, 10)
Ocu-Phrin	(Ocumed)	Solution (2.5, 10)
Phenylephrine HCl	(Iolab)	Solution (2.5, 10)

carinic activity. These tertiary ammonium compounds penetrate the blood–brain barrier (BBB) well, with scopolamine providing more significant CNS effects than atropine (6). Homatropine is a semisynthetic antimuscarinic agent produced by the combination of mandelic acid with the base, tropine (1). The addition of a second methyl group to nitrogen results in the corresponding quaternary ammonium derivatives, methylatropine nitrate, methscopolamine bromide, and homatropine methylbromide, which, while exhibiting reduced CNS permeability, produce significant nicotinic blocking activity and are of little value in ophthalmology (1,6). In contrast, the synthetic congeners cyclopentolate and tropicamide are structurally very different from the natural alkaloids (Fig. 1) and are indispensable in ophthalmic practice due to their rapid onset and relatively short duration of action.

Phenylephrine is a synthetic analogue of epinephrine. It differs from epinephrine only in lacking an OH group in the number 4 position on the benzene ring (1). Its potency as an α-adrenoceptor agonist is less than that of epinephrine.

Pharmacology

Anticholinergic drugs block the actions of ACh and other cholinergic agonists by competing for a common binding site on the muscarinic receptor. This antagonism may be overcome by sufficiently increasing the concentration of ACh at the receptor site of the target tissue. Although three subtypes of muscarinic receptor have been identified pharmacologically (M_1 in sympathetic ganglia and cerebral cortex, M_2 in cardiac muscle, and M_3 in smooth muscle and various glands) and five structural variants have been established by molecular cloning techniques, the anticholinergic agents used in ophthalmology are nonselective (1). Antimuscarinic drugs have little action at the neuromuscular junction except at very high concentrations; however, they may exert significant effects in sympathetic ganglia, which contain the M_1 muscarinic receptor subtype (6).

Adrenergic mydriatics such as phenylephrine act directly on α_1-adrenoceptors but have little or no effect on β-adrenoceptors. A minor component of its pharmacologic

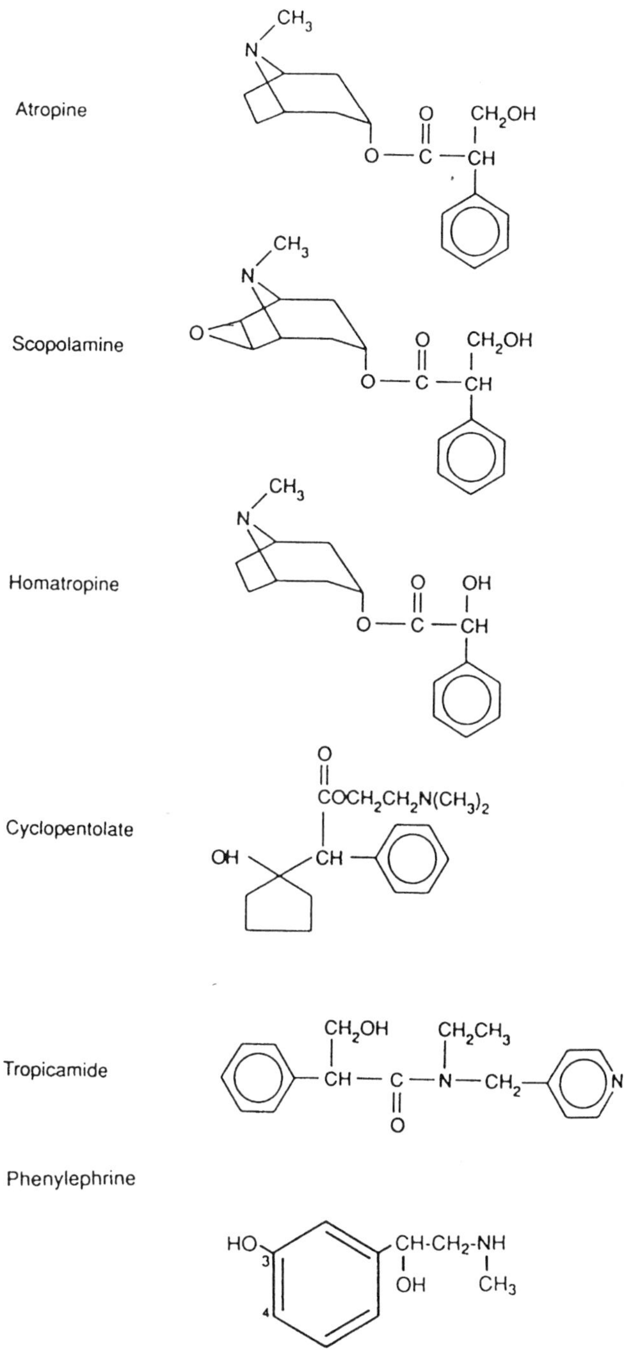

Atropine

Scopolamine

Homatropine

Cyclopentolate

Tropicamide

Phenylephrine

FIG. 60-1. Structural formulas of atropine, scopolamine, homatropine, cyclopentolate, tropicamide, and phenylephrine.

action, as opposed to that of hydroxyamphetamine, may be due to the release of norepinephrine (NE) from presynaptic adrenergic nerve terminals (1).

Clinical Pharmacology

General systemic effects of antimuscarinic drugs relate to the site of parasympathetic neuroeffector inhibition at various organs and include vasoconstriction; decreased sweating; bronchial, salivary, and gastric secretion; inhibition of cardiac vagal tone with tachycardia; CNS depression; and decreased gastric and urinary bladder tonus (1). Ocular effect are mediated by the blockage of postganglionic parasympathetic innervation to the longitudinal muscle of the ciliary body and the iris sphincter, with consequent cycloplegia and mydriasis, respectively. In addition, topically applied anticholinergic agents produce conjunctival and uveal arteriole dilation and reduced permeability of the blood–aqueous barrier (8).

The major systemic consequence of direct activation of α_1-adrenoceptors in vascular smooth muscle (VSM) is increased peripheral vascular resistance and increased blood pressure (BP) (1). In the eye, phenylephrine acts on α-adrenoceptors on the sympathetically innervated iris dilator muscle, arterioles, and Muller's muscle to produce pupillary dilation without cycloplegia, vasoconstriction, and lid elevation (8).

The relative potencies of the commonly used topical antimuscarinic and adrenergic agents, as reflected by the onset of and recovery from mydriasis and cycloplegia, are listed in descending order in Table 2. In general, mydriasis occurs more rapidly, persists longer, and can be achieved at lower concentrations with the anticholinergic agents (6).

The ocular effects of topical atropine, the most potent cycloplegic and mydriatic agent, were first systematically studied by Feddersen in 1844 (9). Onset of mydriasis was observed within 12 minutes of topical application of 1 drop of a 1% solution, reaching a maximum in 26 minutes, with recovery of preinstillation pupillary size by day 10. Cycloplegia began in 12 to 18 minutes and peaked at 160 minutes; full accommodative recovery was achieved by day 8. Although a single drop of atropine may have a prolonged mydriatic/cycloplegic effect in an otherwise healthy patient, eyes with active intraocular inflammation are much more resistant to atropinization and may require more frequent instillation (two to three times daily) together with supplemental 10% phenylephrine to achieve adequate mydriasis (2).

Individual variation in response to topical atropine administration is also related to iris pigmentation; mydriasis and cycloplegia have slower onset and longer duration in patients with dark irides than in those with light irides (2,10). Pigment binding is believed to reduce the bioavailability of initially administered atropine while providing a prolonged release effect of accumulated drug over time to the muscarinic receptors of the iris and ciliary body.

Scopolamine differs from atropine in that it exerts a more potent antimuscarinic action on the iris, ciliary body, secretory glands, and CNS on a weight basis and has a shorter duration of mydriasis and cycloplegia than atropine at dosage levels used clinically (11). After instillation of 0.5% solution of scopolamine, maximal pupillary dilation occurred by 20 minutes and was sustained for 90 minutes and with pupils recovered to preinstillation size by day 8.

TABLE 60-2. *Potency of Mydriatic-Cycloplegic Agents*

Drug	Strength (%)	Mydriasis Maximal (min)	Mydriasis Recovery (days)	Cycloplegia Maximal (hr)	Cycloplegia Recovery (days)
Atropine	1.0	30–40	7–10	1–3	7–12
Scopolamine	0.5	20–30	3–7	$\frac{1}{2}$–1	5–7
Homatropine	1.0	40–60	1–3	$\frac{1}{2}$–1	1–3
Cyclopentolate	0.5–1.0	30–60	1	$\frac{1}{2}$–1	1
Tropicamide	0.5–1.0	20–40	$\frac{1}{4}$–1	$\frac{1}{2}$	$<\frac{1}{4}$
Phenylephrine	2.5–10	20–60	3–6	None	None

Adapted from Brown JH. Atropine, scopolamine and related antimuscarinic drugs. In: Gilman AG, Rall TW, Nies AS, Taylor P, eds. *Goodman and Gilman's the pharmacologic basis of therapeutics.* New York: Pergamon press, 1990;8:161.

Maximal cycloplegia was achieved by 40 minutes, with accommodative recovery by day 3 (12).

Homatropine is approximately one tenth as potent as atropine, with maximal mydriasis occurring within 40 minutes after topical instillation of a 1% solution and recovery in 1 to 3 days (13). Its cycloplegic activity is significantly less pronounced than that of atropine or scopolamine (Table 2).

The onset of maximal mydriasis and cycloplegia after topical administration of either 2 drops of a 0.5% solution or 1 drop of 1% solution of cyclopentolate in white patients has been shown to occur in 20 to 30 and 30 to 60 minutes, respectively, with full recovery of each by 24 hours (4). In contrast, instillation of similar concentrations of drug in black patients or white patients with dark irides produced less effective mydriasis and cycloplegia (13,14). In addition, cyclogel did not alter intraocular pressure (IOP) in normal eyes (14). Its usefulness as an adjunctive agent in management of intraocular inflammatory disease may be limited, however, as it has been shown to be a chemoattractant to inflammatory cells (15). Various other mydriatic agents, including atropine, homatropine, scopolamine, and tropicamide, failed to produce a similar dose-dependent increase in the migration of neutrophils when tested in vitro (16).

Tropicamide is the shortest-acting cycloplegic, with a greater mydriatic than cycloplegic effect (Table 2). It has been shown to provide adequate mydriasis for routine ophthalmoscopy at concentrations as low as 0.25% (17), and pupillary dilation appears to be independent of iris pigmentation (18). Maximum mydriasis has been shown to occur within 25 to 30 minutes of instillation of either a 0.5% or 1% solution, with recovery of preinstillation pupillary size by 6 hours (5). Cycloplegia was also achieved in 30 minutes; however, the effect appeared to be dose-related, with significant differences between the 0.25% and 1% solutions but not among the 0.5%, 0.75%, or 1% concentrations (19).

The mydriatic and cycloplegic efficacy of tropicamide has been compared to that of cyclopentolate, homatropine, and phenylephrine (5). The degree of mydriasis at 30 minutes after instillation of 0.5% or 1% tropicamide was greater than that produced by either 1% cyclopentolate, 5% homatropine, or 10% phenylephrine. Although the maximal cycloplegic action of 1% tropicamide at 30 minutes was more pronounced than that observed with 1% cyclopentolate or 5% homatropine, the effect was not sustained at later timepoints.

Phenylephrine produces maximal mydriasis, with virtually no cycloplegia, in 45 to 60 minutes, depending on the concentration used, with recovery from mydriasis in approximately 6 hours (20,21). Dose–response curves demonstrate an increased mydriatic effect with concentrations of phenylephrine to 5%, but little additional benefit at concentrations approaching 10% (22). Clinical studies comparing pupillary dilation with 1.5% and 10% preparations in patients selected at random and not controlled for age or iris color failed to demonstrate significantly greater mydriasis at the higher concentration of phenylephrine (23,24). Mydriasis varies with iris color and anterior chamber depth; blue eyes with shallow chambers are more responsive than deep chambers and dark irides (25). Finally, topical administration of phenylephrine has been shown to decrease IOP in both normal eyes and those with open-angle glaucoma, although the effect is less pronounced than that produced by epinephrine (26).

Pharmaceutics

The various dosage forms and manufacturers of the most commonly used mydriatic-cycloplegic agents are shown in Table 1. Prolonged exposure of phenylephrine solutions to air, light, or heat may cause oxidation and a consequent brown discoloration. To prolong the shelf life of phenylephrine, an antioxidant, sodium bisulfite, is frequently added to the vehicle, and refrigeration of the solution is recommended (11).

Pharmacokinetics and Metabolism

Topically applied mydriatic agents reach their targets in the eye by diffusing through the cornea, whereas they are absorbed systemically primarily through the conjunctival vessels and nasal mucosa. At a physiologic pH, the pKa values of atropine, homatropine, cyclopentolate, and tropicamide are 9.8. 9.9, 8.4, and 5.37, respectively. A predominance of nonionized molecules exists at lower pKa values, promoting greater diffusibility through the lipid layer of the corneal epithelium and thus greater bioavailability (11), which may explain the more rapid onset and shorter duration of action of tropicamide as compared with the other antimuscarinic drugs.

Prior instillation of a topical anesthetic enhances the mydriatic and cycloplegic effect of anticholinergic agents (27,28). Likewise, the mydriatic response of phenylephrine is facilitated by use of topical anesthetic agents (29). Moreover, these pharmacologic effects are amplified by trauma or procedures such as tonometry or gonioscopy, which can disturb corneal epithelial integrity (30). Gentle lid closure for 5 minutes after instillation of mydriatic drops not only prolongs corneal contact time, but also reduces the action of the nasolacrimal pump, thereby enhancing intraocular absorption while minimizing systemic access through the nasolacrimal duct (31).

The intraocular distribution of atropine has been studied after subconjunctival injection of radiolabeled drug in rabbits (32). Significant radioactivity was present in the cornea, aqueous, and vitreous, concentrations were lower in the iris, ciliary body, and retina 90 minutes after injection, and 75% of the radioactivity had dissipated from the eye in 5 hours.

Anticholinergic drugs are readily absorbed by the gastrointestinal (GI) tract and distributed throughout the body. Atropine has a $t_{\frac{1}{2}}$ of approximately 4 hours, with 50% of a single dose being hydrolyzed in the liver and the remainder excreted unchanged in the urine (1). Phenylephrine, in comparison, is rapidly conjugated and oxidized in the GI mucosa and liver, with only a small fraction being excreted in the urine of normal persons (33).

TABLE 60-3. *Clinical applications of mydriatic-cycloplegic agents*

Dilated funduscopy
Cycloplegic refraction
Pre- and Postoperative dilation
Anterior uveitis
Lysis of posterior synechiae
Secondary glaucomas
Associated with inflammation
Ciliary block glaucoma
Lens subluxation
Suppression of amblyopia
Accommodative esotropia
Diagnostic testing
Horner's syndrome
Provocative test for angle-closure glaucoma

Therapeutic Use

The clinical applications of mydriatic-cycloplegic agents in ophthalmology are numerous (Table 3), with drug selection depending on the indication and the degree of effect desired; e.g., tropicamide 1% alone may provide adequate dilation with minimal cycloplegia and thus obviate residual blurring of vision during routine funduscopic screening (34). However, reflex contraction of the iris sphincter due to exposure to light during prolonged ophthalmoscopy may require the addition of an adrenergic agent to achieve wide mydriasis. The combination of phenylephrine 2.5% and tropicamide 0.5% or 1% or cyclopentolate 0.5% in a single solution or separately is effective in achieving this end. It also provides adequate mydriasis in patients with dark irides and diabetes (who may respond poorly to topical anticholinergics alone) (35). In contrast, cycloplegia for refraction in children aged more than 5 years is often achieved by premedication with atropine 0.5% ointment or solution three times daily for 3 days preceding examination and once on the day of refraction. In adults, 1 drop of 1% cyclopentolate (2% in patients with dark irides) every 15 minutes for one to two doses is frequently sufficient to provide adequate cycloplegia (36).

In the management of uveitis, the choice of mydriatic-cycloplegic agent used in concert with appropriate antiinflammatory therapy depends on the nature, severity, location, and duration of inflammation. These agents are most often used in the presence of a clinically significant anterior chamber inflammatory response irrespective of the location of the primary disease focus (anterior vs. posterior uveitis). The principal goals of therapy include complete control of inflammation while limiting permanent ocular structural damage, specifically, prevention of anterior and posterior synechiae formation, iris and ciliary body blood vessel incompetence, secondary cataract, cystic macula, and phthisis bulbi.

Mydriatic-cycloplegic drugs are particularly valuable in both prevention of posterior synechiae, by keeping the pupil in motion until ocular inflammation has been controlled, and in disruption of synechiae that have already formed (37). The choice of agent, drug combination, frequency, and route of administration depends largely on the severity of uveitis and degree of intraocular pathology. Because the duration of action of mydriatic-cycloplegic agents varies between eyes and with the degree of inflammation, these choices must be made in the context of the individual patient. For example, in patients who present with very mild iridocyclitis and ocular discomfort, 1% tropicamide twice daily in combination with topical corticosteroids may suffice to relieve ciliary spasm without prolonged paralysis of accommodation. In contrast, frequent instillation of atropine 2% may be required in patients with severe ocular pain and a plasmoid anterior chamber. There is little evidence to support the efficacy of mydriatic-cycloplegic agents in reducing either inflammation itself or photophobia in patients with uveitis; rather, aggressive therapy with topical steroids is essential to their mitigation.

We prefer not to use long-acting agents such as atropine and scopolamine routinely, because these drugs cause prolonged paralysis of accommodation, do not keep the pupil moving, and may be associated with unpleasant CNS side effects (scopolamine). However, long-term dilation with these agents may be of value, even during periods of remission, in patients with chronic disease such as juvenile rheumatoid arthritis-associated iridocyclitis and sarcoidosis, in which inflammatory exacerbations are often frequent and severe and may occur without warning (37).

Use of cyclopentolate may be contraindicated in patients with uveitis, since it has been shown to be a chemoattractant to inflammatory cells in vitro (described in the Clinical Pharmacology section) (16). In moderate iridocyclitis, phenylephrine or tropicamide alone provide inadequate protection, because the attenuated mydriatic effect of these drugs is further reduced in the presence of inflammation.

Most cases of active iridocyclitis may be adequately treated supplementally with homatropine 5% at a frequency titrated to the anterior chamber inflammatory response (as much as 1 drop every 2 hours) (37). Alternatively, a combination of phenylephrine 2.5% and tropicamide 1% may be used in a similar fashion to move the pupil during anterior uveitis, or instilled, 1 drop every 20 minutes for three to four doses, to break recently formed or weak posterior synechiae (8). Phenylephrine 10% applied to the cornea, usually preceded by a topical anesthetic, has also been used to break recently formed posterior synechiae; however, this agent must be used with caution because of its potential to produce adverse cardiovascular effects (38). For more tenacious iridolenticular adhesions, frequent applications (one drop every 5 minutes) of a potent mydriatic-cycloplegic (atropine) may be tried.

Should synechialysis fail with the regimens already described, a cotton pledget soaked in a "dynamite cocktail" mixture of various dilating agents may be applied to the topically anesthetized eye in proximity to the area where the synechiae are most extensive and left in place for 10 to 15 minutes. We have successfully used a mixture of equal parts of cocaine 4%, epinephrine 1 : 1,000, and atropine 1%; other investigators have advocated a filtered mixture of 0.4% homatropine, 0.5% phenylephrine, and 1.0% proparacaine in 100 ml sterile water (37). With use of these mixtures, complete synechialysis may not be apparent until the following day. Finally, a small volume (0.25 ml) of the latter mixture may be injected subconjunctivally at the junction of the adhesion and the freely mobile pupil if synechiae still remain (37). Again, attention must be paid to potential untoward cardiovascular effects, particularly in elderly patients, because the mixture contains phenylephrine.

Side Effects and Toxicity

The adverse side effects resulting from topical administration of anticholinergic medications may be local, directly affecting the eye and ocular adnexa, or systemic, due to absorption through the conjunctival vessels and/or nasolacrimal duct.

Atropine

Systemic toxic effects of atropine are dose-dependent, with considerable variation between patients (1). A single drop of a 1% solution provides 0.5 mg drug (39); a lethal dose is contained in 200 drops for adults and in 20 drops for children (1). Signs and symptoms of atropine toxicity include fever, tachycardia, dermal flushing, dryness of the skin and mouth, irritability (the foregoing are particularly common in children), confusional psychosis (especially in the elderly), drowsiness, ataxia, urinary retention, convulsions, and even death (36). Systemic absorption of atropine or of any topically applied solution can be minimized by nasolacrimal occlusion or gentle lid closure for 5 minutes after instillation (described in the Pharmacokinetics section) (31).

The ocular and local side effects of topical atropine administration are numerous and clinically significant. Acute, chronic follicular and/or papillary conjunctivitis and contact dermatitis may arise from direct irritation or hypersensitivity to the drug preparation itself (2,11). Atropine, as well as other topical anticholinergic drugs, increases IOP pressure to some degree in 25% to 30% of eyes with open-angle glaucoma (40). This effect is transient, does not occur in normal eyes, and is believed to arise from a decreased facility of outflow associated with a loss of ciliary muscle tonus (2). In addition, these agents increase the risk of precipitating acute angle-closure glaucoma in eyes with anatomically narrow angles or a plateau iris configuration (25). Finally, atropine causes photophobia and blurred vision due to its prolonged mydriatic effect and paralysis of accommodation. Systemic administration of atropine in conventional doses (0.6 mg) has little ocular effect, but scopolamine in equivalent amounts can cause mydriasis and loss of accommodation (1).

Scopolamine

The ocular side effects of scopolamine are, with the exception of a shorter duration of action, almost the same as those of atropine. Although systemic effects after topical application are fewer, CNS toxicity appears to be more common, particularly in the elderly, with scopolamine use as compared with atropine use (41). Black children are apparently more sensitive to the systemic effect of scopolamine (39).

Homatropine

The side-effect profile of homatropine is indistinguishable from that of atropine (42). However, because it is a less potent drug with a shorter duration of action, it has one fiftieth of the toxicity of atropine and is tolerated in much larger doses than atropine (39). IOP increase in patients with open-angle glaucoma occurs more often with homatropine than with atropine or scopolamine (8).

Cyclopentolate

Transient stinging on instillation is the most common ocular side effect of cyclopentolate, occurring more frequently at higher concentrations (43). Other ocular reactions are similar to those described for atropine.

Likewise, the evolution of systemic toxicity after topical use of cyclopentate is dose-related and parallels that of atropine, except that cyclopentolate is associated with a high incidence of CNS side effects (39). These may occur at any age but occur more often in the very young and in the elderly. In children, CNS effects are particularly common with use of the 2% solution or after multiple instillations of 1% cyclopentolate and include ataxia, restlessness, memory loss, visual hallucinations, psychosis, disorientation, and irrelevant speech (44). Although these reactions are typically transient, possible serious neurologic sequelae may develop, including generalized seizures (45). In addition, GI dysfunction has been reported in premature infants after topical administration of either 1% or 0.5% cyclopentolate (46).

Tropicamide

Because of short duration of action, adverse ocular side effects are rare with topical application tropicamide but may include hypersensitivity reactions, blurred vision, angle-closure glaucoma in the anatomically predisposed, and a slight increase in IOP (8). For similar reasons, systemic toxicity is distinctly uncommon, although psychotic reactions, cardiorespiratory collapse, and a transient episode of unconsciousness and muscular rigidity in a child have been reported (47).

Anticholinergic Overdosage

Treatment of anticholinergic overdosage is both supportive and specific. Adequate hydration and measures to prevent hyperpyrexia may be combined with the specific antidote for CNS toxicity—physostigmine—if these symptoms are severe. A dose of 1 to 4 mg physostigmine salicylate in adults and 0.5 mg in children is administered parenterally and repeated every 15 minutes as necessary (1). Diazepam is a suitable alternative, providing both sedation and control of convulsions, if specific therapy is not available (39).

Phenylephrine

Local adverse reactions to topical phenylephrine include transient pain, lacrimation, keratitis, and allergic dermatoconjunctivitis (48,49). Angle-closure glaucoma in an anatomically predisposed eye, as well as a transient increase in IOP due to the release of pigment granules from the posterior surface of the iris epithelium with obstruction of the trabecular meshwork may occur after therapy with topical phenylephrine (50). This phenomenon is more common in older patients with dark irides and in those with pigment dispersion and pseudoexfoliation syndromes. Lid retraction may be observed because of the adrenergic effect of the drug on Muller's muscle. Rebound miosis has been reported in patients 24 hours after instillation of phenylephrine aged more than 50 years, with attenuation of the mydriatic response on subsequent dosing (22). Corneal stromal edema and endothelial toxicity may occur, particularly when phenylephrine is administered concomitantly with a topical anesthetic in corneas denuded of epithelium (51).

Systemic side effects occur more commonly when stronger concentrations, such as phenylephrine 10%, are instilled repeatedly (25). These reactions include the following: tachycardia, hypertension, reflex bradycardia, angina, ventricular arrhythmia, myocardial infarction, cardiac failure, cardiac arrest, and subarachnoid hemorrhage. Although the overall incidence of severe transient systemic hypertension observed in association with 10% phenylephrine may be low, infants and the elderly appear to be those most susceptible to its administration (52). Adverse cardiovascular effects can be avoided by using a 2.5% solution (48). The risk of systemic toxicity in neonates and infants can be reduced by decreasing the drop volume (53) or by using a solution containing cyclopentolate 0.2% and phenylephrine (Cyclomydril), which has been shown to achieve safe and effective mydriasis in premature infants (54).

High-risk Groups

Both anticholinergic and adrenergic mydriatics present a risk of angle-closure glaucoma in patients with anatomically narrow angles and in eyes with plateau iris configuration (25); therefore, long-acting agents such as atropine and scopolamine are contraindicated in such eyes and shorter-acting agents, including phenylephrine, should be used cautiously if at all. Hypersensitivity to other anticholinergic or adrenergic agents is an absolute contraindication to use of atropine, scopolamine, or phenylephrine.

Patients with Down's syndrome, keratoconus, spastic paralysis, brain damage, and light irides are particularly sensitive to the mydriatic and systemic side effects of anticholinergic drugs; atropine and scopolamine should be used judiciously in such patients (55).

Systemic reactions are more frequent after topical administration of both anticholinergic and adrenergic mydriatics in infants, children, and the elderly. These agents should be used at the minimal effective concentration and not more often than is absolutely necessary in such patients. Of the topical anticholinergic drugs, atropine, scopolamine, and cyclopentolate 2% (especially in children) are the most frequent offenders, with scopolamine and cyclopentolate associated with a preponderance of CNS toxicity in all age groups (36) (described in the Side Effects and Toxicity section).

Phenylephrine 10% should be used cautiously, if at all, in patients previously treated with atropine, those with coronary artery disease, systemic hypertension (especially those receiving reserpine, methyldopa, or guanethidine), orthostatic hypertension, insulin-dependent diabetes, or aneurysms and should be avoided in neonates and in the elderly (56–58). It has been suggested that patients at risk of undue increase in systemic BP or other adverse cardiovascular effects be monitored for 20 to 30 minutes after instillation of even reduced concentrations (2.5%) of phenylephrine drops (59). Other patients at risk of an increased BP response to topical phenylephrine include those treated with monoamine oxidase inhibitors and tricyclic antidepressants (36). β-Adrenergic blocking agents failed to demonstrate such an effect in a controlled study of patients with hypertension (60).

In general, mydriatic agents should be used during pregnancy only when absolutely necessary. First trimester use of atropine and homatropine may cause minor, non–life-threatening malformations, as is the case with phenylephrine, which has been associated with clubfoot and inguinal hernia in particular (61). Parenteral administration of phenylephrine late in pregnancy may induce fetal hypoxia, as manifested by tachycardia (62), and scopolamine administered systemically at term may have adverse fetal effects, as reflected by decreased heart rate variability and deceleration (63).

Whether systemically administered sympathomimetics or anticholinergics are distributed into the breast milk is not known with certainty. Because infants are exquisitely sensitive to anticholinergic agents, breast feeding should probably be suspended if these agents must be applied topically to nursing mothers, and use of phenylephrine, which can precipitate severe hypertension, may be contraindicated (64).

Drug Interactions

Analgesics, antihistamines, monoamine oxidase inhibitors, phenothiazines, and tricyclic antidepressants all promote the activity of anticholinergic agents. Anticholinergic drugs themselves enhance the activity of phenothiazines and diminish that of anticholinesterases and have a variable effect on analgesics (25).

Concomitant use of phenylephrine 2.5% with echothiopate has been suggested during treatment of accommodative esotropia or open-angle glaucoma because this combination prevents the formation of miotic cysts (65). The mechanism by which phenylephrine mediates this effect is unknown. Monoamine oxidase inhibitors and tricyclic antidepressants enhance the systemic BP response of concomitantly administered topical phenylephrine (36) (described in High-risk Groups section). In patients treated with such drugs for whom phenylephrine is deemed a medical priority, psychiatric medications should be discontinued for at least 21 days before topical therapy is initiated (8). Finally, phenylephrine itself diminishes the activity of adrenergic blockers and phenothiazines.

Major Clinical Trials

No high-quality, randomized controlled clinical trials have established the definitive efficacy of mydriatic-cycloplegic agents in reducing or in prevention of the adverse sequelae of intraocular inflammation.

REFERENCES

1. Brown JH. Atropine, scopolamine, and related drugs. In: Gilman AG, Rall TW, Nies AS, Taylor P, eds. *Goodman and Gilman's the pharmacological basis of therapeutics.* New York: Pergamon Press, 1990; 150–165.
2. Havener WA. *Ocular pharmacology.* St. Louis: C.V. Mosby, 1983;475–491.
3. Beitel RJ. Cycloplegic refraction. In: Tasman W, Jaeger EA, eds. *Duane's clinical ophthalmology,* vol. 1. Philadelphia: J.B. Lippincott, 1992;Ch. 41.
4. Priestly BS, Medine MM. A new mydriatic and cycloplegic drug. *Am J Ophthalmol* 1951;34:572–575.
5. Merrill OL, Goldberg B, Zavel S. bis Tropicamide, a new parasympatholytic. *Curr Ther Res* 1960;2:43–50.
6. Liv JHK, Erickson K. Cholinergic agents. In: Albert DM, Jakobiec FA, eds. *Principles and practice of ophthalmology: basic sciences.* Philadelphia: W.B. Saunders, 1994;985–992.
7. Heath P. Neosynephrine hydrochloride. Some uses and effects in ophthalmology. *Arch Ophthalmol* 1936;16:839–846.
8. Pavan-Langston D, Dunkel EC. *Handbook of ocular drug therapy and ocular side effects of systemic drugs.* Boston: Little, Brown, 1991;226–239.
9. Federsen IM. Beitrag zur Atropinvergiftung. Inaug Dissert Berlin; Franke O. 1884, as cited by: Manon J. Cycloplegia and mydriasis by use of atropine, scopolamine and homatropine-paradrine. *Arch Ophthalmol* 1940;23:340–350.
10. Wolf AV, Hodge AC. Effects of atropine sulfate, methylatropine nitrate (metropine) and homatropine hydrobromide on adult human eyes. *Arch Ophthalmol* 1946;32:293–301.
11. Jaanus SD, Pagano VT, Bartlett JO. Drugs affecting the autonomic nervous system. In: Bartlett JD, Jaanus SD, eds. *Clinical ocular pharmacology.* Boston: Butterworths, 1989;69–148.
12. Marron J. Cycloplegia and mydriasis by use of atropine, scopolamine, and homatropine-paradrine. *Arch Ophthalmol* 1940;23:340–350.
13. Gettes BD, Leopold IH. Evaluation of five new cycloplegic drugs. *Arch Ophthalmol* 1953;49:24–27.
14. Abraham SU. A new mydriatic and cycloplegic drug: compound 75 GT. *Am J Ophthalmol* 1953;36:69–73.
15. Nussenblatt RB, Palestine AG. *Uveitis, fundamentals and clinical practice.* Chicago: Year Book Medical Publishers, 1989;137–138.
16. Tsai E, Till GO, Marak GE. Effects of mydriatic agents on neutrophil migration. *Ophthalmic Res* 1988;20:14–19.
17. Gettes BD. Tropicamide, a new cycloplegic mydriatic. *Arch Ophthalmol* 1961;65:48–52.
18. Dillon JR, Tyhurst CW, Yolton RL. The mydriatic effect of tropicamide on light and dark irides. *J Am Optom Assoc* 1977;48:653–658.
19. Pollack SL, Hunt JS, Polse KA. Dose-response effects of tropicamide HCl. *Am J Optom Physiol Opt* 1981;58:361–366.

20. Gambill HD, Ogle KN, Kearns TP. Mydriatic effect of four drugs determined by pupillograph. *Arch Ophthalmol* 1967;77:740–746.
21. Doughty MJ, Lyle W, Trevino R, et al. A study of mydriasis produced by topical phenylephrine 2.5% in young adults. *Can J Optom* 1988; 50:40–60.
22. Haddad NJ, Moyer NJ, Riley FC. Mydriatic effect of phenylephrine hydrochloride. *Am J Ophthalmol* 1970;70:729–733.
23. Smith RB, Read S, Oczypik PM. Mydriatic effect of phenylephrine. *Eye Ear Nose Throat Monthly* 1976;55:133–134.
24. Neuhaus RW, Helper RS. Mydriatic effect of phenylephrine 10% vs. phenylephrine 2.5% (aq.). *Ann Ophthal* 1980;12:1159–1160.
25. Fraunfelder FT. *Drug-induced ocular side effects and drug interactions,* 3rd ed. Philadelphia: Lea & Febiger, 1989.
26. Lee PF. The influence of epinephrine and phenylephrine on intraocular pressure. *Arch Ophthalmol* 1958;60:863–867.
27. Apt L, Henrick A. Pupillary dilatation with single eyedrop mydriatic combinations. *Am J Ophthalmol* 1980;89:553–559.
28. Sinclair SH, Pelham V, Giovanoni R, Regan CD. Mydriatic solution for outpatient indirect ophthalmoscopy. *Arch Ophthalmol* 1980;98: 1572–1574.
29. Jaurequi MJ, Polse KA. Mydriatic effect using phenylephrine and proparacaine. *Am J Optom Physiol Opt* 1974;51:545–549.
30. Marr WG, Wood R, Senterfit L, Sigelman S. Effect of topical anesthetics on regeneration of corneal epithelium. *Am J Ophthalmol* 1957; 43:606–610.
31. Zimmerman TJ, Kooner KS, Kandarakis AS, Fiegler LP. Improving the therapeutic index of topically applied ocular drugs. *Arch Ophthalmol* 1984;102:551–553.
32. Janes RC, Stiles JF. The penetration of C^{14} labeled atropine into the eye. *Arch Ophthalmol* 1959;62:69–74.
33. Hoffman BB, Lefkowitz RJ. Catecholamines and sympathomimetic drugs. In: Gilman AG, Rall TW, Nies AS, Taylor P, eds. *Goodman and Gilman's the pharmacological basis of therapeutics.* New York: Pergamon Press, 1990;187–220.
34. Steinman WC, Millstein ME, Sinclair SH. Pupillary dilation with tropicamide 1% for funduscopic screening. A study of duration of action. *Ann Intern Med* 1987;107:181–184.
35. Huber MSE, Smith SA, Smith SE. Mydriatic drug for diabetic patients. *Br J Ophthalmol* 1985;69:425–427.
36. *AMA drug evaluation.* Chicago: American Medical Association, 1994;2123–2136.
37. Smith RE, Nozik RA. *Uveitis, a clinical approach to diagnosis and management.* Baltimore: Williams & Wilkins, 1989;51–72.
38. Heath P, Geiter CW. Use of phenylephrine hydrochloride (neosynephrine) in ophthalmology. *Arch Ophthalmol* 1949;41:172–177.
39. Potter DE. Drugs that alter the autonomic nervous system function. In: Lamberts DW, Potter DE, eds. *Clinical ophthalmic pharmacology.* Boston: Little, Brown, 1987;297–334.
40. Shaw BR, Lewis RA. Intraocular pressure elevation after pupillary dilation in open angle glaucoma. *Arch Ophthalmol* 1986;104:1185–1188.
41. Freund M, Merin S. Toxic effect of scopolamine eyedrops. *Am J Ophthalmol* 1970;70:637–639.
42. Hoefnagel D. Toxic effects of atropine and homatropine eyedrops in children. *N Engl J Med* 1961;264:168–171.
43. Cramp J. Reported cases of reactions and side effects of the drugs which optometrists use. *Aust J Optom* 1976;59:13–25.
44. Binkhorst RD, Weinstein GW, Baretz RM, Glahane MS. Psychotic reaction induced by cyclopentolate. *Am J Ophthalmol* 1963;56:1243–1245.
45. Kennerdel JS, Wucher FP. Cyclopentolate associated with two cases of grand mal seizure. *Arch Ophthalmol* 1972;87:634–635.
46. Isenberg SJ, Abrams C, Hyman PE. Effects of cyclopentolate eyedrops on gastric secretory function in pre-term infants. *Ophthalmology* 1985;92:698–700.
47. Wahl JW. Systemic reactions to tropicamide. *Arch Ophthalmol* 1969; 82:320–321.
48. Meyer SM, Fraunfelder FT. Phenylephrine hydrochloride. *Ophthalmology* 1980;87:1177–1880.
49. Geyer O, Lazar M. Allergic blepharo-conjunctivitis due to phenylephrine. *J Ocul Pharmacol* 1988;4:123–126.
50. Mitsui Y, Takagi Y. Nature of aqueous floaters due to sympathomimetic mydriatics. *Arch Ophthalmol* 1961;65:626–631.
51. Edelhauser HF, Hine JE, Pederson H, Van Horn D, Schultz RO. The effect of phenylephrine on the cornea. *Arch Ophthalmol* 1979;97: 937–947.
52. Brown MM, Brown GC, Spaeth GL. Lack of side effects from topically administered 10% phenylephrine eyedrops. A controlled study. *Arch Ophthalmol* 1980;98:487–489.
53. Lynch MG, Brown RH, Goode SM, Schoenwald RD, Chien DS. Reduction of phenylephrine drop size in infants achieves equal dilation with decreased systemic absorption. *Arch Ophthalmol* 1987;105: 1364–1365.
54. Isenberg S, Everett S, Parelhoff E. A comparison of mydriatic eye drops in low-weight infants. *Ophthalmology* 1984;91:278–279.
55. Eggers HM. Toxicity of drugs used in the diagnosis and treatment of strabismus. In: Srinivasan DB, ed. *Ocular therapeutics.* New York: Masson, 1980;115–122.
56. Fraunfelder FT, Scafidi AF. Possible adverse effects from topical ocular 10% phenylephrine. *Am J Ophthalmol* 1978;85:862–868.
57. Kim JM, Stevenson CE, Mathewson HS. Hypertensive reactions to phenylephrine eyedrops in patients with sympathetic denervation. *Am J Ophthalmol* 1978;85:862–868.
58. Robertson D. Contraindication to the use of ocular phenylephrine in idiopathic orthostatic hypotension. *Am J Ophthalmol* 1979;87:819–822.
59. Kumar V, Schoenwald RD, Barcellos WA, Chien DS, Folk JC, Weingeist TA. Aqueous vs. viscous phenylephrine. I. Systemic absorption and cardiovascular effects. *Arch Ophthalmol* 1986;104: 1189–1191.
60. Myers MG. Beta adrenoceptor antagonism and pressor response to phenylephrine. *Clin Pharmacol Ther* 1984;36:57–63.
61. Heinonen OP, Slone D, Shapiro S. *Birth defects and drugs in pregnancy.* Littleton: Publishing Sciences Group, 1977;297–313, 345–356.
62. Smith NT, Corgascio AN. The use and misuse of pressor agents. *Anesthesiology* 1970;33:58–101.
63. Ayrumlooi J, Tobias M, Berg P. The effects of scopolamine and ancillary analgesics upon the fetal heart rate recording. *J Reprod Med* 1980;25:323–326.
64. Samples JR, Meyer SM. Use of ophthalmic medications in pregnant and nursing women. *Am J Ophthalmol* 1988;106:616–623.
65. Chiri NB, Gold AA, Breinin G. Iris cysts and miotics. *Arch Ophthalmol* 1964;71:611–616.

Textbook of Ocular Pharmacology,
edited by T.J. Zimmerman, et al.
Lippincott–Raven Publishers, Philadelphia © 1997.

CHAPTER 61

Nonsteroidal Antiinflammatory Drugs

Albert Vitale and C. Stephen Foster

NONSTEROIDAL ANTIINFLAMMATORY DRUGS

Introduction, History, and Source

In the last 20 years, we have witnessed the development of a family of clinically useful aspirin-like, nonsteroidal antiinflammatory drugs (NSAIDs), which are among the most widely prescribed agents in general medicine for treatment of inflammation associated with rheumatic diseases and which have recently become commercially available worldwide as ophthalmic eye drops (1). In ophthalmic practice, these agents are used principally in the prevention and treatment of cystoid macular edema (CME), intraoperative miosis, and postoperative inflammation associated with cataract surgery. In addition, NSAID therapy, especially in conjunction with topical, periocular, or systemic steroids, constitutes an important facet of our approach to the management of patients with uveitis. Specifically, these agents are steroid-sparing and are useful in prevention of disease relapse and macular edema recurrence associated with intraocular inflammation.

Prior to the emergence of corticosteroids, nonsteroidal agents, such as aspirin, were used in treatment of severe intraocular inflammation (2). With the demonstration in the early 1970s of the inhibitory effect of aspirin on the synthesis of prostaglandins (3) (potent inflammatory mediators), other NSAIDs were developed in an effort to provide effective antiinflammatory activity while obviating the dose-limiting side effects associated with corticosteroids. Today, several chemical classes of synthetic NSAIDs exist and have antiinflammatory, antipyretic, and analgesic properties similar to those of aspirin (Table 1) by virtue of their common pharmacodynamics. At the time of this writing, four nonsteroidal solutions have been approved by the Food and Drug Administration (FDA) for ophthalmic use in the United States (Table 2), whereas in Europe and in other parts of the world, NSAIDs have been more widely used in treatment of intraocular inflammation and its sequelae (CME).

A. Vitale: Retina Specialists of Boston and The Massachusetts Eye and Ear Infirmary, Harvard Medical School, Boston, Massachusetts 02214.

C. S. Foster: Immunology and Uveitis Service, The Massachusetts Eye and Ear Infirmary, Harvard Medical School, Boston, Massachusetts 02214.

Official Drug Name and Chemistry

The more commonly prescribed systemic NSAIDs are shown according to chemical class, along with their nonproprietary name, the manufacturer, the trade name, and the typical daily adult dosage in Table 1. The currently available topical preparations are similarly shown in Table 2. Representative structural formulas from each chemical class of NSAID are shown in Figure 1. Although these compounds are heterogeneous, their unifying and defining feature is the absence of a steroid nucleus in their chemical structure (as compared with the chemical structure of hydrocortisone shown in Fig. 1A in Chapter 69, *this volume*). Of the chemical classes enumerated, the salicylates, fenamates, and pyrazolone derivatives are either unstable in solution or too toxic for ocular applications (4). In contrast, the phenylalkanoic acids are water soluble, allowing the formulation of flurbiprofen and suprofen as Ocufen 0.03% (Allergan, Irvine, CA) and Profenal 1% (Alcon, Fort Worth, TX) ophthalmic solutions respectively. These preparations have been approved by the FDA for inhibition of intraoperative miosis during cataract surgery (5,6). Most recently, ketorolac tromethamine 0.5% (Acular, Allergan) has become available as a topical agent for treatment of allergic conjunctivitis (4). Likewise, diclofenac 0.1% (Voltaren, Ciba Vision, Duluth, GA), a water soluble phenylacetic acid derivative, has been approved for treatment of inflammation after cataract surgery (7).

Pharmacology

The mechanism by which all NSAIDs mediate their pharmacologic effects is related in part to the inhibition of

TABLE 61-1. *Systemic nonsteroidal antiinflammatory agents*

Drug class	Drug: Generic	Drug: Trade name	Supplied (mg)	Typical adult daily dose (mg)
Salycilates	Aspirin	Multiple	325–925	650 every 4 hr
	Diflunisal	Dolobid (MSD, West Point, PA)	250, 500	250–500 b.i.d.
Fenamates	Mefenamate	Pronstel (Parke-Davis, Morris Plains, NJ)	250	250 q.i.d.
	Meclofenamate	Meclomen (Parke-Davis)	50, 100	50–100 q.i.d.
Indoles	Indomethacin	Indocin (MSD)	25, 50, 75(SR)	25–50 t.i.d.–q.i.d., 75 b.i.d.
	Sulindac	Clinoril (MSD)	150, 200	150–200 b.i.d.
	Tolmentin	Tolectin (McNeil, Raritan, NJ)	200, 400, 600	400 t.i.d.
Phenylacetic acids	Diclofenac	Voltaren (Geigy, Summit, NJ)	25, 50, 75	50–75 b.i.d.
Phenylalkanoic acids	Fenoprofen	Nalfon (Lilly, Indianapolis, IN)	200, 300, 600	300–600 t.i.d.
	Ketoprofen	Oridus (Wyeth, Philadelphia, PA)	25, 50, 75	75 t.i.d.–50 q.i.d.
	Piroxicam	Feldene (Pfizer, New York, NY)	10, 20	10 b.i.d., 20 q.d.
	Flurbiprofen	Ansaid (Upjohn, Kalamazoo, NJ)	50, 100	100 t.i.d.
	Ketorolac	Toradol (Syntex, Nutley, NJ)	10	10 q.i.d.
	Naproxen	Naprosyn (Syntex)	250, 375, 500	250–500 b.i.d.
		Anaprox (Syntex)	275, 550	275–550 b.i.d.
		Motrin (Upjohn)		
		Rufen (Boots, Whippany, NJ)	200, 300, 400, 600, 800	400–800 t.i.d.
	Ibuprofen	Advil (Whitehall, Madison, NJ)		
		Nuprin (Bristol Meyers, Princeton, NJ)		
Pyrazolons	Phenylbutazone	Butazolidin (Geigy)	100	100 t.i.d.–q.i.d.
		Azolid (USV, Westborough, MA)		
	Oxyphenylbutazone	Tandearil (Geigy)	100	100 t.i.d.–q.i.d.
		Oxalid (USV)		
Para-aminophenols	Acetaminophen	Multiple	80, 325, 500, 650	650 every 4 hr

b.i.d., twice daily; t.i.d., three times daily; q.i.d., four times daily.

cyclooxygenase, the enzyme responsible for conversion of arachidonic acid (AA) to cyclic endoperoxidases (PGG_2, PGH_2), the precursors of prostaglandins, in ocular and nonocular tissues (8) (Fig. 2). Plasma membrane-bound AA is released from phospholipid through the action of phospholipase-A and generates substrate for the cyclooxygenase and lipoxygenase catabolic pathways, with subsequent prostaglandin and leukotriene (LT) generation. Cyclooxygenase inhibition is the specific action of the currently available NSAIDs, although lipoxygenase activity may be affected to some degree by diclofenac. Theoretically, specific inhibition of cyclooxygenase could indirectly enhance the production of LTs by shunting more AA to be metabolized by lipoxygenase. In contrast, corticosteroids, which retard the release of AA by inhibiting phospholipase-A, inhibit both the cyclooxygenase and lipoxygenase pathway products (9). This phenomenon may explain the superior antiinflammatory potency of corticosteroids as compared with that of NSAIDs and may provide the basis for therapeutic synergism when these agents are used together.

The pharmacologic actions of NSAIDs are probably more complex than was previously appreciated, involving more than sole inhibition of cyclooxygenase (1). There appears to be a correlation between the antiinflammatory potency of NSAIDs with the degree of albumin binding, as

TABLE 61-2. *Topical nonsteroidal antiinflammatory agents*

Drug: Generic	Drug: Trade name	Supplied		Typical doses
Flurbiprofen[a,b]	Ocufen (Allergan, Irvine, CA)	0.03%	Solution	One drop every 30 mins, 2 hr preoperatively (total dose 4 drops)
Suprofen[a,b]	Profenal (Alcon, Fort Worth, TX)	1.0%	Solution	Two drops at 1, 2, and 3 hr preoperatively or every 4 hr while awake on the day of surgery
Diclofenal[a]	Voltaren (Ciba Vision, Duluth, GA)	0.1%	Solution	q.i.d.
Ketorolac[a]	Acular (Syntex, Nutley, NJ)	0.5%	Solution	t.i.d.
Indomethacin	Indocid (MSD, West Point, PA)	0.5%–1%	Suspension	q.i.d.

[a]Approved by the Food and Drug Administration for ophthalmic use.
[b]Approved for intraoperative miosis only.

A

Aspirin

B

Mefenamic Acid

C. INDOMETHACIN
[Indocin]

D. DICLOFENAC SODIUM
[Voltaren]

E. FLURBIPROFEN
[Ansaid]

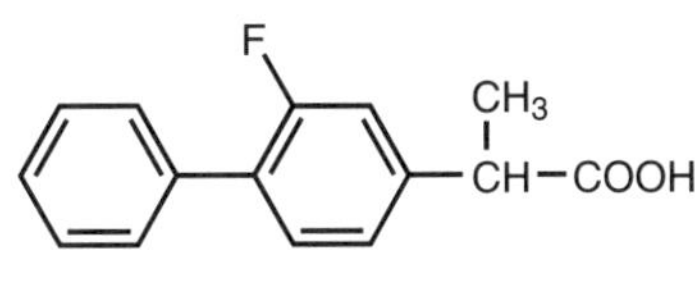

F. PHENYLBUTAZONE

G. ACETAMINOPHEN

FIG. 61-1. Chemical structures of representative nonsteroidal antiinflammatory drugs. **A:** Aspirin (salicylates). **B:** Mefenemate (tenemates). **C:** Indomethacin (indoles). **D:** Diclofenal (phenylacetic acids). **F:** Phenylbutazone (pyrazolons). **G:** Acetaminophen (*para*-aminophenols).

well as a relationship between antiinflammatory activity, NSAID acidity, and the efficacy of inhibition of prostaglandin synthesis. Evidence also shows that NSAIDs have free radical scavenger activity (10), as well as antichemotactic activity, which modulates humoral and cellular events during inflammatory reactions (11).

Clinical Pharmacology

All NSAIDs share, to some degree, antiinflammatory, antipyretic, and analgesic properties; however, there are important differences among individual agents with respect to these activities. For example, acetaminophen is commonly prescribed to reduce fever and mild pain, but is only weakly antiinflammatory and has no effect on platelets and bleeding time. Although the reasons for these differences are poorly defined, they may relate to differential enzyme inhibition in the target tissues (8). Furthermore, the diversity of NSAID pharmacologic activity is directly related to the multifaceted biologic effects of prostaglandins, whose biosynthesis they inhibit.

Prostaglandins are 20 carbon, unsaturated fatty acid derivatives with a cyclopentane ring, present in nearly every

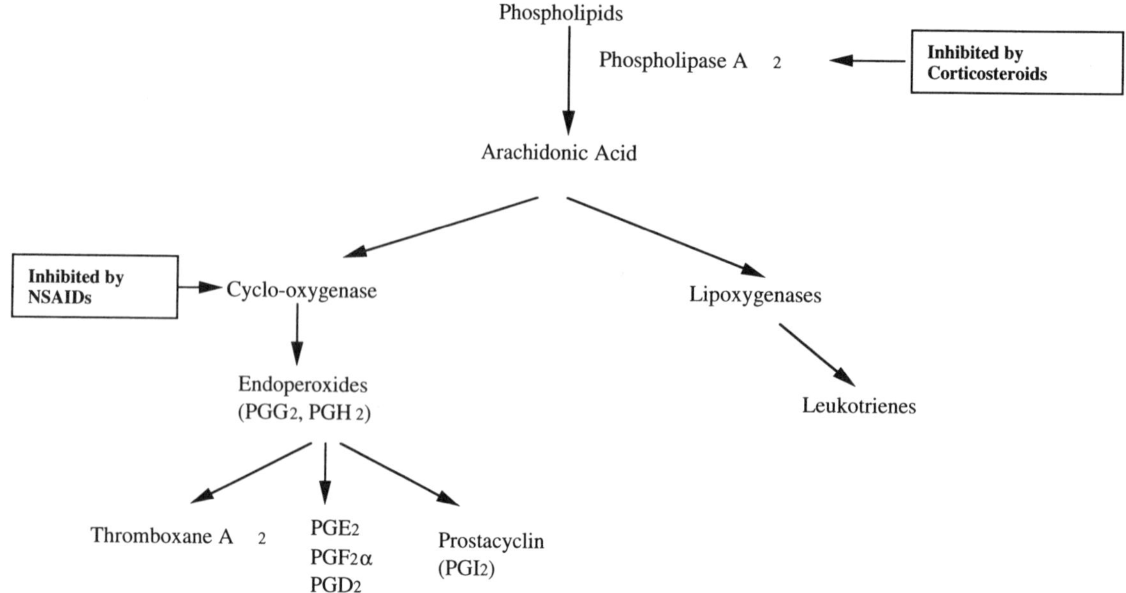

FIG. 61-2. Arachadonic metabolic pathways.

organ, including the eye. In addition to their well-known role in the inflammatory response, prostaglandins are believed to play important roles in the control of pain, body temperature, blood coagulation, intraocular pressure (IOP), lipid and carbohydrate metabolism, and cardiovascular and renal physiology (8).

The link between prostaglandins and the eye dates back to the isolation of a substance termed irin from extracts of rabbit iris tissue nearly 30 years ago (12). This substance, which produced pupillary constriction when injected into the anterior chamber of animal eyes, was later shown to contain prostaglandins (13). In addition to inducing miosis, prostaglandins have a diverse spectrum of action in the eye, increasing inflammation (14), enhancing vascular permeability of blood–ocular barriers (15), and producing conjunctival hyperemia, and changes in IOP (16) (Table 3). Furthermore, increased levels of prostaglandins have been detected in the aqueous humor after trauma (15), cataract surgery (17), and laser iridotomy (18).

The precise mechanism of prostaglandin action is not known. Some prostaglandins display differential effects on various tissues, whereas others behave antagonistically with one another (7). These factors notwithstanding, it is the NSAID-mediated cyclooxygenase inhibition of prostaglandin biosynthesis that is responsible for their therapeutic effects in ophthalmology: the prevention and treatment of CME, intraoperative miosis, and intraocular inflammation associated with cataract surgery and uveitis.

TABLE 61-3. *Ocular effects of prostaglandins*

PGD_2:	Vasodilatation and chemosis
PGE, PGE_2:	Vasodilatation and miosis, increase IOP, capillary permeability, and inflammation
PGE_2:	Decreases IOP, minimal effect on inflammation or miosis

IOP, intraocular pressure.

Adapted from To K, Abelson MB, Neufeld A. Nonsteroidal antiinflammatory drugs. In: Albert DM, Jakobiec FH, eds. *Principles and practice of ophthalmology: basic sciences.* Philadelphia: W.B. Saunders, 1994:1022.

Pharmaceutics

The dosage sizes and typical frequency of administration for adults of the more commonly prescribed systemic NSAIDs are shown in Table 1. Currently available topical preparations are shown in Table 2. All systemic NSAIDs should be taken with food, milk, or antacid.

Pharmacokinetics and Metabolism

All orally administered NSAIDs are readily absorbed from the gastrointestinal (GI) tract, reaching peak serum concentrations in 0.5 to 5 hours (19). A correlation between plasma concentration and therapeutic efficacy has been demonstrated for aspirin and naproxen; however, this relationship has not been established for other NSAIDs (20).

All NSAIDs are highly protein-bound (90% to 99%), especially to albumin and to ocular tissues, and have a small volume of distribution (4). These characteristics may increase the risk of potential adverse interactions with drugs that share a similar high avidity for plasma proteins (e.g., oral hypoglycemic agents and anticoagulants) (20).

The liver is the major site of NSAID metabolism, with the unchanged drug and its metabolites excreted primarily by the kidneys and secondarily in the feces. The plasma elimination half-lives ($t\frac{1}{2}$) of different NSAIDs vary greatly, which probably relates to enterohepatic circulation (4). Therefore, patients with compromised renal or hepatic function are at risk of development of toxic side effects of NSAIDs, even at recommended doses.

Topically applied NSAIDs are distributed throughout the ocular tissues, including the cornea, conjunctiva, sclera, iris, ciliary body, lens, retina, choroid, vitreous, and aqueous humor (21) and provide adequate levels in the latter to inhibit prostaglandin synthesis in animal studies (5,22). Although good ocular penetration is achieved after systemic administration of NSAIDs, topically applied drug appears to provide superior bioavailability in the anterior chamber (23).

Finally, a significant percentage of topically applied NSAID drugs may gain access to the systemic circulation through the nasolacrimal duct (21,24). Although only a small quantity of drug is ultimately absorbed systemically after topical instillation, as is attested by the paucity of systemic side effects associated with this route versus that of oral administration, we should not assume that the topical route is completely devoid of such toxicity (4).

Therapeutic Use

Prevention of Intraoperative Miosis

The single most important risk factor for vitreous loss and zonular breaks during extracapsular cataract surgery with intraocular lens (IOL) implantation is decreasing pupil size (25). Surgical trauma is believed to stimulate production of certain prostaglandins that mediate miosis independently of cholinergic mechanisms (26). Two topical NSAIDs, flurbiprofen 0.03% and suprofen 1%, have been approved by the FDA for use in the United States to ameliorate this problem. Flurbiprofen 0.03%, administered every 30 minutes, beginning 2 hours before surgery, was shown in two double-masked, placebo-controlled, randomized studies to limit intraoperative miosis during anterior segment surgery (5,27). A similarly designed multicenter trial of topical suprofen 1% showed pupillary constriction to be reduced during cataract surgery when 2 drops were administered every 4 hours on the day before surgery and every hour for three doses immediately before surgery (28). Preoperative treatment is crucial since topically applied NSAIDs block the synthesis of prostaglandins rather than their effects on the iris once the prostaglandins are formed. Although these studies clearly show a statistically significant inhibitory effect on intraoperative miosis, the use of topical NSAIDs routinely by all surgeons may not be associated with a clinically significant inhibitory effect (4). The changes in pupil size observed in these studies is small, varies considerably from one surgeon to the next, and significant changes in pupil size in control eyes are larger, in several instances, than in NSAID-treated eyes (1). These findings suggest that surgical miosis may be mediated in part by as yet unidentified endogenous factors independent of surgical technique or prostaglandin pharmacodynamics (4).

Postsurgical Inflammation

Many well-controlled clinical studies provide evidence that NSAIDs topically applied before and immediately after cataract surgery are useful in management of postoperative inflammation (1). Such treatment might serve to obviate the potential untoward side effects of secondary glaucoma, increased risk of infection, and impaired wound healing associated with topical steroid use (see Chapter 59, Corticosteroids, Side Effects and Toxicity, this volume).

Postoperative inflammation, as measure directly (slit-lamp examination) or indirectly (fluorophotometry in detecting perturbation in the blood–aqueous barrier) appears to be reduced by several topical NSAIDs, including indocin 1.0% (29), flurbiprofen 0.03% (30), ketorolac 0.5% (31,32), and diclofenac 0.1% (7) in randomized, double-masked, placebo-controlled comparisons. The treatment effect was observed after both intracapsular and extracapsular surgery, irrespective of IOL implantation and whether corticosteroids were administered concurrently or postoperatively. A good correlation between slit-lamp and anterior ocular fluorophotometry observations was noted and was confirmed by more recent studies in which a laser cell flare meter method was used (4).

Ketorolac 0.5% versus dexamethasone 0.1% (33) and diclofenac 0.1%, 0.5%, and 0.01% versus prednisolone 1% (34) have been compared in randomized, controlled, double-masked studies. These two treatment arms were not statistically different in reducing postoperative inflammation, as judged by slit-lamp examinations for cells, flare, and chemosis; however, topical NSAIDs were superior to topical steroids in reducing the breakdown of the blood–aqueous barrier, as measured by fluorophotometry (4).

These studies suggest that topical NSAIDs may serve as possible substitutes for corticosteroids in management of postoperative inflammation. However, at present, only diclofenac 0.1%, 1 drop four times daily, beginning 24 hours after cataract surgery, has been approved by the FDA for this purpose.

Prophylaxis and Treatment of CME

Common to all disease entities associated with CME is the disruption of the inner or outer blood–retinal barrier (35). Free radicals generated by ultraviolet light, vitreous traction, and inflammation have all been implicated in its pathogenesis and undoubtedly play a central role in the evolution of CME after cataract surgery or that associated with uveitis. The many well-designed clinical studies that have demonstrated a beneficial effect of both topical and systemic NSAID therapy for prevention of angiographic CME and the treatment of chronic symptomatic CME after cataract surgery have been thoughtfully and comprehensively reviewed elsewhere (1,36,37). In the assessment of the therapeutic efficacy of NSAIDs in treatment of CME, the following have been consistently emphasized: (a) the importance of double-masked, randomized, placebo-controlled comparisons in an entity whose natural history is marked by spontaneous remission and recurrences; (b) the differentiation between angiographic and clinically significant CME; and (c) the separation of prophylactic treatment from therapy for established CME.

Of the most frequently cited controlled studies establishing the efficacy of topical NSAIDs in the prophylaxis of angiographic CME after cataract extraction (38–40), only one has demonstrated a statistically significant improvement in Snellen visual acuity (38), an effect that was not sustained longer than 3 months. The use of non-Snellen parameters of visual function and the benefit of prophylactic therapy for more than 1 year have not yet been evaluated. Furthermore, in these studies corticosteroids were administered concurrently in the postoperative period, introducing the potential for therapeutic synergism between the two drugs and thus rendering conclusions with regard to NSAID monotherapy difficult. A recent double-masked, placebo-controlled study demonstrated a statistically significant reduction in postoperative angiographic CME, however, although with no significant improvement in visual acuity, after prophylactic treatment with topical ketorolac 0.5%, 1 drop three times daily, initiated 1 day preoperatively and continued for 19 days postoperatively, without concurrent use of corticosteroids (41).

Finally, two double-masked, placebo-controlled, randomized studies have provided evidence that topical ketorolac 0.5% may improve vision in some patients with CME that has been present for 6 months or more after cataract extraction (42,43). One regimen for the treatment of established CME begins with intensive topical steroids (eight times daily) and topical NSAIDs (four to six times daily) for 2 weeks. If no significant improvement or worsening of CME is observed, systemic NSAIDs are instituted and topical NSAIDs are discontinued (44).

Uveitis

NSAID therapy is an important adjunct in our therapeutic approach to patients with uveitis, particularly when it is used in conjunction with topical, periocular, and systemic steroids. Not only have these medicines been shown to decrease intraocular inflammation after cataract extraction and to be useful in prophylaxis and treatment of CME, but they may also be steroid-sparing, reducing the total amount of corticosteroid required to eliminate inflammation. Such is true of topical NSAID therapy; we believe that these agents do not produce a clinically profound reduction in intraocular inflammation per se, but instead obviate steroid-induced side effects in patients with chronic uveitis by allowing a reduction in the effective dose of steroid. Indeed, 5.0% tolmetin versus 0.5% prednisolone versus saline was compared in a double-masked, randomized, controlled clinical trial of 100 patients with acute nongranulomatous anterior uveitis. No statistically significant difference in "cure" rate was demonstrated at the end of the 3-week study (45). Similarly, 49 patients with acute anterior uveitis randomized to a masked comparison between 1% indomethacin and 0.1% dexamethasone applied six times daily manifested a more marked reduction in inflammation in the steroid group by day 7, with no difference between the two groups at 2 weeks (46).

Similarly, little evidence supports the use of systemic NSAIDs as the sole agent during an episode of acute anterior uveitis. However, in our experience, oral NSAIDs are particularly useful in long-term management of recurrent anterior uveitis, substantially reducing the amount of corticosteroid required to achieve inflammatory quiescence and enabling patients, in many cases, to maintain a steady course without inflammatory exacerbations once steroids have been discontinued. Adjunctive therapy with systemic NSAIDs was shown to reduce the inflammatory activity and allow a reduction in the dose of corticosteroids in a group of children with chronic iridocyclitis (47) and to prevent further attacks of juvenile rheumatoid arthritis-associated iridocyclitis (48).

In cases of posterior uveitis and secondary vasculitis, we find oral NSAID agents effective in eliminating macular edema and preventing its recurrence. Typically, we initially treat patients with a combination of transseptal steroid (Kenalog 40 mg) and an oral NSAID (Voltaren 75 mg twice daily). In some instances, systemic oral prednisone (1 mg/kg/day) is administered every morning for 7 to 14 days, depending on the severity of intraocular inflammation. Steroids are tapered and discontinued once the macular edema has been eliminated and the uveitis controlled; however, the NSAID is continued for 6 to 12 months, barring the occurrence of drug-induced toxicity. Primary retinal vasculitis does not appear to be amenable to oral NSAID therapy. We consider steroids and cytotoxic agents necessary in such cases.

Finally, the safety and efficacy of systemic NSAIDs has been evaluated in a nonrandomized, uncontrolled fashion in a large uveitis population at the Massachusetts Eye and Ear Infirmary in the past 10 years. At the time of this writing, diclofenac (Voltaren) and difunisal (Dolobid) are the safest and most effective agents, with indomethacin (Indocin SR) and naproxen (Naprosyn) ranking close seconds. Piroxicam (Feldene), sulindac (Clinoril), and ibuprofen (Motrin) have been the least effective for therapy of intraocular inflammatory disease and associated macular edema (Table 1). Just as a variation exists in individual responsiveness to any given NSAID in the treatment of rheumatic disease, so too an apparent differential effectiveness exists between one NSAID and another in management of uveitis. We will try three different NSAIDs before declaring that any given patient is unlikely to benefit from this form of therapy.

Other Therapeutic Uses

Oral NSAIDs are the agents of choice for the treatment of episcleritis and for most cases of simple, diffuse, and nodular scleritis, although, as is true of adjunctive therapy in uveitis, sequential trials of several NSAIDs may be required before one that is completely effective is found (49). Topical NSAIDs do not appear to be effective in management of episcleritis (50), and topical steroids prolong the overall duration of the patient's problem, with a greater number of recurrences after discontinuation of therapy, unnecessarily exposing the patient to the potential side effects of such treatment. The treatment of scleritis associated with collagen vascular or connective tissue diseases is more complex, frequently requiring more potent therapy in addition to NSAIDs. For patients with scleritis, in whom a diagnosis of Wegener's granulomatosis or polyarteritis nodosa has been made, or for individuals with necrotizing scleritis associated with rheumatoid arthritis or relapsing polychondritis, immunosuppressive chemotherapy is mandatory (49).

Finally, topical NSAIDs may be useful in management of ocular allergic disorders. Topical flurbiprofen 0.03% and suprofen 1% have been reported to be superior to placebo in treatment of allergic conjunctivitis (51) and vernal conjunctivitis (52), respectively, and Ketorolac 0.5% reduces the pruritis frequently associated with seasonal allergic conjunctivitis (4).

Side Effects and Toxicity

Topical Administration

The most common side effects after topical NSAID administration are transient burning, stinging, and conjunctival hyperemia (4). Despite modifications in the formulation of NSAIDs in an effort to minimize ocular irritation, burning and stinging may still occur, presenting a potential compliance problem. In addition, postoperative atonic mydriasis has been reported in patients receiving topical NSAIDs before cataract surgery (1). The pharmacologic mechanism mediating this phenomenon is poorly defined (53) and its relationship to a similar adverse event after uncomplicated cataract surgery in patients not receiving preoperative NSAIDs has not been evaluated (54,55).

Topical NSAIDs are contraindicated in patients with active dendritic or geographic herpes keratitis (56). Although preliminary studies have not demonstrated an adverse effect of topical NSAIDs on either fungal (57) or bacterial (58) ocular infections, it would be imprudent to assume that such therapy is completely risk-free.

Systemic Administration

Oral NSAIDs have been associated with a wide variety of adverse reactions; those most severe and clinically significant are GI, CNS, hematologic, renal, hepatic, dermatologic, and immunologic. GI irritation is the most common side effect, ranging from nausea, vomiting, and cramps to gastric and intestinal ulceration, with a potential for significant bleeding and anemia (20). The relative risk of developing a clinically significant peptic ulcer is three to eight times greater among patients receiving oral NSAID therapy, particularly among the elderly, and the risk is compounded by the concomitant use of oral corticosteroids, alcohol, and tobacco (59). NSAIDs are believed to inhibit locally protective prostaglandins (PGE_2, PGI_2) responsible for gastric mucin production, thus potentiating the possibility of GI erosion (8). Consequently, antacids and H_2-blocking agents do not prevent NSAID-induced ulcers (60), whereas misoprostol (Cytotec), a prostaglandin analogue, may offer some protection in patients at risk of developing this complication (61).

CNS side effects of NSAIDs include somnolence, dizziness, lightheadedness, confusion, fatigue, anxiety, depression, psychotic episodes, and headache. The latter is a well-known side effect of indomethacin and is reported in more than 10% of patients treated with this drug (20).

Hematologic toxicity is manifested clinically by a prolonged bleeding time. All NSAIDs inhibit platelet production of thromboxane A_2, a potent platelet aggregator (62). Aplastic anemia, agranulocytosis, and related blood dyscrasias have been reported, but are exceedingly rare (20).

NSAIDs have little effect on renal function in healthy persons; however, they may decrease renal blood flow and glomerular filtration in patients with congestive heart failure, chronic renal failure, cirrhosis with ascites, or hypovolemia of any etiology and thus precipitate acute renal failure. In such clinical conditions, renal perfusion is maintained by the vasodilatory effects of locally produced prostaglandin against reflex pressor effects (8). NSAIDs abrogate this prostaglandin-mediated autoregulatory phenomenon (65).

Hepatic reactions occur occasionally, and include hepatitis and abnormal results of liver function tests. Predisposing factors to acute liver injury include impaired renal clearance, large doses, prolonged therapy, intercurrent viral illness, and advanced age (64).

Dermatologic reactions to systemic NSAID therapy commonly include urticaria, exanthema, photosensitivity, and pruritus. More important, potentially serious entities such as toxic epidermal necrolysis, erythema multiforme, and anaphylactoid reactions have been induced by these agents (65).

Metabolic changes, including fluid retention, edema, weight gain, and hypersensitivity reactions, have been reported with all NSAIDs (20). A history of the latter, or allergic reaction to aspirin, to which NSAIDs may exhibit cross-sensitivity, constitutes a definitive contraindication to their use. In addition, patients with the syndrome of nasal polyps, angioedema, and bronchospastic reactivity to aspirin should not be treated with NSAIDs (66).

Overdose

Overdose of NSAIDs, other than salicylates and phenylbutazone, rarely presents a serious problem (67). In general, significant symptoms of NSAID overdose occur after ingestion of 5 to 10 times the average therapeutic dose. Presenting signs and symptoms range from GI upset, nystagmus, drowsiness, tinnitus, and disorientation to seizures, acute renal failure, cardiopulmonary arrest, and coma. The diagnosis is based largely on a history of NSAID ingestion since signs and symptoms are nonspecific and specific serum levels of drug are usually unavailable. Therapy consists of emergency and supportive measures (maintenance of an airway, fluid volume, and treatment of seizures) and decontamination procedures, including induction of emesis, gastric lavage, and administration of activated charcoal and cathartics. Although no specific antidote to NSAID poisoning exists, vitamin K may be used in patients with prolonged prothrombin times. Because NSAIDs are highly protein bound and extensively metabolized, hemodialysis, peritoneal dialysis, and forced diuresis are not likely to be effective (68). In contrast, hemodialysis is very effective in rapidly removing salicylates and correcting acid-base and fluid abnormalities arising as a consequence of aspirin overdose. In addition, sodium bicarbonate is frequently administered to treat the metabolic acidosis and enhance salicylate clearance by the kidneys. Supportive and decontamination measures are similarly critical to management of salicylate overdose.

High-risk Groups

All patients should be educated concerning the signs and symptoms of serious GI toxicity and the measures by which they might be diminished (smoking and ethanol cessation and ingestion of medication with food). Patients at greatest risk of these complications include those with a history of peptic ulcer disease, those treated concomitantly with oral corticosteroids, and the elderly (59).

The risk of NSAID-induced acute renal failure is increased in patients with underlying chronic renal failure, atherosclerosis, hepatic sclerosis (especially with ascites), and volume depletion; such patients require vigilant monitoring of the blood urea nitrogen (BUN), creatinine level, and urinary sediment (8). The elderly, who renal function usually is reduced, should also be monitored closely (69). Furthermore, persons with impaired renal function are at risk of developing hepatotoxicity. Early signs of hepatotoxicity in an otherwise healthy patient are heralded by abnormalities in the liver function tests, especially the ALT level.

Patients with underlying bleeding disorders should use NSAIDs cautiously since NSAIDs impair platelet aggregation and prolong bleeding time. Patients undergoing surgical procedures should discontinue oral NSAIDs 24 to 48 hours preoperatively, whereas, with aspirin treatment 7 to 10 hours are required for recovery of platelet functional activity (20).

The choice of NSAID in children is limited and should be restricted to the drugs that have been tested extensively in this age group, i.e., aspirin, naproxen, and tolmetin (8). Of particular note, administration of aspirin to a child in the setting of a viral febrile illness is contraindicated, because of its association with Reye's syndrome.

No evidence suggests that salicylates have teratogenic effects on the human fetus (70). Although fewer human data are available, other NSAIDs have not been associated with teratogenicity in animal studies (20). Despite these findings, NSAIDs are generally not recommended during pregnancy unless absolutely necessary, in which case aspirin at low doses is probably the safest treatment. Administration of aspirin or any other NSAID during the last 6 months of pregnancy may prolong gestation and labor, increase the risk of postpartum hemorrhage, and promote intrauterine closure of the ductus arteriosus (8). Side effects produced by NSAID therapy during breast feeding are uncommon; however, metabolic acidosis in infants of mothers receiving salicylates has been reported (20).

Drug Interactions

NSAIDs are highly bound to plasma proteins and therefore may displace certain other concomitantly administered drugs from a common binding site, potentiating these actions and producing significant adverse effects. Such is the case with concurrent therapy with warfarin, sulfonylurea hypoglycemic agents, and methotrexate; dosage must be adjusted to prevent potential untoward effects (8). This is particularly important in patients treated with warfarin, because of the intrinsic antiplatelet activity of NSAIDs.

Both NSAIDs and lithium are excreted by the proximal convoluted tubule in the kidney. Their concomitant administration, especially with diclofenac, has resulted in reduced lithium clearance and lithium toxicity (20). Probenecid, which also acts at the proximal convoluted tubule, may also impair NSAID metabolism and excretion.

Concomitant administration of NSAIDs and cyclosporine may produce synergistic nephrotoxicity by reducing renal blood flow. A transient but significant increase in serum creatinine has been observed after combined therapy with these agents (71).

Major Clinical Trials

A summary and discussion of the major clinical trials with regard to the therapeutic efficacy of NSAIDs in ophthalmology appears in the superb therapeutic review article by Flach (1). Many of these studies, as well as others relevant to NSAID therapy in uveitis, are cited and discussed in the Therapeutic Use section.

REFERENCES

1. Flach AJ. Cyclo-oxygenase inhibitors in ophthalmology. *Surv Ophthalmol* 1992;36:259–284.
2. Gifford H. On the treatment of sympathetic ophthalmia by large doses of salicylate of sodium aspirin or other salicylate compounds. *Ophthalmoscope* 1910;8:257–258.
3. Vane JR. Inhibition of prostaglandin synthesis as a mechanism of action for aspirin-like drugs. *Nature* 1971;231:232–235.
4. Flach AJ. Nonsteroidal anti-inflammatory drugs in ophthalmology. *Int Ophthalmol Clin* 1993;33:1–7.
5. *Summary basis of approval for Ocufen® (Allergan's Flurbiprofen) subsequent to new drug application.* Washington, D.C., Department of Health and Human Services, Food and Drug Administration, 1987; 19–404.
6. *Summary basis of approval for Profenal® (Alcon's Suprofen) subsequent to new drug application.* Washington, D.C., Department of Health and Human Services, Food and Drug Administration, 1989; 19–387.
7. Vickers FF, McGuigan LJB, Ford C, et al. The effect of diclofenal sodium ophthalmic on the treatment of postoperative inflammation. *Invest Ophthalmol Vis Sci (ARVO Suppl)* 1991;32:793.
8. Insel PA. Analgesic-antidiuretics and antiinflammatory agents: drugs employed in the treatment of rheumatoid arthritis and gout. In: Gilman AG, Rall TW, Nies AS, Taylor P, eds. *Goodman and Gilman's the pharmacological basis of therapeutics.* New York: Pergamon Press, 1990;638–681.
9. Haynes RC. Adrenocorticotropic hormone; adrenocorticosteroids and their synthetic analogs; inhibitors of the synthesis and actions of adrenocorticotropic hormones. In: *Goodman and Gilman's the pharmacological basis of therapeutics.* New York: Pergamon Press, 1990; 1431–1462.
10. Burne K, Glatt M, Graf P. Minireview: mechanisms of action of anti-inflammatory drugs. *Gen Pharmacol* 1976;7:27–33.
11. Abramson SB, Weissmann G. The mechanism of action of nonsteroidal antiinflammatory drugs. *Arthritis Rheum* 1989;32:1–9.
12. Ambache N. Irin, a smooth muscle contracting substance present in rabbit iris. *J Physiol (Lond)* 1955;29:65–66.
13. Bito LZ. Prostaglandins, other eicosanoids and their derivatives as potential antiglaucoma agents. In: Drance SM, Neufeld AH, eds. *Applied pharmacology in medical treatments of glaucoma.* New York: Grune & Stratton, 1984;Ch. 20.
14. Bhattacherjer P. Prostaglandin and inflammatory reactions in the eye. *Methods Find Eye Clin Pharmacol* 1980;2:17–31.
15. Eakins KE. Prostaglandins and non-prostaglandin-mediated breakdown of the blood-aqueous barrier. *Exp Eye Res* 1977;80(suppl):483–498.
16. Abelson MB, Butrus SI, Kliman GH, Lanson DL, Lorey EJ, Topical arachidonic acid: a model for screening anti-inflammatory agents. *J Ocul Pharmacol* 1987;3:63–75.
17. Miyake K, Sugiyama S, Norismatsu I, Ozawa T. Prevention of cystoid macular edema after lens extraction by topical indomethacin: III Radioimmunoassay measurement of prostaglandins in the aqueous during and after lens extraction procedures. *Graefes Arch Clin Exp Ophthalmol* 1978;209:83–88.
18. Unger WG, Bass MS. Prostaglandin and nerve mediated response of the rabbit eye to argon laser irradiation of the iris. *Ophthalmologica* 1977;175:153–158.
19. Porter RS. Factors determining efficacy of NSAIDs. *Drug Intell Clin Pharm* 1984;18:42–51.
20. *AMA drug evaluations.* Chicago: American Medical Association, 1994;1814–1833.
21. Ling TL, Combs OL. Ocular bioavailability and tissue distribution of ketorolac tromethamine in rabbits. *J Pharm Sci* 1987;76:289–294.
22. Anderson JA, Chen CC, Vita JB. Disposition of topical flurbiprofen in normal and aphakic rabbit eyes. *Arch Ophthalmol* 1982;100:642–645.
23. Sanders DR, Goldstick B, Kraff C, et al. Aqueous penetration of oral and topical indomethacin in humans. *Arch Ophthalmol* 1983;101: 1614–1616.
24. Tang-Lui DD, Liu SS, Weinkam RJ. Ocular and systemic bioavailability of ophthalmic flurbiprofen. *J Pharmacokinet Biopharm* 1984; 12:611–626.
25. Guzek JP, Holm M, Cotter JB, et al. Risk factors for intraoperative complications in 1000 extracapsular cases. *Ophthalmology* 1983;94: 461–466.
26. Cole DF, Unger WG. Prostaglandins as mediators for the responses of the eye due to trauma. *Exp Eye Res* 1973;17:357–368.
27. Keates RH, McGowan KA. Clinical trial of flurbiprofen to maintain pupillary dilation during cataract surgery. *Ann Ophthalmol* 1984;16: 919–921.
28. Stark WJ, Fagadu WR, Stewart RH. Reduction of pupillary constriction during cataract surgery using suprofen. *Arch Ophthalmol* 1986; 104:364–366.
29. Sanders DR, Kraff ML. Steroidal and nonsteroidal anti-inflammatory agents. Effects on postsurgical inflammation and blood-aqueous barrier breakdown. *Arch Ophthalmol* 1984;102:1453–1456.
30. Sabiston MB, Tessler D, Sumersk H, et al. Reduction of inflammation following cataract surgery by flurbiprofen. *Ophthalmic Surg* 1987;18: 873–877.
31. Flach AJ, Graham J, Kruger LP, Stegman RC, Tanenbaum L. Quantitative assessment of postsurgical breakdown of the blood-aqueous barrier following administration of ketorolac iromethamine solution. A double-masked, paired comparison with vehicle-placebo solution study. *Arch Ophthalmol* 1988;106:344–347.
32. Flach AJ, Lavelle CJ, Olander KW, Retzlaff JH, Sorenson LW. The effect of ketorolac 0.5% solution in reducing postsurgical inflammation following ECCE with IOL. Double-masked, parallel comparison with vehicle. *Ophthalmology* 1988;75:1279–1284.
33. Flach AJ, Kraff MC, Sanders DR, Tanenbaum L. The quantitative effect of 0.5% ketorolac tromethamine solution and dexamethasone phosphate 0.1% solution on postsurgical blood-aqueous barrier. *Arch Ophthalmol* 1988;106:480–483.
34. Kraff MC, Sanders DR, McGuigan L, et al. Inhibition of blood-aqueous humor barrier breakdown with diclofenac. A fluorophotometric study. *Arch Ophthalmol* 1990;108:380–383.
35. Jampol LM, Po SM. Macular edema. In: Ryan SJ, ed. *Retina,* vol. 2. St. Louis: CV Mosby, 1994;999–1008.
36. Jampol LM. Pharmacologic therapy of aphakic cystoid macular edema: a review. *Ophthalmology* 1982;89:891–897.
37. Jampol LM. PHarmacologic therapy of aphakic and pseudophakic cystoid macular edema: 1985 update. *Ophthalmology* 1985;92:807–810.
38. Miyake K, Sakamura S, Miura H. Long-term follow-up study of the prevention of aphakic cystoid macular edema by topical indomethacin. *Br J Ophthalmol* 1980;64:324–328.
39. Yannuzzi LA, Landau AN, Turtz AL. Incidence of aphakic cystoid macular edema with the use of topical indomethacin. *Ophthalmology* 1981;88:947–954.
40. Kraff MC, Sanders DR, Jampol LM, Pegman GA, Lieberman HL. Prophylaxis of pseudophakic cystoid macular edema with topical indomethacin. *Ophthalmology* 1982;89:885–890.
41. Flach AJ, Stegman RC, Graham J. Prophylaxis of aphakic cystoid macular edema without corticosteroids. *Ophthalmology* 1990;97: 1253–1258.
42. Flach AJ, Jampol LM, Yannuzzi LA, et al. Improvement in visual acuity in chronic aphakic and pseudophakic cystoid macular edema after treatment with topical 0.5% ketorolac ophthalmic solution. *Am J Ophthalmol* 1991;112:514–519.
43. Flach AJ, Dolan BJ, Irvine AR. Effectiveness of ketorolac 0.5% solution for chronic aphakic and pseudophakic cystoid macular edema. *Am J Ophthalmol* 1987;103:479–486.
44. To K, Abelson MB, Neufeld A. Nonsteroidal antiinflammatory drugs. In: Albert DM, Jakobiec FA, eds. *Principles and practice of ophthal-*

mology: basic sciences. Philadelphia: WB Saunders, 1994;1022–1027.
45. Young BJ, Cunningham WF, Akingbehin T. Double-masked, controlled clinical trial of 5% tolmetin versus 0.5% prednisolone versus 0.9% saline in acute endogenous nongranulomatous anterior uveitis. *Br J Ophthalmol* 1981;26:389–391.
46. Sand BB, Krogh E. Topical indomethacin, a prostaglandin inhibitor, in acute anterior uveitis. A controlled clinical trial of non-steroid versus steroid anti-inflammatory treatment. *Acta Ophthalmol* 1991;69: 145–148.
47. Olsen NY, Lindsley CB, Godfrey WA. Nonsteroidal anti-inflammatory drug therapy in chronic childhood iridocyclitis. *Am J Dis Child* 1988;142:1289–1292.
48. Giordano M. Long-term prophylaxis of recurring spondylitic iridocyclitis with antimalarials and non-steroidal antiphlogistics [German]. *Z Rheumatol* 1982;41:105–106.
49. Foster CS, Sainz de la Maza M. *The sclera.* New York: Springer-Verlag, 1993;299–307.
50. Lyons CJ, Hakin KN, Watson PG. Topical flurbiprofen: an effective treatment for episcleritis? *Eye* 1990;4:521–525.
51. Bishop K, Abelson M, Cheetham J, et al. Evaluation of flurbiprofen in the treatment of antigen-induced allergic conjunctivitis. *Invest Ophthalmol Vis Sci (ARVO Suppl)* 1990;31:487.
52. Buckley DC, Caldwell DR, Reaves TA. Treatment of vernal conjunctivitis with suprofen, topical non-steroidal anti-inflammatory agent. *Invest Ophthalmol Vis Sci (ARVO Suppl)* 1986;27:29.
53. Eakins KE, Whitelock RAF, Bennett A, Martenet AL. Prostaglandin-like activity in ocular inflammation. *Br Med J* 1972;3:452–453.
54. Lam S, Beck RW, Han D, Creighton JB. Atonic pupil after cataract surgery. *Ophthalmology* 1989;96:589–590.
55. Percival SPB. Results after intracapsular extraction: the atonic pupil. *Ophthalmic Surg* 1977;8:138–143.
56. *Physicians' desk reference for ophthalmology.* Montvale, NJ: Medical Economics Data, 1993;236.
57. Fraser-Smith EB, Matthews TR. Effect of ketorolac on *Candida albicans* ocular infection in rabbits. *Arch Ophthalmol* 1987;105:264–267.
58. Fraser-Smith EB, Matthews TR. Effect of ketorolac on *Pseudomonas aeruginosa* ocular infection in rabbits. *J Ocul Pharm* 1988;4:101– 109.
59. Griffin MR, Piper JM, Daugherty JR, Snowden M, Ray LK. Nonsteroidal antiinflammatory drug use and increased risk for peptic ulcer disease in elderly persons. *Ann Intern Med* 1991;114:257–263.
60. Soll AH, Weinstein WM, Kurata J, McCarthy D. Nonsteroidal anti-inflammatory drugs and peptic ulcer disease. *Ann Intern Med* 1991;114: 307–319.
61. Graham DY, Agrawal NM, Roth SH. Prevention of NSAID-induced gastric ulcer with misoprostol, multicentre, double-blind, placebo-controlled trial. *Lancet* 1988;2:1277–1280.
62. Hamburg M, Svensson J, Samuelsson B. Thromboxane: a new group of biologically active compounds derived from prostaglandin endoperoxides. *Proc Natl Acad Sci USA* 1975;72:2994–2998.
63. Clive DM, Stoff JS. Renal syndromes associated with nonsteroidal antiinflammatory drugs. *N Engl J Med* 1984;310:563–572.
64. Rodriguez LAG. The role of nonsteroidal antiinflammatory drugs in acute liver injury. *Br Med J* 1992;305:865–868.
65. Davis LS. New uses for old drugs. In: Wolverton SE, Wilkins JK, eds. *Systemic drugs for skin diseases.* Philadelphia: WB Saunders, 1991; 375–376.
66. Foster CS. Nonsteroidal anti-inflammatory and immunosuppressive agents. In: Lamberts DW, Potter DE, eds. *Clinical ophthalmic pharmacology.* Boston: Little, Brown, 1987;179–181.
67. Meredith TJ, Vale JA. *Non-narcotic analgesics: problems of overdosage.* Drugs 1986;32(suppl 4):177–205.
68. Kim S. Salicylates. In: Olsen KR, ed. *Poisoning and drug overdose.* Norwalk, CT: Appleton and Lange, 1990;261–264.
69. Gurwitz JH, Avorn J, Ross-Degnan D, Lipsitz LA. Nonsteroidal anti-inflammatory drug-associated azotemia in the very old. *JAMA* 1990; 264–471.
70. Byron MA. Treatment of rheumatic diseases. *RMJ* 1987;294:236–238.
71. Harris KP, Jenkins D, Walls J. Nonsteroidal antiinflammatory drugs and cyclosporine. A potentially serious adverse interaction. *Transplantation* 1988;46:598–599.

Textbook of Ocular Pharmacology,
edited by T.J. Zimmerman, et al.
Lippincott–Raven Publishers, Philadelphia © 1997.

CHAPTER 62

Immunosuppressive Chemotherapy

Albert Vitale and C. Stephen Foster

GENERAL CONSIDERATIONS

Although the use of immunosuppressive and biologic agents to inhibit immune reactions is at least half a century old (1), in the past decade, we have witnessed the development of several new modalities and effective treatment strategies for management of inflammatory and immunologic ocular disease. This evolution has been possible largely because we have achieved better insight into the pathophysiology of inflammation and an improved understanding of the immune system's role in the genesis of localized ocular disease as well as the secondary ocular manifestations of systemic diseases and because more potent and selective immunomodulating drugs have been developed. The goal of therapy is suppression of the immune inflammatory response, whether it be due to trauma, surgery, infection, or response to foreign or self-antigens, so that the integrity of ocular structures critical to good visual function is preserved.

Immunosuppressive agents, by definition, suppress development of at least one type of immune reaction: They modify the specific immune sensitization of lymphoid cells (1). However, the precise mechanisms by which these agents achieve their effects remain to be elucidated, for it is often difficult to distinguish between drug-mediated suppression of the immune response itself and suppression of the inflammatory expression thereof. A common feature of this family of drugs is their ability to interfere with the synthesis of nucleic acids and/or protein (Fig. 1). Although these actions are commonly invoked as the major immunosuppressive mechanism because of the exquisite sensitivity of lymphoid proliferation and cytokine elaboration after antigenic stimulation to this type of interference, the effect of immunosuppressive agents cannot be explained by this notion alone (1). This is not surprising, given the extraordinary complexity and interdependence of various immunoregulatory networks.

The immunosuppressive drugs for which sufficient experience and information exists to warrant their use in the treatment of ocular inflammatory conditions are shown in Table 1 according to drug class and include the following: the alkylating agents (cyclophosphamide and chlorambucil), antimetabolites (azathioprine and methotrexate), antibiotics [cyclosporine-A, FK 506, rapamycin (RAPA), and dapsone], and immune-related adjuvants (bromocriptine, ketoconazole, and colchicine).

Because of concerns regarding their low therapeutic index, immunosuppressive agents were, until recently, reserved for treatment of severe, sight-threatening, steroid-resistant uveitis or for use in patients who had developed unacceptable steroid-induced adverse effects. Now, instead of being regarded as merely steroid-sparing, these drugs are often used as first-line agents for a variety of diseases with destructive ocular sequelae such as Wegener's granulomatosis and Behçet's syndrome, for which long-term remission or cure may be achieved. We consider the concurrence of ocular inflammatory disease and polyarteritis nodosa, relapsing polychondritis (especially with renal involvement), or necrotizing scleritis in association with rheumatoid arthritis to be absolute indications for institution of immunosuppressive chemotherapy. The International Uveitis Study Group recommendations include sympathetic ophthalmia and Vogt-Koyanagi-Harada syndrome in this category (2), and we have expanded the list of entities that constitute absolute indications for use of immunosuppressive therapies (Table 2). The patients must be adequately immunosuppressed, yet be spared the potentially serious consequences of drug toxicity (Table 3). In the hands of physicians trained in their use and monitoring, immunosuppressive agents appear to produce fewer serious adverse effects than does chronic use of systemic steroids.

A. Vitale: Retina Specialists of Boston and The Massachusetts Eye and Ear Infirmary, Harvard Medical School, Boston, Massachusetts 02214.

C. S. Foster: Immunology and Uveitis Service, The Massachusetts Eye and Ear Infirmary, Harvard Medical School, Boston, Massachusetts 02214.

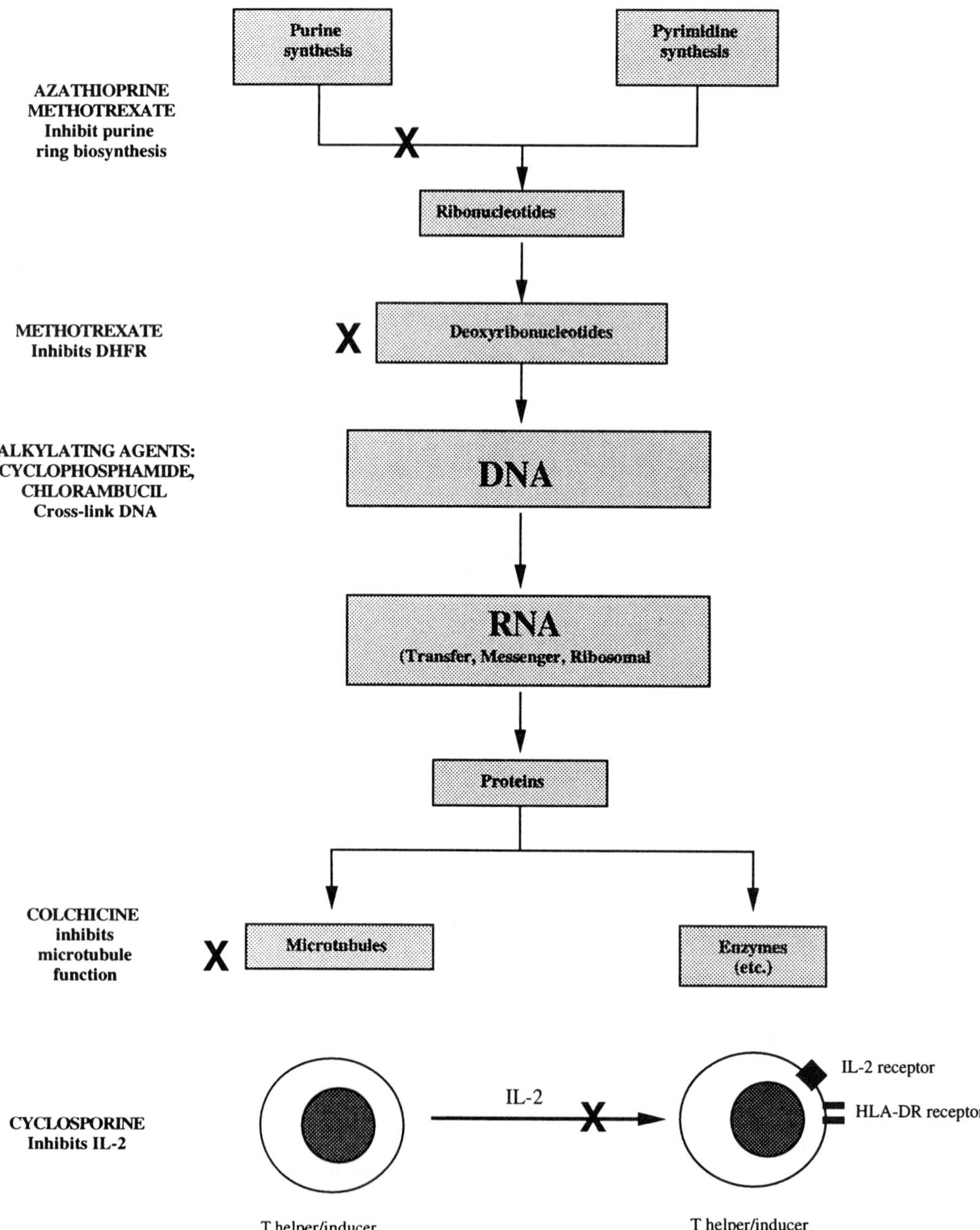

FIG. 62-1. Mechanism of action of immunosuppressive agents used in the treatment of uveitis. (Adapted from Calabresi P, Chabner BA. Chemotherapy of neoplastic diseases. In: Gilman AG, Rall TW, Nies AS, Taylor P, eds. *Goodman and Gilman's the pharmacological basis of therapeutics.* New York: Pergamon Press, 1990;1208.)

TABLE 62-1. *Immunosuppressive drugs: Class, dosage and route of administration*

Class/drug	Dose and route
Alkylating agents	
Cyclophosphamide	1–2 mg/kg/day, p.o., i.v.
Chlorambucil	0.1 mg/kg/day, p.o.
Antimetabolites	
Azathioprine	1–2.4 mg/kg/day, p.o.
Methotrexate	2.5–15 mg every 1–4 weeks, over 36–48 hours, p.o., i.m., i.v.
Antibiotics	
Cyclosporine	2.5–5.0 mg/kg/day, p.o., 5 times daily, topical
FK 506	0.1–0.15 mg/kg/day, p.o.
Rapamycin	
Dapsone	25–50 mg, 2–3 times daily, p.o.
Adjuvants	
Bromocriptine	2.5 mg, 3–4 times daily, p.o.
Ketoconazole	200 mg/1–2 times daily, p.o.
Colchicine	0.5–0.6 mg, 2–3 times daily, p.o.

Immunosuppressive agents represent the final rung in our stepladder approach to the medical treatment of ocular inflammatory disease. The safe use of these drugs begins with exclusion of infectious, mechanical, or other treatable causes of ocular inflammation. Diagnostic studies are then obtained, both based on a careful review of systems and from the physical findings. Whenever possible, biopsy and histologic examination of inflamed tissue are performed (e.g., conjunctival biopsy in patients with ocular cicatricial pemphigoid), because they provide the most reliable guide to the nature of an underlying immunopathologic process. Collaboration with a laboratory expert in the processing and interpretation of such material is essential. The diagnosis, based on the available data and modified as new information is obtained, serves to guide the therapeutic approach. Immunosuppressive chemotherapy is instituted as first-line therapy only when there is an absolute indication for its use. It is rarely necessary for most cases of uveitis.

TABLE 62-2. *General categorization of indications for immunosuppressive chemotherapy*

Indication/disease entity
Absolute
Behçet's disease with retinal involvement
Sympathetic ophthalmia
Vogt-Koyanagi-Harada syndrome
Rheumatoid necrotizing scleritis and/or peripheral ulcerative keratitis
Wegener's granulomatosis
Polyarteritis nodosa
Relapsing polychondritis with scleritis
Juvenile rheumatoid arthritis associated iridocyclitis unresponsive to conventional therapy
Ocular cicatricial pemphigoid
Bilateral Mooren's ulcer
Relative
Intermediate uveitis
Retinal vasculitis with central vascular leakage
Severe chronic iridocyclitis or panuveitis
Questionable
Intermediate uveitis in children
Sarcoid-associated uveitis inadequately responsive to steroid
Keratoplasty with multiple rejections

Informed consent is obtained and documented, and the patient is given an explanation of the potential risks and benefits involved in any therapeutic modality [periocular or systemic steroids, nonsteroidal antiinflammatory drugs (NSAIDs), or immunosuppressive agents] used in the management of patients with progressive, vision-threatening, destructive ocular inflammatory disease. We begin with steroids, and use them aggressively, in the maximally tolerated doses and administer them by all possible routes (topical, periocular injection, systemic). If, despite this approach, the patient's disease is chronic or subject to frequent relapses, we add an oral NSAID to the treatment regimen. If this combination fails to achieve the goal of total quiescence of all ocular inflammation or produces adverse side effects that are unacceptable to either the patient or the physician, the patient is offered the alternative of a systemic immunosuppressive chemotherapeutic drug.

The choice of the immunosuppressive agent is individualized for each patient and depends on a variety of considerations, including the underlying disease, the patient's age, sex, and medical status. (Table 4) Patients are carefully screened for risk factors which might preclude the use of certain immunosuppressive agents (i.e., hepatic disease for methotrexate and renal disease for cyclosporine). Patients are also informed of the proper dosing and intake, potential adverse reactions, and alternatives to immunosuppressive therapy. For example, adequate hydration with oral use of cyclophosphamide substantially reduces the risk of hemorrhagic cystitis, whereas sperm banking is advisable for young patients who are to receive therapy with chlorambucil.

The responsibility for the details of the management of patients requiring immunosuppressive chemotherapy must lie with a clinician who, by virtue of training and experience, is truly expert in the use of these agents and in the recognition and treatment of potentially serious side effects that may arise. A "hand in glove" collaboration between the ophthalmologist and the chemotherapist—usually, in our experience, an oncologist or hematologist—works most effectively for patients requiring such medications.

In contrast to our approach with corticosteroids, with immunosuppressive agents we start with the lowest dose of

TABLE 62-3. *Major adverse reactions of immunosuppresive drugs*

Drug	Adverse reaction
Cyclophosphamide	Sterile hemorrhagic cystitis, myelosuppression, reversible alopecia, secondary malignancies, transient blurring of vision
Chlorambucil	Myelosuppression (moderate but rapid), gonadal dysfunction, secondary malignancies
Methotrexate	Hepatotoxicity, ulcerative stomatitis, bone marrow suppression, diarrhea
Azathioprine	Bone marrow suppression (leukopenia), nausea, secondary infections
Cyclosporine	Nephrotoxicity, hypertension, hyperuricemia, hyperglycemia, hepatotoxicity, nausea, and vomiting
FK 506	Similar to cyclosporine; neurotoxicity
Rapamycin	Unknown
Dapsone	Hemolytic anemia, methemoglobinemia, nausea, mononucleosislike syndrome, blurred vision
Bromocriptine	Postural hypotension, nausea, vomiting
Ketoconazole	Hepatotoxicity, endocrine abnormalities, gastrointestinal upset
Colchicine	Nausea, vomiting, diarrhea, bone marrow suppression

drug and titrate it according to the patient's clinical condition. An adequate therapeutic response and the identification and management of adverse effects is best achieved by careful ocular examination and review of systems at specified intervals to detect subtle changes rather than by exclusive reliance on laboratory results.

TABLE 62-4. *Major indications for specific immunosuppressive drugs*

Drug/indication
Cyclophosphamide
Wegener's granulomatosis, polyarteritis nodosa, necrotizing scleritis associated with rheumatoid arthritis or relapsing polychondritis, Mooren's ulcer, cicatricial pemphigoid, sympathetic ophthalmia, Behçet's disease
Chlorambucil
Behçet's disease, sympathetic ophthalmia, juvenile rheumatoid arthritis (JRA)-associated iridocyclitis
Methotrexate
Sympathetic ophthalmia, scleritis, JRA-associated iridocyclitis
Azathioprine
Behçet's disease, Wegener's granulomatosis, systemic lupus erythematosus, scleritis, cicatricial pemphigoid, JRA-associated iridocyclitis
Cyclosporine
Behçet's disease, birdshot retinochoroidopathy, sarcoidosis, pars planitis, Vogt-Koyanagi-Harada syndrome, sympathetic ophthalmia, idiopathic posterior uveitis, corneal graft rejection
FK 506
Behçet's disease, idiopathic posterior uveitis
Rapamycin
Unknown, adjunct to cyclosporine
Dapsone
Cicatricial pemphigoid, relapsing polychondritis
Bromocriptine
Adjunct to cyclosporine, iridocyclitis, thyroid ophthalmopathy
Ketoconazole
Adjunct to cyclosporine
Colchicine
Behçet's disease

Notwithstanding, periodic complete hemograms, including differential and platelet values, should be obtained in all patients before therapy is initiated and again at 1- to 4-week intervals to monitor for myelosuppression. We avoid depressing the leukocyte count below 3,500 cells/μl or the neutrophil count below 1500 cells/μl, and avoid thrombocytopenia less than 75,000 platelets/μl (3). In addition, liver function tests, urinalysis, blood urea nitrogen (BUN), and serum creatinine should be obtained before initiation of therapy and at intervals of 1 to 4 months, depending on the medication. The frequency of this schedule will depend on the particular agent used and its major toxicity, with more frequent monitoring at the initiation of therapy, during changes in drug dosage, and during episodes of drug toxicity management.

If an adequate clinical response is observed after a minimum of 3 months of treatment at the maximal tolerable dosage or if toxicity precludes continuation of therapy, the medication should be discontinued and consideration given to substituting an alternative immunosuppressive agent. If, instead, a good clinical response is obtained and the patient is free of cellular inflammatory activity in the eye, the drug may be tapered and discontinued in most patients after 1 year of therapy if their disease does not recur.

We have successfully treated a wide variety of uveitic and other ocular inflammatory disorders with immunosuppressive chemotherapy using this stepladder paradigm. Details of the pharmacology of the individual immunosuppressive agents used in this strategy follow.

CYTOTOXIC IMMUNOSUPPRESSIVE DRUGS

The alkylating agents, primarily cyclophosphamide and chlorambucil, and the antimetabolites methotrexate and azathioprine, constitute the two major categories of cytotoxic drugs used in management of ocular inflammatory disease. As a group, the alkylators are more potent agents and consequently are more apt to produce toxic adverse effects.

Alkylating Agents

CYCLOPHOSPHAMIDE

History and Source

Cyclophosphamide belongs to the nitrogen mustard family of alkylating agents and is among the most widely used immunosuppressive chemotherapeutic agents in treatment of autoimmune inflammatory disease. The profound leukopenia and aplasia of lymphoid tissue induced by these agents was first reported in 1919 after sulfur mustard was used as a chemical weapon in World War I (4). The potentially beneficial application of those agents to human disease was first appreciated in the 1940s when nitrogen mustard was administered to patients with lymphoma (5). Roda-Perez (5) in the early 1950s, first reported use of cyclophosphamide for treatment of uveitis of unknown etiology, almost predating the introduction of corticosteroids into ophthalmic practice (6,7). Today, cyclophosphamide plays a primary role in treatment of several potentially lethal systemic vasculitities with destructive ocular involvement (Wegener's granulomatosis and polyarteritis nodosa) as well as several other forms of extraocular and intraocular inflammatory diseases that are poorly responsive to corticosteroids (Table 4).

Official Drug Name and Chemistry

Cyclophosphamide (Cytoxan, Neosar) is 2-*bis* [(2-chloroethyl) amino] tetrahydro-2H-1,3,2-oxazaphosphorine 2-oxide monohydrate and has a molecular weight of 279.1. It is a cyclic oxazaphosphorine (Fig. 2) derived from mechlorethamine with the molecular formula of $C_7H_{15}C_{12}$ $N_2O_2P{\cdot}H_2O$. The biologic activity of this compound is based on the presence of the *bis*-chloroethyl amino group attached to the phosphorus of oxazaphosphorine, and its cyclic structure enhances its chemical stability (8).

Pharmacology

Cyclophosphamide, like many other immunosuppressive agents, is a prodrug and must be converted in vivo by the hepatic microsomal cytochrome P-450 mixed function oxidase system into its active metabolites, phosphoramide mustard and 4-hydroxy-cyclophosphamide (9). These products act through nucleophilic substitution reactions resulting in formation of covalent cross linkages (alkylation) with DNA, thereby mediating their major immunosuppressive activity (Fig. 1). By targeting the 7-nitrogen atom of guanine, cyclophosphamide promotes guanidine-thymidine linkages with resultant DNA miscoding, breaks in single-stranded DNA, and formation of phosphodiester bonds after repair of those breaks, with resultant defective cell function (8). Cross-linkages occur not only between DNA strands, but also between DNA and RNA and between these molecules and cellular proteins, with consequent cytotoxicity (10). The actions of cyclophosphamide are cell cycle-nonspecific.

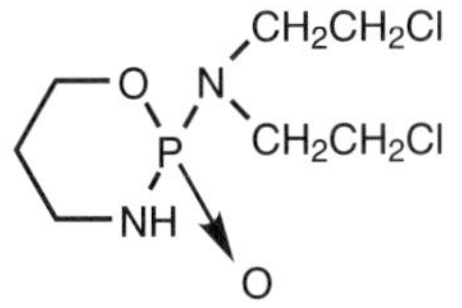

FIG. 62-2. Chemical structure of cyclophosphamide.

Clinical Pharmacology

In doses used clinically, cyclophosphamide has a profound effect on lymphoid cells. Both B- and T-cell function are depressed, although with acute administration of high doses of drug, B cells appear to be more affected (11). In lower doses, or with chronic administration, however, it is likely that cyclophosphamide depresses B- and T-cell populations equally (12,13). The inhibitory effect on the humoral immune system results in suppression of both primary and secondary antibody responses (11,14,16). Cyclophosphamide is also effective in inhibiting cell-mediated immunity, such as the delayed-type skin hypersensitivity (DTH) reaction in both humans and animals (5). It is the only immunosuppressive agent that can induce immunologic tolerance to a particular antigen (10). Development of such tolerance entails complex kinetics and pharmakokinetics, as the drug must be given 24 to 48 hours after antigen priming (15). Although the mechanism of such tolerance is likely to involve the activity of suppressor T cells that develop after antigen priming, low doses of cyclophosphamide in animal models have been shown to enhance immunoreactivity paradoxically by preferentially depressing suppressor T cells, resulting in release from tolerance and the expression of DTH. Higher doses of drug suppressed both T-helper and suppressor T-cell subsets, with consequent blunting of T-cell–mediated humoral and DTH responses, (17–19). Therefore dosage and timing of cyclophosphamide administration apparently are critical to its effect on lymphocyte subsets, which complicates judgments with respect to its clinical use in new applications (10). Although cyclophosphamide has little effect on fully developed macrophages, it does inhibit development of monocyte precursors. Finally, cyclophosphamide has been shown to prevent development of autoimmune disease in the NZB/NZW F_1 mouse model of systemic lupus erythematosus (20).

Pharmaceutics

Cyclophosphamide (Cytoxan, Bristol-Myers Squibb) is supplied as 25- and 50-mg tablets and as a powder in 100,

200, and 500 mg and 1- and 3-g vials (Neosar, Adria, and Cytoxan, Bristol-Myers Squibb) for injection. The drug may be administered orally, intramuscularly, intravenously, intrapleurally, or intraperitoneally. Use with benzyl alcohol-preserved diluents should be avoided.

Pharmakokinetics and Metabolism

Approximately 75% of an oral dose of cyclophosphamide is absorbed from the gastrointestinal (GI) tract, reaching peak plasma levels approximately 1 hour after ingestion, and is widely distributed throughout the body, including the brain (21). The drug undergoes metabolic conversion in the liver into its cytotoxic metabolites, which are approximately 50% bound to serum albumin. The plasma half-life ($t_{\frac{1}{2}}$) of cyclophosphamide is 4 to 6 hours, with 10% to 20% of the native drug, which itself is unbound to plasma proteins, being excreted unchanged in the urine (22). Although the metabolites of cyclophosphamide are oxidized further into inactive products, the acrolein metabolite is believed to play a central role in bladder toxicity (21).

Therapeutic Use

Cyclophosphamide is the treatment of choice for any patient with ocular manifestations of Wegener's granulomatosis or polyarteritis nodosa. Cyclophosphamide, used alone or in combination with systemic steroids, is superior to corticosteroids alone in treating the necrotizing scleritis of Wegener's granulomatosis; with combination therapy, it produces dramatic improvement in patient survival in both disease entities (23–26).

Cyclophosphamide is also the most effective treatment for patients with highly destructive forms of ocular inflammation (peripheral ulcerative keratitis) associated with rheumatoid arthritis; its use correlates positively with survival of those with active systemic and necrotizing ocular disease (28,29).

Although the extraocular manifestations of relapsing polychondritis commonly respond to systemic therapy with dapsone, the necrotizing scleritis and peripheral ulcerative keratitis observed in some of these patients is often more refractory to immunomodulatory therapy than is that associated with Wegener's granulomatosis, polyarteritis nodosa, or rheumatoid arthritis (30,31). In such intransigent cases, we have found that cyclophosphamide, with or without systemic steroid and NSAID therapy is efficacious (32).

Bilateral Mooren's ulcer, although rare, is similarly recalcitrant to conventional therapy, resulting in progressive, relentless, corneal destruction. Foster (33) and Brown and Mondino (34) reported excellent recovery rates and improved prognoses, respectively, in such cases when cyclophosphamide was used.

In patients with active, progressive, ocular cicatricial pemphigoid, cyclophosphamide is used as first-line treatment. Foster (35), in a randomized, double masked, clinical trial, demonstrated that cyclophosphamide, in combination with prednisone, is superior to steroid alone. Typically, the duration of cyclophosphamide therapy is 1 year, with a relapse rate of approximately 20% after discontinuation of therapy (36).

Behçet's disease, affecting the retina or visceral structures, requires immunosuppressive chemotherapy. Either cyclophosphamide or chlorambucil is an appropriate choice for treatment of the posterior uveitis or retinal vasculitis manifestations of this entity. Cyclophosphamide was shown to be superior to steroids in suppressing ocular inflammation in patients with Behçet's disease (37). Similarly, oral cyclophosphamide produced ocular and systemic improvement in a patient with Behçet's disease who had been previously unresponsive to systemic corticosteroids (38). Although chlorambucil may be the single most efficacious agent in management of Behçet's disease, capable of inducing long-term disease remission, intravenous pulse therapy with cyclophosphamide may be a highly effective alternative (39). We and other researchers (40) have shown both agents to be superior to cyclosporine (cyclosporine A, CSA) in management of the posterior segment manifestations of Behçet's disease.

Using our stepladder approach, we have successfully treated many other forms of posterior uveitis with cytotoxic agents, including cyclophosphamide, in patients who have been unresponsive to conventional therapy or who have developed unacceptable steroid-induced side effects (Table 4). Buckley and Gills (41) reported that oral cyclophosphamide was effective in management of 9 patients with pars planitis. Similarly, Wong (42) reported a favorable treatment effect in a small number of patients treated with intravenous cyclophosphamide. More recently, Martenet (43) described a 21-year experience in treating 268 patients with uveitis of various etiologies, including sympathetic ophthalmia, with cytotoxic medication, predominantly cyclophosphamide in combination with procarbazine; visual acuity improved in approximately half of the patients and stabilized in the remainder, with very few treatment failures. The major cause for reduced visual acuity during the study period, even in successful cases, was chronic macular edema and cataract formation. Other than a few isolated cases of azospermia, no important systemic or hematologic complications were observed.

Dosage and Route. The recommended dose of cyclophosphamide for the treatment of ocular disease is 1 to 2 mg/kg/day administered orally or intravenously (Table 1). We prefer that patients take their total daily dose in the morning, instructing them to maintain adequate oral fluids throughout the rest of the day, in an effort to induce frequent voiding. In this way, the risk of hemorrhagic cystitis from prolonged contact of the bladder mucosa with cyclophosphamide metabolites is minimized.

Intravenous administration of cyclophosphamide offers certain advantages over oral administration and is useful in the following clinical situations: (a) It permits rapid induction in patients with severe ocular inflammatory involvement (i.e., fulminant retinal vasculitis in association with Behçet's disease); (b) it avoids prolonged bladder exposure, allowing larger doses, yet less frequent dosing in patients with hemorrhagic cystitis induced from oral intake; and (c) it induces only transient neutropenia, making intercurrent infections less likely.

We administer 1 g/m^2 body surface area of cyclophosphamide intravenously in 250 cc normal saline, piggybacked onto the second half of 1 L 0.5% dextrose in water, infused in a 2-hour period. These infusions are repeated every 3 to 4 weeks, depending on the clinical response and the nadir of the leukocyte count.

Complete hemograms, including platelet levels and leukocyte differentials, and urinalysis must be obtained before initiation of therapy and then again on a weekly basis until the drug dosage, disease activity, and hematologic parameters have stabilized (16). Our goal is to maintain a mild leukopenia: Unlike with many immunosuppressive agents, the level of leukopenia achieved with cyclophosphamide is a reasonable monitor of the adequacy of immunosuppression. We try, however, to avoid a leukocyte count less than 3,500 cells/μl, a neutrophil count less than 1,500 cells/μl, and a platelet count less than 75,000 cells/μl (3). Thereafter, performing hematologic monitoring every 2 weeks and obtaining a monthly serum chemistry profile is appropriate.

Side Effects and Toxicity

A wide variety of toxic effects have been observed (Table 3). As many as 70% of patients experience anorexia, nausea, vomiting, or stomatitis, effects that apparently are dose related (22). We emphasize that for doses we use in the care of our patients with ocular inflammation, the incidence of such side effects is much lower. Five percent to 30% of patients receiving intensive or prolonged therapy experience alopecia, which is usually reversible (21).

The most common dose-limiting toxicity of cyclophosphamide is bone marrow depression, the leukocytes being more significantly affected than the platelets. The nadir of leukopenia usually occurs within 1 to 2 weeks after therapy is initiated; recovery is observed within 10 days of the last dose (44).

A relatively common and well-recognized dose-limiting adverse effect is sterile hemorrhagic cystitis, which results from high concentrations of active metabolites (e.g., aerolein) in the bladder (8). The onset of this complication is variable, occurring as early as 24 hours after initiation of therapy to as late as several weeks after drug discontinuation (44). Should this complication arise, patients must undergo cystoscopy, so that other causes of microscopic hematuria, such as nephritis associated with Wegener's granulomatosis, can be excluded. In addition, the patient's dosing schedule and routine for fluid intake in the afternoon and evening should be carefully reviewed. If hemorrhagic cystitis is confirmed, the bleeding is usually self-limited, with most patients responding to drug cessation, high fluid intake, and bed rest. In severe cases, however, supravesical urinary diversion may be necessary (45). With morning dosing, adequate hydration (2 to 3 L fluid during the day), and frequent voiding, the incidence and severity of this complication may be significantly reduced (35,41).

Cyclophosphamide has been associated with development of secondary malignancies, most commonly acute myelocytic leukemia and bladder carcinoma, in patients with intercurrent neoplastic, rheumatologic, or renal disease who have received cumulative doses in excess of 76 g (46). It has been recommended that patients who have received daily doses in excess of 50 g cyclophosphamide for more than 2 years or who have experienced multiple episodes of hemorrhagic cystitis undergo routine screening, including yearly urine cytology (47). If suspicious or malignant cells are present, biopsy of abnormal areas is mandatory.

Gonadal dysfunction, including azospermia and amenorrhea, has been observed in 60% of patients after 6 months of treatment with cyclophosphamide (48). Because this effect may be irreversible, sperm banking is advisable before initiation of therapy, particularly if protracted therapy is anticipated.

Ocular side effects have been reported, including dry eyes in as many as 50% of patients treated, blurred vision, and increased intraocular pressure (IOP) (49). The mechanism underlying those adverse effects or a causal link to cyclophosphamide therapy itself is poorly defined (16). Other less common adverse effects include cardiac myopathy (usually occurring with large doses), hepatic dysfunction, irreversible pulmonary fibrosis, impaired renal clearance of water with resultant hyponatremia, and anaphylaxis (22).

Overdose. Signs and symptoms of cyclophosphamide overdose are identical to the toxic effects previously discussed herein. No specific antidote exists. Management is generally supportive, with appropriate treatment of concurrent infection, myelosuppression, or cardiac toxicity as indicated.

Recently, a human granulocyte colony-stimulating factor (G-CSF) has become available through recombinant DNA technology. Filgrastim (Neupogen, Amgen) has been shown to be safe and effective in accelerating recovery of neutrophil counts after administration of a variety of chemotherapeutic regimens, and thus decreases the risk of systemic infection (22). Filgrastim may be administered subcutaneously or intravenously at an initial dose of 5 μg/kg/day, as a single daily injection, for neutrophil counts less than 500/μl. The drug should not be initiated until 24 hours after a given dose of chemotherapy and should be discontinued 24 hours before the next cycle of chemotherapy. The dose may be increased by 5 μg/kg/day after 5 to 7 days, with daily administration of filgrastim until the neutrophil count returns to normal levels (i.e., more than 10,000 μl) (22).

High-risk Groups

Clinicians must be vigilant in detecting untoward toxicity or the development of opportunistic infections in any patient treated with cyclophosphamide who is concurrently receiving immunosuppression for an independent reason: previous radiation therapy, tumor cell infiltration of the bone marrow, or previous therapy with cytotoxic agents. Viral infections, especially herpes zoster, tend to occur more readily in neutropenic patients receiving cyclophosphamide (50). Cytotoxic therapy, in general, is contraindicated in patients with focal chorioretinitis, herpes simplex, herpes zoster, Cytomegalovirus, AIDS retinopathy, toxoplasmosis, tuberculosis, and fungal infections (51).

Because the major routes of metabolism and excretion for cyclophosphamide are hepatic and renal, dosage reductions have been recommended for patients with hepatic and renal dysfunction. However, anephric patients treated with full doses of cyclophosphamide failed to exhibit increased hematologic or other toxic side effects (52).

Because cyclophosphamide is a teratogen, causing CNS and skeletal abnormalities in the fetus, contraception is inadvisable during cyclophosphamide therapy. Nursing mothers should be cautioned that the drug is excreted in the breast milk and may exert toxic effects in their infants (50).

The use of cytotoxic drugs (cyclophosphamide, chlorambucil, azathioprine, or methotrexate) in children for treatment of non–life-threatening inflammatory disease is less controversial today than even 5 years ago, due in large measure to the pioneering work of rheumatologists treating children with juvenile rheumatoid arthritis (JRA). Although there is little question about the efficacy of such therapy in children with, for example, JRA-associated iridocyclitis that is unresponsive to steroids and other conventional treatments, the potential risks of delayed malignancy or sterility associated with the treatment must be seriously considered, especially with regard to alkylating agent therapy, because of the age of the patients. We explore the merits and drawbacks of the various treatment options with both the patient and the parents, making the decision of whether or not to use cytotoxic agents on an individual basis. It is hoped that prospective comparative trials in this patient group will clarify the relative risks and benefits of systemic immunosuppressive chemotherapy early in the course of chronic inflammation associated with JRA (10).

Contraindications. Cyclophosphamide is contraindicated in patients with severely depressed bone marrow function and in those with a history of hypersensitivity to the drug.

Drug Interactions

The metabolism of cyclophosphamide is affected by drugs that induce (phenobarbital) or inhibit (allopurinol) the hepatic microsomal mixed function oxidase system (22). Consequently, concurrent administration of allopurinol prolongs the serum $t_{\frac{1}{2}}$ of cyclophosphamide, and chronic administration of high doses of phenobarbital increases its metabolism and leukopenic activity. Chloramphenicol and corticosteroids may inhibit microsomal enzyme metabolism of cyclophosphamide and thus blunt its action, and the effects of agents such as halothane, nitrous oxide, and succinylcholine are enhanced by cyclophosphamide (44). In addition, cyclophosphamide increases the myocardial toxicity of doxorubicin (21). Finally, other immunosuppressive agents may have synergistic immunosuppressive and carcinogenic effects.

Major Clinical Trials

Clinical studies of importance with respect to the efficacy of each of the individual immunosuppressive agents for treatment of noninfectious inflammatory ocular disease are cited and discussed in the Therapeutic Use section.

CHLORAMBUCIL

Chlorambucil was first synthesized in the early 1950s and was subsequently introduced into the clinical world primarily for the treatment of malignant lymphoma (5). Today, it is the treatment of choice for chronic lymphocytic leukemia and primary (Waldenstrom's) macroglobulinemia and is sometimes used to treat the vasculitic complications of rheumatoid arthritis, autoimmune hemolytic anemias associated with cold agglutinins, and Hodgkin's disease (22). Chlorambucil was introduced into ophthalmic practice in 1970 when Mamo and Azzam (53) first reported its efficacy in the treatment of Behçet's disease, and today remains the most frequently used immunosuppressive agent in its management.

Official Drug Name and Chemistry

Chlorambucil (Leukeran) is 2-[*bis* (chlorethyl) amino]-benzenebutanoic acid with a molecular weight of 304.21. Its structure (Fig. 3) as an aromatic derivative of mechlorethamine renders it essentially inert, making it suitable for oral administration (5).

PHARMACOLOGY

Chlorambucil, like cyclophosphamide, is a nitrogen mustard derivative; the two share many similar pharmacologi-

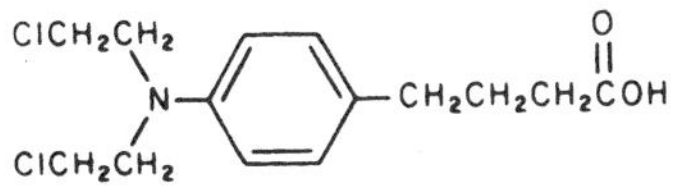

FIG. 62-3. Chemical structure of chlorambucil.

cal properties, including a common mechanism of action (Fig. 1). As an alkylating agent, chlorambucil interferes with DNA replication and RNA transcription, ultimately resulting in disruption of nucleic acid function. These actions are cell cycle nonspecific.

Clinical Pharmacology

Chlorambucil has immunosuppressive properties, exerting its action principally through suppression of B lymphocytes. It is the slowest-acting nitrogen mustard derivative in clinical use, requiring 2 weeks to have an effect (50). Its cytotoxic effects on the bone marrow, lymphoid organs, and epithelial tissues are similar to those of other agents in this class of drugs (8).

Pharmaceutics

Chlorambucil (Leukeran, Glaxo-Wellcome, Research Triangle Park, NC) is available in 2-mg sugar-coated tablets for oral use. The drug should be stored at 59° to 77°F in a dry place.

Pharmacokinetics and Metabolism

Chlorambucil is readily absorbed after oral administration, reaching peak plasma levels in 1 hour, and is distributed throughout the tissues in a fairly homogeneous fashion (44). As an unmetabolized prodrug, chlorambucil is extensively bound to plasma and tissue proteins, with a plasma $t_{1/2}$ of 1 to 5 hours. It is extensively metabolized in the liver to the active principal, phenylacetic acid mustard, which itself retains a $t_{1/2}$ of approximately 2.5 hours (22). Renal excretion is the major route of elimination for this and other metabolites; very little drug is excreted unchanged in the urine or feces.

Therapeutic Use

The efficacy of chlorambucil in the management of ocular or neuro-Behçet's disease has been confirmed by numerous investigators (54–58) since its introduction by Mamo and Azzam (53). Although Tabbara (59) questioned the use of this agent because of concerns about its effect on spermatogenesis, long-term remissions and cures have been reported with chlorambucil in patients with Behçet's disease (60,61). In managing Behçet's disease, we treated 8 of 29 patients with chlorambucil, effecting long-term inflammatory control in all but 1 (39). Although cyclosporine, when used at high doses (10 mg/kg/day), has been reported to produce dramatic and prompt responses in patients with Behçet's disease (62), this dose is now clearly contraindicated because of its nephrotoxicity. At more acceptable, less nephrotoxic doses (5–7 mg/kg/day), cyclosporine may not induce long-standing drug-free remissions and is, in our experience and that of other investigators (63), distinctly inferior to chlorambucil, cyclophosphamide, and azathioprine in the care of the ocular complications of Behçet's disease.

Chlorambucil has also been used successfully in treatment of various other forms of uveitis recalcitrant to conventional therapy (Table 4). Godfrey et al. (64) reported that 10 of 31 patients with intractable idiopathic uveitis improved with chlorambucil. Andrasch et al. (65) conducted a trial in which 25 patients were treated with either azathioprine in combination with low-dose steroids or chlorambucil. All 13 patients with severe chronic uveitis responded to chlorambucil, whereas 10 of them were either intolerant of or failed to respond to azathioprine. Jennings and Tessler (66) have presented data confirming the observations of previous investigators (43,64) which suggest that chlorambucil may be effective in treatment of sympathetic ophthalmia.

Finally, several investigators (64,67,68) have shown intractable JRA-associated iridocyclitis to be responsive to chlorambucil. Although Godfrey et al. (64) reported equivocal results in 1 patient, Kanski (67) described favorable responses in 5 of 6 patients with ocular inflammation associated with JRA who were treated with chlorambucil. Foster and Barrett (68) achieved complete inflammatory control in 3 patients with JRA-associated iridocyclitis, 1 of whom had been unresponsive to systemic and topical corticosteroids, NSAIDs, and methotrexate.

Dosage and Route of Administration. Several dosage regimens have been suggested for oral administration of chlorambucil. Godfrey et al. (64) advocate an initial dose of 2 mg/day, increased by an additional 2 mg/day for a maximal dose of 10 to 12 mg/day or until a favorable clinical response is observed. We prefer to begin with a dose of 0.1 mg/kg/day, titrating the dose based on the clinical response and drug tolerance every 3 weeks, for a maximum daily dose of 18 mg/day (Table 1). Such high doses are used only in cases of severe sight-threatening inflammation in patients who display no untoward reaction to the drug. All patients receiving chlorambucil require vigilant monitoring for potential adverse reactions, particularly myelosuppression, as this complication increases significantly at doses greater than 10 mg/day. Hematologic monitoring is performed as previously described for cyclophosphamide, with similar target parameters for leukocyte, neutrophil, and platelet counts. We advocate increased vigilance in monitoring at approximately 3 months of treatment. A dose-accumulation effect on the bone marrow is common, and dosage must be reduced progressively in the ensuing 3 to 6 months. Liver function tests should be repeated every 3 to 4 months.

Side Effects and Toxicity

Hematologic toxicity is the most prominent adverse effect of chlorambucil therapy (Table 3). Myelosuppression is usually moderate, gradual, and reversible (69). However, abrupt and profound leukopenia, sometimes persisting for months after discontinuation of chlorambucil, may occur, particularly when high doses (10 mg/day) are administered for prolonged times. If leukocyte or platelet counts fall below the target level, the dose of chlorambucil should be reduced. If profound depression occurs, the drug must be discontinued.

Chlorambucil may produce significant gonadal dysfunction. In a group of 10 patients reported by Tabbara (59), 7 developed oligospermia and 3 acquired azoospermia when a dose of 0.2 mg/kg was used. We do not recommend this dose. This effect may or may not be reversible after therapy is discontinued. As with cyclophosphamide, before initiation of therapy with chlorambucil, sperm banking should be recommended to adolescent men and adults who are still planning a family. In women, potentially irreversible ovarian dysfunction resulting in a medication-induced menopause may arise with prolonged therapy (70).

Malignancies, mostly acute leukemia, have been reported in patients with polycythemia vera receiving daily doses greater than 4 mg (71) and in patients with breast cancer who are receiving protracted therapy with chlorambucil (72). Other, less commonly encountered toxicities include gastrointestinal distress, pulmonary fibrosis, hepatitis, rash, and CNS stimulation (44), including seizures in adults and children (33).

Overdose. There is no specific antidote for overdosage with chlorambucil, the signs and symptoms of which mirror its toxicity. As with cyclophosphamide, management is supportive, with appropriate treatment of concurrent infections and myelosuppression with G-CSF as indicated.

High-risk Groups

Chlorambucil is a potential teratogen and has been reported to cause urogenital abnormalities in the offspring of mothers receiving this drug during the first trimester of pregnancy (74). Although no well-controlled studies have been performed in pregnant women, those of childbearing potential should avoid becoming pregnant, and those who become pregnant while receiving chlorambucil should be advised of the potential hazard to the fetus. Whether the drug is excreted in the breast milk is not known.

As with cyclophosphamide, the safety and effectiveness of chlorambucil for the treatment of sight-threatening ocular inflammatory disease in the pediatric age group is controversial and is best considered on a case-by-case basis.

Contraindications. Chlorambucil is contraindicated in patients who have demonstrated either previous resistance or hypersensitivity to it.

Drug Interactions

There are no known drug–drug interactions with chlorambucil, although other immunosuppressive agents undoubtedly have an additive effect.

Major Clinical Trials

Major clinical trials are described in the Therapeutic Use section.

Antimetabolites

METHOTREXATE

History and Source

In 1948, inhibitors of the vitamin folic acid were first reported to produce striking, although temporary, remissions in acute leukemia in children (75). Subsequently, in 1963, the curative potential of chemotherapy in human cancer was demonstrated when methotrexate was shown to produce long-term, complete remissions of trophoblastic choriocarcinoma in women (76). Today, methotrexate is the agent of choice (in combination with mercaptopurine) in the maintenance therapy of acute lymphocytic leukemia (22) and is effective in treatment of a variety of systemic inflammatory conditions, including psoriasis, rheumatoid arthritis refractory to conventional therapy, JRA, Reiter's disease, polymyositis and, in rare cases, sarcoidosis (10,77, 78). The use of methotrexate in management of ocular inflammatory disease has been reported rarely, with the first citation by Wong and Hersh (79) appearing in 1965. Experience with this agent in treatment of non–life-threatening systemic inflammatory disease has grown, and methotrexate is now frequently the first immunosuppressive agent considered for use in cases of pediatric uveitis refractory to more conventional therapy.

Official Drug Name and Chemistry

Methotrexate (Folex, Mexate, Rheumatrex) is 4-amino-N^{10}-methyl pteroylglutamic acid, with a molecular weight of 454.5. Its structure (Fig. 4) is analogous to that of folic acid, differing only in two areas: the amino group in the 4-carbon position is substituted for a hydroxyl group, and a methyl group at the N^{10} position appears instead of a hydrogen atom (80).

Pharmacology

Methotrexate prevents the conversion of dihydrofolate to tetrahydrofolate by competitively and irreversibly binding to the enzyme dihydrofolate reductase (DHFR) (8).

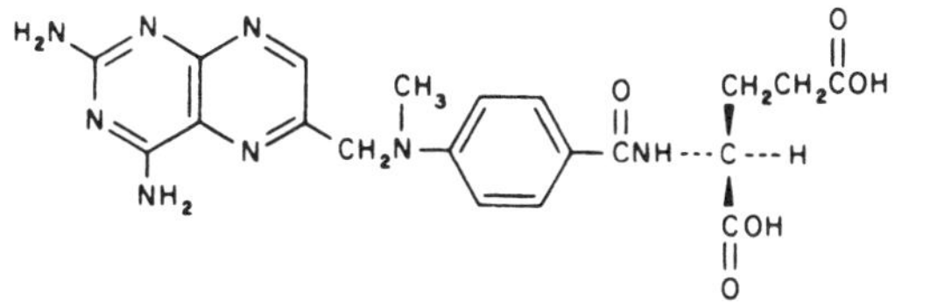

FIG. 62-4. Chemical structure of methotrexate.

Tetrahydrofolate is an essential cofactor in the production of 1-carbon units critical to synthesis of purine nucleotides and thymidylate. In addition, a less rapid, partially reversible competitive inhibition of thymidylate synthetase also occurs within 24 hours after methotrexate administration (8). The net effect is inhibition of DNA synthesis, repair, RNA synthesis, and cell division in a cell cycle-specific (S phase) fashion (Fig. 5).

The blockage of DHFR can be bypassed clinically by use of leukovorin calcium (N^5-formyl-tetrahydrofolate, folinic acid, citrovorum factor), a fully functional folate coenzyme (8). So-called "leucovorin rescue" is achieved, allowing recovery of normal tissues and permitting use of larger doses of methotrexate.

Clinical Pharmacology

Methotrexate has little effect on resting cells; instead, it exerts its cytotoxic actions in actively proliferating tissues such as malignant cells, fetal cells, cells of the GI tract, urinary bladder, buccal mucosa, and bone marrow. By inhibiting DNA synthesis in immunologically competent cells, methotrexate has some activity as an immunosuppressive agent. Both B and T cells are affected (81), and the primary and secondary antibody responses can be suppressed when administered during antigen encounter (82,83). Apparently, it has no significant effect on cell-mediated immunity. Low-dose methotrexate has been shown to depress acute-phase reactants while leaving cellular parameters unaltered (84,85). These observations have led some investigators to suggest that, at these doses, methotrexate acts more as an antiinflammatory agent than as an immunosuppressive agent, possibly explaining its reduced effectiveness in treatment of chronic uveitis and retinal vasculitis as compared to that in treatment of scleritis and orbital myositis (86).

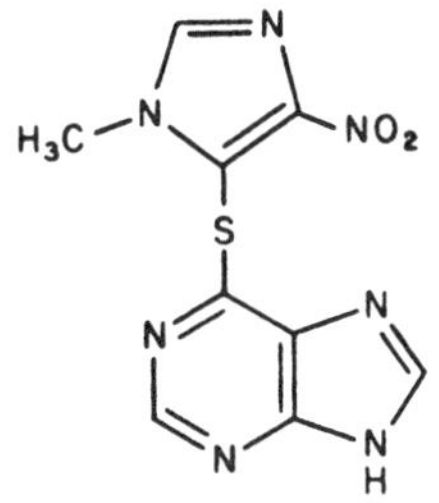

FIG. 62-5. Chemical structure of azathioprine.

Pharmaceutics

Methotrexate (Lederle, Philadelphia, PA) is available in 2.5-mg tablets and as preparations for injection (intravenous, intramuscular, intrathecal) as follows: methotrexate (Lederle) solution, 2.5 and 25 mg/ml; (methotrexate LPF) powder, 20, 50, 100, 250 mg and 1 g; and Folex (Adria) solution, 25 mg/ml.

Pharmakokinetics and Metabolism

Orally administered methotrexate is readily absorbed through a dose-dependent, saturable active transport system, with peak plasma concentrations attained in 1 to 4 hours. The peak plasma concentration after intramuscular injection is 30 minutes to 2 hours. Once absorbed, the plasma concentration of methotrexate undergoes a triphasic reduction: The first phase is the fastest (0.75 hours) and reflects drug distribution throughout the body; the second occurs over 2 to 4 hours and represents renal excretion; the third phase, varying between 10 and 27 hours, is the terminal $t_{\frac{1}{2}}$ of the drug and is believed to reflect the slow release of DHFR bound to methotrexate from the tissues (87).

Approximately 50% of methotrexate is bound to plasma proteins, with the remaining unbound fraction mediating its cytotoxic effects (8). Drug concentrations and duration of cellular exposure are important determinants of these effects and are influenced by factors which might increase the unbound portion (displacement from plasma proteins by other drugs) or prolong drug elimination (renal insufficiency). Methotrexate is transported into cells by carrier-mediated active transport systems and stored intracellularly in the form of polyglutamate conjugates, which may be important determinants of the site and duration of action (22). Methotrexate is believed to be minimally metabolized, with 50% to 90% excreted unchanged in the urine by a combination of glomerular filtration and active tubular secretion (8). The drug does accumulate in the liver and kidney, however, particularly after high doses, prolonged administration, or both. Retention of the drug as polyglutamates for long periods is postulated to play a key role in methotrexate toxicity (80).

Therapeutic Use

Concern regarding the adverse effects of methotrexate may have limited its use in management of ocular inflammatory disease (Table 4). In their initial reports, Wong and Hersh (79,88) reported favorable responses in 9 of 10 patients with steroid-resistant cyclitis who were treated with high-dose (25 mg/m^2) intravenous methotrexate every 4 hours for 6 weeks. Although few serious adverse reactions occurred, inflammatory symptoms recurred in more than half of the patients when therapy was discontinued. Wong (89) successfully used a similar strategy in treating a patient with sympathetic ophthalmia recalcitrant to conventional therapy. Lazar et al. (90) obtained similarly encouraging results in 14 of 17 patients with various steroid-resistant uveitis, including 4 with sympathetic ophthalmia, who were treated with intravenous methotrexate. However, this success was associated with significant drug-induced toxicity, including GI complications, secondary infections, and laboratory evidence of liver damage.

More recently, the reduced frequency and severity of adverse reactions reported with oral or intramuscular low-dose, pulsed (weekly) methotrexate therapy in the dermatologic (91) and rheumatologic literature (92) has been exploited in management of a variety of ocular inflammatory disorders. Methotrexate may be sufficient to control scleritis associated with collagen vascular diseases such as Reiter's syndrome and rheumatoid arthritis, but not in collagen diseases complicated by relapsing polychondritis (32). Uveitic entities, for which once-weekly oral or intramuscular methotrexate may be particularly well-suited include those associated with Reiter's syndrome, ankylosing spondylitis, inflammatory bowel disease, psoriatic arthritis, and JRA (10,68). In retrospective study, 56% of 12 patients with chronic uveitis-vitritis and retinal vasculitis responded to oral low-dose, pulsed methotrexate in combination with corticosteroids (86). In the same study, 9 of 10 patients with inflammatory pseudotumor, orbital myositis, and scleritis showed improvement, with 5 (50%) achieving disease remission.

Dosage and Route of Administration. We initiate methotrexate therapy with a weekly dose of 2.5 mg to 7.5 mg administered orally, intramuscularly, or intravenously, as either a single or divided dose, in a 36- to 48-hour period (Table 1). The dose is escalated gradually as dictated by the clinical response to a maximum of 15 mg/week.

Methotrexate has a delayed onset of action, requiring 3 to 6 weeks to take effect (50). Complete hemograms, with platelet and differential values, should be obtained before the onset of therapy and at intervals of 1 to 4 weeks. Similarly, pretreatment liver function tests, urinalysis, BUN, and serum creatinine should be obtained, and tests should be repeated every 3 to 6 weeks.

Side Effects and Toxicity

Myelosuppression is the major dose-limiting toxicity of methotrexate (Table 3). Leukopenia and thrombocytopenia appear in the first 2 weeks after a bolus dose or short-term infusion, usually with rapid recovery. Although more prolonged and severe myelosuppression is more commonly associated with higher doses, or occurs in patients with compromised renal, liver, or bone marrow function, pancytopenia has been reported with low-dose methotrexate therapy (93). Leucovorin is given in such cases to rescue the bone marrow, optimally in 6 to 8 hours after methotrexate administration, and is continued for 72 hours thereafter (87). Doses equal to or greater than the last dose of methotrexate are administered either intravenously, generally ranging from 10 to 15 mg/m^2, or orally at doses not in excess of 25 mg, every 6 hours. Depending on the serum methotrexate levels at 24 and 72 hours after dosing, leucovorin rescue should be continued until the levels of methotrexate decrease to less than 10^{-8} M (94). Although leucovorin effectively counteracts the toxic side effects of folic acid antagonists such as methotrexate, it also impairs its therapeutic efficacy.

Considerable attention has been focused on methotrexate-induced hepatotoxicity which may develop after short- and long-term use. Acute liver toxicity, manifested by a transient increase in serum transaminases may be evident within a few days of high-dose methotrexate administration. Chronic, low-dose methotrexate therapy, as is commonly used in management of some patients with psoriasis or rheumatoid arthritis, may lead to hepatic fibrosis and, occasionally, to cirrhosis (80). Liver function tests are not reliable indexes of the development of hepatic fibrosis; liver biopsy is the definitive diagnostic procedure. Current guidelines suggest a biopsy before administration of methotrexate in patients at high risk of development of hepatotoxicity (those with obesity, alcoholism, or intercurrent liver or kidney disease) and in all patients receiving a cumulative dose of 1.5 g if further treatment with methotrexate is anticipated (94). The role of routine liver biopsy in the follow-up of patients receiving low-dose methotrexate has been challenged, especially in light of the small numbers of patients who develop clinical, laboratory, and histopathologic evidence of liver disease while treated with this regimen (92,95). Therefore, the clinician must decide, on a case-by-case basis, whether the cost and risk of the procedure outweighs the possibility that biopsy results will dictate a change in the patient's management. We do not treat patients who are at increased risk of development of hepatotoxicity with methotrexate, and we do not monitor patients whom we do treat with liver biopsy.

Pulmonary toxicity, including acute pneumonitis and pulmonary fibrosis, has been reported with both low- and high-dose methotrexate therapy. Pneumonitis presents with a dry nonproductive cough with dyspnea, high fever, and hypoxemia and probably represents either an idiosyncratic reaction or hypersensitivity (96). It usually responds to discontinuation of methotrexate and brief systemic steroid therapy.

GI toxicities include nausea, ulcerative mucositis, and diarrhea, all of which may respond to dosage reduction (97). Alopecia, dermatitis, and acute renal failure due to precipitation of drug in the renal tubules may occur with high-dose regimens (80). To date, no controlled data in humans or animals indicate that methotrexate is carcinogenic (98–100).

Finally, ocular side effects are not uncommon; they include irritation, photophobia, aggravation of seborrheic blepharitis, and epiphoria in 25% of patients (49). These signs and symptoms usually abate with time and do not necessitate discontinuation of drug.

Overdose. The signs and symptoms of methotrexate overdosage parallel its toxic side effects. Leucovorin should be administered as promptly as possible to diminish these effects. General supportive measures, as in management of any drug overdose, should be instituted.

High-risk Groups

Methotrexate is a known teratogen and abortifacient and may cause oligospermia (87). Women of childbearing age treated with this medication must use reliable contraception. In addition, due to concerns regarding the mutagenic potential of methotrexate, both men and women should allow at least a 12-week period to elapse between discontinuation of therapy and attempt at conception. Methotrexate therapy is also ill-advised in nursing mothers because of the potential serious adverse reactions from this drug in breast-fed infants. The safety and effectiveness of methotrexate in the pediatric age group has not been established; however, one study indicates that this agent is well-tolerated in children with JRA (101).

The risk of developing serious liver disease from treatment with low-dose methotrexate increases with age and other factors (92). Decreasing renal and hepatic reserves in the elderly contribute significantly to this problem; therefore, clinicians should use extreme caution in administering methotrexate in this age group. Callen and Kulp-Shorten (80) suggest performing a creatinine clearance in any patient aged more than 50 years for whom methotrexate treatment is considered and that a value less than 50 ml/minute constitutes a contraindication to its use.

Contraindications. Groups in whom methotrexate therapy is contraindicated include pregnant or nursing women; patients with known alcoholism, alcoholic liver disease, or chronic liver disease of any etiology; patients with immunodeficiency states, irrespective of cause; patients with preexisting blood dyscrasias or bone marrow suppression, and any patient with a known hypersensitivity to the drug.

Drug Interactions

Concomitant consumption of salicylates, sulfonamides, chloramphenicol, or tetracycline may increase the fraction of unbound serum methotrexate through displacement from plasma proteins, thereby potentiating the risk of methotrexate-induced adverse effects. Similarly, concurrent treatment with drugs such as NSAIDs or probenecid, which impair renal blood flow or tubular secretion, may delay drug excretion and lead to severe toxicity (22).

Major Clinical Trials

Major clinical trials are described in the Therapeutic Use section.

AZATHIOPRINE

History and Source

Azathioprine was introduced and developed in the early 1960s as a derivative of 6-mercaptopurine (6-MP) in an effort to produce a drug with similar immunosuppressive action but a more prolonged duration of activity (21). Today, 6-MP is rarely used; however, azathioprine remains a mainstay in organ transplant surgery and is one of the most widely used agents in treatment of dermatologic and autoimmune diseases; it is approved by the FDA for use in patients with rheumatoid arthritis. 6-MP and azathioprine were introduced into ophthalmic practice by Newell et al. in 1966 (102) and 1967 (103) and were among the first immunosuppressants used for treatment of ocular immune-mediated disorders.

Official Drug Name and Chemistry

Chemically azathioprine (Imuran, Glaxo-Wellcome, Research Triangle Park, NC) is 6[(1-methyl-4-nitroimidazol-5 ql) thio] purine with a molecular weight of 277.29 (Fig. 5). It is an imidazolyl derivative of 6-MP and is therefore classified as a purine analogue. Both drugs are structurally similar to hypoxanthine, an important precursor in purine metabolism (8).

Pharmacology

Azathioprine is a prodrug which is quickly metabolized in the liver to its active form, 6-MP, which in turn interferes with purine metabolism and ultimately with DNA, RNA, and protein synthesis (Fig. 1). Specifically, 6-MP, through its conversion to thioinosine-5-phosphate, a purine analogue, provides a false precursor, thereby impairing adenine and guanine nucleotide formation (8). DNA metabolism is inhibited in a cell cycle-specific (S phase) manner.

Clinical Pharmacology

Although the immunosuppressive effects of azathioprine probably relate to the disruption of DNA synthesis in immunocompetent lymphoid cells, its action is incompletely understood and cannot be explained by this mechanism alone. The humoral immune response is relatively unaffected by azathioprine when administered in therapeutic, nontoxic doses of 2 to 3 mg/kg/day. However, variable alterations in antibody production can occur when large doses of thiopurine are administered within 48 hours of antigen priming and may induce temporary tolerance when administered in conjunction with large doses of antigen (1).

Azathioprine has been shown to suppress both B and T lymphocytes, the effect of which is relatively more selective for the latter cellular subset (104). In addition, thiopurines suppress the mixed lymphocyte reaction in vivo, depress recirculating T lymphocytes that are in the process of homing, and suppress the development of monocyte precursors and thus the participation of K cells (which themselves are derived from monocyte precursors) in antibody-dependent cytotoxicity reactions (10). Although thiopurines inhibit delayed-type hypersensitivity reactions and prolong renal, skin, and cardiac allografts, they do not affect development of autoimmune disease in New Zealand black mice, which is mainly antibody-mediated (20).

Pharmaceutics

Azathioprine (Imuran, Glaxo-Wellcome, Research Triangle Park, NC) is available as 50-mg tablets for oral administration or as a lyophilized powder equivalent to 100 mg drug for intravenous use. This medication should be stored in a dry place at 59° to 77°F and should be protected from light.

Pharmacokinetics and Metabolism

After oral administration, approximately 50% of azathioprine is absorbed within 2 hours (21). It is rapidly metabolized in erythrocytes and in the liver, where it is cleaved to mercaptopurine and then catabolized to various methylated derivatives. Specifically, xanthine oxidase catalyzes the formation of 6-thiouric acid, the principal metabolite, whereas approximately 10% of azathioprine is cleaved to form 1-methyl-4 nitro-5 thioimidizole (8). Proportionate variation in these metabolites may explain the differences in the magnitude and duration of drug effects among individual patients.

Approximately 30% of both azathioprine and 6-MP are bound to serum protein. Renal clearance accounts for less than 2% of its excretion; neither drug is detectable in the urine after 8 hours (22). Typical doses of azathioprine produce blood levels of less than 1 μg/ml; however, since both the magnitude and duration of its clinical effects correlate with the level of thiopurine nucleotide in the target tissues, blood levels of azathioprine or 6-MP are of little value in guiding therapy (21). Cytotoxicity is enhanced in patients with renal insufficiency because effects may persist long after drug clearance is complete.

Therapeutic Use

Many reports in the ophthalmic literature describe successful control of various corticosteroid-resistant ocular inflammatory diseases and uveitic syndromes with azathioprine, alone or in combination with corticosteroids or other immunosuppressive agents (Table 4). Azathioprine has been effective in treatment of scleritis associated with relapsing polychondritis (RP) (32) and as an adjunctive, second-line agent in control of progressive conjunctival inflammation in ocular cicatricial pemphigoid (35).

Reports of the efficacy of azathioprine in various uveitic syndromes have been variable. Newell et al. (103) treated 20 patients with uveitis of different etiologies and found that azathioprine was most effective in those with pars planitis. Andrash et al. (65) reported that azathioprine, in combination with corticosteroids, was effective in 12 of 22 patients with chronic uveitis. However, azathioprine was discontinued in 4 patients who failed to respond and in 6 with GI distress. In contradistinction, Mathews et al. (105) showed that azathioprine, compared with placebo in a controlled, double-masked trial, was no more effective than placebo in reducing the inflammatory activity of 19 patients with chronic iridocyclitis. Whereas Moore (106), using a combination of azathioprine and corticosteroids, reported successful treatment of sympathetic ophthalmia in a child in 1968, subsequent work by Newell and Krill (103) and Martenet (43) failed to duplicate this experience. In our practice (107), azathioprine has been effective in treatment of JRA-associated iridocyclitis unresponsive to conventional steroid therapy.

In treatment of Behçet's disease, a recent 2-year, double-masked, randomized, controlled study demonstrated that azathioprine (2.5 mg/kg/day) prevented development of new eye lesions and reduced the frequency and intensity of recurrent inflammation in patients with established ocular or systemic disease (108). No serious adverse effects were reported among the 37 treated patients. Foster et al. (39) reported more equivocal results among 8 patients with Behçet's disease. Inflammatory control was achieved in 1 patient treated with a combination of azathioprine and corticosteroids and in 2 patients receiving azathioprine and cyclosporine; however, therapy had to be discontinued in 1 patient who developed severe leukopenia (39). We do not consider azathioprine the most effective drug for treatment of Behçet's disease.

Frequently, we use azathioprine as a steroid-sparing drug, allowing systemic steroids to be tapered to an acceptable level, with eventual discontinuation. Entities for which we have found this approach valuable include multifocal choroiditis with panuveitis, sympathetic ophthalmia, Vogt-Koyanagi-Harada (VKH) syndrome, sarcoidosis, pars planitis, and Reiter's syndrome-associated iridocyclitis.

Dosage and Route of Administration. A single or divided oral dose of azathioprine administered as 2 to 3 mg/kg/day is suggested (Table 1). This amount should be reduced by 25% if allopurinol is administered concomitantly, since allopurinol interferes with the metabolism of 6-MP (8) (described in Drug Interactions section). The clinical response and laboratory parameters should be monitored in the same way suggested for chlorambucil and cyclophosphamide.

Side Effects and Toxicity

The frequency and severity of adverse effects of azathioprine depend on the dose, duration of therapy, and on the nature of any underlying disease (renal, hepatic) that might potentiate toxicity (Table 3). Although reports in the ophthalmic literature suggest that azathioprine is well tolerated, vigilant hematologic monitoring is crucial, because bone marrow suppression with leukopenia and thrombocytopenia are common (44). Typically, myelosuppression is delayed, appearing 1 to 2 weeks after initiation of therapy, and may persist for days to weeks after the drug has been discontinued. Prompt dosage reduction or withdrawal of azathioprine may be necessary if myelosuppression is severe.

Symptomatic GI discomfort (nausea, vomiting, and diarrhea) is the most common side effect and the principal reason for discontinuation of azathioprine therapy (109). Other adverse effects include interstitial pneumonitis, hepatocellular necrosis, pancreatitis, stomatitis, alopecia and, rarely, secondary infections (51).

Azathioprine has been implicated in potentiating the risk of neoplasia, especially leukemia and lymphomas, in transplant patients (110). However, several studies have demonstrated no difference in the overall frequency of malignancy in the general population from that observed in patients with rheumatoid arthritis receiving conventional doses of azathioprine (111,112).

Overdose. Ingestion of very large doses of azathioprine may lead to bone marrow hypoplasia, bleeding, infection, and death. In the single case report of a renal transplant patient who ingested a dose of 7,500 mg azathioprine, the immediate toxic reactions were nausea, vomiting and diarrhea, followed by leukopenia, and mild abnormalities of liver function (113). All laboratory values had returned to normal 6 days after the overdose. In addition to general supportive measures, including induction of emesis and gastric lavage, hemodialysis has been shown to remove 45% of drug in an 8-hour period (114).

High-risk Groups

Azathioprine should be avoided whenever possible in pregnant women because it has been shown to be mutagenic and teratogenic in laboratory animals and to cross the placenta in humans (22). Conception should also be avoided for a period of not less than 12 weeks after discontinuation of therapy. Likewise, use of azathioprine in nursing mothers is not recommended because the drug or its metabolites are transferred at low levels in the breast milk (115). The safety and efficacy of azathioprine in the pediatric age group have not been established. Patients with impaired renal function, especially the elderly or in patients who have just undergone kidney transplantation, may have delayed clearance of azathioprine and its metabolites and require dosage adjustments to avoid toxic sequelae.

Contraindications. Azathioprine is contraindicated in patients with a history of hypersensitivity to the drug or in those who are immunosuppressed and in patients with rheumatoid arthritis previously treated with alkylating agents in whom the risk of neoplasia is potentially high (116).

Drug Interactions

Because allopurinol inhibits xanthine oxidase, thereby impairing the conversion of azathioprine to its metabolites, the dosage of azathioprine should be reduced by 25% in patients treated concomitantly with these medications. Severe leukopenia associated with use of angiotensin-converting enzyme inhibitors in patients receiving azathioprine has been reported (117). The clearance of azathioprine may be affected by drugs that inhibit (ketoconazole, erythromycin) or induce (phenatoin, rifampin, phenobarbital) the hepatic microsomal enzyme system (22).

Major Clinical Trials

Major clinical trials are described in the Therapeutic Use section.

NONCYTOTOXIC IMMUNOSUPPRESSIVE DRUGS

The role of noncytotoxic agents in control of immune-related ocular inflammation has grown in importance and in scope with the development of drugs that mediate immunosuppression by selectively and reversibly targeting cellular subsets in the immune system without producing undue myelosuppression. Cyclosporine is the prototypical example of such an agent; however, several other naturally occurring and synthetic antibiotics (FK 506 and rapamycin, RAPA) show great promise in their capacity to suppress autoimmune uveitis. Other antibiotics, such as dapsone, have been explored for their antiinflammatory effects in treatment of inflammatory/immune diseases with potentially destructive ocular sequelae. Finally, several drugs have been used primarily as adjuvants to immunosuppressive agents, either as a dosage-lowering strategy (bromocriptine or ketoconazole with cyclosporine) or in the prophylaxis of recurrent inflammatory disease (colchicine for Behçet's disease).

Antibiotics

CSA

History and Source

Cyclosporine, also known as CSA, is a fungal metabolite which was discovered by Borel at Sandoz Laboratories (1969–1970) (118). Although the drug was originally isolated from cultures of *Tolypocladium inflatum Gams* and *Clindrocarpon lucidum* as part of a screening program for new antifungal agents, its profound and specific immunosuppressive properties became readily apparent (119). CSA was first shown to be effective in suppressing autoimmune uveitis by Nussenblatt et al. (120,121) and was subsequently applied to treatment of a variety of rheumatic diseases. CSA, and the emergence of similar immune-selective agents, has revolutionized the arena of organ transplantation and holds the promise of more effective and specific treatment of destructive systemic and ocular autoimmune disease. Three excellent reviews of the pharmacology, immunology, and clinical uses of CSA have been published (122–124).

Official Drug Name and Chemistry

Cyclosporine (Sandoz, East Hanover, NJ) is a neutral, hydrophobic, cyclic endecapeptide (molecular weight 1,203 daltons) consisting of 11 amino acids, one of which, the 9-carbon residue at position 1, is unique (125) (Fig. 6). The amino acids at positions 1, 2, 3, 10, and 11 form a hydrophillic active site, with the biologic action of the molecule being very sensitive to changes in stereochemical configurations at these positions (123,125).

Pharmacology

The mechanism by which CSA reversibly inhibits T-cell–mediated (particularly helper T cell) alloimmune and autoimmune responses is not completely understood, attesting to the enormous complexity underlying T-cell activation (Fig. 1). Before being activated, T cells are primed, by virtue of specific immunorecognition with antigen presented by antigen-presenting cells (APC) to express receptors for certain lymphokines (e.g., interleukin-1, IL-1) on their cell surface, which act to promote cellular maturation. Activation takes place through a second series of T-cell recognition events, which result in the synthesis of other lymphokines (e.g., IL-2), which promote clonal expansion and cytoaggressive potential (124). The best evidence obtained thus far indicates that CSA disrupts the transmission of signals from the T-cell receptor (TCR) to genes that encode for multiple lymphokines and enzymes necessary for activation of resting T cells and cytoaggression while leaving the T-cell priming reaction unaffected (125). FK 506 (Fig. 7), although structurally distinct from CSA, is believed to act through a similar molecular mechanism, resulting in the inhibition of T-helper cell activation, lymphokine production, and lymphocyte proliferation. In contrast, RAPA (Fig. 8), although it is a closely related structural analogue of FK 506, exhibits a distinct mode of action, affecting the T-cell activation-proliferation pathway at a later stage, and is discussed separately.

Clinical Pharmacology

After engagement of the TCR with antigen complexed with class I or II major histocompatibility (MHC)-associated peptides on the cell surface, activation of the TCR signal transmission pathway proceeds through the cytoplasma via calcium (CA^{++})-dependent or CA^{++}-independent pathways (126). The latter is initiated through protein kinase C (PKC)-triggered reactions. CA^{++}-Dependent activation eventuates in promotion of specific nuclear transcription factors, such as nuclear factor of activated T cells (NF-AT), which regulate the transcription of genes involved in T-cell activation, such as that for IL-2 (Fig. 9). NF-AT itself consists of two subunits: a cytoplasmic component (NF-ATc), which is translocated into the nucleus under the influence of TCR activation pathways, and a newly synthesized nuclear subunit (NF-ATn). Both components are necessary for the binding of NF-AT to DNA and transcriptional activation of, for example, the IL-2 gene (126).

CSA binds to cyclophilin, a 17-kDa cytosolic protein belonging to a family of proteins termed immunophilins, and is concentrated intracellularly. Similarly, FK 506-binding protein, another immunophilin, binds both FK 506 and

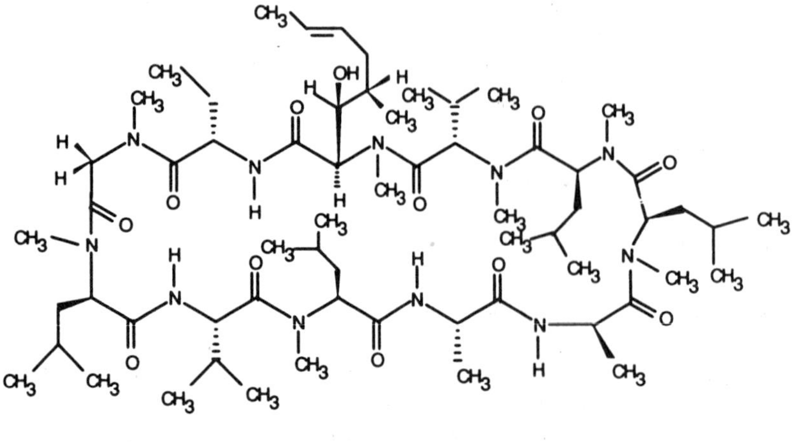

FIG. 62-6. Chemical structure of cyclosporine A.

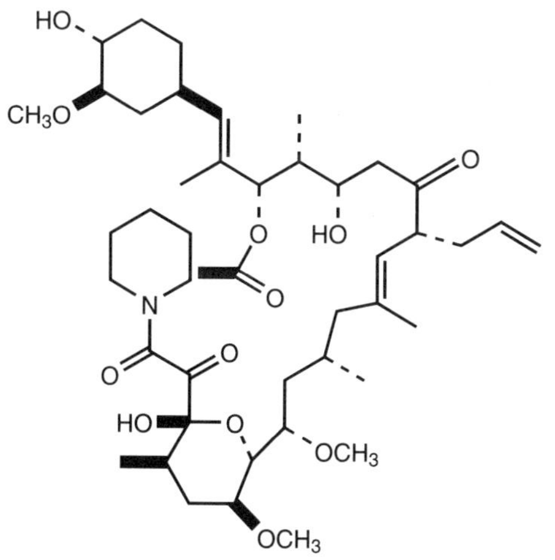

FIG. 62-7. Chemical structure of FK 506.

RAPA. These binding proteins, isoforms of which are present in most mammalian cells, have been shown to have peptidyl proline *cis-trans* isomerase (PPI ase) activity, enzymes that participate in the unfolding of cytoplasmic proteins, exposing their functional conformation (127).

When bound to their respective immunophilins, CSA and FK 506 form a ternary complex with calcineurin, inhibiting calmodulin binding together with the Ca^{++}-activated phosphatase activity of calcineurin (Fig. 9) (128). This results in inhibition of dephosphorylation of the cytoplasmic subunit of NF-AT and thus inhibits its translocation into the nucleus and subsequent activation of transcription of the IL-2 gene (among others) (129). Neither CSA nor FK 506 has impact on the cascade of events that follow T-cell cytokine gene activation.

Therefore, CSA and FK 506 halt the progression of Ca^{++}-dependent T-cell activation early in the cell cycle (from G_0 to G_1) and thus suppress the synthesis of IL-2, IL-3, IL-4, IL-5, tumor necrosis factor (TNF-α) and interferon-γ (IFN-γ), all important cellular immune signals

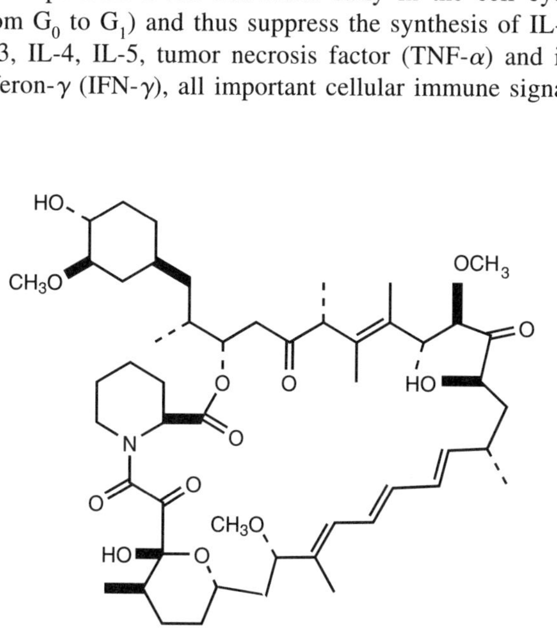

FIG. 62-8. Chemical structure of rapamycin.

(130,131). In addition, both drugs inhibit expression of the IL-2 receptor and may also inhibit IL-1 release from antigen-presenting cells such as monocytes (10).

The actions of CSA and FK 506 are selective, affecting T helper-inducer and cytotoxic subsets preferentially while leaving T suppressor cells relatively uninhibited, thereby setting the stage for suppression of immune responses. These drugs markedly decrease antibody production to T-cell–dependent antigens, inhibit cytotoxic activity generated in mixed leukocyte reactions, and prolong the viability of skin, kidney, liver, heart, and pancreas allografts in experimental animals and in humans (51). They may also mitigate graft-versus-host disease (GVHD) and prolong the life of other transplanted tissues such as the cornea.

Pharmaceutics

Cyclosporine (Sandimmune, Sandoz, East Hanover, NJ) is available for oral administration as a solution containing 100 mg/ml vehicle (12.5% ethanol in olive oil), which is mixed with milk or orange juice immediately before ingestion. It is also formulated as 25-mg and 100 mg (12.7% ethanol) soft gelatin capsules.

For intravenous use, CSA is formulated as a solution containing 50 mg drug and 1 ml vehicle (33% ethanol in polyoxethylated castor oil) and is diluted with 0.9% sodium chloride or 5% dextrose immediately before infusion. CSA for topical use is not commercially available; however, 1% to 2% CSA eye drops may be easily prepared using the oral formulation, a procedure which is described in detail by deSmet and Nussenblatt (124).

Pharmakokinetics and Metabolism

Absorption of CSA from the GI tract is slow and incomplete, the bioavailability varying from 20% to 50% with a mean value of 30% of the oral dose (127). Peak plasma levels are achieved within 3 to 4 hours of ingestion. Administration of CSA with food increases the peak and trough blood concentrations, whereas malabsorption of the drug is common after orthotopic liver transplantation or biliary diversion or in association with inflammatory bowel disease, reduced gastric emptying, and GI motility (22).

The volume of distribution ranges from less than 1 L/kg to 13 L/kg, with most drug being distributed outside the blood volume. Distribution within whole blood is concentration dependent, with approximately 60% to 75% of drug contained in erythrocytes and 10% to 20% concentrated in leukocytes, apparently reflecting the content of cyclophilin in the latter (127). Uptake by both erythrocytes and leukocytes becomes saturated at high concentrations. Approximately 90% of CSA in the circulation is bound to plasma proteins, primarily lipoproteins. Although some drug circulates "free" in the plasma, this fraction does not correlate

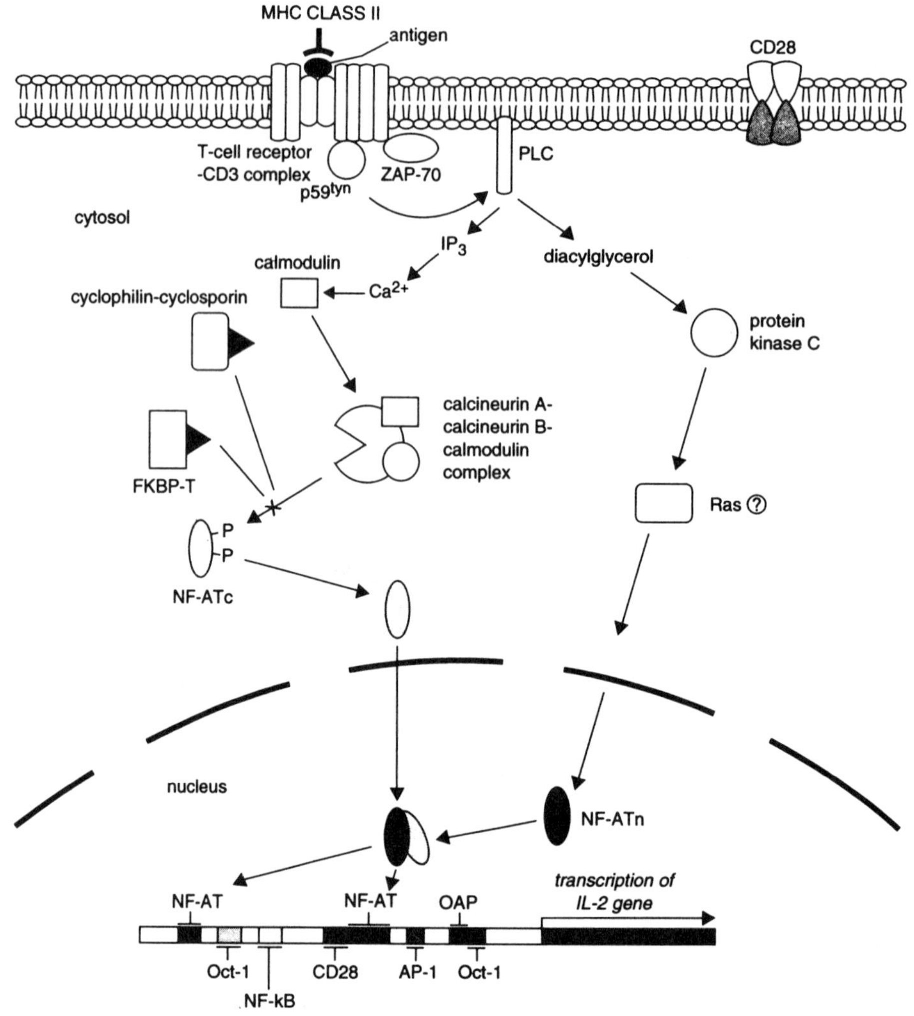

FIG. 62-9. The T-cell receptor signal transduction pathway leading to interleukin-2 (IL-2) transcription. PLC, phospholipase C; IP_3, inositol-1,4,5 triphosphate; $NF\text{-}AT_c$, the cytoplasmic component of the nuclear factor of activated T cells; $NF\text{-}AT_n$, the nuclear component of NF-AT; FKBP, FK 506 binding protein. (From Liu J. FK 506 and cyclosporin, molecular probes for studying intracellular signal transduction. *Immunol Today* 1993;14:293.)

with the total blood level of CSA or with adverse side effects (132).

The extent of tissue deposition varies between patients, with fat having the highest concentration of drug, approximately 10 times that in plasma (122). However, since there is apparently no connection between obesity and the volume of distribution, factors other than the lipophilic nature of CSA, such as the tissue content of cytoplasmic binding proteins, which themselves may accumulate drug for months after discontinuation of therapy, are probably involved (123). High concentrations of CSA are also detected in the liver, kidney, pancreas, adrenal, and lymphoid tissue, whereas very low levels occur in the brain (122).

Ocular bioavailability depends on the route of administration and the integrity of the blood–ocular barriers (124). After systemic administration of CSA in patients with chronic flare, the concentration of drug in the aqueous has been shown to be 40% that of the plasma concentration (133), whereas in experimental animals with uninflamed ocular tissues very poor ocular penetration was achieved (134). Furthermore, in animal models, CSA appears to be concentrated in ocular pigment, and thus might influence intraocular drug concentration (135).

Topically applied CSA penetrates the cornea poorly and fails to achieve therapeutically efficacious concentrations when the epithelium is intact (136,137). However, using collagen shields containing CSA, Chen reported cornea and aqueous concentrations on the order of 10 times that obtained with drops (138). The use of an α-cyclodextrin vehicle was reported to achieve similar concentrations (139). Periocular or intracameral administration of CSA has not been used in humans (140).

CSA is extensively metabolized in the liver by cytochrome P-450, undergoing hydroxylation or demethylation (141). Enterohepatic recirculation occurs, with most of the drug being excreted in the bile and only 6% appearing in the urine. The median $t_{\frac{1}{2}}$ is 6.7 to 8.7 hours (123). CSA clearance varies in individuals, with concomitant administration of drugs that have impact on cytochrome P-450 activity (described in the Drug Interactions section), in patients with hepatic impairment, in the elderly, and in children (described in the High-risk Groups section).

Therapeutic Use

CSA has been used to treat a wide variety of ocular immune-mediated disorders. It appears to be particularly useful in patients with bilateral, sight-threatening uveitis of a noninfectious etiology when both the retina and choroid are involved, who have either become dependent on systemic corticosteroids for the control of intraocular inflammation, or who have become intolerant of conventional therapy with this medication (Table 4).

Nussenblatt et al. of the National Eye Institute were first to report the efficacy of CSA at doses of 10 mg/kg/day in patients with intractable uveitis of various etiologies (including Behçet's disease, birdshot retinochoroidopathy, sarcoidosis, pars planitis, VKH, multiple sclerosis, sympathetic ophthalmia, and idiopathic vitritis) refractory to corticosteroid and cytotoxic agents (62,120,121,142,143). These observations were subsequently corroborated by other investigators in two uncontrolled, nonrandomized trials (144,145) and in treatment of birdshot retinochoroidopathy (146), Behçet's disease (147), and VKH (148). In a recent randomized, double-masked study, Nussenblatt et al. (149) demonstrated that CSA, used as monotherapy, was effective in controlling intraocular inflammation in 46% of 56 patients who were intolerant of steroids; another 35% of patients in the study responded to combined CSA and systemic steroid therapy. In these studies and in two additional double-masked trials (150,151) demonstrating the clinical efficacy of CSA for various forms of noninfectious uveitis, a dose of 10 mg/kg/day was used, a dose now known to be associated with a 100% incidence of untoward nephrotoxic and hypertensive effects. Low-dose CSA therapy (mean maintenance dose 4.0 ± 1.1 mg/kg/day) alone (152) or in combination with corticosteroids (153), has been used successfully in management of noninfectious uveitis, with resultant improvement or stabilization of visual acuity in 85% of patients and a reduction or stabilization of vitreous inflammation in 97% of eyes monitored for as long as 2 years (153,154). Nephrotoxic and hypertensive side effects were less frequent but not completely avoided; nephrotoxicity in older patients with underlying systemic hypertension was particularly troublesome (154). Low-dose CSA therapy (2.5 to 5.0 mg/kg/day) has also been successfully used, alone or in combination with other immunosuppressive agents, in treatment of birdshot retinochoroidopathy with resultant improvement or stabilization of visual acuity in most patients and few drug-induced side effects (155).

In the management of Behçet's disease, initial reports clearly demonstrated the superiority of CSA to colchicine (150) or to the combination of cytotoxic agents and steroids (156) in prevention of ocular inflammatory recurrence when dosage schedules of 10 mg/kg/day were used. However, such high-dose regimens produce unacceptable nephrotoxic side effects, and less toxic doses of 5 to 7 mg/kg/day, in our experience (39) and in that of other investigators (63), are distinctly inferior to cytotoxic agents (azathioprine, cyclophosphamide, and chlorambucil) in management of the posterior segment manifestations and inflammatory recurrences in patients with Behçet's disease.

A recent retrospective study of a small number of patients with severe ocular Behçet's disease (157) showed a trend toward therapeutic success and diminished nephrotoxicity in those treated with a combination of CSA (mean dosage 6.2 mg/kg/day) and prednisone (mean dosage 29.4 mg/day) as compared with treatment with CSA alone (mean dosage 8.6 mg/kg/day). The definitive efficacy and long-term outcome of combined CSA regimens with prednisone and other immunosuppressive agents (e.g., azathioprine) in Behçet's disease and other uveitic entities await critical evaluation in prospective, randomized trials.

Several uncontrolled studies involving small numbers of patients support the efficacy of systemic CSA for treatment of corneal ulceration with or without scleral melting (122,158,159) and for peripheral ulcerative keratitis associated with Wegener's granulomatosis (160,161). Use of systemic CSA was also successful in preventing corneal transplant rejection in high-risk eyes; the overall success rate during the follow-up period was impressive (162,163).

Despite its poor penetration into the eye, topical CSA has been successfully used in treatment of a variety of immune-mediated ocular surface phenomena, including ligneous conjunctivitis (164,165), vernal conjunctivitis (166–168), and high-risk corneal grafts (169,170). Its efficacy for the latter indication should be clarified by the long-awaited results of a multicenter clinical trial, and the usefulness of topical CSA for other oculocutaneous disorders, such as Sjögren's syndrome and atopic keratoconjunctivitis, is currently under investigation.

Dosage and Route of Administration. Our philosophy regarding the care of patients with uveitis in general has been one of complete intolerance of even low-grade inflammation and a limited tolerance of steroid use in patients for whom alternative antiinflammatory medication is a reasonable option, in an effort to limit permanent structural damage to vital ocular structures. For these reasons, in patients who have failed conventional therapy and in whom a reasonable chance for visual rehabilitation exists, we rely on the degree of vitreal and retinal inflammation rather than on visual acuity as the parameters determining the threshold for initiation of CSA therapy, subsequent dosage adjustments, and addition of other steroid-sparing agents. Provided that no contraindication to its use exists (uncontrolled systemic hypertension, abnormal renal or liver function tests, pregnancy, or drug hypersensitivity), we initiate CSA therapy at 2.5 mg/kg/day, once daily, with dosage increments of 50 mg to a maximum of 5 mg/kg/day and titrated to the clinical response (Table 1). If no response is observed at this dosage after 1 month, we will occasionally increase the dosage to 7.5 mg/kg/day for no more than 4 weeks and taper it to 5 mg/kg/day once inflammation has been controlled. If no response is evident after 3 months of treatment, the medication is discontinued. If, on the other hand, a favorable response is achieved, we attempt to taper systemic steroids and maintain the lowest possible dose of CSA that provides an adequate therapeutic effect, while minimizing toxicity, for at least 1 year. In our experience and that of other investigators (144,145), recurrent inflammation is most often associated with attempted reductions of CSA dosage, necessitating a compensatory upward dosage adjustment or addition of a steroid-sparing agent such as azathioprine.

Nussenblatt et al. advocate initial therapy with combined low-dose CSA (2.5 mg/kg/day twice daily) and reduced-dose prednisone (0.2 to 0.5 mg/kg/day) for 2 to 3 months, with subsequent taper of either CSA or steroid, depending on the clinical response and the needs of the patient (124). Not only has this strategy proved effective (149,153,157), but combination therapy with other adjunctive agents such as bromocriptine (171) and ketoconazole (172) has also been advocated to reduce the dosage of CSA necessary to achieve inflammatory control and thus decrease both the risk of untoward toxicity and the cost of therapy (described in section on Adjuvants to Immunosuppressive Therapy).

Ben Ezra et al. (173) have proposed guidelines for use of low-dose CSA in Behçet's disease, the fundamental principles of which have been extended and are shared by most investigators in caring for patients with noninfectious bilateral, intermediate, or posterior uveitis. This entails evaluation and treatment of patients for evidence of untoward renal or hypertensive effects before and during therapy, with vigilant attention paid to increases in the serum creatinine levels more than 30% above baseline and to physical parameters [sustained systolic blood pressure (BP) more than 140 mm Hg or diastolic BP more than 90 mm Hg] which might require dosage reduction or cessation of therapy. Correspondingly, a complete hemogram with differential, serum creatinine, and BUN determinations, urinalysis, and liver function tests should be obtained before therapy is initiated and repeated periodically, together with determination of creatinine clearance, to monitor potential CSA-induced toxic effects.

Although adjusting the dose of CSA according to trough levels may result in a more favorable clinical course than will a fixed dose regimen (123), routine sampling of the trough level is probably not necessary with lower initial drug doses (2.5 to 5 mg/kg/day) if renal function is carefully monitored. In circumstances in which blood monitoring might be judicious (hepatic dysfunction or patient noncompliance), the trough level should be obtained 12 hours after the last dose. More accurate measurements are obtained from whole blood than from serum levels (174,175) and with daily doses of CSA greater than 3 mg/kg/day. Although acceptable trough values for kidney and bone marrow recipients range from 100 to 250 mg/ml (176,177), corresponding values for low-dose regimens used in ocular disease have not been definitively established. Furthermore, reference ranges vary depending on the measurement method used.

Side Effects and Toxicity

Most of the toxic side effects of CSA therapy described in the literature were reported in association with high-dose (10 mg/kg/day) schedules in organ transplant recipients. Although current low-dose regimens (5 mg/kg/day) produce fewer adverse reactions, nephrotoxicity and hypertension are the most common and worrisome events encountered by ophthalmologists, particularly with chronic administration of CSA (Table 3).

Nephrotoxicity is manifested clinically by increased serum creatinine with a disproportionate increase in BUN, preserved urine output and sodium reabsorption, decreased creatinine clearance and, in the extreme, systemic hypertension (178). Dose-dependent CSA alterations in renal hemodynamics, including vasoconstriction of the afferent glomerular arteriole with subsequent decrease in renal blood flow, are believed to produce a reduction in glomerular filtration rate (GFR) (147). Initially, CSA-induced nephrotoxicity is reversible by dose reduction; however, chronic, irreversible, interstitial fibrosis and renal tubular atrophy can occur, particularly in patients treated with high doses or in whom the serum creatinine is allowed to remain at persistently increased levels. Indeed, initial studies with high-dose CSA indicated that nephrotoxicity, as demonstrated by renal biopsy, may precede an increase in serum creatinine, suggesting that serum creatinine underestimates the potential for renal damage and should not be used as the sole marker of renal toxicity (179). Subsequent work has shown that minimal pathologic changes, as evidenced by renal biopsy, are produced when lower starting doses (7.5 mg/kg/day or less) are used (180,181).

Nevertheless, functional changes are still observed, as manifested by an increase in serum creatinine levels and the frequent occurrence of systemic hypertension during the first 12 months of low-dose CSA (mean maintenance 4.0 ± 1.1 mg/kg/day) therapy, alone or in combination with systemic steroids (152–154). Clinicopathologic data from a recent large series of patients with autoimmune or inflammatory disease treated with a maintenance dose of CSA 5 mg/kg/day or less suggests, however, that their functional perturbations are not likely to translate into permanent renal damage provided that the serum creatinine remains within 30% of its baseline value (182). Furthermore, these data indicate that CSA-associated nephropathy may be related more to the maximal dose administered rather than to the cumulative effects of smaller doses. We (155) and other investigators (183) have shown that the potential for serious renal complications may be reduced if initial doses of 2.5 or 5 mg/kg daily are used rather than 7.5 or 10 mg/kg daily and if vigilant attention is paid to renal functional indexes.

Hypertension develops, or is exacerbated, in a dose-dependent reversible fashion in approximately 15% to 25% of patients within the first few weeks of initiation of CSA therapy (184). Hypertension is more common in patients treated with the combination of CSA and steroids than in patients treated with CSA alone (185) and in those with impaired renal function (50). An abrupt increase in systemic BP after prolonged CSA therapy, particularly in obese patients, may signal imminent renal toxicity and should prompt the clinician to obtain a trough CSA level and check the serum creatinine (124). Systemic hypertension promptly responds to dosage reduction in most cases, and its presence, before or during therapy, does not constitute a contraindication to use of CSA, provided that it is aggressively controlled.

Although CSA does not induce leukopenia, it is associated with a normochronic, normocytic anemia in 25% of patients, an increased sedimentation rate in 40% of patients (186), and a mild, dose-dependent increase in the serum transaminases and bilirubin levels (123). Hyperuricemia and gouty arthritis (187) are common among transplant recipients, and increases in total serum cholesterol due to an increased low-density lipoprotein fraction have also been reported in such patients treated with CSA (188).

Lymphoproliferative disease has developed in patients receiving CSA; however, these neoplasms do not appear to be due to the drug itself but rather to immunosuppression in general. The incidence of lymphoma was no greater in patients receiving CSA than in those treated with other immunosuppressive agents in a large clinical series of 5,000 transplant recipients monitored for 5 years (122). Whereas CSA is known to increase serum prolactin levels, causing gynecomastia in men and promoting the growth of benign breast adenomas in women, no definitive association between breast carcinoma and CSA has been demonstrated to date (124).

Other common adverse reactions include paresthesias and temperature hypersensitivity developing within days of initiation of CSA therapy, as well as nausea and vomiting, none of which usually require discontinuation of therapy (109). Hirsutism of mild to moderate degree may develop in 50% of patients during the first few months of therapy, as well as gingival hyperplasia, exacerbated by poor oral hygiene, in as many as 25% of patients (122). Neurotoxicity, as manifested by a fine hand tremor that usually abates during therapy, and a reversible myopathy has been detected in patients after liver transplantation (16,50). An increased risk of opportunistic infections with Herpesviruses, *Candida,* and *Pneumocystis* is a potential complication of immunosuppression with CSA (51).

Ocular side effects due to systemic use of CSA include decreased vision, lid erythema and nonspecific conjunctivitis, visual hallucinations, and conjunctival and retinal hemorrhages secondary to anemia. Topically applied CSA is reasonably well tolerated, although eyelid irritation and burning sensation may occur (49).

Overdose. Experience with overdosage with CSA is minimal. Transient hepatotoxicity and nephrotoxicity, together with hypertension, dysesthesias, flushing, and GI upset may occur, lasting no more than a few days (113). General supportive measures and symptomatic treatment should be instituted, as in all cases of drug overdosage.

High-risk Groups

CSA readily crosses the placenta to the fetus. Although it has been shown to be embryo- and fetotoxic in experimental animals, it is not an animal teratogen, and the limited experience in women thus far indicates that it is unlikely to be a human teratogen (189). Successful pregnancies have been reported in patients receiving CSA, with growth retardation being the most common problem in infants exposed to the drug in utero (189). Nevertheless, CSA should be used during pregnancy only when the potential benefit justifies the risk to the fetus. Because the drug is excreted in the human milk, it is to be avoided in nursing mothers.

Although no well-controlled studies have been conducted in the pediatric age group, CSA has been used successfully in children without undue adverse effects. Higher doses of drug are necessary in children, as the clearance rate in children is 45% higher than in adults (174). The converse is true in the elderly and in patients with hepatic disease in whom drug clearance is slower; therefore, they are at increased risk of development of toxic side effects.

Contraindications. Contraindications to the use of CSA include uncontrolled systemic hypertension, hepatic disease, renal insufficiency, pregnancy, and a history of hypersensitivity to the drug.

Drug Interactions

There are many important drug interactions with CSA. Synergistic nephrotoxicity may occur with concomitant use of aminoglycosides, amphotericin B, ketoconazole, vancomycin, melphan, cimetidine, ranitidine, trimethoprim with sulfamethoxazole, ciprofloxacin, and NSAIDs (22). By inhibiting the local prostaglandin production, NSAIDs potentiate CSA nephrotoxicity by further compromising renal blood flow (50). NSAIDs have been shown to produce a transient yet significant increase in serum creatinine when used with CSA (190), an effect which may prove particularly problematic because of the widespread availability of these drugs.

Because CSA is extensively metabolized by the hepatic microsomal enzyme system, drugs that affect cytochrome

P-450 will alter blood levels of the drug. Medications that have been reported to inhibit these enzymes and thus increase CSA levels include verapamil, diltiazem, ketoconazole, fluconazole, itraconazole, danazol, bromocriptine, metoclopamide, erythromycin, and methylprednisolone (22). Drugs that induce cytochrome P-450, thereby reducing CSA level, include rifampin, phenytoin, phenobarbital, and carbamazepine (22).

Other drug interactions include digitalis toxicity resulting from an apparent reduction in the volume of distribution of digitalis when it is administered with CSA (50), convulsions with concomitant administration of large doses of methylpredisolone, and reversible myopathy with rhabdomyolysis with combined lovastatin and CSA therapy (22).

Major Clinical Trials

Major clinical trials are described in the Therapeutic Use section.

FK 506 AND RAPA

FK 506 and RAPA are among the more promising new immunosuppressive agents that resemble CSA in their effects without producing cytotoxicity. FK 506, now known as Tacrolimus (Prograf, Fujisawa, Deerfield, IL) was recently approved by the FDA for prophylaxis of organ rejection for patients undergoing allogenic liver transplantation. For the sake of simplicity and to avoid confusion, we refer to this drug by its original investigational name, FK 506, because it is referenced as such in the literature.

FK 506 is a macrolide antibiotic which was discovered in 1984 at the Fujisawa Pharmaceutical Company during a routine screening for naturally occurring immunosuppressive agents; it was extracted from the fermentation broth of a strain of soil fungus, *Streptomyces tsukubaensis,* found in the Tsukuba region of Japan (191). This compound was shown to have a spectrum of activity similar to that of CSA in experimental models of transplantation and autoimmunity. Clinical trials with FK 506 were initiated in February 1989 at the University of Pittsburgh, primarily involving liver transplantation and subsequently extended to heart, kidney, and small bowel transplants. Its early success in this arena, with the demonstration that steroids could be tapered more rapidly with FK 506 than with CSA, suggested that FK 506 might be applicable to other clinical conditions as monotherapy (125). Mochizuki et al. were first to establish the efficacy of FK 506 in treatment of uveitis, both in experimental animals and in patients (192).

RAPA is also a macrolide antibiotic that was discovered as an antifungal agent produced by *S. hygroscodicus* and isolated from a soil sample collected from Easter Island (RAPA Nui) (193). Despite its structural similarity to FK 506 and its similar immunosuppressive effectiveness in experimental transplant models, RAPA was discovered to have a mechanism of action distinct from those of FK 506 and CSA. Likewise, because its toxicity may be caused by distinct mechanisms, RAPA may prove useful as the sole agent or provide a strategy for combination therapy with CSA that maximizes immunosuppression and mitigates drug toxicity (125). No information regarding use of RAPA in humans is currently available because the drug is presently undergoing phase I trials. A recent report, however, indicated that RAPA is useful in treatment of autoimmune uveitis in rats (194).

Official Drug Name and Chemistry

FK 506, now known as tacrolimus (Prograf, Fujisawa), is a 822-kDa molecule ($C_{44}H_{69}NO_{12}\cdot H_2O$) (Fig. 7). It is insoluble in water, but readily dissolves in organic solvents such as methanol, ethanol, and acetone (195).

RAPA ($C_{51}H_{79}NO_{13}$) has a molecular weight of 914.2 kDa and shares the unusual hemiketal masked α, β-diketo amide moiety with FK 506, yet has a larger ring structure and a unique triene segment (196) (Fig. 8).

Pharmacology

FK 506 and CSA, although structurally distinct, share many pharmacologic properties, including a similar mechanism of action (Fig. 9). In essence, both FK 506 and CSA, complexed with their respective binding proteins, suppress cell-mediated immunity in a synergistic fashion by inhibiting DNA translation of specific lymphokines (IL-2, IL-3, IL-4, and IFN-8) and the expression of the IL-2 receptor on activated T cells. FK 506, however, is at least 10 times more potent than CSA, both in vitro and in vivo (126). RAPA, on the other hand, blunts the response of T cells and B cells to specific lymphokines rather than inhibiting their production (130,131).

Clinical Pharmacology

Although RAPA and FK 506 share similar immunosuppressive potencies and structural characteristics and even bind to the same immunophilin (FK binding position), they affect immune cells in vitro quite differently. Although not cytotoxic, RAPA differs from FK 506 in that protein synthesis in resting lymphocytes and constitutive DNA synthesis in transformed cells is inhibited (125). Whereas FK 506 and CSA inhibit Ca^{++}-dependent T-cell activation, thereby preventing transcription of early phase lymphokine genes, RAPA blocks both Ca^{++}-dependent and Ca^{++}-independent T-cell activation without preventing the expression of these genes (130,131,197,198). In contrast to FK 506 and CSA, RAPA has no effect on the expression of the IL-2 receptor. In addition, RAPA blocks Ca^{++}-dependent T cell division at a later stage in the cell cycle than does FK 506 or CSA by preventing the advancement of cells into S phase by acting in late G (FK 506), as opposed to blocking cell division at the G_0-G_1 interface (CSA) (197). As a consequence, RAPA inhibits the proliferation of activated T cells even when added 12 hours after stimulation, whereas FK 506 and CSA are effective only if added in the first few hours after T-cell stimulation (127).

On a molecular level, whereas the RAPA-FK binding protein complex is necessary for its inhibitory action, the precise target analogous to calcineurin for FK 506 and CSA has yet to be identified. RAPA does not affect NF-AT translocation, but is believed to inhibit T cell activation in G_1 instead by inhibiting the activity of phosphatase enzymes (198). Whatever the ultimate putative target might be, the common RAPA/FK 506-immunophilin complex interacts with other molecules to create functionally different complexes which mediate the particular suppressive effects for each drug (197).

In essence, RAPA, unlike FK 506 or CSA, does not consistently inhibit the synthesis of IL-2, its receptor, or other lymphokines, but instead acts like a functional antagonist to cytokine action, inhibiting the proliferation of T cells in response to IL-2 and IL-4. Because of their differential actions throughout the cell cycle, FK 506 and CSA exert their action on resting T cells and are unlikely to have an immunosuppressive effect once T cells have been fully activated, whereas the antiproliferative effects of RAPA are independent of the commitment step in T-cell activation (130,131).

Finally, all three agents are immune selective, with the thrust of immunosuppression resulting from inhibition of helper T cell activities. In addition, FK 506 may selectively prevent maturation of helper T cells in the thymus (197), whereas RAPA suppresses a wider spectrum of both T- and B-cell activation pathways (130,131).

The powerful immunosuppressive properties of FK 506 in vivo are manifested by its ability to prolong the survival of a variety of organ and skin grafts in rodents, dogs, nonhuman primates, and humans (195). Moreover, the demonstration that FK 506 can reverse ongoing acute or early chronic liver rejection distinguishes it from CSA (199). Its apparent hepatotropic properties, as compared with that of other agents, are poorly understood, but may explain its early success in liver transplantation. RAPA has also been shown to suppress acute rejection of organ and skin allografts in rodents and in nonhuman primates as well as to mitigate GVH and host-versus-graft (HVG) reactions (197).

Pharmaceutics

FK 506, currently marketed as tacrolimus (Prograf, Fujisawa), is available for oral administration as capsules containing 1 mg or 5 mg anhydrous drug or as a sterile solution for intravenous injection. The latter contains the equivalent of 5 mg anhydrous FK 506 in 1 ml polyoxyl 60 hydrogenated castor oil and dehydrated alcohol. It is supplied as an ampule, which is diluted in either 0.9% sodium chloride or 5% dextrose in water before use.

RAPA is an investigational agent, and attempts to create a single formulation suitable for all routes of administration have not been successful. Because RAPA is extremely insoluble in aqueous physiologic buffers, attempts to deliver the drug orally in a 0.2% carboxy-methylcellulose suspension or parenterally in a Cremophor EL-based vehicle have resulted in variable drug bioavailability in experimental animals (196). To date, RAPA solubilized in a polysorbate/polyethylene glycol (PEG)-based solution, delivered by continuous intravenous infusion, affords the best opportunity to study the intrinsic properties of the drug (195,196).

Pharmacokinetics and Metabolism

FK 506 is variably and poorly absorbed from the GI tract after oral administration. The absolute oral bioavailability may range from 5% to 67% (mean 27%) in transplant patients with various degrees of hepatic function (22). A peak plasma concentration of 0.5 to 5.6 mg/L [as measured by enzyme-linked immunoabsorbent assay (ELISA) using a monoclonal anti-FK 506 antibody] was observed within 0.5 to 8 hours of a single oral dose of 0.15 mg/kg, whereas the concentration detected after intravenous infusion of a similar dose of drug administered in 2 hours ranged from 10 to 24 mg/L (200). Although trough plasma concentrations have been reported to correlate poorly with the dose, apparently a close correlation exists between the area under the FK 506 concentration–time curve and the concentrations of drug in whole blood and plasma (200). Unlike that of cyclosporine, FK 506 absorption is not dependent on the availability of bile in the gut; however, the presence of food may decrease its absorption (22).

FK 506 is widely distributed throughout the bodily tissues, with a large volume of distribution (1,300 L), conferred largely by its highly lipophilic nature (200). In the vascular compartment, the drug is highly bound to erythrocytes, with a mean blood plasma trough concentration of 10 : 1 (22). The differential plasma-erythrocyte distribution of FK 506 is influenced by the drug concentration, hematocrit, and temperature. Plasma concentrations at 37°C are approximately twice those at 24°C; therefore, the plasma and whole blood concentrations of drug are nonlinearly related (200). In plasma, FK 506 is highly bound (88%) to plasma proteins, chiefly albumin.

FK 506 is extensively metabolized in the liver by *N*-demethylation and hydroxylation, with less than 1% of the parent compound being excreted unchanged in the bile, feces, or urine in a 48-hour period (201). Two of the nine metabolites of FK 506 have been shown to retain immunosuppressive activity in vitro (200). The plasma elimination $t_{\frac{1}{2}}$ varies from 3.5 to 40.5 hours (mean 8.7 hours) (22).

Like CSA, FK 506 has a dose-dependent effect on different components of the hepatic mixed function oxidate system, with consequent alterations in its own metabolism induced by drugs that either induce or inhibit cytochrome P-450. Similarly, because of its extensive hepatic metabolism, the plasma concentration, $t_{\frac{1}{2}}$, and clearance of FK 506 are increased in patients with liver disease, whereas patients with renal impairment are not expected to show similar alterations in these parameters (200).

The pharmacokinetics of RAPA remain unknown, due largely to the limited sensitivity of most readily available assays for detection of picogram quantities of drug in the bodily fluids. The development of an ELISA with monoclonal antibodies of sufficient sensitivity may obviate this problem and provide a practical method for routine screening of drug levels (196).

Therapeutic Use

FK 506. Although the therapeutic efficacy and benefits of FK 506 in prevention and reversal of organ transplantation, particularly hepatic, are implicit given its recent approval by the FDA for this purpose, the application of this drug for treatment of other autoimmune phenomena is now under investigation in both animal models and in humans (Table 4). FK 506 has been shown to prevent development of experimental collagen-induced arthritis (202), insulin-dependent diabetes (203), autoimmune glomerulonephritis (204), and experimental allergic encephalomyelitis (EAE) (205) in rats, and to reduce proteinuria significantly and prolong survival in a mouse model [New Zealand black/white (NZB/W) hybrid]of systemic lupus erythematosus (206). Kawashima et al. (207,208) demonstrated that FK 506 suppresses development of experimental autoimmune uveitis (EAU) in rats at doses 10 to 30 times lower than CSA doses when administered either from 0 to 14 days postimmunization with uveitogenic antigen (207,208). Subsequent work has shown the effectiveness of FK 506 in suppressing induction of EAU in primates (209).

Although experience with FK 506 in human autoimmune disease has been limited, both the efficacy and therapeutic potential of this agent have been demonstrated in several entities, including psoriasis (210), nephrotic syndrome (211), and noninfectious uveitis (212). With regard to the latter, Mochizuki et al. (212) recently reported favorable results in an open, multicentered study in which FK 506 was used as monotherapy in treatment of 53 patients (41 with Behçet's disease) with refractory uveitis. The majority (76.5%) were judged to have disease reduction, after dosage adjustments, during the 12-week trial. Visual acuity remained stable or improved in 72.9% of 96 treated eyes, and the number of recurrent ocular inflammatory episodes in Behçet's disease patients was markedly reduced. Furthermore, for reasons that are not clear, FK 506 therapy was effective in 7 of 11 patients who had been refractory to prior treatment with CSA (212).

Dosage and Route of Administration. In the study of Mochizuki et al. (212), the therapeutic efficacy of FK 506 administered orally for refractory noninfectious uveitis was dosage dependent. A daily dose of 0.05 mg/kg/day orally was inadequate in most patients, whereas a daily dose of 0.1 to 0.15 mg/kg/day proved efficacious, with little associated toxicity, and this dose was suggested for appropriate maintenance (212) (Table 1). Higher doses (0.15 and 2.0 mg/kg/day), although more effective than 0.1 mg/kg/day, produced various undesirable side effects, requiring careful monitoring. In addition, it was recommended that FK 506 trough levels be maintained between 15 and 25 ng/ml, as these levels correlate with both therapeutic efficacy and the incidence of adverse side effects. Finally, as with CSA, a complete hemogram, liver function tests, and serum BUN and creatinine determinations performed before, initiation of therapy as well as determination of creatinine clearance, repeated periodically (every 3 to 4 months), are necessary.

RAPA. In addition to its beneficial effects on experimental organ allografts, RAPA, like FK 506, has been shown to be effective treatment of autoimmune disease in experimental animals (129,194,213). Recently, Roberge et al. (194) demonstrated the efficacy of RAPA in preventing development of EAU in rats, dose dependently, when administered for 14 days by continuous intravenous (i.v.) infusion, whether initiated on the day of, or 1 week after, disease induction. At doses of 0.1 and 0.5 mg/kg i.v., RAPA prevented EAU in 12 of 14 rats in each dose group, whereas at a dose of 1 mg/kg, RAPA completely suppressed disease development (194).

The synergistic effect between RAPA and CSA observed in vitro and in rodent and canine models of organ transplantation (129,196) has also been demonstrated in a rat model of EAU (214); in this study, intramuscular (i.m.) injection of CSA (2 mg/kg) prevented the onset of disease in only 3 of the 15 animals, whereas its combination with RAPA (0.01 mg/kg i.v.) prevented development of EAU completely. These observations, together with RAPA's unique immunosuppressive profile, indicate its high clinical potential, particularly in combination with CSA or other immunosuppressive agents, in treatment of autoimmune uveitis. Such combination strategies might provide maximal therapeutic efficacy at the lowest possible dose of either agent and thereby limit the potential toxic consequences of treatment.

Side Effects and Toxicity

FK 506. FK 506 and CSA share similar major side effect profiles (nephrotoxicity, hypertension, neurotoxicity, and hyperglycemia); however, hirsutism, gingival hyperplasia, and coarsening of facial features have not been reported in patients treated with FK 506 (214) (Table 3). The major dose-limiting side effect is chronic nephrotoxicity, the overall incidence, clinical presentation, and pathophysiology of which are essentially the same as those of CSA. Although the GFR appears to be less adversely affected by FK 506 in the long term, its effect on renal structural integrity with prolonged use requires further study (200). Renal impairment developed in 28.3% of 53 patients treated with FK 506 for refractory uveitis, and although this side effect was dose-dependent, transient, and mild in most patients, it was severe enough to require discontinuation of therapy in 3 (212).

Neurologic side effects reported in transplant patients most often occur after intravenous administration and range in severity from minor reactions (headache, paresthesias, tremors, and sleep disturbances) in approximately 20% of patients to major neurotoxicity (expressive aphasia, seizures, akinetic mutism, encephalopathy, and coma), reported in less than 10% (200). In the FK 506 uveitis study, neurologic symptoms, including a meningitislike clinical picture, developed dose dependently after oral administration in 12 of 53 patients and resolved with dosage reduction or discontinuation of therapy (212).

Other adverse reactions reported by Mochizuki et al. (212) in their FK 506 uveitis study included GI symptoms (18.9% of 53 patients) and transient hyperglycemia (13.2% of 53 patients). Among transplant patients, the latter commonly occurs in the perioperative period, with as many as 20% of patients requiring insulin therapy at 6 months; at 1 year, as few as 5.5% are still insulin dependent (200).

Opportunistic bacterial, viral, and fungal infections are potential complications of immunosuppression with either FK 506 or CSA. Although 20% of FK 506-treated transplant patients developed CMV infections at the University of Pittsburgh Medical Center, no patient treated with this agent for nontransplant indications developed such an infection (216). The incidence of posttransplant lymphoproliferative disorders at the same institution in association with FK 506 was reported to be 1.6% (217).

Whereas systemic hypertension may occur with either CSA or FK 506, its incidence is less frequent (216) and discontinuation of antihypertensive therapy is more common with FK 506 (200). In addition, both drugs have been associated with the rare occurrence of hemolytic anemia; however, unlike with CSA, with FK 506 hypercholesterolemia is not a complication of therapy (200).

Overdose. There is little experience with FK 506 overdose. It produces no unique reactions other than the toxic side effects previously described, and treatment consists of general supportive measures as in any case of drug overdosage (218). Due to the extensive plasma protein and erythrocyte binding of FK 506, it is unlikely that hemodialysis would be an effective intervention.

RAPA. Although it may be tempting to extend conclusions regarding drug toxicity in animal models to humans, such an approach is often confounded by significant inconsistencies, as experience with both CSA and FK 506 has shown. For example, the major dose-limiting toxicity of both agents in clinical practice is nephrotoxicity, whereas in animal models therapeutic doses of CSA were relatively nontoxic (196). FK 506, while producing severe anorexia and widespread vasculitis in dogs, is well tolerated in rodents (215) and has a favorable therapeutic index in humans despite intercurrent neurotoxicity and nephrotoxicity (219). Nevertheless, RAPA apparently is not nephrotoxic in animals. Continuous intravenous infusion of drug for 14 days in hypertensive rats produced little alteration in the clinical indexes of renal function (urine output, plasma creatinine, and creatinine clearance), and histologic examination of the kidneys showed significant pathologic changes (196). RAPA administered in a similar manner produced an initial body weight loss in rats during the first week of treatment, with normal weight gain thereafter (194). In a murine model of CMV infection, RAPA produced less susceptibility to primary CMV infection than CSA, and combined CSA-RAPA regimens did not increase the morbidity of hosts carrying latent virus (196).

High-risk Groups

Because of its extensive metabolism by the liver, blood levels of FK 506 may be significantly increased in patients with hepatic impairment, placing them at risk of development of neurotoxicity and nephrotoxicity (215). Likewise, patients with underlying renal disease may require dosage adjustments and risk further compromise in their kidney function as a consequence of FK 506-induced nephrotoxicity. Elderly patients, who may have both reduced renal and hepatic reserves, should be carefully monitored for development of toxic side effects. Because of its hyperglycemic and hypertensive effects, patients with diabetes mellitus and systemic hypertension also require vigilant monitoring and medical control if FK 506 is to be implemented.

FK 506 does not exhibit mutagenic activity in vivo or in vitro. Fetotoxicity has been demonstrated in animals, and teratogenic effects have been observed (126). FK 506 crosses the placenta. Although no well-controlled studies of pregnant women have been conducted, FK 506 during pregnancy has been associated with neonatal hyperkalemia and renal dysfunction (218). Therefore, its use during pregnancy should be reserved for circumstances in which the potential benefit to the mother justifies the risk to the fetus. Because FK 506 is excreted in human milk, it should be avoided during nursing.

Children have undergone successful liver transplantation with FK 506 immunosuppression (200). As with CSA, pediatric patients receiving FK 506 generally require higher doses to maintain adequate blood trough levels.

Contraindications. Anaphylactic reactions have occurred, with use of FK 506, most often in patients receiving injectable preparations of FK 506 containing castor oil derivatives (218). Therefore, FK 506 is contraindicated in patients with a known hypersensitivity to the drug or vehicle. It is further recommended that patients receiving intravenous therapy receive oral drug instead as soon as it can be tolerated.

Drug Interactions

The same potential for synergistic nephrotoxicity previously described for CSA (described in CSA, Drug Interactions section) exists with coadministration of FK 506 and agents with known renal toxic effects. For this reason, CSA and FK 506 should not be used simultaneously (200).

FK 506, like CSA, is metabolized by cytochrome P-450; therefore, drugs that either potentiate or inhibit these enzymes are expected to produce corresponding changes in FK 506 metabolism, with respective decreased or increased blood levels of FK 506 during concomitant administration. Those drugs producing either increased or decreased blood levels of FK 506 because of their effects on the hepatic microsomal enzymes are identical to those previously described for CSA (CSA, Drug Interactions section) (200).

As during treatment with other immunosuppressive agents, vaccinations may be less effective during treatment with FK 506. Use of live vaccines should be avoided (218).

Major Clinical Trials

Major clinical trials are described in the Therapeutic Use section.

DAPSONE

History and Source

Dapsone was first synthesized in 1908 by Fromm and Wittmann; however, not until the 1940s did it gain prominence as the first truly effective therapy for leprosy (220). Today, dapsone is the mainstay of therapy for leprosy for more than 2 million people. In addition, it produces dramatic clinical effects in treatment of both dermatitis herpetiformis and bullous pemphigoid (220). Person and Rogers (221), in the late 1970s, and Rogers et al. (222), in the early 1980s, showed dapsone to be effective in controlling both the systemic and ocular inflammatory activity of cicatricial pemphigoid, a potentially blinding and fatal disease.

Official Drug Name and Chemistry

Dapsone, 4, 4[1] diaminodiphenylsulfone (DDS), molecular weight 248.3, is a synthetic sulfone. Its structural formula is shown in Figure 10.

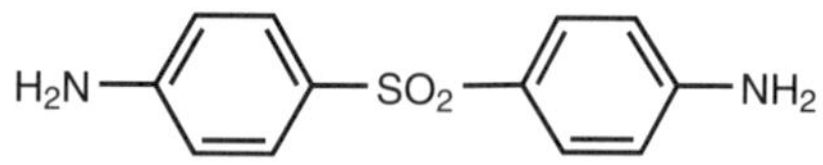

$H_2N-C_6H_4-SO_2-C_6H_4-NH_2$

FIG. 62-10. Chemical structure of dapsone.

Pharmacology

Dapsone has both antimicrobial and antiinflammatory activity, although the mechanisms by which it influences the inflammatory and immune systems are not clear.

Clinical Pharmacology

Antimicrobial Activity. Dapsone has both bactericidal and bacteriostatic activity against *Mycobacterium leprae,* readily penetrating bacterial cells. The mechanism of action is the same as that of the sulfonamides (223); i.e., dapsone competitively inhibits p-aminobenzoic acid (PABA) in the microorganism, thereby interrupting purine and, ultimately, nucleic acid biosynthesis. This inhibition is reversible when the sulfonamide is displaced by excess PABA.

Dapsone is also effective against plasmodia throughout its life cycle and retains full activity against plasmodia that have developed resistance to 4-aminoquinolone antimalarials (224). This may explain the low prevalence of malaria in patients with leprosy who are treated with dapsone (220). In addition, the antibiotic spectrum of dapsone has been expanded to include *P. carinii* infection in patients with AIDS and cutaneous leishmaniasis (225).

Antiinflammatory Activity. Dapsone is believed to mediate its antiinflammatory effects in dermatitis herpetiformis and pemphigoid by a variety of mechanisms. Evidence suggests that dapsone stabilizes lysosomal membranes, decreasing the release of their contents (226,227), and interferes with the myeloperoxidase/H_2O_2/halide-mediated cytotoxic system of neutrophils (227,228). In addition, dapsone has been shown to inhibit the Arthus reaction and adjuvant-induced arthritis in a manner similar to that of corticosteroids and indomethacin (227).

Pharmaceutics

Dapsone (DDS, Jacobus, Princeton, NJ) is supplied as either 25-mg or 100-mg tablets. The drug may be stored at room temperature but should be protected from light.

Pharmacokinetics and Metabolism

Dapsone is slowly, yet almost completely, absorbed from the GI tract, reaching peak plasma levels within 4 to 6 hours of ingestion, and achieves steady-state serum levels in 1 week (225). For inexplicable reasons, higher dapsone blood levels are achieved in women than in men (229).

Dapsone is distributed throughout the total body water and in all tissues; however, it tends to be retained by the skin, liver, kidneys, and muscles (223) but penetrates ocular tissues poorly (225). Dapsone undergoes extensive enterohepatic recirculation and tends to remain in the circulation for a long time, with a mean elimination $t_{\frac{1}{2}}$ of 22 hours (223).

Approximately 70% of dapsone is protein-bound and undergoes acetylation in the liver, the rate of which is genetically determined. Acetylation rate (slow vs. fast) has no impact on the clinical efficacy of the drug or its associated adverse effects (227). Dapsone and its metabolites are conjugated with glucuronic acid in the liver and excreted by the kidneys. Of a single 100-mg oral dose, 90% is eliminated in 9 days, with approximately 90% of the drug excreted in the urine and 10% excreted in the bile (225).

Therapeutic Use

Nonophthalmic uses of dapsone include treatment of leprosy, malaria, dermatitis, herpetiformis, bullous pemphigoid, cicatricial phemphigoid, pemphigus vulgaris, relapsing polychondritis, *P. carinii,* infection in patients with AIDS, and cutaneous leishmaniasis.

Ophthalmic uses of dapsone include cicatricial pemphigoid affecting the conjunctiva (OCP) and scleritis associated with RP (Table 4). Foster (35) confirmed the initial favorable outcomes reported by Person and Rogers (221) and Rogers et al. (222) in their use of dapsone for treatment of more than 130 patients with OCP: The progression of fibrosis was halted in 70% of cases. Dapsone is recommended as the first-line agent for treatment of OCP if the inflammatory activity is not severe, the disease is not rapidly progressive, and the patient is not glucose-6-phosphate dehydrogenase (G6-PD)-deficient (16). A response is usually observed within 4 weeks of initiation of therapy.

Dapsone has also been shown to be useful in treatment of the extraocular manifestations of RP (230,231); however, its efficacy with regard to the ocular manifestations of this disease is uncertain (232). Using dapsone alone, or in combination with NSAIDs or systemic corticosteroids, Huang-Xuan et al. (32) reported a favorable response in 6 of 11 patients with simple or nodular scleritis associated with RP. Dapsone is ineffective in treatment of necrotizing scleritis associated with RP, because this entity is among the most recalcitrant ocular inflammatory diseases to even the most aggressive chemotherapeutic strategies (30).

Dosage and Route of Administration. Dapsone treatment is initiated at 25 mg administered twice daily for 1 week (Table 1). The dose is increased to 50 mg twice daily, with further adjustments depending on the clinical response and drug tolerance, to a maximum of 150 mg/day (35). Slow dosage tapering to a maintenance level should begin once the inflammatory process is brought under control. Average dose reduction time is 8 months (range 4 months to 2.5 years) (51). Depending on the disease process, patients with OCP who fail dapsone therapy or exhibit severe progressive inflammatory disease usually respond to cyclophosphamide (3) (described in Cyclophosphamide, Therapeutic Use section).

Patients with simple or nodular scleritis associated with RP who fail to respond to a combination of NSAID and dapsone have systemic steroids added to their therapeutic regimen—typically 1 mg/kg/day with a rapid taper once the scleritis has completely resolved, with substitution of an alternate-day schedule once the 20-mg/day level has been reached. Steroids are then tapered as previously described (see Chapter 69, Corticosteroids, Therapeutic Use section, this volume). If the scleritis fails to respond to this combination, we add low-dose methotrexate (7.5 to 15 mg/wk) or daily azathioprine (2 mg/kg/day) (30). For necrotizing scleritis associated with RP, we most commonly use the combination of high-dose systemic corticosteroids and cyclophosphamide, resorting in some patients to once weekly pulse therapy with the latter agent (30).

Before therapy is initiated, baseline laboratory studies should be obtained, including a complete hemogram with differential and reticulocyte count, a chemistry profile including serum creatinine and BUN determinations, and liver function tests, urinalysis, and a G6-PD level. Because most patients receiving dapsone experience low-grade hemolysis, and because of its hepatotoxic potential, monitoring the hemogram and reticulocyte count early in the course of therapy, together with the liver function tests, is helpful in assessing whether a slow escalation in the dose is acceptable. We typically monitor the hemogram and reticulocyte count every 2 weeks for the first 3 months of therapy and every 6 weeks thereafter. Renal and hepatic function are monitored monthly during the first 3 months of therapy and then periodically every 3 to 4 months. Methemoglobin levels should be obtained only as clinically indicated (in patients with cardiopulmonary disease or methemoglobin-reductase deficiency) (225).

Side Effects and Toxicity

Dose-related hemolysis and methemoglobinemia are the most frequent adverse effects associated with dapsone therapy (Table 3), the latter occurring in most patients receiving 200 mg or more of drug daily, irrespective of G6-PD levels (233). In normal patients, anemia is usually not apparent until 3 to 4 weeks after initiation of therapy and rarely necessitates drug discontinuation. In contrast, hemolysis is more common and more severe and occurs at reduced dosages and earlier in the course of therapy in patients with G6-PD deficiency (227). Dapsone is believed to mediate this reaction in G6-PD–deficient patients by oxidizing glutathione, the reduced form of which is essential to the protection of erythrocytes from hemolysis. Therefore, determining baseline G6-PD levels is mandatory in all patients for whom dapsone therapy is contemplated. Death resulting from agranulocytosis, aplastic anemia, and other blood dyscrasias has been reported in association with dapsone treatment (234).

Other possible adverse effects of dapsone treatment include a reversible peripheral neuropathy, toxic hepatitis, and cholestatic jaundice, GI intolerance, cutaneous hypersensitivity reactions, and a potentially fatal mononucleosislike syndrome (227,233). The latter occurs rarely and is believed to be a hypersensitivity reaction characterized by fever, malaise, exfoliative dermatitis, methemoglobinemia, anemia, lymphadenopathy, and hepatomegaly with jaundice. Eosinophilia and an increased number of atypical lymphocytes are generally present (225). The condition improves with dapsone discontinuation and institution of corticosteroid therapy.

Overdose. Signs and symptoms of acute dapsone overdosage, appearing minutes to 24 hours after ingestion, include hyperexcitability, nausea, and vomiting (113). Supportive measures, especially emesis induction and gastric lavage, should be instituted. Methemoglobinemia-induced depression, seizures, and severe cyanosis require immediate treatment with methylene blue (MB), 1 to 2 mg/kg i.v., irrespective of the patient's methemoglobin reductase status (235). If methemoglobin reaccumulates, the dose of MB may be repeated in 30 minutes. For nonemergent therapy, MB may be administered orally in doses of 3 to 5 mg/kg every 4 to 6 hours. Because MB reduction is dependent on G6-PD, it is contraindicated in G6-PD–deficient patients (113).

High-risk Groups

Dapsone should be used with extreme caution in patients with G6-PD deficiency or methemoglobin-reductase deficiency, leukopenia, severe anemia, liver disease, and renal insufficiency (225). Elderly patients, who may have compromised hepatic and renal reserves, should likewise be monitored closely.

Dapsone readily crosses the placenta. Although it has been shown to be carcinogenic in laboratory rodents, no teratogenic or fetal abnormalities have been reported in humans (22). Nevertheless, use of this medication in pregnant women has not been adequately studied, and one should not assume that it poses no risk to the fetus. Because dapsone is excreted in the breast milk in significant quantities, it should be avoided in nursing mothers to protect the neonate from potential hemolytic reactions. Dapsone may be safely used in the pediatric age group, in a schedule similar to that used for adults, but in reduced doses (113).

Contraindications. Dapsone is contraindicated in patients with a history of hypersensitivity to the drug or its derivatives, including sulfonamides.

Drug Interactions

Probenecid may prolong the serum $t_{\frac{1}{2}}$ of dapsone by reducing its renal excretion. Concurrent use with rifampin, on the other hand, may reduce the serum concentration of dapsone by as much as 10-fold, as it induces hepatic microsomal enzyme activity and thus dapsone metabolism (22). Concomitant use of dapsone with drugs that can also cause anemia or leukopenia, such as folic acid antagonists and trimethoprim, requires vigilant hematologic monitoring (225).

Major Clinical Trials

Major clinical trials are described in the Therapeutic Use section.

Adjuvants to Immunosuppressive Therapy

Several agents have been used primarily as adjuvants to immunosuppressive drugs: bromocriptine or ketoconazole in combination with CSA as a dosage-lowering strategy and colchicine as a prophylactic agent in management of inflammatory recurrences in Behçet's disease.

BROMOCRIPTINE

History and Source

Bromocriptine, a semisynthetic ergot alkaloid, was initially developed in 1967 as an inhibitor of prolactin secretion and was subsequently shown to simulate directly and compete with specific binding to dopaminergic receptors in various tissues throughout the body (235). Today, bromocriptine is widely used in management of Parkinson's disease and in a wide range of conditions associated with hyperprolactinemia, including amenorrhea/galactorrhea, female infertility, postpartum lactation, and pituitary adenoma. With the demonstration of prolactin's powerful immunomodulatory properties, bromocriptine has been applied as an adjunctive agent in management of noninfectious ocular inflammatory disease in both animal models and in humans (109).

Official Drug Name and Chemistry

Bromocriptine mesylate (Parlodel, Sandoz), molecular weight 654.62, is an ergot derivative of lysergic acid. The addition of the bromine atom to this alkaloid confers its potent dopaminergic activity (236) (Fig. 11).

Pharmacology

The pharmacologic action of bromocriptine is directly related to its stimulation of dopamine receptors in the CNS, the cardiovascular system, the GI system, and the HPA (236). In the HPA, secretion of prolactin from the anterior pituitary is modulated by dopamine (prolactin inhibitory factor), which is synthesized in the hypothalamus and transported to its target by the hypothalamo-hypophyseal portal capillary system (235). Bromocriptine, as a dopamine agonist, thereby inhibits prolactin secretion.

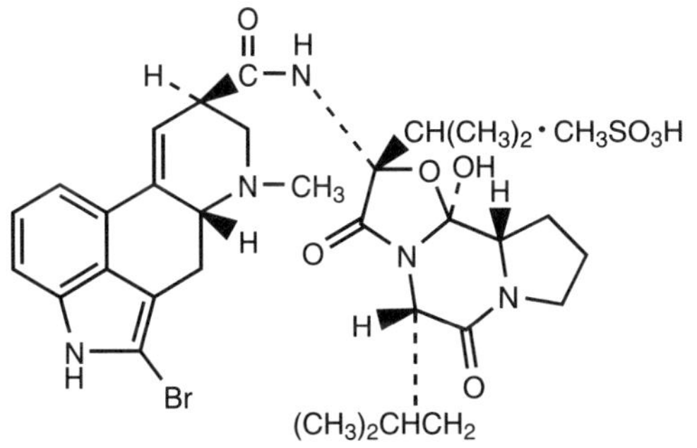

FIG. 62-11. Chemical structure of bromocriptine.

Clinical Pharmacology

Prolactin has potent effects on the immune system. Experimental studies in rats, in which prolactin levels were reduced either by hypophysectomy or bromocriptine administration, resulted in a marked decrease in both the humoral and cellular immune response (237,238). In addition, prolactin stimulates lymphocyte activation, binds to receptors on B cells, and competes with cyclosporine for receptors on T cells (239–241). Palestine et al. demonstrated an enhanced effect of low-dose CSA used in combination with bromocriptine in treatment of experimental autoimmune uveitis (242). This effect was most pronounced in female animals with high prolactin levels, suggesting that the efficacy of a given dose of CSA is enhanced by bromocriptine's inhibition of prolactin secretion.

Pharmaceutics

Bromocriptine (Parlodel, Sandoz) is formulated as 5-mg capsules and 2.5-mg tablets for oral use. It should be stored below 75°F in a light-resistant container.

Pharmacokinetics and Metabolism

Bromocriptine is rapidly absorbed after oral administration, achieving peak plasma levels in 1 to 3 hours, with a positive linear relationship between dose and peak plasma level, over a wide range of doses (235). First-pass metabolism of the absorbed dose is greater than 90%, with the majority (98%) being excreted in the feces and only 2% excreted in the urine (22). The plasma $t_{1/2}$ is 3 hours, and serum prolactin levels remain suppressed for as long as 14 hours after a single dose (235).

Therapeutic Use

No definitive indications for the use of bromocriptine in uveitis have been formulated (Table 4). Bromocriptine alone was reported to be efficacious in treatment of steroid-dependent, recurrent anterior uveitis in 4 patients with associated Parkinson's disease or hyperprolactinemia (243). However, a similar effect was not observed in a small, randomized, double-masked study in which all subjects had pretreatment prolactin levels at the lower border of normal (244). This study suggested that the utility of bromocriptine in recurrent anterior uveitis may be limited to patients with concomitantly abnormal dopamine or prolactin levels.

The effective use of bromocriptine combined with low-dose CSA (4 mg/kg/day) as a dosage-lowering strategy was demonstrated by Palestine et al. in their treatment of 14 patients with bilateral, sight-threatening uveitis of various etiologies (8 with intermediate uveitis, 3 with Behçet's disease, 2 with sarcoidosis, and 1 with idiopathic disease) (171). Not only was vision significantly improved in 8 of 14 patients, but nephrotoxicity was also curtailed, with no increase in serum creatinine during the 6-month follow-up period. However, the long-term efficacy of this particular therapeutic combination is, according to the same group of investigators, inferior to that of orally administered steroid and CSA (140).

Finally, bromocriptine was reported to be effective in treatment of thyroid ophthalmopathy (245–247). Increased pretreatment thyroid-stimulating hormone and prolactin levels were associated with clinical improvement after bromocriptine therapy in many, but not all, cases.

Dosage and Route of Administration. To minimize early adverse side effects, low-dose bromocriptine (1.25 mg) is administered orally, with food, at bedtime. The dose is then gradually increased to 2.5 mg, three or four times daily (16,235) (Table 1).

Side Effects and Toxicity

Early adverse effects, including nausea, vomiting, and postural hypotension, are common with initiation of bromocriptine therapy and may be minimized by ingestion of the medication with food or at bedtime (22) (Table 3). Although tolerance to nausea and orthostatic lightheadedness may develop in 3 to 4 days, rarely a first-dose syncopal phenomenon can occur (235). Other, less common effects observed in patients treated with larger doses include headache, dyspepsia, constipation, nasal congestion, dryness of the mouth, nocturnal leg cramps, depression, impaired concentration, nightmares, peripheral digital vasospasm on exposure to cold, and pleural thickening (22). Dry eye symptoms associated with bromocriptine have also been reported (248).

Overdose. Bromocriptine overdosage may produce nausea, vomiting, and severe hypotension. Treatment consists of supportive measures, especially gastric lavage and administration of intravenous fluids to treat hypotension (249).

High-risk Groups

Teratogenicity and other adverse effects to the mother or fetus have not been associated with use of bromocriptine for induction of ovulation or during pregnancy (235). Nevertheless, because bromocriptine crosses the placenta and may suppress fetal prolactin levels, the drug should be avoided during pregnancy unless indicated. Mothers who choose to breast feed their infants should avoid bromocriptine since it suppresses lactation. The safety and efficacy of this agent has not been established in the pediatric age range. Continued surveillance is necessary for development of any late-appearing adverse effects in the pediatric age group and among children born to mothers treated with bromocriptine during a portion of their pregnancy.

The safety and efficacy of bromocriptine in elderly patients, or in those with renal or hepatic disease, have not been established. Caution must be exercised in administering bromocriptine concurrently with any antihypertensive medication.

Contraindications. Bromocriptine should not be administered to patients with uncontrolled systemic hypertension, toxemia of pregnancy, or a history of hypersensitivity to ergot alkaloids (113).

Drug Interactions

The hepatic clearance of bromocriptine may be reduced by the concomitant administration of erythromycin (22). In addition, the efficacy of bromocriptine may be diminished in patients who are also receiving agents that exhibit dopamine antagonism (i.e., phenothiazines) (113).

Major Clinical Trials

Major clinical trials are described in the Therapeutic Use section.

KETOCONAZOLE

History and Source

The development of ketoconazole marks an important breakthrough in antifungal therapy, as it was the first synthetic, orally effective, broad spectrum antimycotic agent (250). The clinical experience with this drug and its congeners is now extensive. In fact, a clinically significant drug interaction between ketoconazole and systemically administered CSA has been recently exploited in an attempt to minimize the effective dose, toxicity, and cost associated with the latter agent in the therapy of both renal allograft rejection (250) and noninfectious endogenous uveitis (172).

Official Drug Name and Chemistry

Ketoconazole (Nizoral, Janssen, Titusville, NJ), molecular weight 531.44, is an imidazole drug. Modifications of its basic imidazole structure (Fig. 12) have spawned multiple antifungal agents (e.g., clotrimazole, econazole, miconazole, and itraconazole), with each substitution providing drugs with different physical characteristics (251).

Pharmacology

The primary mechanism of action of all imidazoles is inhibition of sterol metabolism. Specifically, ketoconazole prevents ergosterol synthesis by inhibiting the cytochrome P-450 enzyme system that catalyzes the C14-demethylation of lanosterol, the precursor of ergosterol (252). This effect produces changes in the fungal cell membrane phospholipid composition, altering its permeability characteristics and impairing membrane-bound enzyme systems necessary for growth (223). The inhibition of ergosterol biosynthesis in fungi is much more pronounced than that of cholesterol formation in mammalian cells, explaining the differential toxicity of ketoconazole in humans versus fungi (251).

Clinical Pharmacology

Ketoconazole is fungistatic at low concentrations and fungicidal at high concentrations. It is active against candidiasis, pityrosporosis, dermatophytosis, blastomycosis, coccidioidomycosis, cryptococcosis, and histoplasmosis (251).

The inhibitory action of this drug on the cytochrome P-450 system has additional important clinical implications, especially with respect to clinically significant drug interactions, both adverse and potentially therapeutic. Specifically, concomitant administration of ketoconazole with CSA, which is also extensively metabolized by the hepatic cytochrome P-450 enzymes (141), results in increased blood concentrations of CSA that may become toxic if the dose is not adjusted (253,254). Therefore, this interaction provides the rationale for a combined drug strategy allowing reduced yet effective doses of CSA while minimizing the risk of potential drug toxicity.

Pharmaceutics

Ketoconazole (Nizoral, Janssen) is available as 200-mg tablets for oral use and as a 2% topical cream.

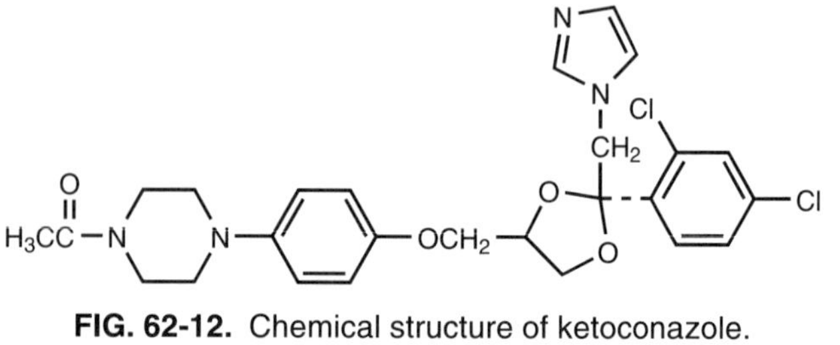

FIG. 62-12. Chemical structure of ketoconazole.

Pharmacokinetics and Metabolism

The absorption of ketoconazole is variable among patients and depends mainly on gastric acidity. Because the optimal solubility of ketoconazole in water requires a pH less than 3, bioavailability is markedly reduced in patients with achlorhydria (especially in the elderly and in patients with AIDS), and in those treated with antacids, H_2 receptor antagonists, anticholinergics, and antiparkinsonian agents (250,252). Suboptimal absorption may be minimized by the administration of ketoconazole 2 hours before these latter agents are administered to patients who require them.

After oral doses of 200, 400, and 800 mg of ketoconazole, respective peak plasma concentrations of 4, 8, and 20 mg/ml are achieved in approximately 2 hours (223,255). The plasma $t_{\frac{1}{2}}$ appears to be dose-dependent, varying from 1 to 2 hours to as long as 8 hours with a dose of 800 mg (223,256).

Ketoconazole is extensively metabolized by the hepatic cytochrome P-450 enzyme system, with the inactive metabolites being excreted by the biliary system and appearing in the feces (252). Very little active drug is excreted in the urine. Approximately 84% of ketoconazole is bound to plasma proteins (mostly albumin), 15% to erythrocytes, and 1% is free (257). Therefore, renal insufficiency, hemodialysis, or peritoneal dialysis have little effect on drug metabolism, whereas preexisting liver disease warrants careful laboratory monitoring, given ketoconazole's inherent potential for hepatotoxicity (251). However, even with moderate hepatic dysfunction, preliminary studies have shown no effect on the concentration of ketoconazole in the blood (223).

Ketoconazole has wide tissue distribution, achieving effective concentrations in keratinocytes, saliva, and vaginal fluid (251). However, concentrations in the CSF are only 1% to 4% of those in the serum at usual therapeutic doses in patients with fungal meningitis (22).

Therapeutic Use

For nonophthalmic purposes, ketoconazole is the drug of choice for treatment of nonmeningeal blastomycosis, histoplasmosis, coccidioidomycosis, pseudoallescheriasis, and paracoccidioidomycosis in otherwise healthy, immunocompetent patients (258). It is also the preferred treatment for chronic mucocutaneous candidiasis and is effective in the control of severe oral and esophageal candidiasis, as well as in severe recalcitrant dermatophyte infections (251).

The combined use of ketoconazole with CSA was initially reported in a group of 18 patients undergoing renal transplant in whom a reduction of 30% in their usual maintenance CSA dose of 8 mg/kg/day was achieved (250). None of the patients developed CSA-associated adverse events during the 13-month follow-up period.

Recently, deSmet et al. (172) of the National Eye Institute demonstrated the efficacy of combination therapy with ketoconazole (200 mg/day) and low-dose CSA (5 mg/kg/day) together with prednisone (0 to 0.5 mg/kg/day) in maintaining inflammatory remission in a double-masked, placebo-controlled study of 10 patients with endogenous uveitis (Tables 1 and 4). These patients, who were all in clinical remission while treated with combined low-dose CSA and prednisone therapy, had their CSA dose initially reduced by 70% in a 3-day period. Four of 6 (66%) control subjects experienced recurrent inflammatory episodes, whereas none of the 4 patients treated with the ketoconazole combination had a relapse of uveitis during the 3-month follow-up period. Furthermore, some patients treated with this combination continued to show improvement in their visual acuity, suggesting that the sustained drug levels of CSA afforded by the addition of ketoconazole are more effective in maintaining remission than are the more dramatic fluctuations in drug concentration produced by the usual treatment schedule (172).

Not only was a much smaller volume of CSA necessary to control inflammation in the ketoconazole-treated group, but toxicity was also limited to a transient decrease in GFR in 2 patients, at 1 month, which promptly returned to a normal rate after further reduction in the CSA dose (172). The researchers suggest that when ketoconazole is added to the therapeutic regimen, the dose of CSA should initially be decreased by 30% of its baseline value and continued at this reduced dose for a minimum of four CSA $t_{\frac{1}{2}}$ (several days), after which time a whole blood CSA level should be obtained (124,172). Further CSA dosage reductions may be indicated if this level remains increased. Initial careful monitoring of the serum creatinine and for clinical signs of acute CSA toxicity is necessary. Maintenance of the whole blood levels of CSA within the lower range of normal (500 to 1,000 ng/L) minimizes CSA-associated toxicity (172).

Side Effects and Toxicity

The most important adverse effects of ketoconazole therapy are hepatotoxicity and those arising from its influence on steroid biosynthesis (Table 3).

Hepatotoxicity. Ketoconazole-induced hepatotoxicity is believed to be due to a metabolic idiosyncracy in susceptible patients (250). The abrupt onset of potentially fatal hepatic dysfunction resembling viral hepatitis occurs in approximately 1 in 15,000 exposed patients, especially middle-aged women, between days 11 and 68 of ketoconazole therapy (259). Both the physician and the patient should have a heightened awareness of this potential complication. Asymptomatic and reversible elevations in the alanine and aspartate aminotransferase levels occur in 2% to 5% of patients (22).

Steroid Synthesis. Although the ketoconazole-mediated inhibition of steroid biosynthesis with regard to cytochrome P-450 enzymes is more pronounced in fungi than in humans, several endocrinologic abnormalities are known to occur in patients treated with this medication. Approximately 10% of women experience menstrual irregularity and a variable number of men report gynecomastia, decreased libido and potency, and oligospermia (223). Doses of ketoconazole as low as 400 mg/day may cause a reversible reduction in free testosterone and estradiol plasma levels, whereas higher doses (600 to 800 mg/day) may transiently inhibit adrenal steroidogenesis by blocking the 11-hydroxylation step of synthesis (22). Hypoadrenalism has been reported, especially with high doses of ketoconazole; therefore, this drug should be avoided in patients undergoing major surgery or in those exposed to other significant stressful conditions (223).

Other less severe but more common side effects include dose-related GI upset (nausea and vomiting), occurring in approximately 50% of patients receiving 800 mg daily (22). An allergic rash occurs in approximately 4% of patients, and pruritis without rash occurs in about 2% of individuals (223).

Overdose. General supportive measures together with gastric lavage with sodium bicarbonate should be instituted in the event of accidental overdosage of ketoconazole.

High-risk Groups

Ketoconazole has been shown to be teratogenic in animal models, producing syndactyly and oligodactyly in the offspring of rats when given at doses of 80 mg/kg/day (10 times the human dose) (22). Because data are insufficient to allow evaluation of the safety of the drug in pregnant women, it should be avoided during pregnancy unless the potential benefit to the mother outweighs the risk to the fetus. Because ketoconazole is excreted in the breast milk, mothers treated with the drug should not breast feed.

Likewise, the use of ketoconazole has not been studied systematically in the pediatric age group. Indeed, no information is available on use of this medication in children aged less than 2 years (113).

The absence of gastric acidity compromises the absorption of ketoconazole. Therefore, reduced bioavailability of drug may complicate therapy in the elderly and in patients with AIDS, both of whom frequently have achlorhydria.

Contraindications. Concomitant administration of ketoconazole with terfenadine or astemizole inhibits their metabolism and increases the plasma levels of both drugs and the active metabolite of the latter, placing the patient at risk of potentially fatal cardiac arrhythmias (113). Ketoconazole is also contraindicated in any patient with a known hypersensitivity to it or any other imidazole drug.

Drug Interactions

Concomitant administration of ketoconazole with coumarinlike agents enhances the anticoagulant effect of the latter (251). The blood level of CSA is increased by ketoconazole. In addition, ketoconazole reduces the clearance of chlordiazepoxide, theophilline, and methylprednisolone (22).

Conversely, concurrent use of ketoconazole with rifampin or isoniazid, or both, results in decreased ketoconazole concentrations (113). Coadministration of phenytoin and ketoconazole produces alterations in the levels of one or both of these drugs (251).

Major Clinical Trials

Major clinical trials are described in the Therapeutic Use section.

COLCHICINE

History and Source

Colchicine, an alkaloid derived from the autumn crocus *Colchium autumnale,* has been used for treatment of acute gout since the 6th century A.D. (260). Colchicine was isolated from colchicum in 1820 and first synthesized in 1965 (261). Although its antiinflammatory properties are best known in management of gout, colchicine is the drug of choice for treatment of familial Mediterranean fever and is effective in a variety of dermatologic and systemic diseases, such as psoriasis and Behçet's disease, which are characterized by neutrophil participation in the lesions (262–264). It is in the prophylaxis of the recurrent ocular and systemic inflammatory manifestations of Behçet's disease that ophthalmologists find colchicine most useful.

Official Drug Name and Chemistry

Colchicine, a phenathrene derivative, is acetyltrimethylcolchicinic acid (Fig. 13). It has a molecular weight of 399.44; the empirical formula is $C_{22}H_{25}NO_6$.

Pharmacology

Colchicine exhibits both antiinflammatory and antimitotic properties, mediated mainly through its inhibition of microtubular formation (260) (Fig. 1).

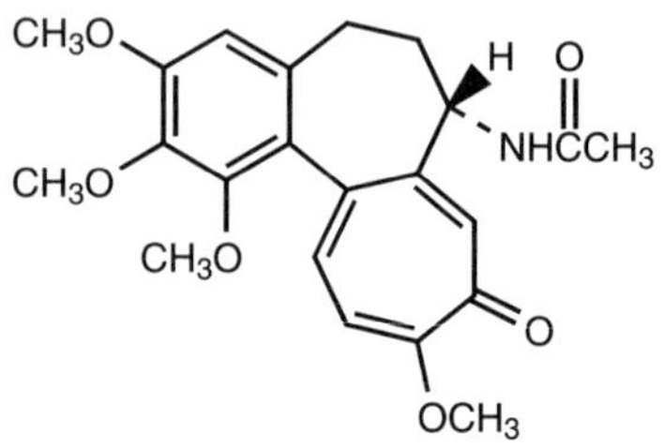

CH_3O CH_3O CH_3O H O $NHCCH_3$ O OCH_3

FIG. 62-13. Chemical structure of colchicine.

Clinical Pharmacology

Colchicine's antiinflammatory characteristics are poorly understood and chiefly involve depression of neutrophil motility, adhesiveness, chemotaxis, and lysosomal degranulation (261). The drug is concentrated extremely well in leukocytes, where it binds to dimers of tubulin, thus preventing the assembly of tubulin subunits. This disrupts the function of the spindle apparatus, arresting mitosis in metaphase, and causes the depolymerization and disappearance of fibrillar microtubules in granulocytes and other motile cells (264–266). In this way, the migration of granulocytes to the site of inflammation, together with release of lactic acid and proinflammatory lysosomal enzymes, is inhibited, thereby breaking the cycle leading to the inflammatory response (260).

Colchicine has also been shown to inhibit release of histamine from mast cell granules in vitro, secretion of insulin and parathromone, and movement of melanin granules in melanophores (262,263). These effects are believed to be due to colchicine's inhibition of granule translocation by the microtubular system (260).

Pharmaceutics

Colchicine (generic) is available as 0.5-mg and 0.6-mg tablets for oral use and as a sterile solution (0.5 mg/ml) for injection. It should be shielded from ultraviolet light exposure to prevent its degradation into inactive products (260).

Pharmacokinetics and Metabolism

Colchicine is rapidly absorbed after oral administration, reaching peak plasma concentrations between 30 and 120 minutes after ingestion (262). After intravenous injection of a 1-mg bolus in normal subjects, the mean elimination $t_{\frac{1}{2}}$ is 601 ± 155 ml/min and the apparent volume of distribution is 2 L/kg (22). Protein binding is minimal.

Large amounts of colchicine enter the intestinal tract in the bile and intestinal secretions, with high concentrations also occurring in the kidney, liver, and spleen. However, the drug is largely excluded from the brain, heart, and skeletal muscle (260). Colchicine can also be detected in peripheral leukocytes for at least 9 days after a single intravenous dose (260).

The drug undergoes hepatic metabolism, most being eliminated in the feces, with 10% to 20% excreted in the urine (262). In patients with hepatic dysfunction, a greater fraction of colchicine is shunted from the liver and excreted in the urine (260).

Therapeutic Use

Colchicine has been proven effective, alone or in combination with other immunosuppressive agents, in controlling the ocular and systemic manifestations of Behçet's disease (263,267–274) (Table 4). In a series of 131 patients with Behçet's disease reported by Mizushima et al. (273), 104 responded to colchicine. Foster et al. (39) used colchicine to treat 19 patients with Behçet's disease, successfully preventing inflammatory flare-ups in 3 patients with mild disease; 15 others required concomitant immunosuppressive therapy. Colchicine was discontinued in 1 patient because of diarrhea.

Because enhanced neutrophil migration is a characteristic feature of Behçet's disease, colchicine is most useful in prophylaxis of recurrent inflammatory episodes (rather than in treatment of active disease) or in the rare patient with mild, unilateral involvement in whom the clinician wishes to defer immunosuppressive therapy (109). In countries where the incidence of Behçet's disease is high, there is no consensus regarding its utility; colchicine therapy is more popular in Japan than in Turkey and is of equivocal value in whites.

Dosage and Route of Administration. The recommended dose is 0.5 to 0.6 mg orally two to three times daily (16,271,273,274) (Table 1).

Side Effects and Toxicity

The most common adverse effect of colchicine therapy is GI upset (Table 3). Although the drug is well tolerated in moderate dosages, the function of the rapidly proliferating epithelial cells in the GI tract is altered such that nausea, vomiting, abdominal cramping, hyperperistalsis, and watery diarrhea can occur at therapeutic doses, especially with 0.6 mg administered three times a day (262). Drugs to control vomiting and diarrhea may be useful; however, to avoid more serious toxicity, colchicine should be discontinued once symptoms of intolerance occur. The intravenous route obviates these GI side effects and produces a faster therapeutic effect; however, extravasation produces inflammation and necrosis of skin and soft tissues (260).

Chronic administration of colchicine can produce leukopenia, aplastic anemia, thrombocytopenia, myopathy, and alopecia (261). Azospermia and megaloblastic anemia secondary to vitamin B_{12} malabsorption have also been described (262). Complete hemogram and platelet counts, together with serum chemistries and urinalyses should be performed before initiation of therapy and periodically (every 3 to 4 months) thereafter.

Overdose. The fatal oral dose of colchicine in adults is approximately 20 mg (22). Signs and symptoms of acute poisoning include fever, hemorrhagic gastroenteritis, extensive vascular damage, nephrotoxicity, muscular depression, and an ascending paralysis of the CNS (260). In addition, a choleralike syndrome with severe fluid and electrolyte disturbances may ensue, together with respiratory distress syndrome, disseminated intravascular coagulation, bone marrow failure and, ultimately shock (261).

Management of acute intoxication is symptomatic and includes general supportive measures; repeated doses of activated charcoal orally, with gastric lavage; maintenance of fluid volume; treatment of hypothermia; administration of vitamin K, fresh frozen plasma, or platelets as indicated for coagulopathy; parenteral nutrition; correction of electrolyte disturbances; and intravenous administration of benzodiazepines if generalized seizures occur (22). Reversible alopecia and rebound leukocytosis are common in patients who survive serious colchicine intoxication (22,262).

High-risk Groups

Colchicine should be administered with great caution in the elderly, especially those with renal, hepatic, GI, or cardiovascular disease (260). Oral colchicine often causes diarrhea before relieving gout in elderly patients (22). Furthermore, diminished hepatic and renal reserves in these patients increases the plasma levels of colchicine, placing them at increased risk of development of chronic toxicity.

Colchicine has been reported to be teratogenic in humans (275) and should not be used during pregnancy (261). Whether the drug is excreted in the breast milk is not known; therefore, caution must be exercised when colchicine is administered to nursing mothers. Its safety and efficacy have yet to be established in children.

Contraindications. Colchicine is contraindicated in patients with severe GI, renal, hepatic, or cardiac disorders, especially in the presence of combined kidney and liver disease (113). A hypersensitivity reaction to the drug also constitutes a contraindication to its use.

Drug Interactions

Colchicine has been reported to induce a reversible malabsorption of vitamin B_{12}, with resultant megaloblastic anemia, presumably by altering the function of the ileal mucosa (262).

Major Clinical Trials

Major clinical trials are described in the Therapeutic Use section.

REFERENCES

1. Bach JF. *The mode of action of immunosuppressive drugs.* Amsterdam: Elsevier North Holland, 1975.
2. Biswas J, Rao NA. Management of intraocular inflammation. In: Ryan SJ, ed. *Retina,* vol. 2. St. Louis: Mosby-Year Book, 1994; 1061–1068.
3. Foster CS, Wilson SA, Ekins MB. Immunosuppressive therapy for ocular cicatricial pemphigoid. *Ophthalmology* 1982;89:340–353.
4. Krumbhaar EB, Krumbhaar HD. The blood and bone marrow in yellow cross gas (mustard gas) poisoning: changes produced in the bone marrow of fatal cases. *J Med Res* 1919;40:497–507.
5. Gery I, Nussenblatt RB. Immunosuppressive drugs. In: Sears ML, ed. *Pharmacology of the eye.* Berlin: Springer-Verlag, 1984;586–609.
6. Roda-Perez E. Sobre un case se uveitis de etiologia ignota tratado con mostaza introgenada. *Rev Clin Esp* 1951;40:265–267.
7. Roda-Perez E. El tratamiento de las uveitis de etiologia ignota con mostaza nitrogenada. *Arch Soc Oftal Hisp-Am* 1952;12:131–151.
8. Calabresi P, Chabner BA. Chemotherapy of neoplastic diseases. In: Gilman AG, Rall TW, Nies AS, Taylor P, eds. *Goodman and Gilman's the pharmacological basis of therapeutics.* New York: Pergamon Press, 1990;1202–1263.
9. Brock N. Oxazaphosphorine cytostatics: past-present-future: Seventh Cain Memorial Award Lecture. *Cancer Res* 1989;49:1–7.
10. Foster CS. Pharmacologic treatment of immune disorders. In: Albert DM, Jakobiec FA, eds. *Principles and practice of ophthalmology, basic sciences.* Philadelphia: W.B. Saunders, 1994;1076–1084.
11. Stockman GP, Heim LR, South MA, Trentin JJ. Differential effects of cyclophosphamide on the B and T cell compartments of adult mice. *J Immunol* 1973;110:277–282.
12. Clements PJ, Yu DTY, Levy J, Paulus HE, Barnett EU. Effects of cyclophosphamide on B and T lymphocytes in rheumatoid arthritis. *Arthritis Rheum* 1974;17:347–353.
13. Fauci AS, Dale DC, Wolff SM. Cyclophosphamide and lymphocyte subpopulations in Wegner's granulomatosis. *Arthritis Rheum* 1974; 17:355–361.
14. Lerman SP, Weidanz WP. The effect of cyclophosphamide on the ontogeny of the humoral immune response in chickens. *J Immunol* 1970;105:614–619.
15. Foster CS. Nonsteroidal anti-inflammatory and immunosuppressive agents. In: Lamberts DW, Potter DE, eds. *Clinical ophthalmic pharmacology.* Boston: Little, Brown, 1987;181–192.
16. Hemady R, Tauber J, Foster CS. Immunosuppressive drugs in immune and inflammatory disease. *Surv Ophthalmol* 1991;35:359–385.
17. Askenase PQ, Hayden BJ, Gershon RK. Augmentation of delayed type hypersensitivity by doses of cyclophosphamide which do not affect antibody responses. *J Exp Med* 1975;141:697–702.
18. Shand FL, Liew FY. Differential sensitivity to cyclophosphamide of helper T cells for humoral responses and suppressor T cells for delayed-type hypersensitivity. *Eur J Immunol* 1980;10:480–483.
19. Tabor DK, Kiel DP, Jacobs RF. Cyclophosphamide-sensitive activity of suppressor T cells during treponemal infection. *Immunology* 1987;62:127–132.
20. Lemmel E, Hurd ER, Ziff M. Differential effects of 6 mercaptopurine and cyclophosphamide on autoimmune phenomena in NZB mice. *Clin Exp Immunol* 1971;8:355–362.
21. Rapini RP, Jordan RE, Wolverton SE. Cytotoxic agents. In: Wolverton SE, Wilkins JK, eds. *Systemic drugs for skin diseases.* Philadelphia: W.B. Saunders, 1991;125–151.
22. *AMA drug evaluations.* Chicago: American Medical Association, 1991;396,1059,1654–1655,1671–1672,1843–1844,1972–1973,189 1–1913,2009–2034,2140–2141,2351–2353.
23. Brubaker R, Font RL, Shepero EM. Granulomatous sclerouveitis, regression of ocular lesions with cyclophosphamide and prednisone. *Arch Ophthalmol* 1971;86:517–524.
24. Foster CS. Immunosuppressive therapy for external ocular inflammatory disease. *Ophthalmology* 1980;87:140–150.
25. Jampol LM, West C, Goldberg MF. Therapy of scleritis with cytotoxic agents. *Am J Ophthalmol* 1978;86:266–271.
26. Fauci AS, Haynes BF, Katz P, Wolff SM. Wegener's granulomatosis: prospective clinical and therapeutic experience with 85 patients for 21 years. *Ann Intern Med* 1983;98:76–85.
27. Fauci AS, Duppman JZ, Wolff SM. Cyclophosphamide induced remissions in advanced polyarteritis nodosa. *Am J Med* 1978;64:890–894.
28. Fosdick WM, Parsons JL, Hill DF. Long-term cyclophosphamide therapy in rheumatoid arthritis. *Arthritis Rheum* 1968;9:151–161.
29. Foster CS, Forstot SL, Wilson LA. Mortality rate in rheumatoid arthritis patients developing necrotizing scleritis or peripheral ulcerative keratitis, effects of systemic immunosuppression. *Ophthalmology* 1984;91:1253–1263.

30. Foster CS, Sainz de la Maza, M. *The sclera.* New York: Springer-Verlag, 1993;299–307.
31. Watson PG, Hazleman BL. *The sclera and systemic disorders.* Philadelphia: W.B. Saunders, 1976;90–154.
32. Huang-Xuan T, Foster CS, Rice BA. Scleritis in relapsing polychondritis: response to therapy. *Ophthalmology* 1990;97:892–898.
33. Foster CS. Systemic immunosuppressive therapy for progressive bilateral Mooren's ulcer. *Ophthalmology* 1985;92:1436–1439.
34. Brown SI, Mondino BJ. Therapy of Mooren's ulcer. *Am J Ophthalmol* 1984;98:1–6.
35. Foster CS. Cicatricial pemphigoid. *Trans Am Ophthalmol Soc* 1986; 84:527–663.
36. Neumann R, Tauber J, Foster CS. Remission and recurrence after withdrawal of therapy for ocular cicatricial pemphigoid. *Ophthalmology* 1991;98:858–862.
37. Oniki S, Kurakazu K, Kawata K. Immunosuppressive treatment of Behçet's disease with cyclophosphamide. *Jpn J Ophthalmol* 1976: 20:32–40.
38. Gills JP, Buckley CE. Cyclophosphamide therapy of Behçet's disease. *Ann Ophthalmol* 1970;2:399–405.
39. Foster CS, Baer JC, Raizman MB. Therapeutic responses to systemic immunosuppressive chemotherapy agents in patients with Behçet's syndrome affecting the eyes. In: O'Duffy JD, Kokmen E, eds. *Behçet's disease: basic and clinical aspects.* New York: Marcel Dekker, 1991;581–588.
40. Fain O, Du LTH, Wechsler B. Pulse cyclophosphamide in Behçet's disease. In: O'Duffy JD, Kokmen E, eds. *Behçet's disease: basic and clinical aspects.* New York: Marcel Dekker, 1991;569–573.
41. Buckley CE, Durham NC, Gills JP. Cyclophosphamide therapy of peripheral uveitis. *Arch Intern Med* 1969;124:29–35.
42. Wong VG. Immunosuppressive therapy of ocular inflammatory diseases. *Arch Ophthalmol* 1969;81:628–637.
43. Martenet AC. Immunosuppressive therapy of uveitis: mid- and long-term follow up after classical cytostatic treatment. In: Usui M, Ohno S, Aoki K, eds. *Ocular immunology today.* New York: Excerpta Medica, 1990;443–446.
44. Dorr RT, Fritz WL. *Cancer chemotherapy handbook.* New York: Elsevier/North Holland, 1980.
45. Berkson BM, Come LG, Shapiro I. Severe cystitis induced by cyclophosphamide, role of surgical management. *JAMA* 1973;225:605–606.
46. Puri HC, Campbell RA. Cyclophosphamide and malignancy. *Lancet* 1977;1:1306.
47. Levine CA, Richie JP. Urological complications of cyclophosphamide. *J Urol* 1989;141:1063–1069.
48. Fairley KF, Barrie JV, Johnson W. Sterility and testicular atrophy related to cyclophosphamide therapy. *Lancet* 1972;1:568–569.
49. Fraunfelder FT, Meyer SM. Ocular toxicity from antineoplastic agents. *Ophthalmology* 1983;90:1–3.
50. Rubin B, Palestine AG. Complications of corticosteroids and immunosuppressive drugs. *Int Ophthalmol Clin* 1989;29:159–169.
51. Pavan-Langston D, Dunkel EC. *Handbook of ocular drug therapy and ocular side effects of systemic drugs.* Boston: Little, Brown, 1991;203–213.
52. Colvin M, Chabner BA. Alkylating agents. In: Chabner BA, Collins JM, eds. *Cancer chemotherapy: principles and practice.* Philadelphia: J.B. Lippincott, 1990;276:313.
53. Mamo JG, Azzam SA. Treatment of Behçet's disease with chlorambucil. *Arch Ophthalmol* 1970;84:446–450.
54. Ben Ezra D, Cohen E. Treatment and visual prognosis in Behçet's disease. *Br J Ophthalmol* 1986;70:589–592.
55. Bietti GB, Cerulli L, Pivetti-Pezzi P. Behçet's disease and immunosuppressive treatment. *Mod Probl Ophthalmol* 1976;16:314–323.
56. O'Duffy JD, Robertson DM, Goldstein NP. Chlorambucil in the treatment of uveitis and meningoencephalitis of Behçet's disease. *Am J Med* 1984;76:75–84.
57. Pezzi PD, Gasparri U, DeLiso P, Catarinelli G. Prognosis in Behçet's disease. *Ann Ophthalmol* 1985;17:20–25.
58. Tricoulis D. Treatment of Behçet's disease with chlorambucil. *Br J Ophthalmol* 1976;60:55–57.
59. Tabbara KF. Chlorambucil in Behçet's disease, a reappraisal. *Ophthalmology* 1983;90:906–908.
60. Abdalla MI, Bahgat N. Long-lasting remission of Behçet's disease after chlorambucil therapy. *Br J Ophthalmol* 1993;57:706–710.
61. Elliot JH, Ballinger WH. Behçet's syndrome, treatment with chlorambucil. *Trans Am Ophthalmol Soc* 1984;82:264–281.
62. Nussenblatt RB, Palestine AG, Chan CC, Ochizuki M, Yancey K. Effectiveness of cyclosporine therapy for Behçet's disease. *Arthritis Rheum* 1985;28:671–679.
63. Chavis PS, Antonios SR, Tabbara KF. Cyclosporine effects on optic nerve and retinal vasculitis in Behçet's disease. *Doc Ophthalmol* 1992;80:133–142.
64. Godfrey WA, Epstein WV, O'Connor GR, Kimura SJ, Hogan MJ, Nozik RA. The use of chlorambucil in intractable idiopathic uveitis. *Am J Ophthalmol* 1974;78:415–428.
65. Andrasch RH, Profsky B, Burns RP. Immunosuppressive therapy for severe chronic uveitis. *Arch Ophthalmol* 1978;96:247–251.
66. Jennings T, Tessler HH. Twenty cases of sympathetic ophthalmia. *Br J Ophthalmol* 1989;73:140–145.
67. Kanski JJ. Anterior uveitis in juvenile rheumatoid arthritis. *Arch Ophthalmol* 1977;95:1794–1797.
68. Foster CS, Barrett F. Cataract development and cataract surgery in patients with juvenile rheumatoid arthritis-associated iridocyclitis. *Ophthalmology* 1993;100:809–817.
69. Clements PJ, Davis J. Cytotoxic drugs: their clinical application to the rheumatic diseases. *Semin Arthritis Rheum* 1986;15:231–254.
70. Sobrinho LG, Levine RA, DeConti RL. Amenorrhea in patients with Hodgkin's disease treated with antineoplastic agents. *Am J Obstet Gynecol* 1971;109:135–139.
71. Berk PA, Goldberg JD, Silverman MN, et al. Increased incidence of acute leukemia in polycythemia vera associated with chlorambucil therapy. *N Engl J Med* 1981;304:441–447.
72. Lerner HJ. Acute myelogenous leukemia in students receiving chlorambucil as long-term adjuvant chemotherapy for stage II breast cancer. *Cancer Treat Rep* 1978;62:1135–1138.
73. Williams SA, Makker SP, Grupe WE. Seizures, a significant side effect of chlorambucil therapy in children. *J Pediatr* 1978;93:516–518.
74. Shotton D, Monie IW. Possible teratogenic effect of chlorambucil on a human fetus. *JAMA* 1963;186:74–75.
75. Farber S, Diamond LK, Mercer RD, Sylvester RF, Wolff VA. Temporary remissions in acute leukemia in children produced by folic antagonist 4-amethopteroylglutamic acid (aminopterin). *N Engl J Med* 1948;238:787–793.
76. Hertz R. Folic acid antagonists. Effects on the cell and patient. Clinical staff conference at NIH. *Ann Intern Med* 1963;59:931–956.
77. Weinblatt ME, Kremer JM. Methotrexate in rheumatoid arthritis. *J Am Acad Dermatol* 1988;19:126–128.
78. Lally EV, Ho G. A review of methotrexate therapy in Reiter's syndrome. *Semin Arthritis Rheum* 1985;15:139–145.
79. Wong VG, Hersh EM. Methotrexate in the therapy of cyclitis. *Trans Am Acad Ophthalmol Otolaryngol* 1965;69:279–293.
80. Callen JP, Kulp-Shorten CL. Methotrexate. In: Wolverton SE, Wilkins JK, eds. *Systemic drugs for skin diseases.* Philadelphia: W.B. Saunders, 1991;152–166.
81. Werkheiser W. The biochemical, cellular, and pharmacologic action and effects of the folic acid antagonists. *Cancer Res* 1963;23:1277–1285.
82. Hersh EM, Carbone PP, Wong VG, Greireich EJ. Inhibition of primary immune response in man by antimetabolites. *Cancer Res* 1965;25:1997–2001.
83. Mitchell MS, Wade ME, DeConti RC, Bertino JR, Calabresi P. Immune suppressive effects of cytosine arabinoside and methotrexate in man. *Ann Intern Med* 1969;70:535–547.
84. Andersen PA, West SG, O'Dell JR, Via CS, Claypool RG, Kotzin BL. Weekly pulse methotrexate in rheumatoid arthritis. Clinical and immunologic effects in a randomized, double-blind study. *Ann Intern Med* 1985;103:489–496.
85. Weinblatt ME, Coblyn JS, Fox DA, et al. Efficacy of low-dose methotrexate in rheumatoid arthritis. *N Engl J Med* 1985;312:818–822.
86. Shah SS, Lowder CY, Schmidt MA, Wilke WS, Kosmorsky GS, Meisler DM. Low-dose methotrexate therapy for ocular inflammatory disease. *Ophthalmology* 1992;99:1419–1423.
87. Olsen EA. The pharmacology of methotrexate. *J Am Acad Dermatol* 1991;25:306–317.
88. Wong VG. Methotrexate treatment of uveal disease. *Am J Med Sci* 1966;251:239–241.

89. Wong VG, Hersh EM, McMaster PRB. Treatment of a presumed case of sympathetic ophthalmia with methotrexate. *Arch Ophthalmol* 1966;76:66–76.
90. Lazar M, Weiner MJ, Leopold IH. Treatment of uveitis with methotrexate. *Am J Ophthalmol* 1969;67:383–387.
91. Weinstein G, Roenigk HH, Mailbach H, et al. Psoriasis-liver-methotrexate interactions. *Arch Dermatol* 1973;108:36–42.
92. Walker AM, Funch D, Dreyer NA, et al. Determinants of serious liver disease among patients receiving low-dose methotrexate for rheumatoid arthritis. *Arthritis Rheum* 1993;36:329–335.
93. Shupack JL, Webster GF. Pancytopenia following low-dose oral methotrexate therapy for psoriasis. *JAMA* 1988;259:3594–3596.
94. Roenigk HH, Auerbach R, Maibach HI, Weinstein GD. Methotrexate in psoriasis: revised guidelines. *J Am Acad Dermatol* 1988;19: 145–156.
95. Phillips CA, Cera PJ, Mangan TF, Newman ED. Clinical liver disease in patients with rheumatoid arthritis taking methotrexate. *J Rheumatol* 1989;16:487–493.
96. Ridley MG, Wolfe CS, Mathews JH. Life-threatening acute pneumonitis during low-dose methotrexate treatment for rheumatoid arthritis: a case report and review of the literature. *Ann Rheum Dis* 1988;47:784–788.
97. Schein PS, Winokur SH. Immunosuppressive and cytotoxic chemotherapy: long-term complications. *Ann Intern Med* 1975;82: 84–95.
98. Balin PL, Tindall JP, Roenigk HH. Is methotrexate therapy for psoriasis carcinogenic? A modified retrospective-prospective analysis. *JAMA* 1975;232:359–362.
99. Rustin GJ, Rustin F, Dent J, Booth M, Salt S, Bagshawe KD. No increase in second tumors after cytotoxic chemotherapy for gestational trophoblastic tumors. *N Engl J Med* 1983;308:473–476.
100. Nyfors A, Jensen H. Frequency of malignant neoplasms in 248 long-term methotrexate-treated psoriatics: a preliminary study. *Dermatologica* 1983;167:260–261.
101. Giannini EH, Brewer EJ, Kuzmina N, et al. Methotrexate in resistant juvenile rheumatoid arthritis. *N Engl J Med* 1992;326:1043–1049.
102. Newell FW, Krill AE. Treatment of uveitis with azathioprine (Imuran). *Trans Ophthalmol Soc UK* 1967;87:499–511.
103. Newell FW, Krill AE, Thompson A. The treatment of uveitis with six-mercaptopurine. *Am J Ophthalmol* 1966;61:1250–1255.
104. Rollingshoff M, Schrader J, Wagner H. Effect of azathioprine and cytosine arabinoside on humoral and cellular immunity in vitro. *Clin Exp Immunol* 1973;15:261–269.
105. Mathews JD, Crawford BA, Bignell JL, Mackay IR. Azathioprine in active iridocyclitis, a double blind controlled trial. *Br J Ophthalmol* 1969;53:327–330.
106. Moore EE. Sympathetic ophthalmia treated with azathioprine. *Br J Ophthalmol* 1968;52:688–690.
107. Hemady R, Baer JC, Foster CS. Immunosuppressive drugs in the management of progressive, corticosteroid-resistant uveitis associated with juvenile rheumatoid arthritis. *Int Ophthalmol Clin* 1992; 32:241–252.
108. Yazici H, Pazarli H, Barnes CG, et al. A controlled trial of azathioprine in Behçet's syndrome. *N Engl J Med* 1990;322:281–285.
109. Nussenblatt RB, Palestine AG. *Uveitis, fundamentals and clinical practice.* Chicago: Year Book Medical Publishers, 1989;116–144.
110. Penn I. Malignancies associated with immunosuppressive or cytotoxic therapy. *Surgery* 1978;83:492–502.
111. Singh G, Fries JF, Spitz P, Williams CA. Toxic effects of azathioprine in rheumatoid arthritis. *Arthritis Rheum* 1989;32:837–843.
112. Castor WC, Bull FE. Review of United States data on neoplasma in rheumatoid arthritis. *Am J Med* 1985;78(suppl 1A):133–138.
113. *Physicians' desk reference.* Montvale, New Jersey: Medical Economics Data, 1994;703–704,1081,1096,2067,2071–2074,2114.
114. Schusziarra V, Ziekursch V, Schlamp R, Siemensen HC. Pharmacokinetics of azathioprine under haemodialysis. *Int J Clin Pharmacol Biopharm* 1976;14:298–302.
115. Coulam CB, Moyer TP, Jiang NS, Zincke H. Breast-feeding after renal transplantation. *Transplant Proc* 1982;14:605–609.
116. Hoover R, Fraumeni JF. Drug-induced cancer. *Cancer* 1981;47: 1071–1080.
117. Kirchertz EJ, Gröne HJ, Rieger J, Holscher M, Scheler F. Successful low dose captopril rechallenge following drug-induced leucopenia. *Lancet* 1981;1:1362–1363.
118. Borel JF. The history of cyclosporin A and its significance. In: White DJG, ed. *Cyclosporin A.* New York: Elsevier Biomedical Press, 1982;5–17.
119. Borel JF, Feurer C, Magnee C, Stahelin H. Effects of the new anti-lymphocyte peptide cyclosporin A in animals. *Immunology* 1977;32: 1017–1025.
120. Nussenblatt RB, Palestine AG, Rook AH, Scher I, Wacker WB, Gery I. Treatment of intraocular inflammation with cyclosporin A. *Lancet* 1983;1:235–238.
121. Nussenblatt RB, Palestine AG, Chan CC. Cyclosporine A therapy in the treatment of intraocular inflammatory disease resistant to systemic corticosteroids and cytotoxic agents. *Am J Ophthalmol* 1983; 96:275–282.
122. Nussenblatt RB, Palestine AG. Cyclosporine: immunology, pharmacology and therapeutic uses. *Surv Ophthalmol* 1986;31:159–169.
123. Kahan BD. Cyclosporine. *N Engl J Med* 1989;321:1725–1738.
124. deSmet MD, Nussenblatt RB. Clinical use of cyclosporine in ocular disease. *Int Ophthalmol Clin* 1993;33:31–45.
125. Sigal NH, Dumont FJ. Cyclosporin A, FK-506, and rapamycin: pharmacologic probes of lymphocyte signal transduction. *Annu Rev Immunol* 1992;10:519–560.
126. Thompson AW, Starzl TE. FK 506 and autoimmune disease: perspective and prospects. *Autoimmunity* 1992;12:303–313.
127. Handschumacher RE. Immunosuppressive agents. In: Gilman AG, Rall TW, Nies AS, Taylor P, eds. *Goodman and Gilman's the pharmacological basis of therapeutics.* New York: Pergamon Press, 1990;1264–1276.
128. Liu J. FK 506 and cyclosporin, molecular probes for studying intracellular signal transduction. *Immunol Today* 1993;14:290–295.
129. Sehgal SN. Immunosuppressive profile of rapamycin. *Ann NY Acad Sci* 1993;685:1–8.
130. Chang JY, Sehgal SN. Pharmacology of rapamycin: a new immunosuppressive agent. *B J Rheumatol* 1991;30(suppl 2):62–65.
131. Chang JY, Sehgal SN, Bansbach CC. FK 506 and rapamycin: novel pharmacological probes of the immune response. *Trends in Pharmacol Sci* 1991;12:218–223.
132. Ryffel B, Foxwell BM, Mihatsch MJ, Donatsch P, Maurek G. Biologic significance of cyclosporine metabolites. *Transplant Proc* 1988;20(suppl 2):575–584.
133. Palestine AG, Nussenblatt RB, Chan CC. Cyclosporine penetration into the anterior chamber and cerebrospinal fluid. *Am J Ophthalmol* 1985;99:210–211.
134. Ben Ezra D, Maftzir G. Ocular penetration of cyclosporine A in the rat eye. *Arch Ophthalmol* 1990;108:584–587.
135. Tabbara KF, Al Sayyed Y. Ocular bioavailability of cyclosporin after oral administration. *Transplantation Proceedings* 1988;20 (2 Suppl 2):656–659.
136. Diaz-Llopis M, Menezo JL. Penetration of 2% cyclosporin eyedrops into the aqueous humour. *Br J Ophthalmol* 1989;73:600–603.
137. Ben Ezra D, Maftizir G, deCourten C, Timonen P. Ocular penetration of cyclosporin A. III. The human eye. *Br J Ophthalmol* 1990; 74:350–352.
138. Reidy JJ, Gebhardt BM, Kaufman HE. The collagen shield. A new vehicle for the delivery of cyclosporin A to the eye. *Cornea* 1990;9: 196–199.
139. Kanai A, Alba RM, Takano T, et al. The effect on the cornea of alpha cyclodextrin vehicle for cyclosporin eye drops. *Transplant Proc* 1989;21:3150–3152.
140. Nussenblatt RB. The expanding use of immunosuppression in the treatment of noninfectious ocular disease. *J Autoimmun* 1992;5: 247–257.
141. Beveridge T. Pharmacokinetics and metabolism of cyclosporin A. In: White DJG, ed. *Cyclosporin A.* New York: Elsevier Biomedical Press, 1982;35–44.
142. Nussenblatt RB, Palestine AG, Chan CC, Breen L, Caruso R. Improvement of uveitis and optic nerve disease by cyclosporine in a patient with multiple sclerosis. *Am J Ophthalmol* 1984;97:790–791.
143. Nussenblatt RB, Palestine AG, Chann CC. Cyclosporine therapy for uveitis: long-term follow up. *J Ocul Pharmacol* 1985;1:369–382.
144. Graham EM, Sanders MD, James DG, Hamblin A, Grochwska EK, Dumonde D. Cyclosporin A in the treatment of posterior uveitis. *Trans Ophthal Soc UK* 1985;104:146–151.

145. Wakefield D, McCluskey P. Cyclosporine: a therapy in inflammatory eye disease. *J Ocul Pharmacol* 1991;7:221–226.
146. LeHoang P, Girard B, Deray G, et al. Cyclosporine in the treatment of birdshot retinochoroidopathy. *Transplant Proc* 1988;20(suppl 4):128–130.
147. Binder AI, Graham EM, Sanders MD, Dinning W, James DG, Denman AM. Cyclosporin A in the treatment of severe Behçet's uveitis. *Br J Rheumatol* 1987;76:285–291.
148. Wakefield D, McCluskey P, Reece G. Cyclosporin therapy in Vogt-Koyanagi-Harada disease. *Aust NZ J Ophthalmol* 1990;18:137–142.
149. Nussenblatt RB, Palestine AG, Chan CC, Stevens G, Mellow SD, Green SB. Randomized, double-masked study of cyclosporine compared to prednisolone in the treatment of endogenous uveitis. *Am J Ophthalmol* 1991;112:138–146.
150. Masuda K, Nakajima A, Urayama A, Nakae K, Kogure M, Inaba G. Double-masked trial of cyclosporin versus colchicine and long-term open study of cyclosporin in Behçet's disease. *Lancet* 1989;1:1093–1096.
151. deVries J, Baarsma GS, Zaai MJW, et al. Cyclosporin in the treatment of severe chronic idiopathic uveitis. *Br J Ophthalmol* 1990;74:344–349.
152. Towler HMA, Cliffe AM, Whiting PH, Forrester JV. Low dose cyclosporin A therapy in chronic posterior uveitis. *Eye* 1989;3:282–287.
153. Towler HMA, Whiting PH, Forrester JV. Combination low dose cyclosporin A and steroid therapy in chronic intraocular inflammation. *Eye* 1990;4:514–520.
154. Towler HMA, Lightman SL, Forrester JV. Low-dose cyclosporin therapy of ocular inflammation: preliminary report of a long-term follow-up study. *J Autoimmun* 1992;5(suppl A):259–264.
155. Vitale AT, Rodriguez A, Foster CS. Low-dose cyclosporine therapy in the treatment of birdshot retinochoroidopathy. *Ophthalmology* 1994;101:782–831.
156. Ben Ezra DE, Cohen E, Chajek T, et al. Evaluation of conventional therapy versus cyclosporine A in Behçet's syndrome. *Transplant Proc* 1988;20(suppl 4):143–146.
157. Whitcup SM, Salvo EC, Nussenblatt RB. Combined cyclosporine and corticosteroid therapy for sight-threatening uveitis in Behçet's disease. *Am J Ophthalmol* 1994;118:39–45.
158. Hoffman F, Widerholt M. Local treatment of necrotizing scleritis with cyclosporin A. *Cornea* 1985;4:3–7.
159. Wiebking WJ, Mehlfeld T. Local treatment of corneal ulcers and scleromalacias with cyclosporin A. *Fortschr Ophthalmol* 1986;83:345–347.
160. Kruit PJ, VanBalen AT, Stilma JS. Cyclosporin A treatment in two cases of corneal peripheral melting syndromes. *Doc Ophthalmol* 1985;59:33–39.
161. Kruit PJ. Cyclosporine A treatment in four cases with corneal melting syndrome. *Transplant Proc* 1988;90(suppl):170–172.
162. Hill JC. The use of cyclosporine in high-risk keratoplasty. *Am J Ophthalmol* 1989;107:506–510.
163. Miller K, Huber C, Niederwieser D, Gottinger W. Successful engraftment of high-risk corneal allografts with short-term immunosuppression with cyclosporine. *Transplantation* 1988;45:651–653.
164. Holland EJ, Chan CC, Kuwabara T, Palestine AG, Rowsey JJ, Nussenblatt RB. Immunohistological findings and results of treatment with cyclosporine in ligneous conjunctivitis. *Am J Ophthalmol* 1989;107:160–166.
165. Rubin BI, Holland EJ, deSmet MD, Belfort R, Nussenblatt RB. Response of reactivated ligneous conjunctivitis to topical cyclosporine. *Am J Ophthalmol* 1991;112:95–96.
166. Ben Ezra D, Pe'er J, Brodsky M, Cohen E. Cyclosporine eyedrops for the treatment of severe vernal keratoconjunctivitis. *Am J Ophthalmol* 1986;101:278–282.
167. Bleik PH, Tabbara KF. Topical cyclosporine in vernal keratoconjunctivitis. *Ophthalmology* 1991;98:1679–1684.
168. Secchi AG, Tognon MS, Leonardi A. Topical use of cyclosporine in the treatment of vernal keratoconjunctivitis. *Am J Ophthalmol* 1990;110:641–645.
169. Goichot-Bonnat L, De Beauregard C, Saragoossi JJ, Pouloquen Y. Usage de la cyclosporine A collyre dans la prevéntion dy reject de greffe de cornée chez l'homme: I. Evolution préopératoire de 4 yeux atteints de kératite métaherpetique. *J Fr Ophtalmol* 1987;10:207–211.
170. Belin MW, Bouchard CS, Frantz S, Chmielinska J. Topical cyclosporine in high-risk corneal transplants. *Ophthalmology* 1989;96:1144–1150.
171. Palestine AG, Nussenblatt RB, Gelato M. Therapy of human autoimmune uveitis with low-dose cyclosporine plus bromocriptine. *Transplant Proc* 1988;20(suppl):131–135.
172. deSmet MD, Rubin BJ, Whitcup SM, Lopez JS, Austin HA, Nussenblatt RB. Combined use of cyclosporine and ketoconazole in the treatment of endogenous uveitis. *Am J Ophthalmol* 1992;113:687–690.
173. Ben Ezra D, Nussenblatt RB, Timchen P. *Optimal use of Sandimmune in endogenous uveitis.* Berlin: Springer-Verlag, 1988.
174. Vine W, Bowers LD. Cyclosporine structure, pharmacokinetics, and therapeutic drug monitoring. *Crit Rev Clin Lab Sci* 1987;25:275–311.
175. Masri MA. Cyclosporine blood level monitoring by three special methods: R1A H^3, R1A I_{125}, and fluorescence polarization: comparison of accuracy, cost, reproducibility and percent recovery. *Transplant Proc* 1992;24:1716–1717.
176. Ball PE, Munzer H, Keller HP, Abish E, Rosenthaler J. Specific ^3H radioimmunoassay with a monoclonal antibody for monitoring cyclosporine in blood. *Clin Chem* 1988;34:257–260.
177. Kahan BD, Wideman CA, Reid M, et al. The value of serial trough cyclosporine levels in human renal transplantation. *Transplant Proc* 1984;16:1195–1199.
178. Kahan BD. Cyclosporine nephrotoxicity: pathogenesis, prophylaxis, therapy and prognosis. *Am J Kidney Dis* 1986;8:323–331.
179. Palestine AG, Austin HA, Balow JE, et al. Renal histopathologic alterations in patients treated with cyclosporine for uveitis. *N Engl J Med* 1986;314:1293–1298.
180. Mihatsch MJ, Steiner K, Abeywickrama KH, Landmann J, Thiel G. Risk factors for the development of chronic cyclosporine-nephrotoxicity. *Clin Nephrol* 1988;29:165–175.
181. Miescher PA, Favre H, Chatelanat F, Mihatsch MJ. Combined steroid-cyclosporine treatment of chronic autoimmune diseases. Clinical results and assessment of nephrotoxicity by renal biopsy. *Klin Wochenschr* 1987;65:727–736.
182. Feutren G, Mihatsch MJ. Risk factors for cyclosporine-induced nephrotoxicity in patients with autoimmune diseases. *N Engl J Med* 1992;326:1654–1660.
183. Nussenblatt RB, de Smet MD, Rubin B, et al. A masked, randomized, dose-response study between cyclosporine A and G in the treatment of sight-threatening uveitis of noninfectious origin. *Am J Ophthalmol* 1993;115:583–591.
184. de Groen PL. Cyclosporine. A review and its specific use in liver transplantation. *Mayo Clin Proc* 1989;64:680–689.
185. Loughran TP, Deeg HJ, Dahlberg S, Kennedy MS, Storb R, Thomas EO. Incidence of hypertension after marrow transplantation among 112 patients randomized to either cyclosporine or methotrexate as graft-vs-host disease prophylaxis. *Br J Haematol* 1985;59:547–553.
186. Palestine AG, Nussenblatt RB, Chan CC. Side effects of systemic cyclosporine in patients not undergoing transplantation. *Am J Med* 1984;77:652–656.
187. Lin HY, Rocher LL, McQuillan MA, Schmaltz S, Palella TD, Fox IH. Cyclosporine-induced hyperuricemia and gout. *N Engl J Med* 1989;321:287–292.
188. Ballantyne CM, Podet EJ, Patsch WP, et al. Effects of cyclosporine therapy on plasma lipoprotein levels. *JAMA* 1989;262:53–56.
189. Briggs GG, Freeman RK, Yaffe SJ. *Drugs used in pregnancy and lactation.* Baltimore: Williams & Wilkins, 1990;174–176.
190. Harris KP, Jenkins D, Walls J. Nonsteroidal antiinflammatory drugs and cyclosporine. A potentially serious adverse interaction. *Transplantation* 1988;46:598–599.
191. Kino T, Hatanaka H, Hashimoto M, et al. FK-506, a novel immunosuppressant isolated from Streptomyces. I. Fermentation isolation. Physico-chemical and biological characteristics. *J Antibiot* 1987;40:1249–1255.
192. Mocizuki M, Masuda K, Sakane T, et al. A multicenter clinical open trial of FK 506 in refractory uveitis, including Behçet's disease. *Transplant Proc* 1991;23:3343–3346.
193. Sehgal S, Baker H, Vezina C. Rapamycin (AY-22, 989), a new antifungal antibiotic. II. Fermentation, isolation and characterization. *J Antibiot* 1975;28:727–732.
194. Roberge FG, Xu D, Chan CC, de Smet MD, Nussenblatt RB, Chen H. Treatment of autoimmune neuroretinitis in the rat with ra-

pamycin, an inhibitor of lymphocyte growth factor signal transduction. *Curr Eye Res* 1993;12:197–203.
195. Thompson AW. FK-506—how much potential? *Immunol Today* 1989;10:6–9.
196. Kahan BD, Chang JY, Sehgal S. Preclinical evaluation of a new potent immunosuppressive agent, rapamycin. *Transplantation* 1991; 52:185–191.
197. Morris RE. Rapamycin: FK 506's fraternal twin or distant cousin? *Immunol Today* 1991;12:137–140.
198. Morris RE. In vivo immunopharmacology of the macrolides FK 506 and rapamycin: toward the era of rational immunosuppressive drug discovery, development, and use. *Transplant Proc* 1991;23:2722–2724.
199. Thompson AW. The immunosuppressive macrolides FK-506 and rapamycin. *Immunol Lett* 1991;29:105–111.
200. Peters DH, Fitton A, Plosker GL, Faulds D. Tacrolimus: a review of its pharmacology and therapeutic potential in hepatic and renal transplantation. *Drugs* 1993;46:746–794.
201. Venkataramanan R, Jain A, Cadoff E, et al. Pharmacokinetics of FK 506: preclinical and clinical studies. *Transplant Proc* 1990;22:52–56.
202. Arita C, Hotokebuchi T, Miyahaka H, et al. Inhibition by FK 506 of established lesions of collagen-induced arthritis in rats. *Clin Exp Immunol* 1990;82:456–461.
203. Murase N, Lieberman I, Nalesnik M, et al. Prevention of spontaneous diabetes in BB rats with FK 506. *Lancet* 1990;336:373–374.
204. Okuba Y, Tsukada Y, Marzawa A, Ono K, Yano S, Naruse T. FK 506, a novel immunosuppressive agent, induces antigen-specific immunotolerance in active Heymann's nephritis and in the autologous phase of Masugi nephritis. *Clin Exp Immunol* 1990;82:450–455.
205. Inamura N, Hashimoto M, Nakahara K, et al. Immunosuppressive effect of FK 506 on experimental allergic encephalomyelitis in rats. *Int J Immunopharmacol* 1988;10:991–995.
206. Takabayashi K, Koike T, Kurasawa K, et al. Effects of FK 506, a novel immunosuppressive drug on murine systemic lupus erythematosus. *Clin Immunol Immunopathol* 1989;51:110–117.
207. Kawashima H, Fujino Y, Mochizuki M. Effects of a new immunosuppressive agent, FK 506, on experimental autoimmune uveoretinitis in rats. *Invest Ophthalmol Vis Sci* 1988;29:1265–1271.
208. Kawashima H, Fujino Y, Mochizuki M. Antigen-specific suppressor cells induced by FK 506 in experimental autoimmune uveoretinitis in the rat. *Invest Ophthalmol Vis Sci* 1990;31:31–38.
209. Fujino Y, Chan CC, de Smet MD, et al. FK 506 treatment of experimental autoimmune uveoretinitis in primates. *Transplant Proc* 1991;23:3335–3338.
210. Jegasothy B, Ackerman CD, Todo S, Fung J, Starzel TE. FK 506—a new therapeutic agent for severe, recalcitrant psoriasis. *Arch Dermatol* 1992;128(6):781–785.
211. McCauley J, Shapiro R, Scantlebury V, et al. FK 506 in the management of transplant-related nephrotic syndrome and steroid-resistant nephrotic syndrome. *Transplant Proc* 1991;23:3354–3356.
212. Mochizuki M, Masuda K, Tsuyoshi S, et al. A clinical trial of FK 506 in refractory uveitis. *Am J Ophthalmol* 1993;115:763–769.
213. Martel RR, Klicius J, Galet S. Inhibition of the immune response by rapamycin, a new antifungal antibiotic. *Can J Physiol Pharmacol* 1977;55:48–51.
214. Martin DF, DeBarge LR, Nussenblatt RB, Chan CC, Roberge FG. Synergistic effect of rapamycin and cyclosporine A on the inhibition of experimental autoimmune uveoretinitis. *Invest Ophthalmol Vis Sci* 1993;34(suppl):1476.
215. Macleod AM, Thompson AW. FK 506: an immunosuppressant for the 1990s? *Lancet* 1991;337:25–27.
216. Fung JJ, Alessiani M, Abu-Elmagd K, et al. Adverse effects associated with the use of FK 506. *Transplant Proc* 1991;23:3105–3108.
217. Reyes J, Tzakis A, Green M, et al. Post-transplant lymphoproliferative disorders occurring under primary FK 506 immunosuppression. *Transplant Proc* 1991;23:3044–3046.
218. *Product Information Package Insert, Prograf*™, Fujisawa USA, Inc., Deerfield, IL, 1994.
219. Shapiro R, Fung JJ, Jain AB, Park P, Todo S, Starzl TE. The side effects of FK 506 in humans. *Transplant Proc* 1990;22:35–36.
220. Wozel G. The story of sulfones in tropical medicine and dermatology. *Int J Dermatol* 1989;28:17–21.
221. Person JR, Rogers RS. Bullous pemphigoid responding to sulfapyridine and the sulfones. *Arch Dermatol* 1977;113:610–615.
222. Rogers RS, Seehafer JR, Perry HO. Treatment of cicatricial (benign mucous membrane) pemphigoid with dapsone. *J Am Acad Dermatol* 1982;6:215–223.
223. Mandell GL, Sande MA. Antimicrobial agents: drugs used in the chemotherapy of tuberculosis and leprosy. In: Gilman AG, Rall TW, Nies AS, Taylor P, eds. *Goodman and Gilman's the pharmacological basis of therapeutics.* New York: Pergamon Press, 1990;1159–1164,1169–1171.
224. Wozel G, Barth J. Current aspects of modes of action of dapsone. *Int J Dermatol* 1988;27:547–552.
225. Geer KE. Dapsone and sulfapyridine. In: Wolverton SE, Wilkin JK, eds. *Systemic drugs for skin diseases.* Philadelphia: W.B. Saunders, 1991;247–264.
226. Barranco VP. Inhibition of lysosomal enzymes by dapsone. *Arch Dermatol* 1974;110:563–566.
227. Lang PG. Sulfones and sulfonamides in dermatology today. *J Am Acad Dermatol* 1979;1:479–492.
228. Stendahl O, Molin L, Dahlgren C. The inhibition of polymorphonuclear leukocyte cytotoxicity by dapsone, a possible mechanism in the treatment of dermatitis herpetiformis. *J Clin Invest* 1978;62: 214–220.
229. Pieters FA, Zuidema J. The pharmacokinetics of dapsone after oral administration to healthy volunteers. *Br J Clin Pharmacol* 1986;22: 491–494.
230. Barranco VP, Minor DB, Solomon H. Treatment of relapsing polychondritis with dapsone. *Arch Dermatol* 1976;112:1286–1288.
231. Martin J, Roenigk HH, Lynch W. Tingwald FR. Relapsing polychondritis treated with dapsone. *Arch Dermatol* 1976;112:1272–1274.
232. Matoba A, Plager S, Barber J, McCulley JP. Keratitis in relapsing polychondritis. *Ann Ophthalmol* 1984;16:367–370.
233. DeGowin RL. A review of therapeutic and hemolytic effects of dapsone. *Arch Intern Med* 1967;120:242–248.
234. Potter MN, Yates P, Slade R, Kennedy CT. Agranulocytosis caused by dapsone therapy for granuloma annulare. *J Am Acad Dermatol* 1989;30:87–88.
235. Vance ML, Evans WS, Thorner WO. Bromocriptine. *Ann Intern Med* 1984;100:78–91.
236. Cedarbaum JM, Schleifer LS. Drugs for Parkinson's disease, spasticity, and acute muscle spasma. In: Gilman AG, Rall TW, Wies AS, Taylor P, eds. *Goodman and Gilman's the pharmacological basis of therapeutics.* New York: Pergamon Press, 1990;474–475.
237. Berczi I, Nazy E, Asa SC, Kovacs K. Pituitary hormones and contact sensitivity in rats. *Allergy* 1983;38:325–330.
238. Berczi I, Nagy E, Asa SL, Kovacs K. The influence of pituitary hormones on adjuvant arthritis. *Arthritis Rheum* 1984;27:682–688.
239. Russell DH, Matrisian L, Kibler R, Larson DF, Poulos B, Magun BE. Prolactin receptors on human lymphocytes and their modulation by cyclosporine. *Biochem Biophys Res Commun* 1984;121: 899–906.
240. Russell DH, Kibler R, Matrisian L, Poulos B, Magun BE. Prolactin receptors on human T and B lymphocytes: antagonism of prolactin binding by cyclosporine. *J Immunol* 1985;134:3027–3031.
241. Russell DH, Larson DF. Prolactin induced polyamine biosynthesis in spleen and thymus: specific inhibition by cyclosporine. *Immunopharmacology* 1985;9:165–174.
242. Palestine AG, Muellenberg-Coulombre CB, Kim MK, Golato MC, Nussenblatt RB. Bromocriptine and low dose cyclosporine in the treatment of experimental autoimmune uveitis in rats. *J Clin Invest* 1987;79:1078–1081.
243. Hedner LP, Bynke G. Endogenous iridocyclitis relieved during treatment with bromocriptine. *Am J Ophthalmol* 1985;100:618–619.
244. Palestine AG, Nussenblatt RB. The effect of bromocriptine on anterior uveitis. *Am J Ophthalmol* 1988;106:488–489.
245. Lopatynsky MD, Krohel GB. Bromocriptine therapy for thyroid ophthalmology. *Am J Ophthalmol* 1989;107:680–681.
246. Kazeen KN, Zinkevich IV, Karaseva JI, Kostareva LN. Short-term results of parlodel treatment of patients with diffuse goiter complicated by endocrine ophthalmopathy. *Probl Endocrinol* 1987;33:3–5.
247. Kolodziej-Maciejewska H, Reterski Z. Positive effect of bromocriptine treatment in Graves' disease orbitopathy. *Exp Clin Endocrinol* 1985;86:241–242.

248. Frey WH, Nelson JD, Frick ML, Elde RP. Prolactin immunoreactivity in human tears and lacrimal gland: possible implications for tear production. In: Holly FJ, Lamberts DE, MacKenn DL, eds. *The periocular tear film in health, disease, and contact lens wear.* Lubbock, TX: Dry Eye Institute, Inc., 1986;798–807.
249. *American hospital formulary service drug information.* Bethesda, MD: Board of Directors of the American Society of Hospital Pharmacists, 1994;2431–2435.
250. First MR, Schroeder TJ, Weiskittel P, Myre SA, Alexander JW, Pesce AJ. Concomitant administration of cyclosporine and ketoconazole in renal transplant recipients. *Lancet* 1989;2:1198–1201.
251. Millikan LE, Schrum JP. Antifungal agents. In: Wolverton SE, Wilkin JK, eds. *Systemic drugs for skin diseases.* Philadelphia: W.B. Saunders, 1991;29–36.
252. Van Tyle JH. Ketoconazole. *Pharmacotherapy* 1984;4:343–373.
253. Gumbleton M, Brown JE, Hawksworth G, Whiting PH. The possible relationship between hepatic drug metabolism and ketoconazole enhancement of cyclosporine nephrotoxicity. *Transplantation* 1985;40:454–455.
254. Anderson JE, Morris RE, Blaschke TF. Pharmacodynamics of cyclosporine-ketoconazole interaction in mice. Combined therapy potentiates cyclosporine immunosuppression and toxicity. *Transplantation* 1987;43:529–533.
255. Daneshmend TK, Warnock EL, Turner A, Roberts CJ. Pharmacokinetics of ketoconazole in normal subjects. *J Antimicrob Chemother* 1981;8:299–304.
256. Huang YC, Colaizzi JL, Bierman RH, Woestenborghs R, Heykants J. Pharmacokinetics and dose proportionality of ketoconazole in normal volunteers. *Antimicrob Agents Chemother* 1986;30:206–210.
257. Heel RC, Brogden RN, Carmine A, Morley PA, Spright TM, Avery GS. Ketoconazole: a review of its therapeutic efficacy in superficial and systemic fungal infections. *Drugs* 1982;23:1–36.
258. NIAID Mycoses Study Group. Treatment of blastomycosis and histoplasmosis with ketoconazole. *Ann Intern Med* 1985;103:861–892.
259. Lewis JH, Zimmerman HJ, Benson GD, Ishak KG. Hepatic injury associated with ketoconazole therapy. Analysis of 33 cases. *Gastroenterology* 1984;86:502–513.
260. Insel PA. Analgesic-antipyretics and antiinflammatory agents: drugs employed in the treatment of rheumatoid arthritis and gout. In: Gilman AG, Rall TW, Nies AS, Taylor P, eds. *Goodman and Gilman's the pharmacological basis of therapeutics.* New York: Pergamon Press, 1990;674–676.
261. Davis LS. New uses for old drugs. In: Wilverton SE, Wilkin JK, eds. *Systemic drugs for skin diseases.* Philadelphia: W.B. Saunders, 1991;364–367.
262. Famary JP. Colchicine in therapy: state of the art and nonperspectives for an old drug. *Clin Exp Rheumatol* 1988;6:305–317.
263. Harper RM, Allen BS. Use of colchicine in the treatment of Behçet's disease. *Int J Dermatol* 1982;21:551–554.
264. Ehrenfeld M, Levy M, Bareli M, Gallily R, Eliakim M. Effect of colchicine on polymorphonuclear leukocyte chemotaxis in human volunteers. *Br J Clin Pharmacol* 1980;10:297–300.
265. Malawista SE. The action of colchicine in acute gouty arthritis. *Arthritis Rheum* 1975;19(suppl):835–846.
266. Pesanti EL, Ayline SG. Colchicine effects on lysosomal enzyme induction and intracellular degradation in the cultivated macrophage. *J Exp Med* 1975;141:1030–1046.
267. Sander HM, Randle HW. Use of colchicine in Behçet's syndrome. *Cutis* 1986;37:344–348.
268. Jorizzo JL, Hudson RD, Schmalstieg FC, et al. Behçet's syndrome: immune regulation, circulating immune complexes, neutrophil migration, and colchicine therapy. *J Am Acad Dermatol* 1984;10:205–214.
269. Gatot A, Tovi F. Colchicine therapy in recurrent oral ulcers [Letter]. *Arch Dermatol* 1984;120:994.
270. Ruah CB, Stram JR, Chasin WD. Treatment of several recurrent aphthous stomatitis with colchicine. *Arch Otolaryngol Head Neck Surg* 1988;114:671–675.
271. Frayha RA. Arthropathy of Behçet's disease with marked synovial pleocytosis responsive to colchicine. *Arthritis Rheum* 1982;25:235–236.
272. Hijikata K, Masuda K. Visual prognosis in Behçet's disease: effects of cyclophosphamide and colchicine. *Jpn J Ophthalmol* 1978; 22:506–519.
273. Mizushima Y, Matsumura N, Mori M, et al. Colchicine in Behçet's disease. *Lancet* 1977;2:1037.
274. Raynor A, Askari AD. Behçet's disease and treatment with colchicine. *M Am Acad Dermatol* 1980;2:396–450.
275. Ferreira NR, Buonicoti A. Trisomy after colchicine therapy. *Lancet* 1968;2:1304.

SECTION VI

Anesthesia

Section Editor: Martin A. Acquadro

OVERVIEW

In 1884, Dr. Karl Koller, an Austrian ophthalmologist, demonstrated that cocaine used as a local anesthetic facilitated eye surgery. Indeed, developments in anesthetic drugs and techniques have paralleled the developments in ophthalmology. Ophthalmologic surgeries are the most common surgeries performed in the elderly, and ophthalmic evaluations of and procedures performed on neonates and children, whether healthy or with a variety of syndromes, are now quite common.

Understanding broad pharmacodynamic and pharmacokinetic principles specific to perianesthetic medications improves our ability to optimize anesthetic and surgical plans for diverse patient populations. The first chapter of this section covers the pharmacology of commonly used anesthetic and perianesthetic medications. The focus is on the various classes of drugs and specific drugs commonly used in the various classes. The second chapter of this section focuses on common clinical anesthetic and pharmacologic considerations for ophthalmic surgery. The emphasis is on utilization of various pharmacodynamic properties of the commonly used anesthetic and perianesthetic drugs to optimize patient safety and surgical conditions in a variety of clinical situations.

Textbook of Ocular Pharmacology,
edited by T.J. Zimmerman, et al.
Lippincott–Raven Publishers, Philadelphia © 1997.

CHAPTER 63

Anesthetic and Perianesthetic Medications

Martin A. Acquadro

This chapter focuses on the pharmacology of commonly used anesthetic and perianesthetic medications. Chapter 64 focuses on common clinical anesthetic and pharmacologic considerations for ophthalmic surgery.

PREMEDICATION GOALS

The goals of premedication of patients may include their diminished anxiety, reduced pain, stability of cardiopulmonary function, and diminished gastric volume and acidity (1). Decisions regarding premedication are based on history and physical examination of the patient; nature of the planned surgery; planned anesthetic; timing of the procedure; preferences of the anesthesiologist, surgeon, and patient; and patient safety. The preoperative interview, with a thorough explanation of technique, medications, and monitoring, is extremely important in establishing rapport with obtaining the confidence of the patient. Egbert et al. (2) demonstrated that a preoperative visit by the anesthesiologist was more effective in diminishing fear and anxiety in patients than was premedication alone without visitation and provided the level of comfort experienced by patients who received both a visit and premedication. Some of the common perianesthetic medications discussed in this chapter and used in ophthalmic surgery are reviewed in Table 1.

MEDICATIONS

Benzodiazepines

Anxiolytics are frequently administered to patients in the preoperative period, and benzodiazepines (BZDs) as a class are most frequently prescribed. The most common are lorazepam (LZP, Ativan) (Fig. 1A), alprazolam (Xanax) (Fig. 1B), clonazepam (CZP, Klonopin) (Fig. 1C), diazepam (DZP, Valium) (Fig. 1D), and midazolam (Versed) (Fig. 1E). The BZDs are not commonly associated with nausea and vomiting, are easy to dose and administer, provide the greatest anxiolytic effect at a dose not commonly associated with cardiopulmonary depression, and can offer variable amounts of amnesia, depending on dose and time. They are effective in raising the threshold for CNS toxicity of local anesthetics, and DZP has been used in treatment of status epilepticus and as a muscle relaxant (3–5). All these medications can be administered orally or parenterally, but midazolam is not available in pill form; the solvent used in parenteral preparations of DZP is painful when injected intramuscularly or intravenously and can result in phlebitis, and LZP and DZP are more likely to have cumulative effects if administered repeatedly (4,5). Midazolam has become a very popular anxiolytic due to its water solubility, rapid onset, short duration of action, and predictable response over a given dose range. It can be administered intramuscularly and intravenously (5). In children, midazolam can also be administered intranasally or be mixed with a chilled sweet syrup base and administered orally.

The anxiolytic BZDs, at higher dosages, can also be used for induction of general anesthesia to take advantage of their amnestic and induction qualities. DZP, and particularly midazolam, do not cause as much cardiovascular depression as the common induction agents, barbiturates, and the propylphenol propofol.

The BZDs share similar pharmacokinetics with regard to metabolism and excretion. In general, they are metabolized by the liver and excreted by the kidneys. One-third of the metabolite of DZP is oxazepam, which explains some of the apparent cumulative effects of DZP (4–8).

Barbiturates

Barbiturates are classified as hypnotic agents. They have no analgesic action and indeed may cause hyperalgesia.

M. A. Acquadro: Department of Anesthesia, Massachusetts Eye and Ear Infirmary, Boston, Massachusetts 02114.

TABLE 63-1. *Perianesthetic medications commonly used in ophthalmic surgery*

Anxiolytics		
Diazepam (Fig. 1D)		
0.03–0.1 mg/kg i.v.	Sedation, amnesia	
0.05–0.15 mg/kg p.o.	Raises CNS threshold	
Midazolam (Fig. 1E)		
0.03–0.07 mg/kg i.v.	Sedation, amnesia	
Hypnotics		
Etomidate (Fig. 3B)		
0.3 mg/kg i.v.	Induction for GA	
Pentobarbital (Fig. 2A)		
100–200 mg p.o.	Aid for sleep	
Propofol (Fig. 3A)		
0.5 mg/kg i.v.	Amnesia, sedation	
1.0–2.5 mg/kg i.v.	Induction for GA	
Secobarbital (Fig. 2D)		
100–200 mg/kg p.o.	Aid to sleep	
Thiopental (Fig. 2B)		
0.3–0.6 mg/kg i.v.	Amnesia, sedation	
2–5 mg/kg i.v.	Induction for GA	
Narcotics		
Alfentanil (Fig. 4C)		
0.15–0.3 mg i.v.	Duration 20 min	Equianalgesic to morphine 1–2 mg i.v.
Fentanyl (Fig. 4B)		
0.1 mg/kg i.m.	Duration 1–2 hr	Equianalgesic to morphine 10 mg i.m.
Meperidine (Fig. 4E)		
75 mg i.m.	Duration 3–5 hr	Equianalgesic to morphine 10 mg i.m.
Morphine (Fig. 4A)		
1–2 mg i.v.	Duration 90 min	
10 mg i.m.	Duration 4–5 hr	
Sufentanil		
0.005–0.01 mg i.v.	Duration 15 min	Equianalgesic to morphine 1–2 mg i.v.

Most commonly, barbiturates are used for three purposes. Barbiturates are used as hypnotic induction agents for general anesthesia; patients become apneic and unable to protect their own airway. At lower dosages, barbiturates are also used as a hypnotic agent, producing amnesia for uncomfortable or anxiety-provoking ophthalmic procedures such as intraconal (retrobulbar) or periconal (peribulbar or periocular) local anesthetic eye blocks, when patients do not require support or protection of their airway. Medications often used for these two purposes include sodium

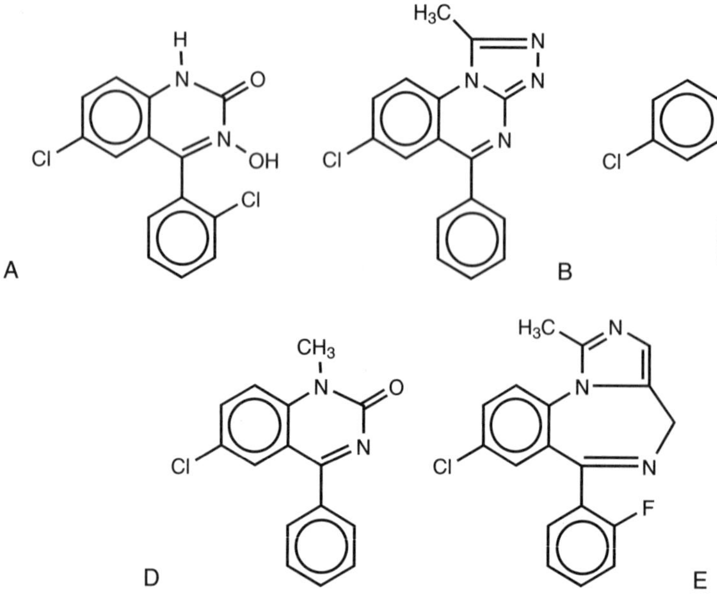

FIG. 63-1.A: Structural formula of lorazepam. **B:** Structural formula of alprazolam. **C:** Structural formula of clonazepam. **D:** Structural formula of diazepam. **E:** Structural formula of midazolam hydrochloride.

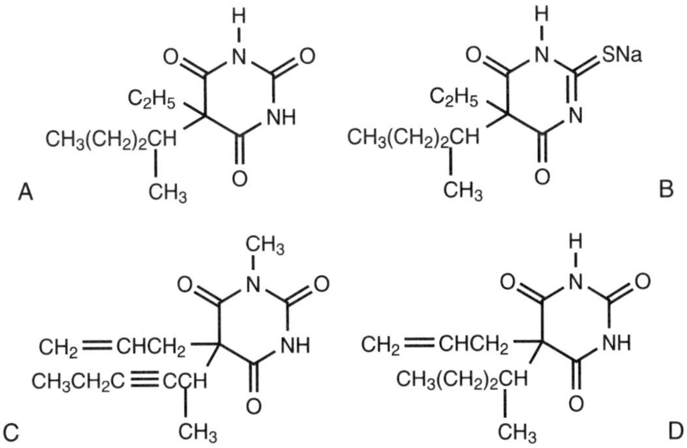

FIG. 63-2.A: Structural formula of pentobarbital sodium. **B:** Structural formula of thiopental sodium. **C:** Structural formula of methohexital sodium. **D:** Structural formula of secobarbital sodium.

pentobarbital (Fig. 2A), sodium thiopental (Fig. 2B), and sodium methohexital (Brevital) (Fig. 2C). A third common purpose of barbiturates is to aid in sleep, particularly on the night before an operation. Pentobarbital or secobarbital (Fig. 2D) in a dose of 100 to 200 mg orally at bedtime is effective. Another common and widely used hypnotic, propofol (Diprivan) (Fig. 3A), is also used as an induction agent for general anesthesia and as an amnestic during local anesthetic blocks. Propofol is also used as a maintenance agent for general anesthesia and as a sedative during conscious sedation for surgery. Propofol is a propylphenol, not a barbiturate. It rarely produces nausea and vomiting, and has antiemetic properties when used in a continuous infusion during pediatric strabismus surgery and, possibly, during adult strabismus surgery (9,10). Sulfur allergy is a contraindication to sodium thiopental. The thiobarbiturate has also been involved in the development of Stevens-Johnson syndrome and erythema multiforme and can precipitate an attack of acute intermittent porphyria. Egg allergy is a contraindication to the use of propofol, as it is maintained in an egg protein emulsification.

The common barbiturates and propofol are cardiovascular depressants, and careful titration in the elderly and in patients with cardiovascular compromise is critical. Barbiturates at low doses causes release of endogenous γ-aminobutyric acid (GABA), but mimics GABA at higher dosages and cause profound CNS depression.

Etomidate (Amidate) (Fig. 3B) is an induction agent for general anesthesia with minimal cardiovascular effects, and is the agent of choice in patients with cardiovascular compromise. Associated nausea and vomiting are rare, and cardiopulmonary depression is minimal. Propofol and etomidate are painful when injected intravenously; prior administration of intravenous lidocaine can diminish the pain along the injected vein. Because propofol has been reported to support rapid microbial growth, it requires aseptic handling and prompt use. Opened, unused propofol should be discarded after 6 hours.

Patients who habitually use barbiturates or alcohol may show tolerance to barbiturates. Induction of hepatic enzymes is associated with barbiturate use, and rapid eye movement (REM) sleep is more likely to be impaired with barbiturates than with benzodiazepines (4–8).

Narcotics

Commonly used narcotics include morphine (Fig. 4A), fentanyl (Fig. 4B), alfentanil (Fig. 4C), and sufentanil (Fig. 4D). A narcotic and nitrous oxide technique is used for general anesthesia but, particularly with morphine, the technique does not always result in complete amnesia. Often an additional drug, such as the inhalation agent propofol or midazolam, will be added. Muscle relaxants are commonly added, because movement is more likely to occur during narcotic nitrous-oxide sedation than during sedation with an inhalation technique. Opioids are associated with analgesia, respiratory depression, mild decreases in

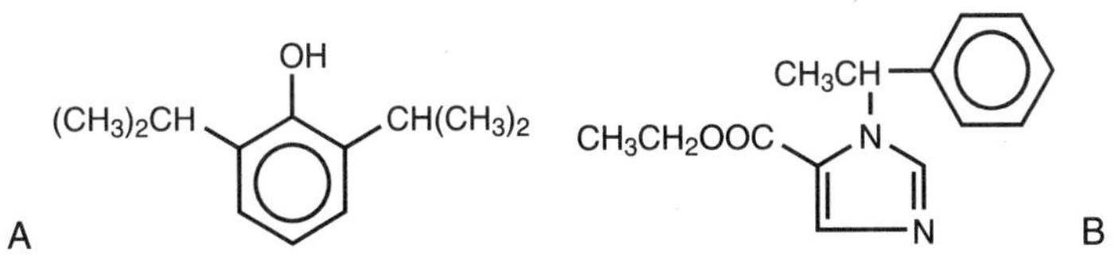

FIG. 63-3.A: Structural formula of propofol. **B:** Structural formula of etomidate.

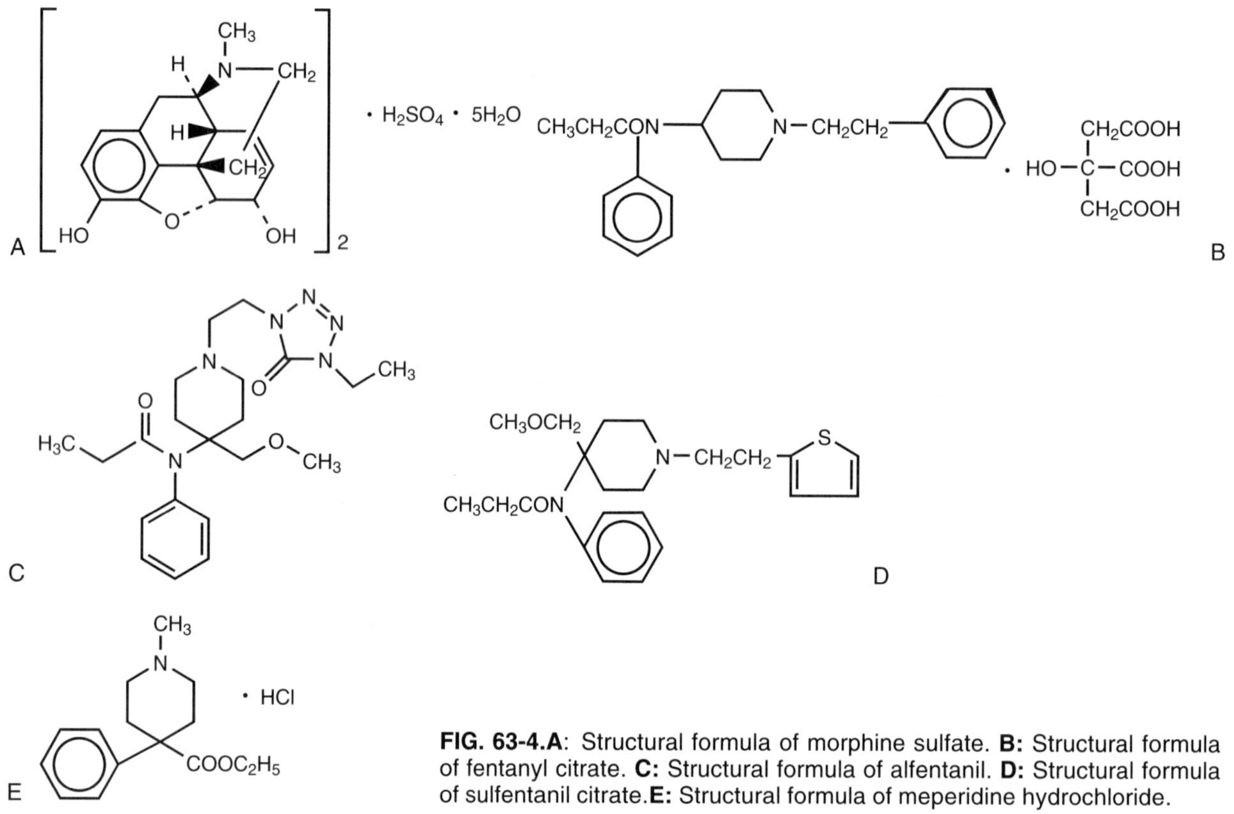

FIG. 63-4.A: Structural formula of morphine sulfate. B: Structural formula of fentanyl citrate. C: Structural formula of alfentanil. D: Structural formula of sulfentanil citrate. E: Structural formula of meperidine hydrochloride.

blood pressure (BP), some delay in emergence, and nausea and vomiting. In ophthalmic general anesthesia, narcotics more often are administered intravenously as supplementation to an inhalation technique, resulting in improved hemodynamic stability, less halogenated agent required intraoperatively, smoother emergence, and less postoperative pain. The patient's respiratory muscles may become rigid during induction of anesthesia with large doses of narcotics, and muscle relaxants may be needed to permit ventilation by the anesthesiologist. Fentanyl has an onset of action in one circulation time, is rapidly redistributed, and has a duration of action of about 30 minutes. However, with large doses, drug can accumulate. Fentanyl is metabolized by the liver and has an elimination half-life ($t_{\frac{1}{2}}$) of 3.5 hours. Alfentanil has one-third to one-fourth the potency of fentanyl, and its duration of action two-thirds shorter. Sufentanil has a potency approximately 10 times that of fentanyl and a duration of action one-half that of fentanyl (4).

Inhalation Anesthetics

The common inhalation anesthetics in wide use are halothane (Fig. 5A), ethrane (Fig. 5B), isoflurane (Fig. 5C), desflurane (Fig. 5D), and nitrous oxide (Fig. 6). The first four are halogenated anesthetics. Nitrous oxide is an inorganic compound.

In general, the halogenated inhalation anesthetics are introduced as maintenance anesthetics after induction with an intravenous agent such as thiopental, propofol, etomidate, or midazolam. In most elective pediatric general anesthesia, however, an intravenous line is started after inhalation induction of general anesthesia with nitrous oxide and halothane. Nitrous oxide is odorless, and halothane is the least irritating of the halogenated anesthetics described herein.

All the halogenated anesthetics cause a dose-related decrease in arterial BP; negative inotropy of the heart; bronchodilation; blunting of hypoxic pulmonary vasoconstriction; reduction of the central respiratory control center

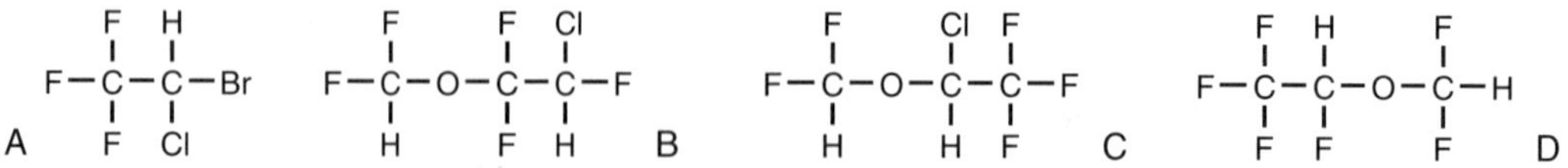

FIG. 63-5.A: Structural formula of halothane. B: Structural formula of enflurane. C: Structural formula of isoflurane. D: Structural formula of desflurane.

N≡N=O

FIG. 63-6. Structural formula of nitrous oxide.

response to carbon dioxide; increase in cerebral blood flow; reductions in renal, splanchnic, and hepatic blood flows; and relaxation of skeletal muscle. Halothane differs from other halogenated agents in that it sensitizes the myocardium more to endogenous and exogenous catecholamines and thus is more likely to induce cardiac arrhythmias. Among the halogenated agents, ethrane, at higher concentrations and during general anesthesia, is most likely to cause seizure activity. With isoflurane, cerebral blood flow is increased slightly, while cerebral metabolism is reduced to a degree only slightly less than that caused by halothane. The cerebral circulation remains responsive to carbon dioxide, and cerebral blood flow, metabolism, and intracranial pressure are reduced by isoflurane and hypocarbia, which makes isoflurane the agent of choice for many neurosurgical procedures.

The hepatic metabolism rates of the halogenated anesthetics are as follows: halothane, 20%; ethrane, 2%; isoflurane, 0.2%; and desflurane, 0.02%. The greatest amount of fluoride ion is released through the kidneys (4). Nitrous oxide can cause predictable surgical anesthesia as a sole agent only when administered under hyperbaric conditions or when given in excess of 80% in oxygen, with the obvious resultant concern regarding hypoxic conditions. Nitrous oxide is of value as an adjuvant to narcotic, hypnotic, anxiolytic, and halogenated agents. Synergism exists between nitrous oxide and other anesthetic agents, allowing a lower required concentration of the associated anesthetic; therefore, unwanted side effects and complications caused by the other agents are fewer. Nitrous oxide is 34 times more soluble than nitrogen in blood, which results in expanding pockets of trapped gas in occluded middle ears, pneumothorax, loops of bowels, lungs, renal cysts, occluded sinuses, and intraocular gas. Because nitrous oxide leaves the blood and enters the alveoli rapidly at the conclusion of anesthesia, one must be careful to minimize or prevent the occurrence of diluted amounts of oxygen in the alveoli by administering 100% oxygen for at least 10 minutes after discontinuing the administration of nitrous oxide (4).

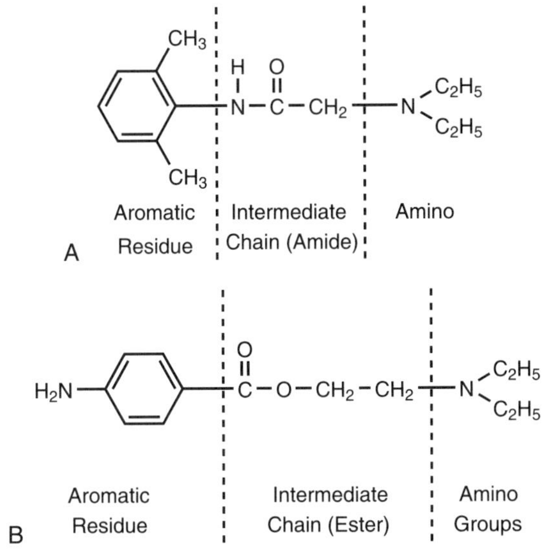

CH_3 H O N–C–CH_2–N C_2H_5 C_2H_5 CH_3

Aromatic Residue | Intermediate Chain (Amide) | Amino

A

H_2N– O C–O–CH_2–CH_2–N C_2H_5 C_2H_5

Aromatic Residue | Intermediate Chain (Ester) | Amino Groups

B

FIG. 63-7.A: Structural formula of lidocaine. **B:** Structural formula of procaine.

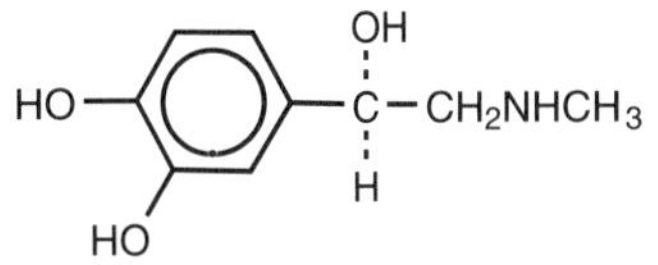

OH HO– C–CH_2NHCH_3 H HO

FIG. 63-8. Structural formula of epinephrine.

Local Anesthetics

Local anesthetics can cause reversible conduction block of sensory and motor nerves. They are chemically classified by their amide (Fig. 7A) or ester (Fig. 7B) link, and this link contributes to their potency. When local anesthetic molecules are deposited near nerve tissue, some of the molecules are removed by the circulation, this process can be reduced slightly by addition of the vasoconstrictor epinephrine (Fig. 8). The anesthetics bind to tissue, ester anesthetics undergo local and systemic hydrolysis by plasma cholinesterase enzymes, and amide anesthetics are metabolized by the liver. The remaining molecules penetrate the nerve sheath. After equilibrium is established in the nerve membrane, depending on the lipophilia of base and cation species, sodium channels are prevented from opening by inhibition of conformational changes that occur with channel activation. The rates and onset of recovery from block are governed by the slow diffusion of local anesthetic molecules in and out of the nerve, not by the much faster binding and dissociation from ionic channels.

Toxicity is related to dosage, method, and site of administration. Unintentional vascular or optic nerve sheath spread to the CNS can result in cardiopulmonary collapse or grand mal seizure. How avidly a drug exhibits tissue and protein binding determines such issues as the volume of distribution of a drug; how much free drug, as opposed to bound drug, is available in circulation; and how long a drug will remain at a receptor site of action, or remain bound to tissue—such as cardiac tissue—and cause prolonged unwanted toxic side effects.

REFERENCES

1. Dripps RD, Eckenhoff JE, Vandam LD. Premedication, transport to the operating room, and preparation for anesthesia. In: Dripps RD, Eckenhoff JE, Vandam LD, eds. *Introduction to anesthesia: the prin-*

ciples of safe practice, 6th ed. Philadelphia: WB Saunders, 1983; 34–44.

2. Egbert LD, Battit GE, Turndorf H, Beecher HK. The value of the preoperative visit by an anesthetist. *JAMA* 1963;185:553–555.
3. De Jong RH, Hebner JE. Diazepam- and lidocaine-induced cardiovascular changes. *Anesthesiology* 1973;39:633–638.
4. Longnecker DE, Marshall BE. General anesthetics. In: Gilman AG, Rall TW, Nies AS, et al., eds. *The pharmacological basis of therapeutics,* 8th ed. New York: Pergamon Press, 1990;285–310.
5. Rall TW. Hypnotics and sedatives; ethanol. In: Gilman AG, Rall TW, Nies AS, et al., eds. *The pharmacological basis of therapeutics,* 8th ed. New York: Pergamon Press, 1990;345–382.
6. Kofke WA, Firestone LL. Commonly used drugs. In: Firestone LL, Lebowitz PW, Cooke, CE, et al., eds. *Clinical anesthesia procedures of the Massachusetts General Hospital,* 3rd ed. Boston: Little, Brown, 1988;590–650.
7. Blazier K. Pain. In: Davison JK, Eckhardt III WF, Perese DA, eds. *Clinical anesthesia procedures of the Massachusetts General Hospital,* 4th ed. Boston: Little, Brown, 1993;582–600.
8. Leong R. Commonly used drugs. In: Davison JK, Eckhardt III WF, Perese DA, eds. *Clinical anesthesia procedures of the Massachusetts General Hospital,* 4th ed. Boston: Little, Brown, 1993;603–651.
9. Weir PM, Munro HM, Reynolds PI, Lewis IH, Wilton NCT. Propofol infusion and the incidence of emesis in pediatric outpatient strabismus surgery. *Anesth Analg* 1993;76:760–764.
10. Ward JB, Niffenegger AS, Lavin CW, et al. The use of propofol and mivacurium anesthetic technique for the immediate post-operative adjustment of sutures in strabismus surgery. *Ophthalmology* 1995; 102:122–128.
11. Ritchie JM, Greene NM. Local anesthetics. In: Gilman AG, Rall TW, Nies AS, et al., eds. *The pharmacological basis of therapeutics,* 8th ed. New York: Pergamon Press, 1990;311–331.

Textbook of Ocular Pharmacology,
edited by T.J. Zimmerman, et al.
Lippincott–Raven Publishers, Philadelphia © 1997.

CHAPTER 64

Anesthetic Considerations for Ophthalmic Surgery

Martin A. Acquadro

PERIOPERATIVE EVALUATION

Patients of various ages, health, and circumstances present for ophthalmic surgery. Preoperative optimization of patient health and proper choices of anesthetic technique and medications contribute greatly to a successful surgical outcome. Ophthalmic surgical patients are often at the extremes of age, at which stages contributing factors of prematurity or advanced age in otherwise healthy persons may include reduced or altered organ system function. Many adult patients present with a variety of systemic diseases, including coronary artery disease, hypertension, diabetes, chronic obstructive pulmonary disease (COPD), liver and kidney disease, and dementia. Preoperative evaluation must be individualized to include the patient's age and health status; history and physical examination; other specialty consultants' opinions regarding baseline health optimization; pertinent laboratory data; the patient's ability to understand language, and ability to communicate; the patient's emotional status; the level of cooperation; the nature of the planned surgery; and the surgeon's requirements and preferences (1). Patients often present with a variety of congenital syndromes, which may complicate a mask airway, placement of an endotracheal tube, or proper hemodynamic management in the setting of abnormal cardiac and vascular disease. A preoperative consultation between the patient and the surgeon well in advance of the scheduled surgery can make the experience a safe and comforting one for all parties involved.

Many ophthalmic procedures can be performed with local anesthesia and sedation. Clinicians must ascertain the experiences of the patient with previous anesthetic agents. The preoperative interview, with a thorough explanation of technique, medications, and monitoring provided to the patient, is extremely important in establishing rapport with and obtaining the confidence of the patient. A study performed by Egbert et al. (2) demonstrated that a preoperative visit by the anesthesiologist was more effective in diminishing patients' fear and anxiety than was premedication alone without visitation, and approached the level of comfort achieved by patients who received both a visit and premedication. Some of the common perianesthetic medications discussed in this chapter and used in ophthalmic surgery are reviewed in Table 1. Patients with hearing aids and dentures benefit from being allowed to retain them when undergoing local anesthesia with sedation. Most medication regimens should not be interrupted; this continuation of medication is part of patient preparation and optimization of baseline health status until the time surgery is performed.

Otherwise completely healthy children with resolving uncomplicated viral upper respiratory infections who do not have a history of other chronic respiratory diseases can often undergo a brief period of general anesthesia with face mask. However, clinical evaluation, interview of the patient and family, physical examination, full knowledge of the contemplated surgery, needs of the surgeon, and overall perioperative safety for the child must be evaluated by an anesthesiologist. Antisialogogues agents that counteract the flow of saliva, can be very helpful in ensuring children's safety during surgery.

GENERAL CLINICAL CONSIDERATIONS FOR OPHTHALMIC SURGERY

Intraocular Pressure (IOP)

Most CNS depressants reduce IOP. These medications include narcotics, barbiturates, neuroleptics, and anxiolyt-

M. A. Acquadro: Department of Anesthesia, Massachusetts Eye and Ear Infirmary, Boston, Massachusetts 02114.

TABLE 64-1. *Perianesthetic medications commonly used for ophthalmic surgery*

Medication and dose		Effects
Antiemetic agents		
Droperidol (Fig. 25)	0.625–2.5 mg i.v.	May prolong sedation; can reduce BP
Metoclopramide (Fig. 23)	0.15 mg/kg i.v.	
Ondansetron (Fig. 24)	4–8 mg i.v.	
Anticholinergic agents		
Atropine (Fig. 2)	0.4–1.2 mg i.v./i.m.	Can cause tachycardia; can cross CNS
Glycopyrolate (Fig. 30)	0.1–0.2 mg i.v./i.m.	Causes less dysrhythmia; does not cross CNS
Scopolamine (Fig. 4)	0.3–0.6 mg i.v./i.m.	Produces more CNS effects; best antisialogogue
H2 Antagonists		
Cimetidine (Fig. 31)	300 mg i.v./i.m./p.o. every 6 hr	Prolongs effects of some medications; can cause confusion
Ranitidine (Fig. 22)	50 mg i.v. every 6–8 hr 150 mg p.o. every 12 hr	

BP, blood pressure, i.v., intravenously; i.m. intramuscularly; p.o., orally.

ics. Inhalation anesthetics reduce IOP in a dose-related fashion (3,4). Several mechanisms of action have been proposed, including depression of the diencephalon, reduced aqueous humor production, increased outflow of aqueous humor, and relaxation of extraocular muscles (3,5,6). Ketamine (Fig. 1) probably reduces or has minimal effect on IOP. However, ketamine is often unsuitable for many types of ophthalmic surgery because it causes nystagmus and blepharospasm (3,7).

Although topical atropine (Fig. 2) is contraindicated in patients with glaucoma, systemic atropine administered in the usual clinical anesthetic dosages has no effect on IOP in either open- or closed-angle glaucoma and is safe for use in patients with glaucoma (6,8).

Hypothermia, hyperventilation (respiratory alkalosis), and metabolic acidosis reduce IOP, whereas hypoventilation (respiratory acidosis) and an increase in carbon dioxide beyond a normal physiologic range, metabolic alkalosis, and hypoxia increase it (3). Trimethonium, despite producing mydriasis, reduces IOP. Other ganglionic blockers, hypertonic solutions, carbonic anhydrous inhibitors, and nondepolarizing neuromuscular blockers reduce IOP. Succinylcholine (Fig. 3), a depolarizing muscle relaxant, increases IOP. Succinylcholine is contraindicated for first time use after an eye has been opened or as a neuromuscular relaxant for intubation without adequate pretreatment, such as intravenous narcotic or lipocaine given prior to the administration of succinylcholine and intubation.

Anesthetic Effects of Ophthalmic Medications

Topical Medications

Many ophthalmic drugs administered topically, systemically, and intraocularly have effects on anesthetic management. Topical medications are slowly absorbed from the conjunctival sac, but are absorbed more rapidly from mucosal surfaces, such as the nasolacrimal duct. Digital pressure over the nasolacrimal duct for 5 minutes can reduce absorption by 67% (9). Gentle closure of the eye can reduce absorption by 65% (10). An overdose of certain topical or systemic eye medications produces adverse effects (AE) in the pediatric and geriatric populations and in patients with myodystrophia or cardiovascular disease.

Atropine administered topically often produces systemic reactions in the pediatric and elderly populations, including tachycardia, flushing, dry mouth and thirst, increase in body temperature, and agitation (in the elderly). Scopolamine (Fig. 4) has a greater propensity to produce CNS excitation and disorientation. Cyclopentolate (Fig. 5) may produce CNS toxicity. Echothiophate iodide (Fig. 6) is a long-acting anticholinesterase that can prolong the actions of ester anesthetics and succinylcholine, which are metabolized by plasma pseudocholinesterase. Effects of echothiophate iodide can last 4 to 6 weeks. Epinephrine (Fig. 7), phenylephrine (Fig. 8), and cocaine (Fig. 9) can cause hypertension, arrhythmias, nervousness, and agitation. Co-

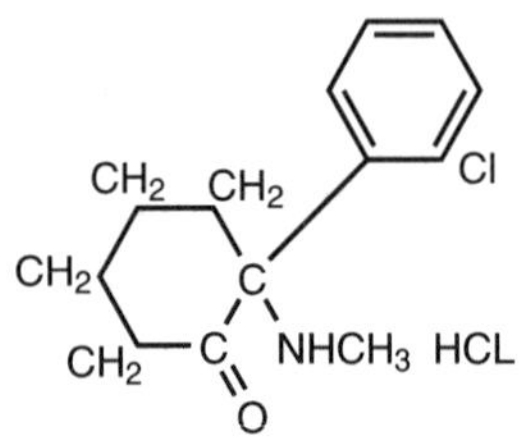

FIG. 64-1. Structural formula of ketamine hydrochloride.

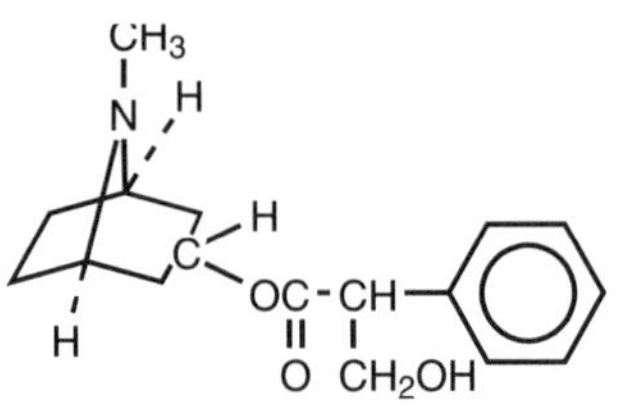

FIG. 64-2. Structural formula of atropine sulfate.

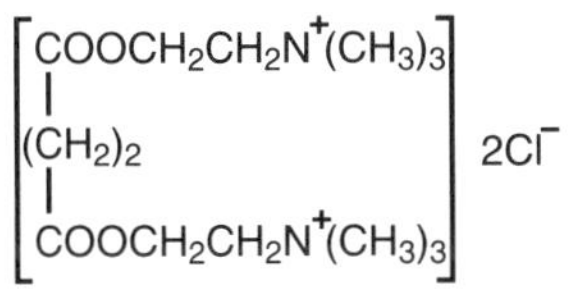

FIG. 64-3. Structural formula of succinylcholine chloride.

caine can also cause a paradoxic coronary vasoconstriction in face of increased myocardial oxygen demand. Timolol (Fig. 10) is a nonselective β-blocker that can have profound effects on patients who have active asthma or who are hypoglycemic. Acetylcholine (ACh) (Fig. 11) can trigger bronchospasm, hypotension, and bradycardia. Patients receiving fluorescein (Fig. 12) may experience nausea, urticaria, respiratory complications involving edema, anaphylactic shock, and myocardial infarction. Several possible mechanisms of action of these agents have been suggested, but none is definitely known (10).

Intraocular Gas

Stinson and Donlon (11) demonstrated that 1 ml air in the presence of 70% nitrous oxide will expand in volume to 2.85 ml in 1 hour because nitrous oxide is 34 times more soluble in blood than nitrogen, which is 79% of air. Sulfur hexafluoride (Fig. 13) is more poorly diffusible, and the volume increase is more impressive, since nitrous oxide is 117 times more diffusible than SF6. Stinson and Donlon (11) have recommended that nitrous oxide be terminated at least 20 minutes before the injection of gas to prevent significant changes in the size of the intravitreous gas bubble (11,12). Furthermore, if reoperation under general anesthesia is necessary, use of nitrous oxide should be avoided for 5 days after placement of an air bubble and for 10 days after placement of sulfur hexafluoride (10). Indeed, Wolf et al. (13) showed that SF6 gas bubbles persist for at least 10 days. Newer intravitreal gases persist as long as 21 to 28 days (12). Octafluorocyclobutane (Fig. 14) has been shown to persist more than 13 days, and perfluoropropane (Fig. 15) has been shown to persist longer than 30 days (10). Use of nitrous oxide should be avoided in any patient who undergoes reoperation within 3 to 4 weeks of intravitreal gas injection (12).

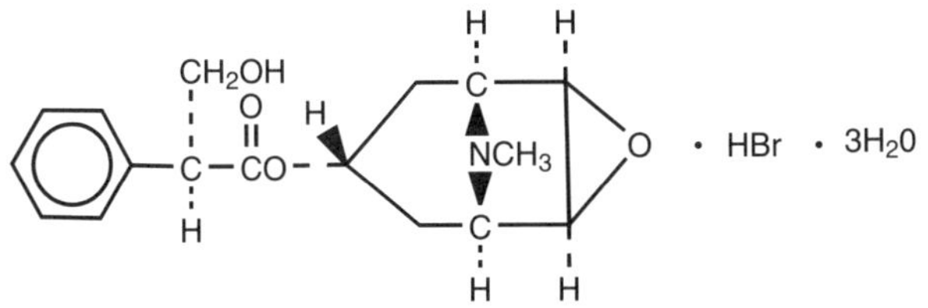

FIG. 64-4. Structural formula of scopolamine hydrobromide.

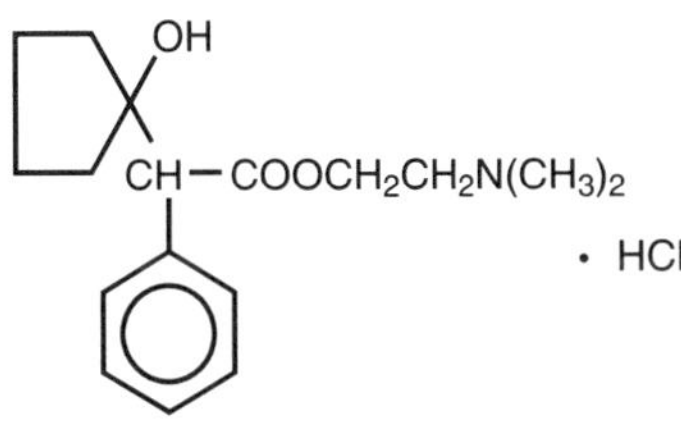

FIG. 64-5. Structural formula of cyclopentolate hydrochloride.

Systemic Medications

Commonly, hypertonic solutions are administered to reduce IOP. Mannitol (Fig. 16) is administered intravenously, has onset in 5 to 10 minutes, shows peak clinical effects in 30 to 45 minutes, and its effects last 5 to 6 hours. Mannitol should be warmed and should be administered through a filter to avoid administration of crystal. Electrolyte abnormalities, particularly hypokalemia, can be made worse. There is the risk of transient hypertension or congestive heart failure caused by rapid expansion of intravascular volume, of myocardial ischemia in patients with poor ventricular function, and of eventual hypotension resulting from rapid diuresis and hypovolemia. Acetazolamide (Fig. 17) is a carbonic anhydrous inhibitor which acts in 5 minutes and has its maximum effect in 20 to 30 minutes. However, administered chronically, it also affects the kidney, with bicarbonate diuresis and large losses of water, potassium, and sodium. Because acetazolamide is a sulfonamide derivative, it may cause allergic reactions, erythema multiforme, Stevens-Johnson syndrome, toxic epidermal necrolysis, and bone marrow depression (10).

SPECIFIC CLINICAL CONSIDERATIONS FOR EYE SURGERY

Local Anesthetic Agents and Complications

Local anesthetic agents are administered either intraconally (retrobulbar) or periconally (peribulbar or periorbital). Pharmacologic complications relate to the amount of anesthetic agent delivered, the amount absorbed intravascularly and its effect on the CNS and the cardiovascular system, and to whether there is direct spread of local anesthetic agent within the optic nerve sheath centrally to

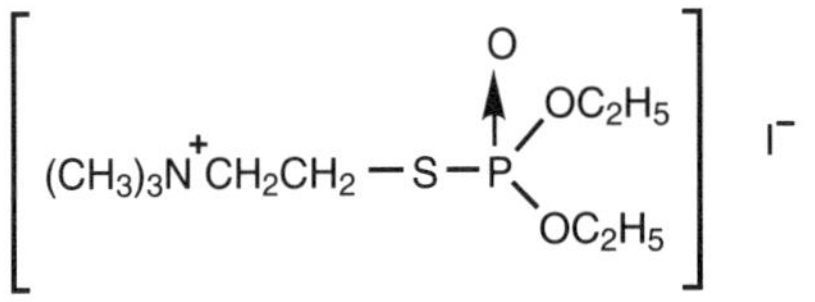

FIG. 64-6. Structural formula of echothiopate iodide.

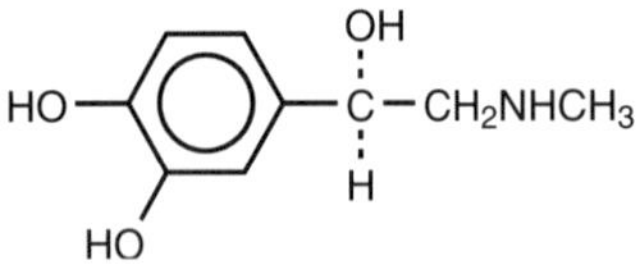

FIG. 64-7. Structural formula of epinephrine.

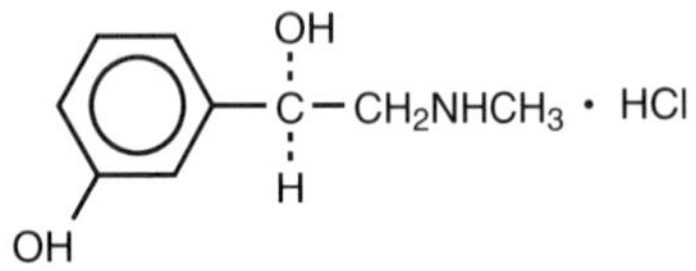

FIG. 64-8. Structural formula of phenylephrine hydrochloride.

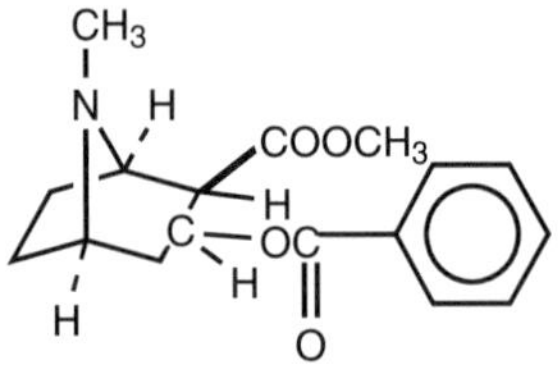

FIG. 64-9. Structural formula of cocaine hydrochloride.

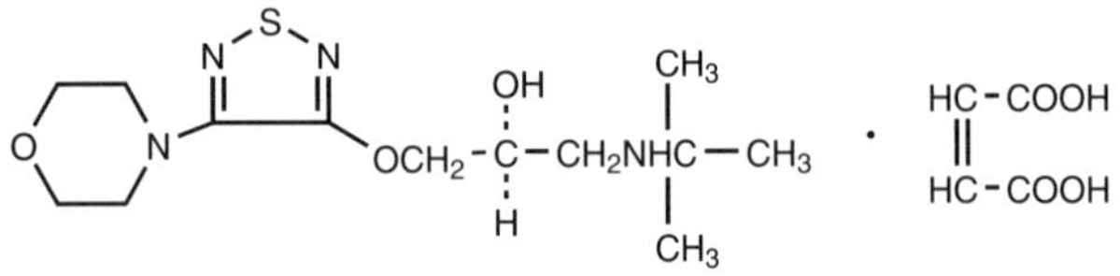

FIG. 64-10. Structural formula of timolol maleate.

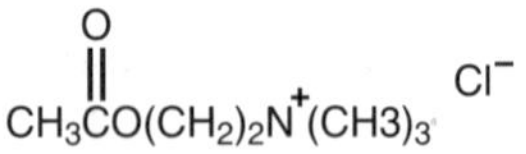

$CH_3CO(CH_2)_2N^+(CH_3)_3\ Cl^-$

FIG. 64-11. Structural formula of acetylcholine chloride.

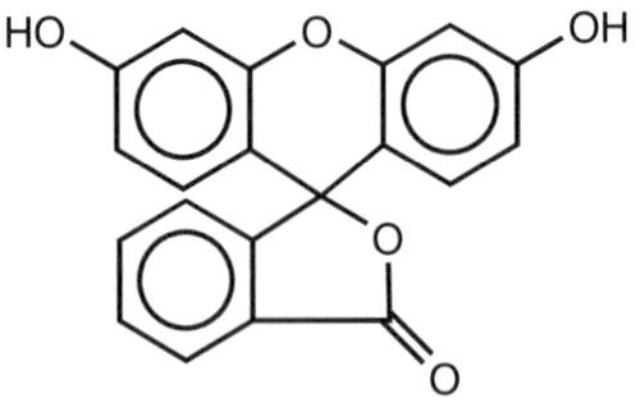

FIG. 64-12. Structural formula of fluorescein.

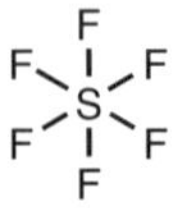

FIG. 64-13. Structural formula of sulfur hexafluoride.

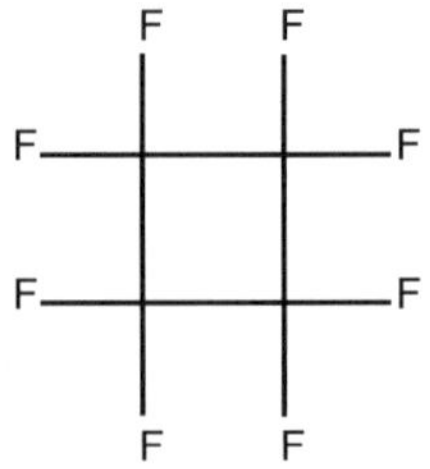

FIG. 64-14. Structural formula of octafluorocyclobutane.

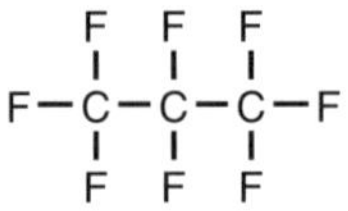

FIG. 64-15. Structural formula of perfluoropropane.

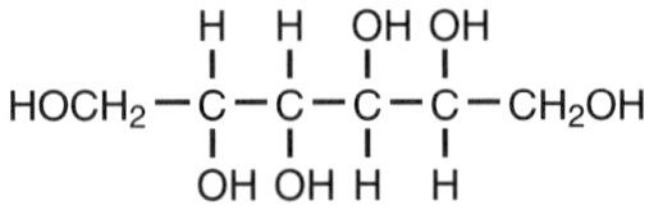

FIG. 64-16. Structural formula of mannitol.

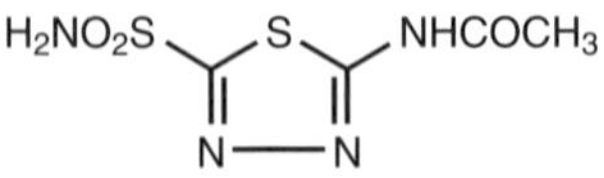

FIG. 64-17. Structural formula of acetazolamide sodium.

the brainstem. Liver disease or poor quality or quantity of plasma pseudocholinesterase may prolong the effect of ester anesthetics. Amides are metabolized directly by the liver. Central spread of anesthetic should be suspected if there is any sign of mental confusion, shivering bordering on convulsant behavior, nausea or vomiting, signs of extraocular paresis or amaurosis of the contralateral eye, dysphagia, sudden fluctuations in cardiovascular vital signs, and dyspnea or respiratory depression. Central spread tends to occur more frequently with intraconal administration, particularly with use of the more traditional Atkinson technique in which, during the inferior orbital injection, the patient looks upward and inward, thereby placing the optic nerve sheath and its vascular and neural contents more in the path of the advancing needle. However, CNS toxicity can also be produced by intravascular absorption. Signs can include drowsiness, personality changes, headache, tinnitus, tingling in the lips and tongue, muscle tremors, or convulsions. The amount of local anesthetic in the blood and available to produce CNS system toxicity depends on site of injection, amount of anesthetic injected, whether or not a vasoconstrictor is used, nature of the particular anesthetic, metabolism of the anesthetic, and degree of ventilation. Hypercarbia resulting from too much sedation can promote CNS toxicity of a local anesthetic. Toxicity of the CNS ranges from excitation to convulsions and is most likely the result of depression of inhibitory or modulatory regions and tracts rather than excitation of the CNS. One must be mindful of the amounts of anesthetic agents administered, particularly when more than one local anesthetic is injected simultaneously. Plasma levels that result in CNS toxicity are 5 to 10 μg/ml for lidocaine (Fig. 18) and 1.5 to 4 μg/ml for bupivicaine (Fig. 19). The plasma concentration of local anesthetic agent that produces CNS toxicity is lower than that which produces cardiac toxicity. However, the difference between plasma levels that produce CNS toxicity and cardiac toxicity is smaller for bupivicaine than lidocaine. It is important to use a minimal concentration of local anesthetic agent, to add the vasoconstrictor epinephrine when possible, to avoid intravascular or optic nerve sheath injections, and not to exceed the toxic level of the anesthetic agent. Maximal dosages of lidocaine injected for a regional technique such as an ophthalmic block are 4 mg/kg or 7 mg/kg with epinephrine; for bupivacaine, the maximal dosage is 2 mg/kg without epinephrine or 3 mg/kg with epinephrine (14).

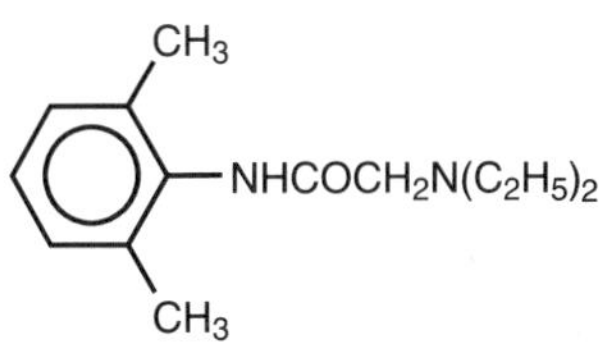

CH_3 / $NHCOCH_2N(C_2H_5)_2$ / CH_3

FIG. 64-18. Structural formula of lidocaine hydrochloride.

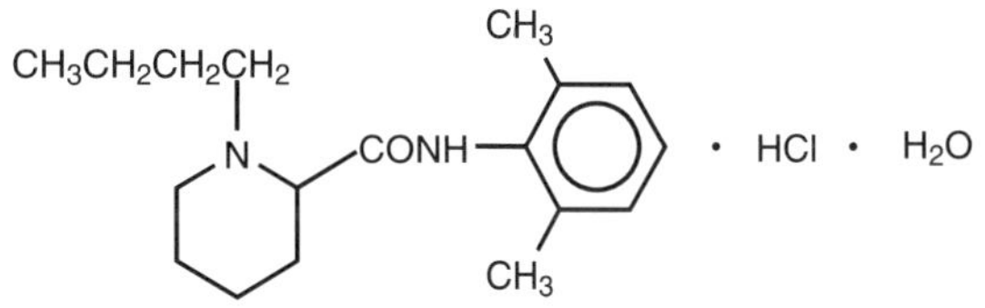

$CH_3CH_2CH_2CH_2$ / N / CONH / CH_3 / CH_3 · HCl · H_2O

FIG. 64-19. Structural formula of bupivacaine hydrochloride.

The addition of epinephrine to produce vasoconstriction and increased anesthetic duration is probably safe for use in cardiac patients. Donlon and Moss (15) demonstrated that 0.06 mg epinephrine (12 ml of 1 : 200,000) produces some systemic uptake, but no untoward clinical effects. Release of endogenous catecholamines may greatly exceed the relatively small amount of injected exogenous catecholamine (15).

MANAGEMENT OF PATIENTS WITH AN OPEN EYE INJURY AND FULL STOMACH

The controversy surrounding the use of succinylcholine, administered alone without proper pretreatment, in the setting of an open eye injury, has existed for several decades. In 1957, two separate articles included communications to the authors concerning the extrusion of intraocular contents from an open eye when succinylcholine was used intraoperatively (16,17). Succinylcholine increases IOP. The mechanism is not known, and the increase in IOP produced by succinylcholine has been demonstrated in intact eye preparations with no muscle attachments (18).

Clinical considerations must balance overall patient safety against any further damage to a ruptured globe. Intraconal or extraconal local anesthetic injections result in increased pressure within the confines of the bony orbit, which translates to extrusion of intraocular contents through the penetrating injury. A general anesthetic is the technique of choice.

After any trauma, patients are considered to have delayed stomach emptying and a full stomach. Patient management includes securing the airway, minimizing the risk of aspiration, and precluding further trauma to the open eye. Any valsalva maneuver, including coughing, bucking, or choking, poses the greatest risk of producing extrusion of intraocular contents and the greatest increase in IOP. The goal of airway management is to secure the airway without valsalva. As compared with other nondepolarizing muscle relaxants, succinylcholine, a depolarizing muscle relaxant, allows the shortest time interval of 60 seconds to reach the optimal time for endotracheal intubation, without bucking or valsalva. At the Massachusetts Eye and Ear Infirmary, either depolarizing or nondepolarizing muscle relaxants are used, depending on the judgment of the anesthesiologist, with regard to securing the airway.

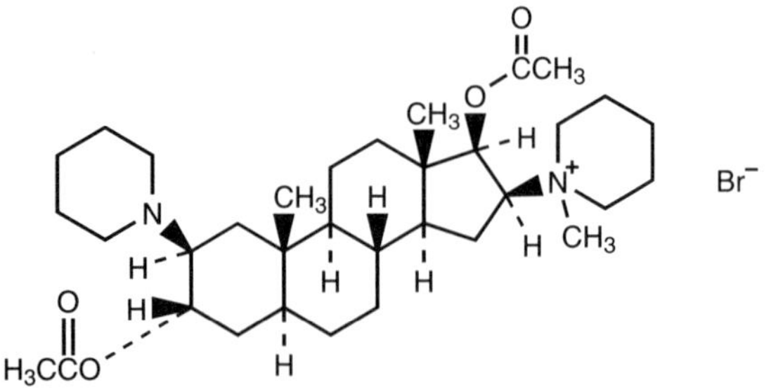

FIG. 64-20. Structural formula of vecuronium bromide.

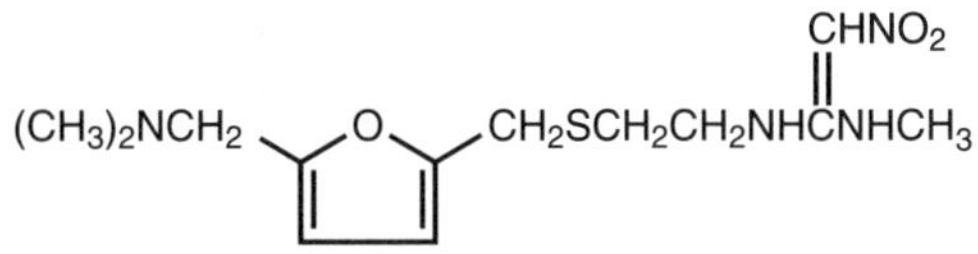

FIG. 64-22. Structural formula of ranitidine hydrochloride.

Grover et al. (19) demonstrated that use of succinylcholine and pretreatment with intravenous lidocaine cause no increase in IOP; they measured baseline intraocular IOP before administering intravenous lidocaine and intravenous induction. Lidocaine 1.5 mg/kg was administered 1 minute before thiopental induction. There was no increase in IOP from baseline after subsequent succinylcholine administration and endotracheal intubation. A potential problem with use of nondepolarizing muscle relaxants, as compared with use of succinylcholine, is the longer time (2 minutes, 30 seconds) necessary to achieve optimal intubating conditions in which there is no chance that coughing, bucking, or any other valsalva maneuver will occur during laryngoscopy and endotracheal intubation. Casson and Jones (20) demonstrated a shortened time of 90 seconds to achievement of intubating conditions with use of high-dose vecuronium (Fig. 20).

At the Massachusetts Eye and Ear Infirmary, we often use a nonparticulate antacid such as bicitra (Fig. 21), an H_2-blocker such as ranitidine (Fig. 22), and metoclopramide (Fig. 23) to achieve improved peristalsis, gastric emptying, and a more competent gastroesophageal sphincter preoperatively. In the operating room, we preoxygenate (denitrogenate) the patient, being careful not to apply pressure with the face mask to the injured eye. Lidocaine 1.5 mg/kg is administered, followed 1 to 2 minutes later by a rapid sequence induction technique with rapid administration of thiopental, succinylcholine, and manual cricoid pressure. After 60 seconds, the patient is in an optimal state for laryngoscopy and endotracheal intubation. An alternative is a modified rapid-sequence induction in which high-dose vecuronium is administered in lieu of succinylcholine, and optimized conditions for laryngoscopy and intubation are achieved in approximately 90 seconds. Nasogastric suction is performed with the patient under deep general anesthesia. Lidocaine 1.0 mg/kg is administered intravenously before the patient is extubated and metoclopramide 0.15 mg/kg is administered if it was not administered preoperatively; use of ondansetron 4 to 8 mg (Fig. 24) or droperidol 0.625 mg (Fig. 25) administered intravenously in the recovery room is considered.

Pediatric patients with penetrating eye injuries often have been crying and coughing and rubbing their injured eye before undergoing surgery. In the interest of safe management of the airway, most anesthesiologists prefer placing an intravenous access before anesthesia is induced, even if the child cries. Often it is safe to administer oral sedation before establishing intravenous access.

Malignant Hyperthermia (MH)

MH is a fulminant hypermetabolic crisis with a mortality of 70% which is triggered by anesthetic drugs. MH was initially described by Denborough in 1960 (20). However, since the introduction of dantrolene, the mortality has decreased to 10% (22). McPherson and Taylor (23) reported MH to be an autosomal dominant disorder in 50% of the families they studied. However, about 20% of families in their study appeared to have either recessive or multifactorial inheritance with variable penetrance (23). There may be more than one aberration in the cellular physiology of MH. The specific mechanism of defect is not entirely clear, but involves inadequate retention and reuptake of calcium by the sarcoplasmic reticulum, resulting in prolonged muscle contraction, heat generated by the restoration of ATP from ADP subsequent to aerobic metabolism, increased muscle energy demands beyond that supplied by aerobic metabolism and therefore supplemented by anaerobic metabolism, lactic acid production, and increased carbon dioxide production. First-degree relatives of patients with MH are at

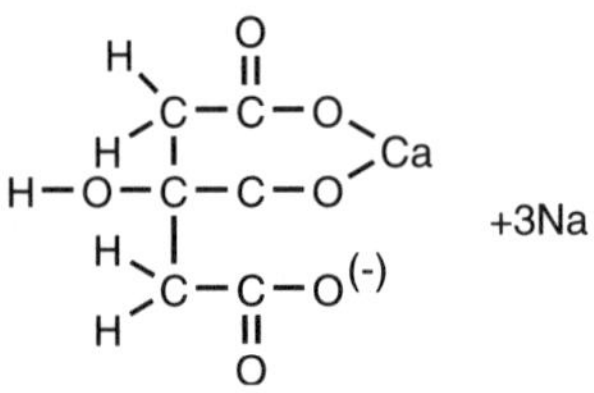

FIG. 64-21. Structural formula of sodium citrate.

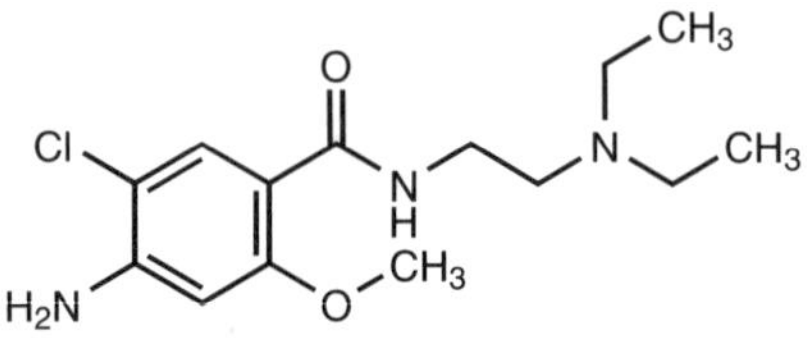

FIG. 64-23. Structural formula of metoclopramide.

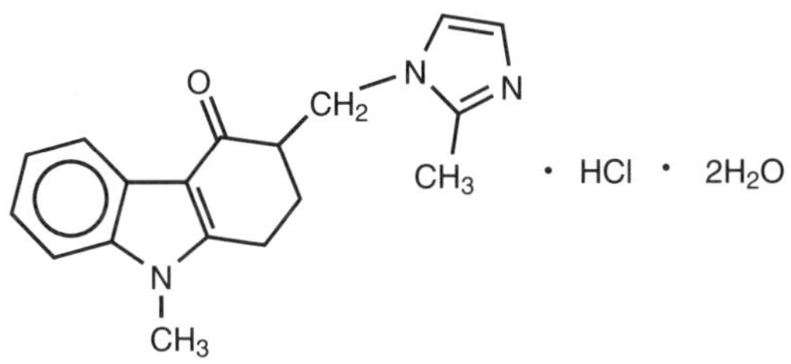

FIG. 64-24. Structural formula of ondansetron hydrochloride.

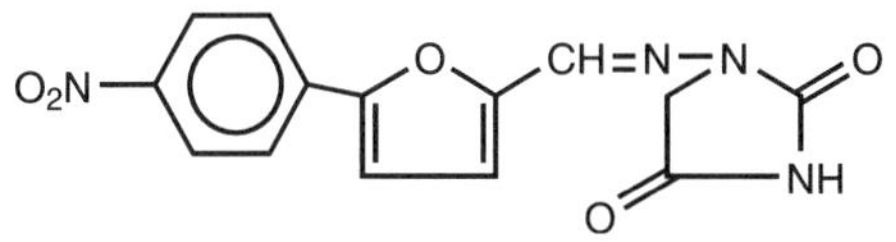

FIG. 64-26. Structural formula of dantrolene sodium.

risk of developing a hypermetabolic crisis under anesthesia. Triggering circumstances and agents include patient fear and inadequate sedation; succinylcholine, which has been involved in 77% of MH cases; halothane, which has been involved in 60% of cases; and all other halogenated inhalation anesthetics. At one time, amide local anesthetics were considered possible triggers of MH; it is now accepted that both ester and amide local anesthetics are safe to use and are not considered MH-triggering agents. In 1985, data from Denmark indicated an MH incidence of 1 in 260,000 anesthetic exposures, but the incidence increased to 1 in 60,000 if the triggering agent succinylcholine was administered, to 1 in 12,000 if the sole presenting nonspecific sign of MH was masseter muscle rigidity, and to 1 in 5,000 if fever and unexplained tachycardia were the sole signs (24). Therefore, the variability in the reported incidence may result from the variability of anesthetics, definitions, and signs of MH (22). MH early warning signs include increased end tidal carbon dioxide, tachycardia, tachypnea, unstable BP, arrhythmias, dark blood in the surgical field, cyanosis, fasciculations or rigidity, metabolic acidosis, fever, hyperkalemia, coagulopathy, myoglobinuria, and elevated creatinine phosphokinase level. Diseases associated with MH include Duchene's muscular dystrophy, central core disease, and neurolept malignant syndrome. Suggestive associations include muscle cramps, increased muscle size with weakness, intolerance to caffeine, and an elevated baseline creatinine phosphokinase level.

Management during an MH crisis includes immediate discontinuation of anesthetic agent; use of a fresh anesthesia machine to ensure that no residual, soluble inhalation halogenated triggering agents can be washed out of plastic and rubber to the patient; hyperventilation with 100% oxygen; administration of dantrolene (Fig. 26), which functions as a muscle relaxant, initially at a dose of 2.5 mg/kg intravenously and increased rapidly to 10 mg/kg to reduce the hypermetabolic state; administration of procainamide (Fig. 27) to 15 mg/kg slowly, if required for arrhythmias; placement of additional large-bore intravenous lines with cooling coils and central and arterial monitoring lines; iced lavage through nasogastric and rectal tubes; correction of acidosis; placement of Foley catheter and administration of liberal amounts of fluid, mannitol, and furosemide (Fig. 28) to maintain urine output; correction of any other metabolic and electrolyte derangements; monitoring for 48 to 72 hours; and administration of additional dantrolene for 48 to 72 hours.

Counseling the patient and family after an episode of MH and deciding whether to perform a halothane-caffeine muscle contracture test are crucial and require consultation with an anesthesiologist.

Management of patients with a known history of MH includes adequate preoperative sedation, the use of acceptable anesthetic agents such as narcotics, nitrous oxide, barbiturates, propofol, ketamine, nondepolarizing muscle relaxants, amide or ester anesthetics, and close monitoring of end tidal carbon dioxide, temperature, and pulse oxymetry (25).

Strabismus Surgery

The propensity for stimulation of the oculocardiac reflex (OCR) to occur is well known. However, prophylactic administration of atropine to prevent slowing of the heart rate (HR) intraoperatively is not a particularly useful treatment. The best treatment is to ask the surgeon to pause in stimulating the OCR. Eventually, the reflex tires. However, if the reflex persists and there is hemodynamic compromise, atropine 0.007 mg/kg intravenous push can be given (12). Succinylcholine is to be avoided if a forced duction test is planned. Administration of a nondepolarizing muscle relaxing agent is appropriate.

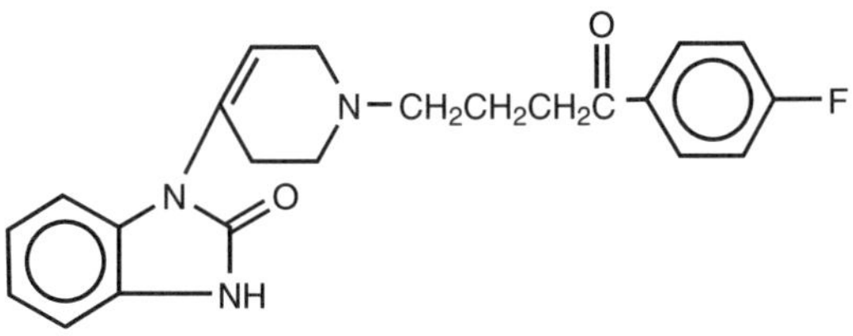

FIG. 64-25. Structural formula of droperidol.

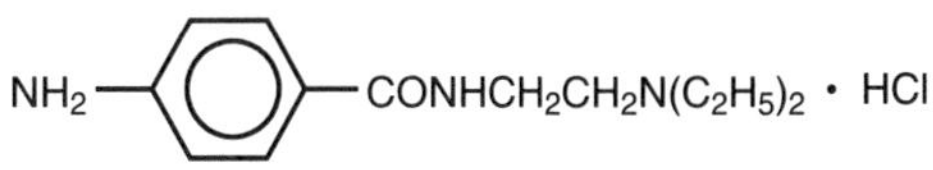

FIG. 64-27. Structural formula of procainamide hydrochloride.

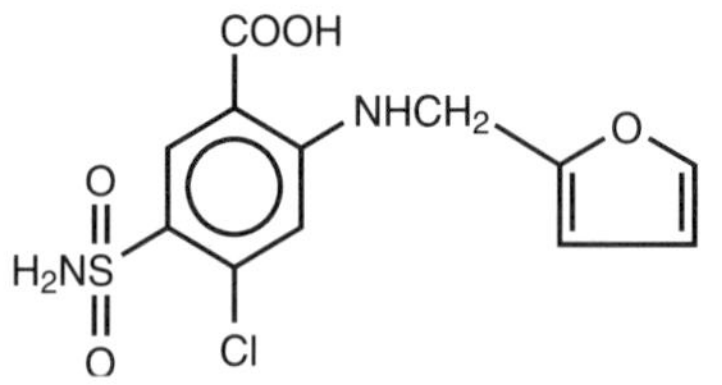

FIG. 64-28. Structural formula of frusemide.

Vomiting after strabismus or eye muscle surgery is common. Abramovitz et al. (26) reported an incidence of 85%; this incidence was diminished to 43% by administration of 0.075 mg/kg droperidol intravenously 30 minutes before the end of surgery. Other investigators recommend administering the same dose of droperidol at the time of induction of anesthesia, which in their study reduced the incidence of vomiting to 10%. Weir et al. (28) demonstrated that a propofol infusion with 66% nitrous oxide and without narcotics was effective in reducing the incidence of vomiting after strabismus surgery to 24% as compared with an incidence of 41% in patients who received halothane alone and an incidence of 64% who received nitrous oxide and propofol, 64% nitrous oxide and propofol infusion in 66% nitrous oxide and narcotics. Recently, at the Massachusetts Eye and Ear Infirmary, we demonstrated a rapid intraoperative wake-up technique for adjustment of adjustable sutures in the operating room using continuous infusions of propofol, mivacron (Fig. 29), and alfentanil in adults with very satisfactory results and a marked decrease in the incidence of nausea and vomiting at 13% (29). Consideration is given to use of lidocaine 1.0 mg/kg intravenously before emergence, use of metoclopramide 0.15 mg/kg if not administered preoperatively and, in the recovery room, use of droperidol 0.625 mg or ondansetron 4 to 8 mg intravenously in adults.

Prematurity

A premature infant may have a history of bronchopulmonary dysplasia, intraventricular hemorrhage, or respiratory and systemic infections. Proper general anesthetic depth is required to achieve smooth ventilation without bronchospasm, and safe management of BP. In premature infants the respiratory control centers are not adequately developed, and the effects of ventilatory depression after administration of anesthetic agents are prolonged. Provision should be made for postoperative 24-hour hospital apnea monitoring in infants of less than 60 weeks postconceptional age. Cardiac output (CO) is the product of stroke volume (SV) and HR. Many patients aged less than 6 months do not have a well-developed sympathetic nervous system that can respond appropriately to laryngeal or surgical stimulation, and their myocardium cannot stretch during longer diastolic filling times, as do those of older patients' hearts, when HR diminishes. Premature infants, neonates, and term infants aged less than 6 months of age are reliant on HR to maintain CO. These patients benefit from administration of atropine 0.01 mg/kg intramuscularly—not less than 0.1 mg total—before induction of anesthesia, for maintenance of CO.

Congenital Syndromes

Congenital syndromes must be factored in the anesthetic and surgical plan for patients of any age. Although use of topical atropine is contraindicated in patients with glaucoma, systemic atropine administered in the usual clinical anesthetic dosages has no effect on IOP in either open- or closed-angle glaucoma and is safe to use in patients with glaucoma (6,8,22).

Surgical treatment of congenital cataracts include intraoperative mydriasis with anterior chamber infusion of epinephrine. Smith et al. (28) did not observe intraoperative arrhythmias in either children or adults receiving halothane anesthesia and anterior chamber instillation of 0.4 to 68 μg/kg.

Preoperative planning of oxygen administration in infants with retinopathy of prematurity (ROP) or in infants who are at risk of developing ROP must acknowledge that oxygen is neither a necessary nor a sufficient cause of ROP. Recommendations are that anesthesiologists keep the

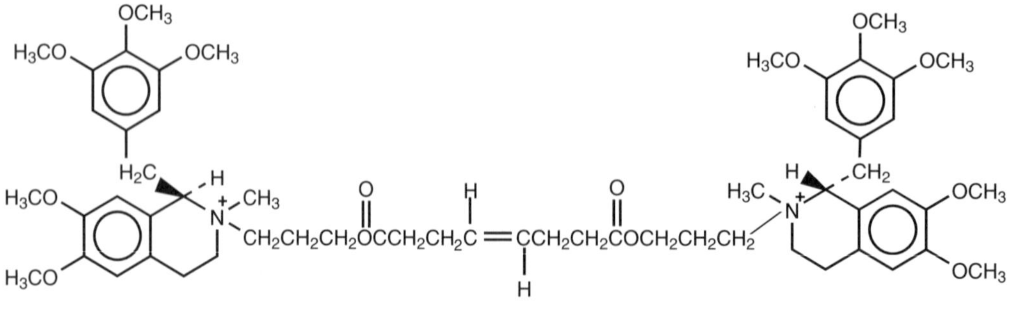

FIG. 64-29. Structural formula of mivacron.

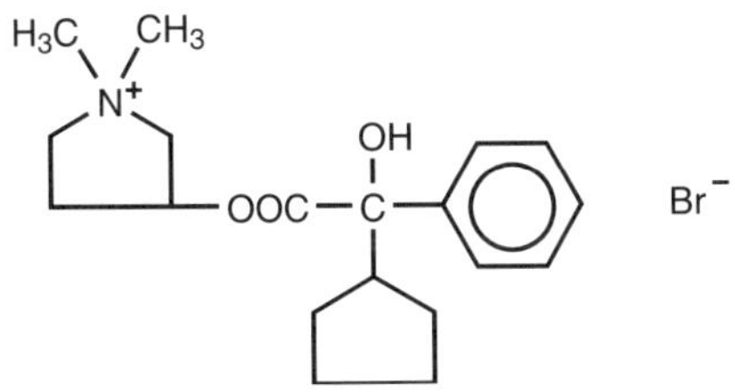

FIG. 64-30. Structural formula of glycopyrrolate.

oxygen saturation at 95% in infants aged less than 44 weeks postconception. However, even with careful titration of oxygen, ROP may still occur because ROP is a multifactorial disease (22). Marfan's syndrome, an autosomal dominant condition, is characterized by cardiovascular, skeletal, and ocular abnormalities. Anesthetic agents should be administered to avoid hypertension, which can result in dissection of the aorta. Congenital myotonic diseases need careful consideration regarding exacerbation of muscle weakness induced by administration of various antibiotic agents, muscle relaxants, muscle relaxant reversal agents, and anesthetic agents.

Riley-Day Syndrome, or familial dysautonomia, is an autosomal recessive condition occurring in Ashkenazi Jewish children, and is characterized by low levels of dopamine β-oxidase. Some symptoms include impaired deglutition, motor weakness, frequent aspiration pneumonitis and postural hypotension. Anesthetic cardiovascular depressants must be administered with extreme caution. Anesthetic cardiovascular depressants must also be administered with caution in patients with Rubella syndrome. Some patients with Von Recklinghausen's disease have an undiagnosed pheochromocytoma and intraoperative hypertension, as well as prolonged response to both depolarizing and nondepolarizing muscle relaxants (22,31).

Patients with type I diabetes tend to be more brittle than patients with noninsulin-dependent diabetes mellitus. In general, patients with type I diabetes are advised to take one-third to one-half their usual dose of intermediate- or long-acting insulin after otaining a fasting blood sugar level. An intravenous infusion of D5W is started and titrated accordingly. Blood sugar levels are monitored in the perioperative period every 1 to 2 hours. Hyperglycemia with blood sugar level greater than 250 mg/dl is treated with small dosages of regular insulin, and blood sugar level less than 100 mg/dL is treated with an increase in the D5W infusion. Patients with type II diabetes receiving oral hypoglycemic agents should discontinue their medication 1 to 2 days preoperatively, depending on the $t_{\frac{1}{2}}$ of the oral hypoglycemic agent, to avoid hypoglycemia in the perioperative period.

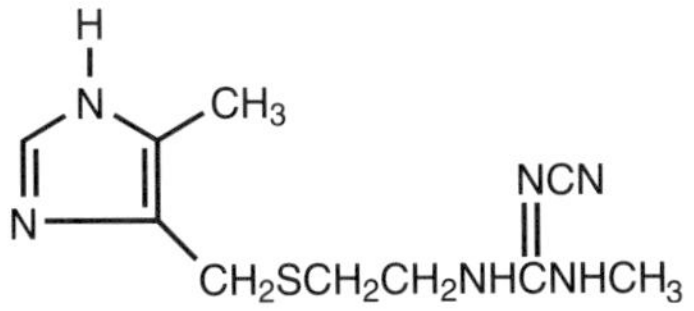

FIG. 64-31. Structural formula of cimetidine hydrochloride.

Patients with congenital syndromes involving abnormal airway or cardiac abnormalities should be examined by the consultant anesthesiologist well in advance of the scheduled surgery. Some syndromes involve relative macroglossia and difficult mask and endotracheal tube management, abnormal cardiac valve function, abnormal cardiac conduction, or abnormal aorta. Infants born with defects as a result of rubella can shed virus for a few months after birth, and health care personnel must be informed.

RECOVERY ROOM CARE AFTER OPHTHALMIC SURGERY

The goals of recovery are safety, comfort, and successful postsurgical healing. All the same preoperative considerations regarding overall health, specific organ system functions, usual medications of the patient, level of cooperation and understanding on the part of the patient, and type of anesthetic technique and medications are of importance in the immediate perianesthetic period of care.

Regardless of whether a local anesthetic agent with sedation or general anesthesia was administered to the patient, the first priority is the safety of patients emerging from anesthesia. Their cardiorespiratory system and mental status must be carefully monitored. The position of the patient requires that a safe airway be maintained until the patient is able to protect his own airway. When deemed safe, head positioning may then conform to the surgeon's instructions.

Generally, narcotic analgesic agents and other CNS depressants are administered carefully to avoid postoperative hypoventilation. The OCR can occur postoperatively during the recovery period, generally as a reaction to ocular pain and swelling. Occasionally it can occur owing to patients' fear or panic. Treatment requires that patients be alert enough to protect their own airway and determination of the cause of OCR. Antiemetic agents include intravenous droperidol 50 μg/kg i.v., metoclopramide 0.15 mg/kg i.v., lidocaine 1.0 mg/kg i.v., and ondansetron 4 to 8 mg i.v. (32). Droperidol may prolong the emergence or recovery period, and, as an α-blocker, may reduce BP. Frequently, hypertension may develop in patients with labile hypertension and can be treated with sublingual nifedipine 10 mg per dose, verapamil, 2.5 mg i.v., hydralazine in 5-mg increments, or esmolol. Coughing can be treated with lidocaine 1 mg/kg or with a narcotic, preferably before the patient emerges from general anesthesia. Pain can be treated with tylenol with codeine or a stronger narcotic (33).

REFERENCES

1. Acquadro MA. Anesthesia for head and neck surgery. In: Davison JK, Eckhardt III WF, Perese DA, eds. *Clinical anesthesia procedures of the Massachusetts General Hospital,* 4th ed. Boston: Little, Brown, 1993;390–401.
2. Egbert LD, Battit GE, Turndorf H, Beecher HK. The value of the preoperative visit by an anesthetist: a study of doctor patient rapport. *JAMA* 1963;185:553–555.
3. McGoldrick KE. Anesthetics and intraocular pressure: management of penetrating eye injuries. In: McGoldrick KE, ed. *Anesthesia for ophthalmic and otolaryngologic surgery.* Philadelphia: WB Saunders, 1992;184–186.
4. Joshi C, Bruce DL. Thiopental and succinylcholine: action on intraocular pressure. *Anesth Analg* 1975;54:471–475.
5. Adler FH. *Physiology of the eye: clinical application,* 5th ed. St Louis: CV Mosby, 1970;249.
6. Duncalf D, Foldes FF. Effect of anesthetic drugs and muscle relaxants on intraocular pressure. In: Smith RB, ed. *Anesthesia in ophthalmology.* Boston: Little, Brown, 1973;21–33.
7. Ausinich B, Rayburn LR, Munson ES, Levy NS. Ketamine and intraocular pressure in children. *Anesth Analg* 1976;55:773–775.
8. Schwartz H, De Roeth A Jr, Papper EM: Preanesthetic use of atropine in patients with glaucoma. *JAMA* 1957;165:144–146.
9. Zimmerman T, Konner KS, Kandarakis AS, et al. Improving the therapeutic index of topically applied ocular drugs. *Arch Ophthalmol* 1984;102:551–553.
10. McGoldrick KE. Anesthetic ramifications of ophthalmic drugs. In: McGoldrick KE, ed. *Anesthesia for ophthalmic and otolaryngologic surgery.* Philadelphia: WB Saunders, 1992;227–234.
11. Stinson III TW, Donlon JV Jr. Interaction of intraocular air and sulfur hexafluoride with nitrous oxide: a computer simulation. *Anesthesiology* 1982;56:385–388.
12. Donlon JV. Anesthesia and eye, ear, nose and throat surgery. In: Miller RD, ed. *Anesthesia,* 3rd ed. New York: Churchill Livingstone, 1990;2001–2024.
13. Wolf GL, Capuano C, Hartung J. Nitrous oxide increases intraocular pressure after intravitreal sulfur hexafluoride injection. *Anesthesiology* 1983;59:547–548.
14. Sweitzer BJ. Local anesthetics. In: Davison JK, Eckhardt WF, Perese DA, eds. *Clinical anesthesia procedures of the Massachusetts General Hospital,* 4th ed. Boston: Little, Brown, 1993;197–205.
15. Donlon JV Jr, Moss J. Plasma catecholamine levels during local anesthesia for cataract operations. *Anesthesiology* 1979;51:471–473.
16. Lincoff HA, Breinin GM, DeVoe AG. The effect of succinylcholine on extraocular muscles. *Am J Ophthalmol* 1957;43:440–444.
17. Dillon JB, Sabawala P, Taylor DB, Gunter R. Action of succinylcholine on extraocular muscles and intraocular pressure. *Anesthesiology* 1957;18:44–49.
18. Kelley RE, Dinner M, Turner LS, et al. Succinylcholine increases intraocular pressure in the human eye with the extraocular muscles detached. *Anesthesiology* 1993;79:948–952.
19. Grover VK, Lata K, Sharma S, et al. Efficacy of lignocaine in the suppression of the intraocular pressure response to suxamethonium and tracheal intubation. *Anaesthesia* 1989;44:22–25.
20. Casson WR, Jones RM. Vecuronium induced neuromuscular blockade. *Anaesthesia* 1986;41:354–357.
21. Denborough MA, Lovell RH. Anaesthetic deaths in a family. *Anaesthesia* 1960;2:45.
22. McGoldrick KE. Pediatric ophthalmic surgery: anesthetic considerations. In: McGoldrick KE, ed. *Anesthesia for ophthalmic and otolaryngologic surgery.* Philadelphia: WB Saunders, 1992;190–209.
23. McPherson EW, Taylor CA. Genetics of malignant hyperthermia: evidence for heterogeneity. *Am J Med Genet* 1982;11:273–285.
24. Ording H. Incidence of malignant hyperthermia in Denmark. *Anesth Analg* 1985;64:700–703.
25. Ryan JF. Malignant hyperthermia. In: Cote CJ, Ryan JF, Todres ID, Goudsouzian NG, eds. *A practice of anesthesia for infants and children,* 2nd ed. Philadelphia: WB Saunders, 1993;417–428.
26. Abramowitz MD, Oh TH, Epstein BS. Antiemetic effect of droperidol following outpatient strabismus surgery in children. *Anesthesiology* 1983;59:579–583.
27. Lerman J, Eustis S, Smith DR. Effect of droperidol pretreatment on postanesthetic vomiting in children undergoing strabismus surgery. *Anesthesiology* 1986;65:322–325.
28. Weir PM, Munro HM, Reynolds PI, Lewis IH, Wilton NCT. Propofol infusion and the incidence of emesis in pediatric outpatient strabismus surgery. *Anesth Analg* 1993;76:760–764.
29. Ward JB, et al. The use of propofol and mivacurium anesthetic technique for the immediate post-operative adjustment of sutures in strabismus surgery. *Ophthalmology* xxxx;xx:xx–xx.
30. Smith RB, Douglas H, Petruscak J, Breslin P. Safety of intraocular adrenaline with halothane anesthesia. *Br J Anaesth* 1972;44:1314–1317.
31. McGoldrick KE. Ocular pahology and systemic diseases: anesthetic implications. In: McGoldrick KE, ed. *Anesthesia for ophthalmic and otolaryngologic surgery.* Philadelphia: WB Saunders, 1992;210–226.
32. Alon E, Himmelseher S. Ondansetron in the treatment of postoperative vomiting: a randomized, double-blind comparison with droperidol and metoclopramide. *Anesth Analg* 1992;75:561–565.
33. Acquadro MA. Recovery room care and problems following ophthalmic and otolaryngologic surgery. In: McGoldrick KE, ed. *Anesthesia for ophthalmic and otolaryngologic surgery.* Philadelphia: WB Saunders, 1992;291–302.

SECTION VII

Ocular Medications for Pediatric Patients

Section Editor: Forrest D. Ellis

OVERVIEW

Ocular medications commonly used in children include mydriatic and cycloplegic agents, topical anesthetic agents, antiglaucoma medications, antiinflammatory agents, antibiotic agents, and antiviral agents. Foundations for the use of ocular medications in children often are not established by controlled clinical trials. Pharmaceutical literature, therefore, often carries required disclaimers to the effect that the safety or efficacy of a particular medication has not been established for children. Controlled clinical trials in children are difficult to conduct and finance because of medicolegal concerns and a low prevalence of medically treatable ocular conditions in the pediatric population (1). Congenital glaucoma, for instance, occurs approximately once in 30,000 live births and is considered a surgical disease, yet many of the few patients with congenital glaucoma do receive various antiglaucoma medications during the course of their postsurgical or interimsurgical management. Administration of such medication to a child might therefore seem inappropriate, but such usage actually is not only common but is considered by clinicians to be mandatory. The Food and Drug Administration (FDA) has recognized that a physician may prescribe a drug product for uses not included in approved labeling and that accepted medical practice often includes drug use that is not reflected in approved drug labeling (2). When vision-threatening disease conditions exist which are known to respond to specific medication available only as "approved" relative to the adult or older child, the thoughtful administration of that medication, weighed against the alternatives, often is appropriate.

Serious or critical side effects of medications, particularly if dose related, may occur in premature infants or newborns or in children with syndromes and metabolic disorders involving major organ dysfunction (3). The clinician considering use of medications "not approved for use in children" does assume additional responsibilities (on the child's behalf) in such cases. Premature infants and neonates may not metabolize medications as expected due to immature organ system function. Indeed, a newborn, especially a premature infant, may have an incomplete diagnostic profile for some time after birth. On the other hand, astute clinicians may be in a unique position to recognize potential systemic drug problems if they have the opportunity to perform an adequate eye examination. Medications known to be nephrotoxic but otherwise appropriate for treatment of a severe ocular infection, for example, might be considered for a patient until an abnormality of the optic nerves, retina, lens, or intraocular pressure (IOP) is noted that alerts the clinician to the possibilities of renal anomalies in that patient (i.e., Warburg syndrome, Lowe syndrome, Senior-Loken syndrome). Under such circumstances, use of a potentially nephrotoxic drug would be contraindicated until these anatomic and physiologic possibilities were investigated. Similar concerns apply to the administration of certain antiglaucoma medications to an infant with pulmonary dysfunction or of vasoactive agents to a patient with congenital cardiovascular disease of undetermined severity.

It is of importance that clinicians examining and treating infants and children for visual disorders may do so with little or no support derived from statistically adequate, controlled clinical trials relative to the age group under treatment. Clinicians must remain alert to known effects and potential side effects of medicines they are using and to signs or symptoms potentially attributable to the medications. Adverse or paradoxical effects should be reported through appropriate means. Until data do accrue from trials and case reports, an informed family, as well as the attending physician, must share the responsibilities inherent in the treatment of patients in these age groups. Fortunately, the incidence of adverse reactions with serious consequences is low.

SPECIAL CONSIDERATIONS REGARDING DRUG DELIVERY TO INFANTS AND CHILDREN

Drug dosages commonly are calculated on a milligram per kilogram basis. Conversion of these weight-based figures to surface area-based figures can be helpful when one calculates dosage for small children (4). High metabolic rates and high surface area/mass ratios sometimes require that small infants and children receive more medication on a milligram per kilogram basis than an adult would receive (5). Surface area, metabolic rate, and fluid volume also predispose the small infant to adverse or exaggerated effects from drugs such as vasoactive agents and β-adrenergic blocking agents.

Certain common ophthalmic preparations must be used with caution or not at all in children with the following dysfunctions:

Cardiovascular dysfunction: Phenylephrine, β-adrenergic antagonists (asthma, dyspnea, arrhythmia)

Pulmonary dysfunction: β-adrenergic antagonists (asthma, dyspnea)

Hepatic dysfunction: Ceftriaxone, carbonic anhydrase inhibitors (liver failure)

Renal dysfunction: Carbonic anhydrase inhibitors, acyclovir (acidosis, electrolyte imbalance, renal failure)

Gastrointestinal tract dysfunction: Cholinomimetics (abdominal cramps, diarrhea, nausea, vomiting); cycloplegic agents (necrotizing enterocolitis suspected in premature infants)

Developmental delay: Cycloplegic agents (temperature elevation, behavior disorders, seizure disorders, respiratory depression)

Until relatively recently, the effects of systemic absorption of medications applied topically to the eye have received relatively little attention in regard to infants. Control of the dose administered to the whole child despite "exact" delivery of a known volume of medication to the eye itself remains a source of concern. Despite methods designed to minimize absorption through the nasolacrimal system and nose, such as occlusion of the puncta, decreasing the drop size (6), or decreasing the concentration of the drug in the drop (7), the precise systemic absorption of topical medication received by a given child is seldom known (8). Blood levels attained by medicines administered to the eye, when measured in investigational protocols, suggest wide variations in the amounts of active agents entering the bloodstream (9). Different clinical methods of drug delivery to the eye and individual variations in absorption rates make precise control of systemic effects difficult to achieve.

REFERENCES

1. Palmer EA. How safe are ocular drugs in pediatrics? *Ophthalmology* 1986;93:1038–1040.
2. *Physicians' Desk Reference for Ophthalmology,* 23rd ed. Montvale, NJ: Medical Economic Data Production Company, 1995.
3. Isenberg S, Everett S. Cardiovascular effects of mydriatics in low-birth-weight infants. *J Pediatr* 1984;105:111–112.
4. Apt L. Pharmacology. In: *The eye in infancy.* St. Louis: CV Mosby, 1994;87–98.
5. Patton TF, Robinson JR. Pediatric dosing considerations in ophthalmology. *J Pediatr Ophthalmol Strabismus.* 1976;13:171.
6. Lynch MG, et al. Reduction of phenylephrine drop size in infants achieves equal dilation with decreased systemic absorption. *Arch Ophthalmol* 1987;105:1364–1365.
7. Wheatcroft S, Sharma A, McAllister J. Reduction in mydriatic drop size in premature infants. *Br J Ophthalmol* 1993;77:364–365.
8. Kumar V, et al. Systemic absorption and cardiovascular effects of phenylephrine eyedrops. *Am J Ophthalmol* 1985;99:180–184.
9. Jennings BJ, Sullivan DE. The effect of topical 2.5% phenylephrine and 1% tropicamide on systemic blood pressure and pulse. *J Am Optom Assoc* 1986;57:382–389.

Textbook of Ocular Pharmacology,
edited by T.J. Zimmerman, et al.
Lippincott–Raven Publishers, Philadelphia © 1997.

CHAPTER 65

Topical Ophthalmic Preparations Used for Infants and Children

Forrest D. Ellis

MYDRIATIC AGENTS

Definitions

Mydriasis: *n.* a long continued or excessive dilatation of the pupil of the eye (1). Mydriatic: *adj.* causing or involving the dilatation of the pupil of the eye (1).

Mydriatic agents dilate the pupil. Pupillary dilation may be desired to enhance the patient's view of the outside world when a partial obstruction of the visual axis exists or, more commonly, to enable the clinician to examine the interior of the eye. Measurement of the refractive error through retinoscopy may be particularly enhanced when mydraiatic agents are used with cycloplegic agents (described herein). Intraocular pressure (IOP)-lowering effects of topically administered sympathomimetic agents have clinical usefulness in children. Mydriatic agents are not effective for relief of pain secondary to spasm of the ciliary muscle.

Mydriatic preparations are derived from compounds that have sympathomimetic activity.

Sympathomimetic: *adj.* simulating sympathetic nervous system action in physiologic effect (1). Catecholamine: *n.* any of various substances (as epinephrine, norepinephrine, and dopamine) that contain a benzene ring with two adjacent hydroxyl groups and a side chain of ethylamine and that function as hormones or neurotransmitters or both (1).

Sympathomimetics are drugs that mimic the action of epinephrine and norepinephrine (which act directly on and produce activity of adrenoceptors). Most sympathomimetic medications used topically act indirectly by causing release of endogenous catecholamines at the neuromuscular junction. Catecholamines act through two principal receptors termed α and β receptors. α Receptors are sensitive to epinephrine, norepinephrine and isoproterenol, in that order; β receptors are more sensitive to isoproterenol, epinephrine, and norepinephrine, in that order (2). β Receptors have now been subdivided into two subtypes, β_1 and β_2. β_1-Receptors have equal affinity for epinephrine and norepinephrine, whereas β_2-receptors have a higher affinity for epinephrine. α-Receptors also have been divided into two subtypes, α_1 and α_2, and these subtypes further subdivided (2).

Sympathomimetic drugs used topically in the eyes of children are epinephrine, dipivefrin, phenylephrine, apraclonidine, hydroxyamphetamine, and cocaine.

Chemical Structure

Epinephrine is 1,2-benzenediol,4-(-1-hydroxy-2-(methylamino)ethyl)-(*R*)-.

Dipivefrin is (±)-3,4dihydroxy-α-((methylamino) methyl) benzyl alcohol 3,4-dipivalate hydrochloride.

The structure of phenylephrine is $C_9H_{13}NO_2$

Aproclonidine is 2-((4-amino-2,6 dichlorophenyl)imino) imidazolidine monohydrochloride.

Hydroxyamphetamine is phenol, 4-(2-amino-propyl)-hydrobromide.

The structure of cocaine is $C_{17}H_{21}NO_4$.

Pharmacology

Epinephrine functions as an α and β agonist without selectivity. It is derived from phenylethylamine, the parent compound from which most sympathomimetic drugs are derived. This compound, a benzene ring with an ethylamine side chain, when modified by the addition of hy-

F. D. Ellis: Department of Ophthalmology, Indiana University, Indianapolis, Indiana 46202.

droxyl groups at the 3 and 4 positions of the ring and at the β position on the side chain, becomes norepinephrine. The addition of a methyl group to the amino group of norepinephrine produces epinephrine, which has increased β_2 activity as compared with norepinephrine.

Dipivefrin, an epinephrine prodrug, is reconverted to epinephrine once inside the eye and therefore has the same mechanism of action as epinephrine. Dipivefrin is formed by esterifying epinephrine with pivalic acid, which serves to enhance penetration of the drug into the eye. Dipivefrin is hydrolyzed back to epinephrine once in the eye and therefore has the same physiologic effects as epinephrine, with nonselective α_1 and α_2, and β activity.

Phenylephrine is a sympathomimetic drug that acts directly on receptors with almost pure α_1 selectivity and very little α_2 activity. Phenylephrine is derived from phenylethylamine by the addition of a hydroxyl group (−OH) at the 3 position on the ring and on the β-carbon and by substitution of a methyl group for the amino group. It is not a catecholamine.

Aproclonidine is a sympathomimetic drug with α_2 selective activity.

Hydroxyamphetamine is a non-catecholamine sympathomimetic drug with an enhanced ability to displace norepinephrine from terminal storage sites; therefore, it is an indirect-acting sympathomimetic agent.

Cocaine is a topical anesthetic agent which has sympathomimetic effects through its ability to block reuptake of norepinephrine at the neuromuscular junction.

Clinical Pharmacology

Epinephrine is a potent sympathomimetic drug with profound cardiovascular activity and without adrenoceptor selectivity. It may increase systolic blood pressure (BP) while reducing diastolic BP. In the eye, epinephrine acts to dilate the pupil and to reduce IOP.

Phenylephrine is less effective but more selective than epinephrine. It acts primarily on α_1-receptors, which in the eye are located in the dilator muscles of the iris. Contraction of these muscles produces pupillary dilation. Phenylephrine is an effective mydriatic but can produce undesirable systemic cardiovascular effects. In infants, these undesirable effects may be those of increased peripheral arterial resistance and decreased venous capacity, leading to increase in BP (3). Heart rate (HR) may slow secondary to baroreceptor stimulation, but cardiac output (CO) may not diminish in response to the slower HR; therefore, marked cardiovascular effects may ensue (2,4).

Clinical Uses of Sympathomimetic Agents in Children

Epinephrine is used to reduce IOP, usually in combination with other drugs. It is an effective pressure-lowering drug, but is not a drug of choice to dilate the pupil. At one time, epinephrine was used in an aqueous solution of 1 : 1,000 concentration as a test for Horner syndrome lesion localization. A sympathetically denervated pupil theoretically would be hypersensitive to epinephrine if a lesion affecting the third neuron existed. A normal pupil or a pupil affected by first- or second-order neuron lesions would not dilate in response to topical 1 : 1,000 epinephrine. However, clinical experience demonstrated that third-order neuron lesions rarely produced a pupil hypersensitive to 1 : 1,000 epinephrine. This test now has been supplanted by use of hydroxyamphetamine (preferred) or weak solutions of phenylephrine. Pharmacologic tests using hydroxyamphetamine can localize the site of the lesion with 84% accuracy and can confirm the localization of a site with 96% accuracy (5).

Pupillary effects of epinephrine are transient, and the potential for cardiovascular side effects is significant in premature infants or neonates. Numerous studies have documented the cardiovascular effects of epinephrine topically administered to the eye. Reports of cystoid macular edema (CME) secondary to administration of topical epinephrine eye drops have not been reported in children.

Phenylephrine hydrochloride is an effective mydriatic agent useful for pupillary dilation either alone or as a supplement to cycloplegic agents (6). It is also used by some surgeons to produce vasoconstriction of conjunctival blood vessels, particularly for strabismus surgery. It is a component of many over-the-counter eye drops used to produce temporary blanching of the conjunctival blood vessels. It may be used together with echothiophate to prevent iris pupillary border cysts, which are sometimes produced when echothiophate is used alone. Phenylephrine eye drops are used to produce dilation of the pupil (they have less potential for producing amblyopia than do cycloplegic agents) in infants with a partial occlusion of the visual axis of one or both eyes such as can be caused by a corneal or lenticular opacity. When used in such a manner, the effectiveness of the medication appears to decrease with prolonged use, although individual variations are common. Local allergic reactions to phenylephrine have been reported to occur with a frequency of about 3% (7).

Phenylephrine hydrochloride is available as eye drops in preparations with concentrations of 1%, 2.5%, and 10%. Frequently, phenylephrine is supplied along with cycloplegic agents in preparations designed to deliver both drugs simultaneously to the eye.

Almost all clinicians treating pediatric patients and many treating adults have abandoned the 10% concentrations of phenylephrine because of the potential undesirable effects on the cardiovascular system (8). Administration of 10% phenylephrine to infants and children is not necessary and therefore is contraindicated (9).

Phenylephrine hydrochloride drops in a concentration of 2.5% is preferred for older children. Premature infants and neonates should not receive even this concentration of medication; instead, should receive a concentration of 1% or less. Phenylephrine hydrochloride in a concentration of 1% is administered with 0.2% cyclopentolate to produce dilation of premature or young infants' eyes, especially for diagnosis and treatment of retinopathy of prematurity (ROP). Premature and newborn infants receiving even small doses of phenylephrine eye drops often develop striking periorbital blanching, which may persist for hours. Duration of action of phenylephrine in the eye is estimated to be 5 to 7 hours.

Horner syndrome occurs in infants and children as a consequence of sympathetic denervation of the eye and face. The effects, usually unilateral, are those of ptosis (sympathetic denervation of Mueller's muscle in the eyelids), ipsilateral flushing and absence of sweating (sympathetic denervation of the vasculature and of the sweat glands [note: the lesion may be third-order neuron but must occur before the separation of sympathetic fibers at the carotid bifurcation]), and miosis (sympathetic denervation of the dilator muscle of the iris). Localization of the lesion to pre- or postganglionic sites can be of diagnostic importance (10). Phenylephrine should dilate a small pupil secondary to Horner syndrome regardless of the site of the lesion because of the direct effect of phenylephrine on the α_1-receptors of the dilator muscles. Therefore, phenylephrine administered after cocaine or hydroxyamphetamine has failed to dilate a Horner pupil can confirm sympathetic denervation of the pupil (by producing dilatation), but does not serve to localize the denervation to either a pre- or postganglionic site. Patients with known first- or second-order neuron lesions have shown "supersensitivity" to topical phenylephrine only in the central neuron lesions (11). The significance of this observation is not known.

Aproclonidine frequently is used in adults for pressure-lowering effects. Its usefulness in children has not been established, although the increasing numbers of laser capsulotomies performed in children after intraocular lens (IOL) implantation suggests that increasing use of this medication can be anticipated.

Hydroxyamphetamine use in the eye is limited to that of localizing the site of a lesion producing a Horner syndrome, although in a 1% concentration it will dilate a normal pupil in a lightly pigmented eye (12). Hydroxyamphetamine has sympathomimetic action mediated by release of norepinephrine vesicles from nerve terminals at the neuromuscular junction and does not have a direct effect on the dilator muscles. This makes it a particularly valuable drug for Horner syndrome localization purposes (5). If a Horner syndrome-producing lesion is preganglionic, release of existing norepinephrine by hydroxyamphetamine will cause pupillary dilatation. A postganglionic lesion results in an absence of norepinephrine at the neuromuscular junction; therefore, no pupillary dilatation occurs when hydroxyamphetamine is applied.

Cocaine is a topically effective anesthetic when applied to the eye or to mucous membranes. Sympathomimetic effects are produced by the prevention of norepinephrine reuptake at the neuromuscular junction, thus prolonging or enhancing the action of norepinephrine which produces pupillary dilation. Rarely, cocaine is used in children's eyes for its topical anesthetic effects (described herein). The commonly used concentrations for children are 4% or less. Ten percent solutions are often used in adults but should be avoided in children (13). Repeated applications of cocaine to the cornea result in the disruption of corneal epithelium, with sloughing of epithelial cells. This ability of cocaine to soften and slough corneal epithelium makes the drug useful as a deepithelializing agent at the time of ocular surgery, e.g., removing opaque epithelium to permit an adequate view of the chamber angle as a prelude to goniotomy or removing epithelium before performance of corneal grafting procedures. Many undesirable and potentially dangerous side effects of cocaine may occur, including hypertension, tachycardia, confusion, arrhythmias, and seizures.

The clinical usefulness of the sympathomimetic activity of cocaine in the eye is to confirm that anisocoria is due to sympathetic denervation. Although originally conceived as a test that would cause pupillary dilation if a first- or second-order neuron was responsible for the Horner syndrome, cocaine does not serve to localize a Horner syndrome to a pre- or postganglionic site. Cocaine will dilate a normal pupil (by blocking norepinephrine reuptake), but will not dilate a Horner pupil (since no norepinephrine is being released at the neuromuscular junction) and may therefore be used to confirm that a Horner pupil is present but not to localize the site of the lesion. Minimal dilation may occur when cocaine is applied to an eye when a first-order neuron lesion is present, but dilation is insignificant and of doubtful clinical value unless to suggest that the sympathetic denervation is incomplete.

Sympathomimetic Agents and Concentrations Available for Topical Use in the Eye

Epinephrine: 0.25%, 0.5%, 1% and 2% drops
Dipivefrin: 0.1%
Aproclonidine: 1% drops
Phenylephrine: 1%, 2.5% and 10% drops
Hydroxyamphetamine: 1% drops
Cocaine: 4% and 10% drops (formulated)

REFERENCES

1. *Webster's Medical Desk Dictionary.* Pease, RW, Jr., ed. Springfield MA: Merriam-Webster, 1986;790.
2. Katzung BG, ed. *Basic and Clinical Pharmacology,* 6th ed. Norwalk, CT: Appleton and Lange, 1995;1046.
3. Isenberg S, Everett S. Cardiovascular effects of mydriatics in low-birth-weight infants. *J Pediatr* 1984;105:111–112.
4. Sindel BD, Baker MD, Maisels MJ, Weinstein J. A comparison of the pupillary and cardiovascular effects of various mydriatic agents in preterm infants. *J Pediatr Ophthalmol Strabismus* 1986;23:273–276.

5. Maloney WF, Younge BR, Moyer NJ. Evaluation of the causes and accuracy of evaluation of pharmacologic localization in Horner's syndrome. *Am J Ophthalmol* 1980;90:394.
6. Carpel EF, Kalina RE. Pupillary responses to mydriatic agents in premature infants. *Am J Ophthalmol* 1973;75:988–991.
7. Vadot E, Piasentin D. Incidence of allergy to eyedrops. Results of a prospective survey in a hospital milieu (in French). *J Fr Ophthalmol* 1986;9:41–43.
8. Van der Spek AF. Cyanosis and cardiovascular depression in a neonate: complications of halothane anesthesia or phenylephrine eyedrops? *Can J Ophthalmol* 1987;22:37–39.
9. Borromeo-McGrail V, Bordiuk JM, Keiter H. Systemic hypertension following ocular administration of 10% phenylephrine in the neonate. *Pediatrics* 1973;51:1032–1036.
10. Brodsky MC, Baker RS, Hamed LM. *Pediatric neuro-ophthalmology,* 1st ed. New York: Springer, 1995;491.
11. Salvesen R, Fredriksen TA, Bogucki A, Sjaastad O. Sweat gland and pupillary responsiveness in Horner's syndrome. *Cephalalgia* 1987;7: 135–146.
12. Heitman K, Bode DD. The paredrine test in normal eyes. A controlled study. *J Clin Neuroophthalmol* 1986;6:228–231.
13. Altman B. Drugs in pediatric ophthalmology. In: Harley RD, ed. *Pediatric Ophthalmology.* Philadelphia: WB Saunders, 1983;82–107.

Textbook of Ocular Pharmacology,
edited by T.J. Zimmerman, et al.
Lippincott–Raven Publishers, Philadelphia © 1997.

CHAPTER 66

Cycloplegic Agents

Forrest D. Ellis

CYCLOPLEGIC AGENTS

Definitions

Cholinergic: *adj.* liberating or activated by acetylcholine (ACh). Cycloplegia: *n.* paralysis of the ciliary muscle of the eye. Cycloplegic: *adj.* producing, involving, or characterized by cycloplegia. Cycloplegic: *n.* a cycloplegic agent. Muscarine: *n.* an ammonium base related to choline. Muscarinic: *adj.* relating to, resembling, producing, or mediating the effects that are produced on organs and tissues by ACh liberated by postganglionic nerve fibers of the parasympathetic nervous system and that are mimicked by muscarine. Nicotinic: *adj.* relating to, resembling, producing, or mediating the effects that are produced by ACh liberated by nerve fibers at autonomic ganglia and at the neuromuscular junctions of voluntary muscle and that are mimicked by nicotine, which increases activity in small doses and inhibits it in larger doses (1).

Cycloplegic agents used in the eyes of children include tropicamide, cyclopentolate, scopolamine, homatropine, and atropine.

Chemical Structure

Tropicamide benzeneacetamide is *N*-ethyl-α-(hydroxymethyl)-*N*-(4-pyridinylmethyl).

Cyclopentolate is 2-(dimethylamino)ethyl 1-hydroxy-α-phenylcyclopentaneacetaate hydrochloride

Scopolamine is benzene acetic acid, α-(hydroxymethyl)-, 9-methyl-3-oxa-9-azatricyclo(3.3.2.O^{2,4})non-7-yl ester, hydrobromide, trihydrate, (7(*S*)-(1α, 2β, 4β,5α,7β)).

Homatropine is benzeneacetic acid, α-hydroxy-,8-methyl-8-azabicyclo(3.2.1)-oct-3-yl ester, hydrobromide, *endo*-(±).

F. D. Ellis: Department of Ophthalmology, Indiana University, Indianapolis, Indiana 46202.

Atropine is benzene acetic acid, α-(hydroxymethyl)-,8-methyl-8-azabicyclo-(3.2.1)oct-3-yl ester, endo-(±), sulfate (2 : 1) (salt), monohydrate.

Pharmacology

Antagonists of muscarinic and nicotinic receptors, the cycloplegic agents have specific receptor blockade affinities. Nicotinic receptor blockade effects are of little use in management of ocular disorders and are not further discussed herein. The antimuscarinic effects of cycloplegic agents, frequently termed parasympatholytic agents, are of paramount importance in management of ocular problems. These drugs are more accurately described as antimuscarinic agents (2). These agents are derived from or are chemically related to the naturally occurring alkaloids in plants and are generically described as tertiary ammonium alkaloid esters of tropic acid. These drugs are easily absorbed through conjunctiva and other mucous membranes.

Cycloplegic agents dilate the pupil through their "parasympatholytic" effects on the constrictor muscles of the iris (cholinoreceptor blockade), leaving the action of the dilator muscles unopposed and therefore creating dilation as well as blocking receptors in the ciliary muscle, thus producing relaxation of accommodation. Drugs in this class act by blocking cholinergics at muscarinic receptor sites. Apparently this is a competitive blockade and is therefore dose dependent (2).

Clinical Pharmacology

Cycloplegic agents are used in children primarily to paralyze accommodation temporarily and secondarily to effect dilation of the pupil. Systemic effects diminish rapidly, but the effects on the pupil dissipate more slowly, lasting hours to days depending on the drug used and the susceptibility of the patient to the medication. Susceptibility appears to be due in large part to the amount of melanin present in the iris (3). More darkly pigmented irides dilate more slowly and recover more rapidly.

Therapeutic Use

Agents are considered in order of their increasing duration of action or paralyzing accommodation.

Tropicamide

Tropicamide is one of the most used topical medications in children. It is a weak cycloplegic agent with a rapid onset of action and few side effects (4). Although accommodation may be paralyzed incompletely, tropicamide remains a useful agent to relax accommodation and dilate the pupil for refractions in children, particularly if distance fixation can be achieved by the child during retinoscopy (5,6). Adverse reactions to tropicamide have not been reported, although confusion or hyperactivity is believed to be occasionally associated with its use.

Cyclopentolate

Cyclopentolate is the cycloplegic agent of choice for relaxation of accommodation in children's eyes. Peak paralysis time of about 45 to 60 minutes allows adequate cycloplegia for most purposes. Persistence of pupillary dilation may last 24 hours in lightly pigmented irides. Cyclopentolate may be toxic to young children, especially to neonates and premature infants. This toxicity is dose dependent and is influenced by the rate and ease of absorption of the drug. Therefore, an intact corneal epithelium and darkly pigmented irides are deterrents to rapid or cumulative absorption of the drug. Side effects include flushing, temperature elevation, hyperactivity, somnolence, delirium, seizures, hallucinations, feeding intolerance, and necrotizing enterocolitis (7).

Gastrointestinal effects are minimized in young infants by withholding feeding before administration of the medication or the ocular examination (8). Hypersensitivity or allergic reaction to the medication may occur (9). Side effects appear to have diminished since most clinicians have abandoned the use of 2% cyclopentolate in favor of 0.5% or 1% solutions, although the 2% strength remains in use.

Homatropine

Homatropine is similar in action to atropine and cannot be used as a substitute when atropine allergy occurs. Because the onset and duration of cycloplegia are shorter in time than that of atropine, homatropine is preferred when a moderate duration of action is desired.

Scopolamine

Scopolamine is substituted for atropine when atropine allergy or hypersensitivity reactions occur or when a moderately long duration of action is desired. Restlessness, psychosis, and hallucinations have been reported.

Atropine

Atropine is the gold standard by which other cycloplegic and mydriatic agents are judged, since it has not only the longest history of use but also the longest and most complete effect on the pupil and on the ciliary muscle. Side effects include follicular conjunctivitis, eczematoid dermatitis, temperature elevation, hypotension, respiratory depression, delirium, and death (10). A significant incidence of contact dermatitis occurs with atropine, possibly as high as 6% (11). Because of the long delay in its onset and its prolonged duration of action, atropine is not used in routine office procedures but is reserved for cases in which dilation of the pupil has not been accomplished by other means or in which prolonged paralysis of the ciliary muscle is desired.

Cycloplegic Agents and Strengths Available for Topical Use in the Eye

Tropicamide: 0.5% and 1% solutions
Cyclopentolate: 0.2% (with phenylephrine 1% as Cyclomydril), 1%, and 2% solutions
Homatropine: 2% and 5% solutions
Scopolamine: 0.25% solution
Atropine: 0.5% and 1% solutions

REFERENCES

1. *Webster's Medical Desk Dictionary.* Pease, RW, Jr., ed. Springfield, MA: Merriam-Webster, 1986;790.
2. Katzung BG, ed. *Basic and Clinical Pharmacology,* 6th ed. Norwalk, CT: Appleton and Lange, 1995;1046.
3. Salazar-Bookaman MM, Wainer I, Patil PN. Relevance of drug-melanin interactions to ocular pharmacology and toxicology. *J Ocul Pharmacol* 1994;10:217–239.
4. Walti H, Daoud P, Broussin B, et al. Cardiovascular and digestive effects of 2 mydriatics in the low-birth-weight newborn infant (in French). *Arch Fr Pediatr* 1987;44:31–33.
5. Egashira SM, Kish LL, Twelker JD, et al. Comparison of cyclopentolate versus tropicamide cycloplegia in children. *Optom Vis Sci* 1993;70:1019–1026.
6. Rosenfield M, Linfield PB. A comparison of the effects of cycloplegics on accommodation ability for distance vision and on the apparent near point. *Ophthalmic Physiol Optom* 1986;6:317–320.
7. Hermansen MC, Sullivan LS. Feeding intolerance following ophthalmologic examination. *Am J Dis Child* 1985;139:367–368.
8. Hermansen MC, Hasan S. Abolition of feeding intolerance following ophthalmologic examination of neonates. *J Pediatr Ophthalmol Strabismus* 1985;22:256–257.

9. Jones LW, Hodes DT. Possible allergic reactions to cyclopentolate hydrochloride: case reports with literature review of uses and adverse reactions. *Ophthalmic Physiol Optom* 1991;11:16–21.
10. *Physicians' Desk Reference for Ophthalmology,* 23rd ed. Sifton DW, ed. Montvale, NJ: Medical Economic Data Production, 1995.
11. Vadot E, Piasentin D. Incidence of allergy to eyedrops. Results of a prospective survey in a hospital milieu (in French). *J Fr ophtalmol* 1986;9:41–43.

Textbook of Ocular Pharmacology,
edited by T.J. Zimmerman, et al.
Lippincott–Raven Publishers, Philadelphia © 1997.

CHAPTER 67

Topical and Local Anesthetic Agents

Forrest D. Ellis

TOPICAL AND LOCAL ANESTHETIC AGENTS

Definition

Anesthetic agents are agents that produce surface anesthesia when applied in drop form to the eye or anesthetize a regional area when administered by injection. Topical or local anesthetic agents which may be used in children include proparacaine, tetracaine, bupivicaine, lidocaine, and cocaine.

Chemical Structure

Local anesthetic agents are weak bases consisting of a lipophilic group connected by an intermediate chain (an ester or an amide) to an ionizable group. Esters generally have a shorter duration of action (1). The agent exists as a larger charged (cationic) and smaller uncharged fraction. The cationic fraction is believed to be the most active but cannot readily transit the cell wall, which it must penetrate to be effective. The uncharged portion of the agent facilitates entry but is less available in the presence of inflammation, during which the pH of tissue fluids is lower and less of this nonionized fraction of the drug is available for diffusion into the cell (1).

Anesthetic agents have effects when applied topically to mucous membranes or when injected into tissues. Local and topical anesthetic agents act reversibly to block axonal conduction of nerve impulses and act on other membranes utilizing sodium channels. Cocaine was the first such agent to be isolated (1860) and was introduced to ophthalmology in 1884 (1,2). Cocaine and the next available topical anesthetic agent, procaine, dominated the local anesthetic scene for the first 80 years, as has lidocaine for the last 50 years. Lidocaine is now considered the standard with which other local anesthetic agents are compared.

F. D. Ellis: Department of Ophthalmology, Indiana University, Indianapolis, Indiana 46202.

Clinical Pharmacology

Local and topical anesthetic agents are selected for use in a given case based on their (lack of) toxicity and on their duration of action. Generally, in the eye, topical anesthetic agents with short duration of action are preferred. Proparacaine is the topical agent generally used for office procedures; tetracaine or cocaine are more likely to be used for surgical procedures. In part, these preferences are due to packaging, costs, and control rather than to physiologic differences among the drugs.

All topical anesthetic agents are potentially subject to abuse by certain patients and are not prescribed for self-administration. Because adverse reactions are potentially more serious in young children, appropriate dosage of these medications is particularly important. Any of the locally administered anesthetic agents will be absorbed systemically and may produce side effects. Excessive absorption of these agents may produce CNS symptoms of dizziness, visual and auditory disturbances, nystagmus, and seizures. A stage of excitement followed by CNS depression and death may result from high blood levels of these agents. When they have been administered as retrobulbar anesthesia, direct penetration of the optic nerve sheath with subsequent optic atrophy, spread to the opposite eye with bulbar signs and transient bilateral blindness, CNS depression, and death have occurred (3). Extraocular muscle penetration has resulted in horizontal and vertical strabismus (4).

All topical and local anesthetic agents depress cardiac activity and excitability, lower blood pressure, and dilate arterioles, except for cocaine which may produce arrhythmias, hypertension, and vasoconstriction. Occasionally, severe or fatal effects occur after doses that would not be expected to be toxic. Route of administration and method of absorption remain speculative in these cases.

Bupivicaine appears to be more toxic than other local anesthetic agents, and several case reports of serious or fatal consequences from bupivicaine have been published.

Prilocaine has produced methemoglobinemia through conversion to the metabolite *o*-toluidine.

Allergic Reactions

Ester types of local anesthetic agents are metabolized to *p*-aminobenzoic acid, which produces allergic reactions in some patients. Amides are not so metabolized and therefore rarely produce allergic reactions.

Therapeutic Use

Topical and local anesthetic agents permit minor surgical procedures to be accomplished without incurring the risks and expense of general anesthesia, but have limited usefulness in children who are unable to cooperate or to understand what is about to occur. Many pediatric ophthalmologists use proparacaine topically as a routine part of the administration of mydriatic or cycloplegic agents and for anesthesia so that intraocular pressure (IOP) can be measured.

Proparacaine Hydrochloride

Proparacaine hydrochloride 0.5% is a popular topical anesthetic agent which often is used in conjunction with topically applied mydriatic and cycloplegic agents, for minor corneal or conjunctival procedures such as removal of foreign bodies, or for diagnostic and therapeutic corneal and conjunctival scrapings. Rapid onset of anesthesia and rapid recovery make this a useful agent for office procedures. Onset of action is within seconds, and duration of action is approximately 35 minutes until the preanesthetized state is regained, but may be prolonged if the cornea is hypesthetic for other reasons (5). Clinically, recovery from a single drop of proparacaine requires approximately 11 minutes (6).

Proparacaine may be used as the anesthetic agent for strabismus surgery in selected adults. Possible side effects of proparacaine use include epithelial keratitis, pupillary dilation, and contact dermatitis. Seizures have been reported to occur after instillation of proparacaine (7). Epithelial changes may be advantageous when proparacaine is used in combination with dilating drops by allowing more rapid transcorneal passage and, through anesthetic effects, reducing reflex tearing otherwise produced by the irritation of mydriatic and cycloplegic agents. The effect of mydriatic and cycloplegic agents applied after the cornea is preanesthetized is prolonged (8). In adults, the rate of onset of cycloplegia was not accelerated by preadministration of proparacaine (9). The effectiveness of proparacaine in enhancing ocular penetration by other drugs such as carbonic anhydrase inhibitors remains controversial, however (10). When used as a deepithelializing agent, proparacaine produced a prolonged keratocyte loss equivalent to that of 100% ethanol. This loss was much greater than the loss produced by scraping the cornea, with use of 4% cocaine or the excimer laser, although the inflammatory response was less with proparacaine than with other agents (11).

Proparacaine is often used as a part of the technique of administering other anesthetic agents, particularly with the advent of peribulbar anesthesia and the cannula technique for administration of retrobulbar anesthetic agents (12,13).

Tetracaine

Tetracaine is a popular topical anesthetic agent which is also available for injection. Tetracaine is packaged for topical delivery in a small sterile dispenser, which makes it popular and cost-effective for surgical procedures. Tetracaine appears to be less desirable than proparacaine in terms of pain on instillation and duration of action; tetracaine is more irritating and its effects last approximately 9.5 minutes, whereas proparacaine's effects last 10.7 minutes (2,6).

Lidocaine

Lidocaine administered by injection is a useful and popular local anesthetic agent used before certain surgical procedures. Its effects last 40 to 60 minutes but can be extended by adding epinephrine to the solution, usually in a dilution of 1 : 200,000. The maximum dose of lidocaine in children is 4.5 mg/kg as a 0.25% to 0.5% solution.

Bupivicaine

Bupivicaine injection is used when prolonged local anesthesia effects are desired. This agent is believed to be more toxic than other popular local anesthetic agents, and several adverse reactions have occurred (3). Because bupivicaine is more toxic in adults, it is seldom used in children unless severe and prolonged pain is expected, such as occurs after cyclocryotherapy. No information is available on effects in children aged less than 12 years. However, 0.5 to 1.0 ml of 0.75% bupivicaine mixed with an equal volume of 1% lidocaine has been used for pain control at the conclusion of cyclocryotherapy in children as young as 5 years of age (0.3 mg/kg for a 5-year-old child weighing 18 kg), without adverse effects (personal experience).

Bupivicaine has been evaluated as a potential topical preparation and appears to have an onset of action similar to that of proparacaine, but is less toxic to the epithelium than proparacaine (14). Bupivicaine is not available as a topical agent.

Cocaine

Cocaine is used for local anesthesia and for vasoconstriction of nasal mucous membranes. Nasal packing may be saturated with cocaine for nasolacrimal intubation or for dacryocystorhinostomy. It may be used to deepithelize the cornea for glaucoma procedures or for lamellar corneal grafts. The epithelial toxicity of cocaine become apparent soon after its introduction as a topical anesthetic agent. In part, subsequent topical anesthetic development was an effort to minimize the epithelial toxicity of cocaine while preserving its anesthetic effects. In vitro studies suggest that cocaine may be less toxic than proparacaine and tetracaine (compared on an equimolar basis), but toxicity in vivo may be increased because of the higher concentrations required to produce the same degree of anesthesia (2). Toxic levels can be reached quickly in children, and caution is advised in its administration, even at lower concentrations. No usefulness for strengths greater than 4% has been established in children.

Available Preparations

Bupivicaine: 0.25%, 0.5%, and 0.75% for injection; also available with 1 : 200,000 epinephrine
Chloroprocaine: 1%, 2%, and 3% for injection
Cocaine: topical; compounded; usual strength 2%, 4%, or 10% solutions
Dyclonine: topical 0.5% and 1% solutions
Etidocaine: 1% for injection; also available as 1% and 1.5% with epinephrine 1 : 200,000
Lidocaine: 0.5%, 1%, 1.5%, 2%, 4%, 10%, and 20% for injection; also available as 0.5%, 1%, 1.5%, and 2% with epinephrine 1 : 200,000
Mepivacaine: 1%, 1.5%, 2%, and 3% for injection; also available as 2% with 1 : 20,000 levonordefrin
Prilocaine: 4% for injection; also 4% with 1 : 200,000 epinephrine
Procaine: 1%, 2%, and 10% for injection
Tetracaine: Topical 0.5% solution; 1% for injection

REFERENCES

1. Katzung BG, ed. *Basic and Clinical Pharmacology,* 6th ed. Norwalk, CT: Appleton and Lange, 1995;1046.
2. Grant RL, Acosta D. Comparative toxicity of tetracaine, proparacaine and cocaine evaluated with primary cultures of rabbit corneal epithelial cells. *Exp Eye Res* 1994;58:469–478.
3. Edge KR, Davis A. Brainstem anaesthesia following a peribulbar block for eye surgery. *Anaesth Intensive Care* 1995;23:219–221.
4. Hamed LM, Helveston EM, Ellis FD. Persistent binocular diplopia after cataract surgery. *Am J Ophthalmol* 1987;103:741–744.
5. Weiss JS, Goren MB. The effect of corneal hypesthesia on the duration of proparacaine anesthetic eyedrops. *Am J Ophthalmol* 1991;112: 326–330.
6. Bartfield JM, Holmes TJ, Raccio-Robak N. A comparison of proparacaine and tetracaine eye anesthetics. *Acad Emerg Med* 1994;1:364–367.
7. Cydulka RK, Betzelos S. Seizures following the use of proparacaine hydrochloride eye drops. *J Emerg Med* 1990;8:131–133.
8. Mordi JA, Lyle WM, Mousa GY. Does prior instillation of a topical anesthetic enhance the effect of tropicamide? *Am J Optom Physiol Opt* 1986;63:290–293.
9. Lovasik JV. Pharmacokinetics of topically applied cyclopentolate HCl and tropicamide. *Am J Optom Physiol Opt* 1986;63:787–803.
10. Bar-Ilan A, Pessah NI. The effects of topical and general anesthesia on ocular drug levels and intraocular pressure lowering activity of topically applied carbonic anhydrase inhibitors. *J Ocul Pharmacol* 1988;4:1–12.
11. Campos M, et al. Keratocyte loss after different methods of de-epithelialization. *Ophthalmology* 1994;101:890–894.
12. Brady MD, Hustead RR, Robinson RH, Becker KE, Jr. Dilution of proparacaine in balanced salt solution reduces pain of anesthetic instillation in the eye. *Reg Anesth* 1994;19: 196–198.
13. Coelho ET, Gomes EB, Martins HS, deSousa B. Prilocaine: an old anesthetic agent and a new ophthalmic procedure. *Ophthalmic Surg* 1993;24:612–616.
14. Liu JC, Steinemann TL, McDonald MB, et al. Topical bupivacaine and proparacaine: a comparison of toxicity, onset of action, and duration of action. *Cornea* 1993;12:228– 232.

Textbook of Ocular Pharmacology,
edited by T.J. Zimmerman, et al.
Lippincott–Raven Publishers, Philadelphia © 1997.

CHAPTER 68

Antiglaucoma Medications

Forrest D. Ellis

ANTIGLAUCOMA MEDICATIONS

Definitions

An antiglaucoma medication is any of a class of medications known to have a beneficial (pressure-lowering) effect on the intraocular pressure (IOP) (1). β-Adrenergic: *adj.* of, relating to, or being a β-receptor. β-blocker: *n.* an agent that combines with and blocks the activity of a β-receptor. α-Adrenergic: *adj.* of, relating to, or being an α-receptor. Cholinomimetic: *adj.* resembling acetylcholine (ACh) or simulating its physiologic action. Carbonic anhydrase: *n.* a zinc-containing enzyme that occurs in living tissue and aids carbon-dioxide transport . . . by catalyzing the reversible hydration of carbon dioxide to carbonic acid (1).

Glaucoma agents which might be used in children include β-blockers (timolol, levobunalol, betaxolol, metripranolol, carteolol), α-agonists, nonselective (epinephrine, dipivefrin), α_2-selective (aproclonidine), cholinomimetics (pilocarpine, physostigmine, carbachol, ecothiophate, isofluorophate), dichlophenamide, methazolamide, dorzolamide).

Chemical Structure

The β-receptor antagonist drugs resemble isoproterenol. α-Agonists (nonselective) are epinephrine or are converted to epinephrine. α_2-Selective agonists are apraclonidine 2-[4(4-amino-2,6,dichlorophenyl) imino]imidazolidine monohydrochloride. Cholinomimetics resemble ACh in structure and function either through direct cholinergic action or through inhibition of cholinesterase activity. Carbonic anhydrase inhibitors are sulfonamide derivatives.

F. D. Ellis: Department of Ophthalmology, Indiana University, Indianapolis, Indiana 46202.

Clinical Pharmacology

β-Blocking agents occupy β-receptor sites and competitively reduce receptor occupancy by catecholamines and other β-agonists. Agents such as timolol and levobunolol are considered nonselective blocking agents, whereas agents such as betaxolol are considered β_1-selective in their affinity for receptor sites. In the eye, pressure-lowering effects of these agents result from decreased aqueous production. These drugs also lower blood pressure and increase airway resistance, particularly in patients with a history of asthma. Effects of different drugs in this class on ocular hemodynamics are under investigation (2).

α-Agonists (nonselective) act through stimulation of α_1- and α_2-receptors, producing increased aqueous outflow and pupillary dilation. α_2-Selective agonists such as apraclonidine act directly and primarily but not exclusively on α_2-receptors. The mechanism of action is not completely understood, but aqueous production is decreased.

Cholinomimetics simulate the action of ACh or inhibit cholinesterase, mechanically opening the spaces of the trabecular meshwork and improving aqueous outflow. Carbonic anhydrase inhibitors block the release of bicarbonate from the ciliary epithelium, which serves to decrease aqueous production.

Clinical Uses

Glaucoma is a major cause of blindness in children and adults. Congenital glaucoma is of the open-angle type, and the anterior chamber is always deep unless another mechanism is responsible for the glaucoma. Although the angle is deep, it is obstructed by amorphous tissue or is underdeveloped. Several hundred complex syndromes have associations with congenital glaucoma. Narrow-angle glaucoma, glaucoma secondary to inflammatory processes, pupillary block glaucoma, and neovascular glaucoma also occur in children. Pupillary block glaucoma probably is increasing secondary to the increasing frequency of implantation of intraocular lenses in children. Several cases have been reported (3).

Congenital or infantile glaucoma is a surgical condition best treated with one or more of a variety of surgical procedures. Medical therapy for childhood glaucoma is used only as a temporizing alternative to surgery or as a supplement to surgery. Because many children with congenital glaucoma have other congenital anomalies with a variety of surgical and anesthetic risk factors, definitive surgery either must be delayed or cannot be performed. In other instances, control of IOP after surgery may be unsatisfactory and topical medications may be used to achieve further pressure-lowering effects. However, β-blockers also produce significant side effects, including alterations in heart rate and rhythm, bronchial constriction, dyslipidemia, and CNS abnormalities, as well as abnormal interactions with other drugs (4).

β-Adrenergic Antagonists

Timolol

Timolol maleate, 0.25% or 0.5% solution, a nonselective β-blocker, is used in children. Lower concentrations are used initially and are adjusted according to response and side effects. The most important side effects of timolol result from systemic absorption. Side effects of timolol common to both adults and children include ocular irritation, depression or mood alteration, arrhythmias, and bronchospasm. Recovery from hypoglycemia in patients with insulin-dependent diabetes is at least a theoretical concern (5).

Clinical data are available regarding the effectiveness and complications of timolol in childhood populations. A study of 100 eyes of 67 patients treated with timolol after one or more surgical procedures demonstrated that 40% of the eyes were spared further surgery, which otherwise would have been required (6). Seventy-eight percent of these eyes had pressure decrease induced with medication, and the drop used was more than 10 mm Hg in 45% of the eyes. Seven patients had demonstrable side effects, including 2 who had asthmatic attacks, 2 who manifested dissociative behavior, and 1 who had bradycardia. Another study demonstrated that approximately two-thirds of patients treated with timolol showed improvement of some degree. Slowing of the resting pulse occurred in some children, and 1 child had therapy discontinued because of side effects of the medication (7). Adverse effects of timolol have been well documented and summarized (8). Significant beneficial effects from timolol in the pediatric population can be expected, generally without serious side effects (9).

Timolol has been tried in children for prevention of progression of myopia, but without demonstrably beneficial results (10,11). Studies have demonstrated a significant reduction in accommodative convergence during the initial 4 minutes of a near-vision task in young adults with emmetropia treated with timolol but not those with myopia (12).

Levobunolol

Levobunolol 0.5% is a nonselective β-adrenergic antagonist similar to timolol. A larger drop size, 50 μl, is delivered, as compared with the 35-μl drop size of timolol. Drop size has potential significance both with regard to systemic absorption in children (and adults) and to cost of the drug (13). Relatively little information exists pertaining specifically to use of levobunolol in children. Adult studies involving young healthy adults suggest significant cardiovascular effects with an increase in mean exercise duration during treatment (14). Information suggests that levobunolol is superior to carteolol in reducing IOP while producing fewer cardiovascular side effects in adults, which suggests that levobunolol might be a better choice for children than carteolol (15). Instances of heart block have been attributed to levobunolol (16).

Single case reports suggest the benefit of occasional use of levobunolol after pediatric pupilloplasty with neodymium (Nd):YAG laser, without side effects (17). Timolol may be better tolerated than levobunolol (18). Blepharitis has been reported (19,20). In a 4-year evaluation of the efficacy and safety of glaucoma treatment with timolol and levobunolol, investigators concluded that levobunolol is relatively effective and relatively safe for long-term (4 years) treatment of glaucoma in adults. Little difference was noted between the effectiveness of 0.5% and 1.0% levobunolol and 0.5% timolol (21).

Betaxolol

Betaxolol 0.5% is a selective β_1-adrenoreceptor antagonist with very weak β-blocking capability (22). As compared with timolol and levobunolol, this drug appears to have fewer bronchopulmonary or cardiac effects. It has negligible local anesthetic effect, but local irritation occurs in 25% to 40% of adult patients (22). The apparent lower propensity for cardiovascular effects in adults might make the drug a better choice for use in children, but no specific data pertaining to children are available.

Metipranolol

Metipranolol is a nonselective β-blocker that has been used in treatment of childhood glaucoma; it has also been applied in treatment of progressive myopia. Myopia treatment remains unproven and controversial, but small studies have suggested possible benefits (23). Serious side effects from metipranolol have been reported in adults, making the choice of this medication for use in children seem unwise. Pulmonary edema was reported in an adult (24). Granulomatous uveitis has been reported in adults (25,26). Other adverse reactions, as well as the reported loss or escape from pressure control in adults, probably makes this drug unsuitable for the pediatric population (27).

Carteolol

Carteolol 1% has nonselective β-blocking capabilities. It is the only drug in this class that has intrinsic sympathomimetic activity (4,28). Whether or not this attribute would make this a more useful or safer drug for children is unknown.

α-Agonists: Epinephrine and Dipivefrin

Epinephrine and dipivefrin produce IOP-lowering effects through unselected α-agonist activity, thereby increasing aqueous outflow. Dipivefrin is a prodrug of epinephrine and passes more readily through the cornea than does epinephrine. Both drugs are available in concentrations stronger than are therapeutically required, making an excess of each drug available to the general circulation, with the potential for adverse cardiovascular effects. Serious cardiovascular side effects of these medications have been reported in children and in adults (29). Zimmerman has suggested that concentrations of 0.05% dipivefrin and 0.5% epinephrine might produce adequate IOP-lowering effects with fewer systemic effects (30). In vitro studies also suggest a cellular toxic effect with higher concentrations of epinephrine (31). As many as 60% of patients receiving dipivefrin and 66% of those receiving epinephrine report side effects (32). When possible, these agents should be avoided or used with caution in infants and young children.

α_2-Selective Agonists

Apraclonidine

Apraclonidine, 0.25% and 0.50% solutions, acts as a selective α_2-agonist, reducing IOP by decreasing aqueous production (33). Apraclonidine has been shown to be an effective pressure-lowering drug with few systemic effects in adults (34). Nevertheless, the incidence of local allergic reactions requiring discontinuation of the drug is high, ranging to 48% (35). As compared with timolol in healthy adult volunteers, apraclonidine did not affect blood pressure or heart rate (as did timolol) but caused a comparable reduction in IOP (36). Present and anticipated use of apraclonidine in children consists of temporary use for postcataract or postlaser capsulotomy IOP control.

Cholinomimetics

Pilocarpine

Pilocarpine (0.25%, 1%, 2%, 4%, 10%), is a direct-acting cholinergic that reduces IOP by stimulating contraction of the ciliary muscle, which opens the trabecular meshwork and thus increases aqueous outflow. In young persons, brow ache is a significant problem, although tolerance may develop. Concentrations must be increased gradually, but higher doses may remain intolerable. Contraction of the ciliary muscle induces transient myopia. Retinal detachment has been reported after pilocarpine drops and, more recently, after use of a sustained-release form of the drug (37–39).

Carbachol

Carbachol (carbamoycholine) is a carbamic acid ester of choline. Carbachol has the same mechanism of action as pilocarpine and the same side effects. Carbachol is resistant to cholinesterase metabolism. Brow ache, ocular irritation, and decreased vision are the most common side effects.

Echothiophate Iodide

Echothiophate iodide (0.03%, 0.0625%, 0.125%, and 0.25%) is an indirect-acting cholinomimetic agent that inhibits ACh metabolism (cholinesterase), producing contraction of ciliary muscle, pupillary constriction, and opening of the trabecular meshwork, thus increasing aqueous outflow. In children, it is more commonly used for diagnosis, stabilization, or temporary treatment of accommodative esotropia, especially when a high accommodative convergence/accommodative ratio (AC/A) is present in a hyperopic child. Doses of 0.125% or less are administered as a single drop daily in each eye.

Side effects of echothiophate therapy include chronic miosis (persisting after discontinuation of the drug), lens opacities, iris cysts (which can be prevented by adding neosynephrine to the preparation), retinal detachment, excess salivation and perspiration, abdominal cramps, diarrhea, vomiting, bronchial constriction, bradycardia, anxiety, and reduced blood cholinesterase levels (40). Cystoid macular edema has been reported in an adult (41). Use of depolarizing muscle relaxants in patients receiving chronic echothiophate therapy may cause prolonged paralysis or postanesthesia apnea. Echothiophate is contraindicated in the presence of uveal inflammation, angle closure glaucoma, and high myopia.

Isoflurophate

Isoflurophate is a potent cholinesterase inhibitor similar in all respects to echothiophate except that it is packaged in ointment form and is preferred by many pediatric ophthalmologists for use in children with hyperopia and high AC/A ratios.

Carbonic Anhydrase Inhibitors

Carbonic anhydrase inhibitors are sulfonamide derivatives that inhibit aqueous production, making them useful in management of pediatric glaucoma. Carbonic anhydrase inhibitors profoundly depress bicarbonate reabsorption by the proximal tubule of the kidney, thus promoting diuresis. The ciliary epithelium of the eye secretes bicarbonate into the aqueous humor in the process of aqueous production. Bicarbonate reabsorption from proximal renal tubules into the bloodstream is blocked by carbonic anhydrase inhibitors; in the eye, the secretion into the aqueous is blocked. Inhibition of bicarbonate secretion reduces aqueous production and reduces IOP.

Parenteral preparations of carbonic anhydrase inhibitors are used only as short-term therapy in infants because metabolic acidosis and electrolyte imbalances are easily produced. Side effects of carbonic anhydrase inhibitors include transient myopia, metallic or unpleasant taste or smell, parasthesias, anorexia, nausea, vomiting, diarrhea, fatigue, renal calculi, Stevens-Johnson syndrome, and aplastic anemia. Carbonic anhydrase inhibitors are contraindicated in patients with reduced sodium or potassium serum levels, severe liver or kidney disease, adrenal failure, or hyperchloremic acidosis. Aplastic anemia has been reported (42).

Topical carbonic anhydrase inhibitors are now available. Alteration of the sulfonamide group to permit penetration of the cornea while minimizing irritation and discomfort has produced a topical agent potentially useful in children. Apparently, increasing ionization of the drug increases the ocular hypotensive effectiveness (43).

Available Preparations

β-Blockers
- Betaxolol: 0.25% drops
- Carteolol: 1% drops
- Levobunolol: 0.5% drops
- Metipranolol: 0.3% drops
- Timolol: 0.25%, 0.5% drops

α-Agonists
- Epinephrine: 0.5%, 1%, and 2% drops
- Dipivefrin: 0.1% drops

α_2-Selective agonists
- Apraclonidine: 1% drops

Cholinomimetics
- Carbachol: 0.75%, 1.5%, 2.25%, and 3% drops
- Pilocarpine: 0.25%, 0.5%, 1%, 2%, 3%, 4%, 5%, 6%, 8%, and 10% drops

Cholinesterase inhibitors
- Physostigmine: 0.25% and 0.5% drops
- Demecarium: 0.25% and 0.5% drops
- Echothiophate iodide: 0.03%, 0.06%, 0.125%, and 0.25% drops
- Isofluorophate: 0.025% ointment

Carbonic anhydrase inhibitors
- Dorzolamide hydrochloride: 2% drops
- Acetazolamide: 125- and 250-mg tablets; 500-mg timed-release capsules
- Acetazolamide sodium: 500 mg powder for injection (parenteral)
- Dichlorphenamide: 50-mg tablets
- Methazolamide: 25- and 50-mg tablets

REFERENCES

1. *Webster's Medical Desk Dictionary.* Pease RW, Jr., ed. Springfield MA: Merriam-Webster, 1986;790.
2. Harris A, Speth GL, Sergott RC, et al. Retrobulbar arterial hemodynamic effects of betaxolol and timolol in normal-tension glaucoma. *Am J Ophthalmol* 1995;120: 168–175.
3. Vajpayee RB, Angra SK, Titiyal JS, et al. Pseudophakic pupillary-block glaucoma in children. *Am J Ophthalmol* 1991;111:715–718.
4. Frishman WH, Fuksbrumer MS, Tannenbaum M. Topical ophthalmic beta-adrenergic blockade for the treatment of glaucoma and ocular hypertension. *J Clin Pharmacol* 1994;34:795–803.
5. Katzung BG, ed. *Basic and Clinical Pharmacology,* 6th ed. Norwalk, CT: Appleton and Lange, 1995;1046.
6. Hoskins HD, Hetherington J, Magee SD, et al. Clinical experience with timolol in childhood glaucoma. *Arch Ophthalmol* 1985;103: 1163–1165.
7. Boger WP, Walton DS. Timolol in uncontrolled childhood glaucomas. *Ophthalmology* 1981;3:253–258.
8. Zimmerman TJ, Leader BJ, Golob DS. Potential side effects of timolol therapy in the treatment of glaucoma. *Ann Ophthalmol* 1981;13: 683–689.
9. Zimmerman TJ, Kooner KS, Morgan KS. Safety and efficacy of timolol in pediatric glaucoma. *Surv Ophthalmol* 1983;28:262–264.
10. Goldschmidt E. Myopia in humans: can progression be arrested? *Ciba Found Symp* 1990;155:222–229.
11. Hosaka A. Myopia prevention and therapy. The role of pharmaceutical agents. Japanese studies. *Acta Ophthalmol Suppl* 1988;185:130–131.
12. Rosenfield M, Gilmartin B. Beta-adrenergic receptor antagonism in myopia. *Ophthalmic Physiol Opt* 1987;7:359–364.
13. Meyer MA, Savitt ML. A comparison of timolol maleate and levobunolol. Length of use per 5-ml bottle. *Ophthalmology* 1994;101: 1658–1661.
14. Weiser BA, Feldman F, Ananthanarayan CR,. Cardiovascular effects of levobunolol eyedrops in healthy subjects. *Can J Ophthalmol* 1991; 26:211–214.
15. Behrens-Baumann W, Kimmich F, Walt JG, Lue J. A comparison of the ocular hypotensive efficacy and systemic safety of 0.5% levobunolol and 2% carteolol. *Ophthalmologica* 1994;208:32–36.
16. Chun JG, Brodsky MA, Allen BJ. Syncope, bradycardia, and atrioventricular block associated with topical ophthalmic levobunolol. *Am Heart J* 1994;127:689–690.
17. Summers CG, Holland EJ. Neodymium:YAG pupilloplasty in pediatric aphakia. *J Pediatr Ophthalmol Strabismus* 1991;28:155–156.
18. Sharir M, Zimmerman TJ, Crandall AS, Mandir N. A comparison of the ocular tolerability of a single dose of timolol and levobunolol in healthy normotensive volunteers. *Ann Ophthalmol* 1993;25:133–137.
19. Schultheiss E. Hypersensitivity to levobunolol (in German). *Derm Beruf Umwelt* 1989;37:185–186.
20. van der Meeren HL, Meurs PJ. Sensitization to levobunolol eyedrops. *Contact Dermatitis* 1993;28:41–42.
21. The Levobunolol Study Group. Levobunolol. A four-year study of efficacy and safety in glaucoma treatment. *Ophthalmology* 1989;96: 642–645.
22. Buckley MM, Goa KL, Clissold SP. Ocular betaxolol. A review of its pharmacological properties, and therapeutic efficacy in glaucoma and ocular hypertension. *Drugs* 1990;40:75–90.
23. Tiburtius H, Tiburtius K. New treatment possibilities of progressive school myopia (in German). *Klin Monatsbl Augenheilkd* 1991;199: 120–121.
24. Johns MD, Ponte CD. Acute pulmonary edema associated with ocular metipranolol use. *Ann Pharmacother* 1995;29:370–373.
25. Akingbehin T, Villada JR. Metipranolol-associated granulomatous anterior uveitis. *Br J Ophthalmol* 1991;75:519–523.
26. Melles RB, Wong IG. Metipranolol-associated granulomatous iritis. *Am J Ophthalmol* 1994;118:712–715.

27. Akingbehin T, Villada JR. Metipranolol-induced adverse reactions: II. Loss of intraocular pressure control *Eye* 1992;6:280–283.
28. Zimmerman TJ. Topical ophthalmic beta blockers: a comparative review. *J Ocul Pharmacol* 1993;9:373–384.
29. Nelson ME, Andrzejowski AZ. Systemic hypertension in patients receiving dipivalyl adrenaline for glaucoma. *Br Med J* 1988;297:741–742.
30. Zimmerman TJ, Sharir M, Nardin GF, Fugua M. Therapeutic index of epinephrine and dipivefrin with nasolacrimal occlusion. *Am J Ophthalmol* 1992;114:8–13.
31. Tripathi BJ, Tripathi RC, Millard CB. Epinephrin-induced toxicity of human trabecular cells in vitro. *Lens Eye Toxic Res* 1989;6:141–156.
32. Mills KB, Jacobs NA. A single-blind randomized trial comparing adrenaline 1.0% with dipivalyl epinephrine (propine) 0.1% in the treatment of open-angle glaucoma and ocular hypertension. *Br J Ophthalmol* 1988;72:465–468.
33. Toris CB, et al. Effects of apraclonidine on aqueous humor dynamics in human eyes. *Ophthalmology* 1995;102:456–461.
34. Nagasubramanian S, Hitchings RA, Demailly P, et al. Comparison of apraclonidine and timolol in chronic open-angle glaucoma. A three-month study. *Ophthalmology* 1993;100:1318–1323.
35. Butler P, Mannschreck M, Lin S, et al. Clinical experience with the long-term use of 1% apraclonidine. Incidence of allergic reactions. *Arch Ophthalmol* 1995; 113:293–296.
36. Coleman AL, et al. Cardiovascular and intraocular pressure effects and plasma concentrations of apraclonidine. *Arch Ophthalmol* 1990; 108:1264–1267.
37. Weseley P, Liebmann J, Ritch R. Rhegmatogenous retinal detachment after initiation of ocusert therapy [Letter]. *Am J Ophthalmol* 1991; 112:458–459.
38. Reichert RW, Shields MB. Intraocular pressure response to the replacement of pilocarpine or carbachol with echothiophate. *Graefes Arch Clin Exp Ophthalmol* 1991;229:252–253.
39. Benedict WL, Shami M. Impending macular hole associated with topical pilocarpine [Letter]. *Am J Ophthalmol* 1992;114:765–766.
40. Manoguerra A, Whitney C, Clark RF, et al. Cholinergic toxicity resulting from ocular instillation of echothiophate iodide eye drops. *J Toxicol Clin Toxicol* 1995; 33:463–465.
41. Halperin LS, Goldman HB. Cystoid macular edema associated with topical echothiophate iodide. *Ann Ophthalmol* 1993;25:457–458.
42. Fraunfelder FT, Fraunfelder FW. Short-term use of carbonic anhydrase inhibitors and hematologic side effects [Letter]. *Arch Ophthalmol* 1992;110:446–447.
43. Brechue WF, Maren TH. pH and drug ionization affects ocular pressure lowering of topical carbonic anhydrase inhibitors. *Invest Ophthalmol Vis Sci* 1993;34:2581–2587.

Textbook of Ocular Pharmacology,
edited by T.J. Zimmerman, et al.
Lippincott–Raven Publishers, Philadelphia © 1997.

CHAPTER 69

Ocular Antiinflammatory Agents

Forrest D. Ellis

OCULAR ANTIINFLAMMATORY AGENTS

Definitions

Antiinflammatory: *adj.* counteracting inflammation. Corticosteroid: *n.* any of various adrenal-cortex steroids. Glucocorticoid: *n.* any of a group of corticoids . . . that are involved . . . in carbohydrate, protein and fat metabolism, that tend to increase liver glyconeogenesis and blood sugar by increasing glyconeogenesis, that are anti-inflammatory and immunosuppressive, and that are used widely in medicine. . . . Anti-histamine: *adj.* tending to block or counteract the physiological action of histamine (1).

Antiinflammatory agents used topically and systemically for children include corticosteroids (dexamethasone, fluorometholone, medrysone, prednisolone), nonsteroidal anti-inflammatory drugs (NSAIDS) (diclofenac, flurbiprofen, ketorolac, suprofen), and antihistamines (levocabastin, lodoxamide).

Chemical Structure

Corticosteroids

All corticosteroids are related to and derived from the parent compound cortisol. All corticosteroids are 21 carbon molecules consisting of a cyclopentoperhydrophenathrene nucleus, three hexane rings, and one pentane ring. Modifications of the basic structure of these agents alters their ability to penetrate the cornea, their antiinflammatory effectiveness, and their duration of action.

F. D. Ellis: Department of Ophthalmology, Indiana University, Indianapolis, Indiana 46202.

NSAIDS

Diclofenac is 2-[(2,6-dichlorophenyl) amino]benzeneacetic acid (a phenylacetic acid derivative). Flurbiprofen is a propionic acid derivative. Ketorolac is a member of the pyrrolo-pyrolle group of NSAIDS.

Antihistamines

Levocabastine is (-)-*trans*-1-[*cis*-4-cyano-4-(*p*-fluorophenyl) cyclohexyl]-3-methyl-4-phenylisonipecotic acid monohydrochloride.

Iodoxamide is *N,N'*-(2-chloro-5-cyano-*m*-phenylene) dioxamic acid tromethamine salt naphazoline: 1H-Imidazole,4,5-dihydro-2-(1-naphthalenylmethyl)-,monohydrochloride.

Clinical Pharmacology

Cortisol derivatives have been important in treatment of ocular inflammatory disease for the past 45 years (2). Corticosteroids were used empirically for years before corticosteroid receptors were identified in the eye. The mechanism of action of corticosteroids involves their ability to enter the cell and alter the production of specific protein products.

Therapeutic Use

Antiinflammatory agents have a wide range of therapeutic applications in the eye. Children may require systemic corticosteroids for a variety of inflammatory and immune-related ocular conditions, including ocular allergies; keratitis; corneal graft rejection; anterior, intermediate, and posterior uveitis; and sympathetic ophthalmia. Oral and parenteral corticosteroids are useful in treatment of optic neuritis, particularly neuromyelitis optica, traumatic optic neuropathy, and myasthenia gravis (3,4).

Children receiving long-term corticosteroid therapy are most likely to receive such therapy for a nonocular (primary) disease, such as a severe form of a collagen vascular disease, rather than a specific ocular process requiring long-term administration of these drugs. Ocular inflammatory diseases generally are treated with intensive, high-dose, short-term therapies, with initial use of corticosteroids and substitution of nonsteroidal agents as the inflammation is brought under control.

Corticosteroids are administered topically, deposited in the subconjunctival or sub-Tenon space, administered directly into lesions such as periocular hemangiomas, or administered orally and intravenously. Systemic corticosteroid therapy can have profound systemic adverse effects in children, and topical therapy can produce serious ocular complications.

Pediatric patients may develop growth retardation, Cushing's syndrome, striae, thinning of the skin, osteoporosis, avascular necrosis of the femoral head, myopathy, mood alteration, fluid and electrolyte imbalance, hypertension, duodenal ulcers, decreased immune response, delayed wound healing, hirsutism, and exacerbation of acne. Pseudotumor cerebri occurs in children, occasionally after corticosteroid discontinuation (5).

In the eye, exacerbation of infectious disease, increased intraocular pressure (IOP), and cataract development occur. Complications and risks of these medications in the eye are related to the potency of the medication as well as to the susceptibility of the patient to the medication. In general terms, dexamethasone is the most potent topical agent and the most risky for use in children, whereas fluorometholone is the weakest topical agent and the safest. Achievement of appropriate response must therefore be accompanied by avoidance of preventable complications.

Intralesional Corticosteroids

Intralesional corticosteroids are used for treatment of capillary hemangiomas and also are used occasionally for treatment of recurrent chalazia. Cutaneous hemangiomas are reported to be present in 3% to 8% of all newborn children. Most such lesions are on the face, but only a portion are located around the eye (6). When the hemangioma involves the eyelid, amblyopia may occur in as many as 43% to 60% of patients and generally is due to induced astigmatism rather than to obstruction of the pupillary axis (6,7). Capillary hemangiomas may be quite large and may involve the nasopharynx and the airway, producing life-threatening complications (8). Ophthalmologists generally consider treating only lesions that are producing astigmatism of a degree expected to cause amblyopia, lesions obstructing the visual axis, or lesions that are ulcerating or are otherwise unacceptable to parents. Cutaneous hemangiomas generally resolve spontaneously, but hemangioma-induced astigmatism and amblyopia will persist unless treated early in the course of their development. Conservative therapy has been emphasized (9). Early treatment may produce a resolution of the astigmatism (7). Treatment with intralesional injection is an accepted form of therapy (10). Serious complications from such therapy, including central retinal artery occlusion, have been reported (11). Other more minor complications such as subcutaneous fat atrophy and skin depigmentation have been reported (12,13). Only the lesions in the periocular area are treated. In some instances, treatment has been combined with laser therapy (14). Other therapies have included α-interferon, topical cortisone cream, and surgical excision (15–17).

For injection of hemangiomas, a mixture of 40 to 80 mg triamcinolone and 6 to 12 mg betamethasone is used; 1 to 2 cc of such a mixture is injected slowly into the lesion, with care taken to avoid intravascular injection or compression of the lesion. The vasoconstricting effect of the corticosteroid is believed to be the mechanism of action. Adrenal suppression can result from this method of administration. Administration of vaccines containing live virus should be avoided for at least 1 week after corticosteroid administration.

Periocular and Systemic Corticosteroids

Corticosteroids administered periocularly or systemically have the same indications, effects, and side effects as those administered by any other route. In children, periocular or systemic administration is generally used for treatment of vision-threatening uveitis.

Topical Corticosteroids

Topical corticosteroids often are indicated for inflammatory conditions of the conjunctiva, cornea, and anterior segment secondary to conditions such as viral stromal keratitis, iritis, corneal and anterior segment injuries, thermal and chemical burns, vernal conjunctivitis, postoperative inflammation, and corneal graft rejection. Topical corticosteroids combined with antiviral agents have been shown to hasten recovery time of viral stromal keratitis (18). Corticosteroids may be administered topically in addition to systemic administration if severe conditions warrant such administration (19). Topical corticosteroids also are used after lamellar and penetrating keratoplasty to control graft rejection, particularly in patients with systemic conditions known to increase the risks of graft failure (20). Corticosteroids are beneficial in treatment of varicella disciform stromal keratitis, although establishing precise dosage can be difficult (21). Side effects of topically administered corticosteroids include increased IOP, delayed wound healing, increased risk of secondary ocular infections, and cataract formation.

NSAIDS

NSAIDS decrease inflammation by inhibiting prostaglandin biosynthesis. No specific pediatric side effects have been reported, but usage of NSAIDS in children has been limited.

Topical administration of ketorolac is indicated for treatment of allergic conjunctivitis (22). This agent has antiinflammatory, analgesic, and antipyretic activity (23). No effect on IOP has been reported. Ketorolac and diclofenac are similar in their effect on pain control and superior to placebo in patients undergoing radial keratotomy (24). Ketorolac was shown to be as effective as dexamethasone in suppressing postoperative inflammation after extracapsular cataract extraction (25). As many as 40% of patients report stinging and burning on instillation of the medication. The potential for cross-reactions to acetylsalicylic acid, phenylacetic acid derivatives, and other NSAIDS exists. Because ketorolac causes ocular irritation, contact lens wearers have been advised not to use this agent.

Ketorolac is available for parenteral administration. Studies have confirmed its antiemetic effectiveness in poststrabismus surgery patients while demonstrating that it was not necessary for pain control (26,27). Renal failure and hyperkalemia have been reported in patients treated with the parenteral form of ketorolac.

Diclofenac is used to control postoperative inflammation. The properties of diclofenac are similar to those of ketorolac, and potential cross-reactions similar to those that occur with ketorolac.

Flurbiprofen and suprofen are indicated for inhibition of intraoperative miosis secondary to intraoperative prostaglandin release and have been shown to be effective for that purpose; however, flurbiprofen administered preoperatively was not effective in controlling postoperative pain (28). Flurbiprofen has been shown to have a favorable influence on cystoid macular edema in adults (29,30).

All these medications may cause ocular irritation and, by inhibiting thrombocyte aggregation, tend to cause increased bleeding from surgical trauma. Patients with bleeding diatheses or those receiving systemic medications that prolong bleeding times should use NSAIDS with caution. Patients with herpetic keratitis should not use NSAIDS, although experimental evidence suggests that flurbiprofen might be beneficial in some instances (31).

Antihistamines

Levocabastine is a selective histamine H_1-receptor antagonist used topically in the eye for relief of allergic symptoms. No significant experience with this agent in children has been reported.

Lodoxamide acts by inhibiting release of mediators by mast cells and appears to be superior to cromolyn sodium in alleviating the signs and symptoms of vernal keratoconjunctivitis (VKC) (32). Studies have shown the efficacy of the mast-cell stabilizer lodoxamide in treatment of VKC. Lodoxamide was superior to cromolyn in alleviating the primary signs and symptoms of VKC (33). Lodoxamide has been shown to be useful in treatment of superior limbic keratoconjunctivitis and allergic keratoconjunctivitis (34,35).

Preparations Available for Topical Clinical Use in the Eye

Corticosteroids
- Dexamethasone suspension and solution: 0.1%
- Dexamethasone ophthalmic ointment: 0.05%
- Fluorometholone suspension: 0.1% and 0.25%
- Fluorometholone ointment: 0.1%
- Medrysone suspension: 1%
- Prednisolone suspension: 0.12%, 0.125%, and 1%

NSAIDS
- Diclofenac solution: 0.1%
- Flurbiprofen solution: 0.03%
- Ketorolac solution: 0.5%
- Suprofen solution: 1%

Antihistamines
- Levocabastine suspension: 0.05%
- Lodoxamide solution: 0.1% solution

REFERENCES

1. *Webster's Medical Desk Dictionary.* Pease RW, Jr. ed. Springfield MA: Merriam-Webster, 1986;790.
2. Gordon DM, McLean JM. Effects of pituitary adrenocorticotropine hormone (ACTH) therapy in ophthalmologic conditions. *JAMA* 1950; 142:1271–1276.
3. Arnold TW, Myers GJ. Neuromyelitis optica (Devic syndrome) in a 12-year-old male with complete recovery following steroids. *Pediatr Neurol* 1987;3:313–315.
4. Beck RW, Cleary PA, Anderson MM, Jr, et al. A randomized, controlled trial of corticosteroids in the treatment of acute optic neuritis. The Optic Neuritis Study Group. *N Engl J Med* 1992;326:581–588.
5. Liu GT, Kay MD, Bienfang DC, Schatz, NJ. Pseudotumor cerebri associated with corticosteroid withdrawal in inflammatory bowel disease. *Am J Ophthalmol* 1994; 117:352–357.
6. Langmann A, Lindner S. Normalization of asymmetric astigmatism after intralesional steroid injection for upper eye lid hemangioma in childhood. *Doc Ophthalmol* 1994;87:283–290.
7. Morrell AJ, Willshaw HE. Normalization of refractive error after steroid injection for adnexal hemangiomas. *Br J Ophthalmol* 1991; 75:301–305.
8. Deady JP, Willshaw HE. Vascular hamartomas in childhood. *Trans Ophthalmol Soc U K* 1986;105:712–716.
9. Motwani MV, Simm JW, Pickering JD. Steroid injection versus conservative treatment of anisometropia amblyopia in juvenile adnexal hemangioma. *J Pediatr Ophthalmol Strabismus* 1995;32:26–28.

10. Kushner BJ. Intralesional corticosteroid injection for infantile adnexal hemangioma. *Am J Ophthalmol* 1982;93:496–506.
11. Shorr N, Seiff SR. Central retinal artery occlusion associated with periocular corticosteroid injection for juvenile hemangioma. *Ophthalmic Surg* 1986;17:229–231.
12. Vazquez-Botet R, Reyes BA, Vazquez-Botet M. Sclerodermiform linear atrophy after the use of intralesional steroids for periorbital hemangiomas: a review of complications. *J Pediatr Ophthalmol Strabismus* 1989;26:124–127.
13. Cogen MS, Elsas FJ. Eyelid depigmentation following corticosteroid injection for infantile ocular adnexal hemangioma. *J Pediatr Ophthalmol Strabismus* 1989;26:35–38.
14. Apfelberg DB, Maser MR, White DN, Lash H. A preliminary study of the combined effect of neodymium: YAG laser photocoagulation and direct steroid instillation in the treatment of capillary/cavernous hemangiomas of infancy. *Ann Plast Surg* 1989;22:94–104.
15. Ricketts RR, Hatley RM, Corolen BJ. Interferon-alpha-2a for the treatment of complex hemangiomas of infancy and childhood. *Ann Surg* 1994;219:605–612; discussion 612–614.
16. Elsas FJ, Lewis AR. Topical treatment of periocular capillary hemangioma. *J Pediatr Ophthalmol Strabismus* 1994;31:153–156.
17. Boyd MJ, Collin JR. Capillary haemangiomas: an approach to their management. *Br J Ophthalmol* 1991;75:298–300.
18. Power WJ, et al. Acyclovir ointment plus topical betamethasone or placebo in first episode disciform keratitis. *Br J Ophthalmol* 1992;76: 711–713.
19. Lennarson P, Barney NP. Interstitial keratitis as presenting ophthalmic sign of sarcoidosis in a child. *J Pediatr Ophthalmol Strabismus* 1995;32:194–196.
20. Lyons CJ, Dart JK, Aclimandos WA. Sclerokeratitis after keratoplasty in atopy. *Ophthalmology* 1990;97:729–733.
21. Martinez J, Lagoutte F, Gauthier L. Post-varicella disciform keratitis. *J Fr Ophtalmol* 1992;15:597–600.
22. Ballas Z, Blumenthal M, Tinkelman DG. Clinical evaluation of ketorolac tromethamine 0.5% ophthalmic solution for the treatment of seasonal allergic conjunctivitis. *Surv Ophthalmol* 1993;38:141–148.
23. Tinkelman DG, Rupp G, Kaufman N. Double-masked, paired-comparison clinical study of ketorolac tromethamine 0.5% ophthalmic solution compared with placebo eyedrops in the treatment of seasonal allergic conjunctivitis. *Surv Ophthalmol* 1993;38:133–140.
24. Epstein RL, Laurence EP. Relative effectiveness of topical ketorolac and topical diclofenac on discomfort after radial keratotomy. *J Cataract Refract Surg* 1995;21:156–159.
25. Flach AJ, Jaffe NS, Akers WA. The effect of ketorolac tromethamine in reducing postoperative inflammation: double-mask parallel comparison with dexamethasone. *Ann Ophthalmol* 1989;21:407–411.
26. Munro HM, Riegger LQ, Reynolds PI. Comparison of the analgesic and emetic properties of ketorolac and morphine for paediatric outpatient strabismus surgery. *Br J Anaesth* 1994;72:624–628.
27. Mendel HG, Guarnieri KM, Sunat LM, Torjman MC. The effects of ketorolac and fentanyl on postoperative vomiting and analgesic requirements in children undergoing strabismus surgery. *Anesth Analg* 1995;80:1129–1133.
28. Fry LL. Efficacy of diclofenac sodium solution in reducing discomfort after cataract surgery. *J Cataract Refract Surg* 1995;21:187–190.
29. Ginsburg AP, Chetham JK, DeGryse RE, Abelson M. Effects of flurbiprofen and indomethacin on acute cystoid macular edema after cataract surgery: functional vision and contrast sensitivity. *J Cataract Refract Surg* 1995;21:82–92.
30. Solomon LD. Efficacy of topical flurbiprofen and indomethacin in preventing pseudophakic cystoid macular edema. Flurbiprofen-CME Study Group I. *J Cataract Refract Surg* 1995;21:73–81.
31. Hendricks RL, Borlknecht CF, Schoenwald RD. The effect of flurbiprofen on herpes simplex virus type 1 stromal keratitis in mice. *Invest Ophthalmol Vis Sci* 1990; 31:1503–1511.
32. Caldwell DR, Verin P, Harsisich-Yonng R. Efficacy and safety of lodoxamide 0.1% vs cromolyn sodium 4% in patients with vernal keratoconjunctivitis. *Am J Ophthalmol* 1992;113:632–637.
33. Santos CI, Huang AJ, Abelson MB. Efficacy of lodoxamide 0.1% ophthalmic solution in resolving corneal epitheliopathy associated with vernal keratoconjunctivitis. *Am J Ophthalmol* 1994;117:488–497.
34. Grutzmacher RD, Foster RS, Feiler LS. Lodoxamide tromethamine treatment for superior limbic keratoconjunctivitis. *Am J Ophthalmol* 1995;120:400–402.
35. Cerqueti PM, Ricca V, Torca MA. Lodoxamide treatment of allergic conjunctivitis. *Int Arch Allergy Immunol* 1994;105:185–189

SECTION VIII

Diagnostic Drugs

Section Editor: Carol F. Zimmerman

To learn how to treat disease, one must learn how to recognize it. The diagnosis is the best trump in the scheme of treatment.

Jean Martin Charcot (1825–1893)

OVERVIEW

Progress in the basic science of ocular pharmacology is fueled by the hope of discovering more effective treatments for disease, with fewer side effects and more convenience. The exciting new discoveries and technology of modern science sometimes obscures one of the most basic tenets of therapy: accurate diagnosis of the disease itself. This section is devoted to those diagnostic agents commonly used in evaluation of ophthalmic disease.

Despite the ever-increasing armamentarium of new drugs, some of the most commonly used mydriatic and cycloplegic agents (described in Chapter 70, this volume) have been used for centuries. Atropine and scopolamine are still useful today. Indeed, the newer synthetic agents such as cyclogyl and tropicamide were developed with similar properties but with fewer side effects and the added convenience of a shorter half-life. Most standard texts treat the mydriatic and cycloplegic agents as one "generic" antimuscarinic or sympathomimetic compound. We hope that readers will find the organization of Chapter 70 by individual drugs useful in locating information unique to the particular agent of interest.

Chapter 71 contains a concise review of iris anatomy and autonomic physiology responsible for control of pupillary size and reactivity. This chapter also presents a general algorithm for the workup of anisocoria. I thank Dr. H. Stanley Thompson for the use of his well-known flow chart. Unfortunately, socioeconomic factors sometimes limit the development and use of some agents. Paredrine, for example, has for years been uniquely helpful in localizing the site of the lesion in Horner's syndrome, but is no longer manufactured. No other drug has proved so useful and safe for this purpose, and we can only hope that some compassionate manufacturer will resume production of this valuable agent, despite its limited application. Ever-increasing regulations also limit the use of cocaine for diagnostic and other indications in some clinical settings.

Even though 90% of patients with myasthenia gravis develop ocular abnormalities, the general ophthalmologist may be unfamiliar with the diagnosis and treatment of myasthenia. This subject is not usually covered in most texts of ocular pharmacology. All readers can appreciate the excellent review by Dr. Wolfe and his colleagues (Chapter 72) of the anatomy, physiology, and pharmacology of the neuromuscular junction and the description of the variety of clinical presentations in this often baffling disorder.

In Chapter 73, Dr. Hogan reviews the "quantum leap" that occurred in the diagnostic arena with the discovery of fluorescein angiography. This discovery was pivotal in our understanding of the retinal circulation and in the characterization of macular and retinovascular disease. The impact of this technique on clinical practice and the development of laser retinal treatment is unquestioned. Yet retinal fluorescein angiography was initially met with skepticism. The original article describing the first potential clinical application was rejected by one ophthalmology journal because it was considered unoriginal and of little significance. As our technology becomes increasingly more sophisticated, fluorophotometry in other ocular tissues is emerging. Among the more promising is indocyanine green videoangiography for the characterization of the choroidal circulation; this technique may improve diagnosis and treatment of choroidal neovascular membranes.

Textbook of Ocular Pharmacology,
edited by T.J. Zimmerman, et al.
Lippincott–Raven Publishers, Philadelphia © 1997.

CHAPTER 70

Mydriatic and Cycloplegic Drugs

Carol F. Zimmerman, R. Nick Hogan, and Trang Diem Le

MYDRIATIC AND CYCLOPLEGIC DRUGS

Drugs used to dilate the pupil act in one of two ways. The agents either inhibit the parasympathetic action of acetylcholine (ACh) at muscarinic receptors in the iris sphincter, or potentiate the sympathetic action of the iris dilator. Clinically, mydriasis facilitates observation of the ocular fundus and is useful in breaking or preventing posterior synechiae associated with ocular inflammation and treating *aqueous misdirection glaucoma.* Drugs such as phenylephrine that produce mydriasis by sympathetic stimulation alone are usually inadequate for indirect ophthalmoscopy because strong light stimulates the parasympathetically innervated iris sphincter and overcomes the mydriasis. Such agents are usually used in combination with parasympatholytic agents (e.g., tropicamide, cyclogyl).

Most mydriatic drugs cause at least some degree of cycloplegia due to their parasympathetic inhibitory effect on the ciliary muscle. Cycloplegia is useful in managing the pain and inflammation of iridocyclitis, for accurate refraction in children, and in treatment of accommodative esotropia and amblyopia. Although all cycloplegic drugs have mydriatic effects, not all mydriatics exhibit cycloplegia.

Although many drugs have mydriatic effects, only those in common use as mydriatic/cycloplegic agents in ophthalmology are discussed in this section. Table 1 compares the properties of these agents.

ATROPINE

History and Source

Atropine is a naturally occurring alkaloid especially prevalent in *Solanaceae* species (*Atropa belladonna* or deadly nightshade, and *Datura stramonium* or Jimson weed, thorn apple) (1,2). The mydriatic and toxic properties of the compound have been known since ancient times. The Hindus use extracts of these shrubs for a variety of medical and ophthalmic disorders. Plineus (23 to 79 A.D.) was said to have used extracts of anagallis, and Galen (135 to 201 A.D.) used extracts of nightshade to dilate the pupils before performance of cataract "couching." Centuries later, Italian women used it to dilate their pupils for beauty; hence, the term "belladonna" (beautiful lady). The drug was also used as a poison; indeed, Linné, the eighteenth century botanist, derived the name *A. belladonna* from "Atropos," the oldest of the Three Fates who cuts the thread of life. Extracts from *A. belladonna* contain atropine as well as the closely related scopolamine (1–3).

Wells, in 1811, first described the cycloplegic and mydriatic effects of the juice of the herb belladonna applied to the eye (4). Atropine in its pure form was first investigated in 1831 by Mein (1). In 1852, Lussana recorded pupillary mydriasis, blurry vision, and loss of near vision as a systemic effect of oral atropine. Lussana (5) and Fedderson (6) attempted the first detailed study of the ocular effects of atropine in 1884, and their data were later confirmed by Wolf and Hodge in 1946 (7).

Atropine is widely used in ophthalmology for treatment of pain associated with anterior segment inflammation, as a means to prevent or break posterior synechiae, and as an aid to refraction. It is also used for "penalization" treatment of amblyopia, and in the treatment of myopia.

Official Drug Name and Chemistry

Atropine is benzeneacetic acid, α-(hydroxy-, 8-methyl-8-azabicyclo[3.2.1]-oct-3-yl ester, endo-($\pm$)-, sulfate (2 : 1) (salt), monohydrate; DL-hyoscyamine sulfate; atropine sul-

C. F. Zimmerman, R. N. Hogan, and T. D. Le: Department of Ophthalmology, UT Southwestern, Dallas, Texas 75235.

TABLE 70-1. *Properties of antimuscarinic and sympathomimetic drugs*

Drug (single drop)	Time of maximum mydriasis	Recovery from mydriasis	Time of maximum cycloplegia	Recovery from cycloplegia
Atropine sulfate 1%	26–40 min	7–12 days	60–180 min	6–12 days
Scopolamine HCl 0.25%	20–30 min	8 days	40 min	3–8 days
Homatropine HBr 2%	10–30 min	1–3 days	30–90 min	1–3 days
Cyclopentolate HCl 1%	30–60 min	1 day	25–75 min	6–24 hr
Tropicamide 1%	20–30 min	3–48 hr	20–40 min	3–6 hr
Phenylephrine HCl 2.5%	15–60 min	3 hr	—	—

fate; atropine. The chemical formula is $(CH_{17}H_{23}NO_3)_2 \cdot H_2SO_4 \cdot H_2O$.

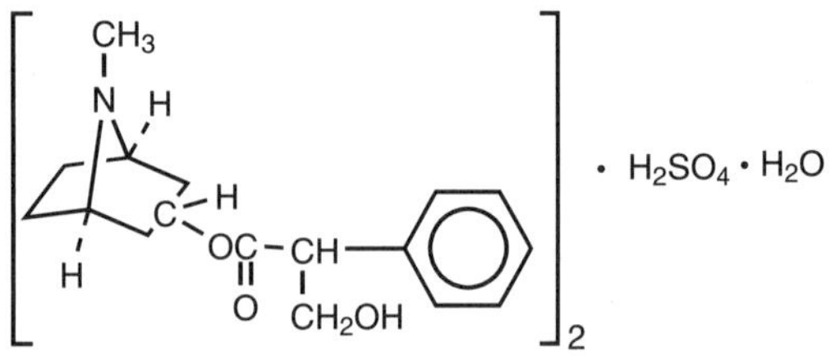

Pharmacology

Atropine is a competitive antagonist of ACh at the parasympathetic, postganglionic, cholinergic nerve endings of smooth muscle, exocrine glands, cardiac muscle, and the CNS. Atropine antagonizes ACh at the muscarinic receptors, with little effect on nicotinic receptors (except at high doses). The drug does not distinguish muscarinic receptor subtypes M_1 (ganglionic), M_2 (cardiac), and M_3 (smooth muscle and glands) (1). The effect may be overcome with sufficient quantities of cholinergic agonists, including pilocarpine, physostigmine, and isoflurophate.

Clinical Pharmacology

In the eye, atropine blocks the response of the iris sphincter and ciliary muscle to ACh, producing pupillary mydriasis and paralysis of accommodation (cycloplegia). The racemic mixture DL-hyoscyamine is used clinically, but only the L-enantiomer is pharmacologically active. Mydriasis begins 12 minutes after topical installation of 1% atropine sulfate, with a maximum effect in 26 to 40 minutes. Full mydriasis lasts 8 hours, and the pupil returns to within 1 mm of preinstallation size in 7 to 12 days. Cycloplegia begins after 12 to 18 minutes, reaching its maximum effect in 180 minutes. Accommodation begins to return in 42 hours and normalizes in 8 days (1,7).

Systemic atropine at standard clinical doses (0.5 to 1.0 mg) causes tachycardia, due to blocking of vagal action of the sinoatrial nodal pacemaker. Tachycardia may be preceded by modest and transient bradycardia. Response is highly variable among individuals and is most marked in healthy young adults. In a study of healthy volunteers, atropine 0.01 mg/kg modestly decreased heart rate (HR) 6 to 15 minutes after intramuscular administration, but this was not statistically significant. A larger dose of 0.02 mg/kg significantly increased HR as much as 39% by 30 to 120 minutes after administration (8). In another study, atropine 1.0 and 2.0 mg intramuscularly increased HR by 15% and 45%, respectively, after 1 hour (9). Administered orally, only the 2.0 mg dose of atropine produced significant tachycardia of 13%. Small doses (0.5 mg or less) may cause modest bradycardia, believed by some investigators to represent central vagal stimulation prior to peripheral muscarinic blockade; more recent data suggest that bradycardia results from blockade of M_1 receptors on the postganglionic parasympathetic neurons, which relieves the inhibitory effects of synaptic ACh on neurotransmitter release (10). Atropine often produces cardiac arrhythmias due to vagal blockade and alteration in the rate of atrioventricular (AV) conduction.

Atropine alone has little effect on the blood vessels and blood pressure (BP). Toxic doses and, rarely, therapeutic doses cause "flushing" due to dilation of the cutaneous vascular bed; the etiology of this phenomenon is unclear, but may be the result of central release of adrenergic vasomotor tonus (11). Atropine blocks the ACh-induced vascular permeability that occurs in iridocyclitis.

Atropine muscarinic blockade in the gastrointestinal (GI) tract reduces gastric and salivary secretion, inhibits gastric and intestinal motility, and delays gastric emptying. Atropine inhibits respiratory secretions and produces bronchodilatation. Intravenous atropine dilates the renal pelvis, ureters, and bladder and decreases bladder and ureteral tone. It has a mild antispasmodic effect on the biliary system. Small doses of atropine inhibit sweating; in larger doses, atropine may cause hyperthermia.

Except for causing modest vagal excitation, atropine has almost no effect on the CNS in therapeutic doses. However, with toxic doses, central excitation causes irritability, restlessness, disorientation, hallucinations, or delirium. With even higher doses, the CNS may become depressed, leading to paralysis, coma, circulatory collapse, and respiratory failure (1).

Pharmaceutics

Atropine is available as the atropine sulfate 0.5% sterile aqueous ophthalmic solution (15 ml) or 1% (5 ml, 15 ml)

(Isopto Atropine, Alcon, Fort Worth, TX; Atropine Care, Akorn, Abita Springs, LA; Atropisol Dropperettes, IOLAB, Claremont, CA; Ocu-Tropine, Ocumed, Roseland, NJ; atropine sulfate, Bausch and Lomb, Tampa, FL; and others). Generic forms are available. Isopto Atropine contains 0.01% benzalkonium chloride, 0.5% hydroxymethylcellulose 2910, and boric acid, sodium hydroxide, and/or hydrochloric acid to adjust pH. Atropine sulfate is available as 0.5% and 1% sterile ophthalmic ointment, 3.5 g with chlorobutanol (chloral derivative), 0.5% white petrolatum, mineral oil, petrolatum and lanolin alcohol, and purified water (Allergan, Irvine, CA; and others). It should be stored in an airtight tight container at 6°–27°C (46–80°F) and protected from freezing. The shelf life (half life, $t_{1/2}$) is 2.7 years at 20°C, pH 7.

Atropine is available as injectable atropine sulfate 0.1 mg/ml; as oral 0.6-, 0.8-, and 1.0-mg tablets, and as a component of numerous antispasmodic oral preparations (diphenoxylate hydrochloride with atropine, Donnatal, Mylan Pharmaceuticals, Morgantown WV; Donnatal, A. H. Robins, Richmond VA; and others.)

Pharmacokinetics

Atropine is well absorbed through the conjunctiva, small bowel, and mucous membranes. Thirty minutes after topical ^{14}C-labeled atropine was instilled into the conjunctiva of rabbits, 2.5% was recovered in the ocular tissues, with the highest concentration evident (1.4%) in the aqueous. Sixty-seven percent was unabsorbed, and the remainder was presumed to be absorbed systemically (12). However, pharmacokinetic and metabolic studies of atropine in animals may not apply to humans who lack atropine esterase. In humans, topical application of 40 μl 1% atropine (0.4 mg) resulted in peak concentration of 860 ± 402 pg/ml at 8 minutes (13).

The pharmacokinetics of atropine is characterized by a fast distribution phase and rapid elimination. Distribution phase $t_{1/2}$ is 1 to 3 minutes (14,15). Peak plasma concentration is reached within 30 minutes of intramuscular (i.m.) injection and is comparable to that achieved with intravenous (i.v.) injection after 1 hour. Absorption of atropine achieved with topical eye drops is at least as rapid as that achieved with intramuscular administration (13). Fourteen to 50% of the drug is protein bound in sera (2,14). Atropine rapidly disappears from the circulation after parenteral administration, with a biexponential concentration–time curve (13,16). Although initial studies using radio-labeled atropine suggested a long $t_{1/2}$ of 12 to 36 hours for atropine, recent techniques of radioimmunoassay (RIA) and radioreceptor assay (RRA) suggest more rapid elimination, with a $t_{1/2}$ ranging from 2 to 5 hours (8,16,17). Pharmacokinetic data vary with the method of assay; RIA measures the racemic mixture DL-hyoscyamine, whereas RRA measures only the active L-hyoscyamine. Higher values for plasma clearance and volume of distribution may be measured by RRA than by RIA due to preferential uptake of the L-isomer by muscarinic receptors. The elimination phase $t_{1/2}$ in younger children (aged less than 2 years) and the elderly is significantly longer than that of adults and older children (14), likely due to an increased apparent volume of distribution in the younger age group and reduced clearance in the elderly. The absorption rate of atropine correlates well with the observed anticholinergic effects. Pharmacokinetic data of parenteral atropine are summarized in Table 2.

Oral atropine is poorly absorbed from the stomach but is well absorbed from the small bowel. Ninety percent of oral atropine is absorbed in this manner (18). Peak effect after oral dosing is 2 hours, but ocular effects may take longer to develop.

The time of maximal mydriasis is 26 to 40 minutes; maximum cycloplegia occurs in 180 minutes (1,7). In-

TABLE 70-2. *Pharmacokinetics of atropine in humans*

Route of administration/age	$t_{1/2}^{a}$ (min)	C_{max} μg/L	t_{max} (min)	$t_{1/2}$ (hr)	V_d (L/kg)	C_l (ml/min/kg)	Reference
Adult (i.m.)		7.5 ± 2.2	8.40 ± 2.2	2.95	3.1 ± 1.9	11.9 ± 3.8	(8)
Adult[b]		2.6 ± 0.5	8.67 ± 2.1	2.43	3.6 ± 2.0	17.3 ± 3.7	(8)
Adult (i.v.)				4.3 ± 1.7	1.7 ± 0.7	5.9 ± 3.6	(16)
Adult[b]				3.7 ± 2.3	3.9 ± 1.5	15.4 ± 10.3	(16)
Age ≤ 2 yr				6.9 ± 3.3	3.2 ± 1.5	6.8 ± 5.3	(14)
0.08–10 yr	2.76 ± 1.8			4.8 ± 3.5	2.2 ± 1.5	6.4 ± 3.9	(14)
16–58 yr	1.68 ± 1.6			3.0 ± 0.9	1.6 ± 0.4	6.8 ± 2.9	(14)
65–75 yr	1.02 ± 0.4			10.0 ± 7.3	1.8 ± 1.2	2.9 ± 1.9	(14)
4–16 yr	1–2			6.5	2.6	5.2–6.4 (0.310–0.384 L/kg/hr)	(15)

0.02 mg/kg dose

C_{max}, maximum plasma concentration; t_{max}, time to C_{max}; $t_{1/2}$, elimination half-life; V_d, volume of distribution; C_l, total clearance; i.m., intramuscular; i.v., intravenous; $t_{1/2}^{a}$, distribution phase half-life; [b]RRA, radioreceptor assay; all other data obtained by radioimmunoassay.

creasing the concentrations of topically applied atropine to more than 1% or increasing drop frequency only increases toxicity, without affecting the degree of cycloplegia. The onset and duration of mydriasis in persons with darkly pigmented irides is longer than that in persons with lightly pigmented irides. Studies using [^{3}H]atropine in rabbits show that the drug is bound to melanin and released from the pigment to act on the muscarinic receptors (19).

The main route of atropine metabolism is hepatic oxidation, conjugation, and hydrolysis. A small fraction (2%) is hydrolyzed to tropine and tropic acid. Metabolic products detected in the urine include atropine, noratropine, equatorial *N*-oxide, tropic acid, and tropine. Urinary excretion is the primary route of elimination of atropine in humans. Half of a single parenteral dose is eliminated in the urine in 4 hours and 77% to 94% is eliminated in 24 hours (16,20). Thirty percent to 50% is excreted in the urine unchanged (20,21).

Therapeutic Use

Atropine provides maximum cycloplegia and is a valuable aid to refraction, especially in younger children with accommodative esotropia or in patients refractory to other agents. Atropine drops or ointment 0.5% to 1% is instilled into the conjunctival sac three times daily for the 3 days before examination is performed. Lesser strengths (0.5%) should be used in fair skinned (blond hair, blue eyes) children and in children aged less than 2 years. Ophthalmic ointment preparations may be used when drops are impractical and may be less toxic than drops. Toxicity may be minimized by compression of the lacrimal sac. Use of atropine should be reserved for patients in whom shorter-acting agents such as cyclopentolate are not adequate. Because of the prolonged duration of cycloplegia and visual impairment it produces, atropine is seldom, if ever, used for cycloplegic refraction in adults.

Atropine 0.5% to 1% daily in eyes with better vision may provide effective penalization therapy for amblyopia, with low risk of occlusion amblyopia (22,23). Cycloplegia may be amblyogenic in neonates, and the risk of amblyopia must be weighed against the benefits of atropine therapy in their treatment (24).

Atropine 1% three times daily reduces ciliary spasm, stabilizes vascular permeability, and prevents posterior synechiae formation in uveitis. The drug should be continued until anterior chamber cells and flare disappear. Atropine may be used as an adjunct to phenylephrine 10% three times daily to maintain mydriasis and break existing posterior synechiae. Inflamed eyes are often more resistant to atropine, and more frequent dosing may be necessary.

Several studies suggest that daily administration of atropine decreases development of myopia, although the effect may reverse when the treatment is discontinued (25,26). Other investigators have been unable to corroborate such claims (23). Atropine 1% at bedtime may be useful in relieving symptomatic myopia in patients with accommodative spasm.

Atropine is used systemically in strabismus and other eye surgery to block the oculocardiac reflex. The drug may be administered as a premedication before surgery or as an intravenous dose during induction of anaesthesia (27). Atropine has long been used as a premedication to general anesthesia to reduce bronchial and salivary secretions. Increasingly, atropine is being replaced by glycopyrrolate, which is a more potent and longer-acting antisialagogue, blocks bradyarrythmias better, and lacks CNS activity.

Atropine is contraindicated in patients with narrow-angle glaucoma, but may be useful in treating malignant (ciliary block) glaucoma (28). It should be used with caution in patients with primary open-angle glaucoma. Atropine is contraindicated in persons with known hypersensitivity to atropine or other antimuscarinic agents.

Side Effects and Toxicity

Blurred vision and photosensitivity are to be expected with use of atropine. Prolonged use of topical atropine may cause local irritation, redness, follicular conjunctivitis, and allergic dermatitis. Symptoms resolve when the drug is discontinued, but may recur with later use. Allergic symptoms caused by topical use usually do not occur when scopolamine, cyclopentolate, or similar agents are substituted.

The side effects of systemic atropine are dose related and variable. At lower doses (0.5 mg), slight bradycardia, dryness of the mouth, and decreased sweating occur. As the dose is increased, HR increases and the pupils may dilate. These effects increase at doses of 2 mg, with frank tachycardia, markedly dry mouth, thirst, flushing, and blurred vision. Even higher doses (5 to 10 mg) produce worsening of these symptoms as well as agitation, difficulty in swallowing, headache, hot dry skin, difficulty in voiding, and reduced GI motility, followed by weak rapid pulse, fever, ataxia, delirium, hallucinations, and coma. Delayed gastric emptying and intestinal distention may be evident in infants. The expression "hot as a hare, red as a beet, dry as a bone, blind as a bat, and mad as a hatter" summarizes the anticholinergic syndrome associated with atropine and related antimuscarinic agents.

Life-threatening side effects include atrial or ventricular arrhythmias and AV dissociation. Atropine toxicity rarely causes death. The fatal dose of atropine is estimated to be 96 to 128 mg in adults (29), although as much as 1 g has been ingested without resulting in death (30). Dosage on a per-weight basis was not reported. In children, the fatal dose is estimated to be 10 mg (29); however, death has been reported with as little as 1.6 mg administered to a 2-year-old boy as topical ophthalmic ointment (31). Three children aged 5', 6' and 8 years survived an oral dose of 600 mg (24.7, 33.9, and 40.7 mg/kg, respectively) without complications (32).

Accidental ingestion may be treated with emesis or gastric lavage with 4% tannic acid. Acute systemic toxicity is treated with 0.2 to 1.0 mg of intravenous physostigmine (0.02 mg/kg in children). The drug is diluted 1 mg per 5 cc normal saline delivered for at least 2 minutes. The dose may be repeated every 5 minutes to a maximum of 2 mg in children and 6 mg in adults. Electrocardiographic (ECG) monitoring should be used during administration of physostigmine, and atropine (1 mg) should be available for treatment of possible bradycardia, convulsions, or bronchoconstriction. For further supportive care, oxygen or mechanical ventilation and treatment of agitation, hyperthermia, dehydration, and urinary retention may be required. Physostigmine may be contraindicated in the presence of hypotension (33,34).

High-risk Groups

Infants, children, and the elderly are particularly at risk of toxicity from systemic or topically applied atropine. One drop of 1% solution contains 0.5 mg atropine; 20 drops of the ophthalmic preparation contains a potentially lethal dose for a child. Pressure should be applied over the lacrimal sac after instillation of the drop, and the medication should not be allowed to run over the face and into the mouth. The hands should be washed after lacrimal occlusion to avoid inadvertent dosing of the fellow eye. The medication should be kept out of reach of children to avoid accidental ingestion. Children with blond hair or blue irides may be especially susceptible to atropine and may require lower concentrations (0.5%). Because cycloplegia may be amblyogenic in neonates, the risk of amblyopia must be weighed against the benefits of atropine therapy in neonates (24).

Atropine readily crosses the placenta; 25% of the corresponding maternal concentration of the drug was detected in the umbilical circulation 2 to 3 minutes after intravenous injection of atropine in the mother (35). Neonates are thus at risk of side effects from systemic administration of the drug to the mother. Mild bradycardia is the most common effect and is usually of no clinical significance. No studies have evaluated the carcinogenic or mutagenic potential for atropine in humans or animals; the drug is not known to be teratogenic. The drug is classified by the FDA as category C; its safety in pregnancy is not established. Atropine is excreted in the breast milk in small amounts, and breast-feeding infants of mothers treated with topical atropine are at potential risk of toxicity.

Increased susceptibility to toxic side effects of atropine has been observed in Down's syndrome (36,37), in spastic paralysis or generalized brain damage ("cerebral palsy") and in the elderly. Atropine has been reported to produce irreversible pupillary mydriasis in patients with keratoconus, but more recent studies have refuted this (38,39).

Atropine is contraindicated in patients with narrow angles because of the risk of angle-closure glaucoma. Topical cycloplegic agents, including atropine, also increase intraocular pressure (IOP) in patients with open-angle glaucoma and in 2% of normal subjects (40). Atropine should be used with caution in patients with chronic open-angle glaucoma. Systemic atropine in patients with glaucoma poses minimal risk due to the low sensitivity of the eye to the systemic drug (41); any effect might be further reduced if the patient is treated with topical miotics. Atropine is contraindicated in persons with known sensitivity to the drug or to the similar drugs scopolamine and homatropine.

Drug Interactions

No interactions of major clinical significance have been reported with atropine; however, its peripheral and central anticholinergic effects may be additive to those of other drugs with anticholinergic side effects, including tricyclic antidepressants, antiparkinsonism drugs, antispasmodic agents, antihistamines, phenothiazines, quinidine, and disopyramide. Significant systemic absorption of atropine may alter the absorption of other drugs due to delayed GI motility. Concurrent use of atropine with cholinergic agents such as isoflurophate, demecarium, and echothiophate may antagonize the miotic and antiglaucoma actions of these drugs.

Major Clinical Trials

Retinoscopy after cyclopentolate was compared to that following atropine 1% in 240 eyes of 120 young esotropic children. Atropine 1% disclosed +.34 diopters (D) more hyperopia than cyclopentolate 1%. However, in a subset of patients (22%), almost all of whom were more than +2.00 D hyperopes, more than +1.00 D hyperopia was disclosed by atropine (42), this implies that atropine is more effective than cyclopentolate in determining the true amount of hyperopia in patients, especially in those with higher degrees of hyperopia.

Optical versus pharmacologic penalization was studied in 160 patients undergoing strabismic or refractive amblyopia. Visual acuity was improved in 76% of eyes pharmacologically penalized with atropine 1% as compared with 78% of eyes optically penalized. Only 8% of patients discontinued the therapy. The study suggested that atropine penalization was an effective method of treatment of amblyopia, with the potential for greater patient compliance than with occlusion therapy; the study did not compare the outcome of atropine penalization with that of occlusion therapy (23).

Reflex bradycardia occurs in 90% of children undergoing ocular surgery, especially strabismus procedures. Premedication with intramuscular atropine 0.01 mg/kg reduced the incidence to 70%; premedication with intravenous atropine at the same dose reduced the incidence to 25%. The mean change in HR in the nonpremedicated group was −30 (±25) beats/min as compared with −17 (±16) beats/min in the group treated intramuscularly and −2 (±15) beats/min in the group treated intravenously (27).

SCOPOLAMINE

History and Source

Scopolamine (hyoscine) is a naturally occurring alkaloid found primarily in the *Solanaceae* shrubs *Hyoscyamus niger* (henbane), *Scopolia carniolica, D. matel* (datura herb), *D. stramonium* (Jimson weed), and *Duboisia myoporoides* (moon flower). It differs from atropine only by the addition of an oxygen bridge which converts tropine to scopine. Although usually extracted from Solanaceae plants, the compound may be synthesized. Scopolamine butylbromide (L-enantiomer) is synthesized for nonophthalmic use.

Use of scopolamine in history parallels that of atropine, recognized for centuries for its ability to dilate pupils to enhance beauty. The Greeks used hyoscyamus to relieve eye pain (1). Vierling (43) and Martelli (44) described the efficacy and duration of scopolamine-induced cycloplegia and mydriasis in 1893, and other reports of its usefulness in clinical refraction soon followed (45).

Official Drug Name and Chemistry

Scopolamine is benzeneacetic acid, α-(hydroxymethyl)-, 9-methyl-3-oxa-9-azatricyclo[3.3.1.0^{2,4}]non-7-yl ester,hydrobromide, [7(*s*)-(1α,2β,4β,5α,7β)]-.; scopolamine hydrobromide; hyoscine; L-scopolamine. Scopolamine and its trihydrate hydrobromide salt occur as the L-isomer (L-hyoscine). The racemic mixture DL-hyoscine is atroscine. The molecular is structure of scopolamine hydrobromide is $C_{17}H_{21}NO_4 \cdot HBr$.

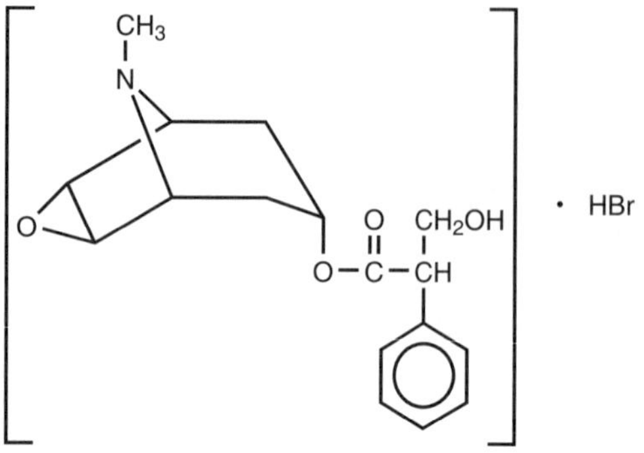

CH3
N
O
O CH2OH
O−C−CH
· HBr

Pharmacology

Scopolamine is a competitive tertiary amine antagonist of ACh at postganglionic muscarinic receptors.

Clinical Pharmacology

Scopolamine blocks the response of the iris sphincter and ciliary muscle to the parasympathetic action of ACh, resulting in mydriasis and cycloplegia. A 0.25% concentration of scopolamine achieves effects comparable to those of 1% atropine, but with a much shorter duration of action. Maximum cycloplegia is achieved in 40 minutes (residual accommodation 1.6 D); recovery begins in 3 days, with full recovery achieved in 8 days. Full mydriasis is achieved in 20 minutes, and lasts 8 hours; full recovery is achieved in 8 days (45).

Scopolamine differs from atropine in many respects. Scopolamine readily crosses the blood–brain barrier (BBB) and, unlike atropine, commonly causes CNS depression at therapeutic doses (described in Side Effects and Toxicity section) (1). Bradycardia at therapeutic doses is common, in contrast to atropine-induced tachycardia (46). Systemic scopolamine, unlike atropine, regularly causes pupillary mydriasis and cycloplegia. Patients who received an intramuscular injection of 0.6 mg atropine showed an average mydriasis of 0.4 mm and lengthening of the near point of 0.8 cm. Patients who received 0.04 to 0.6 mg scopolamine had 1.0 mm mydriasis and lengthening of the near point by 2.7 cm (47).

There is a striking difference between the absorption rate and plasma concentration of scopolamine and the observed clinical effects of the drug. Whereas maximum serum concentrations occur within 10 min after intramuscular injection, peak cardiovascular, sedative, and antisialogogue effects were reached after 1 to 2 hours (48).

Pharmacokinetics

The pharmacokinetics of scopolamine are characterized by rapid absorption and elimination. After intramuscular injection of 0.005 mg/kg, maximum concentration was 1.726 ± 0.486 ng/ml as measured by RRA at 10 ± 10 min (48). The apparent $t_{\frac{1}{2}}$ of elimination was 59 ± 23 minutes. Peak concentration after administration of 0.4 mg i.v. was 2.9 ± 0.24 ng/ml. Levels declined in a biexponential manner with a $t_{\frac{1}{2}}$ of 4.5 ± 1.7 hours. The volume of distribution was 1.4 ± 0.03 L/kg. Systemic clearance was 65.3 ± 5.2 L/hr, but renal clearance was 4.2 ± 1.4 L/hr (49). As with atropine, there is significant transplacental transfer of scopolamine, with the ratio of concentration in the umbilical vein to maternal vein approaching unity (46,48).

Scopolamine is rapidly absorbed after topical application to the eye. Peak plasma concentration 15 minutes after instillation of 0.25% scopolamine in the conjunctival sac is

550 pg/ml (50). Scopolamine is variably absorbed orally, with a bioavailability range of 10.7% to 48.2% and a maximum concentration of 0.53 ±0.11 ng/ml (49).

The metabolism of scopolamine is highly species-specific. In one study, tropic acid was the major metabolite in rabbits and guinea pigs, but significant intraspecies differences in metabolites in rabbits were noted. Aposcopolamine and aponorscopolamine were abundant in guinea pigs. In rats, the major metabolites were *p*-hydroxy-,*m*-hydroxy- and *p*-hydroxy-*m*-methoxy-scopolamine (51). Little information is available about the routes of scopolamine metabolism in humans. Despite its chemical similarity to atropine, only 2.6% ± 1.5% of scopolamine measured by RRA was excreted in human urine as active metabolites; most was excreted as inactive metabolites (46). β-Glucuronide or sulfate conjugation may be an important metabolic pathway (52).

Pharmaceutics

Scopolamine hydrobromide is available as 0.25% solution (Isopto Hyoscine, Alcon) with 0.1% benzalkonium chloride as preservative, vehicle 0.5% hydroxypropylmethylcellulose, sodium chloride, glacial acetic acid, sodium acetate (to adjust pH), and purified water. It is available in 5- and 15-ml drop-tainer bottles. It should be stored at 46° to 80°F and protected from light. Generic preparations are available. It is also available as a patch for transdermal administration for treatment of motion sickness (Transderm Scop, Ciba Pharmaceutical, Summit, NJ) Scopolamine is also found in many antispasmodic preparations (Donnatal, A. H. Robins, Richmond VA; and others).

Therapeutic Use

Indications for scopolamine ophthalmic solution are similar to those for use of atropine (described in Atropine section). The mydriatic effect of scopolamine is similar to that of atropine. Mydriasis for therapeutic or diagnostic evaluation may be achieved with one drop of 0.25% scopolamine as needed. One drop of 0.25% scopolamine is administered 1 hour before cycloplegic refraction in adults and twice daily for 2 days before refraction in children. Scopolamine is less useful than cyclopentolate because of its longer duration. Its cycloplegic properties are slightly less than but comparable to those of atropine (residual accommodation of 1.6 D and 1.9 D, respectively) (45). The duration of scopolamine cycloplegia (3 to 8 days) is shorter than that of atropine (6 to 12 days). Scopolamine may be used as a substitute in patients allergic to topical atropine. To reduce the risk of systemic absorption, pressure should be applied over the lacrimal sac for 2 to 3 minutes after application. The hands should be washed after instillation. One drop of 0.25% scopolamine four times daily or less achieves results similar to those produced by atropine in treatment of ocular inflammation.

Scopolamine is commonly used as a preanesthetic medication to reduce secretions and protect against unwanted vagal activity. It is a common constituent in many preparations for systemic use as an antispasmodic agent, as an aid in radiological and GI endoscopic examinations, and to prevent or treat motion sickness. Contraindications to the use of scopolamine and high risk groups are identical to those for atropine (described in Atropine section).

Side Effects and Toxicity

Anticholinergic symptoms are commonly associated with scopolamine; fatal reactions are exceptionally rare (53–55). The fatal dose in humans has not been established. Symptoms of systemic absorption are identical to those of atropine and include tachycardia, dryness and flushing of the skin, weakness, ataxia, slurred speech, confusion, and hallucinations. Systemic absorption of topical scopolamine may be minimized by compression of the lacrimal sac for 2 to 3 minutes after instillation. Idiosyncratic reactions are more common with scopolamine than with atropine and, unlike atropine, adverse side effects induced by scopolamine commonly occur at ordinary therapeutic doses (1). Local side effects associated with topical use include injection, irritation, follicular conjunctivitis, and eyelid swelling. Treatment of scopolamine overdose is identical to that of atropine overdose (described in the Atropine section).

High-risk Groups

Persons at risk of scopolamine toxicity are the same as those at risk of atropine toxicity.

Drug Interactions

Drug interactions with scopolamine are the same as those described for atropine.

Major Clinical Trials

Cycloplegia and mydriasis with 0.5% scopolamine were studied in 21 patients. The average maximal pupillary diameter was 8 mm, and residual accommodation was 1.6 D as compared with 7.9 mm and 1.9 D produced by 1% atropine. The values for 5% homatropine 1% paredrine were identical to those for scopolamine (45).

The mydriatic effect of scopolamine was equal to that of atropine and homatropine in subjects with dark and light irides and was greater than that produced by sympathomimetic agents. Cycloplegia induced by scopolamine and cyclopentolate was virtually complete and more consistent than that induced by atropine and homatropine (56).

HOMATROPINE

History and Source

Homatropine hydrobromide is a semisynthetic tertiary amine derived from tropine (found in *Solanaceae* plant species) and mandelic acid. It was first used for mydriasis and cycloplegia in 1881 and was considered advantageous because of its relative lack of toxic side effects (57). Numerous studies subsequently documented cycloplegic efficacy comparable to that of atropine, but with a much shorter duration. The drug was often combined with benzedrine, cocaine, or paredrine to enhance and hasten its effect (45,57).

Official Drug Name and Chemistry

Homatropine is benzeneacetic acid, α-hydroxy-, 8-methyl-8-azabicyclo[3.2.1]-oct-3-yl ester, hydrobromide, endo-(±)-.; tropyl mandelate hydrobromide; homatropine hydrobromide. The chemical structure is $C_{16}H_{21}NO_3 \cdot HBr$.

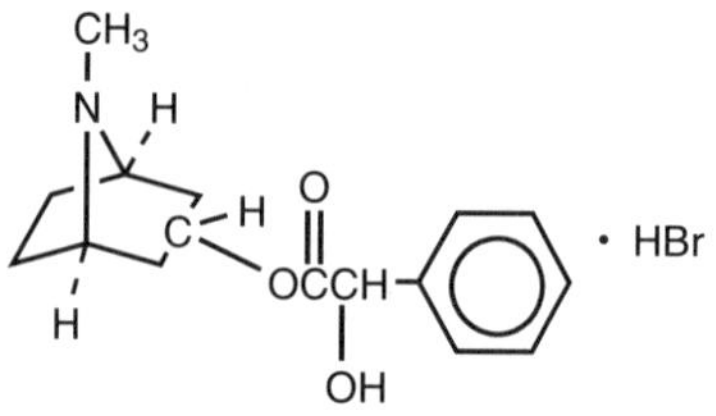

CH_3 N H C H O OCCH OH H · HBr

Pharmacology

Homatropine is a muscarinic antagonist.

Clinical Pharmacology

Homatropine competitively blocks the action of ACh receptors in the iris sphincter and ciliary muscle to produce mydriasis and cycloplegia. Homatropine 2% produces maximum mydriasis in 10 to 30 minutes and maximum cycloplegia in 30 to 90 minutes. Both effects are less than those achieved with atropine. Mean residual accommodation ranges from 0.5 to 2.50 D and is variable among individuals. Recovery from the drug is complete in 1 to 3 days (7,57–59). Homatropine may increase IOP in normal and glaucomatous persons by increasing resistance to aqueous outflow by the trabecular meshwork (40,60).

Pharmaceutics

Homatropine hydrobromide is available as 2% and 5% sterile ophthalmic solution (Isopto Homatropine, Alcon Laboratories; IOLAB) in 5- and 15-ml drop-tainer dispensers. Isopto homatropine contains 0.01% benzalkonium chloride in the 2% strength and 0.0005% benzethonium chloride in the 5% strength in 0.5% hydroxymethylcellulose vehicle, with sodium chloride, polysorbate 80 (in 2% strength), sodium hydroxide and/or hydrochloric acid, and purified water. Homatropine hydrobromide should be stored at 46°to 75°F and protected from light.

Pharmacokinetics

Distribution of homatropine in ocular tissues is not clearly defined. It is likely that homatropine, like atropine, is readily absorbed through the conjunctiva and mucous membranes and rapidly distributed throughout the body. It is poorly absorbed by the cornea because only 0.32% of the drug is non-ionized at physiologic pH (2). The relationship between topical application of the drug and systemic absorption is unknown. Little is known about its metabolism and elimination.

Therapeutic Use

Indications for the use of homatropine are similar to those of atropine (described in Atropine section). To produce mydriasis and cycloplegia in adults, 1 to 2 drops of 2% to 5% solution are instilled into the conjunctival sac and repeated in 5 to 10 minutes. In children, the 2% solution is preferred. Prolonged mydriasis and relatively weak cycloplegia produced by homatropine as compared with other agents (described in Clinical Trials section) make it less desirable as a refractive agent. Homatropine is inferior to atropine for penalization therapy in amblyopia.

Homatropine relieves ciliary spasm, stabilizes vascular permeability, and prevents posterior synechiae in uveitis. One to two drops are used every 3 to 4 hours. Homatropine may be used to treat ciliary block glaucoma and to relax accommodation excess in spasm of the near reflex.

As with other anticholinergic agents, systemic toxicity may result from topical use of homatropine. Systemic absorption may be limited by compression of the lacrimal sac after instillation. Oral use is strictly contraindicated. Individuals with heavily pigmented irides may require larger doses, and the onset of action and time to recovery may be prolonged.

Contraindications to use of homatropine are identical to those to use of atropine. It is contraindicated in narrow-angle glaucoma and in patients with a known hypersensitivity to atropine or other antimuscarinic agents. Chronic-open-angle glaucoma is a relative contraindication, and homatropine should be used with caution in patients with this condition.

Side Effects and Toxicity

Reactions to topical homatropine are identical to, but less common than, reactions to atropine. Toxicity may occur at therapeutic doses, especially in children and the elderly (61,62). At least one fatality has been linked to homatropine; a 7-month-old boy with Down's syndrome died after topical application of an unknown dose of homatropine for ocular examination (63). Symptoms and treatment of homatropine toxicity are identical to atropine (described in Atropine section).

High-risk Groups

Persons at risk of homatropine toxicity are the same as those at risk of atropine toxicity.

Drug Interactions

Drug interactions with homatropine are the same as those described for atropine.

Major Clinical Trials

The cycloplegic and mydriatic properties of 1% atropine, 1% methylatropine, and 1% homatropine were studied in 46 patients. The time to maximum dilation was 40, 50, and 40 minutes, respectively. Atropine produced the greatest pupillary diameter (8.3 mm) and homatropine produced the least (5.9 mm). Residual accommodation was significantly greater with homatropine than with the other agents. Maximum cycloplegia occurred at 5 hours with atropine and metropine, as compared with 25 minutes with homatropine. The onset of recovery from mydriasis for all three drugs was 6 hours (7).

The effect of homatropine on IOP and facility of aqueous outflow were studied in 35 patients with chronic simple glaucoma and 70 normotensive controls. After 2 drops of 5% homatropine, the mean increase in IOP was 2.5 mm (range −2 to +19 mm) in the glaucoma group, as compared with 0.91 mm (range −6 to +3.5 mm) in the control group. The average facility of outflow by tonography decreased 28% in the group with glaucoma and 15% in the normotensive group (60).

TROPICAMIDE

History and Source

Tropicamide is a synthetic derivative of tropic acid, specifically designed for topical use in routine ophthalmic diagnostic procedures. From 1956 to 1958, several investigators described its usefulness as a potent fast-acting and short-lived mydriatic agent. The drug was introduced in the United States by Alcon Laboratories. In 1960, Merrill et al. (64) described the effects of tropicamide in humans. Maximum mydriasis occurred at 30 minutes and exceeded that produced by cyclopentolate and homatropine. Residual accommodation reached a maximum of 1.0 to 1.5 D 30 minutes after instillation. Recovery was complete in 6 hours. There was no effect on IOP and no allergic reaction or irritation. Tropicamide offered obvious advantages over atropinelike compounds, and today it remains among the most widely used topical agents for short-lived mydriasis and cycloplegia.

Official Drug Name and Chemistry

Tropicamide is benzeneacetamide, *N*-ethyl-α-(hydroxymethyl)-*N*-(4-pyridinylmethyl); *bis*-tropamide; tropicamide. The molecular formula is $C_{17}H_{20}N_2O_2$.

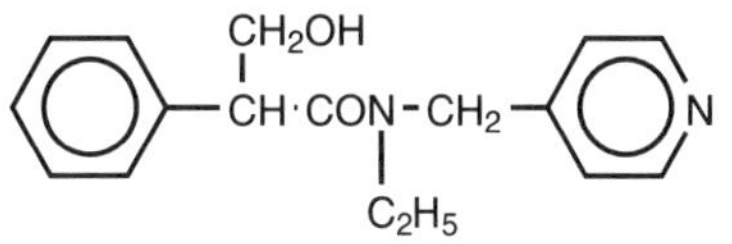

Pharmacology

Tropicamide is a rapidly acting parasympatholytic agent that competes with ACh for the muscarinic receptors.

CLINICAL PHARMACOLOGY

Tropicamide competitively inhibits the action of ACh at the iris sphincter and ciliary body receptors, causing mydriasis and cycloplegia. This effect is dose-related and can be reversed by increasing the concentration of ACh. Tropicamide dilates the pupils to at least 6 mm at concentrations as low as 0.25% (65). The mydriatic effect begins after 5 minutes and reaches a maximum in 25 to 30 minutes. There is no difference in the mydriatic dose-response with 0.25%, 0.5%, 0.75%, and 1% concentrations. The mean maximal mydriasis is 7.7 to 8.2 mm and lasts at least 30 minutes. Accommodation loss is dose dependent; clinically significant cycloplegia occurs only at higher concentrations (0.75% to 1%). A single drop of tropicamide at these concentrations induces a residual accommodation of 1.5 D, as compared with 1.8 and 2.2 D with 0.5% and 0.25%, respectively. The cycloplegic effect begins after 5 minutes and is maximal in 20 to 40 minutes. Complete recovery of accommodation and normalization of pupillary size occur in as little as 3 hours.

Tropicamide, like atropine, has been shown to cause modest bradycardia at rest, probably due to blockade of M_1-receptors on postganglionic parasympathetic neurons. Dynamic exercise in patients treated with tropicamide does not cause clinically significant alterations in cardiovascular function (66).

Pharmaceutics

Commercial preparations of tropicamide contain equal amounts of the L- and D-isomers. The L-isomer has anticholinergic activity 75 times greater that that of its D-counterpart (11). Tropicamide is available as 0.5% and 1.0% sterile ophthalmic solution in 15 ml bottles (Mydriacyl, Alcon, Ft. Worth, TX; Tropicacyl, Akorn, Abita Springs, LA; and Ocu-tropic, Ocumed, Roseland, NJ). The 1.0% solution is available in 3-ml drop-tainers (Mydriacyl) and 2-ml dispensers (Tropicacyl). Generic preparations are also available. Mydriacyl contains 0.5% or 1.0% tropicamide with 0.01% benzalkonium chloride preservative and inactive constituents sodium chloride, edetate disodium, hydrochloride and/or sodium hydroxide, and purified water, adjusted to pH of 4.0 to 5.8. Tropicamide should be tightly sealed and stored at 46° to 80°F (8° to 27°C). It should not be refrigerated.

Pharmacokinetics

Tropicamide is quickly absorbed into the circulation after topical application. Five minutes after instillation of two 40-μl drops into the cul-de-sac, mean peak plasma concentration is 2.8 ± 1.7 ng/ml. The drug disappears quickly from the circulation, with plasma levels of 0.46 ± 0.51 ng/ml at 60 minutes; 120 min after instillation, levels decrease to 240 pg/ml. The apparent equilibrium binding constant of tropicamide to muscarinic receptors in rat brain is 220 ± 25 n*M*. Tropicamide binds to muscarinic receptors with low affinity. It does not bind to tissue as strongly as atropine and occupies only 8% of plasma muscarinic receptors after ocular administration (67). The weak receptor binding and low receptor occupancy may explain the infrequent incidence of systemic toxicity that results from topical use.

Studies in rabbits have shown that transcorneal passage of tropicamide follows first-order kinetics (68). The effect of tropicamide on ocular hemodynamics is negligible. Application of tropicamide 1% to rabbit corneas did not alter ocular blood flow (69). Similarly, a study in human eyes demonstrated no significant change in macular capillary blood flow after instillation of 1% tropicamide (70). Little is known about the metabolic products of tropicamide in humans or animals.

Therapeutic Use

Tropicamide is used exclusively as a topical mydriatic and cycloplegic agent of short duration in ophthalmic diagnostic procedures. For examination of the fundus, 1 to 2 drops of tropicamide 0.5% to 1% are instilled into the cul-de-sac 15 to 20 minutes before examination. Patients with darker irides may require higher doses.

Clinically significant cycloplegia requires higher concentrations; 1 to 2 drops of 1% tropicamide are applied 20 to 30 minutes before refraction. If examination is delayed beyond this time, an additional drop may be applied. The moderate degree of cycloplegia provided by tropicamide is usually sufficient for routine retinoscopy in adults; however, in children in whom a higher degree of cycloplegia is required, more potent agents such as atropine may be required. The combination of tropicamide 0.5% and phenylephrine 2.5% to 10% may provide more effective mydriasis, especially in patients with diabetes who have had laser treatment and other patients who are difficult to dilate (71,72). Tropicamide is contraindicated in patients with narrow angles (prior to the creation of patent iridotomies) and in those with known hypersensitivity to the drug or other atropinelike compounds.

Side Effects and Toxicity

Tropicamide solution is remarkably well tolerated and rarely causes systemic toxicity. Side effects are identical to those of atropine (described in Atropine section). Intravenous and intraperitoneal toxicity in mice reportedly occur at 277 mg/kg and 490 mg/kg, respectively (64). To avoid excessive systemic absorption, digital pressure should be applied on the lacrimal sac for 2 to 3 minutes after drug instillation. Oral use is contraindicated, and care should be taken to avoid accidental ingestion during topical application.

Like other cycloplegic drugs, tropicamide can transiently increase IOP in eyes with open-angle glaucoma and may precipitate angle-closure glaucoma in patients with narrow angles (73,74). The potential systemic side effects of tropicamide are identical to those of other anticholinergic agents (described in Atropine section). Blurred vision and photophobia are common. In children and some adults, tropicamide use has been linked to CNS symptoms, including psychotic reactions, behavior disturbances, sedation, inability to concentrate, fatigue, tachycardia, and cardiorespiratory collapse (1,75).

Allergic reactions, including corneal irritation, severe edema of the eyelids, and rhinitis have occurred with topical use of the drug (75). Generalized urticaria developed after administration of 1% tropicamide in an elderly patient who previously demonstrated erythema multiforme after using scopolamine ophthalmic solution (76). An anaphylactic reaction was reported in a 10-year-old child after ophthalmic instillation of one drop of tropicamide 0.5%. Other investigators suggested that the child, who recovered completely, had only a vasovagal episode or a tonic-clonic seizure (75,77). Despite these reports, tropicamide has an impressive safety record. No adverse effects were reported in 1,000 patients receiving 0.5% tropicamide; 5 of 537 receiving 1% tropicamide had increased IOP of 4 to 12 mm; in all, the increase was transient and judged to be clinically insignificant (78).

High-risk Groups

Tropicamide should not be administered to patients with narrow-angle glaucoma or those with narrow anterior chamber angles before the creation of patent iridotomies. Elderly patients are particularly at risk, due to their higher prevalence of increased IOP.

As with atropine, infants, small children, the elderly, and those with brain damage (including Down's syndrome [36,37]) may be more susceptible to systemic toxicity and CNS disturbances produced by tropicamide use. Potential systemic side effects are identical of those of atropine. Patients who have had previous adverse reactions to atropine or related anticholinergic compounds may be similarly affected by tropicamide (described in Atropine section).

Tropicamide is classified as FDA category C; the safety of tropicamide for use during pregnancy has not been established. There is a potential risk of fetal exposure to tropicamide due to systemic absorption by the mother. The drug should be used only when the indication is clear and the potential benefit to the mother outweighs the potential risk to the fetus. It is not known whether tropicamide is excreted in breast milk.

Drug Interactions

The mydriatic effect of tropicamide may be enhanced by sympathetic agents. The combination of tropicamide 0.5% and phenylephrine 2.5% provided excellent pupillary dilation (8.88 mm, or 3.52 mm greater than baseline) in 30 minutes. The mydriasis lasted more than 7 hours (79). Other studies have shown that lower concentrations of tropicamide (0.25%) and phenylephrine (1.25%) can produce adequate pupillary dilation with minimal risk of side effects (72). The mydriatic effect of tropicamide 0.5% can be completely reversed by thymoxamine 0.5%, but the reversal is incomplete with higher concentrations of tropicamide (80). Dapiprazole reduces pupillary and accommodative recovery time (81).

Tropicamide may interfere with the antiglaucoma and miotic actions of antiglaucoma medications, including echothiophate, isoflurophate, demecarium, carbachol, and pilocarpine; likewise, these agents may interfere with the mydriatic action of tropicamide, which may be useful clinically (1).

Major Clinical Trials

The efficacy of tropicamide in inducing mydriasis and cycloplegia has been well documented in clinical trials (64,65,82,83). In a study of 344 patients, tropicamide 0.5 and 1% provided maximum mydriasis in 30 minutes as compared with cyclopentolate 1%, phenylephrine 10%, and homatropine 5%, which required 60 to 90 minutes. The degree of mydriasis with tropicamide exceeded that achieved with the other agents (64). Whereas dilute tropicamide (0.25% to 0.5%) is satisfactory for mydriasis, adequate cycloplegia required doses of 1% (65,82,83). Merrill et al. (64) and Pollack et al. (65) demonstrated a residual accommodation of 1 to 1.5 D and 1.5 D, respectively, 30 minutes after administration of 1% tropicamide. In a study of 50 patients, Milder (83) found that tropicamide 1% provided inferior cycloplegia to that achieved with homatropine 5%.and cyclopentolate 1% (83). In patients aged less than 20 years, residual accommodation ranged from 3.2 to 6.5 D 30 minutes after instillation. The range of residual accommodation 60 minutes after homatropine 5% instillation was 1.6 to 2.5 D; at 60 minutes after cyclopentolate 1% administration, it was 1 to 1.6 D.

In a study of 20 children aged 6 to 12 years with a mean refractive error of +1.48, Egashir et al. (84) noted no significant difference between cyclopentolate and tropicamide for cycloplegic retinoscopy or distance subjective refraction. Automated refraction disclosed more hyperopia with cyclopentolate (0.14 ± 0.30 D); this was statistically significant but has little clinical importance.

Patients with suspected Alzheimer's disease were shown to have an exaggerated mydriatic response to topical tropicamide similar to that observed in Down's syndrome, which shares some common features with Alzheimer's disease (85). Using tropicamide as a screening test, the investigators identified 18 of 19 individuals with clinically diagnosed or suspected Alzheimer's disease. Other studies have not confirmed this finding (86,87) and cite difficulties in controlling for patient vigilance, iris pigmentation, aqueous fluid dynamics and corneal permeability. Further investigation is needed to determine whether tropicamide will be a useful diagnostic agent for diagnosis of Alzheimer's disease.

CYCLOPENTOLATE

History and Source

Cyclopentolate was first synthesized by Treves and Testa (88) in the early 1950s in a search for an effective antispasmodic agent. Of the synthetic tropine derivatives studied, compound 75 (cyclopentolate) produced rapid and effective mydriasis and cycloplegia. Priestly and Medine (89) reported that 0.5% cyclopentolate produced an average 7 mm mydriasis in 30 minutes, with an average residual accommodation of 1.25 D (as compared with 2.0 D achieved with 5% homatropine). Recovery was complete in less than 24 hours (89). Reports of similar results soon followed (73,90–92). Cyclopentolate was considered the almost ideal mydriatic/cycloplegic agent because of its rapid onset, its production of effective cycloplegia and rapid recovery, and the paucity of resultant systemic or local side effects as compared with those produced by atropinelike drugs. Cyclopentolate has since been widely accepted as the drug of choice for short-term cycloplegia.

Official Drug Name and Chemistry

Cyclopentolate is 2-(dimethylamino)ethyl 1-hydroxy-α-phenylcyclopentaneacetate hydrochloride; cyclopentolate hydrochloride. The chemical formula is $C_{17}H_{25}NO_3 \cdot HCl$.

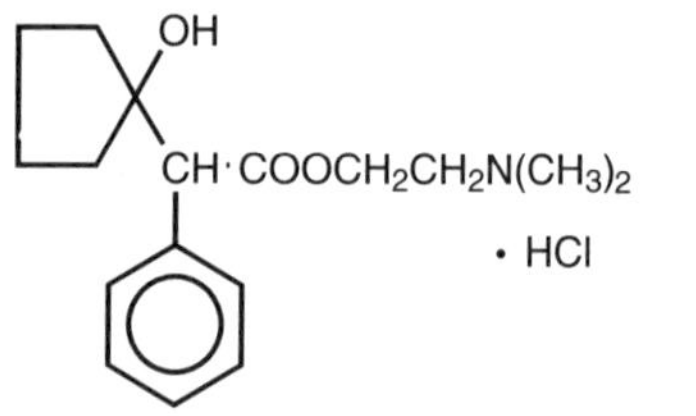

OH

$CH \cdot COOCH_2CH_2N(CH_3)_2$

$\cdot HCl$

Pharmacology

Cyclopentolate is a synthetic tertiary amine antimuscarinic agent.

Clinical Pharmacology

Cyclopentolate competitively blocks the action of ACh at the muscarinic receptors in the iris sphincter and ciliary muscle, producing mydriasis and cycloplegia. Although the compound is present as a racemic mixture in eyedrops, ocular effects are mainly due to the L-isomer (93). One drop of 0.5% to 1.0% cyclopentolate produces maximum mydriasis in 30 to 60 minutes with recovery (to within 1 mm of pretreatment size) achieved in 24 hours. Maximal cycloplegia is achieved in 25 to 75 minutes. Accommodative power recovers to within 2 D of pretreatment power in 6 to 24 hours (1,73,90–92). The dose–response relationship varies with iris pigmentation. In dark irides, the rate of accommodative loss and recovery may be slower and the residual accommodation greater than that observed in light irides (94). This delay in onset and prolonged effect may be due to pigment binding, similar to that observed with atropine (19). Cyclopentolate produced an average residual accommodation of 1.10 D 60 minutes after instillation in white patients, as compared with 1.75 D in black patients (91). In another study, the average residual accommodative amplitude after 0.5% cyclopentolate was 2.4 D in black subjects and 1.3 D in white subjects (92).

Pharmaceutics

Cyclopentolate is available as 0.5%, 1%, and 2% ophthalmic solution USP in 2-, 5-, and 15-ml drop-tainer dispensers (Cyclogyl, Alcon Laboratories, Ft. Worth, TX), as 1% solution in 2 and 15 ml bottles (AK-Pentolate, Akorn, Abita Springs, LA and Pentolair, Bausch and Lomb, Tampa, FL), and as 1% solution in 2-, 5-, and 15-ml dropper bottles (Ocu-Pentolate, Ocumed, Roseland, NJ). Cyclogyl contains 0.01% benzalkonium chloride, boric acid, edetate disodium, potassium chloride (except 2% strength), sodium carbonate and/or hydrochloric acid, and purified water, with a pH range from 3.0 to 5.5. The drug should be stored at 46° to 80°F. Cyclopentolate is also available as 0.2% solution with 1% phenylephrine (Cyclomydril, Alcon Laboratories) in 2- and 5-ml drop-tainer dispensers.

Pharmacokinetics

Cyclopentolate is rapidly absorbed into the system after ocular application (95). Peak plasma concentration of 2.8 ng/ml ± 1.3 occurred 15 ± 11 minutes after topical application of 1% cyclopentolate. Mean elimination $t_{1/2}$ is 112 ± 23 minutes (96). The drug is absorbed through the cornea, conjunctiva, nasal mucosa, and GI tract. A second peak at 2 to 4 hours observed in some subjects may reflect GI absorption from drug swallowed after drainage into the nasopharynx through the nasolacrimal duct. Little is known about the metabolism of cyclopentolate.

Therapeutic Use

For cycloplegia and/or mydriasis in adults, 1 drop of 0.5% to 2.0% cyclopentolate is applied to the conjunctiva 30 to 45 minutes before refraction or ophthalmoscopy. This may be repeated in 5 minutes if necessary. In children, 1 drop of 0.5% to 2.0% is applied, followed by 1 drop of 0.5% or 1.0% in 5 minutes, if necessary. More frequent or stronger doses may be required in patients with dark pigmentation and brown irides. Premature and small infants should receive only a single dose of 0.5%. Use of concentrations greater than 0.5% in small infants is not recommended.

Pressure should be applied to the nasolacrimal sac for 2 to 3 minutes after instillation of the drop to reduce systemic absorption, especially in infants. Children should be monitored for adverse systemic side effects for 30 minutes after application. Feeding should be withheld for 4 hours before drug application to avoid feeding intolerance.

The usual dose of cyclopentolate in uveitis is 1 drop of 0.5% to 2% (0.5% to 1% in children) three or four times daily. Some data suggest that cyclopentolate (unlike atropine, scopolamine, homatropine, and tropicamide) induces a chemokinetic and/or chemotactic neutrophil response (97), and may not be a good choice for treatment of ocular inflammation.

Contraindications to use of cyclopentolate are identical to those for atropine. Cyclopentolate is contraindicated in patients with known sensitivity to the drug or to other antimuscarinic compounds. Relative contraindications to use of cyclopentolate include glaucoma (chronic simple, angle closure, or predisposition to angle closure), Down's syndrome, brain damage, or spastic paralysis. Small infants, children with blond hair and blue eyes, and the elderly may show increased susceptibility to the drug. In these circumstances, the risk of side effects should be carefully weighed against the benefit of treatment.

Side Effects and Toxicity

Local effects from topical application include blepharoconjunctivitis, conjunctivitis, hyperemia, punctate keratitis, burning or stinging, photophobia, and blurring of vision. In most cases, the effects are transient and no treatment is required.

Toxic side effects of cyclopentolate are relatively uncommon and are dose related. Most occur with 1% or 2% strength (75,98,99). Signs of systemic absorption of cyclopentolate are identical to those of atropine toxicity (due to its antimuscarinic action), but occur less frequently (described in Atropine section). Infants may be particularly susceptible to delayed gastric motility, with feeding intolerance. The lethal systemic dose is not established in humans. The intravenous LD_{50} in rats is 32 mg/kg (89).

Treatment of acute systemic toxicity produced by cyclopentate is identical to that used for treatment of atropine toxicity. In children, 0.5 mg intravenous physostigmine is administered slowly. This may be repeated at 5-minute intervals as long as symptoms persist and there are no cholinergic effects, to a maximum of 2 mg. The drug may be administered subcutaneously. In adults, the dose is 2 mg and may be repeated (1 to 2 mg) in 20 minutes if symptoms persist.

High-risk Groups

Neonates, children, the elderly, and individuals with blond hair, fair skin, and blue eyes are particularly susceptible to side effects of cyclopentolate. Persons with Down's syndrome, spastic paralysis, or brain damage may show increased side effects of the drug.

The drug is classified by the FDA as category C; its safety in pregnancy is not established. It is not known whether cyclopentolate is excreted in breast milk. However, the drug is systemically absorbed, and breast-feeding infants of mothers treated with topical cyclopentolate may be at risk of toxicity.

Drug Interactions

Cyclopentolate may antagonize the antiglaucoma and miotic actions of the longer-acting cholinergic antiglaucoma medications (e.g., echothiophate, isoflurophate, demecarium). Cyclopentolate may also antagonize the antiglaucoma actions of carbachol or pilocarpine; these agents may interfere with the mydriatic action of cyclopentolate, which may be of clinical benefit.

Major Clinical Trials

In a study of children, instillation of 3 drops of cyclopentolate 10 minutes apart produced cycloplegia comparable to that of atropine administered for 3 days (100). Atropine 1% ointment applied twice daily for 4 days before retinoscopy produced an average 0.4 D more cycloplegia than that measured 30 minutes after application of cyclopentolate 1%. One versus 2 drops produced no difference in cycloplegia (101).

In a review of data available from 1,035 patients, Gordon and Ehrenberg (91) reported that 2 drops of 0.5% cyclopentolate produced 7 mm mydriasis within 30 minutes of administration as compared with 6.1 mm produced with 0.5% homatropine. Recovery was complete in 24 hours in the cyclopentolate group and in 48 hours in the homatropine group. Residual accommodation with cyclopentolate at 60 minutes was 1.10 D, as compared with 2.00 D achieved with 0.5% homatropine. In black patients, 1% cyclopentolate resulted in a residual accommodation of 1.75 D after 60 minutes as compared with 3.5 D achieved with 5 drops of 2% homatropine (91).

PHENYLEPHRINE HYDROCHLORIDE

History and Source

The vasopressor effects of phenylephrine hydrochloride and related compounds were first demonstrated in adrenal extracts in 1895 (102). Epinephrine, the first active agent isolated, was discovered by Abel in 1899 (103). Other compounds with related structures and pharmacologic effects, including phenylephrine, were subsequently described (104). In 1929, phenylephrine was initially recommended for use as a mydriatic agent in cataract surgery (105). The first extensive evaluation of phenylephrine for ophthalmologic use was conducted in 1936, but side effects of phenylephrine in ophthalmic patients were not systematically studied until 1956 (106,107).

Official Drug Name and Chemistry

Phenylephrine hydrochloride is (-)-*m*-Hydroxy)-α-[(methylamino)methyl] benzyl alcohol hydrochloride; phenylephrine hydrochloride. The chemical formula is $C_9H_{13}NO_2HCl$.

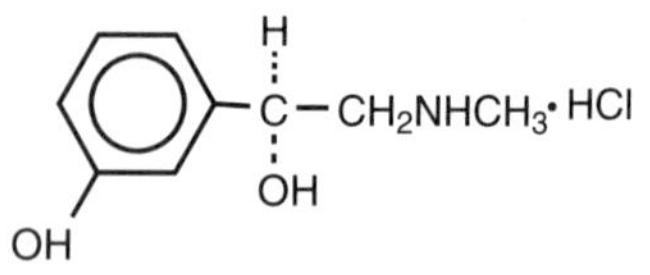

H — C(OH) — $CH_2NHCH_3 \cdot HCl$; OH

Pharmacology

Phenylephrine is a relatively pure α_1-adrenoceptor agonist. It has some weak α_2- and β-receptor agonist properties. Most of its effect occurs through activation of α_1-adrenoceptors, although some indirect effects also occur through release of norepinephrine.

Clinical Pharmacology

The effects of phenylephrine on α_1-adrenoceptors in the eye include local vasoconstriction from the direct action on the arterioles, mydriasis due to simulation of iris dilator muscle receptors, and elevation of eyelids and widening of palpebral fissure from activation of receptors in the palpebral muscles.

Maximum mydriasis occurs 15 to 60 minutes after instillation of 2.5% phenylephrine and after 10 to 90 minutes with 10% phenylephrine. The duration of mydriasis is approximately 3 hours with 2.5% solution and 3 to 7 hours with the 10% solution (108,109). Maximal conjunctival vasoconstriction is attained after 30 to 90 seconds with the 1% solution, and the vasoconstriction can last 2 to 6 hours (106,110).

In a study of the mydriatic dose–response relationship of aqueous phenylephrine HCl, the mydriatic response increased sharply with increasing concentration, reaching a plateau at approximately 2.5% (corresponding to 2 mm mydriasis). Fifty percent of the maximum effect occurred with the 0.5% concentration. Strengths greater than 2.5% did not always produce more mydriasis. Phenylephrine 10% produced maximum mydriasis of 3 mm (110). The study did not take into account the effects of age, iris color, and sex, all factors that had been shown to affect pupillary dynamics (111). The degree of mydriasis is affected by iris color. Darker eyes are more difficult to dilate than lighter eyes because of pigment binding of the drug (56,110–112).

Disruption of the corneal epithelium enhances the effect of phenylephrine by increasing transcorneal absorption. Weiss and Shaffer (113) reported that 30% of patients were dilated with only 0.125% phenylephrine. After tonometry, however, 100% of patients were dilated, indicating that slight alterations in corneal epithelium increase corneal penetration of the drug.

Prior treatment with topical anesthetic agents also enhances penetration of phenylephrine. Mydriasis was noted to increase in eyes pretreated with either proparacaine 0.5%, tetracaine 0.5%, or benoxinate 0.4%, an effect that may be related to changes in the epithelial "barrier" after anesthetic application (114). Ashton et al. (115) demonstrated increased corneal penetration of phenylephrine after pretreatment with flurbiprofen using organ culture methods. This effect may be due to alteration in epithelial barrier function and formation of ion-pairs between drugs, which increases the lipophilicity of phenylephrine.

The α_1-agonist activity of phenylephrine causes vasoconstriction and increase in systolic and diastolic BP that is dose and concentration dependent. In one study, doses of 0.5, 1.0, 2.0, and 4.0 μg/kg/min produced an average increase in systolic BP of 3, 11, 26, and 53 mm Hg, respectively (116). These values correlated to plasma concentrations of 4.1, 11.4, 24.1, and 62.8 μg/L. Blood flow to most vascular beds is markedly decreased, while coronary blood flow is increased. Although chemically similar to epinephrine, phenylephrine lacks the cardiac inotropic and chronotropic actions of epinephrine (117).

Pharmaceutics

Phenylephrine preparations are summarized in Table 3. Phenylephrine Hydrochloride Ophthalmic solution USP (IOLAB Pharmaceuticals, Phoenix, AZ) contains phenylephrine hydrochloride 2.5% or 10%, dibasic and monobasic sodium phosphates, boric acid (in 2.5% strength), phosphoric acid and/or sodium hydroxide to adjust pH, and benzalkonium chloride as preservative in sterile water. Containers should be kept tightly closed to prevent oxidation and should be protected from light and freezing. The solution should not be used if it turns brown or contains precipitate.

Pharmacokinetics

Phenylephrine is rapidly absorbed across the intact corneal epithelium. The peak plasma level of phenylephrine is reached 10 to 20 minutes after topical application (118). Prior instillation of topical anesthetics enhances the rate of drug absorption and may prolong the mydriatic effect (114,115). Damage to the corneal epithelium also increases the absorption rate of phenylephrine. In rabbit eyes, the rate constant for corneal penetration is increased more than 11-fold after the cornea is denuded of epithelium (119). The prolonged phenylephrine mydriasis observed after tonometry is probably due to alteration of the corneal epithelium by this diagnostic procedure (113).

Because phenylephrine is readily absorbed after oral administration but is extensively metabolized by the gut be-

TABLE 70-3. *Ophthalmic drugs containing phenylephrine HCl*

Generic name	Trade name	Manufacturer	Concentration
Mydriatics			
Phenylephrine HCl	AK-Dilate	Akorn	2.5%, 10%
	Mydfrin	Alcon	2.5%
	Ocu-phrin	Ocumed	2.5%, 10%
	Generic	Bausch/Lomb	2.5%
		Iolab	10%
Ocular decongestants			
Phenylephrine HCl	AK-Nephrin	Akorn	0.12%
	Efricel		
	Eye Cool	Danker	0.08%
	Isopto Frin	Alcon	0.12%
	Ocu-phrin	Ocumed	0.12%
	Preferin Liquifilm	Allergan	0.12%
	Relief		
	Tear-Efrin		
	Velva-Kleen		
Combinations			
Phenylephrine HCl plus zinc sulfate	Prefrin-Z	Allergan	Phenylephrine 0.12%
	Zincfrin	Alcon	Zinc sulfate 0.25%
Phenylephrine HCl plus cyclopentolate	Cyclomydril	Alcon	Phenylephrine 1%, Cyclopentolate HCl 0.2%
Phenylephrine HCl plus scopolamine	Murocoll 2	Bausch/Lomb	Phenylephrine 10%, Scopolamine 0.3%
Phenylephrine HCl plus sulfacetamide	Vasosulf	Iolab	Phenylephrine 0.125%, Sulfacetamide 15%

fore absorption, only 40% is systemically bioavailable by this route. Hengstmann and Goronzy (120), using [^{3}H] phenylephrine, measured peak plasma levels of phenylephrine 1 hour after oral ingestion by normal volunteers. After ingestion, only 2.6% of the total dose was present as free phenylephrine, as compared with 16% available after intravenous injection. The volume of distribution was 340 L, and the plasma $t_{\frac{1}{2}}$ was 2 to 3 hours. Total clearance was 2 L/hr. The extent of plasma protein binding is not known (120). Phenylephrine does not cross the blood–ocular barrier, the BBB, or the placenta (108).

Phenylephrine is excreted in the urine almost entirely unchanged (<20%) or as inactive metabolites. The principle routes of metabolism are sulfate conjugation, primarily in the gut, and oxidative deamination by monoamine oxidase in the liver. Forty-six percent of oral phenylephrine is metabolized to phenylephrine 3-*O*-sulphate, as compared with 8% of the intravenously administered drug. Fifty percent of intravenously administered phenylephrine undergoes oxidative deamination to 3-hydroxymandelic acid and 3-hydroxyphenylglycol; the latter compound undergoes sulfate conjugation. Twenty-four percent of an oral dose is metabolized in this manner. At least some of the drug undergoes glucuronidation (120–122).

Therapeutic Uses

Phenylephrine is used as a fast-acting mydriatic agent for ophthalmic diagnostic procedures that do not require cycloplegia. One drop of 2.5% phenylephrine is instilled into the conjunctival sac approximately 20 minutes before the planned procedure is performed. The dose may be repeated in 1 hour as needed. Because sympathomimetic mydriasis alone may be inadequate for procedures in which strong light stimuli are used (indirect ophthalmoscopy) or complete cycloplegia is required, phenylephrine is often used concurrently with antimuscarinic agents. Topical anesthetic agents administered before instillation of phenylephrine may enhance the effect. Persons with darkly pigmented irides may require 10% phenylephrine for effective mydriasis. Drops should not be allowed to run down the face and into the mouth, and pressure should be applied over the lacrimal sac to prevent systemic absorption. Ten percent phenylephrine is contraindicated in neonates, infants, and young children.

Phenylephrine 10% is useful as a topically applied mydriatic agent before performance of intraocular procedures that require a widely dilated pupil and as a postoperative mydriatic to relieve severe ocular inflammation (one drop twice daily) (123).

Phenylephrine is used to prevent or treat posterior synechiae in uveitis. Its potent and short-acting mydriasis causes movement of the pupil that may prevent or arrest synechia formation or break existing synechiae. Its vasoconstrictor effect reduces the hyperemia of uveal inflammation (124). One drop of 10% phenylephrine is applied to the conjunctiva and is repeated in 1 hour if necessary.

Phenylephrine 2.5% may be used to prevent iris cysts associated with use of some drugs such as echothiophate

(124). It should be given concurrently with the causative agent—not more than three times daily. Chronic use of phenylephrine can result in rebound miosis and poor dilatory effect, especially in older patients.

The vasoconstrictor properties of phenylephrine are useful in differentiating benign superficial episcleral congestion from deeper scleral vessel congestion, which may indicate scleritis or iritis (108). One drop of phenylephrine 2.5% is applied to the conjunctiva, and the perilimbal vessels are observed 5 minutes later. Failure of the vessels to blanch is evidence of scleritis or iritis. Dilute phenylephrine 0.08% to 0.12%, 1 drop every 3 to 4 hours, is an effective ocular decongestant (125). However, chronic use may result in severe rebound congestion.

Topical phenylephrine may decrease the intraocular pressure by increasing aqueous outflow facility, and may be useful in the treatment of some secondary glaucomas (124). It may also be used as a provocative test for occludable angles (narrow-angle glaucoma). An increase in IOP of 5 mm or more in response to 1 drop 2.5% phenylephrine strongly suggests the presence of angle-closure glaucoma, although its absence may not exclude the condition (126). This test is no longer favored because occludable angles are currently diagnosed by gonioscopy and are usually safely treated with laser iridotomy.

Phenylephrine is contraindicated in patients with narrow-angle glaucoma and in patients with known hypersensitivity to the drug. Because of the risk of its systemic absorption, the benefit of this drug should be carefully weighed against the possibility of adverse effects in every patient (described in High-risk Groups section). Ten percent solution is contraindicated in neonates and young children and in patients with aneurysms. Phenylephrine is contraindicated in persons with known hypersensitivity to sulfites, which may be present as preservatives in some preparations.

Side Effects and Toxicity

Local reactions to phenylephrine include transient irritation and pain, rebound miosis, bulbar/palpebral conjunctivitis, and periorbital edema. Severe contact dermatitis has also been reported after administration of topical phenylephrine (127).

Conjunctival hypoxia has been reported after 1 drop 2.5% phenylephrine. This may cause potential problems for patients with sickle cell anemia, postoperative patients (reduced wound healing), soft contact lens wearers, and patients treated with epinephrine or related compound for treatment of open-angle glaucoma (128).

Potentially life-threatening side effects include hypertension, tachycardia, ventricular arrhythmia, stroke, myocardial infarction, and subarachnoid hemorrhage. At least 15 cases of myocardial infarction (11 fatal) and 22 other cases of adverse reactions (including severe hypertension, cardiopulmonary collapse, and intracranial hemorrhage) have been reported after application of topical phenylephrine 10% (129). A fatal rupture of a congenital berry aneurysm caused by severe hypertension after one dose of topical phenylephrine was reported in a patient who had been receiving propranolol (130). Patients with preexisting hypertension and cardiovascular or cerebrovascular disease are especially susceptible to adverse effects. Hallucinations can result from chronic overuse of nasal phenylephrine (131). The lethal systemic dose of phenylephrine in humans has not been established; the LD_{50} in rats is 350 mg/kg; in mice, it is 120 mg/kg (phenylephrine hydrochloride, USP, Iolab. Pharmaceuticals, Claremont, CA, package insert, Nov. 1989).

High-risk Groups

The therapeutic benefit of the drug must be weighed against the risks it poses when phenylephrine 2.5% or 10% is used in treatment of patients with coronary vessel disease, advanced atherosclerotic disease, bronchial asthma, hyperthyroidism, hypertension, orthostatic hypotension, insulin-dependent diabetes mellitus, and narrow-angle glaucoma. BP can increase markedly if phenylephrine is absorbed systemically (108,129,132).

Premature infants are at higher risk of adverse effects of phenylephrine (133,134). In a study of 7 preterm infants who received tropicamide 0.5% and phenylephrine 2.5% drops, mean arterial BP increased from a baseline of 41.4 ± 7.9 mm Hg to 51.1 ± 10.4 mm Hg at 8 minutes. The effect began at 2 minutes and continued for 30 minutes. The BP increase may have predisposed these infants to development of intraventricular hemorrhages (134). Phenylephrine 10% is contraindicated for use in infants. Cardiovascular collapse occurred in a 3-week-old girl after topical administration of 1 drop of 10% phenylephrine after induction of general anesthesia with halothane (135).

Patients with open-angle glaucoma may be at significant risk of developing increased IOP after dilation with phenylephrine. In a retrospective study, 32% of patients had an increase in IOP greater than 5 mm Hg and 12% had an increase greater than 10 mm Hg after receiving tropicamide 1% and phenylephrine 2.5%. The concurrent use of miotics was an important risk factor (136). Such an increase in IOP may be harmful in optic nerves already compromised in glaucoma.

Monoamine oxidase inhibitors and tricyclic antidepressants can potentiate the pressor effects of phenylephrine. Patients treated with these medications are at higher risk of adverse side effects, even from topical phenylephrine. Geriatric patients are more prone to the systemic side effects of phenylephrine due to the inherent prevalence of cardiovascular disease and preexisting medical problems.

Phenylephrine is an FDA category C drug; its safety in pregnancy has not been established, and the drug should be used cautiously in pregnant women or breast-feeding women. The presence of phenylephrine in breast milk is probably minimal, but few data are available.

Drug Interactions

Monoamine oxidase inhibitors (e.g., tranylcypromine, clorgyline, phenelzine, furazolidone) prevent metabolism of norepinephrine, leading to increased availability of norepinephrine at the receptor sites. Severe uncontrolled hypertension can occur when phenylephrine is administered concurrently with these drugs (137).

Tricyclic antidepressants (e.g., amitriptyline, nortriptyline, doxepin, imipramine, desipramine) may enhance the pressor effect of phenylephrine. If use of a tricyclic antidepressant is necessary, the dosage of phenylephrine should be reduced (138).

β-Blockers (e.g., propranolol) may enhance the vasopressor effect of phenylephrine by inhibiting vasodilatation. Hypertensive crisis has been reported with concurrent use of these medications (130). β-Agonists and other sympathomimetic agents (e.g., albuterol) can also enhance cardiovascular effects of phenylephrine.

Concurrent use of phenylephrine and guanethidine is not recommended due to increased risk of severe hypertension. Guanethidine exerts its antihypertensive property by inhibiting neuronal uptake of norepinephrine and causes increased hypersensitivity of the adrenergic receptor to catecholamines (139).

Major Clinical Trials

The mydriatic effect of the combination of phenylephrine HCl 5% and tropicamide 0.8% was compared with that of tropicamide 0.8% alone. Although the combination provided fast pupillary dilation, its mydriatic effect did not differ significantly from that of tropicamide 1% alone (140).

The synergistic effect of topical nonsteroidal antiinflammatory drugs (NSAIDS) and phenylephrine in dilating the pupil intraoperatively was evaluated by Gimbel (141) in a trial of 216 patients. Patients undergoing cataract surgery were randomized to receive flurbiprofen, indomethacin with and without epinephrine, epinephrine alone, or placebo. Patients who received the combination of NSAIDS and phenylephrine had less intraoperative miosis than did those who received either drug alone (141).

Lynch et al. (142) examined the effect of a reduced drop size of phenylephrine in 11 premature infants. Phenylephrine drops 8 μl dilated the pupil as well as 30-μl (commercial size), with less systemic absorption (142).

HYDROXYAMPHETAMINE HYDROBROMIDE

Hydroxyamphetamine hydrobromide (paredrine) is a synthetic indirect-acting sympathomimetic that causes pupillary mydriasis by stimulating release of endogenous norepinephrine from intact adrenergic nerve endings in the iris dilator. In normal subjects, hydroxyamphetamine 1% produces a mean increase of pupillary size of +1.96 mm ($\pm$0.61 mm) (143). It has been used in combination with other agents such as homatropine and tropicamide to enhance their mydriatic properties, but it has little or no cycloplegic effect. It is primarily used, however, for pharmacologic localization of lesions causing Horner's syndrome (144). Hydroxyamphetamine hydrobromide, previously available as 1% solution with tropicamide 0.25% (Paremyd, Allergan, Irvine, CA) for mydriasis, has been discontinued. Hydroxyamphetamine is discussed in detail in Chapter 71, *this volume*.

ACKNOWLEDGEMENTS

This work was supported in part by an unrestricted grant from Research to Prevent Blindness, Inc., New York, New York.

REFERENCES

1. Brown JH. Atropine, scopolamine, and related antimuscarinic drugs. In: Gilman AF, Rall TW, Nies AS, Taylor P, eds. *Goodman and Gilman's the Pharmacological Basis of Therapeutics,* 8th ed. New York: Pergamon Press, 1990;150–165.
2. Dollery C. *Therapeutic Drugs.* Edinburgh: Churchill Livingstone, 1991.
3. Loewenfeld IE. Pupillary pharmacology. In: *The pupil,* Detroit: Wayne State University Press, 1993;683–826.
4. Wells WC. Observations and experiments on vision. Cited in Marron J. Cycloplegia and mydriasis by use of atropine, scopolamine and homatropine-paredrine. *Arch Ophthalmol* 1940;23:340–350. *Phil Tr R Soc London* 1811;101:378–380.
5. Lussana F. Dell'azione e delle virtu terapeutiche dell'atropina e della belladonna. Cited in Marron J. Cycloplegia and mydriasis by use of atropine, scopolamine and homatropine-paredrine. *Arch Ophthalmol* 1940;23:340–350. *Ann Univ Med* 1852;140:514.
6. Fedderson IM. Bietrag zur Atropinvergiftung. Cited in Marron J. Cycloplegia and mydriasis by use of atropine, scopolamine and homatropine-paredrine. *Arch Ophthalmol* 1940;23:340–350. *Inaugural Dissertation, Berlin* 1884.
7. Wolf AV, Hodge HC. Effects of atropine sulfate, methylatropine nitrate (metropine) and homatropine hydrobromide on adult human eyes. *Arch Ophthalmol* 1946;36:293–310.
8. Kentala E, Kaila T, Iisalo E, Kanto J. Intramuscular atropine in healthy volunteers: a pharmacokinetic and pharmacodynamic study. *Int J Clin Pharmacol Ther Toxicol* 1990;28:399–404.
9. Mirakhur RK. Comparative study of the effects of oral and I.M. atropine and hyoscine in volunteers. *Br J Anaesth* 1978;50:591–598.
10. Wellstein A, Pitschner HF. Complex dose-response curves of atropine in man explained by different functions of M1- and M2-cholinoreceptors. Cited in Brown JH. Atropine, scopolamine, and related antimuscarinic drugs. In Gilman AF, Rall TW, Nies AS, Taylor P, eds. *Goodman and Gilman's the Pharmacological Basis of Therapeutics.* New York: Pergamon Press, 1990. *Naunyn Schmiedebergs Arch Pharmacol* 1988;338:19–27.
11. Havener WH. Autonomic drugs. In: *Ocular Pharmacology,* St. Louis: C.V. Mosby, 1978;218–328.
12. Janes RC, Stiles JF. The penetration of C14 labeled atropine into the eye. *Ann Ophthalmol* 1959;62:69–74.
13. Lahdes K, Kaila T, Huupponen R, Salminen L, Iisalo E. Systemic absorption of topically applied ocular atropine. *Clin Pharmacol Ther* 1988;44:310–314.
14. Virtanen R, Kanto J, Iisalo E, Iisalo EUM, Salo M, Sjövall S. Pharmacokinetic studies on atropine with special reference to age. *Acta Anaesthesiol Scand* 1982;26:297–300.
15. Pihlajamaki K, Kanto J, Aaltonen L, Iisalo E, Jaakkola P. Pharmacokinetics of atropine in children. *Int J Clin Pharmacol Ther Toxicol* 1986;24:236–239.
16. Aaltonen L, Kanto J, Iisalo E, Pihlajamaki K. Comparison of ra-

dioreceptor assay and radioimmunoassay for atropine: pharmacokinetic application. *Eur J Clin Pharmacol* 1984;26:613–617.
17. Berghem L, Bergman U, Schildt B, Sörbo B. Plasma atropine concentrations determined by radioimmunoassay after single-dose I.V. and I.M. administration. *Br J Anaesth* 1980;52:597–601.
18. Beermann B, Hellström K, Rosén A. The gastrointestinal absorption of atropine in man. *Clin Sci* 1971;40:95–106.
19. Salazar M, Shamada K, Patie PN. Iris pigmentation and atropine mydriasis. *J Pharmacol Exp Ther* 1976;197:79–88.
20. Kalser SC. The fate of atropine in man. *Ann NY Acad Sci* 1995;179: 667–683.
21. Kalser SC, McLain PL. Atropine metabolism in man. *Clin Pharmacol Ther* 1970;11:214–217.
22. von Noorden GK, Milam JB. Penalization in the treatment of amblyopia. *Am J Ophthalmol* 1979;88:511–518.
23. Repka MX, Ray JM. The efficacy of optical and pharmacologic penalization. *Ophthalmology* 1993;100:769–774.
24. Ikeda H, Tremain KE. Amblyopia resulting from penalization: Neurophysiological studies of kittens reared with atropinisation of one or both eyes. *Br J Ophthalmol* 1978;62:21.
25. Gimbel HV. The control of myopia with atropine. *Can J Ophthalmol* 1973;8:527–532.
26. Brodstein RS, Brodstein DE, Olson RJ, Hunt SC, Williams RR. The treatment of myopia with atropine and bifocals. *Ophthalmology* 1984;91:1373–1378.
27. Alexander JP. Reflex disturbances of cardiac rhythm during ophthalmic surgery. *Br J Ophthalmol* 1975;59:518–524.
28. Chandler PA, Grant WM. Mydriatic-cycloplegic treatment in malignant glaucoma. *Arch Ophthalmol* 1962;68:353.
29. O'Connor PS, Mumma JV. Atropine toxicity. *Am J Ophthalmol* 1985;99:613–614.
30. Alexander E, Morris DP, Eslick RL. Atropine poisoning: report of a case with recovery after ingestion of one gram. *N Engl J Med* 1946;234:258–259.
31. Heath WE. Death from atropine poisoning. *Br Med J* 1950;2:608.
32. Mackenzie AL, Piggott JFG. Atropine overdose in three children. *Br J Anaesth* 1971;43:1088–1090.
33. Rumack BH. Anticholinergic poisoning: treatment with physostigmine. *Pediatrics* 1973;52:449–451.
34. Duvoisin RC, Katz R. Reversal of central anticholinergic syndrome in man by physostigmine. *JAMA* 1968;206:1963–1965.
35. Kanto J, Virtanen R, Iisalo E, Mäenpää K, Liukko P. Placental transfer and pharmacokinetics of atropine after a single maternal intravenous and intramuscular administration. *Acta Anaesthesiol Scand* 1981;25:85–88.
36. Harris WS, Goodman RM. Hyper-reactivity to atropine in Down's syndrome. *N Engl J Med* 1968;279:407–410.
37. Sacks B, Smith S. People with Down's syndrome can be distinguished on the basis of cholinergic dysfunction. *J Neurol Neurosurg Psychiatry* 1989;52:1294–1295.
38. Urrets-Zavalía A Jr. Fixed, dilated pupil, iris atrophy and secondary glaucoma: a distinct clinical entity following penetrating keratoplasty in keratoconus. *Am J Ophthalmol* 1963;56:257–265.
39. Geyer O, Rothkoff L, Lazar M. Atropine in keratoplasty for keratoconus. *Cornea* 1991;10:372–373.
40. Harris LS. Cycloplegic-induced intraocular pressure elevations. A study of normal and open-angle glaucomatous eyes. *Arch Ophthalmol* 1968;79:242–246.
41. Tammisto T, Castren JA, Marttila I. Intramuscularly administrated atropine and the eye. *Acta Ophthalmol* 1964;42:408.
42. Rosenbaum AL, Bateman JB, Bremer DL, Liu PY. Cycloplegic refraction in esotropic children. *Ophthalmology* 1981;88:1031–1034.
43. Vierling F. Uber die Wirkung des Scopolamin Hydrobromicum. Cited in Marron J. Cycloplegia and mydriasis by use of atropine, scopolamine and homatropine-paredrine. Arch Ophthalmol 1940; 23:340–350. *Beitr Z Augenheilkd* 1894;13:1.
44. Martelli P. Sulla Scopalamina. Cited in Marron J. Cycloplegia and mydriasis by use of atropine, scopolamine and homatropine-paredrine. *Arch Ophthalmol* 1940;23:340–350. *Arch Ottal* 1893; 1:63.
45. Marron J. Cycloplegia and mydriasis by use of atropine, scopolamine and homatropine-paredrine. *Arch Ophthalmol* 1940;23:340–350.
46. Ali-Melkkilä T, Kanto J, Iisalo E. Pharmacokinetics and related pharmacodynamics of anticholinergic drugs. *Acta Anaesthesiol Scand* 1993;37:633–642.
47. Leopold IH, Comroe JH. Effect of intramuscular administration of atropine, scopolamine, and neostigmine on the human eye. *Arch Ophthalmol* 1948;40:285–290.
48. Kanto J, Kentala E, Kaila T, Pihlajamäki K. Pharmacokinetics of scopolamine during caesarean section: relationship between concentration and effect. *Acta Anaesthesiol Scand* 1989;33:482–486.
49. Putcha L, Cintron NM, Tsui J, Vanderploeg JM, Kramer WG. Pharmacokinetics and oral bioavailability of scopolamine in normal subjects. *Pharm Res* 1989;6:481–485.
50. Lahdes K, Huupponen R, Kaila T, Salminen L, Iisalo E. Systemic absorption of ocular scopolamine in patients. *J Ocul Pharmacol* 1990;6:61–66.
51. Wada S, Yoshimitsu T, Koga N, Yamada H, Oguri K, Yoshimura H. Metabolism in vivo of the tropane alkaloid, scopolamine, in several mammalian species. *Xenobiotica* 1991;21:1289–1300.
52. Kentala E, Kaila T, Ali-Melkkilä T, Kanto J. Beta-glucuronide and sulfate conjugation of scopolamine and glycopyrrolate. *Int J Clin Pharmacol Ther Toxicol* 1990;28:487–489.
53. Watanabe T, Funayama M, Morita M. Fatal anaphylactic shock to hyoscine and diphenhydramine. *Clin Toxicol* 1994;32:593–594.
54. Freund M, Merin S. Toxic effects of scopolamine eye drops. *Am J Ophthalmol* 1970;70:637–639.
55. Young SE, Ruiz RS, Falletta J. Reversal of systemic toxic effects of scopolamine with physostigmine salicylate. *Am J Ophthalmol* 1971; 72:1136–1138.
56. Barbee RF, Smith WO. A comparative study of mydriatic and cycloplegic agents. *Am J Ophthalmol* 1957;44:617–622.
57. Thorne FH, Murphey HS. Cycloplegics. *Arch Ophthalmol* 1939;22: 274–287.
58. Gambill HD, Ogle KN, Kearns TP. Mydriatic effect of four drugs determined with pupillograph. *Arch Ophthalmol* 1967;77:740–746.
59. Gettes BC, Belmont O. Tropicamide: comparative cycloplegic effects. *Arch Ophthalmol* 1961;66:336–341.
60. Christensen RE, Pearce I. Homatropine hydrobromide. Effects of topical application upon the intraocular pressure and aqueous outflow facility values of normal and simple glaucomatous eyes. *Ophthalmology* 1963;70:376–380.
61. Tune LE, Bylsma FW, Hilt DC. Anticholinergic delirium caused by topical homatropine ophthalmologic solution: confirmation by anticholinergic radioreceptor assay in two cases. *J Neuropsychiatry Clin Neurosci* 1992;4:195–197.
62. Hoefnagel D. Toxic effects of atropine and homatropine eyedrops in children. *N Engl J Med* 1961;264:168–171.
63. Walsh FB. *Clinical Neuro-Ophthalmology.* 2nd ed. Baltimore: Williams & Wilkins, 1995;1193.
64. Merrill DL, Goldberg B, Zavell S. Bis-tropamide, a new parasympatholytic. *Curr Ther Res* 1960;12:43–50.
65. Pollack SL, Hunt JS, Polse KA. Dose-response effects of tropicamide HCl. *Am J Optom Physiol Opt* 1981;58:361–366.
66. Pines A, Fisman EZ, Drory Y, et al. Influence of ocular tropicamide on exercise testing. *Cardiology* 1992;81:172–177.
67. Vuori ML, Kaila T, Iisalo E, Saari KM. Systemic absorption and anticholinergic activity of topically applied tropicamide. *J Ocul Pharmacol* 1994;10:431–437.
68. Schoenwald RD, Smolen VF. Drug-absorption analysis from pharmacological data II: transcorneal biophasic availability of tropicamide. *J Pharmacol Sci* 1971;60:1039–1045.
69. Delgado D, Michel P, Jaanus SD. Effect of tropicamide on ocular blood flow in the rabbit. *Am J Optom Physiol Opt* 1982;59:410–412.
70. Robinson F, Petrig BL, Sinclair SH, Riva CE, Grunwald JE. Does topical phenylephrine, tropicamide, or proparacaine affect macular blood flow? *Ophthalmology* 1985;92:1130–1132.
71. Huber MJ, Smith SA, Smith SE. Mydriatic drugs for diabetic patients. *Br J Ophthalmol* 1985;69:425–427.
72. Levine L. Mydriatic effectiveness of dilute combinations of phenylephrine and tropicamide. *Am J Optom Physiol Opt* 1982;59: 580–594.
73. Gettes BC, Leopold IH. Evaluation of five new cycloplegic drugs. *Arch Ophthalmol* 1953;49:24–27.
74. Mapstone R. Dilating dangerous pupils. *Br J Ophthalmol* 1977;61: 517–524.
75. Rengstorff RH, Doughty CB. Mydriatic and cycloplegic drugs: a re-

view of ocular and systemic complications. *Am J Optom Physiol Opt* 1982;59:162–177.
76. Guill MA, Goette DK, Knight CG, Peck CC, Lupton GP. Erythema multiforme and urticaria: eruptions induced by chemically related ophthalmic anticholinergic agents. *Arch Dermatol* 1979;115:742–743.
77. Wahl JW. Systemic reaction to tropicamide. *Arch Ophthalmol* 1969; 82:320–321.
78. Yolton DP, Kandel JS, Yolton RL. Diagnostic pharmaceutical agents: side effects encountered in a study of 15000 applications. *J Am Optom Assoc* 1980;51:113–117.
79. Paggiarino DA, Brancato LJ, Newton RE. The effects on pupil size and accommodation of sympathetic and parasympatholytic agents. *Ann Ophthalmol* 1993;25:244–253.
80. McKinna H, Stewart-Jones JH, Edgar DF, Turner P. Reversal of tropicamide-induced mydriasis by thymoxamine eye drops. *Curr Med Res Opin* 1988;11:1–3.
81. Molinari JF, Johnson ME, Carter J. Dapiprazole clinical efficiency for counteracting tropicamide 1%. *Optom Vis Sci* 1994;71:319–322.
82. Gettes BC. Tropicamide, a new cycloplegic mydriatic. *Arch Ophthalmol* 1961;65:632–635.
83. Milder B. Tropicamide as a cycloplegic agent. *Arch Ophthalmol* 1961;66:70–72.
84. Egashira SM, Kish LL, Twelker JD, Mutti DO, Zadnik K, Adams AJ. Comparison of cyclopentolate versus tropicamide cycloplegia in children. *Optom Vis Sci* 1993;70:1019–1026.
85. Scinto LFM, Daffner KR, Dressler D, et al. A potential noninvasive neurobiological test for Alzheimer's disease. *Science* 1994;266: 1051–1054.
86. Marx JL, Kumar SR, Thach AB, Kiat-Winarko T, Frambach DA. Detecting Alzheimer's disease [Letter]. *Science* 1995;267:1577.
87. Treloar A, Assin M, Macdonald A. Detecting Alzheimer's disease [Letter]. *Science* 1995;267:1578.
88. Treves GR, Testa FC. Basic esters and quaternary derivatives of β-hydroxy acids as antispasmodics. *J Am Chem Soc* 1952;74:46–48.
89. Priestly BS, Medine MM. A new mydriatic and cycloplegic drug. Compound 75 G.T. *Am J Ophthalmol* 1951;34:572–574.
90. Ehrenberg MH, Ramp JA, Blanchard EW, Treves GR. Antispasmodic activity of basic esters and quaternary derivatives of β-hydroxy acids. *J Pharmacol Exp Ther* 1952;106:141–156.
91. Gordon DM, Ehrenberg MH. Cyclopentolate hydrochloride: a new mydriatic and cycloplegic agent. *Am J Ophthalmol* 1954;38:831–838.
92. Milder B, Riffenburgh RS. An evaluation of cyclogyl (compound 75 GT). *Am J Ophthalmol* 1953;36:1724–1726.
93. Smith SA. Factors determining the potency of mydriatic drugs in man. *Br J Clin Pharmacol* 1976;3:503–507.
94. Lovasik JV. Pharmacokinetics of topically applied cyclopentolate HCl and tropicamide. *Am J Optom Physiol Opt* 1986;63:787–803.
95. Kaila T, Huupponen R, Salminen L, Iisalo E. Systemic absorption of ophthalmic cyclopentolate. *Am J Ophthalmol* 1989;107:562–564.
96. Lahdes K, Huupponen R, Kaila T, Monti D, Saettone MF, Salminen L. Plasma concentrations and ocular effects of cyclopentolate after ocular application of three formulations. *Br J Clin Pharmacol* 1993; 35:479–483.
97. Tsai E, Till GO, Marak GE, Jr. Effects of mydriatic agents on neutrophil migration. *Ophthalmic Res* 1988;20:14–19.
98. Jones LWJ, Hodes DT. Possible allergic reactions to cyclopentolate hydrochloride: case reports with literature review of uses and adverse reactions. *Ophthal Physiol Opt* 1991;11:16–21.
99. Caputo AR, Schnitzer RE. Systemic response to eyedrops in neonates: mydriatics in neonates. *J Pediatr Ophthalmol Strabismus* 1978;15:109–122.
100. Gettes BC. Drugs in refraction. *Int Ophthalmol Clin* 1961;1:237–248.
101. Ingram RM, Barr A. Refraction of 1-year-old children after cycloplegia with cyclopentolate; comparison with findings after atropinisation. *Br J Ophthalmol* 1979;63:348–352.
102. Oliver G, Shafer EA. The physiological effects of extracts from the suprarenal capsules. *J Physiol* 1895;18:230–276.
103. Hartung WH. Epinephrine and related compounds: influence of structure on physiologic activity. *Chem Rev* 1931;9:389–465.
104. Barger G, Dale HH. Chemical structure and sympathomimetic action of amines. *J Physiol* 1910;41:19–59.
105. Saint-Martin D. Mydriasis by epinephrine in cataract extraction. *Arch Ophthalmol* 1929;1:141.
106. Heath P. Neosynephrine hydrochloride. Some uses and effects in ophthalmology. *Arch Ophthalmol* 1936;16:839–846.
107. McReynolds WU, Havener WH, Henderson JW. Hazards of the use of sympathomimetic drugs in ophthalmology. *Arch Ophthalmol* 1956;56:176–179.
108. *United States Pharmacopoeia,* 14th ed. Rockville, MD: United States Pharmacopeal Convention, Inc., 1994;2243–2250.
109. Gambill HD, Ogle KN, Kearns TP. Mydriatic effect of phenylephrine hydrochloride. *Am J Ophthalmol* 1970;70:729–733.
110. Haddad NJ, Moyer NJ, Riley FC. Mydriatic effect of phenylephrine hydrochloride. *Am J Ophthalmol* 1970;70:729–733.
111. Antonaci F, Fredriksen TA, Sand T, et al. Electronic pupillometry in healthy controls. Response to sympathicomimetics. *Funct Neurol* 1989;4:91–103.
112. Neuhas RW, Hepler RS. Mydriatic effect of phenylephrine 10% vs. phenylephrine 2.5% (aq). *Ann Ophthalmol* 1980;12:1159–1160.
113. Weiss DI, Shaffer RN. Mydriatic effects of one eighth percent phenylephrine. *Arch Ophthalmol* 1962;12:1159–1160.
114. Lyle WM, Bobier WR. Effects of topical anesthetics on phenylephrine-induced mydriasis. *Am J Optom Physiol Opt* 1977;54:276– 281.
115. Ashton P, Clark DS, Lee VH. A mechanistic study on the enhancement of corneal penetration of phenylephrine by flurbiprofen in the rabbit. *Curr Eye Res* 1992;11:85–90.
116. Martinsson A, Bevergard S, Hjemdahl P. Analysis of phenylephrine in plasma; initial data about the concentration-effect relationship. *Eur J Clin Pharmacol* 1986;30:427–431.
117. Innes IR, Nickerson M. Norepinephrine, epinephrine, and the sympathomimetic amines. In: Goodman LS, Gilman A, eds. *The Pharmacological Basis of Therapeutics,* 5th ed. New York: Macmillan, 1975;477–513.
118. Kumar V, Schoenwald RD, Chien DS, Packer AJ, Choi WW. Systemic absorption and cardiovascular effects of phenylephrine eyedrops. *Am J Ophthalmol* 1985;99:180–184.
119. Antoine ME, Edelhauser HF, O'Brien WJ. Pharmacokinetics of topical phenylephrine HCl. *Invest Ophthalmol Vis Sci* 1984;25:48–54.
120. Hengstmann JH, Goronzy J. Pharmacokinetics of 3H-phenylephrine in man. *Eur J Clin Pharmacol* 1982;21:335–341.
121. Elis J, Laurence DR, Mattie H, Pritchard BNC. Modification by monoamine oxidase inhibitors of the effects of some sympathomimetics on blood pressure. *Br Med J* 1967;2:75–78.
122. Bruce RB, Pitts JE. The determination and excretion of phenylephrine in urine. *Biochem Pharmacol* 1968;17:335–337.
123. Duffin RM, Petit TH, Straatsma BR. 2.5% vs 10% phenylephrine in maintaining mydriasis during cataract surgery. *Arch Ophthalmol* 1983;101:1903–1906.
124. Meyer SM, Fraunfelder FT. Phenylephrine hydrochloride. *Ophthalmology* 1980;87:1177–1180.
125. Abelson MB, Yamamoto GK, Allansmith MR. Effects of ocular decongestants. *Arch Ophthalmol* 1980;98:856–858.
126. Harris LS, Galin MA. Prone provocative testing for narrow angle glaucoma. *Arch Ophthalmol* 1972;87:493–496.
127. Hanna C, Brainard J, Augspager KD. Allergic dermatoconjunctivitis caused by phenylephrine. *Am J Ophthalmol* 1983;95:703–704.
128. Isenberg SJ, Green BF. Effect of phenylephrine hydrochloride on conjunctival PO2. *Arch Ophthalmol* 1984;102:1185–1186.
129. Adler AG, McElwain GE, Merli GJ, Martin JH. Systemic effects of eye drops. *Arch Intern Med* 1982;142:2293–2294.
130. Cass E, Kadar D, Stein HA. Hazards of phenylephrine topical medication in persons taking propranolol. *Can Med Assoc J* 1979;120: 1261–1262.
131. Escobar JI, Karno M. Chronic hallucinosis from nasal drops. *JAMA* 1982;247:1859–1860.
132. Lansche RK. Systemic reactions to topical epinephrine and phenylephrine. *Am J Ophthalmol* 1966;61:95–99.
133. Isenberg S, Everette S. Cardiovascular effects of mydriatics in low-birth-weight infants. *J Pediatr* 1984;105:111–112.
134. Lees BJ, Cabal LA. Increased blood pressure following pupillary dilation with 2.5% phenylephrine hydrochloride in preterm infants. *Pediatrics* 1981;68:231–234.
135. Van Der Spek AF. Cyanosis and cardiovascular depression in a neonate; complications of halothane anesthesia or phenylephrine eyedrops? *Can J Ophthalmol* 1987;22:37–39.

136. Shaw BR, Lewis RA. Intraocular pressure elevation after pupillary dilation in open angle glaucoma. *Arch Ophthalmol* 1986;104:1185–1188.
137. Horler AR, Wynne NA. Hypertensive crisis due to pargyline and metaraminol. *Br Med J* 1965;2:460–461.
138. Boakes AJ, Laurence DR, Teoh PC. Interactions between sympathomimetic amines and antidepressant agents in man. *Br Med J* 1973; 1:311–315.
139. Gulati OD, Dave BT, Gokhale SD. Antagonism of adrenergic neuron blockade in hypertensive subjects. *Clin Pharmacol Ther* 1966;7:510–514.
140. Kergoat H, Lovasik JV, Doughty MJ. A pupillographic evaluation of a phenylephrine HCl 5%-tropicamide 0.8% combination mydriatic. *J Ocul Pharmacol* 1989;5:199–214.
141. Gimbel HV. The effect of treatment with topical nonsteroidal anti-inflammatory drugs with and without intraoperative epinephrine on the maintenance of mydriasis during cataract surgery. *Ophthalmology* 1989;96:585–588.
142. Lynch MG, Brown RH, Goode SM, Schoenwald RD, Chien DS. Reduction of phenylephrine drop size in infants achieves equal dilation with decreased systemic absorption. *Arch Ophthalmol* 1987;105: 1364–1365.
143. Cremer SA, Thompson HS, Digre KB, Kardon RH. Hydroxyamphetamine mydriasis in normal subjects. *Am J Ophthalmol* 1990; 110:66–70.
144. Thompson HS, Mensher JH. Adrenergic mydriasis in Horner's syndrome. Hydroxyamphetamine test for diagnosis of postganglionic defects. *Am J Ophthalmol* 1971;72:472–480.

Textbook of Ocular Pharmacology,
edited by T.J. Zimmerman, et al.
Lippincott–Raven Publishers, Philadelphia © 1997.

CHAPTER 71

Drugs for the Diagnosis of Pupillary Disorders

Carol F. Zimmerman

The size of the pupil is determined by the opposing forces of two smooth muscles, the iris dilator and sphincter. The dilator is radially oriented within the anterior layer of the iris pigment epithelium. It originates in the iris root and inserts approximately 2 mm from the pupillary margin. The dilator is innervated by sympathetic adrenergic neurons. Contraction of the radially oriented fibers enlarges the pupillary aperture. The iris sphincter lies more superficial to the dilator and is circumferentially oriented in a band several millimeters from the pupillary margin. The sphincter is innervated by parasympathetic cholinergic neurons; contraction of the circumferential fibers narrows the pupillary aperture. Abnormalities of pupil size and reactivity are usually caused by disturbances of autonomic innervation. Local lesions of the iris or its muscles are less common.

Physiologic or benign anisocoria of less than 1 mm is observed clinically in approximately 20% of the normal population and was reported in as many as 80% in one study (1). The relative degree of anisocoria remains constant under varying conditions of light and darkness, and the pupils react equally well. Benign anisocoria may not be permanent, and the size of the pupils may even reverse, with the previously larger pupil becoming the smaller. Careful assessment of the pupillary size and reactivity and the identification of focal iris abnormalities are necessary to distinguish benign anisocoria from that associated with nervous system pathology.

THE SYMPATHETIC INNERVATION OF THE IRIS

The sympathetic innervation of the iris dilator consists of a three-neuron pathway (Fig. 1). The first-order or central neurons originate in the hypothalamus and descend through the midbrain tegmentum and pons to course laterally in the medulla. Axons from the central neurons synapse with the second-order or preganglionic neurons in the intermediolateral cell column of the spinal cord at the level of C8-T2 (ciliospinal center of Budge). The preganglionic axons exit the cord through the ventral thoracic root and the white rami communicantes and enter the paravertebral sympathetic chain. The preganglionic axons course in close proximity to the apex of the lung and ascend to the superior cervical ganglion where they synapse with the third-order or postganglionic neurons. The postganglionic axons then ascend with the internal carotid artery to enter the skull; sympathetic fibers for facial sweating and vasoconstriction follow the external carotid artery and its branches to the face. Sympathetic axons in the cavernous sinus are close to the abducens nerve and enter the orbit with the nasociliary nerve. Pupillary sympathetics in the orbit pass through the ciliary ganglion without synapsing and reach the iris dilator muscle through the long ciliary nerves.

C. F. Zimmerman: Department of Ophthalmology, The University of Texas Southwestern Medical Center at Dallas, Dallas, Texas 75235-9057.

HORNER'S SYNDROME

Horner's syndrome, or oculosympathetic paresis, results from ipsilateral interruption of the sympathetic innervation to the eye. Characteristic features include ptosis, miosis, elevation of the lower eyelid with narrowing of the palpebral fissure, and facial anhydrosis. Miosis and slowed dilation result from disruption of the sympathetics to the pupillary dilator muscle. Partial upper eyelid ptosis and elevation of the lower eyelid (inverse ptosis) result from decreased innervation of Mueller's muscle and the lower eyelid retractors. Narrowing of the interpalpebral fissure mimics enophthalmos. Loss of facial sweating occurs if the lesion is proximal to the superior cervical ganglion. Lesions distal to the ganglion spare the sweating and vasoconstrictor fibers. Less consistent features of Horner's syndrome include conjunctival hyperemia, transient ocular hypotony, and increased accommodative amplitudes (2).

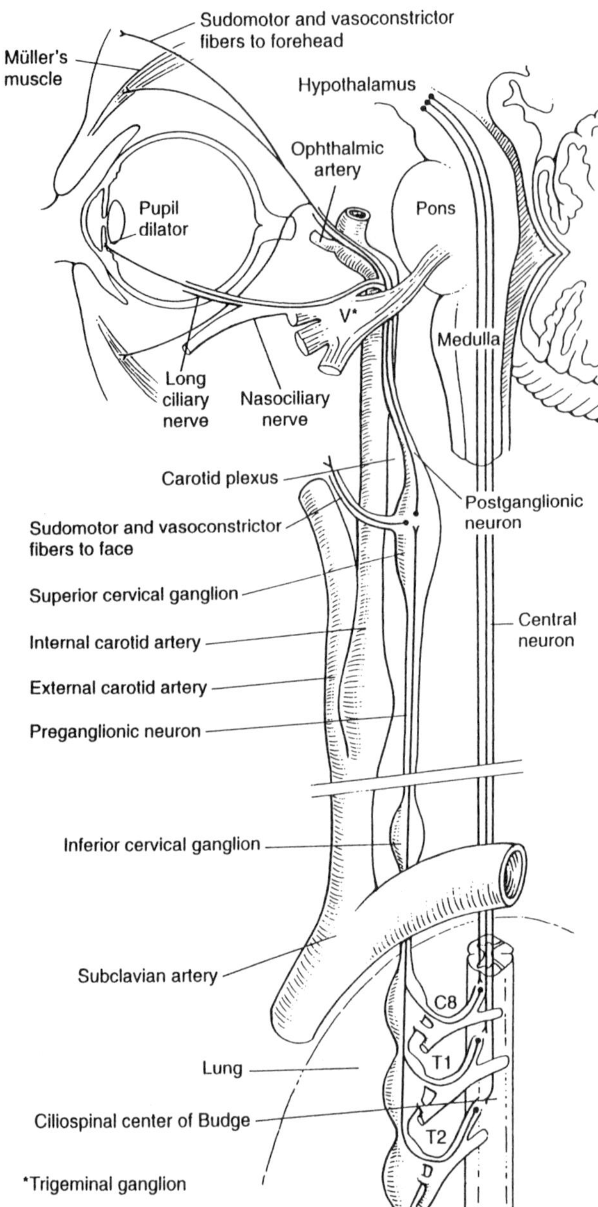

FIG. 71-1. The oculosympathetic pathway. (Redrawn with permission from J.M. Weinstein. *The Pupil.* In: Slamovits TL, Burde R. *Neuro-ophthalmology.* In: Podos SM, Yanoff M, eds. *Textbook of Ophthalmology.* London: Mosby, 1994; 5.1–5.24.)

Heterochromia iridis (difference in color of the two irides) is common in congenital Horner's syndrome and results from defective iris pigmentation by stromal melanocytes, which is under sympathetic control (3). The affected iris is usually a lighter color. Heterochromia iridis is occasionally evident in acquired Horner's syndrome (4).

Lesions of any part of the sympathetic pathway may cause Horner's syndrome. Central Horner's syndrome involves the first-order neuron and is most commonly due to brainstem infarction, particularly occlusion of the posterior inferior cerebellar (lateral medullary syndrome of Wallenburg). Other causes include brainstem hemorrhage, intracranial and intraspinal tumors, syringomyelia, trauma, demyelinating disease, and infection. Horner's syndrome involving the second-order neuron (preganglionic sympathetic paresis) is usually caused by tumors, trauma, or carotid artery dissection (2). Horner's syndrome associated with ipsilateral arm pain raises suspicion of an apical lung tumor (Pancoast's syndrome) (5). Malignant neoplasms are detected in 13% to 35% of patients with Horner's syndrome (6,7). Neoplasms are more likely to be associated with preganglionic Horner's syndrome, with 84% localizing to the first- or second-order neurons. Patients with preganglionic lesions should undergo careful evaluation for cervical or mediastinal neoplasms. Third-order or postganglionic Horner's syndromes are almost always benign, and diagnostic evaluation is seldom necessary (8). Horner's syndrome in childhood is usually due to perinatal injury to the brachial plexus. However, children without birth trauma should be evaluated for cervical or mediastinal tumors, especially neuroblastoma (2,9). Pharmacologic localization of the lesion to the central, preganglionic or postganglionic neuron can be of great use in establishing the etiology of Horner's syndrome (6).

Pharmacologic Tests for Horner's Syndrome

Norepinephrine, the neurotransmitter of the sympathetic postganglionic neuron in the iris, is stored in granules in the postganglionic nerve ending. Sympathetic action potentials are generated by release of norepinephrine, which then diffuses across the postsynaptic cleft to α-adrenoceptors in the iris dilator muscle. The action is terminated by the reuptake of norepinephrine by the presynaptic terminal. The dilator muscle tone is maintained by the equilibrium of norepinephrine release and reuptake.

Cocaine causes pupillary mydriasis by blocking the reuptake of norepinephrine by the postganglionic terminal. More norepinephrine accumulates at the adrenoceptor sites of the dilator muscle, prolonging its action. Lesions at any point along the sympathetic pathway impair the release of norepinephrine at the postganglionic terminal. Because less norepinephrine is released, less can accumulate in the postsynaptic cleft, and pupillary dilation is impaired. Therefore, relatively decreased or absent dilation of the pupil to cocaine, as compared with that of the presumed normal fellow eye, is a positive test and confirms the presence of Horner's syndrome.

Cocaine Test

One drop of 4% to 10% cocaine is placed in each eye, and administration is repeated in 5 minutes. Anesthetic

TABLE 71-1. *Summary of pharmacologic testing of Horner's syndrome*

Pupil	Cocaine 4% to 10%	Hydroxyamphetamine 1%	Epinephrine 0.1%[a]
Normal	Dilation	Dilation	No dilation
Horner's			
Central	No dilation	Dilation	No dilation
Preganglionic	No dilation	Dilation	No dilation
Postganglionic	No dilation	No dilation	Dilation

[a]Pupillary response is similar to that obtained with use of 1% phenylephrine; phenylephrine may be more reliable.

drops or other eye drops should not be used before the test, and mechanical manipulation of the cornea (as occurs with tonometry) should be avoided. The pupils are measured after 45 minutes. If mydriasis has not occurred in either eye after 1 hour (not uncommon with dark irides), an additional drop should be instilled into each eye and the pupils should be observed for 1 to 2 hours. Patients should be warned that urine will test positive for cocaine metabolites for at least 36 hours afterward (10). Postcocaine anisocoria greater than 0.5 mm is considered positive for sympathetic denervation; anisocoria greater than 0.8 mm has a mean odds ratio of 1,050 : 1 and a lower confidence limit of 37 : 1 (11,12). Although a positive cocaine test confirms a Horner's syndrome, it does not localize the lesion in the oculosympathetic pathways.

Hydroxyamphetamine Test

Hydroxyamphetamine is an indirect-acting sympathomimetic which dilates the pupil by stimulating the release of norepinephrine from the postganglionic terminal. Hydroxyamphetamine dilates a normal pupil, as well as one denervated at the level of the central or preganglionic neuron, because the postganglionic terminal retains its store of norepinephrine. A denervated postganglionic neuron has lost its neurotransmitter and reacts poorly to hydroxyamphetamine. Therefore, patients with central or preganglionic Horner's syndrome exhibit normal pupillary mydriasis in response to hydroxyamphetamine, whereas patients with a postganglionic lesion have impaired mydriasis. The hydroxyamphetamine test differentiates a postganglionic lesion from a preganglionic lesion, but there is no known pharmacologic agent that can distinguish a first-order lesion from a second-order lesion.

One drop of 1% hydroxyamphetamine is instilled into each eye and is repeated in 5 minutes. Both pupils are evaluated at 45 minutes. Corneal epithelial trauma, either by drops or mechanical means, should be avoided before the test. Topical cocaine should not be used within 48 hours of the hydroxyamphetamine test (13). Any increase in the anisocoria is positive for postganglionic denervation (8). In a study of patients whose lesions were known, diagnostic specificity was 84% and sensitivity was 96% for postganglionic lesions. Specificity and sensitivity were 97% and 84%, respectively, for more proximal lesions (6). In another study, hydroxyamphetamine showed 93% sensitivity in detecting postganglionic lesions and 90% sensitivity in detecting preganglionic lesions (14). In that study, 1.0 mm anisocoria indicated a 85% probability of a postganglionic lesion, and 1.5 mm indicated a 96% probability of a postganglionic lesion (14). These studies refute earlier claims of 40% sensitivity for postganglionic lesions (15).

A group of patients with congenital Horner's syndrome and known preganglionic neuron lesions failed to dilate with hydroxyamphetamine or demonstrate denervation supersensitivity to phenylephrine; the investigators postulated orthograde transsynaptic degeneration of the postganglionic neuron (9) (Table 1). Pharmacologic testing of Horner's syndrome in infants and young children may be unreliable.

TESTS FOR DENERVATION SUPERSENSITIVITY

Denervation of the postganglionic neuron, but not the central or preganglionic neuron, results in supersensitivity of the iris dilator cells to dilute solutions of direct-acting sympathomimetic agents. Dilute (1:1,000) epinephrine does not dilate a normal pupil, nor does it dilate one with denervation of the central or preganglionic neurons, but it will dilate a pupil with postganglionic Horner's syndrome (16). Epinephrine penetrates the corneal poorly and with considerable individual variability, making the test unreliable. Phenylephrine hydrochloride 1% is considered more reliable (13).

The technique for testing for denervation supersensitivity is identical to that of the cocaine and hydroxyamphetamine tests. As with the cocaine test, care must be taken to avoid corneal epithelial trauma, either pharmacologic or mechanical, before the test. Hydroxyamphetamine is the most reliable pharmacologic agent for localization of Horner's syndrome. The pupillary responses to these diagnostic drugs are summarized in Table 1.

THE PARASYMPATHETIC PUPILLARY PATHWAYS

Pupillary parasympathetic fibers originate in the visceral subnuclei (Edinger-Westphal, anterior median, and the nucleus of Perlia) of the oculomotor nucleus in the dorsal midbrain. They exit the nucleus in the third nerve fasciculus, occupying the superficial and dorsomedial aspect of the third nerve, and enter the orbit through the superior orbital fissure. Preganglionic cholinergic neurons follow the course of the inferior division of the third nerve in the orbit to synapse in the ciliary ganglion, located near the orbital apex medial to the lateral rectus muscle. Postganglionic cholinergic fibers exit the ciliary ganglion in the short ciliary nerves to innervate the pupillary sphincter and ciliary muscle. Interruption of this pathway causes pupillary dilation, poor reactivity, and accommodative paresis.

TONIC PUPIL

Lesions of the ciliary ganglion and/or short ciliary nerves produce tonic pupils. Such pupils are characteristically dilated and react poorly to direct light stimulus, but may contract slowly to near stimuli (pupillary light/near dissociation). Accommodation is usually impaired. Slit lamp microscopy may disclose segmental iris sphincter palsy and slow "vermiform" movements. With time, tonic pupils usually become smaller and may recover accommodation, but they remain poorly reactive to light (2).

Adie's tonic pupil syndrome is the most common cause of internal ophthalmoplegia (17). It occurs in otherwise healthy persons, usually women aged 20 to 40 years. Patients may report mild blurring of the vision, but most are asymptomatic and present with a large unreactive pupil. The condition is unilateral on presentation in 80% of patients and becomes bilateral at a rate of 5% per year. Deep tendon reflexes are absent in 89% (18). The etiology is unknown. Other causes of postganglionic pupillary sphincter denervation are less common; they include ciliary damage from any cause (orbital trauma or surgery), viral infection, orbital or choroidal tumors, and retinal laser photocoagulation or cryotherapy; such denervation may also be part of a more generalized peripheral or autonomic neuropathy (2).

Postganglionic parasympathetic lesions cause denervation supersensitivity to cholinergic agents. Methacholine and pilocarpine are structurally similar to acetylcholine (ACh) and directly stimulate the iris sphincter cells. Parasympathetically denervated pupils constrict to dilute solutions of methacholine and pilocarpine, whereas normal pupils do not. Denervation supersensitivity develops in 80% of patients with Adie's syndrome. In one study, tonic pupils in 64% of patients constricted to 2.5% methacholine and those of 80% constricted to 0.125% pilocarpine. Pupils that fail to constrict with dilute methacholine may constrict to dilute pilocarpine (19).

Preganglionic lesions do not typically produce isolated pupillomotor abnormalities. Other signs of oculomotor nerve dysfunction are invariably present, although they may be subtle. Posterior communicating aneurysms or other compressive lesions may cause early, isolated pupillary dysfunction by compressing the peripherally located pupillary fibers. Such lesions almost always progress to ocular motor or other neurologic deficits. The dilated nonreactive pupil associated with a preganglionic lesion does not typically demonstrate denervation supersensitivity, although exceptions to this rule are well documented (20–22). Although the presence of denervation supersensitivity is extremely useful to diagnosis, careful clinical evaluation is essential to distinguish preganglionic from postganglionic pupillomotor lesions.

PHARMACOLOGIC TESTS FOR PARASYMPATHETIC PUPILLOMOTOR DISORDERS

The diagnosis of the dilated unreactive pupil remains a clinical challenge. Pharmacologic testing is helpful in determining whether the abnormal pupil is due to a postganglionic or preganglionic lesion or to pharmacologic blockade.

One drop of 0.1% or 0.125% pilocarpine is instilled into each eye, and application is repeated in 5 minutes. No drops or diagnostic procedures such as tonometry should be used in the preceding 24 to 48 hours, as this may alter corneal permeability of these agents. The size of both pupils is measured after 45 minutes. A change in the anisocoria greater than 1 mm is considered positive and confirms denervation supersensitivity. Denervation supersensitivity is highly suggestive of, but not pathognomonic for, postganglionic lesions. Mecholyl 2.5% has also been used but is less effective and is no longer commercially available (19).

If neither pupil reacts, the test is repeated using 1% pilocarpine. Equal reaction of both pupils excludes pharmacologic blockade as well as sphincter damage, and a preganglionic lesion must be considered. If anisocoria greater than 1 mm results, pharmacologic blockage is likely. The test may then be repeated using 4% pilocarpine; failure of the pupil to react to 4% pilocarpine is strong evidence of pharmacologic blockade. A logical approach for the clinical and pharmacologic evaluation of anisocoria is shown in Fig. 2.

Individual Drugs

Drugs used almost exclusively for the diagnosis of pupillary disorders are summarized below. Other agents

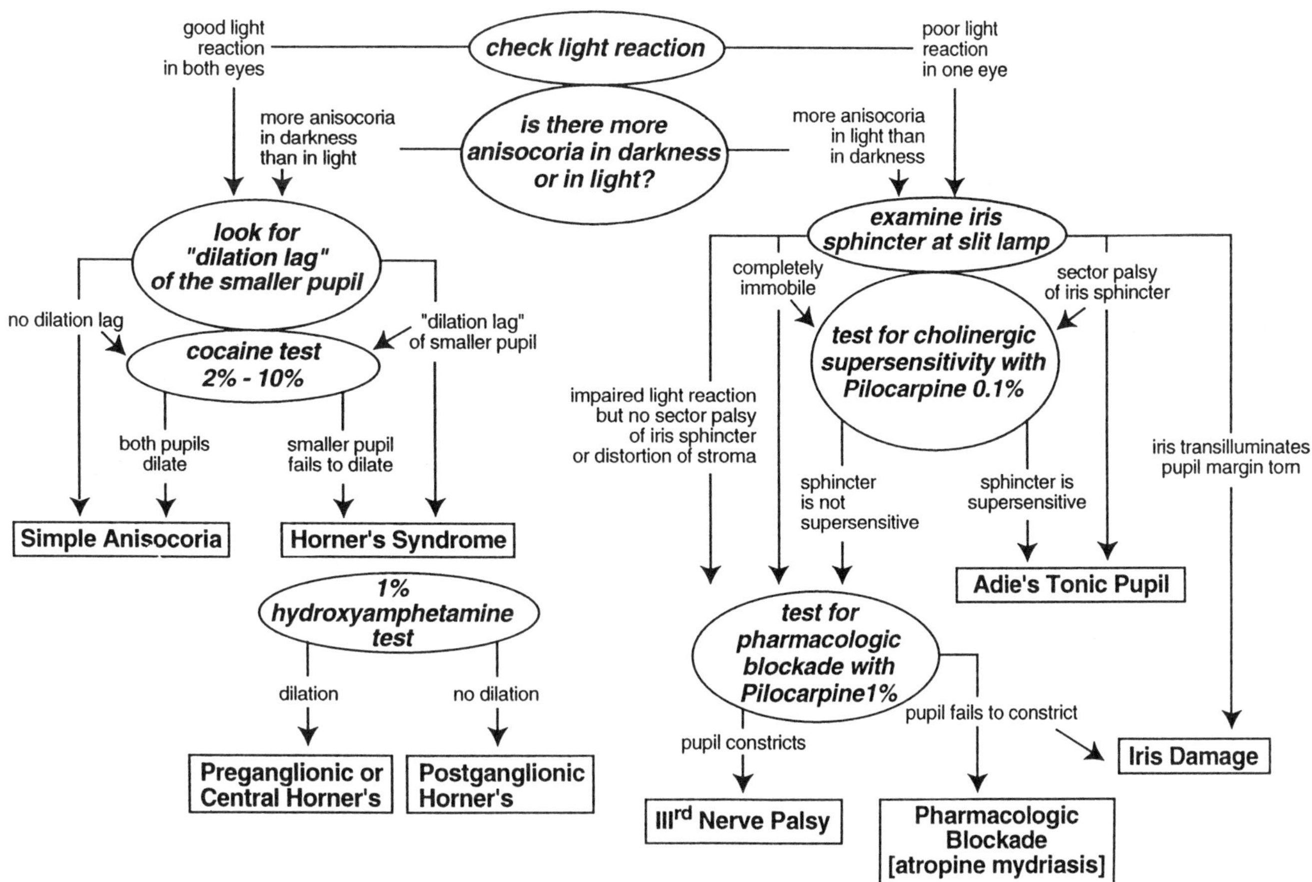

FIG. 71-2. Outline for the evaluation of anisocoria. (Redrawn from Thompson HS, Pilley SFJ. Unequal pupils. A flow chart for sorting out the anisocorias. [*Surv Ophthalmol* 1976; 21:45–48 with permission.])

(pilocarpine, epinephrine, and phenylephrine) are discussed in the sections on Glaucoma and Mydriatics.

HYDROXYAMPHETAMINE

History

Hydroxyamphetamine was first manufactured in Germany in 1913. The drug was shown to produce mydriasis with little or no effect on accommodation or IOP and was introduced as a mydriatic in 1937 (23,24). Its vasopressor effects had been investigated since 1933 (25). The drug was approved for use in the United States in 1938 for mydriasis, as a nasal constrictor, and for treatment of cardiogenic shock and cardiac arrhythmias (26–28). In 1971, Thompson and Mensher (13) observed that topically applied hydroxyamphetamine caused pupillary mydriasis in patients with central or preganglionic Horner's syndrome, but caused incomplete or no mydriasis of the affected pupil if the lesion was postganglionic. The drug's value in localizing the site of the lesion to the preganglionic or postganglionic neuron has since been widely appreciated (6,14,15). Alhough clearly demonstrated to be the most reliable pharmacologic agent for localizing the lesion in Horner's syndrome, hydroxyamphetamine was withdrawn from the market in 1989 (29). The drug was reintroduced in 1993 with 0.25% tropicamide (Paremyd, Allergan, Irvine, CA) as a topical mydriatic combination product, unsuitable for localization of Horner's syndrome. It is no longer available.

Official Drug Name and Chemistry

Hydroxyamphetamine hydrobromide is phenol,4-(2-aminopropyl)-hydrobromide; 2-amino-1(4′-hydroxyphenyl) propane; paredrine. The molecular formula is $C_9H_{13}NO \cdot HBr$ (Fig. 3).

Pharmacology

Hydroxyamphetamine is a synthetic indirect-acting sympathomimetic agent that exerts both α and β activity on smooth muscle (30).

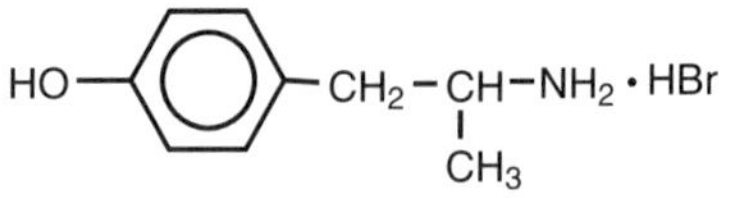

$$HO-C_6H_4-CH_2-CH(CH_3)-NH_2 \cdot HBr$$

FIG. 71-3. Chemical structure of hydroxyamphetamine hydrobromide.

Clinical Pharmacology

When applied topically to the eye, hydroxyamphetamine causes release of endogenous norepinephrine from intact adrenergic nerve terminals. In normal subjects, maximum mydriasis occurs 30–45 minutes after instillation of a 1% to 3% solution and lasts 2 to 3 hours. IOP is not affected (23,31), and there is little or no cycloplegic action (32,33).

The action of hydroxyamphetamine resembles that of ephedrine but without its CNS activity (34). Hydroxyamphetamine has a direct stimulatory effect on the heart and increases systolic and diastolic BP, often with reflex bradycardia. Hydroxyamphetamine has twice the constricting effect of ephedrine on nasal mucosa but exerts little effect on the cutaneous vascular bed (34).

Pharmaceutics

Hydroxyamphetamine is not commercially available in preparation suitable for diagnostic localization of Horner's syndrome. Before 1989, the drug was available as 1.0% solution in distilled water made isotonic with 2% boric acid (Smith, Kline and French, Philadelphia, PA). Hydroxyamphetamine hydrobromide may be compounded by individual pharmacies by prescription. The drug should be stored in airtight containers and protected from light.

Hydroxyamphetamine as 1.0% solution with tropicamide 0.25% (Paremyd, Allergan) for mydriasis is unsuitable for localization of Horner's syndrome and is no longer available.

Pharmacokinetics

The rate of corneal penetration and distribution of hydroxyamphetamine in ocular tissues is not known. Systemic absorption of topical hydroxyamphetamine is considered negligible and clinically insignificant. Hydroxyamphetamine is readily absorbed from the gastrointestinal (GI) tract. The duration of action after oral administration is 90 to 120 min. Ninety-two percent of radiolabeled hydroxyamphetamine is excreted in the urine in 24 hours as the free and conjugated drug (88%) and free and conjugated 4′-hydroxynorephedrine (4%). Ninety-seven percent is excreted after 3 days. The duration of action after intravenous injection is 20 to 30 minutes. Five days after intravenous injection, 75% of the dose is excreted in the urine (30,35).

Therapeutic Use

Hydroxyamphetamine is used principally to localize Horner's syndrome. Topical medications or corneal manipulation (corneal reflex testing, tonometry) should be avoided before the test and at least 48 hours should elapse between attempt at localization and the cocaine test. One drop of 1.0% hydroxyamphetamine is instilled into the conjunctival sac of each eye, and application is repeated in 1 minute. Pupillary size is monitored at 15-minute intervals for 45 min. Failure of the pupil to dilate suggests a postganglionic lesion. Lesions of the central or preganglionic neurons have no effect on pupillary response to hydroxyamphetamine, and the affected pupil will dilate normally.

Hydroxyamphetamine 1.0% may be used with other mydriatics to achieve maximum mydriasis. One to 2 drops is instilled into the conjunctival sac.

The drug may be topically applied as a 0.5% to 1.0% solution to shrink nasal mucosa, but is seldom used for this purpose. Hydroxyamphetamine has been used to treat bradycardia associated with carotid sinus syndrome (60 mg or more), Stokes-Adams attacks (20 to 60 mg, three times daily, t.i.d.), and paroxysmal tachycardia (20 mg hourly for three doses) (34). It is no longer used for this purpose.

Side Effects and Toxicity

Side effects of hydroxyamphetamine as a topical eye drop are similar to those of any mydriatic agent. The drug is relatively contraindicated in patients with narrow-angle glaucoma or in persons with narrow angles in whom acute narrow-angle glaucoma may be precipitated. Evaluation of the anterior chamber angle is advised before use of hydroxyamphetamine in patients with shallow anterior chambers. The drug may increase IOP (due to the mechanical effects of mydriasis), blurring of vision, photophobia, and stinging on instillation. Although allergic conjunctivitis has been reported (32), adverse reactions to ocular use are extremely rare. Potentially, such side effects would be the same as those produced by phenylephrine, including hypertention, headache, nausea, vomiting, palpitations, and cardiac arrhythmias (34). Severe cardiovascular events including fatal myocardial infarction, ventricular fibrillation, hypotension, bradycardia, and syncope have occurred after ocular use of hydroxyamphetamine 1% tropicamide 0.25% solution (Paremyd, Allergan, Irvine CA, package insert, Nov. 1996). Systemic absorption from topical application may be minimized by compression of the lacrimal sac for 2 to 3 minutes after instillation. Hydroxyamphetamine is contraindicated in patients treated with monoamine oxidase inhibitors.

Drug Interactions

Side effects may be additive to those of other sympathomimetic and mydriatic agents.

High-risk Groups

Patients with hypertension, hyperthyroidism, diabetes, narrow-angle glaucoma are at risk of toxicity with use of hydroxyamphetamine. Its safety for use in children and pregnant women is not established.

Major Clinical Trials

Thompson and Mensher (13), studying adrenergic mydriasis in a group of patients with unilateral Horner's syndrome, reported that only patients with intact postganglionic neurons responded to 1% hydroxyamphetamine. Experimental postganglionic Horner's syndrome was induced in one eye by guanethidine, which depletes stores of norepinephrine in the postganglionic nerve terminal. The pharmacologically sympathectomized eye demonstrated marked supersensitivity to dilute phenylephrine after 10 days of treatment and showed no reaction to hydroxyamphetamine after 16 days of treatment (13). Skarf et al. and Czarnecki (36) demonstrated failure of mydriasis with hydroxyamphetamine in rabbits with surgical postganglionic denervation, but normal mydriasis in rabbits with preganglionic lesions (36). In a review of 450 patients with Horner's syndrome, Maloney et al. (6) reported hydroxyamphetamine to have 96% sensitivity in identifying postganglionic lesions and 83% sensitivity in identifying preganglionic lesions. Similarly, Cremer et al. (14) studied 54 patients whose lesions were known with reasonable certainty on clinical grounds. When the difference between the dilation of normal pupil and the Horner's pupil was zero, hydroxyamphetamine correctly identified 88% of known postganglionic lesions, with a sensitivity of 93% (14). These findings are in contrast to those of Van der Wiel and Van Gijn, who reported only 40% sensitivity of hydroxyamphetamine in localizing postganglionic lesions (15).

COCAINE

History and Source

Cocaine is an alkaloid derived from the leaves of the *Erythroxylon coca* shrub in Peru and Bolivia and from *Erythronovogranatense* in Columbia. The coca leaf has been used in South American cultures throughout history for its ability to reduce fatigue and hunger and promote a sense of well-being. Its use as an anesthetic agent in surgery dates back to the ninth century A.D. (37,38).

The alkaloid was first isolated from the coca leaf in 1855 by Friedrich Gaedcke, and the drug was isolated by Albert Niemann in 1860. Although Neimann reported that cocaine anesthetized the tongue, and Von Anrep observed that skin infiltrated with the drug became insensitive to pinprick, Carl Koller is credited with the "discovery" of cocaine as a local anesthetic in 1884 (38,39). He described corneal anesthesia with topical application of cocaine, as well as widening of the palpebral fissures and pupillary mydriasis with minimal effect on accommodation. Cocaine was widely used in ophthalmic surgery and was administered topically and as a subconjunctival injection for corneal procedures, cataract, and strabismus surgery. It was also used to alleviate the pain of iritis and as a mydriatic to break posterior synechiae. Its use rapidly spread to other specialties, including general surgery, otolaryngology, and dentistry. Koller and his contemporary Königstein recognized that cocaine did not dilate the pupils of a patient with Horner's syndrome, but Uhthoff was first to propose its use in neuroophthalmic diagnosis in 1885 (39).

As cocaine's popularity grew in the late 1800s, its highly addictive properties and potential for abuse and toxicity were recognized. With the introduction of other local anesthetic agents, especially procaine in 1905, the use of cocaine has steadily declined. Today, it has very limited use in ophthalmology—as a local anesthetic and for pharmacologic diagnosis of Horner's syndrome.

Official Drug Name and Chemistry

Cocaine is 3-(benzoyloxy)-*N*-methyl-8-azabicyclo[3,2,1] octane-2-carboxylic acid methyl ester; 2*R*-methylcarbonyl-3*S*-benzoyltropine; benzoylmethylecgonine; l-cocaine; β-cocaine; cocaine. The molecular structure is $C_{17}H_{21}NO_4$ (Fig. 4).

Pharmacology

Cocaine is an indirect sympathomimetic agent that inhibits the reuptake of catecholamines at adrenergic nerve terminals (40). Cocaine inhibits nerve conduction without depolarizing the nerve membrane. It inhibits sodium and potassium exchange in nerve fibers and competes with calcium at sites controlling membrane permeability (37). It is a potent local anesthetic owing to its reversible membrane stabilization and vasoconstrictive properties.

Clinical Pharmacology

Cocaine blocks the reuptake of norepinephrine at the sympathetic postganglionic neuron, resulting in pupillary

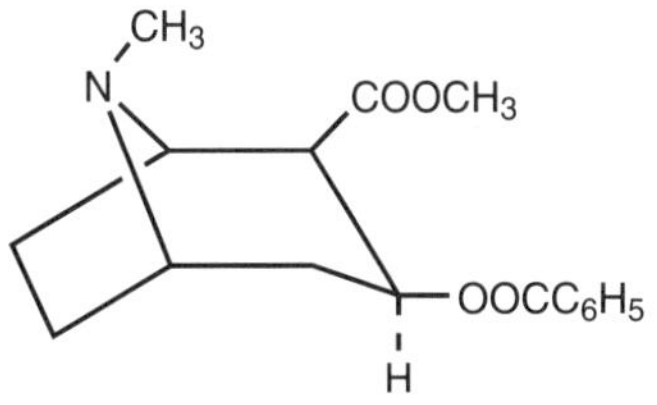

FIG. 71-4. Chemical structure of cocaine.

mydriasis in normal eyes. Denervation anywhere along the three-neuron oculosympathetic pathway impairs release of norepinephrine from the postganglionic nerve terminal; because no norepinephrine is available for reuptake, cocaine cannot cause pupillary mydriasis. Thus, cocaine pharmacologically confirms oculosympathetic paresis, but does not localize the lesion within the neural pathways.

Cocaine blocks the uptake of catecholamines at adrenergic nerve terminals and potentiates the response of sympathetically innervated organs to norepinephrine and epinephrine. The drug causes general CNS stimulation and vasoconstriction and may affect central thermal regulation centers. In small doses, cocaine slows HR by central vagal stimulation; at moderate doses, sympathetic stimulation causes tachycardia and increased BP. Large intravenous doses may cause sudden death from arrhythmias, myocardial infarction, or cardiac failure due to direct depression of cardiac muscle (40).

Cocaine is a potent local anesthetic. It is readily absorbed from all sites of application, but may be limited by vasoconstriction. Inflammation enhances tissue absorption.

Pharmaceutics

Cocaine hydrochloride is available as 4% or 10% aqueous and viscous solution in unit-use glass vials of 4 ml and multidose vials of 10 ml (Roxane Laboratories, Columbus, OH; Astra Pharmaceutical Products, Westboro, MA). It is classified as category II by the Federal Drug Administration (high potential for abuse).

Pharmacokinetics

Most available data apply to cocaine abuse; the rate of corneal penetration and distribution of cocaine in the ocular tissues is not well documented. Cocaine is readily absorbed through the mucosal membranes and GI tract, with similar bioavailability from the two routes. The onset of action after oral administration is 10 to 20 minutes, and the effects last 4 to 5 hours. Peak plasma concentration occurs 50 to 90 minutes after oral administration, reaching plasma levels of 104 to 424 μg/L (41). The effects of intranasal administration occur in a few minutes, reach peak plasma levels in 30 to 60 minutes, and last 30 to 40 minutes (37,42). Bioavailability by the intranasal route varies considerably and may be dose dependent; Jeffcoat et al. (42) report 80% ± 13%, whereas other investigators report lower values of 28% and 60%. Bioavailability after smoking cocaine is 57% ± 19% (range 32% to 77%). Due to its high lipid solubility, cocaine is rapidly taken up by the brain and other tissues. The steady-state volume of distribution in abusers is 1.96 to 2.7 L/kg (41,42). Ninety-one percent of the drug is plasma bound. The elimination $t_{\frac{1}{2}}$ ranges from 31 to 82 minutes, with an average of about 48 minutes, and is similar for all routes of administration (41,43).

Absorption by the intramuscular, topical, and subcutaneous routes may be limited by vasoconstriction. Absorption is enhanced in inflamed or damaged tissues. Systemic absorption from topical application to the eye is considered to be clinically insignificant, but patients may test positive for urinary metabolites for as long as 36 hours after administration by this route (10).

Most of the drug is eliminated in the urine within 24 to 36 hours of administration. Elimination clearance is 2.1 L/min, with nonrenal mechanisms accounting for 98% of total elimination (43). Cocaine is metabolized in humans through two main pathways. Ninety percent of the drug is hydrolyzed by serum and liver pseudocholinesterase to benzoylecgonine, ecgonine methyl ester, and ecgonine (37,44). Benzoylecgonine, the major metabolite, is readily detected in urine by immunoassay (EMIT) (45). A minor oxidative pathway produces norcocaine through *N*-demethylation, which is then oxidized and further metabolized to norcocaine nitroxide by liver enzymes. This compound is believed to be responsible for the hepatotoxicity associated with cocaine use (46). Less than 2% of cocaine is excreted unchanged in the urine (43).

Therapeutic Use

Cocaine is used principally in medicine as a local anesthetic. In dacryocystorhinostomy or other nasolacrimal procedures, cocaine is applied to the nasal mucosa in a gauze-soaked pack or as a nasal spray, not to exceed 3 mm/kg. Cocaine is no longer recommended for corneal or ocular anesthesia. Concomitant use with sympathomimetic agents such as epinephrine and phenylephrine should be avoided (47).

Cocaine is restricted to topical use only; intravenous or internal use is contraindicated. One drop of 4% to 10% cocaine is instilled into the conjunctival sac, and application is repeated in 5 minutes for pharmacologic testing for Horner's syndrome. Cocaine is used rarely as an adjunct to other mydriatic agents to maximize mydriasis, especially to break posterior synechiae, but is not recommended as a general mydriatic agent.

Side Effects and Toxicity

Topical cocaine causes corneal epithelial breakdown, pitting, and sloughing (38). Systemic toxicity from topical application to the eye is not reported.

Systemic toxicity may occur in nasolacrimal procedures, but is uncommon (47,48). Most systemic toxicity results from abuse through intranasal or intravenous use or from smoking the free-base drug. Potentially life-threatening reactions include cardiac arrhythmias or arrest, myocardial infarction, cardiac failure, and depression of respiration. The lethal dose of cocaine in humans is highly variable and not well established. Although the lethal dose is generally considered to be 1200 mg (product package insert), systemic toxicity has been reported with as little as 20 mg (37,47).

Acute overdose may initially cause agitation, skin pallor, hypertension, and tachycardia, followed by respiratory failure, hypoxia, status epilepticus, ventricular arrhythmias and, ultimately, circulatory collapse. Adverse effects also include excitability, confusion, psychosis, disturbed sleep patterns, unconsciousness, nausea, vomiting, abdominal pain, hyperpyrexia, cardiomyopathy, cerebral and spinal cord ischemia and stroke, intracerebral hemorrhage, rhabdomyolysis, and acute renal and hepatic failure (30,37). The treatment of acute overdose includes immediate supportive management to maintain the airway and circulation. Advanced life support may be necessary, and body temperature should be monitored. Intravenous short-acting barbiturates or diazepam should be administered to suppress seizures. Ventricular tachyrhythmia, in the absence of seizure activity, may be managed with lidocaine 1.0 mg/kg. If the cardiac arrhythmia persists or if seizure activity precludes use of lidocaine, propranolol (0.5 to 1.0 mg, to 5 mg) may be used (47).

High-risk Groups

Patients with preexisting cardiovascular or cerebrovascular disease, hypertension, and diabetes are at risk of systemic toxicity. Vasoconstriction and tachycardia may precipitate cardiac ischemia in patients with coronary insufficiency. Cocaine enhances the response to epinephrine, which mobilizes glucose and may lead to hyperglycemia in persons with diabetes. Cocaine lowers the seizure threshold and is contraindicated in patients with seizure disorders. The drug is contraindicated in patients with preexisting neurosis, psychosis, or tendency toward substance abuse. Cocaine is not recommended in neonates, children, or the elderly due to the risk of tachycardia and vasoconstriction.

Cocaine is classified as pregnancy category C; long-term studies to determine the direct effect of cocaine on the fetus have not been conducted (product package insert). Cocaine has been associated with a high rate of spontaneous abortions and complicated deliveries in abusers. Cocaine is transferred transplacentally from the mother to the fetus and has been detected in breast milk. Babies born to cocaine abusers are more likely to have low birth weight and neurologic or neurobehavioral abnormalities (37,49). The drug should be used in pregnant women only if strictly needed.

Drug Interactions

Cocaine potentiates the action of endogenous catecholamine and should be used with extreme caution in patients treated with guanethidine sulfate, reserpine, tricyclic antidepressants, or monoamine oxidase inhibitors. Concomitant use with sympathomimetic agents such as epinephrine or phenylephrine is contraindicated due to the enhanced vasoconstriction. Tricyclic antidepressants are reported to decrease the vasoconstrictive and cardiotoxic effects of cocaine (37,47). The drug should be used with caution with other respiratory depressants such as barbiturates and alcohol.

Major Clinical Trials

Since its recognition as a useful diagnostic agent for Horner's syndrome in the early 1880s, cocaine's efficacy and reliability for this purpose have been essentially unchallenged. Kardon et al. (12) reported that the mean odds ratio of having a Horner's syndrome was 1,054 : 1 when postcocaine anisocoria was greater than 0.8 mm and 77 : 1 when anisocoria was 0.5 mm.

The safety of cocaine in clinical use has been documented in a survey report of 93,004 operations by 741 respondents. Mild reactions occurred in 224 cases (0.24%), and severe reactions occurred in 14 cases (0.015%). No fatalities were reported (48). The efficacy of cocaine as a local anesthetic is discussed elsewhere in this volume.

ACKNOWLEDGMENT

This work was supported in part by an unrestricted grant from Research to Prevent Blindness, Inc., New York, NY.

REFERENCES

1. Lam BL, Thompson HS, Corbett JJ. The prevalence of simple anisocoria. *Am J Ophthalmol* 1987;104:69–73.
2. Miller NR. *Walsh and Hoyt's clinical neuro-ophthalmology,* 4th ed. Baltimore: Williams & Wilkins, 1985.
3. Lepore FE. Diagnostic pharmacology of the pupil. *Clin Neuropharmacol* 1985;8:27–37.
4. Diesenhouse MC, Palay DA, Newman NJ, To K, Albert DM. Acquired heterochromia with Horner syndrome in two adults. *Ophthalmology* 1992;99:1815–1817.
5. Pancoast HK. Superior pulmonary sulcus tumor. *J Am Med Assoc* 1932;99:1391–1396.
6. Maloney WF, Younge BR, Moyer NJ. Evaluation of the causes and accuracy of pharmacologic localization in Horner's syndrome. *Am J Ophthalmol* 1980;90:394–402.
7. Giles CL, Henderson JW. Horner's syndrome: an analysis of 216 cases. *Am J Ophthalmol* 1958;46:289–296.
8. Burde RM, Savino PJ, Trobe JD. Anisocoria and abnormal pupillary light reactions. In: *Clinical Decisions in Neuro-Ophthalmology,* 2nd ed. St. Louis: Mosby Year Book, 1992;321–346.
9. Weinstein JM, Zweifel TJ, Thompson HS. Congenital Horner's syndrome. *Arch Ophthalmol* 1980;98:1074–1078.

10. Bralliar BB, Skarf B, Owens JB. Ophthalmic use of cocaine and the urine test for benzoylecgonine. *N Engl J Med* 1989;320:1757–1758.
11. Friedman JR, Whiting DW, Kosmorsky GS, Burde RM. The cocaine test in normal patients. *Am J Ophthalmol* 1984;98:808–810.
12. Kardon RH, Denison CE, Brown CK, Thompson HS. Critical evaluation of the cocaine test in the diagnosis of Horner's syndrome. *Arch Ophthalmol* 1990;108:384–387.
13. Thompson HS, Mensher JH. Adrenergic mydriasis in Horner's syndrome. Hydroxyamphetamine test for diagnosis of postganglionic defects. *Am J Ophthalmol* 1971;72:472–480.
14. Cremer SA, Thompson HS, Digre KB, Kardon RH. Hydroxyamphetamine mydriasis in Horner's syndrome. *Am J Ophthalmol* 1990; 110:71–76.
15. Van der Wiel HL, Van Gijn J. Localization of Horner's syndrome. Use and limitations of the hydroxyamphetamine test. *J Neurol Sci* 1983; 59:229–235.
16. Foerster O, Gagel O. Die Vorderseitenstrangdurchschneidung beim Menschen. *Z Neurol Psychiatr* 1932;138:1–92.
17. Thompson HS. A classification of "tonic pupils." In: Thompson HS, Daroff R, Frisén L, Glaser JS, Sanders MD, eds. *Topics in Neuro-Ophthalmology.* Baltimore: Williams & Wilkins, 1979;95–96.
18. Thompson HS. Adie's syndrome. Some new observations. *Trans Am Ophthalmol Soc* 1977;75:587–620.
19. Bourgon P, Pilley SFJ, Thompson HS. Cholinergic supersensitivity of the iris sphincter in Adie's tonic pupil. *Am J Ophthalmol* 1978; 85:373–377.
20. Slamovits TL, Miller NR. Intracranial oculomotor nerve paresis with anisocoria and pupillary parasympathetic hypersensitivity. *Am J Ophthalmol* 1987;104:401–406.
21. Coppeto JR, Monteiro MLR, Young D. Tonic pupils following oculomotor nerve palsies. *Ann Ophthalmol* 1985;17:585–588.
22. Jacobson DM. Pupillary responses to dilute pilocarpine in preganglionic 3rd nerve disorders. *Neurology* 1990;40:804–808.
23. Kronfeld PE, McGarry HI, Smith HE. The effect of mydriatics upon the intraocular pressure in so-called primary open angle glaucoma. *Am J Ophthalmol* 1943;26:245.
24. Abbott OW, Henry CM. Paredrine. A clinical investigation of a sympathomimetic drug. *Am J Med Sci* 1937;193:661.
25. Alles GA. The comparative physiological action of DL-β-phenylisopropylamines. I. Pressor effect and toxicity. *J Pharmacol Exp Ther* 1933;47:339–354.
26. Ornston DG. Use of microcrystals of sulfathiazole in otolaryngologic practice. *Arch Otolaryngol* 1945;41:337–342.
27. Altschule MD, Iglauer A. The effect of benzedrine (β-phenylisopropylamine sulfate) and paredrine (β-hydroxy-α-methyl-phenylethylamine hydrobromide) on the circulation, metabolism, and respiration in normal man. *J Clin Invest* 1940;19:497–514.
28. Nathanson MH. Rhythmic property of the human heart. *Arch Intern Med* 1943;72:613–626.
29. Burde RM,Thompson HS. Hydroxyamphetamine. A good drug lost? *Am J Ophthalmol* 1991;111:100–102.
30. Innes IR, Nickerson M. Norepinephrine, epinephrine, and the sympathomimetic amines. In: Goodman LS, Gilman A, eds. *The Pharmacological Basis of Therapeutics,* 5th ed. New York: Macmillan, 1975; 477–513.
31. Tassman IS. The use of paredrine in cycloplegia. *Am J Ophthalmol* 1938;21:1019–1025.
32. Laval J. Allergic dermatitis and conjunctivitis from paredrine hydrobromide. *Arch Ophthalmol* 1941;26:585–586.
33. Thorne FH, Murphey HS. Cycloplegics. *Arch Ophthalmol* 1939;22: 274–287.
34. Blacow NW, ed. *Martindale. The Extra Pharmacopoeia,* 26th ed. London: The Pharmaceutical Press, 1972;17–18.
35. Sever PS, Dring LG, Williams RT. The metabolism of hydroxyamphetamine in man and animals: 4′-hydroxyl[14C] amphetamines (Paredrine). *Trans Biochem Soc* 1973;1:1158–1159.
36. Skarf B, Czarnecki JSC. Distinguishing postganglionic from preganglionic lesions: studies in rabbits with surgically produced Horner's syndrome. *Arch Ophthalmol* 1982;100:1319–1322.
37. Dollery C. *Therapeutic Drugs.* Edinburgh: Churchill Livingstone, 1991;C330–C334.
38. Altman AJ, Albert DM, Fournier GA. Cocaine's use in ophthalmology: our 100-year heritage. *Surv Ophthalmol* 1985;29:300–306.
39. Loewenfeld IE. Pupillary pharmacology. In: *The Pupil.* Detroit: Wayne State University Press, 1993;683–826.
40. Ritchie JM, Cohen PJ. Local anaesthetics. In: Gilman AG, Rall TW, Nies AS, Taylor P, eds. *Goodman and Gilman's the Pharmacological Basis of Therapeutics,* 8th ed. Elmsford: Pergamon Press, 1990.
41. Busto U, Bendayan R, Sellers EM. Clinical pharmacokinetics of non-opiate abused drugs. *Clin Pharmacokinet* 1989;16:1–26.
42. Jeffcoat AJ, Perez-Reyes M, Hill JM, Sadler BM, Cook CE. Cocaine disposition in humans after intravenous injection, nasal insufflation (snorting), or smoking. *Drug Metab Dispos* 1989;17:153–159.
43. Chow MJ, Ambre JJ, Ruo TI, Atkinson AJ, Bowsher DJ, Fischman MW. Kinetics of cocaine distribution, elimination, and chronotropic effects. *Clin Pharmacol Ther* 1985;38:318–324.
44. Stewart DJ, Inaba T, Lucassen M, Kalow W. Cocaine metabolism: cocaine and norcocaine hydrolysis by liver and serum esterases. *Clin Pharmacol Ther* 1979;25:464–468.
45. Mulé SJ, Bastos ML, Jukofsky D. Evaluation of immunoassay methods for detection, in urine, of drugs subject to abuse. *Clin Chem* 1974;20:243–248.
46. Kloss MW, Rosen GM, Raukman EJ. Cocaine-mediated hepatotoxicity: a critical review. *Biochem Pharmacol* 1984;33:169–173.
47. Meyers EF. Cocaine toxicity during dacryocystorhinostomy. *Arch Ophthalmol* 1980;98:842–843.
48. Feehan HF, Mancusi-Ungaro A. The use of cocaine as a topical anaesthetic in nasal surgery: a survey report. *Plastic Reconstr Surg* 1976; 57:62–65.
49. Doberczak TM, Shanzer S, Senie RT, Kandall SR. Neonatal neurologic and electroencephalographic effects of intrauterine cocaine exposure. *J Pediatr* 1988;113:354–358.

Textbook of Ocular Pharmacology,
edited by T.J. Zimmerman, et al.
Lippincott–Raven Publishers, Philadelphia © 1997.

CHAPTER 72

Drugs for the Diagnosis and Treatment of Myasthenia Gravis

Gil I. Wolfe, Richard J. Barohn, and Steven L. Galetta

MYASTHENIA GRAVIS

Myasthenia gravis is an autoimmune disorder characterized by a postsynaptic defect in neuromuscular transmission. It is the most common disease of the neuromuscular junction. The hallmark clinical feature is fluctuating weakness of striated muscle with a propensity to fatigue as the day passes and after exertion (1,2). Ocular symptoms are present in 75% of patients presenting with myasthenia gravis and will eventually appear in 90% (1). Isolated ocular involvement occurs in at least 15% of patients with myasthenia (3). Therefore, it is not unusual for such patients to present to an ophthalmologist. We summarize clinical aspects of ocular myasthenia and review the pharmacology of medications commonly used to diagnose and treat these patients.

Ocular Myasthenia

Extraocular motility defects and unilateral or bilateral ptosis are the main ocular manifestations of myasthenia gravis. In a study of 48 patients with pure ocular myasthenia, 43 (90%) had ptosis and diplopia, and 5 (10%) had isolated ptosis (4). In a large study of 1,487 patients with myasthenia, 202 (14%) had disease restricted to extraocular muscles in a mean follow-up period of 18 years (5). The maximal severity of ocular symptoms was evident during the first year after onset in 70% of the patients and by 3 years in 85%. After a mean follow-up period of 17 years, 68% of the 202 patients with ocular myasthenia had ocular manifestations similar to those in their first 3 years of illness, 14% improved, 14% were in remission, and 5% had worsened. Although corticosteroids may result in a higher rate of clinical improvement and remission, anticholinesterase agents do not alter the natural course of the disease (5,6).

Approximately two-thirds of patients presenting with ocular myasthenia will later have generalized disease. Nearly all patients with ocular myasthenia who develop generalized disease will do so within 2 to 3 years of their initial diagnosis (1,6). As compared with patients with generalized myasthenia, patients with isolated ocular involvement are more often male, more often have negative or low serum antiacetylcholine (ACh) receptor antibody titers, and respond relatively poorly to anticholinesterase therapy (1,7). The estimated prevalence of myasthenia is 1 in every 10,000 to 50,000 people, with women accounting for two-thirds of cases (8). It occurs in all ethnic groups.

Myasthenia gravis should be considered in all patients with extraocular palsies or ptosis and normal pupils (1). The diagnosis is especially likely when weakness of the orbicularis oculi is also demonstrated (8). This muscle is involved in about 25% of ocular myasthenia patients (4).

Ptosis

Ptosis in patients with myasthenia often presents unilaterally, but will eventually involve both eyes in nearly all patients. It may appear in isolation or accompany extraocular palsies. As with motility defects, the ptosis may worsen as the day progresses. A patient may have no levator weakness in the morning and develop ptosis only in afternoon or evening hours. The fatigability may be apparent clinically, with the ptosis developing on sustained upward gaze or after repeated opening and closing of the eyes (8). Ptosis on one side may also worsen when the opposite eyelid is held

G. I. Wolfe and R. J. Barohn: Department of Neurology, University of Texas Southwestern Medical School, Dallas, Texas 75235.

S. L. Galetta: Department of Neurology, University of Pennsylvania Medical Center, Philadelphia, Pennsylvania 19104.

open by the examiner (9). According to Hering's law of equal innervation, manual bracing of the opposite eyelid leads to reduced contraction of the fellow levator palpebrae superioris, thereby aggravating the ptosis in that eye. This phenomenon is known as "curtaining," and in myasthenia it is characterized by a slow, persistent descent of the lid. Cogan's lid twitch also signifies levator weakness. To elicit this sign, the patient looks downward for 10 to 20 seconds and then is asked to saccade back to primary position. The upper eyelid remains elevated for a fraction of a second before drifting downward, generating a twitchlike movement (10). The lid twitch is suggestive, but not diagnostic, of ocular myasthenia.

Motility Defects

Motility defects in ocular myasthenia are usually accompanied by ptosis and encompass the entire range of deficits, from an isolated palsy to complete external ophthalmoparesis. The motility deficits of myasthenia may mimic a pupil-sparing oculomotor nerve palsy or internuclear ophthalmoplegia (11). A clue for clinicians in these settings is the characteristic fluctuation of symptoms in ocular myasthenia, at times even shifting from one eye to the other. Some patients will report diplopia or ptosis only after sustained exertion. The propensity for affected muscles to fatigue may be demonstrated clinically by having patients maintain their eyes in eccentric gaze (12).

Nystagmus

Rarely does nystagmus present as the sole manifestation of ocular myasthenia (7). Nystagmus in myasthenia gravis develops from fatigued eye muscles straining to hold the eyes in eccentric gaze after a saccade. Typically, the nystagmus abates with edrophonium chloride injection and is accentuated by D-tubocurarine (8). Eye movement recordings have demonstrated a variety of other abnormalities, including slow, hypometric, and hypermetric saccades, and small jerking or quivering ocular movements (7,8).

Pupillary Function

Pupillary abnormalities in general exclude the diagnosis of myasthenia gravis. There are, however, scattered reports of iris sphincter involvement in patients with myasthenia. In some cases, anisocoria with sluggish pupillary responses to light has been shown to respond to anticholinesterases (13,14). Prolonged pupillary cycle times and sphincter fatigue on constant light stimulation (15) have also been reported. However, many such patients were studied while treated with anticholinesterases or corticosteroids, which may have contributed to the pupillary abnormalities (8). If present, pupillary dysfunction must be an infrequent, minor component of myasthenia gravis. When iris sphincter dysfunction is prominent, a disorder other than myasthenia gravis should be considered.

THE NEUROMUSCULAR JUNCTION

Familiarity with the pathophysiology, diagnosis, and treatment of myasthenia gravis requires a fundamental understanding of the mechanisms of the neuromuscular junction (Fig. 1). ACh is the natural transmitter of the neuromuscular junction and is synthesized and stored in motor nerve terminals (8,16). Acetylcholine is stored in vesicles, each of which contains a quantum (about 10,000 molecules) of neurotransmitter. At rest, individual vesicles spontaneously release their quantum of ACh at special release sites on the presynaptic membrane. The released neurotransmitter molecules then migrate and bind to ACh receptors located on the postsynaptic membrane, producing a transient increase in the permeability of sodium and potassium ions. The local end-plate depolarization that results is termed a miniature end-plate potential (MEPP). MEPPs have been hypothesized to help maintain resting muscle tone by providing a continuous background of cholinergic stimulation (17).

MEPPs are dwarfed by the larger depolarizations that occur when nerve action potentials (AP) arrive at the presynaptic terminal. These AP rapidly depolarize the presynaptic membrane. The depolarization produces an influx of calcium ions into the motor terminal, leading to exocytosis of a large number of vesicles containing ACh (150 to 200 quanta). The postsynaptic depolarization which results is termed an EPP. Due to a physiologic safety factor, the EPP is normally sufficient to generate an AP along the muscle membrane. Propagation of this muscle AP leads to a cascade of events which drive muscle contraction.

The amplitude of the EPP is directly related to the number of ACh molecules which bind to their receptors. The safety factor normally ensures an adequate number of neurotransmitter-receptor interactions to produce a muscle AP (8). As discussed herein, the immunologic defect in myasthenia gravis directly reduces this safety margin, and muscle weakness ensues.

Neuromuscular transmission is rapid, taking only milliseconds to complete the entire sequence. The process is terminated by diffusion of ACh from the synapse and its rapid hydrolysis by acetylcholinesterase (17).

Pathophysiology of Myasthenia Gravis

A defect in the interaction of ACh with its receptor has been suspected in myasthenia gravis since 1934, when Walker (18) observed that physostigmine, an anticholinesterase, temporarily relieved myasthenic weakness. Later investigators showed that MEPP amplitudes were reduced in patients with myasthenia (19) and that these patients had

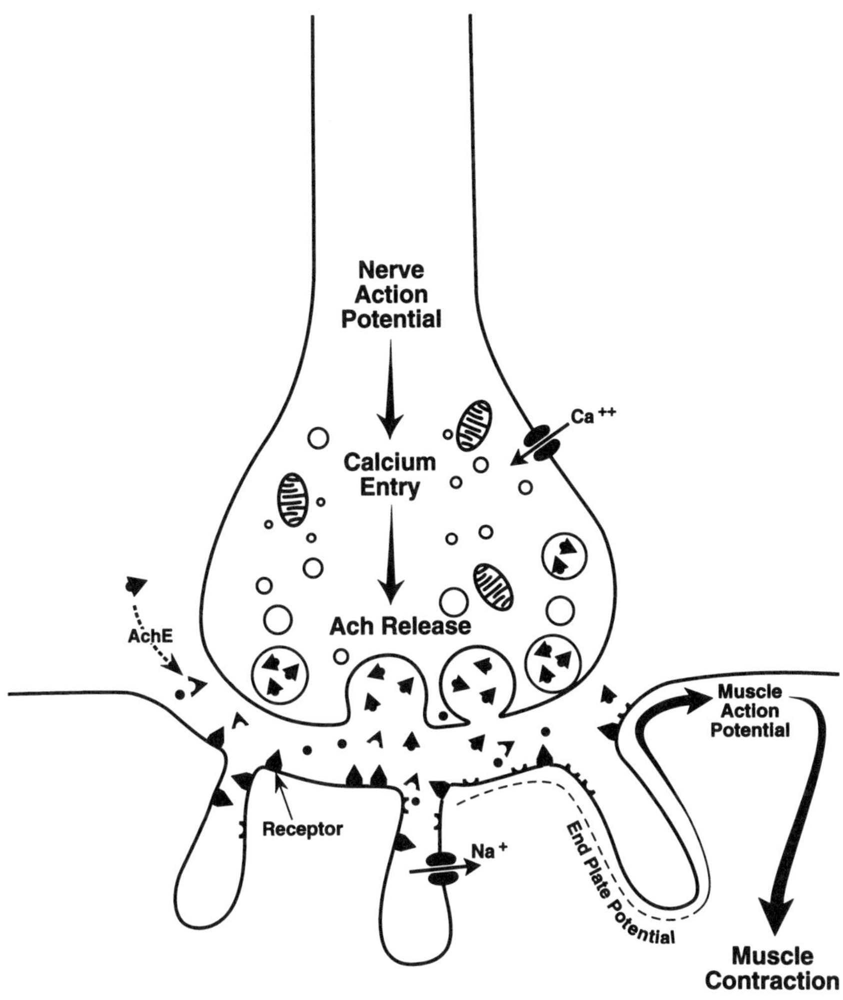

FIG. 72-1. Diagram of the neuromuscular junction. Top: A nerve action potential (AP) arrives at the motor terminal and produces rapid depolarization. The depolarization initiates an influx of calcium ions into the motor axon, leading to synchronized fusion of vesicles containing acetylcholine (ACh) with the presynaptic membrane. Released ACh molecules diffuse across the synapse, bind to their postsynaptic receptors, and generate a localized end-plate potential (EPP). If the EPP reaches threshold, the muscle membrane undergoes an increase in sodium conductance, with subsequent generation of a muscle AP. Propagation of the muscle AP through the muscle fiber culminates in a cascade of events which drive contraction. Neuromuscular transmission is terminated by diffusion of ACh from the synapse and its rapid cleavage by acetylcholinesterase (AChE). (Modified from ref. 7.)

less than one-third the normal number of ACh receptors (20). The association of myasthenia gravis with other autoimmune diseases prompted speculation that an immune disorder was somehow responsible. It is now accepted that myasthenia gravis results from an autoimmune attack on nicotinic ACh receptors by polyclonal IgG antibodies. Antibodies directed against ACh receptors are detected in 80% to 90% of patients with generalized disease and in 50% with ocular myasthenia (7,21,22). In general, antibody titers correlate poorly with the severity of illness, although some relationship may be observed in individual patients.

Anti-ACh receptor antibodies reduce the number of functioning ACh receptors by several mechanisms, which include blocking the receptors, destroying postsynaptic membranes, increasing the rate of receptor breakdown, and impairing synthesis of new receptors (8,16,23,24). The number of functional ACh receptors in involved muscles may be reduced by as much as 70% to 90%. When viewed under the microscope, the complex folding pattern of the neuromuscular junction appears simplified or is destroyed outright.

The thymus gland is believed to play a major role in the autoimmune response of myasthenia gravis. About 12% of patients with myasthenia have thymomas (22), and 70% have thymic hyperplasia (8). Patients with generalized myasthenia improve and may even undergo complete remission after thymectomy. This benefit may reflect the removal of a subpopulation of B lymphocytes which produce the receptor antibody or elimination of a thymic factor which stimulates T cells.

Why Are Eye Muscles Selectively Vulnerable?

Ninety percent of patients with myasthenia have ocular involvement. For several reasons, the extraocular muscles are so commonly affected in this disorder (3). Even slight weakness of an extraocular muscle may produce sufficient misalignment to cause diplopia. Motor units in these muscles fire at much higher rates than those in other skeletal muscles, increasing the likelihood for extraocular muscles to fatigue. Extraocular muscle membranes have relatively fewer synaptic folds and therefore may have a smaller number of ACh receptors. This would reduce the safety margin for neuromuscular transmission at extraocular end plates. Finally, there is growing evidence of antigenic differences between the ACh receptors of extraocular muscle and other skeletal muscle. Anti-ACh receptor antibodies directed against epitopes unique to human extraocular muscle have been identified (25). With conventional radioimmunoassay (RIA), sera from 7 of 17 patients with pure ocular myasthenia were shown to contain antibodies that reacted to extraocular muscle ACh receptors but not to leg muscle ACh receptors. These antibodies were functionally active and caused a reduction in ACh receptors at extraocular muscle end plates. The frequency of ocular involvement in myasthenia may represent a predisposition of the immune system to react against the receptor antigens unique to extraocular muscle (3).

Pharmacologic Diagnostic Studies

Pharmacologic, electrophysiologic and serologic studies are routinely performed to confirm a clinical impression of myasthenia gravis. These diagnostic studies take advantage of the pathophysiologic mechanisms that reduce the safety margin for neuromuscular transmission in the disease.

Routine pharmacologic studies consist of the administration of anticholinesterase agents to inhibit enzymatic hydrolysis of ACh and prolong the availability of the neurotransmitter at the postsynaptic membrane. A positive edrophonium (or Tensilon) test is a reliable indicator of myasthenia gravis, but it is not specific, having been reported in botulism, motor neuron disease, Guillain-Barré syndrome, congenital myasthenic syndromes, and intracranial mass lesions (2).

Before performing the edrophonium test, one must identify a clinical parameter that can be objectively followed for improvement. Daroff (26) has argued that the edrophonium test should be performed only when ptosis or a clinically obvious ophthalmoparesis is present. If these signs are absent, a valid positive endpoint cannot be determined. In addition, a patient occasionally will have a paradoxic response to edrophonium, complicating the interpretation of subjective changes in diplopic images. Quantification of ocular motility defects with Maddox rods, red glass, prisms, and optokinetic nystagmography has been advocated in assessing a patient's response to edrophonium (6). Other investigators have cautioned against use of techniques that rely on subjective measurements of diplopia and do not directly test eye muscle strength.

Edrophonium chloride (Tensilon), a fast-acting, short-lived anticholinesterase, is available in 1-ml ampules and 10-ml vials, each containing a 10-mg/ml solution. After the edrophonium is drawn into a 1-ml tuberculin syringe, a 2- to 3-mg test dose is injected intravenously (i.v.). The patient is carefully monitored for improvement and for idiosyncratic or cholinergic reactions. If there is no response after 1 to 2 minutes, the remainder of the dose is injected. Alternatively, the edrophonium may be administered in 2-mg increments at 30- to 60-second intervals (6). The advantage of this method is that the full 10-mg dose is often not required to produce a positive test. In addition, a positive response may be missed if too much edrophonium is injected. Flushing with normal saline is necessary to ensure delivery of the drug when edrophonium is administered through an intravenous line. Some clinicians recommend administration of a normal saline placebo control, but this is not necessary in most circumstances.

A positive response typically is marked by dramatic improvement in the ptosis or extraocular muscle weakness (Fig. 2). Because of the short action of edrophonium, the test is negative if no response is observed in 3 to 4 minutes. Some patients paradoxically worsen after edrophonium injection and should not be considered to have a positive test (8). Cardiac monitoring with easy access to atropine may be necessary in patients with heart disease or in those prone to bradycardia. Nearly all patients will experience some cholinergic effects such as nausea, lacrimation, salivation, or fasciculations during the test.

Neostigmine, a longer-acting anticholinesterase agent, is an alternative in children who are too uncooperative to monitor for a brief time period or in adults who have diplopia without ptosis. To perform the test in adults, 1.5 mg neostigmine is mixed with 0.6 mg atropine sulfate in a small syringe and injected into the deltoid muscle (1,7). The dose in children is usually 0.04 mg/kg, to a total of 1.5 mg. A positive response is generally evident by 15 minutes and is most obvious 30 minutes after the injection.

Other Diagnostic Studies

Electrophysiologic tests helpful in the diagnosis of myasthenia gravis include repetitive nerve stimulation and single-fiber electromyography (SFEMG). Slow repetitive stimulation of peripheral nerve at a rate of 1 to 5/s depletes immediately available ACh stores (27), further hampering the already reduced safety margin in patients with myasthenia. As a result, motor responses decrease in amplitude on successive stimuli. However, a decremental response is observed in only 50% of patients with isolated ocular myasthenia (4). SFEMG, though technically demanding, is a more sensitive measure for detecting neuromuscular transmission disorders and will demonstrate increased jitter values in more than 80% of patients with ocular myasthenia (2). The sensitivity of SFEMG approaches 100% if the superior rectus or levator palpebralis muscles are studied (28). Neither repetitive stimulation or SFEMG is entirely specific for myasthenia gravis.

Serologic studies will detect antibodies to the ACh receptor in less than half of patients with ocular myasthenia (2). Anti-ACh receptor antibodies were detected in 20 of 44 such patients with pure ocular involvement (4). When positive, antibody titers are significantly lower than levels in patients with generalized disease (4,21).

There is no single test which diagnoses all cases of myasthenia gravis and is 100% specific. Patients with ptosis or clinically obvious ophthalmoparesis should undergo an

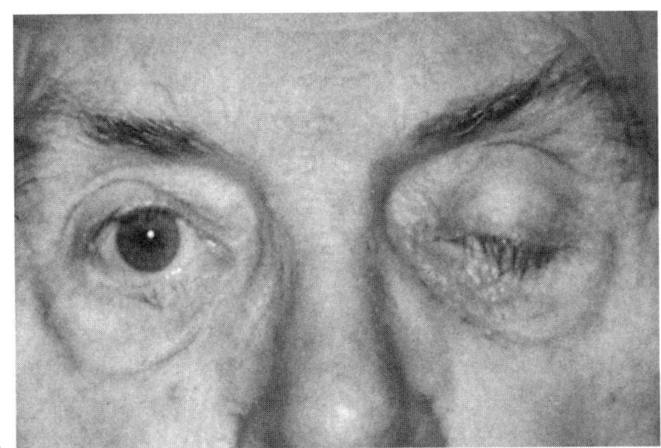

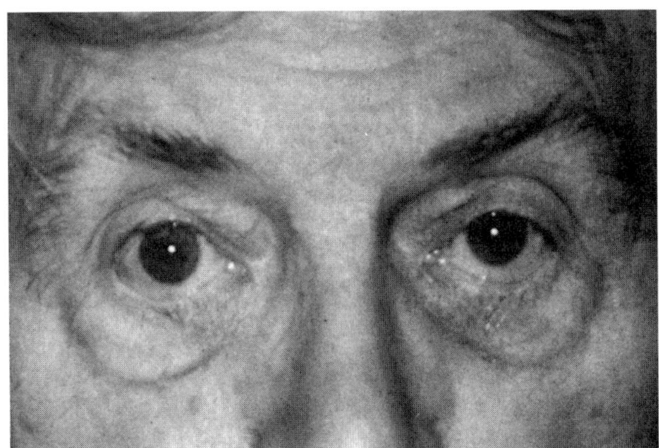

FIG. 72-2. An 80-year-old man with complete left-sided ptosis (**A**) experienced dramatic improvement after edrophonium injection (**B**).

edrophonium or neostigmine test. Serologic testing for anti-ACh receptor antibodies should be performed in all patients with suspected myasthenia. When pharmacologic, serologic, and electrophysiologic studies are combined, a diagnosis will be confirmed in nearly all patients with ocular myasthenia.

Myasthenia gravis is frequently associated with other autoimmune diseases. Therefore, it is prudent to check thyroid function tests and anti-nuclear antibodies in patients with confirmed myasthenia. If systemic corticosteroids are being considered for therapy, fasting serum glucose and a purified protein derivative (PPD) skin test should be performed to check for underlying diabetes mellitus and tuberculosis. Thymic neoplasms or hyperplasia can be detected with computed tomography (CT) or magnetic resonance imaging (MRI) of the chest.

Neonates of myasthenic mothers may develop neonatal myasthenia, a transient disorder characterized by difficulty swallowing, sucking, and breathing. Neonatal myasthenia, presumably due to transplacental transfer of anti-ACh receptor antibodies, has been managed with oral and injectable anticholinesterases. Rarely do these infants require treatment for more than 2 months.

Differential Diagnosis

Bulbar and somatic weakness is present in several other neuromuscular disorders, including congenital myasthenic syndromes, Lambert-Eaton myasthenic syndrome, botulism, and mitochondrial disorders. Grave's disease and intracranial mass lesions can also mimic myasthenia gravis. Occasionally, ocular myasthenia will coexist with thyroid eye disease. In this setting, it is important to determine which disorder is causing most of the symptoms. MRI of the brain should be considered (22) in cases of suspected myasthenia in which disease is restricted to ocular or cranial musculature. Neuroimaging is especially important in patients with atypical presentations or negative diagnostic studies.

Local Treatment

The treatment of ocular myasthenia in patients without generalized disease tends to be conservative. Patients with limited disability may not require systemic therapy and can be managed with local treatment. Ptosis, the most frequent finding, can be managed at times with a crutch attached to an eyeglass frame or with small adhesive tapestrips (6). Although these methods may be uncomfortable or result in some eye irritation due to exposure, they may be preferred by patients who wish to avoid side effects from medication. Ptosis surgery is an option in patients who are refractory to prosthetic and pharmacologic measures but is complicated by corneal exposure and is generally reserved for patients with inactive disease and fixed deficits (6).

No therapy may be necessary in patients with rare, intermittent diplopia. Double vision that is more persistent may be improved with prisms, especially when the deviation is relatively comitant. Patching of one eye is another option in some patients. Due to the fluctuating character of the disease and occasional spontaneous remission, extraocular muscle surgery is rarely recommended in ocular myasthenia (8).

Pharmacologic Therapy

The pharmacologic therapy of ocular myasthenia usually begins with anticholinesterase agents. Pyridostigmine (Mestinon) may improve symptoms in some patients (Fig. 3). However, ocular manifestations of myasthenia respond relatively poorly to anticholinesterases when used alone. The pharmacology of these agents is reviewed in the next section.

The clinical response of ocular myasthenia to systemic corticosteroids is usually more favorable. Although corticosteroids and adrenocorticotrophin (ACTH) were initially considered ineffective in myasthenia gravis, the efficacy of these agents is now well accepted in treatment of patients with either isolated ocular involvement or generalized disease (8). In a large retrospective study, patients with ocular

A 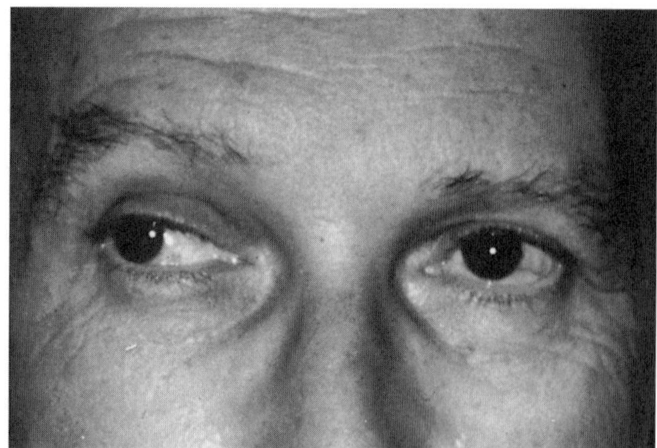

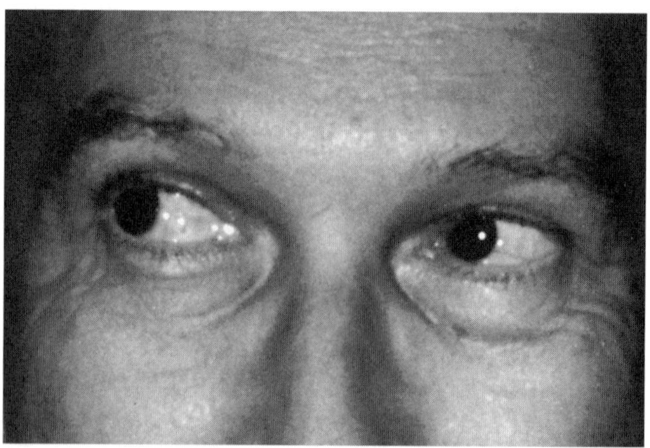 B

FIG. 72-3. A 57-year-old man with a left adduction deficit (**A**) experienced improvement with maintenance pyridostigmine therapy (**B**).

myasthenia treated with corticosteroids had a higher incidence of remission and improvement (5). A typical regimen in patients with ocular myasthenia who have failed anticholinesterase therapy begins with daily oral prednisone at an intermediate dose of 0.5 to 1.0 mg/kg. After patients have demonstrated improvement, an alternate-day schedule is gradually substituted, slowly tapering over a period of several months. An alternative method is to institute prednisone treatment at a low dose of 10 to 25 mg daily or on alternate days, gradually increasing it by 5 mg every 2 to 3 days (22,29). This method reduces but does not eliminate the risk of initial exacerbation and is especially useful in patients with myasthenia with isolated ocular involvement.

In a study of 116 patients with myasthenia treated with prednisone 60 to 80 mg daily, 80% showed marked improvement or no longer had symptoms (30). Patients with pure ocular myasthenia with or without mild limb-girdle weakness demonstrated a slightly better response to prednisone than did patients with more severe disease. Sustained improvement in responders occurred a mean of 13.2 days after prednisone was initiated. More than 90% of responders showed improvement in the first 3 weeks of therapy. The time to maximal improvement ranged from 2 weeks to 6 months (30).

Although some patients will require chronic corticosteroid therapy, a low-dose maintenance schedule that limits adverse side effects can be established in most cases (8). Patients with ocular myasthenia may worsen and, on occasion, even develop generalized disease when corticosteroids are initiated. Therefore, it is best for a neurologist or internist to manage patients who are treated with corticosteroids (1). The pharmacology and side-effects profile of corticosteroids are reviewed in Chapter 59, this volume.

Other immunosuppressive agents such as azathioprine, cytoxan, and cyclosporine are generally reserved for treatment of generalized myasthenia (5,7). Plasmapheresis and intravenous γ-globulin are used to treat patients in myasthenic crisis or in circumstances in which a rapid clinical response is needed.

Indications for thymectomy in myasthenia gravis remain controversial. There is widespread agreement regarding use of thymectomy in patients with suspected thymoma and in those with severe, generalized disease that has responded poorly to pharmacologic therapy (31). Most neurologists do not consider thymectomy in patients with isolated ocular myasthenia because of their limited disability and relatively high rate of remission. However, some researchers consider thymectomy an option for patients with severely disabling ocular symptoms who are refractory to other forms of therapy (31,32).

PHARMACOLOGY OF ANTICHOLINESTERASE AGENTS

General Pharmacology

Anticholinesterase agents act by reversibly inhibiting acetylcholinesterase, the enzyme that rapidly hydrolyzes ACh. By inhibiting breakdown of ACh, anticholinesterases prolong the duration of the neurotransmitter at the motor end plate, thereby increasing the number of neurotransmitter–receptor interactions. The result in myasthenic patients is improved muscle strength with an enhanced response to repetitive nerve stimulation. In addition to inhibiting acetylcholinesterase, these agents have direct actions at some cholinergic receptors, where they act as agonists or antagonists (17). The pharmacologic rationale for their use, however, is to inhibit enzymatic hydrolysis of ACh.

As described earlier, the anticholinesterase edrophonium chloride (Tensilon) is used in diagnosis of myasthenia gravis. Pyridostigmine bromide (Mestinon) and neostigmine bromide (Prostigmin) are mainly used in treatment, administered alone in patients with mild symptoms and as adjunctive agents in patients with more severe disease. The clinical response to cholinesterase inhibitors varies widely among patients. Therefore, individualization of therapy is necessary, with close attention paid to total dosage and timing of administration. The fluctuating nature of the disease may necessitate dosing adjustments, especially in the setting of other illnesses. For instance, medication requirements often increase during infections and other periods of stress. The clinical benefit is usually dose dependent, although cholinergic toxicity occurs at higher doses.

Pyridostigmine is widely regarded as the therapeutic drug of choice because of its longer half-life ($t_{\frac{1}{2}}$) and more favorable side-effect profile. However, the efficacy of the different agents has not been adequately compared in clinical trials (33).

PYRIDOSTIGMINE BROMIDE

History and Source

The earliest recorded use of anticholinesterase compounds dates back to the early 19th century in Western Africa. The native Efik people of Old Calabar used physostigmine derived from crushed Calabar beans as a poison in judicial procedures meant to reveal and destroy witchcraft (34). Rational therapeutic use of anticholinesterase compounds dates back to the second half of the 19th century, when Calabar bean abstract was used as an antidote to atropine poisoning (35) and physostigmine was first used to treat glaucoma (36,37). Walker (18) introduced the use of physostigmine in myasthenia gravis in 1934 when she reported that physostigmine salicylate injections produced dramatic, though temporary, improvement in a 56-year-old woman with generalized disease (18). Soon after the chemical structure of physostigmine was established in 1925, a series of carbamic ester analogues were synthesized and analyzed (38). Today, the synthetic quaternary ammonium compounds pyridostigmine and neostigmine are the mainstays of anticholinesterase therapy in myasthenia gravis because of their limited CNS toxicity.

Official Drug Name and Chemistry

The chemical name of pyridostigmine bromide is 3-hydroxy-1-methylpyridinium bromide dimethylcarbamate (pyridostigmine bromide, Mestinon). The molecular formula is $C_9H_{13}BrN_2O_2$.

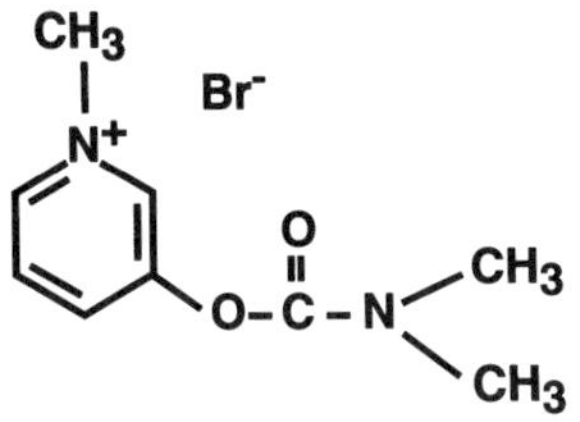

CH_3 Br^- N^+ O O–C–N CH_3 CH_3

Clinical Pharmacology

Pyridostigmine is a reversible inhibitor of acetylcholinesterase. It is an analogue of neostigmine but has fewer side effects, with a lower degree and incidence of bradycardia, salivation, and GI stimulation. Animal studies with use of the injectable drug and human studies with use of an oral preparation demonstrated that pyridostigmine bromide has a longer duration of action than does neostigmine (39).

Pharmaceutics

Pyridostigmine bromide is available in generic form and as the drug Mestinon (ICN Pharmaceuticals, Costa Mesa, CA). Mestinon Injectable is available in 2-ml containers as a 5-mg/ml solution containing 0.2% parabens (methyl and propyl) as preservatives and 0.02% sodium citrate with pH adjusted to approximately 5.0. Mestinon tablets are 60 mg, and Mestinon Timespan tablets (prolonged-release) are 180 mg. Mestinon syrup is 60 mg/5 ml (alcohol 5%). Generic tablets are available in 30-mg form. A 2-mg injection of pyridostigmine is approximately equivalent to 60 mg administered orally (40).

Pharmacokinetics

Pyridostigmine bromide is poorly and variably absorbed from the GI tract. It undergoes extensive hepatic metabolism and is excreted mainly in the urine as inactive metabolites and unchanged drug. The main metabolite is the hydrolysis product 3-hydroxy-*N*-methyl-pyridinium (37). The volume of distribution of pyridostigmine is approximately 1.4 L/kg (33). The plasma $t_{\frac{1}{2}}$ in healthy human subjects was 200 minutes after a 60-mg oral dose and 97 minutes after a 4-mg intravenous infusion (41). The peak plasma concentration was evident 1–2 hours after oral administration and was delayed approximately 90 minutes when the drug was ingested with food. Oral bioavailability was low; the mean value was about 10% (37). However, the oral bioavailability of pyridostigmine was about four times greater than that of neostigmine (42).

Severely impaired renal function prolongs the effect of pyridostigmine and neostigmine (37). The elimination $t_{\frac{1}{2}}$ of pyridostigmine was significantly increased and the plasma clearance was significantly decreased in 4 patients without renal function (43). Approximately 75% of plasma clearance depended on renal function. Pyridostigmine's effects have onset in 30 minutes, with peak activity ranging from 2 to 8 hours. Because its activity decreases slowly, clinicians can achieve sustained blood levels by adjusting the frequency of dosing (8,22).

Therapeutic drug monitoring has not proved useful (33). Mean plasma pyridostigmine concentrations varied widely and did not correlate with dosage in a study of 18 patients with generalized myasthenia (44). Patients with plasma levels greater than 100 ng/ml exhibited cholinergic overstimulation and poor neuromuscular function. Pyridostigmine plasma concentrations tend to be higher in patients with poorly controlled myasthenia than in patients who respond well to the medication. Some therapeutic failures may be due to poor drug absorption (37).

Therapeutic Use

Patients with ocular or generalized myasthenia usually receive an initial oral pyridostigmine dose of 30 to 60 mg every 4 to 6 hours. The dose can be titrated upward on an individual basis to maximize the clinical response, but in general the dose should not exceed 120 mg every 2 hours while the patient is awake. The suggested dose for children is 7 mg/kg daily in five to six doses. Some patients may require intramuscular injections because of poor oral absorption.

The prolonged-release Timespan preparation is not routinely administered during the day because of erratic absorption and effects, but it is useful as a single bedtime dose (24) in generalized patients who are symptomatic at night or on awakening (24,32).

In addition to its use in treatment of myasthenia, pyridostigmine has been used to treat paralytic ileus and postoperative urinary retention. It has been used prophylactically to help protect soldiers from nerve gas agents. Pyridostigmine is believed to be less effective than neostigmine in reversing the action of nondepolarizing neuromuscular blockers (40).

Contraindications to the use of pyridostigmine are known hypersensitivity to anticholinesterase agents or bromides and mechanical obstructions of the GI or urinary tract. It should be used with caution in patients with asthma or cardiac dysrhythmias.

Side Effects and Toxicity

The most common adverse effects of anticholinesterase agents are produced by excessive cholinergic stimulation. Both muscarinic and nicotinic side effects may occur. Muscarinic overstimulation produces nausea and vomiting; abdominal cramping; diarrhea; increased lacrimal, salivary, and bronchial secretions; miosis; and sweating. GI side effects are especially common but can generally be managed symptomatically with glycopyrrolate (Robinul, A. H. Robins, Richmond, VA), loperamide HCl (Imodium, Janssen Pharmaceutical, Titusville, NJ), propantheline bromide (Pro-Banthine, Roberts Pharmaceuticals Corp., Eatontown, NJ), or dephenoxylate HCl with atropine (Lomotil, G. D. Searle & Co., Chicago, IL; others). These anticholinergic agents must be used cautiously, with the realization that they may mask symptoms of impending cholinergic crisis.

Nicotinic toxicity includes muscle cramping, fasciculations, and weakness. Therefore, some few patients with refractory myasthenia may actually worsen when treated with increasing amounts of anticholinesterases. Such a cholinergic crisis may result in death. Prompt discontinuation of anticholinesterase agents is necessary in patients with cholinergic crisis. Atropine sulfate 1 to 2 mg i.v. should be administered to patients in cholinergic crisis, but it reverses only the muscarinic side effects. Atropine doses may be repeated every 10 to 30 minutes until the patient develops anticholinergic effects such as dry mouth, clearing of tracheobronchial secretions, tachycardia, and dilated pupils. In addition to atropine treatment, supportive care is provided, including mechanical ventilation in more severe cases of cholinergic crisis.

High-risk Groups

The safety of pyridostigmine in pregnancy has not been established. Its potential benefit to the mother during pregnancy should be weighed against possible risk to the fetus.

Pyridostigmine crosses the placenta, and very small amounts are present in breast milk. The amount of pyridostigmine per kilogram of body weight ingested by nursing infants of two myasthenic mothers was 0.1% of the maternal dose (45). Pyridostigmine was not detectable in infant plasma. These data suggest that nursing is safe for mothers receiving 300 mg pyridostigmine or less daily (37,42). Anticholinesterase dosing should be reduced appropriately in patients with renal insufficiency. Because neostigmine undergoes more extensive hepatic metabolism than pyridostigmine, neostigmine may be preferred in patients with renal insufficiency.

Drug Interactions

Commonly used drugs known to exacerbate myasthenia gravis are shown in Table 1. Certain antibiotic agents, especially aminoglycosides, have a mild but definite nondepolarizing blocking action at the neuromuscular junction. Aminoglycosides should be used in patients with myasthenia only when there are no other reasonable alternatives (46). Antiarrhythmic and anesthetic agents also interfere with neuromuscular transmission and should be used cautiously, if at all, in patients with myasthenia. D-Penicillamine induces myasthenia gravis, most likely by stimulating or enhancing an immunologic reaction against the neuromuscular junction. This form of myasthenia, which is usually mild and often limited to ocular muscles, remits in most patients within 1 year of drug discontinuation (46). D-Penicillamine should not be used in patients known to have myasthenia.

Early studies suggested that corticosteroids enhance the metabolism of pyridostigmine, but later researchers have failed to identify significant pharmacokinetic interactions between the two drugs (37). Cholinergic drugs theoretically can worsen muscarinic and nicotinic side effects in patients receiving anticholinesterases.

Major Clinical Trials

The efficacy of different anticholinesterase agents has not been compared in careful clinical trials. Of 48 patients

TABLE 72-1. *Drugs that may worsen myasthenia gravis or interfere with neuromuscular transmission*

Antibiotic agents	
	Aminoglycosides
	Erythromycin
	Tetracycline
	Penicillins
	Sulfonamides
	Fluroquinolones
	Clindamycin
	Lincomycin
Anesthetic agents	
	Neuromuscular blocking agents
	Lidocaine
	Procaine
Anticonvulsant agents	
	Phenytoin
	Mephenytoin
	Trimethadione
Cardiovascular drugs	
	β-blockers
	Procainamide
	Quinidine
Rheumatologic drugs	
	Chloroquine
	D-Penicillamine
Miscellaneous	
	Iodinated contrast
	Chlorpromazine
	Corticosteroids
	Lithium

with isolated ocular myasthenia monitored for a mean of 4.5 years, 19 (40%) demonstrated a good response to pyridostigmine (4). Some of these patients received other forms of therapy, including immunosuppressive agents and thymectomy. Corticosteroids were effective in 14 of the 18 patients (78%) treated with them.

Of 13 patients treated only with pyridostigmine, 9 had a good response to therapy. Ptosis was more likely to respond to pyridostigmine than was diplopia (4).

NEOSTIGMINE BROMIDE

History and Source

Neostigmine bromide, a quaternary ammonium derivative, was synthesized shortly after the chemical structure of physostigmine was established in 1925 (38). Its first recorded use in myasthenia gravis was in 1932 (47).

Official Drug Name and Chemistry

The chemical name of neostigmine bromide is (*m*-hydroxyphenyl) trimethylammonium bromide dimethylcarbamate (Prostigmin). The molecular formula is $C_{12}H_{19}BrN_2O_2$ (Fig. 5). A methylsulfate group is substituted for the bromide ion in the parenteral form.

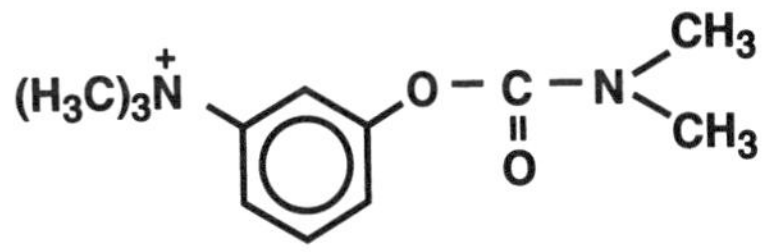

Clinical Pharmacology

Neostigmine is a reversible inhibitor of acetylcholinesterase. The therapeutic response is similar to that of pyridostigmine, but neostigmine has a shorter duration of action and is more potent (33). A 15-mg oral dose or 1 mg i.v. dose of neostigmine is approximately equivalent to a 60-mg oral dose of pyridostigmine. Neostigmine also has direct cholinomimetic effects on skeletal muscle and possibly on autonomic ganglion cells and neurons of the central nervous system.

Pharmaceutics

Neostigmine bromide is available in 15-mg tablets as a generic and as the drug Prostigmin (ICN Pharmaceuticals, Costa Mesa, CA). Generic neostigmine methylsulfate is available as a 0.5- or 1.0-mg/ml solution in 10-ml containers. Prostigmin Injectable is available as a 0.25-mg/ml solution in 1-ml vials, as 0.5 mg/ml in 1- and 10-ml vials, and as 1 mg/ml in 10-ml vials. Prostigmin Injectable is compounded with 0.2% parabens (methyl and propyl) or 0.45% phenol as preservatives and sodium hydroxide to adjust the pH to approximately 5.9.

Pharmacokinetics

Neostigmine bromide, like pyridostigmine, is poorly absorbed from the GI tract. In 3 patients with myasthenia treated with a single 30-mg oral dose, the mean plasma $t_{\frac{1}{2}}$ was 52 minutes. Bioavailability was estimated to be 1% to 2% (42). Protein binding in humans is estimated to be 15% to 25% (40). The apparent volume of distribution varies from 32 to 61 L and is approximately equal to total body water (48). Hepatic metabolism and biliary excretion play more important roles in elimination of neostigmine than in elimination of pyridostigmine. Approximately 80% of a neostigmine dose is excreted in the urine in 24 hours, mainly as unchanged drug and the metabolite 3-hydroxyphenyltrimethylammonium (48).

The activity of neostigmine bromide lasts 2 to 6 hours, similar to that of pyridostigmine. However, once neostigmine reaches a peak level, its activity decreases rapidly. Therefore, it is more difficult to optimize therapy with neostigmine than with pyridostigmine (8).

Therapeutic Use

As with pyridostigmine, the dose and frequency of neostigmine administration must be tailored for individual patients. Whenever possible, it is administered orally, initially at a dose of 15 mg every 3 to 4 hours in adults. The total daily dose usually ranges from 75 to 375 mg. The oral dose in children is 2 mg/kg daily in divided doses. When oral therapy is impractical, intramuscular injections of 0.5 to 2.5 mg have been used in adults, with a total daily dose of 5 to 20 mg. Smaller intramuscular doses have been used to treat children and neonates with myasthenia.

Intravenous use of neostigmine is hazardous and is complicated by severe muscarinic side effects. If neostigmine is used in this form, atropine must be readily available. When neostigmine is used as an alternative to edrophonium in diagnosis of myasthenia gravis, it is administered by intramuscular injection. This diagnostic procedure is described earlier in the chapter.

Like pyridostigmine, neostigmine has been used in treatment of paralytic ileus and postoperative urinary retention. Neostigmine bromide has been administered in eye drops and ointment to reduce IOP in glaucoma (40). Neostigmine is believed to be more effective than pyridostigmine in reversing neuromuscular blockade produced by nondepolarizing muscle relaxants. Nausea and vomiting are common when neostigmine is used postoperatively in this application.

Contraindications to neostigmine use include known hypersensitivity to the drug, peritonitis, and mechanical obstruction of the GI or urinary tract. Neostigmine should be used with extreme caution in patients who have undergone recent intestinal or bladder surgery and cautiously in patients with cardiac dysrhythmias, bradycardia, hypotension, epilepsy, hyperthyroidism, parkinsonism, asthma, and peptic ulcer disease (40).

Side Effects and Toxicity

The side-effect profile of neostigmine is similar to that of pyridostigmine. However, adverse cholinergic effects with therapeutic doses occur more frequently with neostigmine. In cases of cholinergic crisis caused by oral ingestion, the stomach should be emptied by lavage. Ventilatory support should take priority if there is evidence of respiratory failure. Atropine sulfate is administered intravenously in doses of 1 to 2 mg to control muscarinic toxicity. Some investigators advocate use of small doses of D-tubocurarine to manage muscle twitching (40).

High-risk Groups

The safety and effectiveness of neostigmine in children has not been established. Neostigmine is classified as Pregnancy category C. It should be used in pregnant women only if clearly needed. Whether neostigmine is excreted in breast milk is not known. Neostigmine dosage may need to be reduced in patients with renal insufficiency. In one study, the mean serum elimination $t_{1/2}$ in anephric patients was 181 minutes as compared with 80 minutes in patients with normal renal function (49). Neostigmine may be the preferred anticholinesterase in patients with renal insufficiency since it undergoes more extensive hepatic metabolism than pyridostigmine.

Drug Interactions

Drug interactions with neostigmine are similar to those that occur with pyridostigmine. Bradycardia and hypotension have been observed in patients treated with β-blockers who have received neostigmine (40).

EDROPHONIUM CHLORIDE

History and Source

Edrophonium chloride, a synthetic quaternary ammonium anticholinesterase, was introduced as a diagnostic test for myasthenia gravis by Osserman and Kaplan in 1952 (50).

Official Drug Name and Chemistry

The chemical name of edrophonium chloride is ethyl (*m*-hydroxyphenyl)-dimethylammonium chloride (Tensilon). Its molecular formula is $C_{10}H_{16}ClNO$.

Clinical Pharmacology

Edrophonium is similar to other reversible cholinesterase inhibitors, but its action is more rapid in onset and shorter in duration than that of pyridostigmine or neostigmine. In addition, its effect on skeletal muscle is particularly prominent, adding to its usefulness as a diagnostic tool in myasthenia gravis. Patients with ocular myasthenia who respond to edrophonium generally have immediate reduction of their ptosis or diplopia. The response lasts 5 to 15 minutes (33,40).

Pharmaceutics

Edrophonium chloride is available as the drug Tensilon (ICN Pharmaceuticals, Costa Mesa, CA). It is available as a 10-mg/ml sterile solution in 1-ml ampules and 10-ml vials. The solution is compounded with 0.45% phenol and

0.2% sodium sulfite as preservatives and is buffered with sodium citrate and citric acid to a pH of approximately 5.4

Pharmacokinetics

Edrophonium is a short- and rapid-acting anticholinesterase. In a study of surgical patients with normal hepatic and renal function, its mean elimination $t_{\frac{1}{2}}$ after intravenous injection was approximately 110 minutes (51), longer than was previously reported (52). However, edrophonium has a more rapid onset and shorter duration of action than pyridostigmine or neostigmine. When edrophonium was used to antagonize D-tubocurarine blockade, twitch tension rapidly increased to a plateau after 2.9 minutes, as compared with 6.1 minutes with use of neostigmine (51). Except for having a longer distribution $t_{\frac{1}{2}}$, edrophonium had pharmacokinetics similar to those of neostigmine.

Therapeutic Use

Edrophonium chloride's short duration of action limits its use in long-term management of myasthenia gravis. Its rapid onset of action, however, makes it ideal as a diagnostic test for myasthenia gravis. The procedure for a "Tensilon test" is described earlier in this chapter. Edrophonium is also used to differentiate myasthenic crisis from the less common cholinergic emergency, although it is not considered as helpful a test in this application (33). Edrophonium 1 to 2 mg is carefully administered intravenously 1 hour after the last oral anticholinesterase dose (39). The small edrophonium dose is beneficial to patients with a myasthenic exacerbation but further weakens those who are in cholinergic crisis. Because of its brief duration of action, edrophonium is not recommended for maintenance therapy of myasthenia gravis.

As are longer-acting anticholinesterase agents, edrophonium is used to reverse neuromuscular blockade produced by nondepolarizing muscle relaxants. Edrophonium does not reliably sustain its antagonistic effect and is therefore considered less effective than neostigmine in such circumstances (40). However, larger doses of edrophonium appear to eliminate this shortcoming (51).

Contraindications to use of edrophonium are similar to those of other anticholinesterases. In addition, Tensilon solution contains sodium sulfite, which may produce allergic-type reactions and anaphylactic shock. Sulfite sensitivity appears to be uncommon in the general population, but it is more common in persons with asthma (39).

Side Effects and Toxicity

As with other anticholinesterase agents, adverse side effects of edrophonium primarily arise from cholinergic overstimulation. A patient with myasthenia who is in crisis and who is being tested with edrophonium must be carefully monitored for bradycardia, asystole, and other cholinergic reactions. Atropine sulfate and ventilatory support should be readily available to manage cholinergic toxicity. Atropine should also be accessible when edrophonium is used to diagnose myasthenia gravis. The section on pyridostigmine provides a full description of cholinergic side effects and management of cholinergic crisis.

High-risk Groups

The safety of edrophonium in pregnant or lactating women has not been established. When considering the use of edrophonium in such cases, one must weigh potential benefits against possible harm to the mother and child.

Drug Interactions

Because edrophonium is commonly administered to patients receiving other anticholinesterase drugs, the potential of inducing cholinergic crisis should be recognized.

Major Clinical Trials

In a study of 48 patients with isolated ocular myasthenia, 46 demonstrated a positive response to edrophonium injection (4). Of the two patients with false-negative tests, one had mild bilateral ptosis and intermittent diplopia and the other had long-standing unilateral ptosis. The edrophonium relieved only the ptosis in 35% (15 of 43) patients who reported both ptosis and diplopia. The investigators reported a large discordance between a positive response to edrophonium and the subsequent efficacy of oral anticholinesterases. Only 40% of the patients had a satisfactory response to maintenance anticholinesterase therapy (4).

REFERENCES

1. Glaser JS, Bachynski B. Infranuclear disorders of eye movement. In: Glaser JS, ed. *Neuro-ophthalmology,* 2nd ed. Philadelphia: J.B. Lippincott, 1990;361–418.
2. Schmidt D. Myasthenia gravis. In: Lessell S, van Dalen JTW, eds. *Current Neuro-Ophthalmology,* vol. 3. Chicago: Mosby Year Book, 1991; 273–305.
3. Kaminski HJ, Maas E, Spiegel P, Ruff RL. Why are eye muscles frequently involved in myasthenia gravis? *Neurology* 1990;40:1663–1669.
4. Evoli A, Tonali P, Bartoccioni E, Monaco ML. Ocular myasthenia: diagnostic and therapeutic problems. *Acta Neurol Scand* 1988;77:31–35.
5. Grob D, Arsura E, Brunner N, Namba T. The course of myasthenia gravis, and therapies affecting outcome. *Ann NY Acad Sci* 1987;505: 472–499.
6. Weinberg DA, Lesser RL, Vollmer TL. Ocular myasthenia: a protean disorder. *Surv Ophthalmol* 1994;39:169–210.
7. March GA, Johnson LN. Ocular myasthenia gravis. *J Natl Med Assoc* 1993;85:681–684.

8. Miller NR. Myopathies and disorders of neuromuscular transmission. In: *Walsh and Hoyt's Clinical Neuro-Ophthalmology,* 4th ed. Baltimore: Williams & Wilkins, 1985;840–862.
9. Gorelick PB, Rosenberg M, Pagano RJ. Enhanced ptosis in myasthenia gravis. *Arch Neurol* 1981;38:531.
10. Cogan DG. Myasthenia gravis: a review of the disease and a description of lid twitch as a characteristic sign. *Arch Ophthalmol* 1965;74: 217–221.
11. Glaser JS. Myasthenic pseudo-internuclear ophthalmoplegia. *Arch Ophthalmol* 1966;75:363–366.
12. Osher RH, Glaser JS. Myasthenic sustained gaze fatigue. *Am J Ophthalmol* 1980;89:443–445.
13. Herishanu Y, Lavy S. Internal "ophthalmoplegia" in myasthenia gravis. *Ophthalmologica* 1971;163:302–305.
14. Baptista AG, Souza HS. Pupillary abnormalities in myasthenia gravis. *Neurology* 1961;11:210–213.
15. Dutton GN, Garson JA, Richardson RB. Pupillary fatigue in myasthenia gravis. *Trans Ophthal Soc UK* 1982;102:510–513.
16. Drachman DB. Myasthenia gravis: part I. *N Engl J Med* 1978;298: 136–142.
17. Liu JHK, Erickson K. Cholinergic agents. In: Albert DM, Jakobiec FA, eds. *Principles and Practice of Ophthalmology: Basic Sciences.* Philadelphia: W.B. Saunders, 1994;985–992.
18. Walker MB. Treatment of myasthenia with physostigmine. *Lancet* 1934;1:1200–1201.
19. Elmqvist D, Hofmann WW, Kugelberg J, Quastel DMJ. An electrophysiological investigation of neuromuscular transmission in myasthenia gravis. *J Physiol* 1964;174:417–434.
20. Fambrough DM, Drachman DB, Satyamurti S. Neuromuscular junction in myasthenia gravis: decreased acetylcholine receptors. *Science* 1973;182:293–295.
21. Lindstrom JM, Seybold ME, Lennon VA, Whittingham S, Duane D. Antibody to acetylcholine receptor in myasthenia gravis: prevalence, clinical correlates, and diagnostic value. *Neurology* 1976;26:1054–1059.
22. Drachman DB. Myasthenia gravis. *N Engl J Med* 1994;330:1797–1810.
23. Elias SB, Appel SH. Current concepts of pathogenesis and treatment of myasthenia gravis. *Med Clin North Am* 1979;63:745–757.
24. Drachman DB. Myasthenia gravis: part II. *N Engl J Med* 1978;298: 186–193.
25. Oda D. Differences in acetylcholine receptor-antibody interactions between extraocular and extremity muscle fibers. *NY Acad Sci* 1993; 681:238–255.
26. Daroff RB. The office Tensilon test for ocular myasthenia gravis. *Arch Neurol* 1986;43:843–844.
27. Kimura J. Techniques of repetitive stimulation. In: *Electrodiagnosis in Diseases of Nerve and Muscle,* 2nd ed. Philadelphia: F.A. Davis, 1989;184–200.
28. Rivero A, Crovetto L, Lopez L, Maselli R, Nogues M. Single fiber electromyography of extraocular muscles: a sensitive method for the diagnosis of ocular myasthenia gravis. *Muscle Nerve* 1995;18:943– 947.
29. Seybold ME, Drachman DB. Gradually increasing doses of prednisone in myasthenia gravis: reducing the hazards of treatment. *N Engl J Med* 1974;290:81–84.
30. Pascuzzi RM, Coslett HB, Johns TR. Long-term corticosteroid treatment of myasthenia gravis: report of 116 patients. *Ann Neurol* 1984;15:291–298.
31. Lanska DJ. Indications for thymectomy in myasthenia gravis. *Neurology* 1990;40:1828–1829.
32. Sanders DB, Scoppetta C. The treatment of patients with myasthenia gravis. *Neurol Clin* 1994;12:343–368.
33. *Drug Evaluations Annual 1994,* Chicago: American Medical Association, 1994;409–415.
34. Holmstedt B. The ordeal bean of Old Calabar; the pageant of *Physostigma venenosum* in medicine. In: Swain T, ed. *Plants in the Development of Modern Medicine.* Cambridge, MA: Harvard University Press, 1972;303–360.
35. Kleinwächter. Beobachtung über die Wirkung des Calabar-Extracts gegen Atropin-Vergiftung. *Berl Klin Wochensch* 1864;38:369–371.
36. Laqueur L. Ueber Atropin und Physostigmin und ihre Wirkung auf den intraocularen Druck. Ein Beitrag zur Therapie des Glaucoms. *Graefe Arch Clin Exp Ophthalmol* 1877;23:149–176.
37. Aquilonius S-M, Hartvig P. Clinical pharmacokinetics of cholinesterase inhibitors. *Clin Pharmacokinet* 1986;11:236–249.
38. Aeschlimann J, Reinert M. The pharmacological action of some analogues of physostigmine. *J Pharmacol Exp Ther* 1931;43:413–444.
39. *Physicians' Desk Reference,* 48th ed. Montvale, NJ: Medical Economics Production Company, 1994;1050–1058.
40. Reynolds J. *Martindale: the Extra Pharmacopoeia,* 30th ed. London: The Pharmaceutical Press, 1993;1115–1121.
41. Aquilonius S-M, Eckernas S-A, Hartvig P, Lindstrom B, Osterman PO. Pharmacokinetics and oral bioavailability of pyridostigmine in man. *Eur J Clin Pharmacol* 1980;18:423–428.
42. Aquilonius S-M, Eckernas S-A, Hartvig P, Hultman J, Lindstrom B, Osterman PO. A pharmacokinetic study of neostigmine in man using gas chromatography-mass spectrometry. *Eur J Clin Pharmacol* 1979; 15:367–371.
43. Cronnelly R, Stanski DR, Miller RD, Sheiner LB. Pyridostigmine kinetics with and without renal function. *Clin Pharmacol Ther* 1980; 28:78–81.
44. Breyer-Pfaff U, Schmezer A, Maier U, Brinkman A, Schumm F. Neuromuscular function and plasma drug levels in pyridostigmine treatment of myasthenia gravis. *J Neurol Neurosurg Psychiatry* 1990;53: 502–506.
45. Hardell L-I, Lindstrom B, Lonnerholm G, Osterman PO. Pyridostigmine in human breast milk. *Br J Clin Pharmacol* 1982;14:565–567.
46. Howard JF. Adverse drug interactions in disorders of neuromuscular transmission. *J Neurol Orthop Med Surg* 1991;12:26–34.
47. Remen L. Zur Pathogenese und Therapie der myasthenia gravis pseudoparalytica.*Dtsch Z Nervenheilkd* 1932;128:66–78.
48. Somani SM, Chan K, Dehghan A, Calvey TN. Kinetics and metabolism of intramuscular neostigmine in myasthenia gravis. *Clin Pharmacol Ther* 1980;28:64–68.
49. Cronnelly R, Stanski DR, Miller RD, Sheiner LB, Sohn YJ. Renal function and pharmacokinetics of neostigmine in anesthetized man. *Anesthesiology* 1979;51:222–226.
50. Osserman KE, Kaplan LI. Rapid diagnostic test for myasthenia gravis: increased muscle strength, without fasciculations, after intravenous administration of edrophonium (Tensilon) chloride. *J Am Med Assoc* 1952;150:265–268.
51. Morris RB, Cronnelly R, Miller RD, Stanski DR, Fahey MR. Pharmacokinetics of edrophonium and neostigmine when antagonizing d-tubocurarine in man. *Anesthesiology* 1981;54:399–402.
52. Calvey TN, Williams NE, Muir KT, Barber HE. Plasma concentration of edrophonium in man. *Clin Pharmacol Ther* 1976;19:813–820.

Textbook of Ocular Pharmacology,
edited by T.J. Zimmerman, et al.
Lippincott–Raven Publishers, Philadelphia © 1997.

CHAPTER 73

Sodium Fluorescein and Other Tissue Dyes

R. Nick Hogan and Carol F. Zimmerman

TISSUE DYES

SODIUM FLUORESCEIN

History and Source

Fluorescein, a hydroxyxanthene dye, was first synthesized by Adolf von Baeryer (1) in 1871. Its fluorescent properties in solution were immediately recognized, but its application in the diagnosis of ocular disease was not appreciated for some time. In 1882, Pfluger (2) described the first ocular use of fluorescein in an assessment of corneal epithelial integrity. In that same year, Ehrlich noted that intravenously injected fluorescein appeared in the anterior chamber, a phenomenon he used to study ocular fluid dynamics in glaucoma patients (3). Ehrlich's work inspired several other investigators; in 1920 Seidel described his test for aqueous fluid leakage from the anterior segment (4), and in 1957 Goldmann and Schmidt published their classic technique of applanation tonometry using fluorescein as the indicator dye (5).

By the early 20th century, the application of fluorescein for anterior segment diagnosis was well established (6). However, the usefulness of fluorescein in evaluation of posterior ocular structures was not apparent until Burke (7) administered the drug orally in his study of retinal and fundus pathology in 1910. Injected fluorescein was first used in humans in 1960 when McLean and Maumenee studied a choroidal hemangioma; however, they did not obtain photographs (8). Flocks, et al. (9) are credited with producing the first fluorescein angiograph in a cat in 1959.

In 1961, using intravenous (i.v.) fluorescein, Novotny and Alvis (10) began work on visualization of the retinal vasculature. A major technical problem was solved by placing barrier filters in front of the flash tube and camera, thus reducing extraneous light. With this system, they produced the first retinal angiograms of normal humans and of diabetic and hypertensive retinopathy (10). Despite numerous technical modifications to the original photographic prototype, their work remains the backbone of today's modern angiographic process and represented a quantum leap toward better understanding of the pathophysiology and treatment of retinal disease (11).

Jensen and Lundbaek (12) were first to report use of fluorescein angiography in evaluating the vasculature of the iris in diabetic patients. Angiographic changes in diseases of the iris, conjunctiva, sclera, and cornea have since been described (13,14). Other researchers have elucidated the recovery of anterior segment vascular competency after surgery (15,16). Procedures for simple modification of a standard slit lamp have made use of anterior segment fluoroangiography much more practical in the routine clinical setting (17).

Official Drug Name and Chemistry

Sodium fluorescein is dihydroxyspiro[isobenzofuran-1(3H),9-[9H]xanthen]-3-one (uranine yellow). The chemical formula is $C_{20}H_{10}O_5Na_2$. The chemical structure is shown in Fig. 1.

Fluorochemistry

Fluorescein, unlike most organic dyes, exhibits fluorescence. Blue light of 480-nm wavelength excites the fluorescein molecule and shifts the outer electrons to a higher orbit. After 10^{-9} seconds, the electrons return to the ground state, emitting energy as photons at 520 nm (appearing as yellow-green light).

The exact wavelengths of excitation and emission vary with the solvent, fluorescein concentration, and pH. Fluo-

R. N. Hogan: Department of Ophthalmology, Massachusetts Eye and Ear Infirmary, Harvard Medical School, Boston, Massachusetts 02114.

C. F. Zimmerman: Department of Ophthalmology, The University of Texas Southwestern Medical Center at Dallas, Dallas, Texas 75235-9057.

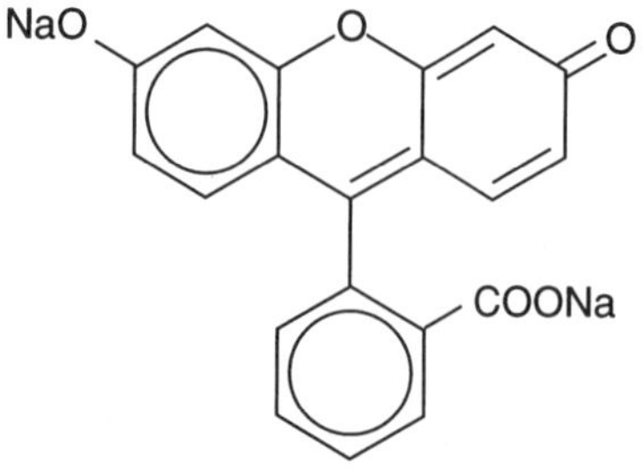

FIG. 73-1. Structural diagram of fluorescein sodium.

rescein at high concentrations forms dimers which absorb their own fluorescent emissions and shift the emission spectrum to a longer wavelength (18), rendering 10% solutions yellow-orange. As aqueous fluorescein concentration decreases, dimerization decreases, and emitted fluorescence levels increase. Therefore, dilution of 2% fluorescein by aqueous humor in the Seidel test causes a brilliant green fluorescence. (4,18) Some investigators believe, however, that this change in fluorescence is due to a shift in the pH to a more alkaline level (19). When the pH of a fluorescein solution is less than 2, the dye is in a cationic form and fluoresces a weak blue-green. When the pH is raised to between 2 and 4, the dye is electrically neutral and brighter blue-green fluorescence is emitted. At pH greater than 5, fluorescein shifts to an anionic form, and the characteristic (and brightest) yellow-green fluorescence appears. Maximal fluorescence occurs at pH 8 (18). However, because the pH of aqueous humor and tears is nearly the same, shifts in fluorescence in positive Seidel tests most likely represent dilutional effects rather than pH effects (14).

Fluorescent properties of fluorescein are also altered by binding with plasma proteins (α_1-lipoprotein, albumin, and hemoglobin) and by metabolic processes (described in section on Metabolism).

Pharmacology

Fluorescein is a relatively inert substance without inherent pharmacologic properties.

Clinical Pharmacology

After topical ocular application of fluorescein, the high lipid content of intact corneal epithelial cells prevents uptake of water-soluble fluorescein molecules. In areas of epithelial cell loss, however, fluorescein passes easily into the corneal stroma, where it diffuses rapidly. If intraepithelial junctions between cells are lost, the same phenomenon occurs. Both these events result in increased levels of fluorescence (20).

After injection, intravascular fluorescein concentration rapidly decreases due to leakage through capillary endothelium into extravascular compartments. This occurs in all organs, except where compartmental barriers exist, as in the brain, in the retina and, to some degree, in the iris. In these tissues, fluorescein can be used to study circulation times, production of capillary ultrafiltrates (fluorophotometry) and abnormal vascular and leakage patterns (21).

Pharmaceutics

Fluorescein is available in topical and injectable forms. The topical preparations are available in liquid form, in liquid form mixed with topical anesthetic agents, or in impregnated paper strips which require wetting to release the agent. The available products are summarized in Table 1.

Aqueous fluorescein is extremely susceptible to a wide variety of bacterial contaminants, especially *Pseudomonas aeruginosa* (22). This problem is circumvented by use of impregnated paper strips (23) or admixture with the anesthetic benoxinate and the preservative chlorobutanol, which have considerable bactericidal activity (24,25) (described in Major Clinical Trials section).

Pharmacokinetics, Concentration–effect Relationship, and Metabolism

Plasma levels of fluorescein are maximal immediately after injection and decrease rapidly in the first 10 minutes, which suggests rapid equilibration of the dye across multiple vascular and extravascular compartments (26). The much slower decrease in plasma concentration thereafter is due to metabolism by the liver and excretion by the kidney. Plasma half-life ($t_{\frac{1}{2}}$) is less than 1 hour (27). Few data are available regarding systemic absorption of fluorescein after topical application.

After injection, fluorescein is bound to plasma proteins and erythrocytes (28). Many investigators have shown that 80% to 90% of fluorescein is bound to proteins, whereas 10% to 20% remains free in solution (29). The rapidity of protein binding has been questioned by Ianacone et al. (30), however, who detected no tritiated fluorescein bound to albumin 10 minutes after standard injection. The binding sites are saturable at greater than 10^{-4} g/ml (31).

Metabolism of fluorescein occurs primarily in the liver by glucuronidation. Fluorescein–monoglucuronide can be detected within 2 minutes of injection. Twenty-five percent of injected fluorescein is removed for metabolism by the liver on the first circulatory pass by glucuronidation (27). Nearly 60% of free fluorescein is metabolized in 30 minutes, and 80% is metabolized in 1 hour (32). Other metabolites include trimethylfluorescein and trimethylfluorescein glucuronide. The overall rate of liver metabolism is 1.5 ml/min/kg (27).

Fluorescein metabolites have only about 4.5% of the fluorescence properties of the free molecule (33), and the observed decrease in fluorescence after injection can be at-

TABLE 73-1. *Topical fluorescein preparations*

Generic name	Trade name	Manufacturer	Concentration
Solutions			
Fluorescein sodium	Fluorescein	Various	2% in 1, 2, and 15 ml
Fluorescein Na with Anesthetic	Fluress	Barnes Hind	0.25% fluorescein Na, 0.4% benoxinate HCl, boric acid buffered povidone and 1% chlorobutanol (preservative)
	Fluorocaine	Akorn	0.25% fluorescein Na, 0.5% proparacaine HCl, povidone and 0.01% thimerosal (preservative)
	Proparacaine-Fluorescein Solution	Bausch & Lomb	0.25% fluorescein Na 0.5% proparacaine HCl
Impregnated Strips			
Fluorescein Na	Fluorets Strips	Akorn	1 mg fluorescein Na
	Fluor-I-Strip	Wyeth-Ayerst	9 mg fluorescein Na, 0.5% chlorobutanol (preservative), polysorbate 80 (surface agent) buffers
	Fluor-I-Strip A.T. (for applanation tonometry)	Wyeth-Ayerst	1 mg fluorescein Na, 0.5% chlorobutanol (preservative), polysorbate 80 (surface agent), buffers
	Ful-Glo	Sola/Barnes-Hinds	0.6% fluorescein Na
Intravenous fluorescein preparations			
Fluorescein Na	AK-Fluor Injection	Akorn	10% and 25% in sterile water
	Fluorescite Injection	Alcon	10% and 25% in sterile water (ampules and syringes)
	Funduscein-10	IOLAB	10% in sterile water
	Funduscein-25	IOLAB	25% in sterile water

tributed in part to intravenous accumulation of these metabolites. Binding to plasma protein quenches the fluorescence of free fluorescein (by 70%) but not the glucuronidated form (31). Therefore, even after binding, nonmetabolized fluorescein has greater fluorescent properties than metabolized fluorescein. As time after injection increases, concentration of metabolized and bound fluorescein moieties increases. Because metabolites of fluorescein are more polar than the free compound, they are less able to cross blood–ocular barriers. This property of fluorescein glucuronide is useful in studies of barrier leakage.

Both fluorescein and fluorescein glucuronide are actively excreted by the kidney (21,32,33). Fluorescein can be detected in urine after the first circulatory pass and is almost completely excreted 6 to 12 hours after injection (26). The elimination rate for fluorescein by the kidney is 1.75 ml/min/kg (27). Urinary fluorescence, however, has been noted as long as 36 hours after injection in patients with normal renal function. Most orally ingested dye is excreted in the urine by 48 hours, although little is known about the pharmacokinetics and metabolism of orally administered fluorescein (21).

Although levels of glucuronidation might be expected to differ in diabetic patients, no significant pharmacokinetic differences in metabolism have been found (33). However, dye elimination is delayed in patients with diabetic nephropathy.

Therapeutic Use

Topical Application

Fluorescein is applied topically by drops or dye-impregnated filter paper. One drop is applied to the inferior cul-de-sac. Paper strips are either prewetted with a sterile wetting agent or applied directly to the inferior cul-de-sac. Slight discoloration of the conjunctiva and eyelids is common, but because fluorescein does not bind chemically to tissues the effect is transient (less than 30 minutes). Residual coloration of the aqueous from diffusion across the cornea into the anterior chamber may be visible for several hours.

Optimal fluorescein concentration depends on the application and information desired. More dilute solutions (0.125%) are used to observe epithelial defects, and more concentrated solutions (2%) are used for detection of aqueous leaks. The highest concentrations (10% to 25%) are reserved for intravenous applications (described below).

Corneal and Conjunctival Epithelial Integrity

Topical fluorescein aids in evaluation of corneal and conjunctival disease, including epithelial edema, punctate erosions, denudation, and ulcerations (34). When viewed with the cobalt-blue filter, fluorescein highlights epithelial defects and corneal irregularities. Controversy exists over the cause of increased fluorescence seen in epithelial defects; it may be due to contact of the dye with a more alkaline corneal stroma (19) or to dilution of the dye in the corneal stroma resulting in less self-quenching and greater relative fluorescence (18). Corneal irregularity may cause pooling of dye and increased fluorescence. Fluorescein also helps identify conjunctival and corneal foreign bodies and evaluate the extent of tissue damage they may cause.

If an infectious corneal ulcer is suspected, fluorescein strips and a preservative-free wetting agent should be used. Benoxinate–fluorescein mixtures have potent antimicrobial activity, which may prevent accurate bacterial culture and identification.

Applanation Tonometry

The most accurate measure of intraocular pressure (IOP) is obtained by Goldmann applanation tonometry using 0.25% fluorescein under cobalt blue illumination (35,36). Measurements made using proparacaine without fluorescein have shown readings from 5.62 to 7.01 mm Hg lower than those measured with benoxinate–fluorescein (37,38). These differences are greater at higher IOP and are probably due to poor visual definition of the applanation mires (14).

Assessment of Leakage of Aqueous Humor (The Seidel Test)

The Seidel test has been widely adapted to detect leaks of aqueous fluid from penetrating injuries of the cornea and conjunctiva after trauma or leaks after anterior segment surgery. One drop of 2% fluorescein is placed in the cul-de-sac. At this concentration, fluorescein is a dark yellow-orange. The ocular surface is then scanned with the cobalt blue filter on the biomicroscope; a rivulet of bright green fluorescence identifies an aqueous fluid leak (39). The dilution of the fluorescein by the aqueous results in a shift of the wavelength of the emission spectrum toward a longer wavelength which, coupled with reduced self-absorption, increases the relative fluorescence level (14,40).

Although 2% fluorescein is optimal, use of 10% and 20% solutions has also been suggested (18). If benoxinate–fluorescein 0.25% is used, aqueous leakage is apparent as lack of fluorescence compared with the surrounding background due to localized dilution beyond the range of perceptible fluorescence.

Use of Fluorescein in Anterior Segment Surgery

Fluorescein, usually 2%, is used to indicate adequate wound closure after trauma surgery and cataract extraction and to evaluate leaks from filtering blebs after glaucoma surgery. Corneal transplant surgeons often instill fluorescein before performing trephination to ascertain if the anterior chamber has been entered. Fluorescein may be used to identify the more fluorescent subepithelial side of free conjunctival grafts during pterygium excision (41). Surgical instrument tips (supersharp blade, calipers) can be dipped in 2% fluorescein to assist in site localization during surgery.

Contact Lens Fitting

Fluorescein is frequently used in fitting hard contact lenses. The lens should be placed in the eye at least 30 minutes before assessment is made. Dilute fluorescein (0.25% or strips) is then placed in the cul-de-sac, and the amount of fluorescence under the lens is evaluated. Because thicker areas of the tear lake under the lens will fluoresce more brightly, the relative distance between the contact lens and the cornea can be assessed over all portions of the lens. A well-fitting lens will have a thin and uniform tear film over the central area of the lens, which gradually thickens toward the peripheral portions of the lens. Other fluorescein patterns might indicate corneal irregularity, astigmatism, or the need for a more loosely or tightly fitting lens. Movement of fluorescein under the lens as the lens shifts with each blink indicates adequate movement of the lens and suggests good corneal oxygen delivery (42).

Fluorescein stains soft (hydrophilic) contact lenses and should not be used in their fitting. Nevertheless, if accidental staining occurs, multiple and separate washings in sterile saline may remove enough of the dye to allow continued use of the stained lens with minimal to no effect on vision. Fluorexon is a fluorescein derivative used to fit soft contact lenses (43). Its larger molecular weight (710 vs. 376 for fluorescein) inhibits penetration into the lens, avoiding staining. Fluorexon, (Fluoresoft, 0.35%, Holles Labs, Cohasset, MA) was recently made available commercially.

Assessment of Lacrimal Production and Drainage Systems

Topical fluorescein is used to evaluate the stability of the tear film as well as the integrity and patency of the lacrimal drainage system. Clinical tests of tear volume (e.g., Schirmer's test) do not ordinarily require fluorescein.

Tear film stability is assessed by observing the "tear break-up time." A wet fluorescein-coated paper strip is applied to the unanesthetized ocular cul-de-sac. The precorneal tear film is then viewed with the cobalt blue filter on the biomicroscope. The time between the last complete blink and the first appearance of a dry spot on the cornea is determined over at least three blinks, and the values are averaged. This tear break-up time is abnormal if it is less than 10 seconds (44). Break-up times less than 10 seconds indicate inadequate or unstable mucinous components of the tears, or "dry eye" (45). Reproducibility of this test is notoriously poor and many factors intrinsic to the test can decrease its inter- and intrasubject reliability (46). Nevertheless, tear break-up time is a useful adjunct to other tests of lacrimal function.

Fluorescein is also used to evaluate the lacrimal drainage system. Classically, these tests have been described as the "Jones I and II tests" (47). The first part of the test (Jones I) is used in patients with suspected obstruction of the drainage system. A drop of 2% fluorescein is placed in the unanesthetized eye. After 3 to 5 minutes, the eye is checked for residual fluorescein in the tear lake. In normal patients, only a small amount of the dye will remain, as the tears drain through a patent ductal system. In patients with obstructed drainage, a larger amount of fluorescein will be retained. If fluorescein is present on a cotton applicator advanced through the nares to the os of the nasolacrimal duct, or on a tissue after the patient is asked to blow his nose, the drainage system is patent or only partially obstructed.

If no dye is seen, the second part of the test is performed (Jones II). A saline-filled syringe attached to a nasolacrimal cannula is advanced through the inferior punctum and lacrimal canaliculus into the lacrimal sac, but not further. A tissue is placed below the nose, and saline is then irrigated. The patient should lean forward to prevent diversion of irrigant into the oropharynx. If fluorescein-stained saline is retrieved from the tissue, a partial obstruction between the lacrimal sac and the nose is present (which required the additional pressure during irrigation of the sac to be overcome). If saline without fluorescein staining is recovered, a "proximal" obstruction exists which did not allow entrance of fluorescein into the sac during the first part of the test. Such an obstruction may be overcome by insertion of the cannula during the second part of the test. If no fluid is recovered from the nose despite adequate irrigation, a complete obstruction within or distal to the lacrimal sac is indicated.

Properly performed, the primary dye test is nearly 100% sensitive (48). An adequate quantity of 2% fluorescein (or at least four wetted strips) should be applied directly to the opening of the punctum and at least 10 minutes should elapse between application of the dye and attempts at recovery.

Intravenous Applications

For standard fluorescein angiography, 5 cc of 10% or 3 cc of 25% solution (7 to 30 mg/kg) is administered intravenously, usually through a "butterfly" catheter into the antecubital vein (21,49). The dose in children is 35 mg/10 pounds body weight for intravenous administration (50). The dye is administered at a constant but rapid speed so that a bright dye front reaches the ocular vessels on the initial circulatory pass. The average transit time from arm to eye in a normal subject is 13 seconds (51,52). Increased arm-to-retina circulation times occur in many disease states, including carotid or ophthalmic artery disease and congestive heart failure with decreased cardiac output, and in conditions of increased central venous pressure or IOP. Local ocular factors such as arterial or venous occlusion may also prolong transit time. Anemia, on the other hand, may shorten transit time (14).

After injection, an initial bright retinal fluorescence is apparent even though the dye concentration is only 0.01% (53,54). Fluorescence intensity fades after about 20 seconds and then reintensifies due to internal quenching of the dye bolus as concentration progressively increases and then decreases with time (53). Photographs are usually taken continuously 2 seconds apart during early arterial (15 seconds), arteriovenous (20 seconds), and venous (30 seconds) phases and then during late phases of the angiogram (10 to 30 minutes) (49).

Fluorescein can also be administered orally. One gram of fluorescein solution is mixed with 200 ml liquid. Peak blood concentration occurs within 30 minutes of ingestion. Because of the long absorption time, differentiation between arterial and venous phases of the angiogram is not possible, limiting study to the late angiographic phase only. Therefore, oral fluorescein is used mostly in evaluation of cystoid macular edema (CME) (41).

The diagnostic advantage of fluorescein angiography is based on its sequestration in vascular spaces unless there is a disturbance of the blood–ocular barrier. Distinct patterns of fluorescence are produced by retinal infection, inflammation, ischemia, and degeneration (55). Fluorescein angiography can also delineate vascular abnormalities, abnormal flow patterns, and generation of new or unusual vessels, as in diabetic neovascularization (49,56). Alterations in the transmission patterns of the dye, either in choroidal or retinal circulatory compartments, have also been used to detect defects in subretinal structure such as choroidal infarcts, retinal pigment epithelium (RPE) tears or degeneration, and choroidal tumors. Detailed analysis of fluorescence patterns is beyond the scope of this text, and the reader is referred to two comprehensive publications (49,57).

Fluorophotometry

Ocular fluorophotometry precisely measures fluorescein concentration in the anterior chamber and vitreous, which may yield information about aqueous humor dynamics (58,59). Fluorophotometric measurements are usually made after standard intravenous injection or, less often, after transcorneal delivery (60). Fluorophotometry is still largely a research tool, but it may have important applications in evaluation of ocular fluid dynamics in diabetes, glaucoma, and uveitis (61–64).

Anterior Segment and Iris Fluorescein Angiography

Fluorescein is injected antecubitally in a manner identical to that used for fundus angiography (65). Five milliliters of 10% fluorescein is injected for evaluation of fine conjunctival or scleral structures at higher magnification; otherwise, if only gross structural changes are studied or if low magnification is used, 0.6 ml of a 20% solution is preferred (66). More rapid sequential photography is required for anterior segment and iris angiography than for fundus angiography.

The normal arm-to-iris circulation time (15 to 20 seconds) is slightly longer than the fundus circulation time (67). Iris vessels are relatively impermeable to fluorescein but appear to leak somewhat more readily than retinal and cerebral vasculature (68) and are more leaky in elderly patients (13). The iris vascular pattern is more difficult to discern in patients with heavily pigmented irises. Specific patterns of neovascularization and leakage in vascular and oncologic disease are delineated in more specialized texts (57,67).

Conjunctival angiography may be used to evaluate scleritis and sclerokeratitis. Alterations in circulation pattern may indicate severity of disease and predict necrotizing processes.

Corneal angiography has been used to investigate neovascular processes in keratitis and after penetrating keratoplasty. Its use is limited, however, because the pattern is obscured as the dye rapidly leaks from neovascular elements into the corneal stroma (57). The use of fluorescein is relatively contraindicated in pregnancy and in patients with known prior allergic hypersensitivity (described in High-risk Groups section).

Side Effects and Toxicity

Topical application of anesthetic–fluorescein combinations causes transient and mild conjunctival stinging in most patients, partly because of the low pH (5) required to preserve antimicrobial activity (69). Severe adverse reactions after topical application are rare, however. Three cases of vasovagal syncope after application of topical benoxinate-fluorescein used in applanation tonometry have been recorded by the National Registry of Drug-Induced Ocular Side-Effects (case reports 404a, 404b, and 421; University of Oregon Health Sciences Center, Portland OR, 1979; personal communication, 1995). The most severe reaction was a single case of grand mal seizure which occurred in a 27-year-old man 60 seconds after instillation of benoxinate-fluorescein. The patient had no history of prior seizures and follow-up neurologic examination was normal (70).

Most patients experience temporary yellow discoloration of their skin and urine after intravenous fluorescein administration. Patients should be advised before undergoing injection that the discoloration may last 1 to 6 hours. A history of abnormal renal function or previous allergic reactions to medications (especially fluorescein) or angiography dye of any kind should be further investigated.

The frequency of reactions to IV fluorescein is summarized in Table 2. Mild reactions occur in approximately 5% of patients (50,71). The most common reaction is nausea in 2.4% to 15% patients (72,73). Nausea occurs within 15 to 30 seconds of injection and abates in 1 to 2 minutes (74). Vomiting is less common (2%). Some investigators report greater incidence of nausea in women than in men, although others report more frequent nausea in men (74,75). The incidence of nausea is directly proportional to the fluorescein concentration (higher concentrations cause more nausea) (76). However, speed of injection may also play a role. In a prospective study, slow injection (5 cc delivered in less than 6 seconds) resulted in 12 times more frequent nausea than did rapid injection (71). The reasons for this remain unclear. Patients who have reacted previously to fluorescein in any way have a 48.6% chance of repeat reactions.

Oral premedication with 50 mg of promethazine 1 hour before fluorescein injections has been reported to reduce the chance of GI reactions in susceptible patients (74). Premedication with 25 mg of promethazine and 25 mg of diphenhydramine reduced the recurrence of nausea and vomiting in patients with previous reactions from 48.6% to

TABLE 73-2. *Frequency of adverse reactions to intravenous fluorescein*[a]

Mild	1:20
nausea, vomiting, extravasation, pruritus[b]	
Moderate	1:63
Urticaria	1:82
Syncope	1:337
Other[c]	1:769
Severe	1:1,900
Respiratory reactions	1:3,800
Cardiac reactions	1:5,300
Tonic-clonic seizures	1:13,900
Death	1:222,000

Modified with permission from L.A. Yannuzzi, et al. *Ophthalmology* 1986;93:611–617(50).

[a]Based on 222,000 angiograms from 2400 respondents to the Fluorescein Angiography Complications Survey.

[b]Differentiation between types of mild reactions was not made.

[c]Includes thrombophlebitis, pyrexia, tissue necrosis, and nerve palsy.

32.1% (71). However, premedication with these agents in patients without previous reactions increased the incidence of adverse reactions from 4.5% to 30%; some reactions may have been reactions to the premedication agents themselves.

Mild allergic reactions to intravenous fluorescein, such as flushing, pruritus, and urticaria occur in 0.5% to 1.25% of patients. Syncope and dyspnea occur in 0.2% to 0.3% (50,71). More severe allergic and idiosyncratic reactions include laryngeal and pulmonary edema (77,78), seizures (79), anaphylactic shock (80), myocardial infarction (81–83), and cardiac arrest (84). Only two patients have died (50); however, severe reaction to fluorescein is estimated to account for one death a year (85,86).

Extravasation of fluorescein may produce pain and irritation at the site of injection, superficial phlebitis, subcutaneous granuloma, and neuritis. Skin sloughing and necrosis may require intensive treatment, with dermatologic consultation and steroid therapy (87–89).

Several mechanisms for fluorescein reactions have been proposed (50). Fluorescein may act as a hapten in triggering histamine release, either directly or through a type I immune hypersensitivity reaction. Histamine is released in the first 3 minutes after fluorescein injection (90). High plasma histamine levels were noted in 15% of patients who developed no adverse reactions and in 66% of those experiencing some form of adverse reaction. Levels remained increased for as long as 10 minutes. Other possible mechanisms include direct vasospastic effects of the injection (91) and reactions to topical agents used to dilate the pupil including phenylephrine (92). Cell-mediated immunity does not play a role in such reactions (77).

Most mild side effects of fluorescein (nausea, vomiting, etc.) subside in minutes, requiring only patient reassurance but no treatment. Extravasation of dye should be treated with cold compresses (49).

Although the full response protocol to cardiopulmonary emergencies is beyond the scope of this chapter, it is imperative that all persons administering fluorescein be able to recognize allergic and anaphylactic reactions and to respond quickly to these potentially life-threatening emergencies. All personnel administering fluorescein must be trained in basic life support (BLS) procedures. Maintaining an airway and respiration is the priority. The patient should be placed supine with feet elevated if possible, and oxygen administered. Vital signs should be monitored. Intramuscular (i.m.) or subcutaneous (s.c.) epinephrine 1 : 1000 at 0.3 ml should be administered (pediatric dose is 0.01 ml/kg of 1 : 1000 s.c.). Intravenous epinephrine 1 : 10,000 at 1.0 ml in 5 minutes is required in hypotensive patients because of decreased peripheral absorption. Epinephrine may be repeated every 5 minutes intramuscularly or every 3 minutes intravenously for a total dose of 5 ml every 15 to 30 minutes and should be used with extreme caution in the elderly and those with history of cardiac or hypertensive problems (93).

After epinephrine is administered, 50 mg diphenhydramine should be immediately injected intramuscularly (intravenously in severe anaphylaxis). A large-bore intravenous catheter should be placed, and fluids should be administered to maintain adequate blood pressure. Depending on the severity of reaction, advanced life support (ALS) may be required.

High-risk Groups

Patients who have had a previous adverse reaction to fluorescein have a 46.8% chance of a repeat reaction (71). In these patients, angiography should be performed only when absolutely necessary and with extreme caution. Whether premedication with antiemetic agents or antihistamines prevents such reactions is not known. If potential allergy is suspected, a skin test may be performed; 0.05 ml fluorescein is injected intradermally, and the site is evaluated for wheal and flare 30 to 60 minutes after injection. Previous hypersensitivity reaction to fluorescein is a relative contraindication.

Fluorescein is unlikely to be used in neonates, but there are no reported contraindications for such use. Fluorescein and its metabolites have been detected in breast milk and, although there are no definite contraindications to its use, the compound should be used with caution in lactating women (21,94).

Fluorescein is classified as FDA pregnancy category C; its safety in pregnancy has not been established. Fluorescein crosses the blood–placenta barrier in humans (95), but has not been proved teratogenic in doses commonly used for angiography (96). A survey of retina specialists indicated no increase in birth anomalies after fluorescein use in pregnant women (97). If fluorescein angiography is necessary for treatment of serious sight-threatening lesions, the data suggest that teratogenic complications are unlikely (21,97). However, because early animal studies indicated possible teratogenic effects, it is still recommended that fluorescein use be avoided during pregnancy, especially during the first trimester. Common side effects (nausea and vomiting) occur with equal frequency in pregnant and nonpregnant women.

Elderly patients are not at greater risk than younger patients of developing side effects (21,98). In one study, the incidence of nausea after intravenous injection was less in the elderly group (9.4% in patients aged less than 50 years and 4.4% in patients aged more than 50 years old) (74).

No clear data on the safety of fluorescein injection in renal insufficiency are available. The incidence of side effects of intravenous fluorescein in patients with renal insufficiency is no greater than that in normal subjects. Even anuric patients presumably clear fluorescein during dialysis, although the relative toxicity of fluorescein in such patients has not been well studied. Decreased dosages, however, may be prudent (49).

Drug Interactions

No known interactions occur between fluorescein and other drugs. Theoretically, interaction with other drugs that bind to plasma proteins could occur. Because of the discoloration of urine by fluorescein, tests that rely on colorimetric assay of substances in the urine may be affected. These include some assays for protein, creatinine, sugars, and urobilinogen (21,49).

Major Clinical Trials

Several studies document antimicrobial activity of fluorescein–benoxinate mixtures. A solution of 0.25% fluorescein sodium and 0.4% benoxinate HCl (Fluress, Barnes-Hinds) was bacteriostatic or bacteriocidal for direct inoculations of *Klebsiella, Pseudomonas aeruginosa, Escherichia coli, Staphylococcus aureus, Proteus vulgaris,* and *Candida albicans.* Kill times for these agents varied from 5 minutes to 24 hours, with most being totally eradicated by 2 hours. When bottles of benoxinate–fluorescein from routine clinical settings were cultured 1 month after opening, no microorganisms were recovered. Similar bottles inoculated with *Pseudomonas* had no growth within 24 hours of inoculation (24,25,69,99).

In contrast, fluorescein–proparacaine mixtures have less antibacterial activity. Significant quantities of *Pseudomonas* and *Staphylococcus aureus* could be cultured from the proparacaine mixtures as long as 2 hours after direct bottle inoculation or after dropper-tip contamination. Benoxinate mixtures, however, were all sterile for these agents within 15 minutes. Although antimicrobial activity is probably related in part to the preservatives chlorobutanol, thimerosal, and povidone present in the mixtures, benoxinate itself has been shown to possess intrinsic bacteriostatic properties (24,69).

Norton et al. (100) described the first major clinical application of fluorescein angiography in the differential diagnosis of posterior ocular disease. Representative cases of benign nevus of the choroid, malignant choroidal melanoma, metastatic choroidal lesions, disciform chorioretinal lesions, low-grade inflammatory lesions, and inactive chorioretinal scars were described in detail. This study of 43 cases was the first attempt at differential interpretation of fluorescein angiographic patterns (100).

In 1968, Gass (101) published his classic series on fluorescein angiography in macular dysfunction due to retinal vascular diseases, including embolic retinal artery obstruction (101), retinal vein obstruction (102), hypertensive and diabetic retinopathy (103,104), retinal telangiectasia (105), and carotid occlusive disease, collagen vascular disease, and vitritis (106). This work established the value of fluorescein angiography in assessment of retinal vascular disorders.

Indocyanine Green (ICG)

The use of ICG as a tool for studying choroidal circulation evolved because of problems visualizing this region with fluorescein. Retinal pigment epithelium blocks both excitation and transmission spectra of fluorescein. In addition, the nonbound portion of fluorescein leaks out of fenestrated choroidal vessels, rendering choroidal circulation more poorly defined than the retinal circulation. In many circumstances, this is acceptable and even advantageous. However, when direct uninterrupted visualization of the choroidal circulation is desired, fluorescein is not appropriate and an alternative is required.

History and Source

ICG is a tricarbocyanine dye first introduced into medicinal use in 1957 by Fox et al. for indicator–dilution studies of cardiac output and circulation (107–109). In 1958, Wheeler et al. (110) demonstrated in dogs that ICG was entirely retained in intravascular compartments and excreted solely by the liver through biliary channels, thus establishing its use for blood flow and hepatic function analysis in humans (111–113).

Direct visualization of choroidal vasculature using ICG was introduced in 1970 by Kogure et al. (114), who developed a method of infrared absorption angiography in monkeys. Kulvin et al. (115) performed the first choroidal ICG angiography in humans in 1970, although their technique required arterial injection and was not practical for routine clinical use. Hochheimer (116) obtained the first intravenous angiograms, but they were of poor clarity as compared with fluorescein photographs. Flower (117) then enhanced image clarity by using bandpass filters for the light source.

In 1976, Orth et al. (118) altered the technique from ICG absorption angiography to ICG fluorescence angiography, thus substantially improving visibility of the choroidal vessels. However, the technique was not sensitive enough to delineate the smaller choriocapillaris (118,119). Better infrared photographic acquisition with use of digital analysis techniques were introduced in 1984 (120). Since then, the clinical usefulness of ICG angiography has paralleled the development of more sophisticated digital equipment. Application of diode laser sources may further enhance the capabilities of this technique by allowing more efficient excitation of ICG at lower light levels in the retina (121). Clearly this is an emerging field with great potential for diagnosis and treatment of choroidal diseases.

Official Drug Name and Chemistry

ICG is anhydro-3,3,33-tetramethyl-1,1-di-(4-sulfobutyl)-4,5,4,5-dibenzoindo-tricarbocyanine hydroxide sodium salt, (Cardiogreen). The chemical formula is $C_{43}H_{47}N_2O_6S_2Na$. The chemical structure is shown in Fig. 2.

Fluorochemistry

The absorption maximum for ICG in water is 770 to 780 nm. The addition of albumin stabilizes the compound and shifts the absorption peak further into the infrared range, with maximum absorption at 805 nm (122). Peak fluorescence occurs at 835 nm.

Pharmacology

ICG is a relatively inert substance without inherent pharmacologic properties.

Clinical Pharmacology

After intravenous injection, ICG is entirely bound to plasma proteins (described in section on Metabolism below). It does not leak out of intravascular compartments where blood barrier systems are intact, making it an ideal agent for studying circulatory systems and blood flow in both normal and abnormal states. Because the emission spectrum of ICG is much different from that of fluorescein and is not blocked by overlying pigment, blood, and lipid, (119) it provides a useful adjunct in diagnosis of choroidal and chorioretinal lesions (123).

Pharmaceutics

Indocyanine green (Cardio-Green [GC], Becton-Dickinson, Cockneyville, MD; Cardio-Green, Akorn, Abita Springs, LA) is a dry powder available in 25- and 50-mg vials containing not more than 5.0% sodium iodide. It is unstable in aqueous form and must be freshly prepared and used within 10 hours of preparation. The diluent provided is "especially prepared" sterile water (pH 5.5 to 6.5) for injection. Reports of incompatibility with some commercially prepared sterile water has been noted (Becton-Dickinson Technical Bulletin no. 02–3042–5, 1990).

Pharmacokinetics, Concentration–effect Relationship, and Metabolism

ICG is rapidly, avidly, and completely bound by plasma proteins after injection (122,124), and distributed within all vascular compartments (112). Baker (124) demonstrated that nearly 80% binds to α_1-lipoproteins rather than to albumin. Blood clearance of ICG occurs almost exclusively through the liver. No significant first-pass excretory effect occurs; only 0.01% of an injected dose is excreted into the bile in the first 3 minutes. However, hepatic clearance of ICG is relatively efficient, with removal rates between 18% and 24% per minute (122). Ninety-seven percent of an administered dose is excreted unchanged in the bile (110,112). No enterohepatic recirculation occurs with ICG (110). The biological $t_{1/2}$ is 2.5 to 3.0 minutes (122).

Because ICG is fully protein bound, it does not easily cross protein barrier systems. Simultaneous measurement of ICG in maternal and fetal blood has shown that ICG does not cross the placental barrier (125). Furthermore, ICG does not cross the blood–brain barrier and cannot be detected in cerebrospinal fluid (126). Although ICG can enter intraretinal cystoid spaces in cases of known neovascularization, no direct data are available on the ability of ICG to traverse the intact blood–ocular barrier (127).

Therapeutic Use

The major use for ocular ICG angiography is in identification of occult choroidal neovascularization (128). However, its application in other chorioretinal problems is increasing. Descriptions of ICG patterns have been published for acute posterior multifocal placoid pigment epitheliopathy (129,130), multiple evanescent white-dot syndrome (131), vortex vein varices (132), central serous chorioretinopathy (133,134), drusen (135), pigment epithelial detachment (136), Harada disease (137) and malignant melanoma of the choroid (138). ICG-retaining choroidal neovascular membranes have been selectively photocoagulated by a diode laser technique (139).

The technique for injection of ICG, either alone or in conjunction with fluorescein angiography, is similar to that used for injection of fluorescein (119,140). ICG is reconstituted from the dry powder using the diluent supplied by the manufacturer (sterile water). The solution is unstable and must be used within 10 hours of mixing. Although in early studies a final concentration of 50 mg/ml and a dose

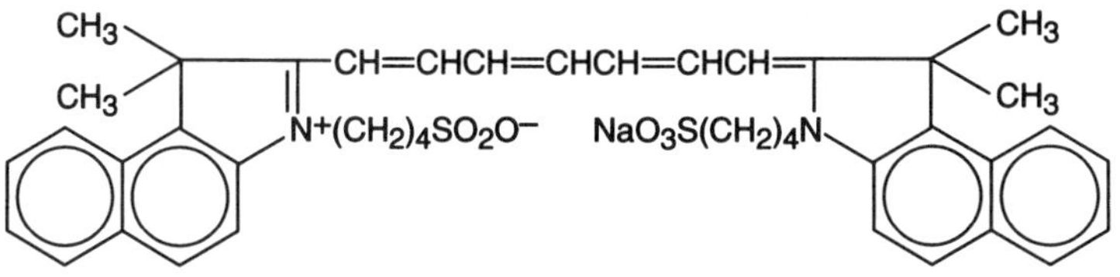

FIG. 73-2. Structural diagram of indocyanine green.

of 3.0 mg/kg were used, this amount is slightly larger than that currently recommended by the FDA. Currently approved dosage is 2 mg/kg in adults. Manufacturers recommend 40 mg ICG dissolved in 2 cc diluent, which is substantially less than the FDA-approved dosage for any patient weighing more than 20 kg (45 pounds) (Indocyanine Green Fact Sheet, Publication no. 3910–10, Akorn Pharmaceuticals, 1993; Becton-Dickinson Technical Bulletin no. 02–3042–5, 1990). The solution is then injected rapidly into the antecubital vein. With use of a three-way stopcock, the vein is immediately flushed with 5 ml saline to decrease hemolysis caused by high residual-dye concentrations.

ICG angiography can be used in conjunction with fluorescein angiography to define the choroidal and retinal circulations separately. Although mixing the dyes in one injection does not alter the physical characteristics of the dye and does not increase toxicity (140), investigators now favor separate injections of fluorescein and ICG administered several minutes apart (141). The order of injections depends on the information desired. ICG is injected first if choroidal lesions are to be studied; fluorescein is injected first if retinal lesions are of interest. ICG may define choroidal lesions better than fluorescein, especially those that underlie hemorrhage (Fig. 3).

The arm-to-choroid transit time for ICG is similar to that of fluorescein (9 to 12 seconds) (142,143). ICG fluorescence appears first in the choroidal arterial system and rapidly flows to the venous system and vortex veins. Macular fluorescence is greatest at the mid-arteriovenous phase. The choriocapillaris should also fill during this phase, but is difficult to capture using anything but the most sophisticated devices with superfast acquisition times (128,143, 144). The entire period from beginning of choroidal filling to beginning of retinal arterial filling is 1.8 seconds (140). Choroidal ICG fluorescence is accessible for only 90 seconds with conventional films, but is visible for several minutes with infrared videoangiography (128). For 10 minutes after injection, background choroidal fluorescence is diffuse and homogenous (143). Yannuzzi et al. (128) reported the value of very-late-phase ICG angiograms at 30 minutes to delineate choroidal neovascular membranes against a relatively dark choroidal background.

Side Effects and Toxicity

The toxicity of ICG is relatively low in mammals. After intravenous injection of ICG in mice, LD_{50} calculations range between 60 and 80 mg/kg. For rats and rabbits, the range is 50 to 70 mg/kg (122). In humans, single intravenous doses of 5 mg/kg have been tolerated without significant toxic effects (145). One patient received 10 mg/kg without untoward effects. No local vascular irritation or phlebitis has been observed after intravenous administration of ICG.

In 1990, a registry for adverse reactions to ocular ICG angiography was established in Boston (86). In 1,923 ICG angiographic procedures, 0.15% of patients experienced mild reactions (nausea, vomiting, extravasation, sneezing, or pruritus), 0.2% developed moderate reactions (urticaria, syncope, other skin eruptions, pyrexia, local tissue necrosis, or nerve palsy), and 0.05% sustained a severe reaction (bronchospasm, laryngospasm, anaphylaxis, circulatory shock, myocardial infarction, tonic-clonic seizure, or cardiac arrest). An additional nonfatal case of severe anaphylaxis with cardiac arrest was recently reported (146). No patients have died after ICG injections for ocular studies (86).

Eighteen cases of severe adverse reactions to ICG used for cardiac studies have been published (86,147). Only 1 of

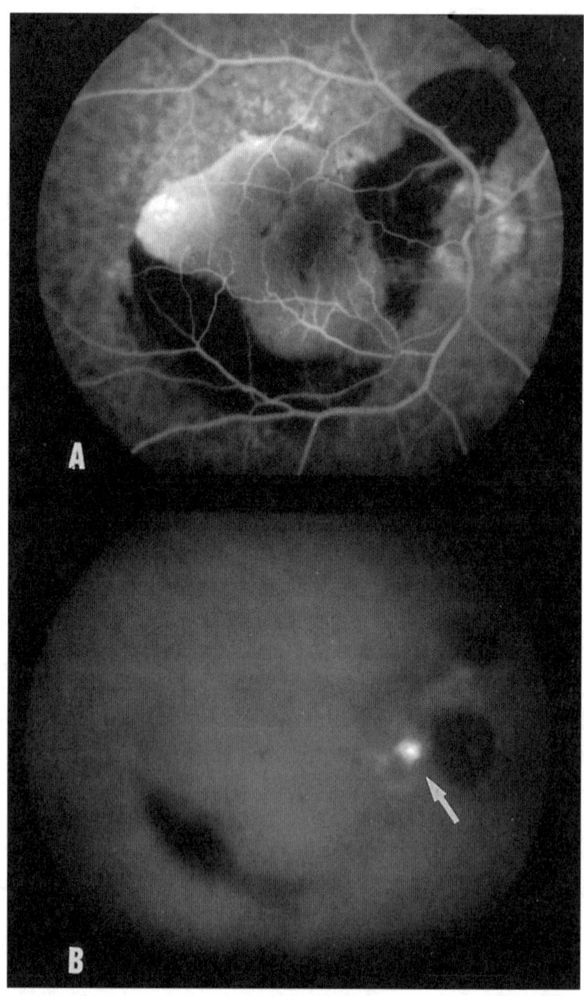

FIG. 73-3. Fluorescent angiograms of occult choroidal neovascularization (CNV) in age-related macular degeneration. **A:** Fluorescein angiogram at early venous phase showing subretinal blood but no obvious CNV. **B:** Indocyanine green videoangiogram at late phase showing a well-defined choroidal neovascular net (arrow) subjacent to overlying subretinal blood. (Photograph courtesy of Richard Hackell.)

the patients had a prior history of drug allergy and the severity of reaction appeared not to correlate with injected dose. However, seven patients had end-stage renal disease and were on hemodialysis (148). For unknown reasons, some patients with renal disease appear to develop an eosinophilia, which manifests as apparent allergic hypersensitivity to ICG (149).

Three fatal anaphylactic reactions to ICG during cardiac catheterization have been reported (150–152). One patient was allergic to penicillin and sulfa drugs. The two other patients had no history of drug allergy; however, one received 36 mg ICG manufactured in Japan, which was slightly different from USP ICG.

The dose of ICG used in ocular angiography is as much as five times more than that used in cardiac output studies (2 mg/kg in ocular studies vs. 25 mg total in cardiac studies). Even so, the higher doses used in ICG angiography appear relatively safe. The overall risk of mild reactions after ocular ICG angiography is 1 : 641, that of moderate reaction is 1 : 480, and that of severe reaction 1 : 1923. The extrapolated risk of death is 1 in 333,333 (86). These data show that ICG produces fewer and less severe adverse side effects than fluorescein. The pathophysiology of these reactions is unclear but may be similar to that for fluorescein and largely idiosyncratic.

No treatment is necessary for mild reactions. For more severe reactions, including possible anaphylaxis, it is identical to that used for treatment of severe reactions to fluorescein (described in Fluorescein section). ICG is contraindicated in patients with a history of allergy to iodine, in pregnant women, and in uremic patients on hemodialysis.

High-risk Groups

ICG should be used in patients with known prior hypersensitivity only with extreme caution. Of the 18 patients in the literature with severe reactions, three had had prior exposure to ICG (151). The dye contains 5.0% sodium iodide and should not be administered to patients with a history of allergy to iodine.

Patients with renal insufficiency, especially those on hemodialysis, are at increased risk of developing adverse reactions. Such patients should probably not be exposed to ICG (148).

There is no information on ICG toxicity in patients with liver disease or jaundice. However, due to hepatic metabolism, there is theoretical concern regarding use of ICG in such patients.

Excretion rates of ICG during pregnancy are decreased to 70% of that in nonpregnant women, possibly because estrogens decrease hepatic excretory functions (122). The FDA has classified ICG as category C; its safety for use in pregnancy has not been established. Iodine-containing contrast materials are generally contraindicated in pregnancy, and it is reasonable that similar restriction be placed on ICG use in pregnancy. However, ICG does not cross the placental barrier (125), and no data on fetal toxicity are available.

ICG is unlikely to be present in breast milk, although there are no data on its recovery in milk of lactating women. Nevertheless, use of ICG in nursing mothers should be avoided. There are no data on adverse reactions to ICG in neonates at concentrations used for angiography. The dose of ICG for blood flow studies in neonates is 1.25 mg/dilution trial, and although increased risk at this dose has been reported, it is considerably less than the dose used in angiography. Dosage for blood-flow studies in older children is 2.5 mg (Becton-Dickinson Technical Bulletin no. 02–3042–5, 1990).

The effect of age on development of adverse reaction has not been examined. There is no physiologic reason to believe that elderly patients with good kidney and liver function would be at additional risk.

Drug Interactions

There are no known drug interactions between ICG and other pharmacologic agents. Fluorescein and ICG have been combined in one injection without interaction or complication (140).

Major Clinical Trials

Two prospective clinical series have shown ICG to be valuable in evaluating ICG in choroidal neovascularization (CNV). Yannuzzi et al. (128) studied a newly developed digital videoangiography apparatus in 129 consecutive patients with exudative age-related macular degeneration (ARMD) and occult CNV. With the aid of ICG angiography, 39% were reclassified as having classic CNV. In only 9% of cases did ICG fail to provide new information. The researchers used these data to guide laser photocoagulation therapy in selected patients. The data support the usefulness of ICG as an adjunct to fluorescein in diagnosis of occult CNV.

This study of Yannuzzi et al. was extended by Guyer et al. (133) to 657 consecutive eyes in patients with suspected occult CNV who were ineligible for laser therapy based on fluorescein data (133). The patients were subgrouped into those with and without RPE detachments. Of the 413 patients without RPE detachments, CNV eligible for laser treatment was detected in 22%. Of the 235 eyes with vascularized RPE detachments, 42% were reclassified as eligible for laser therapy after ICG. Overall, new information leading to potential treatment was obtained in 34.4% of eyes based on ICG angiography. Although the researchers underscore the need for independent confirmation, the data suggest that 1 : 3 patients with occult CNV may be candidates for laser treatment, with use of information obtainable only after ICG angiography (133).

OTHER DYES

In addition to fluorescein and ICG, other agents have been used in evaluation of fundus vascular and mass lesions. Historically, the first dye used was trypan blue, with which Abelsdorf and Wessely (153) delineated retinal vessels in animals in 1909. Sorsby used Kiton Fast Green V in his studies of damaged human retina in 1939 (154). Although various dye stocks have been evaluated for retinal angiographic use, most have proved unsatisfactory in terms of toxicity or practicality (155).

Carboxyfluorescein, a derivative of fluorescein with nearly identical fluorescence parameters, has also been used to analyze retinal vascular systems (156). Carboxyfluorescein is considerably less membrane permeable than fluorescein and thus has advantages in the study of blood–ocular barrier integrity. Liposome-encapsulated carboxyfluorescein was used to study blood flow directly in retinal and optic nerve vasculature and has the advantage of allowing simultaneous measurements in the arteries, capillaries, and veins of the macula and optic nerve (157). Despite the advantages of other agents in certain research areas, fluorescein and ICG are the only dyes currently approved for use in clinical fundus angiography.

Several other dyes are currently used in ophthalmology. Most of these are topically applied and aid in diagnosis of corneal and external eye diseases (14,41,158,159). These include rose bengal (for tear deficiencies), methylene blue (for vital staining of corneal nerves and lacrimal duct irrigation), alcian blue (for differentiation of mucinous deposits), lissamine green (for detection of devitalized cells, especially in vitamin A deficiency), argyrol (as an indicator of adequate surgical preparation), tetrazolium (for evaluation of degenerating cells—similar to rose bengal), bromothymol blue (for evaluation of degenerating cells), trypan blue (for assessment of corneal endothelial viability), and alizarin red S (for assessment of corneal endothelial viability). Use of these agents is described in Chapter 19, *this volume.*

ACKNOWLEDGMENT

This work was supported in part by an unrestricted grant from Research to Prevent Blindness, Inc., New York, NY, and a Heed Ophthalmic Foundation Fellowship Award (to R.N.H.).

REFERENCES

1. Baeryer A. Uber eine neue Klasse von Farbstoffen. *Berl Detsch Chem Ges* 1871;4:555–558.
2. Campbell FW, Boyd TAS. The use of sodium fluorescein in assessing the rate of healing in corneal ulcers. *Br J Ophthalmol* 1950; 34:545–549.
3. Ehrlich P. Uber provocirte Fluorescenzserscheinungen am Auge. *Detsch Med Wochenschr* 1882;8:35–36.
4. Seidel E. Weitere experimentale Untersuchungen über die Quelle und Den verlauf der intraokulären Safströmung: III. Über den vorgang der physiologischen Kammerwasserabsonderung und seine pharmakologische Beeinlüssung. *Graefes Arch Clin Exp Ophthalmol* 1920;102:372–382.
5. Goldmann H, Schmidt T. Uber Applanationstonometrie. *Ophthalmologica* 1957;134:221.
6. Ball JM. *Modern Ophthalmology.* Philadelphia: F.A.Davis, 1916; 875.
7. Burke A. Die klinische, physiologische und pathologische Bedeutung der Fluoreszenz im Auge nach darrieichung von Uranin. *Klin Monatsbl Augenheilkd* 1910;48:445–454.
8. McLean AL, Maumenee AE. Hemangioma of the choroid. *Am J Ophthalmol* 1960;50:3–11.
9. Flocks M, Miller J, Chao P. Retinal circulation time with the aid of fundus cinephotography. *Am J Ophthalmol* 1959;48:3–6.
10. Novotny HR, Alvis DL. A method of photographing fluorescence in circulating blood in the human retina. *Circulation* 1961;24:82–86.
11. Goldberg MF. Twenty-five years of fluorescein angiography. *Arch Ophthalmol* 1985;103:1301.
12. Jensen VA, Lundbaek K. Fluorescein angiography of the iris in recent and long-term diabetes, preliminary communication. *Acta Ophthalmol* 1968;46:584–585.
13. Jampol LM, Rosser MJ, Sears ML. Unusual aspects of progressive essential iris atrophy. *Am J Ophthalmol* 1974;77:353–357.
14. Jampol LM, Cunha-Vaz J. Diagnostic agents in ophthalmology: sodium fluorescein and other dyes. *Handbook Exp Pharmacol* 1984; 69:700–714.
15. Hayreh SS, Scott WE. Fluorescein iris angiography I. Normal pattern II. Disturbances in iris circulation following strabismus operation on various recti. *Arch Ophthalmol* 1978;96:1383–1400.
16. Oliver JM, Lee JP. Recovery of anterior segment circulation after strabismus surgery in adult patients. *Ophthalmology* 1992;99:305– 315.
17. Chandler JW, Sewell JH, Kaufman HE. Anterior segment fluorescein angiography: a simple modification of the Zeiss stereo slit lamp camera. *Ann Ophthalmol* 1975;7:87–92.
18. Romanchuk KG. Fluorescein: physiochemical factors affecting its fluorescence. *Surv Ophthalmol* 1982;26:269–283.
19. Havener WH. Fluorescein and other dyes. In: Havener WH, ed. *Ocular Pharmacology.* St. Louis: C.V. Mosby, 1978; 413–424.
20. Passamore JW, King JH Jr. Vital staining of conjunctiva and cornea. *Arch Ophthalmol* 1955;53:568–574.
21. Dollery C. *Therapeutic Drugs.* Edinburgh: Churchill Livingstone, 1991.
22. Vaughan DG. The contamination of fluorescein solutions—with special reference to *Pseudomonas aeruginosa. Am J Ophthalmol* 1955;39:55–61.
23. Kimura SJ. Fluorescein paper: a simple means of insuring the use of sterile fluorescein. *Am J Ophthalmol* 1951;34:446–447.
24. Duffner LR, Pflugfelder SC, Mandelbaum S, Childress LL. Potential contamination in fluorescein-anesthetic solutions. *Am J Ophthalmol* 1990;110:199–202.
25. Lee H. Prolonged antibacterial activity of a fluorescein-anesthetic solution. *Arch Ophthalmol* 1972;88:385–387.
26. Dollery CT, Hodge JV, Engel M. Studies of retinal circulation with fluorescein. *Br Med J* 1962;2:1210–1215.
27. Grotte D, Mattox V, Brubaker R. Fluorescent, physiological and pharmacokinetic properties of fluorescein glucuronide. *Exp Eye Res* 1985;40:23–33.
28. Palestine AG, Brubaker RF. Pharmacokinetics of fluorescein in the vitreous. *Invest Ophthalmol Vis Sci* 1981;21:542–549.
29. Brubaker RF, Penniston JT, Grotte DA, Nagataki S. Measurement of fluorescein binding in human plasma using fluorescein polarization. *Arch Ophthalmol* 1982;100:625–630.
30. Ianacone CD, Felberg NT, Federman JL. Tritiated fluorescein binding to normal human plasma proteins. *Arch Ophthalmol* 1980;98: 1643–1645.
31. Nagataki S, Matsunaga I. Binding of fluorescein monoglucuronide to human serum albumin. *Invest Ophthalmol Vis Sci* 1985;26:1175–1178.
32. Chen S, Nakamura H, Tamura Z. Studies on the metabolites of fluorescein in rabbit and human urine. *Chem Pharm Bull* 1980;28:1403–1407.
33. Chahal PS, Neal MJ, Kohner EM. Metabolism of fluorescein after intravenous administration. *Invest Ophthalmol Vis Sci* 1985;26:764–768.

34. Norn MS. Micropunctate fluorescein staining of the cornea. *Acta Ophthalmol* 1970;48:108–118.
35. Moses RA. Fluorescein in applanation tonometry. *Am J Ophthalmol* 1960;49:1149–1155.
36. Grant WM. Fluorescein for applanation tonometry: more convenient and uniform application. *Am J Ophthalmol* 1963;55:1252–1253.
37. Roper DL. Applanation tonometry with and without fluorescein. *Am J Ophthalmol* 1980;90:668–671.
38. Bright DC, Potter JW, Allen DC, Spruance RD. Goldmann applanation tonometry without fluorescein. *Am J Optom Physiol Opt* 1981; 58:1120–1126.
39. Seidel E. Nachweis und untersuchung der Kammerwasserstromung an Fistelelaugen mitels der fluoreszein-Probe. In: Abderhalden E, ed. *Handbuch der Biologischen Arbeitsmethoden. Abt. V. Methoden zum Studium der Funktionen der Eizelnen Organe des Tierischen Organismus, Teil 6 (2 Halfte),* Berlin: Urban und Schwarzenberg, 1937;1112–1117.
40. Romanchuk KG. Seidel's test using 10% fluorescein. *Can J Ophthalmol* 1979;14:253–256.
41. Craig EL. Fluorescein and other dyes. In: Mauger TF, Craig EL, eds. *Havener's Ocular Pharmacology.* St. Louis: C.V. Mosby, 1994; 451–467.
42. Stein HA, Slatt BJ, Stein RM. Use and limitations of fluorescein in assessing fitting problems. In: Stein HA, Slatt BJ, Stein RM, eds. *Fitting Guide for Rigid and Soft Contact Lenses.* St. Louis: C.V. Mosby, 1990;234–240.
43. Refojo MF, Miller D, Fiore AS. A new fluorescent stain for soft hydrophilic lens fitting. *Arch Ophthalmol* 1972;87:275–277.
44. Lemp MA, Hamill JR. Factors affecting tear break-up time in normal eyes. *Arch Ophthalmol* 1973;89:103–105.
45. Lemp MA, Dohlman CH, Kuwabara T. Dry eye secondary to mucus deficiency. *Trans Am Acad Ophthalmol Otolaryngol* 1971;75:1223–1227.
46. Vanley GT, Leopold IH, Greff TH. Interpretation of tear film breakup. *Arch Ophthalmol* 1977;95:445–448.
47. Jones LT. The lacrimal secretory system and its treatment. *Am J Ophthalmol* 1966;62:47–60.
48. Wright MM, Bersani TA, Frueh BR. Efficacy of the primary dye test. *Ophthalmology* 1989;96:481–484.
49. Jalkh AE, Celorio JM. *Atlas of Fluorescein Angiography.* Philadelphia: W.B. Saunders, 1993.
50. Yannuzzi LA, Rohrer KT, Tindel LJ, et al. Fluorescein angiography complications survey. *Ophthalmology* 1986;93:611–617.
51. Flower RW, Hochheimer BF. Quantification of indicator dye concentration in ocular blood vessels. *Exp Eye Res* 1977;25:103–111.
52. Smith JL, David NJ, Hart LM, Levenson DS, Tillet CW. Hemangioma of the choroid. *Arch Ophthalmol* 1963;69:51–54.
53. Flower RW, Hochheimer BF. Injection technique of indocyanine green and sodium fluorescein dye angiography of the eye. *Invest Ophthalmol Vis Sci* 1973;12:881–895.
54. Yokoyama Y, Funahashi T, Horiuchi T, Mizuno T. Correlation of the fluorescein angiogram with the dye content in the blood. In: Shimizu K, ed. *Fluorescein Angiography. Proceedings of the International Symposium Fluorescein Angiography, Tokyo, 1972,* Tokyo: Igada-Shoin, 1974;72–76.
55. Orth DH. *Color and Fluorescein Angiographic Atlas of Retinal Vascular Disorders.* Baltimore: Williams & Wilkins, 1984.
56. Norton EWD, Gutman F. Diabetic retinopathy studied by fluorescein angiography. *Ophthalmologica* 1965;150:5–17.
57. Harney BA, Hart JCD, Grey RHB. *Atlas of Fluorescein Angiography.* London: Wolfe, 1994.
58. Coakes RL, Brubaker RF. Method of measuring aqueous humor flow and corneal endothelial permeability using a fluorophotometry nomogram. *Invest Ophthalmol Vis Sci* 1979;18:288–302.
59. Stone RA, Wilson CM. Fluorescein transport in the anterior uvea. *Invest Ophthalmol Vis Sci* 1982;22:301–303.
60. Jones RF, Maurice DM. New methods of measuring the rate of aqueous flow in man with fluorescein. *Exp Eye Res* 1966;5:208–220.
61. Zeimer RC, Blair NP, Cunha-Vaz JG. Vitreous fluorophotometry for clinical research. I. Description and evaluation od a new fluorophotometer. *Arch Ophthalmol* 1983;101:1753–1756.
62. Zeimer RC, Blair NP, Cunha-Vaz JG. Vitreous fluorophotometry for clinical research II. Method of data acquisition and processing. *Arch Ophthalmol* 1983;101:1757–1762.
63. Jackson WE, Chase HP, Garg SK, et al. Vitreous fluorophotometry in insulin-dependent diabetes mellitus. *Arch Ophthalmol* 1990;18: 1733–1735.
64. Nagataki S, Mishima S. Aqueous humor dynamics in glaucomatocyclitic crisis. *Invest Ophthalmol Vis Sci* 1976;15:365–370.
65. Matsui M, Justice J Jr. Anterior segment angiography. In: Justice J Jr, ed. *Ophthalmic Photography.* Boston: Little, Brown, 1995.
66. Watson PG. Anterior segment fluorescein angiography in the surgery of immunologically induced corneal and scleral destructive disorders. *Ophthalmology* 1987;94:1452–1459.
67. Kottow MH. *Anterior Segment Fluorescein Angiography.* Baltimore: Williams & Wilkins, 1978.
68. Rapoport SI. *Blood-brain Barrier in Physiology and Medicine.* New York: Raven Press, 1976;218.
69. Quickert MH. A fluorescein-anesthetic solution for applanation tonometry. *Arch Ophthalmol* 1967;77:734–739.
70. Cohn HC, Jocson VL. A unique case of grand mal seizure after Fluress. *Ann Ophthalmol* 1981;13:1379–1380.
71. Kwiterovich KA, Maguire MG, Murphy RP, et al. Frequency of adverse systemic reactions after fluorescein angiography. *Ophthalmology* 1991;98:1139–1142.
72. Butner RW, McPherson AR. Adverse reactions in intravenous fluorescein angiography. *Ann Ophthalmol* 1983;15:1084–1086.
73. Chazan BI, Balodimos MC, Koncz L. Untoward effects of fluorescein retinal angiography in diabetic patients. *Ann Ophthalmol* 1971; 3:42–49.
74. Schatz H, Farkos WS. Nausea from fluorescein angiography. *Am J Ophthalmol* 1982;93:370–371.
75. Greene GS, Bell LW, Hitching DR, Spaeth GL. Adverse reactions to intravenous fluorescein: evidence for a sex difference. *Ann Ophthalmol* 1765;8:533–536.
76. Wilkerson D, Tate GW, Baldwin HA, Hernsberger PL. Clinical evaluation of fluorescein 25%. *Ann Ophthalmol* 1971;3:42–49.
77. Stein MR, Parker CW. Reactions following intravenous fluorescein. *Am J Ophthalmol* 1971;72:861–868.
78. Hess JB, Pacuraria RI. Acute pulmonary edema following intravenous fluorescein angiography. *Am J Ophthalmol* 1976;82:567–570.
79. Kelley SP, MacDermott NJG, Saunder DC, Leach FN. Convulsion following intravenous fluorescein angiography. *Br J Ophthalmol* 1989;73:655–656.
80. Madowitz JS, Schweiger MJ. Severe anaphylactoid reaction to radiographic contrast media: recurrence despite premedication with diphenhydramine and prednisone. *JAMA* 1979;241:2313–2315.
81. Wesley RE, Blount WC, Arterberry JF. Acute myocardial infarction after fluorescein angiography. *Am J Ophthalmol* 1979;87: 834–835.
82. Deglin SM, Deglin EA, Chung EK. Acute myocardial infarction following fluorescein angiography. *Heart Lung* 1977;6:505–509.
83. McAllister Jr. RG. Hypertensive crisis and myocardial infarction after fluorescein angiography. *South Med J* 1981;74:508–509.
84. Cunningham EE, Balu V. Cardiac arrest following fluorescein angiography. *JAMA* 1979;242:2431.
85. Fraunfelder FT, Meyer SM. *Drug-induced Ocular Side Effects and Drug Interactions.* Philadelphia: Lea & Febiger, 1989;472–474.
86. Hope-Ross M, Yannuzzi LA, Gragoudas ES, et al. Adverse reactions to indocyanine green. *Ophthalmology* 1994;101:529–533.
87. Elman MJ, Fine SL, Sorenson J, et al. Skin necrosis following fluorescein extravasation. A survey of the Macula Society. *Retina* 1987; 789–793.
88. Schatz H. Sloughing of skin following fluorescein extravasation. *Ann Ophthalmol* 1978;10:625.
89. Kratz R, Mazzocco T, Davidson BA. A case report of skin necrosis following infiltration with IV fluorescein. *Ophthalmology* 1980;12: 655–656.
90. Arroyave CM, Wolbers R, Ellis PP. Plasma complement and histamine changes after intravenous administration of sodium fluorescein. *Am J Ophthalmol* 1979;84:474–479.
91. Heffner JE. Reactions to fluorescein. *JAMA* 1980;243:2029–2030.
92. Vaughan RW. Ventricular arrhythmias after topical vasoconstrictors. *Anesth Analg* 1973;52:161–165.
93. Lindzon RD, Silvers WS. Allergy, hypersensitivity, and anaphylaxis. In: Rosen P, Barkin RM, eds. *Emerg Med* St. Louis: C.V. Mosby, 1992;1042–1065.

94. Mattern J, Mayer PR. Excretion of fluorescein into breast milk. *Am J Ophthalmol* 1990;109:598–599.
95. Shekleton P, Fidler J, Grimwade JA. A case of benign intracranial hypertension in pregnancy. *Br J Obstet Gynecol* 1980;87:345–347.
96. McEnerney JK, Wong WP, Peyman GA. Evaluation of the teratogenicity of fluorescein sodium. *Am J Ophthalmol* 1977;84:847–840.
97. Halperin LS, Olk RJ, Soubrane G, Coscas G. Safety of fluorescein angiography during pregnancy. *Am J Ophthalmol* 1990;109:563–566.
98. Fishback DB. Fluorescein circulation time and the treatment of hypertension in the aged. *J Am Geriatr Soc* 1973;21:495–503.
99. Stewart HL. Prolonged antibacterial activity of a fluorescein-anesthetic solution. *Arch Ophthalmol* 1972;88:385–387.
100. Norton EWD, Smith JL, Curtain VT, Justice J. Fluorescein fundus photography: an aid in the differential diagnosis of posterior ocular lesions. *Trans Am Ophthalmol Otol* 1964;68:755–765.
101. Gass JDM. A fluorescein angiographic study of macular dysfunction secondary to retinal vascular disease: I. Embolic retinal artery obstruction. *Arch Ophthalmol* 1968;80:535–549.
102. Gass JDM. A fluorescein angiographic study of macular dysfunction secondary to retinal vascular disease: II. Retinal vein obstruction. *Arch Ophthalmol* 1968;80:550–568.
103. Gass JDM. A fluorescein angiographic study of macular dysfunction secondary to retinal vascular disease: III. Hypertensive retinopathy. *Arch Ophthalmol* 1968;80:569–582.
104. Gass JDM. A fluorescein angiographic study of macular dysfunction secondary to retinovascular disease: IV. Diabetic retinal angiopathy. *Arch Ophthalmol* 1968;80:583–591.
105. Gass JDM. A fluorescein angiographic study of macular dysfunction secondary to retinal vascular disease: V. Retinal telangiectasis. *Arch Ophthalmol* 1968;80:592–605.
106. Gass JDM. A fluorescein angiographic study of macular dysfunction secondary to retinal vascular disease: VI. X-ray irradiation, carotid artery occlusion, collagen vascular disease, and vitritis. *Arch Ophthalmol* 1968;80:606–617.
107. Fox IJ, Brooker LGS, Heseltine DW, Essex HE, Wood EH. A tricarbocyanine dye for continuous recording of dilution curves in whole blood independent of variations in blood oxygen saturation. *Mayo Clin Proc* 1957;32:478–483.
108. Fox IJ, Wood EH. Applications of dilution curves recorded from the right side of the heart of venous circulation with the aid of a new indicator dye. *Mayo Clin Proc* 1957;32:541–550.
109. Fox IJ, Wood EH. Indocyanine green: physical and physiologic properties. *Mayo Clin Proc* 1960;35:732–741.
110. Wheeler HO, Cranston WI, Meltzer JI. Hepatic uptake and biliary excretion of indocyanine green in the dog. *Proc Soc Exp Biol Med* 1958;99:11–14.
111. Weigand BD, Ketterer SG, Rapaport E. The use of indocyanine green in the measurement of hepatic function and blood flow in man. *Am J Dig Dis* 1960;5:427–436.
112. Cherrick GR, Stein SW, Leevy CM, Davidson CS. Indocyanine green: observations on its physical properties, plasma decay and hepatic extraction. *J Clin Invest* 1960;39:592–600.
113. Banaszak EF, Stekiel WJ, Grace RA, Smith JJ. Estimation of hepatic blood flow using a single injection dye clearance method. *Am J Physiol* 1960;198:877–880.
114. Kogure K, David NJ, Yamanouchi U, Choromokos E. Infrared absorption angiography of the fundus circulation. *Arch Ophthalmol* 1970;83:209–214.
115. Kulvin S, Stauffer L, Kogure K, David NJ. Fundus angiography in man by intracarotid administration of dye. *South Med J* 1970;63:998–1000.
116. Hochheimer BF. Angiography of the retina with indocyanine green. *Arch Ophthalmol* 1971;86:564–565.
117. Flower RW. Infrared absorption angiography of the choroid and some observations on the effects of high intraocular pressures. *Am J Ophthalmol* 1972;74:600–614.
118. Orth DH, Patz A, Flower RW. Potential clinical applications of indocyanine green choroidal angiography—preliminary report. *Eye Ear Nose Throat Monthly* 1976;55:15–27.
119. Destro M, Puliafito CA. Indocyanine green videoangiography of choroidal neovascularization. *Ophthalmology* 1989;96:846–853.
120. Hayashi K, Hasegawa Y, Tokoro T. Indocyanine green angiography of central serous chorioretinopathy. *Int Ophthalmol* 1986;9:37–41.
121. Scheider A, Schroedel C. High resolution indocyanine green angiography with a scanning laser ophthalmoscope. *Am J Ophthalmol* 1989;108:458–459.
122. Paumgartner G. The handling of indocyanine green by the liver. *Scweiz Med Wochenschr* 1975;105:1–30.
123. Guyer DR, Puliafito CA, Mones JM, Friedman E, Chang W, Vendoore SR. Digital indocyanine-green angiography in chorioretinal disorders. *Ophthalmology* 1992;99:287–291.
124. Baker KJ. Binding of sulfobromophthalein (SBT) sodium and indocyanine green (ICG) by plasma α1-lipoproteins. *Proc Soc Exp Biol Med* 1966;122:957–963.
125. Probst P, Paumgarner G, Caucig H, Frohlich H, Grabner G. Studies on clearance and placental transfer of indocyanine green during labor. *Clin Chim Acta* 1970;29:157–160.
126. Ketterer SG, Wiegand BD. The excretion of indocyanine green and its use in the estimation of hepatic blood flow. *Clin Res* 1959;7:71.
127. Ho AC, Yannuzzi LA, Guyer DR, Slakter JS, Sorenson JA, Orlock DA. Intraretinal leakage of indocyanine green. *Ophthalmology* 1994;101:534–541.
128. Yannuzzi LA, Slakter JS, Sorenson JA, Ho A, Orlock D. Digital indocyanine green videoangiography and choroidal neovascularization. *Retina* 1992;12:191–223.
129. Yuzawa M, Kawamura A, Matsui M. Indocyanine green videoangiography findings in acute multifocal placoid pigment epitheliopathy. *Acta Ophthalmol* 1994;72:128–133.
130. Dhaliwal RS, Maguire AM, Flower RW, Arribas NP. Acute posterior multifocal placoid pigment epitheliopathy. An indocyanine green angiographic study. *Retina* 1993;13:317–325.
131. Ie D, Glaser BM, Murphy RP, Gordon LW, Sjaarda RN, Thompson JT. Indocyanine green angiography in multiple evanescent white-dot syndrome. *Am J Ophthalmol* 1994;117:7–12.
132. Singh AD, De Potter P, Shields CL, Shields JA. Indocyanine green angiography and ultrasonography of a varix of the vortex vein. *Arch Ophthalmol* 1993;111:1283–1284.
133. Guyer DR, Yannuzzi LA, Slakter JS, Sorenson JA, Ho A, Orlock D. Digital indocyanine green videoangiography of central serous chorioretinopathy. *Arch Ophthalmol* 1994;112:1057–1062.
134. Scheider A, Nasemann JE, Lund OE. Fluorescein and indocyanine green angiographies of central serous choroidopathy by scanning laser ophthalmoscopy. *Am J Ophthalmol* 1993;115:50–56.
135. Scheider A, Neuhauser L. Fluorescence characteristics of drusen during indocyanine-green angiography and their possible correlation with choroidal perfusion. *Ger J Ophthalmol* 1992;1:328–334.
136. Yannuzzi LA, Hope-Ross M, Slakter JS, et al. Analysis of vascularized pigment epithelial detachments using indocyanine green videoangiography. *Retina* 1994;14:99–113.
137. Yuzawa M, Kawamura A, Matsui M. Indocyanine green videoangiographic findings in Harada's disease. *Jpn J Ophthalmol* 1993;37:456–466.
138. De Laey JJ. Diagnosis and differential diagnosis of malignant melanomas of the choroid. *Bull Soc Belge Ophtalmol* 1993;248:6–10.
139. Reichel E, Puliafito CA, Duker JS, Guyer DR. Indocyanine green dye enhanced diode laser photocoagulation of poorly defined subfoveal choroidal neovascularization. *Ophthalmic Surg* 1994;25:195–201.
140. Flower RW, Hochheimer BF. A clinical technique and apparatus for simultaneous angiography of the separate retinal and choroidal circulations. *Invest Ophthalmol Vis Sci* 1973;12:248–261.
141. Avvad FK, Duker JS, Reichel E, Margolis TI, Puliafito CA. The digital indocyanine green videoangiography of characteristics of well-defined choroidal neovascularization. *Ophthalmology* 1995;102:401–405.
142. Hayashi K, De Laey JJ. Indocyanine green angiography of submacular choroidal vessels in the human eye. *Ophthalmologica* 1985;190:20–29.
143. Hayashi K, Hasegawa Y, Miyoshi K, Tazawa Y. Indocyanine green videoangiography of four cases of suspected areolar choroidal atrophy. *Folia Ophthalmol Jpn* 1991;42:105–112.
144. Flower RW. Choroidal angiography today and tomorrow. *Retina* 1992;12:189–190.
145. Leevy CM, Smith F, Longueville J, Baumgartner G, Howard MM. Indocyanine green clearance as a test for hepatic function. *JAMA* 1967;200:236–240.

146. Olsen TW, Lim JI, Capone A, Myles RA, Gilman JP. Anaphylactic shock following indocyanine green angiography. *Arch Ophthalmol* 1996;114:97.
147. Wolfe S, Arend O, Schulte K, Reim M. Severe anaphylactic reaction after indocyanine green fluorescence angiography. *Am J Ophthalmol* 1992;114:638–639.
148. Mitchie DD, Wombolt DG, Carretta RF. Adverse reactions associated with the administration of a tricarbocyanine dye (Cardio-Green) to uremic patients. *J Allergy* 1971;48:235–239.
149. Iseki K, Onoyama K, Fujimi S, Omae T. Shock caused by indocyanine green in chronic hemodialysis patients [Letter]. *Clin Nephrol* 1980;14:210.
150. Garski TR, Staller BJ, Hepner G, Banks VS, Finney RA. Adverse reactions after administration of indocyanine green (Letter). *JAMA* 1978;240:635.
151. Benya R, Quintana J, Brundage B. Adverse reactions to indocyanine green: a case report and review of the literature. *Cathet Cardiovasc Diagn* 1989;17:231–233.
152. Nanikawa R, Hayashi T, Hayashi K. A case of fatal anaphylactic shock induced by indocyanine green (ICG) test. *Jpn J Leg Med* 1978;32:209–214.
153. Abelsdorff G, Wesseley K. Vergleichenphysiologische untersuchengen uber den flussigkeitwechsel des auges in der wirbeitierreihe I. Vogel. *Arch Augenheilkd* 1909;64:65–125.
154. Sorsby A. Vital staining of the retina. *Br J Ophthalmol* 1939;23:20–24.
155. Kikai K. Uber die Vitalarbung des hineren Bulbusabschnittes. *Arch Augenheilkd* 1930;103:541–553.
156. Grimes PA, Stone RA, Laties A, Weiye L. Carboxyfluorescein. A probe of the blood-ocular barriers with lower membrane permeability than fluorescein. *Arch Ophthalmol* 1982;100:635–639.
157. Khoobehi B, Peyman GA. Fluorescent vesical system. A new technique for measuring blood flow in the retina. *Ophthalmology* 1994; 101:1716–1726.
158. Jaanus SD. Dyes. In: Bartlett JD, Jaanus SD, eds. *Clinical Ocular Pharmacology.* Boston: Butterworth, 1984;311–326.
159. Norn MS. *External Eye: Methods of Examination.* Copenhagen: Scriptor, 1974;51–72.

Subject Index

F

Q

R

S